NEED TO KNOW

MEDICAL DIAGNOSES AND RELATED NURSING DIAGNOSES

Mental Health Nursing

Mental Health Nursing

The Nurse-Patient Journey

2nd Edition

Verna Benner Carson, PhD, RN, CS-P

National Director of Restore™ Behavioral Health
for Staff Builders Home Health and Hospice

Formerly
Associate Professor
School of Nursing
University of Maryland at Baltimore
Baltimore, Maryland

W.B. SAUNDERS COMPANY

A Harcourt Health Sciences Company
Philadelphia   London   Toronto   Montreal   Sydney   Tokyo

W.B. SAUNDERS COMPANY
A Harcourt Health Sciences Company

The Curtis Center
Independence Square West
Philadelphia, Pennsylvania 19106

VP, Nursing Editorial Director: Sally Schrefer
Senior Editor: Terri Wood
Senior Developmental Editor: Terri Ward
Copy Editor: Amy L. Cannon
Senior Production Manager: Pete Faber
Illustration Specialist: Fran Moriarty
Indexer: Dennis Dolan

Library of Congress Cataloging-in-Publication Data

Mental health nursing: the nurse-patient journey / [edited by] Verna
Benner Carson.—2nd ed.

p. cm.

Includes bibliographical references and index.

ISBN 0–7216–8053–4

1. Psychiatric nursing.   I. Carson, Verna Benner.
    [DNLM: 1. Psychiatric Nursing.   2. Nurse-Patient Relations.
    3. Psychotherapy—methods.   WY 160 M5493 2000]

RC440.M3546 2000   610.73′68—dc21

DNLM/DLC   99–35203

Excerpts from THE LITTLE PRINCE by Antoine de Saint-Exupery, copyright 1943 and renewed 1971 by Harcourt, Inc. reprinted by permission of the publisher.

MENTAL HEALTH NURSING: The Nurse-Patient Journey   ISBN 0–7216–8053–4

Printed in the United States of America.

Last digit is the print number: 9   8   7   6   5   4   3   2   1

DEDICATION

I dedicate this work to the Lord from whom all good things come. I thank Him for His faithfulness and for the blessings that He showers on me—for health, for the gift of writing, for the call to nursing, but most of all for my husband, John, and our three sons, Adam, Johnny, and Robbie. They make my heart sing.

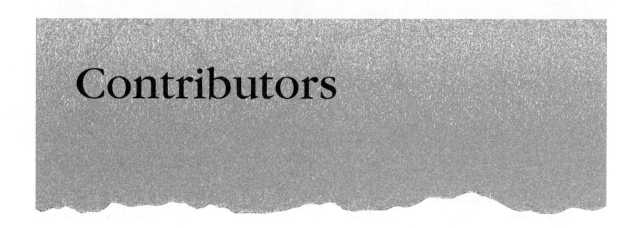

Contributors

Elizabeth Arnold, PhD, RN, CS-P
Associate Professor
University of Maryland School of
 Nursing
Baltimore
Psychotherapist
Town Center Psychiatric Associates
Kensington, Maryland

Judith Buchanan, MHSc, RN
Associate Professor
University of New Brunswick
Saint John, New Brunswick,
 Canada
President
Canadian Federation of Mental
 Health Nurses

**Verna Benner Carson, PhD, RN,
CS-P**
National Director
Restore Behavioral Health Program
 for Staff Builders Home Health
 and Hospice
Fallston, Maryland
Formerly
Associate Professor
School of Nursing
University of Maryland at Baltimore
Baltimore, Maryland

**Carol Distasio, RN, MSN, MPH,
C, CS, HH**
Nurse Psychotherapist
Consultant, Educator, Clinician,
 and Author in Psychiatric, Home
 Health, and Geriatric Nursing
Baltimore, Maryland

Charlotte Eliopoulos, RNC, PhD
President
Health Education Network
Glen Arm, Maryland

Edna Fordyce, EdD, RN, CS-P
Professor Emeritus
Department of Nursing
Towson University
Towson, Maryland

Judy S. Fuhrmann, MS, RN, CS-P
Assistant Professor of Nursing
John Tyler Community College
Chester, Virginia
Private Psychotherapy Practice
Midlothian, Virginia

**Joanne DeSanto Iennaco, MSN,
RNC**
Assistant Professor
Saint Joseph's College
Standish, Maine

Miriam Jacik, MSN, MSPsy
Case Manager
Genesis Health Ventures, Inc.
Kennett Square, Pennsylvania

Carol J. Johnston, MS, RN, CS-P
Adjunct Faculty
University of Maryland
Baltimore, Maryland
Catonsville Community College
Catonsville, Maryland
Director
Utilization Management
Clifton T. Perkins Hospital
Jessup, Maryland
Care Manager
Magellan Behavioral Health
Columbia, Maryland

Sarah Lechner, MSN
Research Coordinator
University of Pennsylvania
Philadelphia, Pennsylvania

Pamela E. Marcus, MS, RN, CS-P
Adjunct Faculty, Nursing
Prince George's Community
  College
Largo, Maryland
Clinical Specialist–Nurse
  Psychotherapist
Greater Southeast Community
  Hospital
Washington, D.C.

Mary Moller, MSN, ARNP, CS
Administrator
Suncrest Wellness Center
Spokane, Washington

Carolyn M. Scott, MS, RN
National Coordinator
Behavioral Health Program
Staff Builders Home Health and
  Hospice
Chicago, Illinois

Nancy Shoemaker, MS, RN
Clinical Specialist
Omni House Behavioral Health
  System
Glen Burnie, Maryland

Nina M. Smith, MEd, RNC
National Associate Director
Restore Behavioral Health Program
Staff Builders Home Health and
  Hospice
Ft. Collins, Colorado

Dianne Taylor, EdD, RN, CS-P
Associate Professor
Psychiatric–Mental Health Nursing
Towson University
Towson, Maryland

Sue Ann Thomas, PhD, RN, CS-P
Professor
Georgetown University
School of Nursing
Washington, D.C.
Partner
Siegel and Thomes Health Care
  Group
Ellicott City, Maryland

Jane Trainis, MS, RN, CS
Clinical Instructor
Towson University
Johns Hopkins University
Baltimore, Maryland

**Katherine J. Vanderhorst,
RN, BSN**
Director
Behavioral Health
Staff Builders Home Health and
  Hospice
Amherst, New York

Daria Virvan, MSN, RN, CS
Nurse Psychotherapist
Town Center Psychiatric Associates
Rockville, Maryland

Mary Ann Wilkinson, EdD, MSN
Adjunct Faculty
Psychiatric Nursing
University of Maryland School of
  Nursing
Baltimore, Maryland
Coordinator
Mental Health Services
MGH Home Health
Olney, Maryland

Evelyn L. Yap, MS, RN, CS-P
Clinical Manager
Behavioral Health
Visiting Nurse Association of
  Maryland
Baltimore, Maryland

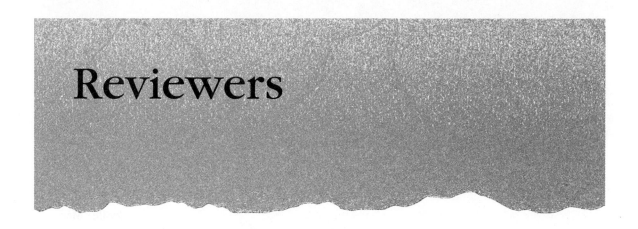

Reviewers

Susan Alden, ND, ARNP, CS
Private Practice
Davenport Medical Center
Davenport, Iowa

Wendy L. Bauer, MSN, RNCS
School of Nursing
Owens Community College
Toledo, Ohio

Janie Cavaroc Brenden, PhD, RNC
School of Nursing
Mississippi Gulf Coast Community
 College
Gautier, Mississippi

Carolyn Pierce Buckelew, BSN, MA, RNCS, NCC
Raritan Bay Medical Center
C.E. Gregory School of Nursing
Perth Amboy, New Jersey

Leona Castor, MSN, MSEd, DED
Department of Nursing
Wilkes University
Wilkes-Barre, Pennsylvania

Karen Espeland, MSN, RN, CARN
College of Nursing
Medcenter One
Bismarck, North Dakota

Gheta G. Grace, MSN, RN
School of Nursing
Alabama Southern Community
 College
Monroeville, Alabama

Denise Marshall, BSN, RN, MEd
School of Nursing
Wor-Wic Community College
Cambridge, Maryland

Wanda K. Mohr, PhD, RNC, FAAN
School of Nursing
University of Pennsylvania
Philadelphia, Pennsylvania

Shirley P. O'Neil, MS, BSN
School of Nursing
Rockford College
Rockford, Illinois

Linda L. Treloar, MA, RN, CS, GNP, ANP-C
School of Nursing
Scottsdale Community College
Scottsdale, Arizona

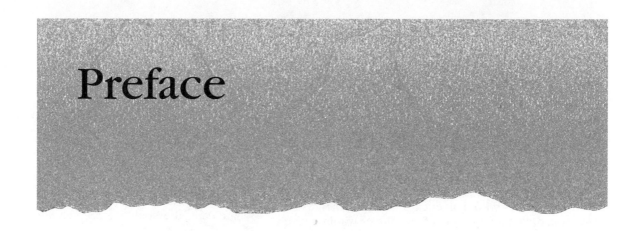

Preface

CHANGE

Change is certain—we can count on it. We don't necessarily embrace it or invite it, but its dependability is absolute. Frequently, we resist change, clinging to what we know—what is comfortable—then when it slips away, we long for what was. So as I reflect on this second edition of *Mental Health Nursing: The Nurse-Patient Journey,* I am struck, almost overwhelmed, by the changes that have occurred in psychiatric nursing, in the way that I practice as a psychiatric nurse, and in my personal life. All of these changes have, in some way, large or small, shaped this second edition. Let me invite you to journey into my universe a bit so that you can appreciate these change events and understand how they have influenced this textbook.

PROFESSIONAL CHANGES

Psychiatric nursing as well as other specialties within health care has been impacted by managed care. Efforts to adjust to and anticipate the continuing implications of managed care require tireless effort and diligence. Practice patterns are shifting. Managed care gives greater emphasis to networks of providers than to individual practitioners. Cost-containment efforts have affected reimbursement, restricted access to care, and tightened authorization of care across the continuum. Increasingly, the line between public and private is blurred as more state and federal programs are turned over to private enterprises. The health care system, which is in constant flux, no longer values the "therapeutic relationship"; it is oriented to Band-Aid interventions and quick fixes. Additionally, the developments within neurobiology and psychopharmacology have been staggering, and they also affect the practice of psychiatric nursing.

All these changes present real challenges, not the least of which is how to credibly integrate holism and the journey into this text when these ideals are devalued by the health care system that you are entering. Add to this the fact that the amount of time allotted for teaching psychiatric nursing has been condensed—a situation that presents faculty members with a serious dilemma. Do they teach the same amount of content in significantly less time, or do they pick and choose what they believe is most relevant, hoping that you are adequately prepared not only to take your NCLEX but also to practice? These are not easy challenges to meet. The solutions that I have arrived at address these issues and prepare you to enter this new and constantly evolving practice arena.

The first strategy I chose was to reduce the size of the textbook to 39 chapters from 46. Content is presented in a more condensed format. There is greater emphasis on specific nursing interventions to guide you as you interact with psychiatric patients. There is more information about managed behavioral care and case management—two entities that daily confront the psychiatric nurse. There is increased depth in the areas of neurophysiology and psychopharmacology. I removed the individual chapters that dealt with psychiatric home care (although it is near to my heart) and community mental health care in recognition that the goal of this textbook is not to prepare you to specialize in either of these practice areas. Most likely, you will have clinical experiences across the continuum of psychiatric care—thus, the addition of a new chapter that addresses the continuum. Another change is the removal of the chapters that dealt with individual, group, and family therapy—again, most of you will not be therapists, and the information was not particularly relevant to you. In place of those chapters are two new ones: 1) Chapter 13: Basic Interventions, which addresses what you will be doing as a student and as a beginning practitioner of psychiatric nursing, and 2) Chapter 14: Advanced Therapeutic Interventions, which provides an overview of individual, family, and group therapies.

PERSONAL CHANGES

I no longer work as a faculty member but have moved into the private sector as the National Director of the Restore Behavioral Health program for Staff Builders Home Health and Hospice. This position allows me to meet and work with nurses across the country. I develop and implement programs that directly affect the provision of psychiatric home care. Although I still teach, my teaching activities focus on improving the practice of psychiatric nurses who deliver care within the home and increasing the understanding of nonnurses within health care regarding contributions made by psychiatric nurses. My experiences outside of academia have changed my views about what you need to be an effective practitioner.

So, although this edition still maintains a comprehensive "why" or theory base for what you do as a psychiatric nurse, it includes a much stronger emphasis on the "what" that you do—with the addition of the specific features that address the "what" of psychiatric nursing.

STABILITY—MY VISION FOR THE TEXTBOOK

I believe the first edition forged new ground for psychiatric nursing. Although the facts of the first edition are similar to the facts found in other psychiatric nursing texts, the holistic focus with a clear incorporation of spirituality and patients' stories made the first edition unique. The second edition maintains that same focus and that same vision. In fact, after traversing through much illness and suffering with my family, I am even more committed than ever before to the importance of spirituality to nursing care. I saw the comfort that my family's own spiritual beliefs brought to them. I saw the healing power that came from nurses who respected spirituality, who created an environment in which spirituality could be freely expressed, and who themselves were spiritual individuals who reached out not only with expertise but also with love.

SPIRITUALITY VERSUS RELIGION

One of the issues that was misconstrued in the first edition concerned the spiritual focus of the textbook. Some people asserted that the book was too religious. This is an issue that warrants clarification. Religion refers to a chosen belief system and membership in an organized faith tradition with all the rites, rules, and rituals that are inherent in that tradition. Spirituality refers to a relationship with a higher power—however that higher power is defined. Spirituality is concerned with how that relationship is translated into values, principles, and choices for living. Spirituality also animates life, allows for the experiences of joy and forgiveness, and allows us to ascribe meaning and purpose beyond the circumstances of our daily lives. For many people, their religion offers them the form through which they express their spirituality. For others, religion holds no meaning yet they are spiritual. And still there are others who are active within their faith traditions but who are not spiritual. As nurses, we need to explore these issues because both religion and spirituality can be critical factors in the healing process. This is supported by a growing body of research, which is discussed in Chapter 1. This book does not exclude anyone's beliefs or present a bias toward any faith tradition. In fact, with the focus on loving and compassionate care, the book is extremely inclusive.

THE STRUCTURE OF THE BOOK

Mental Health Nursing: The Nurse-Patient Journey is organized into seven units:

Unit I: Background for the Journey
Unit II: The Nature of the Journey
Unit III: Guiding the Journey
Unit IV: Travelers Across the Life Span
Unit V: The Wounded Traveler
Unit VI: The Journey and Society
Unit VII: The Journey Forward

Each unit begins with a Traveler's Log, which presents a unique view from a mental health nurse's life.

Unit I: Background for the Journey includes chapters about the beliefs of the contributors to this text, the history of mental health nursing, the mental health system, roles and practice settings for mental health nurses, legal and ethical issues in mental health nursing, and theories that guide the journey of mental health nursing. *Unit II: The Nature of the Journey* includes a state-of-the-art chapter covering neurobiological influences on mental health and mental illness. Another chapter focuses on self-concept, not only from the patient's perspective but also from your perspective, as we look at how patients and nurses reciprocally influence one another. One chapter, unique to this textbook, deals with the attributes and strengths that enable some people to be triumphant survivors in life's journey. A chapter new to this text deals with therapeutic communication skills and the development of therapeutic relationships. Another new chapter reviews the nursing process and presents an overview of its application to psychiatric nursing. The last chapter in this unit deals with the impact of culture on mental health, mental illness, and mental health care.

Unit III: Guiding the Journey covers the therapeutic approaches used in mental health nursing. This unit includes three new chapters: one dealing with basic interventions, another dealing with advanced interventions, and a third dealing with the continuum of care. In addition, we include a chapter dealing with mind-body-spirit therapies, including the use of therapies that stem from an Eastern approach to health and well-being. Last, we offer an in-depth chapter on psychopharmacology.

Unit IV: Travelers Across the Life Span gives an overview of normal developmental tasks and crises from childhood to old age and also explores age-related mental health issues. One new chapter provides an in-depth review of normal childhood and the psychiatric issues of childhood, and another presents a comparable review of adolescence and the psychiatric issues confronting that developmental stage. The chapter about adulthood is a distinctive feature of this textbook. The years covering adulthood, where we generally spend most of our lives, are frequently ignored completely or glossed over in textbooks of psychiatric nursing. To remedy this deficiency, we present in this chapter, an in-depth look at the many challenges and issues that confront the developing adult. Another chapter takes a close look at the unique mental health issues affecting the elderly. The last chapter in this unit covers loss and its impact not only on the journey of the psychiatric patient but also on your own journey as well.

Unit V: The Wounded Traveler is the largest unit in the book. In it you will learn about specific psychiatric illnesses and gain a window into the lives of the patients whose journeys are affected by them. The unit includes chapters about stress and anxiety disorders, schizophrenia, mood disorders, substance abuse, behavioral disorders, dissociative disorders, psychosexual disorders, eating disorders, and psychophysiological disorders. We have also included separate chapters on suicide and cognitive disorders. *Unit VI: The Journey and Society* includes comprehensive coverage of homelessness, violence, rape, and AIDS, four issues with tremendous psychiatric as well as social relevance. *Unit VII: The Journey Forward,* the last unit, looks at improving the journey through total quality management research. Chapter 39, the last chapter in the book, looks forward and anticipates the skills that will be needed to continue to make a difference in the lives of patients, families, and communities.

THE STRUCTURE OF THE CHAPTERS

The chapters of *Mental Health Nursing* follow a consistent structure and include a number of highlighted features to help you focus on and learn content that is critical to your education in psychiatric nursing.

Each chapter begins with a quotation chosen to spark your interest in the subject covered in the chapter. Next, **Learning Objectives** give you a "preorganizing" framework with which to approach your reading of the chapter. A **Key Terminology** list follows, introducing important terms that are highlighted and defined within the body of the chapter. These terms are essential to your understanding of the content of the chapter.

After a brief introduction to the chapter, we then typically introduce a story drawn from general literature, psychiatric literature, or the personal or professional experiences of the contributor. The purpose of this story is to help bring to life the human drama that is mental health nursing and to give you a context for, and a reinforcement of, key content from the chapter. Frequently, we build on these stories throughout the chapter. Additional glimpses into the lives of patients appear as **Case Examples** throughout the book.

Most chapters covering specific psychiatric disorders, and some other chapters as well, include an application of the **Nursing Process.** We use the six-step nursing process specified in the American Nurses Association's 1999 publication, *A Statement on Psychiatric–Mental Health Clinical Nursing Practice and Standards of Psychiatric–Mental Health Clinical Nursing Practice:* assessment, diagnosis, outcome identification, planning, implementation, and evaluation. An addition to many of the chapters is the **Snapshot** feature presenting a Nursing Intervention Specific to . . . . This feature provides you with concrete suggestions regarding how you develop a relationship with a patient suffering with a particular disorder; what you assess; what you teach the patient or caregiver; what skills you want the patient or caregiver to demonstrate; and what other health professionals you include in the care plan.

Many chapters include special boxes called **Medical Diagnoses and Related Nursing Diagnoses.** These boxes present diagnostic criteria for selected disorders from the American Psychiatric Association's *Diagnostic and Statistical Manual of Mental Disorders, Fourth Edition,* (DSM-IV). They also may suggest related North American Nursing Diagnosis Association (NANDA) nursing diagnoses that frequently accompany the psychiatric diagnoses. For each NANDA diagnosis, we provide a definition and an example of how a two-part diagnosis might be written for a specific patient.

Many of the chapters also include highlighted educational material in **Need to Know** boxes (**What Patients Need to Know, What Families Need to Know,** and so on) for you to share with patients and their families. This material is written in question-and-answer form in everyday language especially for use by patients and families.

New to this edition are **Home Care Clinical Practice Guidelines.** These illustrated algorithms present the various steps, stages, medical personnel, and care plan involved in the treatment of a mental health patient in the rapidly growing home care practice setting.

Also new to this edition is a color insert. Full-color examples of brain scan images show the visible differences among the brains of patients.

Throughout the chapters, you will find **Check Your Reading** questions to help you review the content, clarify your thinking, and reinforce your learning as you progress through the chapter. Suggested answers to these questions appear in the Instructor's Manual. All the chapters have a new feature, **What do you think?,** which poses reflective and challenging questions for you to consider. They are different from the **Check Your Reading** questions, which review facts that you have read. **What do you think?** questions ask you to search your heart, your values, and your attitudes and open them up to personal scrutiny.

Many of the chapters, particularly those covering specific mental disorders, conclude with **Case Studies.** These **Case Studies** present a brief case history, then demonstrate the application of the six-step nursing process to the case.

At the end of each chapter, after some brief conclusions, you'll find **Key Points to Remember.** These list-style summaries of key points made in the chapter help you review the content and focus on the critical points of each chapter. After the **Key Points,** we provide suggested **Learning Activities,** most of which are experiential. Completing these activities is a way of making the content of the chapter more meaningful to you. Next you'll find **Critical Thinking Exercises** designed to assist you in thinking creatively and flexibly about situations and in looking beyond the obvious in your problem-solving. The chapters conclude with **Additional Resources,** which provide you with names of organizations and ways to contact them that provide you access to a wealth of information. After the **Additional Resources** are the **References,** followed by a list of **Suggested Readings** that we believe would be particularly helpful to you if you are interested in further exploration of the chapter's content.

At the end of *Mental Health Nursing: The Nurse-Patient Journey,* you'll find three appendices, two of which are new to this edition. Appendix I presents Standard Patient and Family Curriculum With Sample Teaching Tools. Appendix II shows Spiritual Interventions Appropriate for Psychiatric Patients—an addition that seems fitting given the holistic nature of the textbook. In Appendix III, we reprint the complete DSM-IV classification of mental disorders.

I feel privileged to be able to journey with you for a time in your study of mental health nursing. As you read this book and undertake that journey along with me and each of the contributors, we hope that our vision of a shared journey will take hold in your own heart and that you will offer that vision to patients throughout your nursing career.

VERNA BENNER CARSON

Acknowledgments

I am convinced that writing is always fraught with challenges and difficulties. If I could put life on hold and declare a moratorium on personal loss and crisis the process would be easy. However, because that is not possible, I convince myself that the challenges only make the writing richer and more relevant because the writing grows out of real life struggles.

When I look back over the past 4 years, I feel incredibly blessed that despite the personal pain that my family and I have endured, we are all okay—actually, better than okay! As I write this, I am reminded of the prayer *Footprints in the Sand*. In this prayer, a man recounts a dream in which he walked across a beach with the Lord at his side. As he walked, scenes from his life flashed across the skies. In each scene, he noticed two sets of footprints, his and the Lord's. When the last scene of his life flashed by, he looked back over the sands and saw that many times along the path of life, there was only one set of footprints. He turned to the Lord and asked him, "When I decided to follow you, you promised you would always be with me. Why then at the most troublesome times of my life did you leave my side?" The Lord answered him, "My precious child, I never left you during your times of trials and suffering. Where you see only one set of footprints, I was carrying you." I too have been carried and loved, and this has only strengthened my commitment to share this with you and to communicate the importance of integrating the love of God into your theory-based expertise.

My friend and co-editor on the first edition, Dr. Elizabeth Arnold, decided for personal reasons not to share in the editorial role of the second edition. Although I fully accepted and supported her decision, I missed her partnership. Her wisdom, her experience in psychiatric nursing, and her sense of humor were all valuable assets to the first edition and to me personally. We are fortunate that she decided to contribute Chapter 14, Advanced Therapeutic Interventions. Dr. Arnold is one of the most talented nurse psychotherapists I know,

and it would be a loss to you if you did not benefit in some way from her knowledge and expertise.

During the past 4 years, I lost some key members of my personal cheering squad. My mother, Dorothy Benner, was one of God's gentle creations who loved unconditionally. She never judged others or rejected them because of strange or unusual behavior. Everyone she met had a place at her table. She returned to God on December 30th, 1996. My mother-in-law, Mary Carson, died on November 17th, 1998. She was a loving and generous woman, and we were blessed to have her live with us for 6 years. My father, Kenneth Benner, died on February 24th, 1999. He was an extraordinary man—courageous, loving, and unselfish. Although I know he is happy with God and my mother, the missing is terrible. I can in no way minimize the impact of these losses. In fact, their painful reality has been a constant intrusion into the writing of this textbook. However, I feel blessed that these wonderful people were such an important part of my life; their love and support meant the world to me. They were people of deep and abiding faith who taught me that life is a gift, that people need to be loved, and that God must be at the center of my life. Their deaths have only intensified my commitment to the unique vision and mission of this textbook.

I am grateful to each and every one of my contributors. They produced wonderful material according to a tight time schedule. I am grateful to my family; they continue to be my cheering squad, encouraging me when I think I can't write another word, praising my work, offering to help me in a myriad of little and big ways. My husband, John, is my in-house computer expert, who frequently interrupts my work to give me a cup of coffee, a snack, or a back rub, or to tell me some outrageous story that makes me laugh. In addition to my husband, my sister Kathy provided me valuable administrative and typing support in the manuscript preparation. My niece Dawnie handled correspondence, copying, Internet searching, and telephone calls. Reviewers offered invaluable critiques that sharpened the writing and alerted me to material that needed to be clarified, expanded, or deleted. A special thanks to my colleagues at Staff Builders Home Health and Hospice. It would be difficult to find a more affirming and professionally challenging group with whom to work. Steve Savitsky, David Savitsky, Dale Clift, Sandy Parshall, Carolina Conn, Michael Seago, Ding Alonzo, Judy Breckbill, Deb Lytle, Noreen Coyne, and Katherine Vanderhorst represent some of the very best in home care. Mario Marchi, Carolyn Scott, and Nina Smith are members of the Restore Behavioral Health program team, and even though I am their "boss," they are like family to me—they make work fun!

The staff members of W.B. Saunders Company were indispensable throughout the entire process and deserve a special word of thanks. Although I have worked on other projects with Saunders, this is the first time that I have worked with Terri Wood, the nursing editor. Terri believes in me and supports me in very concrete ways to facilitate getting the job done. My developmental editor, Terri Ward, is a friend at the other end of the telephone line. She did a superb job of keeping the book on schedule, offering me suggestions that simplified the process, and handling the unit opening sections, a new feature in this edition.

Thanks also to my production team at W.B. Saunders Company. Amy Cannon copy edited the entire manuscript, ensuring that the material was presented with clarity, consistency, and precision. Peter Faber managed the book's production, working with other members of the production team, with the typesetter, and with the printer to ensure that the quality of the book's manufacturing matched the quality of its contents.

Last, I would like to thank the many patients who allowed us to accompany them on their journeys. From these shared experiences emerged the vision for the book.

VERNA BENNER CARSON

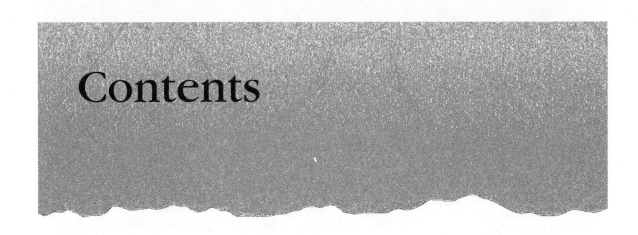

Contents

Color plates follow page 136.

xxii   **Contents**

Unit VI The Journey and Society 973

Unit VII The Journey Forward 1087

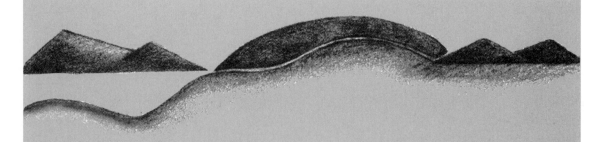

I Background for the Journey

Traveler's Log

To my surprise, I was placed on an inpatient mental health unit for a summer student-nursing internship. The first day my head swam with thoughts and fears about the next 12 weeks. I was afraid that this specialty area would be unappealing. Would I find I was not cut out to be a mental health nurse? My heart pounded as I walked to the unit. I felt as if everyone could hear it pound, and I consciously tried to slow down my breathing. I was apprehensive about the "psych patients" I would meet. My supervisor told me about the unit and the people being treated there. She showed me the desk and gave me a tour. I was struck by how quiet, comfortable, and not-hospital-like it seemed. I saw many people as we toured the unit, and I remember wondering, "Which are patients and which are staff? They all look so normal!"

I was teamed with a nurse to admit a young man who had been forced to leave college because of anxiety attacks. We sat together talking about life in college. He explained that final examinations and athletic competition had been too much and how he feared that he would never find success in life. As I left him, I reflected on how similar his concerns were to my own. After this, I went to a group therapy session in which I saw seven adults reach out to each other for support; my preceptor facilitated their problem-solving. In the course of the hour, they solved potential problems that might have interfered with their successful recovery.

At the end of the day, I met with my supervisor again. She wanted to know what I thought of my first day. I told her I could identify with the patients' problems and that they seemed quite normal. The stereotypes I had held of violent, bizarre people had come crashing down within hours. We talked about the wish that we personally would never be touched by a mental health problem. We reflected on society's wish to think there is something different or "wrong" with those who suffer with mental health problems. I realized that given the histories and circumstances of those I had met that day, anyone might have problems coping. As I walked to my car, I again felt anxious, but my anxiety was no longer related to a fear of psych patients but to the understanding that as human beings, we are all vulnerable to problems with coping.

—Joanne DeSanto Iennaco

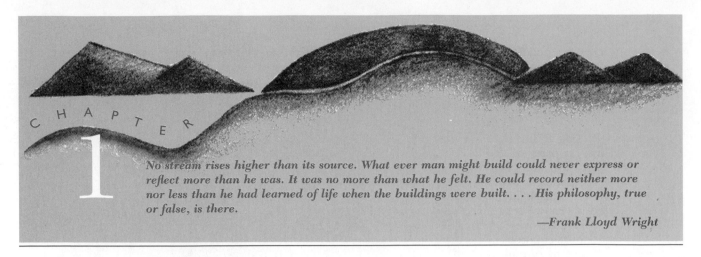

No stream rises higher than its source. What ever man might build could never express or reflect more than he was. It was no more than what he felt. He could record neither more nor less than he had learned of life when the buildings were built. . . . His philosophy, true or false, is there.

—Frank Lloyd Wright

Points of Departure
Beliefs to Guide the Journey

Learning Objectives

After studying this chapter, you should be able to:

1. Talk about a holistic approach to psychiatric patients.
2. Define a world view and give at least two examples of different world views.
3. Discuss the characteristics of a theistic world view.
4. Discuss the relevance of philosophies or world views such as humanism, secularism, behaviorism, and existentialism to psychiatric nursing.
5. Discuss at least two research studies that demonstrate the impact of a theistic world view on mental health.
6. Discuss the metaphor of the "journey" as it relates to the nurse-patient relationship.
7. Talk about the issues that are likely to affect your journey as a student in psychiatric nursing.
8. Describe the Stallwood-Stoll model of human functioning.

Key Terminology

Behaviorism
Existentialism
Holism
Humanism

Monism
Pantheism
Polytheism

Secularism
Theism
World view

AN INVITATION TO THE JOURNEY

This chapter, as well as this textbook, differs from most you have read. I am inviting you to be open to both the didactic and the experiential components of psychiatric nursing and to join me along with my contributors as we journey in psychiatric nursing. Initially, your journey may be colored by conflicting feelings—fear and curiosity, dread and anticipation, repulsion and compassion. For some of you, the journey will be so enjoyable that you will choose to make this your nursing specialty. For others, a different journey in nursing is more suited to your strengths. In any event, your sojourn into this specialty is guaranteed to impact all of your nursing practice and even holds the possibility of transforming you as you come to understand yourself and others better. Psychiatric nursing is about a journey, the nurse-patient journey. Although the journey itself holds incredible paradoxes—joy and sorrow, happiness and sadness, as well as excitement and frustration—it is never boring.

Psychiatric nursing affords us the privilege of accompanying patients on parts of their lives' journeys. As fellow sojourners, we are offered glimpses into the private worlds of patients. Sometimes we are invited into those private worlds in an intimate way, sometimes we are shocked by what we see and learn in the patient's world, sometimes we are overcome with the magnitude of pain the patient has endured and is experiencing, and sometimes we want to run away. Other times we are drawn to offer whatever we can to ease the suffering and to assist the patient in living a fuller, happier, and more productive life. We believe that it is indeed a privilege to be able to work with psychiatric patients. Many times these are the least understood and most poorly treated of all patients in the health care system. Yet these patients have much to teach us about survival, about spiritual strength, about resiliency, and about the importance of being treated with respect, dignity, and compassion.

We have a shared vision for this textbook, and that vision is captured by the image of a journey. Life is a journey, psychiatric nursing is a journey, the nurse-patient relationship is a journey. We know that we are moving forward, but we do not always know where we are going or where the next bend in the road will be. We know that each of our journeys is unique, yet there are times, for brief periods, when we walk with another.

A PERSPECTIVE FOR THE JOURNEY

In addition to our vision of the journey, we desire to convey our beliefs about people and how people should be treated. These beliefs stem from our **world view,** which is a way of looking at the big picture of life and making sense of it. A world view helps us to organize our experiences in a meaningful way and to draw conclusions about the significance of these experiences to our lives. We share this with you because it is important to be straightforward about foundational assumptions. However, it is *not necessary* for you to accept our world view to read and benefit from this textbook. Equally true, it is not necessary for patients to share in our world view to be cared for by us. We can and do respect individuals who hold different world views, and we strive to find areas of commonality.

➤ *Check Your Reading*
1. What is a world view?
   Look at a big picture in life + make sense of it

Our Theistic World View

Before describing our theistic world view, it is important to tell you that it is not a religious world view, although it is spiritual. Perhaps you have never distinguished spirituality and religion, but they are not the same. Spirituality is about experience and what happens in our hearts. Religion attempts to conceptualize that experience through codes, rules, and a system for ordering life. For some individuals, their religion and spirituality are the same. For others, there is little or no relationship between the two. Still other individuals profess a specific religious faith but are not at all spiritual (Carson, 1998).

Sometimes *world view* and *spirituality* are interchangeable terms, and for us, this is true. We operate from a theistic world view. We believe that

1. A loving and benevolent creator God exists.
2. We are created in God's image.
3. God loves us.
4. Our actions toward each other should reflect God's love.
5. Hope of change always exists.
6. We are holistic beings: we have integrated physical, emotional, and spiritual dimensions.

Theism stresses forgiving and treating people with kindness, patience, gentleness, and forbearance. These qualities are essential in psychiatric nursing, where the symptoms that patients display are frequently viewed by society as repugnant and bizarre.

What do you think? Have you ever thought about your own world view? If so, how would you describe it? Is there room in your world view for beliefs of others that might differ or even conflict with your own? How do you respond to individuals whose basic beliefs about the value of life; the value of the individual; the place of integrity, love, justice, and mercy in life differ from your own?

➤ *Check Your Reading*
2. What is a theistic world view? spiritual
3. What are the basic beliefs of a theistic world view? Gods image, actions reflect Gods love, hope of change exists
4. What does a theistic world view stress regarding how we should treat others?
   forgive + treat people = kind, patient, gentle

A Theistic View of People and Patients

We view patients as whole beings **(holism).** We think of patients as more than their symptoms; they are not just people who hear voices, who are anxious, or who dress in bizarre ways but people who have rich life experiences to share with us who happen to manifest a particular psychiatric symptom. Patients are just like us; in fact, one of the most frightening insights for a novice in psychiatric nursing is that we share many similarities with patients. It is always safer to believe that we are qualitatively different from the psychiatric patients for whom we care. Patients are wounded people, just as we are all wounded people, some of us more deeply and seriously than others (Nouwen, 1979).

None of us gets through this life without experiencing sadness, rejection, disappointment, isolation, loneliness, and confusion.

When we are wounded, we hurt all over. When something is wrong, it affects our whole being: mind, body, and soul. Therefore, it is imperative that when we attempt to understand and help, we get the whole picture. We need to know about patients' bodies. Where do they feel tension or heaviness? How have they somatized their pain? Have they neglected their bodies because of intense and crippling sadness? We need to know about their minds. What are their thought processes? Are they confused, coherent, or scattered, or have they shut down their thinking? What have they done to survive? How do they make meaning out of their lives? We need to understand their feelings, which are essentially human expressions that give seasoning to experiences. Are they feeling sad, angry, rejected, or alone? Can they identify and express their feelings? We need to know about their social circle. Who or what provides them with support? We need to know about their spirituality. What impact is their illness having on their spirit? Has their illness impacted or been impacted by their religious faith and practices? We need to know about their families. What part do families play in their healing? These understandings are all essential to piecing together the patient's story.

Another choice we would like to explain to you is why we have decided to use the word *patient* rather than *client* throughout the text. This choice is reflective of foundational beliefs about psychiatric patients. The term *client* is thought to denote a consumer of health care, a full participant in the health care process. It is a term that shifts the focus from psychiatric illness to mental health. But in truth, the term *client* means "someone who is dependent on another for protection" (Levine, 1989, p. 125). People we see in psychiatric hospitals usually refer to themselves as patients as do people we see for psychiatric home care and those we see privately in our own offices. We have been corrected by people who were called clients. It is not uncommon for people to react negatively to the term *client* because it is "cold" and "too businesslike." The term *patient,* on the other hand, means "one who suffers and forbears" (Levine, 1989, p. 125). Somehow, the term *patient* seems more accurate than *client* when describing the person in need of psychiatric services. Frequently, psychiatric patients have suffered not only their own private anguish and turmoil but also the stigma and rejection of society, upheaval and stress in their families, lack of understanding in their places of work, and sometimes the continuation of this suffering within the mental health system.

What *do you think?* When you refer to the people for whom you provide care, do you call them patients or clients? Is the distinction at all important to you? Do you think it matters to those for whom we care?

► *Check Your Reading*

5. What does a theistic world view tell us about people and patients?
6. Why do we need to know patients from physical, social, emotional, and spiritual perspectives?
7. What is the difference between the terms *patient* and *client*?

A Theistic Model of Human Beings

A model of human beings that best describes the interaction of body, mind, and spirit was developed by Jean Stallwood and Ruth Stoll (1975) and is shown in Figure 1-1. The model shows three concentric circles. The largest circle refers to the physical being, with the five senses: seeing, hearing, tasting, feeling, and smelling. The physical or body self is "world-conscious." The next circle is the psychosocial, that part of the person that gives one self-awareness and personality through emotions, intellect, moral sense, and will. The innermost circle, the spirit, is the most difficult to comprehend because of its mysterious and indefinable nature. The spirit is that part of the person that pervades all of the other dimensions. Within this spiritual center lies the potential for consciousness of and relatedness to God.

Because each person is and functions as a dynamic whole and not as three separate dimensions, each dimension influences and is influenced by the others. This flow among the three dimensions of a person is represented on the model by the broken lines that make up the boundaries of the circles. The model also depicts arrows flowing into and out of the three circles. This illustrates the mutually interactive nature of the person with outside influences such as social support, including family and friends; God; and material resources that

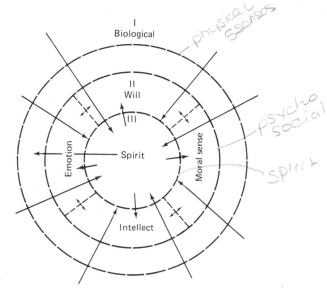

Figure 1-1
The Stallwood-Stoll model of human functioning. (Reprinted with the permission of Simon & Schuster Inc. from CLINICAL NURSING 3/e by Irene L. Beland and J. Y. Passos. Copyright ©1975 Macmillan Publishing Company.)

strengthen or weaken the person. Therefore, when a person is feeling depressed, the experience includes not only sadness but also crying, sleeping and eating problems, slowed thinking, lack of energy, conflict in personal relationships, and a spiritual void expressed as hopelessness and despair about God's place in the person's life.

Any therapeutic approach that deals *only* with the mind or *only* with the body is woefully inadequate. Going back to the example of the person who feels depressed, comprehensive treatment includes using an antidepressant, teaching the causes and effects of depression, encouraging that hope exists because depression is treatable, attending to physical problems, involving family and significant others in care, and discussing ways to alleviate spiritual distress.

> **W**hat do you think? What situations have made you aware of your own interconnectedness? That is, have you had emotional struggles that have resulted in physical and spiritual distress? Have you ever experienced spiritual distress that was expressed through your body and mind? How did you deal with these situations? What helped you and what hindered you in resolving the situations?

> ► *Check Your Reading*
> 8. What do the three concentric circles in the Stallwood-Stoll model of human functioning represent?
> 9. How does the model illustrate the interactive aspects of the dimensions of human beings?
> 10. What implications does the Stallwood-Stoll model have for psychiatric nursing?

A Theistic View of Brain Physiology

You might be wondering where the exploding research on brain physiology and function fits into a textbook that holds a holistic perspective. We believe that this research is highly significant and promises to transform not only the treatment of the psychiatric patient but also the role of the psychiatric nurse. However, we *do not think* that understanding the brain holds the key to eradicating the pain of psychiatric illnesses. If this were the whole answer, we could eliminate most of this textbook and focus exclusively on the brain. We believe that imbalances in brain physiology cause vulnerabilities or predispositions to certain psychiatric illnesses. In some people, the physical imbalance is so overwhelming (such as is the case with an anencephalic infant) that we can do little cognitively, emotionally, spiritually, or physically to alter the outcome for that person. Examples of people in whom physiology dictates destiny, however, probably represent the minority.

Most of us have some physiological vulnerabilities with which we struggle, but we are certainly not defined by those characteristics. The determining factors influencing whether or not we develop an illness include the presence or absence of a loving family, the presence or absence of significant others in our lives who supply us with love and affirmation, the adequacy and safety of our environment, and the adequacy of our diet to meet the demands for a healthy body and mind. Our understanding of the complex nature of human beings is so primitive that we cannot predict how much of one factor or another makes the difference between health and illness. What we do know is that people respond to love; that people can change, if only in small ways; and that the nurse-patient relationship makes a difference.

> ► *Check Your Reading*
> 11. How does a focus on brain physiology "fit in" with a theistic world view?

Other World Views

A theistic world view does not exclude consideration of ideas from other philosophies or world views. Many of the "isms," such as behaviorism, humanism, existentialism, and secularism, are essentially nonreligious in that they make no direct mention of a Supreme Being. Others, such as monism, pantheism, and polytheism, are religious in that they specifically address a Supreme Being or Beings. Although some of these world views make important contributions to our understanding of human behavior, "isms" generally have a narrow focus and are *exclusive* rather than *inclusive* (Carson, 1998).

Behaviorism as a World View. **Behaviorism** suggests that people are no more and no less than the behaviors that they exhibit. Behaviorism focuses on changing behavior through controlled systems of reinforcers. The emphasis is not on free will, choice, personal meaning, or the importance of feelings. In psychiatric nursing, we study behavior; we believe that all behavior is meaningful, and we sometimes draw on techniques to change behavior. But we never lose sight of the fact that people are more than their behaviors.

Humanism as a World View. Let us look at **humanism,** a world view that extols the value and importance of the human being. A humanist attempts to modify behavior and feelings by focusing on a person's innate goodness. The humanist believes that the person is always striving toward the good, that the power to change lies solely within the person, and that it is not necessary to recognize or draw on God in the healing process. Humanism adds much of value to psychiatric nursing, and in this textbook, we draw on humanist thinking. However, because humanism excludes the significance of the transcendent in human activity, it is not as comprehensive a world view as theism.

Existentialism as a World View. **Existentialism** focuses on the analysis of individual existence in a universe that is incomprehensible. The existentialist encourages the person to assume responsibility for freely made choices without any certain knowledge of what is right or wrong. We agree with some of the existentialist's notions: the importance of the person's story and how the person makes decisions when faced with choices. These are essential to understanding and assisting patients; thus, we have included stories as an existential thread throughout the text. But again, existentialism is not the whole story.

Secularism as a World View. **Secularism** is based on the belief that full understanding of the world comes through technical and scientific advances. Secularism in its purest form is, at the least, indifferent to spiritual concerns; often, it overtly rejects as irrelevant spirituality as well as religion and religious considerations.

Monism and Pantheism as World Views. **Monism** suggests that a basic oneness of being exists and that the transcendent force in the universe is not a personal God but rather a universal energy force. A monistic world view leads to a pantheistic world view. **Pantheism** suggests that everything is the same and that there is no difference between what exists in the world and the universal energy. The pantheistic world view leads its followers to the conclusion that all people and things share in the divine energy source and that, essentially, all are God. Both monism and pantheism value relativism rather than absolutes and emphasize striving for balance within within individual lives and the eradication of self. Pantheistic practices include therapeutic touch, acupuncture, chakra analysis, shiatsu (acupressure), Ayurvedic medicine, and polarity therapy. Monism and pantheism undergird much of Buddhism and Hinduism, although there is a broad range of beliefs within these religions.

Polytheism as a World View. **Polytheism** suggests that many gods exist in the universe. In polytheistic religions, sacrifices are frequently made to appease the gods or to appeal to the gods for special favors (Pacwa, 1992). Indigenous religions, as well as some forms of Buddhism and Hinduism, are polytheistic.

What do you think? Does your nursing program have a defined world view? Is it implicit or explicit? Is that world view compatible with your own? If not, how have the differences revealed themselves to you?

➤ *Check Your Reading*

12. Name two nonreligious world views.
13. Describe how humanism affects psychiatric nursing.
14. What contribution does behaviorism make to psychiatric nursing?
15. What does existentialism postulate that has significance for psychiatric nursing?
16. Describe monism, pantheism, and polytheism.
17. Contrast theism with monism, pantheism, and polytheism.

Research Supporting the Positive Impact of a Theistic World View on Mental Health

The National Institute for Healthcare Research focuses on the connection between faith and medicine. It sponsors research and conferences and publishes a quarterly newsletter. The newsletter frequently summarizes research that demonstrates a link between an aspect of health and spirituality and/or religious practice. Box 1-1 includes a summary of some of these research findings.

ISSUES YOU WILL FACE ON THE JOURNEY

The last area that we want to address in this chapter concerns your own journey as a psychiatric nursing student. You face several specific issues as you enter a psychiatric nursing rotation.

Anxiety About the New Situations You Will Encounter

It is not uncommon to feel stress and anxiety about new situations. You may have preconceived ideas about what a psychiatric hospital is like. Perhaps you have seen dramatizations on television or in the movies that have influenced your thinking. Perhaps you have a loved one with a psychiatric illness. Whatever the reasons, nursing students frequently approach the psychiatric experience with an increased stress level. The stress response can adversely affect your behavior. It is helpful to discuss this with your instructor and to seek suggestions to promote relaxation and adaptive thinking.

Threats to Your Role as a Nurse

Another issue confronted by psychiatric nursing students is a threat to their nursing role arising from several characteristics unique to psychiatric nursing: (1) lack of

Box 1–1 ■ ■ ■ ■ ■
Research on the Impact of Religion on Mental Health

In a prospective study of 2812 elderly people in New Haven, Connecticut, religiosity was inversely related to depression and subsequent disability and was directly related to improved functional ability (Idler & Kasl, 1992).

Among 2679 participants in the National Institute of Epidemiological Catchment Area study, frequent church attendees had lower rates of psychopathology than infrequent attendees in three denominations (Koenig, George, Meador, Blarer, & Dyck, 1994).

In a systematic review, Gartner, Larson, and Allen (1991) found that religious commitment was inversely related to suicide in 13 of 16 of the reviewed studies.

professional attire; (2) lack of structure; (3) decisions about whether or not to read the patient's chart; (4) need for self-awareness; (5) fear of being injured and of injuring patients emotionally; (6) fear of rejection; (7) fear of identifying with patients; and (8) frustration over inability to change patients.

Lack of Professional Attire. In a psychiatric setting, staff members generally wear street clothes rather than uniforms, and they usually do not carry professional equipment such as stethoscopes or bandage scissors. Students often cannot tell the patients from the staff and fear that they will be embarrassed by practicing newly formed interview and assessment skills on staff rather than on patients. Stripped of the security afforded by the outward symbols of the nursing role, students are left with the awareness that their main therapeutic tools are their communication and interpersonal skills and their abilities to empathize and problem solve. Again, the result of this role threat is increased anxiety.

Lack of Structure. For students who are accustomed to the lock-step structure of a medical-surgical unit, the lack of structure—or rather the different structure—on a psychiatric unit can be disconcerting. In fact, it may seem that the psychiatric nursing staff does little. This couldn't be further from the truth. Perhaps if we present the role of the psychiatric nurse in a concrete way, we can alleviate some of the anxiety produced by this different structure.

Although there are many ways to conceptualize the psychiatric nursing role, the following four categories of interventions may help you. First, the nurse is focused on developing a relationship with the patient and selecting the appropriate communication techniques to facilitate that development. Second, the nurse is concerned with the patient's health status. This concern is manifested by using assessment skills as well as hands-on interventions, including administering and monitoring medications and treatments. Third, the nurse is responsible for improving the patient's self-care knowledge by teaching about the illness, medication, and other issues. Fourth, the nurse is concerned with improving the patient's self-care skills. This involves teaching the patient specific health-promoting skills, such as keeping a journal; setting up a medication compliance pack; problem solving; and using thought-stopping techniques.

It may not be readily apparent to the novice just how much energy can be expended in these areas. It is important that students get involved in the activities of the unit; involvement promotes fitting in and allows students to discover their place more quickly than students who wait on the sidelines until they feel comfortable with the environment. Students have shared that an article by Clement (1988) entitled "The myths and realities of psychiatric nursing, or I feel guilty when I just sit and talk" helps them cope with the different structure of psychiatric nursing.

Decisions About Whether or Not to Read the Patient's Chart. Reading the patient's chart before meeting the patient is an issue that can be important to the nursing student. There are advantages to reading the chart before meeting the patient, but there are also advantages to reading the chart *after* meeting the patient. For the anxious student, reading the chart is a concrete activity that lessens his or her anxiety and helps to structure the student's time. For less anxious students, meeting the patient without reading the chart allows them to get to know the patient free of bias. Most likely, your instructor will assist you in making the chart-reading decision.

Need for Self-Awareness. We described psychiatric nursing as a journey for you, and indeed it is. The journey into increased self-awareness is exciting and rewarding, but it is sometimes scary. To be an effective helper, each of us needs to know ourselves and to be aware of our own thoughts and feelings, strengths and weaknesses, values, and reactions to people, places, and things. The goal of self-awareness is not to change all that we are—in fact, most students are affirmed in the communication and interpersonal skills they already possess—but rather, the goal is to know and understand ourselves so that we can effectively use the gift of who we are. Students approach the task of increasing self-awareness in many ways. Some find that keeping a journal allows them to freely express who they are without judgment. Others find meditation, prayer, periods of quiet solitude, sharing in groups or individual clinical supervision sessions, and completing process recordings (written verbatim accounts of their nurse-patient interactions) to be effective strategies to enhance self-awareness.

Fear of Being Injured and of Injuring Patients Emotionally. Many students begin the journey into psychiatric nursing afraid that they will be harmed by patients or that they will say the "wrong" thing and cause harm to patients. The fear of physical harm at the hands of the violent patient has been greatly exaggerated by media portrayals of patients as wild and out of control. Likewise, causing irreparable harm to the patient by saying the wrong thing is unlikely. Although part of the focus of a psychiatric nursing course is to strengthen therapeutic communication skills, most patients are very attentive to nonverbal cues and are sensitive to the intent of the nursing student. If you are caring and concerned, most likely you will communicate this message even if your words somehow miss the mark. You might also have fears about your own ability to remain in control if a patient acts in an inappropriate way in front of you. Other students have reported the benefits of anticipating such incidents and thinking about acceptable responses beforehand.

Fear of Rejection. Another concern that students express as they journey into psychiatric nursing is that they will be rejected by patients. It is not uncommon for psychiatric patients to be shy and wary with strangers. What appears to be rejecting behavior on the part of the patient may actually be the patient's fear of approaching new people. Although you may encounter patients who are shy or even hostile and withdrawn, many patients welcome the interest of the nursing student and are receptive to the student's overtures.

Fear of Identifying With Patients. As you journey into psychiatric nursing you may find that you encounter patients with problems, stresses, and conflicts similar to your own. This may frighten you; you may find yourself thinking something like, "There but for the grace of God go I." When confronted with these feelings, it will help you to talk to your instructor, who can help you look at how you have effectively coped with your situation or who can help you see the subtle differences between the patient's situation and your own.

Frustration Over Inability to Change Patients. You may find your journey frustrating because you are unable to complete goals that you have set for a particular nurse-patient interaction. Psychiatric nursing brings you face to face with the truth that you cannot change or be responsible for anyone's behavior but your own. If the patient is not cooperating, you can evaluate your own approach and modify it, but you cannot dictate or control the patient's choice of whether to respond to your approach. This is a hard lesson but one that has implications far beyond psychiatric nursing.

Cost of Your Involvement

The last issue to look at concerning your own journey is the cost of your involvement. We ask you to provide holistic care; we ask you to be kind, empathetic, attentive, and reflective; we ask you to *care* about patients. What we are asking you to do has a cost attached to it. This cost is seldom acknowledged or mentioned. When you get involved with and care about people, you feel their pain and sorrow. You become frustrated, sad, and sometimes angry. To stay healthy, you must find positive outlets to express those feelings. You need to talk about them in a supportive and accepting environment. You need to attend to your own spiritual needs, most importantly your relationship with God, as you understand God. You need to receive supervision to understand the dynamics of the nurse-patient relationship. In other words, you need to take care of yourself—body, mind, and spirit—just as you are teaching patients to take care of themselves. No one—and this is worth repeating—*no one* can continually give without receiving refreshment, nurturance, and inspiriting care. So take care of yourself, not only during your journey into psychiatric nursing but also throughout your nursing career.

➤ *Check Your Reading*

18. Identify two issues that you will face as a nursing student entering a psychiatric nursing rotation for the first time.
19. Describe two of the situations characteristic of psychiatric nursing that may pose a threat to your role as a nurse.
20. Identify two common fears experienced by nursing students entering a psychiatric nursing rotation for the first time.
21. Describe at least three strategies that you can use to cope with the anxiety that you might feel as a novice in psychiatric nursing.
22. What is meant by the "cost of involvement"?

Conclusions

Psychiatric nursing, like all of life, is a journey in which no guarantees exist about what lies ahead. We invite you to join us in the journey of psychiatric nursing and to be open to its possibilities. We invite you to view your role with psychiatric patients as one involving a privileged position of sharing, if only for a brief period, in their journeys.

The psychiatric nursing journey and the life journey on which we have embarked are undergirded by unwavering belief in a theistic world view, a world view that holds forth a creator God who considers us His beloved and calls us into relationship with Him. From this relationship and this world view, we are encouraged to respond to others with the same love that the Creator has poured forth on us. Our journey also has been affected by beliefs from several other world views, including humanism, existentialism, and behaviorism.

Your journey into psychiatric nursing is sure to be affected by multiple other issues, including your own feelings of uncertainty and fear; threats to your role as a nurse, including the lack of both professional attire and structure; indecision about issues such as whether or not to read the patient's chart; the focus on getting to know yourself better; fears of being injured and of causing injury, of being rejected by patients, and of identifying with patients; frustration over your inability to change patients; and, finally, an awareness that the cost of involvement can be high. We hope that you will counter these issues with a sense of your importance as an instrument of healing and with an awareness that you, stripped of the outward acoutrements of nursing, are a powerful force in the patient's attempts to construct a more healthy journey.

Key Points to Remember

- Psychiatric nursing, like all of life, is a journey. We are privileged to accompany patients on parts of their journeys.
- Psychiatric patients, who are frequently the least understood and most poorly treated of all patients, have much to teach us about survival, spiritual strength, resiliency, and the importance of being treated with respect, dignity, and compassion.
- The underlying foundation for this textbook is *not* a specific religion but rather a theistic world view. This world view includes the following beliefs: (1) a loving and benevolent creator God exists; (2) we are created

in God's image; (3) God loves us; (4) our actions toward each other should reflect God's love; (5) hope of change always exists; and (6) we are holistic beings: we have integrated physical, emotional, and spiritual dimensions.

- A theistic world view stresses forgiving and treating people with kindness, patience, gentleness, and forbearance. These qualities are essential in psychiatric nursing.

- A theistic world view suggests that if psychiatric nurses are to make a difference in the lives of their patients, the focus of nursing interventions must be on all the dimensions that make up the person—physical, emotional, and spiritual.

- Stallwood and Stoll identified a theistic model of human beings that demonstrates the interaction of all the dimensions that make up a person.

- A theistic world view is not inconsistent with a focus on the role of neurophysiology in psychiatric illness. However, brain physiology tells only part of the patient's story; the rest of the story draws from many other sources, including the patient's spirituality.

- A theistic model of intervention is holistic. It includes a focus on behaviors, affective processes, sensations, images, thoughts, interpersonal relationships, and spirituality.

- The term *patient* rather than *client* is used throughout the text because *patient* describes the long suffering and forbearance of the person seeking psychiatric care.

- Several nonspiritual world views exist, including behaviorism, humanism, secularism, and existentialism. In this textbook, we draw on behaviorism, humanism, and existentialism, while realizing that they are not as comprehensive as theism.

- Three spiritual world views also exist: monism, pantheism, and polytheism. Monism purports that all in the universe is the same and that the divine is an impersonal energy force. Pantheism extends monism to state that because everything is one and all is the same, then we are all God. Polytheism holds forth a belief in many gods.

- Multiple issues confront you as you begin your journey into psychiatric nursing. These issues include your own feelings of uncertainty and fear; threats to your role as a nurse, including both the lack of professional attire and the lack of structure; indecision about issues such as whether to read the patient's chart; the focus on getting to know yourself better; fears of being injured by and of causing injury to patients, of being rejected by patients, and of identifying with patients; frustration over your inability to change patients; and, finally, an awareness that the cost of involvement can be high.

- The psychiatric nursing role can be conceptualized to have four categories of interventions including those that deal with communication techniques and relationship building; those that deal with monitoring and impacting the patient's health status; those that deal with impacting the patient's self-care knowledge; and last, those that increase the patient's self-care skills.

- The cost of involvement can be offset by the knowledge that you are a powerful instrument of healing for the patient who is struggling to change his or her own story.

Learning Activities

1. Read current journal articles on spirituality in nursing. See if you are able to determine the world view from which the authors are operating. Do you agree with the world view that is presented?

2. Think about your own world view. How do you view the big picture of life? Does God play a role in your world view? Does God play a role in your view of nursing? If so, what is His role? Are you able to consider the world views of others, even when they are different from your own beliefs?

3. How are religion and spirituality different for you? How are they the same? How do they impact on your perception of nursing and your role as a psychiatric nurse?

4. Keep a journal about your own journey into nursing. Focus on the reasons you chose to pursue nursing as a career. What does your journey tell you about your own world view?

5. Think about clinical situations in which patients hold world views different from your own. How do you handle these situations?

6. Think about the issues that you will face as you journey into psychiatric nursing. What resources do you currently use to take care of yourself? What resources do you need to better care for yourself? What are your spiritual resources?

Critical Thinking Exercises

All the students in Professor Smyth's psychiatric clinical laboratory have been asked to think about their life experiences and how these experiences might affect their thoughts and beliefs about the importance of spirituality in psychiatric illness. Sarah's thoughts went to when she was 10 years old, to the day when her mother and brother were taken to the emergency department following an automobile accident with a drunk driver. Ever since that day, she knew she wanted to be a nurse so that she could help others. Sarah was aware of the sadness that overcame her as she remembered how her brother's struggle to live had failed and how her mother continued to struggle with wanting to live. Sarah refused to go to church after the accident. This learning experience was not going to be easy. Sarah had seen the inside of crisis centers all too often.

1. What assumptions can you make about Sarah's belief in God?

2. What evidence suggests that your assumptions are true?

3. What other information do you need to determine if your assumptions are valid?

Sarah was assigned to interview Mr. Jasline, a patient with a history of depression. After talking with him she discovered that he was also in the hospital for detoxification because of his chronic use of alcohol. After the interview, she discussed her feelings about Mr. Jasline with Professor Smyth.

1. How might Sarah's past experiences influence her practice?

2. What are possible responses that Sarah might have to Mr. Jasline?

3. What conclusions can you draw from the data in the above paragraph?

Additional Resources

National Institute for Healthcare Research (NIHR)

www.nihr.org

Log on to find out about the faith-medicine connection: updates on research, conferences, spokesperson presentations, press releases, and products.

References

Carson, V. B. (1998). Spirituality. In J. M. Leahy & P. E. Kizilay (Eds.), *Foundations of nursing practice: A nursing process approach* (pp. 1074-1093). Philadelphia: W. B. Saunders.

Clement, J. A. (1988). The myths and realities of psychiatric nursing or I feel guilty when I just sit and talk. *Imprint, 35,* 40-41.

Gartner, J., Larson, D., & Allen, G. (1991). Religious commitment and mental health: A review of the empirical literature. *Journal of Psychology and Theology, 19,* 6-25.

Idler, E. L., & Kasl, S. V. (1992). Religion, disability, depression, and the timing of death. *American Journal of Sociology, 97,* 1052-1079.

Koenig, H. G., George, L. K., Meador, K. G., Blarer, D. G., & Dyck,

P. B. (1994). Religious affiliation and psychiatric disorder among Protestant baby boomers. *Hospital and Community Psychiatry, 45,* 586-596.

Levine, M. (1989). Beyond dilemma. *Seminars in Oncology Nursing, 5,* 124-128.

Nouwen, H. J. M. (1979). *The wounded healer: Ministry in contemporary society.* New York: Doubleday.

Pacwa, M. (1992). *Catholics and the new age.* Ann Arbor, MI: Servant Publications.

Stallwood, J., & Stoll, R. (1975). Spiritual dimension of nursing practice. In I. L. Beland & J. Y. Passos (Eds.), *Clinical nursing* (3rd ed.). New York: Macmillan.

Suggested Readings

Carson, V. B. (1993). Spirituality: Generic or Christian. *Journal of Christian Nursing, 10*(1), 24-27.

Sire, J. (1988). *The universe next door* (2nd ed.). Downers Grove, IL: Inter-Varsity Press.

Turner, S. (1990, September 24). Lean, green and meaningless. *Christianity Today,* 26-27.

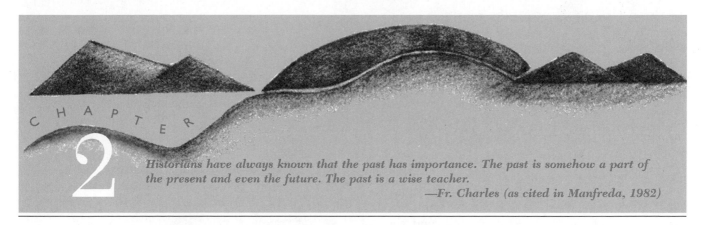

Historians have always known that the past has importance. The past is somehow a part of the present and even the future. The past is a wise teacher.

—*Fr. Charles (as cited in Manfreda, 1982)*

The Wisdom of Past Travelers
Heritage of Psychiatric Nursing

Learning Objectives

After studying this chapter, you should be able to:

1. Describe the contributions of the following people to psychiatric nursing: Harriet Bailey, Clifford Beers, Dorothea Lynde Dix, Dorothy Mereness, Adolph Meyer, Hildegard E. Peplau, Phillippe Pinel, Linda Richards, Benjamin Rush, Harry Stack Sullivan, Euphemia "Effie" Jane Taylor, and William Tuke.

2. Identify the influence of the following U.S. legislation: the National Mental Health Act of 1946, the Hill-Burton Act, the Mental Retardation Facilities and Community Mental Health Centers Construction Act of 1963, the Community Mental Health Center Amendment of 1975, the Community Mental Health Systems Act, the Omnibus Budget Reconciliation Act of 1982, and the Americans With Disabilities Act of 1990.

3. Discuss the influence of World War I and World War II on the care of the mentally ill.

4. Identify important "firsts" in psychiatric nursing: the first psychiatric nurse, the opening of the McLean Training School for Nurses, the first psychiatric nursing textbook, the first psychiatric nursing journal, and the first psychiatric nursing professor.

5. Identify the historical significance of the following hospitals associated with the care of the mentally ill: Bethlehem Hospital, the Eastern Lunatic Asylum, Pennsylvania Hospital, and the McLean Asylum.

6. Discuss the impact of psychobiological therapies on the journey of psychiatric nursing.

7. Identify one effect of deinstitutionalization on the journey of psychiatric nursing.

8. Discuss the significance of the "Decade of the Brain" on the journey of psychiatric nursing.

Key Terminology

Almshouses	Sigmund Freud	Hildegard E. Peplau	Benjamin Rush
Asylums	Jails	Phillippe Pinel	Harry Stack Sullivan
Harriet Bailey	Emil Kraepelin	Private mental hospitals	Euphemia "Effie" Jane Taylor
Clifford Beers	William C. Menninger	Public mental hospitals	William Tuke
Bethlehem Hospital	Adolph Meyer	Linda Richards	York Retreat
Dorothea Lynde Dix	Pennsylvania Hospital		

Portions of this chapter are from the previous edition chapter contributed by Mary Ellen Lashley, PhD, RN, CRNP, CS.

The journey of psychiatric nurses and the patients for whom they have cared has been arduous and rewarding, disheartening and encouraging, despairing and hopeful, buffeted and enhanced by societal forces and events, spanning centuries. In as much as a journey may involve many paths and many steps and be influenced by numerous individuals as well as by predictable and unexpected events, so has been the journey of nurses who have chosen to care for patients suffering from mental illness.

Psychiatric nurses have met their patients in a diversity of settings and under an array of circumstances, some shamefully inadequate, neglectful, and harmful; some barely adequate; and in some fortunate instances, some that were appealing and comfortable places for recovery. Nurses caring for the mentally ill have also been either helped or hindered by colleagues in other nursing disciplines and by other health care providers. Like the patients for whom they have cared, mental health nurses have been misunderstood and ostracized.

Joyce Travelbee (1969), a psychiatric nurse educator, observed that "an aura of mystery" continues to exist regarding the nature of psychiatric nursing (p. 21). She also noted that there was a "still prevalent belief . . . that psychiatric nurses are in some ways peculiar" and a belief that "the longer a nurse works with the mentally ill the more like 'them' she becomes" (p. 22). She characterized psychiatric nursing practice as "a searching, tiring, sometimes tedious but always interesting process" (p. 23).

In this story, Edna Fordyce reflects on her own journey in psychiatric nursing.

Edna Fordyce's Story

My journey in psychiatric nursing began in 1953 when, as a junior nursing student in a diploma nursing program, I commenced my psychiatric affiliation at Rochester State Hospital in Rochester, Minnesota. This was the type of educational setting and curriculum experienced by most nursing students at that time. We spent 3 months on the hospital campus, living in a nurses' residence on the grounds, attending classes, and participating in the care of patients on the various wards of the hospital. Our schedule of classes and assignments to the hospital wards added up to a 40-hour week. Our classes on mental illness and nursing care were conducted by nurse instructors and physicians, most of them psychiatrists. One of our required textbooks was Helena Render's *Nurse-Patient Relationships in Psychiatry*, published in 1947. It is important to note that the modern pharmacological treatment of mental illness had not yet been instituted; at that time, most of the medications used today had not yet been discovered. By comparison with today, knowledge about the causes and treatment of mental illness was not as extensive.

This experience was truly memorable and has influenced my life in many ways, including my career choices. I was challenged by the nursing responsibilities in which we participated. Nursing activities included daily personal care of the patients, playing table games with them on the units, and, when possible, taking them off the wards to activities or for walks on the hospital grounds. And yes, there were dances, held twice weekly, to which we escorted patients and participated with them. For me, dancing meant skipping to the music alongside the patient partner rather than actually dancing.

Assisting With Electroconvulsive Therapy

Every Monday, Wednesday, and Friday, 45 to 50 patients of the nearly 2000 who were hospitalized received the relatively new therapy of electroconvulsive therapy (ECT), sometimes referred to as *shock therapy*. I recall assisting in what seemed like the herding of these folks dressed in white gowns and blue-striped bathrobes through the network of hospital tunnels to receive their treatment. The treatment was given without the benefit of anesthesia, although the drug curare was administered before the treatment to lessen the risk of fractures that could occur during the treatment. When the electric current was administered through electrodes placed on the patient's temples, the patient experienced a grand mal seizure. Hospital staff, assisted by nursing students, held the patient on the bed until the seizure subsided. After the patients awakened, we gave them a glass of milk. When they were steady enough to walk without falling, they were once again herded through the hospital tunnels, back to the nursing wards for bathing and dressing for the day. The red, sleepy faces with blood-tinged eyes remain in my memory even today.

Observing Prefrontal Lobotomies

I also observed the procedure of prefrontal lobotomy, which entailed the cutting of the prefrontal lobe tissues of the brain to calm the violent patient. I was assigned to care for some of these patients postoperatively. The superintendent of the hospital oversaw each procedure and had a reputation for maintaining high standards of care for patients. His leadership was effective in obtaining state legislative support for the resources he requested, such as more modern hospital buildings.

The hospital was one of seven state-supported hospitals in Minnesota. This state was recognized as having made substantial progress in caring for the mentally ill, with considerable credit having been given to Governor Luther Youngdahl (Sareyan, 1994).

Memories of Overcrowding, Seclusion, and Green Lawns

Other memories of those days are still impressed in my consciousness. Paramount is the memory of the overcrowded state of the hospital wards. There were insufficient beds for everyone on each of the 16 wards. For example, one unit with a capacity for 45 patients housed more than 90 patients. This overcrowding necessitated the use of cots at nighttime. After all thepatients were bedded down for the night, we barely had room to pass between the cots to leave the ward after completion of our assigned evening hours. Many hours of seclusion were the daily experience for the most violent and psychotic patients. For others, this form of restraint was a periodic occurrence. I saw no other physical restraints used in the hospital. A few years earlier, a massive bonfire had been held in Minnesota to destroy mechanical restraints such as the canvas camisole restraints *(straitjackets)* so often associated with mental institutions.

The hospital grounds were dominated by a long building of four stories with many wards, characteristic of the Kirkbride architectural plan and frequently the basis of hospital construction from 1854 to 1914 (Baxter & Hathcox, 1994). Several newer but smaller two-story buildings with four wards were also present on the hospital campus. Within these buildings, each ward had semiprivate rooms and well-lighted, spacious dayrooms. The hospital also had its own farm; the fields and green lawn of the hospital grounds were maintained by patients and hospital employees.

Memories of Caring and Commitment

Overall, I saw great kindness demonstrated toward patients by committed hospital staff from the various caregiving disciplines. Head nurses were responsible for each hospital ward. Many of them were registered nurses who had obtained their education from the training school that had previously existed at the hospital. This was a common type of educational program before World War II. Psychiatric aides, along with the nursing students, constituted the nursing staff under the supervision of the head nurse.

One head nurse, whom I greatly admired, was a model of commitment for everyone who knew her. She always assigned herself to be on duty for the special holidays of the year because on these days, she needed to be with her "ladies." The ladies of whom this nurse, Esther Swenson, spoke were among the most disturbed, psychotically ill women hospitalized at this facility.

I am quite certain that neither Esther Swenson nor many of her nurse colleagues could have articulated a theory or framework for their nursing practice, as espoused in contemporary textbooks. However, intuition, common sense, long hours spent with patients, and experience in responding to their behaviors, as well as their personal humanness, provided the basis for their practice of psychiatric nursing. The 3 months of my affiliation passed all too quickly, and soon I was to sadly bid farewell to a special nursing experience.

The words of George Santayana (cited in Church, 1982) seem fitting as I reflect on these experiences as a nursing student: "We must welcome the future remembering that soon it will be the past; and we must respect the past, remembering that once it was all that was humanly possible" (p. 1).

Moving on to a Psychiatric Unit in a General Hospital

After 2 years of general staff nursing, I ventured to assume a position in one of the new psychiatric units then existing in a general hospital; it was one of few. I was in charge of the insulin therapy room (insulin was administered to induce coma, with the intent of interrupting psychotic symptoms) and assisted with ECT. I was also the charge nurse assigned on designated shifts. Although these responsibilities were frightening, my confidence grew with experience. The year was 1956, and the new drug chlorpromazine (Thorazine) had recently been released. My colleagues and I administered this medication with great hopes of alleviating the many symptoms (delusions and hallucinations) patients were experiencing. Other medications, such as additional antipsychotic medications, antidepressants, and lithium, now so familiar, were not yet existent. The sedatives used then (such as phenobarbital) had only limited benefit in alleviating symptoms.

Returning to the State Hospital

After completing baccalaureate studies at the University of Minnesota (1960), I was fortunate to return to the state hospital of my student psychiatric affiliation. This time, with a new bachelor's degree and a little experience, I was the new instructor of nursing for the diploma students from six schools of nursing during their 12-week psychiatric affiliation.

During these years, numerous new medications (both antipsychotics and antidepressants) were approved and administered. Also during this time, psychiatric admissions at the hospital became predominantly voluntary; previously, the majority of patients were admitted as "committed" or "involuntary." Largely because of the new medications, hospital wards now had quieter and calmer atmospheres, and patients were more receptive to interactions and participation in hospital and ward activities.

On to Graduate School

I undertook graduate study at the University of Washington from 1967 to 1968, where my education was partially supported by federal funding that was then available for nurses seeking additional education. My hours of study were devoted to the writings of notable psychiatric authors such as Sigmund Freud, Harry Stack Sullivan, Karen Horney, Viktor Frankl, and others, as well as the emerging nurse theorists specializing in psychiatric nursing such as Joyce Travelbee and Hildegard E. Peplau. *Process recordings* (verbatim accounts of nurse-patient interactions) were written, examined, and reviewed to enhance our relationship and supervision skills.

Teaching the Next Generation of Psychiatric Nurses

Since 1960, I have taught graduate and undergraduate students, and this has been a rewarding experience.

Teaching has allowed me to participate in patient care in a variety of settings and to be involved in the changing forms of treatment for the mentally ill. Psychiatric nursing has opened doors for me to participate in various activities such as mental health counseling in the community. It has also enabled me to contribute to my church family through mental health counseling and other caring ministries, for example the *Stephen Ministry,* a lay caregiving program that is in operation in many Christian denominations. ■

Just as Fordyce's story is unique and spans more than 40 years of momentous change within the profession, many stories exist of other individuals who have contributed to the specialty of psychiatric nursing. In this chapter, you will meet some of them, read of important events, and learn about some of the settings for care that have existed through time. Our journey today has been made possible by the efforts of a myriad of individuals. Their contributions, individually and as a group, have championed the cause of the mentally ill, gained more appropriate care for these often neglected patients, and increased the understanding on which more effective care might be based. Their stories are woven with determination and perseverance, difficulties and triumphs.

However, before we can even look at these stories, we must review a time when there were no psychiatric nurses, psychiatric theories, or medical treatments, yet there were still individuals who were mentally ill. Bailey (1935), a psychiatric nurse and author, stated, "Mental disease is as old as the human race . . ." (p. 1). Alexander and Selesnick (1966), historians of psychiatry, observed,

The mentally ill have always been with us . . . to be feared, marveled at, laughed at, pitied, or tortured, but all too seldom cured. Their existence shakes us to the core of our being, for they make us painfully aware that sanity is a fragile thing. (p. 3)

Grob (1994) viewed the mentally ill as being an "inescapable presence," which has raised many issues and presented dilemmas to society (p. 3).

EARLY TRAVELERS

During the earliest times, behavior that was considered abnormal, such as that of the mentally ill, was attributed to supernatural forces. Evil spirits or punishment from the gods, the devil, or demons was believed to be the cause of diseases, including mental diseases. Alexander and Selesnick (1966) reported that witch doctors or medicine men were the first psychiatrists.

One of the prominent and perhaps most influential physicians of his own time and even to the present was Hippocrates (460–375 BC). According to the nurse historian Donahue (1985, 1996), Hippocrates was thought to be a direct descendent of Asklepios, the chief healer in Greek mythology. Hippocrates prepared a classification of mental disorders (Alexander & Se-

lesnick, 1966). In his "theory of disease," he described body humors (Donahue, 1996, p. 56)—yellow bile, black bile, phlegm, and blood—and attributed human behaviors to excesses of particular humors. For example, the excess of black bile was thought to be responsible for the disease melancholia (depression).

Despite Hippocrates' attributing illness causation to other factors in his writings and teachings, remnants of the early thinking regarding demonology recurred at various times. For instance, witch hunting occurred in Europe and in Colonial America. Those individuals thought to be witches and demons, mostly women, were hunted and killed in horrible ways. The cruel treatment of the mentally ill that occurred (e.g., beatings) was often intended to drive the evil spirits from the people and to restore them to health (Deutsch, 1949).

W*hat do you think?* How do these primitive ideas about psychiatric illness influence current thinking?

➤ *Check Your Reading*
1. In early history, to what did people attribute the cause of mental illness?
2. Who were the earliest "psychiatrists"?
3. What did Hippocrates believe was the cause of depression?

18TH, 19TH, AND 20TH CENTURY TRAVELERS

Phillippe Pinel (1745–1826). "This gentle man taught compassionate treatment of the mentally ill by his own example" (Dolan, Fitzpatrick, & Herrmann, 1983, p. 122). Thus Dolan et al. described the brave French psychiatrist **Phillippe Pinel,** MD. In 1792, Pinel risked his own career in medicine and perhaps his life when, as the chief of the Bicêtre mental hospital in Paris, he released patients from the incarcerating chains and other restraints that confined them. A famous painting depicts his similar actions at the women's asylum at Salpêtrière, also in Paris (Donahue, 1996, p. 169). In describing Pinel's contribution to the care of the mentally ill, Grob (1994) stated the premise of Pinel's treatment was "psychologically-oriented." Pinel developed "what he called *traitement moral,* which in England and America became known as 'moral treatment' or 'moral management'" (Grob, 1994, p. 27).

William Tuke (1732–1822). Meanwhile, in England in the same year that Pinel removed the chains from patients at Bicêtre, **William Tuke,** a successful businessman, established the **York Retreat.** The York Retreat exemplified the humanitarian approach to the mentally ill, which was also the basis of Pinel's actions. William Tuke and his fellow Quaker colleagues (Friends) believed that the tenets of the Quaker faith, which suggest treating people with kindness in a pleasant environment, could bring recovery to the ill. The York Retreat

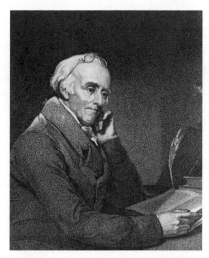

Figure 2–1
Benjamin Rush, MD (1745–1813). (Courtesy of the National Library of Medicine, Bethesda, MD.)

Sunday school teacher at the East Cambridge jail in Massachusetts. There, criminals and "lunatics" were crowded together in dirty, cold prison conditions. Although initially unsuccessful, her first action was to obtain a means to provide some heat for this setting. Her first Sunday visit in 1841 was the beginning of her extensive study of conditions throughout New England, about which she subsequently reported to influential community leaders and legislatures of the respective New England states. Her intention was that the insane people of the community be cared for appropriately. For years she crusaded to obtain facilities for the care of the mentally ill. This eventually resulted in the

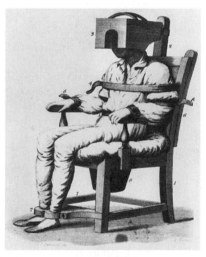

Figure 2–2
The tranquilizer chair devised by Benjamin Rush. (Courtesy of the National Library of Medicine, Bethesda, MD.) hang from ceiling

was administered by three generations of family members according to these basic beliefs. The pioneering efforts of Pinel and Tuke were precursors to the modern day milieu (environmental) therapy (see Chapter 15). The influence of the Quakers, as cited by Grob (1994), was evidenced by the fact that "half of the hospitals in the United States founded before 1824 borrowed heavily from the Quaker example" (p. 29).

Benjamin Rush (1745–1813). In Colonial America, **Benjamin Rush,** MD, was the first American to undertake the serious study of mental illness (Figure 2-1). Rush was also one of the signers of the Declaration of Independence. In addition to being an inventor and physician, he was the author of the classic book on mental illness, *Diseases of the Mind,* which was published in 1812. Benjamin Rush attended patients at the Pennsylvania Hospital in Philadelphia for 30 years (Bailey, 1935).

Rush viewed the physician-patient relationship as a significant factor with curative benefits. Based on his view that mental illness was the result of faulty blood circulation in the brain, he devised methodologies of treatment such as the "tranquilizer chair" (Figure 2-2). The chair hung from the ceiling, and patients were restrained in the chair with heads covered. This form of restraint, although innovative for its time, would not meet with current acceptable practices of medical care. Rush held a humane attitude toward the care of the mentally ill and, based on his many accomplishments, is credited as being the Father of American Psychiatry. Also among his treatment perspectives is evidence of the forerunner of what was later known as *attitude therapy.* Rush advocated that gentleness was necessary for the depressed person and that firmness should be used when manic behavior was present.

Dorothea Lynde Dix (1802–1887). **Dorothea Lynde Dix** (Figure 2-3), a New England schoolteacher and crusader for reform in the care of the mentally ill, was first made aware of the dreadful conditions in which some mentally ill people lived when she was a volunteer

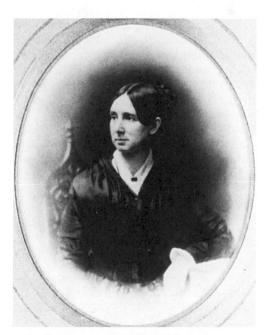

Figure 2–3
Dorothea Lynde Dix (1802–1887). (Courtesy of the National Library of Medicine, Bethesda, MD.) heat

establishment of at least 30 hospitals in the United States, Canada, Scotland, and Japan (Bailey, 1935; Tiffany, 1918). Among these hospitals was the first state hospital in Trenton, New Jersey, and The Government Hospital for the Insane (now Saint Elizabeth's Hospital) in Washington, D.C.

At the outset of the Civil War (1861–1865), when she was more than 60 years of age, Dix arrived in Washington, D.C., to volunteer her services for nursing care and was appointed Superintendent of Female Nurses of the Union Army (1861). This appointment made Dix "the first woman appointed to an administrative position in the federal government" (Flanigan, 1976, p. 13). Dix ardently pursued her efforts. They are all the more impressive because she experienced repeated episodes of illness that left her physically depleted and that had earlier necessitated that she abandon her teaching career. The last several years of her life were spent in an apartment provided for her at the Trenton State Hospital in New Jersey (the first hospital she helped to establish). In concluding his biography of Dorothea Lynde Dix, Tiffany (1918) quoted from a letter by Charles H. Nichols, informing friends of her death: "Thus has died and been laid to rest in the most quiet, unostentatious way the most useful and distinguished woman America has yet produced" (p. 375).

The U.S. Postal Service issued a 1¢ stamp of the Great Americans Series in 1983 in recognition of Dix (Forester & Grandinetti, 1991; Figure 2–4).

Emil Kraepelin (1856–1926). **Emil Kraepelin,** MD, was considered to be one of the most influential psychiatrists during his lifetime. Alexander and Selesnick (1966) stated, "Kraepelin's work is the culmination of the neurophysiological approach" (p. 165). Blazer (1998) called Kraepelin "an unbiased and persistent observer of the symptoms of the patients under his care" (p. 62). The first comprehensive descriptions of mental illnesses were developed from Kraepelin's observations and, according to Blazer, are the basis of the diagnostic system currently in use. The descriptions Kraepelin developed of mood disorders have been preserved and are still being studied and referred to. Kraepelin was a professor of clinical psychiatry in Munich for 19 years.

Sigmund Freud (1856–1939). **Sigmund Freud,** MD, a neurologist who studied with the notable neurologist Jean Martin Charcot, established a practice in Vienna. He originated a perspective of illness and treatment known as the *psychoanalytical approach* as

Box 2–1 ■ ■ ■ ■ ■ ■
Clifford Beers: A Patient's Story

Clifford Beers (1876–1943) suffered from severe bipolar (manic-depressive) illness, with the first episode occurring during his college years. His story is sensitively portrayed in his 1908 book, *A Mind That Found Itself.* In this autobiographical text, he described, with great insight and sobering detail, his experience with mental illness. Beers described his own life story as a "history of a mental civil war, which I fought single-handed on a battlefield that lay within the compass of my skull" (p. 1).

His story illustrates the painful isolation experienced by people with mental illness. He noted, "for more than two years, I was without relatives or friends, in fact, without a world, except that one created by my own mind from the chaos that reigned within it" (p. 28). His story also depicts the cruelty imposed on people with mental illness in an era when little was known about the cause or treatment of such debilitating conditions. In one account, Beers described a violent assault that he endured at the hands of his attendants while he was a patient at a mental institution: "First I was knocked down. Then for several minutes I was kicked about the room— struck, kneed, and choked. . . . (p.161). I soon observed that the only patients who were not likely to be subjected to abuse were the very ones least in need of care and treatment" (p. 164).

Beers was instrumental in bringing into public view the problems within institutions for the mentally ill and the need for greater attention to the causes, treatment, and prevention of mental illness. The National Committee for Mental Hygiene was organized in 1909. Because of his pioneering efforts on behalf of the mentally ill, Clifford Beers became one of only a select few laypeople to be admitted for membership in the American Psychiatric Association as an honorary member. "The death of Clifford Beers, which occurred on July 9, 1943, brought to a close one of the most remarkable careers in modern philanthropy" (Beers, 1943, p. vii).

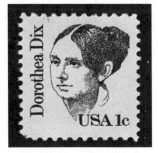

Figure 2–4
The Dorothea Dix 1¢ stamp issued on September 23, 1983, by the U.S. Postal Service as part of its Great Americans Series.

well as a theoretical basis for understanding the formation and development of personality. After his visit to the United States in 1909, when he presented a series of lectures at Clark University in Massachusetts, his controversial ideas generated interest among U.S. psychiatrists. In fact, Freud's influence is still apparent in the teaching and practice of psychiatry in the United States. Although the soundness of Freudian theory is considered controversial by many, Freud's contributions are no less noteworthy. Further discussion of Freud's theory may be found in Chapter 6.

Adolph Meyer (1866–1950). **Adolph Meyer,** MD, was a professor of psychiatry at Johns Hopkins University in Baltimore. He is remembered for developing his biology of the whole personality, or the *psychobiological* perspective of psychiatry, also sometimes referred to as *commonsense psychiatry.* Meyer emphasized that psychiatry is a biological science, and he advocated that a comprehensive study of the individual's history, including his or her life situation, be undertaken. His wife Mary undertook a project of visiting his patients in their homes. Because of this work, she is considered by some to be America's first psychiatric social worker. But perhaps her role was also the prototype of the modern community mental health (CMH) nurse. As Director of the Henry Phipps Psychiatric Clinic at Johns Hopkins University, Meyer was a colleague of Euphemia "Effie" Jane Taylor, the first Director of Nursing Services.

Clifford Beers (1876–1943). **Clifford Beers,** a significant crusader for the mentally ill, wrote of his experiences as a patient (Box 2-1). His first-person account of his mental illness and the circumstances he endured as a patient were to influence many. The Mental Hygiene Movement was a direct outcome of his crusading efforts, which included his autobiography, *A Mind That Found Itself* (1908). Many influential people of that day, including Adolph Meyer, supported and advised Beers in his endeavors (Figure 2-5).

Linda Richards (1841–1930). In September 1872, **Linda Richards,** a young Bostonian, was admitted along with four other young women to the new Training School at the New England Hospital (the first U.S. training school). Richards (1911; Figure 2-6) described her student experiences as follows:

Our days were not eight hours; they were nearer twice eight. We rose at 5:30 A.M. and left the wards at 9 P.M. to go to our beds, which were in little rooms between the wards. Each nurse took care of her ward of six patients both day and night. . . . (p. 10). We wore no uniforms, the only stipulation being that our dresses should be washable. (p. 11)

Further, Richards (1911) reported:

Every second week we were off duty one afternoon from two to five o'clock. We had no evenings out, no hours for study or recreation and no regular leave on Sunday. Only

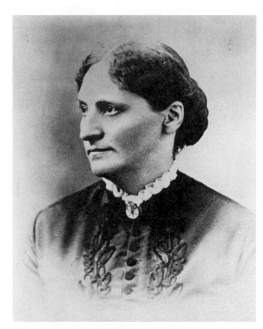

Figure 2–6
Linda Richards (1841–1930). (Courtesy of the National Library of Medicine, Bethesda, MD.)

twice during the year was I given the opportunity to go to church. (p. 11)

We had no textbooks, nor did we have entrance or final examinations. Each nurse was quietly given her diploma as she completed her year of training. (p. 12)

After a rigorous year of study and clinical work, Richards received a diploma from this 1-year program. Because she was the first student to apply to and to enter this new school and the first to graduate (October 19, 1873), Linda Richards is designated as America's first trained nurse. She is also honored as the first psychiatric nurse in the United States.

After her graduation from the training school, Richards became Night Superintendent at Bellevue Hospital in New York for 1 year. She then became Superintendent of the Boston Training School. Richards established and directed the first training school for nurses in Japan (1885-1889). When she returned to the United States, she became Superintendent of Nurses at the New England Hospital for Women and Children. She subsequently held similar positions at Brooklyn Homeopathic Hospital, Hartford Hospital, and University of Pennsylvania Hospital (Dolan, Fitzpatrick, & Herrmann, 1983).

Along with Edward A. Cowles and Mary Palmer, Linda Richards planned the curriculum for the McLean Training School for Nurses, established at the McLean Asylum (later the McLean Hospital Belmont, Massachusetts) in 1882; the opening of the McLean Training School is considered by many to mark the beginning of modern psychiatric nursing (Sutton, 1986). During the latter years of her outstanding career, Richards was Superintendent of Nurses at Taunton Insane Hospital (1899-1903), at Worcester Hospital for the Insane (1903-1906), and at Michigan Insane Hospital (1906-1909). She reorganized or established training schools

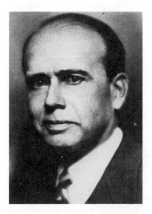

Figure 2–5
Clifford Beers (1876–1943). (Courtesy of the National Library of Medicine, Bethesda, MD.)

for nurses at these hospitals, believing that such educational programs were a necessity. Richards (1911) observed that better care for patients in the state hospitals could be accomplished only by better training for the nurses who worked there. She contended, "It stands to reason that the mentally sick should be at least as well cared for as the physically sick" (p. 108). In fact, more than any other nurse in the early 1900s, Richards was able to assess patients in terms of their physical and emotional needs (Sills, 1973). She believed that the two essential qualities for a good psychiatric nurse were patience and tact and that both of these qualities could be developed as the individual gained experience in the care of the mentally ill.

Former students of Richards described her as kind, enthusiastic, just, and intelligent, with a sense of humor. She had a vigorous personality and was loved by the patients. Doona (1984), a psychiatric nurse and author, observed, "Richards' kindness and gentleness in caring for the mentally ill proved what the new nursing could do" (p. 56). When Sophia Palmer (first editor) and Mary E. P. Davis (first business manager), both former students of Linda Richards, established the *American Journal of Nursing* in 1900, they honored her by "presenting her with the first share of stock in the American Journal of Nursing Company" (Doona, 1984, p. 53).

Harriet Bailey (1875–1953). The first psychiatric nursing textbook, *Nursing Mental Diseases* (1920), was authored by **Harriet Bailey,** BS, RN, a nurse educator and pioneer in psychiatric nursing (Church & Buckwalter, 1980). This textbook was published in 1920 by Macmillan as a clothbound book priced at $1.60. The book remained in print through the fourth edition, which was authored by Bailey in 1939. Church and Buckwalter reported that the book went out of print in 1954 after it had been the standard textbook on mental nursing for 20 years. In the preface of the book, Bailey (1920) stated that the text came about because colleagues had requested that she put her lecture notes together for reference use. In the third edition (1935), the content had expanded from 13 chapters in the original edition to 22 chapters.

During her noteworthy career, Bailey was Assistant Superintendent of Nurses at the Henry Phipps Psychiatric Clinic of Johns Hopkins Hospital in Baltimore and Superintendent of Nurses at Manhattan State Hospital in New York, and she held other prominent responsibilities in nursing. As a psychiatric nurse educator and leader in nursing, Bailey urged that nursing education include mental health nursing. Church and Buckwalter (1980) credited Bailey with being "one of psychiatric nursing's pioneers" and stated that she "championed the cause of psychiatric nursing education above all others" in endeavoring to advance the respectability of psychiatric nursing (p. 60).

Euphemia "Effie" Jane Taylor (1874–1970). **Euphemia "Effie" Jane Taylor** directed the course in psychiatric nursing that was offered at the Johns Hopkins Hospital, where she was appointed as the first Director of Nursing Services at the Henry Phipps Psychiatric Clinic in 1913. Throughout her distinguished

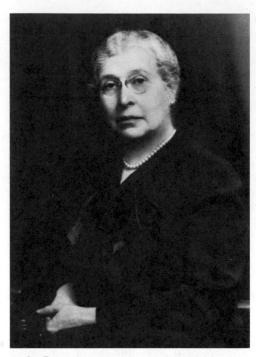

Figure 2–7
Euphemia "Effie" Jane Taylor (1874–1970). (Courtesy of the National Library of Medicine, Bethesda, MD.)

career, Taylor (Figure 2–7) was a proponent for the inclusion of psychiatric nursing in the nurses' educational program. She joined the faculty of the Yale School of Nursing in 1923 and assisted the first dean of the school, Annie W. Goodrich, in founding the new university school. (The Yale School of Nursing was the first autonomous university-based school of nursing to have its own independent budget.) Taylor succeeded Goodrich, becoming the second Dean of the School of Nursing, a position she held for 10 years until she retired in 1944. Taylor was the first psychiatric nurse to be designated Professor of Nursing when she was thus appointed in 1926. At that time, Goodrich observed that Taylor possibly was the only professor of psychiatric nursing in the world (Dolan, Fitzpatrick, & Herrmann, 1983).

Taylor was Superintendent of Nurses at the New Haven Hospital for 11 years. In 1937, she was elected President of the International Council of Nurses, a position she subsequently held for 10 years, including the crucial years during World War II. Buckwalter and Church (1979) observed that Taylor "maintained a strong personal commitment to psychiatric nursing" (p. 125). At the American Nurses Association (ANA) Convention on June 13, 1986, Taylor was inducted into the ANA Nursing Hall of Fame as a "suffragette pioneer in the field of psychiatric nursing" (Convention Preview, 1986, p. 36). "The history of Miss Taylor's many contributions to nursing provides an inspiring example of a humanitarian and nurse, who had a great impact on the development of her profession—nationally, internationally, and specifically in the field of psychiatric nursing" (Buckwalter & Church, 1979, p. 131).

Harry Stack Sullivan (1892–1949). **Harry Stack Sullivan,** MD, emphasized the significance of interpersonal relationships. He considered mental illness to be the result of disturbances in relationships beginning in early childhood or infancy. His treatment approach focused on the restoration of effectiveness in communication and the growth of interpersonal relationships. His perspective, the interpersonal theory of psychiatry, has made a significant contribution to the education and practice of many disciplines. Nurses found the components of this viewpoint applicable to nursing practice, and the basic tenets of this psychiatric perspective became a substantial framework for the subsequent focus on interpersonal relationships in nursing. **Hildegard E. Peplau's** classic publication, *Interpersonal Relations in Nursing* (1952), translated Sullivan's interpersonal perspective into a language that nurses could understand and put into practice. For further discussion of Sullivan's theory, see Chapter 6.

William C. Menninger (1899–1966). **William C. Menninger,** MD, established a 1-year postgraduate course in psychiatric nursing at the Menninger Hospital in Topeka, Kansas, in 1932. Menninger recognized that psychiatric nursing was important in the patient's treatment and chances for recovery (Hall, 1967). He was the 75th President of the American Psychiatric Association and served as Director of the Neuropsychiatric Consultants Division, Office of the Surgeon General, during World War II.

> **W***hat do you think?* If time travel was a reality, which of the early travelers in psychiatry would you like to meet? What would you like to ask them?

➤ *Check Your Reading*

4. What is Phillippe Pinel credited with having done?
5. What did William Tuke do at the York Retreat?
6. Name America's first trained psychiatric nurse.
7. What is the name of the first psychiatric training school?
8. What was the title of the first psychiatric nursing textbook, and who wrote it?
9. Who was the first psychiatric nurse to be designated Professor of Nursing?
10. What did Clifford Beers write?
11. What was the major contribution made to psychiatry by Emil Kraepelin?
12. Dorothea Lynde Dix was a crusader during which war?
13. Who is attributed with inventing the tranquilizing chair?
14. Harry Stack Sullivan is credited with a theory about what?
15. Hildegard E. Peplau wrote a psychiatric nursing textbook dealing with what topic?

CHANGING SETTINGS FOR MENTAL HEALTH CARE

The mentally ill have been housed or cared for in a variety of settings. Sister Charles Marie, a nursing historian and former dean of The Catholic University's School of Nursing, described the progression of settings in this way:

Originally hospitals functioned as shelters for the sick poor. In the latter part of the nineteenth century many state hospitals for the mentally ill were founded and poor farms were established. . . . Seriously ill mental patients who were judged dangerous to society were imprisoned, less harmful persons were allowed to roam about at will. Little thought was given to treatment, rehabilitation or prevention. (Frank, 1959, pp. 151, 152)

Throughout history, the settings for the care of the mentally ill have ranged from **jails** to **almshouses** to **asylums** and to **private** and **public mental hospitals.** Grob (1994) said, the "history of the care and treatment of the mentally ill resembles a seemingly endless journey between two extremes—confinement in a mental hospital versus living in the community" (p. 3). The quality of the settings, including the hospitals, has varied greatly.

One of the most famous or *infamous* hospitals is the **Bethlehem Hospital** in London (Figure 2–8). Donahue (1996) reported that it was founded in 1247 as a priory, and about 1330 its designation was changed to a hospital. Donahue noted that Bethlehem Hospital was the first English institution for the mentally ill. In the 16th century, King Henry VIII dedicated this facility as a lunatic asylum. By the 18th century, deterioration had reached a dreadful point, and the facility became known as the notorious "Bedlam" (Figure 2-9).

The attendants, or keepers of the patients, were allowed to exhibit the boisterous patients for two pence (or one penny) a look. The more harmless patients were used to seek charity on the streets of London. In his

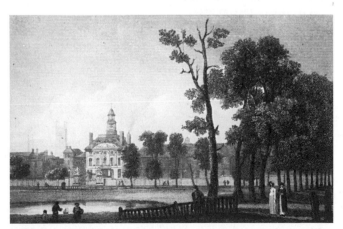

F i g u r e 2 – 8
Bethlehem Hospital, London. (Courtesy of the National Library of Medicine, Bethesda, MD.)

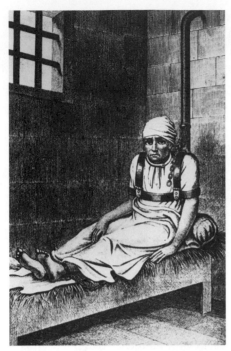

Figure 2–9
A patient, William Norris, in chains at Bedlam, London's notorious Bethlehem Hospital. (Courtesy of the National Library of Medicine, Bethesda, MD.)

writing of *King Lear,* Shakespeare referred to these individuals as the "Bedlam Beggars" (Bailey, 1935, p. 3).

In Colonial America, the prevailing attitude toward the mentally ill was anything but scientific. Many abuses were accorded to those whose illnesses were poorly understood. However, some had a more enlightened view toward the mentally ill. Through the efforts of Benjamin Franklin, patriot, inventor, and humanitarian statesman, the **Pennsylvania Hospital** in Philadelphia was founded in 1751. This hospital became the first general hospital to provide care for the mentally ill in the United States. In 1885, when the first two patients were admitted, one of them was identified as a lunatic (Noyes & Haydon, 1948, p. 360).

Notable reformers such as Phillippe Pinel in France and William Tuke in England (both discussed earlier) represented a humanitarian perspective. The influence of these men was not limited to Europe. Their ideas reached across the ocean and influenced a Baltimore businessman, Moses Sheppard (1775–1857). Sheppard, acquainted with the endeavors in England of Tuke, a fellow Quaker, sought to provide for the mentally ill through his financial bequest, which was used to establish the Sheppard Asylum. The first patient was admitted to this asylum in 1891. The asylum further benefited from a substantial bequest from the estate of Enoch Pratt. Pratt's donation carried with it a stipulation to the Board of Trustees that his name be incorporated into the name of the hospital. Therefore, the asylum's name was changed to the Sheppard and Enoch Pratt Hospital, which has carried on the humanitarian

traditions of Sheppard and Pratt for more than 100 years (Forbush & Forbush, 1986; Figure 2-10).

One of the most historic approaches for care has existed in Gheel, Belgium, since 1851. In this community, mentally ill individuals reside in the homes of residents of Gheel. They maintain some semblance of a normal life while seeing a psychiatrist on a regular basis.

As described earlier, the efforts of Dorothea Lynde Dix were instrumental in the establishment of numerous state mental hospitals during the 1880s. The care of the mentally ill remained within the purview of the state mental health systems until after World War II. At that time, legislation provided funding to include psychiatric units within general hospitals. This trend was furthered by a stipulation in the Community Mental Health Centers Construction Act of 1963 that stated that the services of a general hospital were considered to be incomplete if provisions were not made for the care of the mentally ill. Mobile treatment teams then began providing care to the mentally ill, as did staff in CMH centers. For many, the patient's home is becoming the preferred site for care (see Chapter 15). Day treatment hospitals and community rehabilitation programs are replacing inpatient hospitalization. The settings within the psychiatric care continuum provide the patient with many alternatives for receiving care.

Increasingly, nurses are venturing into private practice, either as solo practitioners or as members of a multidisciplinary group. In addition, psychiatric nurses are taking their skills into nontraditional settings such as schools, nursing homes, industry, and churches.

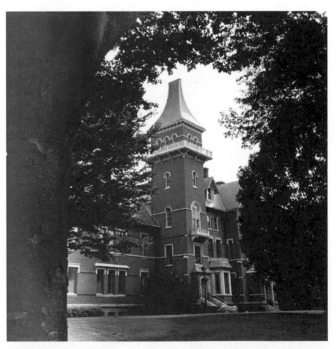

Figure 2–10
The Sheppard and Enoch Pratt Hospital, Towson, MD. (Photograph by Brian K. Glock. Courtesy of the Sheppard Pratt Health System, Towson, MD.)

What do you think? How would you interpret the value of a place like Gheel? Do we have anything comparable in our mental health system?

► *Check Your Reading*

16. Why is Bedlam famous?
17. What is the name of the hospital founded as a result of the efforts of Benjamin Franklin?
18. Why is Gheel, Belgium, famous?
19. Name at least two alternative settings for psychiatric care outside the inpatient unit.

INFLUENCE OF WORLD WARS I AND II ON MENTAL HEALTH CARE

Both World War I and World War II exposed the prevalence of mental illness, especially among the young men of age for induction into military service. During World War I, from 2% to 5% of draftees were rejected because of psychiatric illness (Hall, 1967). Many draftees who were inducted subsequently became ill during active duty in the armed forces. *Shell shock* was the term associated with the psychiatric casualties of World War I. During World War II, 14% of draftees were not eligible for military service because of psychiatric illness. The number of psychiatric casualties during World War II was even higher than those during World War I. Menninger, mentioned earlier, used the term *combat exhaustion* for a mental illness associated with World War I (Hall, 1967). Psychiatric services became overtaxed as casualties increased. Prominent psychiatrists of the time were enlisted to provide leadership in treating these patients. Menninger was one who served with distinction. He and others brought expertise to the treatment of mental illness throughout the military.

Meanwhile, at home, conscientious objectors who declined active duty in the military served their equivalent of military service in some form of public service. The Selective Service established Civilian Public Service units in state mental hospitals beginning in June 1942 (Sareyan, 1994). The individuals assigned to these units served—most as psychiatric attendants—in 61 public psychiatric hospitals and state training schools for the retarded. Their help was sorely needed because staffs in these facilities had been drastically diminished as personnel joined wartime efforts in the military or in assembly plants.

These newcomers to the psychiatric settings were exposed firsthand and for the first time to the dreadful conditions within various hospitals. They were horrified at the undesirable conditions of neglect and overcrowding and at the paucity of treatment (Sareyan, 1994). Not content to ignore or do nothing about these conditions, many put their observations in writing in newspapers and magazines. Albert Maisel (1946), a science writer, wrote an exposé titled, "Bedlam 1946: Most U.S. mental hospitals are a shame and a disgrace," which was published in *Life*, based on the accounts of members of the Civilian Public Service units. These writings, along with others such as *The Shame of the States,* written by Albert Deutsch (1948), exposed the conditions and heightened the public's awareness to what was called, in one author's book title, *Out of Sight, Out of Mind* (Wright, 1947). A novel, *The Snake Pit,* written by Mary Jane Ward in 1946 (1964) and subsequently made into a motion picture by the same name, depicted similar deplorable conditions.

What do you think? Hospital stays are becomingly increasingly shorter; the days of being institutionalized for an indefinite period have passed. No longer can we say that the mentally ill are out of sight, out of mind. Are they better off today? Defend your answer.

► *Check Your Reading*

20. What influence did World Wars I and II have on the treatment of mental illness?
21. What public service did conscientious objectors perform during wartime?
22. What was the impact of *The Shame of the States,* written by Albert Deutsch?

INFLUENCE OF LEGISLATION ON MENTAL HEALTH CARE

The National Mental Health Act of 1946. Following World War II, the National Mental Health Act (July 1946) was enacted by the U.S. Congress to improve the mental health of the nation's people. Several significant provisions of this legislation were realized as funds were established for training personnel in the four core disciplines: psychiatry, nursing, clinical psychology, and social work. From this legislative action, the National Institute of Mental Health (NIMH) was also established (1949), and funds were allocated for research into the causes and treatment of mental illness.

The Hill-Burton Act of 1946. In 1946, the Hospital Survey and Construction Act, also called the Hill-Burton Act, became law. This bill provided federal funding to the states to survey health needs and plan and construct hospitals and other health centers. The federal government paid one third of the cost for the survey and construction; the states assumed responsibility for the other two thirds. The development of psychiatric units in general hospitals was a direct outcome of this funding.

The National Mental Health Study Act. The Joint Commission on Mental Illness and Health was established as a result of the National Mental Health Study Act. This study group's report, *Action for Mental Health,* was published in 1961 (Joint Commission on Mental Illness and Health, 1961). This study highlighted mental illness as the number one public health problem. Two nurses, Kathleen Black and Mary F. Liston, served on the multidisciplinary commission.

The Mental Retardation Facilities and Community Mental Health Centers Construction Act of 1963. With the enthusiastic support of President John F. Kennedy, this legislation became a reality. This bill was designed to facilitate treatment of people with mental illness within their communities. To do so, it is necessary to do the following:

- Save the patient from debilitating effects of institutionalization.
- Return the patient to home and community life as soon as possible.
- Maintain the patient in the community as long as possible.

Aftercare and rehabilitation thus were recognized as essential parts of all service to mental patients, and the various methods of achieving rehabilitation were understood to be integrated into all forms of services, among them day hospitals, night hospitals, aftercare clinics, public health nursing services, foster family care, convalescent nursing homes, rehabilitation centers, work services, and ex-patient groups (Joint Commission on Mental Illness and Health, 1961).

The funding for CMH programs was extended once again in 1970. At this time, Congress, in response to the Joint Commission on the Mental Health of Children, which cited inadequate services for young people, specifically earmarked money to serve youth. In addition, funding was added for drug and alcohol services.

The Community Mental Health Center Amendment of 1975 (P.L. 94-63). By 1975, the federal government amended its original 1963 law and specified that CMH centers must provide 12 services to qualify for federal monies. In addition to the original five services (inpatient care, outpatient care, partial hospitalization, emergency care, consultation and education), the following services were required: specialized services for children and elderly people, screening, aftercare, transitional housing, drug abuse services, and alcoholism treatment.

In 1977, President Jimmy Carter mandated a major reassessment of mental health needs. He established a 20-member President's Commission on Mental Health, which included a nurse, Martha Mitchell, who was Chair of the ANA Division on Psychiatric and Mental Health Nursing Practice. In 1978, the *Report to the President of the President's Commission on Mental Health* was published and focused on strengthening the CMH system as the foundation for the mental health system. This involved improving community support systems, continuing to phase out large public hospitals, establishing a center within NIMH with a focus on primary prevention, and improving the delivery of services to underserved and high-risk populations.

The report also advocated other major changes in the delivery of mental health care. These suggestions included establishing national health insurance that included coverage for mental health; encouraging private insurance carriers to include mental health coverage (including outpatient departments) in their packages; providing funding to increase the number of mental health professionals, especially those who work with children, elderly people, and minorities; developing advocacy programs for the chronically mentally ill; protecting the rights of all people in need of mental health services; increasing support for research related to mental health and illness; providing public health education to increase the public's understanding of mental health and illness; and centralizing the evaluation efforts of governmental agencies.

The Community Mental Health Systems Act of 1980. In 1980, the Community Mental Health Systems Act was passed. It was designed to implement the recommendations of the President's Commission on Mental Health and to coordinate the two-tiered mental health system that had evolved since the original 1963 legislation that mandated the establishment of CMH centers. The most severely disabled of the chronically mentally ill still resided within state institutions; those who were less disabled used the services of the CMH centers. Virtually no coordination existed between these two systems. Consequently, patients "fell through the cracks," so to speak, because of the lack of continuity and communication between the two tiers.

Omnibus Budget Reconciliation Act of 1982 (P.L. 97-35). The programs authorized by this legislation were to be implemented in 1982, but before this could occur, a significant retrenchment by the federal government occurred in terms of its responsibilities in the area of mental health. The 97th Congress essentially repealed the Community Mental Health Systems Act of 1980 with the passage of the Reagan administration's Omnibus Budget Reconciliation Act. This bill moved the authority and administration of mental health programs from NIMH to the individual states. Each state received a block grant to cover alcohol abuse, drug abuse, and mental health services. As of 1984, federal funding for CMH and other mental health care delivery programs was terminated. CMH centers are now mandated to provide only five essential services: outpatient care, partial hospitalization, 24-hour hospitalization and emergency care, consultation and education, and screening services. The continued existence of CMH centers is dependent on state support, private funding, and ability to earn revenue.

The Americans With Disabilities Act of 1990. Most recently, the federal government mandated the elimination of discrimination against those with disabilities (which included those with a mental illness) with the passage of the Americans With Disabilities Act of 1990.

Parity Legislation. In January 1996, Congress passed a National Mental Health Parity Bill. The provisions of this bill, which went into effect in January 1998, included a call for parity between mental and physical illness for annual and lifetime caps in health care plans that provide mental health coverage and inclusion of all businesses with more than 50 employees. This bill excluded parity for alcohol and substance abuse and allowed far-reaching cost-containment measures for mental health care that differ from physical health care and effectively maintain an unequal playing field for those afflicted with mental illness. Although mental health advocates applauded the 1996 legislation and many states have passed parity legislation, the impact of this legislation has been more symbolic than actual, and a great deal of work remains to be done.

Projections into the future promise no dramatic federal funding projects for the care of the mentally ill. The political climate seems to support *smaller* rather than *bigger* when it comes to programs directed at meeting human needs. With so many programs competing for limited funds, the challenge of the mental health system is to try to do more with less.

What do you think? Has legislation significantly improved the lot of the mentally ill? Defend your answer.

➤ *Check Your Reading*

23. What was the name of the bill passed in 1946? What impact did it have on issues of mental health?
24. For what purpose did the Hill-Burton Act provide funding?
25. What was the purpose of the Community Mental Health Centers Construction Act of 1963?
26. What does the Americans With Disabilities Act protect?

INFLUENCE OF PSYCHOBIOLOGICAL TREATMENT ON MENTAL HEALTH CARE

Throughout history, those involved in the treatment and care of people with mental illnesses have been attempting to use various somatic therapies, ranging from the tranquilizing chair to ECT to psychotropic drugs and diet therapy. In 1938, as an alternative to inducing convulsion with drugs (e.g., pentylenetetrazol [Metrazol]), two Italian psychiatrists, Ugo Cerletti and Lucio Bini, established electric shock therapy. Although at times this treatment, now termed *ECT,* has been criticized, it remains valuable for many individuals, particularly those suffering from depression.

The synthesis of chlorpromazine by a French drug firm in December 1950 was a breakthrough in what would become the major treatment mode for mental illness worldwide. Flowers (1998) cited the development of this medication as one of the significant discoveries since 1900. This medication was introduced in the United States in 1954 (The introduction of chlorpromazine, 1976; Swazey, 1974).

A growing number of antipsychotic, antidepressant, antimania, and antianxiety medications have since been widely used to help reduce the need for hospitalization and to generally improve the quality of life for those afflicted with mental illnesses. This has made a tremendous impact on the nation. James Howe, Past President of National Alliance for the Mentally Ill (NAMI), observed that in the 16 years following the introduction of lithium (1970), a drug used to control mood swings, this medication was credited with saving more than $17 billion. The continuing addition of new medications to treat the symptoms of serious mental illnesses has brought new hope and relief to thousands who suffer from the painful consequences of mental illness. One

challenge, as we move forward, is to influence the managed care organizations as well as state and local departments of mental health to include the newest medications in their approved formularies.

➤ *Check Your Reading*

27. What was the name of the first antipsychotic drug introduced?
28. What is ECT?
29. What was the nationality of the physicians who invented ECT?
30. What is the effect of the drug lithium?

INFLUENCE OF DEINSTITUTIONALIZATION ON MENTAL HEALTH CARE

During the 1960s, an enthusiastic and extensive process of moving individuals from the public mental hospitals to the community was undertaken. This process of deinstitutionalization drastically reduced the numbers of patients who were hospitalized. For example, 552,150 patients were in the large U.S. public psychiatric hospitals in 1955 compared with only 109,939 patients in 1985 (Torrey, 1993). Torrey (1997) observed that in 1994, these numbers had further decreased to 71,619. Vermont was exemplary in the organized planning of the transition of individuals from the hospital to the community. In this state, their pioneering rehabilitation program was unusual because community support was present when the process of deinstitutionalization was put into effect (Harding, Zubin, & Strauss, 1987). However, few other states can report such successful transitions. As a result, many mentally ill now live on the streets of our nation. Torrey (1993) reported that one third of the homeless are mentally ill. In the article "Jails: The new mental institutions," the *NAMI Advocate* (1991) reported, "on any given day, the Los Angeles County Jail routinely houses 700 more people with mental illness than does the largest public mental hospital in the country, Pilgrim State in New York . . . Across America, one-third more mentally ill individuals reside in jails than in mental hospitals" (p. 1). Hatfield and Lefley (1987) have observed that the family has become the prominent caregiver for the mentally ill. For an untold number of others, there are simply no caregivers.

What do you think? What provisions has your community made for the long-term deinstitutionalized care of the mentally ill? How would you evaluate access to housing, medical and psychiatric care, psychosocial programs, and psychiatric vocational rehabilitation programs?

➤ *Check Your Reading*

31. What has been the impact of deinstitutionalization on state mental hospitals?
32. What has been the impact of deinstitutionalization on communities?

INFLUENCE OF INTERPERSONAL RELATIONSHIPS ON MENTAL HEALTH CARE

As a result of the benefits derived from the psychiatric medications made available in the 1950s, many patients, for the first time, became able to engage in interpersonal relationships with psychiatrists, nurses, and others, which opened new possibilities for their recovery. The responsibilities and activities of the psychiatric nurse were now expanded. The central focus of nursing literature, nursing conferences, and nursing education in the 1950s and 1960s increasingly became the nurse-patient relationship. Manfreda (1982), a psychiatric nurse and author, said, "The development of interpersonal nursing marked an important milestone in American nursing. From the procedure oriented, to the more involved process of interaction, the emphasis shifted to the Nurse-Patient Relationship" (p. xi).

Manfreda (1982) credited the contributions of anthropologists, psychiatrists, psychologists, and social scientists for their work establishing the roots of interpersonal nursing and wrote of the inspirational practice and writings of the nursing leaders in the 1930s. For example, she noted Helena Render's 1937 description of nurse-patient interaction recordings as a teaching method. Other psychiatric nurse authors included in Manfreda's historical discussion of the roots of interpersonal nursing were Olga Weiss, Elizabeth Bixler Torrey, Hildegard E. Peplau, Sister Kathleen Black, and Gwen Tudor Will.

Psychiatric nursing leaders emerged as authors of significant publications. A classic reference in psychiatric nursing was *Interpersonal Relations in Nursing* (1952) by Hildegard E. Peplau. O'Toole and Welt (1989) reported that Peplau had completed her work on this book in 1948, but "it was not published until four years later because it was considered too revolutionary for a nurse to publish such a book without a physician as co-author" (p. xviii). Box 2-2 tells Hildegard E. Peplau's story.

During the 1960s, other psychiatric nurse authors further contributed to the understanding of nurse-patient relationships. *The Dynamic Nurse-Patient Relationship: Function, Process and Principles* (1961) was authored by Ida Jean Orlando. Orlando's book, which focused on the needs of the patient and on the nurses' deliberative intervention (nursing process), became another classic. Joyce Travelbee, a student of Ida Orlando, later wrote another influential publication, *Interpersonal Aspects of Nursing,* first published in 1966. A further contribution to the nurse-patient relationship literature was *Nurse-Patient Communication* by Garland K. Lewis (1978).

At the 1958 annual convention of the ANA, the 16-mm film *Psychiatric Nursing: The Nurse-Patient Relationship* was premiered (*ANA in Review,* 1958, p. 2; *Psychiatric Nursing,* 1958). The film was produced by the ANA and the National League for Nursing in cooperation with the Mental Health Education Unit of Smith Kline and French (who marketed the antipsychotic medication Thorazine [chlorpromazine]). The

filming took place on the grounds of the New Jersey State Hospital at Greystone Park, with a nursing student portraying a withdrawn patient, "Trudy," who benefits from the nurse-patient relationship, as does the nurse working with Trudy. The nurse learns from the recording and analysis of her nurse-patient interactions. The enduring worth of this fine production has been ensured by its current availability on videotape.

Today, psychiatric nursing educators continue to assign to students the recording and subsequent analysis of their nurse-patient interactions. Thus, as noted by Manfreda (1982), the interpersonal aspects of nursing continue the perspective taught us by Florence Nightingale.

What do you think? How would you respond to the comment, "nursing's focus on the interpersonal relationship is its unique contribution to psychiatric care"?

➤ *Check Your Reading*
33. What impact did the use of psychotropic medications have on the practice of psychiatric nursing?
34. What is the movie *Psychiatric Nursing: The Nurse-Patient Relationship* about?

INFLUENCE OF NURSING PROFESSIONALIZATION ON MENTAL HEALTH CARE

In 1892, Isabel Adams Hampton (later Isabel Hampton Robb) wrote about her vision for the professionalization of nursing. In her textbook, *Nursing Ethics,* published in 1901 (as cited in Dolan, Fitzpatrick, & Herrmann, 1983), she wrote:

The trained nurse, then, is no longer to be regarded as a better trained, more useful, higher class servant, but as one who has knowledge and is worthy of respect, consideration and due recompense. . . . She is also essentially an instructor; part of her duties have to do with the prevention of disease and sickness, as well as the relief of suffering humanity. . . . These are some of the essentials in nursing by which it has come to be regarded as a profession, but there still remains much to be desired, much to work for, in order to add to its dignity and usefulness. As the standard of education and requirements become a higher character and the training more efficient, the trained nurse will draw nearer to science and its demands and take a greater share as a social factor in solving the world's needs. (pp. 277, 278)

Although Hampton Robb alludes to specific defining characteristics of a profession, for further definition it is valuable to examine the work of Abraham Flexner, who in 1915 identified the criteria by which a profession was to be judged. In the years since Flexner wrote his criteria, other models have been proposed that also provide logical characteristics by which to evaluate a profession. However, Flexner's criteria are still relevant

Box 2–2 ■ ■ ■ ■ ■
Hildegard E. Peplau: A Pioneer Nursing Leader and Theorist in Psychiatric Nursing

Hildegard E. Peplau was born in 1909 in Reading, Pennsylvania. She began her nursing journey in the late 1920s as a student at the Pottstown Hospital School of Nursing in Pennsylvania. In her earliest professional years, she assumed positions in general and private duty nursing, operating room supervision and instruction, and college health. Dr. Peplau returned to school at Bennington College to pursue a bachelor's degree in interpersonal psychology. Her field experiences in her program of study and particularly her experiences at the Bellevue Hospital in New York City exposed her to many notable and influential psychiatric leaders of the time, including Dr. Lauretta Bender, Dr. Frieda Fromm-Reichman, and Dr. Harry Stack Sullivan. These significant experiences and relationships greatly influenced her thinking and outlook on psychiatric nursing.

During World War II, Dr. Peplau served in the Army Nurse Corps, both stateside and overseas. Here, she was once again introduced to many new and innovative psychiatric practices. Following World War II, she studied at Teachers College, Columbia University, where she received her graduate degree in psychiatric nursing (and later her doctorate in education). The program in psychiatric nursing included lectures by prominent nurses including Laura Fitzsimmons, then Psychiatric Nurse Consultant to the American Psychiatric Association. Field work included experiences at the New York State Psychiatric Institute, Columbia-Presbyterian Hospital, New York City. Her final examination required her to demonstrate a wet sheet pack.

During these years of practice, Dr. Peplau observed many psychiatric nursing practices that today would be considered highly unusual. For example, nurses were considered to be custodians of patients. Families were excluded from the patient care experience and discouraged from visiting. Patients were considered to be hospital property and were often used to do the maintenance work within the hospital, including groundskeeping, farming, and cooking. The most chronically ill patients were housed in back wards, and ECT, insulin therapy, lobotomy, and hydrotherapy were common treatments employed in the care of the mentally ill. Wards were often in a state of disrepair, with broken furniture, poor lighting, and chipped and peeling paint. Privileges were given to the more docile, agreeable, or entertaining patients. Such privileges included securing a desirable bed location near the radiator in winter or obtaining extra food. Restraints and seclusion rooms were commonly used to manage disruptive behavior.

During World War II, society evidenced a major change in attitude toward the mentally ill, as the number of psychiatric casualties from the war escalated. Dr. Peplau saw the passage of the Mental Health Act in 1946 as a major milestone for change in the practice of psychiatry. Dr. Peplau taught in the graduate program in psychiatric nursing at Teachers College (1948–1952) and later at Rutgers University in New Jersey (1954–1974). Funding through the Mental Health Act paid her salary. Dr. Peplau recalled that one nurse even called her "the kept woman of the government" (personal communication, November 3, 1990).

Changes in Dr. Peplau's professional practice mirrored changes in the field of psychiatric nursing. Her classic text *Interpersonal Relations in Nursing,* published in 1952, espoused her theory of nursing as a therapeutic, psychodynamic, interpersonal process and affirmed the importance of the nurse-patient relationship as a therapeutic and educative instrument in the care of the mentally ill. In 1958, she initiated her own private practice in New York City and evolved her own approach to psychotherapy.

Dr. Peplau saw nursing as a rapidly changing profession, increasing in scope and complexity. Although the biomedicalization of psychiatry, the emphasis on pharmacotherapy, and the proliferation of genetic and brain studies on mental illness causation are important advances, Dr. Peplau affirmed that it is the human, interpersonal process that should be the major domain for nursing research, theory development, and practice. She stated, "Psychiatric problems are, in the main, problems of persons—not primarily of their biology or physiology" (personal communication November 3, 1990).

Dr. Peplau died March 17, 1999, at her home in California.

---

to current practice. Becker (1970) cited Flexner's criteria as including the following:

1. Professional activity is basically intellectual with great personal responsibility.
2. It is based on great knowledge, not routine activities.
3. It is practical rather than theoretical.
4. It has a technique that can be taught, which is the basis for professional education.
5. It is organized internally.

6. It is motivated by altruism, with members working for some aspect of the good of society.

Critically examining each of these criteria allows us to come to a conclusion about the status of all of nursing as a profession and also the status of psychiatric nursing as a professional specialty within nursing. Some of Flexner's criteria, for instance criteria 2 and 4, give rise to debate among nurses. For example, although nurses recognize that education is a requirement to be a nurse, the debate centers on how much preparation constitutes a professional level. Is the associate's degree graduate a professional? What about the nurse who has earned a diploma? In psychiatric nursing, these questions become even more critical because significant differences in the amount of time devoted to mental health and illness content exist across differing educational programs.

Few nurses would argue with the essential truth of the first criterion. Certainly in psychiatric nursing, nurses are confronted with situations that require a great deal of thinking and analysis. The answers to "why" a patient acts in a certain way or "what" will change that behavior cannot be memorized; they must be reflected on. Criterion 3 is accepted without question in nursing. Nursing has always defined itself as a practice profession, which means that theory is gained to enhance practice. Within psychiatric nursing, psychiatric nurse leaders are calling for those in the field to conduct research that is outcome oriented so that nurses can demonstrate the effectiveness of various nursing interventions (McBride, 1986). Criterion 5, which deals with internal organization, is certainly true of both nursing as a whole and psychiatric nursing as a specialty. We have professional organizations that provide internal organization, the ANA provides organization to the profession as a whole, the National League for Nursing provides internal organization to nursing education, and the Society for Education and Research in Psychiatric-Mental Health Nursing and the American Psychiatric Nurses Association provide organization for the specialty of psychiatric nursing. We have standards of practice for the whole body of nursing as well as standards of practice for the specialty of psychiatric nursing. The ANA Statement on Psychiatric Nursing was first formulated in 1963, and in 1994, the Standards of Psychiatric and Mental Health Nursing Practice were revised. The ANA's Code of Ethics serves as another internal organizer and is applicable to the whole body of nursing practice.

The last criterion, which deals with altruistic motivation, is one that hardly needs defense in any nursing specialty. The whole thrust of nursing practice is to alleviate suffering of the individual, family, or other group. Because most nurses never become rich from nursing remuneration, one must ask why else nurses do what they do, if not to make a difference in society.

As a specialty within nursing, psychiatric nurses have a unique body of knowledge. This was first recognized with the establishment, in 1943, of the first university program in psychiatric nursing at The Catholic University of America. In 1967, a clinical focus in psychiatric nursing was included for doctoral students at The Catholic University of America when the Doctorate in Nursing Science was initiated.

Earlier in this chapter, you were reminded of the first psychiatric nursing textbook. Another publication worthy of mention is *Essentials of Psychiatric Nursing* (Taylor, 1994). This book was first published as *Psychiatry for Nurses* in 1940, when it was coauthored by Dr. Louis Karnosh and Edith Gage, RN. After Gage's death, Dr. Dorothy Mereness coauthored the 3rd edition, published in 1949. Mereness became the major author of the 7th edition, published in 1966 as *Essentials of Psychiatric Nursing*. With the publication of the 14th edition in 1994, *Essentials of Psychiatric Nursing* became the only psychiatric nursing textbook to have remained in continuous print for more than 50 years.

Psychiatric nurses credited with contributions to nursing theory include the following: Joyce Fitzpatrick, Madeline Leininger, Betty M. Neuman, Ida Jean Orlando, Hildegard E. Peplau, Joyce Travelbee, Loretta T. Zderad, and Josephine G. Patterson (Fordyce, 1988).

Specialized psychiatric nursing journals have made their appearance since 1963, with the initial publication of the *Journal of Psychiatric Nursing* (name changed to *Journal of Psychiatric Nursing and Mental Health Services* in 1967; since 1981 it has been called *Journal of Psychosocial Nursing and Mental Health Services*). *Perspectives of Psychiatric Care* was first published in 1963 and the journal *Archives of Psychiatric Nursing* was introduced in 1987. The first issue of the *Journal of the American Psychiatric Nurses Association* was introduced in February 1995.

October 1997 marked the inauguration of the networking organization, Alliance for Psychosocial Nursing (*Journal of Psychosocial Nursing and Mental Health Services,* December 1997, p. 6). Another significant event in the specialty occurred with the development of the ANA Certification Program (1973, 1979). Two levels of certification were established, one for the generalist and one for the specialist.

What do you think? What are your reactions to Flexner's criteria?

➤ *Check Your Reading*
35. Where was the first university program in psychiatric nursing established?
36. What was the first psychiatric nursing journal?
37. What are the two levels of certification established by the ANA Certification Program?

INFLUENCE OF FAMILY ADVOCACY ON MENTAL HEALTH CARE

The 1980s and 1990s were increasingly characterized by the voices of consumers and families. The founding of NAMI, in 1979, brought families together for needed support. The membership of this remarkable organization has grown at an amazing rate, making it the fastest growing advocacy group in the United States. Its members have become effective crusaders for expanded resources and for improvements in existing resources for those who are mentally ill. They are also a valuable source of support for family members of the mentally ill (Jones, 1992; Box 2-3).

What do you think? Should a psychiatric nurse be actively involved in NAMI?

➤ *Check Your Reading*
38. What is NAMI?

Box 2–3 ■ ■ ■ ■ ■
The National Alliance for the Mentally Ill: The Story of a Self-Help Organization

NAMI is a national self-help organization devoted to providing support to the families of the mentally ill, promoting public education and research on mental illness, advocating on behalf of the mentally ill, and providing information and referral services. NAMI was organized by families affected by mental illness who wished to promote public understanding of the needs of the mentally ill and to improve social conditions for their mentally ill loved ones. In 1967, Charles and Harriet Shetler of Madison, Wisconsin, shattered by the diagnosis of schizophrenia in their 18-year-old son and feeling blamed by mental health professionals for his illness, began meeting with other families who had similar experiences. They sought mutual support and understanding from one another and fought for improved mental health services in their community. In 1979, Harriet Shetler and the members of her group began to pull together similar support groups throughout the nation. They invited people from across the country to meet with them. From this meeting, it became evident that a united voice was needed to strengthen their position and to ultimately effect needed social change on a national level (McClory, 1986). From this initial assembly of self-help groups, the NAMI movement began.

To a great extent, NAMI's strength and influence are derived from its members' personal experiences with mental illness. The fundamental tenets of NAMI include the belief that mental illness is a biological disease process and not a result of dysfunctional family relationships. Rather than being viewed as the cause of mental illness, the family is seen as central to the support and treatment of the mentally ill member. In addition, laypeople are viewed as integral to the success and leadership of the organization (Hatfield, 1991). James Howe, Past President of NAMI, has a son suffering from chronic mental illness. NAMI has grown to encompass more than 172,000 members and more than 1100 affiliate chapters nationwide (*Facts About NAMI*, 1998).

NAMI is a respected movement in the psychiatric community. In fact, Dr. E. Fuller Torrey, renowned psychiatrist, proclaimed NAMI "the most important thing to happen for people with schizophrenia since antipsychotic drugs were introduced in the 1950's" (McClory, 1986, p. 19).

For more information, contact:
National Alliance for the Mentally Ill (NAMI)
200 North Glebe Road
Suite 1015
Arlington, VA 22203
800-950-NAMI
http://www.nami.org

DECADE OF THE BRAIN

By presidential proclamation, the 1990s were designated the "Decade of the Brain." President George Bush signed the proclamation on July 17, 1990 based on the recommendation of the U.S. Congress, Joint Resolution 174. The goal of this endeavor was to create joint cooperative efforts between public and federal government programs to study the brain with the hope of conquering brain diseases in the decade.

A former director of the NIMH, Lewis L. Judd, MD, reported (1990) that because of the progress in neuroscience, 90% of what was known about the brain in 1990 had been learned in the 10 years since 1980. The new tools of technology, such as MRI (magnetic resonance imaging), PET (positron-emission tomography), and CT (computed tomography), have provided researchers the "microscope" needed to view the brain structure and function. Brain abnormalities are being identified that are associated with several serious mental illnesses.

In *Healthy People 2000* (U.S. Department of Health and Human Services, 1992), national health promotion and disease prevention objectives for the year 2000 associated with psychiatric nursing practice included a 10% reduction in suicide rates, an 18% reduction in adverse effects of stress, a 15% reduction in homicide rates, and a 10% decrease in assault injuries. Other goals addressed reducing the prevalence of mental disorders, increasing treatment for people with major depressive disorders, and increasing use of community support and employee mental health programs. It was also hoped that primary care providers would increase attention to the cognitive, emotional, and behavioral needs of their patients.

Lowery (1992) said, "Psychiatric mental health nursing will need to take stock of itself—its practice, its education, and its research—if it is to successfully prepare for the changes in care of the mentally ill" (p. 13). Lowery and other psychiatric nursing leaders urged that, as attention focused on the biochemical components of illness and treatment, interpersonal and psychosocial needs continued to receive the appropriate level of attention. Many challenges await psychiatric nurses now and in the future. Grob (1994) profoundly stated society's obligation toward those in need of care:

It has often been noted that a society will be judged by the manner in which it treats its most vulnerable and dependent citizens. In this sense, the severely mentally ill have a moral claim upon our sympathy, compassion, and above all, upon our assistance. (p. 311)

What do you think? Do you see psychiatric nursing taking stock of itself as a profession?

Box 2-4 ■ ■ ■ ■ ■ ■
Chronology of Significant Events in the History of Mental Health Nursing

1751 Pennsylvania Hospital (Philadelphia) established through the efforts of Benjamin Franklin; this was the first hospital to make provisions for care of the insane as well as the physically ill

1773 Eastern Lunatic Asylum in Williamsburg, Virginia, established; this was the first public asylum (hospital) in the United States for people of "insane or disordered minds"

1792 York Retreat in England founded by William Tuke

1792 Phillippe Pinel in Paris, France removed the shackles from those held at the Bicêtre

1812 Publication of *Diseases of the Mind* by Benjamin Rush, Philadelphia

1818 McLean Asylum founded in Massachusetts

1841 Dorothea Lynde Dix volunteered at East Cambridge Jail in Massachussetts as a Sunday school teacher, thus embarking on a lifelong crusade for reform in the care of the mentally ill

1873 Linda Richards earned a diploma as the first nurse to complete the 1-year training program at New England Hospital

1882 Training School for Nurses at the McLean Asylum was founded, with the first graduates completing their course of study in 1886

1891 First patient admitted to the Sheppard Asylum (Baltimore)

1900 Initial publication of the *American Journal of Nursing*

1908 Publication of *A Mind That Found Itself* by Clifford W. Beers

1914–1918 World War I, psychiatric casualties of the war and shortage of nurses were evident

1920 Publication of *Nursing Mental Diseases* by nurse educator Harriet Bailey

1926 Appointment of Euphemia "Effie" Jane Taylor as the first psychiatric nurse to be appointed Professor of Nursing

1938 Introduction of ECT, devised by Drs. Ugo Cerletti and Lucio Bini in Italy

1939–1945 World War II, a high toll of psychiatric casualties noted

1940 Publication of *Psychiatry for Nurses* by Louis Karnosh and Edith Gage, RN

1946 National Mental Health Act passed by the U.S. Congress
Hill-Burton Act passed by U.S. Congress

1947 Publication of *Nurse-Patient Relationships in Psychiatry* by Helena Render

1948 Publication of *The Shame of the States* by Albert Deutsch

1949 NIMH established under the provisions of the National Mental Health Act of 1946
Publication of *Psychiatry for Nurses* by Dorothy Mereness and Louis Karnosh

1952 Publication of *Interpersonal Relations in Nursing* by Hildegard E. Peplau

1954 Advent of the use of the antipsychotic medication chlorpromazine (Thorazine) in the United States, synthesized in France, in 1950

1955 National Mental Health Study Act, which established the Joint Commission on Mental Illness and Health

1961 Publication of *Action for Mental Health*, final report of The Joint Commission on Mental Illness and Health

1963 Community Mental Health Centers Construction Act passed by Congress
Publication of *Journal of Psychiatric Nursing* began; in 1967 renamed *Journal of Psychiatric Nursing and Mental Health Services*; in 1981 renamed *Journal of Psychosocial Nursing and Mental Health Services*
Initial publication of *Perspectives of Psychiatric Care*

1966 Enactment of the Medicare Bill

1973 *Standards of Psychiatric–Mental Health Nursing* published Certification of Psychiatric–Mental Health Nurse Generalists established by the ANA

1979 ANA established certification of psychiatric–mental health nurse specialists
NAMI founded

1982 Century Celebration of Psychiatric Nursing, Washington, D.C.

1986 National Alliance for Research on Schizophrenia and Depression founded

1987 Publication of *Archives of Psychiatric Nursing* began

1988 NIMH Epidemiological Catchment Area Study

1990 Americans With Disabilities Act passed by the U.S. Congress
Presidential proclamation by George Bush declared the 1990s the "Decade of the Brain"

1994 Publication of *Essentials of Psychiatric Nursing*, 14th edition, by Cecilia Taylor; originally published as *Psychiatry for Nurses* in 1940

1995 Publication of *Journal of the American Psychiatric Nurses Association* began

1996 National Mental Health Parity Bill passed by Congress

1997 Alliance for Psychosocial Nursing was formed in London
Limited Parity Bill passed by U.S. Congress

1998 January 1 National Mental Health Parity Bill went into effect

Box 2-4 provides a chronology of significant events in the history of mental health nursing.

➤ *Check Your Reading*

39. What U.S. president declared the 1990s the Decade of the Brain?

40. What are the goals of *Healthy People 2000* that are appropriate for psychiatric nursing?
41. What do the acronyms PET and MRI mean?

Conclusions

The historical, social, political, and economic developments of the past century carved the path and provided the inroads that shaped the journey of psychiatric–mental health nursing practice. It is not surprising, then, that the future journey of psychiatric–mental health nursing will be greatly influenced by the stories that are being lived today by nursing leaders and practitioners, consumers, and all people touched by mental illness. It is important for nurses to be involved in shaping the course of their destinies by developing an understanding of both the historical context in which their practice emerges and the present forces and future trends that are likely to shape and further define the position of psychiatric–mental health nursing in the health care delivery system. The issues of homelessness, substance abuse, violence and human abuse, multiculturalism, and national health care reform will likely shape the course of psychiatric–mental health nursing practice well into the 21st century. The psychiatric–mental health nurse can be in an ideal position to address each of these issues through research, education, patient advocacy, and political action to ensure that the path on which nursing journeys is well lit by knowledge, insight, and profound sensitivity for all people who, in one way or another, have been touched by mental illness.

Key Points to Remember

- In earliest recorded history, mental illness was attributed to the anger of the gods, the devil, or demonic possession.
- Hippocrates suggested that bodily humors were responsible for behaviors.
- Phillippe Pinel, a French psychiatrist, unchained mentally ill patients.
- William Tuke established the York Retreat in 1792. The York Retreat was a treatment facility for the mentally ill where kindness and a pleasant environment were viewed as essentials for healing.
- Benjamin Rush, the Father of American Psychiatry, published his book *Diseases of the Mind* in 1812. He advocated gentle and humane treatment for the mentally ill.
- Dorothea Lynde Dix crusaded for more humane treatment of the mentally ill by advocating that psychiatric hospitals be built from public funds.
- Emil Kraepelin developed the first comprehensive description of mental disorders.
- Sigmund Freud developed the psychoanalytical approach to human behavior and the principles of psychoanalysis.
- Adolph Meyer, a professor at Johns Hopkins University, was known for his psychobiological perspective and commonsense psychiatry.
- Clifford Beers, a former mental patient, wrote *A Mind That Found Itself*, a book that detailed his experiences as a patient.
- Linda Richards graduated in 1873 from the Training School at the New England Hospital and became America's first trained psychiatric nurse.
- Harriet Bailey authored the first psychiatric nursing textbook, *Nursing Mental Diseases*, in 1920.
- Euphemia "Effie" Jane Taylor was the first psychiatric nurse to be appointed Professor of Nursing at Yale University in 1926.
- Harry Stack Sullivan developed the interpersonal theory of psychiatry.
- Hildegard E. Peplau used many of Sullivan's concepts and wrote them in a language that was understandable and useable to nurses in their practices.
- William C. Menninger started the first postgraduate school of psychiatric nursing in 1932.
- Over the course of centuries, as public opinion and knowledge about mental illness and the mentally ill waxed and waned, settings where the mentally ill have been cared for have included almshouses, asylums, hospitals, CMH centers, mobile treatment teams, day hospitals, community rehabilitation centers, and private homes. The quality of these settings has varied greatly.
- World Wars I and II focused attention on the large numbers of young men who were unable to serve in the military because of preexisting psychiatric illness and the large numbers of young men who became psychiatrically disabled because of wartime conditions.
- Legislation such as the National Mental Health Act, the Hill-Burton Act, the Mental Retardation Facilities and Community Mental Health Centers Construction Act of 1963, the Community Mental Health Center Amendment in 1975, the Community Mental Health Systems Act, the Omnibus Budget Reconciliation Act, and the Americans With Disabilities Act of 1990 has served to promote the delivery of care to the mentally ill, either through funding for education or research or through funding of construction for new facilities.

- Psychobiological therapies, including psychotropic drugs, have dramatically changed the practice of psychiatric nursing.
- Deinstitutionalization has reduced the number of chronically mentally ill patients residing in large state hospitals but has increased the number of patients who now live on the streets of our nation because of inadequate community resources to provide them with housing and care.

- Interpersonal relationships are a primary focus of psychiatric nursing practice.
- NAMI provides support for families who struggle to cope with a loved one who has a psychiatric illness.
- Research conducted during the Decade of the Brain will increase our understanding of the neurobiological influences on behavior and will shape the future journey of psychiatric nursing.

Learning Activities

1. Interview several nurses to discover their stories. Why did they become nurses? What changes have they witnessed within the profession? In what direction do they see themselves journeying within the profession?
2. Go to the library and read at least one of the books mentioned in this chapter. Get a flavor for a particular historical time and place from the author's descriptions. (See Suggested Readings.)
3. Set up a panel discussion with students portraying different historical figures. Have each character argue for the changes that she or he sees as essential to provide care for the mentally ill.
4. Begin to write your own story about why you chose

nursing. As you journey through nursing as a student and later as a professional nurse, continue to add to your story. Over time, note the patterns and themes that emerge as you weave the tapestry of your life's story.
5. Interview nurses from different educational backgrounds to determine what each believes about the qualifications of a professional. Ask each one if she or he sees herself or himself as a professional nurse. Ask for the reason behind the answer given.
6. View a copy of the videotape In Search of Ourselves (Markowitz, 1998). Identify milestone events recounted in this presentation.

Critical Thinking Exercises

Ms. Fields, a junior nursing student, was writing a paper about the history of psychiatric nursing during her psychiatric–mental health nursing course. She decided to research the influence (if any) that Hildegard E. Peplau had on her current learning about psychiatric nursing. She began to write "Dr. Peplau was a pioneer in the development of psychiatric nursing. She wrote *Interpersonal Relations in Nursing* in 1952, in which she affirms the belief that nurses, through the use of the nurse-patient relationship, can be therapeutic and educative instruments in the care of the mentally ill (Peplau, 1952). Peplau believes that the human interpersonal process needs to be the major concern of the nurse's practice and that 'psychiatric problems . . . are problems of persons—not primarily of their biology or physiology' " (personal communication, November 3, 1990).

1. As Ms. Fields wrote her paper about Dr. Peplau's influence on present day psychiatric nursing, what did she infer about Dr. Peplau's point of view?
2. What assumptions can we make about Ms. Fields's understanding of Dr. Peplau's point of view regarding present-day psychiatric nursing practice?

3. Does Ms. Fields present a precise, clear picture of Dr. Peplau's position?

Ms. Fields continued to write: "Even though Dr. Peplau developed her theory on interpersonal relations in nursing in 1952, psychiatric nursing of today is still greatly influenced by Dr. Peplau's ideas. Although psychiatric nursing care has recently been influenced by the impact of biochemical and genetic knowledge, nursing must continue to recognize the importance of the interpersonal process."

1. What evidence does Ms. Fields present to support her assumptions about Dr. Peplau's point of view regarding psychiatric nursing?
2. What other information does Ms. Fields need to know to clarify her understanding of Dr. Peplau's ideas?
3. If you were to reason from Dr. Peplau's point of view about psychiatric nursing practice, what would you say about psychiatric nursing practice?
4. What other points of view might be considered when practicing psychiatric nursing?

Additional Resources

National Alliance for the Mentally Ill (NAMI)

200 North Glebe Road
Suite 1015
Arlington, VA 22203
800-950-NAMI
http://www.nami.org

References

Alexander, F., & Selesnick, S. (1966). *The history of psychiatry.* New York: Harper & Row.

American Nurses Association. (1994). *Standards of psychiatric and mental health nursing practice.* Kansas City, MO: Author.

Americans With Disabilities Act of 1990, Pub. L. No. 100-336 (1990).

ANA in Review. (1958, Spring). *6*(1).

Bailey, H. (1920). *Nursing mental diseases.* New York: Macmillan.

Bailey, H. (1935). *Nursing mental diseases* (3rd ed.). New York: Macmillan.

Baxter, W. E., & Hathcox, D. W. (1994). *America's care of the mentally ill: A photographic history.* Washington, DC: American Psychiatric Press.

Becker, H. (1970). *Sociological work: Method and substance.* Chicago: Adline.

Beers, C. (1908). *A mind that found itself.* New York: Doubleday.

Beers, C. (1943). *A mind that found itself* (29th ed.) [Preface]. New York: Doubleday.

Blazer, D. G. (1998). *Freud vs. God: How psychiatry lost its soul and Christianity lost its mind.* Downers Grove, IL: Inter-Varsity Press.

Buckwalter, K. C., & Church, O. M. (1979). Euphemia Jane Taylor: An uncommon psychiatric nurse. *Perspectives in Psychiatric Care, 18*(2), 62-66.

Church, O. M. (1982). That noble reform: The emergence of psychiatric nursing in the United States, 1882-1963. *Dissertation Abstracts International, 43-05B,* 1434. (University Microfilms No. AAG8220717.)

Church, O. M., & Buckwalter, K. C. (1980). Harriet Bailey: A psychiatric nurse pioneer. *Perspectives in Psychiatric Care, 18*(2), 62-66.

Community Mental Health Systems Act, Pub. L. No. 96-398 (1980).

Community Mental Health Center Amendment, Pub. L. No. 94-63 (1975).

Convention Preview, Anaheim 86: Effie Taylor to enter ANA Nursing Hall of Fame. (1986). *Journal of Psychosocial Nursing and Mental Health Services, 24*(5), 36.

Deutsch, A. (1948). *The shame of the states.* New York: Harcourt Brace.

Deutsch, A. (1949). *The mentally ill in America* (2nd ed.). New York: Columbia University Press.

Dolan, J. A., Fitzpatrick, M. L., & Herrmann, E. K. (1983). *Nursing in society: A historical perspective* (15th ed.). Philadelphia: W. B. Saunders.

Donahue, M. P. (1985). *Nursing: The finest art.* St. Louis, MO: C. V. Mosby.

Donahue, M. P. (1996). *Nursing: The finest art* (2nd ed.). St. Louis, MO: Mosby-Year Book.

Doona, M. E. (1984). At least as well cared for . . . Linda Richards and the mentally ill. *Image: The Journal of Nursing Scholarship, 16*(2), 51-56.

Facts about NAMI. (1998). Arlington: National Alliance for the Mentally Ill.

Flanigan, L. (1976). *One strong voice: The story of the American Nurses' Association.* Kansas City, MO: American Nurses' Association.

Flowers, C. (1998). *A science odyssey: 100 years of discovery.* New York: Morrow.

Forbush, B., & Forbush, B. (1986). *Gatehouse: The evolution of the Sheppard and Enoch Pratt Hospital, 1853-1986.* Baltimore: The Sheppard and Enoch Pratt Hospital.

Fordyce, E. (1988). Theorists in nursing. In J. Flynn & P. Heffron (Eds.), *Nursing: From concept to practice* (2nd ed., p. 69-87). Norwalk, CT: Appleton and Lange.

Forester, D. A., & Grandinetti, P. M. (1991). A distinguished history on postage stamps in nursing. *The American Philatelist, 105,* 710-717.

Frank, C. M. (1959). *Foundations of nursing* (2nd ed.). Philadelphia: W. B. Saunders.

Grob, G. N. (1994). *The mad among us: A history of the care of America's mentally ill.* New York: The Free Press.

Hall, B. H. (Ed.). (1967). *A psychiatrist for a troubled world.* New York: Viking Press.

Harding, C., Zubin, J., & Strauss, J. (1987). Chronicity in schizophrenia: Fact, partial fact, or artifact. *Hospital and Community Psychiatry, 38,* 479-491.

Hatfield, A. (1991). The national alliance for the mentally ill: A decade later. *Community Mental Health Journal, 27*(2), 95-103.

Hatfield, A., & Lefley, H. (Eds.). (1987). *Families of the mentally ill: Coping and adaptation.* New York: Guilford Press.

The introduction of chlorpromazine. (1976). *Hospital and Community Psychiatry, 27,* 505.

Jails: The new mental institutions. (1991, March/April). *NAMI Advocate, 12*(2), 1, 12.

Joint Commission on Mental Illness and Health (1961). *Action for mental health: Final report, 1961.* New York: Basic Books.

Jones, S. (1992). The family as an advocate for the mentally ill. *Archives of Psychiatric Nursing, 6,* 145-146.

Judd, L. (1990). Putting mental health on the nation's health agenda. NIMH Report. *Hospital and Community Psychiatry, 41,* 131, 132, 134.

Lewis, G. (1978). *Nurse-patient communication* (3rd ed.). Dubuque, IA: William C. Brown.

Lowery, B. (1992). Psychiatric nursing in the 1990's and beyond. *Journal of Psychosocial Nursing and Mental Health Services, 30*(1), 7-13.

Maisel, A. Q. (1946). Bedlam 1946: Most U.S. mental hospitals are a shame and a disgrace. *Life, 40*(5), 102-118.

Manfreda, M. L. (1982). *The roots of interpersonal nursing.* Cromwell: Cromwell Printing.

Markowitz, A. (Writer, Producer). (1998). In search of ourselves (Episode 3 of 5). In Friedman, T. (Series Executive Producer), *A science odyssey: 100 years of discovery* [videotape]. (Available from PBS Home Video, P.O. Box 751089, Charlotte, NC 28275-1089; 800-828-4PBS.)

McBride, A. B. (1986). Present issues and future perspectives of psychosocial nursing theory and research. *Journal of Psychosocial Nursing and Mental Health Services, 24*(9), 27-32.

McClory, R. (1986, July). The history of NAMI. *Ways,* 16-19.

Mental Health Study Act, Pub. L. No. 182.

Mental Retardation Facilities and Community Mental Health Centers Construction Act of 1963, Pub. L. No. 88-164 (1963).

The National Mental Health Act, Pub. L. No. 487 (1946).

Noyes, A., & Haydon, E. (1948). *Textbook of psychiatric nursing* (4th ed.). New York: Macmillan.

Omnibus Budget Reconciliation Act, Pub. L. No. 97-35 (1982).

Orlando, I. J. (1961). *The dynamic nurse-patient relationship: Function, process and principles.* New York: Putnam.

O'Toole, A. W., & Welt, S. R. (1989). *Interpersonal theory in nursing practice: Selected works of Hildegard E. Peplau.* New York: Springer.

Peplau, H. E. (1952). *Interpersonal relations in nursing.* New York: Putnam's.

Peplau, H. E. (1982a). Some reflections on earlier days in psychiatric nursing. *Journal of Psychosocial Nursing and Mental Health Services, 20*(8), 17-24.

Peplau, H. E. (1982b). Historical development of psychiatric nursing: A preliminary statement of some facts and trends. In S. Smoyak & S. Rouslin (Eds.). *A collection of classics in psychiatric nursing literature* (pp. 10-46). Thorofare, NJ: Slack.

Psychiatric nursing: The nurse-patient relationship. [Film]. (1958). Philadelphia: Smith Kline and French; (1990). Reissued on video for the American Psychiatric Nurses Association. (Available from Slack, Inc., 6900 Grove Road, Thorofare, NJ 08086.)

Render, H. W. (1947). *Nurse-patient relationships in psychiatry.* New York: McGraw-Hill.

Richards, L. (1911). *Reminiscences of America's first trained nurse (Linda Richards).* Boston: Whitcomb and Barrows.

Sareyan, A. (1994). *The turning point: How men of conscience brought about major change in the care of America's mentally ill.* Washington, DC: American Psychiatric Press.

Shakespeare, W. *King Lear.* Act 2, Scene 3.

Sills, G. M. (1973). Historical developments and issues in psychiatric mental health nursing. In M. M. Leininger (Ed.), *Contemporary issues in mental health nursing.* Boston: Little, Brown.

Smoyak, S. A. (1997). Alliance for psychosocial nurses, [Editorial]. *Journal of Psychosocial Nursing and Mental Health Services, 35*(12), 6.

Sutton, S. B. (1986). *Crossroads in psychiatry: A history of the McLean Hospital.* Washington, DC: American Psychiatric Press.

Swazey, J. P. (1974). *Chlorpromazine in psychiatry.* Boston: The Massachusetts Institute of Technology.

Taylor, C. M. (1990). *Mereness' essentials of psychiatric nursing* (13th ed.). St. Louis: C. V. Mosby.

Taylor, C. M. (1994). *Essentials of psychiatric nursing* (14th ed.). St. Louis: C. V. Mosby.

Tiffany, F. (1918). *Life of Dorothea Lynde Dix.* Boston: Houghton Mifflin.

Torrey, E. F. (1988). *Nowhere to go: The tragic odyssey of the homeless mentally ill.* New York: Harper & Row.

Torrey, E. F. (1993). The scandalous neglect of the mentally ill homeless. *National Forum, 78*(1), 4-7, 12.

Torrey, E. F. (1997). *Out of the shadows: Confronting America's mental illness crisis.* New York: John Wiley.

Travelbee, J. (1969). *Intervention in psychiatric nursing.* Philadelphia: F. A. Davis.

U.S. Department of Health and Human Services. (1992). *Healthy people 2000: National health promotion and disease prevention objectives.* Boston: Jones and Bartlett.

Ward, M. J. (1964). *The snake pit.* New York: New American Library.

Wright, F. L. (1947). *Out of sight, out of mind.* Philadelphia: National Mental Health Foundation.

Suggested Readings

Beers, C. (1908). *A mind that found itself.* New York: Doubleday.

Bullough, V. L., Sentz, L., & Stein, A. P. (1992). *American nursing: A biographical dictionary* (Vol. 2). New York: Garland.

Church, O. M. (1982). That noble reform: The emergence of psychiatric nursing in the United States, 1882-1963. *Dissertation Abstracts International, 43-05B,* 1434. (University Microfilms No. AAG8220717).

Deutsch, A. (1948). *The shame of the states.* New York: Harcourt Brace.

Deutsch, A. (1949). *The mentally ill in America* (2nd ed.). New York: Columbia University Press.

Flynn, L. M. (1993). Political impact of the family-consumer movement. *National Forum, 78*(1), 8-12.

Grob, G. N. (1994). *The mad among us: A history of the care of America's mentally ill.* New York: The Free Press.

Robb, I. H. (1901). *Nursing ethics.* Cleveland, OH: J. B. Savage.

Smoyak, S. A., & Rouslin, S. (Eds.). (1982). *A collection of classics in psychiatric nursing literature.* Thorofare, NJ: Slack.

Thompson, J. W. (1994). Trends in the development of psychiatric services. *Hospital and Community Psychiatry, 45,* 987-992.

Tiffany, F. (1918). *Life of Dorothea Lynde Dix.* Boston: Houghton Mifflin.

Torrey, E. F. (1988). *Nowhere to go: The tragic odyssey of the homeless mentally ill.* New York: Harper & Row.

Torrey, E. F. (1997). *Out of the shadows: Confronting America's mental illness crisis.* New York: John Wiley.

Wilson, D. (1975). *Stranger and traveler: The story of Dorothea Dix, American reformer.* Boston: Little, Brown.

Wright, F. L. (1947). *Out of sight, out of mind.* Philadelphia: National Mental Health Foundation.

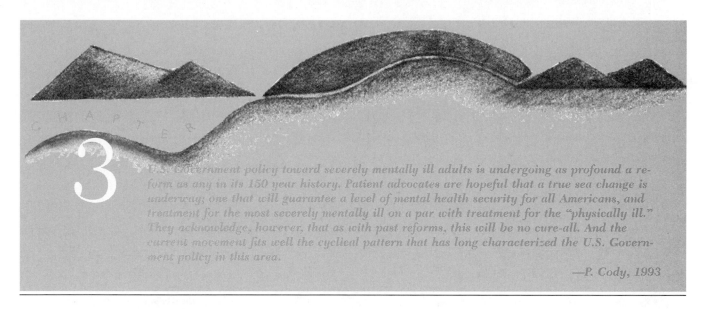

U.S. Government policy toward severely mentally ill adults is undergoing as profound a reform as any in its 150 year history. Patient advocates are hopeful that a true sea change is underway; one that will guarantee a level of mental health security for all Americans, and treatment for the most severely mentally ill on a par with treatment for the "physically ill." They acknowledge, however, that as with past reforms, this will be no cure-all. And the current movement fits well the cyclical pattern that has long characterized the U.S. Government policy in this area.

—P. Cody, 1993

Highways for the Journey
The Mental Health System

Learning Objectives

After studying this chapter, you should be able to:

1. Understand the significance of *Diagnostic and Statistical Manual of Mental Disorders, Fourth Edition* (DSM-IV) and *International Classification of Diseases, Ninth Revision, Clinical Modification* (ICD-9-CM) in the practice of psychiatric nursing.

2. Appreciate the impact on the practice of psychiatric nursing of societal forces such as homelessness, the increasing numbers of aged Americans, unemployment, and the increasing numbers of young people who have both a psychiatric illness and a substance abuse problem.

3. Talk about shifting federal policies toward the care of the mentally ill and the impact that these ever-changing policies have on the care of the mentally ill and on the practice of psychiatric nursing.

4. Define managed behavioral health care.

5. Define primary care.

6. Discuss case management and its impact on psychiatric nursing.

7. Understand how reimbursement policies affect the practice of psychiatric nursing.

8. Discuss the impact of institutional settings on the practice of psychiatric nursing.

9. Discuss practice roles of psychiatric nurses.

10. Discuss the scope of practice of psychiatric nurses.

Key Terminology

Capitation system	DSM-IV	Managed behavioral health	Parity
Carve outs	Health maintenance organi-	care	Practice roles
Case management	zation	Managed care	Preferred provider organi-
Case rate	ICD-9	Medicaid	zation
Deinstitutionalization	ICD-9-CM	Medical cost offset	Point-of-service plan
Discounted fee for service	Integrated delivery system	Medicare	Primary care
			Scope of practice

The journey of psychiatric nursing, like every profession, is shaped and transformed by the forces of history and happenings of the larger society. Some of these influences include social changes, theoretical revisions and innovations, the nation's economic conditions and political ideology, modifications in the health care system itself, and the continuing stigma and misunderstanding that surround the mentally ill. Ignorance characterizes much of the thinking about the mentally ill and holds that the mentally ill are responsible for their illnesses, that they need greater determination, perseverance, and character building to improve their lot in life. This kind of ignorance about the nature of mental illness and the suffering it exacts on patients and loved ones allows those who are not afflicted (including those who control governmental purse strings) to feel justified in the meager and inconsistent support provided for programs to assist the mentally ill.

This chapter examines some of the external forces, which sometimes seem like intersecting highways, and their impact on the journey shared by psychiatric-mental health nurses and their patients. Specifically, we focus on the impact of the *Diagnostic and Statistical Manual of Mental Disorders, Fourth Edition* **(DSM-IV)** and the World Health Organization's *Clinical Modification of the International Classification of Diseases, Ninth Revision* **(ICD-9-CM)**; public policy, including legislation; social changes; reimbursement issues; the role of managed behavioral health care organizations; **practice roles** as well as the **scope of practice;** primary care; and settings where psychiatric care is provided. It is important to recognize the mutually reciprocal relationships that exist among these diverse highways in the mental health system. For instance, social changes do not occur in isolation; they may occur in response to policy changes and vice versa. Examining these forces separately is valuable for study purposes, but true understanding requires recognition of the complexity of these issues.

Herman's story is an account of one man's experience with the mental health system. The story illustrates how a policy change designed to save mental health dollars by downsizing hospitals had a ripple effect on a particular patient, Herman, and on several agencies. See What Families Need to Know: Myths and Realities of Serious Mental Illness.

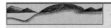 **Herman's Story**

In autumn 1992, Herman was 1 of 20 patients remaining at Greystone State Hospital in rural New England. He and the other patients were the only barrier remaining to the hospital's closure, and the

---

WHAT FAMILIES NEED TO KNOW

Myths and Realities of Serious Mental Illness

Who is affected by serious mental illness?

The three serious types of mental disorders (schizophrenia, manic-depressive disorder, and major depression) affect up to 20% of the population. All three of these disorders are "brain diseases" that affect people of all ages, all races, and all socioeconomic groups. One family in 25 will be directly affected by a serious, chronic mental illness.

What causes serious mental illness?

Serious mental illness is organically based and cannot be cured. However, these disorders are highly controllable with medication and support services. Poor parenting contributes to but is not the cause of serious mental illness.

Are seriously mentally ill people violent or mentally retarded?

People with serious mental illness can be violent but more frequently they are *victims* of violence in our society. People with serious mental illness are not necessarily mentally retarded. Often, they are exceptionally gifted in many areas of intellectual development and creative expression.

What is a split personality?

By *split personality,* most people are referring to a rare mental illness called multiple personality disorder. People with multiple personality disorder have two or more distinct personalities, often of different ages and genders. The mental illness known as *schizophrenia* is not the same thing as a split personality. Schizophrenia is a disorder of a person's thought processes that interferes with the brain's ability to think clearly and logically.

What causes depression?

Serious depression—what mental health professionals call *major depression*—and manic-depressive disorder are considered mood disorders and are caused by chemical imbalances. These imbalances can be corrected dramatically by medication and support services.

Data from National Alliance for the Mentally Ill. (1987). *Serious mental illnesses: Myths and realities.* Arlington, VA: Author.

state mental health bureaucracy was being pushed hard to find them placements and save millions of dollars a year.

On a Pathway to Nowhere

Herman was not a particularly difficult patient; he was something worse—an enigma. In his 2 years at Greystone, he had never assaulted a staff member or another patient or attempted to escape. Despite the fact that he shaved every morning, dressed in a suit on visiting days, and was sometimes mistaken for a physician, he had never been issued a single pass to the hospital grounds.

Herman's admission to Greystone and his behavior inside it did not conform to any of the pathways into or out of a state mental hospital. He did not show symptoms of decompensated schizophrenia or any other major mental illness; therefore, he could not be categorized, put on medication, taught better coping skills, and released. He had been committed because, while trying to kill himself, he had set his apartment building on fire and endangered many lives. His wife, who had left him some months before, told clinicians that he had sexually abused one daughter and beaten other children. He had no memory of the fire or his suicide attempt, and he showed no remorse, grief, or insight into it, despite repeated but gentle questioning by Greystone's clinicians. And so he was stuck at Greystone, categorized as a psychopath and a con artist who had failed to exhibit human responses that could have opened the pathway to his release.

Dilemma With No Easy Answer

When Herman's characterization as a psychopath came face to face with the governor's directive to close Greystone, the state mental health director for the region came to our community care center. He was in a terrible bind. Herman's behavior was still impeccable, but a local forensic psychologist had recently interviewed him and confirmed the diagnosis: a dangerous psychopath. Yet Herman had to go, and soon. The state department of mental health wanted us to design a program for Herman so that they could shut down Greystone without the risk of becoming the subject of a "60 Minutes" exposé depicting the state facility as incompetent for releasing a dangerous psychopath.

The state administrators tried to transfer their quandary to us; now we were in a bind. We obviously could not supply as much security as a state hospital, yet we could not afford to offend the state administrators who were the source of half of our operating budget. As the clinic director and I discussed the matter with state administrators, I realized that all of us—community mental health (CMH) staff, state administrators, and Herman—were stuck together in a "narrative" that seemed to offer no easy answers.

Breakthrough

After much discussion, the director and I agreed to interview Herman for a place in our community support program. The state administrators wanted it to be a routine interview preliminary to discharge, but because our program was voluntary and we had to find out whether we could all get along and work together productively, we insisted on reserving judgment until we met Herman.

Two weeks later, I sat in my office waiting for Herman. As the community care center's forensic psychologist, I faced a crucial decision. Would I define the interview as a formal forensic evaluation, assessing Herman's dangerousness for later submission to the state? Or could it be an informal, confidential encounter in which we got to know each other as two people who might work closely together in the future?

At the last minute—as I greeted Herman in the waiting room—I decided to be informal. I told him about my choice as he settled himself into a chair in my office. He seemed pleased with my decision. I began gently urging him to tell me his story as I completed a family history.

About half an hour later, Herman was telling me about the Christmas holiday just before he tried to kill himself. His wife and family had left him, and he was working hard at restoring an apartment building he owned.

As he talked, I noticed a change in Herman's usually facile manner and self-possessed face. It was as if a sudden wind had blown in, darkening his features. "I really hoped that somehow they would come back and spend Christmas with me," he said, standing staunch in the growing gale. I leaned forward and rolled my chair a little closer to him. I don't remember exactly what I said, but it was something like, "It sounds like that really meant a lot to you."

Herman tried to contain his grief, but it overcame him. He wept, and we sat together for a couple of minutes. Then he collected himself. "Hmmm," he said, dabbing his eyes with a tissue. "Well I'll be damned. I don't know where that came from."

He may not have known where it came from but his tears sure made sense to me. He had shown himself to be a human being with feelings, capable of taking part in a relationship. I decided that Herman would do okay in our community support program. At the same time, I knew that by choosing to believe in a scenario of hope and recovery rather than one of pathology, I was taking a risk.

Move to the Community

A week later, Herman left the state hospital. His wife and family obtained restraining orders against him, and we made agreements to notify the local police when Herman planned visits to the town where they lived. He moved into a supervised apartment shared with another patient and began making his way in the world. You might say that his tears had formed a river that carried him to a new definition of himself, but it was really a lot more complicated than that. His tears solved our agency's problem as well as his own.

Writing a New Story

I struggled to comprehend what had happened and began to understand that together Herman and I had created a new narrative, a new story. The new story, which unfolded as the weeks went on, depicted Herman as a man who had lost a great deal in his life; a man who, with his last shred of pride, had maintained himself in rigid isolation in the state hospital to avoid being categorized as a "mental patient." To break down and show his grief would have assuaged the anxieties of administrators, but for Herman it would have meant joining a club to which he did not choose to belong. He felt he had been unfairly imprisoned and had spent 2 long years in a marathon effort to maintain his integrity.

Later, I met with community support staff who were to deal with Herman every day. I presented them with the two narratives—Herman as a psychopath and Herman as a man choosing to grieve his losses in his own way—and suggested that, although at any given moment either one might appear to have greater truth, they should not "marry" either one. Rather, they should allow Herman to define himself in his new situation to create a new story.

Herman returned weekly for therapy with me for a couple of months, and he now comes in about once every 3 weeks. He keeps himself busy, takes excellent care of his supervised apartment, and cooks elaborate meals for himself and his roommate, a patient with a lower level of daily functioning. He talks about getting a job someday. In 4 months, he has not attempted to contact his family or been in any trouble with the law.

As a humanistically oriented family therapist, I was intrigued to note that it was Herman's grief that provided the bridge to a new narrative. Had he not had the courage to show his feelings, our impasse would have continued indefinitely. What I had supplied was the open space within which a new narrative could be invented. My willful ignorance allowed us to encounter each other as two people who needed to define themselves anew.

As Herman gets more established, he is settling into a fairly rigid approach to life. No miracles have happened, but, to the relief of the state administrators, his new narrative is beginning to have real veracity, and, most importantly, it is offering Herman a chance for a new life. Fortunately, Herman's narrative has a positive ending. This is not always the case when patients are caught in the changing world of mental health care. ∎

Story from Murphy, M. J. (1993). Herman wept, or the battle of narratives: A case study. *The Family Therapy Networker, 17*(3), 77–79.

DIAGNOSTIC AND CLASSIFICATION SYSTEMS AND THEIR IMPACT ON THE JOURNEY

You must be familiar with two diagnostic and classification systems in psychiatric nursing: the ICD-9-CM and the DSM-IV. It is important for you to understand both systems, because together they are used for compilation of statistics and for reimbursement of expenses (Figure 3–1).

DSM-IV

In spring 1994, the DSM-IV was published; it represents the third revision in 15 years; the number of mental disorders included has increased from 106 to 300. The manual, touted by the American Psychiatric Association as scientific, actually intermingles science with social values.

Whether or not the manual is scientific, knowledge and understanding of its contents are essential for psychiatric nurses as well as for other mental health professionals. Insurance companies use the DSM-IV to determine reimbursement for psychiatric services. In order to be paid, providers of psychiatric services must submit reimbursement claims that list an official diagnostic label accompanied by a DSM code number. The DSM-IV is the most cited book in psychiatry and is used by courts, schools, social agencies, and college classrooms to establish diagnoses.

The DSM-IV contains not only nomenclature but also the numerical codes for each of the disorders. The codes correspond with those in the ICD-9-CM in order to facilitate the exchange of scientific data across international and language barriers. A complete DSM-IV classification list appears in Appendix III.

The DSM-IV retains the multiaxial assessment system that appeared in the previous edition. On Axis I, the clinician reports clinical disorders and other conditions

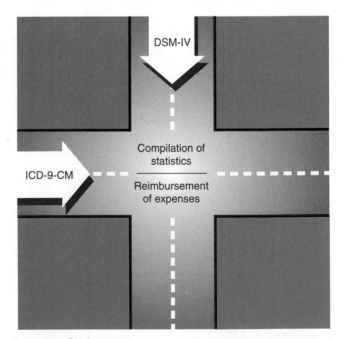

Figure 3–1

The diagnostic and classifications of the *Diagnostic and Statistical Manual of Mental Disorders, Fourth Edition* and the *Clinical Modification of the International Classification of Diseases, Ninth Revision* intersect for purposes of compilation of statistics and reimbursement of expenses.

Box 3–1 ■ ■ ■ ■ ■
Examples of Axis IV Problems (Psychosocial and Environmental)

Problems With Primary Support Group

Death of a family member
Health problems in family
Disruption of family by separation, divorce, or estrangement
Removal from the home
Remarriage of parent
Sexual or physical abuse
Parental overprotection
Neglect
Inadequate discipline
Discord with siblings
Birth of a sibling

Problems Related to the Social Environment

Death or loss of friend
Inadequate social support
Living alone
Difficulty with acculturation
Discrimination
Adjustment to life cycle transition (such as retirement)
Educational problems
Illiteracy
Academic problems
Discord with teachers or classmates
Inadequate school environment

Occupational Problems

Unemployment
Threat of job loss

Stressful work schedule
Difficult work conditions
Job dissatisfaction
Job change
Discord with boss or coworkers

Housing Problems

Homelessness
Inadequate housing
Unsafe neighborhood
Discord with neighbors or landlord

Economic Problems

Extreme poverty
Inadequate finances
Insufficient welfare support

Problems With Access to Health Care Services

Inadequate health care services
Transportation to health care facilities unavailable
Inadequate health insurance

Problems Related to Interaction With Legal System or Crime

Arrest
Incarceration
Litigation
Victim of crime

Based on information from the *Diagnostic and Statistical Manual of Mental Disorders, Fourth Edition.* Copyright 1994 American Psychiatric Association.

---

that may be a focus of clinical attention. On Axis II, the clinician reports personality disorders and mental retardation, and on Axis III, he or she reports general medical conditions. Axis IV is for reporting psychosocial and environmental problems (Box 3–1). On Axis V, the clinician reports on a global assessment of functioning.

The DSM-IV is the language of psychiatry, and if nurses are to communicate with other mental health care providers, they must be able to speak and understand this language. In addition, nurses are frequently involved in coding diagnoses on clinical records or insurance claims. For instance, in settings such as CMH centers and private practice, the nurse is responsible for making the diagnosis and entering it, along with the appropriate statistical code, in the record. In institutions or other settings in which psychiatrists take responsibility for establishing the patient's diagnosis, the nurse may find the diagnosis

recorded in the clinical record. See Figure 3–2 for an example of a completed multiaxial diagnosis.

ICD-9-CM

In 1979, the World Health Organization in Geneva published the *International Classification of Diseases, Ninth Revision,* usually referred to as the **ICD-9.** This manual provides a classification of diseases for use in coding morbidity and mortality data for statistical purposes, and it is used in clinical situations to index hospital records by disease and procedure. However, in the United States, clinicians and others responsible for the care of patients found they needed a classification with more specificity than that provided by the ICD-9. Accordingly, the National Center for Health Statistics convened a steering committee in 1977. What resulted

Axis I: Clinical Disorders

Other Conditions That May Be a Focus of Clinical Attention

Diagnostic Code   DSM-IV Name

296.23   Major Depressive Disorder, Single Episode, Severe Without Psychotic Features

Axis II: Personality Disorders

Mental Retardation

Diagnostic Code   DSM-IV Name

301.6   Dependent Personality Disorder

Axis III: General Medical Conditions

ICD-9-CM Code   ICD-9-CM Name

382.9   Otitis Media, Recurrent

Axis IV: Psychosocial and Environmental Problems

Check:

☑ Problems with primary support group (specify): ___Victim of Child Abuse_____

☐ Problems related to social environment (specify): _____

☐ Educational problems (specify): _____

☐ Occupational problems (specify): _____

☐ Housing problems (specify): _____

☐ Economic problems (specify): _____

☐ Problems with access to health care services (specify): _____

_____

☐ Problems related to interaction with the legal system/crime

(specify): _____

_____

☐ Other psychosocial and environmental problems (specify): _____

Axis V: Global Assessment of Functioning Scale: Score 53 ____ ____ ;   Time Frame: _Recurrent_____

Figure 3–2
Example of a completed multiaxial diagnosis. (Based on information from the *Diagnostic and Statistical Manual of Mental Disorders, Fourth Edition.* Copyright 1994 American Psychiatric Association.)

was the ICD-9-CM, the "CM" standing for *Clinical Modification.* In 1992, the World Health Organization published the ICD-10; it is not currently in official use in the United States. The codes and terms provided in the DSM-IV are fully compatible with both the ICD-9-CM and the ICD-10. The ICD-9-CM names of diseases and codes are used to designate Axis III in the multiaxial system of the DSM-IV.

What do you think? Have you bought into and supported the stigma surrounding the mentally ill? In what ways? How do you see the mentally ill stigmatized? What can you do about it?

➤ *Check Your Reading*
1. What is the DSM-IV?
2. Why does the psychiatric nurse need to understand and be able to use the DSM-IV?
3. What is the ICD-9-CM?
4. Why does the psychiatric nurse need to understand and be able to use the ICD-9-CM?
5. What is the multiaxial system of diagnosis?
6. Name the five axes and explain what each represents.

PUBLIC POLICY AND JUDICIAL DECISIONS AND THEIR IMPACT ON THE JOURNEY

Figure 3-3 summarizes the major changes in public policy and the major judicial decisions that have affected mental health care in the United States.

Public Policy

The National Mental Health Act (1946). With the passage of the National Mental Health Act in 1946, the federal government took an active role in shaping the mental health delivery system, both raising and dashing the hopes of those who are intimately involved with the issues of the mentally ill. Congress has passed laws that expanded the care of the mentally ill but then failed to adequately fund the programs that were mandated.

Community Mental Health Centers Construction Act (1963). The Community Mental Health Act, in 1963, launched a major shift in the delivery of care as well as in attitudes toward the mentally ill. The promise of the 1963 legislation and the reality were quite different.

Often, little or no collaboration occurred between the large state hospitals and the communities. The process of moving patients from the large state hospitals, where many of them resided for extended periods, into communities is referred to as *deinstitutionalization*. These patients were moved into community systems where the care was fragmented and inadequate. System components, such as housing, vocational rehabilitation, leisure activities, access to either free or affordable medical care, and access to transportation, were lacking in 1963. Despite Congress's continued support of the CMH movement throughout the 1970s, serious implementation problems remained.

Rescinding Earlier Legislation (1981). At the request of President Reagan, Congress repealed the earlier CMH legislation and restructured size of community service. The new legislation provided no funds for inpatient care. This represented a major departure from the initial 1963 Community Mental Health Act. CMH centers continue to struggle with insufficient funding and a breakdown of community (Daw, 1993).

Stewart B. McKinney Homeless Assistance Act (1987). The Stewart B. McKinney Homeless Assistance Act was passed in 1987 with the intent of solving the problem (largely caused by the Community Mental Health Act of 1963) of the homeless mentally ill. However, in 1992, an estimated 160,000 people with mental illnesses were living on the streets in the United States. The 1993 report of the Federal Task Force on Homelessness and Severe Mental Illness offered "action steps" to be implemented by various federal departments and agencies to improve the housing, income, health, and mental health status of these people.

The Task Force proposed a strategy for promoting systems integration but not for funding specialized housing. It mentioned transitional facilities without describing how to expand the stock of affordable

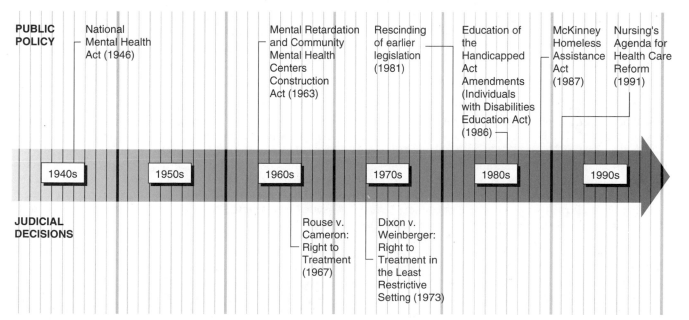

Figure 3-3
Major landmarks in public policy and judicial decisions affecting mental health care.

housing. Bassuk and Buckner (1992) surmised that getting the homeless off the streets was a cosmetic expedient. What was required to solve the problem was a willingness to do the following:

- Care for the disenfranchised among us.
- Include them in the community.
- Provide the housing and community support they need.
- Change ineffective systems.

The Education of the Handicapped Act Amendments (1986). The Education of the Handicapped Act Amendments of 1986 (P.L. 99-457) reflected the public recognition of the needs of developmentally vulnerable children whose mental health has long been neglected in most of the nation.

Included within the purview of early intervention are such elements as prevention, family focus, interdisciplinary cooperation, **case management,** and use of multiple sources of funding. In 1989, each of the states was engaged in a 5-year planning process intended to be fully implemented by 1991. As usual with most new federal initiatives, regulations were delayed, funding was inadequate for achieving all of the goals implicit in the law, and interstate and intrastate coordination was limited.

In 1991, the act was renamed the Individuals With Disabilities Education Act (IDEA). In 1991, Congress enacted P.L. 102-119, Individuals With Disabilities Education Act Amendments of 1991. This law prompted the states and professionals to develop innovative, cost-effective ways to serve children and families. As these early intervention systems for children from birth to age 3 years emerged, it was important for service providers and consumers to meet, identify priorities and resources, collaborate and network, and facilitate plans for change.

However, the public policy is inconsistent even within laws passed by Congress. This is best exemplified by the National Defense Authorization Act for Fiscal Year 1991, which restricts payment by the department for a child's residential treatment to 150 days per calendar year, and in legislation that provides funding for nonresidential but not for residential forms of mental health services, for example, the Children's and Communities Mental Health Systems Improvement Act of 1990 (Wells, 1991). These bills provide powerful illustrations of the impact of inadequate funding on the availability of services.

By 1993, all states were participating in the Education of the Handicapped Act Amendments of 1986 on some level. Because federal funds were insufficient to cover the costs for all children from birth to age 3 years, flexibility was allowed for state programming. Usually, this was determined by the amount of funding the state authorized to combine with the federal funds. Because of limited funding, some states do not serve all young children at risk (e.g., those born to mothers addicted to alcohol and drugs) but serve only those youngsters who have definitive diagnoses.

In addition to services for infants and toddlers, some statewide initiatives exist to develop community alternatives to residential treatment for adults. The goal of such programs is to redirect resources from institutional care to time-limited, patient-centered, and all-encompassing services.

Nursing's Agenda for Health Care Reform (1991). In 1991, nursing proactively developed an agenda for health care reform in anticipation of a public policy change. Krauss (1993) authored *Health Care Reform: Essential Mental Health Services.* The plan addressed needs in the following areas:

1. Primary care mental health services
2. Managed care
3. Universal access to basic mental health benefits packages
4. Structure and financing of the public mental health system for continuous care

What was meant by the term **primary care** mental health services? Millar (1995) described it as broad in scope because it looks at the needs of the whole person, not separating people into mind-body dichotomies. It includes all services necessary for promotion of optimal mental health, prevention of mental illness, health maintenance, management or referral of mental and general health problems, and rehabilitation.

Community Reinvestment Acts. Many states have passed these acts to help move funds from outdated, underused state hospitals into the community for housing, rehabilitation, and community programs. An example is New York, which passed the Community Mental Health Reinvestment Act of 1993. The state shifted an estimated $211 million from the closure of several state hospitals and the downsizing of others to the following services: case management, crisis intervention, psychiatric rehabilitation, supported work programs, consumer self-help and peer advocacy programs, supported housing, and services for the homeless mentally ill.

Mental Health Parity Act (1996). Consumers, families, and advocates have lobbied for years to eliminate insurance discrimination against people seeking mental health care and to achieve **parity** with the coverage accorded other illnesses. In 1996, U.S. Congress approved a law that prods employers to provide more generous mental-health (excluding alcohol and substance abuse) benefits by requiring them to set annual and lifetime coverage benefits similar to those for medical coverage. The law does allow some companies to be exempt: firms with 50 workers or fewer and those that do not offer mental health benefits. It also doesn't prohibit companies from setting employees' copayments and deductibles at a higher level. The law became effective January 1, 1998. By the end of 1998, many states had enacted their own parity legislation. Some of this legislation was even more far-reaching in that alcohol and substance abuse was included.

In an editorial written in June 1998, the editor of *Archives of Psychiatric Nursing,* Judith Krauss, warned psychiatric nurses of the perils involved in the processes of parity and privatization and urged nurses to advocate for the seriously and persistently mentally ill. Krauss's contention was that as mental health advocates seek to push for parity, the public mental health sector and Medicaid push just as hard to get out of the business of providing mental health care. Public providers are moving toward privatizing mental health care under the auspices of large behavioral health companies that are limiting services and utilization and substituting lower cost paraprofessional providers whenever necessary (Krauss, 1998). See What Families Need to Know: Stigma Associated With Mental Illness.

Balanced Budget Act (BBA) (1997). In August 1997, Congress passed the BBA. This was hailed as a monumental achievement of the Clinton administration. However, one of the strategies detailed by the BBA to balance the budget was the enactment of an interim payment system for home care. The interim payment system was designed to reduce projected expenditures for Medicare home health services for fiscal years 1998 and 1999. Medicare reimbursement to home care agencies was rolled back to 1993-1994 limits. By the end of 1998, more than 1500 home care agencies had closed their doors. Long-term patients were particularly hard hit by the BBA. Many agencies, fearing the financial ramifications of exceeding their per beneficiary limit, refused to accept patients who might require many visits over a long period. Included in this group were many of the seriously and persistently mentally ill who benefit from home care services. In addition, Congress removed venipuncture as a qualifying skilled service. This resulted in at least 800,000 beneficiaries' becoming ineligible for home care services; some of them psychiatric patients who were receiving venipunctures for monitoring of lithium or clozapine (Clozaril) levels (Lewin Group, 1998).

Another provision of the BBA of 1997 was that Medicare reimbursement be provided for services conducted by all nurse practitioners and clinical nurse specialists in both rural and urban areas. This change was due largely to lobbying efforts by the American Psychiatric Nurses Association (Streff, 1998).

Judicial Decisions

Judicial decisions have had significant impact on the practice of psychiatry. Specifically, decisions regarding the patient's right to treatment and the patient's right to treatment in the least restrictive setting are discussed.

Rouse v. Cameron: Right to Treatment (1967). This 1967 case in Washington, D.C., focused on the issue of a patient's right to receive adequate treatment. The court held that patients' confinement without treatment was tantamount to incarceration. The court affirmed that the purpose of involuntary hospitalization was treatment, not punishment. If the patient did not receive this treatment, the patient could be transferred, released, or even awarded damages for his or her period of confinement. The court stated that the hospital was not responsible for the success of the treatment but that the hospital was responsible to demonstrate that an honest attempt to provide treatment was made (Birnbaum, 1960).

In 1972, a case decided in Alabama (Wyatt v. Stickney) extended this right to treatment to all mentally

---

 WHAT FAMILIES NEED TO KNOW

Stigma Associated With Mental Illness

What does *stigma* mean in regard to psychiatric patients?

Stigma means "damage to reputation." It is the covert and sometimes overt shame and ridicule our society places on mental illness.

Who suffers from the stigma of mental illness?

Stigma is destructive to families and patients who suffer from mental illness, and it often prevents people from seeking appropriate treatment. It also thwarts funding of research and services for the mentally ill and their families.

Why are mentally ill people so stigmatized?

Some of the symptoms of serious mental illness, such as auditory and visual hallucinations, are frightening

to the general public. It is natural for people to fear what they do not understand. In earlier times, mental illnesses were thought to be caused by possession by evil spirits, and people with mental illness were placed in locked facilities. The public needs to be educated; unfortunately, this process of attitude change is often long and arduous.

What can I do to help reduce the stigma associated with mental illness?

Become educated about the causes of and current treatments for mental illness. Teach others with whom you come in contact what you have learned. Be an advocate. Education is the best way to bring the concept of mental illness out of the Dark Ages and to decrease discrimination.

ill and mentally retarded individuals who were involuntarily hospitalized. The court defined criteria for adequate treatment in three areas:

1. Physical and psychological environments that are humane
2. Sufficient numbers of qualified staff who are able to administer adequate treatment
3. Individualized treatment plans

The impact of the right-to-treatment decisions has had economic reverberations for the states. Adhering to the three criteria for adequate treatment is costly and has required states to reconsider how they allocate resources to the care of the mentally ill.

Dixon v. Weinberger: Right to Treatment in the Least Restrictive Setting (1973). The emphasis on personal freedom produced stringent standards for determination of dangerousness to self or others, which is the criterion for an involuntary admission. The cases behind this right have all asserted that if the patient can function in some setting other than a hospital, then the courts have a responsibility to place him or her in such a setting. This was the ruling in this 1973 case (Dixon v. Weinberger). The judge placed responsibility on the city government of Washington, D.C., and on the federal government to identify patients who could be transferred to the community and to initiate this process, even if it involved creating alternative facilities.

Application of the humanitarian concept of the least restrictive environment while the person is in treatment has not been without problems. In fact, in some instances, the result has been inhumane. Communities have not responded to this right to treatment in the least restrictive setting with adequate support, affordable housing, or meaningful treatment. For the chronically mentally ill who do not pose a threat to self or others yet who have woefully inadequate self-care and survival skills, this decision has often meant that they are vulnerable and living on the streets of our cities. Instances have been reported in which former inpatients died after being placed in group homes and foster homes that had inadequate safeguards. Bachrach suggested that instead of evaluating whether a setting is the least restrictive, we evaluate whether a setting is the "most therapeutic environment" (cited in Schulberg & Killilea, 1992, p. 60).

Gladwell (1993) described the plight of a 40-year-old man (Mr. M) who had been jailed repeatedly, once for 4½ years, but had never been treated for bipolar disorder. The writer emphasized that the Massachusetts law for involuntary commitment has a narrow definition of dangerousness. The law requires that a patient who refuses treatment cannot be forced to accept it unless declared to be legally incompetent. Even with the record showing Mr. M's attempts to kill his parents, he had been denied admission to inpatient care. Each time he appeared in court, an attorney who values liberty over recovery from a serious illness, successfully defended his right to be jailed instead of hospitalized. Mr. M. has a disorder that is treatable, but when Gladwell reported this situation, Mr. M had not received treatment.

What *do you think?* What role should government play in the care of the mentally ill? Should the public system of care be absorbed into private for-profit companies?

➤ *Check Your Reading*

7. What impact did the Community Mental Health legislation of 1963 have on mental health delivery?
8. What happened in 1981 that impacted significantly on the CMH movement?
9. What was the purpose of the Stewart B. McKinney Homeless Assistance Act? Did it achieve its intended purpose?
10. What are the areas addressed in nursing's agenda for health care reform?
11. What was the goal of the Mental Health Parity Law?
12. What does "right to treatment" include?
13. What impact did the judicial decisions regarding "right to treatment in the least restrictive setting" have on the mental health care system?

SOCIAL CHANGES AND THEIR IMPACT ON THE JOURNEY

Figure 3–4 summarizes the major social changes that have affected mental health care in the United States.

The 1960s: A Decade of Change

The late 1960s were characterized by the coming of age of the baby-boomer generation. This generation ques-

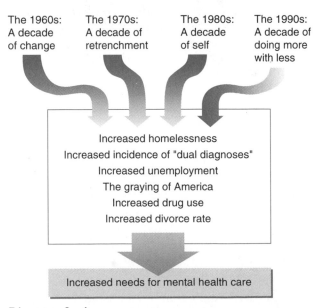

The 1960s: A decade of change

The 1970s: A decade of retrenchment

The 1980s: A decade of self

The 1990s: A decade of doing more with less

Increased homelessness
Increased incidence of "dual diagnoses"
Increased unemployment
The graying of America
Increased drug use
Increased divorce rate

Increased needs for mental health care

Figure 3–4
Influence of social changes on the need for mental health care.

tioned values, structure, and religion; in fact, the whole fabric of U.S. culture was the focus of their examination and rejection. People had a sense that this generation could and would change the world. No doubt many of the issues that they challenged, such as sexual mores and drug use, have left a lasting impact on U.S. society.

During this same time of social and political activism came the ground-breaking Community Mental Health legislation of 1963. Mental health workers were caught up in the feeling that permeated the generation, that change was at hand and that people could make a difference.

The 1970s: A Decade of Retrenchment

As we moved into the 1970s, the high expectations of the late 1960s and early 1970s gave way to resignation, disillusionment, and even depression. The protesters grew up; they married and began raising their own families. They no longer had the rallying points of the 1960s.

Likewise, reality began to filter into the CMH movement. The problems of insufficient funding and planning were increasingly apparent. Many patients who were discharged from state hospitals, as well as those who once would have been admitted to the large hospitals but were now being turned away, ended up living on the streets.

The 1980s: A Decade of Self

The 1980s ushered in a time of materialism and self-focus. *Acquiring, owning, having,* and *buying* were the important words; *serving, giving, caring,* and *sacrificing* were not fashionable or popular ideas in U.S. culture. This focus clearly had an impact on the care of the mentally ill. The clearest evidence of this is the 1981 Omnibus Budget Reconciliation Act, which rescinded many of the earlier legislative mandates for financing CMH treatment.

The 1990s: A Decade of Doing More With Less

In the 1990s, Americans were faced with what seemed to be overwhelming and intractable social problems. The results of the new value system included a mental health system that was woefully inadequate to deal with the mental health fallout of these societal changes. One thing became clear: no human service program, including mental health programs, could expect massive infusions of money to solve problems. We all faced the challenge of doing more with less and of finding creative solutions to devastating problems, one of which continued to be the problem of homelessness.

Increased Homelessness

The ideals of the CMH movement were based on the assumption that patients could live in the community with their families during treatment. Yet experience has shown that a large number of these patients had no families at all or none who would welcome them into their homes. As a result of this false assumption of the CMH movement, many of the chronic mentally ill have become homeless on the streets of our cities.

The increase in the homeless population has an impact on the journey of psychiatric nursing. Some nurses feel called to work with this population and in response to that call either have started nurse-run clinics to serve the homeless or have accepted positions with funded agencies whose focus is to serve this needy population. (See Chapter 34 for a comprehensive presentation of the problems of the homeless.)

An Increased Incidence of Dual Diagnoses

Another group that has required attention is the increasing number of young adults who have both chronic mental illnesses and substance abuse problems. Many elude the grasp of the mental health system or become patients only when in crisis. These patients represent a major challenge to mental health care providers because they do not respond well to established treatments and protocols. Frequently, an integrated approach using inpatient, partial, and outpatient treatment programs, combined with attendance at a nearby college, is an effective strategy for this group.

Increased Unemployment and Changing Employer-Employee Relationship

In 1992, Shore pointed out that during the recession of the early 1990s, the increased numbers of unemployed Americans placed greater demands on the mental health system. Shore urged mental health professionals, who certainly recognize the relationship of unemployment to mental health, to study it, discuss it, and apply their knowledge in practice. He reminded us that people who are usually stable experience intense emotional suffering when they lose their jobs. Imagine, then, the difficulties experienced by people with severe mental disorders when they try to find work in an economy with shrinking job opportunities. The stigma of mental illness often hampers their efforts in tangible ways, even when the job market is favorable, further complicating their personal journey.

In the late 1990s, the employment situation had improved but the work culture and the relationship between employee and employer had changed dramatically. No longer did people take jobs with the expectation of working for one employer for life; rather, jobs were viewed as transitory, with little loyalty between employee and employer. Many people held multiple part-time jobs in order to "put together" the equivalent of a full-time salary and a benefit package (Ferrie, 1998).

Graying of America

In the last waning decades of the 20th century, the population of people older than 65 years increased more than twice as fast as that of people younger than 65. As people live longer, their use of health services, including mental health care services, increases as they contend with the demands and limitations imposed by chronic illnesses. It is estimated that more than 80% of the elderly have chronic diseases, and at least 50% of that number suffer from physical and social limitations as a result of their chronic illnesses. Many psychiatric nurses have responded to the increase in the psychogeriatric population by specializing in the care of this group.

What do you think? From your experiences, how have the societal changes impacted on mental health? What should be done to help people deal with these changes?

➤ *Check Your Reading*

14. Identify the social problem that is directly linked to the Community Mental Health Act of 1963.
15. What characterized the decade that spanned the mid-1960s through the mid-1970s? The mid-1970s through the mid-1980s? The mid-1980s to the present?
16. What impact have drug problems had on the mental health system?
17. How has the graying of America affected the mental health system?
18. What does *dual diagnosis* mean?
19. What is the relationship between unemployment and mental health problems?

FUNDING AND REIMBURSEMENT AND THEIR IMPACT ON THE JOURNEY

Financing is perhaps the most pervasive problem facing the mental health field today, because money, more than any other factor, shapes our service delivery system and our journey.

Mental Health Care Before Insurance

Until the mid-20th century, mental health care providers had few effective treatments for people with mental illnesses. Those who developed acute symptoms either recovered "spontaneously" or went on to become chronically ill. The state hospitals were supported by tax funds requested by the executive branch of state government and appropriated by the state legislators. Much of the initial motivation for developing state hospitals in the 19th century was to reduce costs. The state hospitals were perceived to be cost-effective, preferred treatment settings over smaller, more numerous county institutions (Baker, 1992).

As the population of the United States increased, so did the population in state mental hospitals. Few people had the means to pay for care in private psychiatric hospitals; therefore, the majority of those who developed mental illnesses went to state hospitals. The financial resources of these hospitals was rarely enough to support adequate care. Some had large enough appropriations to provide therapies such as occupational therapy, hydrotherapy, and electroconvulsive therapy to selected patients. Others could barely supply adequate diets and clean, comfortable surroundings.

Current State of Funding and Reimbursement

The U.S. health care system is undergoing dramatic changes in response to rising health care costs. Taxpayers, employers, and employees have decided that health care costs are too high. In response to this, there have been significant changes in reimbursement for health care. These changes have raised serious questions about the quality of health care. In particular, these changes have drastically affected behavioral health care.

The problem of funding adequate services for people with serious mental illnesses was presented by Goldberg (1993). Goldberg (1993) cited a report of the National Institute for Mental Health (NIMH) Advisory Council on the cost and treatment of serious mental illness, approximately 5 million people—or 28% of the adult population—suffer from serious mental illness. A 1992 report of the Congress Office of Technology Assessment, *The Biology of Mental Disorders* (U.S. Congress Office of Technology Assessment, 1992), cited the total costs of serious mental illness for 1991 at $135 billion. According to NIMH, this figure includes 20% of Social Security Insurance, $20 billion per year in direct treatment costs, and another $7 billion for long-term nursing care. In addition, psychiatric problems cost millions per year in lost productivity.

By the end of the 1990s, there was a growing realization that those people with behavioral health problems such as depression, anxiety, and alcohol and substance abuse also use more medical services than those without diagnosed behavioral health problems. A 1995 study in the *Archives of General Psychiatry* by Simon, VonKorff, and Barlow found that depressed patients use medical services so heavily that the direct cost of treating depression accounted for only a small portion of their overall medical expenses. The study also looked at several explanations for their findings, for example, physical illness may lead to depression and

Box 3-2 ■ ■ ■ ■ ■
Community Services Needed by Patients With Severe Mental Illness

- Access to effective and cheap medication
- A permanent place to live with adequate food and support
- Access to periodic emergency inpatient treatment to deal with exacerbations of illness with minimal amount of red tape
- Meaningful and structured daytime activity
- Places to socialize and be accepted
- Access to medical and dental care
- Case management
- A system that recognizes the long-term nature of the illness and the need for continuous, long-term services and support
- Someone to care

depression may make physical suffering worse. A number of studies have examined the issue of **medical cost offset,** which refers to cost savings when brief psychiatric interventions are provided to medically ill patients to augment the medical treatment (Faulkner & Gray, 1995; Kennedy, Polivka, & Steel, 1997; Michelson, Stratakin, & Hill, 1996). In fact, Blue Cross of Massachusetts, in collaboration with the American Psychological Association, released actuarial data demonstrating that the integration of a 16-week group psychotherapy intervention into an overall treatment plan for early-stage breast cancer produced $5.00 savings for every $1.00 spent on psychological services (Healthcare Demand & Disease Management, 1998).

Because of the growing recognition of the total costs of treating behavioral health disorders, there is no doubt that the public mental health system will continue to be seriously affected. The public system will take on a more private look as Medicaid mandates its enrollees into managed care plans and as large behavioral health organizations bid on managing county and state behavioral health "**carve outs.**"

In this same period, families, especially those who are members of the National Alliance for the Mentally Ill (NAMI 1987), continue to make it clear what services are important to them and to their relatives with severe mental illnesses. Box 3-2 presents a list of community services needed by those with severe mental illness.

Because of the changes in access to health care and reimbursement, the traditional delivery system continues to evolve. Table 3-1 compares the traditional delivery system with the evolving managed care delivery system.

TYPES OF REIMBURSEMENT

Private Health Insurance (Fee for Service)

The traditional health plans were fee-for-service plans or indemnity plans that allowed for coverage of almost all medical expenses after the yearly deductibles and copayments for specific services were satisfied. Patients faced few, if any, restrictions on their choices of physicians or places where medical care could be obtained. However, most of these plans limited payment for behavioral health services or offered few or no mental health and substance abuse services.

Medicare and Medicaid

When **Medicare** (federal insurance for those Social Security recipients older than 65 years or for those who are judged to be disabled) and **Medicaid** (federal insurance for those who are judged to be in the lowest

AREA OF CONCERN	**TRADITIONAL**	**MANAGED CARE**
Customer	Individual person	Member population
Reimbursement	Fee for service	Capitation, case rates
Setting focus	Inpatient care	Outpatient care, network of services, community-based care
Prevention services	Episodic care, disease focus	Continuous care, screenings, health promotion (exercise, smoking), disease prevention
Market	Length of stay, number of admissions, procedures	Number of covered lives
Providers	Numerous hospitals, private physicians	Networks, hospital mergers, primary care networks
Trend of services	Duplication	Consolidation
Physician	Patient choice, specialty care	Primary care (family practitioner, general practitioner, internal medicine)
Authorization	None required	Case management, utilization review

T A B L E 3 – 1 Comparison of Traditional and Managed Care Systems

socioeconomic group) became available in 1965, the government predicted that the quality of care in psychiatric hospitals would improve. Medicare covered active treatment of patients older than age 65 for a limited time; it did not cover custodial care. Medicaid covered adult inpatient care under specified circumstances. State hospitals able to meet the standards set by the Health Care Financing Administration to receive Medicare and Medicaid reimbursements saw the Medicare and Medicaid programs as sources of additional funds. However, rather than use this influx of federal monies to improve care, states frequently responded with significant decreases in state appropriations.

Medicare expenditures are increasing at a rate of 10% per year. Because of this, Medicare could be bankrupt soon. Therefore, it is an obvious place for numerous parties to reduce costs. Thus, managed care has been designated as the system that can contain costs for Medicare. Not only is Medicare a target of managed care but also states have begun receiving waivers from Medicaid to develop new delivery systems. Additionally, some states are mandating Medicaid recipients to choose a managed care plan. Many times these plans cover only a particular portion of the mental health benefits necessary for the seriously and persistently mentally ill enrollee. The remaining benefits may be carved out to traditional Medicaid.

Managed Care

Managed care plans integrate the management financing and delivery of health care services to an enrolled patient population in an effort to contain health care costs and increase quality of care (Brennan & Cochran, 1998). The goal of managed care is not simply to lower costs; rather, the goal is to ensure that maximal value is received from the resources used in the production and delivery of health care services in the population.

Some types of managed care plans are directed at a commercial population for whom employers or employees have chosen the plan and other plans are federally funded to serve Medicare and Medicaid recipients. All federally funded plans have the following three characteristics (Brennan & Cochran, 1998):

1. An organized system for providing health care in a geographical area
2. An agreed on set of basic and supplemental health maintenance and treatment services
3. A voluntarily enrolled group of people

Managed behavioral health care is the term that applies to managed care for mental health and substance abuse disorders. Some managed care companies manage their own behavioral health benefits, and some use a large **managed behavioral health care** company. They contract with insurers or employers to monitor the use of mental health benefits. They aim to minimize admissions to inpatient and residential treatment centers; to stimulate the use of alternative, less costly, forms of treatment; and to limit outpatient care to brief forms of therapy. In the late 1990s, several of these large entities merged, with predictions that 5 to 10 large managed behavioral health care companies will serve all in the future.

Managed care comes in several shapes and sizes, from plans that limit a patient's choices of physicians and hospitals to those that allow choice with some additional cost involved. Box 3-3 presents the most common forms of managed care plans that are available.

Nursing supports the concept of managed care as a cost-effective monitoring system for the delivery of mental health services. Nursing also endorses the use of psychiatric–mental health nurses as highly qualified professional participants in both direct and indirect care roles within a managed care system. Krauss (1998) cautioned the nursing profession to continuously monitor managed care systems to ensure that the original objectives of cost-benefit and appropriate quality care are realized.

Managed care uses a number of techniques to control costs and utilization of services. These are defined in Box 3-4.

One of the concerns about managed care is that quality of care is sacrificed for cost containment. Ideally, there is a balance between cost and quality, so that quality is maintained and wasteful expenditures are minimized. We must steward our resources wisely, but there is certainly tension among what seem to be competing values and goals: delivering high-quality care, containing costs, and making a profit. In 1997, many managed care companies received a "report card" in which they were evaluated on a number of variables, including access to care, availability of flexible benefits, timeliness of service delivery, and range of available services. NAMI, independently, gave managed care, in general, low marks for its alleged unresponsiveness to

---

Box 3–3 ■ ■ ■ ■ ■
Most Common Forms of Managed Care Plans

Health maintenance organization (HMO): A health plan that provides coverage for access to health care for its members, including ambulatory care, preventive health care, hospitalization, and catastrophic care. The primary care physician is the gatekeeper to specialist care. HMOs contract to provide care at a fixed yearly rate (*capitation:* fixed per member, per month fee).

Preferred provider organization (PPO): A plan that contracts with physicians and hospitals. The physicians receive a discounted fee for service. The members are encouraged to see a provider in the network and are usually penalized with a higher copayment if they use a provider outside the network.

Point-of-service (POS) plan: This plan falls somewhere between an HMO and a PPO in terms of freedom of choice. There are financial benefits if the enrollee sees a provider inside the network.

Box 3–4 ■ ■ ■ ■ ■
Managed Care Techniques to Control Costs and Utilization of Services

Types of Cost-Control Techniques

Case management: A process of coordinating services; the case manager focuses on coordinating the most efficient and cost-effective treatment to achieve favorable outcomes (Zander, 1998).

Authorization: The managed care company's case manager reviews a patient's status to determine whether the treatment being sought is medically appropriate and necessary and whether the provider is an approved one. If these conditions are met, the patient is given authorization to proceed with services. Most managed care plans require authorization before hospital admission.

Utilization review: The process of determining if services are medically necessary, directing the patient to the most appropriate provider, deciding the most effective intervention, or evaluating the outcome and costs of such services (Corcoran & Vandiver, 1998).

Types of Utilization Review

Prospective utilization reviews: Evaluate the need for services in advance of treatment and may require authorization for a particular service or provider.

Concurrent utilization reviews: Occur during treatment to determine if additional care is required.

Retrospective utilization reviews: Evaluate the course and outcome of treatment in order to assess the quality of care and determine whether reimbursement is authorized.

Record reviews: In-depth reviews of a record to evaluate all aspects of care. Usually this occurs with patients who are hospitalized or require hospitalization.

---

stay. This method is close to what is known as a **case rate,** in which a provider is reimbursed for providing a set service for an episode of care. The funding is based on the number and type of enrollees in the member population.

Under a **capitation system,** a member pays a preset fee per month or for the year. The payer contracts with the providers to share risk because providers receive preset funding for the number of people in the plan that they manage. *Capitation* is a fixed amount of money per person for a specific period, as compared with *reimbursement,* which is based on the actual costs of service. Typically, the managed care company contracts with a network of providers to provide a full continuum of care. By sharing risk with the provider, the managed care company hopes the provider develops a comprehensive, clinically sound plan of care for the enrollee. It also hopes providers use expensive tests and services appropriately and coordinate care within the service network. Because this system has incentives to control costs, there are always questions about whether or not a patient is receiving quality care. Providers should track outcomes; this shows that providers' choices are not only cost effective but also clinically appropriate.

Many plans still pay physicians a **discounted fee for service,** which is a discounted rate for authorized services. Many plans also require that the enrollee pay a copayment when seeing a physician.

Other Reimbursement Issues

The American Nurses Association lobbied for many years for legislation that would authorize direct reimbursement to nurses who provide health care services to federal employees and their dependents. In the 99th Congress, legislation was enacted (Federal Employees Benefits Improvement Act, 1986) that authorized direct reimbursement for nonphysician providers, including registered nurses, in medically underserved areas. By November 5, 1990, direct reimbursement to advanced practice nurses became policy. In the BBA of 1997, reimbursement for clinical nurse specialists was extended to urban as well as rural areas.

> **W**hat do you think? What are your experiences with managed care? Do you think managed care provides high-quality services to the mentally ill? Defend your answer.

➤ *Check Your Reading*

20. What has happened to state funding of psychiatric care over the past 30 years?
21. What impact did Medicare and Medicaid have on the treatment of the mentally ill?
22. What is the purpose of managed care? What are some of the forms of managed care organizations?
23. What procedures does managed care use to control costs and monitor utilization of services?
24. Discuss the most common reimbursement methods in managed care today.

---

the needs of the seriously and persistently mentally ill. A major issue to be determined legislatively concerns the rights of consumers to sue managed care companies over quality-of-care issues.

Reimbursement Methods

Under traditional fee-for-service plans, providers saw a patient, billed the payer, and received a set fee. Managed care uses several methods to reimburse providers. Medicare diagnosis-related groups are a type of prospective payment system that pays a hospital a set amount of money based on diagnosis. The payment fee is set regardless of the actual service provided or the length of

TREATMENT SETTINGS AND THEIR IMPACT ON THE JOURNEY

During the 1990s, due to rising health care costs and changes in reimbursement, providers consolidated and focus turned to maintaining the patient in the least restrictive level of care. There also was an increased focus on providing illness prevention and wellness programs, as well as direct care from the primary care practitioner. Providing a full continuum of care through an integrated delivery system became the goal. An **integrated delivery system** involves all levels of care that are necessary for a given population, including inpatient services, outpatient treatment, primary care networks, home-based services, and long-term care. The traditional system of care was episodic, with little emphasis on illness prevention, whereas the system of care in the 1990s attempted to integrate illness prevention services in order to prevent more costly levels of care.

Private and Public Hospitals

The basic functions of hospitals for the mentally ill are listed:

- Restoration of patients to health so that they can leave the hospital at the earliest possible moment
- Sufficient functional improvement so that patients can live as nearly normal as possible in the institutional setting

Both private and nonprofit psychiatric hospitals offer a wide range of services, including care of children, adolescents, adults, elderly people, and the medically ill. Not every hospital provides every service, but many do. They often provide a continuum of care from admission to residential aftercare. Some offer adult day treatment, partial hospitalization, and outpatient services, as well. Many clinical settings work constructively with families and provide space for family support groups to meet. Often, nurse clinicians function as members of treatment teams. Both graduate nurse generalists and certified specialists are employed as staff members and in leadership positions.

One result of reduced health benefits for mental disorders and of managed care has been a shorter length of stay than in the past. Nurses caring for patients in these hospitals find it necessary to rapidly assess the patient's needs and strengths, to develop an individual nursing care plan that is consistent with the treatment plan, and to start the discharge planning process as soon as the patient is admitted. The nurse, as part of the multidisciplinary team, must offer therapeutic care that effectively promotes relief of symptoms and strengthens healthy coping behavior in the patient.

Specialized Hospitals

The high incidence of chemical dependency (i.e., dependence on alcohol and on drugs such as cocaine, heroin, and other substances) has led to the establishment of hospitals for the treatment of people with these disorders. These hospitals may be public or private. In addition, a few general hospitals have detoxification units for the care of patients who are acutely intoxicated and require a blend of skilled medical and psychiatric treatment for a limited period. Nurses are essential staff members in detoxification units and in hospitals for the treatment of chemical dependency. The treatment programs may rely on nurses to function as group and individual therapists, to work with family members of the dependent person, and to encourage attendance at self-help group meetings such as Alcoholics Anonymous and Narcotics Anonymous. Some of these specialized hospitals have rehabilitation programs; however, others are limited by managed care rules and provide follow-up in outpatient programs. Some health insurance programs will not authorize payment for inpatient treatment until intensive outpatient treatment has been tried and evaluated for effectiveness. Many hospitals have developed treatment programs to fit this model.

Specialized Units Within Hospitals

Geriatric Units. As the U.S. populace has begun to age and life expectancy has increased, many state and private psychiatric hospitals have responded by adding specialized units for the diagnosis and treatment of psychogeriatric patients. Sometimes, however, elderly patients who are in general hospitals for medical or surgical treatments exhibit problematic behaviors as a result of or in response to physical illnesses. Psychiatric liaison nurses may be called to help the staff cope with the patient or to suggest where care be provided, such as in the psychiatric unit or elsewhere.

Child and Adolescent Units. Numerous psychiatric as well as general hospitals have specialized units for children with mental health problems. An estimated 4% of children and adolescents aged 9 through 17 are diagnosed with a severe psychiatric disorder. It is estimated that there are 7.5 million children younger than 18 years who have psychiatric, behavioral, or developmental disorders (Vanderhorst & Benner-Carson, 1998).

Most child and adolescent units have a regimented therapeutic environment for their specialized problems. The units offer a variety of health care disciplines that collectively develop a treatment plan. Also, in conjunction with working with the child, a main focus of the nursing and medical staff is continual assessment of the family and its impact on the child's illness. With managed care, the goal is often to stabilize the children as quickly as possible and treat them in an outpatient setting. In most cases, psychiatrists do not hospitalize a child unless he or she is a danger to self or others or is experiencing a psychotic break. (See Chapter 18 for a more thorough discussion of childhood psychiatric issues.)

Psychiatric Units. Many general hospitals offer psychiatric care, among other services. These units are designed for short-term, acute care. That is, patients are admitted, treated, and released quickly. Patients who require longer periods of hospitalization are generally transferred to a state facility. Hospital psychiatric units play an important role in the maintenance of patients with chronic mental illnesses within the community. These patients periodically experience exacerbations of their symptoms, requiring short-term stays for stabilization.

Forensic Units. Since the 1960s, there has been a significant increase in the number of incarcerated people who suffer from severe mental illness. Gladwell (1993) pointed out that 30,000 seriously mentally ill Americans were locked up in local jails in 1993. Many times they were locked up for vagrancy, stealing, and other aberrant behaviors that were secondary to their mental illness. Rather than receiving treatment for the mental illness, they were treated as criminals. In some communities, the local mental health authority provided resources for some treatment. In others, no treatment was provided, and the patient stayed in jail until the court decided where the patient was to go. Nurses employed in these settings were challenged to use ingenuity in their efforts to provide therapeutic care.

Some states have forensic psychiatry units or hospitals for accused people who are found by the court to be "not guilty by reason of insanity" but are deemed to be "too dangerous to others" to be released. Most state and federal prison systems also have specialized sections for the care of prisoners who develop symptoms of mental illnesses after they have been convicted. Nurses are employed in both settings, and some have developed expertise at providing therapeutically effective care while maintaining a high level of security. Nurses in these settings must be informed about the applicable laws and do their part to ascertain that they follow these laws.

Residential Treatment Centers

Children and adolescents with long-standing behavioral and emotional problems who cannot be effectively managed in their homes are usually referred to residential treatment centers. The children placed in these centers are highly vulnerable, and their needs often outstrip the system's ability to provide for them. Public policy favors placing children and adolescents for short durations, usually not long enough to see a cure. A continuum of care is needed but is not always provided. These children and their families often travel a difficult and painful journey. Nurses who work in such centers are called on to join that journey in a way that connects with troubled children and families to give them affirmation and hope and to help them see alternatives (Wells, 1991).

Outpatient Settings and Community Mental Health Centers

Every state has outpatient facilities for mental health treatment; some are attached to hospitals, and some are freestanding. In addition, all states have mental health centers, each serving approximately 250,000 people, with limited funding from the federal government.

As with the general population, many people with chronic mental illnesses also need medical and dental care. Some centers employ adult–nurse practitioners to provide basic medical care. These nurses refer people with more severe problems to physicians.

Nurses employed in CMH centers often have administrative, case management, and therapeutic assignments. Many are expert at providing individual, group, and family therapy as well as managing a therapeutic milieu. In addition to contributing to the operation of CMH centers, mental health nurses are key providers of crisis intervention, including serving on hotlines for suicide prevention. The nurse's roles contribute to supporting the patient's journey within the community setting.

Since the mid-1970s, adult day treatment and partial hospitalization programs have been used as substitutes for inpatient care. Either of these settings has been included as part of some CMH centers or was operated by private group practices. Nurses are usually members of the staff of adult day programs, working as team members with psychiatrists and with ancillary therapists. (See Chapter 15 for a more complete discussion of the continuum of care.)

Home Care

Behavioral health home care is emerging as an increasingly popular specialty home care program for agencies to offer. The goals of psychiatric home care include the following:

- Complete the continuum of care
- Increase compliance with medication compliance and treatment
- Provide psychoeducation and skills to increase independent functioning
- Maintain patients in their home environments

In two outcome studies (Vanderhorst & Benner-Carson, 1998; Vanderhorst, Benner-Carson, & Midla, 1998) that focused on psychiatric home care, the results demonstrated that short-term and intermittent behavioral health home care is the following:

- Is cost-effective
- Decreases use of costly inpatient hospitals and emergency departments
- Increases medication and treatment compliance

As the use of psychiatric home care is increasing, managed care is recognizing that this modality is a cost-effective and clinically sound alternative that fits nicely into the continuum of behavioral health services.

Private Practice

Since the mid-1970s, increasing numbers of certified specialists in psychiatric–mental health nursing have been entering the private practice of psychotherapy. Some join group practices with other mental health professionals. Some work in solo practices or in one of the therapies covered in Chapter 14. In the early years of psychiatric–mental health nursing, nurses struggled to be recognized as providers of psychiatric–mental health care and to be covered by health insurance policies. A factor in this struggle for recognition was the issue of whether or not to include psychotherapies within the scope of nursing practice. Some state boards of nursing have regulations that specify that psychotherapies *are* within the scope of practice of qualified, certified specialists. In many states, nurses are not only recognized and accepted as providers of mental health care but also reimbursed for their services by third-party payers.

> **W**hat do you think? Is it possible to deliver both cost-effective and quality care? Is there a conflict between the ethics of care and cost containment? What needs to occur to maintain a balance between these two values?

> **➤ *Check Your Reading***
> 25. What is an integrated delivery system?
> 26. Why is the push today to maintain patients in the least restrictive environment of care?
> 27. What is the purpose of inpatient psychiatric treatment?
> 28. What is a forensic unit?
> 29. Name two different types of specialty units for the treatment of psychiatric problems.
> 30. What is a residential treatment center and what does it offer?
> 31. What type of psychiatric nurse can be in private practice?
> 32. Describe the role of the psychiatric nurse in a CMH center.
> 33. Name one change in the health care system that has encouraged the development of psychiatric home care programs.

Conclusions

The journey of psychiatric nursing is affected by the same external forces that affect all of society. This chapter reviewed the impact of the DSM-IV and the ICD-9-CM on psychiatric nursing. Changes in public policy influence the entire mental health care system, including psychiatric nursing. For instance, legislation such as the Community Mental Health Act of 1963 shifted the focus of mental health care from large hospitals to community centers. Likewise, psychiatric nursing's journey shifted from hospital-based nursing, which was many times custodial in nature, to community-based nursing, where nursing practice assumed more independent and therapeutic functions. Legislation has resulted in unexpected and undesirable changes, such as the increase in the number of homeless mentally ill that resulted from inadequate planning and implementation of the 1963 legislation. The 1996 Mental Health Parity Law is a step toward reimbursing and accepting mental illness as we do physical illness.

Social changes from the 1960s onward shifted attitudes toward the care of the mentally ill. These changes have also resulted in increasing numbers of people requiring mental health care from a system with decreasing capacity to meet the needs of all who require assistance. Changes such as the dramatic increase in the homeless population, the proliferation of drug use and subsequent emergence of the dual diagnosis population, unemployment, and the graying of America have strained the mental health care system's ability to respond. Psychiatric nursing's journey is also affected by these changes because nurses have specialized in the care of these subpopulations.

Funding is the most pervasive problem facing the mental health system. Legislative effectiveness has been limited by inadequate funding. Likewise, inadequate funding has contributed to the social changes that have strained the mental health care system. Most Americans have inadequate mental health care coverage, and the public funding for these services has also been seriously curtailed. Medicare and Medicaid, which were anticipated to improve mental health care for those eligible, have made it more challenging by allowing states to have managed care administer these plans. In this age of managed care, we are faced with the realities that HMOs manage care differently and frequently refuse to provide all the care that the seriously and persistently mentally ill may require. Capitation, under which an enrollee pays a per member, per month (or year) fee and providers receive a set amount for a specific time period, is an emerging reimbursement method.

Institutions where psychiatric care is delivered have changed dramatically. In the 1960s, most mental health care was provided in either large state hospitals or exclusive private facilities. This changed with the Mental Retardation Facilities and Community Mental Health Centers Construction Act of 1963, as increasing numbers of CMH centers grew up all over the country. This change has continued with a proliferation of various types of community-based sites developing in response to legislation, judicial precedents, societal changes, and available funding. The mental health care landscape of the 1990s supported an integrated delivery system that encompassed psychiatric hospitals, psychiatric units within general hospitals, residential treatment centers, CMH care centers, outpatient clinics, day treatment programs, home care, and nurse-run private practices, as well as nurse-run clinics.

Key Points to Remember

- The DSM-IV contains the diagnostic criteria for mental illnesses. Nurses must understand and be able to use the DSM-IV for reimbursement and for chart documentation.
- The ICD-9-CM provides a classification of diseases for use in coding morbidity and mortality data for statistical purposes, and it is used in clinical situations to index hospital records by disease and procedure.
- In 1946, with the passage of the National Mental Health Act, the federal government assumed an active role in regulating mental health care in the United States.
- The federal government's role mandated a major shift in the mental health care system when the Mental Retardation Facilities and Community Mental Health Centers Construction Act was passed in 1963, moving the care of the chronically mentally ill from the large state hospitals to the community. However, the CMH movement was underfunded.
- Since 1980, with fiscal and political support for the CMH movement lost, homelessness, drug abuse, and violent crime have increased.
- The Stewart B. McKinney Homeless Assistance Act was passed in 1987 to deal with the growing problem of the homeless mentally ill. The legislation was never funded sufficiently to address the areas of change mandated by the law.
- The Education of the Handicapped Act Amendments of 1986 represented the most far-reaching public legislation ever enacted for disabled and developmentally vulnerable children. As with previous legislation, funding was inadequate for achieving the goals implicit in the law, and interstate and intrastate coordination was limited.
- Nursing developed its own agenda for health care reform, calling for primary care services, managed care, universal access to a basic mental health benefit package, and structure and financing of the public mental health system for continuous care.
- Specific social changes, such as homelessness, can be traced to legislative mandates such as the Mental Retardation Facilities and Community Mental Health Centers Construction Act of 1963. Homelessness, unemployment, increased drug use and the growing number of young people with dual diagnoses, and the graying of America have all contributed to the mental health problems in the United States.
- Funding is probably one of the most pervasive problems facing the mental health field today. Medicare, Medicaid, managed care, out-of-pocket payment, and charity care are the reimbursement sources for mental health care. The increase in managed care plans and the push to curtail health care spending have led to increased consolidation among providers and the formation of networks to coordinate and provide care. Advanced practice certified specialists in psychiatric–mental health services can receive direct reimbursement for psychiatric services.

Learning Activities

1. Call your state legislature and obtain copies of the Nurse Practice Act governing the practice of the certified nurse specialist in adult psychiatric–mental health. What are the boundaries of the nurse's practice in your state?
2. Find out what legislation your state has passed that directly affects reimbursement for mental health services. Does your state's Medicaid program reimburse for mental health services? Does your state have parity legislation that mandates that mental health coverage be equal to other coverage?
3. Do some research into the continuum of psychiatric care in your state. Does your state have state and private psychiatric hospitals, CMH centers, partial hospitalization programs, day treatment programs, psychosocial programs, mobile treatment, and psychiatric home care programs?
4. Find out when your local chapter of NAMI meets and attend one of their meetings. What impact has this organization had on the care of the mentally ill in your area? Consider joining or supporting them financially.

Critical Thinking Exercises

Consider the following statement about the "right to treatment in the least restrictive setting" presented earlier in this chapter. In a 1975 case (Dixon v. Weinberger), it was ruled that if a patient can function in some setting other than a hospital, the courts have a responsibility to place him or her in such a setting. Schulberg and Killilea (1992) commented that the application of the humanitarian concept of the "least restrictive environment" has not been without problems, and at times, it has been inhumane. Communities have not responded with adequate support, affordable housing, or meaningful treatment. The chronically mentally ill, who are not a threat to self or others but who have inadequate self-care or survival skills, are often vulnerable and end up living on city streets. Incidences of patient deaths in group homes and foster homes with inadequate safeguards have been reported.

1. What do you think is the main issue here?
2. What is the point of view of the authors, Schulberg and Killilea, concerning the 1973 ruling related to the right to treatment in the least restrictive setting?
3. What evidence supports Schulberg and Killilea's position?
4. Consider any biases.

Mr. Que, a nurse on the inpatient psychiatry unit, was informed by Mr. Zee, a patient on the unit for 4 hours, that he was leaving the hospital. Mr. Zee was admitted with a history of self-destructive behavior and a recent attempt to physically harm his wife. Mr. Que knows that, according to the law, the patient has a right to refuse treatment. However, he is also aware that it is his professional responsibility to provide the patient with a safe environment.

1. What if Mr. Que decides to let the patient leave?
2. What else could happen as a result of Mr. Que's decision?
3. What is an alternative approach to Mr. Que's letting the patient leave?

Additional Resources

U.S. Department of Health and Human Services (DHHS)

http://www.os.dhhs.gov/

References

American Psychiatric Association. (1994). *Diagnostic and statistical manual of mental disorders* (4th ed.). Washington, DC: Author.

Baker, F. (1992). Effects of value systems on service delivery. In H. C. Schulberg & M. Killilea (Eds.), *The modern practice of community mental health* (pp. 246–264). San Francisco, CA: Jossey-Bass.

Balanced Budget Act, Pub. L. No. 102-119 (1997).

Bassuk, E. L., & Buckner, T. C. (1992). Out of mind—out of sight: The homeless mentally ill. *American Journal of Orthopsychiatry, 62,* 330-331.

Birnbaum, M. (1960). The right to treatment. *American Bar Association Journal, 46,* 499-505.

Brennan, S. J., & Cochran, M. (1998). Home healthcare nursing in the managed care environment. *Home Healthcare Nurse, 16,* 280-287.

Cody, P. (1993). U.S. policy toward the severely mentally ill: A search for humane treatment. *Family Therapy News, 24*(3), 36.

Community Mental Health Reinvestment Act, 1993, S. 6214, A. 8928.

Corcoran, K., & Vandiver, V. (1998). *Managed care and the emergence of cost containment and quality assurance: Maneuvering the maze of managed care* (pp. 1–24). New York: Free Press.

Daw, J. (1993). Community mental health centers face an uncertain future. *Family Therapy News, 24*(3), 9.

Dixon v. Weinberger, 405 F. Supp. 974 (1973).

Education of the Handicapped Act Amendments, Pub. L. No. 99-457 (1986).

Faulkner, M., & Gray, D. (1995). *Behavioral outcomes and guidelines sourcebook: New trends, findings and outcomes,* (Vol. 13, pp. 26–33). New York: Faulkner & Gray.

Federal Employees Benefits Improvement Act of 1986. Public Law 99-251.

Ferrie, J. E. (1998). The health effects of major organizational change and job insecurity. *Social Science Medicine, 46,* 243-254.

Gladwell, M. (1993, May 12). A brush with madness. *The Washington Post, 81,* 88-89.

Goldberg, J. R. (1993). Research snapshot: Severe mental illness. *Family Therapy News, 24*(3), 2.

Healthcare demand & disease management. (1998), *4*(3), 44-45.

Individuals With Disabilities Education Act Amendments. Pub. L. No. 102-119 (1991).

Kennedy, C. W., Polivka, B. J., & Steel, J. S. (1997). Psychiatric symptoms in a community based medically ill population. *Home Healthcare Nurse, 15,* 431-441.

Krauss, J. B. (1993). Executive summary. In *Health care reform: Essential mental health services.* Washington, DC: American Nurses Publishing.

Krauss, J. B. (1998). The perils of parity and privatization. *Archives of Psychiatric Nursing, 12*(3), 129-130.

The Lewin Group. (1998, March). *Implications of the Medicare home health interim payment system of the 1997 Balanced Budget Act.* Fairfax, VA: Author.

Mental Health Parity Act, Pub. L. No. 104-204 (1996).

Mental Retardation Facilities and Community Mental Health Centers Construction Act, Pub. L. No. 88-164 (1963).

Michelson, D., Stratakin, C., & Hill, L. (1996). Bone mineral density in women with depression. *New England Journal of Medicine, 335,* 1176-1181.

Millar, T. P. (1995). An adaptive approach to primary prevention in child psychiatry. *Perspectives in Biology and Medicine, 38,* 256-273.

Murphy, M. J. (1993). Herman wept, or the battle of narratives: A case study. *The Family Therapy Networker, 173*(3), 77-79.

National Alliance for the Mentally Ill (1987). *Serious mental illnesses: Myths and realities.* Arlington, VA: Author.

National Defense Authorization Act for Fiscal Year 1991, Pub. L. No. 101-510 (1990).

National Mental Health Act, Pub. L. No. 79-487 (1946).

Omnibus Budget Reconciliation Act, Pub. L. No. 97-35 (1981).

Rouse v. Cameron, 128 U.S. App. D.C. 283 (1967).

Schulberg, H. C., & Killilea, M. (Eds.) (1992). *The modern practice of community mental health.* San Francisco, CA: Jossey-Bass.

Shore, M. F. (1992). Mental health work in a free-fall economy. *American Journal of Orthopsychiatry, 62,* 162.

Simon, G. E., VonKorff, M., & Barlow, W. (1995). Health care costs of primary care patient with recognized depression. *Archives of General Psychiatry, 52,* 850-856.

Stewart B. McKinney Homeless Assistance Act, Pub. L. No. 100-77 (1987).

Streff, M. B. (1998). Legislative outlook. *APNA News, 10*(2), 4.

U.S. Congress, Office of Technology Assessment. (1995). *The authoritative guide: New developments in the biology of mental disorders.* Piscataway, NJ: Research and Education Association.

U.S. Congress, Office of Technology Assessment. (1992). *The biology of mental disorders* (OTA-BA-538). Washington, DC: U.S. Government Printing Office.

U.S. Task Force on Homelessness and Severe Mental Illness. (1993). *Outcasts on main street: Report of the Federal Task Force on Homelessness and Severe Mental Illness.* (ADM) 92-1904. Washington, DC: U.S. Dept. of Health and Human Services: Interagency Council on the Homeless: Task Force on Homelessness and Severe Mental Illness.

Vanderhorst, K., Benner-Carson, V., & Midla, C. (1998, May). Psychiatric home care: Clinically valid and cost effective. *Caring,* 64–68.

Vanderhorst, K. & Benner-Carson, V. (1998, August). Psychiatric home care: Restoring troubled youth to wholeness. *Journal of Care Management, 4,* 54, 57–60.

Wells, K. (1991). Long-term residential treatment for children. *American Journal of Orthopsychiatry, 61,* 324–326.

World Health Association. (1967). *International classification of diseases: Ninth revision.* Los Angeles: Practice Management Information.

World Health Association. (1979). *International classification of diseases: Ninth revision, clinical modification* (4th ed.). Los Angeles: Practice Management Information.

Wyatt v. Stickney, 344 F. Supp. 373, 375 (1972).

Zander, K. (1998). *The New Definition* (Vol. 9, No. 3). South Natick, MA: The Center for Case Management.

Suggested Readings

Brennan, S. J., & Cochran, M. (1998). Home healthcare nursing in the managed care environment. *Home Healthcare Nurse, 16,* 280–287.

Vanderhorst, K., Benner-Carson, V., & Midla, C. (1998). Psychiatric home care: Clinically valid and cost effective. *Caring, 17*(5) 64–68.

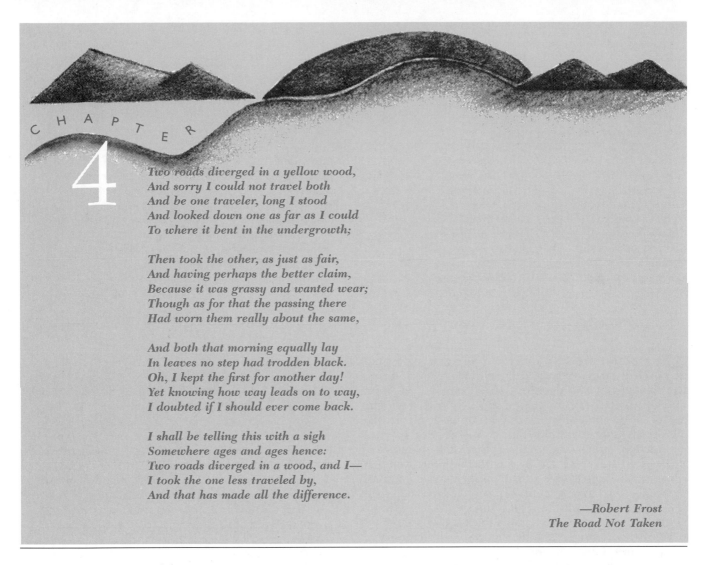

Practice Roles and Settings

Learning Objectives

After studying this chapter, you should be able to:

1. Discuss the scope and implications of the American Nurses Association (ANA) *Standards of Psychiatric–Mental Health Clinical Nursing Practice* (ANA, 1999).

2. Discuss the ANA standards of professional performance.

3. Differentiate direct and indirect care.

4. Define the term *advocate.*

5. Differentiate between the two levels of psychiatric–mental health clinical practice.

6. Define the term *peer review.*

7. Define the term *accountability,* and discuss to whom the nurse is accountable.

8. Discuss the roles of lobbying and networking in collaboration.
9. Define the terms *stress* and *burnout*.
10. Discuss the strategies to deal with burnout and restore spiritual balance.

Key Terminology

Accountability	Direct care	Primary care	Roles
Advocate	Health status	Professional behavior stan-	Secondary prevention
Burnout	Indirect care	dards	Self-care knowledge
Certification	Internet	Psychiatric consultation-	Self-care skill
Certified generalist	Lobbying	liaison nurse	Stewards of resources
Certified specialist	Networking	Psychiatric–mental health ad-	Stress
Clinical specialists	Peer review	vanced practice nurse	Tertiary prevention
Collaboration	Performance standards	Psychiatric–mental health reg-	
Continuing education	Preventive care	istered nurse	

Each of us traverses a different journey into nursing. Even though we may end up walking together on the same path, the decisions that lead each of us to choose first nursing and then a specialty within nursing are as varied and individual as each of us. It is true that all nurses share commonalities. We have a core of knowledge, skills, and values that link us in this profession. But there are just as many differences that separate us. This is true in the specialty of psychiatric nursing—we have a core of knowledge and skills regarding communication and interpersonal relationships, various treatment modalities, and causes of psychiatric disorders. Beyond this core lies a tapestry of unique roles, interpretations of roles, and functions that clearly not only draw from but also expand on the core knowledge and skills. What draws us to particular specialties within nursing is the spiritual aspect of our nursing journey—the meaning that the specialty holds for us and whether we have a sense of vocation or calling to a particular specialty. This chapter examines the richness that exists in psychiatric nursing, the various roles that psychiatric nurses fill, the functions that they perform, the challenges that they face, and the stress inherent in their journeys. In Sheila Spear's story, you get a glimpse into her psychiatric nursing journey.

Sheila Spear's Story

My journey in psychiatric nursing began when I was 15. My mother, a medical-surgical nurse and my inspiration, encouraged me to try nursing. I received training as a "pinkie," which was comparable to a nursing assistant, at one of the hospitals in Baltimore City. I continued in that role for a summer. I was promoted to a nursing assistant and worked at that same hospital during high school and then at a nursing home on summer breaks during my first 2 years of college. Although I was technically doing medical-surgical nursing functions, I was always keen to my patients' emotional, mental, and spiritual needs. I can remember my favorite thing to do was sit and spend time talking with my patients.

My first true psychiatric nursing experience occurred at Delaware State Hospital during my junior year at the University of Delaware. We spent 2 days a week for 8 weeks at the hospital. One of my most vivid memories is seeing the huge gray brick building that had bars over the windows and around the porches as we first drove onto campus. My classmates and I were very nervous, and I guess you could even say scared, when we saw that dreary and stark building. Once inside the building, there was a series of locked doors and a long, empty hallway that led to the units. Each unit had a large day room with gray walls; simple chairs; and, most importantly, patients curled up in chairs, lying on the floor, or pacing. My thought was, "What in the world am I going to be able to do to help these people?"

Timidly, I approached some of the patients because I really wanted to make a difference. I was also expected to do process recordings and care plans to examine patients' mental status and behavior and plan accordingly. Patients enjoyed talking to us. They smiled. They began waiting for us and participated in our dances and sing-alongs. They divulged some of their innermost fears, delusions, and frustrations and seemed calmer after talking. It was after this experience that I knew I wanted to be a psychiatric nurse. I learned about the strength of the human connection and how powerful support, caring, and listening can be.

I then looked into summer jobs and was selected, out of many students, to be a student mental health worker at Sheppard Enoch Pratt Hospital between my junior and senior years of nursing school. I had the opportunity to work on the eating disorders unit. It was there that I learned about milieu therapy, behavior modification, the use of seclusion, and community meetings and still more about the importance of being supportive and consistent with individuals. My favorable experience at Sheppard Enoch Pratt Hospital made firm my decision to continue in psychiatric nursing.

After graduation from nursing school, I was hired at Johns Hopkins Bayview Medical Center for the acute psychiatric unit. I worked there for 6½ years in the role of staff nurse and evening charge nurse. It was during my tenure on the acute psychiatric unit that I learned about the importance of biochemical etiology in the treatment of mental illnesses, sharpened my interpersonal skills with patients, and worked with many strong mentoring nurse clinicians. These nurses encouraged and helped me go back to school, participate in research, begin a family education support group, and volunteer for the Depression and Related Affective Disorders Association. I learned that psychiatric nurses can and do perform a variety of things that are rewarding and beneficial to others.

During graduate school, I was able to sharpen my therapy skills and focused on both family and group therapy. It was during this time that I learned about and gained a great deal from examining my relationships and myself. I continued to be interested in and researched the role of social, spiritual, emotional, and physical support in relation to mental illnesses and treatment.

After graduate school, I became the nursing instructor at a small state psychiatric hospital and enjoyed teaching both staff and patients about mental illnesses, their etiologies and treatments, ways to cope more effectively, and other healthy behaviors. I also started on my journey to my present role, which is working with seriously and persistently mentally ill individuals in their homes and in the community. This, so far, has been my most rewarding nursing. Doing home and community psychiatric nursing has allowed me to work with individuals as whole people. I am able to examine the lives of individuals and really learn how they live, and I help them see and use their strengths, qualities, and resources. I can help them tap into their supports in their communities. I help people realize the goals of returning to school and work, living on their own, having a bank account, and managing their lives. The biggest thing I try to do with patients is to help them to see themselves as individuals with potential rather than as people who are defined by their illnesses. I often say to patients, "You can do whatever you put your mind and heart into, and I will help you."

Psychiatric nursing is a rewarding career and allows me to do many things, but most of all I see myself as a "life coach." ■

Sheila's story is unique and highlights the twists and turns in one nurse's journey through psychiatric nursing. Not every psychiatric nurse chooses community and home-based psychiatric nursing.

CORE PRACTICE ROLES

The practice roles of the psychiatric nurse have evolved over the years (see Chapter 2 for psychiatric nursing's historical journey) from custodians of those who were viewed as deviant to nurses with multifaceted roles that include many functions (Church, 1987; Gregg, 1954). The ANA (1994) described psychiatric–mental health nursing as

. . . the diagnosis and treatment of human responses to actual or potential mental health problems. Psychiatric–mental health nursing is a specialized area of nursing practice, employing theories of human behavior as its science and purposeful use of self as its art. (p. 7)

Box 4-1 summarizes the "phenomena of concern" to psychiatric–mental health nursing.

The ANA recommends the baccalaureate degree as the entry-level educational preparation for psychiatric nursing. Psychiatric–mental health nursing demands knowledge of numerous theories drawing from a variety of sources, including biological, cultural, environmental, psychological, and sociological theories (see Chapter 6 for a complete discussion of theory). In 1994, the ANA published revised *Standards of Psychiatric–Mental Health Clinical Nursing Practice* (Box 4-2).

The standards of care described in the ANA *Standards of Psychiatric–Mental Health Clinical Nursing Practice* give rise to many of the roles of the psychiatric–mental health nurse. These **roles** are illustrated in Figure 4-1.

Each of these eight roles is discussed in these sections.

Provider of Direct and Indirect Care to Patient and Family—Health Status

The ANA (1976) differentiates between direct and indirect care roles. **Direct care** involves all the areas that the nurse assesses and all the actions performed by the nurse for a particular patient and family. Direct care has an impact on the patient's **health status. Indirect care** encompasses all the patient-related activities for which the nurse is responsible but which are delegated to others. Both the direct and indirect care roles require that the nurse use the nursing process, and both roles are undertaken in diverse settings. These settings include community mental health (CMH) centers, inpatient psychiatric settings, patients' homes, private practice, schools, industry, general hospitals, and nurse-run clinics. Box 4-3 describes the role of the psychiatric nurse in an emergency department.

Direct and indirect care requires expertise in

- Psychobiological therapies—electroconvulsive therapy, medications, diet, and exercise
- Psychotherapeutic techniques

The nurse must keep abreast of the latest research regarding treatment strategies. In addition, the nurse uses delegation and supervision skills to ensure that the indirect care is delivered appropriately.

Box 4–1 ■ ■ ■ ■ ■
Phenomena of Concern to Psychiatric–Mental Health Nursing

Actual or potential mental health problems pertaining to
- The maintenance of optimal health and well-being and the prevention of psychobiological illness
- Self-care limitations or impaired functioning related to mental and emotional distress
- Deficits in the functioning of significant biological, emotional, and cognitive systems
- Emotional stress or crisis components of illness, pain, and disability
- Self-concept changes, developmental issues, and life process changes
- Problems related to emotions, such as anxiety, anger, sadness, loneliness, and grief
- Physical symptoms that occur along with altered psychological functioning
- Alterations in thinking, perceiving, symbolizing, communicating, and decision-making
- Difficulties in relating to others
- Behaviors and mental states that indicate the patient is a danger to self or others or has a severe disability
- Interpersonal, systemic, sociocultural, spiritual, or environmental circumstances or events that affect the mental and emotional well-being of the individual, family, or community
- Symptom management and side effects and toxicities associated with psychopharmacological intervention and other aspects of the treatment regimen

Reprinted with permission from *A Statement on Psychiatric-Mental Health Clinical Nursing Practice and Standards of Psychiatric-Mental Health Clinical Nursing Practice,* © 1994, American Nurses Association, Washington, DC.

Box 4–2 ■ ■ ■ ■ ■
ANA *Standards of Psychiatric–Mental Health Clinical Nursing Practice*

Standards of Care

Standard I. Assessment
The psychiatric–mental health nurse collects patient health data.

Standard II. Diagnosis
The psychiatric–mental health nurse analyzes the assessment data in determining diagnoses.

Standard III. Outcome Identification
The psychiatric–mental health nurse identifies expected outcomes individualized to the patient.

Standard IV. Planning
The psychiatric–mental health nurse develops a plan of care that prescribes interventions to attain expected outcomes.

Standard V. Implementation
The psychiatric–mental health nurse implements the interventions identified in the plan of care.

Standard Va. Counseling
The psychiatric–mental health nurse uses counseling interventions to assist patients in improving or regaining their previous coping abilities, fostering mental health, and preventing mental illness and disability.

Standard Vb. Millieu Therapy
The psychiatric–mental health nurse provides, structures, and maintains a therapeutic environment in collaboration with the patient and other health care providers.

Standard Vc. Self-Care Activities
The psychiatric–mental health nurse structures interventions around the patient's activities of daily living to foster self-care and mental and physical well-being.

Standard Vd. Psychobiological Interventions
The psychiatric–mental health nurse uses knowledge of psychobiological interventions and applies clinical skills to restore the patient's health and prevent further disability.

Standard Ve. Health Teaching
The psychiatric–mental health nurse, through health teaching, assists patients in achieving satisfying, productive, and healthy patterns of living.

Standard Vf. Case Management
The psychiatric–mental health nurse provides case management to coordinate comprehensive health services and to ensure continuity of care.

Standard Vg. Health Promotion and Health Maintenance
The psychiatric–mental health nurse employs strategies and interventions to promote and maintain mental health and prevent mental illness.

Advanced Practice Interventions Vh-Vj

The following interventions (Vh-Vj) may be performed only by the certified specialist in psychiatric–mental health nursing.

Box 4–2 ■ ■ ■ ■ ■

ANA *Standards of Psychiatric–Mental Health Clinical Nursing Practice* Continued

Standard Vh. Psychotherapy
The certified specialist in psychiatric–mental health nursing uses individual, group, and family psychotherapy; child psychotherapy; and other therapies to assist patients in fostering mental health, preventing mental illness and disability, and improving or regaining previous health status and functional abilities.

Standard Vi. Prescription of Pharmacological Agents
The certified specialist uses prescription of pharmacological agents in accordance with the state nursing practice act, to treat symptoms of psychiatric illness and improve functional health status.

Standard Vj. Consultation
The certified specialist provides consultation to health care providers and others to influence the plans of care for patients and to enhance the abilities of others to provide psychiatric and mental health care and effect change in systems.

Standard VI. Evaluation
The psychiatric–mental health nurse evaluates the patient's progress in attaining expected outcomes.

Standards of Professional Performance

Standard I. Quality of Care
The psychiatric–mental health nurse systematically evaluates the quality of care and effectiveness of psychiatric–mental health nursing.

Standard II. Performance Appraisal
The psychiatric–mental health nurse evaluates own

psychiatric–mental health nursing practice in relation to professional standards and relevant statutes and regulations.

Standard III. Education
The psychiatric–mental health nurse acquires and maintains current knowledge in nursing practice.

Standard IV. Collegiality
The psychiatric–mental health nurse contributes to the professional development of peers, colleagues, and others.

Standard V. Ethics
The psychiatric–mental health nurse's decisions and actions on behalf of patients are determined in an ethical manner.

Standard VI. Collaboration
The psychiatric–mental health nurse collaborates with the patient, significant others, and health care providers in providing care.

Standard VII. Research
The psychiatric–mental health nurse contributes to nursing and mental health through the use of research.

Standard VIII. Resource Utilization
The psychiatric–mental health nurse considers factors related to safety, effectiveness, and cost in planning and delivering patient care.

Reprinted with permission from *A Statement on Psychiatric-Mental Health Clinical Nursing Practice and Standards of Psychiatric-Mental Health Clinical Nursing Practice,* © 1994, American Nurses Association, Washington, DC.

Box 4–3 ■ ■ ■ ■ ■

Role of the Psychiatric Nurse in an Emergency Department Setting

The psychiatric nurse works collaboratively with emergency department personnel to
- Respond to psychiatric admissions after the emergency department physician has determined that there is need for a psychiatric evaluation
- Perform an immediate psychiatric evaluation including mental status examination

- Communicate findings with the on-call psychiatrist
- Collaborate with emergency department nurses to develop plan of care
- Remain available by telephone to emergency department staff

Modified from Dunn, J. (1989). Psychiatric intervention in the community hospital emergency room. *Journal of Nursing Administration, 19*(1), 36–40.

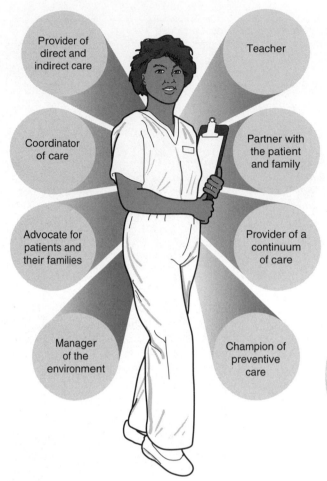

Figure 4–1
Roles of the psychiatric–mental health nurse stemming from the standards of care of the American Nurses Association *Standards of Psychiatric–Mental Health Clinical Nursing Practice.*

Standard Vh from the standards of care focuses on the role of the nurse as psychotherapist and involves the direct care role of the nurse. However, Standard Vh is written for the **certified specialist** (CS) in psychiatric–mental health nursing who has obtained additional education and extensive clinical experience and who participates in ongoing clinical supervision.

Manager of the Environment

The nurse is considered the guardian of the therapeutic environment (see Chapters 13 and 15 for a comprehensive presentation of the psychiatric–mental health nurse's role in managing the therapeutic milieu). The role of managing the environment involves negotiating environmental issues and teaching patients and families to do the same. The nurse assesses potentially stressful characteristics of the environment and develops strategies to eliminate or decrease these stresses. Managing the environment focuses on the global aspects of appearance, ambiance, and safety as well as the micro aspects of orienting new patients to the unit and

assisting each patient to fit into the environment comfortably.

Teacher

The role of teacher is an essential one. It is one of the primary intervention strategies the nurse uses in improving mental health (see Chapter 13 for a comprehensive discussion of the psychiatric–mental health nurse's responsibilities involving patient and family education). Teaching focuses on improving the patient's and family's **self-care knowledge** and **self-care skill** and assisting the patient and family to attain greater facility at living with the effects of mental illness. Some topics that nurses address in their teaching include the following:

- Medication management
- Illness management
- Dealing with emergencies
- Communication skills
- Coping skills

Trends in mental health care include

- Increased emphasis on self-determination of patients
- Involvement of patients and families in care
- Limited government funding to support CMH programs
- Emergence of the intervention model of rehabilitation

These trends highlight the importance of teaching (Chapter 13 describes the teaching role in greater detail [Carson, 1994, 1998]).

Coordinator of Care and Provider of a Continuum of Care

These roles of the coordinator of care and provider of a continuum of care go hand in hand. Nurses' holistic perspective enables them to recognize and appreciate the here-and-now needs, the round-the-clock activities, and the postdischarge needs. This perspective is essential not only in an inpatient unit where multiple therapies and activities must be coordinated but also in the community where the patient and family require a seamless transition into a continuum of care to prevent them from falling through the cracks of the health care system (Barratt, 1989; Carson, 1994, 1998). The nurse's role in facilitating progress within the health care system to progressively less restrictive settings is a role that cannot be understated. The nurse may act as discharge planner in the inpatient unit coordinating various community referrals. At the time of discharge, a CMH or psychiatric–home care nurse may assume case management responsibilities to ensure that the inpatient referrals actually become a reality (see Chapter 13 for a further discussion of case management). Ensuring that this coordination occurs entails

- Advocating for the patient
- Networking with a variety of community resources

- Negotiating the most appropriate services for the patient
- Exercising tremendous patience and a stick-to-it attitude to provide continuity of care

Advocate for Patients and Their Families

Advocacy is a critical role in monitoring local, state, and national legislative trends. With limited resources, funds designated for treatment and rehabilitation of the mentally ill are particularly vulnerable to the legislative process. The advocacy role involves

- Educating patients about their rights and responsibilities
- Negotiating for mental health services
- Influencing legislation on local, state, national, and international levels

The role of **advocate** is especially important in reeducating people who continue to stigmatize and ostracize the mentally ill.

Champion of Preventive Care

As champion of **preventive care,** the nurse supports a wellness focus as opposed to an illness focus. Such a focus (**primary care**) includes health promotion, illness prevention, and protection against disease. Within the scope of preventive care lie many of the following independent functions of the psychiatric-mental health nurse:

- Providing information about mental health issues, such as facilitative communication skills, parenting, stress reduction, principles of mental health, and sex education
- Affecting societal changes that have an impact on mental health (e.g., improved living conditions, greater access to affordable housing, and better education)
- Making appropriate referrals before mental illness occurs
- Teaching patients in inpatient settings strategies to prevent future hospitalizations
- Working with community and legislative groups on issues related to mental health

In addition to championing preventive care, the psychiatric nurse is also involved in both secondary and tertiary prevention. **Secondary prevention** involves those nursing activities directed at reducing actual illness by early detection and treatment of the problem. Screening for anxiety and depression is an example of secondary prevention. **Tertiary prevention** involves those nursing activities that focus on reducing the residual impairment or disability resulting from an illness. Psychiatric rehabilitation is an example of tertiary prevention.

Partner With the Patient and Family on Their Journey

The last role, entering into a partnership with the patient and family on their journey, is the role that synthesizes all the others and draws on the nurse's interpersonal and communication skills (see Chapter 10). This role focuses the nurse on the patient's and family's stories, stories replete with personal struggles and victories. This role allows the nurse to glimpse the special meaning inherent in those stories. Finally, this role allows the nurse to choose the personal gifts and professional skills that assist the patient and family to divert the journey to one of greater health and improved functioning (McBride, 1990).

These roles are always integral to the functioning of the psychiatric-mental health nurse, regardless of the specialty path that is chosen within the field. For instance, in Sheila Spear's story, her description of her role as life coach included all eight of the roles. In the disorders chapters you will see a feature entitled Snapshot View of Nursing Interventions That Facilitate the Patient's Journey Through. . . . This feature summarizes nursing interventions that deal with promoting health status; self-care skills; self-care knowledge; coordinating care; and, through relationship development, partnering with the patient and family through their journey.

*W*hat do you think? How does the description of the psychiatric nurse's core roles fit with your own perception of nursing? How does this information fit into your observations of nursing practice? Can you identify each of these core roles in nurses whom you encounter? If not, which roles are not apparent?

> ➤ *Check Your Reading*
> 1. Define direct care.
> 2. Define indirect care.
> 3. What does it mean to be the "manager of the environment"?
> 4. Give two examples of topics that might be taught by the nurse in his or her role as teacher.
> 5. What is a continuum of care?
> 6. What is involved in being a patient advocate?
> 7. Give two examples of psychiatric nursing functions that are part of preventive care.
> 8. Define primary, secondary, and tertiary care.
> 9. What does it mean to be a partner with the patient and family in their journey?

PRACTICE PATHS

Let's look at some other practice paths chosen by psychiatric-mental health nurses. The ANA delineates two levels of expertise within psychiatric-mental health clinical nursing practice: a basic level, the *generalist;* and an advanced level, the *specialist.* The basic level practitioner is the **psychiatric–mental health registered nurse** (RN), generally a staff nurse. The specialists have selected either adult or child and adolescent psychiatric nursing as their focus. **Certification** involves a formal review of clinical nursing practice and includes educational, practice, and, in the case of the specialist, supervision requirements.

Basic Level: Psychiatric–Mental Health Registered Nurse

The **certified generalist** is a licensed RN with a baccalaureate degree in nursing who has demonstrated clinical skills within the specialty that exceed those of a beginning RN or a novice in the specialty. The generalist has practiced at least 1600 hours within 2 of the past 4 years, is currently working in psychiatric nursing at least 8 hours per week, and has passed the ANA certification examination. The letter "C" placed after the RN (i.e., RN,C) indicates that the nurse is certified as a generalist.

The practice path chosen by the certified generalist is characterized by direct care. In fact, these nurses provide most of the direct care that patients receive during inpatient psychiatric hospitalizations. The setting itself may be specialized to serve the needs of a particular type of psychiatric patient, such as the patient with schizophrenia, the severely and persistently mentally ill patient, or the patient with an eating disorder. Each of these types of patients requires that the nurse integrate all eight roles discussed earlier. The "how" of each role differs with the patient and the setting.

Advanced Level: Psychiatric–Mental Health Advanced Practice Registered Nurse

The title **psychiatric–mental health advanced practice nurse** describes RNs educated at the master's level, at a minimum, who are nationally certified as **clinical specialists** or nurse practitioners in psychiatric and mental health nursing. The preparation of these advanced practice nurses is distinguished by a depth of knowledge of theory and practice, supervised clinical practice, and competence in advanced clinical nursing skills. These nurses have the ability to function independently and to manage complex mental health problems. The doctorally prepared psychiatric-mental health RN in advanced practice has both a master's degree in nursing and a doctorate in nursing or a related field. Nurses with earned doctorates generally follow one of two traditions:

- Advanced development of the clinical aspect of psychiatric nursing with a strong research focus (Doctor of Nursing Science [DNSc])
- Research and theory development in the science of psychiatric-mental health nursing (Doctor of Philosophy [PhD])

The psychiatric-mental health RN in advanced practice has been historically referred to as a CS. The term *advanced practice RN*, which may apply to a nurse anesthetist, clinical specialist, nurse midwife, or nurse practitioner, has emerged in response to the need for uniform titling within the nursing profession. The appropriate designation for advanced clinical practice in this specialty is that of the CS in psychiatric and mental health nursing (RN,CS). In the 1994 ANA *Standards of Psychiatric-Mental Health Clinical Nursing Practice*, the advanced practice nurse is referred to as a CS. The requirements for certification as a specialist include the following:

1. A master's degree or higher degree in nursing with a specialization in psychiatric and mental health nursing (nurses who have master's degrees in other specialty areas may apply to sit for the certification examination if they have a minimum of 24 graduate credits in psychiatric and mental health theory and have received supervision in two psychotherapeutic modalities)
2. Current psychiatric and mental health nursing practice of at least 4 hours per week
3. Clinical experience in at least two psychotherapeutic modalities
4. A minimum of 800 hours of direct patient contact in advanced clinical practice of psychiatric and mental health nursing (half of these hours may be earned through the clinical practicum component of a master's program)
5. A minimum of 100 hours of individual or group clinical supervision/consultation plus references from the supervisors/consultants
6. Successful completion of ANA certification examination

The advanced practice RN in psychiatric-mental health nursing chooses practice paths that include the provision of direct patient care in the form of individual, family, and group psychotherapy, provided in diverse settings including private practices, homes, and clinics. The variety of settings in which the advanced practice RN provides services is mind-boggling and is limited only by the entrepreneurial skills of the individual nurse coupled with the ability to sell the value of her or his clinical skills to an employer. For instance, CSs in psychiatric-mental health nursing work in outreach to the homeless, in psychiatric home care, in prison systems, and on college campuses. They are employed by industry to establish wellness programs. They work in nursing homes to develop and implement programs to manage demented behaviors of the elderly residents. They serve as community advisors regarding programs promoting mental health. They are employed in rehabilitation centers to assist in meeting the psychological problems of patients requiring intensive rehabilitation. They work in school systems from the elementary level through college to provide psychological care and to promote the mental health of young people.

In addition to the practice path involving direct care, the CS is involved in indirect care roles, including teaching, consulting, administering, and conducting research. The **psychiatric consultation-liaison nurse** provides all of these services within the general hospital setting. The story about Barbara illustrates the role of a CS, Wendy, who chose a path in community psychiatry.

As Wendy describes Barbara, she clearly illustrates both the general roles of the psychiatric nurse and the variation of those roles when applied to a specific patient population (Box 4-4).

Since the mid-1970s, increasing numbers of nurses have been obtaining doctoral education in psychiatric and mental health nursing. Their practice paths continue to include the direct and indirect care roles. What exemplifies their practice is a high level of expertise and competence and the scope of influence they bring to bear on professional and community concerns.

A review of the journey of progression within psychiatric–mental health nursing illustrates the movement from novice, to advanced beginner, to competent nurse, to proficient practitioner, and, finally, to expert described by Benner (1984). The novice enters the profession armed with basic education that provides a foundation in the therapies, nurse-patient relationships, and therapeutic communication. The initial experiences and supervision of the psychiatric nurse foster a progression to advanced beginner. At this stage, the nurse has coped with enough real life situations to begin to observe recurrent meaningful patterns in patient behavior, as well as to gain an awareness of personal skills and weaknesses in given patient situations. For instance, an advanced beginner could realistically identify the changes in a patient's verbal activity preceding an aggressive outburst. In Benner's (1984) classification system, the competent nurse parallels the basic level of certification of the psychiatric–mental health RN.

The psychiatric–mental health RN may continue the skill-honing process through additional clinical experience and supervision, continuing education, and graduate education and may move on to the next level of certification, which is that of the CS in psychiatric–mental health nursing. The CS equates to Benner's (1984) proficient nurse. At this level of expertise, the nurse is broadening the scope of practice to include attention to more general issues within the profession.

The highest level of expertise is achieved by the master's prepared nurse with experience and the doctorally prepared nurse, whose position is analogous to Benner's expert nurse. Although still involved in direct care, the focus of the doctorally prepared nurse is on expanding and strengthening theory that is informing the profession and on constituting the foundation of practice for the novice practitioner. This path, from novice to expert in psychiatric and mental health nursing, is an exciting journey (Figure 4-2).

> *What do you think?* Reread Wendy's story about Barbara. Based on Wendy's description, would you characterize her practice as advanced? Defend your answer.

► *Check Your Reading*
10. What are the two levels of expertise within psychiatric–mental health clinical practice?
11. What level of education is required at the basic level of practice?

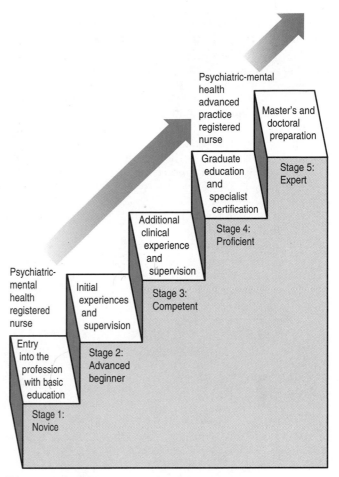

Figure 4–2
The journey from novice psychiatric nurse to expert psychiatric nurse.

12. What level of education is required at the advanced level of practice?
13. What practice role is fulfilled by the basic level psychiatric–mental health RN?
14. Name three of the indirect care roles performed by the CS.

PROFESSIONAL PERFORMANCE STANDARDS AND ROLES

In addition to the standards of care and related roles that directly affect the patient, the psychiatric–mental health nurse is expected to adhere to the standards of professional performance set forth by the ANA (see Box 4-2). **Professional behavior standards** state the behaviors nurses are expected to exhibit when caring for their patients. These standards give rise to the following roles (Figure 4-3):

1. Bearer of professional standards
2. Evaluator of care
3. Lifelong learner
4. Community participant
5. Ethical decision-maker
6. Collaborator
7. Researcher
8. Steward of resources

Box 4-4 ■ ■ ■ ■ ■
Wendy's Story: Working With Barbara

As a nurse at Creative Alternatives from the beginning of this demonstration project, I have seen exciting things happen for all of the members of our program. There is one person who stands out as a great testimony to the strengths of our nontraditional approach and how nurses can function creatively. Her name is Barbara and she is 56 years old.

I was Barbara's therapist in a traditional multidisciplinary team from 1988 to 1993, before her enrollment in Creative Alternatives. She left one of many long state hospital admissions and was placed in the highest level of care in a residential program. There were constant problems and battles with lab work, activities of daily living, agitation, and resistance to help. Her goals were to smoke cigarettes, drink coffee, and watch TV, and she wanted very much to be left alone. Her schizophrenia was generally manifested by tremendous negative symptoms without relief from medications, therapy, or other interventions. She had psychogenic polydipsia with frequent electrolyte imbalance problems that, at times, were life-threatening. In general, she was very unhappy. She had intensely institutional traits and was not interested in gaining independence skills. She wanted to be cared for with the basics and otherwise left alone. She was extremely disheveled, malodorous, and difficult to either connect with or be around. Barbara was very good at cussing people out and distancing herself from others. She spent 3 months on our acute psychiatric unit before we had to transfer her to a state hospital in March 1993 because we were unable to help her. She was mute and without any motivation to return to the community.

It was at this state hospital that Creative Alternatives began to engage members. Barbara was on our list. She and I had a previous relationship of sorts; there was already some trust, which allowed me to take her on the 35-mile trip to Baltimore to look for housing and prepare for discharge. She had gained about 70 pounds and was still generally anxious and apathetic, but she was receptive to discharge. She had been resistant to lab work and medical care at the hospital, but she was aware that she was expected to undergo them to enroll in the project. She was discharged and enrolled in Creative Alternatives in February 1995.

Since her enrollment, her negativity has melted away and revealed increased personality, sensitivity, trust, joy, and confidence. She has lost a lot of her anxiousness and fearfulness in exchange for a sense of inner beauty as well as concern for her appearance. She has been an inspiration for us as staff to look beyond the individuals we first meet to see the future potential. Barbara has already exceeded my wildest dreams, so I strive to keep looking for even more potential that has yet to be realized. One can't reap these successes in short-term relationships. Our history spans approximately 10 years together—4 of which were in this program. Such dramatic changes are slow but inspiring. This once miserable person has blossomed into a truly happy and capable woman who is enjoying life and her accomplishments.

Saying she wanted to use the bus and to work have been huge surprises. Even though she lives in a board and care home where food, medications, and activities of daily living support are provided, it is a drug-infested city neighborhood. She walks with a limp and has a noticeable arm deformity, making her seem vulnerable and dependent. For the first time in her life, she wanted to work. To get to work, she needed to learn how to use the bus and to walk through her neighborhood to get the bus. The drug dealers and regulars in the area know her and are protective of her, and she has always been safe. She learned to take the bus and worked in our thrift store in a training position for 5 months. She is now looking for a more challenging job that she will enjoy.

Barbara has been extremely good with her money, buying clothes and saving surplus funds herself in a bank account. She left Creative Alternatives' office-based system of distributing personal allowance and goes, via bus, to her bank. We are her representative payee and she receives a check from our program for her monthly personal allowance. She budgets cigarettes, toiletry articles, clothing, and other sundries from this money. She is anxious to earn more money, as she did when she worked.

Her family has been extremely pleased by her accomplishments. A couple of years ago, one family member said, "I didn't recognize her, she looks so good." She has now lost all of her excess weight. She has glasses and dentures, wears both, and broadly smiles at her new appearance and changes. Of course, she receives marvelous positive feedback for her strides toward greater independence. She is able to control her fluid intake, so she has gone years without an episode of electrolyte imbalance.

Her health has been a challenge in the midst of all the growth. In the past, having a mammogram or lab work done involved a huge struggle with Barbara. In 1 year, she had three major surgical hurdles. First, she underwent a breast biopsy for a suspicious lump. Fortunately, it was benign. But being unable to take anything by mouth for hours before surgery required lots of diversion. We blew bubbles, shot airplanes, and played games to pass the time, so that it was fun, not torture. Her second medical challenge stemmed from a fall that occurred just before the breast biopsy. She fell at a care provider's home, where it became evident that the care she was receiving was inadequate. She was subsequently moved. Through many medical errors, misread radiographs, and poor follow-up, there was constant advocacy and effort to get her the appropriate care in a timely fashion. She ended up

Box 4–4 ■ ■ ■ ■ ■
Wendy's Story: Working With Barbara *Continued*

with a huge knee deformity, with excessive pain, and in need of a left total knee replacement. I sought out the best doctors possible but gave Barbara options in her care. She had the total knee replacement and constant support with visits, treats, and cigarettes to help with the rehabilitation. Despite poor team communication by the rehabilitation staff, she and her new care provider were trained and faithfully did the exercises at home. At 1 month after surgery, she was already 3 months ahead of the average patient in the recovery process, and she has since had no problems with her knee.

Her third medical challenge involved another surgery. Through work-ups, the chronic problem she had of urinary incontinence was being followed for 1 year in Johns Hopkins Hospital's continence clinic with little change. First urology, then neurology, and finally neurosurgery became involved. She had an extremely unstable C4-5 disk that needed fusion. There was an option not to repair it because there was no pain and she had lived with it for a long time; however, a minor fall or a motor vehicle accident could very well have left Barbara paralyzed. She had a C4-5 anterior cervical diskectomy with fusion done in June 1997 to prevent further neurological problems, stabilize her neck, and reduce further damage to her bladder. She wore a Philadelphia collar for months, and we would not take her anywhere without it.

How did this woman, who hated anything having to do with medical procedures, get through three major surgeries and countless medical appointments? Early after discharge, her treatment plan included an incentive. I would take her and encourage her through appointments, procedures, or whatever she faced, then we would go to lunch and have fun together. We'd sing along, off-tune, to the oldies that played on the radio and laugh at ourselves. Eventually, Barbara started asking, "Don't I have any appointments this week?" which really meant, "Aren't we going out to eat?" Barbara and I have become friends and we enjoy each other. I am more than a nurse, a team leader, or a staff member to her. We have shared in serious challenges, and together we have overcome them. The relationships that staff develop with the members of Creative Alternatives are the key to successful outcomes. I don't mean that we manipulate the members into doing what we want them to do. We treat them as adults, respect their decisions, and provide support and information to explore the rewards and consequences of choices.

In nursing, there has always been an ideal to provide holistic care. At Creative Alternatives, the focus on holistic care is real—not just lip service. We support people by doing whatever it takes in any area of their lives. Psychiatric nurses are the key to the care—we understand the interaction among physical, emotional, and spiritual needs, and we guide others who have less knowledge and experience to be good caregivers.

Bearer of Professional Standards and Evaluator of Care

The roles inherent in **performance standards** I and II (see Box 4-2) really go hand in hand. The psychiatric nurse participates in systematic evaluation of the quality of care and effectiveness of psychiatric nursing practice as well as evaluates and improves his or her own clinical performance. These activities are accomplished through self-evaluation, **peer review,** and formal organizational evaluation of care through a variety of quality or process improvement activities. As a result of the evaluation process, changes are implemented by individuals, units, and organizations to improve care (Zerwekh & Claborn, 1994).

Embedded in the process of evaluation is the concept of **accountability,** which means to be answerable to someone for one's actions. In 1980, Hildegard Peplau wrote an article entitled "The Psychiatric Nurse— Accountable? To Whom? For What?" (Peplau, 1980). Peplau discussed the shift in accountability from personal to public. In the following quote, she stressed the importance of the accountability of the professional nurse to self.

The primary accountability of a professional is here—a matter of integrity—honesty in the moral sense, and purity of motives so that professional aims are pursued. Adherence should be to the purpose of the work with patients, which, stated generally, is to promote health-conducive behavior, and in the process, to aid the release and development of the patient's potential, while safeguarding all patient rights. To accomplish these purposes requires constant evaluation of one's practices, keeping up with and testing new theories, and periodically reviewing clinical data with peers for the possibility of inappropriate action based on faulty inferences. (p. 131)

Peplau continued to say that for nurses, this review must address two questions:

• How does the individual nurse use time while at work?
• Does that nurse's use of time support the interests of patients?

Additionally, nurses are accountable to nurse colleagues at work and in the profession at large. One of the most important kinds of peer review involves nurses' disclosure and assessment of clinical data from nurse-patient relationships in a supervisory review process in

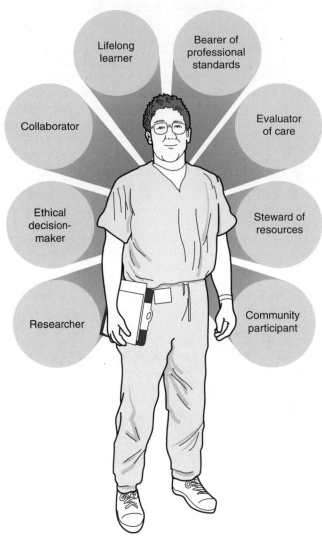

Figure 4–3
Roles of the psychiatric–mental health nurse stemming from the standards of professional performance of the American Nurses Association *Standards of Psychiatric–Mental Health Clinical Nursing Practice.*

spondents in this study identified the following characteristics as essential for the effective supervisor:

- Ability to share knowledge
- Ability to provide feedback
- Personal warmth
- Clinical competence
- Openness to self-examination
- Mentally healthy

Nurses are accountable beyond the work situation to be spokespersons for what nursing is and does. If psychiatric nurses are unable to articulate the health problems that they treat, it is difficult to make a case for nursing's needs before legislators, third-party payers, administrators, other health professionals, and even nurses themselves.

Nurses are accountable to the public to ensure that "they get their money's worth" when nursing services are involved. This means that nurses monitor competencies within the profession, communicate to the public the meaning of the credentialing process, and monitor and report any abuses of patients that they observe.

Although hospital accountability procedures include a review of records to guarantee that each patient has a written individual treatment plan, only the nurse's personal accountability ensures that these plans are actually implemented.

Most importantly, psychiatric nurses are accountable to the patients whom they serve. This accountability means that the nurse must disclose to the patient the

which nurse colleagues openly discuss and comment on each other's work. Peer review in psychiatric nursing is probably more important than in other nursing disciplines. This importance stems from the fact that the focus of psychiatric nursing is understanding human behavior, which always contains a certain amount of ambiguity. The peer review process helps the nurse maintain a therapeutic role with the patient and provides collegial support (Johnson, Richardson, Von Endt, & Lindgren, 1982; Pesut & Williams, 1990). Johnson et al. identified a model for a professional support group in which members meet to receive practical help, share experiences, exchange information, and stimulate new ideas. Figure 4-4 illustrates this model.

In the 1990 study by Pesut and Williams, psychiatric clinical specialists supported the need for continued clinical supervision after master's education. The re-

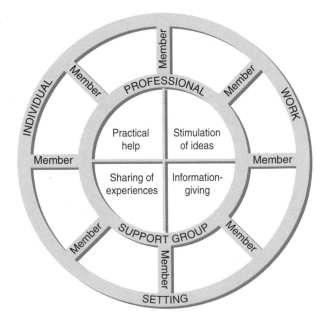

Figure 4–4
The model of a professional support group developed by Johnson and colleagues. (Modified from Johnson, R. M., Richardson, J. I., Von Endt, L., & Lindgren, K. S. [1982]. The professional support group: A model for psychiatric clinical nurse specialists. *Journal of Psychosocial Nursing and Mental Health Services, 20*[2], 9–13.)

purpose of nursing activities, the nature of what is to be done, the mutual responsibilities of nurse and patient, and the expected outcomes. Accountability does not mean that the nurse is responsible for the success of treatment; rather, it means she or he is responsible for the nature of the effort directed toward meeting specified outcomes and for keeping the patient informed regarding the purpose of the work to be done.

Lifelong Learner

The nurse as lifelong learner is engaged in a process of continually expanding her or his base of knowledge, understanding of human behavior, and repertoire of interpersonal skills (Girgenti & Mathis, 1994). **Continuing education,** through formal course work, seminars, in-service programs, symposia, and conferences, is a requisite for staying clinically competent. The psychiatric nurse has multiple resources that facilitate staying abreast of advances in the profession, including many psychiatric nursing journals

- *Archives of Psychiatric Nursing*
- *Journal of the American Psychiatric Nurses Association*
- *Journal of Psychosocial Nursing and Mental Health Services*
- *Journal of Child and Adolescent Psychiatric Nursing*
- *Issues in Mental Health Nursing*
- *Perspectives in Psychiatric Care*

In addition to journals, the **Internet** provides an exciting way to explore information about psychiatric nursing and related specialties and topics (Lim, 1996; Shoech & Smith, 1995). Through the Internet, nurses can be linked with others around the globe and access the latest information on psychiatric medications, mental disorders, mental health organizations, delivery systems, legislation, and conferences and other educational offerings. Some pharmaceutical companies provide continuing education programs through the Internet. The Internet is revolutionizing the way in which nurses stay abreast of changes within the profession.

Community Participant

As community participants, nurses assume responsibility to assist others in acquiring knowledge and skills. This responsibility is met through formal and informal teaching, sharing clinical observations and interpretations with colleagues and other professionals, and encouraging others to continue to seek out knowledge. One of the best ways to be active within the community of psychiatric nurses is to support professional organizations, such as the American Psychiatric Nurses Association. This organization provides leadership to advance psychiatric–mental health nursing practice to improve mental health care for individuals, families, groups, and communities and to shape health policy for the delivery of mental health services. See Additional Resources for a list of professional organizations specific to psychiatric nursing.

Ethical Decision-Maker

The nurse is responsible for providing care that is competent, sensitive, and holistic. Such a responsibility represents a sacred trust between the public and the nursing profession. This trust requires that nurses act morally and ethically in all situations. Boundaries are necessary within the nurse-patient relationship to protect the patient's well-being and safeguard against any patient exploitation, including sexual. The nurse is cognizant of situations in which ethical choices are not black and white but rather more complex, and in such situations, the nurse seeks available resources to assist in the decision-making process (see Chapter 5 for a discussion of ethical issues in greater detail).

Collaborator

The nurse as collaborator recognizes that nursing is only one component of the health care team. As members of the health care team, nurses must work with other team members to ensure that patients receive the highest quality of care possible. In psychiatry, every patient must have an individualized treatment plan that reflects the collaborative efforts of nursing, psychiatry, social work, occupational therapy, recreational therapy, and any other specialties that are involved in the patient's care. Table 4-1 identifies the other mental health team members and their respective roles.

Collaboration goes beyond the level of the individual patient and extends to issues involving programs, units, institutions, communities, and the United States as a whole. Collaboration subsumes the role of advocate described under Core Practice Roles. Nursing is responsible to make its voice heard in policy debates that affect mental health care. Participating in the decision-making process is essential if nursing is to articulate its unique perspective regarding patient care issues. Nursing has a responsibility to be involved in the whole continuum of primary, secondary, and tertiary services related to mental health issues.

Successful collaboration may involve the development of networking and lobbying skills as well. **Networking** includes developing a group of associates whose skills, talents, knowledge, and influence enhance the nurse's own goals. For instance, a CMH nurse's effectiveness as a case manager increases exponentially if he or she has developed a network of resources in the community that can be called on to assist a particular patient.

According to Meisenhelder (1982), networking occurs at three levels. The first is the grassroots level among staff nurses, which promotes cohesiveness, unity, and a base of emotional and professional support. The second occurs at the leadership level, with the common goal of increasing the power of nurses in the

T A B L E   4 – I   Other Members of the Psychiatric Treatment Team

Psychiatrist

Physician who specializes in mental disorders. Responsible for diagnosis and treatment. The psychiatrist may be the team leader or administrator of the inpatient unit. This is especially true in facilities that are philosophically guided by the medical model of treatment.

Clinical Psychologist

Professional whose training and education focused on mental health issues. Provides psychotherapy, plans and implements programs of behavior modification, conducts psychological testing, and conducts research.

Psychiatric Social Worker

Social worker whose preparation involves a 2-year master's program with specialization in mental health issues and supervised clinical practice post-master's. Focuses on assisting the patient and family to cope more effectively and identify appropriate community resources, on assisting the patient to maintain or develop a support system, and on facilitating the patient's transition from inpatient to the community. The psychiatric social worker is also involved in providing psychotherapy and may engage in private practice.

Occupational Therapist

Professional with a baccalaureate degree in occupational therapy. Uses creative and manual techniques to assist patients in working toward specific psychotherapeutic goals. Also, may work with patients to develop independent living skills to smooth the transition between hospital and community.

Creative Arts Therapist

Uses a variety of modalities, including dance, art, poetry, and music, to assist the patient to relate in a more open and honest manner and to increase social interaction and self-esteem.

Recreational Therapist

Plans and guides recreational activities to target the therapeutic needs of patients. Designs activities to facilitate social interaction, healthy recreation, and interpersonal and intrapsychic experiences.

Psychiatric Paraprofessional

Referred to as the psychiatric aide, technician, or attendant. Provides much of the direct care to hospitalized patients, especially in large public institutions. Usually receives on-the-job training directed at increasing interpersonal skills and sensitivities. The psychiatric paraprofessional plays an important role in maintaining the therapeutic environment of many inpatient units; therefore, it is essential that he or she be under the supervision of a professional nurse.

Mental Health/Human Service Worker

Newest addition to the psychiatric team. Receives training at certificate, associate, and baccalaureate levels. Engages patient in psychosocial activities that provide support and social contact. Implements behavioral interventions. Functions under supervision of a professional nurse. The mental health/human service worker's popularity is increasing in light of the growing need for additional mental health workers, inability of the traditional professional services to meet the increasing demands for more personnel, proven effectiveness, and relative economy of employing such a worker.

health care system. The third is the informational networking level, which is absolutely essential for political activism.

Lobbying is a strategy used to influence policy decisions by influencing the policymakers (Bushy & Smith, 1990). Historically, nursing has not been seen as a powerful political force, despite the potential for power inherent in the large numbers of nurses. Given the size of the profession, however, it is conceivable that group power could be exercised through organized lobbying efforts. The purpose of such efforts would be to influence public opinion as well as legislators' opinions through careful analysis and persuasive communication of current issues (Dumas, 1994).

Researcher

The last performance standard of the ANA deals with the nurse as researcher. The inclusion of research as a performance standard strongly reinforces the need to continually strive to develop the profession further. We do not have all the answers. In fact, even with the plethora of published research, psychiatric nursing is in its infancy in defining effective interventions for specific psychiatric disorders.

The research standard covers levels of participation from the nurse who takes part in studies designed by other nurses or health professionals to the nurse who acts as principal investigator in conducting research. Nursing's involvement in research also includes incorporating new research findings into practice and monitoring the protection of human subjects.

Steward of Resources

Increasingly, in this age of managed care, nurses are becoming **stewards of resources,** being forced to examine ways to conserve resources. We are being called on to do more with less

- Staff
- Latitude in how long we can keep a patient in the hospital

- Autonomy in deciding the length of patient treatment in outpatient settings
- Freedom to choose the type of provider that we would like
- Freedom to continue old systems and processes without carefully examining and perhaps restructuring them

Questions such as the following are being directed to nurses on a daily basis:

- What is the best use of the patient's insurance benefits?
- How can we deliver quality care in a cost-effective manner?
- Who is both qualified and cost-effective to provide certain services?

Nurses must be good stewards of all the resources that they manage, including their own time and talents, the material resources of the agencies for which they work, and the insurance and personal resources of the patients and families for whom they care.

What do you think? Write down your thoughts about whether professional performance standards are necessary. Are they enforceable? If so, how? How do you see yourself incorporating them into your own practice?

➤ *Check Your Reading*

15. Define peer review.
16. What does it mean to be accountable?
17. Why is continuing education important?
18. What is the nurse's responsibility as a community participant?
19. What is a collaborator?
20. Define networking.
21. Define lobbying.
22. Give two acceptable levels of research participation for the psychiatric–mental health nurse.
23. What does stewardship involve?

STRESS AND BURNOUT

Understanding Stress and Burnout

Without question, nursing is a stressful profession. **Stress** is part of both the direct and the indirect care roles. Faced daily with the pain and suffering of others, nurses are called on to give comfort, solace, and support even when their own resources for doing so are depleted. In addition to difficult patient issues that cause the nurse stress, administrative issues, such as poor working conditions and unreasonable demands, siphon energy away from the nurse's primary focus, which is the care of the patient. Dawkins, Depp, and Seltzer (1985) suggested the following three reasons for examining stress in nursing:

1. Stress is costly to the individual nurse, resulting in psychosomatic illnesses, impaired mental health, alcoholism, and drug abuse.

2. Stress is costly to the organization, resulting in absenteeism, tardiness, turnover, and sabotage of programs.

3. Stress interferes with the nurse's ability to care for patients adequately.

Most of the research that exists on nursing stress focuses on nurses who work in settings in which physical health is the focus. It is equally important to examine the stress that exists in psychiatric nursing. Dawkins et al. (1985) developed the 78-item Psychiatric Nurses' Occupational Stress Scale and administered it to 43 nurses at one hospital. The findings of this study are of particular interest because 50% of the high-stressor items are produced by administrative and organizational issues. The most stressful item involved not being notified of changes before they took place. Negative characteristics of patients are viewed as relatively nonstressful. Figure 4–5 illustrates some of the stressors encountered by psychiatric–mental health nurses.

Stress can lead to **burnout,** which was defined by Arnold (1989) as an exhaustion of physical and emotional strength. Muldary (1983) suggested that nurses are particularly vulnerable to burnout, resulting in an "erosion of spirit and a general demoralization under conditions perceived as highly stressful" (p. 7).

Arnold (1989) discussed burnout as a spiritual issue for the nurse whose spirit is assaulted and whose life feels fragmented and suggested that there is a need to make whole and to draw life back into balance. The stress that is experienced catapults the nurse into a crisis of meaning. Arnold said malaise of the spirit occurs

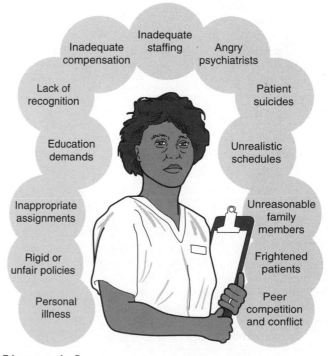

Figure 4–5
Some stressors encountered by psychiatric–mental health nurses.

when the spirit is "pitted against a reality that cannot be changed" or ordered in a meaningful way (p. 326). Box 4–5 lists questions the nurse can use to help maintain or restore balance and wholeness.

Strategies for Dealing With Stress and Burnout

Many strategies have been suggested for dealing with stress and, ultimately, burnout. These strategies focus on changing the external environment in which nurses practice, including establishing an interpersonally supportive environment and educating nurses about ways to deal with conflict, to negotiate, and to manage change (Cronin-Stubbs & Brophy, 1985).

Arnold (1989) suggested a model of dealing with burnout that addresses the inner processes of the nurse and gets at the core of burnout: a spiritual crisis of meaning (Figure 4–6). Incorporated into this model is an A-B-C mnemonic for the mutually dependent processes involved in restoring or maintaining a creatively balanced lifestyle.

Developing Awareness. The first step of the process, developing awareness, involves naming the stressful event and owning one's personal contribution to the situation. By naming a stressful event, we take it from the realm of the intangible and all-pervasive to the concrete and manageable; this is absolutely essential to identifying solutions.

Achieving Balance. The second step, achieving balance, involves recognizing that we cannot have all of our wants satisfied in the ways that we decide are best for us, and it is not possible to meet them all at the same time. Conflicting wants, needs, and responsibilities must be continually balanced. Priorities must be established and reestablished.

Nurses are particularly vulnerable to the self-deceptive belief that they must be all things to all people, and they often allow responsibilities to become dictatorial. As more and more of the nurse's time and

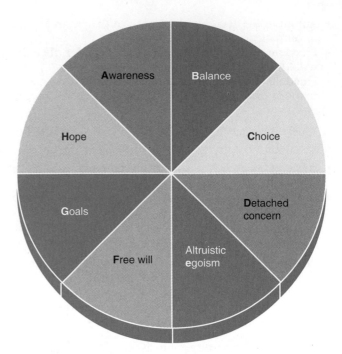

Figure 4–6
Arnold's model of dealing with burnout.

energy are used to address the *shoulds,* there is little time and energy available for the people most significant in the nurse's life. This results in physical exhaustion and spiritual depletion. Countering the effects of imbalance is possible through the following actions:

- Delegating
- Using energy-efficient and time-efficient ways of meeting responsibilities
- Saying "no"
- Establishing priorities
- Setting aside regular, planned time for the people most important in your life
- Taking time for spiritually renewing activities, such as taking walks, reading favorite books, praying, meditating, or spending time with good friends

Making Choices. The third step, making choices, involves looking at alternatives and deciding *what is to be done* as well as *how to think about circumstances.* Choices, such as whether to work a double shift or to study for an upcoming examination and whether to volunteer for one more hospital committee or to attend a child's championship soccer game, are the kinds of choices with which nurses are frequently confronted. It is important that we examine these choices carefully to avoid falling into a pattern of always choosing work over family or everything else over self.

Just as important as choosing to do or not to do particular tasks are the choices that we have regarding how we think about change and situations that are problematic. For instance, sometimes our choice might be to acknowledge that circumstances are beyond our ability to control and to use this experience to further our own growth. Another choice might be to confront

Box 4–5 ■ ■ ■ ■ ■

Questions to Be Used by the Nurse to Help Maintain or Restore Balance and Wholeness

- How do my ordinary activities of daily life fit into my life goals?
- What is missing or what needs to be eliminated to help me achieve balanced wholeness?
- Why is it that I put so much stock in the words and ideas of others and have so little faith in the legitimacy of my own?
- Who defines me—myself or others?

Modified from Arnold, E. (1989). Burnout as a spiritual issue: Rediscovering meaning in nursing practice. In V. B. Carson (Ed.), *Spiritual dimensions of nursing practice.* Philadelphia: W. B. Saunders.

the inner tension and to explore whether there is a way, from our own experiences, to make a difference for others. These two choices allow us to find spiritual meaning in difficult situations. Another choice is to resist the possibilities for change that are inherent in the present circumstances and to focus on the negatives of the situation. This last choice keeps us rooted in the present and mired in the circumstances of change that are threatening.

Developing Detached Concern. The fourth step in achieving spiritual balance is the development of detached concern. This does not refer to distancing ourselves from others but rather to detaching from our own ego involvement. Detached concern allows us to do our best at any given moment without excessive concern about how our performance affects the past or future. The nurse focuses on the here and now and is intent on making the most out of the present situation. Meaning is drawn from the present, and the nurse does not dwell on the past, avoiding *what could have been*; also, the focus is not on the future, in wishful *if onlys.*

Detached concern, with its present orientation, keeps us directed to the only aspect of life that we can truly control. Except in our minds, we can never go back, we can never redo what is done, and we can never predict what will be. We can, however, fully immerse our time and talents in the current situation. By shifting attention away from our own concerns, we are freer to engage in life.

The ability to achieve detached concern can be developed. One practical strategy involves learning to laugh at ourselves and to avoid taking ourselves too seriously. Another strategy involves using quiet reflective time to allow ourselves to appreciate the diverse implications of a situation. Contemplation allows us to see our overinvolvement in a situation and to recognize the places where our own ego and interests blind us to the total realities. Along with meditation, prayer may help allow us to detach our egos from a situation. By turning a problem over to God or a higher power, as defined by the individual, the problem is viewed from a different vantage point, allowing the consideration of other options.

This attitude of detached concern carries with it a "letting go" of preconceived expectations about how life should unfold and how people should behave and instead embraces the possibilities inherent in every situation. This approach to life can be both frightening and freeing.

In psychiatric nursing, detached concern is of particular importance. Patients with psychiatric illnesses frequently say and do things that are hurtful to others. A nurse in close relationship with a patient is also subject to these hurtful behaviors and must have a way of dealing with the hurt that allows continued interaction with the patient. For instance, a patient who is dealing with anger at his family yells at his primary nurse, "Get out of my room, you're just like my wife, I don't want to hear your nagging voice." The nurse without detached concern feels angry and hurt and avoids further involvement with this patient. With detached concern, the nurse acknowledges the immediate visceral reaction to the patient's outburst but is able to avoid interpreting this behavior as a personal assault to self. Instead, the nurse recognizes the outburst as an essential aspect of the patient's healing process and plans to use this to open up discussion with the patient at a later time.

Practicing Altruistic Egoism. The fifth step in achieving spiritual balance quite simply involves extending the altruistic caring that is freely given to others to the care of ourselves. If we have difficulty remembering the last time that we chose to do something for ourselves, it is only a matter of time until our reserve of comfort and empathy, so freely given to others, will be depleted. To take care of self is not self-indulgent, it is necessary. It is absolutely true that we cannot give to others what we do not possess ourselves. Just as healthy bodies require food, water, and rest, healthy spirits require nourishment and respite.

Exercising Free Will. The sixth step toward spiritual balance is the exercise of free will, which helps us stick to deliberately chosen paths. It keeps us focused on our inner struggles and conflicts and helps us avoid quick solutions and escapes to difficult problems. Free will allows us to challenge the belief that we are merely buffeted along by the winds of life without any control over the outcome of our life. The exercise of free will is one of the major antidotes to the spiritual doldrums linked with burnout. Free will informs us that, regardless of the circumstances in which we find ourselves, we have the ability to make committed and deliberate choices; it allows us to live out our convictions despite obstacles and our own wavering certainty. It involves personal responsibility, persistence, and accountability.

Developing Goals. The seventh step toward spiritual balance is learning to develop goals. Without goals, we go through life without direction. Goals allow us to operate from a coherent foundation, organizing efforts and activities in a meaningful way. Setting goals is an active phase of productive living and a powerful strategy for preventing burnout. Goals must be realistic to be helpful. Goals that strive for perfection doom the nurse to failure before any action is undertaken.

Realistic goals require two steps. The first is to focus on our inner gifts that might help us achieve our aims. During this step, it is often beneficial to seek feedback from a friend or advisor who can help us to look at our potential. The second step is to recognize that most goals are not achieved without the help and cooperation of others, including God (however defined). Input from others, such as friends, sharing groups, spiritual directors, mentors, or supervisors, often provides fresh insights and perspectives. The process of sharing also fosters a sense of community, which is supportive of goal achievement.

Fostering Hope. The final step in achieving spiritual balance and preventing burnout is fostering hope. This attribute allows us to experience the possibility of our own worth and to see ourselves fitting into the larger picture of life. Hope is an attitude-oriented as well as an action-oriented way of being. Attitudinally, hope involves expectations of ourselves, others, situations, and God. We always "hope for something better"—a raise, resolution of an interpersonal conflict, relief from pain, healing, even a sunny day. These expectations, subject to change and revision, keep us moving forward. Expectations give direction to our actions and ways of interacting. The possibilities that we see act as guideposts for choices we make. Without hope, we are actors without a director. We lack an image of the possible endings in the drama of life in which we are participating. Without hope, it is difficult to see that what we do has meaning beyond ourselves.

What do you think? How would you respond to the following statement: "It is not the external stress that does you in, it is how you choose

to respond to that stress"? How can you incorporate the "ABCs" of preventing spiritual burnout into your own life? How can you incorporate this information into your work with patients?

➤ *Check Your Reading*
24. What is stress?
25. What is burnout?
26. What makes burnout a spiritual issue?
27. Name at least three of the strategies to deal with burnout.

Conclusions

In this chapter, we have explored the richness of roles, practice paths, and responsibilities of the psychiatric nurse. The journey that takes a nurse into psychiatric nursing, regardless of the specialization of that journey, is never dull or boring. It is a journey that deals with the drama of human destiny: the successes, the failures, and, most importantly, the process of life itself as it plays out. Psychiatric nurses perform a role in the unfolding story of every patient and family with whom they interact. These stories are forever changed because of the nurse's contribution. Serving as a health supportive resource, the nurse guides, assists, affirms, and even cajoles the patient and family in the choices that they make and the paths they choose.

This chapter examined the ANA professional practice and performance standards. These standards provide structure and direction to all that the psychiatric nurse does, including the following eight roles:

- Provider of direct and indirect care
- Manager of the environment
- Teacher
- Coordinator of care
- Provider of a continuum of care
- Advocate for patients and their families
- Champion of preventive care
- Partner with the patient and family

Different practice paths were examined with respect to the two levels of expertise within psychiatric–mental health clinical practice: basic and advanced. Within these practice paths, nurses focus on direct and indirect care roles. These roles also were examined. Last, stress and burnout were considered. Arnold's (1989) approach to burnout as a spiritual issue was presented, and strategies to deal with burnout were explicated.

Key Points to Remember

- The progression into psychiatric nursing represents a spiritual journey for the nurse involved.
- The core practice roles include provider of direct and indirect care, manager of the environment, teacher, coordinator of care, provider of a continuum of care, advocate for patients and their families, champion of preventive care, and partner with the patient and family on their journey.
- The ANA published *Standards of Psychiatric–Mental Health Clinical Nursing Practice* for basic and advanced levels.
- The ANA delineates two levels of expertise within psychiatric–mental health nursing practice.
- The basic level psychiatric–mental health RN possesses a baccalaureate degree, has demonstrated skills, and has met the certification requirements.
- The advanced level psychiatric–mental health RN possesses at least a master's degree, has demonstrated

proficient skills, and has met the certification requirements.
- The ANA published professional performance standards that give rise to specific roles.
- Nursing is a stressful career.
- Stress can lead to burnout, which is a spiritual issue about meaning.
- There are specific strategies for dealing with burnout and restoring spiritual balance, including

Developing **a**wareness
Achieving **b**alance
Making **c**hoices
Developing **d**etached concern
Practicing altruistic **e**goism
Exercising **f**ree will
Developing **g**oals
Fostering **h**ope

Learning Activities

1. Answer the questions posed in Box 4-5. Is your life in balance? If not, why not?
2. Observe the nurses in the settings where you are undergoing your clinical experiences. What roles do you see these psychiatric nurses fulfilling? What roles are not being met? Why do you think that there are some roles that are not being addressed by the nurses that you observe?
3. Call your state nurses' association to inquire about the lobbying practices of nurses in your state. What are they lobbying for? Is the lobbying done by individual nurses, the state organization, or a professional lobbyist hired by the association?
4. As you obtain clinical experience, make note of what areas are "researchable" for the practice of psychiatric nursing.

Critical Thinking Exercises

Miss Pebble, a nursing instructor, wants to increase her students' ability to develop critical thinking skills while they are in the psychiatric clinical experience. During postconference, she asks the students to think about the following:

1. What assumptions about mental illness do you bring with you to the psychiatric setting?
2. What experiences lead you to this point of view?
3. What implications will your assumptions have for your clinical practice—negative and positive?

Miss Pebble presented her students with the following questions:

1. What meaning do you assume the word *insane* has?
2. Can the word have other meanings.
3. Do the alternate meanings (points of view) have implications for your inferences about what the patient is communicating?
4. What inferences can be drawn about the teacher's beliefs about critical thinking?
5. What evidence suggests that the purpose for this exercise is clear? Unclear?

Additional Resources

American Psychiatric Nurses Association (APNA)

1200 19th Street, NW
Washington, DC 20036-2422
202-857-1133
202-223-4579 (Fax)
http://www.apna.org

Association of Child and Adolescent Psychiatric Nurses, Inc. (ACAPN)

1211 Locust Street
Philadelphia, PA 19107
800-826-2950

International Society of Psychiatric Consultation Liaison Nurses (ISPCLN)

7794 Grow Drive
Pensacola, FL 32514
904-474-4147

Society for Education and Research in Psychiatric–Mental Health Nursing (SERPN)

7794 Grow Drive
Pensacola, FL 32514
904-474-9024

References

American Nurses Association, Division on Psychiatric and Mental Health Nursing Practice. (1976). *Statement on psychiatric and mental health nursing practice.* Kansas City, MO: Author.

American Nurses Association. (1980). *Nursing, a social policy statement.* Kansas City, MO: Author.

American Nurses Association, Council on Psychiatric and Mental Health Nursing. (1994). *A statement on psychiatric-mental health clinical nursing practice; and, Standards of psychiatric-mental health clinical nursing practice.* Washington, DC: Author.

Arnold, E. (1989). Burnout as a spiritual issue: Rediscovering meaning in nursing practice. In V. B. Carson (Ed.), *Spiritual dimensions of nursing practice.* Philadelphia: W. B. Saunders.

Barratt, E. (1989). Community psychiatric nurses: Their self-perceived roles. *Journal of Advanced Nursing, 14,* 42–48.

Benner, P. (1984). *From novice to expert.* Menlo Park, CA: Addison-Wesley.

Bushy, A., & Smith, T. O. (1990). Lobbying: The hows and wherefores. *Nursing Management, 21*(4), 39–45.

Carson, V. B. (1994). Doing psych, but talking med-surg language. *Caring Magazine, 13*(6), 32-38, 40-41.

Carson, V. B. (1998). Designing an effective psychiatric home care program. *Home Care Consultant, 5*(4), 16-20, 21.

Church, O. M. (1987). From custody to community in psychiatric nursing. *Nursing Research, 36*(1), 48-55.

Cronin-Stubbs, D., & Brophy, E. B. (1985). Burnout: Can social support save the psych nurse? *Journal of Psychosocial Nursing and Mental Health Services, 23*(7), 8-13.

Dawkins, J. E., Depp, F. C., & Seltzer, N. E. (1985). Stress and the psychiatric nurse. *Journal of Psychiatric Nursing, 23*(11), 9-15.

Dumas, R. (1994). Psychiatric nursing in an era of change. *Journal of Psychosocial Nursing and Mental Health Services, 32*(1), 1-14.

Dunn, J. (1989). Psychiatric interventions in the community hospital emergency room. *Journal of Nursing Administration, 19,* 36-40.

Frost, R. (1971). *The road not taken.* New York: Henry Holt.

Girgenti, J. R., & Mathis, A. C. (1994). Putting psychiatric nursing standards into clinical practice. *Nursing Standards, 32*(6), 39-42.

Gregg, D. (1954). The psychiatric nurse's role. *American Journal of Nursing, 54,* 848-851.

Johnson, R. M., Richardson, J. I., Von Endt, L., & Lindgren, K. S.

(1982). The professional support group: A model for psychiatric clinical nurse specialists. *Journal of Psychiatric Nursing and Mental Health Services, 20*(2), 9-13.

Lim, R. (1996). The Internet: Applications for mental health clinicians in clinical settings, training, and research. *Psychiatric Services, 47,* 597.

McBride, A. B. (1990). Psychiatric nursing in the 1990's. *Archives of Psychiatric Nursing, 4*(1), 21-28.

Meisenhelder, J. (1982). Networking and nursing. *Image, 14*(3), 77-82.

Muldary, T. (1983). *Burnout and health professionals: Manifestations and management.* Norwalk, CT: Appleton & Lange.

Peplau, H. E. (1980). The psychiatric nurse—accountable? To whom? For what? *Perspectives in Psychiatric Care, 18,* 128-134.

Pesut, D. J., & Williams, C. A. (1990). The nature of clinical supervision in psychiatric nursing: A survey of clinical specialists. *Archives of Psychiatric Nursing, 4,* 188-194.

Schoech, D., & Smith, K. (1995). Use of electronic networking for the enhancement of mental health services. *Behavioral Health Care Tomorrow, 4,* 23.

Zerwekh, J., & Claborn, J. C. (1994). *Nursing today: Transition and trends.* Philadelphia: W. B. Saunders.

Suggested Readings

Carson, V. B. (1994). Doing psych, but talking med-surg language. *Caring Magazine, 13*(6), 32-38, 40-41.

Dumas, R. (1994). Psychiatric nursing in an era of change. *Journal of Psychosocial Nursing and Mental Health Services, 32*(1), 1-14.

Girgenti, J. R., & Mathis, A. C. (1994). Putting psychiatric nursing standards into clinical practice. *Nursing Standards, 32*(6), 39-42.

Peplau, H. E. (1980). The psychiatric nurse—accountable? To whom? For what? *Perspectives in Psychiatric Care, 18,* 128-134.

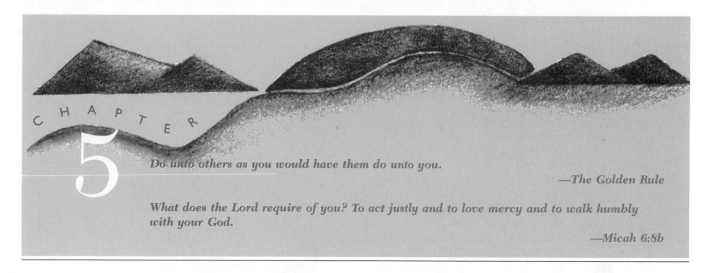

Do unto others as you would have them do unto you.

—*The Golden Rule*

What does the Lord require of you? To act justly and to love mercy and to walk humbly with your God.

—*Micah 6:8b*

Rules That Govern the Journey
Legal and Ethical Issues

Learning Objectives

After studying this chapter, you should be able to:

1. Define the terms associated with legal and ethical issues.
2. Recognize the discomfort created by ethical dilemmas.
3. Analyze practice dilemmas, and name the principles of ethics involved.
4. Claim your own hierarchy of ethical principles, and evaluate ethical decisions in light of your choices.
5. Increase your self-understanding through the analysis of personal ethical choices.
6. Compare and contrast the two types of admission to a psychiatric hospital: voluntary and involuntary.
7. Discuss the concept of involuntary community treatment.
8. Discuss the issue of criminal responsibility in psychiatry.
9. Discuss the concept of patients' rights.
10. List at least three patients' rights.

Key Terminology

Accountability	Conventional level	Malpractice	Postconventional level
Advocacy	Covenant	Moral (ethical) dilemma	Preconventional level
Assault	Emergency hospitalization	Moral distress	Restraint
Autonomy	Fidelity	Moral uncertainty	Seclusion
Battery	Incompetent	Nonmaleficence	Tarasoff decision
Behavior control	Informed consent	No-suicide contract	Therapeutic alliance
Beneficence	Involuntary treatment	Paternalism	Tort
Competent	Justice	Patient rights	Veracity
Confidentiality	Love	Personal boundaries	Voluntary treatment

The journey through psychiatric nursing necessitates understanding the rules of the road. These rules include both legal and ethical issues. Psychiatric nurses are confronted, on a daily basis, with the interface of legal and ethical issues as they attempt to balance the rights of the individual patient with the rights of society. This chapter elucidates those rules.

The world is full of ethical choices, choices in which none of the alternatives seem good. We make choices with a level of ethical uncertainty, and, in the process, we experience ethical distress. Questions arise, such as Did I do the right thing? Was I fair? Could I have been more loving in my actions? Whose rights are important in this issue? Do I have the right to decide? Does anyone have the right to make decisions for another person? Sometimes there is no right answer—only more questions.

The health care industry seems to have more than its share of ethical questions, possibly because of its intimate, life-and-death nature. Nurses routinely make choices that have moral significance, often unbeknownst to anyone except the nurse. In psychiatric nursing, in which the symptoms of the illnesses have an impact on a patient's safety, behavior, thinking, and relating, the ethical issues abound. Because of the choices that psychiatric nurses routinely make, it is necessary to learn about ethics and the law. The nurse's practice is to exemplify the quotations cited at the beginning of this chapter, that is, to choose to act with justice, mercy, and consistent regard and respect for others. The challenge is to discern what is just in a given situation and to determine how to balance justice, mercy, and love.

Mrs. Swanson's Story

Mrs. Swanson was 68 years old when she awoke in a psychiatric hospital, her first admission in her lifetime.

Mrs. Swanson's thoughts raced. "I'm so afraid," she thought. "Why are these people coming into my room? What do they want? Why are they asking me to leave my room and join the group? What group? Why do they speak English? They look like humans. How do they know my name? Maybe the spacemen who kidnapped me are holding me for ransom and are trying to find out what humans are like. I hope they don't hurt me. I'm not going to eat or drink anything. There is no way I am going to let them poison me. I guess I should be grateful that I'm still alive, but I wonder what they plan to do with me. Maybe they'll let me go home. Home!" Mrs. Swanson thought, as tears rolled down her cheeks. "What must my husband be thinking? He must be so frightened, wondering what could have happened to me. He must be looking everywhere for me. If only I could tell him I'm okay. I hope he didn't see them jolt my body and throw me into the spacecraft. I hope he didn't see me leave him, our farm, and our animals behind. How long have I been held captive? I wish someone would give me answers.

"Another woman just entered the door, and she's asking me if she can turn on some lights. Why is she asking me?" Mrs. Swanson wondered. "I'm her prisoner. But the woman is so kind, maybe I had better answer her."

"Please turn the light on," Mrs. Swanson responded. The woman turned on a reading lamp. Mrs. Swanson looked around and saw that she was sitting in a comfortable rocking chair. There was a bed, a chest of drawers, a desk, and a clock. "They must tell time like on Earth, or does it just look similar? I'll wait to see what happens at 12:59," she thought.

"I need to take your vital signs," the young woman said. "Then, how about a shower and breakfast?" Mrs. Swanson shrank back. "Vital signs?" she thought. "Does she think I'm dead?"

"Am I dead?" Mrs. Swanson asked.

"What do you think?" the young woman asked.

Mrs. Swanson considered. "Maybe I am dead," she thought. "But I thought I'd go to heaven."

Mrs. Swanson asked, "Is this heaven?"

"No," the young woman said, and smiled. "This is Memorial Hospital, and you are in the psychiatric unit."

"Memorial in Hudson?"

"Yes. You seem surprised."

"Oh, thank God!" Mrs. Swanson screamed, and she began sobbing. Two other people ran into the room at that point, alerted by her scream. "I'm home!" she shouted. "The spacemen brought me back to earth! You're real! You really are human!"

Mrs. Swanson began shaking, and her chest started hurting. The young woman quickly wrapped the blood pressure cuff around her arm and took a reading. Mrs. Swanson thought, "The shock of the kidnapping and space journey has taken its toll on my body. I'm glad to be in the hospital where people will take care of me." ■

If you were taking Mrs. Swanson's journey, how would you want to be treated? Would you want your nurse to understand your concerns about eating and drinking? Would you expect to be forced to take medication? Would you want your nurse to support your view of reality? This chapter explores the ethical and legal boundaries that guide your journey as a caring professional in relationship with Mrs. Swanson and other psychiatric patients. In addition, patients' rights are addressed.

PRINCIPLES OF ETHICS TO GUIDE THE JOURNEY

As we are faced with ethical dilemmas, we ask ourselves the following questions:

- How can I best care for my patient?
- Is my patient able to make good decisions?
- Do I have the right to make decisions for my patient?

Answering these questions leads us to choices that, we hope, cause the least damage to human integrity. Underlying our choices are a number of ethical principles or the reasons given for the choices that we make. The eight principles of ethics that guide helping relationships follow:

1. Justice
2. Love
3. Beneficence
4. Nonmaleficence
5. Autonomy
6. Paternalism
7. Veracity
8. Fidelity

From a theistic world view, justice and love subsume all the other principles. Not everyone who engages in ethical decision-making, however, does so from a theistic perspective, and an individual's world view influences his or her preferred principles. For instance, a humanist might value the principle of autonomy over other principles.

As you face ethical dilemmas, you are confronted with three tasks. First, you need to define your own world view. Second, you make decisions consistent with that world view. Third, you use professional judgment to appropriately apply the selected principles to your decision-making.

What do you think? When a patient is psychotic, that is, out of touch with reality, should all decisions be made for that person?

► *Check Your Reading*
1. What are the two main ethical principles operating in a theistic world view?
2. Name the eight ethical principles.

Justice as a Guide on the Journey

Justice is the distributive principle concerned with the equitable treatment and fair handling of people. Although justice has always been important in making ethical decisions, the issues of health care reform, managed care, and parity for mental health have brought the principle of justice into focus. Justice is concerned with making right or appropriate decisions about providing or withholding health care from individuals, families, or populations.

The question of what is just is difficult to answer. Is reward or health care given to those in need? To those who can pay for it? To those who have made contributions to society? To those who have the potential to make a contribution? To those who take personal responsibility for their health? Personal and societal values shape the application of justice, and people hold strong opinions. The 1994 referendum in California to deny health care, educational benefits, and other social benefits to illegal immigrants is an example

of the difficulty in deciding what is just. The citizens of California voted that justice is not served by rewarding illegal immigrants with services that they did not earn or for which they did not pay. The courts in California immediately responded by blocking the enactment of the referendum, arguing that it is unjust to deprive any person, illegal immigrant or citizen, of the basic necessities of life.

There are those who advocate for universal access as the new norm for justice but only for basic services. There is no consensus, however, about what constitutes basic services. Some argue that coverage for mental health services is a basic service; some consider such coverage to be optional, additional, or a luxury.

Considerations of justice are important not only for global issues such as health care reform but also in the small, everyday decisions that nurses face. For instance, if a nurse decides that one patient can have a second dinner yet denies another patient dessert, the principle of justice is in operation. As with any just decisions, all onlookers evaluate the rightness or fairness of the decision. Just decisions are difficult to render but are required by the nurse. Because psychiatric patients are most often treated in groups, many patients determine the fairness of a decision. Many of these kinds of decisions are made in consultation with the group of patients affected by the decision and by the person about whom the just action is being determined.

What do you think? Is mental health care a right? What do you think about parity legislation?

► *Check Your Reading*
3. Define justice.
4. Give one example in which justice is the issue in the care of the mentally ill.

Love as a Guide on the Journey

Love, when applied to ethical decision-making, has nothing to do with what the Greeks referred to as *eros,* or desiring something for self, but rather *agape,* meaning a self-giving and sacrificial attitude. Love in this context is different from friendship in that its survival does not depend on reciprocal admiration. Love is an overall moral principle, all-inclusive and exceptionless, that from a theistic world view governs all of our actions. Love derives from a relationship with God that results in service to others (Miller, 1998).

Loving patients is exemplified when you are able to accept a patient unconditionally even though the patient behaves in ways that are undesirable. This does not mean that you accept the behaviors. In fact, the most loving action that you can take is to set limits on behaviors that threaten the patient or other people. An example of such love balanced with limit setting is shown in Case Example 5–1.

■ **CASE EXAMPLE 5-1**
■ **Mimi's Story**

All morning, Mimi screamed obscenities at anyone who even looked her way. Everyone, patients and staff members included, was on edge. Jim, the nurse assigned to Mimi, approached her at a respectful distance and spoke to her. "Mimi," Jim said, "I can see you're upset this morning. We're all concerned about you and how you're feeling, but people are getting upset because of your screaming. I'd like to help you calm down. I'd like to go to the quiet room together and stay with you while you try to calm down. If that doesn't help, then we can try a dose of the medication that the doctor ordered for you. I don't want people getting angry at you, so let's do something to improve the situation." ■

What do you think? Have you ever been challenged to love a difficult person? How did you put this love into practice?

➤ **Check Your Reading**
5. Define love when it is applied to ethical dilemmas.
6. What is the relationship between justice and love as ethical principles?

Beneficence as a Guide on the Journey

Beneficence operates whenever you engage in making decisions for people who are incompetent and do not have the faculties to decide for themselves. Whenever possible, families are included in the operation of beneficence for incompetent people.

Beneficence is active, even aggressive, in promoting good, preventing harm, and removing evil. For instance, when the symptoms of psychiatric illness place a patient at risk, it is your responsibility to actively thwart harmful actions that could lead to suicide or homicide. It is more difficult to deal with thoughts, feelings, attitudes, and negative self-talk that are also harmful but in a more subtle way. The application of beneficence in the subtle situations of harm requires more skillful confrontation.

Nonmaleficence as a Guide on the Journey

Nonmaleficence means that no harm or risk of harm may be inflicted on another. This principle focuses more on the provider than on the patient; you resist being sarcastic, showing irritation, comparing one patient to another in a belittling way, displacing unpleasant feelings onto others, or using patients to meet your own needs. Nonmaleficence requires you to be self-aware; to manage personal behavior, thoughts, and feelings; and to

take responsibility for your actions. Further, exhibiting this level of maturity and mental health is an excellent role model for others.

What do you think? What situations have you observed in which beneficence or nonmaleficence was operational?

➤ **Check Your Reading**
7. Define beneficence.
8. Define nonmaleficence.
9. Give an example of violation of beneficence and nonmaleficence.

Autonomy as a Guide on the Journey

Autonomy means choosing freely and living with the consequences of the choice. This does not mean that people live in isolation and alienation; autonomy is most powerful when operating in community (Danis & Churchhill, 1990; Miller, 1998). You encourage autonomy when you provide the patient with adequate information and the necessary support needed to make choices. Assisting people to choose the right and the good may not generate the choice that you would have made. Supporting the person's choice, however, enables autonomy.

Supporting autonomy does not preclude the patient's right to change a choice. For example, a mother may decide not to sign a permit for psychotropic medication for an adolescent child. That choice may be difficult to make, given the recommendation of the treatment team. But after living with that choice for a week and seeing the continuing pain and aggressive behavior of her psychotic child, the mother may reconsider her choice.

You encourage autonomy by doing the following:

• Giving information
• Helping the patient and family sort through values, observations, facts, and alternatives
• Understanding the immense responsibilities of autonomy
• Supporting patients and families in and through the process

What do you think? How would you respond to someone who argued for autonomy over all other ethical principles? What do you think about the statement, "Your freedom ends where my nose begins"?

➤ **Check Your Reading**
10. What is autonomy?
11. What are some of the conflicts that arise when we respect the patient's autonomy?

Paternalism as a Guide on the Journey

Paternalism is based on the belief that the knowledge and education of the professional authorizes him or her to make decisions for the good of the patient, regardless of the patient's wishes. Paternalism derives from parental protection of and decisions for a child and indicates the nature of the relationship (Levenson, 1986–1987).

A patient who has made a serious suicide attempt provides an opportunity for paternalism. The person who interrupts the attempt commits the first paternalistic act—discounting the patient's decision. The patient does not want to be evaluated for possible psychiatric intervention; therefore, insistence that the person receive evaluation is the second paternalistic act. Telling the patient of the need for a short hospital stay and handing him or her a pen to sign admission papers are paternalistic acts. If the patient decides to go home or leave the hospital when staff members think he or she is still in danger of suicide, paternalism operates through the staff members' decision-making process. Do staff members file involuntary commitment papers and hold the patient for a court hearing? Do staff members manipulate and coerce the patient to stay or to decide tomorrow? Do staff members talk relatives into refusing transportation or housing? These are all acts of paternalism. The purpose is to maintain the life of the person; the actions are consistently taken on behalf of the person (Silvius, 1998). Clinical judgment and team decision-making help you know when to use paternalism, professional standards, legal requirements, and autonomy. Personal and professional conflicts, values, and judgments are inherent in ethical decision-making, as this example in this paragraph shows.

Veracity as a Guide on the Journey

Veracity refers to telling the truth, an obligation that is sometimes difficult to meet in the health care setting. First, patients sometimes ask questions that do not have concrete answers. They want guarantees that symptoms will go away and that they will get better, when there are no such guarantees. It is difficult, at times, to know what is the truth. A parent might ask you, "Is our daughter in control of her behavior and intentionally aggressive?" Or, "Will she ever improve enough to be able to return to college?" A young woman with a history of having been sexually abused may ask you if it is possible for her ever to be a good mother. These concerns call for support and excellent communication skills, but concrete answers are inappropriate. Sometimes, veracity is an obligation that is difficult to fulfill.

Second, other kinds of questions have answers, but you may be uncomfortable answering because you fear that your response may threaten your relationship with the patient. Sometimes the question highlights behavior that you are ashamed of or do not want to acknowledge. The patient may ask, "Are you angry with me?" "Were you talking about me to that other nurse?" "Why are you afraid of me?"

> **W**hat do you think? How would you handle these opportunities for veracity? Have you encountered patient situations where it was difficult for you to be truthful? What was that situation like?

➤ *Check Your Reading*
12. Define paternalism.
13. Define veracity.
14. Give an example of a situation in which paternalism is the preferred principle.
15. Give an example in which patients ask for an answer and veracity is difficult.

Fidelity as a Guide on the Journey

Fidelity is faithfulness to obligations, duties, or observances; it is keeping promises and is akin to veracity. Fidelity is vital in establishing trustworthy relationships with patients and staff members. Following through, being reliable, and telling the truth, regardless of the personal consequences, fit the standard of fidelity.

Fidelity begins with seemingly small incidents. "I'll be back in 15 minutes." "I'll go for a walk with you right after dinner." "I'll sit with you and your husband while you explain your need for your medication." Your work reality is filled with unexpected needs, changes in plans, and multiple priorities. Making commitments to a patient, a family, or a group of patients necessitates follow-through or confidentiality with full understanding of that reality.

There are times when a commitment or promise simply cannot be kept. When you use fidelity, you must tell the patient that the commitment cannot be kept and why (short of violating someone else's confidentiality), and make amends. Amends may be in the form of an apology, an acknowledgment of the other's disappointment, or setting another time to fulfill the commitment.

Fidelity also includes the following:

- Carrying out physicians' prescriptions for patients
- Questioning and refusing to administer inappropriate or unsafe prescriptions
- Documenting, on management reports, why promises could not be kept
- Following through, with consistency, the treatment plan developed by the team or members of the nursing staff on other shifts

Teamwork depends on faithfully following through, as if the commitment were personally made. This kind of team fidelity requires thoughtful consideration of the obligations placed on other staff members when promises are made that other people will have to fulfill.

From the simple definitions and explanations of the eight ethical principles, one can see the overlap and potential conflict among ethical principles, for example, autonomy and beneficence or paternalism and veracity.

➤ *Check Your Reading*

16. What is fidelity?
17. How does fidelity play a part in teamwork on a unit?
18. Give one example of a situation in which it would be difficult to tell a patient the truth.

ETHICAL DECISION-MAKING THROUGHOUT THE JOURNEY

In addition to relying on principles to help you arrive at ethical decisions, we might use one of two different models of ethical decision-making. The first model, developed by Kohlberg, deals with justice; the second model, developed by Gilligan, is based on care.

Lawrence Kohlberg's model of moral development focuses on three levels—preconventional, conventional, and postconventional (Kohlberg & Kramer, 1969). During the **preconventional level,** children respond to rules of society and the labels "good" and "bad." Children act out of an absolute respect for authority rather than out of any respect for or understanding of morality. As children continue to develop, they move into satisfying their own needs rather than being concerned with the needs of others.

Kohlberg's second level, the **conventional level,** is characterized by conformity to the rules expected by family and culture with no thought to consequences. At first, children are totally focused on meeting the "good boy/good girl" expectations to win approval from others. Later in the conventional level, children focus on following fixed rules, on respecting authority and law, and on maintaining the social order.

The third level proposed by Kohlberg, the **postconventional level,** occurs when individuals make a conscious effort to define their own morality apart from outside authorities. Individuals begin the postconventional level when they see themselves as participants in the changing matrix of social obligations and responsibilities. As moral development continues, however, universal ethical principles, such as justice, human rights, and respect for the dignity of human life, become important because the conscience serves as the final arbiter in ethical dilemmas.

Kohlberg's framework highlights justice as the guiding principle for decisions. Moral development is evaluated by the degree of autonomy and accountability of the individual making the judgment, and the highest levels of morality are attained by the individual who independently makes and lives with the consequences of the decision. A criticism of this framework is the emphasis on the individual alone. Because developmental research on Kohlberg's model has included mostly men, the framework is thought to reflect a male socialization in Middle American society.

In studies using Kohlberg's (1969) model, women consistently appear deficient in moral development. Generally, women exemplify the conventional good girl morality, whereas men usually achieve a higher level of moral development, even occasionally moving into the level of autonomous morality. This finding is not surprising to Kohlberg, who believed that men and women see moral problems in the same light. He concluded, however, that the deficient female moral development was a direct function of remaining in the home to help and please others. Kohlberg believed that as women moved into the workplace, they would be confronted with the inadequacy of this moral perspective and progress, like men, toward the higher levels of moral decision-making, in which rules are subordinated to universal principles of justice.

An alternative to the autonomy of the individual making ethical decisions is Gilligan's (1982) perspective of care. Gilligan challenged Kohlberg's assumptions that justice and moral rights are the highest form of moral development. She studied young girls, college women, and housewives to determine how they frame ethical problems and discovered that females tended to focus on conflicting personal responsibilities rather than conflicting rights and justice. Women focused on their responsibilities within the context of family and community and required that other factors as well as justice be considered. The relationship of this framework is considered more "female" in orientation because of the emphasis on caring and mercy.

Gilligan (1982) reminded us that social conditioning is vital in determining the ways in which people conceptualize moral problems, the issues that they perceive as ethical conflicts, and the values that they use to resolve the conflicts. Girls and boys are socialized in different ways. Boys frequently engage in games with rigid rules that they use to resolve interpersonal conflicts. The first step in the process of individuation for a boy involves separating himself from others. A boy's skills at intimacy and relationships are developed later.

Girls engage in less competitive and less structured games with more flexible attitudes toward rules. Girls tend to deal with conflicts by stopping the games and finding alternative activities so as to preserve the relationships. Girls generally identify who they are simultaneously through their relationships.

Gilligan's (1982) perspective is useful to nursing because of the emphasis on obligation, sacrifice, and sensitivity about hurting others. She believed that a moral person is one who responds to need and demonstrates care and responsibility in relationships.

Figure 5-1 emphasizes the importance of social conditioning and social scripting for moral decision-making. The figure does not emphasize the difference in social conditioning experienced by boys and girls. As you look at the figure, however, keep in mind that world view (box A); desire and anxiety (box B); and objects, relationships, and ideals (box C) differ for boys and girls.

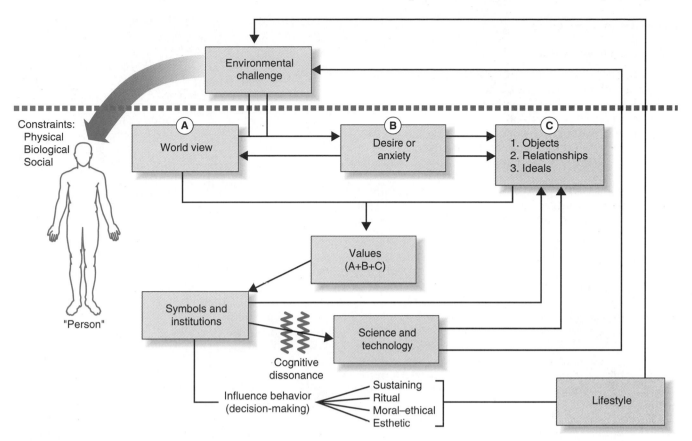

Figure 5-1
Social and environmental factors affecting our moral values. Whether we are a health care consumer or practitioner, we are subject to a variety of personal and environmental influences that condition and color the values we develop and the decisions we make. Below the broken horizontal line are the many personal factors we need to consider. Initially, three elements, A, our fixed or process world view; B, our emerging desires and anxieties; and C, our objects, personal relationships, and ideals, combine to create our personal values. These values are then given social expression in our laws, cultural values, and institutions. But science and technology also have an impact on our symbols and institutions, sometimes in a positive way, sometimes creating a disturbance or challenge (a cognitive dissonance). Filtered through our social institutions and symbols, our personal values are expressed in a particular lifestyle. The way we live as individuals then feeds back and impacts on our social and physical environment. The interaction between our personal lifestyles and the environment feeds back to us as individuals. As a result, we experience physical, biological, and social constraints. But the changing environment also has an impact on our world view and leads to new desires or anxieties. Because this network of interacting factors is constantly changing for each one of us, we should be aware of these factors and how they might affect our decisions in biomedical ethics as well as other issues. (From *Ethical decisions in medicine*. Brody, H. [1976]. Boston. Published by Little, Brown and Company.)

Moral and ethical perspectives may be developed from two perspectives, justice and care. These principles are not really "male" or "female," and the view of them as such serves only to polarize the genders. Although neither perspective is totally adequate in making ethical decisions, most people emphasize one over the other and argue that one model is superior to the other. Truth is most likely found, however, in the tension between justice and care, with neither being superior to the other. Both need to be considered when making ethical decisions. This exemplifies why ethics in real life is not a simple, factual exercise; ethics requires complex judgment, clarity of thinking, and ownership of one's own values.

What do you think? How do we balance justice and care? Where does mercy fit into the picture?

➤ *Check Your Reading*
19. What are the three levels of ethical decision-making as described by Kohlberg?
20. How does Gilligan's theory differ from that of Kohlberg?

LEGAL AND ETHICAL DILEMMAS THROUGHOUT THE JOURNEY

There are multiple legal and ethical dilemmas; they entail a broad spectrum from "is there something wrong in this situation?" to "what is the right thing to do?" Seven legal and ethical dilemmas in the practice of psychiatric–mental health nursing are presented for exploration.

Informed Consent

Informed consent is a

1. Choice based on understanding the situation, outcomes, alternatives, risks, and benefits
2. Choice made freely, without inducement, force, or any other kind of coercion
3. Choice made by a competent person who fully comprehends all the information being given
4. Legal doctrine designed to protect the rights of patients
5. Ongoing consensual process that involves mutual decision-making and ensures that the patient is kept informed at all stages of the therapeutic process (Usher & Arthur, 1998)

The opposite of informed consent is **assault** (threatening to touch or creating a fear of being touched) and **battery** (intentional touching without the person's permission).

How often are you expected to, or expect yourself to, assist a person who does not want assistance? From helping with bathing and toileting to secluding and restraining, members of the nursing staff have multiple opportunities to be uncertain and experience dilemmas and distress (Fowler, 1989) and to act anyway, on behalf of the patient.

The center of the informed consent dilemma is the patient's understanding. Multiple factors influence the patient's ability to process information and apply it to the real-life situation. With older adults, age, education, and cognitive ability can influence understanding of informed consent (Sugarman, McCrory, & Hubal, 1998), and with psychiatric patients, the factors are even more complex.

The symptoms of psychiatric illnesses affect thought, perception, and mood. The disorders interfere with the patient's ability to process information, and interpret data. To compound the problems presented by the psychiatric illness, add the ordinary anxiety with which all people deal daily, top it with the additional anxiety of the situation and its meaning, subtract the person's coping effectiveness, and weigh the patient's true understanding of the information presented.

Let's return to our opening story of Mrs. Swanson. Given her state of mind, was it possible for her to give informed consent? She was under the impression that she was a captive, possibly of benevolent beings. Would she have trusted her captors enough to think they were telling her the truth? She did not think she was ill, so why would she consent to take medication? If she did agree, would her consent have been valid? Similar considerations play a role whenever informed consent is obtained from patients diagnosed with psychiatric illnesses.

An article in *Time* (Willwerth, 1994) entitled, "Madness in Fine Print," addressed the issue of informed consent in relation to enrolling schizophrenic patients, who have information-processing deficits, in experimental research. Willwerth reported that 10 different University of California—Los Angeles, Veterans Administration experiments were under investigation for "ill-informed consent" (p. 62). The investigations focused on the manner in which researchers were informing study participants about the risks involved in their participation. Evidence indicated that some researchers deliberately withheld information about the high risk for psychotic relapse and used coercive techniques to enlist the participation of subjects.

Each person has a set of "meaning questions" that influence the decision. For instance, in the *Time* article, one patient, Harry Cummings, confronted the following meaning questions: "Will these drugs make me better? What if I don't participate—will my veteran's benefits be cut off?" (p. 63). In the example of Mrs. Swanson in our beginning story, her meaning questions might include, "If I eat and drink what they give me, will I get to go home? If I cooperate, will I be able to see my husband again?" Other patients may be confronted with questions such as, "Does this mean I'm crazy? Am I being punished? Am I hopeless? Can I ever get well? Will I be able to get rid of these voices? What if I'm not strong enough to help myself? Will my spouse divorce me? Will I end up hospitalized or homeless? What if I can't hold down a job? What if my insurance is canceled?" And so forth.

Meaning questions, in fact, must be answered honestly and weighed carefully for the patient to come to an informed decision. Unanswered questions, however, and answers that are meaningless to the patient complicate the patient's ability to make an informed decision. Patients who present with psychosis are still able to consent to treatment, but the information must be presented in such a way as to convey understanding of clinical care. You can see why a professional might be tempted to make a paternalistic, even beneficent response and make the decision for the patient. It is easy for those of us who have the education, experience, and distance from the intimacy of the patient's life to convince ourselves that we are in an excellent position to give advice. It is generally not in the patient's best interest, however, to short-circuit his or her decision-making process.

Why not give advice? If clinicians had only education, experience, and objectivity, one might be able to make a case for telling the patient what to do. There are factors, however, that create a subtly coercive environment when advice is given. When you are asked for advice, your expertise is acknowledged. You have the power to influence, and that power carries tremendous responsibility. You can never be absolutely sure that your advice is absolutely objective, free of your own biases. How can you know with certainty what will work in another person's life? Are you aware of all the latest research related to the patient's concerns or all the available options? What if you have a different perception of the patient's illness than the patient does?

The core issue involved with giving advice is power and the misuse of it. We must take care not to abuse the power we have in relationships with patients so that we do not block the patient's ability to choose freely. Patients may need someone to help them arrive at an attribution or give meaning to a specific decision.

Communication skills of listening, reflection, restatement, and so forth are invaluable to this process. In informed consent, the nurse's goal is to help the patient weigh accurate information in light of the meaning of that decision and to choose fully, including being willing to live with the consequences of the choice.

Informed consent is extremely complex. Yet, how much time is given to a patient and family to make a choice and sign the paper? The point is, informed consent is not a goal or an end point; it is a process. At any point, patients may change their minds, may ask more questions, may need someone to listen as the meaning of a decision or condition is explored. Members of the nursing staff are invaluable in this process. The patient's status in the process of informed consent needs to be communicated to the multidisciplinary treatment team so that all those involved may be of assistance in supporting the patient's self-determination and autonomy.

> **W**hat do you think? Have you ever performed an intervention against a patient's will? How did you deal with the issue of informed consent?

> ➤ **Check Your Reading**
> 21. Define informed consent.
> 22. What are the requirements for informed consent?
> 23. What is the risk in giving the patient advice?

Competence

Various medical and psychiatric disorders produce cognitive disturbances that result in temporary or permanent incompetence. This incompetence affects decision-making capacity and ability to give informed consent. Problems exist related to obtaining informed consent, especially in the elderly. Distinction needs to be made between *incapacitated* and *incompetent* and to determine the patient's level of ability to make decisions. A psychiatric illness does not invalidate the patient's ability to give informed consent, but it might influence the degree of judgment the patient has in making decisions (Ahmed, 1998).

An adult is considered mentally **competent** if he or she is able to carry out his or her personal affairs. If the person is not capable of making competent decisions, a special court hearing is needed to declare him or her **incompetent**. To prove incompetence, the following three elements must be present:

1. The person must have a mental disorder
2. The person must have a defect in judgment
3. The defect must make the person incapable of handling personal affairs

If ruled incompetent, a person cannot vote, marry, drive, or make contracts. If competence is regained, another court hearing is necessary to restore legal competency.

> **W**hat do you think? Is every person who experiences psychotic thinking incompetent?

> ➤ **Check Your Reading**
> 24. What is competence?
> 25. What are the three elements necessary to declare incompetence?

Electroconvulsive Therapy

Many issues juxtapose when electroconvulsive therapy (ECT) is discussed: world view (see Chapter 1), body integrity, knowledge base, informed consent, and outcome of treatment, to name a few. If you believe that the brain is a complex memory bank organized like files, the idea of passing a jolt of electricity through those files is absurd. Why disorganize those files? The person may never be able to find and store all the information properly. How does ECT work? For what disorders is ECT used? Have you read the latest studies on the efficacy of ECT? Because the physician recommends ECT for a particular patient, under what circumstances would you communicate concern about that recommendation? To whom would you communicate concern? Case Example 5–2 demonstrates an ethical dilemma involving ECT.

■ **CASE EXAMPLE 5–2**
■ **Wanda's Story**

Wanda, 31 years old and mayor of her city, was admitted to a psychiatric hospital for psychotic depression after a serious suicide attempt. Immediately before her attempt, a friend with whom she was having an affair sent flowers to her office. She was horrified. What would her colleagues think? Her husband and children? She was instantly overwhelmed with guilt over the violation of her marriage vows and impulsively ran her car off a bridge.

Wanda was admitted to an inpatient unit, severely depressed, experiencing psychotic thoughts, and still expressing suicidal ideation. Robert, one of the psychiatric nurses on the unit, began to work with Wanda. They quickly established a therapeutic relationship in which they discussed the affair, guilt, conflict resolution, meaning of the relationship and her marriage, and her belief that she needed to seek forgiveness from God. In addition, Wanda was prescribed fluoxetine (Prozac). Robert provided medication and illness teaching for Wanda.

The psychiatrist recommended ECT. Robert was shocked that this recommendation was offered to the patient because Wanda seemed to be responding. Wanda agreed to the ECT because of her continuing inability to function at home or in her job. Robert, having diagnosed Wanda's condition as "inability to function related to values conflict," questioned the psychiatrist about the recommendation for ECT and expressed reservations regarding Wanda's ability to provide informed consent. The psychiatrist assured Robert that Wanda had given informed consent; with this assurance, Robert supported Wanda's decision.

After the first ECT treatment, Wanda emerged from the psychosis. She had only a vague recollection of the hours of conversation with Robert. Her depression abated, she could think clearly and concentrate, and she wondered why she was in the hospital. Wanda had two more treatments and was functioning as mayor again within a week. ■

Several questions arise from this example. Was Wanda able to give informed consent for ECT? Because she was experiencing a psychotic depression, the ECT treatments were apparently the treatment of choice for Wanda. Because a positive outcome was achieved, is informed consent even relevant? Does the end justify the means?

Although a "cure" or definite positive outcome was achieved, what about caring for Wanda as a person? The issues for Wanda had not changed, although the psychotic depression was resolved. For the nurse, informed consent was the reason for his acquiescence. Wanda's autonomy and right to self-determination were honored, against the nurse's personal choice for Wanda. Beneficence and paternalism could have been the principles emphasized by the nurse, however, and a different process could have occurred. Had Robert continued to be concerned after talking with the psychiatrist, the next step probably would have been for him to read the latest research on ECT. If Robert was still not comfortable with the treatment plan, he could have talked to his supervisor, a clinical specialist, a clinical ethicist, or a patient advocate to help him develop strategies to approach Wanda, her family, and the psychiatrist about ethical issues surrounding the treatment choice.

What do you think? What do you think about ECT?

➤ *Check Your Reading*
26. Explain the reason Robert objected to Wanda's receiving ECT.
27. What are the options open to a nurse faced with an ethical dilemma?

Use of Medication When the Patient Refuses

There are many factors creating **moral distress,** which is knowing the right action but perceiving constraints because of institutional policies, written or unwritten (Fowler, 1989). The patient who signs admission and treatment papers but refuses prescribed medication creates distress for the nurse. The patient is deemed capable of giving informed consent and therefore is capable of giving informed refusal. The patient's condition warrants a fair trial of a particular medication,

and the nurse has considerable manipulative and persuasive powers to use to talk the patient into taking the medication. For Mrs. Swanson, in the opening story of the chapter, the nurse would have had to work hard to get her to take medication she might think was poison. What would help most in alleviating the psychotic symptoms she seemed to exhibit?

When the nurse uses persuasion and manipulation to get the patient to take medication, paternalism is operating. The nurse is acting on what he or she believes is best for the patient, despite the patient's own assessment. Yet, it is not uncommon, after several doses of medication, for a patient to be grateful for the nurse's cajoling and convincing. The patient is now functioning at a near-normal level and is no longer suffering the anguish of psychosis.

The opposite may also be true. Patients may agree to take medication while under constant surveillance. These patients may decide to "cheek" medication (hide the medicine in their cheeks) given by the nurse or quit taking medication immediately after discharge. Even though discharge criteria are met and the patient is functioning much better, paternalism was not useful in producing long-term benefit for the patient. Had beneficence been used, the patient's sense of self would have been reaffirmed, and perhaps a greater willingness to take medications would have been achieved. Research has shown that patients who refuse treatment have negative attitudes toward hospitalization, are more assaultive, are more likely to require seclusion and restraint, and have longer hospitalization stays (Kasper et al., 1997).

What is in the patient's best interest? Ultimately, the patient decides. The nurse-patient relationship creates a context within which the patient's dilemma and the nurse's dilemma in helping the patient may be explored, and the best choice for the patient may emerge. Box 5-1

Box 5-1 ■ ■ ■ ■ ■
Criteria to Be Considered When Medications Are Coerced or Forced

- The patient must be judged to be a danger to self or others.
- The patient must be judged incompetent to evaluate the necessity of treatment.
- The medication administered will be of benefit to the patient.
- All less restrictive means of behavior control have been unsuccessful.
- There is clear and logical documentation of the process and reasons for administration.
- The medications administered are consistent with the diagnosis and behavioral manifestations.
- Medical and nursing assessments have been completed.
- Therapeutic effects and side effects are monitored.

provides criteria to be considered when medications are given.

> ➤ *Check Your Reading*

28. When we use manipulation to convince a patient to take medication, what principle are we using?
29. What characteristics of psychiatric illness interfere with the patient's ability to recognize that he or she needs medication?

Ideals of Practice Versus Reality

In nursing school, as difficult and demanding as it is, students do not experience the real world. Faculty intentionally simplify the students' learning environment by selecting certain experiences, objectives, patients, and settings to facilitate students' learning. This approach serves students well because the complexity of the health care environment may actually overwhelm students and make learning even more difficult. The goal of academic preparation, by graduation, is to expose students to the full range of options in nursing and to enable mastery through application of all that the students have learned.

There are factors, however, that occur with graduation and licensure that cannot be introduced in nursing school:

1. Legal accountability for one's own actions as well as for actions delegated to unlicensed assistive personnel
2. Increase in the number and acuity of patients being served
3. Awareness of the need for additional growth in knowledge base necessitated by choosing a particular setting in which and population with whom to work
4. Awareness of being a novice in nursing, with much to learn
5. Recognition that newly acquired skills need refinement, art, and creativity
6. Awareness of the need to work out relationships with team members representing various levels of expertise, years of socialization, values, and cultures
7. The experience of ongoing work versus the short-term experiences of semesters and changing environments

These are only a few of the variables that new graduates confront. Nursing education provides a foundation of knowledge and the tools to acquire the knowledge and skills that are still needed. There is no way, however, that new graduates enter the work world feeling totally prepared to handle any and all situations.

So what about the ideals of practice versus the reality? If you are practicing ethically, you need to understand that there is no ideal, yet at the same time you must not tolerate abuses in the name of reality. You need to practice with one foot firmly grounded in "what is" and the other foot facing toward "what ought to be" (Zoloth-Dorfman, 1994).

For instance, Joan, a nurse in charge, recognized that today the needs of the patients are greater than the resources—time, staff members, equipment, supplies, medications—available (what is); further, no more resources can be acquired from other sources. Therefore, "what ought to be" cannot be attained in the usual deployment and allocation of resources. Several options are available to Joan.

One viable option in this situation is to change what can be changed: allocation in the usual way. Joan can rearrange the schedule, stagger the use of equipment, assign staff members in different ways, and cancel nonessential tests and treatments (those that can wait until the next shift or next day). This option attempts to resolve a **moral (ethical) dilemma** (an issue in which there is no right or best solution) and decrease moral distress (the psychic pain experienced when no answer is a good one). In the process of living out an option, Joan will probably encounter **moral uncertainty.** For instance, Mr. Kay is having an acute episode of psychosis with paranoid features. In an effort to redeploy resources, Joan assesses that Mr. Kay will probably react suspiciously to the change and not be willing to participate in the added group activities, and his symptoms may escalate in response to the changed environmental stimulation. Should Joan

- Give Mr. Kay an antipsychotic medication on an as needed basis in anticipation of his response?
- Deploy a staff member to be particularly alert to Mr. Kay's needs with the understanding that another patient will receive less individual attention?
- Assign Mr. Kay specific treatment activities that require his spending time away from the group?
- Do nothing special?

And what about individual consideration for each and every patient receiving professional services under the accountability of Joan today? Is there time, need, or purpose to include other members of the team to assist in solving the dilemma of fewer resources? By definition, moral uncertainty has no clear solution. There is no room for Joan to become overwhelmed and immobilized by the ethical issues. Joan is expected to think clearly, clarify her own hierarchy of ethical values, and act consistently on behalf of the patients served in a timely, planned, calm manner. It is no surprise that the person with this level of ethical responsibility must be educated to make such decisions and is held legally accountable for doing so. **Accountability** is defined as taking full responsibility for one's actions.

Being accountable includes understanding the legal aspects of care. If the legally defined duties of care are violated in the course of care, then **malpractice** exists. Claims may be filed against the nurse under the law of negligent tort. A **tort** is a civil wrongdoing for which the injured party is entitled to compensation. Each nurse must consider personal malpractice liability insurance because the individual is held responsible in malpractice claims. To prove negligent tort, the plaintiff must prove a legal duty of care existed, the nurse performed the duty negligently, damages were suffered as a result, and the damages sustained were substantial (Box 5-2).

> **W**hat do you think? Some nurses believe that they are at greater risk for being sued if they carry their own malpractice insurance. How would you respond to this position?

> ➤ **Check Your Reading**
> 30. List three factors that new graduates confront when they leave the school environment.
> 31. What are some of the reality situations that confront the new graduate? Highlight the conflict between the ideal and the real.
> 32. List three ways to avoid litigation.

Good of the Group Versus Freedom of the Individual

Society is organized in families and other groups. All people function in and derive benefit from groups. Much of psychiatric-mental health treatment occurs in groups. Democratic principles emphasize the importance of the individual within the context of the group, which reinforces the nurse's mandate to weigh the rights of the individual against the good of the group. Quite often, the nurse and other members of the treatment team must struggle with two mutually exclusive principles: the greatest good for the greatest number, contrasted with the primacy of the individual. Many of our current social issues bring home this conflict: gun control, smoking, pollution, and domestic violence, to name a few.

In the psychiatric-mental health arena, what is the right thing to do? Some mentally ill people, not harmful

Box 5-2 ■ ■ ■ ■ ■
Defenses Against Lawsuits

- Implement care based on standards of nursing practice
- Know the laws of your state and the specifics of the nurse practice act as it relates to your practice
- Maintain confidentiality of patient information
- Keep accurate and concise nursing records
- Maintain therapeutic boundaries, avoid sexual contact and personal relationships with patients
- Obtain informed consent
- Report potential abuse or neglect
- Ensure adequate supervision of employees
- Document the communication and coordination of patient care
- Observe and record patient activity while on suicide observation per physician order

to themselves or others, choose to live homeless. Sometimes they are arrested for violating society's rights through petty theft, loitering, and pandering. Sometimes they are victims of rape, theft, and murder because of the vulnerability of homelessness. Should they have to live with, and pay for, the consequences? Do they choose homelessness because they are sick and therefore not capable of choosing? If society decides that homelessness is not a choice, where is adequate housing provided? Who pays for the housing? Who forces the person to use the housing provided, and how is that enforced? Does forcing someone to sleep in a shelter constitute false imprisonment? There are many questions and no easy answers.

In a small, relatively simple environment of an inpatient unit, how does the nurse respond to the aimless wandering of one patient into other patients' rooms (the individual's right to privacy)? How does the nurse respond when a patient screams angry obscenities, disturbing the patients in the group session next door (the individual's right to freedom of expression versus the group's right to a safe environment)? In a therapeutic milieu (environment), the nurse is responsible for managing the ambiance of the unit. So what does the nurse do?

It is said that one person's rights end at the next person's nose. How far does that right extend? To olfactory cells in the nose? To one's ears? We do not tolerate physical aggression, but where does the line exist for verbal abuse, emotional abuse, or sexual abuse? Although society, families, churches, legislatures, and courts try to determine general guidelines, the nurse judges, decides, legislates, and acts every hour of the day. The decisions differ from nurse to nurse, setting to setting, situation to situation, and sometimes day to day.

The guiding principle in the struggle of individual versus group rights is this: How can both individual and group rights be affirmed within the context of the individual's and group's responsibilities? The solutions require sensitivity, creativity, commitment, and support. The answers do not come easily. Often, both the individual and the group cannot be affirmed; a choice must be made and the consequences accepted. After such an experience, it helps to talk with a friend, a spiritual advocate, or God. Clarification, illumination, and comfort may emerge (Fowler, 1989). Wisdom and choices may accrue. But there will never be a time when you always know the right thing to do.

> **W**hat do you think? Have you ever struggled to balance an individual's rights against a group's rights? How did you handle or resolve the conflict?

> ➤ **Check Your Reading**
> 33. Identify one conflict in which the nurse must make a choice between the good of the individual and the good of the staff members.
> 34. What is the guiding principle when a conflict between the individual's and group's needs occurs?

Behavior Control

Behavior control once meant only the manipulation of a person's behavior by design. Now, with the institutionalization of biofeedback, meditation, medication, and other variables, behavior control is more complex. The use of food, odors, and pleasurable stimuli; the installation of patient-controlled analgesia units; and the installation of transcutaneous electrical nerve stimulation units to alter mood, pain, and behavior are opportunities to alter, and possibly to control, behavior.

The crux of the issue of behavior control is accountability. The person who controls the behavior is accountable for it. Right behind the issue of accountability is the question of control. Does a person have control (at least 51%) over her or his behavior? At what point is a person in control and accountable?

Coercive behavior controls are **seclusion** and **restraint.** If a patient cannot control himself or herself, staff members exert control to prohibit harm to the self or others. In this situation, behavior control is justified based on the principle of beneficence over autonomy. The protection of self and others is emphasized over the freedom of movement. Chemical restraints (medications) may be viewed by staff members as less coercive than physical restraints but are actually the most restrictive form of restraints and involve the same ethical issues (Parker, 1993).

In order for a staff member to use seclusion or restraint, less restrictive alternatives must have failed. By using early interventions, therapeutic one-to-one verbal support, and medications as required and understanding prodromal signs such as escalating psychotic behavior and nonpsychotic agitation, occurrence of seclusion or restraint decreases. Understanding this therapeutic strategy demonstrates the effectiveness of interactions in safely dealing with aggressive situations and assisting the patient to maintain self-control.

There are more subtle behavior controls, such as rewarding desirable behavior, punishing undesirable behavior, and allowing natural consequences to flow from the person's behavior. We have all been socialized through these processes. These forms of behavior control are formally applied with students, with individuals who are developmentally delayed, and with the chronically mentally ill, to name a few. These methods of reinforcement are considered ethically appropriate, even morally right.

Behavior control is an ethical issue when the person being manipulated or controlled is harmed physically, emotionally, spiritually, financially, or socially by the manipulation. For instance, members of the nursing staff expect all patients to be asleep before evening change of shifts so that fewer staff members are required for the night shift; the evening nurse medicates all patients, as needed, with sleeping medication or antihistamines, turns off the television, and sends everybody to bed an hour before the night shift arrives.

A patient may decide to enter into a **no-suicide contract** with the therapist, choosing to forego suicide as an option, under the specifics of the contract. The therapist-nurse may have encouraged the decision and may have indicated that the therapeutic relationship would be terminated without the contract. The therapist-nurse has used the power of the relationship and will enforce consequences if the patient does not enter into the contract or breaks the contract. This is a form of behavior control. Is it unethical? The patient may believe it is and question the therapist-nurse's fidelity.

Multiple ethical issues arise by the moment, in every relationship, in every setting. Ethical principles that clarify, guide, and comfort the nurse have been presented. For an expert practitioner, the ethical issues do not go away and may, in fact, be more poignant and more distressing than for a novice practitioner with much yet to learn.

What do you think? Do we have the right to control the behavior of another individual?

➤ *Check Your Reading*

35. What is the most restrictive form of constraint?
36. What is the crux of the behavior control issue?
37. Name two types of coercive behavior controls.

LEGAL PARAMETERS FOR THE JOURNEY

In addition to ethics, with its endless questions, there are legal restrictions and obligations with firm boundaries that influence the practice of psychiatric nursing. Some are mandated through laws from state to state; others are mandated by professional and consumer protection groups and acknowledged among professional groups and in courts as being the power of the law.

Voluntary Versus Involuntary Treatment

When people are harmful to themselves or others or cannot take care of themselves properly, they are in need of help. If the person chooses treatment, enters into an active decision-making process with the treatment team, and works to achieve treatment goals, a positive treatment relationship and outcome are likely to result. The illness and ensuing dysfunctional behavior patterns, however, may keep the patient from participating fully in the recommendations made, and the patient may need to grapple with the meaning and purpose of illness as stated earlier. With either situation, the patient may voluntarily agree to accept treatment. This **voluntary treatment** must be based on informed consent.

Some people, however, do not agree to enter into treatment, and the clinicians who have made the determination of need for treatment must make a decision: Is this person imminently dangerous to self or others or unable to take care of fundamental human needs? If either answer is "yes," the clinician has a legal obligation both to protect the person and society and to protect the person's right to freedom. This is the first step of **involuntary treatment,** sometimes called *commitment.* Although the specific protocols and time frames vary from state to state, the guidelines in Box 5–3 capture the legal requirements.

Mary's Story

"Please don't take me. . . . Please, please. I'm not sick, I'm not crazy. You don't understand—they were out to get me. I know that they have been plotting for weeks. They have listened to my conversations through the walls of my apartment; they follow me when I leave. You don't see them but I know they're out there. Please let me go—no—don't put those handcuffs on me—I didn't do anything wrong! Who told you to take me away? I'm not crazy." ∎

Box 5–3 ∎ ∎ ∎ ∎ ∎
Legal Requirements for Involuntary Detention

- When the accountable clinician decides to detain the patient, the papers to notify the court (or its designee) must be completed, the patient needs to know, and family needs to be notified if the patient agrees.
- The hospital/clinic/clinician may not hold a patient against his or her will for any length of time, unless the state has been notified. This allows the state or its designee to oversee the patient's rights, ensure a hearing of the facts, and determine what is in the best interest of the patient and society.
- The state (via judge, court, hearing) determines if the patient may exercise his or her prerogative and refuse treatment or if the patient is to be held involuntarily (against his or her will) for treatment.
- A length of time is determined, after which the patient shall have the right to speak to the court or its designee. Again, the court determines the patient's current status in relation to harm to self or others and ability to care for basic human needs. The patient may be required to remain in treatment involuntarily or may be released from treatment at that hearing.
- At any time before the hearing, the patient may decide to enter into treatment voluntarily or may get better and not have to be forced by the treatment team to continue in treatment. The court is simply notified of the change in patient health status or decision and the hearing is canceled.

Mary is 38 years old. She is diagnosed with paranoid schizophrenia. She is very ill. For 2 weeks her behavior has become increasingly threatening to her neighbors. Finally, her landlord called 911 and reported Mary's behavior to the police who have come to take Mary to the emergency department for an evaluation. Mary is being taken against her will. She is being removed from her apartment in handcuffs. She has not hurt anyone—but she has frightened others with her verbal ranting. People fear Mary; they believe she poses a danger to them.

W*hat do you think?* Does Mary pose a danger to people? Is there a better way to protect both Mary and her neighbors? Are Mary's rights being violated in this situation? How should Mary be treated? How do we balance individual and community rights?

Mary's situation highlights a major difference between psychiatry and other specialties. When a psychiatric patient becomes acutely ill, resulting in difficult and threatening behaviors, the patient may be treated like a criminal rather than like a person who is sick. Contrast this situation with that of a diabetic patient who neglects to manage her or his care and goes into a diabetic coma. We generally do not hold the diabetic patient to the same level of personal responsibility and accountability for self-care management as we do the psychiatric patient who may have far less control over her or his illness.

Mary's admission will probably be an involuntary one; she will be committed. Let's take a closer look at the differences between these two types of admission.

Voluntary Admission

If Mary had gone to her psychiatrist or the emergency department and asked to be admitted because she recognized that her paranoia was increasing, that would be called a "voluntary admission." Seventy-three percent of the 1.6 million annual admissions to psychiatric hospitals in the United States are voluntary. Patients willingly seek help and recognize that they are having difficulty managing life. In these situations, patients lose none of their civil rights; they can still vote, hold onto their driver's licenses, buy and sell property, engage in business affairs, practice their professions, and hold office. Just as these people decided to admit themselves, they can decide to discharge themselves. Certainly, this is the best situation; however, it is not always possible.

Involuntary Admission or Commitment

In situations such as Mary's, in which the patient poses a danger to others, the state can act to force the individual to receive help. The state is able to do this through two legal theories. The first is through police powers, which authorize the state to protect the community from the potentially dangerous acts of the mentally ill, and sometimes the mentally retarded, substance abusers, and mentally disabled minors. Police powers are invoked when the patient is suicidal, is homicidal, poses a danger to others, has a mental illness, and rejects help. The second theory is that of *parens patriae*. Under this theory, the state can provide care for those who are unable to take care of themselves. There is a trend in all the states to use *parens patriae* less frequently than police powers to impose an involuntary hospitalization on an individual. This is due to three issues:

1. Increased emphasis on individual liberty and rights
2. Increased emphasis on mandating treatment in the least restrictive setting
3. Increased budgetary constraints at the state level, which have required many states to get out of the business of caring for the mentally ill

The standards for involuntary commitment vary considerably across states. Because of this, it is essential that you learn what your state requires. Box 5-3 summarizes legal requirements for involuntary hospitalization.

Involuntary hospitalization or commitment carries with it significant stigma. In addition, patients lose their civil rights, including

1. Entering into contracts
2. Voting
3. Driving
4. Serving on a jury
5. Marrying
6. Entering into civil litigation
7. Obtaining a professional license

The decision to involuntarily hospitalize an individual is not one to be made lightly.

Process for Involuntary Hospitalization

Let's go back to Mary and take a look at what led to her being removed from her apartment and what will most likely happen next. Mary's landlord called 911 and lodged a formal complaint against Mary, which the police are required to investigate. The landlord could also have gone to court and entered a sworn petition against Mary. A judge who would determine whether Mary's situation necessitated police intervention would have heard this petition. Once Mary is transported to a medical facility, one or two physicians (depending on the state) will examine her and decide whether Mary requires treatment or can be released. Some states require that one of the physicians be a psychiatrist. The decision to admit can be the result of a medical, a court, or an administrative commitment. Box 5-4 defines these different commitments.

Again, let's return to Mary's situation. After Mary is examined, two physicians, one a psychiatrist, determine that Mary requires short-term hospitalization. There are three types of involuntary hospitalization that they can recommend:

1. **Emergency hospitalization:** Used for acutely ill patients to control an immediate threat to self or others. Usually, emergency hospitalization is limited to 48 to 72

Box 5–4 ■ ■ ■ ■ ■
Medical, Court, and Administrative Commitments

Medical: Physicians decide whether or not to commit patients; used primarily in emergency situations.

Court: Judge or jury decides whether or not to commit in a formal hearing; this method of commitment is used more frequently than the other two because it allows the individual due process of the law and protects the individual against infringements on liberty and rights that are protected by the 14th Amendment of the U.S. Constitution. Although the patient has the right to legal counsel and the right to have counsel appointed if he or she does not have counsel, this right is not always recognized.

Administrative: A tribunal of hearing officers decides whether or not to commit patients..

hours by state law. It allows individuals to be detained in a psychiatric hospital until necessary legal steps can be taken for additional hospitalization.

2. **Short-term hospitalization:** Used for observation, diagnosis, and short-term treatment. Usually, hospitalization is for a designated period, which varies by state. At the end of that period, the patient is reevaluated to determine readiness for discharge; if the patient is not ready, then a petition can be filed for a long-term commitment.

3. **Long-term or formal commitment:** Allows for hospitalization for an indefinite period. Patients maintain the right to consult a lawyer and petition the court to reevaluate their need for continued hospitalization. The patient's situation is reviewed by the court at intervals of 3, 6, and 12 months, at which times the need for continued hospitalization is determined.

What do you think? How would you respond to Mary to ensure that her rights were protected?

➤ *Check Your Reading*
38. Define voluntary treatment.
39. What is required before an involuntary admission can occur?

Involuntary Community Treatment

Patient rights guarantee treatment in the least restrictive environment. As a response to this right, assertive community treatment program models are beginning to recognize that involuntary commitment procedures can be used for people with severe and persistent mental illness who are at risk of harm to self or others (Richmond, Trujillo, Schmelzer, Phillips, & Davis,

1996). Geller (1993) proposed that patients who meet the criteria for outpatient commitment can be successfully treated in the community setting. Outpatient commitment is appropriate if

1. The patient expresses an interest in living in the community.
2. The patient has previously failed in the community.
3. The patient has a degree of competency necessary to understand the stipulations of his or her involuntary community treatment.
4. The patient has the capacity to comply with the involuntary community treatment plan and is not dangerous to self or others.
5. The treatment ordered has demonstrated efficacy when used properly by the patient in question.
6. The ordered treatment can be delivered in the outpatient system, is sufficient for the patient's needs, and is necessary to sustain community tenure, which is the patient's ability to function and remain in the community.
7. The ordered treatment can be monitored by an outpatient treatment facility.
8. The treating agency delivers the ordered treatment and willingly participates in enforcing compliance with those treatments.
9. The public sector inpatient system supports the outpatient system's participation in the provision of involuntary community treatment.

What do you think? What do you think are the dangers and benefits of involuntary community treatment?

► *Check Your Reading*
40. Define involuntary community treatment.
41. Define the type of person who would benefit from this level of care.

Criminal Responsibility: The Insanity Defense

"Not guilty by reason of insanity" (NGRI) and "guilty but mentally ill" (GBMI) are two defenses that generate much public attention. NGRI states that when the person committed the crime, he or she could not tell right from wrong or could not control his or her behavior because of a mental defect or illness. The law holds that the person should not be held criminally responsible for his or her behavior, but the legal test of this can vary from state to state. Insanity, as a legal description, explains a behavior, but it does not excuse it.

Those found NGRI are rarely set free. They are committed at the court's discretion, often to a state mental facility. No discharge or release date is predetermined. The person is released only, again, at the discretion of the court that ordered the commitment.

Montana, Idaho, and Utah have abolished the insanity defense and incarcerate people who have been found GBMI in prison along with other convicted inmates.

Release from commitment is dependent on the patient's being evaluated as likely to not repeat the offense and as safe to be released into the community. Studies have shown that people found NGRI or GBMI, on the average, are held at least as long as and often longer than people found guilty and sent to prison for similar crimes.

What do you think? Why do you think NGRI and GBMI are controversial?

► *Check Your Reading*
42. Describe NGRI.
43. What criteria must be met for release from commitment by reason of insanity?

Nurse Practice Acts

Each state has defined nursing and nursing practice. Although these definitions are conceptual to allow for evolution in knowledge base and practice, they also establish boundaries within which the nurse must practice. Boards established in each state are delegated the responsibility of protecting the public from abuse of nursing practice. Most state practice acts specify the following information:

1. Process to obtain licensure and to practice within that state
2. Definition of the educational requirements for entry into practice
3. Definition of the scope of practice for each level of nursing
4. Process by which board of nursing members are selected
5. Type of situations in which disciplinary action is warranted
6. Details of appeal steps a nurse can take if he or she believes disciplinary steps taken by the board are not fair

What do you think? Why is it important to be familiar with your nurse practice act?

► *Check Your Reading*
44. Identify three types of information included in each state's nurse practice act.
45. What is the purpose of the nurse practice acts in each state?

Boundary Issues

Maintaining appropriate distance while offering oneself for a healing relationship requires considerable skill (see Chapter 10 for a thorough discussion of nurse-patient relationships). How close is too close? When is professional conduct actually alienating? There are at least two participants and several audiences to consider in addressing boundary issues: the patient; the nurse; and the profession's, institution's, and society's standards.

Patients often have damage to their sense of self and where they believe their **personal boundaries** are. Some patients have no sense of boundaries because they have endured repeated personal violations. These patients often intrude into others' personal space by standing too close to others, moving too quickly toward others, touching others' bodies in inappropriate places, or touching others for too long. What is an inappropriate statement or act to most people does not bother these patients at all. They have deficits in boundary awareness and boundary maintenance.

Boundaries may also be closed and rigid, and the person may need an unusually large amount of personal space. Actions or statements that are unusual but appropriate to most people may be highly intrusive to patients with rigid boundaries. Culture also has a profound influence on the awareness and maintenance of boundaries. For instance, in some cultures, people talk loudly and stand close to one another, whereas in other cultures, people have no physical contact.

Members of the nursing staff may have the same deficits in boundary awareness and maintenance. People who migrate to health careers because of experiences in dysfunctional families often have boundary problems. They may be more *or* less tolerant with societal norms related to aggressive language, physical comforting, and signals of intimacy, for instance. In addition, the professions have made a distinction between professional and social relationships; these relationships may not exist in the same time frame, and they have specific principles that guide them (see Chapter 10). The purpose of this distinction is to protect the patient from abuse of power and exploitation in the relationship. In a professional relationship, the good of the patient is the central and sole concern; the needs of the helping person are met separate and apart from the helping relationship.

Ethically, nurses must be alert to the possibility of sexual, emotional, and financial exploitation, both for themselves and for the members of the health care team with whom they work. Box 5-5 lists some common boundary dilemmas that occur in hospitals and other settings.

Boundary violations exist on a continuum. They may be as horrific as rape or emotional battering. They may be as subtle as extra long hugs, accidental brushes against private parts, or the quiet assurance that the staff member is the only one who really understands and can help. Constant awareness, confrontation, and discussion among staff members are absolutely necessary for staff members to maintain professional, helpful relationships with patients.

Boundary violations may occur among staff members as well. Therefore, the same monitoring and diligence are necessary to maintain open communication in the work group. The mildest influence of social relationships in the work group is pairing, which may

Box 5-5 ■ ■ ■ ■ ■
Common Boundary Dilemmas

- The patient's door is closed; the psychiatric technician knocks and quickly opens the door, catching the patient stepping out of the shower.
- The psychiatric technician knocks and is told not to come in; the technician is obligated to document a personal evaluation of the patient's status (at 15-minute checks) and must see the patient. Because the patient answered, shall the technician document personal evaluation or insist on seeing the patient?
  What if the patient says, "I'm fine. I'm trying to take a nap"? What if the patient says, "Leave me alone! Why won't you trust me?"
  What if the patient says, "I'm not dressed"?
- Being attracted to a patient is not uncommon. How does the nurse deal with that?
  What if the patient asks her to meet him at the coffee shop on her break?
  What if the nurse gives her phone number to the patient and offers her support after discharge?
- What if a grandmotherly, nurturing nurse regularly touches, pats, and caresses her patients, giving them all the same amount of attention? Is there potential for boundary violation?

considerably hinder the group's healthy function. Energy needed for patient care is siphoned off into social relationships.

What do you think? How can a patient violate the boundaries of a nurse? How can this be handled while being respectful of the patient?

➤ *Check Your Reading*
46. Give two examples of behaviors that a person with undefined or loose boundaries might display.
47. What characterizes an individual with rigid boundaries?

RIGHTS OF PATIENTS ON THE JOURNEY

People needing psychiatric-mental health services are similar to all people in every other respect: They have the right to life, liberty, and the pursuit of happiness. Because of the stigma of psychiatric illness, however, extra effort is made to ensure that the rights of psychiatric patients are safeguarded. The American Nurses Association (ANA, 1985) code for nurses codifies the rights of psychiatric patients. Other attempts to codify the rights of psychiatric patients include those put forth by the U.S. Mental Health Systems Act (1980) and by the American Hospital Association (1994).

American Nurses Association Code for Nurses

Written in 1976, with subsequent interpretive statements (ANA, 1985), the ANA code for nurses establishes baseline expectations for all registered nurses without exception. The following items are included in the code:

Item 1: "The nurse provides services with respect for human dignity and the uniqueness of the patient, unrestricted by considerations of social or economic status, personal attributes, or the nature of health problems." This item requires the nurse to act consistently on behalf of all patients. If ethically distressed, the nurse may refuse to provide a particular treatment or may have the patient transferred to another nurse's care. These are not options, however, if the nurse is distressed over the patient's condition (such as AIDS), personal attributes (such as a rape conviction), or socioeconomic status (such as homelessness). Nurses are committed to caring for all people.

Item 2: "The nurse safeguards the patient's right to privacy by judiciously protecting information of a confidential nature." Confidentiality is a mandate of the profession, with legal consequences in the case of patients with AIDS or chemical dependency. Probably because the stigma of these illnesses is great, these patients are specifically protected at a higher level of legal sanction. All patients, however, have the right to "tell their story," in their own way, to a person of their own choice. Psychiatric records are histories of intimate, sometimes damaging information; therefore, confidentiality includes medical and other written and electronic records. Telephone answering devices, cellular phones, computers, and facsimile machines must also be used with utmost caution.

Item 3: "The nurse acts to safeguard the patient and the public when health care and safety are affected by the incompetent, unethical, or illegal practice of any person." When nurses suspect or confirm impaired practice in themselves or another, they have an ethical obligation to act to safeguard individual patients and society as a whole. Within an organization, there are ethics and clinical practice committees that encourage and receive such information. The state board of the profession to which the clinician belongs is also an excellent source for assistance in dealing with a clinician who jeopardizes the safety and health of patients. The state board is the next step when an employer refuses to accept or investigate a legitimate concern for practice.

Item 4: "The nurse assumes responsibility and accountability for individual nursing judgments and actions." The nurse, by virtue of legal license and ethical obligation, is held responsible for consistently acting on behalf of patients, including respecting the autonomy of patients.

Item 5: "The nurse maintains competence in nursing." Case Example 5–2 illustrated the ethical dilemma that may occur when the nurse has not maintained a current knowledge base and clinical judgment in the specific area of practice. The example was outdated knowledge related to ECT.

Item 6: "The nurse exercises informed judgment and uses individual competence and qualifications as criteria in seeking consultation, accepting responsibilities, and delegating nursing activities to others." Health care is expensive, chaotic, and rapidly changing. The nurse is expected to act on behalf of the patient by using all appropriate resources. Assistive personnel are a wonderful resource when used appropriately. Willingness to take on new responsibilities is expected when the nurse has adequate knowledge and clinical judgment to perform the new responsibilities. Anyone expecting the nurse to increase responsibilities should also be aware of the ethical mandate to help the nurse demonstrate competency.

Item 7: "The nurse participates in activities that contribute to the ongoing development of the profession's body of knowledge." The nurse participates in developing clinical protocols, testing new ways of practice, and writing nursing care plans.

Item 8: "The nurse participates in the profession's efforts to implement and improve standards of nursing." The nurse must be aware of the standards and any updates in order to implement and improve the standards of nursing. Membership in the state nurses association provides ready access to the latest information on standards development and implementation. Standards are implemented in a variety of ways. Nurses and institutions have different ways to implement standards. Sharing various methods of implementation helps everyone improve standards. For instance, some agencies use case managers, others use clinical pathways, and others use standards of care. Some nurses focus on the nature of the nurse-patient relationship to encourage participation in treatment. Other nurses may identify and use the patient's internal motivators. Others may work on goals and encourage the patient to actively pursue these goals.

Item 9: "The nurse participates in the profession's efforts to establish and maintain conditions of employment conducive to high-quality nursing care." The environment within which a nurse practices influences the quality of care provided. For instance, one agency may be highly structured, and the nurses there may work primarily with policies, procedures, and protocols. Another agency may have little structure and may expect the nurse to practice at a high standard, regardless of education or experience. When conditions adversely affect the work of the practice environment, the nurse has an ethical responsibility to communicate and suggest solutions.

Item 10: "The nurse participates in the profession's efforts to protect the public from misinformation and misrepresentation and to maintain the integrity of nursing." Misinformation exists about various diseases and their effects, the vulnerability of the community to the effects of mental illness, and the contribution nursing makes to health care. A nurse's responsibility goes far beyond a particular practice setting and patient or family group. The obligation includes embracing the community's understanding of health and the myriad factors that influence it. For example, being involved in the local parent-teacher organization and being involved in the passage of legislation for public health endeavors are ways to influence community health. Failure to fulfill this obligation adversely affects society's relationship with nursing.

Item 11: "The nurse collaborates with members of the health professions and other citizens in promoting community and national efforts to meet public health needs." Nurses are aware of the necessity to address issues related to health and health care on the community, state (provincial), and national levels. The code requires each nurse to participate in some way beyond his or her employment to help meet the health needs of the public.

Other Attempts to Codify the Rights of Psychiatric Patients

One attempt to codify the rights of psychiatric patients is the Bill of Rights for Patients included in the U.S. Mental Health Systems Act (1980) (Box 5-6). Another attempt to codify those rights was developed by the American Hospital Association (1994) (Box 5-7).

> ➤ *Check Your Reading*
> 48. Name at least four rights of psychiatric patients.
> 49. What is the purpose of the ANA Code for Nurses?

THREE IMPORTANT PROCESSES AFFECTING THE THERAPEUTIC RELATIONSHIP

The three processes to be explored here strengthen the nurse's role in any setting; in addition, there are other significant processes. These were chosen because of their significance in the therapeutic relationship between psychiatric patients and nurses. The three processes are confidentiality, therapeutic alliance, and advocacy.

Confidentiality

A therapeutic relationship (see Chapter 10) absolutely requires that the nurse handle intimate communications with utmost respect, almost with awe. To trust another

---

B o x 5 – 6 ■ ■ ■ ■ ■
Mental Health Systems Act Recommended Bill of Rights for Patients

- The right to appropriate treatment in settings and under conditions most supportive of and least restrictive to personal liberty
- The right to an individualized, written treatment plan
- The right to ongoing participation in the planning of services and the right to a reasonable explanation of general mental condition, treatment objectives, adverse effects of treatment, reasons for treatment, and available alternatives
- The right to refuse treatment except when the patient poses imminent danger to self or others

---

person is a gift, which, for psychiatric patients, must be earned. **Confidentiality** of information is basic to the relationship. Ethical dilemmas develop, however. The patient asks you if you can keep a secret; another says you must promise not to tell after the information is already shared. With whom may the information be shared? Guidelines for maintaining confidentiality in psychiatric–mental health nursing are presented in Box 5-8.

The one exception to confidentiality relates to the **Tarasoff decision** (*Tarasoff v. Regents of the University of California,* 1976) (Box 5-9). In the Tarasoff case, a California court clearly established the therapist's duty to use reasonable care to protect a known, intended victim of a patient's threats. The court ruled that this duty might be discharged by either warning the prospective victim or taking other reasonable steps under the circumstances. Many state and some federal courts have agreed with the California ruling that a Tarasoff-type duty to warn exists for mental health care professionals. The extent of this duty to warn, however, and how it may be discharged varies from state to state.

> ➤ *Check Your Reading*
> 50. What does it mean to keep information confidential?
> 51. Name two of the conflicts that arise from the issue of confidentiality.
> 52. What is the implication of the Tarasoff decision?

Therapeutic Alliance

Although much has been said about boundary maintenance and prohibition of sexual or exploitative behavior, the other side of boundary maintenance, the **therapeutic alliance,** has not been mentioned in an ethical context. The nurse is obliged to attempt to reach the patient, to make a connection that is healthy and encouraging, and to journey for a while with that person.

Box 5-7 ■ ■ ■ ■ ■
A Patient's Bill of Rights

Introduction

Effective health care requires collaboration between patients and physicians and other health care professionals. Open and honest communication, respect for personal and professional values, and sensitivity to differences are integral to optimal patient care. As the setting for the provision of health services, hospitals must provide a foundation for understanding and respecting the rights and responsibilities of patients, their families, physicians, and other caregivers. Hospitals must ensure a health care ethic that respects the role of patients in decision making about treatment choices and other aspects of their care. Hospitals must be sensitive to cultural, racial, linguistic, religious, age, gender, and other differences as well as the needs of people with disabilities.

The American Hospital Association (1994) presents *A Patient's Bill of Rights* with the expectation that it will contribute to more effective patient care and be supported by the hospital on behalf of the institution, its medical staff, employees, and patients. The American Hospital Association encourages health care institutions to tailor this bill of rights to their patient community by translating and/or simplifying the language of this bill of rights as may be necessary to ensure that patients and their families understand their rights and responsibilities.

Bill of Rights°

1. The patient has the right to considerate and respectful care.
2. The patient has the right to and is encouraged to obtain from physicians and other direct caregivers relevant, current, and understandable information concerning diagnosis, treatment, and prognosis.
3. Except in emergencies when the patient lacks decision-making capacity and the need for treatment is urgent, the patient is entitled to the opportunity to discuss and request information related to the specific procedures and/or treatments, the risks involved, the possible length of recuperation, and the medically reasonable alternatives and their accompanying risks and benefits.
4. Patients have the right to know the identity of physicians, nurses, and others involved in their care, as well as when those involved are students, residents, or other trainees. The patient also has the right to know the immediate and long-term financial implications of treatment choices, insofar as they are known.
5. The patient has the right to make decisions about the plan of care prior to and during the course of treatment and to refuse a recommended treatment or plan of care to the extent permitted by law and hospital policy and to be informed of the medical consequences of this action. In case of such refusal, the patient is entitled to other appropriate care and services that the hospital provides or transfer to another hospital. The hospital should notify patients of any policy that might affect patient choice within the institution.
6. The patient has the right to have an advance directive (such as a living will, health care proxy, or durable power of attorney for health care) concerning treatment or designating a surrogate decision maker with the expectation that the hospital will honor the intent of that directive to the extent permitted by law and hospital policy.
7. Health care institutions must advise patients of their rights under state law and hospital policy to make informed medical choices, ask if the patient has an advance directive, and include that information in patient records. The patient has the right to timely information about hospital policy that may limit its ability to implement fully a legally valid advance directive.
8. The patient has the right to every consideration of privacy. Case discussion, consultation, examination, and treatment should be conducted so as to protect each patient's privacy.
9. The patient has the right to expect that all communications and records pertaining to his/her care will be treated as confidential by the hospital, except in cases such as suspected abuse and public health hazards when reporting is permitted or required by law. The patient has the right to expect that the hospital will emphasize the confidentiality of this information when it releases it to any other parties entitled to review information in these records.
10. The patient has the right to review the records pertaining to his/her medical care and to have the information explained or interpreted as necessary, except when restricted by law.
11. The patient has the right to expect that, within its capacity and policies, a hospital will make reasonable response to the request of a patient for appropriate and medically indicated care and services. The hospital must provide evaluation, service, and/or referral as indicated by the urgency of the case. When medically appropriate and legally permissible, or when a patient has so requested, a patient may be transferred to another facility. The institution to which the patient is to be transferred must first have accepted the patient for transfer. The patient must also have the benefit of complete information and explanation concerning the need for, risks, benefits, and alternatives to such a transfer.

Box 5–7 ■ ■ ■ ■ ■

A Patient's Bill of Rights *Continued*

12. The patient has the right to ask and be informed of the existence of business relationships among the hospital, educational institutions, other health care providers, or payers that may influence the patient's treatment and care.

13. The patient has the right to consent to or decline to participate in proposed research studies or human experimentation affecting care and treatment or requiring direct patient involvement, and to have those studies fully explained prior to consent. A patient who declines to participate in research or experimentation is entitled to the most effective care that the hospital can otherwise provide.

14. The patient has the right to expect reasonable continuity of care when appropriate and to be informed by physicians and other caregivers of available and realistic patient care options when hospital care is no longer appropriate.

15. The patient has the right to be informed of hospital policies and practices that relate to patient care, treatment, and responsibilities. The patient has the right to be informed of available resources for resolving disputes, grievances, and conflicts, such as ethics committees, patient representatives, or other mechanisms available in the institution. The patient has the right to be informed of the hospital's charges for services and available payment methods.

The collaborative nature of health care requires that patients, or their families/surrogates, participate in their care. The effectiveness of care and patient satisfaction with the course of treatment depend, in part, on the patient fulfilling certain responsibilities. Patients are responsible for providing information about past illnesses, hospitalizations, medications, and other matters related to health status. To participate effectively in decision making, patients must be encouraged to take responsibility for requesting additional information or clarification about their health status or treatment when they do not fully understand information and instructions. Patients are also responsible for ensuring that the health care institution has a copy of their written advance directive if they have one. Patients are responsible for informing their physicians and other caregivers if they anticipate problems in following prescribed treatment.

Patients should also be aware of the hospital's obligation to be reasonably efficient and equitable in providing care to other patients and the community. The hospital's rules and regulations are designed to help the hospital meet this obligation. Patients and their families are responsible for making reasonable accommodations to the needs of the hospital, other patients, medical staff, and hospital employees. Patients are responsible for providing necessary information for insurance claims and for working with the hospital to make payment arrangements, when necessary.

A person's health depends on much more than health care services. Patients are responsible for recognizing the impact of their life-style on their personal health.

Conclusion

Hospitals have many functions to perform, including the enhancement of health status, health promotion, and the prevention and treatment of injury and disease; the immediate and ongoing care and rehabilitation of patients; the education of health professionals, patients, and the community; and research. All these activities must be conducted with an overriding concern for the values and dignity of patients.

*These rights can be exercised on the patient's behalf by a designated surrogate or proxy decision maker if the patient lacks decision-making capacity, is legally incompetent, or is a minor.

Reprinted with permission of the American Hospital Association, copyright 1994. AHA. (1994). *Values in conflict: Resolving ethical issues in health care* (2nd ed.). Chicago: American Hospital Association.

There are days when nurses may treat that obligation as an unreasonable burden or an unrealistic expectation. The nurse who chooses to be in psychiatric–mental health nursing also chooses to be available to patients for healthy therapeutic relationships. Dealing with countertransference, cultural differences, and personality differences are necessary in nursing if you are to be available for patients (see Chapters 8, 10, and 12).

Using the power inherent in the nurse-patient relationship for the sole and specific good of the patient is necessary. Is insistence on payment for service or not sharing one's phone number in the best interest of the patient? In the best interest of the nurse? Maybe both, but you are obliged to be brutally honest with yourself about real motives and desires. Psychiatric nurses find it useful to be supervised by a supportive, objective professional who has more experience and who can assist the nurse to look at these issues.

▶ *Check Your Reading*

53. What is a therapeutic alliance?

Advocacy

The primary role of **advocacy** is to protect the patient's rights and interests. Fortunately, the entire team as well

Box 5–8 ■ ■ ■ ■ ■
Guidelines for Maintaining Confidentiality in Psychiatric–Mental Health Nursing

- Do not promise to keep a secret. Secrets are appropriate in a social relationship but not in a therapeutic one.
- Do promise to respect the person's confidence and to share it only with members of the team who need to know. For instance, share information with members of the direct care staff that the patient intends to commit suicide tonight. Share financial concerns and medication problems with the multidisciplinary team. Share with the supervisor a revelation that a team member was perceived to be making sexual advances toward the patient.
- Be careful to neither deny nor confirm someone's presence in the mental health system. This includes the patient's friends in the community who say, "Oh, Mary, my best friend, is at your clinic. How is she doing?" Or the nurse's spouse may ask how a coworker is faring on a unit at the hospital. A child may want a specific example, including defining characteristics, of how the nurse-parent helped somebody that day. Each of these is problematic in relationship to confidentiality.
- Be careful with medical and electronic records. Do not read the charts or listen to reports about people for whom you will not be providing services. To do so in curiosity is not to be indulged as a professional.

Box 5–9 ■ ■ ■ ■ ■
Exceptions That Allow for Release of Information Without the Patient's Consent

- Emergency situations when acting in the patient's best interest
- Court-ordered release by subpoena duces tecum (except in the case of alcohol or substance abuse)
- Court-ordered evaluation or report
- Criminal proceedings
- Reporting crimes, threats, or suspected abuse or neglect
- Agency legal counsel
- The coroner
- Commitment proceedings
- Acting to protect third parties (Tarasoff decision)
- Reports required by state law

as society has a role to play in advocacy: What hurts one hurts all; what helps one is an encouragement to all. A strict advocacy role requires one to rise above fear of reprisal and assertively speak for the patient or insist that the patient be heard. Anyone who assesses that the patient's rights may be in jeopardy is required to make that situation known. Many ways exist to communicate a concern that the patient has not been heard. Ethics committees exist as patient advocates in a complex environment. Administrators often have open-door policies in relation to ethical issues; many institutions have policies protecting an employee who speaks out on behalf of a patient.

Once the institution has heard and responded and a conclusion is reached, you have acted appropriately. This action is appropriate whether or not the decision is the one you would have made or the decision you thought the patient wanted made. The obligation continues beyond the walls of the organization, however, if you know some deception has occurred and the patient's best interest was not at the heart of the decision.

Another important factor related to advocacy is relationship. Advocacy is difficult to do honestly and accurately in the absence of a trusting, helpful, therapeutic relationship. In any relationship, each person has responsibilities and accountabilities. **Covenant** may be a more appropriate way to think about the obligation to protect a patient's rights and interests, that is, placing the role of advocacy in the context of the relationship in which both people have role responsibilities to each other (Bernal, 1991).

Advocacy is one of many responsibilities, and you must ethically weigh the consequences of acting on one responsibility to the detriment of another. For instance, advocating for the patient's right to refuse medication may escalate the patient's symptoms of ambivalence and reinforce the patient's refusal, even though the medication has had demonstrated effectiveness for this patient in the past.

Working in institutional settings with others caring for the same patients also makes advocacy difficult. There may be relatively little agreement among the 24-hour nursing staff members, for instance, about a patient's insistence that he sleep nude. Institutional and hierarchical structure may create difficulty for the nurses who desire to be advocates (Bernal, 1991).

Advocacy is necessary, but all team members have an ethical obligation to protect the patient's wishes and desires. Only rarely must one act independently and in isolation.

> **W**hat do you think? Could you advocate for the patient's right to choose behaviors that are morally reprehensible to you?

▶ *Check Your Reading*
54. What is the purpose of advocacy?

Conclusions

Ethics is the way one thinks about and discusses moral problems. Ethical principles that guide nursing practice are justice, love, beneficence, nonmaleficence, autonomy, paternalism, veracity, and fidelity. Two theoretical frameworks are the primary models used to discuss ethics. Kohlberg's theory is an individual developmental model that, at its highest level, culminates in justice. Gilligan's framework of care is a model possibly more comfortable for nurses that, at its highest level, culminates in mercy. The best ethical decisions, however, are probably made when both principles (justice and caring) are applied.

Common ethical dilemmas facing psychiatric–mental health nurses involve the application of ethics principles: use of informed consent, use of ECT with unsuitable patients, coercion in medication use, ideal practice contrasted with the realities of practice, or group and individual rights in conflict. Legal guidelines, including the process for involuntary admission, freedom from coercion, nursing practice acts, and boundary issues, are important in psychiatric nursing practice.

Patients, although ill, maintain their constitutional rights. They have the right to use the telephone and to have access to mail and personal property. Patients also have rights to privacy, care, and participation in treatment planning. In addition, patients have the right to treatment in the least restrictive environment that will provide adequate therapeutic structure, support, and benefit. The nurse's role in ethics includes confidentiality, therapeutic alliance, and advocacy.

Throughout the chapter, more questions were posed than answers given. Such is the nature of ethics. To struggle with ethical uncertainty, to confront ethical dilemmas, and to live with ethical distress are part of the awesome responsibility of nursing.

Key Points to Remember

- Eight principles guide ethical decision-making: justice, love, beneficence, nonmaleficence, autonomy, paternalism, veracity, and fidelity.
- Kohlberg postulated a theory of moral development that has three levels: the preconventional level, in which external rules determine right and wrong actions; the conventional level, in which family's and community's rules are accepted and used to determine right and wrong; and the postconventional level, in which the individual uses his or her own conscience to arrive at decisions. Justice is emphasized in Kohlberg's theory.
- Gilligan postulated a theory regarding the moral development of women. Gilligan believes that women approach moral issues from a perspective of care and mutually connected and responsible relationships. This perspective of care provides an alternative to Kohlberg's model.
- There are many ethical dilemmas facing the psychiatric nurse. Informed consent, the use of ECT with unsuitable patients, use of medication when the patient refuses, the ideals of practice versus the reality, the good of the individual versus the good of the group, and behavior control were among the ethical dilemmas presented.
- Legal parameters provide firmer boundaries for practice than those provided by ethical principles.
- Patients can voluntarily admit themselves to a psychiatric facility, or if they are a danger to self or others, they may be involuntarily admitted or committed to an inpatient facility.
- Nurse practice acts define the boundaries of practice within each state.
- Boundary issues are important between the nurse and the patient as well as among staff members.
- Psychiatric patients maintain all their civil liberties.
- The ANA code for nurses specifies baseline expectations for all registered nurses.
- There are three processes inherent in the nurse's ethical responsibilities: confidentiality, therapeutic alliance, and advocacy.

Learning Activities

1. Think about some clinical situations that have placed you in ethical conflicts. What were the conflicting issues? What principles did you use to resolve the conflicts?
2. When you find yourself in difficult situations in which the answers are neither clear nor easy, what principles do you tend to rely on most of the time?
3. The principle of autonomy is an important one in U.S. society because of the value we place on individual rights. Does a person have the right to take his or her own life? Support your answer using ethical principles.
4. When you see or read about a homeless person who has a psychiatric illness, what is your reaction as to your own or society's responsibilities? What principles are you using in your response?
5. How does your own world view (e.g., theistic, pantheistic, humanistic, secular) affect your own ethical decision-making?

Critical Thinking Exercises

Do you think that there should be parity in mental health coverage? Would your opinion change if you or a loved one needed mental health services? If these services are not included among basic services, how do you think they should be paid for? Who should pay for them? How does the principle of justice apply to your answer?

Mr. Thomas, a student nurse in his 2nd day of the psychiatric rotation, reads a nurse's note about a patient that he is about to be assigned to. It reads: *Patient Mr. Z was actively hallucinating and delusional all day. Refused nurse's attempts to talk to him.*

1. What can Mr. Thomas infer from the note about Mr. Z's behavior?

2. Does the note paint a clear and precise picture of Mr. Z's behavior?

3. What are alternate ways of conceptualizing a note about Mr. Z to bring more focus to an overall picture of his behavior?

Later in the day, Mr. Z becomes violent, and the student observes the staff members forcibly subduing the patient while administering an injection of a major tranquilizer. Mr. Z is yelling, "You can't do this to me, I have rights."

In this situation

1. What are the patient's rights, and are they being violated?

2. What ethical principles might be in conflict in providing therapeutic care for Mr. Z?

3. What suggestions would you have about balancing Mr. Z's rights with those of the group?

4. What ethical principles would be involved?

Additional Resources

American Academy of Psychiatry and the Law

P.O. Box 30
One Regency Drive
Bloomfield, CT 06002
860-242-5450
http://www.emory.edu/AAPL/index.html
For further information about insanity defense contact this organization.

References

Ahmed, M. B. (1998). Psychological and legal aspects of mental incompetence. *Texas Medicine, 94*(3), 64-67.

American Hospital Association. (1994). *Values in conflict: Resolving ethical issues in health care* (2nd ed.). Chicago: Author.

American Nurses Association. (1985). *Code for nurses with interpretation statements.* Kansas City, MO: Author.

Bernal, E. W. (1991). The nurse as patient advocate. *Hastings Center Report, 22*(4), 18-23.

Danis, M., & Churchhill, L. R. (1990). Autonomy and the common weal. *Hastings Center Report, 21*(1), 25-31.

Fowler, M. D. M. (1989). Ethical decision making in clinical practice. *Nursing Clinics of North America, 24,* 955-965.

Geller, J. (1993). On being "committed" to treatment in the community. *Innovations Research, 2*(1), 23.

Gilligan, C. (1982). *In a different voice: Psychological theory and women's development.* Cambridge, MA: Harvard University Press.

Kasper, J. A., Hoge, S. K., Feucht Haviar, T., Cortina, J., & Cohen, B. (1997). Prospective study of patients' refusal of antipsychotic medication under a physician's discretion review procedure. *American Journal of Psychiatry, 154,* 483-489.

Kohlberg, L., & Kramer, R. (1969). Continuities and discontinuities in childhood and moral judgment. *Human Development, 12*(2), 93-120.

Levenson, J. L. (1986-1987). Psychiatric commitment and involuntary hospitalization: An ethical perspective. *Psychiatric Quarterly, 58,* 106-112.

Mental Health Systems Act, Pub. L. No. 96-398, § 9501 (1980).

Miller, A. B. (1998). Dissecting the dilemma. *Journal of Christian Nursing, 15*(4), 7-9.

Parker, J. G. (1993). Chemical restraints and the child psychiatric patient—a question of autonomy or veracity? Unpublished manuscript.

Richmond, I., Trujillo, D., Schmelzer, J., Phillips, S., & Davis, D. (1996). Least restrictive alternatives: Do they really work? *Journal of Nursing Care Quality, 11*(1), 29-37.

Silvius, P. G. (1998). Deciding to die. *Journal of Christian Nursing, 15*(4), 14-15.

Sugarman, J., McCrory, D. C., & Hubal, R. C. (1998). Getting meaningful informed consent from older adults: A structured literature review of empirical research. *Journal of the American Geriatric Society, 46,* 517-524.

Tarasoff v. Regents of the University of California, 17 Cal. 3d., 425, 551. p. 2d 334 (1976).

Usher, K. J., & Arthur, D. (1998). Process consent: A model for enhancing informed consent in mental health nursing. *Journal of Advanced Nursing, 27,* 692-697.

Willwerth, W. (1994, November 7). Madness in fine print. *Time.*

Zoloth-Dorfman, L. (1994). First person plural: Community and method in ethics consultation. *Journal of Clinical Ethics, 5*(1), 49-54.

Suggested Readings

American Hospital Association. (1994). *Values in conflict: Resolving ethical issues in health care* (2nd ed.). Chicago: Author.

Curtin, L. L. (1994). Morals: From Bobbit to Kevorkian. *Nursing Magazine, 25*(6), 42-43.

Myers, S. (1990). Seclusion: A last resort measure. *Perspectives in Psychiatric Care, 26*(3), 24-28.

Sabin, J. E. (1994). Managed care: A credo for ethical managed care in mental health practice. *Hospital and Community Psychiatry, 45,* 859-860.

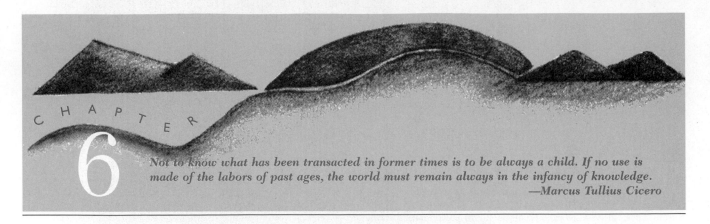

Not to know what has been transacted in former times is to be always a child. If no use is made of the labors of past ages, the world must remain always in the infancy of knowledge.
—*Marcus Tullius Cicero*

Guideposts
Theories That Structure the Journey

Learning Objectives

After studying this chapter, you should be able to:

1. Identify the nature and role of theories as guideposts for the journey.
2. Describe the historical contributions of classical Greek scholars to mental health nursing.
3. Identify the contributions of science and psychology to mental health nursing.
4. Specify the role of psychoanalytic theory in mental health nursing.
5. Compare and contrast ego developmental, humanistic, and existential models of psychology.
6. Describe selected tenets of behavioral theory.
7. Analyze the role of nursing theory in mental health nursing.

Key Terminology

Archetypes	Ego psychology	Operant conditioning	Self-reinforcement
Behavioral models	Existential models	Psychoanalytic therapy	Social learning theory
Collective unconscious	Humanistic psychology	Psychology	Superego
Conditioning	Id	Psychosocial crisis	Theory
Dynamism	Metaparadigm	Reinforcer	Unconscious
Ego	Nursing theory	Self-efficacy	

To provide quality professional care, as opposed to mere comfort, kindness, and concern, a framework for understanding personality and mental health is imperative. Psychiatric nurses practice from a comprehensive theory base, derived from the disciplines of philosophy, medicine, psychology, sociology, education, and, of course, nursing. Using the journey metaphor, theory serves as the essential signpost to guide the way while

also pointing out the hidden roads a professional traveler might chance on. Theories direct the traveler by mapping out established routes to reach the desired destination.

The theories presented in this chapter do not represent an exhaustive study of all theoretical viewpoints used in mental health nursing. Rather, the goal of this chapter is to provide the psychiatric–mental health nurse with a representative sample of the dominant theories that have shaped current thinking about personality and the best ways to treat mental disorders, beginning with those of the early Greek scholars. Each of the theorists grappled with the essential nature of personality, and had to reexamine and modify old assumptions to fit evolving paradigms about personality and treating mental disorders. Each scholar's theory helps the psychiatric nurse discover the unifying elements between the past and present in ways that directly affect clinical practice. Through each theorist's contribution to the human journey, the authors hope that the richness of psychiatric-mental health nursing can be realized; it is a specialty that is necessary to our scientific understanding of people with or without mental illness.

Theory development does not emerge solely from a scientific base; it also significantly reflects the reality of the theorist's personal journey. Each theoretical model reflects careful thinking about the phenomena, the theoretical perspective commonly beginning on a personal note that reflects the author's formative life experiences. These parallel perspectives—theoretical and personal—provide structure and integrity to each cognitive model. Betty Neuman's systems model, presented in the first story, is no exception.

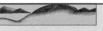 ## Betty Neuman's Story

The real roots of the Neuman systems model are embedded in my early childhood years. My view of the world was shaped by the simple events of farm life. There was reverence, dignity, and respect for all life. When human needs arose in our rural community, my parents were always the first to offer food, clothing, or solace of various kinds. My mother, a self-taught midwife, delivered babies in the area. Although we had limited financial resources, we never felt poor. I was aware at an early age of the importance of God in my life and of having my needs met holistically. After church on Sundays, neighborhood youths would visit to play games and sing religious songs while my mother played the organ.

My parents were organic farmers, and we never lacked wholesome food. Long distances precluded regular medical care, so much of our medicine was from herbs that my mother harvested from the woods, following directions passed down from American Indians who had once lived in the area. In these early, formative years, creativity, caring, and self-reliance in problem solving were automatic, and our developmental needs were satisfied. An unconscious expectation was patterned for a holistic view of people, and environmental influences were seen as manageable. This background, in addition to a knowledge of systems theory and an avid interest in human behavior, formed an important base for the development of the systems model in 1970.

Impact of Early Professional Experiences

Another major factor was experiential. Obviously, my background in psychiatric nursing was important as a starting point for considering the relevant relationships in client data. In addition, other important experiences contributed to the development of the Neuman systems model. Through role modeling the teaching and practice of mental health consultation for graduate students at UCLA from 1967 to 1973, I learned the value of working with other disciplines. I always requested, from the clinical agencies in Greater Los Angeles, the presence of practitioners from the other health care disciplines involved with each case presentation, and I worked collaboratively with them to resolve issues in problem cases. This experience was invaluable. As a result of that collaboration, I found that the "total" data were available to help me consider the nature of patient variables, referred to in the model as "interacting variables."

Consultation with interdisciplinary resources (visiting nurse associations, public health departments, teen posts, jails, and schools) had the effect of strengthening my belief in patients as holistic beings, subject to both internal and external forces. The importance of exploring all aspects of the patient's condition, of identifying the adequacy of resources, and of supporting and integrating care with other disciplines to reinforce existing patient strengths became clear to me. Without a blending of all these efforts to resolve the patient's problem, the effectiveness of the nurse was reduced. I learned the importance of the influence of one variable on another. For example, it became clear that psychological difficulties could cause or contribute to physical problems, or vice versa. Without a spiritual commitment, motivation and hope for wellness are reduced. Making explicit the relationships among the variables in the model was exciting and challenging. At the time, however, I had only intuitive knowledge and not a graphic model for describing these connections.

An Opportunity to Formulate Ideas

In 1970, there was an opportunity to formalize my ideas. I was assigned the task of developing and coordinating an entry-level graduate course related to four variables affecting mental health: physiological, psychological, sociocultural, and developmental. The purpose of the course was to provide students with a breadth of understanding before they selected a clinical specialty track focusing on one of these four variables. My persistent concern was how to make individual lectures interesting and meaningful for the students. The model came into being in 1970 and was readily accepted by the teaching faculty as a tool for conveying their lecture content. The model set the variables into a broader, holistic, systems perspective that allowed faculty to place their content within the broader human context of variable interactive relationships and possibilities. From this content, faculty made assumptions and generated hypotheses.

Refining the Model

Rae Jeanne Young, a close colleague and the course co-coordinator, had a definite impact on the model; together, we struggled to clarify the model's concepts with and for the students. The richness of student and faculty input enhanced the robustness of the model. Evaluation over a 2-year period proved the value of the Neuman systems model, earlier referred to as the "total person approach to patient problems" (Neumann & Young, 1972). Unfortunately, the course itself did not continue after I resigned from UCLA in 1973. The Neuman systems model, however, has gained in strength as it continues to influence current applications in practice, education, and research.

Incorporating the Spiritual

In 1975, my first consultation for the model occurred at Neumann College in Aston, Pennsylvania, as faculty engaged in curriculum revision. Although the original model subsumed the spiritual variable under the sociocultural variable, I recall being excited about discussing with faculty the treatment of the spiritual concerns of patients. (The spiritual variable was not made explicit initially because in the secular environment at UCLA, it was not dealt with as a nursing concern.) Were I to redo the model, I would place spirituality as a central, dominant variable, satisfying further my belief that all input first comes through to the mind and then to the body.

The Neuman systems model satisfies my lifelong quest for "caring" in considering all aspects of a patient's condition within the environment. To be holistic is to "care"; "to help each other live," which is my motto, is to care. ∎

Betty Neuman's story speaks eloquently of how theory development in the human sciences is deeply rooted in its author's own human experience, not as a tangential appendage but as a unifying element at its core.

As we begin our examination of theories, it is important to remember that no one theoretical framework can adequately describe the complexity of the human being or the multidimensional nature of behavior. Given this qualification, each respective conceptual model represents the particular world view of its originator and highlights significant factors to explain human functioning. The student will find it necessary to extract the critical concepts from all of the presented theories and to begin to synthesize them into a broader framework that has personal meaning. These theoretical understandings both govern and direct psychiatric-mental health nursing practice.

WHAT IS A THEORY?

Basically a **theory** consists of concepts that represent "a concise summary of thoughts related to a phenomenon" (Meleis, 1991, p. 12). Each concept provides a symbolic shorthand for describing an abstract reality. For example, the concept of anxiety in Peplau's model symbolizes a fairly wide range of behaviors, spanning both physiological and psychological aspects of the phenomenon. When one hears the term *anxiety,* behaviors associated with anxiety are brought to mind as a gestalt, without much further explanation. Thus, *theories never represent absolute truths but rather portray an abstract representation of a phenomenon and a conceptual tool to describe it in an organized way.*

Theories develop within a historical context that not only necessarily builds on but also challenges classic ways of thinking about a subject. Changes in theoretical perspective usually represent a major paradigm shift in thinking. The new way of thinking creates an intellectual upheaval and a radical new interpretation of the relative truths that shape scientific thinking about a defined subject. For example, the behavioral approach to the treatment of mental illness represents a major deviation from Freudian thinking about the role of the unconscious in shaping behavior and as the focus of psychological treatment.

In some instances, theory fills a vacuum in thinking about a subject. For example, Florence Nightingale's *Notes on Nursing* (1860) provided the first serious documentation of nursing as a professional form of caring about other human beings. Wundt's establishment of the first school of psychology performed a similar service for psychology.

The real strength of having a theoretical base for practice is that it provides a systematic way of ordering knowledge about a subject. This allows the knowledge to be shared with others in deepening a common understanding of the phenomena under scrutiny, for example, nurses learn from the same text in planning and implementing actual nursing care. Theoretical knowledge provides a framework for considering the nature of human behavior and the best ways to treat maladaptive functioning. It allows a researcher to classify observations about a phenomenon in a precise way. This process is a necessary prerequisite for generating hypotheses capable of being tested experimentally.

THEORIES FROM DISCIPLINES OTHER THAN NURSING

Contributions From the Early Greek Scholars

Uniquely human emotional, psychological, and cognitive processes have fascinated great thinkers since the earliest days of civilization. Tracing its roots to ancient times (before the time of Christ), current concepts of psychiatric-mental health nursing emerged originally from the writings of ancient Greek scholars, who spoke of the *whole person,* consisting of mind, body, and spirit, both interrelated and irreducible. At the time, this was a paradigm shift from the previous theory of the mind as influenced solely by magical spirits from external sources. These early Greek scholars challenged this long-standing but crippling world view of the mind and introduced humans' natural resources as a factor in affecting behavior. Along with Hippocrates, a physician contemporary of the classical Greek philosophers, Socrates, Plato, and Aristotle (Hall & Lindzey, 1970; Fancher, 1990) distinguished themselves as the original scholars of the mind.

Socrates

One of the first Greek scholars to explain the nature of the mind was Socrates (470–399 BC). Socrates was the son of a sculptor and a midwife. Socrates was obsessed with searching "his own mind and the minds of his fellow citizens in an attempt to discover the essence of man and of goodness" (Rader, 1969, p. 10). His pursuit of meaning developed into the Socratic method, a form of question and answer carried on between two or more people or within oneself, as the primary method of investigation. The singular goal of the Socratic method was to discover the truth. The process involved collecting all available data and, through critical examination, determining not only the essential nature of the data but also how they fit with other pieces of data. The contemporary cognitive processes of active listening and critical thinking are basically an outgrowth and extension of *Socratic Questioning* (Paul, 1993). Socrates' famous statement, "An unexamined life is not worth living," is widely quoted today as a rationale for seeking self-awareness.

Plato

Plato (ca. 427–347 BC) was a member of one of the finest families in Athens. His career was shaped by the work of Socrates; he began to write his famous dialogues designed to complete the work of Socrates (Rader, 1969). Plato speculated that character and intelligence are inherited. He argued that the soul was imprinted with special knowledge and that these inherent notions would manifest themselves when a relevant external event or stimulus triggered them into awareness. Sigmund Freud (1914–1964) credits Plato's book, *The Nature of Soul*, with anticipating his own groundbreaking work on dream interpretation.

Plato described the soul—or the *psyche* as the Greeks called it—as the center of will, self-motion, and knowing. Organized into three kinds of operation—reason, passion, and appetite—Plato believed that the logical psyche, or rational soul, dominated the psyche. The role of the rational soul was to process information and solve problems and to permit the planning and implementation of decisions. Unchecked, human appetites threatened the balance of effective living, entrapping a person in intemperate behaviors. Ideally, reason prevailed over appetite, augmented by passion, as the "spirited" element. Plato viewed the spirited element of the soul as being "akin to our 'sense of honor,' manifested in indignation, which takes the side of reason against appetite but cannot be identified with reason, since it is found in children and animals and it may be rebuked by reason" (Plato, quoted in Rader, 1969, p. 682). Freud's later ideas about the structure of personality are recognizable byproducts of this earlier philosophical understanding.

Aristotle

Aristotle (384–322 BC) was the son of a court physician of King Amyntas II of Macedonia. He pursued a career as a philosopher, initially as a member of Plato's school, but subsequently founded a school of his own, the Lyceum, which he presided over for 12 years (Jaeger, 1934). Similar to his teacher Plato, Aristotle identified the soul as the center of mental activity. He argued, however, that experience comes from the external world through the senses rather than as innate knowledge as proposed by Plato. Aristotle defined three aspects of the soul, which he characterized as vegetative, sensitive, and rational. To him, the most primitive was the vegetative soul. He envisioned the vegetative soul as being responsible for nourishment and reproductive functions. The sensitive soul was more sophisticated and was thought to control movement, sensation, memory, and imagination. Aristotle contended that the rational soul operated at a higher level. He believed that it was designed to orchestrate reasoning, consciousness, and ethics. The rational soul was exclusive to humankind. In contrast to Plato (who envisioned the soul as imprinted with special knowledge), Aristotle described this soul as a blank slate—a *tabula rasa*—to be filled and molded, based on the individual's experiences and subsequent reactions.

Aristotle proposed that an individual exercises judgment based on experience. This judgment consists of the impact of the physical sensations on the soul, with the mind acting as the agent of interpretation for the activities of life. By linking the soul with actions of the physical being, Aristotle made an important contribution to the study of psychology. He removed much of the mysticism previously associated with the soul and its function, thus opening the door for serious scientific investigation. In making a conceptual leap from undefinable causes to mind-body causality of mental disorders, Aristotle anticipated the psychosomatic interest of modern science in explaining human behavior. Because of Aristotle's innovative ideas, the Greek term *psyche,* which simply means the mind, is now part of the common vernacular.

Hippocrates

A physician and contemporary (460–377 BC) of early Greek philosophers, Hippocrates suggested a link between body type and characteristic behaviors. He based his assumptions on an ancient Greek theory that the physical universe consists of four basic elements: air, earth, fire, and water. Revered as the "father of medicine," Hippocrates hypothesized that the body consists of four corresponding humors: blood, black bile, yellow bile, and phlegm. At a time when mental illness generally was interpreted as the presence in a person of evil spirits or supernatural forces, Hippocrates placed it within the context of disease by claiming that imbalances in the body humors caused the symptoms of mental illness. For example, he asserted that excess black bile accounted for the development of depressive symptoms. Galen (ca. 129–200 AD), another Greek physician, later proposed a general topology of physique and disposition, by suggesting that overabundance of any of these humors accounted for characteristic personality traits. The terms *sanguine* (hopeful), *melancholic* (sad), *choleric* (hot-tempered), and *phlegmatic* (apathetic) continue to describe mood even though these ancient psychophysiological theories have long since been discarded (Leibert & Spiegler, 1982).

Hippocrates understood that health required the presence of certain positive physiological and environmental conditions. He recognized that the mind and body interact as a whole. In fact, he instructed his patients on how to harness the power of their minds to heal their bodies—a radical concept that is currently being reconsidered by many modern-day healers. The relevance of these early scholarly thoughts about consciousness and the structure of the mind to psychiatric nursing practice is summarized in Table 6–1.

Contributions From Early Scientists

René Descartes

Two unlikely scientists contributed in different ways to our current understanding of behavior. The first was René Descartes (1596–1650), a Renaissance scholar, who upheld the idea that mind and body were connected through a complicated mechanism between soul and brain as follows (Descartes, 1931):

Thus, when the soul desires to recollect something, this desire causes the gland, by inclining successively to different sides, to thrust the spirits towards different parts of the brain until it comes across the part where the traces left there by the object we wish to recollect are found. (article 42)

Although his ideas may sound somewhat naive today, they were revolutionary in Descartes' era, and, more important, they clearly demonstrate an initial understanding of the interactive role that body, mind, and soul play in regulating behavior. The role of the unconscious, although implied rather than explicit, is explained as memory traces.

Charles Darwin

In 1871, Charles Darwin (1809–1882) startled Victorian society with a radically different explanation of the mind. He challenged previous philosophical views of humans (and the mind) as having an invariate existence by introducing a more naturalistic theory. Instead of viewing the human organism as a fixed object, Darwin was convinced that it should be considered as an adaptive organism, capable of change. He highlighted the importance of function and adaptation with his theory of evolution—or "survival of the fittest"—forever

T A B L E 6 – I Relevance of the Ancient Greek Philosophers to Psychiatric Nursing Practice		
PHILOSOPHER	**CENTRAL TENETS**	**RELEVANCE TO PSYCHIATRIC NURSING PRACTICE**
Socrates	Socratic questioning and dialogue between people can help them in their search for truth.	Active listening helps to elicit the truth. Critical thinking, in which nurse and patient examine a problem carefully, consider the presence of faulty assumptions, review the evidence and the ideas of everyone concerned, and draw conclusions based on the evidence, is an effective problem-solving strategy.
Aristotle	The mind, body, and soul are interrelated and cannot be understood separately.	Nurses take a holistic approach to patient care.
Hippocrates	Mental disorders must be seen in the context of disease.	Thorough knowledge of the biochemical factors involved in mental illness, the use of pharmacological interventions, and the use of dynamic approaches to mental illness are required in the treatment of mental disorders.
	The mind has power to control the functions of the body.	Through such interventions as imagery, biofeedback, and relaxation techniques, nurses can help patients achieve more control over the reactions of their bodies.
Plato	Free will exists.	Nurses empower patients, foster their self-control, and educate them about the power of positive thinking, self-reliance, and confidence.
	Interpretation of one's reality varies with one's individual perceptions.	Nurses assess patient perceptions and help patients to become aware of their perceived realities. Nurses also help patients to see how this version is influenced, enhanced, and undermined. Nurses can employ strategies to facilitate self-promoting perceptions.
	Habits are repetitive, positive and negative behaviors that become automatic.	Nurses recognize that considerable effort is required to change behavior when modification is necessary. They recognize the importance of short-term and long-term goals.

Chapter 6 Guideposts 105

altering the way humankind viewed the process of growth and change (Fancher, 1990).

Darwin borrowed extensively from earlier schools of thinking. Despite the fact, however, that both Galileo and Descartes centuries before had pointed out similar observations, he received the official credit for describing the first set of assumptions about the adaptation of an organism to its environment. In his book *On the Origin of Species,* Darwin (1871, 1873) laid out an impressive thesis that within any given population, those best able to adapt to their environment have the greatest likelihood of surviving. He stressed the importance of direct observation in describing human behavior, pointing to its validity in studying animal behavior.

Darwin also received credit for focusing on individual differences as important determinants of behavior. He speculated that people with more highly adaptive gene pools were better physically equipped to survive. This became the genesis of his theory of evolution by natural selection.

According to Darwin, mental traits similarly conform to the principles of evolution. He argued that emotions were inherited and served an adaptive purpose. Furthermore, he placed great significance on the usefulness of physical gestures that accompany all emotional reactions. For example, the wide-eyed expression of surprise heightened one's visual field, permitting the person to see an item of interest more vividly. In this manner, Darwin connected emotional expression directly to a physiological response in the nervous system. He considered that humans were influenced both by conscious rational thought and by the unconscious, or instincts. Darwin postulated that instincts were left over from an animalistic past.

Darwin believed that all life forms are basically motivated by two distinct drives: the will to survive and the desire to reproduce. Freud later elaborated on the idea of unconscious instincts to develop his own thesis on the libido and thanatos as basic instinctual drives present in every human being. So in many ways, Darwin's work is considered a precursor of the psychoanalytic approach to the study of behavior, without which Freud's ideas might not have achieved such broad acceptance.

Darwin's theory of evolution has many far-reaching implications for nursing practice. Genetic make-up and adaptive functioning indicate that human physiology can predispose one to either successful or unsuccessful psychological functioning. An evolutionary perspective also challenges the nurse to consider the importance of individual differences in planning care. That conscious thought enters into expression of behavior, but is supplemented by unconscious instincts, provides the nurse with a clearer understanding of the nature of unconventional behaviors.

The Advent of Psychology as a Formal Discipline

The discipline of **psychology** emerged in the late 19th century, essentially as a byproduct of philosophy and experimental physiology. By 1896, the field was well established as a respected academic science. Two forward thinkers—Wilhelm Wundt of Germany and William James of the United States—were largely responsible for this recognition. They are considered the "psychological popes of the old and new worlds" (Fancher, 1990, p. 239).

Wilhelm Wundt

Generally credited with establishing modern psychology as a science, Wilhelm Wundt (1832–1920) graduated from the University of Tübingen medical school in Germany. Wundt disliked private medical practice, however, and instead chose to work as a physiologist in an academic setting. In 1879, Wundt opened an experimental laboratory in Leipzig, the first of its kind, to research the conscious experiences of adults. His research centered around examining the association between sensory nerve stimulation and subsequent motor nerve response. With the aid of an instrument known as the "thought meter," he determined that stimulation did not lead to an immediate reaction. Instead, a period of time elapsed in midsequence, and Wundt concluded from these studies that thoughts occurred at this juncture.

Wundt identified the central nervous system as the force behind thinking and attention—the process whereby thoughts take form. By isolating the connection between conscious thoughts and the central nervous system, Wundt had, in effect, begun the study of the interrelationship between physiology and mental functions. Wundt realized that his assumptions implied the mind possessed its own inborn creative sources. Furthermore, Wundt understood that the mental mechanisms it sheltered would extend beyond attention into many alternative and diverse functions. For his method and overall contributions to the field, Wundt is identified as the "father of experimental psychology" (Fancher, 1990).

From his research, Wundt became aware that there was another aspect of mental functioning that was inaccessible by experimental or physiological means. This area was larger than individual consciousness and encompassed social consciousness. Ethnic, cultural, religious, and social dynamics fell into this realm of psychology and helped explain other important determinants of behavior and personality.

Underlining both subtypes (the physiological aspect of psychological functioning and the social implications) is the notion that exploration of conscious experiences is critical to understanding mental health behaviors. Introspection is an essential conduit for accessing these experiences and providing information about psychological processes. Wundt believed the processes of sensation and voluntary movement are of paramount importance. At this intersection, psychology and physiology meet. Wundt defined internal sensations as the psychological state that one experiences. Therefore, an internal sensation is a feeling or a mood. This reaction occurs within the individual intrapsychically.

Wundt defined voluntary movement as the actual muscular action that is generated by a psychological impulse, in other words, the behavioral action taken as a direct consequence of the psychological state. Both feeling states (also known as affect and action) are identified as critical psychological expressions. Although Wundt's theory was later rejected as being too narrow, he retains his place in the history of psychology as its first experimental scientist. By insisting on an empirical method for the study of behavior, Wundt created the important link between an experimental and a social psychology and established the legitimacy of psychology as a science.

William James

William James (1842–1910) is considered a pioneer of American psychology. He was an American philosopher who published the first textbook in psychology in 1890, a two-volume treatise on *Principles of Psychology*. Two years later, he revised his original work into *Psychology: The Briefer Course* for classroom use (Alport, 1892–1985). James was born in New York City and raised in privileged circumstances as the eldest son of five children, in a family in which education and intellectual pursuits were highly valued. Although financially secure, his father suffered from severe anxiety and struggled with feelings of insecurity, unfulfillment, and indecisiveness. Ultimately, his father resolved these issues independently.

The younger James (Fancher, 1990) was undoubtedly influenced by both his family atmosphere and their values. He cherished opportunities for learning but, like his father, was prone to emotional difficulties. In fact, James battled serious bouts of depression, anxiety, and ambivalent feelings about his self-worth during much of the first half of his life. James attended Harvard University and Harvard Medical School, concentrating his studies on physiology. Unfortunately, during James' course of study, family conflicts, coupled with his own failing physical health, led James to thoughts of suicide. Instead of killing himself, however, James opted to continue his education in physiology abroad.

In Germany, in 1867, James first encountered Wilhelm Wundt's article on physiological psychology—an article that was to change the course of his life and work. When James read about Wundt's work, he was struck by the interplay between physiology and psychology and began to incorporate those concepts into his own work.

James returned to Harvard, but he became despondent again. He felt pessimistic and anxiety-ridden, until a chance reading about free will, written by French philosopher Charles Renouvier (1815–1903), inspired him to empower himself. Renouvier defined free will in terms of self-control. He stated that by maintaining a thought, one exerts free will. Stimulated by his new sense of empowerment, James began to use free will to modify his thoughts and attitudes. Fascinated by the concept of free will, he read profusely on the subject and eventually came on the work of a British philosopher, Alexander Bain (1818–1903). Bain wrote at length about habit and emphasized the importance of voluntary repetition as the means by which actions become habitual and thus automatic. As James successfully applied both Renouvier's and Bain's ideas in coping with his own personal crises, he was able to harness his personal creative power, and he began to believe in its efficacy. Motivated by his enhanced knowledge of free will and the successful resolution of his own crisis, James formulated a new set of principles of psychological theory (Fancher, 1990).

The essence of James' theory is rooted in the ideas of the classical Greek scholars discussed earlier. Similarly to Socrates and Aristotle, James believed that the search for truth about human beings lies in having an open mind and a systematic reasoned approach to examining the meaning of human behavior. James, however, expanded their notion of the verification process beyond the dimensions of the individual soul to include its integral link with the larger schema of human experiences. He described the subjective life of a person as a "stream of thought consciousness. . . . It is nothing jointed, it flows. A 'river' or 'stream' are metaphors by which it is most naturally described" (James, 1890–1950, p. 239). James viewed human beings as choice makers and saw attention to the task as a necessary prerequisite for dispelling tangential interests and associations.

James understood that people are influenced by many factors in the formation of their free will actions, and he viewed free will as a correlate of full attention to difficult tasks. Through self-examination, James became aware of his own motivators. He surmised that human behavior was clearly associated with the interpretation of one's reality. James emphasized the significance of perceptions and presumed that a psychological belief in oneself fueled creative energy. He hypothesized that autonomy and determination are human resources that facilitate the implementation of free will.

As James pursued this line of inquiry, he considered the significance of behavior and how it might develop. He described habit as essential for a stable society. Although habits could be either good or bad, they provided predictability to behavior. James accepted Bain's sequence of habit formation as *voluntary repetition* (Fancher, 1990, p. 247), in which a person, acting on her or his own volition, repeats a behavior until eventually that behavior becomes permanently imprinted into the nervous system. In this way, the behavior becomes automatic. Once a habit is established, it is difficult to undo.

Many of the innovative ideas of James, a powerful writer, about the "science of mental life" are still valid today. His chapter on habit, with its practical maxims of maintaining focus, permitting no exceptions, and continuous practice, provided a pragmatic lead into our current understanding of how behavioral therapies work. The idea that one has free will and can make reasoned choices that affect feeling and behavior reaches into the heart of many behavioral-cognitive approaches to change. His lectures on the nature of pragmatism, proposing it as a reality-based and action-oriented approach to behavioral decisions (James, 1907) is a recognizable forerunner of contemporary reality-based theories of therapeutic approaches to behavioral change.

James spearheaded the development of psychology as a professional discipline in the United States. He taught the first psychology courses at a university level and brought the message of this new discipline to the general population in the United States. Because he was able to apply so many of the concepts he wrote about from his own personal journey, his theory has an especially powerful ring of truth to it. Table 6–2 summarizes the relevance of these early psychologists to psychiatric nursing practice.

What do you think? Each of us constructs our own theories about human behavior. These theories grow out of our own experiences. What are your theories about the relationship between thoughts, feelings, and actions? What determines how individuals behave? Is behavior determined by genetics, physiology, environment, or an interplay among all of these factors? What personal experiences have shaped your theories?

➤ **Check Your Reading**
1. How does theory reflect the personal journey of the theorist?
2. What are some of the contributions the early Greek scholars made to the development of psychology?
3. In what ways did Wundt and James mark the journey of psychology as a profession?

Psychodynamic Theories

Sigmund Freud

Freud's (1856–1939) groundbreaking theory of personality structure and development and his insistence on

psychological treatment of behavioral symptoms revolutionized thinking about mental health disorders. His discovery of unconscious motivation represented a monumental breakthrough in the treatment of emotionally disturbed people. Freud believed that the vast majority of mental disorders were not organic in origin but rather developed as the result of unresolved emotional conflicts in childhood. His psychodynamic formulations grew out of personal observations regarding his own behavior, his family, and friends as well as those of his patients.

Freud was born in Freiberg, Moravia (Czechoslovakia). His father recognized his academic talents early and encouraged Freud to develop them. As a youngster, he was interested in history and humanities, with a tendency toward law. Freud's life, however, took a completely different direction as a result of a chance scientific reading he encountered just before completing high school. He found the article so compelling that he made a spontaneous decision to enroll in the University of Vienna's medical school.

Although Freud never intended to enter private medical practice, he had no choice in the matter. As a Jew in an anti-Semitic environment, he was denied opportunities in academic settings. Consequently, Freud established a practice in neurology. He continued to pursue his research and publication, however, which earned him respect and attention—but drew sharp criticism because of the radical nature of his ideas.

Among the patients Freud treated were *hysterics*—people who were suffering despite the absence of a physiological cause. Many physicians of the day refused to treat these patients, believing them to be malingerers or impostors. As a student of Jean-Martin Charcot

---

TABLE 6–2 Relevance of the Early Psychologists to Psychiatric Nursing Practice

PSYCHOLOGIST	CENTRAL TENETS	RELEVANCE TO PSYCHIATRIC NURSING PRACTICE
Wilhem Wundt	There is an association between sensory nerve stimulation and motor response.	Nurses take a holistic approach to patient care.
	Neurological and physiological status affect mental status. There is a link between mood, behavior, and mental function.	Nursing assessment and potential intervention must track this sequence to promote successful function.
	Conscious thought occurs and originates in the central resources. Each person has innate creative resources.	Nurses must assist patients in becoming aware of their thoughts and in benefiting from their inner resources.
William James	Free will exists.	Nurses empower patients, foster their self-control and educate them about the power of positive thinking, self-reliance, and confidence.
	Interpretation of one's reality varies with one's individual perceptions.	Nurses assess patient perceptions and help patients to become aware of their perceived realities. Nurses also help patients to see how this version is influenced, enhanced, and undermined. Nurses can employ strategies to facilitate self-promoting perceptions.
	Habits are repetitive, positive and negative behaviors that become automatic.	Nurses recognize that considerable effort is required to change behavior when modification is necessary. They recognize the importance of short-term and long-term goals.

(1825–1893), a famous French psychiatrist, Freud understood the genuineness of their symptoms and considered them worthy of his care. Freud learned from Charcot how to perform hypnosis, and although his results were mixed, his experiences provided the impetus to consider other psychological methods of treatment. Then Josef Breuer (1842–1925), a Viennese doctor and an old friend of Freud's, offered a supplemental treatment to hypnosis. Breuer had begun talking with a hysterical patient about her symptoms and their origin while she was under hypnosis. This strategy effectively cured her and became known as the *cathartic method*. Freud employed talk therapy (cathartic method) as a primary means of treating individuals with mental symptoms and later added the concept of free association with dramatic results in his patients. His writings spanned more than 40 years and included 23 volumes, which had an influence not only on the psychiatric community but also on the development of literature, art, and social ideologies (English & English, 1958; Strachey, 1964). For example, impressionist and surrealist art often contains unconscious symbolism as well as reality. In literature, fairy tales are said to reflect the unconscious, and the presence of the unconscious is also found in the stream of consciousness method of writing and in drawing.

Freud offered the psychiatric world a systematic way of looking at the structure and function of personality. Although psychiatry today has broadened, refined, and even refuted Freud's original ideas about individual behavior, the essence of his pioneering contributions remains as a powerful foundation for current thinking about human personality. Current psychiatric terminology, including the unconscious, defense mechanisms, repression, transference and countertransference, the concept of resistance, interpretation, and the stages of psychosocial development, initially were defined by Freud. Popular contemporary terms such as *anal retentive* personality, *Oedipus complex, tip of the iceberg, erogenous zones,* and *Freudian slips* (of the tongue) trace their origins to Freud. Among the many psychological concepts that still hold true today is Freud's most important: his insistence that all behavior is motivated, and much of it is not within the person's conscious awareness.

THE DYNAMICS OF THE PERSONALITY

Freud described the dynamics of personality in terms of basic instincts and anxiety. Instincts arise internally, whereas anxiety, although also a state of tension, derives from external sources. Freud identified two basic drives or instincts in human beings: *libido* was defined as the pleasure principle in the life drive. *Thanatos,* derived from the Greek word meaning death, incorporated human beings' destructive instincts. A person's libido seeks satisfaction through sex and satisfying hunger or thirst needs. Thanatos represents a person's aggressive drive to kill or be killed. The life instincts provide energy for human survival and reproduction. Destructive behaviors toward self or others are better explained by the instinctual energy associated with thanatos (Hall & Lindzey, 1970). The three structures of the mind, that is,

id, ego, and superego, use the psychic energy represented in humans' instinctual drives to regulate all living processes.

Freud believed in psychic determinism: all behavior, no matter how random it may appear, has an identifiable cause both created and interpreted by an individual's personal history and experiences. He held that the earlier unresolved conflicts a child had with significant adults continued to have an impact on the person's life until they could be brought into conscious awareness. Although current thinking challenges Freud's insistence that "remembering repressed traumatic situations is the ultimate goal" (Alexander, 1959, p. 322) of therapy, there is no question that helping patients talk about unresolved conflicts, past as well as present, is beneficial.

Anxiety, a concept described later in this chapter and discussed in Chapter 23, has the dual functions of warning a person of an approaching physical or psychological threat and motivating a person to take action. When anxiety reaches an intolerable point and cannot be resolved easily by the ego, the ego employs defense mechanisms to ward off the perceived danger in the person's environment. Although everyone uses ego defense mechanisms to some degree, the ego's persistent inability to master the situation, to harness difficult emotions, or to control dangerous impulses usually results in psychiatric symptoms. Freud identified three types of anxiety: objective, neurotic, and moral anxiety. With objective anxiety, the threat is real and external to the person experiencing it. Neurotic anxiety occurs when there is conflict between the id and ego, whereby the ego is unsuccessful in quelling the urges of the id. According to Freud, neurotic anxiety can present as free-floating, phobic, or panic. Free-floating anxiety is a vague, nebulous dread without an objective stimulus. Phobic anxiety is characterized by a specific irrational fear about a displaced object, for example, fear of heights, fear of crowds, claustrophobia. Murder, suicide, and violence often are undesired outcomes of panic. Freud defines moral anxiety as anxiety emerging from conflicts between the ego and the superego, in which a person fears punishment by his or her conscience for actions taken.

THE STRUCTURE OF THE PERSONALITY

Freud originally identified a topographical theory of how the mind functions and described the landscape of the mind as having three distinct mental processes. He considered the conscious part of the mind to be the tip of the iceberg. It represented all of the material a person was aware of at any given moment in time. Just below the surface of awareness is the preconscious. Although the preconscious does not lie within a person's awareness, material contained in this layer of the mind can be retrieved rather easily through conscious effort. By contrast, the **unconscious** consists of all of the repressed memories, passions, and unacceptable urges lying deep below the surface. The vast realm of the unconscious has a forceful, unseen effect on the conscious thoughts and behaviors of a person. Recognition of the contents of the unconscious usually cannot be retrieved by an individual through personal efforts. With the skillful intervention of a therapist, however, it is possible to bring unconscious material into conscious awareness.

Later, Freud taught that personality is composed of three major systems: the id, ego, and superego. Although they are distinct systems, the three work closely together. Generally, behavior is the result of this interaction. Rarely does one system function to the exclusion of the others. Ideally, the three systems work as a team, under the rational administrative leadership of the ego. Because only so much energy is available to any person, the three systems often compete with one another for dominance. One system can overpower the effectiveness of the other two systems. For example, an overly responsible person governed by the superego may have great difficulty experiencing the fun and conviviality a person with a better balance of id might. The patient with antisocial disorder frequently experiences serious difficulty getting in touch with the superego and lacks the ego stability that most mature, responsible adults possess. Although not incompatible with Freud's earlier topographical model, his structural view of how the mind functions is not totally comparable either. Rather they represent two different approaches to the study of personality functioning (Marmer, 1994).

Id. At birth, an infant is all id, motivated by instinctual drives of hunger and thirst. As the mind's most primitive system, it is from the id that the ego and superego later evolve. The **id** is considered the source of all psychic energy, providing vital empowerment to both the ego and the superego. The validity of Freud's argument about the energy effect of the id is evidenced in the renewal of strength most people feel after a good vacation or recreational respite.

Freud believed that all inherited and instinctual psychological processes reside in the id. He considered it to be the "true psychic reality" because the id is aware only of emotional perceptions. It is not privy to the constraints of an objective reality. Consequently, the laws of logic do not apply to thoughts stimulated by the id. The pleasure principle is its guiding force.

Whenever tension is experienced, the id is driven to reduce this tension instantly in an attempt to return to a tension-free, or pleasurable, state. The pleasure principle has two methods of reducing tension: reflex action and primary process. *Reflex action,* as the name implies, is inherent and automatic. Gagging is a reflex. The human body has many such reflexes, such as crying and laughing, which successfully alleviate certain forms of tension.

Not all tension, however, can be reduced or removed through reflex action. This is particularly true of psychic or emotional tension, commonly called anxiety. Naturally, the remaining tension causes frustration. Freud labeled as *primary process* the energy discharge of mental impulses, occurring without delay and uninhibited by any reality factors. Through primary processes, the id attempts to diminish tension by creating an image of the object that would rectify the uncomfortable situation. For example, the mirages of water that people

experience in the desert enable them to experience in their minds the reality of plentiful water. This mental image is known as *wish-fulfillment.* The id perceives the mental image of water to be synonymous with the actual fluid because it knows only subjective reality. Primary process is seen in the images of small children, with the ego rupture of feelings present in severe mental illness, with autistic thinking, and in dreams.

Wish-fulfillment cannot sustain the individual because one obviously cannot drink imaginary water. Therefore, primary process alone does not suffice to reduce tension. To successfully accommodate to changes in the environment, external reality must be considered, which requires the development of secondary processes grounded in truth. Secondary psychological processes mark the emergence of the ego; they are associated with the preconscious and conscious elements of personality.

Ego. Freud conceptualized a higher level of functioning that he classified as secondary psychological processes and assigned to the ego. He viewed the **ego** as the "executive of personality" because it controls the gateways to actions, selects the features of the environment to which it will respond, and decides which instincts will be satisfied, and in what manner (Hall & Lindzey, 1970, p. 34).

The ego has a regulatory function (the *reality principle*), which allows a person to delay gratification and to consider environmental factors that are either favorable or unfavorable to the discharge of mental impulses. It determines the response needed by an individual to negotiate with the objective world of reality. The essential difference between the ego and the id is that the id knows only subjective experience, whereas the ego can differentiate between subjective reality, memory images, and objective reality. Through secondary processes, an individual is able to recognize the reality factors of a situation and to make conscious decisions based on all of the evidence.

The ego is charged with the mission of self-preservation. Governed by the reality principle, it nevertheless derives from the id and is never entirely free from it. The reality principle puts the desires of the id on hold to tolerate the tension, until a satisfactory outlet for tension reduction is produced. Reality becomes the utmost priority but only by visualization of an object that can reduce tension. This kind of teamwork makes it possible to arrive at the ultimate goal of tension reduction, thereby gratifying the id as well.

Secondary processes provide the energy to plan a course of action and to test this action in an effort to determine the validity of the plan. The hungry man thinks about where he can eat dinner and then seeks that destination. This process is known as *reality testing* because the individual is attempting to factor in reality to implement a plan for tension reduction. It is the ego that coordinates the expression of self, with attention to the various demands from id, superego, and reality.

Superego. The superego is the last portion of personality to be developed. It represents the ideal rather than the real, seeking perfection, as opposed to pursuing pleasure or engaging reason. The **superego** represents the moral component of personality and incorporates the child's view of his or her parents' values and ideals. Consequently, it internalizes and absorbs these messages on morality and righteousness. The goals of the superego (Hall & Lindzey, 1970) are to

- Curb the impulses of the id, especially the sexual and aggressive ones
- Influence the ego to endorse moralistic goals
- Strive for perfection

Two subsystems operate in the superego: the conscience and the ego-ideal. The conscience corresponds to the child's version of what his or her parents have condemned. The child makes these interpretations based on what led to punishment or disapproval. Memory images activated by a person's conscience create guilt associations and inhibit behavior or destroy the temptation to act it out permanently. Conversely, the ego-ideal internalizes what the parents consider morally good—the standards of virtue. When standards imposed by the superego are realized, a person feels the pride of achievement. Similar to the id, however, the superego is irrational and relies on the ego for reality testing.

Ordinarily, personality is successfully integrated under the supervision of the ego. The ego is capable of exerting this influence because it is most effective in tension reduction, which is to say it is fueled with the greatest amount of psychic energy. Difficulties in mentally healthy functioning occur when the ego fails to maintain control of the psychic energy, allowing the id or superego to prevail instead. Too much superego influence is as detrimental to personal growth as being controlled by id. Eric Berne later popularized Freud's concepts of id, ego, and superego in applying them to a theoretical framework of communication in the psyche as child, adult, and parent, respectively.

DEVELOPMENTAL STAGES

Freud is believed to be the first theorist to propose developmental stages of personality (Fancher, 1990; Freud, 1960, 1969; Hall & Lindzey, 1970; Smith & Vetter, 1982). Freud described five psychosexual stages of development (described further on), ending in adolescence, but he emphasized the significance of early childhood experiences. According to Freud, personality is largely determined by 5 years of age. Each developmental stage makes a contribution to the development of a mature personality and involves focusing on a particular bodily zone (mouth, anus, genitals), referred to as an *erogenous zone*. Each erogenous zone represents a vital function, readily observable as a focus of attention in the behaviors of the child. Freud argued, however, that the pleasure associated with the erogenous zone exceeded that of mere need satisfaction. Freud referred to the first three stages of psychosexual development (oral, anal, and phallic) as pregenital stages to distinguish them from the genital stage, in which energy associated with egocentricity gets transformed into genuine love of others.

Oral Stage. Freud's first stage of psychosexual development, referred to as the *oral stage,* occurs from birth through approximately the 1st year of life. During this time, the infant sucks to nourish himself or herself—not only as a vital function but also to pacify or comfort the self. The infant puts everything in its mouth, even its own body parts. Because the process of eating for the infant also includes being held, there are psychological as well as physical satisfactions associated with the oral stage of personality development. Naiveté, in believing anything one is told; biting sarcasm; and belligerence are all examples of adult personality traits reflective of difficulties stemming from this stage (Hall & Lindzey, 1970). The way an alcoholic often drinks directly from the bottle mimics behaviors from this early stage of development.

Anal Stage. Freud identified the second stage of psychosexual development as the *anal stage.* Extending from 18 months of age until approximately age 3, the anal stage focuses on voluntary regulation of excretion, emphasizing body control and mastery. For the first time, the child becomes aware that his or her instinctual impulses are controllable as the task of toilet training becomes an issue. Emotional trauma associated with toilet training can result in later emotional dysfunctions. Expulsive traits (such as temper tantrums and slovenliness) or retentive traits (such as withholding and stubbornness) may develop as a result. The term *anal retentive* is sometimes used to describe people with an excessive need to retain control and not let go of details.

Phallic Stage. Freud's third stage of psychosexual development, the *phallic stage,* usually lasts from 3 to 5 years of age. The genitalia become the focal body point during this period, as the child discovers erotic pleasure when the genitals are touched. Autoerotic behavior and its associated pleasures coincide with the Oedipus complex, which Freud believed to be his greatest discovery (Hall & Lindzey, 1970). In this complex, named after the King of Thebes who murdered his father and married his mother, the young child feels attachment for the parent of the opposite sex and experiences hostility toward the parent of the same sex. Freud believed that a little boy suffered from castration anxiety, fearing that his father would cut off his penis. Resolution of the Oedipus complex allows a boy to identify with his father and later to develop attachment for women other than his mother. The counterpart of the Oedipus complex in little boys is the Electra complex in little girls. Once a little girl discovers she does not have a penis, she develops what Freud referred to as penis envy. She views her mother as a threat to her relationship with her father. To resolve the conflict, little girls play with their dolls and substitute the wish for a baby for the wish for a penis. The Electra complex is resolved by the little girl's identification with her mother, which frees her to achieve her own sexual identity. Freud's ideas about castration anxiety and penis envy seem outrageous in a modern age in which men and women are viewed as more equal, and a person is thought of as a whole person. His assertion that "anatomy is destiny" no longer has the ring of truth. Freud was quite correct, however, in assuming that a person's successful negotiation of future relationships with the opposite sex had their roots in the level of acceptance children feel early from opposite-sex and same-sex parents.

Latency Stage. Freud did not pay much attention to the *latency stage* other than to say that it is a rather prolonged childhood period of quiescence. He considered it to be unremarkable from a psychodynamic perspective. Occurring between 7 and 13 years of age, the child's sexual impulses are repressed until adolescence, when hormonal changes reactivate them, and they burst forth with great intensity. Latency, however, is important from the perspective that the child is developing the skills needed to make the transition from a full home environment to one that includes the broader perspective of school and playmates. During the latency stage, children develop relationships with peers, allowing them to develop the self-confidence needed to compete and collaborate with others outside of the family unit. Usually, the child in the latency stage shows great interest in peers of the same sex and little interest in peers of the opposite sex.

Genital Stage. Freud's final stage of psychosexual maturity, the *genital stage,* begins in adolescence and extends into adulthood. In this stage, the adolescent redirects self-love into attachment to others. Successful passage through this period of development allows the transformation of the child with pleasure-seeking tendencies to assume deliberately the mantle of a "reality-oriented, socialized adult" (Hall & Lindzey, 1970, p. 53). Earlier stages of development are integrated into the personality with the final outcome incorporating elements from all of the previous stages. Healthy completion of these stages enables the mature adult to maintain tolerable levels of anxiety and to employ tension-reduction techniques proficiently. Individual personality is the outcome of this complex process. Table 6–3 contrasts Freud's psychosexual stages of development with Erik Erikson's psychosocial stages.

PSYCHOANALYTIC TECHNIQUES

Considered the Father of Psychoanalysis, Freud carefully laid out a method of treating behavioral symptoms by psychological rather than physical means. His thoughts about the value of talking about painful issues are the basis for most counseling practices today. Freud viewed the patient's remembrance of repressed memories as the goal of **psychoanalytic therapy** and the method by which this material is elicited by the analyst as catharsis and free association. The therapeutic goal of the cathartic method was to have the patient explore bothersome symptoms in depth. As patients relived in their minds the nature of their symptoms and put them into words, they were able to draw out the emotionally laden memory associated with the symptom. This cathexis enabled the patient to experience an emotion that had been previously denied. Once a patient achieved insight about the origin and nature of the repressed feelings, the symptom lost its power.

TABLE 6–3 Comparison Between Freud's Psychosexual Stages and Erikson's Psychosocial Stages

AGE	ERIKSON'S PSYCHOSOCIAL STAGES	PRIMARY PERSON ORIENTATION	STRENGTHS	QUALITIES	FREUD'S PSYCHOSEXUAL STAGES	JUNG'S PSYCHOSOCIAL ORIENTATION
0–2	Trust vs. mistrust	Mother	Hope	To receive, to give	Oral	Largely unconscious
2–4	Autonomy vs. shame/doubt	Father	Will power	To control, to let go	Anal	
4–6	Initiative vs. guilt	Basic family	Purpose	To make, to play act	Oedipal	Beginning ego consciousness
6–12	Industry vs. inferiority	Neighborhood, school	Competence	To make things, to put things together	Latency	
13–19	Identity vs. identity diffusion	Peer groups	Fidelity	To be one's self	Puberty	Individual consciousness
Young adult	Intimacy vs. isolation	Partners in marriage, friendship	Love	To share one's self with another	Genital	Social adaptation, achievement
Adult	Generativity vs. self-absorption	Children, community	Care	To take care of, to create		Inner reflection, individuation
Old age	Integrity vs. despair	Humankind	Wisdom	To accept being, to accept not being		Self-knowledge of the meaning of one's existence

From Arnold, E., & Boggs, K. (1995). *Interpersonal relationships: Professional communication skills for nurses* (p. 13). Philadelphia: W. B. Saunders; adapted from THE LIFE CYCLE COMPLETED: A Review by Erik H. Erikson. Copyright © 1982 by Rikan Enterprises, Ltd. Reprinted by permission of W. W. Norton & Company, Inc.

Freud (1960, 1961, 1969) later refined his psychoanalytic technique to include free association. Free association requires full and honest, uncensored disclosure of thoughts and feelings as they come to mind. Freud understood that free association led the patient on a path to the pathological ideas that caused pain. He encouraged his patients to share everything, without evaluating the merit of their responses. By listening to people's associations, Freud came to the conclusion that talking about difficult emotional issues had the potential to heal the emotional wounds of mental illness.

Within the therapeutic relationship, Freud described a relatively rigid therapeutic intervention method in which the patient had to fit a certain mold of activity. He observed, however, that not all patients fitted the mold. During the course of therapy, certain patients developed emotional blocks that got in the way of full catharsis. Those patients who refused or were unable to comply with full catharsis were considered resistant. Freud held that this was because of transference distortions. Each patient brings into the therapeutic situation certain beliefs and feelings associated with past experiences that can color or distort the way in which the person experiences the current reality. For example, a person may have had bad experiences with authority figures in the past and therefore relates to authority figures in the present as being inflexible or critical even when there is no evidence of the therapist having such characteristics. These unconscious distortions interfere with the work of the therapy and influence the ways in which the patient perceives the therapist.

Freud noticed also that the behaviors of the analysand (patient) and the therapist had a reciprocal effect on one another. When the therapist responds with his or her own feelings, this behavior reflects the therapist's distortions of the situation. These perceptual distortions constitute countertransference reactions and also disrupt the flow of the therapy. Transference and countertransference reactions are discussed in more detail in Chapter 10.

RELEVANCE TO NURSING

Freud's theory has relevance to psychiatric nursing practice at many junctures. First, it offers a comprehensive explanation of complex human processes and suggests that many diverse sources stemming from the person's past affect personality. Freud's theory of the unconscious is particularly valuable as a baseline for considering the multidimensional nature of behavior. By becoming familiar with these diverse conscious and unconscious influences, a nurse can develop and begin to formulate a hypothesis about the root causes of patient suffering. The id, ego, and superego represent different, often conflicting, needs coexisting within each person's psyche. Understanding the structural nature of the mind allows the nurse to respond more appropriately when obvious conflicts emerge in the nurse-patient relationship.

Freud's conceptualizations of transference and countertransference find their way into many therapeutic interactions. A professional nurse requires constant self-awareness to avoid confusing his or her own intrapsychic conflicts with that of the patients.

Clinical interventions derived from psychodynamic thought are vast. Individual talk sessions with patients that emphasize attentive listening and focus on underlying themes are important tools of healing in psychiatric care. Although the current emphasis in treatment is on the here and now, sensitivity to understanding the meaning of a patient's conversation usually results in improved patient care.

Carl Jung

Jung (1875-1961) was born in Switzerland, the only child of a minister and his wife. He initially entered the University of Basel, seeking a degree as a philogist, but became more interested in medicine and psychiatry. Consequently, he obtained a degree in medicine from the university and began working at a psychiatric clinic in Zurich.

Jung initially was impressed with Freud's work, and he viewed him as an important mentor. In turn, Freud admired the brilliance of Jung's thinking and shared many ideas with him. Then in 1914, Jung broke all contact with Freud because of his opposition to Freud's insistence that sexual energy was the driving force in humans. Jung then developed his own method of psychoanalysis, referred to as *analytical psychology,* which had a strong emphasis on dream interpretation and self-disclosure (Jung, 1916).

Jung built on Freud's ideas, but he differed with Freud on several fundamental issues. Instead of viewing libido as the pleasure principle, Jung characterized it as psychic energy, "the total force which pulses through all the forms and activities of the psychic system and establishes a communication between them" (Jacobi, 1951, p. 89).

THE STRUCTURE OF THE PERSONALITY

Like Freud, Jung believed in the unconscious. But he took the concept a step further to embrace a **collective unconscious,** which he defined as comprising a person's racial and cultural heritage and consisting of universal images held by all humans. He categorized the latter as archetypes. According to Jung, the collective unconscious was the foundation for the entire personality structure. Usually, it is unconscious, but it can rush uninvited into consciousness during a psychotic break, presenting as a primary process with chaotic material and distorted feelings that are frightening to the individual experiencing them. Jung defined a *personal unconscious,* consisting of memories that once were conscious but are no longer remembered. He agreed with Freud that conscious awareness was a much smaller part of the personality, frequently governed by elements of the unconscious until they were drawn into conscious awareness through therapy.

One of Jung's most important concepts was that of **archetypes.** Jung defined an archetype as "a universal thought form (idea) which contains a large element of emotion" (Hall & Lindzey, 1970, p. 85). He contended that archetypes represent experiences that have existed for a long time in the collective unconscious. Their energy continues to have an influence on present generations. Examples of commonly recognized archetypes include the earth mother, birth, death, the magician, unity, and the wise old man.

Of particular importance in the study of personality are the archetypes that influence interpersonal behavior. Some become so important to the structure of personality that they evolve into systems of their own and have a dramatic influence on behavior. Four of the most important include *persona, shadow, anima-animus,* and *the self* (Fordham, 1953). Jung defined the *persona* as the social mask people wear to meet the varying demands of social situations. The persona can include physical appearance, gestures, and manner of verbal presentation, all designed to satisfy the social needs of a situation. When the persona represents the essential nature of a person, all is well. When it is at odds with a person's personality, a persona can severely restrict the full expression of self.

Jung observed a paradox about personality structure, in that within each person's psyche many different elements, some light and some dark, coexist (Jung, 1973). For each path a person chooses, there is the one that was not chosen. Recognition of the shadow side of self is not a disavowal of choices made but rather a completion of all that was involved in making the choice so that the person recognizes that there was a choice and on what basis it was made (Moore, 1992). Jung defined the *shadow* as the inferior side of the psyche, the part that is disowned by an individual, only to reappear in dreams or to find itself personified in another person. For example, Adrienne develops a particular intense dislike for Jackie without really knowing why the feeling is so intense. Jung (1973, 1975) would suggest that the feelings occur because Adrienne's unconscious recognizes qualities in Jackie that she also possesses but does not want to acknowledge consciously. Becoming aware of one's shadow side permits more leverage in interpersonal relationships and offers an opportunity to integrate all qualities productively into one's personality.

Jung also proposed the existence of a *worldwide shadow,* accounting for much of the evil in the world that cannot be attributed to personal choice. According to Jung, every person is capable of both terrible wrongs and courageous right actions, given the right set of circumstances. To ignore or minimize the presence of evil in the world is a dangerous proposition, examples of which are found in the many people each year who are duped into giving away their life savings for falsely advertised good causes.

Jung insisted that division of psychological characteristics as being "male" or "female" was an artificial distortion of psychological reality that did both genders a disservice. According to Jung, both men and women contain the opposite characteristics—aggressiveness in women, tenderness in men—as integral parts of their personality. He labeled these characteristics *anima* (emotional characteristics traditionally associated with women) and *animus* (rationalizing characteristics traditionally associated with men). Men and women are most human when they are able to acknowledge and act on the paradox of having both types of characteristics coexisting within a unified self.

Jung considered *the self,* which he envisioned as embodying a person's longing for unity and wholeness, as the personality's most important structural system. Symbolized in the form of a circle, with neither beginning nor end, the self represents the core of the personality. Jung described the two primary orientations of self as *extroversion,* in which a person enjoys full participation in the outer world, and *introversion,* in which a person is mainly oriented toward the inner world. The extrovert makes decisions spontaneously and is happiest in a crowd. Extroverts are uncomfortable with a lack of action. By contrast, the introvert needs time to reflect before making decisions and prefers the company of one or two people to being in large crowds.

Jung also identified four psychological functions that help account for the way a person processes information and makes decisions: thinking, feeling, sensing, and intuition. Although everyone has all four psychological functions available for use, Jung proposed that people use one more than the other three. He identified the one used most often as the superior function and the least differentiated as the inferior function. Evidence of the inferior function is found in dreams and fantasies (Hall & Lindzey, 1970). Jung's descriptions of the four common archetypes and four fundamental psychological functions formed the basis for the Meyers-Briggs Temperament Scales used extensively today in career and marital counseling.

Jung believed that the goal of personality development was self-realization. This was to be accomplished through individuation, which he described as developing a strong sense of self as apart but always in connective harmony with community (transcendent function). The self could find fulfillment through symbolic meaning, achievement, and religious experiences (Jung, 1958). Personal accomplishments in work and relationships could be forms of self-expression leading to individuation. In the process of achieving selfhood, Jung believed that humans were transformed from purely biological creatures into spiritual individuals. Although his description of the collective unconscious could be interpreted as a somewhat pantheistic world view, Jung was a deeply spiritual man, and he believed that spirituality was a necessary part of mental health (Jung, 1933).

RELEVANCE TO NURSING

Many of Jung's concepts are relevant in the nursing care of mentally ill patients. He introduced the idea of humans' cultural heritage as being an important dimension of self. He spoke of the self as being central to unity and wholeness. Jung's insistence that men and women, although different, also possess characteristics that can aid in their understanding of one another is extremely helpful in promoting more satisfying gender roles. He offered an explanation for the common tendency in individuals to project their undesired characteristics onto others and to reject their existence in themselves. Understanding the origin of people's irrational thoughts about others and their biases can aid in a more compassionate approach toward patients.

Interpersonal Psychodynamic Theory: Harry Stack Sullivan

Sullivan's (1894–1949) interpersonal model evolved in opposition to psychoanalytic theory's strong emphasis on reducing personality to biological drives. Harry Stack Sullivan was trained in psychodynamic methodology and championed the interpersonal model. (Hall & Lindzey, 1970; Smith & Vetter, 1982; Sullivan, 1954, 1972). Although he recognized the Freudian concepts of psychic energy, anxiety reduction, and the unconscious, Sullivan rejected other fundamental aspects of Freud's theory. His theory is classified as a *psychodynamic* (interpersonal) one because it is based on human relationships. Sullivan proposes that personality cannot be studied apart from the social and cultural influences on behavior, and his theory draws on knowledge from anthropology and sociology in addition to psychology. Sullivan viewed any unit of behavior that a person demonstrated in a relationship as a **dynamism,** which he defined as an energy transference. A dynamism could be one of fear, intimacy, hostility, or lust. Sullivan viewed personality as a tension system in which tensions emerged and had to be relieved. He identified two basic sources of tension: needs and anxiety.

Rather than looking at instinctual drives as the driving force behind behavior, Sullivan's theory centers around the concept of anxiety as an interpersonally determined experience. He viewed the pursuit of biological satisfaction and the pursuit of emotional security as the motivators for most behavior. Satisfaction needs encompass the fundamental biological demands necessary for survival, that is, the need for nourishment, rest, sex, freedom from loneliness, and so forth. These needs are present immediately and require the infant to interact with others. Presumably, as a result of these positive interactions, need fulfillment occurs. The developing human benefits concurrently from attachment to others and from the tenderness this provides (security needs).

Security needs are psychological. They refer to the need to avoid anxiety and to feel safe and accepted. Psychological security leads to a sense of well-being and belonging, congruent with the social norms and value systems of a person's community. According to Sullivan, a person becomes mentally ill when the person's self-system compromises the capacity to meet his or her needs for physiological satisfaction or psychological security.

According to Sullivan, anxiety develops from real or imagined threats to the self. The degree of anxiety is proportional to the amount of threat it stimulates. Anxiety is to be avoided at all costs. It first develops in infancy when there is a breakdown in the mother-child interaction.

THE SELF-SYSTEM

Sullivan portrayed the self-system as an important dynamism, which operates to prevent an individual from experiencing anxiety. In the process of becoming a mature human being, a person develops three personifications of the self-concept: the "good me," the "bad me," and the "not me," to ward against anxiety. Ideally the good me, in which the person experiences the self as good and worthwhile, predominates in the personality structure. The good me evolves out of the child's security and knowledge of the mother's approval. The bad me develops from observations of behaviors that the mother does not like and serves as a deterrent against behaviors that would earn disapproval. The not me portion of self-concept relates to activities and behaviors that are so ego-alien they must be disowned by the individual as not being a part of self. Sullivan believed that not me manifestations of behavior are present in psychosis and in delusional thinking.

Sullivan suggested that personality functioning was actually best determined through observation of particular modes of interpersonal behavior. He identified three cognitive processes:

- Protaxic thinking (instinctual perceptions)
- Parataxic thinking (cause-effect relationships are established)
- Syntaxic thinking (consistent with Freud's secondary processes)

In infancy, only the protaxic mode exists, but as the child develops and interacts with important interpersonal figures, thinking progresses to a higher level (Marmer, 1994). Ideally, therapy supports syntaxic thinking processes as a way of establishing the validity of and organizing information obtained through lower modes of cognitive functioning.

Sullivan's interpersonal model disputes the notion that cognitive insight alone brings about therapeutic change. Instead, his model stresses the nature and quality of the interpersonal relationship as the primary basis for healing. Furthermore, Sullivan firmly believed that the social attempt to separate these phenomena defeats the point. According to Sullivan, the essence of personality lies at this juncture and is best understood in its relation to the current interpersonal encounter.

Although the interpersonal therapist takes a patient history as background data, the major thrust of therapeutic intervention takes place through a corrective emotional experience that examines components of the self-system used to defend the individual against the emergence of anxiety. Once the patient becomes aware of components in the self-system that are not working or are dissociated from memory, the process of therapy takes on a reeducation focus. By directly experiencing a healthy authentic relationship with a helping person, working through difficult interpersonal problems, and learning better communication strategies, the patient is better able to establish healthy relationships with other people. Each relationship between a professional helping person and a patient is founded on respect and equality.

RELEVANCE TO NURSING

Sullivan's theory is the foundation for Hildegard Peplau's theory of interpersonal relationship. His thought that therapy should basically be used as a forum to educate patients and to assist them in gaining personal insight is the basis for Peplau's use of the nurse as an "educative instrument." It was Sullivan who first used the term *participant observer,* meaning that professional helpers cannot be isolated from the therapeutic situation if they are to be effective. The nurse must interact with the patient as an authentic human being. Mutuality, respect for the patient, unconditional acceptance, and empathy, proposed as essential characteristics in modern therapeutic relationships, were important aspects of Sullivan's theory of interpersonal therapy.

Sullivan also demonstrated that a psychotherapeutic environment is an invaluable treatment tool. His idea of a psychotherapeutic milieu evolved around an accepting atmosphere, which provided numerous opportunities for practicing interpersonal skills and developing relationships. Group psychotherapy, family therapy, and educational and skill training programs as well as unstructured periods can be incorporated into the design of a psychotherapeutic environment to facilitate healthy interactions. This method is now being used in virtually all residential and day hospital settings.

> **W**hat do you think? As you read about these various theorists, can you identify ways in which their concepts have been accepted into the general culture? How has your thinking been influenced by Freudian or Jungian thought? Do you accept the concept of the unconscious? If so what does that acceptance do to beliefs regarding free will or personal responsibility?

▶ Check Your Reading

4. In what ways might psychoanalytic theory principles influence an assessment of a psychiatric patient?
5. What do you consider to be Carl Jung's most important contributions to the study of personality?
6. In what ways does Sullivan's interpersonal theory challenge the ideas of the psychoanalytic model?

Ego Theory: Erik Erikson

Erik Erikson's (1902–1994) original work on personality development (1950, 1982) forms the foundation for understanding psychological growth and development. He was born in Frankfurt, Germany (Smith & Vetter, 1982). Erikson's formal education ended with the completion of high school. Instead of attending college, he traveled throughout Europe, eventually landing in Vienna. He accepted a position at the day care center Anna Freud had created for the children of student psychoanalysts, and it was here that his fascination for

observing and documenting human development at different points in the life span began. Erikson studied under Sigmund Freud's instruction, completing his education in 1933. He soon became one of the first child psychoanalysts in the United States.

Erikson practiced **ego psychology** because he focused on the ego. His vision of the ego differs from Freud's original concept of a fixed object. In Erikson's theory, the ego is separate and liberated from the id, developing across the course of the complete life cycle. In fact, Erikson contended that ego development is influenced by family, social, and even environmental factors. He described his theory as based on the epigenetic principle, in which sequential maturation occurs according to a biological time pattern, and maintained that "eight basic strengths emerge as we go through life, each the outgrowth of a time-specific developmental confrontation" (Erikson, 1988, p. 74). In contrast to epigenesis in the embryo, however, "where a strength is not adequately developed according to the given sequence for its scheduled period of critical resolution, the supports of the environment may bring it into appropriate balance at a later period" (Erikson, 1988, p. 75). Thus, life cycle psychological theory has a more hopeful note for successful resolution of psychosocial tasks.

Erikson (1982) described the human life cycle as a series of eight ego developmental stages, spanning from birth to death. Each stage presents a **psychosocial crisis** whose goal is to integrate both physical maturation and societal demands. At each maturational juncture, the person either masters the psychosocial crisis effectively (and thus strengthens his or her ego), or the inverse occurs. Each step forward involves a disconnection with previous ways of thinking about the self and a loss of the comfort associated with the previous sense of self. Consequently, each psychosocial crisis creates anxiety. Although Erikson's stages of ego development follow the chronological pattern Freud proposed, they incorporate and focus on psychosocial factors to a much larger extent.

1. *Basic trust versus mistrust* occurs in infancy. Initially, the newborn is completely dependent on others to meet its needs. Gradually, the infant acquires limited control by relying on the five senses. General trust is learned when the infant's needs are tended to satisfactorily and consistently. Self-trust is formed when the infant is able to rely on his or her inputs. Conversely, the infant learns to mistrust a withholding, inconsistent world that thwarts self-reliance. Trust is a critical issue with Erikson, and he emphasizes its importance in therapeutic relationships. *The interpersonal strength is hope.*

2. *Autonomy versus shame and doubt* coincides with toddlerhood, which starts before a child reaches 2 years of age. During this stage, muscular development advances, allowing rudimentary language, ambulation, and bodily control. The child who is encouraged to take more responsibility for self is better able to feel and act independently. Shame and doubt emerge when parents

inhibit their child's natural striving for independence by somehow undermining it. *The interpersonal strength is will.*

3. *Initiative versus guilt* takes place in early childhood. The central issue here revolves around the child's attempts to pursue and obtain a goal, to achieve a sense of purpose. This stage corresponds to Freud's Oedipus complex. Mastery requires the child to identify with the parent of the same sex and to adopt parental values to mold the superego. Guilt is experienced if the child's own directives are shunned. *The interpersonal strength is purpose.*

4. *Industry versus inferiority* occurs during latency. At this phase, interactions outside the family structure assume increasing significance. The child is challenged to comply with social values, establish friendships, and acquire new skills, all of which can lead to feelings of competency. Failure at this endeavor, however, leads to feelings of inferiority. *The interpersonal strength is competence.*

5. *Identity versus role confusion* is the crisis associated with adolescence. The struggle here is to find oneself in the midst of turmoil. Mastery involves integrating a sense of personal identity, based on sexual maturity, individuation from the family, meaningful peer relationships, and decisiveness about ambitions in life. *The interpersonal strength is fidelity.*

6. *Intimacy versus isolation* is the first of the three adult stages. It occurs as a person seeks mature love, closeness, and sharing with another. Mastery of this psychosocial stage results in a capacity for being in a sustained, intimate relationship. *The interpersonal strength is love.*

7. *Generativity versus stagnation* occurs during middle age (30–60 years of age). The central issue in this stage is work and productivity. The emphasis here is on generativity, that is, a genuine regard for improving society by one's own efforts. This requires a concern for others. Stagnation is rooted in a lack of this concern, which leaves the individual void of meaningfulness and searching for that elusive quality. *The interpersonal strength is caring.*

8. *Ego integrity versus despair* entails a review of one's accomplishments. A positive evaluation leads to ego integrity, whereas a negative appraisal causes despair. Despair relates to feelings of loss and dissatisfaction with one's inability to uphold his or her values. *The interpersonal strength is wisdom.*

Erikson's stages of ego development are also discussed in Chapters 18 through 21. Erikson's contributions to the understanding of human development are significant. He expanded on previous theories of human development and included the influence of social and cultural factors as relevant antecedents and supports for personal growth. Erikson forced psychological attention on developmental crises in adulthood and the interactions needed to resolve them. Erikson's theory of ego development is a hopeful one because people always carry within them the potential to rework a previous psychosocial stage in a more personally satisfying way.

RELEVANCE TO NURSING

Nurses use Erikson's model as an important part of patient assessment. Analysis of behavior patterns, using Erikson's framework, can identify age-appropriate or arrested development of normal interpersonal skills. A developmental framework helps the nurse know what types of interventions are most likely to be effective. For example, children in Erikson's initiative versus guilt stage of development respond best if they actively participate and ask many questions. Elderly patients respond to a life review strategy that focuses on the integrity of their life as a composite of experience. In the therapeutic encounter, individual responsibility and the capacity for improving one's functioning are addressed. Treatment approaches and intervention strategies can be tailored to support the patient's developmental level.

Humanistic Theories

Humanistic psychology arose in protest to the psychoanalytic school of thought, which the proponents of humanistic psychology believed explicitly excluded human potential and the possibility of choosing life patterns supportive of personal growth. Humanistic frameworks emphasize a person's capacity for self-actualization. They seek to understand behavior from the patient's perspective, as he or she subjectively experiences it.

Abraham Maslow

Maslow (1908–1970) is considered the "father of humanistic psychology." In 1962, he suggested that humanistic psychology represented the third force in psychology, the first two being psychoanalysis and behaviorism (Bugental, 1967). Maslow conceptualized human motivation as a *hierarchy of dynamic processes (needs)* that are critical for the development and growth of all humans. Central to his theory is the assumption that humans are active rather than passive participants in life, striving for self-actualization. Maslow (1968) focuses on human need fulfillment, which he describes in six incremental stages, beginning with physiological survival needs and ending with self-transcendent needs (Figure 6–1). Although these needs are present in all humans, the behaviors that emanate from them differ according to a person's unique biological make-up and environmental factors. Maslow describes humans' more basic needs as D-motives or deficiency needs, meaning that they are so basic to existence that they must be resolved to reduce the tension associated with them. Because they have the greatest strength, needs at a lower level must always be satisfied before a person turns his attention to higher-level needs. As an example, a homeless person is not going to be interested in joining a support group to get more in touch with his or her feelings and experience the joy of belonging when issues of basic survival remain unresolved. Maslow describes self-esteem and self-actualization as "B-motives," or "being needs", reflective of growth motivation.

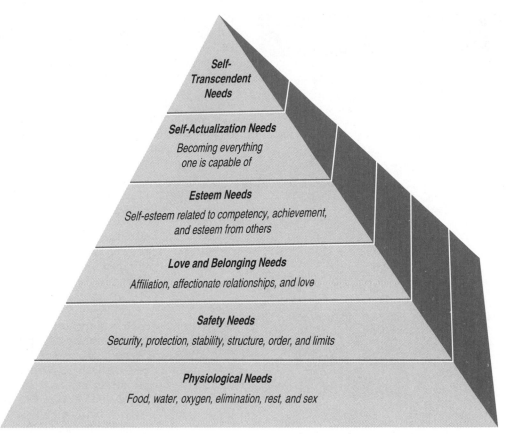

Figure 6–1
Maslow's hierarchy of needs. (Adapted from Maslow, A. H. [1972]. *The farther reaches of human nature.* New York: Viking.)

As basic deficiency needs are met, a person turns attention to personal growth needs to develop his or her human capacity to the fullest extent possible. Maslow's (1968) emphasis on being needs or growth needs is about human potential. He suggests looking at a person's strengths rather than at personality deficits. A person's striving for personal growth leads one to realize one's fullest expression of talents and personality assets, "the human being at his best" (Maslow, 1963). Self-actualized people develop a problem-centered approach to life, identify with humankind, and transcend their environment. They develop a philosophical outlook on life rather than being overwhelmed by every life event. Most important, they can distinguish the means from the end and act in an ethical manner that brings inner peace. According to Maslow, the self is the inner core of personality, holding some characteristics in common with others and possessing other characteristics not held by many others. Using a case study method, Maslow arrived at his description of self-actualized people by studying the behaviors of remarkable people such as Thomas Jefferson, Abraham Lincoln, Eleanor Roosevelt, and Albert Einstein as well as the behaviors of those Maslow himself came into contact with and admired (Maslow, 1970). Behaviors associated with a self-actualized person are presented in Table 6–4. Maslow's theory of self-actualization has influenced the field of psychiatry in providing a rationale for the development of sensitivity and encounter groups, which help people

get in touch with who they are in the moment and their human potential.

RELEVANCE TO NURSING

The value of Maslow's model in nursing practice is twofold. First, the emphasis on human potential and the patient's strengths is key to successful nurse-patient relationships. The second value lies in establishing what is most important in the sequencing of nursing actions in the nurse-patient relationship. For example, attempting to collect any but the most essential information when a patient is struggling with drug withdrawal is inappropriate. Following Maslow's model as a way of prioritizing actions, the nurse would meet the patient's physiological need for stabilizing vital signs and pain relief before collecting general information for a nursing database.

Carl Rogers

Rogers (b. 1902) is clearly one of the most prominent humanist psychologists. He was born in Oak Park, Illinois, and grew up in a family environment that stressed hard work and religious commitment. After college and a stint in the seminary, he transferred to Columbia University, where he received his PhD in 1931. His theory evolved from observations in his clinical work with psychiatric patients, but his work has been extended to the field of education as well as psychology.

TABLE 6–4 Behaviors Associated With a Self-Actualized Person	
CHARACTERISTIC	**BEHAVIOR**
Realistic orientation	Can see the world and the people in it accurately and without value orientations; not given to unrealistic wishful thinking
Spontaneity	Behavior marked by simplicity and naturalness
Acceptance of self and others	Has a positive self-concept and an uncritical acceptance of self and others
Close relationships with others	Values people and is valued by others; relationships are deep and meaningful
Autonomous thinking	Has strong convictions and is able to act on them; does not depend on the approval of others
Appreciation of life	Is glad to be alive and appreciates what life brings; enjoys life at its fullest
Creativity	Is able to solve problems in creative ways
Consideration of and respect for others	Respects and values individual differences

Adapted from Maslow, A. (1956). Self actualizing people: A study of psychological health. In C. Moustakas (Ed.), *The self: Explorations in personal growth*. New York: Harper & Row.

Carl Rogers (1961) defined the self as

the organized, consistent, conceptual gestalt composed of perceptions characteristic of the "I" or "me" and the perceptions of the relationships of the "I" or "me" to others and the various aspects of life together with the values attached to these perceptions. (p. 200)

He developed a person-centered model of psychotherapy that emphasizes the uniqueness of the individual. First described in his classic text, *Counseling and Psychotherapy* (1942), Rogers believed that all humans have an innate potential to develop and make full use of their talents and personality characteristics. Rogers (1963) referred to this natural guidance system, unique to each individual, as the actualizing tendency. With the actualizing tendency as a natural guide for personal growth, people live their lives in ways that promote personal satisfaction as well as growth and development. When people disregard their actualizing tendency in favor of trying to please others and receive approval, they develop symptoms. They forget what they know to be true about themselves and consequently become confused and unable to evaluate behaviors that can lead to personal growth.

Rogers' person-centered model of psychotherapy is based on the premise that people have within themselves everything they need for understanding and changing their attitudes and behaviors. A person-centered counseling approach is designed to reestablish the person's actualizing tendency as the natural guide for behavior. Certain conditions or attitudes of the therapist offered to the patient, such as unconditional positive regard, empathy, and congruence, are regarded as necessary and sufficient conditions for successful therapy results (Rogers, 1942). These therapist-offered conditions allow patients to experience their unique, true feelings in a safe, supportive interpersonal environment. Rogers speaks of *congruence,* which means that the therapist acts in an authentic manner, as the first critical condition for successfully helping people. The therapist allows the patient to see the therapist as he or she is in the relationship without needing to hide behind a role. The openness of the therapist is in direct opposition to the psychoanalytic approach, in which the person of the therapist is unavailable to the patient.

The second necessary condition for successful therapeutic outcome is *unconditional acceptance* and *positive regard.* By providing a climate of unconditional positive regard, patients are able to experience whatever feeling they have without fear of reprisal or disapproval. *Empathetic understanding* is the third critical attitude and occurs when the therapist is able to experience the feelings and personal meanings as if they were happening to the therapist and is able to communicate that understanding to the patient. When the patient feels understood, he or she is freer to self-disclose at a deeper level, and it becomes easier to listen more accurately to the inner self.

RELEVANCE TO NURSING

Rogers' humanistic model encourages nurses to look at each patient as a unique human being, a person who feels, knows, and experiences life in a special way. His theory portrays people as being basically good with an inherent potential for self-actualization. Rogers's necessary conditions for a successful therapeutic outcome provide a valuable structure for understanding personal attitudes the nurse needs to have to facilitate change in the patient. Rogers' (1963) insistence that "man does not simply have the characteristics of a machine, he is not simply a being in the grip of unconscious motives, he is a person in the process of creating himself, a person who creates meaning in life" (p. 82) has a powerful influence on the conduct of the nurse-patient relationship. The attitudes of unconditional positive regard, empathetic understanding, and genuineness achieved through self-awareness are foundational concepts in effective nurse-patient relationships. A person-centered nursing approach recognizes the uniqueness of the individual and tries to engage the patient as an equal collaborator in the journey toward mental health.

Existential Theories

Yalom (1980) speaks of existential models of human behavioral therapy as an orphan looking for a home, as there is no single model associated with existentialism. Instead, existential theories attempt to define what it means to be fully human and to find meaning in existence. Focused on personal freedom, authenticity, anxiety, meaning, and death, existential models were heavily influenced by secular and religious philosophers such as Heidegger (1962), Kierkegaard (1844–1957), and Tillich (1952). Martin Buber's (1970) description of an I-Thou relationship designed to enhance awareness and acceptance of the uniqueness of each human being is a natural outgrowth of these earlier writings. Buber believed that "relation is reciprocity" (p. 58). Whether or not the other person fully appreciates the deed is not as important as the person's extending the soul's creative power to another with his or her whole being. In that extension of self lies the possibility of a human connection capable of transforming the meaning of the experience between two people. Theoretical concepts related to the I-Thou relationship are found in Chapter 10.

Existential models essentially view mental illness as occurring when a person loses contact with his or her essential humanness and is unable to establish human relationships with others based on honesty. Basically, the person is living a lie, and the meaning of life centers around the anxiety needed to maintain an inauthentic way of being. These people suffer from feelings of intense isolation from others and a chronic sense of emptiness. They have lost faith in themselves and have difficulty learning from and accepting the natural limits of their life circumstances.

Taking personal responsibility is key to existential therapy approaches. The existential therapist would argue against using a specific set of therapeutic strategies, preferring instead to develop a meaningful relationship in which both participants are fully present in the immediacy of the moment. Existential therapists encourage their patients to shed the lies that hide the reality of their existence and to develop human relationships that reflect and support their personal integrity.

Existential models view anxiety as an important wake-up call motivating people to take charge of their lives and to make needed changes. People are free to make decisions that enable them to find real meaning in their lives and to discard maladaptive or unsatisfying life patterns. A person is the architect of his or her own destiny and free to choose the person he or she wishes to become. If a person chooses to abdicate the responsibility for authentic living, the result is anxiety, depression, and guilt. Existentially based concepts are found in the theoretically based psychotherapies of Ludwig Binswanger, Rollo May, Viktor Frankl, William Glasser, and Irving Yalom. Two representative frameworks are presented here.

Viktor Frankl

Frankl was born in 1905, a Jewish man who spent 3 years in a concentration camp, losing his wife, mother, father, and brother during this tragic time. He observed that some people in the concentration camp were able to sustain their personal integrity and to emerge strengthened despite losing all that they held dear and suffering intense emotional pain. Their sense of self-respect and personal integrity remained untouched. From this experience, Frankl developed *logotherapy* (*logo*, taken from the Greek word for "meaning"), a form of support designed to help people who have lost their reason for living to reclaim their sense of self-respect. Logotherapy is a future-oriented therapy, focused on one's need to find meaning and value in living as the most important life task. "Everyone has his own specific vocation or mission in life; everyone must carry out a concrete assignment that demands fulfillment. . . . Each man is questioned by life; and he can only respond by answering for his own life; to life he can only respond by being responsible" (Frankl, 1969, pp. 170–171).

Strategies proposed by Frankl include dereflection and paradoxical intention. *Dereflection* involves helping patients to refocus their attention away from anxiety-producing stimuli. For example, the therapist might encourage a man fearful of impotency to concentrate on his partner's pleasure rather than his performance. *Paradoxical intention* involves instructing a patient to exaggerate the behavior that is causing distress. For example, Frankl described a case in which a bookkeeper experienced such anxiety when he tried to write legibly in his ledger that he was in danger of losing his job. Frankl encouraged him to deliberately write with an illegible scrawl. Ironically, he found he was unable to do this when it became a conscious act, and the symptoms that caused him so much distress vanished quickly. This technique has been used successfully with obsessive-compulsive behaviors found in individuals and families.

William Glasser

Glasser, a psychiatrist, developed his model of reality therapy as an outgrowth of his work with patients in a variety of clinical settings. He proposes that "unhappiness is the result and not the cause of irresponsibility" (Glasser, 1965). *Reality therapy* is a highly pragmatic model that focuses on the here and now as the only reality to be considered. Glasser proposed that there is no way a person's past can be rewritten, so it is fruitless to consider it. Blaming personal failures on external circumstances, lack of opportunity, poor family relationships, or virtually any other circumstances is not acceptable. Instead the reality therapist encourages the patient to rewrite his or her life script and to consider definite plans based on the personal responsibility and self-discipline needed for a different outcome. The therapist becomes the therapeutic ally, but it is ultimately up to the patient to develop a functional understanding of reality. Strategies focus on what the patient does and not on what the patient feels. The approach is a positive one in which the therapist conveys the belief that the patient can influence his or her feelings and has the capability to develop a more successful pattern of living. Persistent refocusing on progress, taking the next step, and considering practical issues needed for successful resolution of difficult life problems help patients develop the positive attitudes needed for successful living.

> **What do you think?** As you read about these various theories, is there one that fits your own world view more than another? Are you comfortable with pieces from a variety of theories? Which approach best captures your own theories and approaches to dealing with and understanding people?

➤ *Check Your Reading*

7. Why might Erikson's theory remain so relevant today?
8. How does humanistic theory enhance the personal journey of the patient?
9. In what ways do humanistic and existential models parallel and diverge from each other?

Behavioral Theories

Behavioral approaches to therapy initially were developed as a protest response to Freud's assumption that a person's destiny was carved in stone at an early age. By contrast, a behaviorist considers personality as what people do and not who they are. Behavioral models postulate that personality consists of learned behaviors. Consequently, personality is synonymous with behavior. If you change the behavior, you change the personality.

Behavioral models originated from lessons learned in experimental animal laboratories during the 19th century, first with Pavlov's dog experiments and later in the 20th century with Skinner's research on rat behavior. These behavioral theorists developed their observations of animal behavior into systematic applications of learning principles that could be applied to humans. Used in education as well as in psychiatric settings to manage problem behaviors, behavior modification, programmed learning, biofeedback, and token economies are commonly used techniques based on behavioral models. Behavioral models emphasize the ways in which observable behavioral responses are learned and can be modified in a particular environment. Three of the most influential behavioral theorists were Ivan Pavlov, James Watson, and B. F. Skinner. Their models focus on a belief that it is possible to influence behavior through a process referred to as conditioning. **Conditioning** involves pairing a behavior with a condition that reinforces or diminishes the behavior's occurrence.

Ivan Pavlov

Pavlov (1849–1936) was a Russian physiologist who won the Nobel Prize for his outstanding contributions to the physiology of digestion, which he studied through his well-known dog experiments. From incidental observations of the dogs, he noticed that they were able to anticipate when food would be forthcoming, and they would begin to salivate even before actually experiencing the meal. Pavlov labeled this process *psychic secretions.* He hypothesized that the psychic component was a learned association between two events: the presence of experimental apparatus and the serving of meat.

Pavlov (1928) formalized his observations of behaviors in dogs in a theory of classical conditioning. He observed that the dog salivated naturally whenever it was presented with food but did not have a similar reaction to the sound of a tuning fork, an unconditioned stimulus. By repeatedly sounding the tuning fork when the dog was presented with food, the dog began to associate salivation with both the food and the tuning fork. Pavlov was able to "condition" the dog's response so that the dog continued to salivate when the tuning fork was rung without food being present.

In *classical conditioning,* a neutral stimulus (such as the bell tone) is repeatedly paired with a stimulus that innately elicits a response (such as food triggering salivation). Through this process, the neutral stimulus is transformed into a *conditioned stimulus.* The eliciting stimulus (in this case, the meat) is called the *unconditioned stimulus.* Repetitive pairing of the two causes the establishment of a predictable pattern, and subsequently learning occurs. Classical conditioning sometimes is referred to as *respondent conditioning* because the subject is basically a passive agent. Respondents are responses that result from specific, identifiable stimuli. They may be learned responses (as in the case of an animal wincing when a tone is heard that has been repeatedly paired with a shock) or unlearned (such as when a physical reflex is provoked and produced).

Pavlov introduced the term *reinforcement* in describing the dog's selective response to a given stimulus. Although he considered his scientific observations to represent physiological responses, rather than psychological, his ideas formed the foundation for the development of behavioral therapies and are widely used in educational settings.

James B. Watson

Watson (1878–1958) was an American psychologist who developed the school of thought referred to as behaviorism (Watson, 1919, 1928). He was strongly influenced by Pavlov's conditioning principles and began to apply these principles to human beings. Watson placed a strong emphasis on the role of the social environment in shaping behavior. He is best known for his experiments with little Albert. The experiment consisted of standing behind the child, who liked animals, and making a loud noise with a hammer every time the child reached for the animal (a large white rat). After a number of repetitions, little Albert became afraid of the white rat and later of all furry animals and objects, without the presence of the loud noise.

B. F. Skinner

Skinner (1904–1990) was part of a second wave of behavioral theorists who expanded the notion of stimulus-response behavioral approaches to learning to include the concept of reinforcement (Fancher, 1990; Hall & Lindzey, 1970; Skinner, 1987; Smith & Vetter, 1982). He earned his college degree as an English major, but he did not find satisfaction with literature. Although literature described the way people functioned, it could not explain why they did so. Through his reading, however, Skinner happened on the writings of prominent behaviorists. Here he began to find potential answers to the questions that haunted him about the psychology of behavior. Skinner attended Harvard graduate school in psychology and was recognized there as an outstanding student. At Harvard, Skinner concentrated his studies on behavioral change—specifically, behavioral learning and behavioral modification. In addition to his studies of rat behavior at the university, Skinner raised his second daughter, for the first 2½ years, in an air-conditioned box, which he called a baby tender. The baby tender was marketed commercially, but needless to say it never caught on with the public.

Skinner is generally recognized as one of the prime movers behind the behavioral movement in mental health. Like Freud, he believed that all behavior is determined. He differed, though, with Freud about its origin. Skinner proposed that human behavior is supported by reinforcement contingencies and that it is possible to predict and control the behavior of others through an understanding of the nature of humans' reinforcers. In taking this stand, he also distanced himself from Pavlovian thinking, which viewed behavioral change as a simple stimulus-response connection. Skinner added a second principle of learning that includes motivation and social reinforcement (Woodward, 1982; Figure 6–2).

Skinner based his theory on his research with rats, in which he was able to elicit responses. Using the famous Skinner box, he demonstrated that if he reinforced a rat with food for pressing a lever when a light would go on and did not reinforce the rat when the light was off, the rat "learned" to press the lever so that it would get the food. He labeled the light as a *discriminative stimulus,* meaning that it was the paired association of the reinforcer with behavior and not the stimulus itself that caused the rat to press the lever. The discriminative stimulus acts as a cue for the desired behavior. Examples in everyday life include the bell that signals students to leave class, traffic lights, and business bonuses. Behavior modification, a form of treatment used extensively with patients suffering from a wide range of disorders, such as retardation, sexual dysfunction, enuresis, violence, and autism; chronically ill patients; and adolescents with behavior problems, emphasizes Skinner's basic premise that all behavioral responses, being learned, can also be unlearned.

Skinner labeled the most important segment of his theory **operant conditioning.** Operant conditioning refers to the manipulation of selected reinforcers to elicit and strengthen desired behavioral reinforcers. Reinforcers refer to the consequences of the behavior. Skinner believed that a person performs a behavior (discharges an operant) and receives a consequence (reinforcer) as a result of performing the behavior. The consequence makes it more or less probable that the person will repeat the behavior. If the consequence is positive, the chances of repetition increase. Negative consequences have a deterrent effect on behavior. For example, the use of disulfiram (Antabuse) discourages people from drinking because it causes physical effects if the person tries to drink while on the medication. Absence of reinforcement also decreases behavior. Thus, if a person typically gets attention by making a joke and no one laughs at it, this particular behavior tends to decrease because it is not being reinforced. At the heart of Skinner's theory is the proposition that reinforcement ultimately determines the existence of behavior.

Skinner defined **reinforcers** as anything that increases the occurrence of a behavior. The value of a reinforcer lies in its meaning to a particular individual. A reinforcer for one person may not have any effect as a reinforcer on another. According to Skinner, there are two types of reinforcers: (1) *primary reinforcers,* which are of survival importance, such as food, water, and sex; and (2) *secondary (conditioned) reinforcers,* such as money, material goods, and praise.

Change is measured by counting the rate of occurrence related to a specific behavior. The clinician uses cumulative written records to assess an individual's rate of response. Beginning with a thorough analysis of target behaviors, the goal of behavioral therapy is to change the respondent's behavior by providing positive reinforcement (token, gift, or praise) if a behavior is accomplished or negative reinforcement (withdrawing sanctions or verbal disapproval) if the behavior ceases to exist. Complex behaviors usually need to be broken down into smaller steps. This allows for *shaping* behavior, which consists of progressively reinforcing the smaller steps needed to achieve a certain behavior.

RELEVANCE TO NURSING

Skinner's behavioral model provides a concrete method for modifying behaviors or replacing them. Behavior management and modification programs based on his principles have proved to be successful in altering targeted behaviors. Programmed learning and token economies represent extensions of Skinner's thoughts

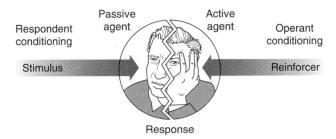

Figure 6–2
Respondent conditioning versus operant conditioning.

on learning. The efficacy of behavioral models is easier to test empirically because the data are straightforward. Behavioral methods are particularly effective with adolescent acting-out behaviors and many forms of chronic mental illness.

Albert Bandura

Bandura (b. 1925) attempted to rectify the oversimplification of a two-factored behavioral theory by developing a model based on social learning through imitation (1962, 1977). **Social learning theory** conceptualizes psychological functioning as an integration of both environmental conditions and personal attributes. This integration is ongoing and reciprocal. In 1977, Bandura wrote a book, *Social Learning Theory,* in which he postulated that people do alter their behavior in response to situational changes. He also proposed that people learn best by observation, by watching others perform, and by the subsequent modeling of behavior. Bandura based his conclusions on research findings that not all behavioral responses could be accounted for by connective cues between stimulus-response, or response reinforcement. Instead, he observed that behavioral change occurred in many instances as a result of external social discriminative cues that influenced behavior. For example, in many societies, aggressive behaviors are not modeled, or socially reinforced, for little girls as they are for little boys as being particularly desirable ways of acting.

Bandura believed that human behavior is best explained by considering it as a reciprocal interaction continuously occurring between the organism and behavioral, cognitive, and environmental influences. He proposed that people observe which behaviors are rewarded or punished and "vicariously" embrace the implications of the modeling stimuli they witness. In addition to external reinforcement, people engage in **self-reinforcement,** whereby an individual reinforces himself or herself in the absence of an actual reinforcer. Bandura believed that symbolic, vicarious, and self-regulatory processes are instrumental in determining the precise behavioral action one assumes. For example, a student notices that another student has completed his or her homework assignment. This knowledge stimulates the first student to complete his or her own work.

This vicarious learning is much more efficient because instead of repeatedly trying new behaviors and judging the effect of such actions, humans possess the ability to witness another's actions and outcomes. Through this experience, the person learns modes of behavior that can help him or her avoid potentially dangerous responses and speed up the acquisition of new or advantageous behaviors.

MODELING

Bandura considered modeling an important principle of learning. Modeling affects learning because of the information it provides the individual. Cognitive functions are the critical components in this process. The

actual learning and the activation of the system occurs in a four-step process:

1. Attentional processes
2. Retention
3. Motor reproduction
4. Motivation

Attentional Processes. The quality of one's attentiveness to and accurate perception of an observed behavior has obvious implications for its success as a learning experience. The attentional processes circumscribe what is focused on in the observation. Certain factors affect the attentional process. These include personal attributes of the model, such as how charismatic and capable he or she is. The behavior itself influences attentiveness. The degree of relevancy it bears to the observing individual's life circumstance and the complexity of the behavior are two factors that play a part in the process.

Retention. The second process in the sequence is retention. Retention refers to the ability to recollect the information. Symbolic representation through imagery or language allows the experience to be coded in memory, thereby creating a method for the observer to continue benefitting from past observational experiences.

Motor Reproduction. Motor reproduction is identified as the third phase. It is not necessarily achieved, however, immediately following retention. In fact, for most complex skills, practice is usually required before reactment can be perfected. Self-corrective measures can be used to make improvements, but sometimes confounding variables (such as physical limitations or incomplete data collection of the observation itself) permanently preclude the development of the desired behavior.

Motivation. The last process is motivation. Social learning theory recognizes the fact that not all learned behavior is executed. Performance of the behavior at some future date is linked to the reinforcement it will produce. People favor development of behaviors that have no negative consequence.

SELF-EFFICACY THEORY

In addition to his contributions related to observational learning and modeling, Bandura (1977, 1978) proposed a theory of self-efficacy that also has relevance for psychiatric nursing. **Self-efficacy** refers to a person's belief or expectation that he or she has the capacity to effect a desired outcome through his or her own personal efforts. Bandura (1977) suggested that all psychotherapeutic strategies should have the common goal of "creating and strengthening expectations of personal efficacy" (p. 193). He submitted that perceptions of self-efficacy affect motivation in rather profound ways and that people tend to avoid those situations that challenge their perceptions of self-efficacy. The stronger the belief that a person will be able to master a difficult situation, the more active the person's personal efforts are likely to be, and the more persistent he or she will be in achieving the goal.

RELEVANCE TO NURSING

Social learning theory has blended cognitive functioning with environmental factors, in an attempt to balance inner and outer resources and to offer a more comprehensive conception of human behavior. Nursing practice incorporates techniques from operant and classical conditioning to assist individuals in changing their own behavior or to use these principles for more effective parenting. Also the patient's education in relation to cognitive processes highlighted in this theory can be explained to enhance client understanding about skill development and motivation.

What do you think? Reflect on your own behavior. How much of what you do can be explained through a stimulus-response model? How much could be explained through Bandura's self-efficacy theory. Can you think of situations in your own life that are similar to the experiment with little Albert?

➤ *Check Your Reading*

10. What are some of the differences between behavioral and social learning models?
11. How would you differentiate between a respondent conditioning and an operant conditioning strategy?
12. What do you see as the value of behavioral models for psychiatric nursing?

Biological Theories

The advent of psychopharmacology presented a major challenge to the previous psychodynamic approaches to mental illness. Since the early 1950s, clinicians have increasingly noted that psychoactive chemicals could significantly alter the symptoms of major thought disorders, depression, and anxiety disorder. Medications having differential effects on various neurotransmitters helped restore brain function, allowing patients with mental illness to continue their journey productively, with greater satisfaction and with far less emotional pain. The observations of clinicians working with mentally ill patients led to significant scientific research regarding the ways in which brain chemistry and physiology might explain these effects. The biopsychiatric treatment of mental illness refuted the idea of mental illness as being determined by social conflicts with significant others. Instead, the theoretical stance in a biochemical model of mental illness is that people have a natural predisposition that places them at particular risk for mental illness. Inborn chemical features of reactivity make an individual susceptible to particular disorders, given the appropriate level of stress.

A biological model of mental illness focuses on neurological, chemical, biological, and genetic issues. A biological perspective seeks to understand how the body and brain interact to create emotions, memories, and perceptual experiences. From a biological view-

point, hereditary factors and biochemical influences in the brain govern how messages are transmitted within the body as well as how moods and motivation get activated. Biological models explain how these factors interact and contribute to human functioning. There have been tremendous breakthroughs in understanding and identifying the significant role that neurotransmitters and chemical imbalances play in mental health. Owing to the wealth of knowledge in this area and its importance in understanding the biological factors in mental illness, Chapter 7 is devoted to this topic.

The danger in accepting a purely biological theory of mental illness is that, when carried to an extreme, it suggests social control of behavior through modification of the brain's biochemistry and refutes the idea of personal responsibility for behavior. A biological model defines mental illness as an individual disorder. Such a theory ignores the measureless influences of social, environmental, cultural, economic, and educational factors that play a role in the development and treatment of mental illness.

Blending the Non-Nursing Theories

Ideally, different theoretical perspectives complement one another and enrich the therapeutic journey. They address the complex nature of biopsychosocial and spiritual meaning and value in a person's life. No one theory adequately reveals the complexity of human behavior. A multidimensional view of each human being can provide the kinds of information needed, the method of assessment most applicable to an individual patient's problem, and the types of intervention most likely to achieve desired therapeutic outcomes. For example, medication may significantly reduce troublesome symptoms and allow a relationship to develop. The relationship may provide a patient with the capacity for insight, the most direct route to a more productive and satisfying life. Other patients with similar symptoms but lacking insight or simply wanting symptom relief might benefit from a behavioral approach.

Each psychological theory perspective emphasizes a particular psychological lens for making sense of human beings and their behavior. Consider depression as an example. A psychoanalytic perspective would explore depressive symptoms as being related to repression of earlier hostility and aggressive drives. Taken from a behavioral perspective, a clinician would focus on understanding the antecedent conditions for the development of symptoms and would prescribe behavioral strategies to eliminate the symptom. A social learning theorist might consider the depressive symptoms as representing learned helplessness. Interventions would teach the patient constructive ways to manage life differently. The clinician with a biological perspective would understand a person's depressive symptoms as a misfiring of neurotransmitters. This clinician would orchestrate a medical approach to symptom management by prescribing antidepressants or electroconvulsive therapy to correct the chemical imbalance. By contrast, a humanistic perspective would emphasize a person's individual strengths and human potential. Understanding a person's subjective experience of the depressive symptoms and their relationship to events in the present would be a primary focus of intervention. Psychodynamic approaches to the treatment of depression would focus on the relationship between nurse and patient, whereas an existential approach would emphasize personal responsibility for discovering the meaning of the person's current circumstances in light of the larger journey.

The decision to use a particular theoretical approach should reflect the individualized situation of the patient and the comfort of the clinician in applying that theoretical perspective. Woodward (1982) suggests that "theoretical differences and priority debates are a conspicuous characteristic of normal scientific practices rather than a deviation from them" (p. 408). Taken in this spirit, students are encouraged to select those concepts and ideas that enrich their discussion and application of theoretical and historical perspectives to the study and practice of psychiatric nursing.

NURSING THEORIES

Value of Theoretical Frameworks in Nursing

Although theory from other disciplines adopted and modified by nursing is critical to the understanding of psychiatric–mental health nursing, this knowledge is incomplete without specific attention paid to nursing theory. Donaldson and Crowley (1978) defined a *discipline* as "a unique perspective, a distinct way of viewing all the phenomena, which ultimately defines the limits and nature of its inquiry" (p. 113). The discipline of nursing has a unique body of knowledge, specifically ordered to inform its members of the content and process needed for effective nursing. Governing this unique body of knowledge are theories of nursing representing a number of world views about the discipline of nursing and its particular domain of knowledge. General theories of nursing lay out the domain of the profession, establish the boundaries of nursing practice, provide a basis for research, and serve as a guide for curriculum development (Arnold & Boggs, 1999).

Psychiatric–mental health nursing is recognized as a subspecialty within the larger discipline of professional nursing. McCracken (1994) noted that "programs grounded in theory are more likely to be clinically consistent and organized" (p. 44). The theoretical foundations of professional and psychiatric nursing practice provide the nurse with confidence in his or her ideas and direct actions taken in therapeutic relationships. By blending theory with the nurse's own personal style (i.e., therapeutic use of self), nurses can implement the nursing process in creative ways that truly reflect both the art and the science of psychiatric nursing.

Meleis (1991) claimed that "the primary use of theory is to guide research" (p. 21). Certainly, this is a valid use

of theory and particularly important in understanding a science of such complexity and inferred knowledge. Theories are as much designed to raise essential questions about phenomena as to answer them. Research opens up new opportunities for understandings never before considered. Through research and empirical testing of theoretical concepts, scholars verify theoretical knowledge, enrich current understandings with new findings, and refute past wisdom. Critical thinking about theoretical perspectives as well as reflective dialogue and debate among scholars about the validity of a theory cannot help but stimulate creativity, self-awareness, and development of cognitive competence.

Theory development in nursing has provided opportunities for nurses to describe, empirically test, and evaluate the nature of professional nursing practice. Theory development in nursing has provided opportunities for nurses to test empirically and describe the nature of nursing practice and its impact on patient outcomes in the professional literature. Moreover, graduate students in universities throughout the United States and abroad have provided ideas, struggled to understand the language and meaning of concepts, critiqued ideas, and developed important research studies to support the validity of nursing theory. Thus, nursing theories have a special integrity springing from the commitment and continuous refinement of major propositions and ideas by nursing's primary and contributing authors. Although difficult to prove pragmatically, there is little question that nursing theory has played an important role in helping nurses define their identity as members of a professional discipline.

What Is Nursing Theory?

Nursing theory represents the unique systematic study of nursing experience. Each theoretical perspective evolves from a broader structural base of nursing knowledge, beginning with a **metaparadigm,** or world view, of what constitutes the phenomena of concern in professional nursing. Nursing's metaparadigm consists of four elements: person, environment, health, and nursing. Nursing is included as a separate dimension so that the activities of professional nursing are identifiable as being quite distinct from those of other disciplines. These four elements of concern to nursing are found in each theorist's presentation, although the way in which they are described differ according to the theorist's orientation.

Nursing knowledge proceeds from the general to the more specific in a structural hierarchy that begins with a metaparadigm, develops into conceptual models, and completes its structural mission with the construction of theories that can be tested empirically. *Conceptual models* represent abstract word images of each theorist's thinking about the nature of person, environment, health, and nursing. Corresponding to the concepts (main ideas) in the model are assumptions, defined as the values, ideas, and principles of the theorist. Conceptual models cannot be tested empirically because they do not spell out the relationships between the different concepts. Conceptual models often contain single belief statements, referred to as postulates, which expand the meaning of a concept. Conceptual models in nursing sometimes are categorized as developmental, systems, interactionist, and more recently, caring as a way of describing their primary focus.

Nursing theories represent the most tangible and specific description of nursing knowledge. They can be tested empirically because they specifically define the relationships among concepts, assumptions, and postulates found in a particular nursing model. Key concepts of selected nursing theories are presented in Table 6-5. For a more complete explanation of the conceptual

TABLE 6–5 Key Concepts of Selected Nursing Theories

THEORIST	GOAL	COMPOSITION	VIEW OF HEALTH	VIEW OF THE ENVIRONMENT	NATURE	PURPOSE
Peplau	Equilibrium	System with physiological, psychological, and social components	Forward movement of the personality	Significant others	Therapeutic interpersonal process	Helping people to meet needs and develop
Johnson	Balance	Behavioral system with seven subsystems	Equilibrium	External inputs	External force toward balance	Restoration, attainment, or maintenance of system stability
Orem	Constancy	Whole with physical, psychological, interpersonal, social aspects	Meeting self-care needs	External forces	Systems that address self-care requisites	Help people to meet self-care needs
Roy	Equilibrium	System with biopsychosocial components	Adaptation	External conditions	Manipulation of stimuli to foster coping	Promotion of adaptation
Rogers	Increased complexity of pattern	Indivisible energy field	Increasing innovativeness of patterning	Contiguous, continuously interacting energy field	Promotion of repatterning	Facilitating health potential
Zderad and Patterson	Self-awareness	Holistic being with meaning and choice	Choice and responsibility, wholeness	Peak life events	Genuine encounter	Affirmation of validation of human experience
Neuman	System stability	Holistic being with physiological, psychological, sociocultural, spiritual variables	Equilibrium	Internal and external stressors	Stress-reducing activities	Promotion of equilibrium
Watson	Sense of inner harmony	Integrated and inseparable spiritual, mental, and physical spheres	Unity and harmony	Energy field external to the person	Transpersonal caring	Promoting harmony
Leininger	Individual/social well-being	Composite of individual, cultural, and social components	Improving human condition	Contextual factors (patient's culture)	Transcultural caring	Improving healthy conditions or lifeways
Parse	Process of becoming	Open being	Process of becoming	Energy field in continuous interaction with the person	Interpersonal processes	Improving quality of life

Adapted from Leddy, S., & Pepper, J. M. (1993). *Conceptual bases of professional nursing* (3rd ed., pp. 174–175). Philadelphia: J. B. Lippincott.

theory models in nursing practice, see the original works of the theorists and nursing theory texts identified in the references at the end of the chapter.

Early Nursing Theorists

"The journey from the days of Florence Nightingale to modern nursing has been long, hard, and bumpy" (Meleis, 1991, p. 49). It is only within the last 40 years that a body of knowledge distinctly labeled as *nursing,* linked to but separate from what nurses do, has been established and confirmed through research. Even more recently, nurses have declared professional nursing to be a distinct, autonomous health discipline and have insisted that their work be valued as skilled nursing care.

Theory development in nursing began with Florence Nightingale's (1860) observations in her classic work, *Notes on Nursing.* Modern nursing theory development in which a body of knowledge labeled distinctly as professional nursing did not emerge as a serious endeavor until the 1950s. Early theorists believed that until nurses could define the boundaries and activities of professional nursing, the profession would continue to be defined by others. Consequently, academic nursing leaders, such as Virginia Henderson, Dorothea Johnson, Hildegard Peplau, and Dorothy Orem, developed theoretical models designed to direct nursing practice and to establish the domain of a body of knowledge referred to as professional nursing. They provided a simple but clear linkage between abstract concepts and what nurses actually do. Since that time, other nursing theorists, such as Myra Levine, Martha Rogers, Imogene King, Sister Callista Roy, Madeline Leininger, Jean Watson, Betty Neuman, and Rosemarie Rizzo Parse (Meleis, 1991), have joined the ranks of serious nursing scholars in developing theories about the body of knowledge that is uniquely nursing.

Evolution of Theory Models in Psychiatric Nursing

The theoretical journey to psychiatric nursing as a subspecialty emerged as a reality in the 1950s, first with Peplau's interpersonal relationship theory in 1952. The 1960s saw the proliferation of nursing theories and the development of several models with special applicability to psychiatric nursing, namely Josephine Paterson and Loretta Zderad, Ida Orlando, Sister Callista Roy, Joyce Travelbee, and Ernestine Wiedenbach). What these theoretical models had in common was a special focus on the nurse-patient relationship. They emphasized the relationship as a human experience with meanings that could be understood and validated. Within the relationship, the person of the nurse engages with the patient as a holistic being, "not as an additive summation, but rather as a gestalt" (Paterson & Zderad, 1988, p. 25). The nurse uses self as a primary therapeutic agent who walks with the patient, listens empathetically to the patient's report of his or her experience, and actively enters the patient's world as a fellow human traveler (Travelbee, 1961). Meleis (1991) noted, "Properties of interaction as validation (Wiedenbach), meeting (Orlando), being totally present and relating (Paterson and Zderad) are delineated and defined by this group of theorists."

"Caring" Models

Current models of relevance to psychiatric nursing have developed around a caring mode of involved interaction with patients (Marriner-Tomey, 1994). According to these theorists (e.g., Watson, Leininger, and Neuman), the essence of nursing is caring. Benner and Wrubel (1989) characterized caring as the foundation of excellence in nursing practice. There is little argument that caring is critical to understanding psychiatric–mental health nursing.

In a caring relationship, Montgomery and Webster (1994) stated that there is a deep subjective involvement with the patient that contains "existential or spiritual significance." Nurses, using a caring model, "value feelings, intuition, and other forms of subjective participation in the client's world" (p. 293), in addition to more scientific understandings of a mentally ill patient. The nurse assumes the role of participant observer, as originally spoken of by Sullivan in a psychological framework, and Peplau (1952) from the nursing perspective. Nursing interventions are designed to acknowledge the shared humanity of nurse and patient while supporting the natural healing resources within the patient in developing creative solutions to difficult problems of living.

"Relationship" Models

Although principles of communication and relationship lend themselves to implementation of all nursing frameworks, those that specifically focus on interpersonal relationships include Peplau, Travelbee, Orlando, and Wiedenbach (Marriner-Tomey, 1994). The nursing theory framework chosen for the study of the nurse-patient relationship in this book is that of Hildegard Peplau.

Hildegard Peplau

Hildegard Peplau (b. 1905) was the first nurse to identify psychiatric nursing both as an essential element of general nursing and as a specialty area that embraces specific governing principles (Peplau, 1952). She was the first nurse theorist to describe the nurse-patient relationship as the foundation of nursing practice (Forchuk, 1991). In shifting the focus from what nurses do "to" patients to what nurses do "with" patients, Peplau (1989) engineered a major paradigm shift from a model focused on medical treatments to an interpersonal relational model of nursing practice. She identified ways in which the nurse makes specialized use of a professional relationship to identify and intervene therapeutically in psychosocial nursing problems.

Peplau (1987) viewed nursing as a developmental educative instrument designed to help individuals and communities use their capacities in living more productively. Her theory is mainly concerned with the processes by which the nurse helps patients make positive changes in their health care status and well-being. Observation, interpretation, and intervention form the essence of a nurse-patient relationship. Raw data must be interpreted and transformed into a meaningful explanation, acceptable in meaning to the nurse and patient.

A transformation process occurs as the nurse observes and listens to the patient and develops impressions and general ideas about the meaning of the patient's situation. These inferences are validated with the patient for accuracy. Illness is viewed as a unique opportunity for experiential learning, personal growth, and improved coping strategies for living (Peplau, 1982a, 1982b).

The dynamic nursing approach proposed by Peplau is not that of a passive spectator-observer. Peplau advocates being participant observers in therapeutic conversations. She insists that nurses must observe not only the behavior of the patient but also their own behavior. Data are collected by interacting directly with the patient. Nurses have a keen awareness not only of their own role and what is appropriate but also of the roles the patient may be projecting on them: friend, parent, protagonist, or sex object. Because none of these roles are useful in providing nursing care to patients, Peplau asserts that the social and personal needs of the nurse should not be a part of the nurse-patient conversation.

In Peplau's classic text, *Interpersonal Theory of Nursing,* developed around the concept of the nurse-patient relationship, the nurse-patient relationship is laid out as a dynamic learning experience in which personal-social growth can occur. Peplau (1952) outlined four developmental phases of the nurse-patient relationship: orientation, working (comprising identification and exploitation), and resolution.

When Peplau first presented her theory of *interpersonal nursing* in 1952, the model quickly became the accepted foundation of psychiatric nursing practice. A nurse herself, Peplau was determined to professionalize the practice of nursing. Her theory had its foundations in Freud's psychoanalytic drive-reduction model described earlier. Peplau placed considerable emphasis, however, on the importance of the interpersonal relationship, which she identified as the communication process that occurs between patient and nurse. She believed that by analyzing the interpersonal interactions occurring within the nurse-patient relationship, the nurse could enhance a patient's personal growth. Every interaction with a patient presented another opportunity for the patient to experience a positive relationship and to gain personal insights.

There are four crucial elements inherent in Peplau's model:

1. Mutuality
2. Phasic relatedness
3. Anxiety gradient
4. Uniqueness

Mutuality is the reciprocal process that occurs between nurse and patient. Through meaningful, shared verbal encounters, the nurse and patient work together to achieve identified health goals. The nurse's clinical skill, creative capacity, and style have a powerful effect on the quality of the therapeutic experience and considerable influence on what the patient will learn. Likewise, because the nurse is a person involved in this reciprocal process, he or she also grows with each interaction.

Phasic relatedness refers to the contrived, purposeful, therapeutic relationship that the professional nurse has with a patient. There are sequential steps to phasic relatedness that range from initiation to termination. Specifically, these steps are known as orientation, identification, exploitation, and resolution. The nurse must have self-awareness to participate effectively in this process. The role involves using the actual relationship and its unique dynamics to help the patient in seeking interpersonal experiences that offer alternative outcomes. For example, the nurse can provide feedback and help patients improve their effectiveness in communication and coping. Thus, each interaction has the potential to be educative.

The *anxiety gradient* is a critical aspect in Peplau's theory. Anxiety is present in all relationships and manifests itself in the nurse-patient relationship as well. Peplau proposed that anxiety-producing events actually awaken past unmet needs. Peplau envisioned the nurse's role as aiding the patient in the management or alleviation of anxiety. This requires that the professional first address the current anxiety and assist the patient in coping with it effectively (based on deliberate problem-solving techniques), as opposed to automatic responsive behavior rooted in defense mechanisms.

Peplau (1982a, 1982b, 1982c) outlined simple steps to accomplish this goal, the first of which is to support the patient in *identifying and labeling his or her anxiety* accurately. The sufferer may be unaware that he or she is experiencing anxiety. Anxiety, however, is observable. Thus, by assessing the patient for evidence of anxiety and asking if he or she feels uncomfortable, nervous, or anxious, the nurse fosters self-recognition, and can validate that feeling.

In the second step, the patient is encouraged to *identify strategies to relieve the experience of anxiety.* This is achieved by questioning the patient about how he or she soothes the self to reduce the tension. Often, such inquiries necessitate repetitive questioning by the nurse until an adequate response is presented. This process empowers the patient by connecting successful stress-reducing techniques with anxiety.

With strategies to relieve anxiety, in step 3 the patient is ready to consider the facts and circumstances that provoke him or her. In other words, the patient attempts to *determine the precipitating causes of anxiety.* The primary aim, however, is to highlight the description of the anxious experience and provide the nurse with enough data to speculate about the cause. Again the nurse assists the patient to ascertain these data by asking probing questions about the particulars of these anxiety-producing situations. Successful completion of the third step leads to step 4, which entails the patient gaining *personal insight* into the precipitating cause of anxiety. *Uniqueness* is the final element in Peplau's model. The content and characteristics of the nurse-patient relationship are unique. Each relationship is an original one that cannot be duplicated, although patterns may emerge, so that the process can be replicated in other settings. This uniqueness addresses the collaborative effort inherent in the relationship and the significance of each member. Both play an important role in ensuring that this relationship will be educational, growth producing, and successful.

Ida Orlando

Ida Orlando (b. 1926) focused on *patient participation* in the nursing process. According to her theory, the patient assumes a central role. The patient collaborates in the nursing assessment to identify patient assets and health needs. Once this is ascertained, the nurse and patient must distinguish between those needs that he or she can meet autonomously and those that require assistance.

The nurse's role is to offer any assistance necessary to meet the patient's unfulfilled needs. Special attention, however, is paid to the patient's sense of adequacy or well-being, with effort directed at increasing the patient's competencies, thereby strengthening health. *Patient validation* in both assessment and evaluation is crucial. It is imperative that the patient validate the fact that these needs are actually being met to his or her satisfaction (Andrews, 1983). The patient can be viewed as an integral member of the health care team, involved in and responsible for the treatment plan and its implementation. Patient validation of its efficacy provides a valuable outcome standard to ensure the delivery of quality care.

> **W**hat do you think? How do nursing theories impact on your nursing activities?

➤ *Check Your Reading*
13. Why should nurses be concerned with nursing theory?
14. How would you describe the structure of nursing knowledge?
15. What is meant by a "caring" relationship in psychiatric nursing?
16. What do you see as Hildegard Peplau's contribution to psychiatric nursing?

Conclusions

In this chapter, we have examined a variety of mental health theories. No one theory adequately describes the richness or the uniqueness of a human being. No theory adequately identifies the multidimensional determinants or aspects of human behavior. Nevertheless, theoretical frameworks provide a systematic way of understanding and communicating about human personality and behavior.

The evolution of psychiatric nursing has its roots in the theories of ancient Greek scholars. Later, scientists such as Descartes and Darwin added to our understanding of the human mind by describing mind-body connections and identifying the mind's developmental aspects. Freud is recognized as the father of psychoanalysis. In addition to describing the structure of the mind, he introduced the concept of talking about painful emotional issues as the means of resolving them. Jung added another dimension to the study of behavior by establishing the concept of shadow and the paradox of men and women each having characteristics typically associated with the opposite sex. Sullivan broadened early psychoanalytic thinking by proposing personality development as an interpersonal phenomenon, and Rogers took it a step further by describing a person-centered approach to psychotherapy. Existential models focus on the here and now relationship occurring between the therapist and patient. By contrast, behavioral models view personality as behavior that can be learned and unlearned, and biological models focus on the physical basis and function of neurotransmitters in mental illness.

All of these theories are relevant to the study of personality and human behavior. It is critical for nurses to integrate these concepts with the concepts held about nursing as a profession. Now that you have been exposed to an overview of some of the more important theorists of relevance to psychiatric nursing, it becomes your challenge to incorporate these concepts into a holistic framework to guide you on your clinical journey.

Key Points to Remember

- Psychiatric nurses practice from a comprehensive theory base, derived from the disciplines of philosophy, medicine, psychology, sociology, education, and, of course, nursing.
- Theories never represent absolute truths but rather portray an abstract representation of a phenomenon and a conceptual tool to describe phenomena in an organized way.
- Theory consists of concepts that represent "a concise summary of thoughts related to a phenomenon." Each concept provides a symbolic shorthand for describing an abstract reality.

- Theories develop within a historical context that necessarily builds on but also challenges classic ways of thinking about a subject. Changes in theoretical perspective usually represent a major paradigm shift in thinking.
- Current understandings of psychiatric–mental health nursing emerged originally from the writings of ancient Greek scholars. Their masterful voices spoke of the "whole person," consisting of mind, body, and spirit, both interrelated and irreducible.
- Darwin highlighted the importance of function and adaptation with his theory of evolution—or "survival of the fittest"—forever altering the way humankind viewed the process of growth and change. He believed that those best able to adapt to their environment have the greatest likelihood of surviving.
- Wundt created the important link between an experimental and a social psychology and established the legitimacy of psychology as a science.
- James spearheaded the development of psychology as a professional discipline in the United States. He taught the first psychology courses at a university level and brought the message of this new discipline to the general U.S. population.
- Freud believed that the vast majority of mental disorders were not organic in origin but developed as the result of unresolved emotional conflicts in childhood. All behavior, no matter how random it may appear, has an identifiable cause.
- Freud taught that personality is composed of three major systems: the id, ego, and superego.
- Jung developed the notion of the collective uncon-scious, consisting of humans' cultural and ethnic heritage. Within the unconscious exist universal archetypes, the most important of which include persona, shadow, self, animus, and anima.
- Sullivan proposed that personality cannot be studied apart from the social and cultural influences on behavior.
- Erikson described a theory based on the epigenetic principle and consisting of eight psychosocial developmental stages.
- Maslow's theory of self-actualization focuses on basic needs, which he described as six incremental stages of personal growth needs.
- Rogers developed a person-centered model of psychotherapy that emphasizes the uniqueness of the individual.
- Existential models focus on taking responsibility, personal freedom, authenticity, anxiety, meaning, and death.
- Behavioral models consider personality as what people do and not who they are; they propose that personality consists of learned behaviors.
- Bandura proposed a social learning theory that conceptualizes psychological functioning as an integration of both environmental conditions and personal attributes.
- Biological models of mental illness focus on neurological, chemical, biological, and genetic issues.
- Nursing theory represents the unique systematic study of nursing experience. The four elements that make up its metaparadigm are person, environment, health, and nursing.

Learning Activities

1. To help you develop a personal philosophy of psychiatric nursing, complete this exercise at the beginning of your psychiatric nursing rotation and refine it at the end. After reading this chapter, develop your own philosophical perspective on how you want to approach the study of psychiatric patients and their behavior. Include all of the ideas that you believe to be important in interacting with and treating psychiatric patients. Give a thoughtful, personal rationale for why you believe your approach is appropriate. Provide a short paragraph about the personal influences that have contributed to your philosophical approach to psychiatric nursing. After completing the exercise, consider how difficult it was for you to develop your personal philosophy of psychiatric nursing. As you heard the philosophies of other students, did any of their ideas broaden or suggest new perspectives in your thinking?

2. To help you develop an appreciation for the process of Socratic questioning, think of a clinical situation or human dilemma in which the process of critical thinking, using a Socratic questioning method, might apply. Specify the nature of the problem in a concise problem statement. Identify the underlying assumptions and the stakeholders (anyone involved with the problem). Get their perceptions of the problem through asking questions about who, why, what, where, and how the problem exists. Develop a solution that is rational and meets the dimensions of the problem. Seek evidence for the beneficial effects of implementing the solution you choose, and identify the consequences (including negative ones) related to its implementation. Validate your conclusions with the stakeholders you identified. As you share your critical thinking problem with your classmates, ask for their reactions and for further suggestions or modifications to your thinking.

3. To help you develop an appreciation for the meaning of a peak experience, respond to the following instructions by Maslow (1968):

I would like you to think of the most wonderful experience or experiences of your life; happiest moments, ecstatic moments, moments of rapture, perhaps from being in love, or from listening to music or suddenly "being hit" by a book or painting, or from some great creative moment. First list these. And then try to tell me how you feel in such acute moments, how you feel differently from the way you feel at other times, how you are at the moment a different person in some ways. (p. 71)

- Share your answer with the other students. Identify commonalities in the experience of special or peak moments. Identify common themes about differences in experience of feelings. How could you use this exercise in your practice of psychiatric nursing?

Critical Thinking Exercise

Consider the following passage from this chapter:

Freud's theory has relevance to psychiatric nursing practice at many junctures. First, it offers a comprehensive explanation of complex human processes and suggests that many diverse sources stemming from the person's past affect personality. Freud's theory of the unconscious is particularly valuable as a baseline for considering the multidimensional nature of behavior. By becoming familiar with these diverse conscious and unconscious influences, a nurse can develop and begin to formulate a hypothesis about the root causes of patient suffering. . . . Understanding the structural nature of the mind allows the nurse to respond more appropriately when obvious conflicts emerge in the nurse-patient relationship.

1. What is the point of view of the authors?
2. What assumption(s) are the authors making?
3. What inference(s) can you draw from the authors' statement about Freud?

While in the clinical area, the head nurse is overheard telling another nurse that she thinks that Freud was a male chauvinist and thinks that his ideas about women are not useful in today's world.

1. What assumptions can the student make about the two different statements about Freud?
2. What inferences can you draw about the head nurse's belief system?
3. What do you think are the reasons the head nurse made her statements about Freud?
4. How would you test your assumptions about the head nurse's reasons?

References

Alexander, F. (1959). Current problems in dynamic psychotherapy in its relation to psychoanalysis. *American Journal of Psychiatry, 116,* 320-323.

Alport, G. (Ed.). (1985). *William James' psychology: The briefer course.* Notre Dame, IN: Notre Dame Press.

Andrews, C. M. (1983). Ida Orlando's model of nursing. In J. J. Fitzpatrick & A. L. Whall (Eds.), *Conceptual models of nursing: Analysis and application* (pp. 47-65). Bowie, MD: Robert J. Brady.

Arnold, E., & Boggs, K. (1999). *Interpersonal relationships: Communication skills for nurses.* Philadelphia: W. B. Saunders.

Bandura, A. (1962). Social learning through imitation. In M. R. Jones (Ed.), *Nebraska symposium on motivation.* Lincoln, NE: University of Nebraska Press.

Bandura, A. (1977). *Social learning theory.* Englewood Cliffs, NJ: Prentice-Hall.

Bandura, A. (1978). Reflections on self efficacy. In S. Rachman (Ed.), *Advances in behavior research and therapy* (Vol. 1). Oxford, England: Pergamon Press.

Benner, P., & Wrubel, J. (1989). *The primacy of caring: Stress and coping in health and illness.* Menlo Park, CA: Addison-Wesley.

Buber, M. (1970). *I and thou* (W. Kaufmann, Trans.). New York: Scribner's.

Bugental, J. (1967). *Challenges of a humanistic psychology.* New York: Harper & Row.

Darwin, C. (1871). *On the origin of species.* New York: Appleton.

Darwin, C. (1873). *The expression of the emotions in man and animals.* New York: Appleton.

Descartes, R. (1931). *The passions of the soul.* In (G. R. T. Ross, Trans.), *The philosophical works of Descartes* (Vol. 1). Cambridge, England: Cambridge University Press.

Donaldson, S. K., & Crowley, D. M. (1978). The discipline of nursing. *Nursing Outlook, 26,* 113-120.

Encyclopedia Americana. (1974). (International edition, Vol. 2, pp. 288-292). New York: Americana.

English, H., & English, A. (1958). *Comprehensive dictionary of psychological and psychoanalytic terms.* New York: Longmans, Green.

Erikson, E. H. (1950). *Childhood and society.* New York: Norton.

Erikson, E. H. (1982). *The life cycle completed.* New York: Norton.

Erikson, J. (1988). *Wisdom and the senses: The way of creativity.* New York: Norton.

Fancher, R. E. (1990). *Pioneers of psychology.* New York: Norton.

Field, W. E. (1979). *The psychotherapy of Hildegard E. Peplau.* New Brunfels, TX: PSF Publications.

Forchuk, C. (1991). A comparison of the works of Peplau and Orlando. *Archives of Psychiatric Nursing, 5*(1), 38-45.

Fordham, F. (1953). *An introduction to Jung's psychology.* London: Penguin.

Frankl, V. (1969). *The will to meaning.* Cleveland, OH: New American Library.

Freud, S. (1964). On the history of the psychoanalytic movement. In J. Strachey (Ed.), *The standard edition of the complete psychological works of Sigmund Freud* (Vol. 14). London: Hogarth Press.

Freud, S. (1960). *The ego and the id* (J. Strachey, Trans.). New York: Norton.

Freud, S. (1961). *The interpretation of dreams* (J. Strachey, Ed. and Trans.). New York: Scientific Editions.

Freud, S. (1969). *An outline of psycho-analysis* (J. Strachey, Trans.). New York: Norton.

Glasser, W. (1965). *Reality therapy.* New York: Harper & Row.

Hall, C. S., & Lindzey, G. (1970). *Theories of personality.* New York: John Wiley.

Heidegger, M. (1962). *Being and time.* New York: Harper & Row.

Jacobi, J. (1951). *The psychology of C. G. Jung* (Rev. ed.). New Haven, CT: Yale University Press.

Jaeger, W. (1934). *Aristotle: Fundamentals of the history of his development.* Oxford, England: Clarendon Press.

James, W. (1907). *Pragmatism: A new name for some old ways of thinking* (Lectures II and VI). New York: Longmans, Green.

James, W. (1950). *Principles of psychology* (Vol. 1). New York: Dover.

Jung, C. G. (1916). *Analytical psychology.* New York: Moffatt, Yard.

Jung, C. G. (1933). *Modern man in search of a soul* (W. S. Dell & C. F. Baynes, Trans.). New York: Harcourt Brace Jovanovich.

Jung, C. G. (1958). *Psyche and symbol.* Garden City, NY: Doubleday.

Jung, C. G. (1973). *Memories, dreams, reflections* (A. Jaffé Ed., R. Winston & C. Winston, Trans.). New York: Pantheon Books.

Jung, C. G. (1975). *Letters.* G. Adler & A. Jaffé (Eds.) (R. F. C. Hull, Trans.). Bollington Series XCV:2. Princeton, NJ: Princeton University Press.

Kierkegaard, S. (1957). *The concept of dread.* Princeton, NJ: Princeton University Press.

Leibert, R., & Spiegler, M. (1982). *Personality: Strategies and issues.* Homewood, IL: Dorsey Press.

Marmer, S. (1994). Theories of the mind and psychopathology. In *The American Psychiatric Press textbook of psychiatry.* Washington, DC: American Psychiatric Association Press.

Marriner-Tomey, A. (1994). *Nursing theorists and their work* (2nd ed.). St. Louis, MO: C. V. Mosby.

Maslow, A. H. (1963). Self-actualizing people. In G. B. Levitas (Ed.), *The world of psychology* (Vol. 2). New York: Braziller.

Maslow, A. H. (1968). *Toward a psychology of being* (2nd ed.). Princeton, NJ: Van Nostrand.

Maslow, A. H. (1970). *Motivation and personality* (Rev. ed.) New York: Harper & Row.

McCracken, A. (1994, April). Special care units: Meeting the needs of cognitively impaired persons. *Journal of Gerontological Nursing,* 41-46.

Meleis, A. L. (1991). *Theoretical nursing: Development and progress* (2nd ed.). Philadelphia: J. B. Lippincott.

Neuman, B., & Young, R. (1972). A model for teaching total person approach to patient problems. *Nursing Research, 21,* 264-269.

Nightingale, F. (1860). *Notes on nursing: What it is and what it is not.* Philadelphia: W. B. Saunders.

Paterson, J., & Zderad, L. (1988). *Humanistic nursing.* New York: National League for Nursing.

Paul, R. (1993). *Critical thinking* (2nd ed.). Santa Rosa, CA: Critical Thinking Foundation.

Pavlov, I. P. (1928). *Lectures on conditioned reflexes* (W. H. Gantt, Ed. and Trans.). New York: International Publishers.

Peplau, H. E. (1952). *Interpersonal relations in nursing.* New York: Putnam's.

Peplau, H. E. (1982a). Therapeutic concepts. In S. A. Smoyak & S. Rouslin (Eds.), *A collection of classics in psychiatric nursing literature* (pp. 91-108). Thorofare, NJ: Slack.

Peplau, H. E. (1982b). Interpersonal techniques: The crux of psychiatric nursing. In S. A. Smoyak & S. Rouslin (Eds.), *A collection of classics in psychiatric literature* (pp. 276-281). Thorofare, NJ: Slack.

Peplau, H. E. (1982c). Some reflections on earlier days in psychiatric nursing. *Journal of Psychosocial Nursing and Mental Health Services, 20*(8), 17-24.

Peplau, H. E. (1987). Interpersonal constructs for nursing practice. *Nursing Education Today, 7,* 201-208.

Peplau, H. E. (1989). Future directions in psychiatric nursing from the perspective of history. *Journal of Psychosocial Nursing, 27*(2), 18-28.

Rader, M. (1969). *The enduring questions: Main problems of philosophy* (2nd ed.). New York: Holt, Rinehart & Winston.

Rogers, C. R. (1942). *Counseling and psychotherapy: Newer concepts in practice.* Boston: Houghton Mifflin.

Rogers, C. R. (1961). *On becoming a person.* Boston: Houghton Mifflin.

Rogers, C. R. (1963). Toward a science of the person. *Journal of Humanistic Psychology, 2,* 72-92.

Skinner, B. F. (1987). Whatever happened to psychology as the science of behavior? *American Psychologist, 42,* 780-786.

Smith, B. D., & Vetter, H. J. (1982). *Theoretical approaches to personality.* Engelwood Cliffs, NJ: Prentice-Hall.

Strachey, J. (Ed.). (1964). *The standard edition of the complete psychological works of Sigmund Freud.* London: Hogarth Press.

Sullivan, H. S. (1954). *The psychiatric interview.* New York: Norton.

Sullivan, H. S. (1972). *Personal psychopathology.* New York: Norton.

Tillich, P. (1952). *The courage to be.* New Haven: Yale University Press.

Travelbee, J. (1961). *Intervention in psychiatric nursing* (p. 12). Philadelphia: F. A. Davis.

Watson, J. (1919). *Psychology from the standpoint of a behaviorist.* Philadelphia: J. B. Lippincott.

Watson, J. (1928). *The ways of behaviorism.* New York: Harper.

Woodward, W. (1982). The "discovery" of social behaviorism and social learning theory, 1870-1980. *American Psychologist, 37,* 396-410.

Yalom, I. (1980). *Existential psychotherapy.* New York: Basic Books.

Suggested Readings

Erikson, E. H. (1950). *Childhood and society.* New York: Norton.

Forchuk, C. (1991). A comparison of the works of Peplau and Orlando. *Archives of Psychiatric Nursing, 5*(1), 38-45.

Forchuk, C., Beaton, S., Crawford, L., Ide, L., Voorberg, N., & Bethune, J. (1989). Incorporating Peplau's theory and case management. *Journal of Psychosocial Nursing, 27*(2), 35-38.

Hall, C. S., & Lindzey, G. (1970). *Theories of personality.* New York: John Wiley.

Marriner-Tomey, A. (1994). *Nursing theorists and their work* (2nd ed.) St. Louis, MO: C. V. Mosby.

Neuman, B. (1992). *The Neuman systems model* (2nd ed.). Norwalk, CT: Appleton-Century-Crofts.

Peplau, H. E. (1987). Interpersonal constructs for nursing practice. *Nursing Education Today, 7,* 201-208.

Rogers, C. R. (1961). *On becoming a person.* Boston: Houghton Mifflin.

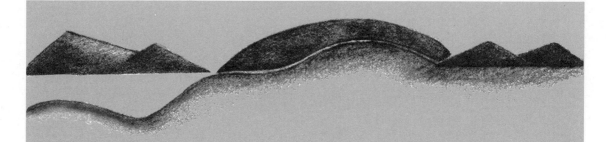

II The Nature of the Journey

Traveler's Log

Every second, people reach out for help. Although their wounds may not be visible, they are deep: fractured minds and souls trying to cope with the stressors of the 21st century. Burdened by an illness and the stigma of being different, how do we reach them? We approach them using the art and science of nursing, hoping to ease their pain. Teaching new coping stategies, better decision-making skills, symptom management, medication compliance, relaxation techniques, and journaling are just some of the ways we can help.

Psychiatric nursing offers unique opportunities in a variety of settings. It is about learning the complexities of the mind as it is influenced by the outside forces that complete the mosaic of our lives. Therapeutic communication remains paramount to the nurse-patient relationship. Counseling, teaching, structuring the milieu to promote a healing environment, rolemodeling appropriate behaviors, and firm, respectful limit-setting provide opportunities for growth. It is uplifting and inspiring to know that we have an integral part in their recovery. We are enlightened as we see the person heal. As we learn more about the brain and the environmental conditions that mold us, we are better able to intervene and instill hope to those so troubled. I challenge you to join this journey that has been so rewarding for me.

—Jane Trainis, RN, MS, CS

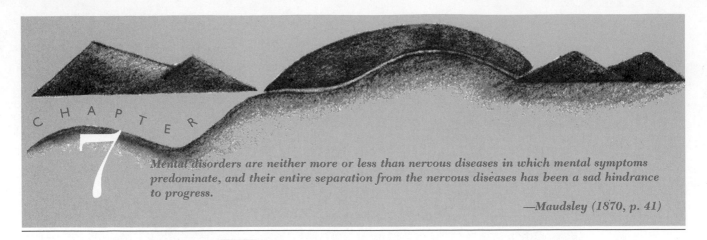

C H A P T E R

7

Mental disorders are neither more or less than nervous diseases in which mental symptoms predominate, and their entire separation from the nervous diseases has been a sad hindrance to progress.

—Maudsley (1870, p. 41)

Physical Dimensions of the Journey
Neurobiological Influences

Learning Objectives

After studying this chapter, you should be able to:

1. Identify the significant contributors to the development of biological psychiatry.
2. Describe the gross structures of the brain.
3. Explain the cellular organization of the neuron.
4. Discuss the effect of membrane permeability on neuronal transmission.
5. Identify the major neurotransmitters and their effects on neuronal transmission.
6. Explain the importance of the neuroendocrine cascade.
7. Identify the laboratory tests used for diagnostic evaluation of psychiatric patients.
8. Discuss the importance of biological psychiatry to the understanding of the cause of selected mental illnesses.
9. Identify the implications of biological psychiatry on the practice of psychiatric nursing.

Key Terminology

Action potential	Dopamine hypothesis	Monozygotic	Sensitization
Basal ganglia	Endocrine system	Motor homunculus	Somatosensory area
Brain imaging	GABA (γ-aminobutyric acid)	Neuroscience	Synaptic plasticity
Catecholamine hypothesis	Kindling	Neurotransmitters	Ventricular system
Dizygotic	Limbic system	Psychobiology	

In the field of neurobiological psychiatry, the journey to uncover the causes of mental illness has encompassed many decades of exploration and much mysticism. Hopes have been raised for the discovery of a distinct biological basis for the major mental illnesses only to have those hopes squelched by contradictory evidence. However, as technology continues to improve, more and more is being uncovered about the biological factors that contribute to the development of mental illnesses, and we find ourselves on the threshold of even greater understandings.

This chapter will help you understand the neurological and biological revolution in psychiatry. The enormous body of knowledge in neurobiological research has provided convincing evidence for understanding the possible causes of mental illnesses and the efficacy of various treatments of psychiatric disorders (Lieberman & Rush, 1996). Psychiatric nursing is faced with the major challenges of integrating the implications of this research and redefining the practice to meet the needs of the mentally ill. The psychiatric nurse has an integral role in the provision of holistic care to patients; he or she integrates the scientific theories and develops therapeutic interventions and outcome indicators of care so that the severely and persistently mentally ill have opportunities to lead independent, functional lives. Mr. A's story is a good example of a patient's first visit with a psychiatrist.

Mr. A's Story

Mr. A is 22 years old, white, and single. His elderly parents accompany him and they appear quite concerned over Mr. A's physical and mental status. They report that he has been unemployed for some time and that he does not seem to have any desire to find another job so that he can continue to support himself. They fear that he will never leave home. They say that he has always been "a little different" and added that he has always had "spells" during which he seems dizzy, looks over to one side as if hallucinating, and chews.

Mr. A is alert, oriented, appropriately groomed, casually dressed, and well mannered, and he walks with a steady gait. His speech is intense and clear but full of detail, and his statements detail mostly his impressive qualifications and achievements in life. The patient presents in a stern, humorless manner. Although he denies any delusions or hallucinations, he exhibits an extreme preoccupation with his weight and the effects of environmental pollution on the inner city. At the end of the hour, Mr. A continues to talk about irrelevant issues and the psychiatrist finds it difficult to terminate the interview.

A physical examination showed no abnormalities. A neurological examination, routine laboratory tests, an EEG, and a CT scan were all within normal limits.

What do you think? Does Mr. A have a mental illness? What is your impression of Mr. A's behavior? What advice would reassure Mr. A's parents regarding his physical and mental health? What advice would decrease Mr. A's parents' concerns about his future?

The discussion about neurobiological psychiatry that appears later in this chapter provides you with information and strategies to help you understand the nature of

Mr. A's illness and provides some treatment options to implement once a diagnosis has been made. However, it is important to know that psychiatry is based on the science of neurology and incorporates many disciplines including anatomy, physiology, genetics, biochemistry, physics, immunology, pharmacology, psychiatry, electronics, and computer science. Clinicians who specialize in **neuroscience** may also collaborate in the delivery of health care with professionals from other disciplines such as nurses, social workers, psychologists, pharmacists, and clergy. Neuroscience encompasses a set of related disciplines, such as neurology and psychiatry, that investigate the relationship between brain structure and function and human thoughts, feelings, and behaviors.

This chapter addresses the biological influences in neuropsychiatry, including the internal and external factors affecting mental illness across an individual's lifetime. We begin with an overview of biological psychiatry and its related neurological disciplines, followed by discussions of diagnostic procedures and etiological implications of neurobiological psychiatry on some major mental illnesses. Finally, we review and critique the literature on the biological revolution in psychiatry and explain the implications of psychobiology on the practice of psychiatric nursing.

OVERVIEW OF NEUROBIOLOGICAL PSYCHIATRY

Historical records reveal that understandings about the nature of mental illness have been influenced by political, social, philosophical, and spiritual factors. Ancient society reacted to mental illness with fear, shame, guilt, and embarrassment. At times, treatments of the suffering individual were inhumane. For example, the mentally ill were often exhibited like zoo animals or tortured and burned to death (Andreasen, 1984). The afflicted were not viewed as suffering from brain disease; rather, their illnesses were attributed to ill manner, and attitude or even demon possession.

However, even though most ancient people failed to connect mental illness to physical causes, the foundation of biological psychiatry actually dates back to early times (Trimble, 1996). The great thinkers Plato and Aristotle were convinced that the mind had a relationship with the brain and the heart. Hippocrates, in classical times, believed that aberration in mental functioning was due to the imbalance of body humors (blood, phlegm, black bile, and yellow bile). At that time, depression was believed to be related to an excess of black bile.

In the 17th century, the French philosopher René Descartes declared that the mind was a nonmaterial thing, entirely separate from the physical tissues found inside the head. He argued that the brain was related to sensation and movement, whereas the mind was the soul (Trimble, 1996). Thus, *spirit* became an important aspect in disease theory. Despite its early beginnings in Europe, the biological approach to psychiatry arrived in the United States at a relatively late date, the 1970s.

By the end of the 18th century, Whytt's (1765) experiments in England on the nervous system led to the publication of his book, *On Nervous, Hypochondriacal or Hysterical Diseases,* the first important treatise on psychiatric diseases. Meanwhile, the interest in the brain of several neurological scientists in Europe continued, and more discoveries related to the functions and the structure of the brain were hypothesized. Broca, in 1861, completed his findings on the localization of aphasia, which he specified to the left frontal convolution of the brain (injury in this area left a person nearly mute but able to understand). Another important neurologist at that time was Wernicke (1874), who proceeded to identify that damage to the superior temporal region left a person speaking fluently without the ability to understand. This finding was hailed as impressive and was named the *localization theory.*

After this discovery, Jackson reported on the laterality functions of the hemispheres of the brain. He differentiated the right and left physiology of the hemispheres (Trimble, 1996). The mapping of the brain was aided by the staining techniques of Golgi, which produced much improved visualization of the cells under the microscope. While the neurologists in Western Europe were investigating the different important areas in the brain, in Germany, Emil Kraepelin's (1896) contribution to psychiatry was the description and classification of the specific types of major psychiatric illnesses. He differentiated manic-depressive disorder from dementia praecox (later renamed *schizophrenia* by Eugene Bleuler). His writings attest to his firmly held views that mental illness was probably due to an unrecognized physical factor. Similarly, Freud made significant contributions to neurology and anatomy and wrote his monograph on aphasia. However, Freud continued to focus primarily on psychoanalysis rather than biological links to mental illness.

In the United States, Freud's psychoanalytical theories, not Kraepelin's biological psychiatry, became the central framework for practitioners. The United States, in 1910, adapted the intrapsychic explanations and psychoanalytical theories of Freud. In addition, a group of behavioral scientists hypothesized about the general laws governing behavior. John B. Watson founded behaviorism and defended behavior as the proper focus of psychology. While psychoanalysis and behaviorism dominated U.S. thinking, a biological focus characterized European research.

Adolf Meyer, another important influence in the early years of the 20th century, proposed the concept of **psychobiology.** Meyer's approach focused on the integration of the individual's life experiences using psychological and biological data derived from the person's life chart. This biopsychosocial approach to diagnosis and treatment evolved as a major psychiatric model for practicing clinicians (Sabshin, 1988). Meyer was responsible for U.S. thinking shifting away from the psychological models of mental illness toward a more holistic model.

In the 1950s, the treatment of psychiatric patients changed radically as a result of a series of chance discoveries in the pharmacological arena. For example, the discovery of the antipsychotic properties of chlorpromazine, the antidepressant action of monoamine oxidase inhibitors, and the tricyclic antidepressants changed the practice of psychiatry and offered new hope to those afflicted with mental illnesses. About 10 years later, in the 1960s, the practice of biological psychiatry was limited to the prescription of nonspecific medications and treatments such as electroconvulsive therapy and lobotomy. However, the neurochemical era had begun and was followed by major discoveries in neuroimaging in the 1970s. Several books were published regarding the use of imaging techniques to visualize the structure of the brain. However, evidence to support the causative factors of mental disorders was inconclusive due to failure of the studies to identify the specific loci of the disorders. Additional research has shown that human experience, adaptation, and gene selection influence brain growth and development (Rhawn, 1996).

Since the late 1970s, significant developments in neuroscience and biological psychiatry have markedly increased the understanding of the structural and functional changes in the brain and the symptoms of mental illness. The recognition that mental illnesses are diseases affecting the brain led to further study of the biochemical foundations of thought, mood, affect, emotion, and behavior known as *psychobiology* (Bushness & DeForge, 1994; Hill, 1991; McEnany, 1991). Other subspecialties that have contributed major insights to psychiatry are shown in Box 7-1.

The major areas of psychobiological research in the 1990s included **brain imaging** techniques, the role of neurotransmitters and neuronal receptors in the formation of behavior, the psychobiology of emotion, the theory of brain plasticity, the role of molecular genetics in the etiology of mental illness, and the theories of longevity and aging (Jazwinski, 1996; Kirkwood, 1996). Brain imaging techniques are methods of visualizing the brain with the use of routine radiographs and by using "radioopaque" substance to outline the deeper structures not easily visible on the radiograph. The explosion of knowledge in neuropsychiatry demonstrated a need for the integration of the research findings to identify, specifically, the causes of mental illnesses.

Box 7–1 ■ ■ ■ ■ ■
Other Subspecialties That Contribute to Psychiatry

- **Neuroanatomy:** The study of brain structure
- **Neurophysiology:** The study of brain function
- **Neurochemistry:** The study of chemical processes that control the brain function
- **Neuroendocrinology:** The study of the relationship between glandular function and brain function
- **Neuropharmacology:** The study of the effects of drugs on the brain

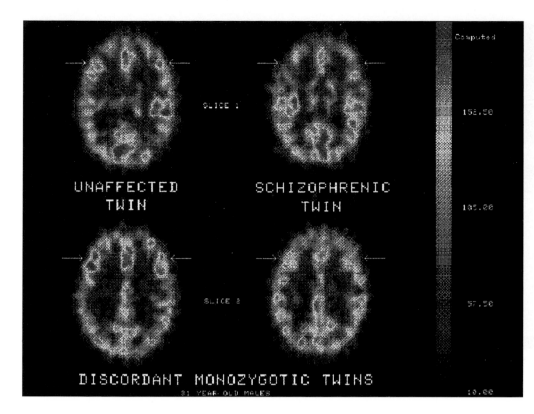

Figure 1
PET scans of blood flow in identical twins, one of whom has schizophrenia, illustrate that individuals with this illness have reduced brain activity in their frontal lobes when asked to perform a reasoning task that requires activation of this area. Schizophrenic clients also perform poorly on the task. This suggests a site of functional impairments in schizophrenia. (From Karen Berman, MD, courtesy of National Institute of Mental Health, Clinical Brain Disorders Branch.)

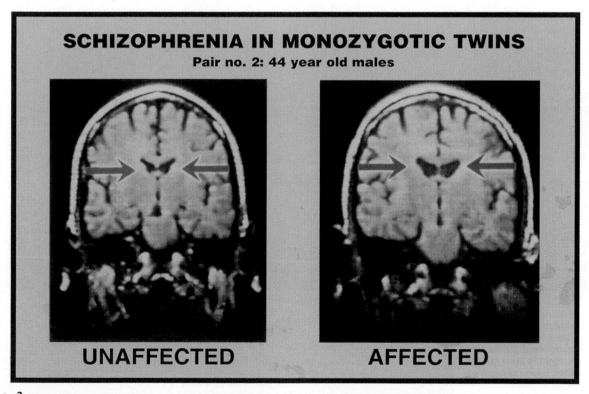

Figure 2
Loss of brain volume associated with schizophrenia is clearly shown by MRI scans comparing the size of ventricles (butterfly-shaped, fluid-filled spaces in the midbrain) of identical twins, one of whom has schizophrenia *(right)*. The ventricles of the twin with schizophrenia are larger. This suggests structural brain changes associated with the illness. (From Daniel Weinberger, MD, courtesy of National Institute of Mental Health, Clinical Brain Disorders Branch.)

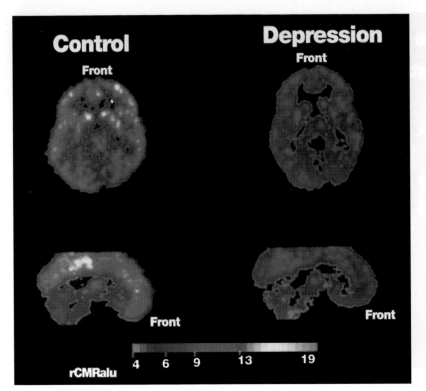

Figure 7

PET scans of the brain of a person without depression *(L)* and the brain of a person with depression *(R)* reveal reduced brain activity *(darker colors)* during depression, especially in the prefrontal cortex. (From Mark George, MD, National Institute of Mental Health, Biological Psychiatry Branch.)

Other important advances in contemporary psychiatry included the discoveries in genetics and molecular biological studies of neuroreceptors. The research supporting the role of neurochemicals in the formation and enactment of behavior extended to other related disciplines in neuropsychiatry, for example, the collaborative studies on cognitive neuroscience (Andreasen, 1997). The "Decade of the Brain" of the 1990s heightened the understanding of the biological dimension of emotion and led to additional research in this area. The journey continues with the hope that the specific cause of mental disorder will finally be identified. Let's return to the case of Mr. A.

The psychiatrist learned from Mr. A's parents that his mother developed toxemia when she was pregnant with Mr. A and experienced a difficult delivery. At 14 months, Mr. A had been hospitalized with a high fever and seizures. In school, Mr. A was often accused of not paying attention, and even his parents described him as a daydreamer.

Despite Mr. A's normal EEG findings, the psychiatrist decided to further evaluate the reason for the subtle signs and symptoms that Mr. A. was manifesting. In addition, the physician recognized that EEGs fail to detect a deep temporal lobe seizure focus in about 50% of patients. Diagnostic specificity of the EEG is enhanced by sleep deprivation and the use of sphenoidal or nasopharyngeal recording electrodes. Indeed, after completion of this additional procedure, Mr. A was accurately diagnosed with temporal lobe epilepsy. Without this differential diagnostic procedure, the diagnosis of temporal lobe epilepsy might have been missed and the psychiatrist might have established schizophrenia as the diagnosis for Mr. A. ■

Psychiatric nursing, especially in the United States, is moving from the study of the "troubled mind" to the "broken brain" and the brain-behavior connection. The journey began with one essential step, the understanding of the brain. The most recent pathway is the brain-cognition-behavior connection.

What do you think? As you reflect on the case of Mr. A, are your own preconceptions about the nature of mental illness challenged? If so, in what ways?

➤ *Check Your Reading*
1. What sciences are involved in biological psychiatry?
2. What did Descartes teach regarding the mind and body?
3. What did the behaviorists hope to map?
4. What does the term *neuroscience* encompass?
5. What new areas of research directly affect the biological revolution in psychiatry?

NEUROANATOMY

Brain

Macrostructure

As a psychiatric nurse, it is essential for you to have a comprehensive knowledge of the normal structure and functions of the brain to enable you to effectively plan the nursing care of the mentally ill. In this portion of the chapter, we discuss the gross anatomy of the brain and the functions of the vital systems that make a person human. You are referred to other texts on basic anatomy and physiology to learn more about these areas. Our intention is to enhance your knowledge of the central nervous system (CNS).

The nervous system is divided into the CNS and the peripheral nervous system (PNS). The CNS is made up of the brain, which is encapsulated in the skull, and the spinal cord, which lies within the vertebral canal. The PNS is composed of 31 pairs of spinal nerves and 12 pairs of cranial nerves (Keltner & Folks, 1993).

The brain is an impressive and complex organ that has a major role in regulating behavior and mental processes. It weighs approximately 3 lb and looks like a shapeless, creamy, pinkish fat mass. Its surface is covered with fissures, or wrinkles, called *sulci,* and the ridges are called *gyri.* The surface is darker than the rest of the brain due to the unmyelinated (uninsulated) cells that support the area commonly called the *gray matter* or the *cerebral cortex.* Most of the brain is made up of myelinated (insulated) cells commonly called the *white matter.* The *glial cells,* in the white matter, are the building blocks of the myelin sheaths, and their purpose is to insulate the nervous system. A few areas of gray matter also invade the deeper layer within the white matter. The brain tissue is soft, delicate, and fragile; however, it is covered with a tough, fibrous sac called the *dura mater,* which is filled with cerebrospinal fluid (CSF) that protects the sensitive mass from hostile forces.

The main portion of the brain (cerebrum) is divided into two globular halves, the left and right cerebral hemispheres. Both hemispheres connect with the spinal cord and the vertebrae, transmitting messages to and from the brain. The afferent nerve bundles travel to the brain, and efferent nerve bundles travel away from the brain. A thin strip of white matter called the *corpus callosum* attaches the left and right hemispheres to each other. Figure 7–1 shows the gross structure of the brain and Box 7–2 lists major components of the brain.

Surface Structure

The cerebral hemisphere is divided into four lobes named after the corresponding bone in the skull: the frontal, parietal, occipital, and temporal lobes (Kingsley, 1996). The hemispheres are sometimes referred to as the *telencephalon,* or *endbrain,* because they are the most developed of the brain structure. See Figure 7–2 for a view of a hemisphere.

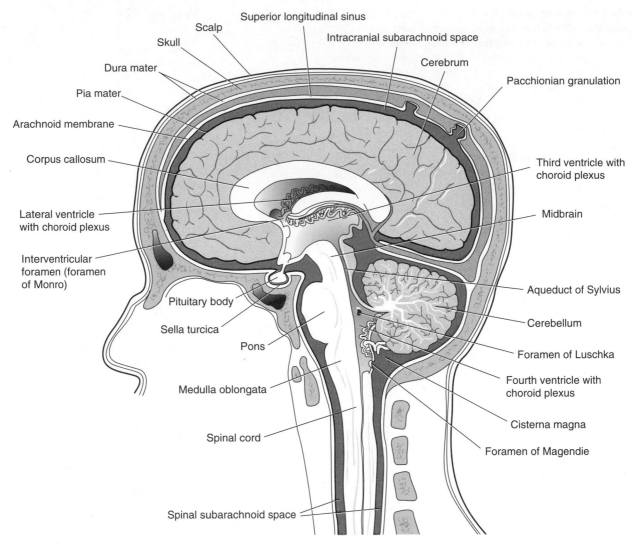

Figure 7–1
The macrostructure of the brain.

The frontal lobe (cortex) is the largest of the five lobes, beginning at the front of the brain and reaching back to the central sulcus. The area between the central and the precentral sulcus is known as the *motor area* and is responsible for controlling body movement. The frontal lobe is the seat of intellectual functioning, judgment, reasoning, and abstract thought. It also plays an important role in modulation of emotional experience, expression of mood, social maturity, and inhibition of unacceptable behavior.

Penfield mapped the motor area between 1940 and 1950. He reported, in detail, the relationship between parts of the cortex and specific muscle groups; his graphic depiction of this relationship is often called the **motor homunculus** (Figure 7–3). Motor homunculus relates to specific muscle groups that are controlled by parts of the cortex of the brain.

Motor control is highly lateralized. The left side of the brain governs the right side of the body, and the right side of the brain governs the left side of the body. This discovery sparked interest in the laterality of the hemispheres of the brain (Table 7–1).

The parietal lobe extends from the central sulcus to the lateral fissure of Sylvius. Midway deep between the frontal and the parietal lobes is the corpus callosum, which holds a massive collection of axons interconnecting the two hemispheres (Kingsley, 1996). The parietal lobe receives and evaluates most sensory information (except smell, hearing, and vision). It also modulates spatial orientation. The **somatosensory area** occupies part of the parietal lobe that controls sensations from the arms and legs.

The occipital lobe lies posterior to the parietooccipital sulcus, extending to the wall of the temporal lobe. It contains the primary visual receptive area responsible for storing visual information and interpreting visual responses. A disruption in this site may lead to illusions and hallucinations.

The temporal lobe is prominent laterally because it juts out and forward, with the deep sylvian fissure separating it from the frontal lobe. It receives and evaluates olfactory and auditory input and plays an important role in memory. It is also associated with abstract thought and judgment. Damage to Wernicke's

Box 7–2 ▪ ▪ ▪ ▪ ▪
Summary of Major Components of Brain

I. Cerebrum (forebrain): Largest portion of brain
  A. Cortex: Gray matter rich in neurons and a complex network of axons and dendrites; forms the corrugated surface of the four lobes of the cerebral hemispheres
  B. Frontal Lobes: Important in emotional expression, mood, planning, motivation, control of voluntary motor functions, and speech
  C. Parietal Lobes: Important in receiving and evaluating sensory information
  D. Temporal Lobes: Important in receiving and evaluating auditory and olfactory input; influences memory; involved in abstract thought and judgment
  E. Occipital Lobes: Important in receiving and evaluating visual input
II. Diencephalon: Widespread connections throughout brain; involved in the majority of sensory, motor, and limbic pathways
  A. Thalamus: Influences affect, foresight, mood, and general body movements, and is associated with strong emotions such as rage and fear; all sensory information is relayed through the thalamus
  B. Pineal Gland: Involved in the reproductive cycle; secretes melatonin; may be involved in the sleep–wake cycle
  C. Hypothalamus: Major control center for the pituitary; involved in regulation of homeostasis and autonomic, endocrine, emotional, and somatic functions; involved in regulating feeding and drinking behavior; regulates temperature, cardiac function, gut motility, and sexual activity; involved in coordinating sleep–wake cycle; regulates the stress response
IV. Cerebellum (little brain): Involved in cognitive, behavioral, and affective functions; full range of sensory inputs go through cerebellum; involved in processing sensory information, and it is part of the motor system
V. Brain Stem: Connects the brain to the spinal column; home of cranial nerve nuclei; controls autonomic functions such as breathing and cardiovascular functions
  A. Midbrain: Contains ascending and descending nerve tracks; center of the visual cortex; involved in regulation of reflex movement of eyes and head; assists in unconscious regulation and coordination of motor activities; part of the auditory pathway; contains part of the basal ganglia (substantia nigra) where dopamine is manufactured

  B. Pons: Contains ascending and descending nerve tracks; relays information between cerebrum and cerebellum; reflex center; most norepinephrine manufactured in locus caeruleus
  C. Medulla Oblongata: Conduction pathway for ascending and descending pathways; controls conscious muscular movement; involved in balance, coordination, and modulation of sound impulses from the inner ear; center for important reflexes such as heart rate, breathing, swallowing, vomiting, sneezing, and coughing
  D. Reticular Formation: Core of brain stem; controls sleep–wake cycle; plays a role in maintaining alertness, arousal, consciousness; contributes to bodily functions such as respiration and cardiac rhythms
VI. Basal Ganglia: Controls muscle tone, activity, and posture; coordinates movements of large muscles; inhibits unwanted muscular activity; when there is a problem, results in extrapyramidal syndrome
VII. Limbic System: Involved with subjective emotional states, aggression, rage, submission, sexual behavior, mood, memory, pleasure, and learning
  A. Hippocampus: Involved in turning short-term memory into long-term memory; contains large amounts of neurotransmitters
  B. Amygdala: Generates emotions from thoughts and perceptions
  C. Fornix: Connects the hippocampus to the hypothalamus
VIII. Ventricles: Each cerebral hemisphere contains a large cavity called the lateral ventricle; a smaller midline cavity, the third ventricle, is located in the center of the diencephalon between the two halves of the thalamus; the fourth ventricle is the area of the pons and the medulla oblongata and connects with the central canal of the spinal cord, extending nearly the full length of the spinal cord
IX. Spinal Fluid: Cerebral spinal fluid bathes the brain with nutrients and cushions the brain within the skull; exits through the blood stream
X. Neurons: Groups of brain cells that are arranged in networks and communicate with each other through neurotransmission that leads to all human activity including body functions, intelligence, consciousness, creativity, memory, and emotional expression

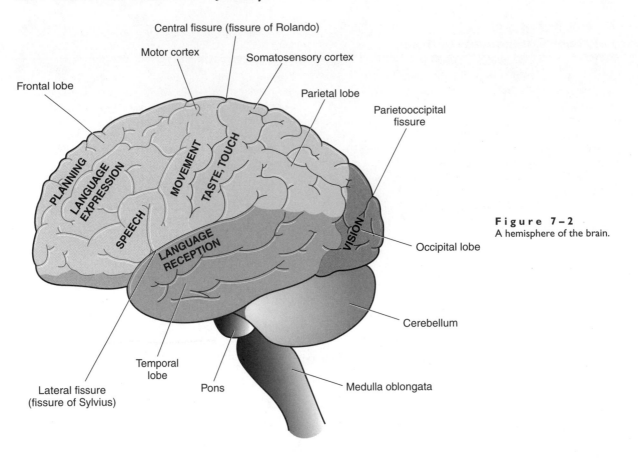

Figure 7-2
A hemisphere of the brain.

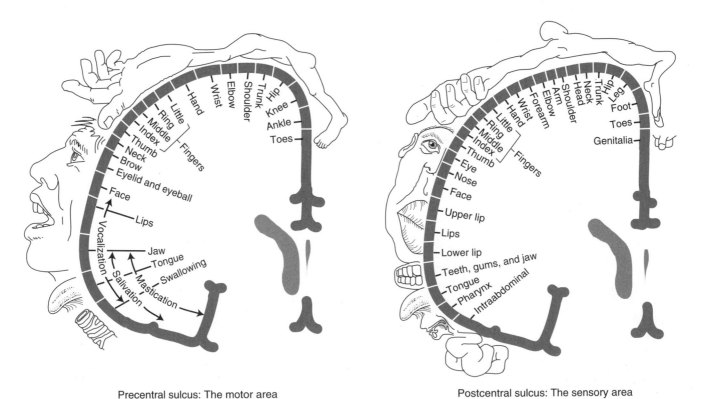

Precentral sulcus: The motor area

Postcentral sulcus: The sensory area

Figure 7-3
The motor homunculus and the somatosensory homunculus.

TABLE 7–1 Functions of the Hemispheres of the Brain

LOBE	LEFT HEMISPHERE	RIGHT HEMISPHERE
Frontal	Control of motor behavior Perception Broca's area (speech) Concentration Abstract thinking Global orientation Identification of objects (upside down)	Control of motor behavior Perception Concentration Abstract thinking Global orientation
Parietal	Simple solving of math problems Reading and writing Identification of symbols Naming of simple objects Demonstration of object use Recognition and naming of body parts Orientation to right and left	Ability to copy
Temporal	Reading and writing Wernicke's area Memory Naming of simple objects	Repetition of rhythms and musical tones
Occipital	Identification of hidden objects	Identification of camouflaged objects

area, which is in this region, results in receptive or sensory aphasia.

Within the brain, two important structures bridge the major pathways between the higher cortex and the lower group of neurons: the diencephalon, or interbrain, and the basal ganglia, or lower nerve knot. The diencephalon consists of small masses of gray matter made up of cell bodies of neurons. It is widespread and holds important connections with the sensory, motor, and limbic pathways. It serves as the relay station between the lower brain centers and the higher cortical centers. The thalamus and the hypothalamus are the most important structures of the diencephalon.

The thalamus is the major pathway for sensory and motor impulses to and from the cerebral hemisphere, and it is the modulator of emotions and behavior, especially fear and rage. All sensory impulses and many other anatomical loops relay in the thalamus.

The hypothalamus is the major control center for the pituitary gland; the hypothalamus maintains homeostasis and regulates autonomic, endocrine, emotional, and somatic functions. It also regulates feeding and drinking behavior, temperature, cardiac function, gut motility, and sexual activity and coordinates the sleep–wake cycle.

The pineal gland is also located within the diencephalon. It is an endocrine gland involved in the reproductive cycle. In darkness, it secretes melatonin; melatonin is involved in gonadal functioning. The pineal gland may be involved in the sleep–wake cycle, but its exact effects are not clear.

The basal ganglion is made up of several deep gray matter structures located bilaterally in the cerebrum, diencephalon, and midbrain. It regulates muscle tone, activity, and posture and coordinates large-muscle movements. Disruption in this area results in extrapyramidal syndromes. The relationship between the basal

ganglia and the limbic system is discussed later in the chapter.

The midbrain, pons (bridge), and medulla (marrow) oblongata are sometimes grouped together and called the *brain stem*. This portion of the brain is the most primitive and is primarily concerned with the capacity for survival. It regulates heartbeat, respiration, and other vital functions. It receives information from the remainder of the body through the spinal cord and cranial nerves. It is also the area where dopamine as well as most of the brain's norepinephrine is manufactured.

The cerebellum, or "little brain," is sometimes considered a part of the midbrain. It is a relatively large and intensely foliated structure that serves as a major modulator of movement, and it is involved with equilibrium, muscle tone, postural control, and coordination of body movement. It receives a full range of sensory inputs and sends these inputs to various sites in the brain stem and thalamus (see Figure 7–1).

► *Check Your Reading*

6. What differentiates white matter from gray matter?
7. What structure connects the right hemisphere with the left?
8. Afferent tracts travel in which direction? In which direction do efferent tracts travel?
9. What are the functions of the frontal, parietal, occipital, and temporal lobes?
10. What function does the somatosensory area serve?
11. Disruption in the occipital lobe may lead to what?
12. What is the function of the structures of the diencephalon?
13. What is the role of the thalamus?
14. What does the hypothalamus regulate?

15. What does the brain stem regulate?
16. The cerebellum is involved with which function of the body?

Inner Structure

Limbic System

Another brain system that appears in both the frontal and the temporal lobes but is not visible from the outer brain is the **limbic system,** or border system (Figure 7-4). It is connected to a variety of gray matter centers that are deep inside the brain. The components of the limbic system are the following: the olfactory nerves, the olfactory bulbs and tracts, the septum, the amygdala, the parahippocampal gyrus, the hippocampus, the fimbria-fornix, and the preoptic area (Keltner & Folks, 1995).

The limbic system is an important modulator of emotions and may be one of the systems that play a role in the development of mental illness. The cortical part of this system consists of the cingulate gyrus, which arches back around the corpus callosum, connects with the parahippocampal gyrus in the temporal lobe, and curves under to form the uncus, or hook. Subcortical portions include the septal region near the septum pellucidum,

or translucent divider; the fornix; and the mammillary bodies (see Figure 7-4).

The paired mammillary bodies regulate the processes of learning and memory. Toward the front are the two optic tracts that carry fibers from the nerve cells lining the back of the eyeball. These tracts cross, as do many other tracts in the brain. Their place of crossing is called the *optic chiasm*. Just above the optic tract is the olfactory tubercle, a cranial nerve collecting information about the smell of things. In the middle of all of these structures is the thalamus. There are actually two thalami, one on each side of the brain, and they are usually fused in the midline by the massa intermedia. Arching above the thalamus is the fornix, part of the limbic system, and below it are the structures of the hypothalamus.

The components and connections of the limbic system contain most of the elements that define the individual's personality, cognitive style, and patterns of behavior. Information from the external environment is collected through the hippocampus of the temporal lobe, frontal lobe, cingulate gyrus, and olfactory bulb. The thalamus and septal nuclei serve as transmitters to pass information from major structures, such as mammillary bodies, hypothalamus, amygdala, and hippocampus. Damage to either the septal nuclei, mammillary bodies, amygdala, and hippocampus or a combination

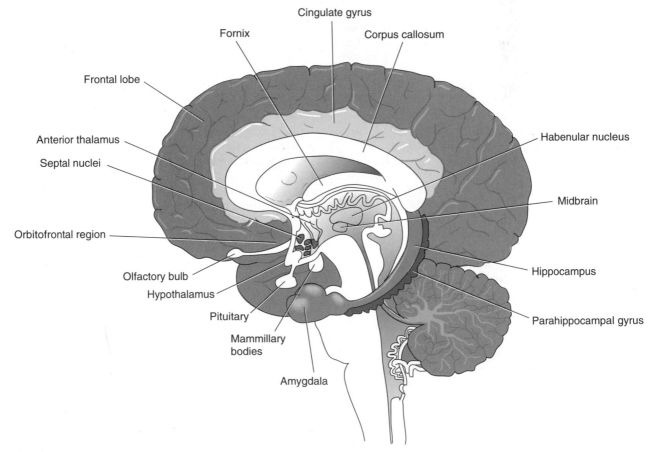

F i g u r e 7 – 4
The structures of the limbic system.

thereof, produces loss of the ability to learn new information and to store the information in long-term memory. Some types of mood disorders are thought to be related to the hyperarousal of the hypothalamic-pituitary-adrenal axis (HPAA).

Other structures, such as the cingulate gyrus and the frontal lobe, are known to be involved in the ability to think creatively and make decisions. These structures also modulate the ability to start and stop various behaviors. Neuroscientists believe that the key to understanding many aspects of mental illness may originate within the limbic system and its connections (Benes, 1993).

Basal Ganglia

The **basal ganglia** lie within the primitive motor system, sometimes referred to as the *extrapyramidal system.* Within this system, the chain of command runs from specific regions in the frontal and parietal cortex, down through the caudate and putamen, to the globus pallidus, and on to the thalamus. Feedback loops occur throughout the system.

The basal ganglia are considered modulators of movement and integrators of sensory information. The basal ganglia share with the limbic system a particular neurotransmitter, dopamine, which is considered important in the development of schizophrenia. Some neuroscientists believe that the study of the basal ganglia may improve the understanding of schizophrenia. Also, the structures of the basal ganglia tend to be selectively damaged in some important diseases. For example, Huntington's chorea is characterized by a "broken" caudate nucleus. Parkinson's disease results from the death of nerve cells in the substantia nigra (black substance), a gray matter center that is part of the basal ganglia but located in the midbrain. Both of these diseases of the basal ganglia have symptoms similar to those of some common mental illnesses.

Ventricular System

The **ventricular system** consists of four fluid-filled cavities buried deep within the brain. There are two lateral ventricles, one within each hemisphere. Each of the lateral ventricles has projections into the frontal lobe, the occipital lobe, and the temporal lobe. The frontal and temporal horns of the lateral ventricles are connected to the much smaller midline third ventricle, which is surrounded on each side by the two thalami. The third ventricle extends down and is connected to an even smaller fourth ventricle, which then flows into a fluid-filled column that runs through the center of the spinal cord. The ventricular system is filled with CSF (see Figure 7-1).

The ventricular system is of interest to neuroscientists for several reasons. First, when brain cells are damaged or die, the substance of the brain grows smaller, and the ventricles enlarge to fill the empty space within the skull; thus, ventricular enlargement provides a useful index of brain atrophy or shrinkage. Also, the

ventricles are major landmarks that can be seen clearly with CT scans. Finally, ventricular enlargement has been noted in some patients with schizophrenia and dementia.

> ➤ *Check Your Reading*
> 17. What is the role of the limbic system?
> 18. What mental disorder may be associated with hyperarousal in the HPAA?
> 19. What mental disorder is associated with dysfunction of the basal ganglia?
> 20. Why is the ventricular system of interest to neuroscientists?

Microstructure

The nervous system is the most complicated and complex structure ever to influence human beings. There are only three types of nerve cells: neurons, glial cells, and Schwann's cells. The nervous system replicates a small number of simple structures and modifies the specificity of the interconnections among the neurons (Kingsley, 1996). Currently, neuroscientists believe that the neurons are responsible for formulating and transmitting all the messages of the brain. The glial (glue) cells are thought to be cementing, supporting, and nourishing structures for the neurons. The brain has been estimated to contain 10 trillion cells of which 90% are glial cells.

Neurons differ in shape and appearance depending on their purpose. *Afferent neurons* are specialized to receive messages, whereas *efferent neurons* send out messages. All neurons are secretory cells that produce an extensive amount of proteins and are basically bound by the cell membrane. Figure 7-5 shows the structure of a neuron. The main work center of the neuron is the cell body, which contains the nucleus of the cell. *Dendrites* are tiny fibers that extend from the cell body and enable the surface to process the synaptic connections that need to occur (Kingsley, 1996).

In addition to the dendrites, the cell body sends out a long, tubular projection called the *axon.* Many axons are covered with myelin, which is produced by glial cells in the CNS and Schwann's cells in the PNS. The axons are the "wires" of the nervous system. Although some axons are relatively short, others may be as long as 1 m. This organization of axons permits electrical impulses to travel from the cell body to the end of the nerve fiber and to the next configuration. The end of the axon branches into as many as 1000 terminals.

The neuronal communication is carried out either by electrical conduction or by chemical processes. The axon is filled with and surrounded by a fluid containing a high concentration of electrically charged substances called *ions,* such as sodium (Na^+), potassium (K^+), and chloride (Cl^-). When a message arrives at the axon, an **action potential** occurs; this is also known as the *depolarization process.* This electrical event is created by the ionic reaction between the elements in the membrane.

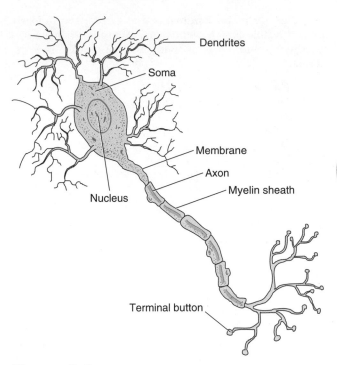

Figure 7-5
The structure of a neuron.

Receptors are cell membrane proteins that react to specific neurotransmitters. These proteins are programmed to receive messages and to bind with particular types of neurotransmitters. Scientists have discovered that these receptors are complex and perform multiple functions. In addition, the receptors may change the permeability of the membrane, and they may communicate outside of the cell to send messages. Specific enzymes quickly inactivate neurotransmitters that are not bound to receptors. For example, norepinephrine is inactivated by the enzyme monoamine oxidase, and dopamine is inactivated by dopamine β-hydroxylase.

Some drugs may increase or decrease the sensitivity of particular receptors. This may either explain the mechanism of action of the drugs or account for their side effects. For example, prolonged use of antipsychotic drugs may eventually lead to oversensitivity of receptors, thereby causing *tardive dyskinesia* (a movement disorder characterized by involuntary rolling of the tongue or twitching of facial or other small muscles).

The permeability of the membrane forming the axon changes, and this change causes positively charged sodium ions to flow in to the intracellular area from the extracellular surface while the potassium ions exit to the external surface. The larger the axon, the faster the message can travel. Figure 7-6 shows a membrane potential. Membrane potential is the critical mechanism underlying the control of the distribution of ions and the regulators of electrical charges across the neuronal membrane. A number of factors influence this process, such as the quality and the nature of the channels, the external events, and the permeability of the membranes.

When the electrical impulse traveling down the axon reaches its presynaptic terminal, it spreads out in hundreds of nerve terminals that communicate with the dendrites and cell bodies of other neurons. The communication point between the neurons is called the *synapse* (junction). Finally, a series of chemical events occurs following the electrical conduction. Figure 7-7 shows an axon and a synapse.

At the end of the nerve terminal are synaptic vesicles that look like small clumps of sacs. These sacs contain chemical substances called **neurotransmitters.** These function as chemical messengers. When an impulse reaches the presynaptic terminal, it is accompanied by calcium ions (Ca^{2+}). These ions enhance the movement of synaptic vesicles toward the presynaptic membrane. Once the vesicles reach the presynaptic membrane and receive a strong positive charge, the sacs surrounding the packets of neurochemicals burst, and neurochemicals flow into the synaptic cleft. Released neurotransmitters in the synaptic cleft interact directly with receptor molecules in the postsynaptic membrane.

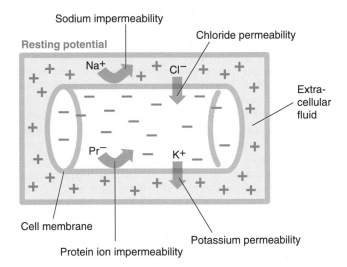

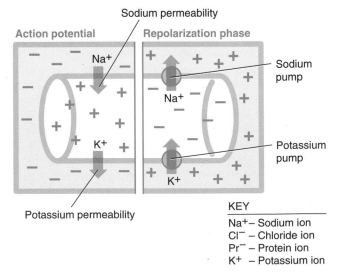

Figure 7-6
A membrane potential.

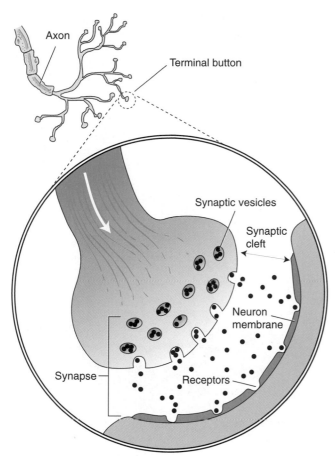

Figure 7-7
An axon and a synapse, shown enlarged.

Other psychoactive drugs, such as diazepam (Valium), may bind to the modulating component in the **GABA (γ-aminobutyric acid)** receptor, preventing it from functioning appropriately and giving GABA free rein as an inhibitor.

Several second messenger systems in the postsynaptic structures also appear to be involved in neuronal transmission through ion systems. Much of the work in neuroscience since the late 1980s has been focused on identifying neurotransmitters and their receptor sites and on better understanding these second messenger systems.

➤ *Check Your Reading*

21. What are the functions of the cell body, axon, and dendrites?
22. Describe the ionic changes that occur in the cell during an action potential.
23. What is the function of the neurotransmitter?

Neurotransmitters

The brain's chemistry is unique, complex, and highly organized. It is supported by billions of nerve cells with trillions of synapses that make organized neurotransmission possible. Data demonstrate that mental disorders result from problems in the regulation of a specific neurotransmission system. The psychiatric nurse must be familiar with the dynamics of neurotransmitters not only because of the physiological effects that they exert in the body systems but also because of the influence they exert on rehabilitation of the patient with mental illness.

The process of transmitting information in neuronal pathways must follow the basic properties of neurotransmission. Receptors respond through excitation at postsynaptic sites or inhibition at presynaptic sites (the conversion into action by a second messenger system modulating the target protein), and, finally, the inactivation of neurotransmitters by enzymatic breakdown or reuptake back into the neuron.

Current research in neuroscience involves identifying and charting locations of neurotransmitters in the brain and learning how they interact with receptor sites in other neurons. There are four major types of neurotransmitters linked with psychiatric illness (Table 7-2):

1. Biogenic amines, including norepinephrine, dopamine, serotonin, and melatonin
2. Cholinergic neurotransmitters, including acetylcholine
3. Amino acids, including glutamate and GABA
4. Neuropeptides, including endorphins, enkephalins, and substance P

Let's take a closer look at these neurotransmitters. Figure 7-8 shows three of these neurotransmitter systems.

TABLE 7-2 Neurotransmitters in the Brain			
CHOLINERGIC NEUROTRANSMITTER	**BIOGENIC AMINE**	**AMINO ACID**	**NEUROPEPTIDE**
Acetylcholine	Dopamine	γ-Aminobutyric acid (GABA)	Endorphin
	Norepinephrine	Glycine	Enkephalin
	Serotonin	Glutamate	Neurotensin
	Histamine		Vasoactive intestinal peptide
	Melatonin		Cholecystokinin
			Substance P

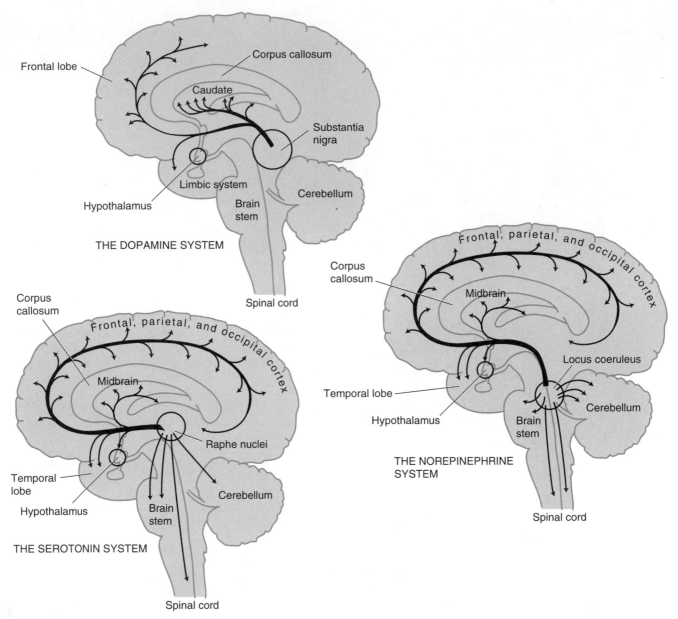

Figure 7-8
The dopamine, norepinephrine, and serotonin systems. (Redrawn from THE HUMAN BRAIN COLORING BOOK by Marian C. Diamond. Copyright © 1985 by Coloring Concepts, Inc. Reprinted by permission of HarperCollins Publishers, Inc.)

Acetylcholine

One of the first neurotransmitters identified in the brain was acetylcholine. It is found predominantly in the amygdala, hippocampus, caudate and putamen, nucleus accumbens, cortex, thalamus, and brain stem. It has two receptor subtypes: nicotinic and muscarinic. *Nicotinic receptors* exert a stimulatory effect through their actions on ion channels and are known to improve learning and memory. *Muscarinic receptors* are either stimulatory or inhibitory; they are associated with memory dysfunction and some adverse effects of antipsychotic medication known as anticholinergic effects (e.g., dry mouth). The primary role of acetylcholine in the brain is to facilitate cognitive function or to modulate another neurotransmitter. Alzheimer's disease is a classic example of a disorder resulting from loss of cholinergic neurons in the hippocampus and entorhinal cortex. Although treatment options for patients with Alzheimer's disease are limited, research has demonstrated some improvement in memory through the administration of cholinesterase inhibitors to increase the available acetylcholine in the synapse.

Dopamine

Dopamine is an inhibitory neurotransmitter found in the mesolimbic, nigrostriatal, and mesocortical areas. The pathways project from the substantia nigra to the caudate nucleus and putamen. Increased dopamine is associated with pleasurable feelings of reward and increased locomotion; however, movement is retarded when there is a deficit of available dopamine. There are two families of dopamine: D_1 and D_2. D_2 is the most investigated dopamine family due to its link with schizophrenia. The antipsychotic medications are believed to work at the D_2 receptor family. Research on new antipsychotic medications points to a dysregulation in both D_2 and serotonin systems as critical in the physiology of schizophrenia.

Norepinephrine

This neurotransmitter is diffusely distributed throughout the PNS and CNS; is located in the locus caeruleus; and has projections to the midbrain including the amygdala and the septum, and to the entire cerebral cortex. It has two receptor subtypes, α and β. The β-receptors are implicated in various cardiac disorders and hypertension, and knowledge of the side effects of this receptor is important in preventing further adverse effects of some psychotropic agents. Norepinephrine plays a role in the regulation of awareness of external environment, attention, memory, arousal, and learning. Research from neurochemical and pharmacological studies indicates that norepinephrine is involved in some types of depression, anxiety, and attention-deficit hyperactivity disorder.

Serotonin

This neurotransmitter has been the subject of multiple research investigations on the cause and treatment of mental illness. Serotoninergic neurons originate in the raphe nucleus and project into the cortex, hippocampus, thalamus, and cerebellum. Serotonin is synthesized by dietary tryptophan, inactivated by a reuptake mechanism, and degraded by monoamine oxidase. On the one hand, serotonin is believed to have a role in psychosis, depression, aggression, violent suicide attempts, and impulsivity. On the other hand, fearfulness, inhibition, anxiety, and obsessive-compulsive disorder are linked with excess serotonin. Serotonin is further processed in the pineal gland, resulting in the production of melatonin. Melatonin is implicated in affective disorders, which are frequently characterized by abnormal sleep–wake cycles.

Neuropeptides

More than 50 peptides are known to be present in the limbic system. They are prominently identified in the hypothalamus, amygdala, septum, nucleus accumbens, cortex, and hippocampus. These neuropeptides have endocrine functions, and researchers are interested in the opiate-like peptides (endorphins and enkephalins) associated with reducing pain, as well as neurotensin, vasoactive intestinal peptide, cholecystokinin, and substance P.

Amino Acids

The amino acids are divided into excitatory and inhibitory classes. Glutamate, an excitatory amino acid, is important because it is toxic when levels are high; glutamate is believed to be involved in brain development. GABA is the major inhibitory class found in the cortex, thalamus, substantia nigra, caudate, and cerebellum. It has specific binding sites for benzodiazepines, which are used to treat anxiety and seizure disorders.

➤ *Check Your Reading*

24. In cases in which some drugs used to treat depression and schizophrenia inhibit the acetylcholine system, what is the effect called?
25. What is the physiological mechanism involved in Alzheimer's disease?
26. What neurotransmitter is involved with the development of schizophrenia?
27. What two neurotransmitters are implicated in the development of depression?
28. What neurotransmitter is implicated in cardiac disorders?

NEUROPHYSIOLOGY

To understand the brain more fully, you must know not only the anatomical structures but also how various parts are related to one another to perform various functions or tasks. This is the scope of the branch of neuroscience called *neurophysiology.*

Sensory System

The *sensory system* is the link between the external and internal environments by way of sensory and motor fibers. The specific area where all physical sensations are processed is located in the somatosensory region, in front of the parietal cortex, just behind the motor strip that forms the rear border of the frontal cortex. Bodily sensations such as heat, cold, pain, and pressure or touch are processed in this region.

Some information received from the senses or generated by thought is integrated and processed in other parts of the brain, for example, motor cortex for voluntary movement. The intricate bundle of nerve fibers receives all the impulses, and the information is processed throughout the brain in a highly integrated fashion. Similar processes occur with the auditory and visual system; however, the information is collected initially by the specific sensory receptor, for example, the optic nerve for vision, and then sent to the thalamus and finally to the somatosensory region (Clayman, 1995).

Language System

The ability to speak differentiates human beings from the rest of the animal species. The language system, located in the left hemisphere of the brain, consists of

- Broca's area in the frontal lobe
- Auditory cortex and Wernicke's area in the temporal lobe
- Angular gyrus in the parietal lobe
- Visual area in the occipital lobe

Any disruption or damage to these centers or the nerve fiber pathways may result in a language abnormality called *aphasia.*

Some patients with schizophrenia suffer from abnormalities in the language system. For example, the patient may use *neologism* (private words or phrases that have special meaning to the speaker) and not be understood by others. In response to a query by the nurse, for example, the patient may respond, "ethiuel tanigram."

Memory System

The memory center has widely diffuse storage areas that are symmetrically found on both sides of the brain. The following structures are involved in the consolidation of memory: hippocampus, mammillary bodies, septal region of the limbic system, and part of the thalamus. When damage occurs on only one side, memory usually remains intact, but bilateral lesions lead to a complete memory deficit.

Neuroscientists have differentiated three types of memory. The first one is *sensory memory,* such as brief recognition of a sound. When this event is retained and interpreted, it becomes *short-term memory* that may be stored for a few minutes. Finally, consolidation of the event by attention, repetition, and association of ideas converts the memory to *long-term storage.* Recollection depends on how effective the consolidation of memory is (Clayman, 1995).

Frontal System

The frontal lobes serve as the primary senior executives of the brain. Scientific findings of the 1990s revealed that the frontal system exerts a number of important functions necessary for the normal personality and for social and emotional maturity of the individual. Specifically, the frontal lobes mediate information throughout the neuroaxis via the cortex, thalamus, cingulate gyrus, limbic system, and reticular formation. For example, the lobes maintain and shift attention; exert organizational control; anticipate consequences; consider alternatives; plan; formulate goals; and shape, direct, and modulate personality and emotional functioning (Rhawn, 1996).

Attempts are being made to refine the charting of the frontal system and to clearly connect the frontal lobes with the manifestations of such major mental illnesses as schizophrenia and affective disorders. Research clearly suggests that there is malfunction in the frontal lobe of patients diagnosed with schizophrenia (Rhawn, 1996). These patients often display bizarre, socially inappropriate, unpredictable, and impulsive behaviors. They also tend to have difficulty initiating spontaneous behavior, through either speech or social interactions. Similar to patients with frontal lesions, they may have poor grooming or hygiene. It is difficult to determine whether these symptoms arise from abnormalities in the frontal system itself or whether the symptoms may be caused by a breakdown in communication between the frontal system and other systems. In addition, there is considerable overlap in functional lesions so that the abnormality may not be confined to one specific region of the frontal lobe.

> ➤ *Check Your Reading*
> 29. What type of information does the sensory area collect?
> 30. What abnormality is linked with damage to Broca's area?
> 31. Which area permits recognition of language in auditory form?
> 32. In what illnesses is frontal lobe dysfunction suggested?
> 33. What are the three types of memory?

Neuroendocrine System

The CNS regulates the **endocrine system,** with the hypothalamus as the command center. It secretes specific neuroregulatory hormones or releasing factors that can activate or inhibit the function of the anterior pituitary gland (known as the *master gland*). The pituitary gland is surrounded by brain tissue and is directly impacted by the brain's chemical activity. In turn, the pituitary gland directs the functioning of the other endocrine glands (Fogel, Schiffer, & Rao, 1996).

The endocrine system includes the thyroid gland, the adrenal glands, the part of the pancreas that produces insulin, and the sexual glands (testes in males and ovaries in females). The hypothalamus; the adrenal, sexual, and thyroid glands; and pituitary communicate with each other with the help of chemical messengers called *hormones* traveling through the bloodstream. The feedback loop mechanism between the hypothalamus and the organs of the endocrine system also monitors the pituitary gland. For example, feedback loops regulate the production of estrogen from the ovaries, androgen (testosterone) from the testes, corticosteroids from the adrenal glands, and thyroid hormone from the thyroid gland. In addition to all of these functions, the hypothalamus, with the pituitary as intermediary, is the center for the regulation of aggression, appetite, thirst, water balance, and growth rate. Figure 7-9 illustrates the neuroendocrine cascade:

- Hypothalamic-pituitary-thyroid axis
- Hypothalamic-pituitary-adrenal axis (HPAA)
- Hypothalamic-pituitary-gonadal axis

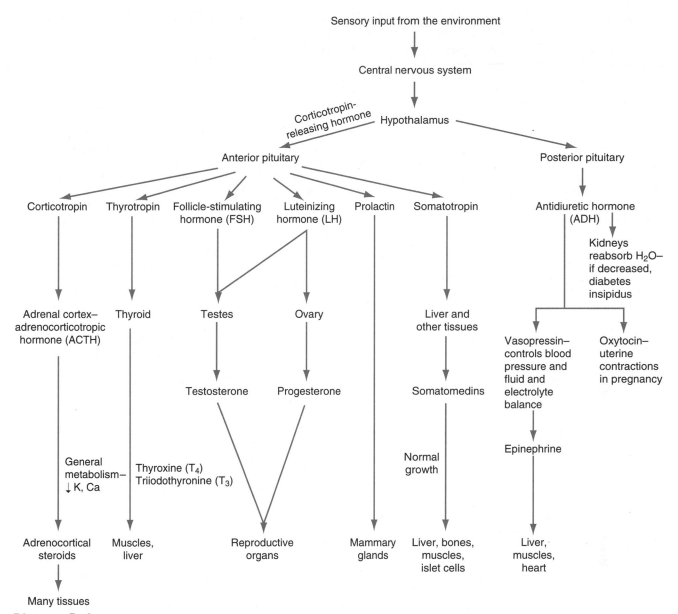

Figure 7–9
The neuroendocrine cascade.

Biochemical changes in the brain initiate a cascade of effects that ripple through the endocrine systems. These effects can be measured peripherally through specific laboratory tests, which are often referred to as biological markers for psychiatric illness. Although these biological markers are promising, their current use in clinical practice is limited. They are expensive, time consuming, sometimes uncomfortable, and not specific or consistent enough to guarantee precise diagnoses. For instance, research during the mid- to late 1990s (Thase, Frank, & Kupfer, 1993) suggested that patients with mood disorders may be suffering from an imbalance in the HPAA. Many of the symptoms of mood disorder are consistent with these types of neuroendocrine abnormalities because they involve changes in appetite, sleep regulation, and adaptability to stress and change. This knowledge, however, does not point consistently to the most efficacious clinical intervention.

➤ *Check Your Reading*
34. What are hormones?
35. Which structure is known as the command center of the neuroendocrine system?
36. What changes occurring in depression are consistent with neuroendocrine abnormalities?

Psychoimmunology

Research that explores the interaction between the immune system and the CNS is in its infancy. However, preliminary findings reveal that these two systems share similar characteristics. For instance, both systems have the capacity for memory. The immune system and the CNS affect each other, and the effect is bidirectional in nature (Hayes, 1995).

Findings demonstrate that white blood cells (WBCs) are directly affected by the nervous system. WBCs have receptors for the neurotransmitters dopamine, serotonin, and acetylcholine as well as for a number of hormones (Kaplan & Sadock, 1995). Low levels of norepinephrine stimulate proliferation of T cells (a specific kind of WBC); conversely, high concentrations of norepinephrine inhibit T cell proliferation. Immune response is inhibited by an increase in serotonin, whereas a decrease in serotonin enhances immune response. These findings suggest that the immune system is directly responsive to abnormalities in the brain's neurotransmitter systems, which are related to mental illness. Furthermore, these findings suggest that the structures that create WBCs, including the thymus, bone marrow, lymph nodes, and spleen, are responsive to the nervous system and thus to changes in the body's psychological state of arousal. Research has demonstrated the reduction of WBCs following the death of a spouse and during the course of depression. Additional research may clarify the interactive role played by the immune system and the CNS in shielding the body from pathogens and preventing psychiatric symptoms.

What do you think? What is the relationship between stress and illness? Does stress cause mental illness? If stress is a causative factor, what is the interaction between the brain and the experience of stress?

NEUROBIOLOGICAL LABORATORY TESTS

The rapid advancement in neuroscience laboratory and imaging techniques has illuminated the importance of biological markers in the diagnosis, treatment, and prognosis of patients with functional psychiatric disorders. The goal to identify biological markers that possess the specificity and concreteness of findings such as glucosuria (used to identify diabetes) remains elusive for psychiatric disorders. In most investigations, a variety of tests are available to evaluate mental disorders, such as brain imaging techniques; blood, urine, and CSF measures of neuroendocrine and neurotransmitter function; and sleep EEG to evaluate the electrical activity of the brain. However, many of these tests are associated with varying degrees of discomfort, expense, and risk of adverse effects. In addition, some neuroimaging techniques have a number of limitations. The psychiatric nurse must be prepared to intervene when necessary to alleviate the discomfort of the procedure and to advocate for patients who might encounter emotional discomfort, pain, and side effects of the procedure.

A later scientific development centers on the relationship of the mind and brain in the study of mental illness, known as *psychopathology*. Even though neuroscience has progressed in several areas of subspecialties in which major theories have evolved, there is no decisive resolution regarding the relationship of mind and brain. For instance, research on synaptic plasticity (Jefferey & Reid, 1997; Ruppin, Reggia, & Horn, 1996) promises exciting findings regarding the cognitive machinery behind beliefs and memory and how beliefs and memories are represented within associated neural networks. This research focuses on two major fields of interest. The first is the creation of artificial neural network models constructed according to biologically inspired principles. The second is the hope that these artificial networks will not only provide solutions to unsolved problems in engineering and computing but also shed light on brain function and the molecular biology within the brain that underlies synaptic plasticity. **Synaptic plasticity** refers to the fact that in cases in which neurons are closely associated and one neuron is repeatedly involved in exciting or firing another neuron, over time that connection is strengthened so that the first neuron is able to excite the second neuron more effectively. This research is preliminary and has not resulted in therapeutic applications. However, preliminary findings suggest greater understanding of the persistence of hallucinations and delusions in schizophrenia as well as the occurrence of post-electroconvulsive therapy amnesia in depressed patients.

Electroencephalography

EEG has been used diagnostically in psychiatry for many years. A similarity has been noted in symptoms of patients with temporal lobe epilepsy and some psychiatric diagnoses. Specifically, when the abnormal focus is on the left side, patients tend to be obsessional, be humorless, be concerned with religious ideas, and have a low libido. These patients closely resemble patients with a diagnosis of obsessive-compulsive personality disorder.

Since the 1980s, neuroscientists have been focusing on the electrical activity of the brain during sleep. Empirical research indicating that sleep patterns of patients with insomnia are disturbed supports laboratory sleep studies of patients with subjective complaints of insomnia. This is apparent in non–rapid eye movement (REM) abnormalities in the depressed patient, such as prolonged sleep latency in 90% of depressed patients, increased wakefulness, and early morning awakening. These findings point to a chronic state of sleep arousal in depressed patients. They spend less time in stages 3 and 4 of the sleep cycle, which are the refreshing slow-wave stages of sleep, and more time in stage 5, or REM sleep. They also tend to have a higher mean sleep temperature and flattened sleep curve. This indicates that the individual is in an active waking state instead of sleeping.

What do you think? A patient tells you, "I have been very depressed—I can't get enough sleep. I feel like I am in bed all the time, but I never feel rested." How would you respond?

Brain Imaging Tests

Computed Tomography

The use of CT has had a major impact on the practice of neurology and psychiatry. This tool was introduced in the early 1970s because previous testing with brain angiography and traditional radiographs failed to provide direct visualization of the brain tissue. The CT scan can provide computer-generated "slices" of the brain, which can be stacked by the computer, resulting in a three-dimensional image (Trimble, 1996). A fine beam of x-rays is projected through the patient's head while it interacts with the detector, and the computer records the proportions of x-rays absorbed by brain tissues of different densities (Trimble, 1996).

Some researchers are recommending that CT scans be performed on patients with any of the following conditions: dementia, psychosis, movement disorder, depression, anorexia nervosa, and schizophrenia. However, because the test is costly and does not allow a high degree of differentiation among diagnoses, these recommendations are not generally authorized by managed care companies. Not all patients with the aforementioned diagnoses have abnormal CT scans, whereas patients with other diagnoses such as mania may also have abnormal CT scans (Begley, Wright, Church, & Hager, 1992). The results of CT scans indicate that some types of schizophrenia may be due, in part, to abnormalities in the limbic system.

Radiologists and psychiatrists working together have developed a method of measuring lateral ventricular volume that adjusts for overall brain size. This method is called *ventricular-brain ratio.* Most studies have found that ventricular enlargement usually occurs in the early phase of schizophrenia (Fogel et al., 1996) and that the degree of enlargement correlates with the severity of symptoms. Similar studies also reveal an increase in the ventricular-brain ratio in depressed patients, especially those with late life depression associated with dementia (Alexopolos, Young, & Shindledecker, 1992). One exciting area of research in biological psychiatry involves the correlation between structural brain pathology and the negative symptoms of schizophrenia. The negative symptoms of schizophrenia include affective flattening or blunting, poverty of speech, blocking, poor grooming, lack of motivation, deficits in cognition, social withdrawal, and anhedonia. The implications of this research include the development of a more refined system of classification of schizophrenia and further advances in the prescription of certain types of psychopharmacological medications.

Magnetic Resonance Imaging

MRI is another technique used for diagnostic evaluations. Tissue images obtained from MRI are used to rule out conditions such as hydrocephalus, cerebral vascular accidents, tumors, and personality disorders. Future advances in this technology are projected to include the use of complimentary functional MRI to evaluate regional cerebral blood flow and cerebral metabolism (Fogel et al., 1996). Figure 7–10 is an example of MRI of the left hemisphere of the brain of monozygotic female twins.

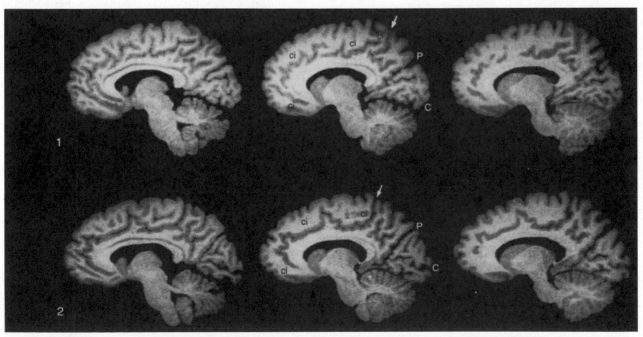

Figure 7–10
MRI of the left hemisphere of the brain of monozygotic female twins. (From Steinmetz, H., Herzog, A., Huang, Y., & Hackländer, T. [1994]. Discordant brain-surface anatomy in monozygotic twins [Letter]. *New England Journal of Medicine, 331,* 951–953. Copyright © 1994 Massachusetts Medical Society. All rights reserved.)

Positron Emission Tomography and Single Photon Emission Computed Tomography

Positron emission tomography (PET) involves the introduction of radioactive substances that are taken up by the brain. This is accomplished through the injection of glucose labeled with the fluorine-18 positron. Because glucose is the fuel that provides brain cells with nourishment, it serves as a useful substance to differentially identify metabolism in the various parts of the brain. Radiation is emitted from those parts of the brain that are most active and therefore take up the largest amounts of isotopes.

Different aspects of brain functioning can be evaluated with PET including cerebral blood flow, brain oxygen consumption, brain glucose metabolism, and CNS neurotransmitter receptor function, but a PET scan is expensive. During the 1990s, PET began to be used to study brain function in affective disorders, schizophrenia, and childhood autism. Investigators have used PET scans to compare normal subjects with schizophrenic and autistic patients, and the scientists have determined that patients with autism and schizophrenia may have less frontal brain activity while they are at rest (Begley et al., 1992). Other studies have used tagged neurotransmitters and psychoactive drugs in the brains of patients with mental illnesses and neurodegenerative disorders. These tags are specific labels used to identify those transmitters being studied.

Single photon emission computed tomography (SPECT) is similar to PET but uses more stable substances and detectors to visualize blood flow than PET uses. Both allow investigators to study brain metabolism and cerebral blood flow. SPECT has been used often with radiopharmaceutical imaging, particularly in testing brain muscarinic acetylcholine receptors and in testing blood perfusion of patients with Alzheimer's disease. Additionally, it has been used extensively with normal volunteers in an attempt to delineate brain areas associated with the acquisition and utilization of different types of knowledge.

Superconducting Quantum Interference Device Brain Mapping

The superconducting quantum interference device (SQUID) senses tiny changes in magnetic fields. When neurons fire, they create an electrical current. These electrical fields induce magnetic fields, which indicate neuronal activity. In this way, brain action can be mapped through the depiction of magnetic fields, thus the use of the term *SQUID brain mapping*. Although this technique is more sophisticated than PET, it is expensive and limited to research applications.

Brain Electrical Activity Mapping

Brain electrical activity mapping (BEAM) uses CT techniques to display data derived from EEG. It maps brain electrical activity that can be sensory evoked by a specific stimulus, such as a sudden sound or a flash of light, or cognitively evoked by specific mental tasks.

Although most of the above-mentioned techniques lack the ability to detect subtler functional differences that occur at the network and chemical levels in disorders such as schizophrenia, they have taken our journey to understanding mental illnesses quantum leaps forward. When the results of these techniques are coupled with neuropsychological testing and observations regarding deficits in an individual's cognitive, sensory, or language functions, it is possible to make links to specific areas of the brain responsible for these functions. This knowledge will, in turn, point to even greater understanding regarding the causes of mental illnesses, as well as possible curative interventions.

What do you think? A couple you know is getting married. The woman has a first cousin who is schizophrenic. She asks you, "Are there any tests that I can have that will tell me if I will have a child with schizophrenia?" How would you respond?

➤ *Check Your Reading*

37. How do CT scans construct an image?
38. In the use of the CT scan in schizophrenic patients, what are researchers attempting to correlate?
39. What abnormalities have been found on PET in some patients with schizophrenia and autism?
40. In what area of research has SQUID been used?

Neurochemical Tests

In contrast to brain imaging techniques, neurochemical research focuses on the chemicals that reside in the brain and that are known to influence the individual's emotional and mental conditions. Samples of blood, urine, and CSF are analyzed to determine the levels of brain chemicals being circulated. Blood tests are also used to determine drug levels for titration with some psychoactive drugs, such as the antidepressants nortriptyline (Pamelor) and desipramine (Norpramin), and drugs used to treat bipolar disorder, such as lithium and carbamazepine (Tegretol).

Tests of Neuroendocrine Function

For years, clinicians have noticed that patients experiencing depression display symptoms similar to people with diseases of the thyroid and adrenal glands. Some of those symptoms include fatigue, change in appetite, and insomnia. Studies have identified that in major depression, there are neuroendocrine abnormalities, specifically abnormalities of cortisol production (Sachar et al., 1973). The dexamethasone suppression test (DST) is one laboratory study developed in the 1970s and still used occasionally today.

Dexamethasone Suppression Test

The DST was designed to determine if the communication system between the brain and the adrenal glands is dysfunctional. The patient is given a small dose (1 mg) of the synthetic steroid dexamethasone, a synthetic hormone similar to cortisol, and blood levels are assessed at different intervals. As the level of this substance in the blood is elevated, the hypothalamus in normal individuals reads the plasma cortisol level as high. The hypothalamus stops sending corticotropin-releasing hormone to the pituitary gland and, in return, the pituitary gland stops sending adrenocorticotropic hormone to the adrenal glands. In this way, taking the dexamethasone tablet suppresses the HPAA, and within 12 hours, the blood levels of cortisol drop low. This is considered normal suppression.

In some patients with major depression, their systems fail to suppress the dexamethasone, and their plasma cortisol levels remain high. The DST is said to be abnormal. The DST is considered a possible test for depression, but it is not used routinely.

Thyrotropin-Releasing Hormone Stimulation Test

The thyrotropin-releasing hormone (TRH) test measures thyroid function. In individuals with a normal functioning thyroid, the hypothalamus produces TRH. In response, the pituitary secretes thyroid-stimulating hormone (TSH). If the hypothalamus fails to secrete TRH, the thyroid function is reduced. The procedure involves injecting the patient with an intravenous bolus of TRH. Blood samples are drawn and TSH is measured at specific intervals. In a normal response, TSH increases two times the baseline in 30 minutes; in about 40% of patients with major depression, there is a blunted TSH response.

> **What do you think?** A patient is acting in a really strange manner. His diagnosis is schizophrenia. You overhear another nurse say, "He acts bizarre just to get attention; I hate it when we have a mental patient on our unit." Based on what you know about the biological basis of mental illnesses, how would you respond to this nurse?

► *Check Your Reading*

41. What is the neuroendocrine abnormality in major depression?

IMPLICATIONS OF NEUROBIOLOGICAL PSYCHIATRY

The explosion of knowledge in neurobiological psychiatry since the 1970s still leaves us with no clear answer to the question: "What causes mental illness?" The answer to the question may depend on various internal and external factors that contribute to human nature.

Even with the advances in neuropsychiatry, mental illnesses tend to carry an aura of guilt and moral responsibility. Confusion still exists due to the dichotomy between the mind and the body; hence, a disease of the mind must be categorically different from a disease of the body. The word *mind* refers to those functions that reside in the brain; this includes mental or emotional processes. Mental illnesses manifest as diseases of the mind that arise from the brain. However, the search for the cause of mental illness continues, and for every new development in neuroscience and psychiatry, psychiatric nursing is challenged to redefine its goals to meet the needs of the mentally ill.

> **What do you think?** As you review the findings presented in this chapter, what is your position regarding the stigma that surrounds patients affected with a brain disease? How would you respond to a person who made a derogatory remark about an individual with schizophrenia?

Let's turn our attention to the three major psychiatric illnesses and apply the biological findings to each one of these disorders. As you read this, keep in mind that the research continues to change what we know in each of these situations. It is imperative that you understand the current state of knowledge and that you keep abreast as new findings are integrated into the diagnosis and treatment of schizophrenia, depression, and anxiety.

Schizophrenia

Schizophrenia is a serious psychiatric illness with a worldwide lifetime prevalence of 1%. It is a major cause of long-term disability (Fogel et al., 1996). Although research continues to show progress in the study of schizophrenia, the complexities and the range of symptoms present in this disorder thwart efforts to specifically identify the causes of the illness.

In fact, the evidence from a variety of studies suggests that schizophrenia is not a single disease but a group of related symptoms that are classified as a single syndrome. One type, referred to as *florid* or *positive schizophrenia*, is characterized by prominent "positive" symptoms, such as delusions and hallucinations. This type tends to respond well to traditional antipsychotic medication treatment. Perhaps this type of schizophrenia is neurochemical. Another type, characterized by predominant "negative" or defect symptoms, such as blunted affect and impoverished speech, may be due to diffuse structural damage to the brain as evidenced by ventricular enlargement. In some individuals, there has been lessening of these symptoms with use of the newer atypical antipsychotic drugs. Let's examine the story of Mark in Case Example 7-1.

CASE EXAMPLE 7-1
Mark's Story

Mark is 34 years old, single, formerly a Yale scholar, ill for almost 12 years with schizophrenia. He was apprehended by the police for striking an elderly woman and was sent to the emergency room. Mark's chief complaint is "That ugly woman. She and the rest of them deserve more than that for what they put me through."

Mark has been continually ill since the age of 22. His difficulty started during his 1st year of law school. During that year he had become more and more convinced that his classmates were making fun of him. His girlfriend broke off their relationship because his behavior became too difficult for her to handle. Mark believed that a supernatural force had been involved with his girlfriend. He called the police and asked for their help in solving the problem. He was asked to leave law school and seek psychiatric help.

Mark maintains that his apartment is the center of a large communication system that involves all the residents, neighbors, and those "homosexuals" in the neighborhood. He complained of the radio in his room continually broadcasting reports accusing him of homosexuality. He wrote long, incoherent letters to his family which included odds and ends of English history, politics and other scholarly writings he recalled of his scholarly years. ■

Adapted from Spitzer, R. L., Gibbon, M., Skodal, A. E., Williams, J. B, & First, M. B. (1989). *DSM-III-R Casebook*. Washington, DC: American Psychiatric Press.

Neurochemical Factors

Over the years, there have been many theories regarding the neurochemical basis of schizophrenia; however, the findings remain inconclusive because most of the studies yielded inconsistent results. The most widely accepted theory concerning neurochemical abnormalities in schizophrenia is the **dopamine hypothesis.** According to this hypothesis, schizophrenia is due, in part, to an excess of dopamine neurotransmission (Fogel et al., 1996). As indicated in Figure 7-8, dopamine is an important messenger in many parts of the limbic system, responsible for controlling emotion and personality. The first evidence in support of this hypothesis came from the development of neuroleptic drugs, which block D_2 receptors (dopamine), thereby improving the positive symptoms of schizophrenia. These receptors seem to occur in increased numbers in the basal ganglia and limbic systems of patients suffering from schizophrenia. The second major finding relates to amphetamine and other aminergic agents, which increase the activity of dopamine and other catecholamines that can provoke a psychotic state or worsen the symptoms of some patients, particularly those who are treatment resistant (Fogel et al., 1996).

Among the other brain chemicals that have been implicated in schizophrenia research are serotonin, norepinephrine metabolites, dopamine metabolites in the CSF such as homovanillic acid, and neuropeptides. The implications of these studies remain unclear, but the results show loss of affected neurons. Pharmacological developments using newer atypical antipsychotic drugs are promising and may lead to a better understanding of the cause of schizophrenia.

Brain Imaging

The most notable structural pathology demonstrated with brain imaging in schizophrenia is the obvious ventricular enlargement located in the deep subcortical region. This is presumably due to brain shrinkage secondary to neuronal death. The rate of ventricular enlargement in schizophrenic patients ranges from 10% to 50% (Suddarth, Christison, & Torry, 1990). Several replicated studies using MRI technology revealed similar findings, especially in the temporal lobe of the brain where small areas of distinct damage were found. This explains the probable source of hallucinated voices that plague many schizophrenic patients.

Genetic Factors

Genetic research has shown that mental illness may be influenced by genetic transmission. Early studies of the relatives of schizophrenics summarized by Slater (1968) indicated that although the disorder occurs in only about 1% of the population, parents of schizophrenics had the disease 3.8% of the time, siblings 8.7%, and children 12%. These data support the idea that the rate of schizophrenia is clearly higher for individuals with a first-degree or second-degree relative with the disorder. Kallman (1946) examined comparative rates of psychiatric disorders in **monozygotic** (identical) twins compared with same-sex **dizygotic** (fraternal) twins, reared together or apart. He found a concordance rate of 86% for monozygotic twins raised either together or apart and a 50% concordance rate for dizygotic twins. Other studies have identified rates of 50% for monozygotic twins, 10% to 15% for dizygotic twins, 10% for siblings, 15% in cases in which one parent is schizophrenic, 35% in cases in which both parents are schizophrenic, 2% to 3% in cases in which a second-degree relative is affected, and 1% in cases in which there is no affected relative.

The most recent genetic hypothesis centers on the vulnerability of trinucleotide repeat amplification—a mutation theory in which specific DNA occurs more than once when genes are copied in schizophrenia. For example, if one child carrying a gene for schizophrenia happens to have more trinucleotide repeats than others, this child could be pushed over the threshold into mental illness (Akbarian et al., 1995).

Neuroimmunology: Viral Theory

Another hypothesis is that schizophrenia may be due to a viral illness occurring early in life and producing some type of mild encephalitis, or brain inflammation, that predisposes an individual to the development of schizophrenia. This idea has been supported, in part, by studies of virus-like agents found in the CSF of some schizophrenics and the observation that more schizophrenics are born during the winter months when viral diseases are more prevalent (Wright, Takei, Rifkin, & Murray, 1995).

Psychiatric Nursing Implications

The implications for psychiatric nursing focus on many critical issues of care, specifically on managing the patient with this disability and handicap. Schizophrenia can involve massive disruptions of thinking, perception, emotion, and behavior. Mark's story is a classic example of this illness. Successful psychiatric nursing care involves alleviating the suffering of the patient and those around him or her; encouraging the patient to take the medications that alleviate symptoms; and helping the patient function better cognitively, emotionally, and socially.

Schizophrenia may lead to progressive neurological and psychological impairments that generally impact the person's capacity to restore and maintain his or her ability to perform functional activities. It is important that the nurse continuously assess the patient's cognitive abilities, self-care knowledge and skills, strengths and weaknesses, and ability to focus his or her attention on the goals of the treatment plan. Reality testing is necessary in rehabilitation. Although the illness itself follows a specific neurologic and psychiatric deterioration, hope always exists that the patient's condition may stabilize or the patient will learn new skills to compensate for what he or she has lost secondary to the disease.

Current research indicates that neuronal growth or regeneration can be actively facilitated by the appropriate physical and mental exercises necessary to stimulate the neuronal circuitry. The scientific studies on brain-derived neurotrophic factor, a growth factor for substantia nigra (dopamine site), and neurotrophin 3 showed that synaptic transmission in the hippocampus increases with exercise, which results in enhanced neuronal growth, function, and survival (Kang & Schuman, 1995; Neeper, 1995). Additionally, environmental and behavioral interventions may be implemented to take advantage of residual areas of strength or unimpaired functions and to compensate for the patient's impairments. For example, strategies such as the use of appointment books, memory books, and other cues may be useful for those with memory impairment. Patients and caregivers require teaching and support regarding many tasks of daily living that may require the use of these tools.

The psychiatric nurse's goal must include a life management plan for the patient. Such a plan includes coordinating those involved in the patient's care: the professionals of various disciplines, the patient's family, and the patient's significant other. The nurse reinforces all that is done by others and works with the patient to continually revise the plan to meet his or her changing needs. The plan must include health promotion to prevent further exacerbation or decompensation of either schizophrenia or other concurrent medical illnesses.

What do you think? The argument about whether nature or nurture determines who we are and what we become has raged for centuries. How would you respond to this age-old question? How do counseling and psychotherapy fit into a paradigm that emphasizes biological causation?

➤ Check Your Reading

42. There is a higher incidence of schizophrenia in which type of twins?
43. The viral theory of the cause of schizophrenia is supported by what evidence?

Mood Disorders

Since the 1990s, more advanced neurobiological, psychiatric, and pharmacological research has demonstrated better understanding of mood disorders. Despite the underlying conflicts with the classification of depressive illness, specialists have identified the two primary mood disorders as major depressive disorder and bipolar 1 disorder. Major depression is considered a more severe, unrelenting syndrome. More than 15 million people in the United States have it each year, and the economic costs of depression are estimated to be $30 billion annually in the United States (Wortman, 1997). Let's examine Case Example 7–2.

■ CASE EXAMPLE 7–2
■ Mrs. B's Story

Mrs. B is a 50-year-old woman who sought consultation because of increasing feelings of sadness, "nervousness" and of thoughts about killing herself. During the preceding month she had lost interest in her work as a legal secretary, spent more time in bed, and called in sick frequently. She reported that she had difficulty sleeping throughout the night and had lost 20 pounds. She was fully alert and cooperative but easily tearful. Her motor behavior was slow, and her nervousness decreased in frequency. Her affect was restricted and her mood was sad.

Mr. B related that this is the first time in their 24-year marriage that Mrs. B has acted in this manner. He stated that his wife refuses to go out socially because she wants to rest but he never sees her sleeping. He said that he forces her to eat and became frightened when she stated that she wanted to die. He insisted that she see a mental health professional. ■

Adapted from Tomb, D. A., & Christensen, D. D. (1987). *Case Studies in Psychiatry for the House Officer.* Copyright © 1987, Williams & Wilkins.

Neurochemical Factors

There are three basic monoamine hypotheses of depression specifically related to the neurotransmitter assigned to the system:

1. The **catecholamine hypothesis** includes dopamine and norepinephrine and the serotonin hypothesis. Indolamine is the amino molecule for serotonin wherein it is metabolized into 5-hydroxyindole acetic acid in the brain. The catecholamine hypothesis describes the deficiency of norepinephrine in the brain.

2. The dopamine hypothesis is based on the pharmacological evidence that certain neuroleptic agents block dopamine receptors and thus are effective antimanic agents and may be antidepressants as well (Trimble, 1996).

3. The serotonin hypothesis is similar to norepinephrine findings respective to a decreased amount of serotonin in the brain.

Another theory of depression relates to the modulatory effect of the monoamines during reuptake in the synapse. Any disruption during the reuptake process may result in depression.

A number of methods are used to examine the presence of adequate amounts of neurotransmitters in the system. Laboratory test of urine MHPG (3-methoxy-4-hydroxyphenylglycol, the metabolite of norepinephrine) is one method of measuring the amount of norepinephrine in the urine. Lower MHPG in the urine is indicative of depression.

In studies of direct assay of norepinephrine and mass spectroscopic assay of MHPG, researchers hypothesized that the locus coeruleus is implicated in depression. The report suggested that there are increased levels of CSF and plasma norepinephrine and increased urinary MHPG in patients with major depression (Bushness & DeForge, 1994).

In addition to catecholamines, GABA and acetylcholine transmissions have been studied in relation to mood disorders. Based on pharmacological data, it has been postulated that patients with major depression possess a hyperresponsive cholinergic (acetylcholine) system, whereas decreased GABA levels in the CSF and plasma are found in depressed patients.

These hypotheses suggest the possibility that there may be subgroups of depressive illnesses. Developments may lead to the differential prescription of antidepressant drugs based on neurochemical findings.

Neuroendocrine Factors

Investigation suggests that depressed patients may have a dysregulation of endocrine functions in the brain through secretions of hormones from the hypothalamus to the pituitary gland. Some depressed patients produce large amounts of cortisol and are unable to suppress it normally. These phenomena appear to identify a defect in the HPAA. Challenge tests with insulin and TRH suggest that defects do not lie in target organs but are probably at the level of the hypothalamus or higher.

Brain Imaging

The results of imaging research into mood disorders have been inconclusive. Although CT and MRI scans have demonstrated larger ventricles and reductions in cortical mass in patients with affective disorders than in the control group, the clinical significance of these findings remains obscure. PET scans demonstrate different metabolism rates and cerebral activity in depressed and manic patients than in controls (Thase, Frank, & Kupfer, 1993).

Genetic Factors

The affective disorders have an important genetic component, particularly in bipolar illness (Trimble, 1996). Genetic studies have consistently shown that the relatives of people suffering from mood disorders have a much higher rate of mania and depression than occurs in the general population. For example, about 20% of the parents of patients with depression also have depression, and the rate in brothers, sisters, and children is even higher—possibly as high as 30%. The rate tends to be higher in female relatives than in male relatives. This parallels the higher incidence of depression diagnosed in females. The spouses of people suffering from depression also have a relatively high rate of depression—about 20%.

Twin studies also indicate that 65% of monozygotic twins have concordance for the illness as compared with only 14% of dizygotic twins. On the other hand, linkage studies of bipolar disorder have not revealed reliable genetic markers due to lack of replicated investigations of the association of chromosome 11 with bipolar illness (Trimble, 1996)

Circadian Rhythm Hypothesis

Several features of mood disorders suggest abnormalities in circadian rhythms. These include the inherent cycles of depression, the pronounced abnormalities in rest-activity cycle, the length and timing of sleep stages, and the clinical responsiveness to experimental alterations in circadian organization. Changes in both non-REM and REM sleep in patients with mood disorder seem to reflect a pathological state of arousal.

Benca, Obermyer, Thisted, and Gillin (1992) conducted a metaanalysis of sleep disorders in more than 7000 patients. The results showed reduced total sleep time in most patients and an increase in REM in those with affective disorder (Trimble, 1996).

In addition, a subcategory of mood disorders, seasonal affective disorder (SAD), has been identified. SAD seems to point to the importance of circadian rhythms in the cause of depression. People with SAD have an apparent reaction to changes in environmental factors, such as climate, latitude, and light.

Kindling and Behavioral Sensitization Hypothesis

Another model that attempts to account for the cyclical pattern of mood disorders is the kindling-sensitization hypothesis. Electrical **kindling** refers to the phenomenon of repeated stimulation by low-level electrical impulses followed by increased responsiveness to stable low doses of stimulation over time, resulting in seizures (Andreasen, 1997).

Sensitization refers to the effect of repeated stressors on behavioral outcomes. For instance, repeated exposure to inescapable shock may produce a progressive increase in behavioral and neurochemical abnormalities. In this model, kindled limbic seizures or the sensitization of the limbic system may account for many features of mood disorders. This could then explain the predisposition for depression caused by stressful early childhood experiences, the gradual worsening of episodes over time, and the decreasing amount of time between depressive episodes.

Psychiatric Nursing Implications

Depression is one of the most common clinical problems encountered by health providers. Often, the signs and symptoms of depression are not recognized and the cost of this illness to patients, their families, and society is significant. Only about half of all persons with major depression ever receive specific treatment.

Mood disorders are clearly complex in their etiology. Current research points to major dysregulation of neurotransmitter systems as well as of brain mechanisms that regulate sleep–wake cycles and other biological rhythms. It is increasingly apparent that depression is not a "one treatment fits all" disorder but requires diverse treatments—both with medications and with other approaches. For instance, the SAD patient may benefit from phototherapy; some depressed individuals may respond to sleep deprivation. This diversity in treatment approaches makes it essential for psychiatric nurses to keep abreast of the latest research findings and to remain in the forefront of interpreting the clinical implications of these findings.

W*hat do you think?* The battle continues to rage over whether psychiatric illnesses should have parity with medical illnesses in terms of insurance coverage. Is there a difference between psychiatric and medical illnesses? If so, what are the differences? How would you respond to individuals who said they did not want to pay increased insurance premiums for illnesses that were "all in a person's mind"?

➤ *Check Your Reading*

44. Which factors in mood disorders point to changes in circadian rhythms?
45. What symptoms of mood disorders support a kindling-sensitization model?

Anxiety Disorders

Dramatic advances in neuroscience research have illuminated new hopes for treatment, cure, and even prevention of anxiety disorders. Although it is clear that environmental factors play an important role in the production of anxiety disorders, research has also demonstrated that major biological mechanisms have etiological significance (Case Example 7–3).

■ **CASE EXAMPLE 7–3**
■ **Ben's Story**

A 30-year-old married electrician, Ben, was brought in on a stretcher to the emergency room. He was breathing quite rapidly, trembling, and saying, "I am going to die, I'm going to die." He complained of air hunger, tightness in his throat and chest, and coldness and numbness in his hands and feet. Ben admits that he often experiences a dry mouth and throat and that his concentration is affected by all these uncontrollable sensations. He states that these

feelings have remained almost constant for the last 2 years. He also has many worries, including the fear of infidelity on the part of his wife, and the fear that he is not a good father. These fears appear to be unwarranted. His heart rate is 120 per minute, respiration 34 per minute, blood pressure is 140/86 mm Hg. All his laboratory tests and other physical findings are within normal limits. ■

Adapted from Spitzer, R. L., Gibbon, M., Skodal, A. E., Williams, J. B., & First, M. B. (1989). *DSM-III-R Casebook*. Washington, DC: American Psychiatric Press.

Neurochemical Factors

Numerous neurochemical studies have been conducted to identify the neurotransmitters and neuropeptides that mediate the behavioral responses associated with anxiety disorders. A major focus in a number of clinical studies has been the relationship of stress to anxiety. Available data support the hypothesis that there is a relationship between central norepinephrine and anxiety and that the locus coeruleus, which produces 70% of the brain's norepinephrine, is the crucial factor in the regulation of anxiety. The research points to the role of norepinephrine in the development of an anxiety disorder; however, it does not seem to be the cause of the illness.

Another theory of anxiety centers on GABA, which is cited as the neurotransmitter involved in the regulation of anxiety. GABA and benzodiazepine receptors actually are part of the same molecular complex. It is known that benzodiazepine enhances and prolongs the action of GABA so that any alterations in the system support the hypothesis that GABA has a role in the regulation of anxiety (Fogel et al., 1996). Benzodiazepine receptors are widely distributed throughout the cerebral cortex, cerebellum, amygdala, hippocampus, and dentate gyrus.

A development in the treatment of one type of anxiety disorder, panic disorder, has been identified. Scientists at Yale discovered that patients with panic disorder tend to develop chemical sensitivity to the brain's neuroadrenergic system, which releases norepinephrine. They demonstrated that long-term high levels of anxiety lead to actual physical changes in the brain wherein the brain's own survival processes eventually damage its own cells. The victims have a significantly smaller hippocampus, the area that plays a crucial role in memory. The findings were confirmed by MRI and PET (Wortman, 1997).

There is also evidence linking serotonin transmission in the midbrain to panic attacks. Patients experiencing panic may actually have hypersensitive serotonin receptors. The fact that the selective serotonin reuptake inhibitors (SSRIs), drugs that potentiate the regulation of serotonin, are effective in treating panic and obsessive-compulsive disorders, points to a major role for serotonin in the etiology of anxiety disorders.

Brain Imaging

Imaging research, using CT and MRI scans, has demonstrated brain atrophy or underdevelopment in patients with panic disorder. Brain activity has also been shown to be abnormal in patients with panic disorder. The clinical significance of these findings is unclear.

Genetic Factors

Evidence is steadily accumulating that a predisposition to develop anxiety disorders may also be partly hereditary. Early studies, based on review of patient records and family histories, suggested that relatives of people with anxiety disorders have a high incidence of anxiety disorders (about 20%) compared with the general population rate of 5%. Female relatives are affected about twice as often as male relatives.

Torgerson (1990) compared 32 monozygotic and 53 same-sex dizygotic twins in Norway and concluded that hereditary factors were significant in panic disorder but not in generalized anxiety disorder. This suggests that there may be a significant genetic component to a predisposition to panic disorders, but the data on anxiety disorders are still equivocal.

Psychiatric Nursing Implications

Normal anxiety is sometimes difficult to differentiate from pathological anxiety. Growth and change as a result of experiencing something new and untried usually accompany normal anxiety. By contrast, pathological anxiety is an inappropriate response to a given stimulus. The psychiatric nurse must understand the difference between such forms of anxiety so that appropriate interventions can be offered.

The nurse's role includes teaching the patient and family that the anxiety associated with panic attacks is related to a dysregulation of the fight-or-flight response and may be due to a combination of genetic vulnerability and the individual's response to stressful life events. The teaching must include the facts that a variety of interventions exist, including the use of medication and cognitive strategies, that are effective in treating panic. This information provides the patient and family with a sense of control over a situation that is incapacitating and apparently uncontrollable.

What do you think? When a individual is diagnosed with a mental illness, how much personal responsibility does he or she bear for his or her actions?

➤ *Check Your Reading*

46. How do antianxiety drugs work within the body?
47. Patients with panic disorders share some biochemical similarities with what other type of illnesses?

Conclusions

Psychiatric nurses must understand neuroscience and be able to translate the findings into clinically appropriate interventions. The education of nurses has always required a foundation in both the social and the natural sciences. The shift in the current understanding of neurobiological and psychiatric nursing is another step in our journey to practice holistically in advocating, caring, and rehabilitating the mentally ill. Our previous knowledge of psychodynamic and social models enhances our basic knowledge of therapeutic interventions that are crucial in the management of patients who are affected by debilitating and progressively devastating mental disorders. The journey to psychiatric and mental health nursing has begun.

Key Points to Remember

- The term *neuroscience* encompasses a set of related disciplines that share the common goal of understanding the relationship between brain structure and function and human thoughts, feelings, and behavior.
- New areas of brain research affecting the revolution in biological psychiatry include brain imaging, understanding the biological dimensions of emotion, the role of neurochemicals in the formation and enactment of behavior, shifting knowledge of brain plasticity after birth, and understanding molecular genetics.
- Myelination differentiates white matter from gray matter.
- The corpus callosum connects the right hemisphere with the left.
- Afferent tracts travel to the brain.
- Glial cells are the supporting, cementing, and nourishing structures for the neuron.

- The cell body is the work center of the neuron. The axons are the wires of the nervous system. The dendrites increase the ability of the neuron to receive information.
- During an action potential, the permeability of the membrane forming the axon changes, causing positively charged sodium ions to flow into a cellular space.
- The function of the neurotransmitter is to send the message chemically.
- An anticholinergic effect occurs when some drugs that are used to treat depression and schizophrenia inhibit the acetylcholine system.
- It is believed that dopamine is involved in the development of schizophrenia.
- Norepinephrine and serotonin are implicated in the development of depression.

- Serotonin has been linked with aggressive behavior.
- The frontal lobe is the seat of intellectual functioning. The parietal lobe receives information about various bodily sensations and synthesizes and elaborates sensory impulses. The occipital lobe receives and sends out information. It contains the primary visual area. The temporal lobe receives auditory impulses, stores memory patterns for symbolic sounds, receives and transmits gustatory impulses, and receives and transmits olfactory input.
- Disruption in the occipital lobe may lead to illusions and hallucinations.
- Diencephalon structures serve as relay stations between the lower brain centers and the higher cortical centers.
- The thalamus is the major pathway for sensory and motor impulses to and from the cerebral hemispheres and the modulator of emotions and behavior.
- The hypothalamus regulates hormonal function.
- The brain stem regulates the activities of the heart, respiration, and other vital functions.
- The cerebellum is a major modulator of movement.
- The role of the limbic system is to modulate emotions.
- The pineal gland partially regulates the sleep–wake cycle.
- The paired mammillary bodies function in the process of learning and memory.
- Depression may be associated with hyperarousal in the HPAA.
- The basal ganglia function as modulators of movement and integrators of sensory information.
- Schizophrenia may be associated with basal ganglia dysfunction.
- Huntington's chorea and Parkinson's disease involve basal ganglia structures.
- The ventricular system is of interest to neuroscientists because ventricular enlargement provides a useful index of brain atrophy, and ventricles are major landmarks seen on CT scans. Ventricular enlargement has also been noted in some patients with schizophrenia and dementia.
- Damage to Broca's area leads to difficulty in speaking fluently.
- Wernicke's area permits recognition of language in auditory form.

- In schizophrenia, there is a possibility of frontal lobe dysfunction.
- The command center of the neuroendocrine system lies in the hypothalamus.
- Changes in appetite, sleep regulation, and adaptability to stress and change occurring in depression are consistent with neuroendocrine abnormalities.
- CT scans beam x-rays through the body to construct an image.
- CT and MRI identify structure, whereas PET identifies function.
- Some patients with schizophrenia and autism have been found to have impairment of prefrontal cortical functioning, or *hypofrontality* on PET scans.
- SQUID has been used with normal volunteers to delineate areas associated with the acquisition and utilization of different types of knowledge.
- Some people with major depression experience abnormalities in cortisol production.
- Patients with temporal lobe epilepsy resemble patients with obsessive-compulsive disorder.
- Patients with major depression may experience prolonged sleep latency, increased wakefulness, and early morning awakening.
- There is a higher incidence of schizophrenia in monozygotic twins than in dizygotic twins.
- The viral theory of the cause of schizophrenia is supported by a virus-like agent found in the CSF of some schizophrenics and the observation that more schizophrenics are born during the winter months, when viral diseases are more prevalent.
- Norepinephrine, serotonin, acetylcholine, and GABA have been studied in relation to mood disorders.
- The HPAA is implicated in the inability of the neuroendocrine system to suppress cortisol.
- Inherent cycles of depression, the pronounced abnormalities in rest–activity cycle, and the length and timing of sleep stages are all factors in mood disorders that point to changes in circadian rhythms.
- The gradual worsening of occurrences of illness over time and the decreasing amount of time between episodes are symptoms of mood disorders supporting a kindling-sensitization model of etiology in affective disorders.
- The benzodiazepine receptor facilitates the GABA system.

Learning Activities

1. Draw and diagram an axon and a synapse.
2. Draw and diagram a neuron.
3. Make a chart showing the disorders of schizophrenia, depression, and anxiety. For each of the disorders, identify the major neurotransmitters involved, the area of the brain most implicated, and the results of the brain dysfunction.
4. As you proceed through your psychiatric clinical experience, formulate both a psychodynamic and a biological explanation for each of your patients' diagnoses. Once you have done that, go back to the formulation and show the interaction of environment, experience, and biology.
5. Do you think that spirituality has a role in biological psychiatry?

Critical Thinking Exercises

Mr. Norman, an 18-year-old, was admitted to the crisis center after he was found running down the street naked at 2:00 in the morning. He was diagnosed as having an acute psychotic episode. Mr. Alder, a nurse with 30 years of experience with psychiatric patients, tells his new graduate nurse, Ms. Newman, about the way patients' families used to be informed about the treatment and causes of schizophrenia. He states that he was taught that families were to blame for causing the illness, particularly the mother, who was reported to give out mixed messages. Today, we are taught that biology and chemistry play an important role in the development of major psychiatric disorders.

1. What inference can Ms. Newman draw about Mr. Alder's beliefs about nursing practice?

2. What are the consequences of attributing the etiology of mental illness to biological factors?

Mr. Alder approaches Mr. Norman's mother and father to give them information about their son's condition. He tells them about their son's medications and their actions. He also tells them that it is important that they know about the illness so that they can support their son and help him to reach his highest level of functioning. Ms. Newman notices that Mr. Norman's parents are attentive and listening to Mr. Alder's instruction.

1. What information would the nurse want to include in discussing Mr. Norman's illness and care?

2. What is an alternative to the above approaches?

Additional Resources

American Psychiatric Association (APA)

Division of Public Affairs
1400 K Street, NW
Washington, DC 20005
202-682-6220

Source of current information about specific psychiatric disorders and treatments.

Brainscape

http://beast.cbmv.jhu.edu:8000/projects/brainscape/brainscape-4.html

National Alliance for the Mentally Ill (NAMI)
200 North Glebe Road
Suite 1015
Arlington, VA 22203-3754
800-950-NAMI or 703-524-7600

Members are entitled to regular updates regarding current research in psychiatry. NAMI maintains an extensive library of pamphlets, books, posters, videotapes, and audiotapes, which are available to members at a low cost and cover a wide variety of topics in psychiatry.

Neurophysiology

http://williamcalvin.com/neuro-uw.html

Neurosciences on the Internet

http://www.neuroguide.com

Society for Neuronal Regulation (SNR)
Neurofeedback Archive

http://www.snr-jnt.org/NFBArch/nindex.htm

References

Akbarian, S., Kim, J. J., Potkin, S. G., Hagman, J. O., Tafazzoli, A., Bunney, W. E., Jr., & Jones, E. G. (1995). Gene expression for glutamic acid decarboxylase is reduced without loss of neurons in prefrontal cortex of schizophrenics. *Archives of General Psychiatry, 52,* 258-266.

Alexopolos, G. S., Young, R. C., & Shindledecker, R. D. (1992). Brain computed tomography findings in geriatric depression and primary degenerative dementia. *Biological Psychiatry, 31,* 591-599.

Andreasen, N. (1984). *The broken brain: the biological revolution in psychiatry.* New York: Harper & Row.

Andreasen, N. (1997). Linking mind and brain in the study of mental illnesses: A project for a scientific psychopathology. *Science, 275,* 1586-1593.

Begley, S., Wright, L., Church, V., & Hager, M. (1992, March 27). Mapping the brain. *Newsweek,* 48-54.

Benca, R. M., Obermeyer, W. H., Thisted, R. A., Gillin, J. C. (1992). Sleep and psychiatric disorders: A meta-analysis. *Archives of General Psychiatry, 49,* 651-668.

Benes, F. M. (1993). Neurobiological investigations in cingulate cortex of schizophrenic brain. *Schizophrenia Bulletin, 19,* 537-550.

Broca, P. (1861). Remarques sur le siege de la faculté du langage articulé, suivies d' une observation d' aphemie. *Bulletin de la Societé d'Anatomie, 36,* 330-357.

Bushness, F. K. L., & DeForge, V. (1994). Seasonal affective disorder. *Perspectives in Psychiatric Care, 30*(4), 21-25.

Clayman, C. (1995). *The human body: An illustrated guide to its structure, function, and disorders.* London: Dorleng Kindersley Limited.

Fogel, B., Schiffer, R., & Rao, S. (1996). *Neuropsychiatry.* Baltimore: Williams & Wilkins.

Giannini, A. J. (1986). *The biologic foundations of clinical psychiatry.* New York: Elsevier.

Glod, C. (1996). Recent advances in the pharmacotherapy of major depression. *Archives of Psychiatric Nursing, 10,* 355-364.

Hayes, A. (1995). Psychiatric nursing: What does biology have to do with it? *Archives of Psychiatric Nursing, 9,* 216-224.

Hill, L. (1991). The neurophysiology of acute anxiety: A review of the literature. *CRNA: The Clinical Forum for Nurse Anesthetists, 2*(2), 52-61.

Jazwinski, S. M. (1996). Longevity, genes, and aging. *Science, 273,* 54-59.

Jefferey, K., & Reid, I. (1997). Modifiable neuronal connections: An overview for psychiatrists. *American Journal of Psychiatry, 154,* 156-164.

Kallman, E. (1946). The genetic theory of schizophrenia. *American Journal of Psychiatry, 103,* 309-322.

Kaplan, H. I., & Sadock, B. J. (Eds.). (1995). *Comprehensive textbook of psychiatry* (6th ed.). Baltimore: Williams & Wilkins.

Kang, H., & Schuman, E. (1995). Long-lasting neurotrophin-induced enhancement synaptic transmission hippocampus. *Science, 267,* 1568.

Keltner, N., & Folks, D. (1993). *Psychotropic drugs.* St. Louis, MO: Mosby-Year Book.

Kingsley, R. (1996). *Concise text of neuroscience.* Baltimore: Williams & Wilkins.

Kirkwood, T. B. (1996). Human senescēnce. *Bioessays, 18,* 1009-1016.

Kraepelin, E. (1896). *Psychiatrie* (5th ed.). Barth, Leipzig (R. M. Barclay, Trans.) Edinburgh: E & S Livingstone.

Lieberman, J., & Rush, A. (1996). Redefining the role of psychiatry in medicine. *American Journal of Psychiatry, 153,* 1388-1397.

Maudsley, H. (1870). *Body and mind.* London: Macmillan.

McEnany, G. W. (1991). Psychobiology and psychiatric nursing: A philosophical matrix. *Archives of Psychiatric Nursing, 5,* 255-261.

Neeper, S. (1995). Exercise and brain neurotrophins. *Nature, 373,* 109.

Rhawn, J. (1996). Neuropsychiatry, neuropsychology, and clinical neuroscience: Emotion, evolution, cognition, language, memory, brain damage, and abnormal behavior (2nd ed.). Baltimore: Williams & Wilkins.

Ruppin, E., Reggia, J. A., & Horn, D. (1996). Pathogenesis of schizophrenic delusions and hallucinations: A neural model. *Schizophrenia Bulletin, 22*(1), 105-123.

Sabshin, M. (1990). Turning points in twentieth-century American psychiatry. *American Journal of Psychiatry, 147,* 1267-1274.

Sachar, E. J., Hellman, L., Roffwarg, H. P., Halpern, F. S., Fukushima, D. K., & Gallagher, T. F. (1973). Disrupted 24-hour pattern of cortisol secretion in psychotic depression. *Archives of General Psychiatry, 28,* 1926.

Slater, E. (1968). A review of earlier evidence in genetic factors in schizophrenia. In D. Rosenthal & S. Kety (Eds.), *The transmission of schizophrenia: Proceedings of the second research conference of the Foundations Fund for Research in Psychiatry,* (pp. 15-26). Oxford: Pergamon Press.

Suddarth, R. L., Christison, G. W., & Torry, E. F. (1990). Cerebral anatomical abnormalities in monozygotic twins discordant for schizophrenia. *New England Journal of Medicine, 322,* 789-794.

Thase, M., Frank, E., & Kupfer, D. (1993). Biological processes in major depression. In E. Beckman & W. Leber (Eds.), *Handbook of depression.* New York: Guilford Press.

Torgerson, S. (1990). Twin studies in panic disorder. In J. Ballenger (Ed.), *Neurobiology of panic disorder.* New York: Alan R. Liss.

Trimble, M. R. (1996). *Biological psychiatry* (2nd ed.). New York: John Wiley.

Wernicke, C. (1874). *Der aphasische symptomen complex: Eine Psychologische Studie auf Anatomischer Basis.* Breslau, Germany: Cohn & Weigert.

Whytt, R. (1765). On nervous, hypochondriacal or hysterical diseases. Edinburgh: Becket and Du Hondt.

Wortman, M. (1997, Fall/Winter). Brain chemistry. *Yale Medicine,* 3-11.

Wright, P., Takei, N., Rifkin, L., & Murray, R. M. (1995). Maternal influenza, obstetric complications, and schizophrenia. *American Journal of Psychiatry, 152,* 1714-1720.

Suggested Readings

Andreasen, N. (1997). Linking mind and brain in the study of mental illnesses: A project for a scientific psychopathology. *Science, 275,* 1586-1593.

Bushness, F. K. L., & DeForge, V. (1994). Seasonal affective disorder. *Perspectives in Psychiatric Care, 30*(4), 21-25.

McEnany, G. W. (1991). Psychobiology and psychiatric nursing: A philosophical matrix. *Archives of Psychiatric Nursing, 5,* 255-261.

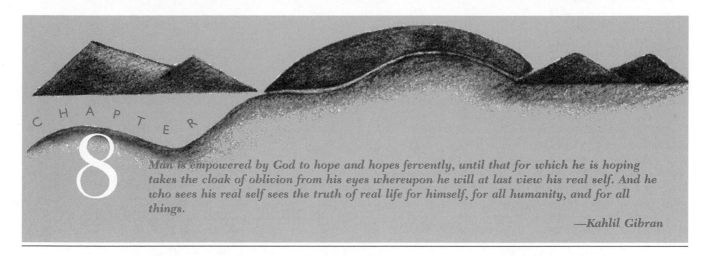

Man is empowered by God to hope and hopes fervently, until that for which he is hoping takes the cloak of oblivion from his eyes whereupon he will at last view his real self. And he who sees his real self sees the truth of real life for himself, for all humanity, and for all things.

—Kahlil Gibran

Shared Attributes of Every Traveler
Self-Concept

Learning Objectives

After studying this chapter, you should be able to:

1. Define self, self-concept, and all of the interrelated dimensions of self-concept.

2. Describe the key factors that influence the development of the self and self-concept.

3. Discuss the reciprocal relationship between human needs according to Maslow and the progression through the developmental stages according to Erikson.

4. Explain how human beings are more alike than they are different and how sharing our humanness can affect another's self-concept.

5. Begin to examine the processes involved in the development and incorporation of the professional self into one's self-concept.

Key Terminology

Birth order	Ideal self	Purpose	Self-efficacy
Body image	Meaning	Role	Self-esteem
Cognitive processes	Perceptual processes	Role conflict	Self-respect
Developmental tasks	Personal identity	Self	Sibling position
Emotional processes	Personality	Self-awareness	Social self
Gender identity	Physical self	Self-concept	Spiritual self
God-consciousness	Psychological self	Self-confidence	Thinking
Hierarchy of basic needs			

Pat Benner (1984) stated in her book *From Novice to Expert: Excellence and Power in Clinical Nursing Practice,*

Nursing students enter a new clinical area as novices; they have little understanding of the contextual meaning of the recently learned textbook terms. But, students are not the only novices: any nurse entering a clinical setting where she or he has no experience with the patient population may be limited to the novice level if the goals and tools of patient care are unfamiliar. (p. 21)

In the following stories, you are introduced to Sarah and Glen, both nursing students, both novices as they enter into the realm of psychiatric nursing. Let's take a look at how Sarah and Glen view themselves, their strengths, their weaknesses, and their fears and anticipations about psychiatric nursing.

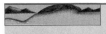

Stories of Two Nursing Students

Sarah and Glen, two senior nursing students, are sitting in their apartment attempting to complete a written assignment before their 1st clinical day in a psychiatric facility. The directive given in class was, "Go home, think about who you are, and write down in a journal all that you know about yourself, your strengths, weaknesses, any special qualities, even how you see yourself physically. What is there about you that will affect how you relate to the patients whom you will meet during the upcoming semester?" The following journals were written.

Sarah: Nursing Student

"Who am I? I am Sarah Smith! I am 20 years old. I am 5′11″, weigh 120 pounds, and my parents think I'm too thin. But my own opinion is that I could lose a few pounds. I am a nursing student in my last semester of school. I should graduate in June if I can finish this psych thing and get through it as fast as possible. I'm more of a med-surg type of person and am scared to death of entering a psych facility. What will I do all day without IVs [intravenous lines] to check, shots to give, or treatments to do? I'm not much of a talker. I've always been a thinker and a doer. My mother always said, 'If you want something done, ask Sarah to do it.' My dad left when I was 3 years old. He was an alcoholic! This communication stuff really has me concerned; I'm just not good at it. I'll just have to see how this semester goes. Why do we have to write this stuff anyway?"

Glen: Nursing Student

"I am Glen. I am 19 years old, the younger brother of two older sisters. I was born in Minnesota, and I'm Irish Catholic. I can't wait to go to the psych hospital. I have been waiting for this experience since I decided to come to nursing school. Med-surg was OK, but I kept getting into a time crunch because I wanted to talk with my patients instead of doing all the tasks that were assigned—like bed-making, washing out my patients' elastic stockings, and the like. We always seemed to get into wonderful conversations about their feelings, and I just couldn't leave. The problem was, I was always late for postconference, and I usually got a message from my instructor that I forgot to complete all of my assignments. I felt terrible! Maybe now that I'm going to psych I can finally listen to people's feelings and not worry about doing things. God knows, I had enough practice listening to all of my sisters' problems. Oh! I almost forgot . . . I am 5′10″ tall, and I weigh 170 pounds. (I think I'm huggable!) I hope my patients like me! I wonder what psych patients are like? I wonder if I can do as well as I think I can?" ∎

How are these two students going to do in their "psych rotation," as they call it? Will both succeed? Will one have an easier time than the other? Will their experiences be the same? What will they need to learn to have a meaningful experience? What will they need to do to have a positive experience? Will they have to learn the same things? What challenges will each face during this stage of growth and development as people and as professionals? Who are the patients with whom they will work?

What do you think? As you read Sarah's and Glen's stories, what thoughts come to your mind? Take a minute and jot down your story.

To connect with another human being, one must clearly define the "self" that is being offered. In this chapter you explore the development of the self and concepts related to self. Questions are asked that will stimulate thinking about the self. Such thinking begins the journey toward understanding each individual's uniqueness. Once the personal self is explored, the professional self that is "becoming" can emerge, so that caring, kindness, and commitment can be shared with peers and patients as each searches for meaning and understanding in his or her experiences.

Sarah and Glen are about to embark on an incredible journey into their selves and the selves of others. They may be surprised to find that they are more similar to their patients than they ever believed was possible.

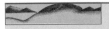

Stories of Two Patients

Ray

Ray came into the hospital because of depression. Although only 26 years of age, he felt older than his years. Although Ray was well groomed and attractive, his shoulders were bent and his eyes were sad. He appeared to be burdened with the weight of many sorrows. Initially, he attributed his sadness to a work situation in which he had been passed over for a promotion. But as his story unfolded, it became apparent that the missed promotion was only his most recent disappointment:

"I am the oldest of three brothers. I used to tell myself that my family was loving and close. That's what we always told each other. But I have slowly come to realize that our only family bond was the well-kept secret that Mom is an alcoholic. My father avoided our home situation by working two jobs. I remember having to care for my younger brothers when my mother was too drunk and my dad was gone. I think that's why I am so responsible now—almost too responsible. I seldom laugh or see the lighter side of things. When I let myself think about it, I feel angry that somehow I got cheated out of being a kid. I remember that when I went away to college, my mother gave me a hug. She felt like a board. I'm sure that I was just as stiff with her. Can you believe that I don't know how to hug? What do you do when someone hugs you? Hug them back or what? These may seem like dumb questions, but we just didn't hug one another in my family.

"I never really fit in with my family, in school, or with kids my own age. Maybe it was because I was too busy acting grown up. My parents never told me I was doing a good job, and my brothers resented me for being the boss. The fact that I didn't get the promotion stirred up a lot of old and painful feelings for me."

Mary Ann

Mary Ann was seen in outpatient therapy to monitor her serum levels of lithium, a medication that she had been taking for several years. Mary Ann had been diagnosed with bipolar disorder, characterized primarily by manic episodes. Her story reveals that, despite her illness, she had a happy childhood:

"I am the middle sister. I have a pretty good relationship with both of my sisters. Oh yeah—we argue. Don't all sisters? But when I need someone to talk to, I usually go to one of them. We have an interesting family. Some people would say we have a high craziness factor. I prefer to think of us as flamboyant. I'm not the only manic-depressive. My older sister has the same thing, only she tends to get depressed. I prefer my symptoms—especially when I am not out of control. I have so many ideas. I write and draw and dance. The arts are really my thing.

"I had my first manic episode right after high school graduation. I really freaked out. I got wilder throughout the summer. I messed with drugs and had sex with anyone. By the end of the summer, I was depressed and tried to kill myself by jumping from a tree. I ended up with a really bad fracture of my arm. I spent some time in a psych hospital and was released. But I had to get sick several more times before I was diagnosed with manic-depression and started taking lithium.

"During the past 10 years, I would take my medication for a while, then I would begin to feel good and stop the medication. And I would always get sick again. When I get sick, my main symptom is wild sexual behavior. When I don't take my medication, I am 5'3" tall and weigh 120 pounds; I weigh 160 pounds when I do take my medication. I want to understand my illness and put it into the larger picture, if you know what I mean. I am beginning to think of my illness as both a gift and a burden." ■

What do you think? Which nursing student would be better suited to work with which patient? What are the commonalities involved between student and patient? What are the differences? What are the identifiable strengths within each of the students that fit with the patients' strengths? We examine these issues as we move through the chapter.

In the stories just cited, both students and patients have a great deal to offer each other, once the initial hesitancies are overcome. When students are anticipating their first psychiatric experiences, they often express fears about personal safety and concern about perceived inadequacies in communicating with patients. Questions such as "What if they are out of control?" and "What if I say something to set them off?" characterize their initial concerns. As the psychiatric experience progresses, the nature of the students' fears changes. The focus shifts to an awareness that similarities exist between the patients and themselves, and new fears emerge that are related to the students' own mental health such as "Could I end up like this?" "Am I all that different?" and "What makes me healthy and them sick?" Although these concerns may be frightening, the recognition that patients are not so different signals a transition in the students' thinking. This transition allows students to understand patients and begin to assume the "helper" role.

Patients also have fears, such as "sounding like I'm crazy," "being seen as weak and ineffective," and "finding no one to understand me." As students and patients begin to experience each other, the fears dissipate and the similarities of the human experience take hold.

What do you think? What are your fears and concerns about your psychiatric nursing experience?

► *Check Your Reading*
1. What are two of the initial concerns students have when they begin a psychiatric clinical experience?
2. What are two common fears of patients as they reveal themselves to nurses?
3. Why is it important for nurses to know themselves?
4. How can nurses use their own story to help themselves relate to others?
5. Is psychiatric nursing the only discipline that requires self-knowledge? Explain.

JOURNEY TOWARD SELF-UNDERSTANDING

In the students' journals at the beginning of the chapter, Sarah and Glen describe themselves as they begin their psychiatric nursing experience. Is their self-knowledge adequate? Is this all they need to know about themselves in order to be able to contribute to the growth of others?

Sarah's and Glen's initial journal entries are certainly a beginning toward self-awareness, but as they progress, they will need to question more deeply to discover more knowledge about self. Additional questions are shown in Box 8–1.

Questions such as those in Box 8–1 are asked by everyone at some point—in fact, they may be asked many times in the course of a lifetime. The answers, although not easy to find, are essential for the development and understanding of the self. Box 8–2 provides questions to encourage self-awareness in the nurse-patient relationship.

Like the students and patients described in this chapter, each of us has a unique story to tell about who we are and how we became that person. In each story, there are similar threads that link us with every other human being. These threads are the shared humanity that allows us to enter and understand another person's lived experiences.

We are all holistic beings with integrated biological, psychosocial, and spiritual natures. The experiences that influence our development differ from one to another. Regardless of how our experiences differ, each of us develops a self-concept and body image, attains certain levels of self-esteem, and assumes roles of our own and of others' choosing. These similarities are explored in the remainder of this chapter.

Self and Self-Concept

Robinson (1974) stated that the self is "the part of the human being that knows himself (herself) as 'I.' It is the

---

Box 8–2 ■ ■ ■ ■ ■
Questions to Encourage Self-Awareness in the Nurse-Patient Relationship

- Can I *be* in some way which will be perceived by the other person as trustworthy, dependable, or consistent in some deep sense?
- Can I be expressive enough as a person that what I am will be communicated unambiguously?
- Can I let myself experience positive attitudes toward this other person—attitudes of warmth, caring, liking, interest, respect?
- Can I be strong enough as a person to be separate from the other?
- Am I secure enough within myself to permit him his separateness?
- Can I let myself enter fully into the world of his feelings and personal meanings and see these as he does?
- Can I receive him as he is? Can I communicate this attitude?
- Can I act with sufficient sensitivity in the relationship that my behavior will not be perceived as a threat?
- Can I free him from the threat of external evaluation?
- Can I meet this other individual as a person who is in the process of *becoming,* or will I be bound by his past and by my past?

Reprinted from Rogers, C. R., Vol. 37, 1958. © ACA. Reprinted with permission. No further reproduction authorized without written permission of the American Counseling Association.

Box 8–1 ■ ■ ■ ■ ■
Questions That Encourage Self-Awareness

- Who am I, really?
- Do I know me?
- Does my physical appearance reflect the me that I want to express?
- What cultural influences have had an impact on me?
- What am I?
- What do I do?
- Which roles do I fulfill?
- Where am I spiritually?
- Whom would I like to be?
- How do I feel about me?
- How do I feel about other people?
- What do I have to offer to others?

---

thinking, knowing, feeling part of the human organism which deals with the world" (p. 19). Miller and Keane (1992) described the self as "the complete being of an individual comprising both physical and psychological characteristics and including both conscious and unconscious components" (p. 1348).

To deal with reality both alone and within relationships, we must be able to view the self, reflect on the self, and understand the self (Dufaulf, 1990; Jerome & Ferrard-McDuffie, 1992). As Peck (1978) put it, "to know the world, we must not only examine it, but we must simultaneously examine the examiner" (p. 51). For self-understanding to be consistent, self-examination must be a lifelong activity. To know who we are, we must possess self-knowledge and self-awareness. **Self-awareness** is made up of all of those things that we know about ourselves—where we invest our energies, where we devote our time, where we derive our satisfactions, where we meet our greatest frustrations, what we strive for, what we consider to be "us."

According to Arnold and Boggs (1995), "Self-concept is the term given to the part of the self that lies within conscious awareness—self-concept encompasses all that a person perceives, knows, values, feels, and holds to be true about his or her identity" (p. 33). Therefore, it is stated that the self possesses conscious and unconscious components, whereas the **self-concept** is made up of the conscious components only. The self-concept possesses a unified nature, yet is differentiated into a constellation of unique dimensions, each with its own diverse functions. Embedded into the self-concept are physical, psychological, social, and spiritual dimensions, which characterize the inner state of an individual and allow that individual to relate to the environment in a unique way (Figure 8–1).

The **physical self** includes the development of a body image and an understanding of physiological functioning. The **psychological self** makes up our personal identity and forms the umbrella for **cognitive processes, perceptual processes,** and **emotional processes.** The **social self** is represented by the many different roles that we assume in presenting ourselves to others. The **spiritual self** allows us the opportunity to connect with God and to find **meaning** and **purpose** in our individual experiences. The **ideal self** is the "me I think I ought to be" or "the me that I would like to be." Our ideas about who we *actually are* make up the self-concept or perceived self, whereas our ideas about who we *should be* form our ideal self. **Self-esteem** can be defined as the individual's personal judgment of his or her own worth. Individuals arrive at this judgment by analyzing how well they match up to their own standards and how well their performances compare with those of others (Arnold & Boggs, 1995). Self-esteem is how we feel about what we know about our self; a person's self-esteem is the key to behavior. Self-esteem influences thinking processes, emotions, desires, values, and goals (Dugas, 1983). "Typically, we constantly compare our perceived self to our ideal self, and the wider the gap between the two, the lower our level of self esteem" (Sanford & Donovan, 1984, p. 8) (Figure 8–2).

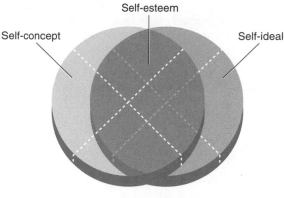

High self-esteem

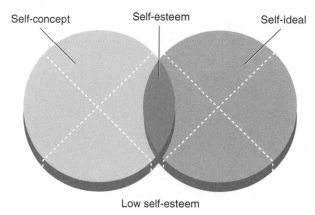

Low self-esteem

Figure 8–2
Relationships among self-concept, self-ideal (ideal self), and self-esteem.

Although the self-concept is a dynamic phenomenon able to respond creatively to novel situations encountered over the life span, it is also a stable and internally consistent representation of who we are. The stability of self-identity is essential in forming meaningful interpersonal relationships based on reciprocal trust.

Development of the Self and the Self-Concept

The self and the self-concept (self-image), with all of their interrelated components, begin to develop during infancy and continue to develop over the course of our lifetimes. The awareness of self begins as vague physical sensations from inner and outer stimuli that become firmed up as we grow, develop, and begin to interact with others. Many of our experiences of self are named and defined by others. As we begin to learn language, we adopt the words that others have used to describe who we are and how well we do what we do. Therefore, much of our self-concept is made up of what we are told by significant others.

"People are not born with the beliefs and images that determine their self image. Children learn self-image by interacting with their environment, family, and reference groups" (Strassen, 1992, p. 38). Oftentimes, as we grow, we need to learn how to objectively compare

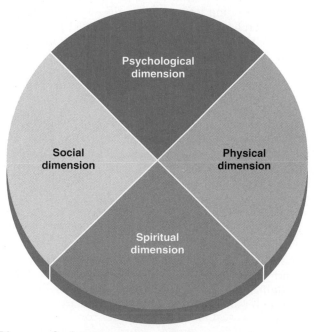

Figure 8–1
The four dimensions of self-concept.

what we have been told about ourselves with what we begin to see for ourselves so that we can see the real talents, abilities, and self-worth that we possess.

> **What do you think?** What influences in your life have contributed to your self-concept? Describe the gap between your perceived self and your ideal self. What perceptions and judgments of significant others have you incorporated into your self-concept?

➤ *Check Your Reading*
6. Define the self.
7. How is the self different from the self-concept?
8. What is self-esteem?
9. What are the dimensions of the self-concept?
10. What happens to self-esteem when the self-concept and the ideal self are far apart?

Physical Self

"What do I look like?"
"Does my body look like other human bodies of the same age and the same gender?"
"Am I pleasing to the eye?"
"Do I need to be concerned about any particular part of myself that can be seen by others?"
"Am I short?"
"Am I taller than most people?"
"Am I muscular?"
"Am I thin?"
"What do I need to do to look more desirable?"

The picture that each of us creates concerning our physical self is called **body image** (Rieser, 1992). Once we recognize the fact that we are separate physical beings—separate from our mothers and separate from the environment—we begin our journey of trying to find out if we're OK when compared with others.

Both our outward appearance and our inner workings, sensations, and sounds represent the necessary processes and sometimes warning signals concerning our physiology. The outward appearance of each human being is generally the same: a head, a trunk, and extremities. Physical differences are present in some people because of genetic or birth alterations, traumatic injury, or illness; however, the majority of individuals have the same general appearance.

The physical self represents the boundary between the inner self, or who we believe we are, and the environment around us. As we learn to dress, or hide our physical boundary from the world, we begin to choose costumes that reflect our feelings of security (Fisher, 1974). Fisher noted that research findings suggest "that the greater a person's uncertainty about the protection provided by his own body border, the more he will seek compensatory ways of reaffirming that border" (p. 22). "In other words, when an individual doubts his boundaries, he may try to reinforce them by making them more visually vivid through the use of attention-getting clothing" (p. 23).

Similarities in the Physical Self

On a macroscopic level, the physical self functions in a similar fashion across individuals. Each of us has a heart that acts as a pump to send oxygenated blood to hungry tissues; each of us has a brain where thought is centered; and each of us has a digestive system that delivers nutrients to the rest of our organs and other body parts. However, on a microscopic level, differences exist in physiological functioning that have a direct impact on self-concept and **personality.** For instance, an individual's ability to deal with stress is probably directly related to the levels of neurotransmitters found in the brain. Some research certainly supports this theory in relation to the schizophrenic patient or to the child with attention-deficit disorder (see Chapters 18 and 24). Although the hormones, enzymes, and neurochemicals may differ in amount (i.e., too little in some, too much in others) and may fluctuate at different times in certain individuals, the basic inner life processes are close in kind when we are considered to be healthy.

Differences in the Physical Self

In addition to recognizing that human bodies are similar, we learn that our own bodies are unique. We learn that some of us are athletic, some are graceful, some move like the wind, and some are clumsy. We learn that we come in different shapes, sizes, colors, and sexes, but the most significant factor is the way we view our physical selves. Each of us relates to others based on how we feel about our physical selves.

Culture and the Physical Self

Culture also influences how we feel about our physical selves. Depending on what a given culture values, individuals reflecting the desired norm feel good about the self, whereas those who are different from what is desired feel inferior and unattractive. Fontaine (1991) pointed out that the desired "ideal woman" has changed considerably from before the 19th century to the present:

In Western culture, prior to the nineteenth century, the female reproductive figure, plump with full breasts, was the erotic ideal.... In 1966, the cultural ideal took a sudden turn to a thin, skeleton image.... The current ideal woman is to be lean, strong, and graceful.... The pressure continues to be on women to control and master their bodies. Self-discipline, compulsive exercising, and continuous dieting are equated with goodness and beauty. (p. 670)

Fontaine stated in her article that "men are less dependent on body size and shape as a primary definition of masculinity" (p. 669). However, men are increasingly affected by cultural pressures to look "good."

What do you think? Reflect back on Sarah's and Glen's journal entries at the beginning of the chapter. Do they contain any clues that body image is an issue with either student? Do you feel that Sarah is influenced by cultural pressures? Does it sound as if Glen is experiencing the same pressures, or does he seem to value different physical characteristics?

The Four "Body Spaces"

Each physical self demands its own personal *body space,* which is the amount of distance with which most people are comfortable in different social settings. According to Hall (cited in Dugas, 1983), body space is also much affected by culture. Four body spaces have been identified in the literature: intimate distance is considered to be 3 to 18 inches; personal distance is 18 inches to 4 feet; social distance is 4 to 12 feet; and public distance is more than 10 to 12 feet (Figure 8–3).

Each of us has a personal preference related to how close another person is allowed to be to us without our experiencing discomfort. The nurse spends a considerable amount of time performing nursing skills within the intimate or personal space of another. It is imperative that nurses be aware of their personal reactions when entering another's space and, in turn, that they attempt to identify the subjective experiences of those whose space is entered.

What do you think? Would Ray and Glen experience the same level of comfort while interacting within the intimate space range? What do you think might happen if Glen put his arm across Ray's shoulders? How about Sarah and Mary Ann? Can you visualize the discomfort and anxiety that might be generated between these students and patients as a blood pressure is obtained or a physical assessment is performed?

Developmental Stages and Body Consciousness

Body consciousness seems to be heightened during specific stages of development and during specific events. The toddler is conscious of body parts and body products, being protective of what is his or hers. It is well known that body integrity and wholeness are important issues during the toddler and preschool years (Arnold & Boggs, 1999). For instance, when blood must be drawn from a toddler, it is imperative that it be done quickly and that a bandage be placed on the puncture site immediately so that the child does not think he or she will "deflate" or "lose all of the air from inside," as one toddler described it.

Adolescence is another developmental stage during which body image is of utmost concern. Adolescents undergo dramatic changes as they move toward physical maturity. An increase in height and weight, secondary sexual characteristics, acne, growing pains, and production of new body fluids are incredible changes that occur within a short time.

It has been stated that adolescent girls report high levels of anxiety, insecurity, and self-consciousness about their bodies as they struggle with their developing identity. Much more so than boys, adolescent girls' positive or negative self-esteem is directly related to satisfaction or dissatisfaction with their physical appearance. (Fontaine, 1991, pp. 669–670)

Is it any wonder that anorexia nervosa and bulimia have become so prevalent?

Aging causes heightened body awareness when we see the beginning of facial wrinkles, thinning or graying of hair, and the spontaneous eruption of liver spots. Millions of dollars are spent attempting to make it all go away when the truth is that it won't go away. We may be able to postpone the signs of aging, but, as time goes by, the changes are noticed. If we are able to incorporate the changed body image into our conscious acceptance, we can give up the masquerade, stop buying hair dye and wrinkle and thigh cream, and spend our money on things that can add *zest* to our lives as we age.

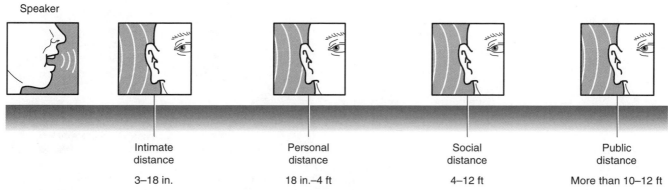

Speaker

Intimate distance
3–18 in.

Personal distance
18 in.–4 ft

Social distance
4–12 ft

Public distance
More than 10–12 ft

Figure 8–3
The four body spaces.

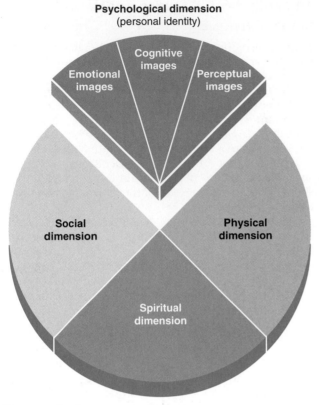

Psychological dimension
(personal identity)

Cognitive images

Emotional images

Perceptual images

Social dimension

Physical dimension

Spiritual dimension

Figure 8–4
The three components of our psychological dimension, or personal identity.

As can be seen, many changes take place during the normal course of development that affect body image and, ultimately, self-concept. Think about the anxieties that develop concerning body integrity, body function, and body image with the onset of illness, the need for surgery, or a sudden, traumatic injury. Even medications can cause alterations in the physical self that disrupt the body image. Psychotropic drugs used to treat psychiatric illness often cause physical changes as well as altered subjective sensations. Fluid retention, weight gain, posture and gait changes, and physical rigidity are side effects that often accompany psychotropic drugs. These side effects are so disturbing that some patients will discontinue their medication once their thinking clears. They often find themselves in a Catch-22 predicament: "What is worse, my real body and the illness, or relief from the illness and awful changes to my body?"

What do you think? What is your body image? What factors have contributed to it? How does your body image impact on your relationships?

➤ *Check Your Reading*
11. Define body image.
12. Define body space and identify the four body spaces.
13. Describe the importance of identifying and understanding feelings associated with the perfor-

mance of nursing skills in a patient's intimate space.
14. Cite one influence that culture has on the physical self.
15. Give two examples of developmental processes that affect the physical self.

Psychological Self

Personal identity is composed of perceptual, cognitive, and emotional images that we have of ourselves. Figure 8–4 illustrates the components of personal identity. Taken together, these images form a unified sense of who we are. This aspect of the self is viewed as the internal regulator of all self functions. It has both a *conscious realm,* that of which we are aware, and an *unconscious realm,* the mental data of which we are unaware. Our perceptual, cognitive, and emotional processes interpret all data received by the senses. Each of these processes is examined.

Perceptual Processes

Perception is the experience of sensing, interpreting, and comprehending the world in which we live. *Perception* is basically how we make sense of what we experience. Two people can interpret the same event in entirely different ways. The old adage of whether a person sees the glass as half full or half empty is an example of how one event can be interpreted in two different ways (Figure 8–5).

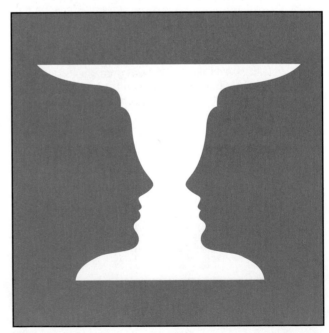

Figure 8–5
"Is the glass half empty or half full?" The answer depends on your perceptions. Likewise, whether you see two faces or a vase in this figure depends on your perception. (From the Westinghouse Learning Corporation Self-Instructional Unit 12. Perception, 1970.)

In our initial stories, both Ray and Sarah came from families in which alcoholism was a problem. We can be assured that the alcoholism affected both of them, but we can be just as sure that they possess unique perceptions of how it affected each of their lives.

How we perceive situations influences how we think and feel about ourselves, others, and the world that we inhabit. We each have an inner world, which consists of how we perceive reality. The external world is also present, where reality objectively exists. Our inner reality may be consistent with the external reality or it may be different. When the inner reality is close to the external reality, the person is said to be "grounded in reality" or "reality oriented." When these realities are at great odds with each other, the person is said to have a "distorted perception of reality." A distorted perception of reality may occur in a limited area of the person's life, and, as such, the impact also may be limited. Or the distortion can affect all aspects of thinking and behavior, as noted in hallucinations and delusions. A person is said to have a mental illness when he or she loses a sense of reality and no longer interacts with the real, objective world.

Development of Perceptual Processes. The earliest roots of our self-perception develop in our relationship with our parents and continue to be modified and formed by relationships and experiences with others. The infant incorporates an awareness of similarities and differences between the parents and also an awareness of their reactions to his or her behavior. Parents who show delight in their infant are laying the groundwork for a healthy self-identity in their child. On the other hand, parents who are stressed and unable to focus on the child's behavior communicate different messages to the developing self of their child. These earliest parental experiences cannot be overly emphasized. Infants who experience a broad and positive array of interpersonal experiences with their parents are better equipped to develop a broad array of interpersonal skills and self-understandings. This foundation translates into a strong sense of self-worth as well as openness to others.

Refer back to the patient and student stories. Both Ray and Mary Ann experienced significant emotional problems. Ray's earliest experiences taught him that he was different and didn't fit in, whereas Mary Ann learned that she was special, and she was able to view her illness as a biological problem rather than a personal deficiency in her self-identity. As a child, Sarah missed her father's affirmation but used that experience to become a responsible doer in her family. Glen, fortunate in his parent's approval and support, developed into a champion listener.

> **W**hat do you think? How have your experiences with your parents influenced who you are today?

The perceptual dimension of self is not fixed or static and continues to develop and increase in complexity. As the child's world expands to include experiences with siblings, friends, adults, and teachers, the inner reality of the child grows to include the feedback received from these people. The richer and more varied a child's early experiences, the more developed the perceptual processes. Generally, the child's outward behavior is a direct reflection of self. As a result of continued reinforcement of behavior, the child develops a more consistent view of self, and behavior becomes more predictable.

Individuals who develop healthy perceptual abilities are able to view a situation in broad terms and to contemplate alternative explanations for events. Their inner reality represents a minimum of distortion with the external reality. They are able to evaluate new information and to conclude that former perceptions are no longer valid. They are able to view the effects of their behaviors and to revise attitudes and actions that seem inappropriate. Their behaviors reflect a healthy balance between dependence and independence. They are able to extend themselves to others as well as to reach out for assistance.

Other experiences, such as illness, affect a person's developing perceptual abilities. Either physical, psychological, or spiritual suffering can limit people's abilities to perceive without significant distortions. Developmental changes such as older age can narrow perceptions due to physical and social limitations. Drugs, both prescribed and illicit, can also affect perceptual abilities.

Impact of Perceptual Processes on Self-Concept. In healthy development, the self-concept corresponds closely with confirmed, factual perceptions. In less than healthy development, the self-concept is hemmed in by unresolved conflicts and misinformation. When confronted with new information, the individual is unable to perceive it and integrate it into his or her self-concept without significant distortion. Once these false perceptions are established as "true," they can become self-perpetuating (Bandura, 1977). For example, people who perceive themselves as unintelligent seek out experiences and engage in behaviors that support this perception. This unhealthy process can be seen as a pattern used not only in relatively unimportant ways but also in significant areas of life. For instance, Ray never received affirmation for being a delightful little boy. Instead, he received the message that he was never good enough as a son, brother, or friend because he didn't fit in with others' expectations. He accepted their conclusions and distorted all experiences through his perceptual curtain of disapproval. Successes in other areas of his life were perceived as good luck and were never fully integrated into his self-concept.

In contrast, Mary Ann's self-perception reflected a high-spirited, creative, and fun-loving child. Parents, siblings, friends, and teachers validated this perception. When she became ill, she was able to view her illness as a part of herself, but certainly not all of who she was. She was able to maintain her initial positive self-image.

This does not mean that perceptual processes cannot change and that the self-concept is destined to remain the same. Fortunately, distorted perceptual processes, although resistant to change, can be corrected through healthy interpersonal relationships. For example, when a nurse and patient each share their perceptions of a given situation, discrepancies can be explored in a nonjudgmental dialogue. This process allows the patient to validate his or her perceptions with the nurse's perceptions or to challenge, analyze, and explore the misperceptions.

What do you think? Can you think of any self-perceptions that reflect distortions? Can you think of any personal events that have greatly influenced your current self-perceptions? Write down your thoughts.

➤ *Check Your Reading*

16. Define personal identity.
17. What is perception?
18. How do our perceptual processes develop?
19. In what way does perception relate to the self-concept?
20. What does it mean that someone is reality oriented?

Cognitive Processes

Thinking is an active and creative mental process stimulated by internal and external conscious data. The process involves three steps:

1. Creating mental images from perceived data
2. Drawing conclusions about these images and the meanings they hold for us
3. Organizing these images into thoughts that are useable and retrievable

One of our uniquely human capacities is that we can think about our own thinking and reflect on and evaluate the effectiveness of this process.

Some aspects of our cognitive abilities are physiologically dependent on our genetic inheritance and on our unique neurological functioning. However, the process of cognition is most commonly viewed as belonging to the psyche. The cognitive self includes not only the innate intelligence of the individual but also a constellation of all past remembered events, educational experiences, and thinking style. The self-concept of a healthy individual is reflected in clear, logical, and rational thinking. Conversely, disease, trauma, and drugs can significantly impair cognitive processes by interfering with brain function.

Development of Cognitive Processes. Although many learning theorists have attempted to explain the development of cognitive processes, Jean Piaget (1952, 1970) offered the most comprehensive developmental explanation. Piaget defined intelligence as a dynamic trait that is always related to an individual's adaptation to the environment under the existing circumstances (Hergenhahn, 1982). Piaget identified four stages of cognitive development:

1. Sensorimotor stage
2. Preoperational thinking stage
3. Concrete operations stage
4. Formal operations stage

The stages are characterized by a progression from simple to complex and from concrete to abstract thinking. Table 8-1 provides the characteristics of each stage.

Influences on Cognitive Processes. Because cognitive processes derive from both physiological and psychological structures, alteration in either can have an effect on cognitive functioning. Mary Ann's manic episodes were directly related to changes in her brain physiology. These changes dramatically inhibited her ability to reason logically and to act rationally. Similar changes in cognitive functioning can result from hypoglycemia, pain, hormonal changes, and particular drugs. Likewise, strong emotions and psychological stress can result in a temporary diminution of cognitive abilities. Sensory deprivation, such as that which occurs in intensive care units, also can result in impaired cognitions and therefore altered thought processes with resultant misperceptions.

Evaluative Aspect of Cognitive Processes. Bandura (1977) defined an aspect of cognition that allows us to evaluate what we can do. He called this quality **self-efficacy,** which he defined as our ability to perform specific tasks based on what we know. Our perceived self-efficacy may or may not correspond to reality. That is, we may believe we are more or less capable than the facts of our actual performance indicate. Take the story of Ray, who believed he was a failure as a son and brother. Yet, to an objective outsider, Ray might appear to be exemplary in both areas because of his responsible behavior.

What do you think? How would you describe your self-efficacy? How did Sarah and Glen

T A B L E 8 – 1 The Stages of Cognitive Development According to Piaget	
STAGE	**CHARACTERISTICS**
Sensorimotor (0–2 y)	Development proceeds from activity to imagining and solving problems through the senses and movement.
Preoperational (2–7 y)	The child moves from knowing the world through sensation and movement to prelogical thinking and finding solutions to problems.
Concrete operational (7–11 y)	The child moves from prelogical thought to solving concrete problems through logic.
Formal operation (11 y–adulthood)	Logical thinking is expanded to include solving abstract and concrete problems.

Data from Piaget, J. (1952). *The origin of intelligence in children.* New York: International Universities Press.

describe their own self-efficacy as they were beginning their psychiatric nursing experience?

> ➤ *Check Your Reading*
> 21. How is intelligence defined by Piaget?
> 22. What are the stages of cognitive development according to Piaget?
> 23. What are two influences on the cognitive process?
> 24. Define self-efficacy and perceived self-efficacy.
> 25. Where else might the nurse find patients who are experiencing impaired thought processes?

Emotional Processes

The *emotional* or *affective self* consists of the spontaneous feelings that we experience in response to life. These reactions provide the "icing on the cake" and the "spice of life." Without feelings, we would go through the motions of living in a gray, dull mist without experiencing the emotional peaks and troughs that color all that we do. On the positive side, we would experience no sadness over loss, but conversely, we would have no joy over gain. Life would be flat.

Feelings are spontaneous. We cannot control how we feel about a certain event, but we can control how we express those feelings. Much of the work of nurses is to encourage patients to become aware of their feelings, to discover the meanings behind their feelings, and to make active choices about how they will respond. "Being in touch with our feelings is the only way we can ever become our highest self, the only way we can become open and free, and the only way we can become our own person" (Viscott, 1976, p. 22).

Incorporated into the emotional aspect of self-concept is self-esteem. As stated previously, *self-esteem* is the measure of how a person feels about what is seen and known about the self. According to Sanford and Donovan (1984), there are two categories of self-esteem: global self-esteem and specific self-esteem. "Global self-esteem is the measure of how much we like and approve of our perceived self as a whole. Specific self-esteem is the measure of how much we like and approve of a certain part of ourselves" (p. 9).

W*hat do you think?* As you review Glen's journal, how does he rate his abilities as a listener? What does that say about his specific self-esteem? What about his specific self-esteem regarding his abilities to complete task-oriented activities? How would you rate his overall global self-esteem? What about Sarah? What does she tell us about her specific and global self-esteem?

Two other concepts are related to self-esteem (emphasis added).

*One is **self-confidence**, the feeling that one is a competent person with the ability to accomplish things. The other is **self-respect**, the feeling that what one is doing or has done is right according to the value system held. (Dugas, 1983, p. 662)*

Virginia Satire, a noted author and a family therapist during the 1970s, has successfully taken the abstract concept of self-esteem and solidified it into concrete terms to enhance understanding through visualization. Satire pictured the self-esteem of each of us as a "huge, black iron pot which stood on three legs." As she worked with families, she was able to get them to describe their level of self-esteem by referring to "low pot" or "high pot." As she stated in her book *Peoplemaking,*

[A] female family member may say, "My pot is high today," and all would know that she felt on top of things, full of energy and good spirits, and secure in the knowledge that she really mattered. Another family member might say, "I feel low pot," which meant that she felt tired, bored, or bruised, not particularly lovable. (1972, p. 21)

Satire went on to explain that "the crucial factor in what happens both inside people and between people is the picture of individual worth that each person carries around with him or her—their pot" (p. 21).

Sanford and Donovan (1984) identified necessary requirements for the development of a solid foundation of self-esteem. Their research pointed out that in our early years, we need to acquire the following five traits to ensure positive feelings about the self:

1. *Sense of significance:* "I count in this world."
2. *Sense of competence:* "I can do it."
3. *Sense of connectedness to others balanced by a sense of separateness from them:* "I can disagree with a loved one and still know we are connected."
4. *Sense of realism about ourselves and the world:* "I have a good sense of what my capabilities and weaknesses are."
5. *Coherent set of ethics and values:* "I have a set of standards that influences my behavior and from which I evaluate the behavior of others."

However, as important as it is to develop these requirements early in life, self-esteem continues to develop over a lifetime. This allows us to make up for some of the early deficiencies.

Self-esteem affects everything that we do in life. Positive self-esteem enables us to meet life's demands with a sense of confidence. Negative self-esteem leads us to doubt our abilities to perform; it gives us a sense that we do not have what it takes and never will. Because the development of self-esteem is a lifelong process, if any of the early requirements are lacking, they can be cultivated over time (Husted, Miller, & Wilczyski, 1990; Klose & Tinius, 1992; Mixson, 1989). In fact, we experience times in life when our ideals are in question or in transition, and our self-esteem plummets or is shaky as a result. At other times, we may face challenges that demand a reevaluation of who we are and who we want to become. Self-esteem fluctuates during these times as the self-concept becomes less than clear. These opportunities for growth have potentially positive outcomes, but the process can be quite painful and disorganizing. Again, let's look at what Sanford and Donovan (1984) said:

Some women have low self-esteem because of something we call self-concept dislocation—which occurs when a major event in a person's life forces her to change the way she looks at and thinks about herself, sometimes radically. A woman who has recently had a mastectomy or gotten divorced will probably go through self-concept disloca-tion—it is not only triggered by unhappy experiences. Anytime a woman makes a major change in her life—whether by getting married, going back to school, having a baby, or changing jobs—her concept of herself will be forced to change, and she may have difficulty adjusting to the new image she has of herself. (p. 17)

Men, too, must face similar periods (i.e., retirement, birth of first child, death of wife, divorce, and job change, to name a few) during their development when they must adjust their self-concept and therefore experience fluctuating self-esteem. Box 8–3 contrasts people with high and low self-esteem.

What do you think? Can you think of times in your life when your self-esteem was very high? Very low? What was happening during those situations in which your self-esteem fluctuated? Can you think of areas in which your specific self-esteem is high? Low? What about your global self-esteem? How does your self-esteem impact on your perfor-mance as a nursing student?

➤ *Check Your Reading*
26. What is the difference between global and specific self-esteem?
27. Define self-confidence and self-respect.
28. What traits are necessary for the development of self-esteem?

29. What is the emotional self?
30. What is the effect of positive self-esteem on behavior, thinking, and goals?

Social Self

One aspect of self is defined by the roles that we assume. This dimension of self, the social or public self, represents the ways that we are known by others (Baumeester, 1986). Some of these roles are gender related, such as male, female, daughter, son, mother, father, lover, or spouse. A **role** is defined as a socially expected behavior pattern associated with an individu-al's function—such as student, friend, parent, or boss—in various social groups, and is greatly affected by the culture in which we are raised.

Family Role

Usually, our first social group is that of our *nuclear family*—or family of origin.

Coming into a family is much like walking in on a party that has been going full blast for some time. There is no guarantee that we will be welcomed, that we will "fit in" with what is already going on, or that we will even understand what is going on. (Sanford & Donovan, 1984)

What is fairly certain, however, is that preformed expectations exist of where and how we fit in.

Each role carries different expectations. Family roles always mean pairs, as you cannot take the role of a wife without a husband, or father without a son or daughter. Beliefs about what each role means can differ. It is

Box 8–3 ■ ■ ■ ■ ■
Characteristics of People With High Versus Low Self-Esteem

High Self-Esteem	**Low Self-Esteem**
• Expect people to value them	• Expect people to be critical of them
• Are active self-agents	• Are passive or obstructive self-agents
• Have positive perceptions of their skills, appear-ance, sexuality, and behaviors	• Have negative perceptions of their skills, appear-ance, sexuality, and behaviors
• Perform equally well when being observed as when not watched	• Perform less well when being observed
• Are nondefensive and assertive in response to criticism	• Are defensive and passive in response to criticism
• Can accept compliments easily	• Have difficulty accepting compliments
• Evaluate their performance realistically	• Have unrealistic expectations about their perfor-mance
• Are relatively comfortable relating to authority figures	• Are uncomfortable relating to authority figures
• Express general satisfaction with life	• Are dissatisfied with their lot in life
• Have a strong social support system	• Have a weak social support system
• Have a primary internal locus of control	• Rely on an external locus of control

From Arnold, E., & Boggs, K. (1999). *Interpersonal relationships: Professional communication skills for nurses* (3rd ed.). Philadelphia: W. B. Saunders.

important for each family member to find out the expected behavior that correlates with each role within the family system (Satire, 1972).

Each of us fills roles that are *ascribed,* such as family position or gender, and roles that we *assume* or choose. Toman (1969) studied the importance of **birth order,** or **sibling position,** within the family of origin and its implication for relationships outside the family system. For example, being the youngest sister of brothers would allow the female child to have vast experience with older brothers but no real day-to-day living experience with older sisters or younger siblings. As a result, it could be hypothesized that as an adult, she would tend to feel most comfortable when interacting with older men, like her brothers, but less comfortable when dealing with women.

> **What do you think?** Glen is the youngest brother of two older sisters. Would this give him an advantage over Sarah in working with Mary Ann? Based on birth order experience, how do you think Sarah could relate to Ray? Look at your own family. How has your own birth order influenced your relationships?

How can three children in the same family and from the same biological parents be different in talents, abilities, behaviors, and total personalities? This is a question frequently asked. However, if one looks at what is going on within the family during the birth of each child, one can see some obvious answers. The parents are different ages as each child enters the family. The demands are different with the addition of each child. The challenge of integrating a new family member is different each time another sibling arrives. In some ways, each child who enters a family has a different set of parents.

How about the element of individual recognition that is consciously or unconsciously considered by each sibling: "What must I do differently than my brothers and sisters to be recognized?" The development of each child's unique set of behavioral traits is an interesting phenomenon to observe. For example, one child may come forth as the intellectual giant, one child may have no time for intellectual pursuits but may devote timeless energies to the athletic role, and the third child may travel in the direction of the artistic one. It is almost as though each child knows there is a unique place that must be found where individual abilities will be praised.

Gender Role

Gender identification is another factor that must be considered when examining roles. "**Gender identity,** or sex role, is the expectation of appropriate male and female behavior found in the attitudes and beliefs of a particular society" (Strassen, 1992, p. 3) (emphasis added). Traditional socialization of women has involved teaching them to focus on listening, nurturing, affiliating, and being sensitive to the needs of others. The sex role socialization for men has traditionally emphasized competition, aggressiveness, leadership, power, and task completion (Strassen, 1992).

In recent years, a considerable effort to move away from the traditional values and move toward gender equality is an obvious trend with a desired outcome for society as well as each individual. Traits would not be ascribed to one gender or the other but rather be considered universal. The "masculine take charge attitude" could be adopted by both men and women during situations in which aggressiveness and power are needed, and the "feminine characteristics" could come to the forefront in both sexes during situations that call for care, concern, and a more humanistic approach. In *Passages,* Sheehy (1974) said that this blending of characteristics normally takes place after the midlife crisis. The ideal, however, would be that this dual nature could be expressed earlier in our lives.

Since the women's liberation movement began in the 1960s, women have experienced a devaluation of their roles as wives and mothers. Many women have moved into the work force and now juggle many roles, trying to fulfill them all. Consequently, it is not uncommon for women to feel enormous pressure and **role conflict** when they cannot resolve the compelling demands on their time. Role conflict may occur at any time when multiple demands place women in situations in which they have to choose one role function to the detriment of another.

Men also have experienced tremendous role confusion since the demand for equality between the sexes has emerged. Behaviors that were once discouraged are now expected, such as showing gentleness, expressing tenderness, sharing feelings, and exhibiting domestic talents, while males are expected to maintain the "masculine characteristics," especially in the work setting. Much work still remains to be done in the area of blending female and male characteristics.

Other Roles

Glen clearly stated in his journal entry that he experienced role conflict when he was faced with talking with his patients and tending to their emotional needs or pleasing his instructor and staff members with task-oriented patient care duties. Glen knew that both were important but that others could perform the tasks, and few individuals might respond to the human side of the patient care situation. For Sarah, her previously held family role of doer influenced how she thought she could present to her patients in the psychiatric setting. Sarah needs to learn how to sit and listen to stories rather than do for her patients.

There are roles that we assume throughout life, some more willingly than others. Many people choose the roles of spouse and parent, whereas others choose the single life without children but meet their affiliative or parental needs in aunt, uncle, mentor, or teacher roles.

Oftentimes, people find that the circumstances of their life force them to assume roles that they really do not like and would not choose.

Reflect on Ray's story. In his family, the expectations of him as the oldest son were rigid. He was expected to carry out the functions that had been abdicated by his parents. He shouldered responsibilities that far exceeded his emotional maturity.

The child in this condition usually ends up with all the responsibilities and none of the privileges of the new role. To take on a new role, he leaves his real role behind, and this becomes a very lonely and unsure place to be. (Satire, 1972, p. 167)

In other families in which roles are more fluid, a child might be expected to do extra work to help out if a parent were ill, but this would clearly be a temporary situation. Other roles that people find themselves in that are not of their choosing are widow, single parent, divorcée, victim of violence, and psychiatric patient. No matter what the role, stereotypical expectations and stigma will be involved (Herd, 1994). As one patient wrote:

*We are human
Just as you
We like the same
Things you enjoy to do
Don't dismiss us
By turning up your nose
Your eyes may be open
But the mind is closed
Don't speak to us as though
We are unaware
If you let us respond
You'll find we are
Very much there
Mental illness is
Illness of the mind
Which is no excuse
To treat us unkind
Because one day
You may wake up
With thoughts unclear
Like us. You'll want
Someone to care*

—*Valerie Gough*

Some roles must be earned, such as those that accompany education and formal certification. Registered nurses, physicians, physical therapists, and occupational therapists must complete extensive academic and clinical education before sitting for licensure. Social workers, ministers, and counselors must complete an internship before actual practice to cultivate the skills necessary to fulfill their roles.

Roles carry with them expectations, prescribed functions, and boundaries. Sometimes the expectations, functions, and boundaries are flexible; other times they are rigid. On the one hand, some parents identify what they want their child's occupation or profession to be before he or she is born. The child has little to say about the direction of his or her life. He or she just lives out the script that is written. On the other hand, some parents provide their child with many opportunities to examine vocational opportunities and support the child's independent choices. Judith Viorst (1986), in her book *Necessary Losses,* stated:

[S]tudies show that children know exactly which role the parent unconsciously assigns to them. . . . Perhaps we can measure a family's health by the freedom it gives us not to accept the assignments. (p. 253)

A common nursing diagnosis for people assigned to uncomfortable or inappropriate roles is Personal Identity Disturbance. Related diagnoses are as follows:

1. Altered family processes
2. Altered parenting
3. Anticipatory grieving
4. Decisional conflict
5. Dysfunctional grieving
6. Hopelessness
7. Ineffective individual coping
8. Parental role conflict
9. Powerlessness
10. Situational low self-esteem
11. Sleep pattern disturbance

Box 8–4 lists questions that you might ask a patient in an assessment interview centered on role relationships.

Box 8–4 ■ ■ ■ ■ ■
Questions to Ask in an Assessment Interview Centered on Role Relationships

Family
- Can you tell me something about your family?
- How would you describe your family unit (e.g., age, sex, health status of members)?
- Who assumes responsibility for decision-making?
- What changes do you anticipate as a result of your illness (condition) in the way you function in your family?
- Who do you see in your family as being most affected by your illness (condition)?
- Who do you see in your family as being supportive of you?

Work
- Can you tell me something about the work you do?
- In general, how would you describe your satisfaction with your work?
- Can you tell me something about how you get along with others on your job?
- What are some of the concerns you have about your job at this time?

Social
- How do you like other people to treat you?
- To whom do you turn for support?
- If _____ is not available to you, who else might provide social support for you?

From Arnold, E., & Boggs, K. (1999). *Interpersonal relationships: Professional communication skills for nurses* (3rd ed.). Philadelphia: W. B. Saunders.

What do you think? As you reflect on your own family life, examine how roles were assigned. What roles did you assume? What roles were prescribed for you? Were roles fluid or fixed? How have those early role experiences influenced you today?

➤ *Check Your Reading*
31. Define role.
32. What is role conflict?
33. Of what importance is sibling position?
34. What is gender identity?
35. Give an example of an ascribed role. An assumed role.

Spiritual Self

The spiritual self functions to help the individual connect with God, find meaning, and make sense from life's circumstances. Within the spiritual self reside beliefs about the universe and our place in it and feelings of transcendence, joy, hopefulness, and love. The spiritual self is expressed through behaviors of selflessness, commitment, moral decisions, choice, self-discipline, and honesty and reverence for God, a higher power, or however this transcendent being is defined by the person. The spiritual self allows the individual to interpret events from a broader perspective than self, taking in the big picture and allowing transcendence of the bonds of ego and personal desires. The spiritual self that strives for meaning seems to be a universal phenomenon, regardless of religious beliefs or convictions.

Spiritual Self and World View

The aspect of spirituality that allows for **God-consciousness** varies across different world views. From a Judeo-Christian world view, spirituality is shaped by the belief in a personal God who is involved in the daily activities of His children. Such a belief might be expressed in behaviors of service, prayer, and stewardship, which are interpreted as God's will. Conversely, spirituality from an Eastern world perspective is shaped by a belief in an impersonal energy or life force that permeates the universe. This type of spirituality might be expressed in meditation, mystical experiences, and striving for peace, harmony, and a disappearance of self. For others, spirituality might be shaped by a belief that people control their own destiny. Such a spirituality might be expressed in humanistic values.

Spiritual Self and Morality

The spiritual self is also the seat of morality. This aspect of the self is thought to develop out of the earliest interaction between the child and parents and significant others. Initially, a child feels that any behavior that makes her or him feel good must be good, and if it produces discomfort or sadness, it is bad. The child's main concern is her or his own pleasure. This state of affairs is short lived. To fit into society, the child needs to learn which behaviors are acceptable and which are not. The parents have the task of defining what is good behavior and what is not. Regardless of whether parents do this consciously or unconsciously, directly or indirectly, they begin the process of shaping the child's behaviors by giving affection for behaviors that are pleasing and withholding affection when the child's behavior is displeasing to them. Over time, the child learns that what is good pleases her or his parents, and what is bad displeases them. These early learnings provide not only the basis for personal integrity but also a structure for wrestling with moral dilemmas.

Development of the Spiritual Self

Although spiritual development has some parallels with psychosocial development, the milestones are not as clear-cut or predictable. In fact, it is not unusual for an individual to be spiritually unaware and suddenly experience a spiritual event that transforms his or her life. But generally speaking, a level of cognitive development and emotional maturity are requisite for dealing with the tough questions that accompany spiritual growth. According to Carson (1998, p. 1076), questions such as the following may be asked:

"Is there something beyond me that gives order to the universe?"
"Where do I stand in relationship to God?"
"Does my life have a purpose? If so, what is it? Is it discernible?"
"Is my purpose in life related to God?"
"Are there ethical principles that go beyond my immediate concerns that should guide my actions?"
"Is there something beyond death? If so, what?"
"What is the meaning of suffering?"

Spiritual Distress

Sometimes the distress that we see in people is misdiagnosed as psychological when it more correctly stems from a spiritual crisis of loss of faith or meaning. The road to spiritual maturity is certainly not an easy one; the answers to the questions are not readily available. Individual faith traditions hold out resources for truth. For the Christian, the scriptures are seen as God's word. For the Jew, the Torah is studied by scholars for understanding of God's word. For the Muslim, truth is found in the Koran. Much of spirituality resides in faith, which by definition is a belief in that which we cannot see. Ultimately, the spiritual aspect of the self views life as a mystery to be lived and not a problem to be solved (Carson, 1998).

The presence of a spiritual self allows the individual to transcend immediate circumstances with the realization that a truth exists that is larger than, but encompasses, self and serves to illuminate and give meaning to individual experiences. Spiritually developed people are less self-involved and more focused on meeting the needs of others through acts of kindness, charity, and service (Carson, 1998).

Mary Ann interpreted her illness as a "burden and a gift." This interpretation allowed her to view her illness as having a significance beyond her suffering. She saw in her illness possibilities that transcended her psychic pain and lack of control and moved her into the realm of creativity and artistic expression. Ray, on the other hand, was so tied to seeking approval that he was unable to view not receiving the promotion as anything but failure. Only through therapy did he allow his spiritual self free reign to begin to ask such questions as "What does this mean for my life?" and "Is there something more that I should be taking from this event other than my feelings of despair?"

What do you think? How does your spiritual self get expressed? How does your spiritual self influence your nursing? How does your spiritual self influence relationships?

➤ *Check Your Reading*

36. Define the spiritual self.
37. What is the universal aspect of the spiritual self?
38. In what way does a world view affect the spiritual self?
39. How does morality develop within the spiritual self?
40. What role does cognitive development serve in the growth of the spiritual self?

JOURNEY TOWARD MENTAL HEALTH OR MENTAL ILLNESS

All individuals have the same basic needs that require satisfaction for physiological and psychological homeostasis to be maintained. As we saw in Chapter 6, Maslow (1970) pointed out these requirements in his **hierarchy of basic needs.** According to Maslow, each of us must meet basic needs before we are able to meet needs at a higher level of development. In Maslow's hierarchy of needs, physiological needs are the most basic and include requirements for food, water, and air. Safety needs come next, and they pertain to our requirement for a secure physical environment. Love and belonging needs include the desire for relationships and connectedness with other people. Esteem needs refer to the desire to be recognized as worthwhile and valuable, and self-actualization needs include the desire for self-fulfillment as individuals realize their potential (Box 8–5; see also Figure 6–1).

In addition to the commonality of needs, we believe that individuals must systematically pass through specific physical and psychological developmental levels for maturation to occur. Erikson (1963) identified the *eight stages of man* that represent the developmental challenges faced by all (Table 8–2; see also Table 6–3).

A reciprocal relationship seems to exist between basic needs and **developmental tasks.** Basic needs must be met, to a certain degree, for a person to deal

---

Box 8–5 ■ ■ ■ ■ ■
Characteristics of a Self-Actualized Person

- A quality of genuineness
- A passion for living
- Ability to get along well with others
- A strong sense of personal worth
- A view of life situations as an opportunity, not a threat
- Ability to experience each moment fully
- Moments of intense emotional meaning, "peak experience"
- Full acceptance of self and others
- Identification with fellow human beings
- High sense of responsibility with a strong desire to serve humanity
- Integrity of purpose

From Arnold, E., & Boggs, K. (1999). *Interpersonal relationships: Professional communication skills for nurses* (3rd ed.). Philadelphia: W. B. Saunders.

---

with developmental tasks, and the developmental tasks must be dealt with and somewhat mastered for the basic needs to be met. If there is a deficiency in one area, there may be a deficiency in the other (Figure 8–6).

Look at the issue of trust. If an infant's basic physiological needs are met, trust can develop. If the basic needs are not met in a timely fashion, trust will not develop as solidly as hoped. On the other hand, the child needs to interact with caregivers or basic needs may not be met positively.

Add to these stresses the normal life situations and life crises that confront us at various times plus biological factors, family position, environment, and cultural influences, and it can be seen that innumerable stimuli can cause a threat to self. With the challenges presented within the developmental levels, stress is evident, and anxiety is generated.

On the one hand, if successful coping strategies are developed to reduce the anxiety, the stress will be decreased, and the individual will gain new ways of coping and interacting with the world. Adaptation will have taken place, and the individual, in time, will be successfully prepared to move on to the next developmental level and its inherent tasks.

On the other hand, if the individual cannot successfully maneuver and accomplish the developmental tasks or if basic needs are either not met at all or inadequately met, anxiety increases, along with the use of exaggerated coping mechanisms. The individual becomes less able to perceive objective reality and accomplish the task at hand. Disequilibrium ensues, resulting in maladaptive behavior (Figure 8–7).

If a person does not accomplish a major developmental task, he or she cannot successfully move on to the next challenge or phase without experiencing some degree of intrapsychic conflict. The individual may be able to go forward physically and intellectually, but

TABLE 8 – 2 Erikson's Eight Stages of Man

AGE	STAGE	PRIMARY PERSON ORIENTATION	STRENGTHS	QUALITIES
0–2 y	Trust vs. mistrust	Mother	Hope	To receive, to give
2–4 y	Autonomy vs. shame or doubt	Father	Will power	To control, to let go
4–6 y	Initiative vs. guilt	Basic family	Purpose	To make, to play act
6–12 y	Industry vs. inferiority	Neighborhood, school	Competence	To make things, to put things together
13–19 y	Identity vs. identity diffusion	Peer groups	Fidelity	To be one's self
Young adult	Intimacy vs. isolation	Partners in marriage, friendship	Love	To share one's self with another
Adult	Generativity vs. self-absorption	Children, community	Care	To take care of, to create
Older adult	Integrity vs. despair	Humankind	Wisdom	To accept being, to accept not being

Adapted from THE LIFE CYCLE COMPLETED: A review by Erik H. Erikson. Copyright © 1982 by Rikan Enterprises, Ltd. Reprinted by permission of W. W. Norton & Company, Inc.

certain aspects of the personality are put on emotional hold; further emotional development is arrested at a level short of maturity. The discomfort that results can range from slight to moderate to total personality disintegra-tion, depending on the level of inadequate problem resolution. The behavior demonstrated by the individual alerts others that difficulties are present and that specific needs have not been met.

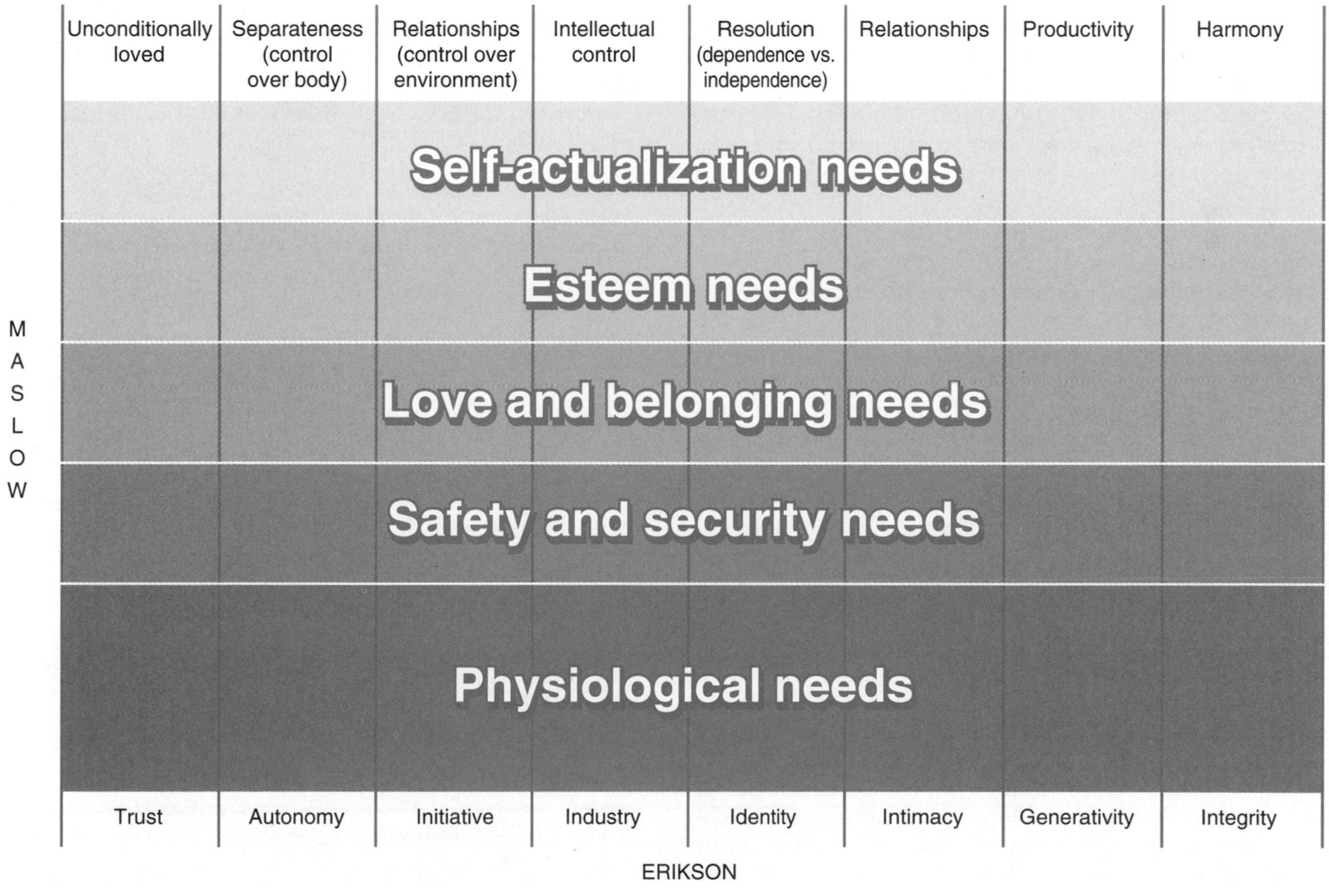

Figure 8 – 6
Relationship between Maslow's hierarchy of needs and Erikson's developmental tasks.

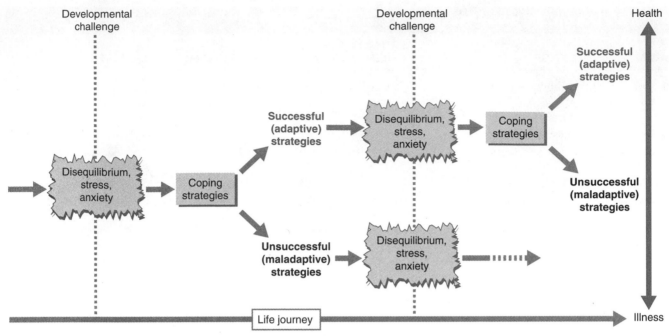

Figure 8–7
Relationship between successful coping and achievement of developmental tasks.

As an individual meets basic needs, makes developmental adjustments, establishes familial and social roles, and faces crisis situations, he or she establishes his or her own unique coping style. The individual who has frustrated needs, inadequate developmental adjustment, and inadequate means of dealing with crises also develops a coping style. As a pattern of coping develops, a characteristic way of relating to the world emerges. Usually, each of us has a mix of coping responses, some of which are growth producing and some of which are not. If a person has too many unhealthy styles, his or her life experiences become limited, and the person's ability to meet his or her needs and cope with stresses may be lessened. This person is said to experience a disturbance in homeostasis as a result of a threat to self and an alteration in the perception of reality. His or her view of the world becomes distorted, and the individual may communicate inappropriately and inadequately. The psychic discomfort felt by the individual is demonstrated through various mental health problems, such as adjustment disorders, psychophysiological manifestations, psychotic disorders, or behaviors indicative of sensory deprivation.

However, if the individual is able to cope successfully with the threat to self, homeostasis is restored; the individual's self-concept, coping abilities, and self-esteem are affirmed; and the individual continues the journey, better prepared to deal with the next stressful event. A positive self-concept, essential to mental health, develops from more than success at coping. In fact, a positive self-concept develops from the cumulative effect of positive, growth-enhancing experiences with others in which we are affirmed for who we are. Mentally healthy individuals possess self-concepts that reflect balance among all the dimensions of self. The balance established is unique to each person and

endows the healthy self with a special integration and wholeness not found in anyone else. The totality of the self-concept is more than the sum of its parts and represents a remarkable organized system in which dimensions are integrated and function in a reciprocal fashion.

Robinson (1983) said that mental health can be described as

a dynamic state in which thought, feeling, and behavior, that is age appropriate and congruent with the local and cultural norms, is demonstrated. It is characterized by the use of behaviors that alter stressors and promote problem resolution. (p. 74)

The mentally healthy individual is able to select from among his or her talents, skills, thoughts, and feelings and use these components of self to work toward goal attainment.

Most of us fit somewhere between mental health and mental illness, depending on life challenges and coping abilities. If we look at the health–illness continuum and apply the same continuum to mental health and mental illness, it would look like Figure 8–8.

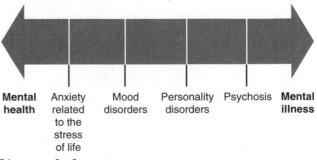

Figure 8–8
The continuum of mental health and mental illness.

The amount of difficulty an individual experiences in coping with daily living and the quality of relationships with self, others, the environment, and God determine where the person falls along the continuum. The placement is based on factors such as the type, number, frequency, and rigidity of the coping maneuvers or defense mechanisms needed to help the individual feel secure; availability of support systems; and innate resiliency.

Refer back to the story of Ray, the patient who was depressed because he was passed over for a job promotion. His self-system was threatened; he felt anxious and unsure of his place in his job. He tried to rationalize that he would receive the next promotion. When this approach failed him, he sought professional assistance to alleviate his depression. When Ray felt depressed, the emotional, perceptual, and cognitive processes of his psychological self were certainly involved. In addition, his physical self suffered from sleeplessness and loss of appetite. His spiritual self questioned his worth and the meaning of his life, and his social self withdrew from interpersonal exchanges. Ray's response to stress was holistic, and Ray's experience highlights this in all aspects of the self.

What do you think? How would you describe your own coping style? Do you think that individuals should be taught coping skills in school? Is it sufficient to trust that life experiences will lead to the development of coping skills?

Personality Development

As the self develops, a personality emerges that reflects an individual's automatic response to the outside world. Personality is composed of all the behavioral traits and attitudinal characteristics by which we are recognized as individuals. Personality reflects an enduring pattern of behavior that is considered to be both conscious and unconscious and reflects a means of adapting to a particular environment and its cultural, ethnic, and community standards.

To examine our personalities, we need to examine the customary ways in which we automatically perceive, think, feel, and react to the world. Sarah and Glen can ask themselves the following questions, which will shed light on their personalities:

"Do I think in concrete or abstract terms?"
"Do I deal with facts and specifics, or do I like to look at the whole picture when facing a situation?"
"Am I an auditory learner, a visual learner, or a doer who reflects on what I experienced in order to learn?"
"Do I rely on my intuition, or do I depend on logical deductions to choose my interaction with the world?"
"Do I like to plan my activities and follow them to the letter, or do I like to leave things open ended, praising myself for the ability to be flexible?"

These are questions that emerge when one looks at personality tendencies:

"How do I primarily relate to the world?"
"Do I get my major satisfactions from working with others or working and thinking alone?"
"Do I feel more fully understood in a group of people, or do I get more satisfaction from spending moments by myself?"

One of the formal investigative methods used to answer these questions is the Myers-Briggs Type Indicator. Drawing from the initial work by Carl Jung (see Chapter 6), a humanistic psychologist who made significant contributions to science and philosophy, Katharine Briggs and Isabel Briggs Myers developed a tool that could "show how we like to look at things and how we like to go about deciding things" (Myers & Myers, 1993, cover page). The Myers-Briggs Type Indicator is used in business and education all over the world to investigate personality preferences. The results can identify whether an individual is primarily an *introvert* or *extrovert;* a *sensor* or an *intuitive person* by nature; a *feeler* or a *thinker* when it comes to making decisions; a *judger* or a *perceiver;* or one who wants things planned and organized or open ended and free floating.

These categories are general but show an individual's preferred, and usually automatic, method of meeting the world. *Preferred* is the key word. The nonpreferred way of approaching the world can be developed within each individual so that a broader view of the world is seen and more breadth is added to an individual's usual way of looking at and dealing with the world. Under stress, the preferred and automatic interactions identified are again called into play. The authors state on the front of their Form G Self-Scorable Myers-Briggs Question Booklet,

[K]nowing your own preferences and learning about other people's can help you understand where your special strengths are, what kinds of work might be enjoyed, and how people with different preferences can relate to each other and be valuable to society. (Myers & Myers, 1993, cover page)

A view in contrast to that offered by the Myers-Briggs Type Indicator is offered by Sire (1990), who suggested that as soon as we label ourselves and each other, we limit our possibilities as human beings. We begin to believe that *we are the label* rather than holding the view that the label describes an aspect of who we are. Sire suggested as an alternative to personality inventories such as the Myers-Briggs that we cultivate self-awareness to understand ourselves and relationship skills to understand others.

Sarah and Glen are facing a new challenge as they prepare to meet their patients. As a result, each will experience some degree of threat to self just because the experience is a new one. The way that each interprets the stress of this new experience will determine which coping mechanisms will be called into play. If they are able to remember past situations in which success was the outcome, they should be able to face the challenge in a positive, growth-producing manner. If the threat becomes overwhelming, defensive behaviors will emerge, and the integration of new behaviors will not be possible. If each has the support of other students and understanding faculty members, they should be able to look at the past self, the present self, and the ideal professional self and learn how to become willing and able to experience others, that is want to enter into another's world and learn skills to enable them to enter into another's world with some confidence.

When they meet their patients, Sarah and Glen will be asked to do what all psychiatric nurses are asked to do: assess their patients, identify problem areas that need to be addressed, and focus on their patients' strengths. The students will be asked to formulate goals and devise interventions that will be dependent on the nature of the problem and the patients' special characteristics and talents.

The most important tool that each student has is himself or herself, as expressed in its own unique way, to therapeutically bring about change in others. The students will learn theories to back up their approaches and techniques for therapeutic communication. They will learn nursing diagnoses that are commonly given to patients with psychiatric disorders, and they will learn some general interventions that can be used to try to establish trust, foster hope, and help patients feel as though they are supported and connected with another person.

In the psychiatric arena, nurses are called on to "use the self" therapeutically. This demands that the nurse know who she or he is personally and that she or he intertwine that personal self with the knowledge and skills required by the specialty to gain experience that will allow the professional self to develop. Becoming an expert is dependent less on time and more on experience and the refinement of "head" knowledge through encounters with many practical situations that add depth, nuances, and shades of difference to theory (Benner, 1984).

Expert nurses grow to the point that their perceptual abilities give direction to the nursing care that is delivered.

The expert nurse often describes her perceptual abilities as "a gut feeling" or "a sense of uneasiness" or "a feeling that things are not quite right." Experts dare not stop with vague hunches, but neither do they dare to ignore those hunches that could lead to early identification of problems and the search for confirming evidence. (Benner, 1984, p. xix)

Thus, the transition from student or novice to expert practitioner requires time, experience, and risk-taking. The nurse must understand that he or she may not have all of the answers in a situation or may not be totally sure of all the right moves. Instead, the nurse must trust in his or her limited theory-based abilities and be willing to share his or her humanness to facilitate connectedness with others.

Psychiatric nurses learn to trust that patients often know what is needed to remedy a situation. Furthermore, if patients are given the opportunity to put forth their story, they are frequently able to articulate the problem to the point at which options become evident. For the nurse, the key to this process is to allow herself or himself the opportunity to be "present" to the patient, even when the answers are not apparent.

If students have the privilege of working with an expert nurse in the field of psychiatric nursing, they will be able to see where they are traveling as they journey toward the development of a professional image. One such expert nurse is Diane, whose story appears here. Once a student-novice, Diane is now a seasoned psychiatric nurse with many years of experience with different types of patients. Her journey illustrates how an expert nurse sees her role and her professional responsibilities and how her professional self merges with her personal self. It is actually difficult to identify where Diane's personal self stops and her professional self begins because they have intertwined to form one being—one self.

Diane's Story

Someone asked me an interesting question the other day. The question was, "Why did you choose psychiatric nursing as your specialty?" As I reflected back on my career, I found that I was drawn to the human side of every patient care situation within which I became involved.

When I worked on a medical unit, I was touched by the loneliness and anxiety experienced by patients and their families as they faced the crises of hospitalization and physical illness.

As I used highly technical skills in the trauma center to treat patients surrounded by machines, tubes, and monitors with limited family contact, I realized the patients needed someone to help them understand the meaning of their experiences, regardless of their level of consciousness or their abilities to interact.

As I came in contact with individuals experiencing psychiatric difficulties, I realized that, just like the trauma patient surrounded by machines that interfered with human interaction, the psychiatric patient was armed with behaviors that kept others at a distance, therefore accentuating loneliness rather than allowing the interactions that would reinforce his or her humanness.

I learned in school that we are all more alike than different. I knew that if I could understand the limits, losses, and changes experienced by individuals and their families and if could break through the loneliness experienced, then, hopefully, I could provide an opportunity for connectedness and could help others realize that they could gain control over their situations.

Everything that I do now focuses on listening to stories about the human condition and about what patients long for and attempting to involve them in activities whereby they can realize their strengths as well as their problems. They can also learn how to relate to others so that they can gain control over their lives.

> The core of mental illness, it seems to me, is loneliness and powerlessness. I feel that if I can help others relate in some way to the world around them, then I have intervened successfully. ∎

Diane seems to know that the nurse is a person, not just that the person is a nurse. Sarah and Glen have much of their journey still before them. As they continue to journey, they will frequently return to many of the questions on which they reflected as they began their psychiatric clinical experience. Their selves will continue to change and expand as they encounter and process new experiences. They will find that just as life is a journey, so too is the discovery of one's own self as well as the discovery of another's self.

➤ *Check Your Reading*
41. What is the importance to mental health of meeting basic needs?
42. What happens if an individual fails to accomplish a major developmental task?
43. What are the characteristics of mental health? Mental illness?
44. What is necessary for a novice nurse to become an expert?
45. To use the self therapeutically, what is required of the nurse?

Conclusions

In this chapter, you have examined the self, self-concept, and all the interrelated ideas that are under the umbrella of the self. You met Sarah and Glen, two nursing students getting ready to embark on two journeys, which included stops where they could view their own selves as well as the selves of psychiatric patients. You met Ray and Mary Ann, two patients with different psychiatric problems. Ray expressed a self that was riddled with uncertainties and feelings of inferiority. Mary Ann's self, despite struggling with a bipolar disorder, was strong and confident. You read about the factors that contribute to the development of the self. You were presented with an array of other concepts such as self-esteem; ideal self; personality; and cognitive, psychological, spiritual, and social selves. We hope you have gained a better understanding of not only what makes you *you* but also what makes me *me*. The process of becoming *I* or *you* is wonderfully complex. However, understanding the process is critically important for nurses who must know themselves and be able to know others.

Key Points to Remember

- Knowing oneself is essential to using oneself therapeutically.
- Moving from novice nurse to expert nurse requires time as well as experience, through which theory gets refined with practice.
- The self is the part of the human being that knows himself or herself as *I;* it includes the thinking, knowing, and feeling part of the individual that deals with the world, and it involves physical as well as psychological characteristics and conscious and unconscious components.
- Self-concept is the conscious knowledge, perceptions, feelings, and thoughts that an individual has about the self.
- Self-esteem is the person's judgment of personal worth.
- Self-awareness is what the person knows about the self.
- Self-concept includes the physical, psychological, social, spiritual, and ideal self dimensions.
- Physical self includes body image or how a person views her or his physical appearance.
- Physical self represents the boundary between inner self and the external environment.
- Physical self is influenced by cultural norms.

- Physical self demands its own body space. Four body spaces are identified in the literature: intimate, personal, social, and public spaces.
- Development influences the physical self.
- Personal identity is composed of perceptual, cognitive, and emotional images that we have of ourselves.
- Perception is how we make sense out of what we experience.
- A person who is reality oriented is one whose inner reality is close to external reality.
- Perceptual processes are affected by early parental interactions.
- Perceptual processes influence the development of the self-concept.
- Piaget defined intelligence as a dynamic trait that is always related to an individual's adaptation to the environment under existing circumstances.
- The cognitive self includes our innate intelligence, as well as all past remembered events, educational experiences, and thinking style.
- Equilibration (homeostasis or Steady State) is the driving force to maintain harmony between the self and the environment.
- Disequilibrium is the experience of disharmony between the self and the environment.

- Piaget identified four stages of cognitive development: sensorimotor stage, preoperational thinking, concrete operations, and formal operations.
- Cognitive function is influenced by physiological as well as psychological factors.
- Self-efficacy is the aspect of cognition that allows us to evaluate what we can do.
- Self-esteem is part of the emotional or affective self.
- Self-esteem consists of global and specific self-esteem.
- Five traits are necessary for the development of self-esteem: (1) a sense of significance; (2) a sense of competence; (3) a sense of connectedness to others balanced by a sense of separateness from them; (4) a sense of realism about ourselves and the world; and (5) a coherent set of ethics and values.
- The social self refers to the roles that we fill.
- Role is defined as a socially accepted behavior pattern associated with an individual's function in various social groups.
- Each role carries expectations.
- Roles can be ascribed or assumed.

- Sibling position influences roles in a family.
- Gender identity is an important factor when considering roles.
- The spiritual self allows us to develop God-consciousness and to make sense from life's circumstances.
- The spiritual self that strives for meaning seems to be a universal phenomenon.
- Spiritual self is shaped by different world views.
- Spiritual self is the seat of morality.
- Spiritual development may parallel psychosocial and cognitive development, but this is not always true.
- Frequently, spiritual distress is misinterpreted as psychological distress.
- Mental health depends on having basic needs met and on accomplishing developmental tasks.
- Personality refers to an enduring pattern of automatic responses to the world. It is a pattern of behavior that is both conscious and unconscious and is a means of adapting to a particular environment and its cultural, ethnic, and community standards.

Learning Activities

1. Refer to the beginning of the chapter and reread the questions to which Sarah and Glen responded in their journals. Write your response to those same questions.
2. What are your unique characteristics?
3. What personal qualities will facilitate or hinder your experience in psychiatric nursing?
4. Reflect on a time when your self-concept was threatened. How did you cope with that situation? How did it influence your self-esteem?
5. How has your family life influenced your perceptual abilities?

6. Can you identify any cultural factors that have affected your self-concept? Your body image? Roles that you have assumed?
7. How has your spiritual self influenced your decision to become a nurse?
8. What is your sibling position? How has your sibling position influenced your abilities to get along with others?
9. What factors have an impact on your cognitive abilities?
10. How close is your ideal self to your self-concept?

Critical Thinking Exercises

Jules is a 24-year-old high school math teacher who was admitted to the psychiatric unit following his physical assault on and verbal threats to "finish off" teacher A. The verbal and physical assault followed an assembly during which teacher A won the Best Teacher of the Year Award. Jules believed that he deserved the award and asked his parents to attend the awards ceremony because he wanted to finally show his parents that he had done something that would make them proud of him. Jules is the third son of four boys of parents who are both biochemists. His mother is a laboratory researcher, and his father is a college professor. Both his older brothers have degrees in biochemistry and are employed at prestigious companies. His younger brother will graduate from Yale next year with a 4.0 average. When his parents noticed that their son was not the recipient of the award and because they were very late for an important conference, they left the ceremony

early, leaving a note of apology to their son about their reason for leaving.

1. Under what assumptions about his concept of self is Jules operating?

2. What inferences has Jules drawn about his parents' image of him?

3. To what conclusions has Jules come about his self-worth in relation to his siblings?

After 4 days, nurse Whyet talks to Jules about his actions. Her purpose was to assess his self-esteem. Ms. Whyet asks him what he likes about himself. His response is, "My parents think I'm not as smart as the rest of my family. I feel like I'm never good enough." Nurse Whyet notices that he is very upset and attempts to make him feel better. She states, "Of course you're good enough. Being a math teacher is a very important job." Jules states, "I guess you're right."

1. What assumption can you make about Ms. Whyet's

knowledge about the development of a concept of self?

2. What alternative responses might be used?

Additional Resources

National Association for Self Esteem (NASE)

http://self-esteem-nase.org/

References

Arnold, E., & Boggs, K. (1995). *Interpersonal relationships: Professional communication skills for nurses* (2nd ed.). Philadelphia: W. B. Saunders.

Arnold, E., & Boggs, K. (1999). *Interpersonal relationships: Professional communication skills for nurses* (3rd ed.). Philadelphia: W. B. Saunders.

Bandura, A. (1977). *Social learning theory.* Englewood Cliffs, NJ: Prentice-Hall.

Baumeester, R. (1986). *Public self and private self.* New York: Springer-Verlag.

Benner, P. (1984). *From novice to expert: Excellence and power in clinical nursing practice.* Menlo Park, CA: Addison-Wesley.

Carson, V. (1989). *Spiritual dimensions of nursing practice.* Philadelphia: W. B. Saunders.

Carson, V. B. (1998). Spirituality. In J. M. Leahy & P. E. Kizilay (Eds.), *Foundations of nursing practice: A nursing process approach.* Philadelphia: W. B. Saunders.

Dufaulf, M. A. (1990). Personal and work resources as variables associated with role mastery in the novice nurse. *Journal of Continuing Education in Nursing, 21,* 78.

Dugas, B. (1983). *Introduction to patient care: A comprehensive approach to nursing* (4th ed.). Philadelphia: W. B. Saunders.

Erikson, E. (1963). *Childhood and society.* New York: Norton.

Felker, D. (1974). *Building positive self concepts.* Minneapolis, MN: Burgess.

Fisher, S. (1974). *Body consciousness.* New York: Aronson.

Fontaine, K. L. (1991). The conspiracy of culture: Women's issues in body size. *Nursing Clinics of North America, 26,* 669-676.

Herd, F., Jr. (1994). Studying mental illness: A student's perspective—how stigma could impair familial functioning in a supportive role. *Journal of Psychosocial Nursing and Mental Health Services, 32*(6), 50-51.

Hergenhahn, B. R. (1982). *An introduction to theories of learning* (2nd ed.). Englewood Cliffs, NJ: Prentice-Hall.

Husted, G. L., Miller, M. C., & Wilczyski, E. M. (1990). 5 ways to build your self esteem. *Nursing, 90, 20*(5), 152, 154.

Jerome, A. M., & Ferrard-McDuffie, H. R. (1992). Nurse self awareness in therapeutic relationships. *Pediatric Nursing, 18,* 153-156.

Klose, P., & Tinius, T. (1992). Confidence builders: A self esteem group at an inpatient psychiatric hospital. *Journal of Psychosocial Nursing and Mental Health Services, 30*(7), 37-38, 59.

Maslow, A. (1970). *Motivation and personality* (2nd ed.). New York: Harper & Row.

Miller, B. F., & Keane, C. B. (1992). *Encyclopedia and dictionary of medicine, nursing, and allied health* (5th ed.). Philadelphia: W. B. Saunders.

Mixson, K. (1989). How to enhance our self esteem. *Advancing Clinical Care, 4*(6), 98.

Myers, P., & Myers, K. (1993). *Myers-Briggs type indicator.* Palo Alto, CA: Consulting Psychologists Press.

Peck, M. S. (1978). *The road less traveled.* New York: Simon and Schuster.

Piaget, J. (1952). *The origin of intelligence in children.* New York: International Universities Press.

Piaget, J. (1970). *Structuralism.* New York: Basic Books.

Rieser, P. A. (1992). Educational, psychological and social aspects of short stature. *Journal of Pediatric Health Care, 6,* 325-334.

Robinson, L. (1974). *Liaison nursing: Psychological approach to patient care.* Philadelphia: F. A. Davis.

Robinson, L. (1983). *Psychiatric nursing as a human experience.* Philadelphia: W. B. Saunders.

Sanford, L., & Donovan, M. E. (1984). *Women and self esteem.* New York: Penguin Books.

Satire, V. (1972). *Peoplemaking.* Palo Alto, CA: Science and Behavior Books.

Sheehy, C. (1974). *Passages: The predictable crises in adult life.* New York: Bantam Books.

Sire, J. (1990). *Discipleship mind.* Downers Grove, IL: Inter-Varsity Press.

Strassen, L. (1992). *The image of professional nursing.* Philadelphia: J. B. Lippincott.

Toman, W. (1969). *Family constellation.* New York: Springer.

Viorst, J. (1986). *Necessary losses.* New York: Ballantine Books.

Viscott, D. (1976). *The language of feelings.* New York: Pocket Books.

Suggested Readings

Berenblatt, M., & Berenblatt, A. J. (1994). *Make an appointment with yourself: Simple steps to positive self-esteem.* Deerfield Beach, FL: Health Communications, Inc.

Bracken, B. (1996). *Handbook of self-concept,* New York: Wiley.

Dufaulf, M. A. (1990). Personal and work resources as variables associated with role mastery in the novice nurse. *Journal of Continuing Education in Nursing, 21,* 78.

Herd, F., Jr. (1994). Studying mental illness: A student's perspective—how stigma could impair familial functioning in a supportive role. *Journal of Psychosocial Nursing and Mental Health Services, 32*(6), 50, 51.

Jerome, A. M., & Ferrard-McDuffie, H. R. (1992). Nurse self awareness in therapeutic relationships. *Pediatric Nursing, 18,* 153-156.

Johnson, H. M. (1986). *How do I love me* (2nd ed.). Salem, WI: Sheffield.

Johnson, H. M. (1989). *A workshop on self-esteem.* Salem, WI: Sheffield.

Klose, P., & Tinius, T. (1992). Confidence builders: A self esteem group at an inpatient psychiatric hospital. *Journal of Psychosocial Nursing and Mental Health Services, 30*(7), 37–38, 59.

Mruk, C. (1995). *Self-esteem: Research, theory and practice.* New York: Springer.

Price, B. (1990). A model for body-image care. *Journal of Advanced Nursing, 15,* 585.

Seward, B. L. (1994). *Managing stress: Principles and strategies for health and wellbeing.* Boston: Jones and Bartlett.

Vaillant, G. (1993). *The wisdom of ego.* Cambridge, MA: Harvard University Press.

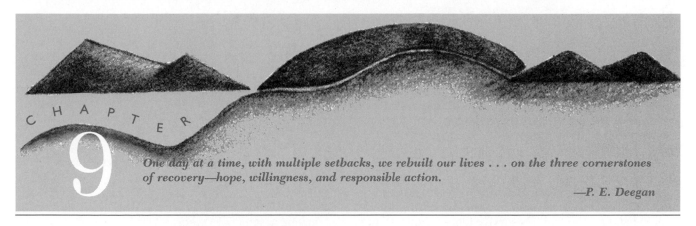

CHAPTER

9

One day at a time, with multiple setbacks, we rebuilt our lives . . . on the three cornerstones of recovery—hope, willingness, and responsible action.

—*P. E. Deegan*

Unique Attributes of Successful Travelers
Personal Strengths

Learning Objectives

After studying this chapter, you should be able to:

1. Describe at least four characteristics of a triumphant survivor.

2. Explain the implications of control, challenge, and commitment as they relate to hardiness.

3. Describe the five themes of resilience.

4. Note the five domains of empowerment and the interventions that nurses can perform to promote personal strengths.

5. Recognize the importance of hope, humor, social support, and spirituality for the patient and family on their journey toward survivorship.

6. Explain at least two strategies that develop personal strengths in the nurse who is caring for patients and families trying to overcome mental health problems and significant loss and grief.

Key Terminology

Despair	Grief	Mental illness	Self-reliance
Empowerment	Hardiness	Perseverance	Survivorship
Equanimity	Loss	Recovery	
Existential aloneness	Meaningfulness	Resilience	

Have you ever wondered about people who have overcome significant illness or loss? Have you ever asked yourself, "How did that person do that?" Have you ever thought, "I'm not sure I could do as well if that happened to me?" Why is it that some overcome difficulties, while others do not? What attributes make the journey successful? Some people manage to triumph over the odds. Others settle for less or lose interest in life, failing to make a go of it. Why is it that some family members weather the turmoil of family crises without overwhelming emotional difficulty, whereas others find it difficult to function? Some survive; others do not or take longer to get on their feet again. What makes the difference?

This area has been the focus of popular (Blum, 1998) and nursing literature, especially relative to survivorship and cancer patients. But, can it also be applied to patients and families experiencing mental health problems, as well as those dealing with loss and grief? Some think it can be applied because with current improvements in the treatment of mental illness, individuals are joining the mainstream of the community, sometimes for the first time. Their assimilation demonstrates that they can be survivors too.

Do nurses play a part in this human drama? Yes, they do. Nurses deal with many survivors in their work settings, especially as the delivery of health care shifts more and more to the community. However, for nurses to help patients and families survive illness and loss, they need to understand the human spirit and the many psychosocial aspects affecting the lives of these individuals. Nurses must have the skills, sensitivity, and understanding to promote a successful journey for the patients and families who are experiencing mental health problems or dealing with loss and grief.

This is the story of a real person, an actual survivor of a mental health problem, who exemplifies the attributes of survivorship, hardiness, and resilience. Ways in which the nurse can promote personal strengths in patients and families are discussed by examining the stages of overcoming grief and loss. Some implications for coping with mental health problems are also noted. Interesting frameworks used in two mental health settings in which nurses practice and promote empowerment are presented. Ways in which nurses can further intervene and participate in the patient's journey of survivorship through the use of hope, humor, social support, and spirituality are also reviewed. The conclusion of this chapter explores strategies for nurses to develop their own personal strengths while they promote strengths in the patient and the family.

 **Vickie's Story**

Vickie is a survivor. Even in her darkest times, she expressed determination to get through her difficulties. A psychiatric nurse who has known Vickie for nearly 20 years remembers the front that Vickie once maintained—laughing and smiling even when she was discouraged. Vickie so hoped that people would like her.

Childhood

Vickie's childhood was stormy. When she was 14 years old she was removed from an abusive home; at 18 she ran away from another abusive situation and showed up in Maryland on the doorstep of an aunt whom she barely knew. This extended family knew her only as "Bill's daughter." Vickie's life continued to be stormy. In the beginning, she struggled, mostly on her own.

Young Adulthood

Vickie was no stranger to problems and crises. Her alcohol abuse and reliance on marijuana worsened behavior that was already rebellious. She remembers her 20s as a time fraught with attempts at self-destruction. Episodes of overdosing and cutting herself included an incident of slashing her own throat. In addition, Vickie could be verbally abusive to those who tried to get close to her. At times, she was absolutely convinced that no one liked her.

For 10 years, Vickie remained unstable and struggled to survive. Because of her threatening and bizarre behavior she was hospitalized repeatedly, diagnosed as schizophrenic, medicated with a variety of psychotropic medications, and monitored by the community mental health (CMH) service.

Referral to Way Station

At one point, Vickie was referred by a CMH nurse to a psychosocial program called Way Station, located in Frederick, Maryland. The agency provided supervised housing, among other mental health services. Vickie was admitted to the program. But she was not yet ready to behave appropriately. Eventually, the program leaders asked her to leave.

Vickie recalls that her "forced expulsion" greatly affected her. She thinks she was beginning to see life's possibilities but was unwilling to let others know that she wanted to change. Ultimately, she did negotiate her return to the program, but she first tried to live with her parents again. The atmosphere was still not supportive, so she returned to Maryland.

Crisis

When Vickie was 28 years old and again a client of Way Station, she made a serious suicide attempt that left her comatose and in an intensive care unit for 2 weeks. During this time, Vickie again came in contact with CMH nurses, as well as the hospital nurses. Together with the nurses at Way Station, these community nurses provided a continuity of caring.

In addition, the caring response from workers and other clients at Way Station began to have an effect on Vickie. She felt sad. Probably for the first time in her life she allowed herself to experience that feeling. She realized that she had hurt them by disregarding herself. She discovered that they really did care about her.

A New Diagnosis

It was at this time that Vickie's diagnosis was changed to multiple personality disorder. The health care team gradually reduced Vickie's medications, and today she manages with small doses of antianxiety and antidepressant agents. With psychotherapy, Vickie has been able to reconnect her feelings with her body and no longer feels numb or neutral. She had lived that way for too long, she says. "Now a big part of me loves living. I'm learning new ways and I want people to like me for who I really am," she exclaims.

Moving Away From Way Station

Gradually, Vickie is moving away from Way Station. She no longer lives in supervised housing. At age 33, she lives with a friend, and they share in the management of their home. She is going to school to gainadditional job skills and plans to seek a part-time job when she completes her résumé. "I get scared thinking about working full time, but I know how to climb out of the hole, and I don't have to feed those dark thoughts. I'll fake it till I make it!" she proclaims. The local chapter of Civitan, a national civic organization, has invited Vickie to join their membership. "Because they think so much of me, they asked me to be secretary," she said with a big smile. "It's a way for me to give back." Civitan facilitates worthy community projects, and Way Station has benefitted from the organization's fundraising. This opportunity pleases Vickie. Her interest in doing for others is a characteristic of a triumphant survivor.

Vickie has progressed from a life of rejection and chaos to one of acceptance and order. She continues to have her ups and downs, but her ability to survive has been due, in part, to her personal attributes and to the caring of many people during these years.

ATTRIBUTES OF SUCCESSFUL TRAVELERS

Survivorship

Stearns (1988), a professor of psychology, has written about **survivorship** after interviewing hundreds of clients who have experienced personal crises that involve major illnesses and traumatic losses. She concluded that specific characteristics describe triumphant survivors and provide them with a strength that supports them through tragedy and trauma. These characteristics include

1. Staying active through times of trouble
2. Living each day moment by moment
3. Proceeding with a sheer determination to get to the next step
4. Overcoming helplessness
5. Getting beyond the suffering and initial sense of entitlement
6. Connecting with significant others to gain strength from the relationships
7. Avoiding destructive or negative contacts while healing
8. Developing a network of individuals and groups consisting of friends, family, and community connections, which provides a healthy social support system that upholds them during recovery

Nurses practice in settings where they can encourage patients and families to overcome difficult times as they proceed toward survivorship. In this vein, Stearns (1988) pointed out that survivors look for encouragement wherever they are and demonstrate courage in a number of ways. Nurses can be alert to signs of courage.

They can be sensitive to a patient's requests for help, notice his or her willingness to grow and change, and coach his or her curiosity about the meaning of each circumstance. Ultimately, survivors become involved in helping others. They get beyond being a victim or feeling helpless and take control of their future. Then, life can become "a story yet to be completed" (Stearns, 1993, p. 10). Triumphant survivors make decisions that shape the years to come and promote their recovery. Nurses are capable of promoting a healthy future for patients and their families who are overcoming emotional or physical trauma or illness.

Likewise, Vickie encountered nurses in her community throughout her years of recovery. Nurses in the emergency department and mental health nurses at Way Station encouraged her to overcome despair and get on with life. As a survivor, Vickie has gone beyond the victim stage and taken responsibility for her future. As she has moved toward mental health, she has gradually been able to set appropriate boundaries for herself without relying on Way Station staff members to direct her. Consequently, she exemplifies the traits of survivors in many ways.

Hardiness

Hardiness, as a personality characteristic, has been defined in the nursing literature as an "inherent health-promoting factor in a stress laden environment" (Bigbee, 1985, p. 55). Individuals who are hardy are thought to be able to resist illness when experiencing stressful life events. A composite of control, commitment, and challenge relates to the presence of hardiness (Kobasa, 1979). Three hypotheses that relate these concepts to people under stress and have significant implications for the interventions that nurses perform with patients and families are the following (Kobasa, 1979):

- Those who have a greater sense of control over what occurs in their lives remain healthier than those who feel powerless in the face of external forces.
- Those who feel committed to the various areas of their lives remain healthier than those who are alienated.
- Those who view change as a challenge remain healthier than those who view it as a threat.

Nurses can recognize individuals who may be at risk for illness when stress is experienced. Interventions for those who feel out of control, hopeless, and hostile can be planned to reduce tension, thereby controlling the effects of a stressful environment. Helping patients gain more control over their environment allows them to access "personal hardiness" and move toward "hardy health behaviors" (Tartasky, 1993, p. 228).

In *Surviving Mental Illness,* Hatfield (1993) reported that individuals who have experienced a **recovery,** not a cure or a return to a premorbid state, claim a "kind of readaptation to the illness that allows life to go forward in a meaningful way" (p. 184). Survivors stress the benefit of encouragement from family and health care providers who emphasize their personal strengths. These positive strokes promote survivors' sense of accomplishment and usefulness.

By devising their own strategies to control symptoms and promote stability, survivors are able to activate the control aspect of hardiness. Therefore, with a growing "acceptance of the illness, the maintenance of a hopeful attitude and the right kind of support," patients and families can be challenged to survive the odds (Hatfield, 1993, p. 184).

Although the information about hardiness and **mental illness** is limited, the caring nurse can access the "coping self that is responsive to positive stimuli and open to change" (Hatfield, 1993, p. 187). Hatfield went on to point out that empathic listening and supportive psychotherapy can help a schizophrenic patient "process his or her experience of the disease and its consequences" (p. 187). Certainly, Vickie was counseled at length about her behavior, which moved her toward better control of herself.

Similarly, Lambert and Lambert (1987) believed that nurses can demonstrate commitment by helping patients examine themselves and experience the results of their behavior, challenging them to grow and seek new opportunities. Emphasizing personal strengths can promote self-esteem and enhance self-control. In these ways, nurses can promote the components of hardiness (i.e., control, commitment, and challenge).

It is apparent that the nurses and staff members of Way Station challenged Vickie to see the value of exercising healthy self-control. She has made a commitment to life and those who care about her. Even though she is sometimes fearful, she loses the fear and takes risks to go on, accepting the challenge of the moment and the future.

Resilience

The ability to bounce back following a crisis or significant loss is an interesting phenomenon. Kadner (1989) defined **resilience** as an "ability to recover from or adjust easily to misfortune or change" (p. 20). Wagnild and Young (1990) recognized resilience as the ability to be flexible and adaptable, characteristics that are important for recovery.

Nurses can enhance resilience and promote survivorship by demonstrating an understanding of the ways in which patients and families conceptualize stressful life events. There are five underlying themes that represent successful adjustment after significant **loss** (Wagnild & Young, 1990, p. 252):

1. Equanimity
2. Perseverance
3. Self-reliance
4. Meaningfulness
5. Existential aloneness

Equanimity implies an ability to view life with a wide-angle lens, accepting the sad times with the happy times, thus enabling one to eventually experience major life events with a positive focus.

But, more than that, it takes a persistence to keep on struggling in spite of hard times and discouragement. Sometimes **perseverance** means being "bull-headed and stubborn . . . simply going through the motions . . . it would take time to get over their losses" (Wagnild & Young, p. 254).

Furthermore, those who exhibit resilience believe in themselves and their abilities. **Self-reliance** requires a search for resources within oneself to handle day-to-day activities. Major changes may need to occur, and strength to carry out changes comes from within.

Those who find that life has a purpose and think that what they have to offer is valuable can adjust to their losses by gaining meaning from their experiences. **Meaningfulness** can revive an outlook on life and change a seemingly negative situation into a time of growth and opportunity.

Recognizing that some experiences in life must be handled alone acknowledges an **existential aloneness.** Wagnild and Young (1990) described this as a "realization that each person's life path is unique" (p. 254). Aloneness can be an opportunity for "creativity, comfort, and self-acceptance" (p. 254). A woman who was widowed expressed herself by saying "I'm me again, just me" (p. 254). In like manner, Vickie pointed out, "I value more and more the time that I can now spend alone."

These themes are typical of resilience found in patients and families who bounce back, despite difficult life situations. The nurse can view this concept philosophically while relating to patients. By giving genuine support, nurses allow patients opportunities to express feelings and show their inner strengths. Actively listening to patients as they explain their life stories enables patients to look at their situation in new ways. Nurses who reflect confidence in patients' abilities and resourcefulness are promoting resilience.

Vickie is resilient as a result of others having confidence that she could rise above her difficulties. With the encouragement of nurses and others who worked with her through the years, she has come to realize that she has an ability to bounce back when a setback or loss occurs.

What do you think? How would you rate yourself on resiliency? What experiences have tested your abilities to bounce back? What have you learned from your personal experiences that could help others?

➤ *Check Your Reading*

1. Name three attributes of successful travelers.
2. List three characteristics of what Stearns called triumphant survivors.
3. Name the three components of hardiness.
4. List the five themes that constitute resilience.

DEVELOPING PATIENTS' PERSONAL STRENGTHS

Helping Patients Overcome Loss and Grief

It is essential that nurses, patients, and families recognize that survivorship is a journey of recovery that (1) is accomplished in stages; (2) takes time; and (3) includes suffering. Onega (1991) raised questions about the concept of suffering and asked whether the suffering of those experiencing a serious mental or physical illness is the same as the suffering of those experiencing **grief** that is associated with death and dying. The suffering seems similar. Chapter 22 discusses loss and grief and provides helpful ways nurses can respond.

Empowering Patients

The healing process of recovery takes place as patients become empowered to accept changes in themselves and their circumstances. Taking as much responsibility as they can handle comfortably and trusting those individuals involved in their care contribute to recovery. Such a philosophy has been the ARTWorks paradigm of the ALI/LifeSkills Program, which is in the psychiatric treatment settings of the Washoe Medical Center in northeast Reno, Nevada. Acceptance, responsibility, and trust are the concepts basic to the paradigm that promotes **empowerment** of the patient (Bowler, 1991).

The basic assumption of the Nevada program is that "people need not be ruled by their circumstances, but can choose how they experience their environment" (Bowler, 1991, p. 23). The paradigm is best summarized as follows:

- Acceptance of what is
- Responsibility for one's experience of what is
- Trust in one's self and the ability of others to make appropriate choices in the face of what is

These concepts define the Nevada program as a "healing health care environment" and the nurse a "healing agent" (p. 23). Nursing staff members use the paradigm principle as they plan and carry out their practice. The nursing program there includes nurse-led classes, community meetings, and group therapy sessions. Nurses are encouraged to "develop diverse skills through case management and program facilitation" for a complex client population, including people with addiction problems and those with mental illnesses.

Nurses were among those who helped Vickie take responsibility for both her dysfunctional and healthy behaviors. "When they let me fall out of their net, reality would hit. Then I had to take responsibility for myself and put my life back together." Gradually, Vickie established a different experience as she was given the opportunity to try out different behaviors.

By allowing her to experiment with a variety of approaches toward accomplishing her goals, the nurses in Way Station empowered Vickie, much as the nurses in the Nevada program empower their clients (Figure 9-1).

Bowler (1991) pointed out that clients in the Nevada program devise their own treatment plans, grounded in the 12-step philosophy of recovery. In addition, staff members and clients are encouraged to nurture themselves, along with others, thereby empowering those involved in the Nevada program to love and care for self and others in a way that is liberating and enriching.

In light of this notion, Bowler (1991) believed that psychiatric–mental health nurses cannot "create an environment of personal transformation for clients unless they can also experience their own empowerment and commitment to a greater vision" (p. 21). She called on nurses to relinquish the victim role; to avoid blaming the system or the administration for what is wrong; and to learn to care for themselves. Applying the principles of the ARTWorks paradigm helps nurses create their own experience. The ALI/LifeSkills program teaches that

trust, acceptance, vision, forgiveness, apology, responsibility and action help individuals attain a better quality of life when applied in one's day-to-day affairs . . . as the satisfying practice environments are, in reality, within themselves. (p. 23)

Empowerment is envisioned somewhat differently in a Midwest CMH center where a community support

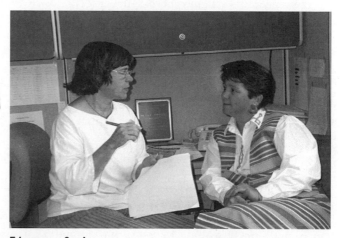

Figure 9-1
Francy and other Way Station nurses empowered Vickie to accomplish her goals.

B o x 9 – 1 ■ ■ ■ ■ ■
Levels of Empowerment

- **Participating:** Exists when patients have a place to be themselves and to become involved, even if it means just being with others, drinking coffee, having a smoke.
- **Choosing:** Exists when the individual is free to choose among a variety of options, implying self-control and taking responsibility for one's behavior.
- **Supporting:** Includes caring, relating, accepting, coaching, and sharing. Friendship is a very important aspect of this level. Here, patients can help each other.
- **Negotiating:** Is a time for mutual respect and feelings of near equality and cooperation, as well as readiness to take a stand on issues.
- **Personal Significance:** Exists when an individual is able to describe the impact of empowerment to personal experience.

service serves patients who are primarily schizophrenic and manic-depressive. Empowerment is a major theme of their work; for example, there is a patient-run drop-in center. Connelly, Keefe, Kleinbeck, Schneider, and Cobb (1993) analyzed four levels of empowerment experienced by these patients as process domains: participating, choosing, supporting, and negotiating. A fifth domain, personal significance, describes the effects of empowerment on the person. Box 9–1 defines these domains.

Through her journey of survivorship, Vickie has had opportunities to experience each of these domains. One cannot mistake her sense of empowerment and her feelings of personal significance now that she is on her own. Because she was given choices about treatment goals and options, she experienced the staff members' support. "They were right beside me, even when I made a mistake. That became a tool to help me grow."

In yet another setting, "the ability to use one's self in the therapeutic process in the service of empowering the client" was described by Hammond (1988) as part of an empowerment treatment model, which she developed while she was a therapist working with women (p. 75). Her principles have implications for mental health nurses because these principles promote survivorship. Some of Hammond's procedures and strategies are shown in Box 9–2.

Hammond (1988) believed that these interventions contribute to her functioning as a role model for patients. "Openness, the capacity to feel, the ability to be action-oriented, and the reorganization of self-identity

from victimization to empowerment" are all important characteristics for the clinician (p. 80).

On the other hand, Keith (1991) encouraged survivors, their families, and health care providers to "assume responsibility for creating their own balance" when striving for an environment of survivorship (p. 113). Assuming responsibility for their own balance provides participants with an atmosphere in which they can own success or failure. She stressed that if professionals think they must fix it for patients, they deny patients independence and the opportunity to determine their destiny, environment, and life. Like Stearns (1988), Keith believed that determination to take responsibility for self promotes recovery; patients need to take an active, aggressive, and sometimes defiant role in their own healing to recover.

Nurses can be empowering facilitators by helping patients to see that "they are not their illness" (Keith, 1991, p. 114). Allowing individuals to express their feelings and validate their emotions gives them the opportunity to access resources within themselves and others to "fight the battle" (p. 114). When the healing process is allowed to proceed, hope can begin to be experienced.

Instilling Hope

Deegan (1988) described hope as "the turning point which must be followed by a willingness to act . . . not . . . absence of pain or struggle . . . a transition from anguish to suffering . . . leading forward to a new future" (p. 14). On the other hand, Stotland (as cited in Raleigh, 1992) defines hope as "an expectation of goal attainment modified by the importance of the goal and the probability of attaining it" (p. 443). When patients

B o x 9 – 2 ■ ■ ■ ■ ■
Nursing Strategies: Empowerment

- **Establishing Mutual Identification Points:** Owning and expressing common or shared experiences with the client to facilitate joining, which can serve to model an example of survival
- **Acting as a Power Agent:** Taking advantage of opportunities to influence other relevant systems in which the client participates, such as making telephone calls on the client's behalf and advocating whenever possible
- **Validating Strengths:** Identifying and relabeling behaviors to indicate the existence of strengths or competencies
- **Self-Disclosure:** Timely and appropriate self-revelations to serve as examples of skill teaching
- **Skill Teaching:** Such as in child management, assertiveness, relaxation, organization of support groups, and résumé writing to foster self-reliance, mastery, and competency

Box 9 – 3 ■ ■ ■ ■ ■
Nursing Strategies: Hope

- Get busy doing something
- Pray or undertake religious activities
- Think about other things
- Talk to others

believe change is possible, they experience hope and willingness to try to work toward recovery. Therefore, "I'm willing to try . . . I am hopeful . . . I discover that I can do" become part of the process of recovery, as explained by Deegan (p. 14).

But where does hope come from, especially when life is grim and hopeless? Raleigh (1992) stated that patients experiencing chronic illness report that the most common sources of hope are family, friends, and religious beliefs. Box 9–3 lists a number of strategies to alleviate hopelessness.

Others helped "by visiting me . . . listening to me . . . talking to me" (p. 446). The findings in Raleigh's study are similar to Stearns' (1988) and to her work with those surviving loss and grief. Both authors proclaimed the value of being active and having personal relationships, especially family and friends.

The informed nurse is in a position to encourage patients to seek visits from family and friends and become involved in meaningful activities. However, family and friends are not always available, for reasons of location, inconvenience, or emotional distance. Quite often, emotional cut-off exists when a family member is mentally ill, leaving the mentally ill individual without that resource for hope. Nurses sometimes act as temporary family for patients until they can become reunited with their families or develop new social connections.

Vickie was without an emotionally close family in the earlier days of her journey; thus, nurses and staff members at Way Station became her family. They spent time with her, talked to her, and listened to her. Their efforts encouraged her to see that they cared for her beyond her problems, for they had confidence in her strengths and ability to survive.

Raleigh (1992) reminded nurses that their companionship and willingness to listen fosters hopefulness. In addition to encouragement, nurses work with a patient to set realistic goals that are readily attainable, based on the patient's progress and current motivation. Creativity and imagination may be in order as nurses brainstorm with the patient about the next horizon. Accomplishment of even little steps provides patients with a sense of "I can do it."

Using Humor

The road toward survivorship is a bumpy one. There are pits and potholes along the way. Humor can absorb some of the shock and grease the wheels of the vehicle that carries survivors.

Sumners (1988) described the therapeutic use of humor in the recovery of substance abusers. Her ideas have implications for anyone recovering from a mental health problem who is persevering to survive his or her difficult experiences. In the process of recovery, humor is a valuable coping skill that nurses can encourage clients to use constructively and appropriately. More specifically,

Humor helps to cushion the pain of self-revelation, to initiate, reestablish, and maintain relationships, and to enable the individual to own and express a full range of emotions without damaging others. (p. 177)

Individuals overcoming substance abuse experience different types of humor throughout the stages of their recovery. During each stage, humor functions to alleviate stress and feelings of anger, anxiety, frustration, and tension. Extinguishing these feelings with substances can be one way to cope, but humor, an "emotion-focused coping strategy," is a healthier alternative (Sumners, 1988, p. 173).

It is of interest that the types and functions of humor used in recovery from substance abuse depend on the stage of recovery. Sumners (1988) described the following recovery stages: drinking or drug use and transition, early recovery, and ongoing recovery. Table 9–1 illustrates the types of humor and their functions during these stages.

TABLE 9 – 1 The Types and Coping Functions of Humor Used in Each Stage of Recovery From Substance Abuse

STAGE OF RECOVERY	TYPES OF HUMOR	COPING FUNCTIONS
Drinking and transition	Attacking, sarcasm, tendentious wit, ridicule, jokes	Relief of anger, hostility, anxiety, aggression, expression of negative feelings
Early recovery	Jokes, self-disparaging, storytelling, practical jokes, puns, absurdity	Detachment, promotion of inclusion in group, social relationships, tension relief, problem solving, communication
Ongoing recovery	Irony, satire, jokes, intellectual play, stories	Acceptance of life's paradox, enhancement of feelings of relatedness to humanity, building and sustaining relationships

From *Issues in Mental Health Nursing, 9,* 169–179. Sumners, A. D. (1988). Taylor & Francis, Inc., Washington, DC. Reproduced with permission. All rights reserved.

It is apparent that the type of humor used changes as a patient progresses toward recovery. Initially, he or she has negative feelings, expressed with sarcasm or ridicule. Exploring the underlying themes of the humor can reveal unexpressed feelings. Consequently, humor can be a way to safely let go of the unexpressed feeling in a socially acceptable manner; laughter, rather than the abused substance, releases the tension. Previously, numbing sensations with substance abuse served as a way of coping. However, humor is a more constructive way to deal with negative feelings.

As recovery progresses and social supports expand, addicted clients find that humor breaks the ice in social situations and reduces isolation, especially as they become members of support groups or actively participate in the community. Circumstances that used to be threatening become less overwhelming, even humorous, as perspectives change and thinking shifts beyond self-centeredness (Sumners, 1988).

Nurses are in unique positions to use humor in their practice settings because of their consistent presence and rapport with patients and families. Warner (1984) pointed out that self-disclosure and humor are two interventions that can be a part of the dynamic process between nurse and patient and instrumental in changing social withdrawal to reintegration.

Humor therapy can include patient assignments to "find a joke you like, dislike, find offensive, find funny, etc. . . ." (Warner, 1984, p. 19). The spontaneous behaviors that result can be most enlightening. Skilled psychiatric nurses can monitor the process positively in a group situation. In addition, they can encourage patients to share humorous life events, discuss individually funny excerpts from a group session or the inpatient unit, mirror humorous techniques, and provide positive or negative feedback that is "cushioned by humor" (p. 20).

At some point, Vickie began to see the futility of her addictive behaviors, perhaps as others humored her by sharing their similar experiences in trying to cope with substance abuse. Because of the numerous fun activities at Way Station, Vickie and others like her were able to have experiences that relieved the intensity of their past situations, brought them closer to those who shared similar fears, and created a new self-acceptance. An improved sense of well-being was apparent to those who participated in the fun.

In addition, Vickie came to realize that she was not the only one who had to deal with substance abuse and mental health problems. Others in the group had overcome addiction. People were there to guide her with a sense of humor. She could laugh at herself, as well as others, much like McKenzie (1982), who used "the tool of humor to laugh over situations that formerly made me tense" (p. 19).

Even though McKenzie was a survivor of schizophrenia rather than substance abuse, the functions of humor

seemed similar and helped her cope with her illness and circumstances.

However, the nurse is urged to be cautious when using humor with the mentally ill. The possibility of misunderstanding can be a stumbling block to which nurses need to be sensitive. In any situation, humor can be used negatively, possibly in a sarcastic or a passive-aggressive manner that is not appropriate or therapeutic. However, refocusing on positive interpersonal communications can be a way of restoring relationships, should humor be used negatively.

Similarly, Vickie knows that laughter is an important element in the lives of the members of the psychosocial program at Way Station. Members of the program and staff members experience times that are lighthearted and even silly. An annual retreat for members of the program and staff members alike is an example of a time of laughter. Activities are geared to promote interaction that is appropriately self-disclosing and social. The sharing of games, skits, singing, and meals has an equalizing effect that humanizes staff members and creates an enjoyable atmosphere of closeness and fun. In this relaxed setting, survivors can discover their strengths and risk new ways of coping. When the road to recovery is greased by the good humor of those who understand what survivors are dealing with, the journey can be more tolerable.

Engaging Social Support

Social support can be a cushion for both individuals and their families who are on the bumpy road of dealing with mental health problems, loss, and grief. Anthony (1993) emphasized that "a common denominator of recovery is the presence of people who believe in and stand by . . . persons one can trust to 'be there' in times of need" (p. 18). Social support, which facilitates recovery, can originate from a variety of sources beyond family and friends, including acquaintances, clubs, sports, churches, and self-help groups.

Jennie Forehand, a Maryland legislator, pleaded with her audience at a Depression and Related Affective Disorders Association symposium at Johns Hopkins University to "never give up" on a family member who is struggling with mental health problems (Walgrove, 1994, p. 4). She pointed out that the agony she experienced when a member of her family was hospitalized for psychotic depression was typical of the families she had come to know as a result. Families endure the disruption of their lives along with the patient. Striking the balance between the family maintaining their own sense of self and providing the necessary support for the patient's recovery is a significant challenge.

Caplan (1974) explained support systems as "social aggregates that provide individuals with opportunities for feedback about themselves and for validations of their expectations about others" (pp. 4–5). In addition, social support systems help individuals deal with their emotions, give them guidance, and promote their competence. Nurses, in their working relationships with patients and families, have many opportunities to interact meaningfully in a manner that provides encouragement and support. Offering the belief that a patient is capable of accomplishing even small objectives promotes competence that can inspire him or her to press on to overcome other obstacles.

Vickie had such a relationship with her therapist at Way Station. "She never threw me away," she exclaimed, as she told of how people stood beside her, even when she made a mistake! She was allowed to choose her own goals toward recovery. Sometimes she didn't trust or she disliked those trying to help her, but they still negotiated with her, offering her choices.

Deegan (1988), a clinical psychologist and a recovered mentally disabled person, claimed that the love and support of others was paramount in her recovery. She recalled those who loved her and did not give up, even when she gave up. Although they were powerless to make her better, they did not abandon her; some suffered with her. "They remained hopeful, despite the odds. Their love . . . was like a constant invitation . . . to be something more than all this self-pity and despair" (p. 14).

Fluctuations between dependence and independence in relationships are common experiences that patients recognize, as indicated by a mental health patient who was interviewed by the Canadian Mental Health Association (Hatfield, 1993):

What you need is to have a lot of support, even at the beginning. You just need someone to help you get through the rough spots. . . . Here, they're pushing for you to be independent and on your own, but at the same time, they're supporting you. If something happens that you can't handle, they're here. (p. 138)

As mentioned, self-help groups provide a meaningful outlet for patients to gain self-esteem and confidence. In Hatfield (1993), Leete said, "we offer each other . . . support and encouragement, friendship . . . draw strength and hope. . . . The realization that it can be done is one of the most useful aspects of any support group" (p. 126). Frese (1994) spoke about his experience of coping with schizophrenia and pointed out that "recovering persons benefit greatly from associating with others with similar disabilities" (p. 5).

The National Alliance for the Mentally Ill (NAMI) is a well-known resource for patients and families. Not only is NAMI a self-help network but it also functions as a strong political organization that represents the interests of the mentally ill and their families. Local chapters throughout the country are available to provide support. (To locate a local NAMI affiliate, see Additional Resources.)

Nurses working with mental health patients are in a position to refer individuals and their family members to an accessible and appropriate support group, such as NAMI. It behooves the caring nurse to be knowledgeable about local support and self-help groups so that referrals can connect patients with support groups that foster survivorship. To become more fully aware, the nurse might consider going to a meeting, as some groups welcome attendance by mental health professionals.

Addressing Spiritual Issues

Traveling the road of survivorship while dealing with issues of loss, grief, or other mental health problems is a lonely trek. When **despair** sets in, patients believe that no one cares. Questions surface, such as "Where is God?" "Why is this happening to me?" "What is the purpose of this suffering?" and nurses may feel at a loss about what to say.

Addressing spiritual issues when a patient is extremely anxious or possibly psychotic can create considerable anxiety for the inexperienced clinician. The anxiety of the spiritual crisis may be compounded by the patient's cognitive confusion that is brought on by an acute psychotic episode. In addition, mental health programs are not focused on meeting patients' spiritual needs (Miller, 1990). Consequently, spirituality, an important aspect of the personality, is often neglected and the needs of the whole person are not taken into consideration.

Accessing the spiritual nature of the mentally ill patient can provide an opportunity for his or her personal growth. The reach toward a greater and higher power can lift the individual out of the pit of despair and aloneness. Sullivan (1993) reported the words of one informant in a study of spirituality and the mentally challenged:

It put the worries off on someone else. I feel that there is someone else out there that has the power to help. . . . This world can be a bit frightening when you just think about the reality of it. You feel just like an ant at a picnic. . . . It (spirituality) just makes you feel more secure. (p. 129)

Another informant in the above study expressed that there was a limit to the depths of despair as it related to periods of psychiatric hospitalizations:

I knew that there was a way out and that God was always watching or taking care of me and that in the end result He had it in control—and so I didn't have to do anything stupid or desperate. . . . I might go through heck but He wasn't going to let me go to the bottom. (p. 129)

Sullivan (1993) found that the participants "spoke of their spirituality providing continual direction for them" (p. 131). For example, another comment was "The faith that you have in God makes a lot of difference in how you feel about things around you" (p. 131). The spiritual dimension of the person is an important part of his or her feeling like a whole person, a person who is connected in mind, body, and spirit.

How do nurses fit into this area of survivorship? Can their relationships contribute to positive change in the lives of patients and families? Nurses need to recognize that spiritual beliefs are a significant resource for coping and learning to live with pain, whether it be physical, emotional, or mental. "A dynamic spiritual belief system enables us to trust that somehow tomorrow will not be beyond our capacities" (Stoll, 1989, p. 194).

Nurses can strengthen the patient's and family's spirituality by supporting the "use of coping strategies such as prayer, music reminiscence, devotional reading, church attendance, physical exercise and journaling" (Stoll, 1989, p. 205). When the nurse and the patient share the same faith, they may have an occasion to share a time of prayer or a favorite scripture reading. Patients may be encouraged by the nurse's assurance of continued prayer on their behalf. Carson (1983) described the calming influence of prayer with an agitated male patient who was placed in seclusion. Because of the trust and rapport that she shared with him, the patient was responsive to this intervention and benefited from the reassurance of God's love. Fortunately for the patient, an understanding nurse was available and was comfortable in addressing his spiritual need.

What do you think? Knowing yourself, what qualities do you possess that may foster a patient's empowerment, hope, and spirituality?

► *Check Your Reading*

5. List three of the six strategies for helping your patients to develop their personal strengths.
6. Define empowerment.
7. Define hope.
8. Describe how humor is typically used during each stage of recovery from substance abuse.
9. Explain the importance of social support for people with mental illness.
10. Describe appropriate ways in which a nurse can strengthen the spirituality of patients and their families.

DEVELOPING PERSONAL STRENGTHS

Recognizing Attributes Typical of Nurses

Nurses also have characteristics of survivorship, hardiness, and resilience. These attributes propel them through the years of education and the juggling act of career and family. Determination and perseverance are predominant strengths that exemplify commitment. However, control can be an issue.

Nurses tend to be the eldest sibling or a big sister or big brother in the family (Toman, 1961). As the oldest, being in either authority or control can become the favored position. This stance can hinder the nurse-patient relationship. Without self-awareness, nurses, in their eagerness to be good caretakers, can take over for patients. Inadvertently, nursing interventions may stifle patients' efforts to accomplish actions on their own. This limits the patient's sense of control and diminishes the opportunity to develop commitment. It becomes the nurse's challenge to be sensitive to patients' needs by fostering their independence and encouraging responsibility.

Nurses who foster resilience in patients and families are often like cheerleaders who can genuinely encourage self-reliance and an attempt to find meaning, even in difficult circumstances. Taking the time to listen to the stories of patients' lives can help patients put events into perspective and make sense out of temporary chaos as they recover from illness or loss.

Again, the ability to empower patients means avoiding problems created by fostering helplessness. Individuals can learn to believe they are incapable or helpless if they are not readily involved in the decision-making process or are simply told what to do. Asking questions that provide the patient and family the opportunity to think about what's next or where they are going from here can stimulate their involvement.

The ability to maintain a calm presence, despite an anxiety-provoking situation, is an important attribute that all nurses need to develop. But sometimes nurses do become anxious and focus prematurely on rescuing patients from stress. When that happens, patients do not access their potential for growth during crisis and become or continue to be dependent. Understanding the balance between allowing dependency while encouraging independence requires considerable sensitivity, patience, and skill. Managing these variables while dealing with one's own anxiety is a juggling act with which nurses are well acquainted.

Dealing With Constraints Imposed by the Health Care System

Unfortunately, the inherent stress of the health care system places constraints on the eager nurse who wants to be sensitive to the needs of individual patients. System dictates to do more with less frequently place nonprofessional staff members in positions of spending more time with patients than the professional nurse. Meanwhile, professional nurses are expected to accept the ramifications of too few staff members, long shifts, and increased documentation. In addition, they are called on to supervise staff members and delegate patient care to others while they themselves have limited opportunity to be with their patients. Finding ways to have quality time with patients requires creativity in time management.

The atmosphere created by these constraints can lead to authoritarian management, serious tension, and morale problems that are conducive to acting-out behaviors by patients, as well as by staff members. Morrison (1990) believed that when staff members overly value being in control, violent behavior in psychiatric inpatient settings results. Tensions mount because of "a rigid rule structure and strict adherence to a role that defines staff behaviors" (p. 36). Morrison (1990) also points out that nonprofessional nursing staff members are more likely to need to be authoritarian, especially with patients, than are professional staff. Power struggles can then result between patients and staff members, as well as among staff members themselves.

In retrospect, Vickie points out that she appreciated staff members' willingness to allow her to experience the consequences of her disruptive behavior. They did not allow themselves to become involved in a power struggle with her. Most likely, her behavior was anxiety provoking for staff members, but they did not pressure her to comply. Instead, they set limits for her. Although the pain of her initial dismissal from the program at Way Station was anxiety provoking, she recognized that she returned more motivated to explore the available growth-producing activities such as job training, symptom management, and leisure activities. Despite the rules, she felt the benefit of the staff's acceptance of "who she was," even though they were compelled to carry out a policy that made her uncomfortable. The calm manner in which they dealt with her promoted her recovery. She knew she could return and give it another try. ■

Managing a balance of control and autonomy can be a fragile strategy for the professional nurse-manager. The integrity of patients and staff members alike is involved if staff members overreact to constraints that are too tight. Nurses need to contain their anxiety and think about what is best for those in their care and under their supervision. It can be especially challenging for the nurse-manager when patients or staff members test limits and act out. When management begins to lose control, patient safety and progress are jeopardized and dysfunctional behavior is enabled.

What do you think? How will you deal with your own anxiety to best assist patients to move toward greater independence?

► *Check Your Reading*
11. Describe a danger of the nurse's being the eldest sibling, a big brother, or big sister.
12. What management style can result from a health care system that requires you to do more with less?
13. What are the dangers of such a management style?

Conclusions

Promoting the attributes of the successful traveler is a challenge for the nurse. Like recovering from physical problems, the notion of survivorship can be applied to those dealing with mental health issues, including grief and loss. Nurses can promote the traits of the triumphant survivor in patients and their families by fostering personal strengths that relate to hardiness (control, commitment, and challenge) and the themes of resilience (equanimity, self-reliance, existential aloneness, perseverance, and meaningfulness). By understanding the significance of grief and loss, the nurse can provide reassurance that recovery is a process of progress toward survivorship. Over time, resolution of a significant loss, whether it be the death of a family member, the effects of a mental or physical illness, or the disappointment of a major event, does occur.

Also, nurses can be involved in empowerment as they encourage patients to accept themselves, take responsibility for their own experience, and trust in themselves and others. A treatment setting that allows participating, choosing, supporting, and negotiating fosters that kind of atmosphere. And nurses who remember the importance of instilling hope, using humor, accessing social support, and

inspiring the spirit promote survivorship. Interventions can be planned with these areas in mind.

The nurse who promotes survivorship is also a survivor. Caring for others in a meaningful way requires attributes of survivorship, hardiness, and resilience. Because nurses work in stressful environments, it is important that they have a clear sense of personal goals and needs to prevent the discouragement of burnout.

Finally, nurses promoting the successful journey of a mental health client, like Vickie, help to instill the feelings of pride and accomplishment.

Vickie has maintained stability and sobriety for an extended period. She is looking forward to greater independence. She continues to complete and revise her goals for the future. "I did it," she exclaims. "I survived!"

One wonders whether she feels like The Little Engine That Could. After pulling an especially heavy load up a hill, he kept saying, "I think I can, I think I can." When he made it to the top, he exclaimed, "I knew I could, I knew I could."

Nurses are partners with patients and families experiencing mental health problems, including loss and grief. They provide encouragement while patients and families struggle to reach the top of "their hill." When they look back and realize what they have survived, they can proudly tell the story of their journey to others, much the same as Vickie has. Then their journey can become a source of strength for others who are chugging along their own uphill road.

Key Points to Remember

- Patients and families experiencing mental health problems, including loss and grief, can be survivors and can resume life with meaning, sometimes in new ways.
- Hardiness and resilience are characteristics of survivors who successfully travel life.
- Nurses can encourage hardiness and resilience by being sensitive to the balance of allowing appropriate dependency and promoting timely independence.
- Patients and families need to recognize that overcoming mental health problems, including loss and grief, is a process that can be worked through. Knowing the stages provides nurses a way of acknowledging progress.
- Nurses can be instrumental in the empowerment of patients and families to accept themselves as they are and to take responsibility to make healthy choices for themselves.
- Hope can be a turning point for those discouraged by mental health problems. Sometimes nurses can instill hope by the interventions they use.

- Humor, when used therapeutically, can be a shock absorber and can grease the wheels on the journey of the successful traveler. Nurses can promote humor in the treatment setting that helps patients see themselves in humorous ways that reduce their anxiety.
- Social systems can be cushions that support individuals and families who are experiencing mental health problems. A substantial support system enhances recovery. Nurses are in positions to encourage the development and expansion of social support.
- Spirituality is a reach for the beyond, an attempt to connect with a power, beyond oneself, that can direct.
- Acknowledging the importance of spiritual beliefs facilitates the acceptance of the whole person (mind, body, and spirit) who is recovering and moving toward survivorship.
- Nurses can be successful travelers on their own journeys. Attributes of survivorship, hardiness, and resilience enhance their ability to be survivors too.

Learning Activities

1. Ask an individual you admire who has lived through a major disappointment or loss what he or she did to survive the experience.
2. Visit a senior citizen center and interview a group of men and women. Ask them what has helped them to remain in control of their lives in spite of aging and health problems.
3. Obtain permission to attend a support group for the mentally ill (e.g., NAMI) or alcoholics (e.g., Alcoholics Anonymous); attend and listen to the members share their stories.
4. Talk to a senior member of your family and ask him or her what helped him or her the most to survive hard times in the past.

Critical Thinking Exercises

Nick Gowen, a nurse cotherapist involved in his first outpatient group with multiple abusers, noticed the approach his cotherapist Jamie Johnson was using. Mr. A, a patient who was a cocaine abuser, told a story about how he wrecked the family car. When Mr. A got out of the car, he looked back at it and it reminded him of a Crackerjack box. As he was telling the story, he joked and laughed about how only crackers jump from Crackerjack boxes. Mr. Gowen thought that the incident was very serious and told Mr. A that it was no laughing matter. Mr. A looked at Mr. Gowen and said, "Don't be a stick in the mud. It's a big joke that I'm still alive."

1. What inference can be made about Mr. Gowen's stance regarding laughter in a therapeutic group?
2. Explore ways that Mr. A could have interpreted Mr. Gowen's comment.

3. What assumptions can the reader make about Mr. Gowen's comment?

As the group continued, Ms. Johnson looked at Mr. A and stated, "Share with us your feelings about what is so funny about your accident." Mr. Gowen wondered why Ms. Johnson was allowing this discussion to continue because it was obvious that Mr. A was in a state of denial about his responsibility for his drug abuse.

1. What assumptions can be made about Ms. Johnson's approach?
2. What can be inferred about what Ms. Johnson thinks about Mr. Gowen's comments?
3. What other information is needed to determine if your assumptions are valid?

Additional Resources

National Alliance for the Mentally Ill (NAMI)
800-950-6264
http://www.nami.org

help! A Consumer's Guide to Mental Health Information
http://www.icomm.ca/madmagic/help/help.html

References

Anthony, W. A. (1993). Recovery from mental illness: The guiding vision of the mental health service system in the 1990s. *Psychosocial Rehabilitation Journal, 16*(4), 11-23.

Bigbee, J. (1985). Hardiness: A new perspective in health promotion. *Nurse Practitioner, 10*(11), 51-56.

Blum, D. (1998, June). Finding strength: How to overcome anything. *Psychology Today, 31*(3), 32-38, 66-67, 69, 72-73.

Bowler, J. B. (1991). Transformation into a healing health care environment: Recovering the possibilities of psychiatric nursing. *Perspectives in Psychiatric Care, 27*(2), 21-25.

Caplan, G. (1974). *Support systems and community mental health.* New York: Behavioral Publications.

Carson, V. B. (1983). Prayer in a psychiatric setting. In J. A. Shelly & S. D. John (Eds.), *Spiritual dimensions of mental health* (pp. 93-97). Downers Grove, IL: Inter-Varsity Press.

Connelly, L. M., Keefe, B. S., Kleinbeck, S. V., Schneider, J. K., & Cobb, A. K. (1993). A place to be yourself: Empowerment from the client's perspective. *Image: Journal of Nursing Scholarship, 25,* 297-303.

Deegan, P. E. (1988). Recovery: The lived experience of rehabilitation. *Psychosocial Rehabilitation Journal, 11*(4), 11-19.

Frese, F. J. (1994). Coping with schizophrenia requires effort. *The Menninger Letter, 2*(3), 4-5.

Hammond, V. W. (1988). Conscious subjectivity or use of one's self in therapeutic process. *Women and Therapy, 6*(4), 75-81.

Hatfield, A. B. (1993). *Surviving mental illness.* New York: Guilford Press.

Kadner, K. D. (1989). Resilience: Responding to adversity. *Journal of Psychosocial Nursing, 27*(7), 20-25.

Keith, S. J. (1991). Surviving survivorship: Creating a balance. *Journal of Psychosocial Oncology, 9*(3), 109-115.

Kobasa, S. (1979). Stressful life events, personality, and health: An inquiry into hardiness. *Journal of Personality and Social Psychology, 37*(1), 1-11.

Lambert, C. E., & Lambert, V. A. (1987). Hardiness: Its development and relevance to nursing. *Image: Journal of Nursing Scholarship, 19,* 92-95.

McKenzie, C. (1982). Recovery. In H. Shelter & P. Straw (Eds.), *A new day: Voices across the land* (pp. 18-20). Arlington, VA: National Alliance for the Mentally Ill.

Miller, J. B. (1990). Mental illness and spiritual crisis: Implications for psychiatric rehabilitation. *Psychosocial Rehabilitation Journal, 14*(2), 29-47.

Morrison, E. F. (1990). The tradition of toughness: A study of nonprofessional nursing care in psychiatric settings. *Image: Journal of Nursing Scholarship, 22*(1), 32-38.

Onega, L. L. (1991). A theoretical framework for psychiatric nursing practice. *Journal of Advanced Nursing, 16,* 68-73.

Raleigh, E. D. (1992). Sources of hope in chronic illness. *Oncology Nursing Forum, 19,* 443-448.

Stearns, A. K. (1984). *Living through personal crisis.* Chicago: Thomas More Press.

Stearns, A. K. (1988). *Coming back: Rebuilding lives after crisis and loss.* New York: Random House.

Stearns, A. K. (1993, January 20). Coming back from crisis and loss: Traits of the "triumphant survivor." Paper presented at Taylor Manor Hospital, Ellicott City, MD.

Stoll, R. I. (1989). Spirituality and chronic illness. In V. B. Carson (Ed.), *Spiritual dimensions of nursing practice* (pp. 180-214). Philadelphia: W. B. Saunders.

Sullivan, W. P. (1993). It helps me to be a whole person: The role of spirituality among the mentally challenged. *Psychosocial Rehabilitation Journal, 16,* 124-134.

Sumners, A. D. (1988). Humor: Coping in recovery from addiction. *Issues in Mental Health Nursing, 9,* 169-179.

Tartasky, D. S. (1993). Hardiness: Conceptual and methodological issues. *Image: Journal of Nursing Scholarship, 25,* 225-229.

Toman, W. (1961). *Family constellation.* New York: Springer.

Wagnild, G., & Young, H. M. (1990). Resilience among older women. *Image: Journal of Nursing Scholarship, 22,* 252-255.

Walgrove, N. J. (1994). A family member's perspective. In W. Resnick (Ed.), *Smooth sailing: Reviews of the 1994 Mood Disorders Symposium* (pp. 4-5). Baltimore: Depression and Related Affective Disorders Association.

Warner, S. L. (1984). Humor and self-disclosure within the milieu. *Journal of Psychosocial Nursing, 22*(4), 17-21.

Suggested Readings

Connelly, L. M., Keefe, B. S., Kleinbeck, S. V., Schneider, J. K., & Cobb, A. K. (1993). A place to be yourself: Empowerment from the client's perspective. *Image: Journal of Nursing Scholarship, 25,* 297-303.

Gibson, C. H. (1991). A concept analysis of empowerment. *Journal of Advanced Nursing, 16,* 354-361.

Hatfield, A. B. (1993). *Surviving mental illness.* New York: Guilford Press.

Lambert, C. E., & Lambert, V. A. (1987). Hardiness: Its development and relevance to nursing. *Image: Journal of Nursing Scholarship, 19,* 92-95.

Stearns, A. K. (1984). *Living through personal crisis.* Chicago: Thomas More Press.

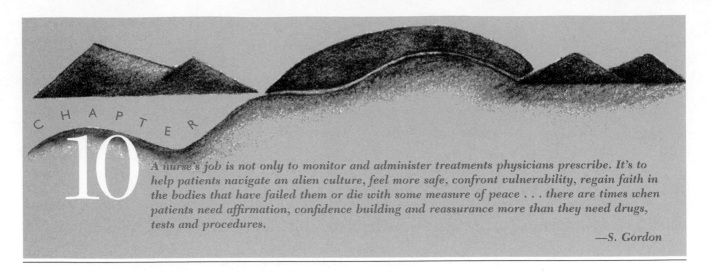

A nurse's job is not only to monitor and administer treatments physicians prescribe. It's to help patients navigate an alien culture, feel more safe, confront vulnerability, regain faith in the bodies that have failed them or die with some measure of peace . . . there are times when patients need affirmation, confidence building and reassurance more than they need drugs, tests and procedures.

—*S. Gordon*

The Vehicle for Healing
Communication as Part of a Therapeutic Relationship

Learning Objectives

After studying this chapter, you should be able to:

1. Identify the role and importance of interpersonal relationships in mental health.

2. Compare and contrast social and therapeutic relationships.

3. Describe the theoretical frameworks and structural components on which therapeutic relationships develop.

4. Describe therapeutic communication as an essential component of therapeutic relationships in psychiatric nursing.

5. Outline the basic responsibilities of the nurse developing therapeutic communication with psychiatric patients.

6. Describe other strategies, along with active listening, that promote and enhance therapeutic communication.

7. Identify some barriers to communication in the nurse-patient relationship.

8. Discuss some of the tasks associated with each phase of the therapeutic relationship: preinteraction, orientation, working, and termination.

Key Terminology

Acceptance	Countertransference	Mutuality	Therapeutic (active) listening
Advocacy	Empathy	Nonverbal communication	Therapeutic relationship
Authenticity	Focused questions	Open-ended questions	Trust
Boundaries	Humor	Orientation phase	Verbal communication
Caring	Metacommunication	Preinteraction phase	Working phase
Clarification	Minimal encouragers	Redirection	
Closed-ended questions	Modeling	Termination phase	

This chapter is about nurse-patient relationships and the process of communication that flows through those relationships as they occur in mental health clinical settings. The chapter centers on the question, "How does the nurse-patient relationship bring together the nurse's and patient's humanness as fellow travelers in a healing encounter that benefits the patient?" Occurring as a stepping stone in the river of life, the relationship can bear the patient to a different and, it is hoped, more satisfying place. This chapter identifies the work of the therapeutic relationship, distinguishes between social and therapeutic relationships, and describes the theoretical frameworks and structural components that guide therapeutic relationships. It explores therapeutic communication as an essential component of the therapeutic relationship and discusses strategies for improved communication that enhance the nurse-patient relationship. Having knowledge of the essential elements and the phases of a therapeutic relationship helps the nurse to understand the basic structure and process of the relationship in mental health settings.

Without question, the quality of a person's interpersonal relationships is an essential element of mental health. The basic work of psychiatric nursing is to help people develop a sense of self through a healing professional relationship. No single approach is applicable to every individual. Each journey is unique, requiring special interventions tailored to meet the individual needs of the patient. How the nurse experiences the patient as a fellow human being is fundamental to a successful relationship.

The Story of the Little Prince

The tale of *The Little Prince* by Antoine de Saint-Exupéry illustrates the essential nature of the bonding required in a therapeutic relationship. In this children's tale, a flower and a fox instruct a young prince on the real meaning of relationship. "I cannot play with you," the fox said. "I am not tamed. . . ."

"What does that mean—tame?" "It is an act too often neglected," said the fox. "It means to establish ties." "To establish ties?" "Just that," said the fox. "To me you are still nothing more than a little boy who is just like a hundred thousand other little boys. And I have no need of you. And you, on your part, have no need of me. To you, I am nothing more than a fox like a hundred thousand other foxes. But if you tame me, then we shall need each other. To me, you will be unique in all the world. To you, I shall be unique in all the world." "I'm beginning to understand," said the little prince. . . .

The fox gazed at the little prince, for a long time. "Please tame me!" he said. "I want to, very much," the little prince replied. "But I have not much time. I have friends to discover, and a great many things to understand." "One only understands the things that one tames," said the fox. "Men have no more time to understand anything. They buy things all ready made at the shops. But there is no shop anywhere where one can buy friendship, and so men have no friends any more. If you want a friend, tame me. . . ."

From de Saint-Exupéry, A. (1943). *The little prince* (K. Woods, Trans.) (p. 80). New York: Harcourt Brace.

This chapter is also about the process of "taming" or establishing ties within the nurse-patient relationship. Without relationships to validate and make sense of one's personal experience, a person finds the world untrustworthy and one's own place in it uncertain.

INTERPERSONAL RELATIONSHIPS

Interpersonal Relationships and Mental Illness

Mental illness affects the self in ways that invariably compromise interpersonal relationships. The mentally ill patient develops maladaptive communication styles and interpersonal defenses that seriously cripple interpersonal relationships (Hagerty, Lynch-Sauer, Patusky, & Bouwsema, 1993).

Mental illness assaults personal meanings and thereby creates a profound disruption in the ability to make connections with others. Loneliness and isolation result and patients do not experience relationships as supportive and nourishing.

Peplau (1952) believed that mental illness represents an opportunity for personal growth and insisted that all people have within them the capacity to overcome ineffective ways of relating with others. The value of a therapeutic relationship in mental illness is that it provides the patient with an "experience of being understood and of being related to another human being" (O'Toole & Welt, 1989, p. 11).

The healing of mental illness usually takes more than medicine (Gebbard, 1992). Interpersonal relationships play a major role in the assessment and treatment of psychiatric symptoms. Patient education, an increasingly important dimension of psychiatric treatment, is far more successful when it is delivered by a knowledgeable health professional within the context of a trusting relationship. Thus, the therapeutic relationship forms "both the context and the means through which change occurs" (Fox, 1993, p. 111).

Social Relationships Compared With Therapeutic Relationships

Moving from the concept of a social relationship to a therapeutic relationship requires a thorough understanding of the similarities and differences between social and therapeutic relationships. Principles of relationships with psychiatric patients, regardless of diagnosis, originate with our understandings of what constitutes successful interpersonal relationships in everyday life.

Elements Common to Both

There are clear similarities between the qualities of successful relationships in everyday life and in psychiatric settings:

1. Acceptance
2. Respect
3. Genuineness
4. Mutual appreciation
5. Honesty

As any relationship develops, each person typically reveals more of who he or she is as a person, regardless of specific content. Both social and therapeutic relationships require similar levels of courtesy and respect for the person. Both depend on a sense of "mutuality, trust and partnership in a common situation" (Friedman, 1985, pp. 11–40). Therapeutic relationships depend on many of the same conversational techniques to facilitate the discussion. Theoretical and conceptual perspectives, however, establish the parameters of therapeutic relationships and clearly distinguish therapeutic relationships from all other types of relations between people.

Elements That Differ

There also are differences between therapeutic relationships and everyday relationships:

1. Purpose
2. Focus
3. Responsibility
4. Degree of self-disclosure
5. Level of personal involvement

Table 10–1 summarizes some of the differences between a social and a therapeutic relationship.

THERAPEUTIC RELATIONSHIPS

Definition of Therapeutic Relationships

A **therapeutic relationship** represents a time-bound alliance between nurse and patient, consciously entered into and characterized by respect, acceptance, empathy, and genuineness. Therapeutic relationships build on the premise that the resources for healing reside within the patient. Therapeutic relationships with the mentally ill can be complex because patients often struggle with issues of trust, and it is essential to earn that trust before the patient is able to take advantage of the help offered.

Therapeutic relationships embrace both the art and the science of nursing practice. Over time, nurses develop a style and philosophy of relationship development that reflects their personal values and beliefs about relationships and how they should interact with their patients. As with all other relationships, the unique nature and quality of the relationship depend on the particular qualities and commitment levels of its participants. The shifting demands of the interpersonal situation create challenges and opportunities for practicing new behaviors. How successfully you adapt communication principles to meet the individualized needs of patients represents the *art* of psychiatric nursing. Application of theoretical knowledge to development of the relationship process and achievement of expected treatment outcomes constitutes the *science* of psychiatric nursing. Both perspectives are equal and integral elements of successful nurse-patient relationships.

Nurse and patient bring into the relationship their own personalized perceptions of the world, community, and self. These perceptions greatly influence the meaning of the relationship, readiness to engage, and motiva-

---

TABLE 10–1 Some Differences Between a Social and a Therapeutic Relationship

SOCIAL RELATIONSHIP	THERAPEUTIC RELATIONSHIP
Encounters and interactions are spontaneous, with or without definite purpose.	Encounters and interactions have a definite health-related purpose.
Goals of relationships vary, and goal achievement may or may not be identifiable.	Goals of relationships directly link to achievement of health-related outcomes.
Relationships can last indefinitely, and there are no set criteria for ending them.	Relationships are time limited and terminate when outcomes are achieved.
Relationships ideally take into consideration the needs of both participants.	Focus of relationships is always on the patient and health-related needs and concerns.
Participants share responsibility for the structure and conduct of relationships.	Nurse assumes responsibility for the structure and conduct of relationships.
Self-disclosure is spontaneous and expected of both participants.	Self-disclosure by the patient is encouraged; self-disclosure by the nurse is limited.
Mutuality and personal involvement are limited only by the needs and desires of the participants and may include physical intimacy.	Mutuality and personal involvement in partnership are limited to meeting the identified goals of the relationship; physical intimacy is prohibited.

tion to maintain the relationship. Within the context of the relationship, nurse and patient agree to work together for a designated period to promote the patient's health and well-being. Therapeutic relationships provide a stable, safe place for self-exploration and mutual discussion because the focus, time, place, and responsibilities of the participants are laid out from the onset of the relationship and are carried through to its termination.

Typically, therapeutic relationships with mentally ill patients progress through distinct sequential phases, originally described by Peplau (1952) as orientation, working (identification and exploration), and termination (resolution). Phases of the relationship typically overlap, and, ideally, they reinforce the patient's progressive movement toward health.

Not all therapeutic relationships progress as a linear advance toward a desired outcome. Instead, the nurse and patient travel down a winding path, sometimes bumpy, sometimes smooth, at times uninteresting, and at other times embellished by human drama. The desired outcomes are off in the distance, known but not always readily visible. Although some therapeutic relationships extend for weeks or months, others take place over the span of an 8-hour work shift, and still others take place in a single 1-hour session.

Helping Process. The essence of a therapeutic relationship is the helping process. This process provides resources to help patients get in touch with their personal strengths in order to help themselves. The desired outcome for the relationship is not to change the person's personality but rather to enable the individual to make whatever changes are necessary to improve his or her quality of life. This is consistent with Peplau's (1992) belief that "the nurse does not have the power to change the behavior of patients" (p. 14).

Requirements for Establishing and Maintaining Growth-Producing Relationships. Establishing and maintaining growth-producing relationships require time, effort, and constant attention. In a therapeutic relationship, each person takes a position toward the other and the experiences as they unfold. Although nurses may have general knowledge of human behavior, each person stands as an individual personality, unique among human beings. Individual differences among patients exist. These must be accepted by the nurse.

What do you think? As you reflect on your own relationships, what are your strengths in relating to others? In what ways have your social relationships differed from therapeutic relationships with patients? Can you have a social relationship with a patient? Defend your answer. Have you ever been tamed? What does that mean to you?

➤ *Check Your Reading*
1. What is the essence of a therapeutic relationship and how do such relationships develop with psychiatric patients?
2. How do social relationships and therapeutic relationships differ?

Use of Self in Therapeutic Relationships

In contrast to many other forms of nursing practice in which knowledge of technical equipment and psychomotor skills are measures of competence, the basic tools and competencies of the nurse in psychiatric nursing center on the therapeutic use of self. *Therapeutic use of self* refers to the nurse's presence, "a physical 'being there,' and psychological 'being with' a patient for the purpose of meeting the patient's health care needs" (Gardner, 1992, p. 191). To effectively use the self as a tool, you should have a basic understanding of communication principles and an adequate knowledge base of common therapeutic disorders and interventions (Arnold & Boggs, 1995, 1999). Equally important is self-awareness (Rogers, 1951). Your knowledge of personal response patterns, strengths, and limitations can influence the interaction in positive ways because the more you know, the more leverage you have in responding.

Lack of self-awareness can pose serious problems in relationships. Therapeutic relationships with mentally ill patients symbolize an act of trust: the patient believes that you will continue the journey even in the face of serious obstacles. Sometimes patients behave in ways that are socially unacceptable; these behaviors may be personally offensive and in deep conflict with your social value system. In no other setting are you as likely to become the immediate target of idealizing, hostile, critical, dependent, and rejecting behaviors as in therapeutic relationships with the seriously mentally ill. Although it is possible to recognize the behavior as part of the mental disorder intellectually, it is not always easy to have the same understanding and acceptance emotionally. Without self-awareness, it becomes humanly impossible to accept the patient as a person regardless of his or her behavior. Yet this is exactly what needs to occur for healing. The nurse must become the patient's therapeutic ally: confronting when necessary, confirming always, being a steadfast companion on the journey to mental health.

Another reason for self-awareness in relationships with the mentally ill lies in the roller coaster effect of patient emotions that occur unpredictably and with regularity. It's important for you to be aware that you don't create these feelings, but that you may be the target for them as the patient displaces onto you emotions from past events and relationships.

Self-awareness helps keep the relationship honest. The process of self-reflection compels nurses to get in touch with their own value positions so that they do not project these positions onto others or reject those who do not share similar values. True acceptance of patients just as they are depends on your awareness of your own attitudes and behaviors in the relationship.

The effective use of self, coupled with self-awareness, helps the nurse to sort out unconscious feelings of **countertransference** and reduces the possibility of behaviors such as overprotection, manipulation, domination, or sexual attraction from compromising the work of the relationship. A byproduct of self-awareness

Primary Benefits of Self-Awareness in the Nurse-Patient Relationship

- Can help you respond therapeutically to difficult patient behaviors
- Facilitates full acceptance of patients
- Helps establish needed caring objectivity
- Makes it easier to separate what belongs to the patient and what belongs to you
- Increases your self-confidence, which enhances the quality of interactions

is self-confidence, which enhances your credibility as a helping person. Box 10-1 summarizes the primary benefits of self-awareness in the nurse-patient relationship.

Self-awareness actually begins unconsciously with a person's internal organization of life experiences. In the course of everyday living, people develop working models of how they should act, how they expect other people to act, and what they consider to be normal behavior. Rarely do people with major mental illnesses fit these working models. Their behaviors are erratic, unusual, and not easily understood. Self-awareness and the effective use of self in the therapeutic relationship must develop from a conscious and continuous reflection on your behavior and its possible impact on the patient and an understanding of how the patient's behavior influences you. Rogers (1958) posed 10 questions, outlined in Box 10-2, that you can use for self-reflection before beginning a patient-centered relationship. Each question directs you to look inward, to travel beyond technical competency to an understanding of the human connections between self and other.

Frameworks to Guide Therapeutic Relationships

Theoretical frameworks guide nursing practice and provide direction for interventions built on strong scientific rationales. Chapter 5 outlines theoretical models that serve as guides in mental health nursing. Three models of interpersonal process are briefly summarized here.

Nursing Framework

Hildegard Peplau (1952) conceptualized the relationship as an alliance between a helping professional and a patient, characterized by significant emotional bonds and connections. Essential to the development of the therapeutic relationship are specific caring behaviors.

First, professional knowledge and skills are required to work with the mentally ill patient. Included in your toolbox are an extensive understanding of the pathophysiology and pharmacology related to the treatment of mental illness. When combined with assessment, communication, teaching, and ethical and legal principles, these tools provide you with the knowledge base required of a psychiatric nurse.

Peplau (1952) stated that the second caring behavior is the need for attentiveness to the patient's experience. Third is the essential quality of positive connectedness that goes beyond the mere exchange of information and involves an emotional attachment of genuine interest to the patient's story. In every aspect of the relationship, you are a participant as well as an observer. Your attitudes, behaviors, and words must support the patient and give credence to the importance of the relationship. Otherwise, the patient's situation can never be fully explored.

The particular value of Peplau's model (1952) lies in her descriptions of the types of relationships desired in psychiatric nursing and in her careful delineation of the

Questions for Self-Reflection Before Beginning a Patient-Centered Relationship

- What are the personal and professional strengths that I bring to this relationship?
- In what ways could my personal life circumstances potentially get in the way of establishing or maintaining this relationship? In what ways might they be helpful?
- Can I understand that each patient's symptoms are a form of communication telling me something about his or her emotional pain?
- Can I comprehend how difficult it is for a patient who is hurting to share his or her deepest pain or to recognize self-imposed psychosocial-spiritual alienation from self and others?
- Can I grasp the characteristics of some patients with whom one intervention works and of those for whom another intervention works?

- What criteria will I use to know when to support a vulnerable patient and when to confront self-destructive behavior?
- How will I be able to maintain therapeutic neutrality and empathy in the face of intense emotions directed toward me or the patient's self-destructive behaviors?
- How do I sustain optimism and hope when progress is slow or seemingly nonexistent with the chronically mentally ill patient?
- How can I sincerely demonstrate confidence in my patient's capacity to develop a different meaningful way of life and to manage his or her own affairs?

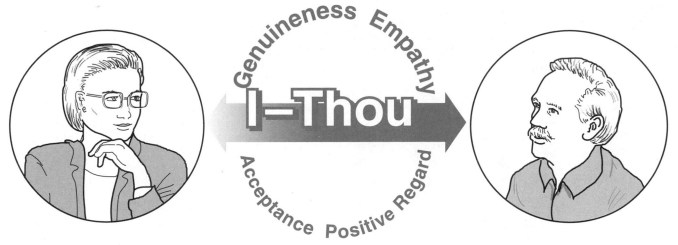

Figure 10-1
Buber's characteristics of a therapeutic relationship.

developmental stages of the therapeutic relationship (orientation, working [identification and exploitation], and resolution [termination] phases). Although Peplau articulated this model in the early 1950s, her model still provides the matrix for understanding relationships in psychiatric nursing as well as most other areas of professional nursing.

Psychological Framework

Carl Rogers' (1951) patient-centered model of therapeutic relationships is useful in several ways. His theory has a distinctly humanistic orientation (see Chapter 5). From the therapist's perspective, the model focuses on the patient as a person in the here and now; from the patient's perspective, the model focuses on how the patient feels he or she is subjectively experienced by the helping person in the relationship. Rogers insisted that people are capable of realizing their highest potential, a view consistent with nursing's goal to help the patient reach his or her optimal level of psychosocial functioning and personal independence. Rogers viewed the patient as an active participant as well as a recipient of care. He suggested that when given the appropriate feedback and encouragement, patients automatically seek self-actualization of their potential. Rogers considered attitudes held by the professional as conditions that are "necessary and sufficient" for therapeutic change. He labeled these empathy, genuineness, unconditional acceptance, and positive regard.

Existential Framework

Martin Buber's (1970) model emphasized the need for the nurse-patient relationship to be one of equal and respectful partnership, which Buber described as an "I-Thou" relationship. In this type of relationship, each participant experiences and values the other as a unique human being surrounded by a distinctive environmental background and possessing an original set of personal strengths, behaviors, and problems. The essence of an I-thou relationship is the mutual discovery of the other person's characteristic humanness (Figure 10–1). Buber suggested that actions performed with another and the experience of that other as a valued unique human being confirm his or her humanness in a meaningful way. Buber used the term *confirming communication* to refer to comments that recognize the individuality of the person and the term *disconfirming communication* to mean comments that fail to acknowledge the unique existence of the other. Nurses can unintentionally disconfirm psychiatric patients by discounting their comments as unimportant, by not picking up on themes, and by assuming they cannot take responsibility. Nurses confirm their patients each time they make a special effort to acknowledge and respond to their individualized needs. Even calling the patient by name confirms his or her unique individuality.

The specific helping skills you use differ with each therapeutic relationship. According to Buber, the basic assumptions of a therapeutic relationship are

- It is an I-thou relationship.
- Certain conditions of unconditional acceptance and positive regard, genuineness, and empathy are necessary for successful outcomes.
- The natural progression of the relationship follows definable stages that are valid for all relationships.

Conceptual Components of Therapeutic Relationships

No matter how skilled the nurse is in applying communication principles, the nature of the nurse's personal involvement is most important and is most likely to be remembered by the patient as the critical factor in treatment. Casement (1991) suggested that the patient's emotional experience of the relationship can be as important as the cognitive insights he or she gains about resolving mental conflicts. Rieman (1986) identified feeling valued as a unique human being, being listened to, and having one's thoughts and feelings understood by another human being as the most significant curative factors identified by patients in a phenomenological study of nurse-patient behaviors.

> **What do you think?** As you read over the three conceptual models of relationships, is there one that resonates with you? Have you ever participated in a therapeutic relationship in which you were the patient or recipient of services and someone else was the professional helper? If so, were the concepts described in the models apparent to you? How did you feel? Was the relationship helpful to you? If so, in what ways? If it was not helpful, why not?

► Check Your Reading

3. How does Peplau conceptualize the therapeutic relationship with mentally ill patients?
4. Describe Rogers' patient-centered model of therapeutic relationships.
5. What is the essence of Buber's approach to relationships with patients?

Use of Therapeutic Communication

Within the context of every nurse-patient relationship, the nurse accompanies the patient as a guide on a time-limited, exploratory journey that, ideally, leads to the patient's discovery of the inner self and its potential for healing emotional wounds. Therapeutic conversations represent the points of interpersonal connection, through which patients are able to tell the story of their journey and the nurse is able to provide encouragement, support, and resourceful information. As patients speak of their immediate experiences and the life events that led up to their current circumstances, they give voice to their fears, feelings, beliefs, hopes, desires, and private realities.

Mental illnesses create significant barriers to the development of common language. They affect the meaning of words and behaviors. Consequently, it is more difficult to use communication as meaningful points of intersection in the usual sense with these patients. They frequently live in fantasy worlds constructed of distorted and hidden meanings that defend them against being hurt, and their words serve as barriers instead of bridges to relationships. Research has shown that psychiatric patients have lessened interpersonal flexibility in their relationships, and their communication tends to miss its mark as a point of intersection. They report their experiences in ways that do not readily produce shared meanings. Mentally ill patients tend to generalize, embellish, delete, distort, omit data, or make shifts in their narratives so that it becomes difficult for others to follow their original experience. Additionally, they do not communicate on a feeling level as easily as mentally healthy people. Table 10-2 demonstrates common speech patterns found in chronically mentally ill patients.

TABLE 10–2 Common Speech Patterns Found in the Chronically Mentally Ill

PATTERN	DEFINITION	FOUND IN
Poverty of speech	Tendency to speak very little, to use one-word answers or phrases	Schizophrenia, depression, and acute situational stress
Pressured speech	Rapid speech with little change in intonation between ideas	Manic-depressive disorders, crisis situations, and anxiety disorders
Flight of ideas	Rapid switching from one idea to another, with little connection between them	Manic-depressive disorders and crisis situations
Thought blocking	Sudden stopping in the middle of a sentence, especially when it involves an anxiety-provoking thought	Global anxiety in most mental disorders, schizophrenic responses to internal stimuli, and cognitive mental disorders
Halting speech	Slow speech with little change in vocal intonation between ideas	Depressive and cognitive disorders and mental retardation
Circumstantial speech	Speech in which the details presented in the message and main point of the conversation have little or no relation to one another	Disorders involving emotionally difficult content, schizophrenia, and cognitive mental disorders
Loose associations	Speech in which there is an absence of logical connections between thoughts and ideas	Schizophrenic disorders
Echolalia	Repeating or echoing the sender's comments	Schizophrenic disorders
Confabulation	Filling in the blanks, replacing data with fantasy	Cognitive mental disorders
Word salad	Words put together that do not go together or make sense	Schizophrenic disorders
Neologisms	Nonsensical linking together of sounds	Schizophrenic disorders
Double bind	Two conflicting elements linked together in the same message	Dysfunctional communication

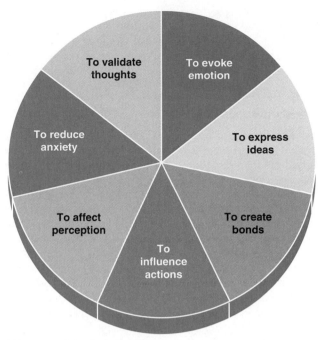

Figure 10-2
Some uses of words.

Before defining and discussing, in more depth, therapeutic communication, it is important to consider the types of communication used by the nurse as well as the patient.

Types of Communication

A major nursing role is to motivate patients to explore the vast potential of communication responses available to them. Nurses can then help patients develop the communication tools needed to reflect on their experiences in ways that enhance their development of critical life skills. Communication is divided into three distinct categories:

1. Verbal communication
2. Nonverbal communication
3. Metacommunication

Verbal Communication. Verbal communication refers to words, oral and written. Most people consider verbal and written communication to be the primary means of sharing experiences. People not only respond to the verbal communication of others but also affect it through the words they use. Thus, words have an action-oriented function as well as an information role. Figure 10-2 displays some of the many uses of words.

It is possible to misunderstand the meaning of a message or the intentions of the sender. Message confusion created by stress, distraction, or cultural interpretations can limit full comprehension, whereas cognitive disorders, psychosis, depressive negativity, or anxiety can more seriously modify the objective meaning of a message.

Nonverbal Communication. Nonverbal communication, according to Mehrabian (1972), accounts for at least 93% of the message transmission between people

(55% transmittal through body cues and another 38% through metacommunication). Only 7% of a person's message is actually transmitted through words. People use a wide variety of nonverbal behaviors to enhance, disguise, negate, or modify their verbal messages. In fact, the meaning of communication is interpreted primarily through nonverbal, rather than verbal, communication (Crowther, 1991). Nonverbal communication modifies spoken words in a variety of ways:

• By reinforcing or contradicting them
• By emphasizing or diminishing their importance
• By identifying or underlining the emotion associated with them

The expression of nonverbal behaviors can be conscious or unconscious. Some behaviors are within the person's control, for example, handshaking, smiling, and nodding one's head. Other behaviors are clearly not within the person's control; blushing, facial tics, shaking, sweating, and heart palpitations are primarily involuntary physiological responses that communicate meaning.

Nonverbal communication behaviors can send several conflicting messages at the same time. For example, smiling while pulling back from the other person in an interaction or looking at one's watch can send mixed signals, even though the body posture and words may indicate attention. When the nonverbal component of the message contradicts the verbal, most people tend to pay more attention to the nonverbal behaviors because they are less likely to be under the voluntary control of the sender (Taylor, Meyer, Rosegrant, & Samples, 1989). Unfortunately, nonverbal communication behaviors are also more likely to be misinterpreted. Validation of the meaning of nonverbal behaviors is always essential. Nonverbal behaviors of openness, presence, and attention in the form of eye contact and an interested, friendly facial expression invite the patient to participate in the relationship as much as the actual words.

Metacommunication. Metacommunication is communication *about* the communication or lack thereof. Watzlawick, Beavin, and Jackson (1967) suggested that one cannot *not* communicate. Even when words are not spoken, people communicate with one another in a myriad of ways. As an integral but implicit part of the message, metacommunication represents the interpersonal bridge between the verbal and nonverbal components of communication. Metacommunication relates to expectations, influence of emotions, attention, and bias of attitudes and values. Metacommunication is emotionally based and emphasizes the relationship aspect, rather than the content, of the message.

Metacommunication aids the receiver in accurately interpreting the emotional meaning of the content. Examples of metacommunication include speech patterns and vocalizations.

Definition of Therapeutic Communication

Therapeutic communication is defined as a form of communication with a health-related purpose that develops as a continuous interaction between nurse and patient, both of whom contribute to its nature and progression. Therapeutic communication principles derive from theoretical models of social communication. Table 10–3 summarizes important differences between social and therapeutic communication. Therapeutic communication becomes a dialogue in which the nurse helps patients look at information from different perspectives and then helps them to develop appropriate responses to the irrational beliefs, thoughts, and feelings that imprison them.

Purpose of Therapeutic Communication

The primary purpose of therapeutic communication is to help patients come to know themselves in ways that allow them to recognize possibilities in their lives and to alter ineffective life patterns (Wachtel, 1993). The nurse's role in the communication process is to help patients transform vague, tangential, or distorted statements into clear, concrete, workable statements that have a common meaning to both. The nurse uses these mutually developed statements as the basis for therapeutic intervention. In the course of discussion, patients learn to make sense out of the ways in which they behave. The nurse enlists the patients as collaborators in the process of self-discovery and uses words, actions, and knowledge to help patients develop a more positive view of themselves and more adaptive ways of interacting in the world (Havens, 1986).

Responsibilities of the Nurse in Therapeutic Communication

The primary responsibility for the structure and conduct of the relationship lies with the nurse. It is the patient's role to do most of the talking. You are responsible for creating the type of interpersonal environment needed for full disclosure of difficult issues and feelings. This includes maintaining boundaries, making sure therapeu-

tic conversations are purposeful and related to identified health-related goals, documenting important information, and developing relevant interdisciplinary care plans with other health team members.

Role of Self-Disclosure in Therapeutic Communication

Self-disclosure can be a highly effective communication tool, if it is used appropriately. Self-disclosure by the nurse of relevant but neutral personal experiences, observations, and feelings is an informational source that the patient can appreciate within a shared human encounter. Appropriate self-disclosure draws the participants together in a mutual experience, enhances trust, and provides a more equal relationship (Ivey, 1988).

Guidelines determine the suitability of self-disclosure. For optimal effectiveness, the nurse's self-disclosure must fit the demands of the situation and the needs of the patient. Sharing personal information that is not directly related to the goals of the relationship serves to distract from rather than enhance goal achievement. Self-disclosures that are pertinent but suggestive of behaviors that the patient cannot achieve not only miss their mark but also can increase anxiety. Similarly, data of an intensely personal experience, even though relevant, may make the patient uncomfortable. For example, sharing a rape experience or an abuse experience may not be appropriate, even though the patient initially brings up the topic.

With self-disclosure, the needs of the patient should be the focus of conversation. You also need to be sensitive to each patient's readiness, vulnerability, and cultural background before sharing personal information. The nurse's self-disclosure of personal feelings about the patient may be appropriate in certain circumstances. In general, this type of self-disclosure should be more about the behavior or clearly evidenced personal characteristics of the patient. Using "I statements" and

---

TABLE 10–3 Important Differences Between Social and Therapeutic Communication

SOCIAL COMMUNICATION	THERAPEUTIC COMMUNICATION
Communication can occur at any time and is not time limited.	Communication occurs within designated time frames and terminates when therapeutic goals are achieved.
Responsibility for the structure and conduct of the conversation is the responsibility of both parties.	Responsiblity for the structure and conduct of the conversation is ultimately the nurse's.
Communication is spontaneous and not necessarily goal directed.	Communication is purposeful and directed toward mutually established goals.
The needs and concerns of both partners can receive equal consideration.	The focus of the conversation is always on the needs and concerns of the patient.
The purpose is for both parties to achieve greater intimacy in the relationship.	The purpose is for the patient to achieve greater self-understanding from the relationship.
Self-disclosure of the details of private life is acceptable for both parties.	Self-disclosure of the nurse's private life is limited and acceptable only under certain circumstances.
Social decorum and adherence to the rules of etiquette are expected.	Conversation does not always reflect adherence to the rules of social etiquette.
Can continue spontaneously at any time, depending on the desires of the participants.	Formally terminates with the end of the session or relationship.

verbs that express your feelings are particularly appropriate, for example, "I think you have made significant progress during your hospitalization, particularly with (give examples)." Statements such as "One of the things I like best about you is your dry sense of humor" or "Right now, I am feeling that you are trying to shut me out by closing your eyes and appearing to sleep" give patients information about the way their behavior affects others. Personal feelings of a deeper nature, either positive or negative, are not appropriate to share. Evaluative self-disclosures such as "I'm very proud of you," "You're my favorite patient," or "I'm so disappointed that you couldn't stay sober over the weekend" are more closely related to the nurse's ego than the patient's behavior. They tend to diminish the patient and compromise your effectiveness.

> **W**hat do you think? Do you think it is appropriate for nurses to share personal information with patients? If so, under what circumstances? When would it be inappropriate?

Preparing the Details for a Therapeutic Interaction

The physical setting, timing, and therapeutic approach all can influence the sending and receiving of effective communication.

Physical Setting

Self-disclosure occurs most easily in a private setting. Usually, it is best to use the same room for each session, away from the mainstream of activity. If there are limited options when choosing the most appropriate place for an interaction, picking the quietest place within the large day room is the place to start. The patient's bedroom is usually not an appropriate place because this is the patient's personal space.

Interactions that take place from a side by side sitting position rather than directly face to face are sometimes easier for the mentally ill patient to tolerate. Communicating from a position in which both participants are at eye level with each other is more effective than conducting the conversation from unequal physical stations (Argyle, 1975). If more than the patient is to be involved, you as the nurse should decide whether the patient is to be the primary informant. Others are asked to hold their comments until they are asked. If the interview is a family-group experience in which all participants can contribute equally, the session should be structured with this expectation.

Time

Time is an important variable to consider when planning for a therapeutic interaction. Determining the amount of therapy that can be accomplished in the time available, checking resources that may be required, and leaving enough time for summarizing the session are all important considerations. The initial interview will take longer than subsequent sessions because you and the patient are unfamiliar with each other. The length and timing of the interventions are dependent on the degree of development of the relationship and the current circumstances.

Timing is important from two perspectives. First is the issue of allowing enough time for the person's message to be fully articulated. This involves approaching your patient gently and allowing the patient to tell stories in his or her own manner. Second, in working with a mentally ill patient, it is particularly important to avoid overloading his or her "circuits" because processing information may take longer than in patients who are not mentally ill. Presenting one idea at a time and waiting until the patient demonstrates some readiness to hear your messages, especially when significant change is required, are important.

Therapeutic Approach

Focusing on the therapeutic approach is another consideration. Successful communication is dependent on your ability to learn your patient's language, to reflect accurately on the nature of his or her feelings, and to verbally convey words and ideas in a conversational format that is easily understood by the patient. You need to draw on a broad spectrum of verbal and nonverbal behaviors to respond effectively to the often disjointed conversations of a mentally ill patient.

CONVERSATIONAL FLEXIBILITY

Conversational flexibility takes many forms because patients come from many walks of life and with a variety of life experiences. The patient's readiness, educational level, and ability to assimilate new information are also determinants in structuring the relationship and planning the most appropriate interventions.

PATIENT'S BEHAVIOR

Another important consideration in choosing a therapeutic approach is the patient's behavior. For example, the patient's mood may fluctuate within the same conversation, beginning with congeniality, moving into anger, and ending in tears. Pauses, silences, and even the pacing of messages can provide cues to the types of modifications you need to make in response to a patient's behavior. By carefully observing the patient, you can notice subtle changes, such as the patient's voice tightening, quavering, or catching with discussion of emotionally difficult material. These observations help you to know when to press for more information, when to back off because the patient is not ready to deal with the material, and when to make an observation about the patient's emotional expression.

CULTURAL INFLUENCES ON COMMUNICATION

Learning the patient's interpersonal language and style becomes even more of a challenge when nurse and patient are of two different cultures (Campinha-Bocote, 1988; Narayan, 1997) (See Chapter 12 for a more complete discussion of culture.) Culture has a powerful effect on language, not only on the words but also on the structure and nuances of communication. Language has a basic structure and a strong linkage to the reality it seeks to explain, which sometimes is not readily translatable into another language. Words in different languages may mean the same thing, or they may mean something completely different. Grammar, vocal tone, verbal inflections, and body language may be understood by one culture as having one meaning and may have the opposite meaning in another culture. For example, eye contact in Western cultures signifies openness and connection. In some Eastern cultures and with American Indian patients, direct eye contact is viewed as a sign of disrespect or aggression. For Mexican and black patients, averting the eyes is a normal behavior when a person is listening, particularly if the person is receiving a reprimand. It does not signal lack of attention. Nodding the head and simultaneously smiling usually means agreement with the speaker's ideas in Western cultures, but it is simply a polite gesture in Asian cultures. Hall (1966), in his multicultural research of space use, noted that Americans typically stand closer to each other than people from England or Germany, whereas Middle Eastern cultures typically permit even closer interpersonal contact.

The cultural impact on language expression varies within the culture as well as among cultures. One person may choose to retain many parts of his or her original culture. Another may take on the aspects of the new culture or may integrate the new with the old. Others may reject or deny their cultural origins. Consideration of a person's cultural background should include attention to the individual expression of cultural beliefs as well as to common expectations for cultural behaviors.

Culture influences behavior in terms of a shared knowledge, belief system, and values that transcend location and time. A person's cultural heritage is traceable through its origins to ethnic roots, historical and political ideology, religion, family, social class, and occupation. Some cultures prescribe a limited range of behaviors and frames of reference for behavior. For example, Asian patients typically use a formal way of relating, with strict formal codes of conduct. Americans tend to relate with more equality in language style among men and women than those of Asian and Hispanic descent.

Frequently, communication conflicts arise because of differences in fundamental cultural beliefs or because of cultural stereotyping, which increases during times of stress. Table 10–4 provides examples of culture-bound mental illnesses.

What do you think? Because culture is such an important consideration, should we make every attempt to provide the patient with caregivers of the same cultural background? Defend your answer.

➤ *Check Your Reading*
6. Define the meaning and purpose of therapeutic communication.
7. Discuss some rules for self-disclosure that the nurse should know and follow.
8. In what ways does culture influence therapeutic communication?

Strategies for Therapeutic Communication

Therapeutic communication strategies consist of two distinct categories, both of which are equally necessary in conversations with patients:

1. Therapeutic listening
2. Verbal and nonverbal intervention strategies

Therapeutic listening skills have been identified as the most important communication tool that nurses use with psychiatric patients. Verbal intervention strategies develop from information obtained through active listening. Without nonverbal interventions to complement and support verbal interaction, the message is only half heard. Nonverbal intervention strategies, such as touch and body language, ideally complete nurses' verbal interventions (Arnold & Boggs, 1995).

Using Active Listening

Kemper (1992) defined the process of **therapeutic (active) listening** as

an interpersonal, confirmation process involving all the senses in which the therapist attends with empathy to

TABLE 10–4 Culture-Bound Mental Illnesses	
CULTURAL GROUP	**CULTURE-BOUND ILLNESS**
Hispanic	*Susto* (soul loss): Caused by a severe fright. When the fright occurs, the spirit captures the soul of the victim. Symptoms include anorexia, apathy, depression, and withdrawal.
African American	*Voodoo illness:* Caused by a supernatural magical hex from which the person cannot escape. Symptoms include nausea, vomiting, diarrhea, or bizarre behavioral symptoms. Carried to an extreme, it can result in voodoo death.
Asian	*Hsieh-ping:* A trance state created by the possession of the victim's body by dead relatives.

Adapted from Campinha-Bacote, J. (1988). Culturological assessment: An important factor in psychiatric consultation-liaison nursing. *Archives of Psychiatric Nursing, 2,* 2410–2450.

TABLE 10-5 Characteristics of Active Listening

Active listening is purposeful. It can provide patients with feedback about themselves of which they are unaware.

Active listening requires attentiveness. Patients' messages are decoded from auditory cues, observations of behaviors, and attention to underlying themes.

Active listening is focused. Focused listening requires full concentration on behaviors and spoken words, without the element of judgment.

Active listening is personal and about shared experiences. This requires observation for verbal and nonverbal content, and congruence between the spoken and feeling dimensions of the message.

Active listening is a process of dialogue. As the patient's story is told, the events of his or her human journey unfold, and with the facts, feelings are helped to emerge.

the patient's verbal and nonverbal messages to facilitate the understanding, synthesis and interpretation of the patient's situation. (p. 22)

Therapeutic listening consists of an active interpersonal give-and-take response process. All of the active listening strategies presented in this chapter are designed to achieve the dual outcome of getting enough information for a comprehensive understanding of the patient's real message and acknowledging the person who is speaking. Active listening responses are deliberately designed to expand, clarify, and verify the content of the message and the intentions of the sender. Table 10-5 outlines some of the principal characteristics of active listening.

Facilitating Active Communication

Active communication responses help bring the patient's story to life. The story of the journey is sometimes told in a voice filled with earnestness, passion, and authenticity; other times, the narrative slowly unfolds, sounding curiously limp and narrow. Usually it is a complicated story, and if you listen well, it is possible to recognize and understand the patient's story as a richly complicated and intriguing account of a human being. Therapeutic conversations provide points of intersection through which patients can enlarge and better understand their self-reflections.

For the process of active communication, nurses usually ask questions, use minimal encouragers, and use clarification for data collection. **Clarification** entails asking the patient to expand and elaborate on incomplete or inadequate data or to make conflicting responses clearer. These strategies encourage the patient to move into deeper content and can expand the patient's awareness of important material. Listening responses should directly relate to the patient's comments. Phrasing your response in the patient's vocabulary and at the patient's developmental level of understanding facilitates ease of dialogue and, consequently, greater understanding.

USING MINIMAL ENCOURAGERS
Minimal encouragers are defined as simple leads into a conversation that provide the patient with cues through body actions; vocalizations; or short phrases, such as "go on" or "let's hear more," to continue talking.

They demonstrate personal interest in what the patient is saying without biasing the patient's responses. For example, you might use eye contact to demonstrate that the patient has your full attention. Looking directly at someone when he or she is speaking conveys concentration to most Americans. Maintaining eye contact decreases distraction from other thoughts. Leaning forward also indicates interest. Vocalizations such as "um" and "ah" and nonverbal encouragers such as nodding and smiling result in increased information flow because they send a nonverbal message of approval that positively reinforces the speaker.

ASKING QUESTIONS
If nurses are to understand their patients, they need to ask questions about what they are hearing and validate the accuracy of their inferences. The nurse uses questions as a primary listening response to elicit more information, demonstrate empathy, and show respect for the patient's thoughts and feelings. Questions have an implicit value in that they allow a patient, in providing answers, an opportunity to think things through out loud. As patients hear themselves speak, they develop different understandings, and new insights can emerge. Hearing immediate feedback from the nurse, coupled with the nurse's skillful use of questions to elicit deeper understanding and greater detail, often helps patients solve their own problems with minimal verbal intervention from the nurse. Excessive use of questioning, however, can interrupt the flow of the conversation. As much as possible, the patient should take the lead in telling his or her story.

Three types of questions, open-ended, closed, and focused, help develop the patient's story.

Open-Ended Questions. **Open-ended questions** are similar to those asked on an essay test and frequently begin with "What?" "How?" "When?" "Why?" "Can you tell me?" or "Can you give me an example?" Open-ended questions give the patient the most latitude in answering. The patient has the opportunity to answer the question as he or she chooses, which may more accurately reflect the patient's immediate concerns. Sometimes, it is appropriate to use a cluster of open-ended questions to get full details about a situation:

Nurse: "You say you feel as if you aren't able to do your work. Can you give me an example of what you mean?"

Patient: "I just can't seem to concentrate, and I can't anticipate the next step."

Nurse: "How does that seem to occur?"

Patient: "There are some days when I go into work and I just can't get anything done. I know what I want to do, but I just can't seem to get my brain in gear."

Nurse: "What is it like when your brain isn't in gear?"

Patient: "I feel confused, and I start projects, but then something distracts me and I don't finish my work."

Closed-Ended Questions. By contrast, **closed-ended questions** are those that directly ask for a specific answer. They offer the receiver a narrow range of response options: "Yes" or "No," "Either this or that," for example. Closed-ended questions are similar in format to multiple-choice tests, in which there is a limited scope of predetermined answers from which to choose. Although closed-ended questions are restrictive, they are quite useful in some situations. For example, they can reinforce an implicit assumption:

Nurse: "So, when you are with your drinking buddies, you really feel like you belong?"

Closed-ended questions can be used to focus the patient on two conflicting parts of an ambiguous statement:

Nurse: "I'm still not clear; are you saying that your parents are opposed to your giving up your job or that they just don't care?"

Focused Questions. A third type of questioning involves focused questions. **Focused questions** are partially open-ended questions that directly ask about specific parts of the data. Used to target information, focused questions are more limited than open-ended questions, but they require more than a simple "Yes" or "No," "Right" or "Wrong" answer. For example, instead of using a closed-ended question to follow up after a patient says that he has trouble "anticipating the next step," the nurse might ask him, "What happens when you try to anticipate the next step?" or "Are there any situations in which anticipating the next step is easier [harder] than others?"

Advantages to All Types of Questions. There are advantages to using all three types of questions. Open-ended questions encourage the most spontaneous answers. Closed-ended questions are useful when immediate information is needed in a situation or when the patient's responses characteristically are so tangential that no information is forthcoming. Closed-ended questions sometimes provide a comfortable lead-in for patients who have trouble being verbally expressive. Focused questions bring forward details about more general information.

In general, questions should begin with items or issues that are nonthreatening and easy to answer. You might open the dialogue with a patient by asking, "How can I help you?" or "Can you tell me a little about what brought you into the hospital?" or simply "Where would you like to start?" Although questions are an important listening response strategy, they should be used judiciously and tactfully. Otherwise, the dialogue can sound more like an inquisition to the patient.

Other techniques of active listening that invite active communication are restating, reflecting, paraphrasing, clarifying, using silence, and summarizing. These are outlined in Table 10–6, with definitions and examples of how to use them.

W*hat do you think?* How do you respond to questions? Does it depend on the type of

TABLE 10–6 Common Strategies for Active Listening

STRATEGY	DEFINITION	SAMPLE STATEMENT
Restating	Repeating part or all of the patient's statement, often with an introductory phrase about the purpose of the restatement	"Let's see if I understand: [followed by the patient's statement]." "Are you saying that: [followed by the patient's statement]."
Reflecting	Identifying the feelings associated with the patient's statement	"It sounds as if you feel bad that your mother didn't visit." "You sound very discouraged."
Paraphrasing	Selectively rewording part of the patient's message to reflect your understanding	*Patient:* "I feel like I don't have a niche anywhere." *Nurse:* "It's hard to figure out where you fit in?"
Clarifying	Directly asking the patient for information not contained in the original message	"Can you give me an example of what you mean by . . . ." "In what ways . . . ?"
Using silence	Deliberately pausing briefly in the dialogue	
Summarizing	Making a statement that synthesizes the meanings of several messages	"Today we talked about . . . ." "So it sounds as if you would find it difficult to ask your parents for the money for several reasons . . . ."

question? Does it depend on who the questioner is? Are there some questions that you find effective in eliciting conversation? How will you integrate active listening and active communication techniques into your nursing "bag of tricks"?

➤ *Check Your Reading*

9. What are some of the characteristics of active listening?
10. Explain how using minimal encouragers and questions can facilitate more active communication on the part of the patient.
11. What are the three types of questions used during therapeutic interactions?

USING THERAPEUTIC VERBAL INTERVENTIONS

Therapeutic verbal interventions require a proactive role in helping patients learn new behaviors. When the patient demonstrates reduced involvement in the treatment process, movement toward identified goals seems stalled, the patient becomes resistant, or the patient seems to have exhausted his or her personal resources, you will have to use this more proactive approach. Examples of these verbal interventions are outlined next.

Reinforcing Strengths. It is important to work from the patient's strengths and to minimize problem areas. People grow more from developing their strengths than from developing an awareness of their weaknesses (Ivey, 1988). The patient's strengths can include personal characteristics. Cooperation with treatment, persistence in the face of adversity, a sense of humor, and intellect are all examples of positive assets that the patient can use to facilitate personal change (Ferguson & Campinha-Bacote, 1989).

Although people learn from negative feedback, constructive feedback is more likely to be received favorably if an acknowledgment of the patient's strengths accompanies it. Including the patient's strengths in the feedback forces the patient to consider the healthier side of the personality as an ally in counteracting the more uncertain maladaptive aspects of behavior.

Confronting and Setting Limits. At times, patients may, because of their illness and feelings of low self-esteem, become hostile, verbally abusive, or seductive. When such a situation occurs, the nurse needs to set appropriate limits. For example, you might say, "Jack, I'm not trying to give you a hard time, but I think it is important for us to both work toward the same goal. How do you think we might do that?" or "Josette, your urine revealed alcohol and drug use. I'm worried that you won't be able to continue with the program if you have another such urine test. What do you think we should do?" Clear limits always must be placed on destructive or divisive self-expressions that threaten self or others. Scapegoating, excessive blame of self or others, emotional withdrawal, and aggressive threats to self or others need to be addressed directly and contained, if necessary (Cotton, Drake, Whitaker, & Potter, 1983).

Patients need reassurance that the staff members will decisively move to contain any self-destructive behaviors. It is helpful to identify, in a calm, matter-of-fact tone, the underlying emotions, fantasies, and fears that destructive self-expressions evoke. (Chapter 35 describes specific techniques for communicating with violent patients in psychiatric settings.)

Giving Constructive Feedback. Nurses use constructive feedback to help people change distorted patterns of thinking, feeling, and behavior. The purpose of feedback is to help a mentally ill patient realistically appraise his or her situation and the role the patient plays in maintaining or changing it. Used therapeutically, feedback can strengthen a person's resource pool in meeting difficult challenges by suggesting alternative options. Feedback can be used to correct misunderstandings or to provide facts about behaviors in need of change.

Feedback may have to be conveyed with strong language. The manner in which you deliver constructive feedback and the tact with which you address the patient's problems are critical. You should present reasonable consequences and practical feedback to the patient that take into account not only the behavior of the patient but also the context, intent, and alternative explanations for the situation. It is important to find out the precise nature of the problem before proceeding with the feedback.

Redirecting. **Redirection** is a communication strategy in which you refocus the patient from a tangential train of thought to a more precise discussion of the topic at hand. The strategy is useful when

- The patient has obvious self-destructive or divisive expressions of feeling, and talking about the feelings does not reduce anxiety.
- You and the patient are stuck in a cycle of repetitive dialogue, with no forward movement toward identified goals.

People tend to talk about those things that bring them pleasure and to avoid topics that cause them discomfort. By changing the conversational flow to the areas the patient needs to discuss, you can both broaden and deepen the patient's perspective on important life issues.

Redirecting the conversation should not force the issue or corner the patient. Rather, the strategy calls the patient's attention to feelings and issues that might not otherwise be available to him or her.

Modeling. **Modeling** occurs as a conscious demonstration of a behavior. Through role-playing and direct verbal intervention or through actions designed to shape the patient's behavior, the nurse models effective behaviors.

Role-playing is an active, conscious form of modeling in which the patient practices desired patterns of behavior with you before employing them in real-life situations. This communication strategy is particularly useful with patients who have social skill deficits.

Another form of role-playing for the patient who is reluctant to engage fully in the therapeutic process is for you to walk him or her through the steps verbally. For example, the nurse might say to the patient, "I wonder if you could just talk me through how you are going to keep your temper in check the next time you really feel frustrated?" As the patient talks, the nurse can identify potential difficulties with the plan, reinforce positive behaviors, and develop more appropriate coping techniques with the patient.

Modeling of appropriate feelings must be done gently, with respect for the feelings of the patient and the context of the situation.

Humor. **Humor** is a resource both nurse and patient use to ease an overly intense moment, put situations into perspective, and share connected moments. Humor cuts through defensiveness. Typically, humor is contagious and can provide new insights. It allows people to see themselves more objectively and at a distance.

Offering Information. This can be a part of the therapeutic verbal intervention used with psychiatric patients. The goal of offering information is to help patients learn new things and, through knowledge, attain competency. Information is more likely to be retained if it is understandable and acceptable to the patient. Box 10–3 identifies important elements of offering information to the patients.

> ***What do you think?*** As you learn about various communication strategies, how would you evaluate your own communication ability? Are you an effective communicator? Do you give constructive feedback? Are you comfortable with setting limits and confronting? What skills do you need to practice? Can you think of situations in which humor was helpful? In which it was not helpful? What were the differences?

➤ *Check Your Reading*

12. Of the therapeutic verbal interventions just outlined, in what situations would the nurse confront and set limits with the patient?
13. Name at least three important elements to remember when attempting to offer information to patients.

Barriers to Therapeutic Communication

Barriers to communication can occur both within the patient and within the nurse.

BARRIERS WITHIN THE PATIENT

Communication does not achieve its desired outcomes when the patient is not committed to making changes in behavior. In attempting to discover the barriers to communication within a given patient, the nurse needs to answer the following questions through the assessment:

1. Is the patient emotionally invested in wanting to make changes?
2. Does change lie within the patient's control?
3. Does the patient have the cognitive ability to hear and understand the meaning of the message?

4. Does the patient have the capacity to pay attention for the required length of the conversation, or is he or she experiencing hallucinations, delusions, or attention deficits?
5. Is the patient able to think clearly and critically about the information presented?

You, the psychiatric nurse, must enlist the patient's interest. When the topic under discussion has personal relevance, the patient is more inclined to pay close attention. The patient is likely to discount or not listen to topics that have little meaning to him or her or that he or she interprets negatively.

Internal sensory inputs, such as hallucinations, illusions, and delusions, may decrease the patient's ability to process information. They are mentioned in this chapter as a barrier to communication and are also referred to in Chapter 24, which addresses thought disorder.

BARRIERS WITHIN THE NURSE

When student nurses begin to interact with psychiatric patients, they usually experience anxiety about what they will say and how the patient is likely to respond. It is important for the student to know that the person behind the symptom almost always benefits from having a human encounter marked by respect, even if the communication is less than perfect. The key to communicating successfully with patients is to be extremely patient and to seek ways of demonstrating, through words and actions, that the patient is a person of value.

Mistakes in communication are a concern to the nurse. It is important to remember the following:

1. The patient responds to your communication as a whole.
2. Communication takes place within the larger context of a caring relationship.
3. Communication is a process and not an event; misunderstandings will arise and can be corrected.

Box 10–3 ■ ■ ■ ■ ■

Important Elements of Offering Information to Patients

- Assess what the patient already knows, patient readiness, and patient ability to learn.
- Use familiar terminology.
- Build on what the patient already knows.
- Present one idea at a time in a logical sequence.
- Provide concrete examples of abstract ideas.
- Repeat important ideas and concepts.
- Provide time for practice.
- Use return demonstrations and validation to evaluate comprehension.
- Provide positive reinforcement and corrective suggestions.
- Give the patient written instructions when needed.

TABLE 10-7 Common Errors That Nurses Make in Communicating With Patients

ERROR	DESCRIPTION	EXAMPLES
Giving unsupported (false) reassurance	Using pseudocomforting phrases in an attempt to offer reassurance	"It will be okay." "Everything will work out."
Giving advice	Making a decision for a client; offering personal opinions; telling a client what he should do; using phrases such as "ought to," "should do"	"I feel you should, . . ." "If I were you I would . . ."
Making false inferences	Making an unsubstantiated assumption about what a client means; interpreting his or her behavior without asking for validation; jumping to conclusions	"What you really mean is you don't like your doctor." "Subconsciously, you are blaming your husband for the accident."
Moralizing	Expressing your own personal values about what is right and wrong, especially on a topic that concerns the client	"Abortion is wrong." "It is wrong to refuse to have that operation."
Value judgments	Conveying your approval or disapproval about the client's behavior or about what he has said; using words such as "good," "bad," or "nice"	"That really wasn't a nice way to behave." "She's a good patient."
Using social responses	Making polite superficial comments that do not focus on what the client is feeling or on what he or she is trying to say; using clichés	"Isn't that nice?" "Hospital rules, you know." "Just do what the doctor says." "It's a beautiful day."

Modified from Arnold, E., & Boggs, K. (1995). *Interpersonal relationships: Professional communication skills for nurses* (2nd ed., p. 225). Philadelphia: W. B. Saunders.

Often, the working through of misunderstandings creates the strongest potential for healing. It's not as important to be a perfect communicator as it is to be a sensitive professional human guide who is committed to understanding and helping a human traveler who temporarily has lost his or her way. Communication is an art and as such requires practice and attention to detail. Some of the more common errors nurses make in communicating with their patients are presented in Table 10-7.

NURSING INTERVENTIONS TO MINIMIZE BARRIERS TO THERAPEUTIC COMMUNICATION

To avoid barriers in communication, you can

1. Do reality checks of your personal biases in communication. If you note bias, you can seek supervision to correct attitudes and perceptions that get in the way of the relationship.

2. Make statements of observations about behavior rather than inferences.

3. Reflect only what you observe and then only within the context of your competency level.

4. Focus listening responses and feedback on the ideas and feelings that the patient shares.

5. Focus feedback on the behaviors rather than the person.

6. Use description rather than evaluation statements about the patient or his or her actions.

7. Frequently validate the accuracy of observations and interpretations of data.

*W*hat do you think? What are your concerns regarding talking to psychiatric patients? How will you handle that experience?

► *Check Your Reading*

14. List at least three barriers to communication the nurse might encounter with a psychiatric patient.

15. What are some common errors nurses can make when communicating with psychiatric patients?

16. Identify one nursing intervention that could minimize the barriers to therapeutic communication created by the nurse?

Establishing Boundaries

Boundaries mark a symbolic separation between people that makes it possible for them to experience their own reality in a unique way and to understand the nature of others. People with well-defined boundaries know who they are and what is important to them. People with loose boundaries usually have difficulty separating their issues and needs from those of others. Boundaries surround social relationships with invisible lines drawn to define space, time, and type of appropriate interaction. They spell out the limits of behavior in relationships. Boundary violations found in everyday life include sexual harassment, moving too close to a person, sharing confidential information, entering a person's room, going through a person's possessions, and taking advantage of a person's inability to say "no" to unreasonable demands.

Personal and interpersonal boundaries are an issue with mentally ill patients, who have either nebulous boundaries or fixed boundaries that do not allow other people to know them. Boundaries are particularly important for the seriously mentally ill, who feel they are vulnerable to attack and misunderstanding any time they actively engage in a relationship with another person. Boundaries are extremely important in therapeutic relationships because they help establish the patient as separate from the nurse and the nurse as neither controlling nor controllable by the patient. Patients appreciate interpersonal boundary limits that are realistic, negotiated in advance, and matter-of-factly enforced with adequate firmness and respect for their personal integrity. Box 10–4 presents guidelines for the development of appropriate boundaries in nurse-patient relationships.

Factors That Enhance Therapeutic Relationships

ADVOCACY

Advocacy is a broad concept that Peplau (1952) recognized as an essential role for the psychiatric nurse. Mentally ill patients need nurses to speak for them. Often, these patients cannot identify their personal problems or communicate their needs effectively. Tanner, Benner, Chesla, and Gordon (1993) described advocates "as persons who stand along side of and empower patients and their families to have a voice when they are weak and vulnerable" (p. 278). Nurses advocate for their patients when they speak on behalf of the mentally ill to ensure adequate access to needed mental health services. Coaching patients to define themselves and to articulate their needs step by step is a form of advocating for the full potential of the patient.

CARING

The therapeutic relationship between nurse and patient in mental health settings is first and foremost a significant human relationship, of which the hallmark is caring. **Caring** is an intangible interactive process with physical, psychosocial, and spiritual dimensions that finds expression through actions designed to promote the health and well-being of patients. Caring represents a gift of self. In a study of patient perceptions of caring behaviors, Brown (1993) found that patients valued personalized care, in which their individualized needs were addressed.

Caring behaviors can develop only in a climate of respect for the uniqueness of the other. Respect for each person represents a perspective of caring that many psychiatric patients have not experienced as a part of their journey before meeting the nurse. The interventions are simple. Patients experience caring by being treated as people worthy of being taken seriously, by having their thoughts and feelings listened to with compassion, and by receiving competent attention to their needs from a professional person—with no strings attached.

Complicating the issue of what caring means to the patient is the realization that the concept varies from culture to culture. For example, a Vietnamese patient would view sharing with the family unit as important, whereas an American patient would view sharing with

---

Box 10–4 ■ ■ ■ ■ ■

Guidelines for the Development of Appropriate Boundaries in Nurse-Patient Relationships

Do	Do Not
• Establish set times for the relationship sessions.	• Give the patient private information about yourself.
• Begin and end sessions on time.	• Give or exchange personal phone numbers with a patient.
• Call the person by his or her given name.	• Give gifts (your presence and your interest are the best gifts).
• Protect the patient's right to privacy and confidentiality.	• Arrange to see the patient at times or in places other than those dictated by treatment.
• Give the patient full information about the disorder and medications.	• Discuss the correctness or value of the therapeutic interventions of other health team members with the patient.
• Safeguard the patient from becoming too vulnerable in the relationship.	• Bend the unit rules for a patient without careful consideration and without consultation with others involved in the patient's care.
• Provide security from harmful behaviors to self or others.	• Accept gifts from a patient (an exception might be a small token made in occupational therapy).
• Prewarn the patient about the end of sessions and the therapeutic relationship.	• Give information about an adult patient to others not directly involved in his or her care, without the patient's permission.
	• Make promises that you cannot keep to a patient.

Box 10–5 ■ ■ ■ ■ ■
Strategies to Enhance Mutuality

- Search for common ground in understanding issues.
- Acknowledge the patient's autonomy.
- Use the relationship to create shared experiences of reality.
- Point out patient strengths.
- Comment on changes in patient behaviors.

the therapist as important. Developing openness and respect for feelings, values, and experiences of all patients, regardless of race, color, creed, or medical condition, are essential caring behaviors.

In a therapeutic relationship, you model how to have a caring, nonexploitative relationship with another human being. The therapeutic relationship is a powerful, rich resource of healing possibilities.

MUTUALITY
Mutuality involves inclusion and connection; it implies equal partnership in achieving a goal. The concept of mutuality offers many unique opportunities to validate and affirm another human being. Both Rogers (1965) and Buber (1957) formally recognized the importance of mutuality in their theories about the nature of the therapeutic relationship. They emphasized that people can change and can take responsibility for themselves with appropriate support. According to Rogers, mutuality requires a search for common ground in understanding issues. The patient presents his or her perceptions of reality, and you bring additional understandings to the situation.

Buber defined the concept of mutuality as being based on the premise that two people in a relationship recognize and respect the separateness, uniqueness, and need for self-growth in the other as well as in himself or herself. Mutuality is not emotional fusion with a patient. It requires an acknowledgment of the independence of the other. Mutuality helps to humanize a highly structured relationship by creating a shared experience of the patient's story and human potential. As a participant-observer in a patient's human journey, the nurse is in a unique position to point out the patient's strengths as they emerge in the relationship.

Ongoing feedback is an important aspect of mutuality that may be key to effecting change and promoting well-being in patients. Box 10–5 summarizes the strategies that the nurse uses to develop and enhance mutuality.

UNCONDITIONAL ACCEPTANCE
It is easier to respect people whose ideas and values parallel our own. Many people, including nurses, base their evaluations of others on their individual characteristics, values, or ideological positions.

Rogers (1965) defined unconditional **acceptance** as the capacity of the nurse to affirm the patient's humanity and to validate his or her life experience without questioning its validity or judging it in any way. This does not mean that you condone all patient behaviors or allow the patient to act out in ways that are damaging to self or others. It does mean that you must strive to understand all human behavior as a form of communication and to recognize that the patient behind the behavior is communicating in the only way he or she has available or can be comfortable communicating at that time.

Novice nurses find it most difficult to accept differences in culture, lifestyle, sexual orientation, life decisions, and values, and they find it hard to have the services they are offering refused or sabotaged.

EMPATHY
In contrast to sympathy, which stops at an expression of feeling, **empathy** represents a mutual interpersonal process in which the nurse is able to capture the inner struggle of the patient, bring together different aspects of the patient's situation in a meaningful way, and communicate that understanding in a way that is understood as truth by the patient (Zderad, 1969).

Empathy allows you to access the inner world of the patient. By paying close attention to key words and phrases the patient uses, you can reflect them back with the same effect with which they were originally expressed. For example, following a patient's description of deep sadness related to the recent suicide of her son, you might empathetically comment, "I don't think there is anything more difficult in life than having to face the death of your child." Box 10–6 identifies nursing behaviors associated with the process of empathy.

Box 10–6 ■ ■ ■ ■ ■
Nursing Behaviors Associated With the Process of Empathy

- Want to know and understand the patient as a person.
- Go beyond appearances and superficial assessments; listen actively to understand fully the patient's message, intent, and associated feelings.
- Ask the right questions and wait for the meaning to reveal itself.
- Place yourself momentarily in the patient's position and experience what it would be like to walk in his or her shoes.
- Step back and reflect on what you are hearing, observing, and intuitively thinking concerning what the patient is revealing to you; develop an appropriate response.
- Share your observations with or reflect your feelings to the patient.

➤ *Check Your Reading*

Box 10–7 ■ ■ ■ ■ ■

Steps for Promoting Reciprocal Trust in the Nurse-Patient Relationship

- · Listen with intent to what the patient is saying.
- · Curb any preconceptions about the patient.
- · Solicit the patient's perspective.
- · Validate your conclusions.
- · Identify specific patient competencies that can help the patient manage particular problems associated with chronic illness.

From Thorne, S. E., & Robinson, C. A. (1988). Reciprocal trust in health care relationships. *Journal of Advanced Nursing, 13,* 782-789. Published by Blackwell Science Ltd.

AUTHENTICITY

The aim of a therapeutic relationship is to help a person discover or recapture a genuine sense of self. The nurse models authenticity by *being* genuine. **Authenticity** means being real with the patient, not hiding behind the mask of professionalism. Although intimate aspects of your life are not shared with the patient, what is brought into the relationship are your natural feelings and attitudes. Authenticity depends on common sense about what is appropriate in any given situation. Take caution, however, when being straightforward. You need to present the truth with compassion and an awareness of the impact a genuine comment may have on the patient. Choosing moments when the patient is receptive and delivering difficult comments with tact and respect for the patient's dignity can preserve the therapeutic relationship while bringing to it the authenticity it needs.

TRUST

The foundation of the nurse-patient relationship is **trust.** How nurses interpret their roles and present them to others affects the trust patients have in them, as nurses. Mental illness makes it more difficult for patients to trust their own reality. They lack confidence in their own behaviors, their feelings, and their competence in mastering difficult life situations. If people cannot trust themselves, it becomes almost impossible for them to trust others. Consequently, the mentally ill patient may find it difficult to trust your intentions and actions.

Trust is a mutual process. It begins with your own confidence in your skills and includes the firm belief that the patient is capable of changing his or her behavior (Thorne & Robinson, 1988). Box 10-7 outlines ways to promote trust that the nurse might use.

What do you think? How have you experienced caring, mutuality, unconditional acceptance, empathy, and authenticity? What have these qualities meant to you? Can you think of situations in which you did not experience these qualities? What were those experiences like?

➤ *Check Your Reading*

17. What are some guidelines for establishing appropriate boundaries in nurse-patient relationships?
18. How do caring and mutuality enhance therapeutic relationships?
19. How does Rogers view unconditional acceptance in relationships with patients?
20. List three nursing behaviors that characterize empathy.
21. Why is trust so important to the relationships that nurses form with their mentally ill patients?

Structuring Therapeutic Relationships

The relationship itself consists of three interrelated and overlapping phases. Although the progression through the sequential phases of the relationship is linear, patients return to previous phases during times of stress.

Preinteraction Phase

The **preinteraction phase** is the only part of the therapeutic relationship in which the patient is not actively involved. Box 10-8 identifies the relevant tasks of the preinteraction phase.

Orientation Phase: Assessment and Diagnosis

The **orientation phase** of the therapeutic relationship is particularly important because it sets the stage for the entire therapeutic interaction to follow. The orientation phase begins with the establishment of the relationship as a safe harbor for self-disclosure and for learning new behaviors and ends with the establishment of a therapeutic contract that specifically defines the nature of the actions needed for desired outcomes. Box 10-9 summarizes the tasks of the orientation phase of the relationship.

ESTABLISHING THE RELATIONSHIP AS A SAFE HARBOR

Desired outcomes for the orientation phase involve the instillation of hope and a commitment to continue with the relationship. During the orientation phase, the conceptual threads of trust, empathy, acceptance, and

Box 10–8 ■ ■ ■ ■ ■

Tasks of the Preinteraction Phase

- · Establish goals for the professional relationship.
- · Create a supportive physical environment.
- · Work out the details of timing.
- · Coordinate the goals of the relationship with the expected outcomes of the treatment plan.
- · Share the goals for the relationship with the health care team.

Box 10–9 ■ ■ ■ ■ ■
Tasks of the Orientation Phase

· Establish the relationship as a safe harbor.
· Encounter the patient.
· Establish role responsibilities.
· Develop rapport.
· Collect assessment data.
· Validate assessment data.
· Formulate appropriate diagnoses.
· Develop a therapeutic contract.

nothing. Words are the source of misunderstandings. But you will sit a little closer to me, every day."

From de Saint-Exupéry, A. (1943). *The little prince* (K. Woods, Trans.) (p. 84). New York: Harcourt Brace.

genuineness are particularly important in helping patients experience the relationship as a safe harbor. The nurse who uses a respectful proactive approach, moves slowly, and demonstrates unswerving perseverance and commitment generally is most successful (Forchuk & Brown, 1989).

ENCOUNTERING THE PATIENT
The orientation phase of the nurse-patient relationship begins with the first encounter (Forchuk, 1992). Your introduction needs to be receptive and compassionate. Body movements, facial expression, and vocal tone are as important as the actual words. As with other beginnings, it is appropriate to use customary amenities: shake hands and tell the patient your name. Asking the patient what he or she prefers to be called signals your desire to know this person as a unique individual. For example, "Hi, I'm Carole Monagle, and I will be your student nurse today. What do you like to be called?"

It is important to realize that when the nurse and patient encounter each other for the first time, they meet as strangers (Peplau, 1952). Neither really understands the other. It is critical that you understand just how vulnerable the mentally ill patient feels in the beginning of a relationship in which it is expected that the patient will self-disclose personal details of his or her life. Chronically mentally ill patients who have experienced multiple or long hospitalizations usually require more time in the orientation phase (Forchuk, 1992).

The goal of the orientation phase is to establish a working alliance and to gain enough relevant assessment data to begin to develop a care plan. First, the trustworthiness of the travelers who are to make the journey together must be established. The fox instructs the Little Prince on the best way to begin the process of relationship.

"What must I do to tame you?" asked the little prince. "You must be very patient," replied the fox. "First you will sit down at a little distance from me—like that—in the grass. I shall look at you out of the corner of my eye, and you will say

The time needed to accomplish the goals of the relationship varies from patient to patient and from situation to situation.

ESTABLISHING ROLE RESPONSIBILITIES
You need to identify your role, the kind of information you will be seeking, and the time you will be spending with the patient. The purpose statement includes what your role is as a helping person, when and under what circumstances the relationship will take place, and why the relationship may prove beneficial. For example:

I will be meeting with you for an hour, beginning at 10:00, and asking you some questions about yourself. We can spend the time talking about things that are of interest and concern to you. People often find that when they talk about what is important to them, it helps to sort out things and develop better ways of handling problems. What you say to me of a personal nature will be kept confidential, unless it might be harmful to yourself or others.

Discovering the patient's ideas about why he or she is seeking treatment and what the patient would like to gain from the relationship reinforces a sense of partnership. It is important to ask open-ended questions about what brought the patient to the hospital (clinic) or what made the patient seek treatment. Once the reason for seeking health care has been established, a second question—"What would you like to get out of our working together?"—provides information about the patient's expectations.

DEVELOPING RAPPORT
Even while introducing yourself to the patient, you begin to observe patterns of communication, for example, whether or not the patient seems interested. A goal of the orientation phase is to put the patient at ease. The patient's comfort is crucial to the success of the therapeutic process. Create an accepting atmosphere that nurtures and supports the patient's self-revelations (Havens, 1989). Responding to patients as people first and as patients second enhances the possibility of establishing meaningful rapport in the orientation.

Although testing behaviors can occur at any time in the relationship, they emerge initially when the patient begins to experience the possibility of closeness. *Testing behaviors* are those actions and words that threaten to sabotage the relationship. These behaviors are purely defensive. A flexible approach is required to protect the relationship from the patient's destructive psychological patterns. For example, the psychotic patient may get up abruptly and leave the interview. You might respond in a moderate tone, "This may not be a good time for us to talk, but I would like to talk with you. Would you mind if I came back a little later?"

Unacceptable testing behaviors, such as abusive verbal interactions, flagrant disregard of boundaries, and serious acting-out, cannot be tolerated. The manner in which they are addressed, however, makes a difference in the patient's reaction to limit-setting.

Casual conversation about neutral topics, important in the beginning of most relationships, is particularly important with the psychiatric patient. It allows the patient to become more comfortable and to experience the nurse as a person.

COLLECTING ASSESSMENT DATA

Once initial rapport is established, you can move into asking for basic information that will form the initial database.

It is important to start where the patient is, by carefully listening to the patient's personal story. A psychiatric diagnosis tells you something about the particular symptoms the patient presents. The nursing diagnosis specifies the particular dynamics and functional patterns in need of nursing intervention. Personal data about one's life journey, developed from the story told by the patient, produce unique information that helps you individualize nursing interventions.

When collecting data, try to obtain a comprehensive picture of the patient that includes an understanding of the reasons for seeking treatment and basic characteristics of the patient's personality development, personal resources, strengths, and limitations. A history of the patient's normal functioning and personal strengths is as important to assess as the problem areas (Havens, 1984). Too often the patient's many areas of normal functioning are overlooked in favor of considering the patient's dysfunctional behavior patterns.

Although data about the patient's mental disorder and functional ability may be developed quickly, personal assessment data often unfold only as the patient's trust level increases. When collecting data, you need to seek the truth with care.

How the patient answers provides valuable data about ways of thinking, ability to make choices, level of knowledge, interests, and personal strengths.

In most cases, the initial interview does not elicit all of the information needed for the assessment. Try to address assessment questions of major importance.

If there is reason to suspect the patient's reliability as a historian, significant others can supply information. Relying exclusively on patient information without soliciting the perceptions of significant others can distort and limit history-taking, particularly with organically impaired or substance-abusing patients. At times, information is sought from significant others to establish the family as part of a team approach to treatment.

VALIDATING ASSESSMENT DATA

An important part of data collection is validation. To be certain that what you observe is indeed an accurate perception of the patient's reality, you should verify your perceptions with the patient and significant others. Effective validation of the patient's experience requires that nurses

- Describe the observed patient behaviors (verbal and nonverbal)
- Verbalize their own perceptions about the behavior's intended meaning, especially if the inference is made about hidden feelings
- Remain nonjudgmental

FORMULATING APPROPRIATE DIAGNOSES

Once the database is complete, the next step is to analyze and synthesize the data into a unified whole from which you begin to formulate nursing diagnoses that relate to and support the psychiatric diagnosis. The problem and need statements embodied in the psychiatric and nursing diagnoses become the basis for deciding what type of nursing intervention is required and what referrals are necessary.

The nursing diagnosis identifies the specific functional behaviors and their hypothesized causes that are in need of nursing intervention. Both perspectives are essential as central organizing ideas about the most effective treatment approaches for each patient. Ideally, the nursing diagnosis is congruent with the *Diagnostic and Statistical Manual of Mental Disorders, Fourth Edition* psychiatric diagnosis, the patient's personal story, and the reasons the patient is seeking treatment.

DEVELOPING A THERAPEUTIC CONTRACT

Once nursing diagnoses are established to the mutual satisfaction of nurse and patient, introduce the idea of a therapeutic contract. A *therapeutic contract* is a verbal or written agreement between the patient and the nurse that supports the aims of the relationship and concretely spells out role expectations and goals. It is a dynamic process statement, requiring negotiation and updating, as the original circumstances change. Each therapeutic contract is unique from a content perspective because it is tailored to meet the individualized needs of the patient. Simple therapeutic contracts consist of information about the nature of the relationship; the place, time, and frequency of sessions; and the length of the relationship, if known. Rules that the patient is expected to follow, such as giving notice if he or she cannot attend sessions, taking no drugs or alcohol, and paying for missed appointments, are included, when appropriate.

Written therapeutic contracts are particularly appropriate with adolescents with problem behaviors and with patients who are acting out or experiencing loss of impulse control, and they serve as an integral part of the nursing care plan. They also are used to deter the patient from self-harm when there is reason to believe that the patient is so inclined.

Contracts should be written in clear, concrete language, leaving little room for differences in interpretation. The terms should be discussed thoroughly and modified, if necessary. Figure 10–3 shows a sample therapeutic contract. Once trust is established and the therapeutic contract is in place, the working phase of the relationship is ready to begin.

I, _____ , agree that I will attend all group meetings on the unit. If I am going to miss a meeting, I will notify the charge nurse prior to the scheduled meeting. I understand that if I miss a meeting without prior notification, for one week I will lose my privileges to go off the unit. I will complete this contract by _____ .

_____
(Nurse's signature)

_____
(Patient's signature)

_____
(Date)

Figure 10–3
A sample therapeutic contract.

What do you think? Are therapeutic contracts necessary in areas of nursing other than psychiatric nursing? Explain your answer.

➤ *Check Your Reading*

22. What are the nurse's tasks during the preinteraction phase?
23. What are important points for the psychiatric nurse to remember when encountering a patient for the first time and attempting to develop rapport?
24. What is the function of a therapeutic contract, and how would you use it in the clinical area?

Working Phase: Outcome Identification, Planning, and Implementation

The **working phase** is the action phase of the relationship. Assessment data continue to be incorporated into an evolving plan of care, but the focus in the working phase is on goal-setting and implementation of planned interventions.

The working phase offers you an opportunity to engage fully in the process of taming or establishing stronger ties. You and the patient begin to understand each other as you both strive toward achieving treatment goals. Box 10–10 summarizes the tasks of the working phase.

IDENTIFYING EXPECTED OUTCOMES AND PLANNING ACHIEVABLE SHORT-TERM GOALS

Once the problems have been identified, you and the patient develop achievable working objectives to meet overall treatment goals. Long-term goals (expected outcomes at time of discharge) direct the development of short-term goals (objectives needed to achieve expected outcomes). Expected outcomes related to the development of social skills and those skills needed for independent living are most appropriate for chronically mentally ill patients. Short-term goals can relate to the reduction of symptoms associated with the mental illness and the sequential steps needed to achieve expected outcomes. For example,

Expected Outcome
Mr. Jones will not experience any anxiety attacks by time of discharge.

Short-Term Goals
• Mr. Jones will keep a daily journal of his behavior and environmental factors noted before experiencing each anxiety attack.
• Mr. Jones will do his breathing exercises when he observes signs of increasing anxiety: flushing, rapid heart rate, panic feelings.
• Mr. Jones will verbalize his anxiety to the nurse.

Short-term objectives can change as the patient masters each behavior needed for goal achievement or finds that it is not effective. As the relationship develops, you help the patient clarify and refine goals (Bulechek & McCloskey, 1992).

Expected outcomes should be clear, realistic, and achievable. Overambitious goals create frustration for the mentally ill patient. Signs that the goals are overwhelming for the patient include withdrawal, regression, return of symptoms, or bizarre behavior. The patient is telling you by behavior rather than through words that he or she cannot achieve the goal. It may be that the task goes beyond the patient's personal sense of mastery. When this occurs, it helps to redefine the goal as smaller sequential steps. For example, grooming can be sequenced in simple incremental steps, such as taking a daily shower, using deodorant, brushing the hair, wearing a tie, and so forth. Each small success makes the next step possible. When simplifying a task, it is best to ". . . try the simplest intervention first . . ."

Box 10–10 ■ ■ ■ ■ ■
Tasks of the Working Phase

· Identify expected outcomes.
· Plan achievable short-term goals.
· Develop realistic solutions using a problem-solving approach.
· Work through resistances and transference.
· Implement the chosen interventions.

When you hear the sound of hoofbeats, think first of horses and not zebras'" (Anderson & Stewart, 1983, p. 42).

Goal-setting is a mutual, interactive process to which you bring information about resources and behavioral dynamics and the patient brings critical personal data that affect goal achievement. Assessment of patient strengths becomes significant because the strengths are the building blocks for the actions needed to achieve identified goals. You need to involve the patient as much as possible in developing relevant treatment goals. As Gerhart (1990) suggested, "persons, despite their mental illness, are often capable of making meaningful decisions relating to their care and the way in which they conduct their lives" (pp. 55–56). Self-determination enhances self-esteem. When the patient helps the nurse develop mutually acceptable treatment goals, it ensures that these goals fit both the patient and the situation. Moreover, active participation by the patient promotes greater self-awareness and personal ownership of treatment goals and the behaviors needed to achieve them.

DEVELOPING REALISTIC SOLUTIONS USING A PROBLEM-SOLVING APPROACH

During the working phase, relationship skills as well as problem-solving skills take form. For many patients, analyzing a problem situation and reaching an effective solution are not behaviors they typically engage in with any ease. The working phase thus becomes a carefully guided experience, ordered around the patient's interests and capabilities. A five-step problem-solving process, summarized in Box 10–11, identifies the actions needed to achieve therapeutic patient outcomes.

Define the Problem or Conflict. The patient should assume primary responsibility for developing a workable problem statement with the assistance of the nurse. Stating the problem in concrete behavioral terms puts boundaries around it and serves as the basis for developing the most appropriate strategies to solve it.

Analyze the Nature of the Problem or Conflict. Questions you might use to help the patient analyze the problem or conflict include the following:

1. *How* do you view your problem?
2. *What* are you feeling right now?
3. *What* resources do you have to resolve the problem?
4. *Who* else is or may need to be involved?

Box 10–11 ■ ■ ■ ■ ■
A Five-Step Problem-Solving Process

1. Define the problem or conflict.
2. Analyze the nature of the problem or conflict.
3. Consider alternatives and their consequences.
4. Weigh the advantages and disadvantages of each alternative.
5. Take action on the decision.

5. *How* will you feel and behave when the problem has been resolved?
6. *What* do you expect will be different in your life and how you feel about yourself if the problems were resolved?

Consider Alternatives and Their Consequences. Looking at alternatives stimulates creative thinking. Included in the process of looking at the alternatives are the following questions:

1. What are all of the possible ways that the problem might be resolved?
2. What are the consequences of taking each action, pro and con?

During this part of the problem-solving process, you can use a technique referred to as *brainstorming.* Brainstorming is a problem-solving strategy in which participants verbalize any thoughts they have about a situation. They consider new information and all possibilities. The goal becomes identification of as many solutions as possible for a particular problem.

Weigh the Advantages and Disadvantages of Each Alternative. Once all possible alternatives have been discovered, the next step is to evaluate the advantages and disadvantages of each option and decide on one, the one with the best fit. Every effort should be made to let the patient explore all of the possible consequences of each idea. You guide the process. The most important gift that you can give to a patient is to help him or her solve problems with the least amount of assistance; otherwise, the patient never learns the process of problem solving as an independent agent. There is often a temptation to tell the patient what you think he or she should do. It is difficult to refrain from giving advice. Once the patient chooses the most promising alternative, the patient is ready to take action on his or her decision.

Take Action on the Decision. The ultimate goal of this problem-solving step is to develop a shared vision as to what needs to be done. Once the patient has decided on a particular alternative, the next step is the patient's course of action. Actions that follow a logical, incremental sequence are easiest to implement and provide the most satisfaction.

When deciding on the most appropriate actions, it is important to build in the possibility of early success. Success builds morale and reinforces motivation. When there are small successes, the work itself becomes a source of satisfaction and a motivator for further efforts. Frequent feedback is important during the action segment. Through consistent dialogue, improvements can be made, new facts revealed, and original plans enhanced or revised. Many of the actions may involve practicing new skills. Step by step rehearsal promotes mastery, and feedback encourages.

WORKING THROUGH RESISTANCES AND TRANSFERENCE

Resistances. The next segment of the working phase involves dealing with potential and actual problems that threaten the relationship (Anderson & Stewart, 1983).

Rapid, steady progress in achieving treatment goals is not as common in mentally ill patients as it is with physically ill patients. The course of treatment is likely to be slower and less dramatic. Mental illnesses are chronic disorders characterized by periods of exacerbation and intervals of remission. Consequently, temporary setbacks are a relatively common occurrence.

When such setbacks occur, and they will occur, you need to linger awhile with the puzzlement until the next part of the patient's story gradually reveals itself and makes sense of what has come before. You must patiently go with the patient's flow and support any of his or her efforts to remain centered and forward moving. Recognizing slips and symptom return as temporary setbacks and stating this to the patient can be helpful. Providing feedback, supplying information about different options, and helping the patient make choices about courses of action enhance the patient's sense of autonomy and self-esteem. Also, you can identify small improvements as evidence of the patient's effort and remind the patient that the journey is a process, not an event. Making eye contact, combing hair, using make-up, making a comment, going to a house of worship, attending the ward movie, and saying "Hello" are important signals of increased engagement that should be acknowledged. Patients with less regressive behaviors often demonstrate increased self-discipline, willingness to examine their behaviors, and increased patience and courage in taking risks or in making small decisions. By noticing these behavioral changes, you can reinforce the patient's motivation for constructive change.

Withdrawal is a common form of resistance in the nurse-patient relationship. Patients frequently move away from taking conscious actions in anxiety-producing situations. Although this behavior helps the patient reduce his or her anxiety temporarily, it undermines the possibility of success in achieving goals. Peplau (1987) suggested that the work cannot continue until the patient becomes aware of his or her behavior and how it is sabotaging progress. Your task with withdrawal behaviors is to make the patient aware (Buber, 1957; Busch, 1987).

The goal is to help the patient reduce anxiety to a more moderate level. Recognizing and naming the anxiety are critical interventions. Short phrases rather than long commentaries should be used when you observe withdrawal in a patient. Acknowledging that the content is anxiety producing—"This must be very difficult for you to accept"—makes the patient aware that there is a reason for the withdrawal.

Transference. The emergence of strong feelings and behavioral attitudes during the course of the relationship is referred to as *transference* when they occur in the patient and *countertransference* when they occur in the nurse. At times, transference can be helpful, but it can also threaten the relationship. Transference reflects emotions transposed from the past onto the present situation.

Transference becomes known as *projective identification* when unconscious and disowned characteristics of previous relationships are projected onto the present relationship and reacted to or relived as if the two relationships were the same. Transference sabotages the goals of the relationship to the extent that the nurse and patient respond to it and, in the process, ignore the issues for which the patient sought treatment. Transference is easy to see when it is blatant; for example, the patient thinks the members of the nursing staff are police officers out to harm him or her physically. Transference also occurs in subtle behaviors, recognizable only with frequent self-reflection, collegial consultation, and comparison with data known about the patient. Examples of transference include either overvaluing or undervaluing the nurse's expertise, exhibiting hostility, offering flattery, or being obsequious.

Whenever transferences appear, you need to address them before proceeding with problem solving. You can briefly describe your reaction to the patient's behavior, asking the patient about the feelings you stir up or whether the behaviors directed toward you are similar to those directed toward significant others.

Another strategy is the use of simple questions about the nature of an observation as you do, for example, when you notice resistance or belligerence in a patient. You can follow up with an exploration of how past relationships may be influencing the patient's perception of the present one. If the transference seems to occur in relation to material discussed during the interaction, evidenced by a change in expression, you might note the change: "I notice your facial expression changed just then. Can you tell me what was going on in your mind just now?" Appropriate observations and responses to transference establish and sustain trust.

Countertransference refers to the psychiatric nurse's personal feelings about the patient. Countertransference can be positive or negative. It can be useful when it serves to resonate the patient's feelings and alert you to the patient's underlying needs. It can be dangerous when you identify so strongly with the patient that there is an unconscious collusion with the patient's pathology. For example, if you believe that only you have an intuitive understanding and calming effect on the patient, there is an emotional overinvolvement that is not good for the patient or you.

Nurses can become aware of countertransference by attending to exaggerated feelings about the patient or an uneasiness about the relationship. Behaviors suggestive of countertransference include thinking about the patient frequently outside of the clinical situation, feeling anger or pride in relation to the patient's behaviors, allowing the patient to act out without commenting on it, and recognizing any personal feelings that do not legitimately belong in a therapeutic relationship. When countertransference emerges, you should explore the following questions:

1. What is similar about this situation (feeling) and others I have experienced?
2. Does this person remind me of someone else or of myself?
3. How have I responded to such feelings in the past?
4. What is my part in the development of these uncomfortable feelings?
5. What is needed to resolve these feelings?

Talking with a knowledgeable colleague usually puts the situation in perspective. With strong countertransference, it may be necessary to transfer care of a particular patient to another primary caregiver.

Termination Phase: Evaluation

The **termination phase** of the relationship parallels the evaluation phase of the nursing process (Peplau, 1952). It refers to the resolution of the nurse-patient relationship. In this phase of the relationship, nurse and patient review all that the patient was able to accomplish during the course of the relationship. Box 10-12 summarizes the tasks of the termination phase.

Ideally, the seeds of termination are sown in the first encounter, when you inform the patient that the relationship is time limited. References to termination should be made enough in advance to allow for thorough discussion of feelings related to ending the relationship.

EVALUATING PATIENT PERFORMANCE

During termination, you and the patient review what he or she was able to accomplish during the relationship. The discussion can start with the behaviors that first attracted the patient's attention and proceed through discussion of changes in the patient's motivation, attention to task, and behavior. Discussion of both positive and negative behaviors is meaningful.

EVALUATING ACHIEVEMENT OF THE EXPECTED OUTCOMES

Ideally, nurses prepare themselves as well as the patient for termination by reviewing what has already been accomplished in the relationship. In the last few sessions, you should ask the patient to identify high and low points for him or her and to provide a summary of his or her progress toward goals. Achievement of therapeutic goals requires examination of all outcomes, logically and step by step. If the goals were partially achieved, you can help the patient identify what still needs to be done.

EVALUATING FUTURE NEEDS

The termination phase blends the events of the past with the realities of the present and the potential for the future. In assessing future patient needs, you help the patient consider what it will be like for him or her after

discharge. This information is used to help the patient anticipate potential problems and possible solutions for handling them successfully.

MAKING APPROPRIATE REFERRALS

Because of the constraints on length of stay in the hospital setting, most patients require referral for follow-up treatment. You can play an important role in helping patients determine their needs for service and in assisting them to access services appropriately.

DEALING WITH COMMON BEHAVIORS ASSOCIATED WITH TERMINATION

In the termination phase of the relationship, it is normal for the patient to demonstrate a number of regressive behaviors that can be disturbing to you if they are not understood. Typical behaviors include return of symptoms, anger, withdrawal, and minimizing the relationship. Some patients complain of a new and terrible symptom in hopes of convincing you to remain involved with them. Usually, maladaptive termination behaviors subside gradually. Recognizing that these symptoms are normal reactions to loss with mentally ill patients and usually temporary decreases the nurse's anxiety.

Ending a significant relationship can create sadness in both the nurse and the patient. In *The Little Prince,* the fox explains why this is so.

So the little prince tamed the fox. And when the hour of his departure drew near— "Ah," said the fox, "I shall cry." "It is your fault," said the little prince. "I never wished you any sort of harm; but you wanted me to tame you." . . . "Yes, that is so," said the fox. "Then it has done you no good at all!" "It has done me good," said the fox, "because of the color of the wheat fields." And then he added: "Go back and look again at the roses. You will understand now that yours is unique in all the world. Then come back to say goodbye to me, and I will make you a present of a secret." . . . And he went back to meet the fox. "Goodbye," he said. "Goodbye," said the fox. "And now here is my secret: It is only with the heart that one sees rightly; what is essential is invisible to the eye." ∎

From de Saint-Exupéry, A. (1943). *The little prince* (K. Woods, Trans.) (pp. 86–87). New York: Harcourt Brace.

Therapeutic relationships, because they confirm the essential nature of another human being, are carried in the heart, even after they end. Although ending any meaningful relationship is painful and sad, the experience of being valued, often a first-time experience for the mentally ill patient, makes the sadness bearable for the patient. Seeing patients progress to higher levels of functioning and knowing that you, the nurse, played a role in their evolving maturity makes the sadness bearable for you.

Gift giving is not an uncommon patient desire in the final stages of a meaningful relationship (Carson, 1999).

Box 10–12 ■ ■ ■ ■ ■
Tasks of the Termination Phase

- Evaluate patient performance.
- Evaluate achievement of the expected outcomes.
- Evaluate future needs.
- Make appropriate referrals.
- Deal with common behaviors associated with termination.

Often, too, you may want to give the patient a gift. The patient may request to continue the relationship through the exchange of phone numbers or may ask you to keep in touch through holiday or birthday cards. These attempts to hold on to the meaning of the relationship need to be recognized as normal. In social relationships, gift giving and phone number exchanges are appropriate and commonplace. Gift giving in a professional relationship, however, needs to be approached with deep caution. Extending the boundaries of the relationship to include gifts, phone number exchange, or additional visits to "see how the patient is doing" are inappropriate.

In turning down a material gift, you need to acknowledge the value of all that you have received from a patient, thus reinforcing the worth of the patient and of the relationship that you have shared. There is no one answer about whether gifts should or should not be exchanged. Although the answer is not simple, it does involve being true to what you know and feel about the patient, assessing the meaning of the gesture, and using your best professional judgment.

> **W**hat do you think? Do you think that termination must involve a final goodbye? Defend your answer.

➤ Check Your Reading

25. What specific tasks are involved in the working phase of a therapeutic relationship?
26. Why would teaching the steps of problem solving be important to psychiatric patients?
27. What are some of the behaviors the nurse would see during the termination phase?
28. How would you characterize the differences between transference and countertransference feelings? In what ways are they related to each other?
29. What would be the best approach in handling the issue of gift giving in the termination phase?

Conclusions

Each nurse-patient relationship represents a human encounter with the potential to heal, to support, and to provide guidance in negotiating the human journey. This chapter presents a framework for understanding the structure and conceptual components of the nurse-patient relationship. Psychological and nursing frameworks relevant to the study of therapeutic relationships identify and define boundaries, caring, respect, empathy, genuineness, authenticity, and trust as key conceptual elements threaded throughout the relationship. Nurses are in an excellent position to develop qualitative research studies exploring the nature of each of these key elements and how they contribute to the healing process in psychiatric nursing. In an era in which health care is increasingly dehumanized with bureaucracy, human encounters in psychiatric nursing become extremely significant.

Key Points to Remember

- A therapeutic relationship represents a time-bound alliance between nurse and patient, consciously entered into and characterized by respect, acceptance, empathy, and genuineness.
- The value of a therapeutic relationship is that it provides the mentally ill patient with an "experience of being understood and of being related to another human being" (O'Toole & Welt, 1989, p. 11). A therapeutic relationship offers the patient hope and the possibility of discovering that he or she has meaning, even if at the time it is to only one other person, the therapist.
- Social and therapeutic relationships differ in their (1) purpose, (2) focus, (3) responsibility, (4) degree of self-disclosure, and (5) level of personal involvement.
- The conceptual components of the relationship—boundaries, caring, advocacy, unconditional acceptance, mutuality, authenticity, and trust—are the essential foundation on which patients begin to restructure their images of themselves and the nature of their journey.
- Therapeutic communication is a special form of communication that has a health-related purpose and develops as a continuous flow of interaction between nurse and patient, with input from both contributing to its nature and progression. Therapeutic communication serves as the primary means through which all nursing interventions occur.
- Therapeutic listening skills, defined as "an interpersonal, confirmation process involving all the senses in which the therapist attends with empathy to the patient's verbal and nonverbal messages to facilitate the understanding, synthesis, and interpretation of the patient's situation," have been identified as the most important communication tool that the nurse uses with psychiatric patients (Kemper, 1992, p. 22).
- Active listening requires more than simply hearing the content of a patient's message and responding to it. Active listening is focused listening. The process of active listening involves making sense of the sender's message and attaching meaning to it.
- Active communication skills include the use of minimal encouragers, appropriate questions, restatement, paraphrasing, reflection, clarification, silence, summarizing, and validation.

- Verbal interventions take a proactive role in helping patients learn new behaviors. Verbal interventions build on the patient's strengths. They include confronting, constructive feedback, redirecting, modeling, humor, and giving information.
- Boundaries are defined as "a dynamic line of demarcation separating an individual's internal (body, mind, and spirit) and external environments and varying in permeability and flexibility" (Scott, 1988, p. 24).
- Advocates are defined as people "who stand along side of and empower patients and their families to have a voice when they are weak and vulnerable" (Tanner et al., 1993, p. 278). Advocacy is a moral responsibility of the nurse designed to maximize patients' self-integrity and personal dignity when they are unable to do this for themselves.
- Caring is an intangible, interactive process with physical, psychosocial, and spiritual dimensions that finds expression through actions designed to promote the health and well-being of patients. Caring is knowing that you would understand and care for another and daring to prove it.
- Mutuality, in its most complete dimension, involves inclusion. A connected relationship is one in which the nurse views the patient first as a person and second as a patient.
- Unconditional acceptance is the nurse's capacity to affirm the patient's humanity and to validate his or her life experience without questioning its validity or judging it in any way.
- Empathy is an interpersonal process in which the nurse is able to capture the inner struggle of the patient, bring together different aspects of the patient's situation in a meaningful way, and communicate that understanding to the patient in a way that is understood as truth by the patient. It is both an attitude and a communication strategy in which the nurse's role as participant-observer is particularly relevant.
- Authenticity or genuineness refers to being real in therapeutic relationships. Although intimate aspects of the nurse's life are not shared with the patient, what is brought into the relationship are the nurse's natural feelings and attitudes.
- The concept of trust involves a person's inner confidence that another person respects, understands, and responds fairly to that person. Trust is a mutual process. It begins with the nurse's confidence in his or her skills and includes the firm belief that the patient is capable of changing his or her behavior.
- The structure of the therapeutic relationship consists of a preinteraction phase, which does not include the patient, and three sequential stages: the orientation, working, and termination phases.
- The goal of the preinteraction phase is to develop a safe environment for the development of the relationship. Specific tasks include identifying professional goals, establishing the physical setting, and working through arrangements with other members of the interdisciplinary health care team.
- The primary goal of the orientation phase is to establish a working alliance with the patient and to gain enough relevant assessment data to begin to develop a care plan. Specific tasks include defining the purpose of the relationship, establishing the role responsibilities of both participants, developing a rapport needed to accomplish the work, collecting relevant assessment data, identifying appropriate psychiatric and nursing diagnoses, and establishing a therapeutic contract.
- The working phase is the action phase of the relationship. Peplau originally subdivided the working phase into two components: the identification phase, in which the patient explores the nature of the problem and its associated feelings, and the exploitation phase, in which the patient maximizes use of all appropriate resources to resolve the problem.
- The termination phase of the relationship parallels the evaluation phase of the nursing process. Evaluation of the effectiveness of the problem-solving approach can include evaluating the patient's performance, determining if the problem has been satisfactorily resolved, reviewing what has been learned in this situation that could prove useful in future situations, and analyzing the positive and negative behaviors that occurred during the problem-solving process.
- The emergence of strong feelings and behavioral attitudes during the course of the relationship are referred to as transference feelings when they occur in a patient and countertransference feelings when they occur in the nurse.

Learning Activities

1. Before you enter the psychiatric unit, think through all of the images and ideas you have about mentally ill patients. What are your concerns? How do you think you will respond to the patients? What do you expect to find on the unit? How do you think the patients will respond to you? Be as honest as possible; there are no right or wrong answers. Write your answers to these questions and share them with your classmates. After you have worked in the psychiatric unit, compare your initial and preconceived ideas with what it was actually like. In what ways have your perceptions changed? If there are changes, to what do you attribute them? Again, there are no right or wrong answers.

2. Identify a situation in which a communication breakdown occurred. Describe the situation in enough detail that it can be role-played (i.e., who was involved, the exact conversation as you remember it, the physical setting, and the timing). In your narrative, use a third person format to describe the events as

they occurred, even if you were personally involved. Using the information in the chapter and in your class discussion, analyze the reasons for the communication breakdown. Discuss how this communication might be improved with some of the principles discussed in the chapter. Role-play with a partner: (1) the communication breakdown scenario and (2) use of active listening and verbal interventions to achieve a different outcome. Discuss in class or with a small group the different reactions of the participants. Consider how you could use this learning with psychiatric patients.

3. John Antione is a 28-year-old schizophrenic single man, newly admitted to the hospital. He appears unshaven, with unkempt hair and loose clothing. He has a distinct body odor. Your instructor thinks working with this patient would be a good challenge for you. Have one student role-play the patient and another the nurse.

4. In small groups of three or four students, apply the five-step problem-solving format (see Box 10–11) to one of the following patient problems.

5. Carol Black was recently admitted to the inpatient unit with suicidal ideation and severe depression following her husband's decision to leave her. Her husband wants to have joint custody of the children so that he does not have to pay child support, and he wants to sell the house. Carol suspects but does not know that there is another woman. She has not worked in 10 years and feels betrayed because she always did what her husband wanted and has never had a life of her own.

6. Jeri Slovak has adult attention-deficit disorder and learning disabilities that compromise her ability to complete written assignments on time. All her life she has felt vulnerable about her inability to organize her life and has defended herself by not telling anyone of her disability. Her college teachers are annoyed with her because she is obviously bright. They think she is either lazy or seriously mentally disturbed. She has been advised that unless she cleans up her act, she will be dismissed from the college program.

7. Pat Calhoun has a severe borderline personality disorder. When she becomes very anxious, she develops psychotic delusional thinking patterns. She believes that the world is coming to an end and that she must collect ammunition and guns to protect herself. She has involved her 8-year-old son in helping her stockpile the ammunition and regularly takes all of her three children to a shooting range. Recently, Pat's husband lost his job and her oldest daughter was involved in an auto accident. Pat's anxiety is at a very high level.

Critical Thinking Exercises

Ms. Miller, a student nurse, is writing a process recording concerning her patient Mr. Tallon. She knows that she must show her instructor that she understands the concept of therapeutic communication and give examples of how her responses were therapeutic. She begins to write: *Mr. Tallon said that he was very upset about his wife's desire to obtain a divorce. When he spoke, his voice was emotionless, his hands folded, his eyes were downcast, and he smiled at me.*

1. What inference can be drawn about Ms. Miller's understanding of the communication process?
2. Is Ms. Miller's description of Mr. Tallon clear?
3. What evidence leads you to this conclusion?

Ms. Miller continues to write: *After I talked with Mr. Tallon for 20 minutes, I decided to comment on the difference between what he said and how he acted. He responded, "You women are all alike; you always find fault with everything."*

1. What assumptions is the patient making about Ms. Miller?
2. What inference can the nurse draw about Mr. Tallon's response?
3. What might have happened if different questions were asked?

Mr. Kain, a student nurse, begins to write a contract with Mr. Herman concerning his plan of care. The contract reads: *Mr. Herman will meet with his nurse at least one time each day to discuss his plans for the day. He will notify his nurse if he has any feelings that frighten him. He will participate in one activity each afternoon.*

1. Is the contract clear and precise?
2. What other information (evidence) do you need to determine whether the contract is therapeutic?
3. What assumptions is Mr. Kain making about contracts?

Mr. Kain sits down with Mr. Herman and reviews the content of the contract. His purpose is to give more structure to Mr. Herman's daily routine. He tells Mr. Herman that it is important for him to participate with others. Mr. Herman signs the contract and keeps a copy for himself. When Mr. Kain leaves the room, Mr. Herman crumples the contract and throws it in the garbage can.

1. What assumption did Mr. Kain make?
2. What point of view is Mr. Herman taking?
3. Consider alternative assumptions about this interaction.

Additional Resources

There is no specific Internet address that provides information specifically about the nurse-patient relationship and communication. However, these addresses are relevant.

American Psychiatric Nurses Association (APNA)

http://www.apna.org

National Institute of Mental Health (NIMH)

http://www.nimh.nih.gov

References

Anderson, C., & Stewart, S. (1983). *Mastering resistance: A practical guide to family therapy.* New York: Guilford Press.

Argyle, M. (1975). *Bodily communication.* Madison, CT: International Universities Press.

Arnold, E., & Boggs, K. (1995). *Interpersonal relations: Communication skills for nurses* (2nd ed.). Philadelphia: W. B. Saunders.

Arnold, E., & Boggs, K. (1999). *Interpersonal relations: Communication skills for nurses* (3rd ed.). Philadelphia: W. B. Saunders.

Brown, A. (1993). A conceptual clarification of respect. *Journal of Advanced Nursing, 16,* 354-361.

Buber, M. (1970). *I-thou* (W. Kaufmann, Trans.). New York: Scribner's.

Buber, M. (1957). Distance and relation. *Psychiatry, 20,* 107-104.

Bulechek, G., & McCloskey, J. (1992). *Nursing interventions.* Philadelphia: W. B. Saunders.

Busch, P. (1987). Therapy with the uninvolved client. *Journal of Psychosocial Nursing and Mental Health Services, 25*(11), 21-25.

Campinha-Bacote, J. (1988). Culturological assessment: An important factor in psychiatric consultation-liaison nursing. *Archives of Psychiatric Nursing, 2,* 2410-2415.

Carroll, L. (1881). *Alice's adventures in wonderland.* New York: Bantam Books.

Carson, V. B. (1999). The experience of grief: Losses and endings in nurse-client relationships. In E. Arnold & K. Boggs (Eds.), *Interpersonal relationships: Professional communication skills for nurses* (3rd ed.). Philadelphia: W. B. Saunders.

Casement, P. (1991). *Learning from the patient.* New York: Guilford Press.

Cotton, P., Drake, R., Whitaker, B., & Potter, J. (1983). Dealing with suicide on a psychiatric in-patient unit. *Hospital and Community Psychiatry, 34*(1), 510-559.

Crowther, D. (1991). Metacommunications: A missed opportunity? *Journal of Psychosocial Nursing, 210*(4), 13-16.

de Saint-Exupéry, A. (1943). *The little prince* (K. Woods, Trans.). New York: Harcourt Brace.

Ferguson, S., & Campinha-Bacote, J. (1989). Humor in nursing. *Journal of Psychosocial Nursing, 27*(4), 210-34.

Forchuk, C. (1992). The orientation phase of the nurse-client relationship: How long does it take? *Perspectives in Psychiatric Care, 28*(4), 1-10.

Forchuk, C., & Brown, B. (1989). Establishing a nurse-client relationship. *Journal of Psychosocial Nursing and Mental Health Services, 27*(2), 30-34.

Fox, R. (1993). Elements of the helping process: A guide for clinicians. New York: Haworth Press.

Friedman, M. (1985). Healing through meeting and the problematic of mutuality. *Journal of Humanistic Psychology, 25*(1), 11-40.

Gardner, D. (1992). Presence. In G. Bulchek & J. McCloskey (Eds.), *Nursing interventions: Treatment for nursing diagnoses* (pp. 111-118). Philadelphia: W. B. Saunders.

Gebbard, G. (1992). Psychodynamic psychiatry in the decade of the brain. *American Journal of Psychiatry, 149*(8), 991-998.

Gerhart, U. (1990). *Caring for the chronic mentally ill.* Itasca, IL: F. E. Peacock.

Hagerty, B., Lynch-Sauer, J., Patusky, K., & Bouwsema, M. (1993). An emerging theory of human relatedness. *Image, 25,* 2101-2106.

Hall, E. (1966). *The hidden dimension.* New York: Doubleday.

Havens, L. (1984). The need for tests of normal functioning in the psychiatric interview. *American Journal of Psychiatry, 141,* 1208-1211.

Havens, L. (1986). *Making contact: Uses of language in psychotherapy.* Cambridge, MA: Harvard University Press.

Havens, L. (1989). *A safe place: Laying the groundwork of psychotherapy.* Cambridge, MA: Harvard University Press.

Ivey, A. (1988). *Intentional interviewing and counseling* (2nd ed.). Monterey, CA: Brooks/Cole.

Kemper, B. (1992). Therapeutic listening: Developing the concept. *Journal of Psychosocial Nursing, 30*(7), 21-23.

Mehrabian, A. (1972). *Non-verbal communication.* Chicago: Aldine.

Narayan, M. C. (1997). Cultural assessment in home health care. *Home Healthcare Nurse, 15,* 665-670.

O'Toole, A., & Welt, S. (Eds.). (1989). Interpersonal theory in nursing practice: Selected works of Hildegard E. Peplau. New York: Springer.

Peplau, H. (1952). *Interpersonal relations in nursing.* New York: Putnam's.

Peplau, H. (1987). Interpersonal constructs for nursing practice. *Nurse Education Today, 7,* 201-208.

Peplau, H. (1992). Interpersonal relations: A theoretical framework for application in nursing practice. *Nursing Science Quarterly, 5,* 13-18.

Rieman, D. (1986). The essential structure of a caring interaction: Doing phenomenology. In P. L. Munhall & C. J. Oiler (Eds.), *Nursing research: A qualitative perspective* (pp. 86-108). Norwalk, CT: Appleton-Century-Crofts.

Rogers, C. R. (1951). Patient centered therapy: Its current practice, implications and theory. Boston: Houghton-Mifflin.

Rogers, C. R. (1958). The characteristics of the helping relationship. *Personnel and Guidance Journal, 37*(1), 68-72.

Tanner, C., Benner, P., Chesla, C., & Gordon, D. (1993). The phenomenology of knowing the patient. *Image, 25,* 273-283.

Taylor, A., Meyer, A., Rosegrant, T., & Samples, B. T. (1989). *Communicating* (5th ed.). Englewood Cliffs, NJ: Prentice-Hall.

Thorne, S. E., & Robinson, C. A. (1988). Reciprocal trust in health care relationships. *Journal of Advanced Nursing, 13,* 782-789.

Wachtel, P. (1993). *Therapeutic communication.* New York: Guilford Press.

Watzlawick, P., Beavin, J. H., & Jackson, D. D. (1967). *Pragmatics of human communication.* New York: Norton.

Zderad, L. (1969). Empathetic nursing: Realization of a human capacity. *Nursing Clinics of North America, 4,* 655-662.

Suggested Readings

Benner, P., & Wrubel, J. (1989). *The primacy of caring: Stress and coping in health and illness.* Menlo Park, CA: Addison-Wesley.

Connelly, L., Keele, B., Kleinbeck, S., Schneider, J., & Cobb, A. (1993). A place to be yourself: Empowerment from the client's perspective. *Image, 25,* 291–303.

Hagerty, B., Lynch-Sauer, J., Patusky, K., & Bouwsema, M. (1993). An emerging theory of human relatedness. *Image, 25,* 2101–2106.

Kalisch, B. J. (1973). What is empathy? *American Journal of Nursing, 73,* 1548–1553.

Lego, S. (1980). The one to one nurse-patient relationship. *Perspectives in Psychiatric Care, 18,* 611–689.

Peplau, H. (1987). Interpersonal constructs for nursing practice. *Nurse Education Today, 7,* 201–208.

Peplau, H. (1992). Interpersonal relations: A theoretical framework for application in nursing practice. *Nursing Science Quarterly, 5,* 13–18.

Zderad, L. (1969). Empathetic nursing: Realization of a human capacity. *Nursing Clinics of North America, 4,* 655–662.

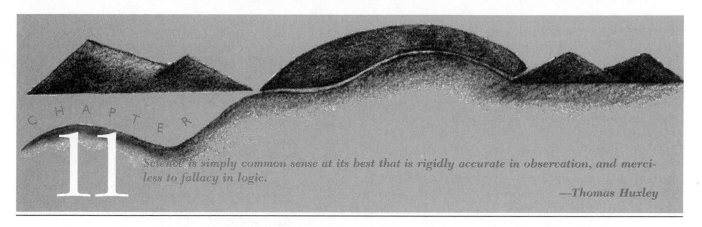

Science is simply common sense at its best that is rigidly accurate in observation, and merciless to fallacy in logic.

—Thomas Huxley

The Map of the Journey
The Nursing Process

Learning Objectives

After studying this chapter you should be able to:

1. Discuss the importance of the nursing process to the practice of psychiatric nursing.

2. Define the steps of the nursing process.

3. Discuss the essentials of a comprehensive assessment, using the five dimensions from the American Nurses Association (ANA) standard for assessment.

4. Identify the steps in nursing diagnosis derived from approved North American Nursing Diagnosis Association (NANDA) and *Diagnostic and Statistical Manual of Mental Disorders, Fourth Edition* (DSM-IV) diagnoses.

5. List the criteria for realistic expected outcomes for patients.

6. Describe one theoretical approach to organizing the nursing care plan.

7. Name the seven psychiatric interventions defined by the ANA for the basic level of psychiatric nursing.

8. Compare and contrast formative and summative evaluations.

9. Apply the entire nursing process to a given patient situation.

10. Explain how the nurse uses the initial nursing interview to establish a therapeutic relationship.

11. Describe how discharge planning begins in the assessment phase of nursing care.

12. Identify at least four reasons why nursing documentation is important at each step of the nursing process.

Key Terminology

Assessment
Cognitive assessment
Data collection tool
Diagnosis
Diagnostic and Statistical Manual of Mental Disorders, Fourth Edition (DSM-IV)

Discharge planning
Documentation
Emotional assessment
Evaluation
Expected outcomes
Formative evaluation
Implementation
Interventions

North American Nursing Diagnosis Association (NANDA)
Nursing process
Physical assessment
Planning
Prioritization
Self-awareness

Sociocultural assessment
Spiritual and philosophical assessment
Standardized rating scales
Standards of Psychiatric–Mental Health Clinical Nursing Practice
Summative evaluation

Whenever you meet a patient for the first time, it is like starting a new journey for you and the patient. The journey holds not only the promise of discovery as you and the patient learn about each other but also the promise of continued self-discovery for you as a professional psychiatric–mental health nurse.

There is an underlying basic "map" for each nurse-patient journey, and that is the nursing process. The **nursing process** provides a scientific framework for the delivery of professional nursing care. As defined by the American Nurses Association (ANA), the nursing process consists of six steps:

1. Assessment
2. Diagnosis
3. Outcome identification
4. Planning
5. Implementation
6. Evaluation

Although the six steps can be described separately, in actual nursing experience they are interactive and flow in a continuous manner throughout the episode of care (Ryan-Wenger, 1990; Sheehan, 1991). Figure 11-1 illustrates the dynamic interrelationship among these steps.

The nursing process has been acknowledged as nursing's scientific method (Townsend, 1991). As with any scientific method of inquiry, the foundation is a problem-solving approach (Hurst, Dean, & Trickey, 1991; Table 11-1). Use of this process provides a systematic and individualized method of fulfilling the goals of nursing (Atkinson & Murray, 1990; Sheehan, 1991):

- To help the patient to promote and maximize his or her level of health

TABLE 11-1   Principles of Problem-Solving Used in the Nursing Process

STEP IN NURSING PROCESS	PRINCIPLE OF PROBLEM-SOLVING
Assessment: data collection	Observation
Diagnosis: formulation of nursing diagnoses	Definition of the problem
Outcome identification	Formulation of hypotheses
Planning: deciding what will be done, who will do it, and where and how it will be done	Planning of an approach
Implementation: carrying out the nursing actions	Testing of hypotheses and solutions
Evaluation: determining the success of the process and the outcomes	Formulation of conclusions

- To maintain the highest level of functioning
- To prevent illness and the sequelae of illness

In each patient's journey, this nursing process is carried out in the context of the therapeutic nurse-patient relationship. From the initial interview on the day of admission until the discharge instructions on the day of discharge, the nurse uses the therapeutic relationship to facilitate the patient's involvement in his or her own care. By demonstrating respect for the patient's autonomy and integrity, the nurse encourages him or her to actively participate in decisions about the treatment plan. This deliberate approach requires thought, knowledge, and experience (Arnold & Boggs, 1995; Sundeen, Stuart, Rankin, & Cohen, 1994; Wilkinson, 1992). Figure 11-2 illustrates the interaction between the nursing process and the nurse-patient relationship. Review Chapter 10 for more in-depth discussion of the therapeutic relationship.

To provide professional care, you must have a sound knowledge base and be able to think critically. The ANA has written generic standards that apply to all nurses, the *Standards of Clinical Nursing Practice* (1991). As you already know from your introductory nursing courses, standards are authoritative statements that describe the responsibilities for which the nurse is accountable. They provide direction for nursing practice and the framework to evaluate the quality of that practice. On your journey, the 1991 generic standards are the "atlas," providing the larger perspective for the nursing process "map." The 1994 ***Standards of Psychiatric–Mental Health Clinical Nursing Practice*** (ANA) provide the "regional" perspective for the journey; they are specific to psychiatric nursing. These standards appear in Chapter 4 and can be reviewed to see their relationship to the nursing process.

This chapter focuses on the six steps of the nursing process applied to psychiatric nursing. You are introduced to one patient, and her story is used to illustrate

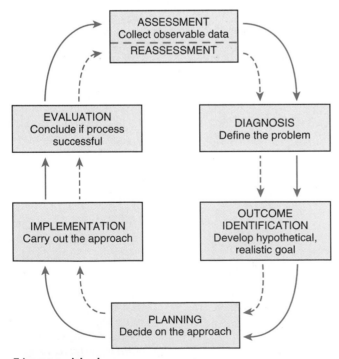

Figure 11-1
Six interactive steps of the nursing process. (Modified from McCaffrey, M., & Beebe, A. [1989]. *Pain: Clinical manual for nursing practice.* St. Louis: C. V. Mosby. Reprinted with permission of C. V. Mosby Company and J. B. Lippincott Company.)

each step. Special attention is given to the **assessment** phase of the process because it is the first step and because it must be repeated continuously for effective nursing care. There is also an emphasis on nursing documentation, which is necessary to implement individualized care and to evaluate the quality of that care.

What do you think? How are the steps of the nursing process similar to or different from the approach you generally use to solve problems? What are the values of using a systematic approach to problem solving?

> ➤ *Check Your Reading*
>
> 1. What is the purpose of the nursing process?
> 2. How is the nursing process related to problem solving?
> 3. What are the steps of the nursing process?
> 4. What are the authoritative statements on nursing practice called?
> 5. What do the *Standards of Psychiatric–Mental Health Clinical Nursing Practice* describe?
> 6. How do the 1994 standards of care for psychiatric nurses relate to the nursing process?

Mrs. Ryan's Story

Mrs. Ryan is a 46-year-old, white, married, Roman Catholic woman who has been admitted to a university-affiliated psychiatric hospital. She has two school-age children and is a full-time homemaker. Her husband reports that prior to admission, Mrs. Ryan had stopped eating and taking her medication and had begun to stay up all night pacing and talking to herself.

A Rough Beginning

On admission, Mrs. Ryan was disheveled and restless, and she alternated between refusing to answer questions and answering them incoherently. She had been hospitalized previously with a diagnosis of paranoid schizophrenia.

Because of Mrs. Ryan's intense physical activity and her inability to communicate verbally, the psychiatric nurses were unable to complete most of the nursing assessment. An assessment by the social work department, usually coordinated with the patient and family, was deferred because of Mrs. Ryan's disorganization.

The 1st Week of Hospitalization

During the 1st week of hospitalization, Mrs. Ryan took her medication and followed simple directions related

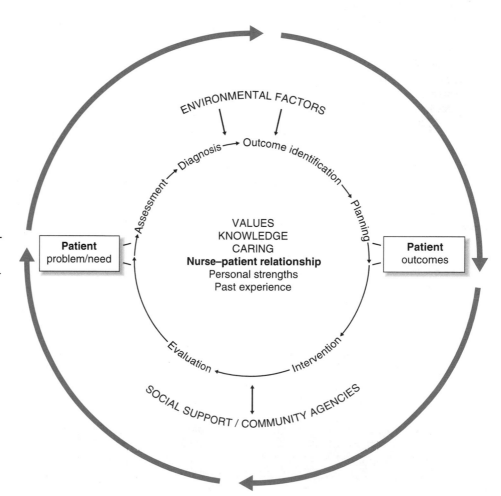

Figure 11–2
Significance of the nurse-patient relationship in the nursing process. (From Arnold, E., & Boggs, K. [1995]. *Interpersonal relationships: Professional communication skills for nurses* [2nd ed.]. Philadelphia: W. B. Saunders.)

to the activities of daily living. She dressed herself, butwith uneven buttoning and unmatched clothing, pushing away nursing staff who tried to assist. She needed supervision during meals and showers because she would not stay long enough to complete the tasks. She was able to toilet independently, and she began to sleep up to 6 hours. Mrs. Ryan often threw water on her face and hair and mumbled while looking at herself in the mirror.

The 2nd Week of Hospitalization

There was no change in Mrs. Ryan's behavior during the 2nd week of hospitalization. Her physicians, therefore, increased her medication, and she began to nap during the day. When she wasn't napping, Mrs. Ryan paced alone in the hallway, talking softly to herself, or she isolated herself in her private room and did not interact with other patients on the ward. When her husband visited and brought her clothes or other items, she avoided him. He spent the visit times quietly sitting by himself in the dining area.

The nurses concluded that Mrs. Ryan was still too psychotic to try to complete the nursing assessment. They considered her too agitated to participate in group meetings and activity therapy.

The 3rd Week of Hospitalization

By the 3rd week of hospitalization, Mrs. Ryan was pacing less. The night nurse reported that Mrs. Ryan cried at night and often said something that sounded like, "Who will feed the children?" Mrs. Ryan's psychiatric team discussed the observation, and they asked her if she was concerned about her children, but she refused to answer. Superficial conversations with Mr. Ryan gave the impression that he was managing the household adequately.

The 4th Week of Hospitalization

At the end of the 4th week of hospitalization, there was no significant improvement in Mrs. Ryan's verbalization or hallucinations. She appeared to listen to staff members, but her answers to questions were incomprehensible. Every night she continued to cry. The staff began to give up hope for a quick recovery, calling her case "chronic." She participated minimally in the activities of the unit, and because she was not threatening to herself or others, she received a decreasing amount of attention from the nursing staff.

A consulting psychiatrist who visited weekly commented on Mrs. Ryan's lack of progress and encouraged the team to reevaluate her treatment plan. The treatment team then reviewed its assessment and noted how incomplete it was in the dimension of social-family issues. They agreed to hold a family meeting with Mr. Ryan to gather more history.

Mr. Ryan was cooperative, and his wife sat through most of the session and seemed to listen. As the team discussed family patterns and issues, Mr. Ryan admitted he had a history of alcoholism and had had arguments with his wife over money prior to her hospitalization. One week, he said, he had spent his whole paycheck before buying groceries or paying bills. Ever since his wife's hospitalization, he was staying sober, and the Ryan children were being cared for by a neighbor. Mr. Ryan reassured his wife that the children were safe, and the social worker arranged for them to visit briefly on the following evening.

Breakthrough

Within days of that family meeting, the staff noticed a change in Mrs. Ryan. She started to respond with a few words to questions about daily activities. Over the next few weeks, she made steady progress in her ability to communicate her needs and wishes. She requested a decrease in medication because she felt sedated. She asked to go to the beauty parlor on her first leave of absence because she looked "so horrible."

Mrs. Ryan was discharged after a 2-month stay. When she left, she was a quiet, soft-spoken woman with an ordinary appearance who thanked the staff for helping her return to her family and home. ∎

NURSING PROCESS

Assessment

As the first step in the nursing process, assessment starts as soon as the nurse-patient interaction begins. In the nurse-patient journey, this interaction differs from getting to know someone in a social situation. Instead of developing a spontaneous relationship based on mutual interests and a shared focus on each other, the nurse becomes acquainted with the patient through planned and structured approaches designed to focus on the patient.

As Mrs. Ryan's case illustrates, it is a challenge to get to know a person whose thought processes and communication skills are severely impaired. A comprehensive nursing assessment requires multiple skills in verbal and nonverbal communication. You must call on creativity and sensitivity as you attempt to gather information on the patient's present status, past history, and health care expectations. The patient is your first and primary source for information, but do not underestimate the value of secondary sources including family and significant others, health team members, records, and results from various tests and laboratory procedures. Especially when the patient cannot provide clear answers, as happened with Mrs. Ryan, additional sources must be used as soon as possible to clarify the database.

Your focus is to gather complete biological, psychological, cognitive, sociological, and spiritual information of the patient. This includes current physical assessment data and health history, and descriptions of behaviors, emotions, and coping patterns. Important sociological factors are cultural and ethnic variables; relationships with family, friends, and other groups or support systems; and involvement in work or school. The patient's religious affiliation and spiritual beliefs are also significant data. All of the information will be used to develop the nursing care plan for one individual, including the beginning of the discharge plan.

Realistic **discharge planning** requires knowledge of the patient's level of functioning prior to this episode of care, including the presence or absence of a support system. The nursing assessment contributes to the treatment team's database, used to define the desired behaviors expected for this patient before discharge.

Later in this chapter, the assessment phase is reviewed to explore all of its dimensions in more detail. For now, refer to Box 11–1 to review significant assessment data from Mrs. Ryan. Once the data are sorted, the nurse is ready to move on to the next phase of the nursing process in which the data are analyzed and nursing diagnoses are formulated (Johnson, Stone, Larson, & Hromek, 1992).

Documentation. In every work setting, the admitting nurse documents assessment data on a specific nursing tool or as part of a multidisciplinary form. Often, the nurse is the first professional to interview the patient and family, if available. It is crucial to record all information accurately, legibly, and promptly whether it is handwritten or in a computerized system. Other nurses will use the database to plan and implement immediate nursing care; the physician and members of other disciplines will also use the data to develop the initial treatment plan, including the criteria for discharge. With the decrease in length of stay at every level of care in recent years, the assessment stage must be

Box 11–1 ■ ■ ■ ■ ■
Example of Nursing Assessment Data for Mrs. Ryan

Biological/Physical	**Cognitive**
Decreased sleep, decreased eating, decreased grooming	Auditory hallucinations, paranoia, incoherent speech

Psychological/ Emotional	**Sociological/ Sociocultural**
Anxious, suspicious, noncompliance with medication	46-year-old white, married, female, mother of two

Spiritual

Roman Catholic

Incomplete Database—Patient is unable to verbally communicate needs and goals. Continue to attempt to complete and use secondary sources including previous record, family, and team member evaluations.

shortened. For example, if Mrs. Ryan were admitted to a hospital today, her length of stay would be closer to 2 weeks instead of 8 weeks, with discharge to a partial hospital program. Later in this chapter, one example of a nursing assessment tool is presented.

W*hat do you think?* How would you approach Mrs. Ryan? What would you say to her? What would you do to initiate a therapeutic relationship? Have you ever dealt with patients like Mrs. Ryan before? What are your thoughts and feelings about embarking on a journey of getting to know patients like Mrs. Ryan?

➤ *Check Your Reading*

7. During the assessment phase, what is the focus of the nurse?
8. What or who is the primary source for data collection?
9. Name the secondary sources for information.
10. What is included in the psychological assessment?

Diagnosis

The purpose of nursing **diagnosis** is to "name" the patient's problems. Once a problem is accurately defined and named, the possible solutions become more obvious. Naming focuses our thinking and problem-solving skills.

The basic-level psychiatric nurse identifies nursing problems by using the nomenclature specified by the **North American Nursing Diagnosis Association (NANDA).** Use of the NANDA diagnostic labels (Box 11–2) is considered within the scope of practice of the basic-level psychiatric nurse. The advanced practice psychiatric nurse uses NANDA diagnoses as well as medical diagnoses from the psychiatrist's resource book, *Diagnostic and Statistical Manual of Mental Disorders, Fourth Edition* (DSM-IV). DSM-IV lists the specific behavioral criteria used to substantiate each psychiatric diagnosis. Once the medical diagnosis is given, the nurse can derive multiple nursing diagnoses related to the specific problem behaviors shown by one patient.

Nursing diagnoses are defined as clinical judgments about individual, family, or community responses to actual and potential health problems. Nursing diagnoses are used to describe an individual patient's condition, to prescribe nursing interventions, and to delineate the parameters for developing outcome criteria. The focus is on human responses to an actual or potential unmet health need. These responses may relate to a disease process, to a complementary concern along the health-illness continuum, or to some other need not connected to the identified medical diagnosis.

As a psychiatric nurse, you compare information collected during the assessment against documented norms of health and wellness. Taking into account the patient's individual variations (related to demographics, background, experience, and situation), you can make inferences about the patient's problems and needs.

Box 11-2 ▪ ▪ ▪ ▪ ▪

North American Nursing Diagnosis Association–Approved Nursing Diagnoses

This list represents the NANDA-approved nursing diagnoses for clinical use and testing for 1999.

Activity Intolerance
Activity Intolerance, Risk for
Adaptive Capacity: Intracranial, Decreased
Adjustment, Impaired
Airway Clearance, Ineffective
Anxiety
Aspiration, Risk for
Body Image Disturbance
Body Temperature, Risk for Altered
Breastfeeding, Effective
Breastfeeding, Ineffective
Breastfeeding, Interrupted
Breathing Pattern, Ineffective
Caregiver Role Strain
Caregiver Role Strain, Risk for
Communication, Impaired Verbal
Community Coping, Ineffective
Community Coping, Potential for Enhanced
Confusion, Acute
Confusion, Chronic
Constipation
Constipation, Perceived
Constipation: Risk for
Coping: Ineffective Individual
Death Anxiety
Decisional Conflict (Specify)
Decreased Cardiac Output
Defensive Coping
Denial, Ineffective
Diarrhea
Disorganized Infant Behavior
Disorganized Infant Behavior, Risk for
Disuse Syndrome, Risk for
Diversional Activity Deficit
Dysfunctional Ventilatory Weaning Response
  (DVWR)
Dysreflexia
Dysreflexia: Risk for Autonomic
Energy Field Disturbance
Environmental Interpretation Syndrome, Impaired
Family Coping: Compromised, Ineffective
Family Coping: Disabling, Ineffective
Family Coping: Potential for Growth
Family Process: Alcoholism, Altered
Family Processes, Altered
Fatigue
Fear
Fluid Volume Deficit
Fluid Volume Deficit, Risk for
Fluid Volume Excess
Fluid Volume Imbalance: Risk for
Gas Exchange, Impaired
Grieving, Anticipatory
Grieving, Dysfunctional
Growth and Development, Altered
Health Maintenance, Altered
Health Seeking Behaviors (Specify)

Home Maintenance Management, Impaired
Hopelessness
Hyperthermia
Hypothermia
Incontinence, Bowel
Incontinence, Functional
Incontinence, Reflex Urinary
Incontinence, Stress
Incontinence, Total
Incontinence, Risk for Urinary
Individual Coping, Ineffective
Infant Feeding Pattern, Ineffective
Infection, Risk for
Injury, Risk for
Knowledge Deficit (Specify)
Loneliness, Risk for
Management of Therapeutic Regimen: Community,
  Ineffective
Management of Therapeutic Regimen: Families, In-
  effective
Management of Therapeutic Regimen: Individual,
  Effective
Management of Therapeutic Regimen (Individual)
  Ineffective
Memory, Impaired
Noncompliance (Specify)
Nutrition: Less than Body Requirements, Altered
Nutrition: More than Body Requirements, Altered
Nutrition: Potential for More than Body Require-
  ments, Altered
Oral Mucous Membrane, Altered
Organized Infant Behavior, Potential for Enhanced
  Pain
Pain, Chronic
Parental Role Conflict
Parent/Infant/Child Attachment, Risk for Altered
Parenting, Altered
Parenting, Risk for Altered
Perioperative Positioning Injury, Risk for
Peripheral Neurovascular Dysfunction, Risk for
Personal Identity Disturbance
Physical Mobility, Impaired
Poisoning, Risk for
Post-Trauma Syndrome
Post-Trauma Syndrome: Risk for
Powerlessness
Protection, Altered
Rape-Trauma Syndrome
Rape-Trauma Syndrome: Compound Reaction
Rape-Trauma Syndrome: Silent Reaction
Relocation Stress Syndrome
Role Performance, Altered
Self Care Deficit
  Bathing/Hygiene
  Dressing/Grooming
  Feeding
  Toileting

Box 11–2 ■ ■ ■ ■ ■
North American Nursing Diagnosis Association–Approved Nursing Diagnoses Continued

Self Esteem, Chronic Low	Spiritual Well-Being, Potential for Enhanced
Self Esteem Disturbance	Suffocation, Risk for
Self Esteem, Situational Low	Sustain Spontaneous Ventilation, Inability to
Self Mutilation, Risk for	Swallowing, Impaired
Sensory/Perceptual Alterations (Specify) (Visual, Auditory, Kinesthetic, Gustatory, Tactile, Olfactory)	Thermoregulation, Ineffective
	Thought Processes, Altered
Sexual Dysfunction	Tissue Integrity, Impaired
Sexuality Patterns, Altered	Tissue Perfusion, Altered (Specify Type) (Renal, Cerebral, Cardiopulmonary, Gastrointestinal, Peripheral)
Skin Integrity, Impaired	
Skin Integrity, Risk for Impaired	
Sleep Pattern Disturbance	Transfer Ability: Impaired
Social Interaction, Impaired	Trauma, Risk for
Social Isolation	Unilateral Neglect
Sorrow, Chronic	Urinary Elimination, Altered
Spiritual Distress (Distress of the Human Spirit)	Urinary Retention
Spiritual Distress: Risk for	Violence: Risk for Self-Directed or Directed at Others

Diagnoses listed in alphabetical order. Modified from 1999 NANDA listing, which lists by taxonomy. Modified from North American Nursing Diagnosis Association (1999). *NANDA nursing diagnoses: Definitions and classification 1999-2000* (pp. 1–7). Philadelphia: NANDA.

Using logical decision-making to apply knowledge and critical thinking, you then analyze the data. This analysis logically progresses from the data to the identification of the nursing diagnosis (Wilkinson, 1992). Box 11–3 shows the steps in this process.

A nursing diagnosis describes an existing or high-risk problem and requires a three-part statement:

1. The health problem
2. The etiological or contributing factors
3. The defining characteristics

The health problem consists of the behavior disruption, or potential disruption, that you have identified and can be improved through nursing intervention. It is the

Box 11–3 ■ ■ ■ ■ ■
Steps in Logical Decision-Making for Arriving at Nursing Diagnoses

1. Identify the patient's behavioral, biological, psychosocial, and spiritual responses to stress.
2. Categorize the data into functional groups.
3. Identify missing data and any incongruencies.
4. Identify any patterns.
5. Compare the data to theoretical information, norms, and standards.
6. Identify basic needs and concerns, taking into account the patient's strengths and limitations.
7. Identify any causal relationships.
8. Identify the applicable nursing diagnoses.

patient's unmet need. The etiological factors include the stressors that contributed to the problem; these can be thought of as the probable causes of the problem. The defining characteristics describe signs and symptoms; these reflect the objective and subjective data for the nursing interventions (Alfaro, 1990; Carpenito, 1995; Doenges & Moorehouse, 1992; Gordon, 1994).

Let's look back at the assessment data (see Box 11–1) and Box 11–4 for Mrs. Ryan to derive nursing diagnoses. Once the nursing diagnoses are identified, the next step is the **prioritization** of the problems in order of importance. Highest priority is given to those problems that are life-threatening. Next in priority are those problems that are likely to cause destructive changes. Lowest in priority are those issues that are related to normative or developmental experiences (Sundeen et al., 1994). Psychiatric nurses often use Maslow's hierarchy of needs to help them prioritize nursing diagnoses (see Chapter 6).

At this point, the nurse validates the identified problems with the patient (if possible) and discusses the next steps on the journey (Freund, 1993), which include establishing the desired outcomes and planning the interventions to accomplish these goals.

Documentation. It is important to document nursing diagnoses or problems in the patient record, whether it is part of the nursing care plan or part of the multidisciplinary treatment plan. Standardized nursing forms may list common NANDA diagnoses for psychiatric patients, but these need to be individualized for each patient. The nurse's charting system may be based on using the nursing diagnosis as a focus. The data, action, and response (DAR format) includes descriptive data, the nursing actions, and the patient's response (Townsend, 1991).

Box 11-4 ■ ■ ■ ■ ■
Mrs. Ryan

Medical Diagnosis

Schizophrenia, paranoid

Nursing Diagnoses

Sleep Pattern Disturbance related to Anxiety as evidenced by pacing at night without sleep.

Altered Thought Process related to hallucinations as evidenced by staring and verbal responses to unseen beings.

Noncompliance with medications related to paranoia as evidenced by relapse with psychotic symptoms.

Altered Nutrition: Less than Body Requirements related to preoccupation with hallucinations as evidenced by eating fewer than two meals per day.

What do you think? Why should a psychiatric nurse have excellent physical as well as psychiatric assessment skills? What would you say to someone who said that psychiatric nurses only talk to patients?

➤ *Check Your Reading*

11. What is the definition of the nursing diagnosis?
12. From what are nursing diagnoses derived?
13. What are the steps in logical decision-making?
14. What is the name of the group that develops the approved list of nursing diagnoses?
15. What are the three parts to a nursing diagnosis statement?
16. How are nursing diagnoses and the psychiatric diagnoses in DSM-IV related?

Outcome Identification

To ensure that the nurse-patient journey is moving in the right direction, the nurse identifies specific goals or **expected outcomes** with criteria for measurement. Expected outcomes are the patient behaviors that the nurse anticipates will occur as a result of nursing interventions, indicating the resolution of or progress toward the patient's problem or unmet need.

There are seven criteria for writing a scientifically sound expected outcome (Hickey, 1990; Redman, 1993); the outcome should be

1. Patient centered
2. Singular
3. Observable
4. Measurable
5. Time limited
6. Mutual
7. Realistic

By including all these elements, the statement of an expected outcome provides information that can be readily evaluated. It designates *who* (the patient) will *do what* (the single behavior to be observed) *how, how much, how often,* and *to what degree* (criteria for measurement), and *when and where* (situational parameters). The nurse encourages the patient to participate as much as possible in setting these goals to ensure that they are mutually agreeable and realistic.

There is at least one expected outcome for each nursing diagnosis, which can also be thought of as the long-term goal. When this outcome is achieved, the problem is considered to be resolved. Because long-term success may take some time, and the patient or nurse may grow discouraged, it is advisable to identify a series of short-term goals that lead to fulfillment of the longer-term expected outcome. You need to recognize that not all long-term goals will be met before discharge: success with short-term goals will be interpreted as evidence of an effective treatment plan that can continue in a less intensive setting. Refer to Box 11-5 for an example of some of Mrs. Ryan's expected outcomes.

When you plan care in this manner, you and your patient can experience increments of success while moving toward your shared destination. Once realistic goals have been developed, the planning step of the process begins.

Documentation. Documenting expected outcomes is very important to steer the nurse-patient journey. By aiming for each preestablished short-term goal as a landmark, the nurse ensures that the trip goes as planned with minimal detours. Without clearly defined outcomes as described earlier, the patient and nurse could stray into territory or issues that are beyond the scope of the particular level of care. All short-term goals must lead the patient in the direction of the final long-term goal, that is, meeting the discharge criteria and moving on to a less restrictive level of care.

What do you think? If a patient is delusional or hallucinating, can you establish mutuality for goal setting? Is it possible to respect a patient's autonomy while setting goals for him or her? If one of the treatment goals is to increase the patient's adherence to a medication regimen and the patient refuses to take medications, how should this be handled? What are your feelings about these kinds of situations, which are not unusual in psychiatric nursing?

➤ *Check Your Reading*

17. What is the purpose of nursing outcomes?
18. What are the criteria for writing an expected outcome?
19. How are short-term goals related to expected outcomes?

Planning

In this stage, you will choose nursing interventions appropriate to an individual's identified problems with specific expected outcomes. To develop a nursing care plan, you must make deliberate decisions about your actions based on your level of practice. ANA defines the *basic* level of psychiatric nursing to include the following categories of interventions:

1. *Counseling*—Communication and interviewing techniques to help patients modify behavior, including teaching new behavior.
2. *Milieu therapy*—Therapeutic use of environment.
3. *Self-care activities*—Helping the patient assume responsibility for the activities of daily living.
4. *Psychobiological interventions*—Medications and other interventions that affect the patient's physiological processes.
5. *Health teaching*—Giving information to decrease a knowledge deficit.
6. *Case management*—Coordination of multiple health services and ensuring continuity of care.
7. *Health promotion and health maintenance*—Enhancement of mental health and prevention of mental illness with clients at-risk for problems.

The psychiatric nurse with an *advanced* level of practice also uses the following interventions:

1. Psychotherapy
2. Prescription of pharmacological agents
3. Consultation

Refer to Chapter 14 for more in-depth discussion of each of these categories.

Many references are available to provide standardized approaches to care that you can tailor to your particular patient situation (see Table 11–2). You can also base your interventions on a nursing intervention classification (NIC) system to ensure that your actions are supported by nursing research and accepted standards of practice (McCloskey & Bulechek, 1992).

One conceptual approach to organize your plan of care focuses on three areas of concern: (1) ongoing monitoring of the patient's level of health, including physical and emotional factors; (2) providing the patient with information to improve his or her level of self-care; and (3) teaching the patient skills to increase his or her level of self-care. For example, in the case of Mrs. Ryan, health problems requiring close monitoring included

1. Disturbed eating pattern
2. Disturbed sleeping pattern
3. Response to hallucinations
4. Response to delusions
5. Increased anxiety level
6. No concurrent medical illnesses to monitor (i.e., if she had had diabetes or hypertension, symptoms of those problems would also have needed ongoing evaluation)

In relation to her knowledge deficits, she needed teaching regarding

1. Illness: Schizophrenia
2. Medication: Purpose, action, and side effects
3. Relapse prevention: Medication compliance, use of social support, healthy habits including eating, sleeping, exercise, and identification of precipitating factors

With regard to her skill deficits, she needed education about

1. Personal care: Eating, bathing, and grooming
2. Cognitive skills: Use of calendar and clock and use of daily or weekly medication container
3. Coping skills: Self-awareness of symptoms of stress, relaxation techniques, setting realistic goals, and controlling response to hallucinations
4. Communication skills: Recognizing feelings, verbal expression of feelings, and assertiveness training

Box 11–5 ■ ■ ■ ■ ■

Example of Long-Term and Short-Term Expected Outcomes for Mrs. Ryan

Long-Term Goal

1. By day 14, the patient will resume usual sleep pattern of 6 hours per night × 3 days.
2. By day 10, the patient will verbalize that she is not hearing voices × 24 hours.

Short-Term Goal

1A. By day 3, the patient will sleep 4 hours × 1.
1B. By day 7, the patient will sleep 6 hours × 1.
2A. By day 2, the patient will respond nonverbally to the nurse by shaking her head yes or no.
2B. By day 5, the patient will verbalize yes or no to simple questions about ADLs.
2C. By day 7, the patient will report decreased frequency of hearing voices.

ADLs, activities of daily living.

A plan of care with interventions to improve the patient's health status and to address deficits in self-care knowledge and skills provides a strong foundation for realistic, achievable patient outcomes. Actual and potential problems are recognized and the whole patient can be treated, targeting physical as well as emotional symptoms. Once you have made a comprehensive plan, you are ready for the next stage of the process, implementation.

Documentation. Whether or not you use a standardized nursing care plan, it is desirable for the admitting nurse to initiate the care plan. As described previously, you are the one who has gathered the most data and interacted with the patient for the longest time since admission. You have already observed the patient's response to yourself and the new environment. Hopefully, the patient has begun to trust you and the treatment team that you represent. Documenting your mutually agreed-on plan is the best way to ensure that the patient will receive that specific care. When nursing staff follow through on your initial plan, the patient's trust is reinforced, facilitating his or her engagement in the treatment process.

> **W**hat do you think? How do you approach the issue of improving a patient's self-care knowledge or skill if the patient is delusional, hallucinating, or generally uncooperative with the plan of treatment?

> ➤ *Check Your Reading*
> 20. How might nursing interventions be categorized in a nursing care plan?
> 21. What are the interventions available to the psychiatric nurse at the basic level of practice?
> 22. What intervention includes communication and interviewing?

Implementation

Implementation refers to all of the nursing actions that the nurse takes to facilitate the patient's achievement of identified patient outcomes. As noted previously, the interventions that you will use in psychiatric nursing depend on your level of practice.

Using the care plan described for Mrs. Ryan as the example, the psychiatric nurse with the basic level of practice would have implemented the following interventions: counseling, milieu therapy, self-care activities, psychobiological interventions, and health teaching.

1. *Counseling* techniques include all of the daily communication with the patient to monitor her health problems and to encourage her verbalization; it also includes teaching to improve her communication and coping skills.

2. *Milieu therapy* involves daily explanation of the hospital ward routine and establishing a consistent schedule for meals, activities, medication, and sleep.

3. *Self-care activities* include all of the assistance needed to help Mrs. Ryan perform activities of daily living, delivered in a manner to preserve her dignity and

to increase her independence as soon as possible. It is notable that the patient's level of functioning must be continuously reevaluated because it will vary over the course of treatment (Johnson et al., 1992). In fact, changes in nonverbal behavior may be the first signs of progress.

4. *Psychobiological interventions* comprise the administration of all medications with observation for effectiveness and side effects. Changes in dosage for psychotropic medication are directly related to nursing staff reports of behavior changes indicating progress or reports of side effects.

5. *Health teaching* addresses all of the other teaching needs or deficits identified in the patient's knowledge and skills. The content and timing for all teaching must be appropriate to the patient's readiness to learn. For example, medication teaching may take place informally at each medication time on a one-to-one basis starting on the 1st day. Teaching about healthy habits as part of relapse prevention could be done in a group later in the hospital stay after the patient's thinking is clearer.

Once you have begun to implement your nursing care plan for an individual patient, you are ready for the final step in the nursing process, evaluation.

Documentation. Ongoing documentation of nursing observations and interventions usually makes up the majority of the chart in most settings. There are various systems for charting progress based on nursing process. One method records steps of the nursing process in each note, the APIE system: *A* for *a*ssessed information; *P* for the *p*roblem; *I* for the *i*ntervention used; and *E* for *e*valuation of the outcomes. Another approach is the problem-oriented record (POR) system. There is a multidisciplinary list of problems to which the nurse refers in a SOAPIE format note: *S* for *s*ubjective patient data about the problem; *O* for *o*bjective data about the problem; *A* for the nurse's *a*ssessment; *P* for the nurse's *p*lan; *I* for the *i*ntervention used; and *E* for *e*valuation of the outcome. More recently, the format for the patient record uses checklists, flowsheets, and limited narrative to streamline the chart. Carson (1994) developed a charting system for psychiatric home care to link the clinical notes to the care plan with the emphasis on patient outcomes for each visit (Figure 11-3).

> **W**hat do you think? How would you address milieu issues in environments other than the inpatient unit? What would your role be regarding milieu in an outpatient clinic?

> ➤ *Check Your Reading*
> 23. What is the focus of milieu therapy?
> 24. What is the aim of self-care interventions?
> 25. What is involved in psychobiological interventions?
> 26. What deficits are the focus of health teaching interventions?
> 27. What is the APIE method for documenting nursing progress notes?
> 28. What is the SOAPIE format for problem-oriented charting?

PSYCHIATRIC NURSING CLINICAL NOTE

PATIENT NAME: _Carl DeBeers_   DATE: _3/5/96_

GOALS THIS VISIT (MUST BE TAKEN FROM CARE PLAN) _Assess the level of activity the pt. is capable of assuming._

Ascertain the duties the HHA will need to assume.

REASON HOMEBOUND (CHECK ALL THAT APPLY)
_____ DISORIENTED
_____ BEHAVIOR POSES RISK TO SELF/OTHERS
_____ USES ASSISTIVE DEVICE TO AID MOBILITY (CANE, WALKER, WHEELCHAIR, BRACES)
_✔_ LIMITED ENDURANCE RELATED TO MEDICAL DX (BECOMES SOB WITH MILD EXERTION)
_____ JUDGMENT IMPAIRED — REQUIRES 24-HOUR SUPERVISION
_✔_ LEAVING HOME IS NOT POSSIBLE WITHOUT TAXING EFFORT
_✔_ LEAVING HOME IS DEPENDENT ON ASSISTANCE FROM OTHERS
_____ AGORAPHOBIC

VITAL SIGNS (IF APPLICABLE)   BP _156/100 sitting   146/100 standing_ P _88_   TEMP _____   RESP _24_ WT_____

ASSESSMENT: CHECK IF ASSESSED; RECORD ONLY SIGNIFICANT CHANGES
MENTAL STATUS:

ORIENTATION _✔_	MEDICATION _____
MEMORY _✔_	EFFECTIVE _✔_
THOUGHT PROCESS _Focused on multiple symptoms_	SIDE EFFECTS _✔_
THOUGHT CONTENT _____	COMPLIANT _✔ Compliant_
EMOTIONAL TONE _"Hyper"_	ACTIVITIES OF DAILY LIVING
SUICIDAL/HOMICIDAL	ACTIVITY AND REST _✔ Limited by dyspnea on exertion_
IDEATION _____	NUTRITION/ELIMINATION _✔_
INTENT _Denies_	HYGIENE/APPEARANCE _✔_
PLAN _____	DIVERSIONAL ACTIVITIES _✔_
JUDGMENT/SAFETY _✔_	SOCIALIZATION _✔_

PATIENT BEHAVIOR/INTERACTION _Expending energies in various directions_
CAREGIVER BEHAVIOR/INTERACTION _____
EMERGENCY/CRISIS INTERVENTION SINCE LAST VISIT:
YES _____   (DESCRIBE) _____
NO _✔_

COMPLIANCE WITH FOLLOW-UP APPOINTMENTS:
YES _____   DATE _3/2/96_   FREQUENCY _Seen in clinic for complaints of left rib pain_
3/4/96   To have chest film and angiogram. To see psychiatrist — Dr. Pearl
NO (ELABORATE) _____

ANY ADDITIONAL ASSESSMENT:
INTERVENTIONS: (IDENTIFY WITH CAREPLAN CODE AND INTERVENTION NUMBER: NEW INTERVENTIONS SHOULD BE ADDED TO CAREPLAN AND DESCRIBED HERE)

INTERVENTIONS	PATIENT/CAREGIVER OUTCOMES	EVALUATION
#3A-D	Medication teaching on Desyrel. Compliant with meds	U.T., G.C.
#10A, B, C #5B, C	Using neighbors for hospital rides, shopping. Detests the dependence	U.T., G.C.
#6B, F, G	Puts little energy into meal preparation–using dietary supplements	U.T., G.C.
#7A-D	Sleeping can be a problem–discussed relaxation techniques	P.T., G.C.
#12A, E, F	Activities have ↑ anxiety–poor understanding of relaxation	P.T., G.C.
#15I, K, H	Bedtime routine lacking	U.T., G.C.

HHA SUPERVISION (EVERY 14 DAYS):

VERBAL ORDERS NEEDED (IF SO, COMPLETE ORDER SHEET AND MODIFY CAREPLAN)

SIGNATURE: _Miriam Jacik, R.N._   REVISIT: _3/5/96_

GOALS FOR NEXT VISIT: _Teaching on addictive behaviors, decreasing cigarettes in light of ↑ COPD_

CODE FOR PATIENT/CAREGIVER OUTCOMES:		CODE FOR EVALUATION OF GOALS:	
UNDERSTOOD TEACHING	= UT	GOALS BEGUN	= GB
UNDERSTOOD PART OF TEACHING	= PT	GOALS CONTINUING	= GC
DOES NOT UNDERSTAND TEACHING	= NOT	GOALS MET	= GM
LESS DEPRESSED	= LD	GOALS REVISED	= GR
MORE DEPRESSED	= MD		
LESS ANXIOUS	= LA		
MORE ANXIOUS	= MA		
FOLLOWED THROUGH WITH NURSE'S SUGGESTIONS	= FLU		

Figure 11–3
A completed example of one of Carson's Psychiatric Nursing Clinical Notes. (Modified from Carson, V. B. [1994]. *Bay Area psychiatric home care manual.* Baltimore: Bay Area Health Care.)

Evaluation

The last step of the nursing process is **evaluation,** but that does not mean that it is an ending. Remember the dynamic nature of the nursing process represented in Figure 11–1. Evaluation means continuous monitoring of the patient (Is he or she accomplishing the expected outcomes?) as well as monitoring the effectiveness of nursing interventions (Should the intervention continue or be revised?). As the patient shows changes over time, new data lead to reassessment and the cycle of the nursing process starts all over again.

Two types of evaluation—formative and summative—can be used. **Formative evaluation** includes reassessment of all aspects of the nursing process as you are implementing care to analyze the patient's responses. The success or failure of a nursing intervention may be due to any number of factors that occur throughout the nursing process (Harris & Gillien, 1992). In performing a formative evaluation, ask yourself these questions:

1. Is the assessment adequate and accurate?

2. Are the nursing diagnoses correctly stated to deal with the patient's needs?

3. Are the expected outcomes properly focused and written in a manner that facilitates evaluation of the achievement of expected outcome?

4. Are the planned interventions adequately thorough, based on sound principles, and efficiently implemented?

5. Can anything else be done if the interventions have not helped the patient to achieve the expected outcome?

6. Can the expected outcomes and short-term goals

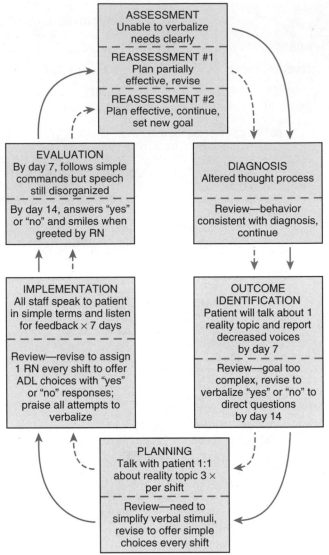

Figure 11–5
Nursing process related to Mrs. Ryan's thought process. ADL, activities of daily living.

be modified to be more applicable to this patient at this time?

7. Can other, more relevant nursing diagnoses be considered?

8. Should any elements of the plan of care be discontinued? Why?

Refer to Figures 11–4 and 11–5 for examples of formative evaluation of the nursing process for two of Mrs. Ryan's problems.

A **summative evaluation** is one in which you make a concluding statement about the entire nurse-patient journey. The summative evaluation includes information from the formative evaluation, as well as recommendations for future nursing care, as appropriate. The summative evaluation is most helpful when you are planning for the patient's discharge from care. It encompasses the status of all identified nursing diagnoses, the patient's current functional status, and recommended actions and referrals. A summative evaluation greatly assists in providing continuity of care.

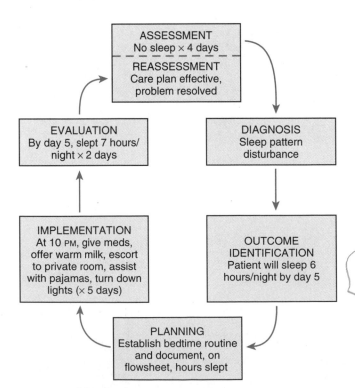

Figure 11–4
Nursing process related to Mrs. Ryan's sleep.

Documentation. As described in the implementation section, evaluation is partially documented in each progress note written by all of the professional staff. Periodically, though, the primary nurse or nurse case manager needs to review all notes and return to the nursing care plan for formal modification. Achievement of short-term and long-term goals is recorded along with dates. When outcomes are not being accomplished, there is reassessment of each step of the nursing process, as noted previously for revisions. Remember, you and the patient designed these expected outcomes as landmarks for the journey. Failure to reach them may indicate you have wandered off the desired path, or perhaps you set up a course that is too steep to follow. Redefining the problem, the outcome, or the intervention must be done promptly in order to maximize the benefits for the patient for this episode of care. As always, the nurse's evaluation is shared with the treatment team and also has an impact on the third-party payer, who is literally counting days of treatment by measuring the patient's outcomes. On discharge, you complete a discharge summary for the record (summative evaluation) and discharge instructions for the patient to summarize significant recommendations for aftercare.

W*hat do you think?* Are there other nursing situations in which an ongoing evaluation as well as a final evaluation would be useful? In what ways does evaluating as you go along help to keep your care focused? Should the patient be involved in the evaluation process? If so, how would you involve Mrs. Ryan?

➤ *Check Your Reading*
29. What is formative evaluation?
30. What is summative evaluation?

ASSESSMENT REVISITED

Now that you have reviewed all six steps of the nursing process, it is important to reinforce the significance of the beginning step in the cycle, that is, assessment and reassessment. As indicated earlier, the nursing database forms the baseline against which behavioral changes in the patient can be measured, indicating the effects of treatment. Nurses are not the only ones interested in this baseline description: other members of the health care team review this information as they formulate their impressions and treatment recommendations; also, third-party payers use initial nursing observations to determine if the patient qualifies for the particular level of care. Reassessment data collected by the nurse are used to revise the nursing care plan, to modify the multidisciplinary treatment plan, and to justify continued treatment to the third-party payer.

In order to produce an accurate and timely nursing assessment, you will use a formal interview with a structured **data collection tool.** The language used in any data collection tool reflects the theoretical frame-

work of its author. Many nursing theorists (e.g., Dorothy Orem, Sister Callista Roy, and Madeline Leininger) have defined the areas of concern for nursing attention in different ways. (For more detail on nursing theories, see Chapter 6.)

One example of a holistic nursing assessment tool is presented here to illustrate significant dimensions as defined by the ANA Psychiatric–Mental Health Nursing Standards. Before explaining the parts of the tool itself, four significant aspects of the initial interview are highlighted.

NEED FOR ATTENTION TO THE ART OF NURSING

First, the unique perspective of nursing, as compared with other health care professions, is its focus on the whole individual with his or her particular problems and potential health problems, along with his or her particular responses. As you assess a patient, you must avoid following the medical model of seeking patterns of behavior and symptoms merely to establish a diagnosis and treatment plan (Salisbury, 1985). Although you are collecting information, you are also starting a therapeutic journey with a unique individual. You need to use simple, clear communication with the patient, and avoid the specialized jargon so characteristic of medical assessment tools (Henderson, 1987). Such jargon poses an unnecessary roadblock to the nurse-patient journey.

NEED FOR SELF-AWARENESS

Second, you need to understand the possible influence of subjective reactions during the interview. You must develop **self-awareness** in order to recognize your personal biases and to reflect on your behavior throughout the conversation. Farrell (1991) noted that "assessment packages are only as good as the data collecting agent" (p. 1062). In all communication situations, both participants experience subjective responses. Relating to a patient who may be resistant or unable to verbalize clearly brings out various reactions in the nurse. These reactions must be acknowledged to differentiate your own responses from those of the patient, so that the data which you document is truly objective. At the same time, an experienced nurse learns to use her or his feelings as a barometer to what is happening in the nurse-patient relationship. For example, if the nurse feels anxiety only in the presence of a particular patient, it is probably indicative of some sort of stress in that relationship.

NEED FOR CONSIDERATION OF PATIENT PERCEPTIONS

Third, you must try to place a central focus on the patient's point of view to demonstrate respect as you initiate the nurse-patient relationship. Throughout the dialogue you listen attentively and accept the patient's

TABLE 11–2 Standardized Rating Scales and Their Use

USE	SCALE (S)
Depression	Beck Inventory
	Hamilton Depression Scale
	Montgomery-Asburg Depression Inventory
	Zung Self-Report Inventory
Anxiety	Modified Spielberger State Anxiety Scale
	Sheehan Patient-Related Anxiety Scale
Obsessive-compulsive behavior	Yale-Brown Obsessive-Compulsive Scale (Y-BOCS)
Mania	Mania Rating Scale
Schizophrenia	Scale for Assessment of Negative Symptoms
Abnormal movements	Abnormal Involuntary Movement Scale (AIMS)
	Simpson Neurological Rating Scale
	CLAMPS Abnormal Movement Scale
General psychiatric assessment	Brief Psychiatric Rating Scale (BPRS)
	Global Assessment of Functioning Scale
Cognitive function	Mini-Mental State Examination
Assessment of children	Connors Parent Questionnaire
	Connors Teacher Questionnaire
	Children's Behavior Inventory
	Children's Psychiatric Rating Scale

report in a nonjudgmental way. The message given to the patient both verbally and nonverbally is that he or she is a partner in solving the problem. Barker (1987) proposed that the interviewer proceed through five steps to really learn about the patient's view of self and the problem:

1. Identify the problem
2. Measure the intensity and frequency
3. Clarify relation to various situations
4. Listen to the patient's explanation or theory about the cause of the problem
5. Listen to the patient's view of any patterns related to the problem.

NEED FOR STANDARDIZED RATING SCALES

Finally, you may be expected to use **standardized rating scales** in addition to the nursing assessment tool. There are several advantages to incorporating these test results into the initial assessment. The test provides an additional, measurable observation for the database that can be used by the nurse or the team in evaluating

outcomes. Also, nurses and patients alike report satisfaction with the use of instruments: nurses feel that they are learning more about the patient and patients enjoy increased contact with the nurse. Table 11-2 lists standardized rating scales that are useful in mental health assessment and indicates how they are used. Some of these rating scales appear in the appropriate disorders chapters in Unit V.

What do you think? How would you introduce a patient to the idea of using standardized assessment tools? How do you feel about interviewing a psychiatric patient? How might your feelings affect the outcomes of the interview?

➤ *Check Your Reading*
31. Name three reasons for the nurse to collect ongoing reassessment data.
32. Why is it important for the nurse to talk in simple, clear terms during the interview?
33. Why must the nurse be explicit about subjective impressions when interviewing the psychiatric patient?
34. Describe two techniques used by the nurse to demonstrate respect for the patient.
35. Identify three advantages to the nurse in using standardized rating scales.

CONDUCTING THE ASSESSMENT

The following 11 sections explain the sample psychiatric nursing assessment tool that is found in Figure 11-6. Remember, you are evaluating a whole person who is a complex system. Even though emotional and physical subsystems are described separately, in reality, there is always interaction between them. For example, physical problems may produce considerable psychological symptoms, and psychological distress can produce significant physical changes. (For more extensive discussion on the anatomy and physiology of the brain that correlates with psychiatric disorders, see Chapter 7.)

Patient Identification

After you introduce yourself and explain the purpose of the interview, it is important to ask the patient all of the basic questions listed in section I and to obtain a full set of vital signs. This initial information exchange provides a brief neutral zone in which the patient and nurse can observe each other and begin their journey. Although the nurse may be analyzing the patient's orientation and general appearance, the patient is deciding if the nurse is trustworthy based on verbal and nonverbal signs of respect. The setting should be as quiet and private as possible. One small but important detail is to ask the patient his or her name preferenceso that staff use it. Without a preference, the patient

I. PATIENT IDENTIFICATION

Date and time of admission _____ By _____ , R.N.

Name _____ Age _____ Sex _____ Race _____

Address _____ Phone _____

Significant other _____ Relation _____

Legal status _____ Referred by _____

Prefers to be called _____

Vital signs: BP_____ T _____ P _____ R _____ Ht _____ Wt _____

II. CHIEF COMPLAINT

Reason for seeking treatment _____

Recent history re: concerns _____

Any suicidal or aggressive ideation _____

Any history of suicidal or aggressive behavior _____

Any family history of suicide or violence _____

III. MEDICATION HISTORY (complete Medication Profile)

IV. HISTORY OF PRIOR PSYCHIATRIC TREATMENT

Date(s), by whom, type _____

Compliance with treatment _____

Effect of treatment _____

Goals for current treatment _____

V. EMOTIONAL ASSESSMENT

Mood: Anxious ☐   Depressed ☐   Euphoric ☐

            Hostile ☐   Labile ☐   Other ☐

Describe (verbal and nonverbal signs) _____

Affect: Sad ☐   Elated ☐   Labile ☐

            Flat ☐   Inappropriate ☐   Other ☐

Describe (verbal and nonverbal signs) _____

Coping patterns–describe usual behavior when feeling:

Anxious _____

Sad _____

Angry _____

VI. COGNITIVE ASSESSMENT

Orientation: Person ☐   Place ☐   Time ☐

                 Describe alteration _____

Memory: Immediate ☐   Recent ☐   Remote ☐

                 Describe deficit(s) _____

Attention: Alert ☐   Lethargic ☐   Distracted ☐

                 Other ☐   Describe other _____

Fund of information: Last three presidents _____

Concentration: Serial 7s _____

Judgment: What would you do in a crowded movie theater if you smelled smoke? _____

Abstract thinking: Similarities (apple/orange) _____

                    Proverb (glass houses) _____

Figure 11–6
A psychiatric nursing assessment tool.

Illustration continued on following page

VI. CONTINUED

Perception: Hallucination ☐   Illusion ☐

                      Describe _____

Communication: Verbal _____

                          Nonverbal _____

                          Any physical impairment   No ☐   Yes ☐   Describe _____

Thinking: Logical ☐   Coherent ☐   Blocking ☐

                         Loose associations ☐   Disorganized ☐   Circumstantial ☐

                         Grandiose ☐   Paranoid ☐   Delusional ☐

                         Describe _____

Self-concept: Strengths _____

                         Weaknesses _____

Insight: Recognizes need for help   Yes ☐   No ☐

                 Accepts responsibilty for self   Yes ☐   No ☐

                 Describe _____

VII. PHYSICAL ASSESSMENT

General appearance (bruises, scars) _____

Current medications (add to Medication Profile) _____

Previous illness/surgery/accident (include date) _____

Current diet _____

Any problem with: Head/neck ☐   Integumentary ☐   Musculoskeletal ☐

                               Mouth/throat ☐   Respiratory ☐   Cardiovascular ☐

                               Nose/ears ☐   Neurological ☐   Genitourinary/reproductive ☐

                               Eyes ☐   Gastrointestinal ☐   Pain (score 1–10) ☐

                               Endocrine ☐

Describe symptoms and treatment _____

Use of: Cigarettes   No ☐   Yes ☐ _____

                Caffeine   No ☐   Yes ☐ _____

                Alcohol   No ☐   Yes ☐ _____

                Drugs   No ☐   Yes ☐ _____

ADLs (activities of daily living)

Activities:	Independ.	Needs assist.	Fully depend.
Ambulating	☐	☐	☐
Toileting	☐	☐	☐
Transfer	☐	☐	☐
Personal care	☐	☐	☐
Feeding	☐	☐	☐

Complete bedrest   ☐ Yes   ☐ No
Bedrest and bathroom   ☐ Yes   ☐ No
Up as tolerated   ☐ Yes   ☐ No
Transfer bed/chair   ☐ Yes   ☐ No
No restrictions   ☐ Yes   ☐ No
Weightbearing   ☐ Full   ☐ Partial   ☐ Non
Other _____

Describe abnormal findings/teaching or referral needs _____

IADLs (instrumental activities of daily living)

Activities:	Independ.	Needs assist.	Fully depend.
Preparing light meals	☐	☐	☐
Preparing full meals	☐	☐	☐
Light housekeeping	☐	☐	☐
Personal laundry	☐	☐	☐
Handling money	☐	☐	☐
Using telephone	☐	☐	☐
Errands	☐	☐	☐

Describe abnormal findings/teaching or referral needs _____

_____

_____

Figure 11–6 *Continued*

VII. CONTINUED

ABUSE ASSESSMENT

TRIADS (type, role of offender, intensity, autonomic symptoms, duration, style) _____

VIII. SOCIOCULTURAL ASSESSMENT

Living situation (spouse or significant other, children, home, responsibilities) _____

Support system (family, friends, agencies) _____

Occupation/income _____

Education _____

Community involvement _____

Current economic/legal/environmental stressors _____

Ethnic background _____

Cultural beliefs related to current problem/treatment _____

IX. SPIRITUAL AND PHILOSOPHICAL ASSESSMENT

Spiritual beliefs _____

Participation in religious practices _____

Beliefs related to current problem _____

Beliefs related to current treatment _____

Most important life values _____

X. ADDITIONAL ASSESSMENT

Input from significant other/secondary source _____

Patient reaction to interviewer _____

Interviewer reaction to patient _____

XI. PROBLEM IDENTIFICATION AND NURSING DIAGNOSIS (refer also to Medication Profile)

Prioritize the three most immediate needs by placing a number beside the appropriate description:

Emotional ☐ _____ Physical ☐ _____ Spiritual ☐ _____

Cognitive ☐ _____ Sociocultural ☐ _____ Discharge planning ☐ _____

Risk factors present (check all that apply):

Danger to self ☐   Danger to others ☐

Elopement ☐   History of noncompliance ☐

History of adverse medication reaction ☐ _____

Concurrent medical problem ☐ _____

Other ☐ Explain _____

If unable to complete full database, explain _____

(Follow-up as necessary and write date and initials in each section when completed.)

Figure 11–6 *Continued*

Illustration continued on following page

III. MEDICATION PROFILE

Name _____ Age _____ Sex _____ Date of admission _____

Admission vital signs: BP _____   T _____   P _____   R _____   Ht _____   Wt _____

Allergies _____

Medication	Reason	Date started	Dose	Effect	Side effects/adverse reactions
I. Current prescriptions					
1.					
2.					
3.					
4.					
5.					
6.					
7.					
8.					
9.					
10.					
II. Current over-the-counter (weekly)					
1.					
2.					
3.					
4.					
5.					
III. History of prescriptions					
1.					
2.					
3.					
4.					
5.					

Figure 11–6 *Continued*

is always addressed by his or her formal title. Last in this section, complete the vital signs. These data cannot be overlooked because the vital signs may be the first clue about a concurrent physical problem that the patient may not verbalize clearly (Dreyfus, 1987; Holmberg, 1988).

Chief Complaint

This portion of the database requires much patience and encouragement on the part of the nurse as the patient begins to discuss potentially painful material. It is necessary to determine why the patient is seeking help at this point in time to allow the nurse to identify the precipitating event.

Questioning about suicidal and aggressive risks must be done in a matter-of-fact tone of voice. As the patient responds, the nurse has the opportunity to give information about hospital or agency procedures (e.g., precautions, privilege levels, and so forth). The nurse can also indicate that this problem is not totally unique and that other patients with similar concerns have been helped by treatment. It is imperative that the nurse record exactly what the patient says about his or her perception of the problem, regardless of what the nurse may know from secondary sources. The patient's perceptions are the key to planning appropriate early interventions, and acceptance of his or her viewpoint engages the patient in planning for self-care (Wheeler, 1989; Whyte & Youhill, 1984). See Box 11–6 for sample interview questions to assess for suicidal or homicidal thoughts.

Box 11–6 ■ ■ ■ ■ ■
Sample Interview Questions to Assess for Suicidal or Homicidal Thoughts

Suicidal Thoughts

- You say you are feeling very sad. Many times, when people feel sad they think about hurting themselves. Have you thought of hurting yourself?
- Are you thinking of hurting yourself now?
- If you would harm yourself, have you thought about how you would do it?
- Do you have a plan for hurting yourself?
- I would like to know what you are thinking and planning. I want to be able to protect you from hurting yourself, and I know that sometimes just talking about your ideas might make you feel less like hurting yourself.
- Have you thought of what life would be like if you were dead? What thoughts have you had?
- What has kept you from acting on these thoughts in the past?

Homicidal Thoughts

- You describe feeling uptight and angry. Have you thought of hurting someone else when you are feeling this way?
- Could you describe your hostile feelings to me?
- What have you done to control these feelings in the past?

Medication History

The patient's use of medications is another crucial topic for you to explore because nursing staff members are involved in medication administration, and early treatment with an unknown patient poses certain risks. Ask the patient to recall as clearly as possible the names, dosage, and effects of all psychotropic medications. If a side effect or allergy is reported, a full description of the reaction is written because patients frequently use the term "allergy" when they mean minor side effect.

Studies have shown a high incidence of medication complications in patients receiving neuroleptics. It is estimated that 75% of all patients receiving antipsychotic medication suffer from extrapyramidal symptoms (see Chapter 17 for a complete discussion of medication issues). For elderly patients, 17% of readmissions to hospitals may be due to adverse drug reactions (Blair, 1990). Because neuroleptic medication side effects range from minor (e.g., a tremor) to life-threatening (e.g., neuroleptic malignant syndrome), it is a serious nursing responsibility to try to prevent a recurrence in a susceptible patient. Prevention or prompt treatment of side effects not only minimizes patient distress during

current treatment but also has an impact on the patient's future medication compliance. It is believed that one third of schizophrenic patients on neuroleptics experience akinesia (stiffness in moving muscles, decreased motor activity) or akathisia (restlessness, inability to sit still), and they also have a relapse rate of 50% during the 1st year after hospitalization, largely because of noncompliance with medications (Blair, 1990; Michaels & Mumford, 1989).

Not to be forgotten in this section is the patient's use of over-the-counter drugs or prescriptions for medical problems. In a state of emotional distress, patients may not produce a complete medical history, but they may tell you the names of prescription drugs they have been taking for medical problems. Many prescription medications used to treat medical problems may produce psychiatric symptoms, especially in the elderly. An accurate medication profile may hold the key to differential diagnosis. Refer to Table 11–3 for examples of commonly used drugs with the potential for psychiatric symptoms (*Medical Letter,* 1998).

History of Prior Psychiatric Treatment

It is important to get specific dates and effects of previous treatment to plan for the most effective current approach. As the patient describes his or her past care, you assess for patterns of compliance and begin to set

TABLE 11–3 Examples of Drugs That Cause Psychiatric Symptoms

MEDICATION	REACTIONS
β-Adrenergic blockers	Depression, psychosis, anxiety
Anticholinergics and atropine	Disorientation, hallucinations, paranoia, agitation
Anticonvulsants	Agitation, confusion, depression
Antihistamine, H₁ blockers	Hallucinations
Baclofen	Hallucinations, anxiety, confusion
Caffeine	Anxiety, psychosis, confusion
Calcium channel blockers	Depression
Cephalosporins	Euphoria, delusions
Cimetidine (Tagamet)	Confusion, psychosis, aggression
Corticosteroids	Psychosis, mania, depression
DEET (Off)	Mania, hallucinations
Digitalis glycosides	Depression, mania, hallucinations
Fluoroquinolone antibiotics	Psychosis, agitation, depression
Narcotics	Anxiety, dysphoria, hallucinations
Ranitidine (Zantac)	Confusion, psychosis, aggression
Salicylates	Agitation, confusion, paranoia
Thiazide diuretics	Depression, suicidal ideation

DEET, diethyltoluamide.

realistic goals for treatment. Specifically, if the patient reports leaving treatment prematurely, either by elopement (running away) or by signing out against medical advice, this signals a potential risk for this admission. At the same time, it allows the patient to detail his or her dissatisfaction or disappointment with past treatment and encourages the setting of goals for this episode. Incorporating the patient's goals into the multidisciplinary treatment plan is one of the most important contributions made by the nurse.

> **W**hat do you think? Can you think of one good reason why it is essential to know about over-the-counter drugs that the patient is using? What factors might keep the patient from sharing this information with you?

> ► *Check Your Reading*
> 36. What risk factor can be detected with routine vital signs?
> 37. Why does the nurse record the patient's perceptions of the problem?
> 38. What questions must be answered in a medication history?
> 39. What is the primary reason for relapse in psychiatric patients?

Emotional Assessment

Even if the patient is unwilling or unable to discuss his or her coping patterns, much of the **emotional assessment** can be completed from previous observations. Again, record the exact words and actions that lead you to select a particular descriptive term. (For definitions and examples of terms commonly used to describe assessment findings, see Table 11–4.)

These behavioral snapshots compose the baseline picture against which comparisons are made to assess progress and to determine discharge criteria. If the patient can describe coping patterns, this information allows the nurse to support strengths and to identify areas of weakness in need of teaching.

Cognitive Assessment

Similar to the preceding section, **cognitive assessment** has already started before these questions are asked, and certain parts can be completed without further inquiry. It is vital, however, that you use precise questions to assess the patient's level of cognition because deficits are not always self-evident. The questions related to orientation, memory, attention, fund of information, judgment, and abstract thinking are derived from the Mini-Mental State Examination (MMSE). Studies have shown the MMSE to be an effective screening tool in identifying cognitive impairments, especially in the elderly (Rovner & Folstein, 1987).

Similar to the clues that the nurse finds with routine vital signs, early detection of cognitive problems may signal an untreated medical condition. Delirium may be caused by a simple urinary tract infection or a much more serious abnormality. "Clinically, delirium can be the most conspicuous presenting feature of a potentially lethal medical condition such as myocardial infarction or pneumonia, particularly in an elderly person" (Lipowski, 1992, p. 335). Treatment of the delirious patient is different from treatment of a physically healthy patient with psychosis.

The interview of the hallucinating patient requires additional attention to detail. Hallucinations may be present in a variety of conditions, including schizophrenia, mood disorders, and alcoholism. Not all hallucinations are considered unpleasant to the patient, and sometimes he or she hears multiple voices in dialogue that represent the positive and negative sides of an issue. With prolonged hallucinations, many patients develop coping mechanisms to control them, for example, wearing headphones, pacing, singing, humming, listening to loud music, and wearing earplugs. If a patient is distracted and seems to be paying attention to internal rather than external stimuli, it may mean that the patient is hallucinating. Hallucinations can be auditory (hearing voices), visual (seeing things that others do not see), or olfactory (smelling things that others do not smell). If you think that your patient is hallucinating, inquire about (Williams, 1989)

1. The type of perception
2. How long it has been present and when it started
3. How much the patient believes it is real
4. The major emotional theme (i.e., is it harmful or helpful to the patient?)
5. The presence of any commands and the patient's response
6. What coping strategies the patient uses to control the hallucinations

This knowledge is helpful in planning interventions that will support the patient's constructive coping patterns. It is important to recognize that it is not always possible to eliminate hallucinations in some patients; rather, the goal may be to help the patient to adapt to the impairment.

Physical Assessment

The abbreviated format used here for **physical assessment** is based on the assumption that the patient is receiving a physical examination and appropriate diagnostic tests as part of the admission procedure. If not, then the nurse needs to communicate with the patient's physician to compare her or his findings with the results of the most recent physical examination. Early identification of medical problems is essential to clarify the psychiatric diagnosis, to identify coexisting medical conditions, and to provide appropriate medical treatment. Psychiatric patients are at increased risk for inadequate treatment of physical problems. Psychiatric

T A B L E I I – 4 Terms Commonly Used to Describe Assessment Findings

TERM	DEFINITION	EXAMPLE
Affect		
Flat	Affect without any expression of feelings; unresponsive to varied topics or surroundings over time	Patient discusses the weather and her mother's death without any change in facial expression or tone of voice.
Inappropriate	Affect does not match the feeling or topic being discussed	Person laughs when speaking of being afraid.
Labile	Affect rapidly changes from one mood to another	During the course of a conversation, person cries and then laughs.
Blocking	Involuntarily interrupting speech or train of thought	Patient begins to answer question but pauses at odd points while speaking.
Circumstantiality	Pattern of speech in which irrelevant details are included with relevant details in describing an event, but follows through on one topic	Person describes his dinner but also describes what he was wearing and a phone call.
Compulsion	An irresistible urge to repeatedly perform an act that may be contrary to one's usual standards due to extreme anxiety if the act is not completed	Person washes her hands five times each hour.
Confabulation	Fabrication of events or situations to fill in gaps in memory, usually in a plausible way	Patient explains his black eye with elaborate story about a fight but his wife reports that he was home all evening.
Delusion	A fixed belief that is defended intensely despite its being illogical or unrealistic; paranoid with excessive suspiciousness; or grandiose with exaggerated view of self-worth	Patient believes the hospital food is poisoned and she only eats food in sealed containers, or patient believes that he is an alien with supernatural powers.
Echolalia	Automatic but meaningless repetition of another person's words	In response to question: "Are you afraid?", patient answers: "Afraid, afraid, afraid."
Echopraxia	Imitation of another person's body movements	Patient sits opposite the interviewer and copies the hand position and leg movements of the interviewer.
Flight of ideas	Rapid stream of talk describing multiple topics unrelated to each other	Patient states, "I feel fine, the trees are green, the chairs are broken."
Hallucination	Sensory perception that does not result from real, external stimulus; most commonly auditory or visual but may be tactile, olfactory, or gustatory	Patient hears voice of a relative talking about her or sees bugs on her hands.
Ideas of reference	Believing that statements or behaviors of others are related to oneself even when no realistic connection exists	Patient believes talk show host is talking about him.
Illusion	Misinterpretation of an external sensory stimulus, usually visual or auditory	Person sees clothing on a chair and thinks it is a cat.
Loose associations	Pattern of speech in which the connections between ideas are so vague that, to the listener, they do not seem to follow any logical sequence	Patient talks about medication, then switches to describe a cat, and then changes the subject again.
Neologism	Word invented by a person with a meaning specific to that person	A crying patient says, "My bermin hurts" but does not explain what that is.
Obsession	Involuntary preoccupation with a particular thought or idea that seems irrational	A thin patient is preoccupied with fear of getting fat.
Perseveration	Involuntary persistence or repetition of an idea or response	Patient keeps repeating one phrase over and over.
Tangentiality	In conversation, the tendency for a response to digress from the original topic	When asked about sleep, the patient replies, "I sleep fine but my mother used to say that I sleep too much, she always criticizes me."

illnesses frequently impair cognitive processes, which in turn results in impaired communication and social skills. These deficits pose a barrier to seeking help, verbalizing symptoms, and following through on treatment recommendations. Some studies point to a high incidence of cardiovascular and endocrine disorders in psychiatric patients that may go untreated without careful assessment (Holmberg, 1988).

As noted earlier, many medical conditions can produce significant psychiatric symptoms. If these underlying problems are not identified, the patient will not respond to usual psychiatric treatment and may develop further medical complications. See Table 11-5 for some examples of common problems (Skuster, Digre, & Corbett, 1992; Talley, 1997).

Many times, a patient who has been reluctant to talk about emotions and thoughts will freely tell the nurse about physical complaints or difficulties in performing daily activities. In such cases, the nurse may decide that it is more productive to shift the conversation to physical issues before completing other sections of the database. It is important to inquire about every subsystem and activity listed. Especially in evaluating activities of daily living (ADLs) and instrumental activities of daily living (IADLs), the nurse must determine the need for referral to rehabilitation team members for treatment and discharge planning.

Two specific risk factors that may be uncovered by a thorough assessment of physical issues are risk for HIV infection and history of or current physical abuse. It is important to question knowledge of safer sex practice for all sexually active patients. Despite potential controversy related to staff or patient beliefs about contraception, precautions for safer sex are now frequently included as part of general health teaching for patients in hospital settings and nearly always involve the nurse (Davidhizar & Cosgray, 1990).

Signs of physical or sexual abuse may become apparent during evaluation of physical or social factors. The presence of physical injuries or a history of frequent accidents may signal an abusive relationship. Early detection allows for appropriate referral to the team social worker for family evaluation and recommendations for community resources in discharge planning. Descriptions of conflict in the family of origin can hint at past abuse. If child abuse from the past is reported, it is important to gather information to assist in treatment. One strategy for collecting this information is the TRIADS system (Burgess, Hartman, & Kelley, 1990): *t*ype of abuse, *r*ole of relationship of the offender, *i*ntensity of

abuse, *a*utonomic response, *d*uration, and *s*tyle of abuse (access and pattern).

> ► *Check Your Reading*
> 40. What problems may be found through use of the Mini-Mental State Examination?
> 41. What specific information is gathered about hallucinations?
> 42. Name two risk factors that may be identified during the physical assessment.

Sociocultural Assessment

As illustrated in the case of Mrs. Ryan, performing a full **sociocultural assessment** with both the patient and significant others can have an impact on the course of treatment. Observations of the individual in a treatment setting, out of context with his or her usual social system, always present an incomplete picture. Data related to the patient's living situation and usual level of interpersonal activity are necessary to

- Understand the whole person
- Develop realistic treatment goals
- Clarify the presence or absence of the support system, which is relevant for successful discharge planning

Pressing financial or legal problems may need immediate attention to allow the patient to attend to even more abstract therapeutic goals. Appropriate referrals to other members of the treatment team or community resources need to be initiated as soon as the need is identified.

The patient's particular cultural or ethnic background contains further keys to treatment. It is essential for you to ask explicitly about the patient's values and beliefs related to

- What caused the present problem
- What will make it better

If the patient's or family's beliefs are at odds with the proposed treatment plan, increased risk for premature withdrawal from care or treatment failure exists.

Specific cultures have their own customs or traditional methods for healing, and increased awareness of these beliefs can facilitate selection of congruent treatment approaches. For example, American Indians traditionally believe in the use of the *talking circle* to resolve problems (i.e., a group sits together in a circle, and everyone offers a prayer without interrupting each other). Thus, an American Indian may benefit more from group therapeutic approaches than from a primary one-to-one relationship. At the same time, cultural belief systems may affect the patient's performance on testing instruments that were standardized with mainstream cultural values. For instance, it is culturally natural for an Inuit girl or woman to feel that she needs help with decision-making. Concluding that she is dependent and needs to increase assertiveness skills would be culturally inappropriate treatment (Campinha-Bacote, 1988; Manson, Walker, & Kivlahan, 1987).

Your awareness of your own cultural biases is essential to objectively evaluate and accept the patient's

TABLE 11-5 Examples of Physical Problems Causing Psychiatric Symptoms	
ILLNESS/CONDITION	**PSYCHIATRIC SYMPTOM**
Cancer	Depression, delirium
Electrolyte imbalance	Delirium
Hearing abnormality	Auditory hallucinations
Hyperthyroidism	Anxiety, confusion
Hypothyroidism	Depression, psychosis
Huntington's chorea	Depression, hallucinations
Parkinson's disease	Depression, dementia
Pernicious anemia	Depression
Urinary tract infection	Delirium

belief system. Studies evaluating the treatment effect of matching the patient and therapist according to race and ethnic background have had mixed results. Although similarity between the patient and therapist may make the therapist more of a role model to the patient, it does not necessarily improve the patient's general level of functioning. It seems that patient-therapist congruence in defining the problems and setting treatment goals is more important than matching their sociocultural backgrounds (Flaskerud, 1990). Chapter 12 offers suggestions for other cultural assessment inquiry.

Spiritual and Philosophical Assessment

Just as knowledge of sociocultural factors plays an important role in understanding the individual and formulating realistic treatment goals, a **spiritual and philosophical assessment** is also important to complete. The presence and intensity of faith in God, degree of religious commitment, and sense of purpose and meaning, along with basic life values, strongly affect the patient's potential for recovery. Specific religious beliefs may be directly linked to the patient's view of the cause of illness and the direction for treatment. For example, it is common for people suffering from mental illness to seek assistance from a clergyperson or spiritual leader before or concurrently with seeking professional help. It is important that the mental health team recognize the importance of this spiritual support and avoid minimizing it in any way. Box 11–7 offers specific questions to use in a spiritual and philosophical assessment.

The patient with a Judeo-Christian background may view his or her illness as a form of suffering for past sins. The patient may seek forgiveness as well as insight as a means of recovery and may respond well to insight-oriented one-to-one discussions. Prayer may be as much a part of his or her healing as therapy (Hutton & Parkinson, 1993).

If the patient is unable to discuss spiritual issues during the initial assessment, it is valuable to follow-up with these questions at a later time. This assessment not only allows the nurse to support positive beliefs and personal religious practices but also identifies the patient at increased risk, who feels hopeless and disengaged from any relationship with God.

Additional Assessment

This separate section is provided primarily for pertinent information from the family or other secondary sources regarding the patient's present behavior and past history. As noted earlier, these data supplement but do not substitute for the knowledge gained directly from the patient. Whenever a significant difference exists between the patient's and others' perceptions, you must respond first to the emotional needs of the patient to maintain the therapeutic relationship. For example, a patient arrives on the unit highly anxious, stating that he is being chased by enemy agents; but

---

Box 11–7 ■ ■ ■ ■ ■

Questions to Use in a Spiritual and Philosophical Assessment

Concept of God

- Is religion or God important to you? If so, can you describe how?
- Do you use prayer in your life? If so, does prayer benefit you in any way?
- Do you believe God or a deity is involved in your personal life? If so, how?
- What is your God or deity like?

Sources of Strength and Hope

- Who are your support people?
- Who is the most important person in your life?
- Are people available to you when you are in need?
- Who or what provides you with strength and hope?

Religious Practices

- Is your religious faith helpful to you?
- Are any religious practices meaningful to you?
- Has your illness affected your religious practices?
- Are any religious books or symbols helpful to you?

Meaning and Purpose

- What gives your life meaning and purpose?
- What makes you get up out of bed every morning and do what you have to do?
- Do you feel that your life makes a difference? If so, in what ways?
- In what ways has your illness had an impact on your meaning and purpose?

Modified from Carson, V. B. (1989). *Spiritual dimensions of nursing practice.* Philadelphia: W. B. Saunders.

---

the police report that he was arrested for stealing food from a convenience store. Your initial intervention addresses the patient's feelings of fear and suspiciousness rather than focusing on socially appropriate behavior.

You also consider data collected by other health team members. For instance, if the patient has had psychological testing, the results of these tests are important pieces of data. Psychological tests provide information on personality styles, thought processes, and intellectual abilities. Tests might include the Minnesota Multiphasic Personality Inventory, the 16 P-F personality test, or the Rorschach Ink-Blot Test.

Also included in this section is an explicit opportunity for the nurse to record subjective reactions during the

**Generic Clinical Pathway for Nursing Process
for All Psychiatric Diagnoses**

Patient Enters Mental Health System} Private practice, community-based service, home care, partial hospitalization, inpatient unit

↓

Initiation of therapeutic relationship

↓

Assessment Process Begun} Interview and observation} patient demographics; chief complaint; medical history; medication history; psychiatric history; emotional assessment; cognitive assessment; physical assessment; sociocultural assessment; spiritual and philosophical assessment; additional assessment → sources} patient, secondary sources, e.g., family; other professionals; medical record → medical testing} laboratory tests} blood, plasma and serum; urine; steroid hormones; polypeptide hormones; thyroid hormones; hematology; cerebrospinal fluid, Pap smear → neuropsychological testing → brain imaging techniques

↓

Diagnosis} Name health problem + etiological or contributing factors + defining characteristics

↓

Outcome Identification} Patient centered; singular; observable; measurable; time limited; mutual; realistic

↓

Planning} Who should meet the need? → nurse; psychiatrist; internist; psychologist; licensed clinical social worker; psychiatric occupational therapist; recreational therapist; and/or mental health aide or technician

What interventions are appropriate for specific patient?

What is needed for discharge planning?

Implementation} Counseling, milieu therapy; self-care activities; psychobiological interventions; health teaching

↓

Evaluation} Formative; summative

Figure 11–7
Generic clinical pathway for nursing process for all psychiatric diagnoses.

interview. These observations acknowledge the importance of the nurse's continuous self-evaluation during the assessment interview and may be useful in interpreting the data.

> *W̲hat do you think?* How would you support a patient's spiritual beliefs? What would you say to a patient who responded to your inquiries regarding spiritual beliefs with the statement, "I have discovered that I am God"? How would you respond to a patient who said, "Medication will not help me, nothing will help me. This illness is God's punishment for all the awful things I have done in my life"?

➤ *Check Your Reading*
43. Identify three reasons to complete the sociocultural assessment.
44. What is the biggest risk if the patient's culture clashes with the treatment plan?
45. Does the patient have to have the same background as the therapist in order to gain therapeutic benefit?
46. What effect does the patient's spiritual belief system have on his or her recovery?

Problem Identification and Nursing Diagnoses

The final section of the questionnaire documents your professional judgment about all the data collected and deserves thoughtful attention. All problems and potential problems are identified using each major dimension, that is, emotional, cognitive, physical, sociocultural, and spiritual. In addition, any needs related to discharge planning are summarized, including self-care deficits, support system, or referrals to other disciplines. The needs are prioritized to indicate at least the top three concerns that require immediate nursing attention. Risk factors are deliberately repeated to ensure that they are addressed in the initial treatment plan. Lack of completion of the full database calls for explanation and continued attempts until all information is obtained (See Figure 11-7).

DOCUMENTATION

A final word is called for regarding nursing **documentation.** Thus far, the emphasis has been on individual recordkeeping that reflects the use of the nursing process and provides a legal record of the care that you provide (Town, 1993; Townsend, 1991). As a professional nurse, though, you also have accountability for evaluating the overall quality of nursing care for your agency. All health care settings are required by regulatory agencies to perform continuous quality improvement functions; that is, they must show ongoing evidence of monitoring and evaluation of all aspects of patient care (Girgenti & Mathis, 1994; Town, 1993). This body of evidence relies on chart reviews conducted by professional staff to measure patient outcomes against established standards of care. You may be called on to participate in nursing peer review or a multidisciplinary committee for quality review. In both cases, your goal is to apply your critical thinking skills in an objective evaluation process that leads to creative recommendations to improve patient care.

Conclusions

The nursing process is a systematic, dynamic, interpersonal, interactive framework for problem-solving in the delivery of nursing care. The skilled and knowledgeable use of this map can help you provide quality psychiatric nursing care throughout your journey with patients who are facing mental illness. A thorough nursing database serves four vital functions.

1. It defines the focus of nursing care for one particular patient, allowing for a comprehensive nursing care plan.

2. It serves as a means of communication with nurses and other colleagues who read the database (or conclusions) as they collect and compare their own data.

3. It interjects the input of nurses into the multidisciplinary treatment plan, advocating for recognition of the patient's own goals.

4. It may serve as justification for treatment to the third-party payer.

As you meet each new patient, another journey begins. Initially, you try to gather as much subjective and objective information as possible from a stranger who presents with impaired communication skills. At the same time, you begin to develop a therapeutic relationship with the patient to provide a basis for trust and hope in treatment. Ongoing assessment leads you to a fuller appreciation of the patient as a unique person with unique strengths, fears, hopes, and goals. Along the way, you discover more about yourself, enhancing your professional and your personal growth.

Key Points to Remember

- The nursing process is nursing's problem-solving approach.
- The nursing process includes six steps: assessment, diagnosis, outcome identification, planning, implementation, and evaluation.
- The ANA *Standards of Clinical Nursing Practice* and the *Standards of Psychiatric–Mental Health Clinical Nursing Practice* are authoritative statements that describe the responsibilities for which all nurses are accountable.
- The *Standards of Psychiatric–Mental Health Clinical Nursing Practice* identify specific interventions appropriate to the basic level practitioner and the certified specialist.
- The focus of assessment is comprehensive and holistic data collection.
- The patient is the primary source of data.
- Psychiatric patients may be limited in their abilities to give an accurate history.
- The initial interview is the first step in the assessment process.
- The assessment phase of the nursing process establishes the foundation for nursing diagnoses, the development of the nursing care plan, and the beginning of discharge planning.
- Nursing diagnoses represent clinical judgments about individual, family, or community responses to actual and potential health problems.

- The nursing diagnosis includes the health problem, the etiological or contributing factors, and the defining characteristics.
- Nursing diagnoses are often related to medical diagnoses, but rather than listing symptoms, nursing diagnoses focus on the human response patterns and suffering of the patient.
- Through prioritization, the psychiatric nurse ranks nursing diagnoses in order of their importance.
- Expected outcomes should be patient-centered, focused on one behavior, observable and measurable, time-limited, mutual, and realistic.
- Interventions for the basic level psychiatric–mental health nurse include counseling, milieu therapy, self-care activities, psychobiological interventions, health teaching, case management, health promotion, and health maintenance activities.
- Interventions for the certified specialist in psychiatric–mental health nursing include psychotherapy, prescription of pharmacological agents, and consultation.
- Evaluation continues throughout the entire nursing process.
- Formative evaluation covers all aspects of the nursing process *as the nurse is providing care.*

- Summative evaluation draws conclusions about the effectiveness of the entire nurse-patient interaction.
- Assessment involves the art of nursing, as relationship and communication skills facilitate data collection.
- Assessment necessitates that the nurse continually evaluate his or her own reactions, values, and beliefs.
- Subjectivity can be controlled through the use of structured questions, observations, and standardized assessment tools.
- Standardized assessment tools enhance data collection; the results are used in treatment planning, and nurses and patients experience satisfaction with using standardized instruments.
- The 1994 standards of psychiatric–mental health nursing published by the ANA provide a framework for comprehensive assessment.
- The assessment tool documents data about patient identification, chief complaint, medication history, psychiatric history, emotional and cognitive assessment, physical assessment, sociocultural assessment, spiritual and philosophical assessment, additional assessment, problem identification, and nursing diagnoses.

Learning Activities

1. Pair up with a classmate and practice collecting data from each other, using the assessment form provided in this chapter or another tool that your instructor selects. Identify which sections are the most personal and difficult to discuss.
2. Form a small work group with two or three other students. Using Mrs. Ryan's story, develop a comprehensive list of nursing diagnoses for Mrs. Ryan.

3. Using the list of nursing diagnoses that your team developed in activity no. 2, prioritize the list and provide the rationale for your decisions.
4. Using Mrs. Ryan's story, develop a nursing plan to address nursing diagnoses, noncompliance with medication, and altered nutrition.

Critical Thinking Exercises

Mrs. James was admitted to the psychiatric diagnostic unit with difficulty concentrating, headaches, and sleeplessness. Past history shows two depressive episodes following surgery for cervical cancer 2 years earlier. Although her admitting diagnosis is depression, an MRI scan of her head was ordered because of her medical history. The patient fears that her cancer has returned. She tells her nurse that if they find another tumor she will kill herself.

1. What is the patient's point of view?
2. What assumptions is the patient making?
3. What inferences can the nurse draw from the patient's statement?

The head nurse believes in the Kantian imperative of always telling the truth and informs the patient that her cancer has spread without preparing her for the bad news.

1. What assumption is the nurse making about the truth?
2. What conclusions has she drawn about the patient's belief system?
3. What evidence suggests that the nurse's conclusion to inform the patient may be faulty?

Additional Resources

American Nurses Association Nursing World

http://www.ana.org

Canadian Nurses Association

http://www.can-nurses.ca

References

Alfaro, R. (1990). *Applying nursing diagnosis and nursing process* (2nd ed.). Philadelphia: J. B. Lippincott.

American Nurses Association. (1991). *Standards of clinical nursing practice*. Washington, DC: American Nurses Publishing.

American Nurses Association, Council on Psychiatry and Mental Health Nursing. (1994). *A statement on psychiatric and mental health clinical nursing practice and standards of psychiatric-mental health clinical nursing practice* (p. 25). Washington, DC: American Nurses Publishing.

American Psychiatric Association. (1994). *Diagnostic and statistical manual of mental disorders, Fourth Edition*. Washington, DC: Author.

Arnold, E., & Boggs, K. (1995). *Interpersonal relationships: Professional communication skills for nurses* (2nd ed.). Philadelphia: W. B. Saunders.

Atkinson, L. D., & Murray, M. E. (1990). *Understanding the nursing process* (4th ed.). New York: Macmillan.

Barker, P. (1987). Assembling the pieces. *Nursing Times. 83*(47), 67.

Blair, D. T. (1990, March). Risk management for extrapyramidal symptoms. *Quality Review Bulletin,* 116.

Bower, P., Mead, N., & Gask, L. (1997). Primary care and mental health problems. *Nursing Times, 93*(18), 58.

Burgess, A. W., Hartman, C. R., & Kelley, S. J. (1990). Assessing child abuse: The TRIADS checklist. *Journal of Psychosocial Nursing, 28*(4), 7.

Campinha-Bacote, J. (1988). Culturological assessment: An important factor in psychiatric consultation-liaison nursing. *Archives of Psychiatric Nursing, 2,* 244.

Carpenito, J. (Ed.). (1995). *Nursing diagnosis: Application to clinical practice* (6th ed.). Philadelphia: J. B. Lippincott.

Carson, V. B. (1989). *Spiritual dimensions of nursing practice*. Philadelphia: W. B. Saunders.

Carson, V. B. (1994, June). Doing psych, but talking med-surg language. *Caring,* 32–41.

Davidhizar, R., & Cosgray, R. (1990). The use of Orem's model in psychiatric rehabilitation assessment. *Rehabilitation Nursing, 15*(1), 39.

D'Ercole, A., Skodol, A., Struening, E., Curtis, J., & Millman, J. (1991). Diagnosis of physical illness in psychiatric patients using axis III and a standardized medical history. *Hospital and Community Psychiatry, 42,* 395.

Doenges, M. E., & Moorehouse, M. F. (1992). *Application of nursing process and nursing diagnosis: An interactive text*. Philadelphia: F. A. Davis.

Dreyfus, J. K. (1987). Nursing assessment of the ED patient with psychiatric symptoms: A quick reference. *Journal of Emergency Nursing, 13,* 278.

Farrell, G. A. (1991). How accurately do nurses perceive patients' needs? A comparison of general and psychiatric settings. *Journal of Advanced Nursing, 16,* 1062.

Fawcett, J. (1994). Psychiatry isn't a primary care specialty? *Psychiatric Annals, 24,* 521.

Flaskerud, J. H. (1990). Matching client and therapist ethnicity, language and gender: A review of research. *Issues in Mental Health Nursing, 11,* 321.

Freund, B. (1993). Validating nursing diagnoses: An approach to reinforce nursing process with BSN-completion students. *Journal of Nursing Education, 32*(3), 140–141.

Gadde, K. M., & Krishman, K. R. R. (1994). Endocrine factors in depression. *Psychiatric Annals, 24,* 521.

Girgenti, J., & Mathis, A. (1994). Putting psychiatric nursing standards into clinical practice. *Journal of Psychosocial Nursing and Mental Health Services, 32*(6), 39–42.

Gordon, M. (1994). *Nursing diagnosis: Process and application* (3rd ed.). New York: McGraw-Hill.

Harris, J., & Gillien, E. (1992). Psychiatric-mental health nursing specialist process evaluation criteria. *Nursing Management, 23*(2), 54, 55, 58.

Henderson, V. (1987). Nursing process—a critique. *Holistic Nursing Practice, 1*(3), 7.

Hickey, P. (1990). *Nursing process handbook*. St. Louis, MO: C. V. Mosby.

Holland, J. (1996). Psychiatry and primary care: Closing the gap. *International Journal of Psychiatry and Medicine, 26*(2), 109.

Holmberg, S. (1988). Physical health problems of the psychiatric client. *Journal of Psychosocial Nursing, 26*(5), 35.

Hurst, K., Dean, A., & Trickey, S. (1991). The recognition and non-recognition of problem-solving stages in nursing practice. *Journal of Advanced Nursing, 16,* 1444–1455.

Hutton, A. P., & Parkinson, A. R. (1993). Theoretical bases for nursing diagnosis in mental health nursing. In R. P. Rawlins, S. R. Williams, & M. N. Johnson (Eds.), *Nursing process in psychiatric nursing.* St. Louis, MO: C. V. Mosby.

Johnson, P. A., Stone, M. A., Larson, A. M., & Hromek, C. A. (1992). Applying nursing diagnosis and nursing process to activities of daily living and mobility. *Geriatric Nursing, 13*(1), 25–27.

Kelley, J. (1994). The nurse solution: Primary care, prevention, case management. *South Dakota Nurse, 36*(2), 1.

Lipowski, Z. I., (1992). Update on delirium. *Psychiatric Clinics of North America, 15,* 335.

Manson, S. M., Walker, R. D., & Kivlahan, D. R. (1987). Psychiatric assessment and treatment of American Indians and Alaska natives. *Hospital and Community Psychiatry, 38*(2), 165.

McCloskey, J. C., & Bulechek, E. M. (1992). *Nursing intervention classification (NIC)*. St. Louis, MO: C. V. Mosby.

McConnell, S., Inderbitzen, L., & Pollard, W. (1991). Primary health care in the CMHC: A role for the nurse practitioner. *Hospital and Community Psychiatry, 43,* 724.

Michaels, R. A., & Mumford, K. (1989). Identifying akinesia and akathisia: The relationship between patient's self-report and nurse's assessment. *Archives of Psychiatric Nursing, 3*(2), 97.

North American Nursing Diagnosis Association. (1995). *NANDA nursing diagnoses: Definitions and classification 1995–1996.* Philadelphia: NANDA.

Redman, B. (1993). *The process of patient education* (7th ed.). St. Louis, MO: C. V. Mosby.

Rovner, B. W., & Folstein, M. F. (1987, January 30). Mini-Mental State Examination in clinical practice. *Hospital Practice,* 99.

Ryan-Wenger, N. M. (1990). A nursing process methodology. *Nursing Outlook, 38*(4), 190–193.

Salisbury, D. (1985, March 6). Don't waste the process. *Nursing Times,* p. 42.

Sheehan, J. (1991). Conceptions of the nursing process among nurse teachers and clinical nurses. *Journal of Advanced Nursing, 16,* 333–342.

Skuster, D. Z., Digre, K. B., & Corbett, J. J. (1992). Neurologic conditions presenting as psychiatric disorders. *Psychiatric Clinics of North America, 15,* 311.

Some drugs that cause psychiatric symptoms. (1998). *Medical Letter, 40*(1020), 21.

Sundeen, S. J., Stuart, G. W., Rankin, E. A., & Cohen, S. A. (1994). *Nurse-patient interaction: Implementing the nursing process* (5th ed.). St. Louis, MO: C. V. Mosby.

Talley, S. (1997). Physical diagnosis for advanced psychiatric nurse practitioners. Part I: Assessment and differential diagnosis. *Journal of the American Psychiatric Nurses Association, 3,* 146.

Town, J. (1993). Changing to computerized documentation—plus! *Nursing Management, 24*(7), 44–46, 48.

Townsend, M. (1991). *Nursing diagnoses in psychiatric nursing* (2nd ed.). Philadelphia: F. A. Davis.

Umbricht, D., & Kane, J. (1996). Medical complications of new antipsychotic drugs. *Schizophrenia Bulletin, 22,* 475.

Wheeler, S. Q. (1989). ED telephone triage: Lessons learned from unusual calls. *Journal of Emergency Nursing, 15,* 481.

Whyte, L., & Youhill, G. (1984, February 1). The nursing process in the care of the mentally ill. *Nursing Times,* p. 49.

Wilkinson, J. (1992). *Nursing process in action: A critical thinking approach*. Menlo Park, CA: Addison-Wesley.

Williams, C. A. (1989). Perspectives on the hallucinatory process. *Issues in Mental Health Nursing, 10,* 99.

Worley, N., Drago, L., & Hadley, T. (1990). Improving the physical health—mental health interface for the chronically mentally ill: Could nurse case managers make a difference? *Archives of Psychiatric Nursing, 4,* 108.

Suggested Readings

Burgess, A. W., Hartman, C. R., & Kelley, S. J. (1990). Assessing child abuse: The TRIADS checklist. *Journal of Psychosocial Nursing, 28*(4), 7.

Carson, V. B. (1994, June). Doing psych, but talking med-surg language. *Caring*, 32-41.

Hurst, K., Dean, A., & Trickey, S. (1991). The recognition and non-recognition of problem-solving stages in nursing practice. *Journal of Advanced Nursing, 16,* 1444-1455.

Johnson, P. A., Stone, M. A., Larson, A. M., & Hromek, C. A. (1992). Applying nursing diagnosis and nursing process to activities of daily living and mobility. *Geriatric Nursing, 13*(1), 25-27.

Savage, P. (1991). Patient assessment in psychiatric nursing. *Journal of Advanced Nursing, 16,* 311.

Seymour, J., Saunders, P., Wattis, J. P., & Daly, L. (1994). Evaluation of early dementia by a trained nurse. *International Journal of Geriatric Psychiatry, 9*(1), 37-42.

Town, J. (1993). Changing to computerized documentation—plus! *Nursing Management, 24*(7), 44-46, 48.

VanCott, M. L. (1993). Communicative competence during nursing admission interviews of elderly patients in acute care settings. *Qualitative Health Research, 3,* 184-208.

Zimmerman, M. (1993). A five-minute psychiatric screening interview. *Journal of Family Practice, 37,* 479-482.

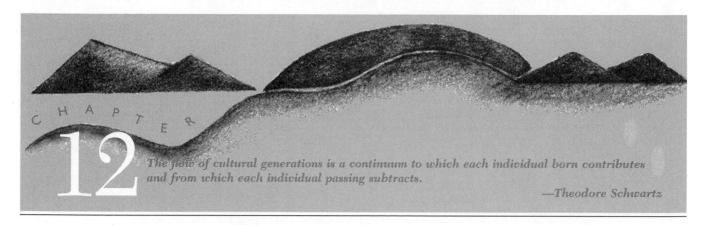

The flow of cultural generations is a continuum to which each individual born contributes and from which each individual passing subtracts.

—*Theodore Schwartz*

Travelers From Many Lands
The Impact of Culture

Learning Objectives

After studying this chapter, you should be able to:

1. Define the components of culture.

2. Discuss the differences between stereotypes and levels of prejudice.

3. Assess the importance of ethnic identity to patients and their extended families.

4. Recognize the significance of beliefs, perceptions, and values as facilitating or impeding help-seeking behavior.

5. Develop a frame of reference when interpreting cultural support systems.

6. Acquire the knowledge and skills needed to intervene appropriately for the patient's culture and difficulties.

7. Assess your journey to various cultures.

Key Terminology

Culture	Ethnic identity	Race	Stereotype
Culture-bound syndrome	Ethnocentrism	Racism	Transcultural identification
Ethnic competence	Prejudice		

Nursing is a journey to many cultures, for every patient is a mosaic of cultural conditioning. Culture represents the interplay between individuals and their society. Patterns of behavior are learned, shared, organized, and transmitted by groups and individuals (Linton, 1945). Inherent in every culture are beliefs and values; behavior that is esteemed; and taboos, roles, and relationships that give meaning to human encounters.

Every culture has norms or standards of behavior that are considered reasonable and normal rather than disabling and abnormal. The diversity of patients seeking mental health care requires that caregivers have an understanding of cultural relativity and be able to view behaviors of other groups without judgment.

Nurses bring their own hierarchy of values and subjective views of the world to the art of healing. Every human being embraces a system of values, private or public, admitted or tacit (Harris, 1972). Thus, understanding terms such as *ethnic identity, culture,* and *stereotyping* is basic to the delivery of helpful and healing services. As professionals, the greatest challenge is to provide care that is culturally relevant to various ethnic groups.

This chapter offers you an explanation of terms that will help you describe and understand culture: *stereotyping, prejudice, ethnic identity, racism, race, culture-bound syndromes, ethnic competence, ethnocentrism,* and *transcultural identification.* Each term identifies a concept that equips you to become a culturally sensitive nurse—one who can meet patients wherever they are on their journeys.

Thao's Story

Try to imagine a country scarred and broken by war. Intellectuals and professionals had to hide their identity to survive. A generation of citizens was forced to embrace an ideology foreign to their ancient traditions.

Imagine a young woman with three small children whose husband was sent to a reeducation camp. His "crime" was that he had been a military officer in South Vietnam. Now he was doomed to years of torment and forced manual labor and tedious hours of indoctrination, his sentence indeterminate. Imagine the restless nights, the myriad questions endured by his young wife and family. Would he resist reeducation? Could he endure the indefinite years of isolation from family and friends? Would he survive the harsh prison environment? What would be the consequences for the family?

Thao's Decision to Leave

In the late 1970s, Saigon was still an important hub for making connections to political taskmasters and for mastering the intricacies of escape. Thao, the young wife and mother, valued family, tradition, dignity, and education, but none of these could be realized without freedom. If she remained in Saigon, her three children—Leong, age 6; Fong, age 5; and Pguong, age 4—would never have an opportunity to live freely and follow the ancient traditions. Thao realized her close-knit family and neighbors had come to the same conclusion. Because the Communists wanted to rid Vietnam of ethnic Chinese, Thao and some of her family and friends, along with more than 150 people, plotted their escape by obtaining false papers.

Imagine the grief of bidding goodbye to family members who elected to stay behind to care for the elderly and be a living presence in their ancient land. Imagine this young wife unable to have a final embrace with her spouse or even risk telling him of the escape plan. Imagine three wide-eyed youngsters who could not be told of the proposed journey nor take any childhood mementos with them. The journey had to be planned with no hint of deception to the new regime, which had eyes and ears everywhere.

The Family's Escape

The secret escape meant that 150 people had to travel in little groups, by bus and by foot, to reach the coast where a boat waited to take them to an unknown destination. Imagine sitting in a crowded bus, peering out windows to etch in one's memory the last scenes of home. How many times had their hearts pounded with fear, anxiety, and sadness? Would their fake papers be discovered? What if one of them became too ill to continue? Finally, they arrived in the coastal town where a sea of humanity surged relentlessly toward unstable boats. The exit price was exact—12 oz of gold for each person stepping onto the boat.

Imagine the boat finally chugging toward open sea—its occupants fearing pirates, rape, starvation, and death. Imagine seeing the shoreline of one's beloved country fade in the mist, obscured by tears of regret and loss. Imagine being a well-educated professional who now had to endure a refugee camp in Indonesia. For months, Thao tried desperately to contact relatives in California—to no avail. Engulfed in hopelessness, Thao wondered, "Was I stupid? Will this camp be the rest of my life?" Finally, a sensitive immigration officer and a staff member with the Refugee High Commission in Indonesia learned of Thao's situation.

Thao sighed with relief and pent-up grief when she was informed in late 1979 that she and her children would be admitted to the United States as refugees. Imagine stepping off the plane in Norfolk, Virginia, in December 1979. There was a chill in the air; there were no familiar faces, sights, sounds, or scents. Everything was different.

Life in a New Land

Imagine exchanging upper middle-class status for a working-class life: working full-time and striving to hold part-time jobs to support not only the family in the United States but also loved ones left behind. Imagine searching for stores selling traditional foods, having no temple in which to worship, and having no extended community in which to celebrate festivals. Imagine trying to make children practice their native language when no neighbor or classmate could speak Vietnamese. Imagine getting word that your husband lay very ill and medication would not be provided because he had not demonstrated that he was reeducated.

Imagine the daily struggle to be a good person, a good neighbor, a good citizen, and a success by American standards. Throughout these years, Thao maintained her modest decorum, inspired her children to excel in their studies, and offered prayers to bless those left behind. Today, Thao jokes about retiring as she works as a culture broker for the latest wave of refugees. Her three children attend universities on scholarships. Leong wants to be a medical doctor; Fong is studying to be a psychologist; and Pguong is looking toward a career in international journalism. Their lives are now full of hope. For Thao and her children, the longing to see loved ones in Vietnam has been answered: a local television station that documented the family odyssey is providing them a journey home.

UNDERSTANDING CULTURE-RELATED TERMS

Culture

Culture refers to the beliefs, behaviors, foods, dress, music, and traditions that give a group its distinctiveness. Members of a cultural group share a consensus of beliefs, social norms, and ways of responding to life. Group members view the world through a common lens shaped by religious tenets, life philosophy, history, and lived experiences.

Cultures are made vibrant by both continuity and change. In Asia, for example, the elderly have traditionally been respected, and the ancestors celebrated. Social transformation, however, has diminished family support, even among the family-oriented Chinese (Heok, 1994). Cultures are not fixed but are subject to growth. Economic conditions, media influences, war, famine, and political upheavals can change even those cultures that have protected themselves from outside influences, as the Chinese have.

Who has the knowledge to interpret or judge another's culture? Serving others as a nurse means developing universal love for and acceptance of all people. Universal love is not only psychologically possible but also essential, the only complete and final way to love (de Chardin, 1967). Understanding another's culture may be a lifelong task. Patience, persistence, effort, and real caring are necessary elements if you are to begin the journey of understanding a fellow traveler's culture.

What do you think? Is it possible to act accepting without actually loving the patient?

➤ *Check Your Reading*
1. What is culture?
2. What external influences change cultures?

Stereotyping

A **stereotype** is an exaggerated belief or fixed idea about a person or group and is sustained by selective perception and selective forgetting. Stereotyping leads to tunnel vision, myths, and "isms" about an individual or a group of people. For instance, the term *old age* has different cultural interpretations. Chronological peers are not always psychological peers. In the United States, a 65-year-old, active and in good health, may contemplate taking on a second or even third career; another person of the same age, in poor health and with diminished hope, may act like a person decades older. Yet age 65 is commonly seen as the retirement age in the United States.

Stereotypes related to age, race, gender, and religion abound, resulting in rigid preconceptions that are used to label people. As a nurse, you need to engage individuals in the wholeness of their humanity. You must look beyond the surface, the label, and the diagnosis, and tap into the essence of the patient. What keeps the patient hoping? What brings comfort and joy? What causes anxiety, depression, isolation? What experiences have shaped the patient's personality? How does the patient's culture define mental health and mental illness?

Concern about stereotyping also raises questions about the role of ethnicity, social class, gender, help-seeking patterns, bias in psychiatric diagnosis, and involuntary commitment in minority populations (Good, 1993). These factors are intertwined with stereotyping and practitioner bias. Labels in mental health imply that precise distinctions can be made between "normal" and "abnormal" behavior. There are, however, serious questions of cultural relevancy and ethics in nursing care. Clinical assessment is a complex task. Interviews and other assessment tools may not be culturally fair, compounding the problems of transcultural nursing.

Brink (1990) defined *transcultural nursing* as "the fusion of nursing and anthropology in both theory and practice." Brink offers an antidote to labeling:

If nurses, whatever their specialty, would view every patient care situation as a study sample of one, collect data on that case, and compare all cases at the end of a year's period, then generalizations could be made on the basis of that comparative data, and each nurse would have added to the body of nursing literature in that field. (p. 34)

The issue of labeling and labeling theory is also central to Cohen's reevaluation of cross-cultural research. Cohen (1992) cited Waxler's work, which found that specific social and cultural variables influenced the molding of mental illness in Sri Lanka:

The first factor was the Sinhalese family, described as being large, tolerant, and relatively strong; mentally ill members were neither alienated nor rejected, but rather cared for and given positive social support. The second factor was the treatment system in which there were many choices and all care was short-term. (p. 60)

Sinhalese culture mediates on the patient's behalf, thus eliminating the negative effects of labeling. The complications of labels such as *insane* or *schizophrenic* are long term: "Once a person is designated abnormal, all of his other behaviors and characteristics are colored by that label" (Rosenhan, 1990, p. 181).

As travelers trying to understand other cultures, we might recall the words of St. Paul: "I don't understand myself at all. The good that I would do, I do not, and that which I would not, that I do" (Romans 7:15). The desire to avoid stereotypes and labeling must commence with a desire to transform the dark corners of your being into areas of light (Catoir, 1990).

What do you think? Is anything wrong with giving someone a psychiatric diagnosis?

➤ *Check Your Reading*
3. How do stereotypes perpetuate "isms"?
4. Other than age, what characteristics are subject to stereotyping?

Prejudice

Prejudice is a preconceived idea or attitude that can be negative, formed before the facts are known, and sustained by overgeneralizations. Prejudice represents a bias without reason, resisting all evidence. Two essential ingredients of prejudice are (1) an attitude of favor or disfavor and (2) an erroneous belief.

Allport's (1979) classic book, *The Nature of Prejudice,* offered insight into levels of prejudice.

- *Antilocution* is talking about a targeted group of people with like-minded people or joking to demean members of a group that is ethnically or culturally different.
- *Avoidance* is an intentional way of behaving designed to forestall, inhibit, or diminish contact with others who are viewed as different.
- *Discrimination* is active exclusion of people who are different by contrived rules or regulations.
- *Physical attack* is violent touching that results from heightened emotions, inadequate facts, and closed minds in which hatred and division are nurtured.
- *Extermination* is the deliberate and systematic destruction of a racial, political, or cultural group as demonstrated by forced sterilization, lynchings, pogroms, massacres, and genocide.

As the levels of prejudice intensify, the targeted people "develop social formation which appears to the surrounding oppressive culture to be excessive or pathological" (Lerner, 1972, p. 465). The coping mechanisms of the targeted group may be extreme withdrawal and fearfulness.

Prejudice against those with mental health problems also exists worldwide. The misconceptions persist that such people are incurable and dangerous and to blame for their conditions. Former friends avoid the patient. Discrimination, subtle or overt, occurs in employment, particularly in professional or political careers. In societies with low tolerance for people with mental illness, cases of physical attack and extermination have been documented, especially during great upheavals, such as war and famine.

W*hat do you think?* Do you think sterilization for mentally ill people is a good idea?

➤ *Check Your Reading*
5. How do levels of prejudice differ in intensity?
6. What prejudices are held toward the mentally ill?

Race and Racism

Race broadly distinguishes individuals or groups on the basis of appearance. Judging others simply on appearance leads to erroneous decision-making, false assumptions, and denial of the uniqueness of each person. **Racism** is a belief that one racial or ethnic group is inferior to another, justifying unequal treatment. Understanding a specific individual or group in relation to other groups for Burke (1986) implied an investigation of five aspects of race:

1. *Prejudice* on an individual level is evidenced by an attitude of derogation, avoidance, discrimination, or attack on another person.
2. *Institutional racism* is supported by a belief in racial superiority of one group over another. Constraints are initiated and power is controlled by one group.
3. *Individual orientations to racism* can lead to specific behaviors:
   - A position of superiority based on fear
   - A do-good position with token gestures
   - A nonreactor position owing to overwhelming anxiety
   - A catastrophic reaction, justifying a position by angry and irrational means
   - An apathetic position, in which an individual goes along with the status quo
4. *Reactions of those affected by racism* include the ways fears, frustrations, and antagonisms affect mental health and adjustment.
5. *Symbolic racism* emerges in the labels *desirable* and *undesirable* and perpetuates rigid patterns of relating between individuals and groups.

Rack (1982) contended that racism may be used as a metaphor for illness. A health professional who makes interpretations may be responding to racial stereotypes. Cultural differences in the manifestations of distress and the way such manifestations are interpreted represent diagnostic pitfalls for the psychiatric nurse and may be linked to racism.

W*hat do you think?* Are there fundamental differences among people from different races?

➤ *Check Your Reading*
7. Define and discuss the various levels of racism.
8. Identify two ways in which racism might interfere in psychiatric nursing.

Ethnocentrism

Ethnocentrism is the making of one's own view the center or focal point for decisions. It implies an acceptance of one's culture as superior and relegates other individuals and groups to a position of inferiority. Individuals or groups are judged or rated against the standards of the ethnocentrist's world view. Although all individuals have a vested interest in their own cultural perspective, effectively providing nursing care to patients from other cultures means eliminating or diminishing the inherent bias of an ethnocentric viewpoint.

➤ *Check Your Reading*
9. Define ethnocentrism.
10. What are the implications of ethnocentrism when providing nursing care to those whose culture is different from your own?

Ethnic Identity

Ethnic identity encompasses the perception and inner sense of affiliation with a group that shares a racial, national, linguistic, or cultural background. Ethnic identity provides the security of knowing that one belongs, a sense of roots. How often have you heard the comment, "He is so Americanized," meaning an immigrant has outwardly conformed to the dominant culture? Understanding another person's deep sense of ethnic identity is not easy in a world in which labeling is based on cursory introductions. Consider the following poem by Paul Laurence Dunbar (1872–1906) entitled *We Wear the Mask:*

We wear the mask that grins and lies,
It hides our cheeks and shades our eyes,—
This debt we pay to human guile;
With torn and bleeding hearts we smile,
And mouth with myriad subtleties.

Why should the world be overwise,
In counting all our tears and sighs?
Nay, let them only see us, while
We wear the mask.

We smile, but, O great Christ, our cries
To Thee from tortured souls arise.
We sing, but oh, the clay is vile
Beneath our feet, and long the mile;
But let the world dream otherwise
We wear the mask.

Ethnicity is linked with an individual's social identity and includes history, language, and religion. Terms such as *ethnic group* and *ethnicity* describe a self-awareness possessed by the people to whom the terms are ascribed. Members of an ethnic group think and behave similarly.

➤ *Check Your Reading*
11. What is the significance of ethnic identity?
12. What is included in the understanding of the term *ethnicity?*

Transcultural Identification

Transcultural identification is the degree to which a particular group modifies its customs and activities to blend with the dominant culture. Modification of a group's customs, however, can lead to blurring or even rejecting a group's original cultural values.

Considerable ethnic variation exists within many ethnic groups—differences attributed to level of ethnic identity, acculturation, family influences, gender-role socialization, religious and spiritual influences, immigration experiences, and linguistic skills (Lee & Richardson, 1991). New immigrants are often faced with conflicting choices: to acculturate their children and grandchildren into the dominant culture, fostering acceptance, or to nurture ethnic pride in their descendants. Regardless of how close-knit a family or ethnic group appears to be, you must be able to evaluate how fluently different generations can speak to each other in their native tongue. Increasingly, grandchildren cannot communicate with their grandparents. The mediator and translator may be the bilingual parent (Quintanilla, 1991).

You need to be tuned into the multiple losses and compromises engendered by immigration; one's country, culture, human attachments, family traditions, and ability to communicate are all threatened. Loss occurs not only by death but also by leaving, being left, changing, letting go, and challenging the status quo. Loss is viewed differently by different cultures. Often, this information about a patient must come from a family member who has shared the journey and understands the complexity of losses and the patient's uniqueness.

The following American phrases illustrate transcultural conflicts: "The early bird catches the worm." "He who hesitates is lost." "God helps those who help themselves." "The squeaky wheel gets the grease." "Tell it like it is." "Do it." "Just say no." These American expressions focus on decisiveness, independence, and a take-charge way of approaching life (Hanson, Lynch, & Wayman, 1990). Many other cultures operate from a different set of beliefs: "Find your enjoyment in renunciation." "What God wills." "The nail that stands up gets pounded down." "Emptying the heart of desires." "It can't be helped." These beliefs underscore a nonattachment to fame, worldly success, and control, and an acceptance of fate as the appropriate means of dealing with life's challenges.

Patterns of kinship, education, religion, economics, and politics are interrelated with the lifeways of a particular group. When the geographical boundaries, social institutions, lines of authority, and family life patterns are significantly altered or completely eradicated, as they are for refugees, change has a profound impact on behavior (Boritz-Wintz, 1994). The trauma of being a refugee requires adaptation to meet a four-phase adjustment process:

1. *Culture shock* is the severe anxiety generated by being in a new culture with unfamiliar language and social norms.

2. *Social isolation* occurs when new refugees are housed where rent is affordable, not necessarily where their compatriots live.

3. *Status inconsistency* is a common experience. Many refugees who held professional credentials have to update or even requalify for licensing in a new country, without the benefit of fluency in their adopted language.

Often they are forced to work jobs that they are overqualified for in order to make ends meet.

4. *Cultural conflicts* invariably occur when the woman is employed and the man, who is the head of the household, is unemployed or working in a marginal job. Here the culturally competent nurse can be an educator and mediator, an advocate and a link to support networks such as mutual assistance associations (MAAs).

What do you think? Should immigrants make more of an effort to become American?

➤ *Check Your Reading*
13. Discuss how variations in transcultural identification can lead to conflicts for both individuals and families.
14. Identify three losses that occur with transcultural identification.

Ethnic Competence

Ethnic competence means acting in a manner congruent with the behavior and expectations of a particular culture. Yet competence does not imply complete mastery of the nuances of all cultures, especially when time is limited. Rather, it commences with respect; sensitivity; and a willingness to observe, listen to, and learn from others whose backgrounds differ from one's own.

A wide range of conceptual frameworks and models is available for use in intercultural situations (Mahon, 1997). Some models focus on the individual (Griffith-Kenney & Christensen, 1986); others adopt a group orientation (Hofstede, 1980). Dobson (1991) developed a detailed transcultural health visiting schema emphasizing similarity and reciprocity in using cultural frames of reference.

As early as 1978, Leininger argued that the Western criteria used in separating "normal" from "abnormal" may not be used by other cultures. Synthesizing and applying the findings of anthropological studies, Leininger (1978) formulated a culturological assessment paradigm based on such aspects as life patterns, values, norms, expressions, taboos, myths, and health–illness systems.

Leininger's theory of cultural care incorporates decades of transcultural research. She believes cultural care goes beyond values, beliefs, and practices. Care is embedded in language; religion; kinship and social patterns; and political, legal, educational, economic, technological, ethnohistorical, and environmental components or institutions of a culture. (See Suggested Readings, Leininger [1997], for insights about the future of transcultural nursing care.)

Developing ethnic or cultural competence is an ongoing task, a perpetual learning process (Taoka, 1997). As Campinha-Bacote (1994, p. 1) put it, "The Culturally Competent Model of Care encourages psychiatric nurses to see themselves as always in the process of becoming culturally competent, rather than being

culturally competent." A culture continues to condition and shape coping styles and concepts of health and illness. Your role includes observing and learning.

What do you think? Is it realistic to expect a nurse to have extensive knowledge of many other cultures?

➤ *Check Your Reading*
15. Name two components of Leininger's culturalogical assessment paradigm.
16. What is ethnic competence?

Culture-Bound Syndromes

A **culture-bound syndrome** is intrinsically ethnocentric and restricted to a specific people and locale. Such syndromes usually involve displays of extreme behavior incongruent with traditional Western psychiatry classifications. Anorexia nervosa and agoraphobia are regarded by many as examples of Western culture-bound syndromes (Dein, 1997). Simons and Hughes (1985) believed that culture-bound syndromes raise issues about the differential contribution of biological and cultural factors in causing and shaping mental disorders. Therefore, when interpreting behavior, you must also consider that culture's ways of expressing normality.

The *Diagnostic and Statistical Manual of Mental Disorders, Fourth Edition* (1994) includes, in Appendix I, a glossary of culture-bound syndromes. For example, *amok* is characterized by a sudden frenzy and is a fully elaborated cultural complex found in Malaysia, Indonesia, and the southern Philippines. In Polynesia, it is called *cafard* or *cathard*; similar patterns are seen in Puerto Rico (*mal de pelea*) and among the Navajo (*iich'aa*). *Ataques de nervios* refers in Hispanic cultures to uncontrolled hysterical outbursts, often with a dissociative component, following a stressful occurrence in the family. Similarly, *bilis* and *colera* or *muina* describe acute physical disturbances resulting from extreme rage. Some other syndromes described follow:

Boufée delirante (West Africa and Haiti): A brief psychotic outburst

Brain fag (West Africa): Fatigue from studying too hard

Dhat or *Jiryan* (India and Pakistan): A fixed belief that sperm is leaking from the body in the urine; the patient may not complain of anxiety about potency but of generalized weakness, malaise, and depression

Koro (Malaysia): The delusional fear that the penis will retract into the abdomen and cause death; called *suo yang* in China

Latah (Malaysia): An exaggerated or hysterical fearfulness with trancelike behavior

Taijin kyofusho (Japan): A morbid fear that one's body is offensive to others

Many culture-bound syndromes are not included in the glossary. For example, *Windigo psychosis,* reported among Cree, Ojibway, and other Algonquian-speaking

Native Americans, appears to be a form of severe depression in which culturally determined fears of cannibalism color the depressive delusions (Angell, 1997), and *piblokto,* reported among Inuit women, has features of agitated depression and fugue-like withdrawal. In *old hag* (Newfoundland), the victim awakens terrified, unable to move, with a sensation of weight on the chest. Other culture-bound syndromes are identified in Chapter 10.

Although many researchers have recorded and attempted to explain culture-bound syndromes, Lefley (1990) concluded that culture-bound syndromes do not seem to fit a universal behavior pattern. The meaning of illness is therefore defined from a particular cultural perspective. Al-Issa (1982, p. 67) contended that "cultural variables may resist measurement and comparison across cultures because it is difficult to isolate them from the context and meaning in which they are embedded."

What *do you think?* Are Western diagnoses more real than these culture-bound syndromes?

➤ *Check Your Reading*
17. What issues are raised by the term *culture-bound syndrome?*
18. Identify three culture-bound syndromes.

MAJOR CULTURAL VARIABLES AFFECTING MENTAL HEALTH CARE

Health care delivery is culture bound and laden with beliefs, values, practices, and ramifications (Simond, 1996). Eliason (1993) and West (1993) went so far as to contend that nursing practice and theory cannot be ethical unless nurses consider cultural factors and incorporate them into the plan of care. Understanding all of these elements and their relevance helps make one culturally competent.

Culture affects all aspects of communication, including concepts involving time, space, touch, and tone of voice. These concepts are clues to accepted norms for daily functioning and important in rendering nursing care.

Time

Time is endowed with different meanings in various cultures. Hall and Whyte (1990, p. 51) identified five aspects of time:

1. Appointment time
2. Discussion time
3. Acquaintance time
4. Visiting time
5. Time schedules

Each of these concepts of time has relevance in providing nursing care.

Throughout much of Asia, for example, because of traffic congestion, it is not unusual for individuals to be several hours late for an engagement but still believe they are on time. Also in Latin America, a 45-minute delay or wait is not unusual. Thus, if you want a patient from those geographical areas to keep an appointment by American time standards, you may need to ask the patient to come earlier.

Discussion time in American culture actually means making your point quickly and efficiently. In Asian and Latino cultures, however, details are important. Therefore, the patient may try to explain the context and symptoms associated with the illness and the role the family is playing in the healing process. Listening to the patient conveys respect and patience and signals that you are cognizant of the patient's culture.

Acquaintance time is the period needed by the patient and family to size up the professional providing health care service. Hall and Whyte (1990) wrote:

[I]n Central America, local custom does not permit a salesman to land in town, call on the customer and walk away with an order, no matter how badly your prospect wants and needs your product. It is traditional there that you must see your man at least three times before you can discuss the nature of your business. (p. 53)

Applying this insight to psychiatric nursing, you might question how often a patient has been labeled *resistant* when the patient actually was looking for clues to establish rapport. Rapport is conveyed by demonstrating awareness of some aspects of the patient's culture and by your own body language and sense of caring. Caring is almost universally recognized in a warm, polite, attending caregiver. Cultures around the world emphasize the importance of acquaintance time. Box 12–1 provides examples.

Treatment of a loved one, particularly in a foreign country, brings significant concern. The psychiatric nurse should use acquaintance time not only for dialogue but also for validating cultural concepts about mental health, mental illness, and treatment. You can then inform the patient about accepted psychiatric modalities currently used in the United States and Canada. We cannot assume that individuals from other cultures, regardless of socioeconomic level, are familiar with American standards of mental health care or that these standards are amenable to their own values and beliefs.

"Visiting time involves the question of who sets the time for a visit" (Hall & Whyte, 1990, p. 53). In India, a person who says "come over and see me . . . see me anytime" means just that. You have crossed a boundary and are now friends. For the psychiatric nurse, this acceptance may facilitate follow-up with a patient. Americans live by schedules, yet Hall and Whyte (1990, p. 54) wrote "not only is our idea of time schedules no part of Arab life but the mere mention of a deadline to an Arab is like waving a red flag in front of a bull."

Time has significance in all cultures. For each ritual surrounding life events that signify the passing of time,

Box 12-1 ■ ■ ■ ■ ■
Acquaintance Time Across Cultures

In Arab cultures, the time required to get something accomplished depends on relationships. Trusting a loved one to the care of a psychiatric nurse, particularly a non-Arab, may require extensive application of acquaintance time to build trust and rapport.

In Japanese culture, time is used to test patience. If you cannot demonstrate patience, you have lost the opportunity to build cultural bridges.

In African American and West Indian cultures, relationships are valued and built over time. Individuals from these cultures are not driven by the actual clock time; the quality of the relationship propels trust and confidence in the health care provider.

Hispanics see time in terms of *mañana* (tomorrow), the exception being a family member's or friend's crisis. In this case, it is important to respond immediately.

In Ethiopia, the time required for a decision is directly proportional to its importance.

such as births, weddings, funerals, and mourning, there is protocol. For instance, in remembrance of a loved one, Filipinos perform family prayers for nine evenings following the person's death. For many, particularly those with strong traditions of ancestor worship, inability to comply with expected cultural norms honoring the deceased may lead to mental health problems.

W*hat do you think?* Is it possible to accommodate other cultures' attitudes toward time in the climate of managed health care?

➤ *Check Your Reading*
19. What is appointment time and what is its potential impact on a nurse-patient relationship?
20. What significance does acquaintance time have for the development of a nurse-patient relationship?

Space

Space is an integral component in communication. Space connotes personal boundaries and conveys culture-specific meanings. Americans and Canadians, for the most part, consider 2 ft to be a comfortable or respectable distance when talking to another adult. Typically, Hispanic Americans and people of Arab culture converse at a more intimate distance, less than 1 ft. To them, this is comfortable and implies an authentic, personal conversation.

Asians are sensitive to each other's personal space and to rules concerning physical contact. They feel comfortable conversing with others who stand 5 to 6 ft away. For African Americans, intimates may engage in close contact; outsiders are expected to stay at least an arm's length away. West Indians maintain little space between friends when communicating; the outsider needs to look for a signal that invites closeness.

Touch

Americans generally are uncomfortable with physical touch. In Arab and Hispanic cultures, however, communication typically includes an embrace, particularly between men. Contact between men and women in Arab culture is prohibited; in Latin America, physical contact may extend to a kiss on the hand of the woman.

Hall and Whyte (1990, pp. 50-51) noted that a handshake in Latin America, particularly between two men, is seen as cold and impersonal. The *doble abrazo,* in which two men embrace by placing their arms around each other's shoulders, is the accepted norm of greeting. Touching the shoulders of a Javanese, however, is seen as a humiliation and an unpardonable breach of traditional etiquette.

W*hat do you think?* Should a nurse follow another culture's norms of touch or maintain a professional consistency?

➤ *Check Your Reading*
21. Give two examples of different cultural views of space.
22. Give two examples of different cultural views of touch.

Voice Tone

The human voice also carries cultural connotations. In American culture, speaking distinctly in a well-moderated and self-controlled tone is the desirable norm. Hall and Whyte (1990) noted, however, that a cool, logical approach to conversation may be regarded by Middle Easterners with suspicion. In the Middle East,

[F]rom childhood, the Arab is permitted, even encouraged, to express his feelings without inhibition. Grown men can weep, shout, gesture expressively and violently, jump up and down—and be admired as sincere. (Hall & Whyte, 1990, p. 49)

Throughout much of Asia, respect and communication are enhanced by speaking in polite but soft tones. Being gregarious or making self-referent statements is not well accepted in traditional Asian societies. One demonstrates manners and humility by listening more than speaking.

Dress and Clothing Color

Much of the world still adheres to distinct uniforms for nurses. A patient from such a geographical region may have difficulty relating to an American nurse in an institution that no longer requires uniforms. You may want to explain to the patient how to recognize "the nurse" (e.g., a specific badge).

In some Asian countries, white is associated with funerals. In many African countries, red symbolizes witchcraft and death. Good mental health in the United States has often been associated with the ability to coordinate the color of one's wardrobe; in Africa, the Caribbean, and the South Pacific, bright, multiple colors are the accepted norm of dress.

Gestures

Many gestures are subtle and easy to overlook. Although many Americans use small hand gestures for emphasis, people of Italian and Hispanic background feel comfortable making extensive hand movements to make a point. To an Arab, however, a quick wave of the hand or showing the sole of one's shoe is considered a violation of basic courtesy.

Words and Terms of Address

Words do not easily translate across cultures but must be understood from a group's frame of reference. You may therefore need to work not merely with a translator but with a culture broker, someone who has an insider's view of the patient's culture (Jezewski, 1995). For example, *old* in Iraq means 40 years and older; for unmarried women, more than 30 is old. In India, people older than age 60 are considered old. Hatton (1992) distinguished between translators and interpreters who also appraise tasks, patients, providers, or information and have considerable power. The culture broker is more than a translator; this person has ascribed or achieved acceptance in two distinct cultures.

Terms of address for an elderly patient vary across cultures. European Americans and African Americans generally use the term *grandmother* or *grandfather* or some variation. Filipinos have specific terms: *lolo* is equivalent to grandfather; *lola* is equivalent to grandmother. *Na ang bultok* means "all white hair already." In Chinese, the middle-aged generation says "old Mr." or "old Mrs." as a sign of respect, whereas the younger generation says "old big." Knowing the accepted form of address for a patient can enhance communication.

> **W***hat do you think?* How does the use of an interpreter or culture broker fit in with the need for confidentiality?

➤ *Check Your Reading*

23. Give an example of how voice tone and gestures differ across cultural groups.

24. How might the American practice of nurses' wearing street clothes rather than uniforms affect someone from another cultural group?

25. Why is it important to know different terms of address in different cultures?

Perceptions of Mental Illness

The stigma attached to seeking mental health treatment appears to be universal. Throughout much of Asia, mental health problems are viewed as imbalances in the body. In Africa and much of the Caribbean, a person with mental illness is viewed as suffering from a spell. Even in the United States, researchers have found that perceptions of elder abuse and help-seeking patterns differ among African American, white, and Korean American elderly women (Moon & Williams, 1993). These differences underscore cultural distinctions in communication, education, diagnosis, and intervention.

Decision-Makers

When the patient is elderly, you need to consult culture-specific informants and decision-makers. For the African American patient, the key decision-maker is often the eldest daughter. In Filipino culture, the eldest child, whether son or daughter, makes the decisions. Among the Vietnamese, the eldest son is traditionally vested with decision-making power, although disruption of family patterns because of war may warrant that the child geographically closest to the parent make decisions. Traditionally, in Chinese culture the eldest son and his wife are expected to be caregivers and decision-makers; likewise, among Hispanic Americans, the eldest son is expected to care for elderly parents.

In many cultures, the mental health or subsequent mental illness of a member of that culture demands a communal response. Although Native Americans sometimes seek services from Western practitioners and the Indian Health Service, the power of the group and the use of ancient rituals in the healing process are widely respected. Islanders of the South Pacific conform to communal decision-making and a prescribed course of action for dealing with mental illness.

Religion

The role of religion varies across cultures and significantly affects the meaning ascribed to good and evil, suffering and salvation. Fervent Catholics rely on God's greatness and prayers to see them through a crisis, whereas Buddhists accept suffering as a reality of life. In Orthodox Judaism, all events of daily life are greeted with an appropriate blessing. Judaism is steeped in ritual for all occasions, with the most solemn blessing uttered at the synagogue service by the officiating rabbi (Catoir, 1992). Rey (1997, p. 159) strongly recommended that a therapist learn about a family's "religious history, values, ritual and community" to improve treatment.

Newbold (1991) asserted that nursing is a ministry:

[P]eople need people, not only to meet their own needs but to be needed by others. The relationship of patient and nurse is unlike any other, and part of its uniqueness is the intimacy with which one relates to a person. (p. 98)

What do you think? What do you think of the statement "nursing is a ministry"?

➤ *Check Your Reading*

26. Give an example of how a culture understands mental illness.
27. Give two examples of how religion affects people across cultures.

SPECIFIC CULTURAL GROUPS

European Americans

European Americans comprise a heterogeneous group. They hold varying beliefs, have divergent immigration patterns to the United States, and present with different forms of mental illness. The 1990 U.S. Census provided data about ethnic background. Respondents represented more than 100 groups. Nearly 100 million Americans claimed their ancestors came from the British Isles; 45 million were of German background; 8 million were French; 7 million were Polish; still many others came from other European nationalities. Similar to all groups, European Americans share specific communication patterns, as summarized in Box 12–2. Several European American groups are detailed next. Be aware that there are also several other less numerous but unique people—for example, Roma or Gypsies, Old Order Amish, and Hutterian Brethren—with singular lifestyles and unique needs (Bodner & Leininger, 1992; Brunt, Lindsey, & Hopkinson, 1997; Buccalo, 1997; Burger, 1996).

Irish Americans

More than 20 million Americans claim Irish heritage. Some have experienced problems associated with alcoholism and concomitant depression. Relentless stereotyping, discrimination, and poverty have led the Irish to develop a strong sense of identity and cohesion, especially in the first and second generations. This ethnic group has traditionally emphasized a strong oral tradition, the development of mythology, and a complex style of communication in which a question may be answered by asking another question.

Traditionally, Irish women have been expected to be strong and nurturing. There is a high tolerance for Irish men to gather in the pub. Mothers cater to sons, thus reinforcing a dependency role. Research (Al-Issa, 1982) suggested a high incidence of schizophrenia among Irish people.

Mental illness creates a sense of shame for the Irish American patient and family. Although psychiatric facilities have existed for more than a century both in

Box 12–2 ■ ■ ■ ■ ■
Communication Patterns Among European Americans

Making eye contact during speaking is a sign of attention and respect.

Getting to the point quickly is valued more by Northern Europeans than by Southern Europeans. Southern Europeans are more gregarious and engage in unhurried small talk.

Relative distance between two speakers in conversation is farther apart than with people from Latin or Arab cultures.

Public behavior is expected to be modest and emotionally restrained, especially among Northern or Eastern Europeans. Emotional displays are seen as irresponsible or in bad taste.

Southern Europeans (e.g., Spaniards and Italians) are more prone to show their emotions, and hand gestures are more often used to make a point in a conversation than is the case with Northern Europeans.

Hand-holding, hugging, and kissing between men and women in public is acceptable.

A slap on the back denotes friendliness.

It is customary to shake hands with people of the opposite sex.

the United States and in Ireland, a family might hide a problem in a loved one by keeping the person confined to one part of the house and seeking cure through prayer.

Irish Americans, particularly first and second generation, are overwhelmingly Catholic. Catholicism postulates that God is love; it offers hope but demands commitment. The psychiatric nurse working with a patient of Irish ancestry needs to address religious beliefs and practices. A pervasive sense of guilt and self-punitiveness is often experienced by an Irish patient who has mental illness. The hopeful message of Catholicism, which focuses on love and forgiveness, is helpful to the patient trying to overcome mental illness: "[The Church] . . . is a refuge for sinners, a comforter of the afflicted and a source of spiritual nourishment on the journey of life" (Catoir, 1992, p. 57). The 12-step recovery programs used by groups such as Alcoholics Anonymous are compatible therapeutic tools for this ethnic group.

➤ *Check Your Reading*

28. Give two characteristics of Irish Americans that affect their risks for mental illness.
29. What is the role of religion in the life of many Irish Americans?

Italian Americans

Most Italian Americans are descendants of people who immigrated to the United States from the southern part of Italy. Italians maintain strong family ties. Regionalism is also important, and Italians often want the listener to know they are Neapolitans, Calabrians, or Venetians. For the psychiatric nurse, it is important to recognize these regional differences.

Although Catholicism is a factor in the lives of most Italians, according to Sowell (1981), religious institutions are viewed distantly, sometimes cynically, by southern Italians. Italians believe that the well-being and honor of the nuclear family are to be preserved at all costs. Although strong family ties can reinforce good mental health, family bonds that are tenuous, critical, or hostile can lead to depression. So too, when religion is seen as external control, a sense of helplessness may propel the Italian American toward depression. For Sicilians, their spirituality is less concerned with conformity to rules for personal salvation than with placating the capricious power of Satan, "the evil eye" (Sowell, 1981). For the nurse working with an Italian American patient, assessment of family relationships, religious beliefs, and degree of emotional expression is important.

Jewish Americans

Jewish people came to the United States and Canada from many European countries, among them Spain, Portugal, Germany, Austria, Russia, and Poland. As a result, they adhere not only to Judaism but also to the cultures from which they emigrated.

In Western Europe, those who practiced their religion could still be identified as French or German; in Eastern Europe, being a Jew was a separate identity isolated from the dominant culture. Nurses who are unfamiliar with the history of the Jews in Europe should become sensitized to issues related to the Holocaust. A study by Kennedy, Kelman, Thomas, and Chen (1996) found that, for reasons the study was unable to identify, elderly Jewish people are more likely to be depressed than elderly people of other religious groups.

Three branches of Judaism exist today. Orthodox believers follow the Talmudic teachings concerning Kosher (dietary) rules, Sabbath observance, and strict adherence to ancient rituals. Conservative Judaism follows prescribed holy days yet reinterprets Talmudic teachings for contemporary practice. Reform Judaism has discontinued some Talmudic practices and stresses adaptability, morality, and belief in God.

Judaism stresses that God has endowed every person with physical, intellectual, and emotional gifts. Individuals are expected to develop these gifts in harmony with all people. All branches of Judaism believe that one's actions become a living memorial in death. Harmonious relationships, good deeds, and praying for forgiveness for wrong deeds are the challenges Judaism presents to its adherents. Individuals are not passive but continuously shape attitudes, memories, and outcomes by the good they do or fail to do.

Over the centuries, the Jewish community has developed a strong ethnic identity as well as elaborate support systems to address the needs of its members, including those with mental illness. This network is important for the psychiatric nurse meeting a Jewish patient's needs. Adherents of Orthodox and Conservative Judaism tend to prefer treatment by a professional who espouses their religious beliefs. The psychiatric nurse needs to understand the significance of specific practices such as Kosher diet, ritual baths, head coverings for women, and prescribed prayers.

What do you think? Have the media shaped your ideas about European American ethnic groups?

➤ **Check Your Reading**
30. What is the role of the family in the mental health of Italian Americans?
31. Why is knowledge of the Jewish community important to assist people with mental illnesses?

African Americans

African Americans believe acceptance must be earned by being sincere and trustworthy. Brusque questioning can cause a patient to be resistive. A commonly held belief is that a person should not share personal information with outsiders. Therefore, professional help is more likely to be accepted if the nurse has earned the respect and trust of the pastor and extended family. Communication patterns among African Americans are summarized in Box 12–3.

African Americans gain strength from their nuclear and extended families, neighbors, close friends, lodge brothers, sorority sisters, and church. For example, a study found that African American women, at high risk for depression due to stressful life events, were less likely to be depressed if they had adequate social support (Warren, 1997). Each family has a *power source,* a person who has control and who sets the rules. You need to identify this significant power source because this individual may influence the patient's acceptance or rejection of treatment interventions.

Some African Americans harbor a pervasive distrust of "the system." You cannot presume an automatic bond between African American nurses and patients. If the nurse promotes a sense of empowerment in the African American patient, advocacy and culture brokering become part of the professional's expanded role (Jezewski, 1993). When access to health care is limited or biased or fails to validate the African American patient's feelings and experiences, you must function as both an advocate and a culture broker. The culture broker's status facilitates a bond with the minority patient and enhances the patient's ability to operate in the dominant culture.

What do you think? Should an African American patient be cared for by a person of color whenever possible?

Box 12-3 ■ ■ ■ ■ ■

Communication Patterns Among African Americans

Touching of one's hair by another person is often considered offensive.

Indirect eye contact is preferred during listening and direct eye contact is preferred during speaking as signs of attentiveness and respect.

Public behavior may be emotionally intense, dynamic, and demonstrative.

A clear distinction is made between *arguing* and *fighting*. Verbal abuse is not necessarily a precursor to violence.

Asking "personal questions" of someone one has met for the first time is seen as improper and intrusive.

Interruption during conversation is usually tolerated. Competition for the floor is granted to the person who is most assertive.

Conversations are regarded as private between the recognized participants. Butting in is seen as eavesdropping and is not tolerated.

Use of the expression "you people" is seen as pejorative and racist.

➤ *Check Your Reading*

32. Why might a culture broker be useful for an African American patient?
33. Why is trust so important in the African American community?

Hispanic Americans

Hispanic is a government designation applied to all people who speak Spanish and identify themselves as belonging to the Latin culture. Some Hispanic people prefer to be called Latino:

People from Central and South America and Mexico, although preferring to identify according to their national origin, such as Dominican or Colombian, are more responsive to the term Latino. (Arredondo, 1991, p. 143)

In actuality, Hispanic Americans vary widely in expressing their culture. In addition, their health care expectations and help-seeking behavior may differ depending on their country of origin and social class. Mufford (1992) found that 50% of Hispanic Americans were born in the United States, with the rest coming from about two dozen other countries. Well-educated, upper-class immigrants may experience situational anxiety, whereas refugees from strife-torn Central America may suffer significant depression. Some Hispanic people work as migrant laborers and have myriad needs related to the harshness of their working and living conditions (Artemis, 1996). Although only about 5% to 10% of Hispanics use folk medicine, including herbs and spiritual healers (Mufford, 1992), you need to elicit this information with sensitive interviewing skills.

Because Hispanics represent nearly 10% of the U.S. population, with Mexican Americans constituting the largest subgroup, an understanding of basic Hispanic cultural beliefs is paramount. Loyalty to the family takes precedence over that to social institutions or individual preferences. *Compadrazgo*, or kinship through godparents, is an important feature of family life. Children learn early about unquestionable parental authority and loyalty. Respect and cooperation define social relationships and obligations. Typical communication patterns are summarized in Box 12-4.

Comas-Diaz (1989) believed that mental illness among Hispanics is a family affair because of the cultural emphasis on kinship, relationships, and identification of each patient with a namesake. Comas-Diaz recommended that nurses explore the myths and stories attributed to the ancestor for whom the patient was named. The death of a loved one can lead to the culture-bound syndrome *susto*, or loss of the soul, expressed in paralyzing grief.

Gender roles are clearly defined in Hispanic culture. This clear role definition is a source of conflict for those who question fixed roles, and, as in all group-centered cultures, the individual who embraces different values or communication styles may end up estranged. "The victim of mismatch feels alienation from individuals, groups and cultures, and institutions that play an important part in his or her life" (Ramirez, 1991, p. 3). Individuals who do not fit in their own culture may exhibit symptoms of depression and an inability to cope. Depression may be referred to as *nervios* or *ataque de nervios* (Juarbe, 1998).

Folk healing, more commonly known as *espiritualismo* or *espiritismo,* is practiced among some Hispanic Americans. Its core beliefs are soul voyaging, altered

Box 12-4 ■ ■ ■ ■ ■

Communication Patterns Among Hispanic Americans

Hissing to gain attention may be acceptable.

Touching often occurs between people during conversation.

Avoiding direct eye contact is sometimes a sign of attentiveness and respect; sustaining direct eye contact may be interpreted as a challenge to authority.

Relative distance between two speakers in conversation is closer than with Northern European Americans.

Official or business conversations are preceded by lengthy greetings, pleasantries, and other talk unrelated to the point of business.

Box 12-5 ◼ ◼ ◼ ◼ ◼
Communication Patterns Among Asian Americans

Vietnamese Culture

Touching or hand-holding between men may be acceptable.

Hand-holding, hugging, and kissing between men and women are unacceptable.

A slap on the back is insulting.

It is not customary to shake hands with people of the opposite sex.

A verbal outburst is unacceptable.

Chinese Culture

Respect is always accorded to an older person.

Patience should be demonstrated.

Speaking in a quiet manner helps promote communication.

Indian Culture

The older person takes the lead in conversation.

Public displays of affection are taboo.

Eyes are generally cast down when listening.

Cambodian and Thai Culture

Feet are the lowest point of the body, spiritually; people do not point their feet at each other nor do they step over each other's feet or legs.

The husband is greeted before his wife, his wife before their children, and the older children before the younger children.

Verbal or nonverbal assent (nod, smile) does not necessarily signify agreement with what is said. It may be done so as not to embarrass the speaker by saying that he or she made little sense.

Shaking hands is not customary. Greeting involves placing the hands, palms together, near the face. Do not try this way of greeting; it may seem patronizing or insulting if the hands are held at an inappropriate height. Shaking hands may be attempted as American ways are learned, but any awkwardness is based less on shyness than on feeling unaccustomed.

The head is the most important part of the body, where the spirit resides; do not touch a Cambodian or Thai child or adult on the head.

Use Mr., Mrs., or Ms. and then the given name, which is usually noted last (as in Smith, Sam). Do not use only the given name. It may indicate an intrusion or lack of respect.

---

states of consciousness, and the presence of spirit-beings who can enter a person's body. According to Kearney (1978),

[I]n *espiritualismo*, trance states include *videncia*, the ability to "see" spirit phenomena with the eyes shut and at a distance; *clarividencia*, the ability to "see" spirit phenomena with opened eyes; and *oído*, the ability to "hear" spirit-beings. (p. 21)

Religion remains a key factor in the lives of most Hispanics. Help-seeking behavior may include praying, offering novenas, making pilgrimages, and directly seeking a priest's or pastor's advice. These religious leaders are usually significant supports.

The work of Rivera (1988) is particularly helpful for the psychiatric nurse working with the Hispanic patient. Rivera found that explaining mental illness as a physiological imbalance that can be corrected by medication is amenable to the Hispanic family's belief system. An educational problem-solving approach helps mobilize all the family in a concerted effort to assist the ill member. Mental health literature consistently indicates that Hispanic Americans desire treatment from a health professional who shows *personalismo,* or formal friendliness; *simpatía,* or warmth and concern; and *respeto,* or respect for the person and culture (Erzinger, 1991).

Good communication demonstrating these qualities can be the beginning of a helping relationship.

What do you think? Should people living in the United States learn to speak English?

➤ *Check Your Reading*
34. What are the three qualities that Hispanic Americans look for in a mental health professional?
35. What are the core beliefs of *espiritismo?*

Asian Americans and Pacific Islanders

Asia is a continent of millions of peoples. Its geography includes towering mountains and majestic rivers. Asian class and caste systems define relationships, and religious movements, such as Buddhism, Islam, Hinduism, and Confucianism, have a profound impact on every aspect of life. Kuo and Kavanaugh (1994, p. 551) made the point that mental health and mental illness are "artificial concepts among people who do not . . . treat mind, body and spirit separately." Communication patterns common among Asian Americans are summarized in Box 12-5. It is important for the nurse to know that Asian Americans generally respond to lower doses of antipsychotic medications than do white people and are sensitive to adverse side effects (Dein, 1997).

Indian Peoples

India is a heterogeneous country with 31 states and 930 million people speaking 15 major languages and hundreds of dialects. India is predominantly Hindu. Hinduism, probably the world's oldest religion, asserts that people consist of *atman,* which is an extension of the cosmic *Brahman,* or universal energy, atmosphere, life, or soul. Accordingly, individuals continue to experience rebirth until they recognize the truth. Present unhappiness is caused by ignorance, selfish attachments, and seeking earthly happiness. The individual seeking *nirvana* (oneness with the universal energy) must lead a good life, have spiritual discipline, and eliminate earthly attachments.

The Hindu religion exerts great influence on how individuals interpret suffering and human existence. The laws of *karma* (action) and *samsara* (reincarnation) were first articulated in the *Upanishads* (Hindu scriptures). "Every individual deed or action was viewed as Karmic input that would inevitably lead to an output in kind, good deeds ripening as good fruit, evil deeds as evil" (Wolpert, 1991, p. 83). Therefore, according to the law of *karma,* depression is viewed as an atonement for some misdeeds in life. Depression results in fewer suicides in India than in Western countries. Rao (1986) reported that both religious injunctions and social stigma may mitigate against completion of suicide attempts.

Rao (1986) wrote that disorders of the mind are mentioned in the *Upanishads,* and that mental illness is estimated to affect some 2 to 7 people per 1000 in India. Although many consult indigenous healers, who include shamans, depression is more often diagnosed through somatic complaints. In India, culture-bound syndromes are common. Sexual neurosis and *koro* (see under Culture-Bound Syndromes) are two; another is *possession syndrome,* in which a patient dissociates from reality. Supernatural or religious frenzy is often the climax of possession.

Rao (1986) found schizophrenia to be distributed across all socioeconomic groups and castes, with the catatonic form (characterized by psychomotor retardation or excitability) the most common expression of this illness. Rao noted that catatonia could be attributed to low linguistic competence, whereas patients with highly developed linguistic skills exhibited more delusional symptoms. For the nurse caring for patients from India, a precise understanding of their educational level, religious beliefs, and family and communal support system is important. If an Indian person becomes mentally ill while residing in another culture, the illness may not correlate with Rao's findings because the patient will have experienced a new set of environmental and social factors.

Southeast Asians

The term *Southeast Asian refugee* masks differences among Vietnamese, Cambodians, and Laotians. The Vietnamese are generally better educated than the other groups, many having had years of exposure to French culture. Before the fall of Saigon in 1975,

> [S]everal thousand military officers, governmental officials, the well-to-do, and the educated escaped to Thailand, from whence some made their way as refugees to the United States. . . . The more heterogeneous "second wave" of refugees who started arriving in 1978 can be divided into the "boat people" from Vietnam and the "land people" from Kampuchea and Laos. (Chan, 1991, pp. 155, 157)

These second wave refugees were poorer and less educated than the 1975 group.

Most Cambodian and Laotian refugees came from rural areas. Some were Catholic, but more were Buddhist and animists. (Animism attributes spirit and awareness to all material entities.) For the psychiatric nurse, understanding the different circumstances endured by refugees and the functional support systems they have created is important. If the patient is a refugee, focus on the circumstances of his or her journey to the United States or Canada. Many have endured great trauma and never received mental health treatment after their arrival. For some, experiences cause late-life flashbacks of earlier trauma and depression.

For the boat people of Asia who arrived in the United States in the 1980s and 1990s, MAAs have become a network for kinship, survival, and adjustment. The acknowledged leaders within the MAA are generally refugees who are bilingual and accepted for their leadership skills.

As a result of the 1987 Amerasian Homecoming Act, an influx of new Asian immigrants and refugees entered the United States. Amerasians, the offspring of American fathers and Asian mothers, have endured years of hostility in Southeast Asia, being stereotyped as the "dust of the earth." They arrive with dreams of being reunited with an American parent, dreams that are seldom fulfilled. They also come to the United States with little formal education, few job skills, and significant identity confusion. Many, however, have mastered street survival skills.

Often, Amerasians enter the mental health system soon after arrival because of anxiety, severe depression, and suicidal ideation. Years of emotional pain, social dissonance, culture conflicts, poor sense of self-worth, and inability to trust or appreciate emotional intimacy mean that the psychiatric nurse confronts many challenges in helping the Amerasian patient. You can help Amerasian patients tell their stories, accept themselves, let go of the past, and move on by assisting them to establish focused, achievable goals.

Buddhism, the religion of many Southeast Asian refugees, postulates that suffering is integral to human existence. Suffering is caused by desire, self-indulgence, or craving and leads to an unending cycle of birth, growth, decay, death, and rebirth. The Noble Eightfold

Path to eliminate desire and suffering and attain nirvana is achieved by

1. Right views
2. Right aims or intent
3. Right speech
4. Right conduct or action
5. Right means of livelihood
6. Right effort
7. Right mindfulness
8. Right meditation or contemplation

Because Buddhism talks about abandoning the self, this religious tenet contradicts the Western psychiatric emphasis on self-worth and self-acceptance. Traditional Asian healers are successful because they are concerned with the whole patient and family—an important approach for psychiatric nurses to emulate.

Chinese Americans

China is an ancient civilization. Its people have emigrated to all corners of the globe, often suffering discrimination in their new homelands. As a result, tight-knit communities of Chinese people have stressed loyalty to one's family and clan and support of MAAs as survival mechanisms.

When meeting a Chinese patient, determine whether that patient was born in China or is a second- or third-generation Chinese living in the United States or Canada. Chen (1996), Finn and Lee (1996), and Tabora and Flaskerud (1994) all produced helpful writings about the implications of cultural differences for nurses caring for patients of Chinese ancestry.

Tseng (1986), in tracing the development of Chinese psychiatry, noted that Chinese medicine has been in existence for more than 3000 years, with herbal medicine frequently prescribed. In China, however, the development of modern Chinese psychiatry and treatment of mental illness has evolved only since the late 1950s. Traditional Chinese medicine considered weakness, exhaustion, emptiness, deficiency, and disharmony to be the reasons for illness. After the Cultural Revolution, Chinese psychiatry was revised, and psychological factors were emphasized as the exclusive causes of mental illness. This orientation still persists in China.

The "overseas Chinese" were subject to discrimination and lived their own separate cultural and social existence, in ethnic enclaves. The Chinese reaction to discrimination was withdrawal, timidity, and anxiety. Overseas Chinese developed Chinatowns complete with community organizations to meet the needs of citizens, including the needs of patients with mental illness. Second- and third-generation Chinese living in the United States retain strong loyalty to family values and ethnic identity. This group has a high percentage of college-educated individuals who are increasingly more integrated into the dominant culture, both occupationally and residentially.

The religious traditions of Taoism and Confucianism have long been practiced by the Chinese. "Taoism holds that everything should be done according to Tao, the natural way; all else is madness" (Bradley, 1963, p. 135). Over the centuries, Taoism became a religion of superstition and magical control; a powerful clan of Taoist priests provided amulets, potions, and incantations. Confucian belief stresses the tradition of ancestor worship, filial piety, benevolent love, duty, wisdom, integrity, and propriety.

Understanding the hierarchy of all relationships is important when helping a Chinese American patient. "The son is inferior to his father and owes *Hsiao,* respect and obedience, to him. So, too, the wife is inferior to her husband and owes him corresponding *Hsiao;* the younger brother, servant, and citizen owe *Hsiao* to elder brothers, master and emperor" (Bradley, 1963, p. 144).

Japanese Americans

Individuals of Japanese origin suffered prejudice and discrimination in the United States, especially in the form of mass internment during World War II. This experience shapes the attitudes of many Japanese Americans today. Among the Japanese Americans, *Issei* are first generation; *Nisei* are second generation; and *Sansei* are third generation. "As of 1942, the average age of Issei males was fifty-five, while that of Nisei was only seventeen" (Sowell, 1981, p. 170). Many in the third generation are militant about correcting past injustices against their ethnic group. The Issei consider the Sansei generation "too American"; hence, there are some intergenerational strains.

Strong family and communal values with emphasis on education, self-control, and pressure to conform have resulted in little social pathology. Fear of failure, however, is an inherent motivator among Japanese, and thus a potential stressor. The Japanese American is expected to conform to family expectations and community norms. The psychiatric nurse needs to understand that individualism is frowned on, even today.

Shinto is the indigenous religion of Japan. It is estimated that 70 million of Japan's 95 million people are adherents of Shinto. Shinto has been influenced by Buddhist and Confucian practices as well as the religious thought of India. The basic concept of deity in Shinto is the concept of *Kami,* meaning something holy or connected with the spirit world. Two main causes of evil and misfortune for individuals, according to Shinto myths, are polluting actions, such as hanging a man's clothes on a hook intended for a woman's clothes, and displeasing the ancestors (Bradley, 1963). When working with Japanese American patients, you need to explore religious beliefs, the Kami as lived daily, and the degree of stress imposed by the need to conform.

Filipino Americans

Although the Philippines have been strongly influenced by the cultures of Spain and the United States, the inherent values of Filipinos remain strongly oriented toward group and church. About 90% of Filipinos are Catholic; the remainder are Muslim or Protestant. More than 800 dialects are spoken in the Philippines. Some

Filipinos are proud of their Spanish origins; others adhere to the influences of Chinese culture; and those who identify themselves as Muslim are strongly influenced by the tenets of Islam.

Since the 1940s, the Philippines have had mental health practitioners, psychiatrists, and psychiatric nurses, yet professional help is sought only after a crisis. A widely inculcated belief is that the extended family can provide the listening ear and guidance needed to resolve a psychological conflict. Filipinos may also consult *psychic surgeons,* who perform bloodless operations to relieve somatic complaints (Dein, 1997). Belief in the preservation of the family's good name and the power of prayer are strong behavioral determinants. As a nurse journeying with a Filipino patient, be aware of this and other cultural beliefs.

Filipinos as a group are sensitive and may be reluctant to ask questions for fear of appearing aggressive or embarrassing the health care provider. They respond better if you speak softly and unhurriedly and demonstrate an interest in the concerns of the family. A cardinal rule is not to say or do anything to embarrass the patient or the family.

Pacific Island Peoples

The Pacific Islands have seen European, Asian, and American influences, yet the significance of the social group remains a strong force for approval or disapproval. The Admiralty Island, for example, situated about 150 miles north of New Guinea, came under German and Australian influence, yet retained their own powerful social stigmas. Romanucci-Ross (1978) provided insights into anger, shame, and suicide in these islands:

A person can be shamed to illness in several ways. A woman, for example, was seen by her husband's brother as she was in a treetop and her genitals were exposed to his glance. In another instance, a man was not paid by his wife's temporary consort for a sexual encounter. Both were undisputed reasons for shame suicide. (p. 129)

Communication patterns among Pacific Island peoples are summarized in Box 12–6.

In most of the Pacific Islands, strong group mores also involve belief in spirits, rituals, and the equivalent of the

Box 12–6 ■ ■ ■ ■ ■
Communication Patterns Among Pacific Islanders

Facial expressions show signs of trust and openness.

Roles are ascribed, with elders permitted to take the lead in conversation.

Refusing to accept hospitality offered through food or beverage is an insult.

Friendship is based on reciprocity.

Native American medicine man or woman. The social definition of insanity in the Admiralty Islands is similar to that in India. If a woman goes against her husband's wishes or is too gregarious, she may be labeled mentally ill.

Dobson (1991) contended that in many cultures, the individual is seen as an integral part of the social group to which he or she belongs, especially in Samoa and the Fiji Islands, where health needs are an inherent aspect of group and community functioning. Al-Issa (1982, p. 9) indicated that the low rates of schizophrenia in the South Pacific "seem to be consistent with a cultural framework that provides communal decisions and clear-cut paths of action for individuals who are predisposed to schizophrenia." The competent transcultural nurse must recognize that attitudes are socially learned and often result in marked cultural differences in what is considered acceptable behavior.

W*hat do you think?* What do you do as a health care provider when what you believe is best for an Asian individual is not what's best for the family?

➤ *Check Your Reading*

36. How might depression be understood in Hinduism?
37. What is the inherent conflict in the beliefs of American psychiatry and Buddhism?
38. Contrast the American and Japanese views on individualism.
39. What is the role of the Filipino extended family in responding to mental illness?

Native Americans

Native Americans come from at least 10 different cultural areas (e.g., California, Northeast, Plains, Southeast, Southwest, Arctic), more than two dozen language families (e.g., Algonquian, Siouan, Iroquoian, Eskimaleut), and numerous tribes (e.g., Shawnee, Seminole, Crow, Blackfoot, Apache, Navajo). Communication patterns among Native Americans are summarized in Box 12–7.

Approximately 1.9 million Native Americans live in the United States, and there are 554 federally recognized tribes or nations. Each of these entities has unique customs, traditions, histories, and social organizations. There are still as many as 200 tribes, such as the Meherrin and Eno-Occaneechi, working to be federally recognized. Older adults may prefer the collective term *American Indian* (Kramer, 1998).

To understand the mental health issues of Native Americans, you must know that the historical relationship between Native American tribes and the U.S. government has created dependency and identity confusion. Services offered by the government have sought to acculturate the Native Americans into the dominant society (Trimble, 1988).

Box 12–7 ■ ■ ■ ■ ■
Communication Patterns Among Native Americans

Native Americans are generally reserved.

They do not engage in small talk, touching, hugging, or demonstrative displays of emotion.

They are comfortable with periods of silence.

To develop rapport, the nonindigenous communicator should know something of the group's real history and not succumb to media stereotypes.

Sharing food and drink is a common form of hospitality.

Roles are formalized, with chiefs, elders, and shamans having a special place of respect.

When a significant decision needs to be made, the above-named people need to be included.

There is a formal hierarchy surrounding roles and status that should be observed.

The decision to leave or stay on an Indian reservation generates many conflicts between urban and reservation Native Americans. The approximately half million urban Native Americans are more likely to be migratory, to become invisible in the dominant culture, and to have less contact with traditional support systems—all factors leading to increased stress, anxiety, and depression (Sage, 1991). Native American children raised in urban areas often lack traditional role models to develop self-esteem and assert their sense of identity. Such children often have more strained intergenerational ties, especially with grandparents still residing on reservations. There is considerable pressure from the family and the tribe to remain in contact and to return for visits. On a reservation, all members of a tribe know their genealogy, and even a person of mixed blood participates in traditional tribal ceremonies or seeks the service of a medicine man or woman.

Native Americans experience high rates of unemployment and poverty and inadequate preventive medical care. Studies (Cheadle, Pearson, Wagner, Psaty, Diehr, & Koepsell, 1994; Grossman, Kreiger, Sugarman, & Forquera, 1994) continue to document the prevalence of risk-taking behavior, especially alcohol and drug abuse, and suicide, even among Native Americans who have achieved a higher socioeconomic status. Complicating the picture are an upsurge in youth violence (Bewin, 1998) and a sudden influx of casino-generated wealth to a small number of tribes (Egan, 1998). Cheadle and colleagues (1994) suggested investigating other social and environmental influences to understand the factors that precipitate mental illness.

Although alcoholism has long been linked with depression and suicide, O'Nell (1993), in working with Flathead Indians residing on a reservation, discovered that for the tribe, depression and consequent drinking may have positive connotations. Similarly, it is a mark of maturity to feel profound loneliness when separated from loved ones, to feel sorrow for the pain one has caused others, and to feel pity for those who have nothing.

Depression, therefore, can be a positive expression of belonging in this milieu. To be sad is to be aware of human interdependence and the gravity of historical, tribal, familial, and personal loss. To be depressed, and that includes tearfulness and sleep and appetite disturbances, is to demonstrate maturity and connectedness to the Indian world. A carefree attitude is often thought of as indicative of immaturity. (O'Nell, 1993, p. 461)

Drinking is seen as a positive expression of sociability, a reaffirmation of the bonds of friendship and kinship. Not drinking may be interpreted as a slight against family and friends. O'Nell also noted that it is inappropriate in the Flathead Indian community to ask direct questions about painful or shameful experiences.

Although the precise meaning of customs, rituals, and taboos remains specific to each group, Native Americans tend to be reverent and use ritual before undertaking activities. They experience an intimate relationship with the natural world and see themselves as extensions of nature. Native American religions involve the belief that the universe is suffused with preternatural forces and powerful spirits. Tribes generally have a shaman or medicine man or woman who is thought to intercede with the spirits through ritual, magic, incantations, sacred objects, or herbal remedies. All tribes emphasize wholeness and balance, each with its own understanding of equilibrium within its oral history and religion.

Ritual purification through the use of sweat lodges is widely accepted on reservations and in urban areas. The sweat lodge is a symbol of Native American religion and identity and is used by all Native American groups. Its "common purpose is to bring the individual closer to the elemental forces of life, and to express unity between all humans, animals, the earth, and the physical forces in the universe" (Walker, Lambert, Walker, & Kivlahan, 1993, p. 565). Because the medicine man or woman conducts the sweat lodge ceremonies, you should view this person as a collaborator in the healing process.

An interview with a Native American patient may evoke an unexpected response pattern. Native American culture emphasizes symbols and periods of silence. Therefore, making chitchat may only increase anxiety. Demonstrating reverence for the environment and knowledge of sacred symbols such as sacred pipes, medicine wheels, and eagle feathers promotes rapport. Never touch a medicine bag or amulet.

Manson, Walker, and Kivlahan (1987) advocated group therapy for Native Americans to clarify issues surrounding identity and the conflicts associated with feelings of being an outsider. Family therapy, too, has been beneficial because elders can be role models, reinforce positive values, and reduce the patient's sense of stigma and isolation (Attneave, 1969).

Inuit and Aleut Peoples

Within the Arctic area, the Eskimaleut language family is used by two groups with ancestral links: the Inuit, or Eskimo, and Aleut peoples. The name *Eskimo* means "eaters of raw meat" in the Algonquian language. This name was used by whites; people to whom it is applied prefer the name *Inuit,* which means "people" in their own language. In Canada, the Eskimos are officially called *Inuit* by the government. Lefever and Davidhizar (1991) wrote of the diversity of Inuit, some living in Canada and others in Alaska, Greenland, and Russia.

The most important support for the Inuit and Aleut peoples continues to be the extended family. Marriage is highly regarded. Children are welcomed and viewed as an assurance of care and support in old age. Among the Inuit, a person of importance is called *tsumatag,* "he who thinks" (Waldman, 1985). In the difficult Arctic environment, Inuit traditionally have created special partnerships with nonfamily members. "Sharing partners" participate in the preparation of food gathered through hunting and fishing; "song partners" perform religious rituals together.

Similar to other Native Americans, Inuit carve beautiful objects out of wood, bone, and ivory for their religious rituals. Many customs prevail for giving birth, cutting the umbilical cord, naming a child, celebrating a good fishing catch, and burying the dead. As in some Asian cultures, Inuit stress respect and the burning of lamps to honor the dead. Inuit draw strength from nature, as the poem *Words to a Sick Child* (Bierhorst, 1983, p. 41) suggested:

Go up to the mountain
From the summit of the mountain you shall seek health,
You shall draw life.

Hysteria occurs with high incidence among Inuit (Davis, 1986). In reviewing the work of earlier researchers, Abel, Metraux, and Roll (1987, p. 55) noted that "antic hysteria is an acute dissociative reaction," probably precipitated by the harsh environment. The climate, the struggle for food, and the preservation of a traditional way of life are made particularly difficult because Inuit possess little capital, and large corporations remain eager to exploit minerals, oil, and gas in their natural environment.

Similar to other native peoples, the Inuit are comfortable with periods of silence, with formal handshakes, with less need for personal space, and with reliance on nonverbal communication. Lefever and Davidhizar (1991) emphasized that "the nurse who understands Eskimo culture will look for nonverbal clues, such as watching the face for raised eyebrows (indicating 'yes') or a wrinkled nose (indicating 'no')." Although Inuit seldom contradict others publicly, their apparent agreement may simply be an acknowledgment of the speaker's words.

For the psychiatric nurse, examining the patient's support system and degree of felt interdependency may be a helpful starting point. Also, learn if the patient has used herbs or consulted a shaman. Determine the patient's relationship to the extended community. In turn, the community's endorsement of you does much to encourage the patient to seek and accept help.

What do you think? How do you see the concept of the reservation fitting into the modern world?

> ➤ *Check Your Reading*
> 40. What effect might chitchat have on a Native American?
> 41. How is depression viewed in the Flathead Indian culture?
> 42. How is drinking viewed within the Flathead Indian culture?
> 43. What is a sweat lodge?
> 44. What is the role of the shaman in Native American cultures?

West Indian and Caribbean Peoples

West Indians are strongly influenced by African traditions and remnants of British, Spanish, Dutch, or French culture, depending on the island of origin and family traditions. Communication patterns among West Indians are summarized in Box 12-8. West Indians frequently speak their thoughts aloud. Children at play quickly dash to cover their heads when it rains, not because they fear getting wet but because they want to keep neatly groomed hair. Superstitions—including belief in *jumbies* (spirits) and some vodoun beliefs—abound in the Caribbean and modify behavior in countless ways. Yet you cannot assume that every patient from the Caribbean holds these beliefs. If serious mental illness is present, however, patients may report that the spirits have taken control.

Unusual behavior may be attributed to weather, nutrition, or a physical illness. Some West Indians seek

B o x 1 2 – 8 ■ ■ ■ ■ ■
Communication Patterns Among West Indians

The communication style is laid back and indirect.

Conversation may ramble before one gets to the heart of the matter.

A non–West Indian should not touch a West Indian because this is considered impolite.

Making direct inquiries without first engaging the person in conversation may give the appearance of impatience.

Smiling and joking are acceptable ways of communicating.

healers experienced in herbs. The great array of herbs for sale at the open-air market in St. Thomas, U.S. Virgin Islands, attests to their extensive use by people from every socioeconomic class.

The family remains the key element to helping the patient explore emotional problems and engage in treatment. Sharing the degree or depth of distress may be especially difficult with a nurse from a different ethnic or cultural group.

McCartney (1971), a native Bahamian, wrote in *Neuroses in the Sun* of the remnants of social, racial, and color prejudice. "Racial prejudice is an aspect of our culture that is as universally decried as it is deeply ingrained in our minds" (p. 53). The effects of conquest and colonialism often create a long-term sense of inferiority, a rejection of authority, and a struggle for identity, especially for those of mixed racial ancestry trying to accept all of their inheritance. You need to recognize that racism is an issue for some patients. McCartney (1971) noted that some individuals from the Caribbean who had

never given much thought to their social value in terms of colour experience some very painful shocks when confronted with the racial value system of an alien society. The psychic damage resulting from this . . . is hard to assess. (pp. 64–65)

Although psychiatric hospitals exist throughout the Caribbean, the stigma of mental illness is sometimes expressed in antagonism toward the mentally ill person and the search for a cure through a spiritualist or an *obeah* practitioner.

Religion is both a social and a spiritual resource in much of the Caribbean. Belief in the supernatural is found in Puerto Rican *espiritismo*, Afro-Cuban *santería*, and Haitian *vodoun*. Each of these religions has prescribed rituals for cleansing people who believe their condition is due to malevolent spirits (Lefley, 1990). In these cultures, you may need to involve not only the family but also a traditional healer, exorcist, or priest as educator, consultant, and cotherapist. Weiss (1992) suggested that

strong disapproval of folk healing by Christian clergy and by Protestant fundamentalist mental health works caused patients and family members (of immigrants from Santo Domingo in the Caribbean) to deny such involvement. (p. 241)

Espiritismo and the Afro-Cuban religions share a view that supernatural entities may possess a living person and that the patient may present with symptoms of paranoia. Weiss (1992) found that when patient's kin consulted healers, it was usually at the point "when patient's illness was especially difficult to manage at home" (p. 248). Both the family and the patient might refer to the patient "as being on the brink of spiritual growth and, at worst, as succumbing to spiritual vulnerabilities or to the evil intent of persons or forces beyond the circle of intimates" (p. 249).

When journeying with a person from the West Indies or the Caribbean, you should recognize that European, American, Indian, and African beliefs are interlaced with religious rituals and folklore. Before attempting to diagnose a patient, you need to know if the patient attributes the distress to being hexed or possessed by evil spirits. For patients who think they have had a hex put on them, ask by whom and why. Try to ascertain if healers or herbalists have been sought. The answers to these questions may reveal the respondent's perception of your role and intention. The patient's trust must be earned.

What do you think? Would consulting an exorcist be colluding with a patient's delusion?

➤ *Check Your Reading*

45. How might someone from the Caribbean explain mental illness?
46. What role does the family play in the treatment of a West Indian patient with a mental illness?

COMMUNICATION FOR CULTURAL UNDERSTANDING

Learning about a patient's culture involves more than filling out forms and asking questions. It must be a journey to acquire perspective; to promote understanding; and to facilitate respect, trust, and the building of a relationship. Learning does not happen without time and effort. It implies that you have first taken the time to study the patient's culture and then to engage the patient and family without making significant cultural mistakes.

Among the immediate variables that may affect communication are (Hofling, Leininger, & Bregg, 1976):

- The patient's behavioral symptoms and presentation or the degree to which in the patient's culture he or she may be considered mentally ill
- The psychiatric nurse's personality, sensitivity, and ability to be a transcultural communicator
- The degree to which the psychiatric nurse deemphasizes the use of medical jargon and speaks to the patient in a tone and manner that create rapport; use of culture-specific idioms or phrases possibly helpful
- The environment for treatment and the emotional climate created by verbal tone and nonverbal signals
- Time as a factor in contributing to the patient's readiness to relate to the psychiatric nurse

Ask yourself the following questions before beginning an intervention with a patient from another culture:

- Do I hold a theoretical orientation about the cause of a patient's mental illness that is in opposition to this patient's religious or cultural beliefs?
- What nonverbal signals do I send that may provoke anxiety, fear, or resistance?
- Does the mental health environment, beginning with the manner in which I receive the patient, signal that the patient's culture is important? Does the decor

include reassuring pictures, artifacts, and bilingual signs?

- Do I assume that someone who speaks with an accent is uneducated?
- Do I pay attention to the impact of my personal style on particular patients?

Learn cross-cultural communication—the dos and don'ts that can provide you with communication tools (Taylor, 1989). See Box 12-9 for communicating strategies across cultural groups.

Doing a Cultural Assessment

Because nurses do not usually have the luxury of taking the hours a truly thorough cultural assessment would demand, it is extremely helpful to complete a checklist of important items during a first interview. Many ethnocultural assessment tools are available (Campinha-Bacote, 1995; Lipson, Dibble, & Minarik, 1996; Morris, 1996). The checklist in Table 12-1 is from Narayan (1997).

Providing Culturally Sensitive Therapy

In providing therapy for a patient from a culture different from your own, you will want to keep in mind everything you know and are learning about that person's background, upbringing, and cultural milieu. As an example, Kendall (1996) pointed out that while

psychotherapy for European Americans has traditionally emphasized the individual and the interior self, African Americans' experiences are embedded in communal activities, which involve the church, neighborhood, and family, necessitating a different approach.

We have seen that because of shame, patients from many cultures will be reluctant to discuss psychiatric symptoms. Once trust has been earned, it may be necessary to ask specifically about such things as depression or posttraumatic stress. The way in which you do this matters. Lipson, Dibble, and Minarik (1996), in a handbook for culturally sensitive nursing care, provided culture-specific explanations and terminology for depression. For example, Native Americans may be comfortable speaking in metaphors, calling depression "heart problems"; South Asians consider *dil uddas bona* to be a sign of spiritual unhappiness and may welcome a therapy that includes meditation or yoga exercises.

But despite such differences and the anxiety that can be generated in a cross-cultural encounter, your capacity to truly *be with* another can bridge cultural gaps. For although the nature of the therapy offered may change to adapt to the needs of various patients, there are therapeutic cornerstones that should be common to any approach: respect, caring, and empathy. As Carl Rogers (1982) said,

To be with another in this way means that for the time being you lay aside the views and values you hold for yourself in order to enter another's world without prejudice. (p. 31)

Box 12–9 ■ ■ ■ ■ ■
Suggestions for Effective Communication

Speak slowly, audibly, and distinctly and use terminology that patients from other cultures can understand.

Use simple words and avoid jargon.

Listen as much as you speak; do not interrupt because this can be seen as rude.

Allow extra time to communicate with someone whose first language may not be your own. Trying to understand one another may require extra effort and time.

Respect silence; do not fill every gap in the conversation.

When you experience frustration or sense conflict or misunderstanding in a cross-cultural situation, stop and ask yourself if the conflict is due to a cultural difference. Try to see a common basis of understanding.

Adapt your style to the demands of a situation. Speak the patient's "language."

Do not make judgments about people based on their accents or language fluency.

Be open and sensitive as to how you give feedback.

Know who in the family is the appointed head or decision-maker.

Understand the "hot buttons" that can lead to conflict:
- Slang
- Racial and ethnic epithets
- Verbal and nonverbal behavior that does not meet accepted cultural norms, including definite pronouncements about a culture that is not your own

Identify and network with the traditional culture brokers and healers.

Ask the patient if he or she uses herbs and what the expected benefits are.

Learn to identify culturally relevant rituals.

Stress the patient's strengths and demonstrate respect and caring.

T A B L E   1 2 – 1   Cultural Assessment Checklist

Patient Identified Cultural/Ethnic Group/Religion

Social Customs

Typical greeting	What is the proper form of address? Is a handshake appropriate? Are shoes worn in the home?
Social customs before "business"	What constitutes social exchanges? Are refreshments part of the social custom?
Direct or indirect communication patterns	

Non-Verbal Patterns of Communication

Eye contact	Is eye contact considered polite or rude?
Tone of voice	What does a soft voice or a loud voice mean in this culture?
Personal space	Is personal space wider or closer than in the American culture?
Facial expressions, gestures	What do smiles, nods, and hand gestures mean?
Touch	When, where, and by whom can a patient be touched?

Client's Explanation of Problem

Diagnosis	What do you call this illness? How would you describe this problem?
Onset	When did the problem start? Why then? What started the problem?
Cause	What caused the problem? What might other people think is wrong with you?
Course	How does the illnes work? What does it do to you? What do you fear most about this problem?
Treatment	How have you treated the illness? What treatment should you receive? Who in your family or community can help you? Traditional practitioners?
Prognosis	How long will the problem last? Is it serious?
Expectations	What are you hoping the nurses will do for you when we come?

Nutrition Assessment

Pattern of meals	What is eaten? When are meals eaten?
Sick foods	
Food intolerance and taboos	

Pain Assessment

Cultural patterns of coping with pain

Patient's perception of severe pain, appropriate treatments

Medication Assessment

Patient's perception of "Western" medications

Possible pharmacogenetic variations

Psychosocial Assessment

Decision-maker

Sick role

Language barriers, translators

Cultural/ethnic community resources

From Narayan, M. C. (1997). Cultural assessment in home care. *Home Healthcare Nurse, 15*(10), 665.

Conclusions

Culture permeates every aspect of human behavior. It shapes perceptions and response patterns. No two cultures are exactly alike, and even within ethnic and cultural groups, differentiation and specificity mean that the competent nurse needs to consider individual patient needs before intervening. Not all researchers agree on the role culture plays in creating psychopathology, which is a universal phenomenon. But cultural beliefs and expecta-tions shape levels of tolerance and support networks and can facilitate or hinder help seeking.

Spirituality or religion exists worldwide. Every religion postulates a set of beliefs, rituals, and practices that can empower or diminish the individual. Clergy representing many religious traditions, native healers, and medicine men and women have roles in the healing of spiritual and emotional wounds.

Although the competent psychiatric nurse may not know every culture in detail, an understanding of cultural diversity leads to nursing care that is sensitive to the patient while promoting the patient's well-being within the norms of the ethnic group.

Key Points to Remember

- Every culture has norms or standards of behavior.
- Cultural relevancy means seeing differences without making value judgments.
- In the journey to another's culture, nurses need to be aware of their own values and subjective world views.
- Cultures undergo both continuity and change.
- Stereotypes perpetuate "isms" and fixed patterns of labeling others.
- Prejudice operates on different levels of severity. Patients who have suffered prejudice may appear more guarded because of their experiences.
- Ethnic identity encompasses the deepest core of being. It encapsulates the individual and provides a sense of affiliation and roots.
- Transcultural identification is the modification of customs and activities so that a particular group can more easily blend with the dominant culture. Language, dress, and gender-role socialization frequently change; such changes may ignite intergenerational conflict.
- Ethnic competence means acting in a manner that is accepted, expected, and congruent with the members of a particular culture.
- Space, time, and color are imbued with different cultural meanings.
- Beware of viewing all members of a given ethnic and cultural group as the same.
- Assessing not only where the patient was raised but also the parents' backgrounds promotes cultural relevancy.
- American emphasis on independence, self-help, and individual rights can clash with both cultural beliefs and religious tenets that stress interdependence, passivity, group norms, divine punishment, fatalism, and destiny.
- Distinguish between an immigrant and a refugee. Immigrants usually plan departure from their homeland. They do not always leave their country due to poverty but may simply want to live abroad and return home to retire. Refugees flee from political, economic, and social upheavals.
- Verbal and nonverbal communication is a significant part of the journey to another's culture. Persistent study, patience, and listening can facilitate acceptance by others of another culture.
- You are on a journey that requires you to change and grow.

Learning Activities

1. Read an ethnic journal and determine what values are being conveyed. How do the values differ from your own? Ethnic journals and magazines include but are not limited to *Ebony, Irish-American, Chinese Studies for Pupils,* and *Hispanic-American.*
2. Visit a refugee resettlement office. Who works there? What messages does the environment suggest? How would you feel if you were a refugee seeking services in a new country? What would be your first priorities?
3. Ask a friend from another ethnic or cultural group if you may come to a religious service or cultural celebration.
4. Think about the world of cultural diversity. About which groups of people do you know least? What do you need to do to be a competent psychiatric nurse as you journey toward understanding the cultures of others?

Critical Thinking Exercises

Ms. Sandra Banes, a community mental health nurse, visited Mrs. Jardee, a Filipino woman who had just lost her husband of 25 years. Ms. Banes was told by Mrs. Jardee's youngest daughter that the mother had not eaten since the funeral 3 days before. When Ms. Banes talked to Mrs. Jardee, who was lying in bed reading her Bible, she complained of back pain while crying incessantly. After assessing Mrs. Jardee, Ms. Banes decided to talk to Mrs. Jardee's daughter about possible hospitalization. When she attempted to approach the daughter about this decision, the daughter said that she could not help her. Ms. Banes was unsure what to make of this response.

1. What assumption(s) can be made about Ms. Banes' understanding about cultural influences in decisions of health care?
2. What evidence do you have to support your assumptions?
3. Consider any bias.

Ms. Banes was concerned and decided to talk to the daughter about the other children in the family. The daughter told the nurse that her older sister had gone to help the younger brother and his wife choose a new school for their children.

1. What other information does Ms. Banes need to know to help Mrs. Jardee?

2. What are your reasons for saying this?

3. What conclusions (if any) can you draw about the outcome of this situation?

References

Abel, T. M., Metraux, R., & Roll, S. (1987). *Psychotherapy and culture.* Albuquerque, NM: University of New Mexico.

Al-Issa, I. (1982). Does culture make a difference in psychopathology? In I. Al-Issa (Ed.), *Culture and psychopathology.* Baltimore: University Park Press.

Allport, G. W. (1979). *The nature of prejudice.* Reading, MA: Addison-Wesley.

American Psychiatric Association. (1994). *Diagnostic and statistical manual of mental disorders* (4th ed.). Washington, DC: American Psychiatric Association.

Angell, G. B. (1997). Madness in the family: The "windigo." *Journal of Family Social Work, 2,* 179-196.

Arredondo, P. (1991). Counseling Latinos. In C. C. Lee & B. L. Richardson (Eds.), *Multicultural issues in counseling: New approaches to diversity.* Alexandria, VA: American Association for Counseling and Development.

Artemis, L. (1996). Migrant health care: Creativity in primary care. *Advanced Practice Nursing Quarterly, 2*(2), 45-49.

Attneave, C. L. (1969). Therapy in tribal settings and urban network intervention. *Family Process 8,* 192-210.

Bewin, J. (Reporter). (1998, March 17). Crime on reservations, I. *All Things Considered.* Washington, DC: National Public Radio.

Bierhorst, J. (Ed.). (1983). *The sacred path: Spells, prayers and power songs of the American Indians.* New York: Quill.

Birket-Smith. (1971). *Eskimos.* New York: Crown.

Bodner, A., & Leininger, M. (1992). Transcultural nursing care values, beliefs and practices of American (USA) Gypsies. *Journal of Transcultural Nursing, 4*(1), 17-28.

Boritz-Wintz. (1994). Problematic issues in cross-cultural psychotherapy: Emotional conflicts occuring during acculturation. *Journal of Multicultural Nursing, 1*(2), 6-11.

Bradley, D. G. (1963). *A guide to the world's religions.* Englewood Cliffs, NJ: Prentice-Hall.

Brink, P. J. (1990). *Transcultural nursing: A book of readings.* Prospect Heights, IL: Waveland Press.

Brunt, J. H., Lindsey, E., & Hopkinson, J. (1997). Health promotion in the Hutterite community and the ethnocentricity of empowerment. *Canadian Journal of Nursing Research, 29*(1), 17-28.

Buccalo, S. (1997). Window on another world: An "English" nurse looks at the Amish culture and their health care beliefs. *Journal of Multicultural Nursing & Health, 3*(2), 53-58.

Burger, J. M. (1996). When the Gypsies come: An insider's view into a mysterious culture. *Journal of Christian Nursing, 13*(4), 4-9.

Burke, A. W. (1986). Racism, prejudice and mental illness. In J. L. Cox (Ed.), *Transcultural psychiatry.* London: Croom Helm.

Campinha-Bacote, J. (1994). *The process of cultural competence in health care: A culturally competent model of care.* Wyoming, OH: Transcultural C.A.R.E. Associates.

Campinha-Bacote, J. (1995). The quest for cultural competence in nursing care. *Nursing Forum, 30*(4), 19-25.

Caplan, N., Whitmore, J. K., & Choy, M. H. (1989). *The Boat People and achievement in America: A study of family life, hard work and cultural values.* Ann Arbor, MI: University of Michigan Press.

Carnevali, D. L. (1983). *Nursing care planning: Diagnosis and management* (3rd ed.). Philadelphia: J. B. Lippincott.

Catoir, J. T. (1990). *God delights in you.* New York: The Christophers.

Catoir, J. T. (1992). *World religions.* New York: Alba House.

Chan, S. (1991). *Asian Americans.* Boston: Twayne Publishers.

Cheadle, A., Pearson, D., Wagner, E., Psaty, B. M., Diehr, P., & Koepsell, T. (1994). Relationship between socioeconomic status, health status and lifestyle practices of American Indians: Evidence from a Plains reservation population. *Public Health Reports, 109,* 405-413.

Chen, Y. D. (1996). Conformity with nature: A theory of Chinese American elders' health promotion and illness prevention processes. *Advances in Nursing Science, 19*(2), 17-26.

Cohen, A. (1992). Prognosis for schizophrenia in the Third World: A reevaluation of cross-cultural research. *Culture, Medicine and Psychiatry, 16,* 53-75.

Comas-Diaz, L. (1989). Culturally relevant issues and treatment implications for Hispanics. In D. R. Koslow & E. P. Salett (Eds.), *Crossing cultures in mental health.* Washington, DC: Sietar International.

Davis, B. D. (1986). Culture and psychiatric nursing: Implications for training. In J. L. Cox (Ed.), *Transcultural psychiatry.* London: Croom Helm.

de Chardin, P. T. (1967). *On love.* New York: Harper & Row.

Dein, S. (1997). ABC of mental health: Mental health in a multiethnic society. *British Medical Journal, 315,* 473-476.

Dobson, S. M. (1991). *Transcultural nursing.* London: Scutari Press.

Egan, T. (1998, March 8). New prosperity brings new conflict to Indian Country. *New York Times,* pp. A1, A24.

Eliason, M. J. (1993). Ethics and transcultural nursing care. *Nursing Outlook, 41,* 225-228.

Erzinger, S. (1991). Communication between Spanish-speaking patients and their doctors in medical encounters. *Culture, Medicine and Psychiatry, 15,* 91-110.

Finn, J., & Lee, M. (1996). Transcultural nurses reflect on discoveries in China using Leininger's sunrise model. *Journal of Transcultural Nursing, 7*(2), 21-27.

Fiske, A. P. (1993). Social errors in four cultures: Evidence about universal forms of social relations. *Journal of Cross-Cultural Psychology, 24,* 463-494.

Good, B. J. (1993). Culture, diagnosis and comorbidity. *Culture, Medicine and Psychiatry, 16,* 427-446.

Griffith-Kenney, J. W., & Christensen, P. J. (Eds.). (1986). *Application of theories, frameworks and models* (2nd ed.). St. Louis, MO: C. V. Mosby.

Grossman, D. C., Krieger, J. W., Sugarman, J. R., & Forquera, R. A. (1994). Health status of urban American Indians and Alaska natives. *Journal of the American Medical Association, 271,* 845-850.

Hall, E. T., & Whyte, W. F. (1990). Intercultural communication: A guide to men of action. In P. J. Brink (Ed.), *Transcultural nursing: A book of readings.* Prospect Heights, IL: Waveland Press.

Hanson, M. J., Lynch, E. W., & Wayman, K. I. (1990). Honoring the cultural diversity of families when gathering data. *Topics in Early Childhood Special Education, 24*(1), 112-131.

Harris, S. J. (1972). *The authentic person.* Niles, IL: Argus Communications.

Hatton, D. C. (1992). Information transmission in bilingual, bicultural contexts. *Journal of Community Health Nursing, 9*(1), 53-59.

Heok, K. E. (1994). *Ageing and old age.* Singapore: Singapore University Press.

Hofling, C. K., Leininger, M. M., & Bregg, E. (1976). *Basic psychiatric concepts in nursing* (2nd ed.). Philadelphia: J. B. Lippincott.

Hofstede, G. (1980). *Culture's consequences. International differences in work-related values.* Beverly Hills, CA: Sage.

Jezewski, M. A. (1993). Culture brokering as a model for advocacy. *Nursing and Health Care, 14*(2), 78–85.

Jezewski, M. A. (1995). Evolution of a grounded theory: Conflict resolution through culture brokering. *Advances in Nursing Science, 17(3)*, 14–30.

Juarbe, T. (1998). Puerto Ricans. In G. Lipson, S. L. Dibble, & P. A. Minarik (Eds.), *Culture and nursing care: A pocket guide.* San Francisco, CA: University of California San Francisco Nursing Press.

Kearney, M. (1978). Spiritualist healing in Mexico. In P. Morley & R. Wallis (Eds.), *Culture and curing: Anthropological perspectives on traditional medical beliefs and practices.* London: Peter Owen.

Kendall, J. (1996). Creating a culturally responsive psychotherapeutic environment for African American Youths: A critical analysis. *Advances in Nursing Science, 18*(4), 11–28.

Keefe, S. E. (1992). Ethnic identity: The domain of perceptions of and attachment to ethnic groups and cultures. *Human Organization, 51*(1), 35–43.

Kennedy, G. J., Kelman, H. R., Thomas, C., & Chen, J. (1996). The relation of religious preference and practice to depressive symptoms among 1,855 older adults. *Journals of Gerontology. Series B, Psychological Sciences and Social Sciences, 51*, 301–308.

Kramer, J. (1998). American Indians. In J. G. Lipson, S. L. Dibble, & P. A. Minarik (Eds.), *Culture and nursing care: A pocket guide.* San Francisco, CA: University of California San Francisco Nursing Press.

Kuo, C., & Kavanaugh, K. H. (1994). Chinese perspectives on culture and mental health. *Issues in Mental Health Nursing, 15*, 551–567.

Lee, C. C., & Richardson, B. L. (1991). Promise and pitfalls of multicultural counseling. In C. C. Lee & B. L. Richardson (Eds.), *Multicultural issues in counseling: New approaches to diversity.* Alexandria, VA: American Association for Counseling and Development.

Lefever, D., & Davidhizar, R. E. (1991). American Eskimos. In J. N. Geiger & R. E. Davidhizar (Eds.), *Transcultural nursing assessment and intervention.* St. Louis, MO: Mosby–Year Book.

Lefley, H. P. (1990). Culture and chronic mental illness. *Hospital and Community Psychiatry, 41*, 277–286.

Leininger, M. (1978). Culturological assessment domains for nursing practices. In M. Leininger (Ed.), *Transcultural nursing: Theories, concepts, practices.* New York: John Wiley.

Lerner, G. (Ed.) (1972). *Black women in white America.* New York: Random House.

Linton, R. (1945). *The cultural background of personality.* Westport, CT: Greenwood Press.

Lipson, J. G., Dibble, S. L., & Minarik, P. A. (1996). *Culture and nursing care: A pocket guide.* San Francisco, CA: San Francisco Nursing Press.

Mahon, P. Y. (1997). Transcultural nursing: A source guide. *Journal of Nursing Staff Development, 13*, 218–222.

Manson, S. M., Walker, R. D., & Kivlahan, D. R. (1987). Psychiatric assessment and treatment of American Indians and Alaska natives. *Hospital and Community Psychiatry, 38*, 165–173.

McCartney, T. O. (1971). *Neuroses in the sun.* Nassau, Bahamas: Executive Printers.

McKenzie, S. C. (1980). *Aging and old age.* Glenview, IL: Scott, Foresman.

Moon, A., & Williams, O. (1993). Perceptions of elder abuse and help-seeking patterns among African-American, Caucasian-American and Korean-American elderly women. *The Gerontologist, 33*, 386–395.

Morris, R. I. (1996). Bridging cultural boundaries: The African American and transcultural caring. *Advanced Practice Nursing Quarterly, 2*(2), 31–38.

Mphande, L., & James-Myers, L. (1993). Traditional African medicine and the optimal theory: Universal insights for health and healing. *Journal of Black Psychology, 19*(1), 25–47.

Mufford, C. (1992, October). A cure of many colors. *New Physician,* 14–19.

Narayan, M. C. (1997). Cultural assessment in home care. *Home Healthcare Nurse, 15*(10), 663–670.

Newbold, C. (1991). To walk with each other. In G. F. A. Pierce (Ed.), *Of human hands.* Minneapolis, MN: Augsburg.

O'Nell, T. D. (1993). Feeling worthless: An ethnographic investigation of depression and problem drinking at the Flathead reservation. *Culture, Medicine, and Psychiatry, 16,* 447–469.

Primeaux, M. (1977). Caring for the American Indian patient. *American Journal of Nursing, 77*, 91–94.

Quintanilla, M. (1991, June 9). The language gap. *Los Angeles Times,* p. E1.

Rack, P. (1982). *Race, culture, and mental disorder.* New York: Tavistock.

Ramirez, M. (1991). *Psychotherapy and counseling with minorities.* New York: Pergamon Press.

Rao, A. V. (1986). Indian and Western psychiatry: A comparison. In J. L. Cox (Ed.), *Transcultural Psychiatry.* London: Croom Helm.

Rey, L. D. (1997). Religion as invisible culture: Knowing about and knowing with. *Journal of Family Social Work, 2,* 159–177.

Rivera, C. (1988). Culturally sensitive aftercare services for chronically mentally ill Hispanics: The case of the psychoeducational/treatment model. *Fordham University Hispanic Research Center Research Bulletin, 11.*

Rogers, C. (1982). Empathic: An unappreciated way of being. In Rubenstein, H. & Bloch, M. H. (Eds.), *Things that matter.* New York: Macmillan.

Rosenhan, D. L. (1990). On being sane in insane places. In P. J. Brink (Ed.), *Transcultural nursing: A book of readings.* Prospect Heights, IL: Waveland Press.

Sage, G. P. (1991). Counseling American Indian adults. In C. C. Lee & B. L. Richardson (Eds.), *Multicultural issues in counseling: New approaches to diversity.* Alexandria, VA: American Association for Counseling and Development.

Schwartz, T. (1976). Relations among generations in time-limited cultures. In T. Schwartz (Ed.), *Socialization as cultural communication.* Los Angeles: University of California Press.

Shuman, R. B. (Ed.). (1970). *A galaxy of black writing.* Durham, NC: Moore.

Simond, M. M. (1996) Case analysis: Cross-cultural conflict in the psychiatric setting. *Journal of Multicultural Nursing and Health, 2(3),* 38–40.

Simons, R. C., & Hughes, C. C. (Eds.) (1985). *The culture-bound syndromes: Folk illnesses of psychiatric and anthropological interest.* Boston: D. Reidel.

Sowell, T. (1981). *Ethnic American: A history.* New York: Basic Books.

Tabora, B. & Flaskerud, J. H. (1994). Depression among Chinese Americans: A review of the literature. *Issues in Mental Health Nursing, 15,* 569–584.

Takaki, R. (1993). *A different mirror: A history of multicultural America.* Boston: Little, Brown.

Taoka, K. N. (1997). Cultivating the seeds of cultural competence is a growth process. *ONS News, 12*(8), 8.

Taylor O. L. (1989). The effects of cultural assumptions on cross-cultural communication. In D. R. Koslow & E. P. Salett (Eds.), *Crossing cultures in mental health.* Washington, DC: Sietar International.

The cultures of illness. (1993, February 15). *U.S. News and World Report,* pp. 73–76.

Trimble, J. E. (1988). Stereotypical images, American Indians and prejudice. In P. Katz & D. Tylor (Eds.), *Eliminating racism: Profiles in controversy.* New York: Plenum Press.

Tseng, W. S. (1986). Chinese psychiatry: Development and characteristics. In J. L. Cox (Ed.), *Transcultural psychiatry.* London: Croom Helm.

Waldman, C. (1985). *Atlas of the North American Indian.* New York: Facts on File.

Walker, R. D., Lambert, M. D., Walker, P. S., & Kivlahan, D. R. (1993). Treatment implications of comorbid psychopathology in American Indians and Alaska natives. *Culture, Medicine, and Psychiatry, 16,* 555–572.

Warren, B. J. (1997). Depression, stressful life events, social support and self-esteem in middle class African American women. *Archives of Psychiatric Nursing, 11*(3), 107–117.

Weiss, C. I. (1992). Controlling domestic life and mental illness: Spiritual and aftercare resource used by Dominican New Yorkers. *Culture, Medicine, and Psychiatry, 16,* 237–271.

West, E. A. (1993). The cultural bridge model. *Nursing Outlook, 41,* 229–234.

Williams, D. R. (1994). The concept of race and health status in America. *Public Health Reports, 109*(1), 26–41.

Wolpert, S. (1991). *India.* Berkeley, CA: University of California Press.

Suggested Readings

Brink, P. J. (Ed.). (1990). *Transcultural nursing: A book of readings.* Prospect Heights, IL: Waveland Press.

Eliason, M. J. (1993). Ethics and transcultural nursing care. *Nursing Outlook, 41,* 225-228.

Geiger, J., & Davidhizar, D. (1991). *Transcultural nursing assessment and intervention.* St. Louis, MO: Mosby-Year Book.

Leininger, M. (1991). *Culture care diversity and universality: A theory of nursing.* New York: National League for Nursing Press.

Leininger, M. (1997). Future directions in transcultural nursing in the 21st century. *International Nursing Review, 44*(1), 19-23.

West, E. A. (1993). The cultural bridge model. *Nursing Outlook, 41,* 229-234.

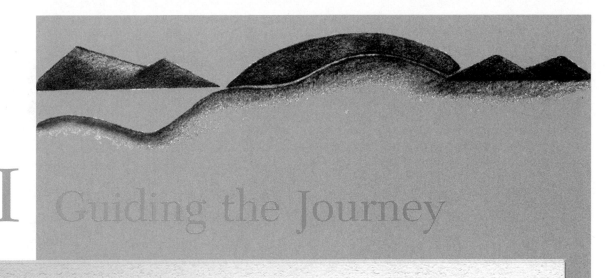

III Guiding the Journey

Traveler's Log

My practice as an independent clinical specialist in psychiatric nursing began in an unusual place, the coronary care unit. As a new graduate, I loved the personal care and close relationships that developed between nurse and patient in this unit. What I did not like was the amount of preventable illness I witnessed. It seemed a little late to begin teaching about health and lifestyle change after damage was done. I wanted to work with these patients before injury occurred.

My journey led me to establish a group practice that specializes in psycho-physiological disorders. My practice is filled with patients with physical illnesses who are seeking help to modify their behaviors. The joy of my work is forming close, personal relationships with my patients and planning with them the changes in their lives. I work with their families also because change in any one person in a family system affects the entire family. I work with my patients and their families to ensure their success and improve their level of wellness.

As a nurse, I have a strong background in physiology, pharmacology, and medical treatment of diseases. My patients are diagnosed with hypertension, congestive heart failure, cancer, migraine headaches, chronic pain, and other disorders. I have the time to get to know each of them as they share their lives with me. We then plan to enhance their personal well being and that of the entire family. We are not working to cure the disease, but to promote a healthy lifestyle.

—Sue Thomas, PhD, RN

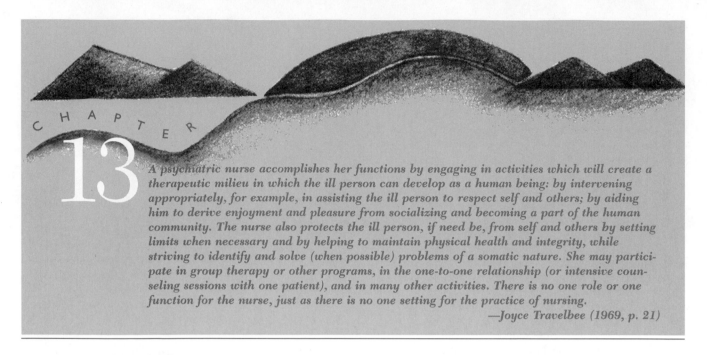

A psychiatric nurse accomplishes her functions by engaging in activities which will create a therapeutic milieu in which the ill person can develop as a human being: by intervening appropriately, for example, in assisting the ill person to respect self and others; by aiding him to derive enjoyment and pleasure from socializing and becoming a part of the human community. The nurse also protects the ill person, if need be, from self and others by setting limits when necessary and by helping to maintain physical health and integrity, while striving to identify and solve (when possible) problems of a somatic nature. She may participate in group therapy or other programs, in the one-to-one relationship (or intensive counseling sessions with one patient), and in many other activities. There is no one role or one function for the nurse, just as there is no one setting for the practice of nursing.

—*Joyce Travelbee (1969, p. 21)*

Basic Interventions

Learning Objectives

After studying this chapter, you should be able to:

1. List at least three basic psychiatric nursing interventions.
2. Describe the teaching-learning process in psychiatric nursing.
3. Define crisis intervention.
4. Describe the process of crisis intervention.
5. Define behavioral therapy.
6. Apply behavioral techniques to the care of the mentally ill patient.
7. Define supportive interventions.

Key Terminology

Active learning	Critical incident debriefing	Objective	Reinforcement schedule
Affective domain	Demonstration	Observational learning	Response
Behavioral therapy	Developmental (maturational)	Operant conditioning	Return demonstration
Classical conditioning	crisis	Passive learning	Self-management
Cognitive-behavioral therapy	Extinction	Patient education	Situational crisis
Cognitive domain	Health education	Positive reinforcement	Stimulus
Crisis	Learning	Psychomotor domain	Supportive interventions
Crisis intervention	Learning style	Punishment	Variable interval schedule
Crisis sequence	Modeling	Readiness	Variable ratio schedule
Crisis state	Negative reinforcement	Reinforcement	

The journey that we have traversed in developing this textbook has drawn on the clinical and teaching experiences of each of the contributing authors, insights gained from literature and research, the comments of faculty members who have adopted the textbook, and, most importantly, thoughtful responses provided to us from students who have used the previous edition of the text. The most consistent student responses have been the following:

- Tell us exactly what the psychiatric nurse does.
- Give us this information in one chapter so that we do not have to search the whole book.
- Make the examples concrete so that we can see the application.

We have tried throughout the text (e.g., the Snapshot of Nursing Interventions to Facilitate a Patient's Journey Through a Specific Psychiatric Problem) to make concrete what is abstract. This chapter represents another major thrust in that direction. The content you are about to read is not only a major revision of this textbook but also a dramatic veering away from the traditional approaches used in other textbooks. This chapter defines and describes the specific interventions used by psychiatric nurses as they work with the mentally ill. Examples are provided so that you can clearly see how these interventions are applied to clinical situations. Let's begin with the story of Leon (whose story is also mentioned in Chapter 24), a patient I had the pleasure of working with in home care in 1995. I will take you through the whole process of care so that you can see exactly what interventions I used to help Leon. Then we will examine in depth the "how to" of specific interventions including teaching, behavioral therapy, and crisis intervention.

Leon's Story

Leon was 35 years old. He was diagnosed with paranoid schizophrenia when he was 18. Leon lived alone in an apartment complex designated for individuals with various types of disabilities. Leon's appearance was a bit off-putting—he was very tall and muscular with a stern affect that could turn "threatening" in a moment's notice. Although he had a few casual acquaintances who lived in his apartment building, his main support was his elderly mother who lived a few blocks away. Leon saw his mother several times a week. They frequently shared dinner, they sang in the choir in a local Baptist church, and they attended church together whenever Leon was well enough to go.

Leon had been referred to home care by a research agency where he had volunteered to participate in a clozapine (Clozaril) project. The physician at the research agency had ordered many nursing interventions appropriate to Leon's condition, such as serum blood draws to monitor Leon's white blood cell

(WBC) count, supportive interventions, teaching about clozapine, and ongoing monitoring of his physical and mental status, specifically his psychotic behavior.

My initial assessment of Leon revealed a very bright man who had experienced his first schizophrenic episode when he was an 18-year-old college freshman. In the years since that first episode, he had been in and out of hospitals, including several prolonged stays in the state hospital system, and he had been arrested for assaultive behavior toward others. Despite a history of having been placed on multiple varied medication regimens, his experience with threatening voices was never totally controlled. When I first met him he was being weaned off of fluphenazine decanoate (Prolixin Decanoate) 25 mg, administered intramuscularly every other week, and oral fluphenazine HCl (Prolixin) taken three times a day. To Leon's credit, he had learned many coping strategies to deal with his troublesome voices. He learned that if he prayed, the voices were less distracting; he also found that talking out loud helped (although this behavior drew the stares of onlookers). Additionally, my assessment revealed an insightful, deeply spiritual, and very motivated man. In addition to Leon's diagnosis of schizophrenia, he had insulin-dependent diabetes. Although his knowledge of schizophrenia was extensive, his knowledge about diabetes and how to manage his diet was sketchy. When I did a physical assessment on Leon I found that his weight was 175 lb, his vital signs were within normal limits, and his diet was poor. He relied heavily on refined carbohydrates (junk food) and foods with high fat contents; the first time I visited his apartment he had fried a pound of bacon and was frying the eggs in the bacon grease. His blood sugar self-monitoring was erratic at best; his method of managing his diabetes was to increase his insulin if he knew he would be eating carbohydrate-rich food.

During our initial interview, I discovered that Leon had not only volunteered for the clozapine research project but also enrolled in a work-study program at a community college. He had registered for 16 credit hours of course work and 20 hours of work. This would be a daunting schedule for the most resilient! I shared my observation with Leon that this was a lot to take on and suggested a slower approach. His response will stay with me forever. He said, "Verna you don't understand. I got sick when I was in college. All my friends have moved on—they are married with children, they have careers, they have lives. But look at me, where am I? I am a diagnosed schizophrenic—I have a history of hospital stays—I have been arrested lots of times. I am no further along than I was when I was 18; in fact, I have taken steps backward. This may be my last opportunity to do something with my life." Leon's heartfelt response was not one that could be countered with rational arguments but rather with acceptance. He was sharing the meaning of having schizophrenia with me. I needed to find ways to support his decision. I said to him that we would keep a close eye on his stress level and his response to the medication change and find ways to support him as he took on some major challenges.

OVERVIEW OF BASIC INTERVENTIONS

How often I have heard students say, "Psych nurses just sit and talk." Think about that statement in light of Leon's needs. Leon required all of the following interventions:

1. Relationship building, including ongoing supportive interventions
2. Health status assessment and somatic intervention: *physical* (psychiatric nurses are frequently the first to assess that the patient has an untreated or undiagnosed physical need), including nutrition, blood sugar levels, WBC count, and vital signs; *psychosocial,* including social support systems, caregiver burden, and environmental issues; *psychiatric,* especially psychotic thinking; and *spiritual,* including religion, degree of religious commitment, and sense of meaning and purpose in life
3. Advocacy
4. Teaching
   - Self-care knowledge, including teaching regarding medication (i.e., clozapine); disease management (i.e., diabetes, American Diabetes Association diet); and family issues regarding communication
   - Self-care skills, including teaching Leon how to monitor his blood sugar and stress levels; how to plan, buy, and prepare an appropriate diet; how to control stress through stress management techniques; ways to expand his coping and problem-solving skills and to deal with crises; how to maintain his spiritual well-being; and how to expand his social support system
   - Behavioral modification of maladaptive responses
   - Crisis intervention, which became important as care continued
5. Case management and consultation
6. Discharge planning

Talking was an important intervention, but it was hardly the only intervention.

What do you think? How do these basic interventions reflect standards of practice? As you study psychiatric nursing, how do you see nurses operationalizing these interventions?

➤ *Check Your Reading*
1. What does health status assessment include?

2. What kinds of topics are taught under self-care knowledge?
3. What kinds of skills are taught under self-care skill?

Relationship Building

The foundation of all skilled interventions, regardless of whether the clinical situation is a psychiatric one or not, is the nurse's ability to develop a relationship with the patient based on respect, compassion, empathy, mutuality, and genuineness. The process of relationship building, with its own directions and map, is fully discussed in Chapter 10 and parallels the implementation of the nursing process. A good relationship is by nature a supportive one. **Supportive interventions** include

- Offering encouragement
- Affirming the other
- Ego-building
- Inspiring hope
- Taking the other's perspective
- Being faithful
- Balancing truthfulness with care
- Being able to see the other's potential
- Accepting the other as he or she is while encouraging movement toward his or her potential

The following exchange with Leon provides you with a concrete example of a supportive intervention:

Leon: "Going to school may be my last chance to make something of myself. I need to know that I'm more than a paranoid schizophrenic."

Nurse: "I can see how important this is to you, Leon. As we work together, we can focus on ways to help you succeed. I think there are strategies I can teach you that will help you deal with the stress of school and work. But I also want you to know that in my eyes you *are* more than the disease of schizophrenia. I'm humbled by your honesty, your insight, your willingness to try something new, and your spiritual integrity."

The nurse's response is accepting of Leon's position, hopeful that there are strategies that can help Leon cope, and affirming of Leon's value as an individual—someone who has much to give.

Health Status Assessment and Somatic Intervention

Assessment, both initial and ongoing, of a patient's health status is one of the psychiatric nurse's major interventions. Our ability to engage in disciplined observation based on knowledge and validated with the patient whenever possible is invaluable. This skill allows us to objectify subjective experiences and to intervene appropriately. Health assessment, covered in depth in

Chapter 11, is the building stone for the whole nursing process. Leon required assessment of his

- Psychiatric status, especially evidence of changes in psychotic thinking
- Adherence to medication schedule
- Response to medications
- Coping skills
- Blood sugar levels
- WBC count
- Nutritional status
- Social support
- Stress management skills
- Spiritual needs
- Knowledge level and learning style

In addition to assessment activities, health status assessment can include direct somatic interventions. For instance, in Leon's case, he was insulin dependent. He knew how to administer his insulin, but he did not know how to use a glucometer to check his blood sugar levels. This was a skill that I performed and also taught him to do. Because many psychiatric patients have concurrent medical conditions, the psychiatric nurse must be able to address these needs with appropriate and competent physical interventions. For instance, a psychiatric nurse might be responsible for teaching coping skills, teaching about the effects of an antipsychotic medication, performing catheter care, and administering a vitamin B_{12} injection.

Advocacy

Being an advocate for an individual psychiatric patient or for a group of patients is an important role. Advocacy that is focused on the individual may involve defending or explaining behaviors that seem incomprehensible to others. Advocacy might involve getting an extension on a rent payment because the patient was too psychotic to pay the bill on time. Or advocacy might take the form of negotiating for a resource not otherwise available to the patient. Advocacy that is focused in a broader sense might involve lobbying or letter writing to influence legislation or policies that could adversely impact on health benefits that are available to the mentally ill. Whatever form advocacy takes, it is a way of aiding, standing up for, and embracing the cause of the individual or a group of individuals dealing, in this case, with psychiatric illness.

Advocacy for Leon involved negotiating with the research team to supply Leon with bus tokens so that he could travel to school and to the research center without financial hardship and to provide Leon with a stipend to offset other costs associated with being in school.

Another advocacy intervention undertaken on Leon's behalf involved offering a group educational program at the apartment complex where Leon lived.

The purpose of the program was to foster greater acceptance and support among the residents and, as a result, expand Leon's base of support. The discussion focused on (1) how various disabilities can make an individual seem "different" and less acceptable; (2) how those disabilities do not determine who the person is; (3) the fact that everyone has needs for friendship, acceptance, and people with whom to share their lives; (4) strategies for reaching out to each other; and (5) role playing of these strategies. This intervention focused on advocacy and involved teaching (discussed later) and group work (fully discussed in Chapter 14).

Teaching: Self-Care Knowledge, Self-Care Skill, Behavioral Modification, and Crisis Intervention

Teaching is a critical intervention for the psychiatric nurse and is at the heart of much of what we do, including cognitive therapy (see Chapter 14), behavior modification, and crisis intervention. Ways to empower patients and families and to communicate the deepest respect for them include providing them with knowledge about disease management; medication and medication management; specific skills such as those involved in problem-solving, coping, and responding to emergencies; using available community resources; making environmental changes to improve the milieu of a home; making lifestyle changes that improve health; staying well physically, emotionally, and spiritually; and managing the vagaries of a chronic illness. However, as important as teaching is, we are not born teachers; teaching is a skill that must be practiced and honed with experience. Patient-family education is discussed at length later in this chapter.

Behavioral modification, which is discussed at length later in the chapter, requires a special kind of teaching in which specific problematic behaviors are targeted for change. Although crisis intervention is part of self-care skill instruction, it also has its own theory and as such is discussed later in this chapter. However, it is important to recognize that crises occur to all of us. They are characterized by

- Their unanticipated but dramatic entry into our lives
- Their unique meaning (something that might be a crisis for me might be something you respond to with a shrug of your shoulders and an "Oh well")
- Their drain on our coping abilities and other resources
- Their consuming nature

The nurse's role is to decrease the patient's anxiety, to assist the patient in finding solutions, to facilitate the expansion of the patient's coping repertoire and support system, and to communicate hope. After all, most crises are self-limiting and as Orphan Annie said, "The sun will come out tomorrow," a perspective that has a way of taking the life and death quality away from most crises. In Leon's case, he presented with a crisis several weeks into our relationship.

Leon had failed his first examination—not by a lot: he missed a passing grade by 2 points. However, he reacted as if he had received a 0 on the test. When I arrived at his apartment for our visit, he was pacing, he was yelling at his voices, he had an angry look on his face, and papers were all over the living room. When I asked him what had happened to cause his upset, it took at least 20 minutes for him to calm down enough to tell me about the test. He was convinced he was a failure, the voices were telling him so. There was no hope and nothing that could be done to change his situation, after all, he was, in his words, "a crazy schizophrenic" and he was ready to withdraw from school altogether.

My first response was to listen. My second response was to gently bring in reality to our conversation and his thinking. I asked him to tell the voices to stop bothering him because they were telling him lies that only served to bring him down. I reminded him that it was the first examination he had taken since he was 18 years old, that he missed passing by only 2 points, and that there were still 3 more examinations and other assignments that would determine his final grade. I had to repeat this message several times before he could begin to hear me. I added that I believed I could help him devise a plan to improve this situation and be successful. He was clearly too upset to take any action himself. I told him that I was going to call the school and find out what resources were available to assist students. I made that telephone call and found out that the school provided a myriad of supports including learning assessments to determine the preferred way of learning (auditory, visual, tactile, kinesthetic), note takers, tape recorders to record lectures, tutors, and a test file of old examinations given by every instructor.

I made the first appointment for Leon to go to the Learning Resource Center at school. It took a good bit of encouragement for him to even commit to keeping the appointment. In fact, before I left that day I wrote out a contract that he signed and agreed to follow through. I left him with clear and direct instructions for dealing with any anxiety that threatened to derail him in his thinking and his resolve. The instructions included taking his medication; going for a walk; calling his mother; praying and reading Scripture; singing; and joining the other residents for dinner rather than eating by himself. Leon was able to follow through with the immediate instructions and he was able to use the available resources at school to address his school performance.

Case Management and Consultation

There are different ways to think about case management. One approach is to consider the case manager not only to be the coordinator of all providers and care-related issues but also to be the gatekeeper of the patient's health care benefits. In this role, the case manager frequently acts as a broker or an agent who attempts to get the most benefits for the least amount of money. Ideally, the case manager acts as a good steward of limited resources.

The other approach is to view case management primarily from a clinical perspective, in which the primary provider is actively involved in giving care as well as coordinating care among formal clinical providers and among an informal set of individuals such as family members, teachers, neighbors, and others. This type of case manager might be communicating with providers of community-based resources such as transportation services, food banks, churches, and recreation facilities that impact on the patient's life and recovery. This form of case management does not involve being a financial gatekeeper but rather an excellent provider, communicator, and consultant.

In Leon's case, with his permission, I was in weekly contact with the research physician, sharing my observations regarding Leon's responses to his weaning from fluphenazine, his responses to clozapine, and other issues such as school demands that might impact on Leon's ability to complete the research project. ■

Discharge Planning

Effective discharge planning begins (just as termination does) during the first nurse-patient encounter. As you collect the initial information about the patient and what the patient's current needs are and anticipated needs will be, you are also thinking about what the patient will need to sustain the accomplishments that you hope to achieve within the relationship. For instance, with Leon, I was immediately struck by how limited his social support system was. His main support was his elderly mother who was not in good health. Although he participated in a church and in the church choir, he remained aloof from any involvement with anyone other than his mother, fearing that he would be rejected by others because of his differentness. Within the apartment complex, he had some casual acquaintances but no one on whom he could really count if he needed help. One of my long-term goals was to expand that social support system so that on discharge, Leon would be surrounded by several strong supports on whom he could depend. I also knew that he had not accessed community resources that could improve the quality of his life. For instance, he did not use available transportation services, he did not participate in a food co-op in his apartment complex that sold food at a substantial discount, and he did not participate in social activities sponsored by the apartment complex, even though he was a talented man with a beautiful singing voice and great sense of humor. Assisting him to expand his reach into the community and into the available resources of his living environment became goals to work toward so that at discharge, Leon would be better connected and supported.

We have looked at an overview of basic interventions. Now let's turn our attention to an in-depth examination of patient-family education, behavioral therapy, and crisis intervention.

> **W**hat do you think? Someone makes the following comment, "He's probably a mental patient—I would stay away from him if I were you." How could you respond from a position of advocacy?

> ➤ *Check Your Reading*
> 4. Give an example of a supportive intervention.
> 5. When does discharge planning begin?
> 6. Give two characteristics of crises.
> 7. Describe two approaches to case management.

PATIENT-FAMILY EDUCATION

Because teaching is an important intervention for the psychiatric nurse, let's take a close look at patient and family education, and then we will apply this to Leon. **Patient education** is a process of deliberately creating cognitive, affective, behavioral, and psychomotor changes (Redman, 1993). **Health education** involves the dissemination of information to foster a state of well-being of mind and body so that the individual can strive toward achieving the highest level of functioning. Mutual responsibility and collaboration between patient and caregiver mark this process. **Learning** is a dynamic process that results in the acquisition of new knowledge and behaviors on the part of the learner. **Active learning** involves the investment of time and energy in activities that lead to the acquisition of the desired knowledge and skills. **Passive learning** occurs when the learner absorbs or internalizes information, without active participation, that is conveyed by others.

Learning takes place through formal and informal modes of education. Education involves teaching, defined as "activities that allow the teacher [facilitator] to help students learn" (Redman, 1993, p. 8). Teaching communicates specific knowledge about a given subject in a manner desired to facilitate learning. The multidimensional process of learning is influenced by the social and cultural context of the learning. The individual's past experiences, perception of the current situation, and appraisal of his or her "need to know" interact to create the sense of readiness to learn.

Theoretical Perspectives on Learning

Learning involves a change in the journey, either through the broadening of the knowledge base or through the development of new motor skills. Different theoretical approaches provide insight into the dynamics of learning (Table 13–1).

Principles of Learning

Although learning is an individualized experience, 16 general principles should be considered when planning any educational endeavor. Each principle influences how the learning progresses and how the educational endeavor is organized. These principles of learning are summarized in Box 13–1.

Adult Learning

In addition to the principles of learning (see Box 13–1) that guide educational endeavors, specific attributes of adult learners are also important. Adult learners use reasoning and reflectively critique situations. In addition, because most adult learners have many other responsibilities, time constraints impinge on the learning process.

Adult learners want pragmatic information to solve real-life problems. What is taught must be relevant and applicable to their concerns. Patients must be kept at the center of all learning activities and must perceive the value of spending time in learning new information. Otherwise, they become passive participants in the learning process.

Adult learners have had many experiences from which to draw to enhance the relevance of new skills and information. Providing examples that demonstrate the usefulness of the new information in real-life situations facilitates the learning process. In addition, providing opportunities for practice and feedback enhances the learning process and improves competence related to any new skill or integration of information.

TABLE 13–1 Educational Theories	
THEORIES	**MAJOR CONCEPTS AND FEATURES**
Behavioral	Classical conditioning Operant conditioning Reinforcement
Psychosocial	Unfreezing Moving Refreezing
Cognitive	Meaning and appraisal of event Storing information Retrieving information
Social cognitive	Impact of significant others Modeling behaviors and attitudes Expectations

Box 13-1 ■ ■ ■ ■ ■
Principles of Learning

1. Life experiences contribute to the resources for further learning.
2. Individual beliefs, values, and attitudes affect the perception of the need to learn.
3. Social and cultural context strongly influence perception.
4. The learning process is stimulated by the person's perception of both the problem and the need to learn.
5. Priority given to learning is influenced by perception, beliefs, values, attitudes, and experiences.
6. Motivation to act depends on the person's perceived susceptibility to and severity of the problem.
7. A person will engage in learning activities if that person believes a solution exists.
8. Belief in one's ability to carry out activities toward a solution is influential in motivation to take action.
9. Stages of cognitive development influence the organization of learning processes and activities.
10. Learning progresses from simple to complex.
11. Cognitive, affective, and psychomotor learning activities have different levels.
12. Individuals have a preferred method to access information (visual, auditory, kinesthetic, olfactory, gustatory).
13. Individuals use different strategies to learn (modeling, trial and error, problem-solving).
14. In any single situation, different people will be at different points in the learning process.
15. In different situations, the same person will be at different points in the learning process.
16. Learning involves change, and change can be stressful to a person (ranging from motivational to overwhelming levels).

Adult learners are accountable for their own learning. Your role as an educator is to be a motivator and facilitator for the patient, so that the patient can discover the new insights and skills that accompany learning.

What do you think? In what ways do you see adult learning principles incorporated into your educational endeavors as a learner?

➤ *Check Your Reading*
8. Identify two characteristics of adult learners.
9. Who is accountable in adult learning?

Motivation

Motivation describes the combination of factors that stimulate, drive, direct, and maintain any behavior. Motivation may originate from within the person or from external factors. It is at the root of the learner's willingness to engage in the educational endeavors and to internalize learning. Evidence of motivation at any point is called **readiness** (Redman, 1993).

Early in the learning process, the learner's values, attitudes, beliefs, perceptions, and needs are motivational factors to address. During learning, ongoing stimulation of the learner's interest and emotional (affective) experiences stimulate motivation. Once the learner has developed a sense of competence, motivation becomes more internal. Success breeds more success.

Motivation and readiness to learn are factors that you must consider. Internal motivation lasts longer than external motivation. Reaffirming the learner's internal motivations strengthens the learning process and the interaction between learner and instructor. Incentives also help motivate the learner.

What do you think? How would you evaluate Leon's motivation?

➤ *Check Your Reading*
10. What is readiness?
11. How do readiness and motivation affect learning?

Education About Serious Mental Illness

Serious mental illness is debilitating to both patient and family and disruptive in almost every aspect of their lives. To deal with these life situations and solve problems, all involved need a sound foundation of relevant information. The seriously mentally ill person may be incapable of making relevant decisions or solving problems. This means these responsibilities often fall on a family member, especially with increasing numbers of the mentally ill cared for outside hospital settings (Moller & Murphy, 1997, 1998).

Providing the family and patient with a solid knowledge base within the limits of each patient's capabilities assists in developing reasonable and realistic expectations. This knowledge base becomes important for planning and carrying out the strategies of care for the patient; the knowledge guides the journey. Teaching programs for the psychiatric patient and family are applicable in acute treatment situations and in management of chronic mental illness. Such programs support the treatment and rehabilitative efforts of care.

The Biopsychosocial-Spiritual Model

A number of different models for understanding mental illness are found in the literature. Each model offers a method of examining information and organizing one's thoughts. If the model is restrictive, the approaches that flow from it are limited. If a combination of models is used, the process is expanded.

One model frequently used by nurses for organizing educational endeavors is the biopsychosocial model. This model encompasses biological, psychological, and sociological theories. Adding a spiritual component makes the model more holistic, thus forming the biopsychosocial-spiritual model.

The basic tenet of biological theory is that psychiatric disorders are diseases caused by biological or neurochemical imbalances within the brain. Psychological theory holds that psychiatric illness is due to psychodynamic interactional factors. Sociological theory suggests that behavioral disorders result from social learning experiences. Spiritual component focuses attention on the essential being of the individual, the role of the transcendent in the person's life, and the spiritual qualities and belief systems that the person holds.

The combined biopsychosocial-spiritual model allows you to account for a variety of factors that contribute to the development, manifestation, and outcomes of any one mental disorder. In addition, this model suggests a multifaceted treatment approach.

Variables That Limit Learning

Psychiatric patient education is tailored to the specific needs of patients. A comprehensive, structured, time-limited program helps each participant assimilate the information, regardless of the form of the teaching. The teaching may be formal or informal and may use any approach. Often, the group learning approach is chosen to facilitate patient interactions and support, especially when the education is for family members or groups of both patients and family members.

The characteristics of the person suffering from the mental illness have an impact on the educational endeavor and its content. Symptoms such as hallucinations make it difficult for the person with schizophrenia to deal with educational stimuli. An individual in the manic phase of a bipolar disorder cannot focus on information. Consider each person's illness experience, readiness to learn, temperament, style of learning, and academic ability, especially when providing patient education to someone diagnosed with a mental illness. Generally, education is delayed until the psychotic symptoms are no longer a problem.

Choices in Educational Content

In developing a learning plan for a person with a mental illness or for the family, you need to do a thorough assessment of the patient's learning needs and choose the approach and methods of teaching. A learning plan, with specific lesson plans for each segment, must then be developed. Implementation requires the artful use of nursing, interpersonal, and communication skills. Evaluating the participants' responses to and progress with an educational plan allows you to modify and revise it.

BROAD CONTENT AREAS AND THEMES

When you develop the learning plan for the mentally ill person and, possibly, the family, organize the content around the major concerns expressed. The teaching sessions provide answers to the questions patients and family members most frequently raise: What is wrong? What caused it? Will the patient get better? What treatments are available? What else can be done? Who can or will do it?

You organize relevant content based on these concerns, including different diagnoses; associated symptoms; probable causes; and treatment options, including specifics about medications, prognosis, and problems involved in living with serious mental illness. You spend much time discussing each patient's experiences and how he or she can learn to live effectively. Including certain themes throughout the sessions further enhances the learning experience of both patient and family. These themes include

- Control of illness versus cure
- Balance between rights and responsibilities
- Illness-monitoring techniques

When these themes are woven throughout the sessions, they reinforce the content presented in previous sessions. Appendix I includes a curriculum outline and selected sample teaching resources that can be used to plan a patient-family educational program. Appendix II includes information about spiritual interventions.

DETAILED CONTENT

The organization of content varies greatly among learning programs. You need to develop a care plan to organize an educational endeavor for psychiatric patients. Read Deedra's Journey, then see Figure 13–1.

Deedra's Journey

Deedra first sought help because she was "really sad all of the time," she "couldn't cope," she suffered from "insomnia," and she was having recurring thoughts of "just quitting . . . ending it all." She had many of the classic symptoms of depression. She said she wished that she could control her feelings. She was frightened that she was "really losing her mind and couldn't stop what was happening to her."

Deedra reported that when she was growing up, her mother had been very moody and withdrawn; Deedra felt that she could never really please her mother. Her father worked two jobs and, when he was home, spent most of his time with her brothers. Although things were "strict at home," she reported that she had a "normal" upbringing. She had three brothers, two older and one younger. After leaving

ASSESSMENT

Assessment data are as follows:

- *Readiness: The patient expresses a desire to learn how to control and to deal with her diagnosis of depression*
- *Learning Style: Assimilation — concepts and details*
- *Resources: Post–high school education; likes to learn; successful legal secretary; motivated at this time*
- *Obstacles: Minimal emotional support from spouse; prefers totally quiet environment — needs to learn how to work with others in the area*

DIAGNOSIS

DSM-IV Diagnosis: *Depression*

Nursing Diagnosis: *Knowledge Deficit related to depressive disorder, treatment, and medications*

OUTCOME IDENTIFICATION, PLANNING, AND IMPLEMENTATION

Expected Outcome 1: *By discharge, the patient will understand depression as a disease process and will understand the coping skills necessary to avoid relapse, cope better, and gain a sense of control.*

Short-Term Goal *(See Educational Lesson Plan.)*	Nursing Interventions *(See Educational Lesson Plan.)*	Rationales

EVALUATION

Formative Evaluation: *Deedra enjoys the educational approach. She is a quick learner who scored 100% in a quiz related to depression. Deedra is able to state the reasons for taking her medications and to explain the dosage schedule and side effects.*

Summative Evaluation: *Deedra has achieved greater insight into her responses to stress. She has begun to try new coping skills but continues to need support in the area of relationships. I am recommending that she attend a social support group.*

Figure 13–1
A sample care plan with an educational lesson plan for Deedra.

home, the members of her family of origin seldom communicated, except for holiday greetings.

Deedra was an "above-average student." She said she liked to learn but that it put a lot of pressure on her. She said that if she brought home a grade that was not an "A," she felt she was a disappointment to her parents. She won a scholarship to a local business school, which she attended after graduating from high school.

As Deedra was growing up, she had few friends. She "didn't date much," and after graduation, she lost all contact with her high school acquaintances. Deedra reported that she had had one good friend, but the friend's husband was transferred and they had moved about 6 months before she sought treatment. During the initial interview, Deedra stated that she did not have anyone she considered a "real friend."

EDUCATIONAL LESSON PLAN*

PATIENT: _Deedra_   DATE: _3/5/99_

TOPIC: _Depression_

SHORT-TERM GOAL	CONTENT OUTLINE	METHODS/STRATEGIES	TIME FACTORS
After the 1:1 session, the patient will: 1. Identify behaviors associated with depression	Define depression. List behaviors. Describe the cycle of negative thoughts and feelings.	Didactic	10 minutes
2. Identify one positive feeling	Explore the desired positive feelings. Explore the feelings with the patient. Identify trigger events. Explore potential resources.	Discussion	15 minutes
3. Identify a thought that she can "stop"	Describe negative thought ruminations. Demonstrate the thought-stopping technique.	Discussion Role play	15 minutes 10 minutes
4. List a "replacement" thought that is neutral	Identify replacement thoughts. List alternatives.	Discussion Journal (homework)	5 minutes 15 minutes qod

*This is a partial lesson plan.

Figure 13-1 Continued

At the time she sought treatment, Deedra was 31 years old and had a job as a legal secretary for a prestigious law firm. She looked young for her age; she was underweight and pale, stating that she "did not eat properly," and she suffered from chronic headaches and pains due to work-related wrist problems. She reported that she often felt "so down and out" that she had trouble functioning and had been missing many days from work. For hours, she would sit in the family room, staring out the window.

Like many working women, Deedra felt the pressures of multiple role demands. She had been married at the age of 21 to a man whom she described as "very stern and rigid." Although she and her husband shared a "loving relationship," they "seldom did anything together any more"; she experienced no pleasure from their intimate relations. She knew she was having trouble keeping up with the things she needed to do around home and work, but the more she thought about it, the more guilt-ridden and immobilized she

became. She spent hours thinking about her problems and how she had disappointed her family. She said that she was neither a good wife nor a good mother to her 10-year-old daughter. Deedra said that she just couldn't deal with her daughter, her husband, her work, or her life. She was "so tired of being so tired."

The treatment plan for Deedra included individual psychotherapy with the certified nurse specialist, antidepressant medication, and patient education to start as soon as she was off suicide precautions. Deedra began treatment with her nurse psychotherapist, meeting three times a week. To facilitate her treatment progress, the nurse psychotherapist incorporated education about depression and coping skills into their sessions. To better provide this educational information, the nurse psychotherapist and the staff members collaborated in their treatment efforts, reviewing patient education information and learning theories. ■

A useful resource to help you develop a detailed lesson plan is *Educating Patients and Families About Mental Illness: A Practical Guide* (Bisbee, 1991). Always remember that the specific needs of the participants may require you to present information in small increments over a longer period than you first planned. At other times, the participants may be ready for more information than you initially planned to present. Having each lesson plan fall within specific time constraints helps you accomplish the entire learning plan within the time allotted. Learning to strike a balance between the desired content and the actual flow of the learning session is a skill that develops with experience.

FAMILY EDUCATION

In addition to the content taught to the patient, several other areas need to be addressed when planning teaching sessions for family members of the mentally ill patient. Family members need to review not only the rights and responsibilities of the patient but also the rights and responsibilities of family members in various relationships to the patient. Acknowledging these rights and responsibilities facilitates a partnership in treatment among the patient, the patient's family, and the health care providers.

Another area of focus is the many roles a patient may assume within the family: sick role, disabled role, recovering role, and well role. The role of the family in treatment, illness management, and rehabilitation are other areas for discussion and teaching. Monitoring the progress of treatment requires learning about relapse and its prevention (Daley, Bowler, & Cahalane, 1992). Encourage the family to learn skills to maintain a therapeutic living environment. In most cases, these skills include managing medication, promoting a healthful lifestyle, and coping and stress management techniques for the caregiver.

Another focus of family education is managing behaviors, including establishing concrete plans for how the family members should cope with the behaviors manifested by the patient. In addition, teaching the family to anticipate potential emergencies is useful. Practicing these coping and emergency plans and contingency plans using role playing or drills helps the family learn the skills needed to manage behavioral aspects of the illness.

Often, the family is called on to teach the patient general activities of daily living (ADLs), including personal skills such as hygiene, grooming, and household care; social skills; and vocational skills. Teach the family members their role in facilitating skills development and strategies for skill building.

Nursing Process

Patient education does not mean handing out instruction sheets. Rather, it involves a process similar to the nursing process.

Assessment

To clarify the exact learning needs of the individual, conduct a thorough assessment. *Do not* assume that you know what the patient needs. Always assess.

LEARNING NEEDS

First, identify "what" the patient needs. Use direct conversations, interviews, questionnaires, and observations to gather information.

LEARNING STYLES

Assessing the **learning style** of the patient tells you "how" this patient learns. Among the styles of learning are those identified by Kolb (DeCoux, 1990): convergent, divergent, assimilation, and accommodation.

People who have a convergent learning style like a single solution to a problem. They prefer to learn by reading information, reading handouts, studying diagrams, and watching specific demonstrations.

Those who have a divergent learning style prefer learning situations that involve group discussions, brainstorming, and individual problem-solving activities.

People with an assimilation learning style like to study theories, detailed interactional models, and diagrams as well as diaries or experiential recordings, which can then be used to create a model.

Learners with the accommodation learning style rely heavily on information from other people and enjoy taking part in preplanned experiments or carrying out the steps of a planned activity. Written directions and procedures, lectures with some directed question and answer sessions, and a specific demonstration with return demonstration suit this learner. See under "Implementation," later, for a definition of return demonstration.

LEARNING READINESS

Assessing readiness shows you "when" the best learning moment may occur.

What do you think? What is your learning style? What impact does your learning style have on your ability to glean the most from various educational endeavors? In your experience, what types of teaching best coincide with your learning style?

▶ *Check Your Reading*
12. What is a learning style?
13. What are the four learning styles identified by Kolb?
14. What are the areas that we assess in regard to a potential learner?

Diagnosis

The specific nursing diagnosis provides the basis and direction for the health teaching that follows. According to Arnold (1999), the nursing diagnosis should specify whether the patient's knowledge deficit is related to lack of exposure or experience, cultural values, misinformation, lack of interest or motivation, unfamiliarity with support resources in the community, or lack of confidence in the health care system.

Outcome Identification

The first step in developing an education plan is determining the long-term outcome, or goal, for the educational endeavor. The major goal helps in developing objectives.

An **objective** is a behavioral statement that guides the learning process and establishes the parameters for evaluating the success of the learning. Examples of precise behavioral terms for identifying learning objectives are shown in Box 13-2.

An objective states the expected behaviors of the patient, not the teaching activity. The objective identifies *who* is required to do *what behavior,* in *what situation,* and *when, how often,* or *how much.*

An additional organizing principle in writing any learning objective is specifying the level of behavior. Behaviors can be divided into three large groupings called domains:

1. **Cognitive domain** deals with intellectual abilities.
2. **Affective domain** deals with psychological aspects such as values, attitudes, feelings, interests, and general appreciation.
3. **Psychomotor domain** encompasses motor skills.

An example of the levels of the cognitive domain, based on the classic work of Bloom and Krawnthol (1984), appears in Box 13-3.

Planning

When the patient has several specified needs, the most immediate concerns are prioritized and addressed first. Planning in this situation requires you to select initial approaches and alternatives to teach the information and assist the patient to meet the objectives. Your plan identifies the parameters of implementation and establishes specific learning sessions. These learning sessions must include time for feedback and reinforcement of the patient's newly acquired information and skills. In addition to the planned sessions, a teaching moment sometimes arises during the day. To capitalize on such opportunities and further the learning, all the people who have significant interactions with the patient should know the educational plan. One method of communicating the specifics of an educational endeavor is to use an educational lesson plan form that contains the essential information (see Figure 13-1).

W*hat do you think?* Is it practical to develop a teaching plan for every teaching encounter you have with a patient?

> ► *Check Your Reading*
> 15. What is an objective?
> 16. What is included in an objective?
> 17. How do we arrive at goals for teaching?

Implementation

Before teaching, you need to decide which of the following teaching approaches to use: individual, such as a one-on-one lecture or a self-study program; a small group approach; or large group approach. Your choice depends on the needs of the patient, content to be learned, environment, time constraints, and economic limitations. Next, you select strategies and techniques to implement the educational plan (Box 13-4). No single technique is best in all situations, and incorporating several techniques tends to enhance the learning experience.

One instructional technique is an individual lecture, a didactic explanation. Lectures provide the opportunity to transmit information and explore for understanding. Reinforcing and praising the patient are important. Adding a discussion session following the lecture reinforces the learning process.

Box 13-2 ■ ■ ■ ■ ■
Commonly Used Behavioral Terms for Identifying Learning Objectives

Administer	Construct	Initiate	Recall
Analyze	Contrast	Institute	Recognize
Apply	Demonstrate	Instruct	Record
Assess	Describe	Interpret	Report
Calculate	Design	Label	Select
Categorize	Develop	List	State
Choose	Differentiate	Measure	Synthesize
Classify	Discuss	Order	Tabulate
Compare	Evaluate	Organize	Tally
Compare and contrast	Explain	Perform	Translate
Compile	Formulate	Predict	Volunteer
Conduct	Identify	Prepare	Write

Box 13-3 ■ ■ ■ ■ ■

Taxonomy of Cognitive-Behavioral Domain Summarized

1.00 Knowledge of Recall/Remembering Information

1.10 Knowledge of specifics
1.11 Knowledge of terminology
1.12 Knowledge of specific terms
1.20 Knowledge of ways and means of dealing with specifics
1.21 Knowledge of conventions
1.22 Knowledge of trends and sequences
1.23 Knowledge of classification and categories
1.24 Knowledge of criteria
1.25 Knowledge of methodology
1.30 Knowledge of universals and abstractions
1.31 Knowledge of principles and generalizations
1.32 Knowledge of theories and structures

2.00 Comprehension—Lowest Level of Understanding

2.10 Translation
2.20 Interpretation
2.30 Extrapolation

3.00 Application—Use of Abstractions in Particular and Concrete Situations

4.00 Analysis—Breakdown Into Constituent Elements; the Relative Hierarchy of Ideas or Relationships Are Expressed

4.10 Analysis of elements
4.20 Analysis of relationships
4.30 Analysis of organizational principles

5.00 Synthesis—Putting Together Elements to Produce a Whole

5.10 Synthesis of a unique communication
5.20 Synthesis of a plan or set of operations
5.30 Synthesis/derivation of a set of abstract relations

6.00 Evaluation—Judgment About the Value of Material/Methods for a Given Purpose

6.10 Judgment of internal evidence
6.20 Judgment of external criteria

Adapted from *TAXONOMY OF EDUCATIONAL OBJECTIVES book 1: Cognitive Domain* by Benjamin S. Bloom. Copyright 1956 by Longman Inc. Copyright renewed 1984 by Benjamin S. Bloom and David R. Krathwohl. Reprinted by permission of Addison-Wesley Educational Publishers Inc.

Box 13-4 ■ ■ ■ ■ ■

Teaching Techniques

Individual lecture and explanation
Individual discussion
Demonstration and return demonstration
Self-study programs
Workbooks
Journal writing and review
Group lecture
Discussion groups
Role playing
Games and simulation
Computer-based instruction

A group lecture format can also be used for instruction. When you present information to a group, the following hints may prove helpful:

• Try to anticipate the questions that may be asked.
• Incorporate audiovisual tools such as transparencies or slides.
• Realize that teaching the actual class is likely to take longer than interacting with a single individual.
• Be advised that advanced preparation and practice of the content presentation is recommended.

Similar to group lecture, group discussion techniques are used to allow learners to exchange ideas, opinions, and feelings about content areas.

Another technique is using the question and answer format to stimulate discussion and problem-solving. Independent thought and the learner's abilities to think through situations are reinforced using this technique.

If it is important for the patient to learn a new procedure, **demonstration,** in which the patient is shown a procedure and **return demonstration,** in which the patient performs the procedure as demonstrated, are invaluable learning techniques. The key to the effectiveness of demonstration and return demonstration is that practice is supported without threat of failure. The learner is able to explore ideas, make mistakes, and rectify them in learning the correct procedures.

Independent learners who have good reading skills and enjoy written materials may profit from self-directed learning techniques. Develop a self-study educational piece that focuses on a few succinct learning objectives. Workbooks allow learners to systematically use, review, and apply information. Still another approach, journal writing, provides learners with a chance to express their thoughts and feelings on a variety of topics. Clarify the purpose of keeping a journal, and give directions for keeping a journal. Reviewing the journal entries with the patient is the most important part of journal learning. Through this discussion, the learner gleans the meaning of what he or she has written.

Role playing that is purposeful simulation of a life event allows groups to actually participate in and learn from structured situations. Each participant is assigned a role. Some participants actually role-play, while other participants are observers. The instructor spends a few minutes with each learner to ensure that everyone understands his or her part. Observers are specifically alerted as to what behaviors to notice during the role play. After the role play, always debrief participants and allow them to discuss the exercise and share their perceptions.

Another learning technique is the use of games. Games allow patients to review material and work through a simulated situation. Each game is designed to accomplish a particular objective. Each participant is given rules and information about that objective. When the game is over, participants discuss what they learned from the experience.

Special techniques that use advanced technology can also be used to enhance the learning experience. Computer-based instruction can range from specific learning modules to interactive video presentations that require patients to respond at certain points. The potential applications of technology to learning techniques is endless. The cost of equipment and necessary hardware and software, however, can be restrictive.

Choosing a teaching technique that best suits the learning objectives for the individual participant is of utmost importance in successful educational endeavors. Likewise, you must enter into each teaching situation prepared and committed to facilitate the learning process.

> **W**hat do you think? Which teaching techniques do you find most conducive to your own learning?

> ➤ *Check Your Reading*
> 18. List at least five different teaching strategies.

Evaluation

The last part of the educational process is evaluating whether or not the learning objectives have been met. The most simple evaluation method is to review each objective for the measurement criteria. To check the patient's retention and understanding of information that has been presented, you can construct a test. A well-constructed test measures the patient's progress, diagnoses difficulties, and determines the effectiveness of teaching. Using a pretest and a posttest is a way to test knowledge acquired. The pretest can provide you with information about what the learner already knows, thus allowing for the most efficient use of the instruction time. In some situations, an oral test may be preferable, especially for those individuals who have reading problems or test anxiety that severely compromises their ability to perform on a written test.

Evaluating the learner's performance of procedures using psychomotor skills requires a different form of testing. Usually, simulations and demonstrations of the skill are used to evaluate the learner's ability to perform.

In addition to evaluating the patient's accomplishments, ask each patient for feedback related to content organization, learning environment, and instructor effectiveness, and ask for suggestions for change. This overall evaluation is often accomplished using a participant feedback form with questions that either are open-ended or allow the learner to rate each area from poor to excellent. These evaluations provide data that can be useful in modifying or strengthening educational efforts.

BEHAVIORAL THERAPY

Behavioral therapy is not just a teaching approach. With its basis being the stimulus-response patterns of conditioning and reinforcement, behavioral therapy is also a therapeutic modality. **Behavioral therapy** addresses *observable* behavior; thoughts and emotions are not addressed because they cannot be directly observed. **Cognitive-behavioral therapy** recognizes learning as an internal process that cannot be observed directly because change occurs in a person's ability to respond in a particular situation. According to the cognitive view, the change in behavior that behaviorists call learning is a reflection of internal change. Thus, in contrast to the behaviorists, cognitive-behavioral psychologists studying learning are interested in such intangible factors as knowledge, meaning, intention, feeling, creativity, expectations, and thought, not just observable behavior.

Bandura (1971), a leader in developing social-cognitive theory, suggested that people "know" more than their behavior indicates (see Chapter 6). The social learning theory places special emphasis on the important roles played by vicarious, symbolic, and self-regulatory processes. The major difference between traditional operant models of behavioral therapy and social learning theory is the thesis in the social learning model that the subject is able to perform a response without it actually being reinforced. Reinforcement, however, can affect the level of response rate and its intensity.

Bandura (1986) is responsible for much of what we know about **observational learning,** which takes place when one sees others rewarded or punished for their actions. Observational learning also occurs when an observer simply copies behavior of a model whom he or she admires. When using observational learning as a behavioral strategy, consistent modeling of the desired behaviors along with positive reinforcement is essential.

Bandura postulated that an individual's learning of a new behavior is contingent on four variables: attention, retention, motor reproduction, and incentive. To learn a behavior through **modeling,** the individual's attention first must be directed toward the target behavior of the model. Second, the individual must have the intellectual capacity to retain an image of the modeled behavior. Third, the patient must have the physical capacity to reproduce the behavior. Finally, the individual must see some value in learning the behavior.

Behavioral methodologies are based on three theoretical approaches to learning. These focus on the ways learning occurs. All three approaches can help facilitate the patient's journey.

Learning Through Simple Association

Also known as contiguity, the theory of learning through simple association grew out of the work of Thorndike (1913) who, using cats as his subjects, described the law of effect. Whenever two sensations occur together over and over again, each becomes associated with the other. Later, when only one of these sensations (a stimulus) occurs, the other (a response) is remembered. *Contiguity* is the association of two events in the mind, which occurs because of their repeated pairing. Thorndike defined **stimulus** as an event that activates behavior and **response** as an observable reaction to a stimulus. Much of our learning in school is done through deliberate and repeated pairing of a stimulus and a correct response. This principle of contiguity is the one on which all other behavioral approaches are based.

Classical Behavioral Conditioning

Classical conditioning is credited to Pavlov, a Russian scientist in the 1920s (see Chapter 6), who used cues to stimulate desired behavioral change. Using dogs as his subjects, Pavlov demonstrated that they could learn to respond automatically to a stimulus that once had no effect on them. He noted that whenever the dogs were given food, they salivated. He then started playing a tuning fork along with the presentation of the food. After he paired the tone with the food repeatedly and then only played the tone, the dogs salivated without the presentation of the food.

One needs only to look at personal experiences to recall situations in which desirable results came from conditioning. If you have been successful in school, you are likely to anticipate new learning experiences eagerly. You might also remember undesirable results from conditioning.

Pavlov used a process called *cueing*, in which a stimulus "sets up" a desired behavior. During the conditioning process, generalization, or responding to similar stimuli in the same way, also takes place. Finally, the individual demonstrates discrimination, or the ability to respond differently to similar stimuli, after behavioral treatment.

Discrimination occurs, in part, because of another process, **extinction**, a gradual disappearance of a learned response. If a conditioned stimulus is presented repeatedly but is not followed by the unconditioned stimulus (e.g., Pavlov's tone is presented but no food is given), the conditioned response (e.g., salivating after the tone) finally goes away, or extinguishes. Another technique for stopping an undesirable behavior is through the use of *satiation*, repeating a problem behavior beyond the point of interest or motivation. For example, one of the most successful programs to help smokers quit involves satiation at the beginning of the program. Smokers are directed to smoke to the point that they become physically ill or repulsed, and later, when they crave cigarettes, they are reminded of the feelings they experienced during the period of satiation. Box 13–5 provides general guidelines for using classical conditioning strategies.

Operant Conditioning

Operant conditioning was introduced as a treatment modality for people in the late 1960s but was viewed with considerable distaste by those in the mental health fields, who deemed it mechanistic and inhumane. Skinner (1953) is generally credited with developing operant conditioning (built on the principles of classical conditioning) as it is currently used in education and treatment. The term *operant* refers to any voluntary behavior. Skinner's work, originally using pigeons, demonstrated that many behaviors are not simple responses to stimuli but represent deliberate actions, or operants. According to Skinner, these operants are affected by

---

B o x 1 3 – 5 ■ ■ ■ ■ ■

Guidelines for the Use of Classical Conditioning Techniques in Psychiatric Settings

- Associate positive, pleasant events with desired behaviors.
- Create a comfortable, nonthreatening environment.
- Avoid competitive and other undesirable situations.
- Choose situations in which limited negative effects will occur.
- Encourage the patient to volunteer to go into the situation.
- If fears are too strong for immediate participation, devise small steps toward the goal (use shaping).
- Help the patient recognize differences and similarities among situations.
- Demonstrate how to discriminate, to respond differently to similar stimuli.
- When appropriate, teach how to generalize, to respond to similar stimuli in the same way.
- Tell the patient that no positive reinforcement will be given unless the desired behavior occurs and that aversive stimuli will occur following undesired behavior (e.g., tell the patient that pushing the button on the patient-controlled-analgesia apparatus will stop pain—providing positive *and negative* reinforcement—and that forgetting to press it will allow pain to recur [aversive stimulus]).

what happens after them, that is, whether or not they are rewarded (reinforced):

Antecedent ⇒ Behavior ⇒ Consequences or A ⇒ B ⇒ C

Operant conditioning largely focuses on controlling behavior by controlling consequences. Three types of operant conditioning are relevant: reinforcement, punishment, and extinction.

Reinforcement

Reinforcement is any behavioral consequence that strengthens behavior. The strengthening can occur as a reward—**positive reinforcement.** In everyday life, positive reinforcement is used to modify people's behavior in a number of ways. For example, some freeways now have special lanes for high-occupancy vehicles, reinforcing (strengthening) the behavior of car-pooling. Drivers who wish to travel to work faster can engage other people in car-pooling and therefore take advantage of the special lane to enjoy the consequence of arriving at work more quickly. The bonuses and merit raises that employees earn for high productivity and the high grades earned by students for superior work are other examples of positive reinforcement.

Another form of reinforcement is **negative reinforcement,** a consequence that strengthens desired behavior by removing an aversive stimulus. Negative reinforcement is an important behavioral strategy that is effective in removing habitual reinforcers for an undesired behavior. If you have been reinforced negatively—that is, avoided the aversive stimulus—you are likely to repeat a desired action when again faced with a similar situation. Negative reinforcement is an important component of behavioral choice in everyday situations. For example, if you have a toothache, any response—for example, taking aspirin—that alleviates the pain (negative reinforcer) is more likely to recur when a toothache recurs. Thus, you "escape" from the unpleasant situation.

Punishment

Unfortunately, the line between negative reinforcement, which strengthens desired behavior, and punishment is sometimes crossed, and one danger in using behavioral strategies is that this distinction is not made. **Punishment,** which reinforces behavior in a disapproving and nonconfirming manner, actually weakens the potential for desired behavior change. For example, it is common in the grocery store to observe a parent criticizing a child for whining or running around. Usually, the child does not respond well to this intervention. The behavior continues because what the child really wants is to leave the store. The child's behavior is being reinforced, but the desired outcome (from the parent's perspective) frequently is not achieved. We seldom hear a parent say to a child, "Gee, you were really good in the store today. You sat quietly in the cart and were very pleasant!"

Using positive reinforcement rather than punishment not only is preventive but also helps to improve the self-image of the other person. Although primary reinforcement strategies eliminate punishment or aversive stimuli because they are not of value for most patients, punishment and aversive stimuli are useful in eliminating certain types of symptoms, as is described later in the chapter.

A special type of aversive reinforcement is the use of "time outs," which essentially remove the patient from the environment and from participation in earning points or tokens for behavior. If time outs must be applied, it is useful to give the patient opportunities to have appropriate behaviors strengthened with other forms of reinforcement.

Extinction

Extinction is a behavioral strategy to decrease the frequency of an undesirable behavior by *ignoring* it. However, when a targeted behavior is first ignored, it may actually increase in frequency as the patient attempts to obtain the previous reinforcement. Additionally, behavior that has been reinforced irregularly and behaviors in which the difference between the external reinforcer of behavior and the absence of that reinforcer is minimal are harder to extinguish. Also, if few alternatives to the target behavior are available, it is more likely to be resistant to extinction procedures. If the behavior is continuously ignored, it decreases over time and eventually is eliminated.

Box 13-6 lists guidelines related to operant conditioning.

What do you think? In what ways is your behavior impacted by operant conditioning? Classical conditioning?

► *Check Your Reading*
19. What role does behavioral learning play in everyday life?

Box 13-6 ■ ■ ■ ■ ■
Guidelines for Operant Conditioning Strategies

- Make sure that only positive behavior is reinforced.
- Make sure reinforcement is truly reinforcing (Premack's principle).
- Give sufficient reinforcement for attempts at tackling new material or trying new skills.
- Use teaching, demonstrating, or modeling to help establish new behaviors.
- When necessary, use shaping to establish a new behavior.
- Gradually decrease reinforcement on an unpredictable schedule to encourage persistence after new behaviors are established.

Principles of Application

There are a number of steps in the application of behavioral principles.

Assessment

The assessment process consists of several substeps.

GENERAL ASSESSMENT

The first step involves gathering general information about the behavioral problem, called the general assessment (see Chapter 11). When considering behavioral techniques, you need to collect assessment information from

- *Patient self-report.* The patient may state, "I become so anxious at a party that I stammer, blush, and sweat." From the patient's perspective, knowledge is power. An accurate assessment of specific behaviors gathered with the patient's cooperation makes him or her responsible for the behavioral change and serves as the foundation for recording progress toward desired behaviors that make sense and are easily understood.
- *Administration of appropriate tests.* Examples include the Subjective Units of Distress Ratings (SUDS), the Beck Depression Scale, and others that are mentioned throughout this book.
- *Ratings of others.* Consider soliciting information from family, friends, and other professionals.
- *Direct observation of patient behaviors.* Note explicit descriptions of a behavior and the number of times it is observed during a 24-hour period. This is particularly useful when patients are either cognitively or emotionally unable or unwilling to identify target behaviors. Patients should be carefully observed around the clock for at least 2 weeks, if possible, to see (1) what they do that they should not do; (2) what they *prefer* doing (potential positive reinforcers); (3) what they do not do that they should do; and (4) what they do not like (potential aversive stimuli and basis for reinforcement). Videotapes are useful direct observation tools.

Detailed interviews and observations provide information about environmental factors that may be subtly reinforcing undesirable behavior. For example, the father of an adolescent with an eating disorder carefully watched what his daughter ate and was concerned and tender with his daughter around this issue, but he spent little time with her otherwise. The implicit message his daughter received was that her eating disorder got her the attention she so badly needed and that this attention was unavailable without her behavioral symptoms. Neither the father nor the daughter was consciously aware of how her father's behavior actually reinforced her symptoms.

DEFINING PROBLEM BEHAVIOR

The second step involves defining the problem behavior. You can think of behavior as being sandwiched between two sets of environmental influences: those that precede it (its antecedents) and those that follow it (its consequences).

TARGETING BEHAVIORS

The third step considers only behavioral activities that interfere with the patient's functioning and are amenable to change. Behavioral therapies are not concerned with insight or motivation. Problem behaviors are identified as discrete actions and are counted precisely over an identified period. These data are then recorded as numbers or are graphed to form the baseline, which is particularly useful when the behavioral changes are small and might go unnoticed without such precision. It is also important to record behaviors occurring spontaneously in the environment that appear to evoke or maintain the behavior. Many patients, including children, like to self-monitor their behavior and work with their charts.

Box 13–7 presents the steps involved in identifying target behaviors.

Target behaviors must be described in specific, clear, observable, and measurable terms as behavioral units. Let's revisit Leon for a moment. He struggled with the requirements of being a student; he failed his first examination. A behavioral description such as "Leon lacks effective study skills" provides little information to either nurse or patient about the exact nature of the patient's undesirable behavior. It would be almost impossible to measure progression toward goal achievement with such baseline data. Instead, a behavioral problem statement such as "When Leon returns from school, he immediately puts the television on and the radio; he reviews his notes in blocks of 3 to 5 minutes with the television and radio blaring in the background" describes Leon's behavior in specific terms that can be measured easily. Such a statement allowed the tutor at the school's learning resource center to know immediately what behavior to target with Leon.

Lazarus (1976) described a patient-therapist dialogue related to targeting a patient's headache behaviors, as shown in Case Example 13-1.

Box 13–7 ■ ■ ■ ■ ■
Guidelines for Targeting Behaviors

- Distinguish between behavioral and nonbehavioral causes of the problem. Is the behavior contributing to the problem, or is the problem due to some factor outside the client's control?
- List behaviors the client must exhibit to follow the recommendations.
- Rank each behavior listed in order of importance (e.g., smearing of feces is more important to address than negative social behaviors).
- Rank each behavior according to the extent to which it is changeable (e.g., lack of language is changeable but only to the extent of the patient's capability to learn).

■ CASE EXAMPLE 13–1
■ Jim's Story

As you read the exchange between the therapist and Jim, note several tasks accomplished by the therapist in order to target the behavior in need of change. First, he engages Jim's interest and actively involves him in the process of looking at his behavior in an analytical manner. He proceeds sequentially to establish baseline data by asking Jim to note what is occurring just before the behavior (antecedent conditions), to record the frequency of the behavior, and to specify its severity. The therapist also engages Jim in observing the consequences, both positive and negative, of the baseline targeted behavior. In one encapsulated conversation, the therapist covers all the essential elements necessary for targeting a behavior in need of change and developing the basis for intervention.

Therapist: "Does anything in particular bring on these headaches? For instance, do you notice them more at certain times or in certain places?"

Jim: (Pause) "I can't say I do. No, not really."

Therapist: "Well, will you keep tabs on these headaches? What I want you to do is to make a note each and every time you have a headache. Will you record the time of day, where you are, and more or less what you were doing just before the headache came on? Jot down exactly what you were doing, feeling, and thinking. I'd like you to do this very thoroughly. Will you do it?"

Jim: "Sure. You want to see if there is some pattern?"

Therapist: "Right. Also, let's get a baseline. Let's see exactly how many times you have a headache over a period of 2 weeks. Could you also make a notation as to the severity of each attack?"

Jim: "Like 'mild,' 'moderate,' or 'severe?'"

Therapist: "Right. And would you keep track of how many aspirins you take? By the way, can you tell me what the consequences are when you do have a headache?"

Jim: "How do you mean?"

Therapist: "I mean, does it spoil your fun? For instance, do you cancel appointments or not go out?"

Jim: "Well, my wife was mad at me only last night because we had tickets for a show and my head was splitting and I opted out."

Therapist: "Do you like shows? Especially the one you missed last night. Were you honestly looking forward to it?"

Jim: (Laughs) "Well, I'll have to put it to you this way. If it had been a poker game, I just might have made it." ■

Developing Nursing Diagnoses

In describing a nursing diagnosis amenable to behavioral intervention, you need to specify the precise behaviors to be changed. For example, a patient with mental retardation may present with a nursing diagnosis of Ineffective Individual Coping, but the precise behaviors associated with the diagnosis may be quite different. Nursing diagnoses might be

- Ineffective Individual Coping related to mental retardation, as evidenced by episodic verbal outbursts,

physical aggression toward peers when stressed, and property destruction
- Ineffective Individual Coping related to mental retardation, as evidenced by inability to dress self, use toilet, or practice personal hygiene

Goal-Setting and Outcome Identification

The treatment outcomes (goals) focus on the problem presented in the nursing diagnosis; the particular objectives to achieve those outcomes focus on the symptoms (evidence). The behavioral goals for the first diagnosis would center on helping this patient assume better control of his or her anger and its associated behavior. Interventions would concentrate not only on providing positive reinforcements or rewards for behavior control but also on manipulating the environment so that trigger events (antecedents) would occur less often. Negative reinforcement might be necessary in the form of time outs. With the second nursing diagnosis, the goals would shift to consideration of the tasks needed for ADLs associated with personal hygiene. Then the behavioral nursing interventions and reinforcement would concentrate on assisting the patient to take individual responsibility for his or her personal needs.

> **W**hat do you think? Given what you have read about behavioral interventions, what does the following statement mean to you: "The only person's behavior that you can change or control is your own"?

➤ *Check Your Reading*
20. Why is it important to precisely define target behaviors?
21. What sources of data might you use in targeting behaviors, and how would you decide which was the most appropriate?

Choosing Reinforcement: Planning

The planning phase of behavioral management focuses on identifying behavioral reinforcers that have meaning to the patient, communicating with other health team members about the elements of the treatment plan to ensure continuity, and developing an appropriate reinforcement schedule.

IDENTIFYING BEHAVIORAL REINFORCERS
One of the most rewarding and challenging techniques you will develop is to be able to anticipate what a patient will do in a given situation and to introduce an alternative activity that will be just as satisfying (if not more satisfying) to the patient in time to prevent the inappropriate behavior. For example, I suggested to Leon that he use television viewing and radio listening as rewards for studying. This allowed him to study more effectively and to enjoy watching television more because he felt that he had earned it.

TYPES OF REINFORCERS

Reinforcers can be tangible items or social activities. Tangible reinforcers take the form of tokens to be exchanged for actual goods (such as candy), privileges, or opportunities when the patient does a desired activity. Social reinforcers, such as praise, approval, and affection, are equally effective for many patients. Leon literally glowed when he received praise. With social reinforcement, it is essential to provide feedback about the behavior or the mastery of a task rather than praising the patient as "being good." Behavioral principles associated with social reinforcement are presented in Box 13–8.

PREMACK'S PRINCIPLE

In some situations, a more preferred activity can serve as a reinforcer for a less preferred activity. This phenomenon was first described in 1965 by David Premack, who asserted that a high-frequency behavior (preferred activity) can be especially effective as a reinforcer for a low-frequency behavior (a less preferred activity). The Premack principle is sometimes referred to as "Grandma's rule": First do what I want you to do; then you may do what you want to do. For example, patients can earn tokens for appropriate behavior (low-frequency behavior), which entitle them to purchase time, objects or treats, or special privileges (high-frequency behavior). Telling Leon that he could watch as much television as he wanted but that he had to study first is an example of using the Premack principle.

IDENTIFYING AND CONTROLLING ANTECEDENTS

Antecedents are those behaviors or circumstances that contribute to the problem or make it more likely to occur. *Environmental manipulation* is a simple intervention often used to change inappropriate behavior. A child who is easily distracted can be helped to concentrate by being placed in a quiet corner with a partial screen. "Baby-proofing" a house prevents accidents. It is possible to use distraction to reduce stimuli for a patient who is threatening property destruction or harm to others before the behavior actually occurs.

By observing a patient closely, you can modify the environment to support his or her functional well-being.

Box 13–8 ■ ■ ■ ■ ■
Basic Principles of Social Reinforcement

- Be sure the patient understands and is able to do the target behavior (consider the patient's limitations).
- Be clear and systematic when giving praise following each occurrence of the target behavior.
- Reward specific, genuine achievement.
- Give recognition to the patient's effort and ability, which will raise self-confidence.
- Do not give undeserved praise.

TABLE 13–2 Types of Reinforcement

SCHEDULE	DEFINITION
Continuous	Reinforcement given after each behavioral response
Intermittent	Reinforcement given randomly after some, but not all, behavioral responses
Variable ratio	Reinforcement given after a certain percentage of responses
Variable interval	Reinforcement given after a certain time interval of response

For example, the colors in a room and the arrangement of the furniture contribute toward the comfort of those sitting there, thus modifying their behavior. Environmental manipulation is a preventive technique that psychologically healthy people use often, and it can be taught to others. Engaging patients in painting a room, rearranging the furniture, or even thinking about such activities can encourage them to use their creative abilities, become more self-reliant, and raise their levels of self-esteem.

In the clinical setting, the environment can be manipulated to support patients in regaining control over their behaviors. Seclusion or time outs may be effective when a patient's behavior threatens appropriate functioning on the unit.

DETERMINING SCHEDULES OF REINFORCEMENT

Too much positive reinforcement tends to *stop* desired behaviors. A **reinforcement schedule** determines the frequency with which reinforcement occurs. Although continuous reinforcement is an advantage initially, the patient needs to develop internal motivation and performance satisfaction that cannot occur if the reinforcement remains solely external. Reinforcement schedules are described as continuous, intermittent, and variable ratio or variable interval, as summarized in Table 13–2.

The critical principle in determining schedules of reinforcement is that the reinforcements must be applied in a systematic manner and that the reinforcers must be clearly linked to behavior performance. An intermittent schedule of reinforcement tends to have the strongest and longest-lasting effect on behavior because of the anticipation of a reward, even when it is not immediately forthcoming. Once a desired behavior is established and a reward is expected, the reinforcement should be withdrawn using a variable ratio schedule or a variable interval schedule. Desired behavioral responses are reinforced frequently but not with each occurrence. Ultimately, the desired behavior should occur consistently because the person never knows when reinforcement might occur.

Two methods are used in applying reinforcement on a variable basis. The first, a **variable ratio schedule,** involves systematically reinforcing a behavior based on a varying number of responses. Usually, the response ratio is known to the nurse but not to the patient and is lengthened gradually—for example, every three times, then every five. The other method, a **variable interval schedule,** is similar but is based on time rather than response ratio. It refers to the reinforcement of behavior based on selected, varying intervals. Using a variable ratio schedule, the therapist may decide to give positive reinforcement after every 5th, then 10th, then 7th, then 12th desired response. The patient who cannot predict the time of reward for desirable behavior is more likely to continue at a high level. Using a variable interval schedule, the therapist reinforces the desirable behavior at unpredictable (to the patient) intervals.

BEHAVIORAL CONTRACTING

Contracting was first introduced in Chapter 10 as the transition point into the working phase of the nurse-patient relationship. In behavioral therapy, the contract represents a negotiated agreement between the nurse and patient. In this contract, the reinforcement contingencies for demonstrating appropriate behavior are clearly identified in advance.

Patient expectations should be stated objectively, specifically, and clearly in positive terms, with the level of behavior expected—for example, "Jane will brush her teeth after every meal." If the behavioral expectation simply reads, "Jane will brush her teeth," then she could brush them once a day and receive the reinforcement. Some behavioral contracts also include a bonus system for sustained excellent performance. Figure 13–2 shows a sample behavioral contract.

> *What do you think?* Is behavioral therapy more or less "humane" than the traditional "talking" therapies?

➤ *Check Your Reading*
22. What is the Premack principle? How would you apply it?

Treatment Applications: Implementation

The basic tools used in the implementation phase vary in direct application, but they all require learning principles involved with shaping, modeling, fading, flooding, reinforcing, and cueing. Distraction and substitute gratification help to shape behavior of lower-functioning patients.

SHAPING AND MODELING

Shaping is a technique used by the therapist to reward behaviors that are approximations of the desired behavior. The therapist initially models or demonstrates the desired behavior. Then the therapist gradually increases expectations as the patient masters smaller approximations toward the goal until the goal is met. The reinforcers are used to encourage behavioral responses in the desired direction.

Shaping is particularly effective when the patient needs to learn a complex behavior that is either difficult or new to his or her behavioral repertoire. Shaping allows the nurse the flexibility of breaking down the

---

This is a contract between *Jack McLaughlin* and *Jennifer Jones, RN* , which begins on *January 19, 2000* and terminates on *discharge from Unit 3B* and consists of the following terms:

Jack McLaughlin will (1) attend all scheduled activities on the unit; (2) approach the nurse and ask for help when feeling out of control; (3) not display any physical or verbal aggression toward others on the unit.

If *Jack McLaughlin* fulfills his contract from Monday through Friday each week, he will be granted a weekend pass. However, if he fails to complete the contract, this privilege will be withheld.

Date *January 18, 2000*

Patient's signature *Jack McLaughlin*

Nurse's signature *Jennifer Jones, RN*

Figure 13–2
A sample behavioral contract.

Box 13-9 ■ ■ ■ ■ ■
Guidelines for Implementing Shaping Procedures

- Break the target behavior down into a series of smaller increments.
- Reinforce each of these smaller behaviors as they occur.
- Gradually link two or more desired steps together before reinforcement.
- Gradually require *all* of the smaller behaviors to occur so that the target behavior occurs before reinforcement.
- Gradually require longer periods of attending to the task before reinforcement.

terminal outcome into smaller segments without losing the overall intent. As the patient masters each step, another is added to the protocol, and the patient must perform the additional step to earn the reward. Guidelines for shaping behaviors are presented in Box 13–9.

CHAINING AND FADING

Chaining is a behavioral technique that involves unifying or "chaining" together individual behaviors in a progressively more complex skill or task expectation. For example, the seriously mentally ill patient may have significant difficulty eating in a socially acceptable manner, but with chaining, each subset of behavior can be taught and reinforced sequentially. Logical sequencing and immediate reinforcement aid the internal processing required to learn the behavior.

Fading is gradually phasing out stimulus prompts related to achievement of a desired behavior as the patient is able to accomplish it without the prompts. For example, once the patient spontaneously puts clothes away without prompting, discontinue the reminders.

FLOODING AND RESPONSE PREVENTION

Flooding, gradually increasing exposure to anxiety-provoking situations within the context of a therapeutic relationship, and response prevention are used to treat obsessive-compulsive disorder (OCD) (e.g., compulsive hand-washing and neck-posturing). Repeated incremental exposure to anxiety involves actual contact with the feared stressor. Instead of facing it alone and without reflection, however, the patient is encouraged to talk about his or her fears, face them with support, and, through exposure with no untoward consequences, reduce their power and thus reduce their symptoms.

CUEING

Cues are prompts that set up the desired behavior. For example, as a cue, the nurse may set a timer or rise from sitting, simultaneously reminding the patient that their time together is almost over. Alternatively, as a cue, the nurse may say, "Our time together is almost over." Such

techniques not only help the patient prepare for the transition but also prevent negative reactions.

Cueing can be taught to patients and can be generalized to other situations. For example, patients can be instructed to recognize events that trigger panic attacks and to employ deep breathing or thought replacement to counter their effects. Cues such as alarms or visual reminders help prompt appropriate responses in dementia victims. Thus, the nurse, by holding the patient's hand along the journey, can teach the patient to provide his or her own cues and prompts, thereby controlling some of his or her emotional responses. Teaching the patient to use mental images, listen to music, or self-talk (e.g., "I am not afraid," "I can breathe deeply") may prove effective.

DISTRACTION

Distraction is a behavioral strategy whereby you can prevent or change inappropriate behavior by simply distracting the patient's attention. Mentally healthy individuals often use distraction deliberately as a way of restoring emotional balance. For example, a person might think, "I feel really down in the dumps today. I think I'll go for a walk [read, garden, call a friend]." Using distraction can significantly change a person's mood. Again, the therapist can teach coping skills. The emotionally deprived patient has a limited coping repertoire.

SUBSTITUTE GRATIFICATION

Emotionally deprived patients are unable to see that they have alternatives. The grossly obese person who eats to alleviate feelings of emptiness is one example. The need for oral gratification is strong and goes back to infancy. One often hears obese people say, "Eating is my only joy." Such a situation illustrates the classic vicious circle in which the more one eats the more one feels negative about oneself. Many other scenarios cause similar feelings and processes. Similar substitute gratification can be used as a deliberate strategy to positively affect behavior.

What do you think? How has your behavior been shaped? What cues do you respond to? How do you use distraction?

► Check Your Reading

23. What are three basic tools of behavioral therapy?
24. Which basic tool of behaviorism might be most appropriate for patients with lower levels of functioning?

Treatment Applications Based on Behavioral Approaches

TOKEN ECONOMY

Token economies grew in popularity in the 1960s and 1970s, especially in treating children and adolescents with behavior problems, and tokens are still used in many inpatient settings for children and adults. With a total milieu approach, the patient earns tokens for demonstrating designated behaviors. The use of a token system is based on the principle of generalized reinforcers. The token serves as a primary reinforcer with more than one secondary reinforcer available for patient selection. Having more than one reinforcer as backups allows much flexibility in using the Premack principle to change reinforcers in line with the patient's desires and encourages personal decision-making.

Tokens also lessen the danger of *reinforcer satiation,* which occurs when a primary reinforcer no longer has meaning for a patient. For example, a patient may tire of a certain candy or not want to go out for recess during the winter months. Moreover, tokens can be assigned different values. As behavior improves, more complex behaviors can be required to earn a token, or the value of an individual token can be reduced. The use of a token system also has the advantage of directly teaching the patient the value of delayed gratification because the token is given at the time of behavior performance, but the exchange of the token for a tangible item or privilege generally occurs later. Box 13–10 outlines the steps in implementing a token economy.

SOCIAL SKILLS TRAINING

Social skills training is a learning process in which people learn functional ways of interacting. When discussing social skills training, first ask, "What distinguishes people who are socially skillful (competent) from those who are not?" The socially competent person demonstrates abilities in

- Obtaining and maintaining the attention of others
- Using others as resources in socially acceptable ways

Box 13–10 ■ ■ ■ ■ ■
Steps in Implementing a Token Economy

1. Decide on the token, and the value of each token. Specify the behaviors that will earn tokens and their token value (a written list is helpful).
2. Decide on the backup reinforcers. Backup reinforcers are most effective when they reflect use of the Premack principle in their selection.
3. Determine the cash value for each backup reinforcer, with the most highly valued by the patient assigned the greatest cash value.
4. Establish exchange times.
5. Explain the token system to the patient and allow for questions.
6. Carefully monitor the relevance of the system, the patient's response, and the possible complications such as other patients stealing tokens. These factors, plus the consistent application across patients, are sometimes overlooked, but they are important to the success of the technique.

- Expressing both affection and hostility toward others
- Leading and following peers
- Competing with others
- Expressing pride in something he or she has done or is doing or in something he or she possesses
- Communicating
- Thinking (i.e., senses dissonance or discrepancies in the environment; anticipates consequences of his or her actions or plans; deals with abstractions, such as numbers, letters, and rules; takes another person's perspective; and makes interesting associations between something he or she sees or hears and something from his or her experience, whether real or imaginary)
- Planning and executing activities requiring several steps by using resources effectively
- Attending to two things at once (e.g., concentrates on the task at hand yet is aware of what is going on around him or her)

The person who is socially incompetent because of mental illness, retardation, or poor role modeling lacks most of these characteristics and is unable to function smoothly in society because of feelings of low self-esteem, isolation, and anger. Such people often resort to violent behavior as a way to express feelings. Violence prevention programs include social skills and anger management training. Many schools have anger management and conflict resolution training for staff members, students, and parents. Typical problems addressed in a behavioral context can include disruptiveness, poor self-management, social withdrawal, emotional control, and low achievement.

One model for social skills training is a cognitive-problem-solving approach in which interpersonal and problem-solving skills are taught. The goal is to look at alternative solutions, means-ends situations, consequential-causal thinking, and sensitivity to interpersonal problems. The person learns to ask, "What is my problem?" "What am I supposed to do?" "What is my plan?" and "How do I do it?"

Another model for social skills training uses a combination of behavioral techniques, verbal cues, self-talk, and family inclusion in environmental manipulations for patients who have difficulty in social settings (Uomoto & Brockway, 1992). Modeling, role playing, rehearsal, and positive reinforcement, used alone or in combination with pharmacotherapy, have been found to be effective in increasing positive social behavior and in reducing displays of depressive affect.

Behavior management through social skills training is used as both a primary and a secondary prevention strategy. A study reported by Vanderhorst and Carson (1998) detailed the outcomes of psychiatric home care delivered to children and adolescents. In this study, the parents were taught behavioral management and communication skills (e.g., listen and communicate, praise and support acceptable behavior, set appropriate limits, encourage mutual respect, interact consistently, and respond effectively when limits are exceeded).

AVERSIVE BEHAVIORAL REINFORCERS IN TREATMENT

Punishment is anything that weakens or suppresses behavior. Today, aversive procedures are widely used to treat such behaviors as alcoholism, sexual deviation, shoplifting, hallucinations, violent and aggressive behavior, and self-mutilation. Punishment is sometimes the treatment of choice when other, less drastic measures have failed to produce the desired effects. Three paradigms for using aversive techniques are

1. Pairing of a maladaptive behavior with a noxious stimulus (e.g., pair the sight and smell of alcohol with electric shock), so that anxiety or fear becomes associated with the once-pleasurable stimulus
2. Punishment (e.g., applied after the patient has had an alcoholic drink)
3. Avoidance training (e.g., the patient avoids punishment by pushing a glass of alcohol away within a certain time)

Some other examples of aversive procedures are electric shock; nauseating and vomitory chemicals; noxious odors; verbal aversion, such as descriptions of disturbing scenes; costs or fines (in a token economy), and denial of positive reinforcement (isolation).

Before initiating any aversive protocol, the therapist, treatment team, and society *must* answer the following questions: "Is this in the best interest of the patient?" "Does its use violate the patient's rights?" and "Is it in the best interests of society?" Ongoing supervision, support, and evaluation of those administering the aversive therapy *must* occur.

For example, a bitter-tasting substance on the fingers of nail-biters, a mild aversive treatment, has been found effective (Silber & Haynes, 1992). Behaviors such as thumb-sucking, hair-pulling, and nose-picking have responded to mild aversive therapy, which was found most effective when the cooperation of the patients played an integral part in the treatment program.

> **W**hat do you think? What are the risks of using aversive therapy or punishment?

► *Check Your Reading*

25. How does a token economy work?
26. List five criteria that you might use to distinguish between a socially competent and a socially incompetent person.
27. How has cognitive theory been integrated with behaviorism?
28. In what situations are aversive reinforcers likely to be used?

Behavioral Strategies in Self-Management

Self-Management

Those in the health care fields are increasingly aware that to increase the possibility of success they need to help patients move toward greater **self-management.** Thus, although behavioral therapy is still often used in its simple forms, many current protocols use complicated, multifaceted models, such as one distributed by The Midwest Center for Stress and Anxiety (see Additional Resources), that include any combination of the following: audiotapes, coaching videotapes, workbook, homework assignments, healthy self-talk strategies, phone support services, and pharmacological interventions (Bassett, 1997).

Biofeedback

Biofeedback and related techniques help patients learn to control hypertension, headaches, dysmenorrhea, and chronic orofacial pain. At the Management of Stress Response Clinic at the University of Washington, for example, patients are taught to take their own blood pressure, and they participate in 14 biofeedback sessions (3 electromyography, 3 autonomic nervous system, and 7 pulse wave velocity sessions). Throughout each session, blood pressure is monitored. Quieting responses and muscle relaxation are taught, along with coping and cognitive skills. Lifestyle factors such as diet and exercise are monitored. Finally, patients are instructed to follow the same protocol when they are discharged, and they are followed for 6 months. At the 6-month point, they return to the clinic for three group sessions about hypertension.

Desensitization

Desensitization is part of a standard behavioral approach in which patients develop behavioral tasks customized to their specific fears. First, the fear is broken down into its components by exploring the particular stimulus cues the patient presents. For example, certain situations may precipitate a phobic reaction, whereas others do not. Crowds at parties may be problematic, whereas similar numbers of people in other settings do not cause the same distress. Or a person may have an avoidance reaction with dogs or with certain types of dogs but not with other animals.

Second, patients are incrementally exposed to what they fear. For example, visual presentations of flying can significantly decrease fear of flying. A fear of flying might be tackled with an 8-week educational program held in a busy airport. The process involves a combination of techniques, including relaxation and systematic desensitization.

Third, patients are instructed how to design their own hierarchies of fear. In the fear of flying example, patients develop a set of statements representing the stages of the flight, order the statements from most fearful to least fearful, and use relaxation techniques to reach a level of relaxation; then they progress through the list.

Fourth, patients practice these techniques every day. With cognitive restructuring, patients are encouraged to think about the effects their belief systems have on their feelings and actions and how these can be changed as a result of the desensitization. They draw up charts containing their old belief systems and their new belief systems. Group support is provided throughout the course of treatment.

Desensitization and modeling in dentistry help to decrease the anxiety of juvenile patients. Before treatment, the child is shown a video demonstrating all aspects of the examination. Music and sounds are on the soundtrack, along with a woman's voice. Evaluating the children includes heart rate monitoring, dentist's subjective observations, parents' observations, children's comments, and behavioral rating scale.

Guided Mastery

Guided mastery has been used in conjunction with desensitization to help people with cardiopulmonary disease manage dyspnea. Through guided mastery patients learn to relax and follow step-by-step instructions. They also learn coping skills, which provide an increased sense of self-mastery. While patients exercise on a treadmill at increasing levels of speed and grade, they experience greater than usual levels of potentially fearful stimulus (dyspnea) in a monitored, safe environment. They are then instructed to take long steps and to relax their shoulders, arms, and hands. Being able to determine the treadmill speed and grade gives patients a feeling of control over the level of dyspnea. Desensitization, used with guided mastery, includes supervision, which provides the patient with constant monitoring. Supervision is oversight by a therapist who monitors level of anxiety and dyspnea. Patients learn that they can tolerate greater intensity of dyspnea at higher levels of exercise than they previously thought they could (Carrieri-Kohlman, Douglas, Gormley, & Stulbarg, 1993).

Applied Relaxation

Relaxation training was originally developed by Jacobson in 1938. Using his progressive relaxation techniques, the therapist gives systematic muscle relaxation instructions in a calm, even tone. Once these techniques are learned, the patient can use them whenever he or she feels anxious and tense. They have also been used as part of a protocol to decrease fear of blushing and trembling (Scholing & Emmelkamp, 1993) and to treat panic disorders (Ost, Westling, & Hellstrom, 1993).

Behavioral Strategies in Preventive Psychiatry

Behavioral techniques can facilitate our collective journey by preventing major health problems for large numbers of people. Because vascular diseases and cancer are currently the major contributors to morbidity and mortality, chronic health problems are considered lifestyle diseases warranting nationwide intervention. For example, excessive smoking and drinking are considered "volitional" acts and present a major challenge to public health and behavioral medicine professionals. Since the late 1970s, population-based behavioral modification programs using cognitive educational techniques (frequent offerings of printed materials and public service presentations on television) for addictive conditions and for chronic disease control have been attempted. Conditions such as high blood pressure, high cholesterol, and obesity have also been targeted, but results of such campaigns are hard to document. Attitudes toward smoking, however, have changed remarkably. Many restrictions have been placed on smoking. However, information indicates that young people are increasingly taking up smoking. Attempts at cancer prevention involve encouragement to obtain early screening (e.g., mammograms, fecal smears).

High birth rates among unmarried adolescents plague the United States, and there is an increasing awareness that babies are adversely affected by their mothers' high-risk lifestyles. In an attempt to design programs to change such behavior, the U.S. Department of Health and Human Services; the Public Health Service; and the Alcohol, Drug Abuse, and Mental Health Administration are focusing on raising awareness and developing community resources.

What do you think? How effective are population-based behavioral strategies?

CRISIS INTERVENTION

The last of the basic interventions to be explained is crisis intervention, mentioned earlier in the chapter in relationship to Leon.

Theoretical Perspectives

Eric Lindemann

In 1944, Lindemann published a classic article on bereavement that later evolved into a model for considering the nature and resolution of crisis in broader terms. He studied 101 patients who were in crisis as a result of personal loss. Lindemann became convinced that appropriate therapeutic intervention could help patients disengage from disconcerting ties to the deceased and develop new patterns of interaction. He believed that the same interventions that were helpful in bereavement would prove just as helpful in other types of stressful events, and he proposed a crisis intervention model as a major element of preventive psychiatry in the community.

Gerald Caplan

Caplan (1964, 1974), a colleague of Lindemann, received credit for describing the sequence of the crisis state and for defining crisis intervention as a distinct form of preventive psychiatric therapy. Caplan believed that crises

- Represent transitional periods in a person's life characterized by emotional and cognitive disequilibrium
- Force a person to reappraise previously held values and beliefs
- Occur when a person is faced with a potentially insoluble problem that has personal meaning
- Usually have antecedents that are identifiable

The crisis state is self-limiting, usually lasting 4 to 6 weeks. It is most accessible for treatment during the peak of the crisis, and it can be resolved successfully or incline the person to the development of a mental disorder. An inability to resolve a crisis successfully makes a person more vulnerable to difficulties in resolving other life crises.

Caplan described four phases of escalating tension that lead to the **crisis state:**

1. Increased tension related to the impact of an identifiable stressor
2. Failure of normal problem-solving strategies
3. Mobilization of more vigorous and aggressive strategies
4. Tension escalation to the breaking point and readily observable emotional disorganization

Caplan's ideas revolutionized previously held concepts of therapeutic intervention by suggesting the need for community-based intervention for basically healthy people in active crisis. His approach stressed that the focus of intervention should be *problem-centered* rather than self-centered. This change in focus reframed the crisis state as a problematic issue in need of a solution rather than the consequence of a fatal flaw or personality defect in need of correction.

Caplan (1974) recognized the important role nurses play in crisis intervention. He stated, "I felt that among health professionals nurses were particularly well suited to stimulate such support and to act as bridges of communication and as mediators between their patients and other professional and non-professional agencies" (p. 215).

Erik Erikson

Erikson (1963, 1968) viewed developmental (maturational) crisis points as critical to normal healthy personality development. Erikson used an eight-stage model of human ego development (see Chapter 6) and proposed that personality growth could be divided into distinctive psychosocial developmental periods, or life stages. Each psychosocial crisis marks the transition to the next life stage. Although the critical demands of life differ from stage to stage, they are relatively similar for all members of a given society.

Although developmental crises are directly related to social expectations, they also are age related. Psychosocial development emerges from a ground plan that uniquely defines each person's personality. In the beginning, the ground plan is not within the individual's

conscious awareness, but it develops with greater clarity as the result of interactions with others and significant life experiences. A *crisis point* occurs when the self-understandings a person previously used to negotiate life no longer are sufficient to meet life's social demands.

Solutions to the tasks contained within each developmental phase are established as formative seeds in previous phases, worked on in the present phase, and refined in subsequent ones. For example, the adolescent's focus on identity actually began much earlier when he or she, as a child, engaged in social role behaviors during play and later developed fundamental skills in peer relationships with schoolmates. Following adolescence, identity becomes more complex and distinctive, as the individual increasingly incorporates social roles and life experience into his or her personal identity. In old age, mature adults reflect back on the meaning of their lives and share their insights with the younger generations.

The central thread in Erikson's (1968) conceptualization of psychosocial crisis was the process of *identity consciousness,* ". . . which is always changing and developing; at its best it is a process of increasing differentiation, and it becomes ever more inclusive as the individual grows aware of a widening circle of others significant to him, from the maternal person to 'mankind'" (p. 23). Although Erikson specified solutions to developmental crises in the extreme, for example, identity versus identity diffusion (see Chapter 6), he intended successful resolution to be framed as a balance between these two polarities. Table 13–3 identifies situational stressors that commonly occur during different stages of life. By understanding common situations occurring during transitional stages, such as marriage, first pregnancy, and retirement, you can help people anticipate developmental passages and provide special help to these people and their families with the psychosocial needs that characteristically emerge at this time.

Donna Aguilera

Aguilera (1994) and Aguilera and Messick (1974) provided a nursing framework for understanding the nature of balancing factors related to crisis and crisis intervention. They identified *balancing factors* as related to the

- Patient's realistic perception of the problem
- Number and quality of social supports
- Caliber of coping mechanisms relevant to the resolution of the problem

Your assessment should focus on the presence or absence of these balancing supports in developing a relevant treatment plan. If a person has several balancing factors, it is much easier for him or her to resolve a crisis than if the person demonstrates lack of insight, has deficient coping skills, and has limited social supports.

Aguilera (1994) identified *supportive relationships,* defined as social support, as being important balancing factors. Social supports can include family, neighbors,

TABLE 13-3 Situational Stressors That Commonly Occur During Different Stages of Life

DEVELOPMENTAL STAGE	STRESSOR
Trust vs. mistrust	Rejection by primary caregiver Physical illness or trauma Hospitalization or separation from a parent
Autonomy vs. shame and doubt	Illness or trauma requiring restraint Rigid toilet training Loss of a parent
Initiative vs. guilt	Physical injury Entering school Loss of a parent
Industry vs. inferiority	Peer or teacher conflicts Dyslexia Moving or changing schools
Identity vs. role confusion	Teenage pregnancy Graduation from high school Entering college First job Loss of a parent
Intimacy vs. isolation	Unwanted pregnancy Separation, divorce, or death of partner Birth of a child
Generativity vs. stagnation, self-absorption	Illness of self or family member Care of compromised parents Children leaving home Layoffs from employment Changes in job responsibilities
Ego integrity vs. despair	Death of spouse, family members, or friends Failing senses, disability Retirement or financial difficulties Neglect or abuse by adult children

friends, clergy members, and health professionals; supportive relationships can occur with informal and chance encounters as well as with longer-term relationships with professionals and significant others. A taxicab driver, sympathetic teacher, or even a stranger can provide a casual remark or brief opportunity to share human pain. Individuals without the support of an extended family or friends are more prone to developing a crisis.

The presence or absence of coping skills is an important balancing factor. The presence or lack of personal resources in terms of attitudes, creativity, intelligence, money, health, and interpersonal relationship skills can significantly influence the threat, de-

velopment, and treatment of a patient in crisis. Successful past coping with difficult situations provides the foundation for developing new initiatives with the current crisis.

The Aguilera/Messick model is useful as an assessment framework for evaluating the impact of a crisis event in functional terms (Figure 13-3). It also serves as a nursing theory-based guidepost for identifying where the intervention needs to focus.

What do you think? Reread the story of Leon's crisis when he failed his first examination. How would you evaluate Leon's balancing factors?

▶ *Check Your Reading*

29. What do you see as the value (if any) of using theoretical frameworks in crisis situations?
30. What implications does Caplan's model have for preventive psychiatry?
31. How would you use Erikson's model to help a patient in crisis?
32. In what ways is the Aguilera/Messick model useful in crisis intervention?

Nature of Crisis

A crisis is both an occurrence and a psychological state precipitated by a hazardous event. The hazardous event, labeled a *critical stressor,* creates great emotional upheaval and temporary personality disorganization. A **crisis** is a serious or decisive state, a turning point. The word *crisis* is a derivative of the Greek word meaning "decision," but the Chinese provide two alternative definitions for it: "danger" and "opportunity." Characteristic of all definitions of crisis is the notion that something extraordinary has happened that requires a person to make a decisive paradigm shift in responding to abnormal circumstances. By definition, if a person knows how to cope with the crisis easily, it is not classified as a true crisis. Crisis is experienced as unexpected, uncontrollable, and a personal threat to self-concept, and it usually involves a loss of something important to the individual. When a person experiences a crisis, he or she typically knows little about how to do the things that he or she has to do to meet the needs of the situation and function appropriately. Moreover, what the person does need to know about coping with the crisis situation must be learned in a relatively short period.

The term *crisis state* is used to describe personal responses—physical, emotional, spiritual, and behavioral—to a crisis situation. In order to help someone deal with a crisis, it is critical to know the crisis "from the inside," that is, the personal way in which each person experiences a particular situation.

Thus, your assessment validates the suffering experienced and collects data. Pay attention to the meaning of

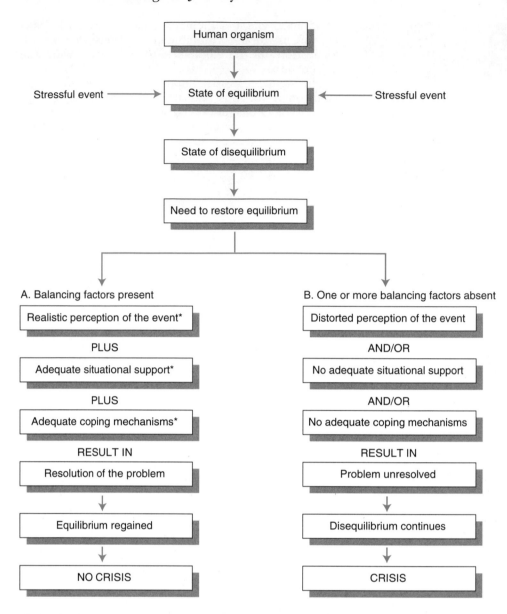

Human organism

Stressful event → State of equilibrium ← Stressful event

State of disequilibrium

Need to restore equilibrium

A. Balancing factors present

Realistic perception of the event*

PLUS

Adequate situational support*

PLUS

Adequate coping mechanisms*

RESULT IN

Resolution of the problem

Equilibrium regained

NO CRISIS

B. One or more balancing factors absent

Distorted perception of the event

AND/OR

No adequate situational support

AND/OR

No adequate coping mechanisms

RESULT IN

Problem unresolved

Disequilibrium continues

CRISIS

*Balancing factors

Figure 13–3
The Aguilera/Messick model, which is useful for assessing the functional impact of a crisis. (Redrawn from Aguilera, D. [1994]. *Crisis intervention: Theory and methodology* [7th ed.]. St. Louis, MO: Mosby–Year Book.)

the event to other significant people involved in the event. A simple, empathetic understanding of the position each family member holds, as you inquire about the nature of the crisis event, helps to organize the family into a self-supporting network, which can help restore the balance in a temporary state of emotional disequilibrium.

Elements Contributing to the Onset of a Crisis State

Caplan (1964) identified five interactive elements that typically contribute to the development of a crisis state. These elements are listed in Box 13-11 and are illustrated in the Case Examples 13-2 and 13-3.

■ **CASE EXAMPLE 13–2**
■ **Mrs. Dittman's Story**

The parents of Margaret Dittman, a hospitalized 4-year-old newly diagnosed with leukemia, insist on being involved with all aspects of her care. They make frequent trips to the hospital, attend support group meetings, and interact frequently with hospital staff members. The staff members view the family as a model of successful coping. One day, however, the mother's emotional reserve seems to "snap." Her coping structure, which up until this point was strong enough to prevent a crisis state, becomes ineffective. Both she and others around her are aware of a significant change in her behavior that resembles symptoms of a psychiatric problem. This mother, however, is simply experiencing a crisis state stemming from exhaustion—a nonpathological emotional response to overwhelming stress. ■

Box 13–11 ■ ■ ■ ■ ■
Five Elements That Typically Contribute to the Development of a Crisis State

1. A critical stressor
2. Vulnerability
3. Failure of previous coping strategies
4. Intolerable tension
5. Lack of social support

Consider Case Example 13-2. The initial strategies you should use with this mother are to support her obvious investment in her child's well-being, to validate her current feelings as a nonpathological response to an overwhelming turn of life events, and to assist her in expressing her concerns and negative feelings. You should also help both parents understand what is happening to their child and use the Aguilera/Messick model to help them shift the weighting of balancing factors in a more positive direction.

Prolonged, unrelieved excessive tension leaves a person in a dangerous condition. In its early stages, excessive tension can be brought under control with the standard crisis intervention strategies described later in this chapter. Unfortunately, without help, a crisis can result in a lower level of functioning, for example, alcohol or drug abuse, chronic psychological symptoms, or social isolation. In its most extreme form, an active crisis state can precipitate a brief reactive psychosis that warrants a specific psychiatric diagnosis. The symptoms produced by a brief reactive psychosis are florid, out of character for the patient, and quite frightening for both patient and staff members. Stabilizing the patient with medication and ensuring a secure, protected environment are essential before using more traditional crisis intervention strategies. One way to distinguish between a brief psychotic state and other forms of pathology is by reviewing past history and current drug use.

■ CASE EXAMPLE 13–3
■ Gretchen's Story

"Admission to a psychiatric hospital was not easy. I did not want to be there, but I felt I had no choice. Walking into the hospital made me feel ill at ease and embarrassed. I was very grateful to have a friend with me to ease the emotional pain. The unit was supposed to be open, but it was locked at the time of my admission. Realizing I was to be held behind locked doors made me feel very humiliated. I also felt like a prisoner, an outcast of society. This was the beginning of the stripping of my personhood—my body and soul.

"I was taken to a small, bare room that looked like a jail cell. It had three chairs and a desk. There were no pictures on the walls, flower arrangements, or anything to make me feel welcome. The room seemed very small and needed a coat of paint. It was here that I was "interrogated." Form after form was presented to me to sign. It was difficult, at best, to keep the forms straight. I signed eight forms, one of which was called "Patient's Rights," which I was told would be good to read some time. After signing all of the forms, the psychiatric technician left and the primary nurse entered to get my history. While she was obtaining my history, my suitcase was taken out of the room.

"At the completion of the history-taking, I was shown to my room. On the way, I had to stop at the desk to have my purse gone through. It made me sick. I wanted to cry. I felt like a very bad person who couldn't be trusted. At the time, I also noticed that many things had been removed from my suitcase. I felt like I had been punched in the stomach or assaulted. Things taken away from me included all aerosols, glass bottles, and electrical appliances such as blow dryer; my embroidery, because it was in a plastic bag; mirrors, tweezers, needles, keys, and even my pillow. Taking my pillow seemed to be the last straw. Everything had been taken from me. I felt angry at these people for taking my things. I felt very alone because I knew none of the patients or staff members. I was upset because no one seemed to know that I was a person—a nurse with a doctoral degree. I was on the wrong side of the desk. Then I felt embarrassed. I shouldn't be here. I was a respectable person, but no one seemed to know or care.

"When I got to my room, I was shocked not to have a bathroom or telephone. Again, I felt like I had been hit in the stomach. Tears, tears, tears—they just wouldn't stop. My roommate came and introduced herself. She was nice. Another patient on the "welcome committee" oriented me to the unit and told me about community life. She also seemed nice and was helpful to me. A physician came and wrote an order so that I could have my pillow. As I lay awake that first night, crying, I wondered how I had ever gotten here. What had I done to deserve this punishment? Why couldn't anyone see me and know how scared I felt?" ■

Maintaining continued casual contacts that are caring and respectful of the patient as a unique person can reduce the incidence of inpatient crisis states. Cardell and Horton-Deutsch (1994) noted that selected research studies support the hypothesis that "patients who felt uncared for and/or misunderstood by the staff reported continued or increased suicidal ideation" (p. 369).

Risk Factors for the Development of a Crisis State

No one is immune to developing a crisis state. Given the right (or wrong) set of circumstances, everyone is capable of experiencing the startling and profound disequilibrium associated with crisis. Nevertheless, there are risk factors that enhance the probability of a person's life events or circumstances resulting in a crisis state. These risk factors include the following:

Overwhelming Nature of the Crisis

Generally, disasters that are naturally occurring events, often called "acts of God," are somewhat less overwhelming to the victims than crises that are precipitated by the careless or wrongful acts of human beings. People accept more readily their lack of control over natural disasters, whereas human made disasters seem preventable.

Concurrent Stressors

Concurrent stressors increase the possibility of crisis. For example, an elderly person with limited financial and social resources may suffer a greater sense of depression and demoralization following a disastrous flood than a younger or richer person. For this elderly person, the tragic event parallels a time of life that characteristically involves many losses and fewer options. Compounding the sense of loss may be a lack of resiliency; the adaptive process and physical stamina needed to respond effectively to the crisis are lacking.

Lack of Previous Life Experience With Similar Stressors, Physical and Emotional State, Age, and Developmental Stage

These elements all contribute to the individual's coping responses. For example, a popular teenage athlete who experiences the loss of a significant relationship or fails expectations in the first semester of college may be at high risk for a crisis state. His less noticed friend, for whom disappointment is a more natural part of the journey, may weather a similar loss with greater equanimity.

Lack of Success Coping With Similar Stressors

Knowing that one has survived a crisis makes the next one a little easier, whereas unsuccessfully resolving a past crisis can heighten the current one's intensity.

Repeated Stressors Without Relief

Holmes and Rahe (1967) developed a research tool to prove their hypothesis that individuals have limited tolerance for repeated stressors. Their *Schedule of Recent Experiences* (Figure 13-4) is used to describe common life change events that qualify as crises; each was given a quantitative weighting. Their schedule is based on the premise that the number and nature of significant life crises over a short period directly correlate with the development of physical illness. The larger the number of serious life events, the more likely the development of a stress-related physical illness within a 3-year period.

Chronic Stress

A lifetime of chronic illness or a dysfunctional family background makes a current crisis more difficult. Each new situation takes a toll that is qualitatively different than suffering from an isolated crisis incident. Intense feelings from previous stressful encounters typically are pushed from memory or minimized as people struggle to survive while dealing with the chaos of the current crisis. Although their beat is faint, these memories of stressful encounters keep intruding, creating and magnifying the rhythms of the current crisis situation.

Physical and Emotional Depletion

It is more difficult for people to maintain a balanced perspective when they are tired, in pain, or distracted by physical symptoms. Drugs and alcohol cloud and distort the meaning of a situation, causing some to be overlooked as potential crises and creating bizarre or numbed, responses to others.

The presence of concurrent psychiatric symptoms makes realistic assessments of a crisis situation less probable.

Crisis as an Opportunity

In the throes of a crisis state, it is difficult to think of it as having a positive value, yet it can be a significant turning point in a person's life journey. First, a crisis state has the capacity to propel a person into an entirely different mode of thinking; it sets an inner revolution of meaning into motion and encourages a reorganization of priorities. For these reasons, you can work more intensively with the person involved, and the possibility for personal growth in a shortened period is much higher. Second, a crisis often brings to light earlier unresolved and related problems that suddenly become available and amenable to treatment. Without the crisis to magnify the problem areas, many people live with chronic problems that exist in a lesser intensity. Thus, crisis intervention has important implications for preventive psychiatry (Case Example 13-4).

■ C A S E   E X A M P L E   1 3 – 4
■ Norma's Story
■
■ Norma Byron's youngest daughter was recently diagnosed
   with anorexia nervosa. The girl was hospitalized in her first
   semester of college. This illness served as an impetus for
   Norma to scrutinize more closely her own seriously dysfunctional marriage. Contributing to the marriage problems were Norma's chronic depression and her husband's need to control. Neither partner was good at expressing

Forty-three common life events are listed in the order of their importance. Total score predicts likelihood of developing a serious illness within the next two years. Scores of more than 300 indicate a high probability (80%) of developing a serious illness within the next few years. Scores between 150 and 300 have a 51% probability, and scores of less than 150 within a year have a 37% probability of developing a major physical or psychological illness.

Life Event	Your Value Score	Life Event	Your Value Score
1. Death of spouse	100 _____	23. Son or daughter leaving home	29 _____
2. Divorce	73 _____	24. Trouble with in-laws	29 _____
3. Marital separation	65 _____	25. Outstanding personal achievement	28 _____
4. Jail term	63 _____	26. Spouse begins or stops work	26 _____
5. Death of a close family member	63 _____	27. Starting or finishing school	26 _____
6. Personal injury or illness	53 _____	28. Change in living conditions	25 _____
7. Marriage	50 _____	29. Revision of personal habits	24 _____
8. Fired at work	47 _____	30. Trouble with boss	23 _____
9. Marital reconciliation	45 _____	31. Change in work hours, conditions	20 _____
10. Retirement	45 _____	32. Change in residence	20 _____
11. Change in family member's health	44 _____	33. Change in schools	20 _____
12. Pregnancy	40 _____	34. Change in recreation	19 _____
13. Sex difficulties	39 _____	35. Change in church activities	19 _____
14. Addition to family	39 _____	36. Change in social activities	18 _____
15. Business readjustment	39 _____	37. Mortgage or loan under $10,000	17 _____
16. Change in financial state	38 _____	38. Change in sleeping habits	16 _____
17. Death of close friend	37 _____	39. Change in number of family get-togethers	15 _____
18. Change to different line of work	36 _____	40. Change in eating habits	15 _____
19. Change in number of arguments with spouse	35 _____	41. Vacation	13 _____
20. Mortgage over $10,000	31 _____	42. Christmas	12 _____
21. Foreclosure of mortgage or loan	30 _____	43. Minor violation of law	11 _____
22. Change in work responsibilities	29 _____		Total _____

Figure 13–4
The Holmes-Rahe Schedule of Recent Experiences. (The scale gives complete wording of the items.) (Reprinted from *Journal of Psychosomatic Research*, 11, Holmes, T. H., & Rahe, R. H., The social readjustment rating scale, 1967, with permission from Elsevier Science.)

feelings that could be heard by the other. Norma and her husband now have the opportunity, in coping with the crisis of their daughter's illness and with appropriate help, to resolve a longstanding dysfunctional communication pattern that otherwise might not have surfaced with such clarity. ∎

From Williamson, J. (1990, Summer/Fall). Reaching children at greatest risk. *Child World*, 35, 65–69.

You can be a valuable resource by joining the patient as a professional ally in a therapeutic process designed to help him or her explore, learn from, and resolve serious life events. Ideally, successful resolution of a crisis leads to greater self-awareness of what is truly important about the journey.

Types of Crises

Crises are typically classified, for description purposes, as situational or maturational (developmental). Situational crises occur unpredictably, whereas maturational crises are identifiable in relation to predictable stages of human development.

Situational Crises

Characteristically, a **situational crisis** is a random event that comes without warning and is entirely nondiscriminatory in its choice of victim. The critical stressor can occur as an unbalancing community, personal, or family circumstance. Situational crises include disasters, community crises, personal crises, and family crises.

Disasters occur as natural or human-caused large-scale events, affecting large numbers of people simultaneously. Melick, Logue, and Frederick (1982) suggested,

[A] disaster is not a single event occurring in the life of an individual; rather it is a series of events preceding and following impact whose sequelae are likely to be experienced over time by exposed individuals, and by the community in which the disaster occurred. (p. 624)

Although disasters always pose personal dilemmas for individual members of a community, the initial focus of crisis intervention is on restabilizing the whole community. Most disasters are reported extensively in the press and immediately generate an outpouring of sympathy and social and practical support from strangers as well as those involved with the victims. Examples of disasters include airplane crashes, earthquakes, war, nuclear power plant accidents, forest fires, hurricanes, droughts, and floods. Governments classify disasters as federal major disasters or federal emergency disasters, depending on their magnitude and severity, for federal relief purposes.

In 1957, Tyhurst studied individual responses to community disaster and was one of the first psychiatrists to propose that a state of crisis does not represent a psychiatric illness. According to Tyhurst, a crisis offered a unique opportunity for personal growth, no matter how severe the symptoms might appear. He described three identifiable phases of adjustment in the **crisis sequence:**

- *Period of impact:* This activates a psychological state of shock; the feeling of wholeness is irrevocably shaken and a sense of unreality is felt.
- *Period of recoil:* This represents an emotional retreat from the event in the form of denial, feelings of hopelessness, and limited attention to working through the problem.
- *Posttraumatic period:* The time when a person begins to integrate the crisis experience into the larger tapestry of life in a productive way.

During a disaster, crisis intervention strategies that directly support and empower the efforts of the local citizenry are most productive for two reasons: (1) they use personal resources available in the group to their advantage, and (2) they serve to help the community reestablish a sense of personal control at a time when typically there is a general feeling of helplessness. Attempts by the professional helper to provide direct assistance are often viewed as an intrusion during the period of *altruistic community,* characteristic of disaster crisis situations.

A community crisis may or may not reach disaster proportions. It may represent a more personalized situational crisis affecting one person or a small segment of the community. An individual's crisis can capture the attention of an entire community if it symbolizes behaviors that potentially can alter the journey for other members. The abduction of a child, a brutal murder, or the discovery of a public official's misconduct are all examples of individual crises that instantly affect an entire community almost as if they are personal experiences. For example, in 1998, there were multiple instances of children killing other children within public school settings. These murders created crises not only for the families involved but also for the local communities and the nation at large, who were faced with the symbolic meaning of these events. Families confronting relocation and urban renewal typically describe their situation as a major community crisis. Faced by a common difficulty, the community tends to draw more closely together. Crisis intervention, both generic and individual, helps families and communities adjust to new roles and shifts in position or status.

Other situational crisis states emerge from personal situations—unexpected externally created circumstances or personal illness that affects a single person or a smaller nucleus of family and friends. For example, an auto accident, a divorce, a rape, a terminal medical diagnosis, or a severe illness in a previously healthy individual can instantly create a state of psychological shock that is potentially overwhelming for the individual or family. Other examples of personal crises are found in Box 13-12. Consider the meaning that each of these personal crisis situations might have on lifestyle, sense of identity, and role relationships.

An individual family member in crisis can precipitate a family crisis that is separate from but related to the individual's crisis. For example, an individual family member who is jailed, dies, or is hospitalized creates financial and emotional consequences for all family members. Other critical stressors that can directly affect normal family functioning, regardless of the family member, include a move to a different geographical area; bankruptcy; marriage; care for elderly parents; delinquency; illegitimacy; a move home of adult children; spousal, child, or elder abuse; and serious illness.

The relationship between individual crisis and family crisis is a reciprocal one. Admitting a loved one to a nursing home, initiating commitment proceedings for a mentally ill relative, and enduring the criminal trial of a family member present critical stressors to all family members as well as to the individual. Sometimes, a family crisis erupts to reveal an underlying psychodynamic problem within the family. For example, as one drug-abusing child is admitted to a treatment center, a second child assumes the delinquent or drug-abusing

Box 13-12 ■ ■ ■ ■ ■
Examples of Personal Crises

Mrs. Jackson's husband died suddenly of a heart attack 6 weeks ago. They had been married for 24 years.

Maria Porter became engaged at Christmas. Her fiancé was involved in an auto accident over New Year's and it looks as though he will be a paraplegic.

Mr. Francis went to the doctor with double vision last week. He learned that he has Graves' disease and that there is a strong possibility that he will be completely blind in 2 years.

Mr. Maxwell has been fired from his job as middle manager after 18 years of employment with the same company.

Mrs. Braxton has become increasingly frail and can no longer live by herself. She must move in with her daughter and her family.

Mrs. DiNola's husband has been diagnosed with Alzheimer's disease. She is 51 years old and has just started a new job.

role in the family. In many instances, the identified patient in crisis actually is either acting out or reacting to the larger context of a crisis in the family. Thus, a crisis provides not only the family's initial entry into the health care system but also a unique opportunity for individual personal growth within the family context. Many of the same strategies used to treat individuals in crisis are extended to the treatment of family members as a collective unit.

In assessing and responding to family crisis, it is important to explore, with the family members, their beliefs about the crisis and its impact on the family. You can obtain this information through conversations about how the family members handle problems, their expectations of each other, and the meanings of such a crisis in their family. Interventions in a family crisis need to consider the family instead of the individual as the decision-making unit, and it is important to regard all family members' viewpoints as important. Knowledge of family strengths, previous coping strategies, perception of the problem, and resources available in the crisis period provides a baseline of data from which to select the most appropriate interventions (Case Example 13–5).

■ **CASE EXAMPLE 13–5**
■ **Martha's Story**

Martha Miller is a 75-year-old widow living on the East Coast of the United States. She has osteoporosis and was successfully treated for colon cancer about 2 years ago. She describes herself as a loner who likes to read and prefers to live by herself. She does not have a good relationship with her daughter, who lives in the area, and she is pained about their estrangement. Recently, Mrs. Miller fell and broke her ankle. Her son, who had suggested that she move near him in California, is now insisting on it. She must decide whether to move near her son or continue to live in a house in which she finds it increasingly difficult to care for herself. Although she has a good relationship with her son, she has a strained relationship with her daughter-in-law, and she fears that living near the couple would not be a good situation. ■

In Case Example 13-5, it is obvious to everyone that Mrs. Miller needs a different level of care than is available to her now. She realizes she is unable to cope effectively by herself, but she is disturbed and unclear as to whether leaving her home and moving across the country is the answer. Although she may not appear to be particularly anxious because her style is to internalize her anxiety, and although the solution seems perfect because her son wants to take care of her, Mrs. Miller is experiencing a crisis state. It is hard for her to sort out what is best in the situation, and she feels an emotional paralysis that prevents her from choosing an appropriate behavioral solution.

As a first step, you need to help Mrs. Miller organize her dilemma in verbal terms. Moreover, her daughter, son, and daughter-in-law may not have thought through what is in their own interests as thoroughly as they have thought about their concern for their mother. This means that a significant part of the intervention process is to explore Mrs. Miller's relationships with her daughter, son, and daughter-in-law in more detail. Also, find out what other possible supports exist in her community.

Do not assume that Mrs. Miller's problems will be helped by direct problem-solving. Your role is to help her regain a sense of control by converting experiences and vague perceptions into words and subsequently validating them with the individuals involved. By helping Mrs. Miller reflect on what has happened and what needs to be done, you can assist her in asking the right questions and building bridges with her adult children that ultimately will prove more beneficial for her and her family than your direct problem-solving.

Families typically resolve crisis states by making important changes in the way they function or approach a crisis situation. But they often need help from you to fully understand the nature of the problem and what it entails for the family. Good intentions are not enough, and you play an important role in helping families organize their immediate situation into workable terms and in assisting them to generate creative alternatives in difficult situations. Table 13–4 identifies relevant family interventions for different behavioral symptoms.

Developmental (Maturational) Crises

The other major categorization of crisis is a **developmental (maturational) crisis.** These crisis states relate to normal periods of maturational transition, as described by Erikson (1963, 1968), and they are typically associated with age-related life events. They tend to arise more gradually than situational crises and can usually be resolved without professional intervention (see Table 13–3).

Typical markers associated with the emergence of developmental crises (e.g., marriage, first job, first home, first baby, children entering school, leaving home, caring for aging parents, retirement, divorce, death of a child) create potentially overwhelming feelings. Anticipatory guidance, recognition, and educational support are early interventions that help an individual recognize and pass through a transitional crisis state successfully. Ironically, many people do not recognize age-stage developmental crises as they go through them, and, consequently, they experience them as strange and unnatural. Explaining that many parents have difficulty with their children's teenage years or that teenagers often appear rebellious and immature because they are trying to establish their own sense of identity helps parents understand difficult behaviors from a different perspective. A simple discussion of normal adolescent rapid swings of mood and behavior is a highly effective strategy in many cases.

When a situational crisis is superimposed on a normal developmental psychosocial crisis point, professional assistance may be necessary. Examples include mastectomy during perimenopause, birth of a special-needs child to an adolescent mother, cancer diagnosis in a teenager or young adult, or early loss of a parent or spouse. Sometimes, the only understanding comes from

TABLE 13-4 Relevant Family Interventions for Different Behavioral Symptoms

SYMPTOM	INTERVENTIONS
Anxiety, shock, fright	Giving information that is brief, concise, explicit, and concrete Repetition of information and frequent reinforcement—encourage families to record important facts in writing Ascertain comprehension by asking families to repeat back to you what information they have been given Provide for and encourage or allow ventilation of feelings, even if they are extreme Maintain constant, nonanxious presence in the face of a highly anxious family Inform families as to the potential range of behaviors and feelings that are within the "norm" for crisis Maximize control within hospital environment, as possible
Denial	Identify what purpose denial is serving for families (e.g., is it buying them "psychological time" for future coping and mobilization of resources?) Evaluate appropriateness of use of denial in terms of time; denial becomes inappropriate when it inhibits families from taking necessary actions or when it is impinging on the course of treatment Do not actively support denial but do not dash hopes for the future (e.g., "It must be very difficult for you to believe your son is nonresponsive and in a trauma unit") If denial is prolonged and dysfunctional, more direct and specific factual representation may be essential
Anger, hostility, distrust	Allow for ventilation of angry feelings, clarifying what thoughts, fears, and beliefs are behind the anger; let them know it's "OK" to be angry Do not personalize families' expressions of these strong emotions Institute family control within the hospital environment when possible (e.g., arrange for set time(s) and set person(s) to give them information in reference to the patient and answer their questions) Remain available to families during their venting of these emotions Ask families how they can take the energy in their anger and put it to positive use for themselves, for the patient, for the situation
Remorse and guilt	Do not try to "rationalize away" guilt for families Listen and support their expression of feeling and verbalizations (e.g., "I can understand how or why you might feel that way; however . . .") Follow the "howevers" with careful, reality-oriented statements or questions (e.g., "None of us can truly control another's behavior"; "Kids make their own choices despite what parents think and want"; "How successful were you when you tried to control _____'s behavior with that before?"; "So many things have happened for which there are no absolute answers")
Grief and depression	Acknowledge families' grief and depression Encourage them to be precise about what it is they are grieving and depressed about; give grief and depression a context Allow families appropriate time for grief Recognize that this is an essential step for future adaptation—do not try to rush the grief process Remain sensitive to your own unfinished business and hence comfort or discomfort with families' grieving and depression
Hope	Clarify with families what their hopes are, individually, and one another Clarify with families what their worst fears are in reference to the situation—are the hopes or fears congruent? Realistic? Unrealistic? Support realistic hope Offer gentle factual information to reframe unrealistic hope (e.g., "With the information you have or the observations you have made, do you think that is still possible?") Assist families in reframing unrealistic hope in some other fashion (e.g., "What do you think others will have learned from _____ if he doesn't make it?" "How do you think _____ would like for you to remember him/her?")

From Kleeman, K. (1989). Families in crisis due to multiple trauma. *Critical Care Nursing Clinics of North America, 1*(1), 25.

the spiritual aspect of oneself (Case Example 13-6). Symptoms of a maturational crisis are typically categorized in the *Diagnostic and Statistical Manual, Fourth Edition,* as one or more "additional conditions that may be a focus of clinical attention," as follows:

V62.3   Academic Problem
V62.2   Occupational Problem
313.82 Identity Problem
V62.89 Phase of Life Problem

■ **CASE EXAMPLE 13-6**
■ **Edward's Story**

Edward, once a vigorous athlete and an active man who swore he would never work behind a desk, was injured in an accident that left him completely paralyzed from the neck down. His fast-paced, perfectionistic lifestyle was suddenly changed. He recalls the following thoughts as he was being taken into the emergency room 15 years ago: "I felt as if God were speaking to me: 'You take control of the physical circumstances. I'll cover everything else.' I had a special feeling of warmth and security in my body." One week after the accident, Edward had an experience "that was like starting my life all over, being born again. I had to throw out everything I knew before starting all over again from scratch." Among the major changes that Edward says he made were developing a more compassionate and trusting sense of others, an appreciation of beauty in the world, and "a deeper, more enhanced dependence on God in controlling things we don't understand." ■

From Miller, W., & C'deBaca, J. (1994). Quantum change: Toward a psychology of transformation. In T. Heatherton & J. Weinberger (Eds.), *Can personality change?* (p. 269). Washington, DC: American Psychological Association. © 1994 by the American Psychological Association. Reprinted with permission.

What do you think? In general, does spirituality impact an individual's ability to confront a crisis? Would spirituality impact the crisis state?

➤ *Check Your Reading*

33. How do the characteristic elements of a crisis interact with one another to create a crisis state?
34. In what ways is knowledge of risk factors helpful in assessing patient needs and planning appropriate nursing interventions?
35. What are the fundamental differences between a situational and a maturational crisis?

Intervening in a Crisis

By definition, a person in a crisis state requires immediate action to resolve the problem. It cannot be tolerated indefinitely. The time frame generally associated with crisis intervention is 4 to 6 weeks.

The American Nurses Association (1994) specified **crisis intervention** as a basic level psychiatric–mental health nursing clinical practice function:

Psychiatric–mental health nurses provide direct crisis intervention services to persons in crisis and serve as members of crisis teams. Crisis intervention is a short-term therapeutic process that focuses on the resolution of an immediate crisis or emergency through the use of available professional personnel, family, and/or environmental resources. (p. 15)

Orientation Phase

As with other forms of interpersonal relationships in psychiatric nursing, the orientation phase in crisis intervention parallels the assessment phase of the nursing process. Initially, you are concerned with three tasks:

1. Triage assessment of the patient for medical and psychiatric emergency
2. Engagement of the patient in the treatment process
3. Development of a comprehensive database to serve as the foundation for planning and intervention for the patient

The focus of the assessment is more immediately and closely associated with crisis resolution. The crisis, perception of hazardous events leading to the state of crisis, and accompanying feelings are the primary concerns. Looking only at the immediate facts of a situation and not considering the patient's perceptions, risk of lethality or violence, sources of social support, or previous coping mechanisms suggests a failure to recognize the many levels of observation required in crisis situations. Exploring underlying personality dynamics is useful only as it relates to the immediate crisis.

TRIAGE ASSESSMENT OF MEDICAL AND PSYCHIATRIC CONDITIONS

Crisis interventions in the emergency department and initial stages of treatment typically require a first-level assessment of the patient's acuity level and emergency medical management of critical physical and psychiatric symptoms before proceeding to a second-level therapeutic response. The crisis state is one of urgency and racing emotions. A sense of intolerable tension invades the entire person, physically, psychologically, and spiritually. Profound anxiety takes over and narrows perceptions. The person is unable to focus on much other than the object of the crisis and its immediate impact on self. For some people, the only solution they see is taking their own life or that of another. Before proceeding with a standard psychiatric interview, you need to evaluate the patient's physical condition, potential for self-harm, and potential for harm to others.

The first consideration in a triage assessment is to identify or rule out physical causes of toxicity and to treat the patient's symptoms appropriately. Failure to recognize the physical symptoms of overdose or drug toxicity can result in permanent damage or death. Patients with cognitive disorders precipitated by alcohol-induced or drug-induced intoxication present a frightening appearance in the emergency department. Typically, patients with cognitive disorders present with symptoms of delirium. Confused and disoriented to time and place, these patients may appear drowsy and stuporous or agitated and belligerent, depending on the cause of the delirium. Symptoms of tachycardia, elevated blood pressure, sweating, and dilated pupils should alert you to the presence of respiratory or cardiac decompensation and *must always be treated as a first-order medical emergency.* Questions about drug use, dosage, and last intake are important. Because of the confused state of these patients, relatives or significant others may provide information about patients' past history and events leading up to arrival in the emergency department that make for a more informed and accurate diagnosis.

After assessing cardiac and respiratory status and physical stabilization, proceed with a mental status examination. Begin with an appraisal of the patient's appearance, gait, movements, and speech. Making the patient comfortable while asking the person accompanying the patient questions may prove more fruitful than asking the patient directly. It is possible to help the organically impaired patient feel more relaxed by offering a glass of water or a visit to the restroom. A calm, understanding, and sympathetic attitude is much more productive than approaching the patient with an initial show of strength.

It is important to set realistic limits, particularly with a belligerent patient, who can be highly provocative and attention grabbing. A patient like this is more easily handled in a smaller room, apart from the mainstream of activity, where distracting stimuli that can further disorganize or anger the patient can be limited. A key factor in first-level assessment, particularly if the person appears disorganized or impulsive, is lethality potential. Chapter 31 provides a detailed explanation of suicidal assessment and interventions.

The second factor to consider in a triage assessment is potential for harm to others. Symptoms cover a wide variety of behaviors ranging from abuse (verbal, sexual, physical) to physical maiming and homicide. Chapter 35 details specifics regarding risk assessment for violence and appropriate interventions.

ENGAGING THE PATIENT

The first contact between you and the patient in a crisis situation sets the stage for all that follows. In acute crisis situations, do not forget to introduce yourself by name, to specify your role, or to acknowledge the patient by name, as a unique individual. There is a tendency to respond to the acuteness of the situation rather than to the patient as a person. Yet simply taking the time to introduce yourself, call the patient by name, and describe your role directs the patient to the type of information you need and the kind of help the patient can expect from you. You can begin the first session by introducing yourself and identifying your role with a simple statement such as "Mrs. Tisedale, I'm Marcia Cohen, the crisis intake nurse tonight. My job is to help people sort out the events, thoughts, and feelings in crisis situations, in order to help them come to terms with what has happened. Won't you have a seat over here?"

As you can see in this statement, your first priority is to put the patient at ease and to establish the direction of assessment and intervention. Make every effort to reduce the patient's anxiety. Simple informal and inviting gestures, such as extending a hand for a handshake, offering to take the patient's coat, providing a comfortable chair, and offering a glass of water, enhance comfort. Next, focus on establishing the interview as a collaborative process, which is not always easy when the patient is acutely anxious.

Crisis intervention is an art as well as a skilled nursing function. Although the concept of patient uniqueness is paramount in considering any treatment approach, it sometimes loses its significance in serious crisis situations because the situation is serious. Yet a patient in severe crisis, in particular, needs to know that his or her unique needs are of concern to the caregivers. This knowledge, in itself, has a calming effect because the patient feels that there is a possibility of joining with an expert to solve a problem that is mutually understood. The interview should begin where the patient is and with the patient's description of what brought him or her to seek treatment. No two people are exactly alike, and although their presentation of symptoms in crisis may appear similar, it is important to look beyond the superficial to each person's interpretation of the unique meaning of the situation.

Typically, a patient in crisis is scared, confused, and anxious. How you respond, what you say, and the manner and tone of your delivery serve to increase or decrease the patient's anxiety. A calm, even voice can secure the patient's attention much better than a more excited tone. Language and content need to be suited to the maturity and readiness of the patient. In fact, anything that adds to the human qualities of crisis intervention enhances its effectiveness.

Ideally, the interpersonal climate in a crisis situation is one that is free flowing and changing while being highly focused on here-and-now problem resolution. Make every effort to ask only those questions that are relevant and directly related to the situation under discussion. It is important to encourage the patient to speak personally about what he or she is experiencing and about the particular issues the patient feels are critical to resolving the crisis.

The therapeutic approach in a crisis situation is much more structured than in other forms of nurse-patient relationships, with much closer time linkage between assessment and intervention. A delicate balance exists between helping the person in crisis to express his or her feelings and structuring the encounter in ways that bring about quick resolution of the crisis state. Obviously, it is important to convey empathetic understanding for the patient's predicament and to encourage the patient to talk about perceptions of the experience. Simply sharing the events and associated feelings can reduce the patient's tension significantly. Time is limited, however; consequently, intervention to stabilize the patient necessarily begins as a part of the assessment phase.

It is not always easy to engage the patient in meaningful dialogue before trust is established. Extreme patience, understanding, and empathy for the patient or family's sense of lost control, helplessness, and powerlessness are necessary. During a crisis, a patient typically demonstrates a cognitive rigidity resulting in unreasonable demands, constricted problem-solving, tunnel vision, and overreaction. It is not uncommon for patients and their families to display confusion and project anger onto the health care system and specific health care providers as defensive maneuvers to reestablish personal strength. If you realize that this behavior may be the only way a person can feel control in a situation experienced as potentially overwhelming and ego shattering, you are able to react with acceptance rather than anger or frustration.

Another characteristic of the crisis state is decreased perceptual attention. People simply do not hear much of the information given to them. Although they may appear attentive and respond appropriately, their anxiety typically prevents full comprehension. Consequently, frequently repeating information, asking the patient to invite a trusted family member or friend to listen with him or her to instructions and explanations, and providing written instructions can prove quite helpful. Having a trusted person with him or her increases the patient's potential for providing fully informed consent in crisis situations. In general, the more involved the patient is in the interview process, the better the quality of the assessment data. Initial efforts to reduce or compensate for excessive anxiety make this possible. Although the specific interviewing strategies and formats depend on the patient's individual needs, the patient is more likely to be compliant with treatment suggestions and to experience the mutuality in the relationship if he or she is involved and less anxious.

Follow-up between sessions helps reduce the sense of helplessness. A flexible policy whereby the patient can contact the crisis center or receive support by phone if the tension becomes intolerable is useful. Few patients abuse this type of consultation.

Finally, in the early stages of a crisis state, many patients want to make binding but impulsive and unwise decisions that they would never make in ordinary circumstances. Discourage this behavior because often other facts come to light, feelings change, and possibilities may emerge that were not apparent in the initial stages of a crisis situation. You can be quite helpful by directly making a statement such as, "I know you are upset right now, but it usually works better to postpone any decisions about major changes until we can get your situation stabilized and the air clears a little bit. Let's look at your situation and see if we can understand what is going on that we can do something about."

An important element of the orientation phase is the instillation of hope. Although it is most important to recognize the profound impact of a crisis, you can portray the crisis as an opportunity to reclaim the essential parts of the human journey:

At times, it is appropriate to identify specifically to patients after an overdose that there must have been a part of them that wanted to die (e.g., the part that led them to take the pills), or else they wouldn't be talking to you, but there also must be a part that wanted to live (e.g., the part that warned a relative to look for them) or else they wouldn't be talking to you. It may be useful to tell patients explicitly that "I want to work with the part of you that wants to live. I'm glad that part of you will have another chance." (Hillard, 1990, p. 119)

As many as one third of the patients presenting in psychiatric crisis in the emergency department are repeaters who use the emergency department as their first-line intervention in crisis situations. Often drawn from the poorest socioeconomic groups, these patients are frequently alcoholic, schizophrenic, homeless, or without significant social supports. Usually, they lack insight, despite the greater majority of them being in psychiatric treatment. This population requires a special set of skills because resistance to treatment and an unwillingness to engage in a treatment process that requires suspension of immediate gratification or resolution of their problem preclude easy engagement of the patient. They need to be taken seriously because they can unintentionally commit suicide.

The patient may present with vague medical symptoms or attribute the symptoms' origin to an accident or medical disorder. For example, a patient, diagnosed with a borderline personality disorder (see Chapter 27), presented in the emergency department, having "fallen down the stairs in her house." She suffered a concussion and a broken nose. What she neglected to tell the staff members was that she had been drinking heavily and that this incident was one of many in which she entered the health care system with physical symptoms reflective of self-mutilation and passive self-destructive acts.

Frequently, chronic psychiatric patients, presenting with medical emergencies, forget to tell the staff members that they are in ongoing active treatment. Or they may tell the crisis intervention team information they feel uncomfortable sharing the level of their stress with their primary therapist. For this reason, all information gathered in the emergency department should be shared with the patient's primary therapist. Consistency and follow-through with frequent and thorough sharing of information are crucial to the successful management of frequent emergency department users. The goals of treatment should focus on resolving the immediate crisis and strengthening the treatment already in progress.

DEVELOPING A COMPREHENSIVE DATABASE

Before you can take any action, you must understand the nature of the crisis and its personal meaning to the patient. Most crisis situations have a factual component and a critical emotional impact. The experience of a crisis has a shattering effect on all the patient's previous assumptions, and often he or she may be genuinely baffled in attempting to understand what has happened and why. Because of the large parts role perception and experience play in development of a crisis state, the patient's unique account of the crisis is extremely important as a starting point. In addition to providing the nurse with necessary baseline data, developing an explanation of how the crisis came to be helps the patient make sense of the change in his or her reality. A good place to begin is with identification of the precipitating factors. You can structure your comments in a simple way, such as, "Jean, I know this is a very difficult situation for you. I wonder if you could start at the beginning, and tell me a little of what led up to your coming to the emergency department [crisis center, hospital unit]."

Verbally putting the information sought in order in a logical, sequential manner, starting with the triggering circumstances, helps the patient stay focused on important relationships between the event and corresponding feelings. Guidelines for general assessment questions are presented in Box 13–13.

You validate the patient's experience by accepting the verbal account and neutralizing emotions through discussion. This is important at a time when the patient's confidence in personal abilities is at a low point.

In the course of telling the story of a crisis, you can help the patient develop a realistic perception of the crisis. A concrete problem definition provides an inner contact with the personalized meaning of a crisis, which is essential to its resolution. Frequently, a patient understands only diffuse outlines of the problem. The patient's perceptions are so clouded by anxiety that it is almost impossible to sort out the actual events in ways

Box 13-13 ■ ■ ■ ■ ■

Guidelines for Asking General Assessment Questions

Begin With the History of Presenting Symptoms

- When did the symptoms begin?
- How are they described by the patient?
- What else is going on simultaneously in the patient's life?
- Is there any evidence of a psychiatric emergency (suicidal ideation, hallucinations)? (If the patient is suicidal, does he or she identify a plan?)
- What medication is the patient taking at this time (dosage, time of last intake)?
- Is the patient currently using recreational drugs (marijuana, hallucinogens, cocaine, alcohol, amphetamines)?
- Is the patient currently in treatment with a therapist?
- Is this the first emergency department visit?

Inquire About Relevant History and Coping Mechanisms

- Has the patient had other similar crisis events?
- Is there a patient or family history of mental illness or drug abuse?

- Has the patient or anyone in the family ever attempted suicide?
- Has a family member or significant person in the patient's life ever experienced a similar crisis?
- How has the patient coped with difficult life situations in the past (past medical and psychiatric evaluations, hospitalizations, treatments)?
- Is there a history of any previous neurological disease or dysfunction?

Assess the Patient's Level of Social Support

- To whom does the patient turn in times of stress?
- Who are the people important and accessible in the patient's life at the present time?
- What is the patient's perception of these people's willingness to be involved with the current crisis?
- If the patient is in treatment, what is the patient's perception of the contract, availability, and therapist involvement?
- What is the nature of the home environment?
- What is the nature of the patient's work and social environments?

that permit realistic solutions. Actively listening for verbal cues and watching for nonverbal cues regarding important points and feelings helps communicate interest and compassion. A comprehensive patient assessment in an emergency situation focuses on the patient's stated complaints, your observations regarding level of functioning, and others' reports, for the purpose of developing a succinct and realistic problem statement. Assessing the risk factors described earlier in the chapter provides insight into the factors that contributed to the development of the crisis state. The problem statement is validated with the patient and forms the basis for developing relevant nursing diagnoses.

In a crisis situation, the patient's thoughts become jumbled, and you can become caught up in the patient's anxiety; therefore, pacing the narrative is essential. There is a tendency in emergency situations to make assumptions or to become overactive. Although it is important to ask for clarification to obtain an accurate and complete understanding of the patient's situation, it is critical to not anticipate the story. Because, in the final analysis, only the patient can resolve his or her crisis in his or her own way, it is important that the patient relive the story of the crisis in his or her own way. Moreover, how the patient relates the story and what the patient feels are important provides you with useful information that would not become available through a more programmed approach to information collection.

Active listening strategies, previously identified in Chapter 10, form the basis for gathering data, defining the problem, and identifying personal strengths. When you lack information about a key part of the problem, it is critical to seek clarification by asking for concrete details.

Using the patient's verbal and nonverbal cues to paraphrase and reflect back key ideas and themes helps the patient stay focused and expand on the story. Whenever possible, use the patient's own words in responding because this feedback reinforces the reality of the person describing his or her experience.

Pacing also involves monitoring the patient's statements so that therapeutic suggestions parallel the patient's level of understanding and acknowledgment. For example, the parents of a newly admitted trauma victim may not be ready to hear the full extent of their son's injuries in the initial sessions. It is critical to be aware of and stay with the patient or family's level of readiness and understanding, rather than to impose a suggestion that may be objectively correct but may not be a good "fit" with the patient's perception of the problem or potential solution.

Therapeutic suggestions and verbal interventions should be concise, empathetic, and related only to the crisis, the patient's perceptions, and his or her feelings surrounding the events. This can be done in one or two sentences. Longer explanations are often not heard because of the patient's anxiety. Periodically summarizing what you understand and what you tell the patient reinforces or corrects key points.

The patient's personal strengths help you decide individualized nursing interventions. When a person feels out of control, typically there is limited self-awareness of personal strengths. Building from a person's strengths reinforces the positive elements that are already present as personality characteristics in working with difficult life issues. Strengths might include the ability to communicate thoughts and express feelings, the ability to perform more than one family role, and the willingness to look at the crisis as an opportunity for change.

Working Phase: Diagnosis, Outcome Identification, and Planning

Nursing diagnoses identify the functional deficits found in crisis situations that are amenable to nursing intervention. Box 13-14 presents the North American Nursing Diagnosis Association (NANDA)-approved diagnostic stems for problems commonly experienced by patients in crisis. Once you have enough information to formulate relevant nursing diagnoses, you can direct the conversation toward the concrete difficulties that need to be resolved first. Doing something about the problem

reduces the sense of helplessness. Emphasizing immediate concerns and thinking aloud about issues in need of more immediate resolution versus issues to address later help focus the client and foster self-monitoring of the tasks needed to resolve the crisis (Case Example 13-7).

■ CASE EXAMPLE 13-7
■ Ann's Story

■ Ann Bartholomew is a 19-year-old single woman who has been living with her boyfriend for the past year. She has a part-time job as a stripper in a local bar. Her parents have "disowned" her because they don't approve of her lifestyle, and the money she brings in from her job is insufficient to support her needs. Moreover, Ann is addicted to marijuana and uses cocaine and alcohol on a fairly regular basis.

Ann just found out that her boyfriend has been cheating on her, and she feels that she can't live without him. Her boyfriend accompanied her to the emergency department after finding that she had just ingested a large amount of alcohol and smoked a large quantity of marijuana. Her parents are concerned about her current condition and have agreed to participate in her treatment.

Ann is initially triaged as a medical-psychiatric emer-

Box 13-14 ■ ■ ■ ■ ■
NANDA Diagnostic Stems for Problems Commonly Experienced by Patients in Crisis

Anxiety
Acute Confusion
Altered Nutrition: Less Than Body Requirements
Altered Parenting
Altered Role Performance
Altered Thought Processes
Decisional Conflict (Specify)
Defensive Coping
Dysfunctional Grieving
Energy Field Disturbance
Hopelessness
Impaired Environmental Interpretation Syndrome
Impaired Home Maintenance Management
Impaired Social Interaction
Ineffective Community Coping
Ineffective Denial
Ineffective Family Coping: Disabling
Ineffective Individual Coping
Ineffective Management of Therapeutic Regimen: Community

Ineffective Management of Therapeutic Regimen: Families
Ineffective Management of Therapeutic Regimen: Individuals
Powerlessness
Rape-Trauma Syndrome
Rape-Trauma Syndrome: Compound Reaction
Rape-Trauma Syndrome: Silent Reaction
Relocation Stress Syndrome
Risk for Injury
Risk for Self-Mutilation
Risk for Violence: Self-Directed
Risk for Violence: Directed at Others
Self-Esteem Disturbance
Sensory/Perceptual Alterations (Specify: Visual, Auditory, Kinesthetic, Gustatory, Tactile, Olfactory)
Sleep Pattern Disturbance
Spiritual Distress (Distress of the Human Spirit)

From North American Nursing Diagnosis Association. (1999). *NANDA nursing diagnoses: Definitions and classification 1999-2000.* Philadelphia: NANDA.

gency. She is evaluated as a moderately low suicide risk who can be treated on an outpatient basis once her condition is stabilized. Her suicide risk is increased because of

drug use, but her lack of a plan, her gender, and the willingness of the family to be involved in treatment lower it. The plans for Ann's care are as follows. ■

Nursing Interventions	Rationales
1. As a means of reducing lethality without hospitalization, obtain from Ann a commitment to treatment and a contract that she will not do anything self-destructive.	1. Even though the nurse evaluates Ann as a moderately low suicidal risk, her methods for coping do not give much evidence of prethought, range of options, or constructive problem-solving. The contract will help her think before acting.
2. Prioritize problem areas as a way of helping Ann to distinguish between major and minor life events needing immediate solutions.	2. In crisis situations, most people have trouble prioritizing their problems or taking charge. A sharp focus on the circumstances needing prompt attention reduces the sense of disorganization and makes the problem areas more manageable.
3. Provide direct intervention with the drug abuse problem.	3. Drug abuse enhances the chances of an unintentional suicide and clouds the clarity of thinking needed to resolve the crisis.
4. Set short-term goals directly related to the resolution of specific parts of the identified problem areas.	4. Successfully coping with the manageable parts of the crisis helps patients feel more capable, and the learned coping skills enable them to respond more effectively.
5. Ann's current crisis situation is more intense because of underlying personal and family dynamics that increased her vulnerability. Providing ongoing support to work through these issues will reduce the likelihood of similar crisis episodes.	5. Refer Ann for case management and mobilization of community resources.

Planning care for patients takes into careful consideration the three elements that Aguilera (1994) considered balancing factors: (1) realistic assessment of the crisis event, (2) coping resources, and (3) sources of personal support. For many patients, a realistic perception of the crisis event eludes them. Your role is to help establish some sense of order in the current chaos and to begin to identify appropriate resources. Simple interventions to contact family or to involve community agencies early in the patient's care can greatly reduce anxiety for both patient and family. You can help patients clarify who could be important to them at this time and how to access them appropriately.

The goal of crisis intervention is to restore the patient to precrisis functioning. Goals that the patient finds acceptable, affordable, accessible, and appropriate to the resolution of the crisis are most likely to be successful (Beckingham & Baumann, 1990). You play an important role in structuring interventions that emphasize patient mastery. Crisis intervention depends on developing a mutual understanding of the problem and the strategies most likely to resolve it. Consequently, you need to be aware of the patient's response and should use frequent validation (see Chapter 10) as a listening response strategy. Planning to include the family and other support systems in the resolution of a crisis offers one of the greatest modifiers of unfortunate circumstances. Selection of behavioral tasks should focus first on immediate, present areas of change needed because these most often also affect the final resolution of the crisis situation.

Another consideration is choosing tasks that are easiest for the patient to implement. This strategy provides patients with ready-to-use successful coping strategies and empowers them to risk trying harder tasks. When it is obvious that the patient is not familiar with or able to grasp the entire sequence of events needed to achieve a

goal, a useful strategy is to break goals down into small achievable segments. Steps involved in reaching the proposed solution should fit both the problem and the resources available to the patient.

What do you think? Reread Ann's story. In what ways does a crisis intervention approach differ from an individual therapy approach?

► *Check Your Reading*
36. How does the assessment phase in crisis intervention differ from that in other types of therapeutic relationships?

Implementation

All interventions are deliberately structured to stabilize the patient immediately, with more extensive intervention planned for a later time. Once the problem is defined, you and the patient mutually review possible alternatives; you explore and anticipate potential consequences, then the patient prioritizes all possible decisions that could be undertaken, using the criteria (acceptable, affordable, and accessible). Just as in other relationships with patients, avoid the temptation to tell the patient what to do. Instead, prompt the patient to consider alternatives, pose questions to stimulate broader thinking about a topic, provide information the patient does not have, and simply be emotionally present as the patient struggles with difficult life issues. Unless the patient presents a danger to self or others, the locus of control should remain with the patient. The objective in providing advice is to help the patient postpone impulsive decision-making when he or she is not in full charge of his or her faculties. Your role in the working phase is to take the least directive posture possible and to encourage the patient to identify the best next step. This means looking at what must be done this day or in the next week, rather than focusing on the ultimate outcome. For the patient to have cognitive mastery over the current situation is the overriding goal of successful crisis intervention.

By contrast with purely insight and behavioral interventions, the emphasis in crisis intervention is on developing concrete strategies to reduce the impact of the stressor. Structuring the environment to maximize patient control and to minimize conflict often reduces tension immediately. The object of this intervention is to provide prompt external support to prevent further chaos or to reduce the patient's stress by removing a tangible stressor in the environment. For example, you might take the patient to a quiet, low-stimuli environment. In the community, the simple intervention of encouraging a young mother to engage the babysitting services of a teenager for several hours a day, thereby providing some respite from child care, can make a potential crisis more manageable.

As you become aware of the patient's strengths, it is important to reinforce these strengths. Simple statements such as, "This is difficult, but I think you are capable of coping with it," or encouraging the patient who is berating his or her current coping skills to wait until he or she is in a better position to make realistic judgments about self-worth reframes the current crisis as a temporary setback rather than a permanent condition. Asking questions about how the patient dealt with previous stresses helps the patient recall past mastery of difficult times, and recognizing previous achievements helps sustain motivation when current outcomes are uncertain. Taking credit for managing small tasks in the immediate situation and taking initial steps toward problem-solving encourages the patient to take the best next step.

Encouraging the patient to talk about emotionally charged events generally promotes emotional relief and reduced distress. In crisis, some patients need permission to express their feelings because they feel shameful, whereas others are simply unaware of the feelings being experienced. You can directly state that unusual and disturbing feelings are a normal part of the crisis state and use active listening to help the patients define the issues as they perceive them. It is important not to discourage crying or feeling angry, unless the expression of feelings is out of control or threatening; then, the feelings may need to be harnessed and redirected toward a more productive outcome. Closely related to encouraging expression of feelings is the concept of normalizing feelings. Frequently, people in crisis feel they are "losing it" or "falling apart" because the distress is so great and the feelings are so strange. Your assurance that crisis precipitates a wide range of reactions can be consoling to the patient. Another strategy to help the patient normalize the situation is to focus fully on the immediate problem and to help the patient develop concrete minisolutions for the immediate concerns.

Earlier in the chapter, a realistic perception of the crisis event was identified as a critical balancing factor for resolving a crisis. You can play an important role in correcting distortions by gently guiding patients to consider alternative explanations and in reducing the sense of blame that frequently accompanies a crisis situation. Sometimes, the crisis is intensified by distorted perceptions, fears, and beliefs about its origin and who is responsible for its development. For instance, a patient may take full personal blame for a situation in which he or she may have played a minor part and that was actually caused by many factors.

Another common feeling is helplessness. Also common are perceptions of being a victim destined to be battered by life circumstances. Statements such as, "If I had done it differently, this wouldn't have happened," or "My life is not worth anything unless I have this job [this girlfriend, this promotion]," indicate this feeling. For example, a young man who had done well with a bank as a computer programmer was laid off suddenly. Intellectually, he recognized that he was one of many laid off by the bank in a period of recession. Emotionally, he struggled with the perception that even if you did a wonderful job and gave everything to the organization, you could be eliminated with the stroke of a pen. Although partially correct in his assumption, he narrowed his perception of this critical life event to reflect his sense that he, as an individual, was at fault rather than simply that he was in the wrong place at the wrong time.

Your listening responses help the patient define central concerns and provide him or her with a unique opportunity to challenge the correctness of such assumptions. In implementing this intervention, you need to be aware of psychosocial differences in how people perceive and respond to crisis. Special consideration of difficulties in language, information processing, or cultural norms that interfere with a mutual understanding of the crisis acknowledges human diversity, which is always present in crisis situations. For example, a young Mexican patient told her physician that she slept in the same bed with her father. This "fact" was recorded as an incestuous relationship when, in reality, it was quite common for children to sleep in the same bed as their parents, and the fact was culturally but not pathologically significant.

When a patient exercises defenses in an adaptive manner, it is important to provide an immediate reinforcement that links the behavior with a particular result. For example, you might tell a patient who decided to call the police instead of beating up his disorderly son, as he normally does, "Making that phone call was a really good thing to do. You dealt with the problem without getting yourself in trouble." In this situation, you explicitly link the patient's reframing of a defensive posture as an adaptive response to an outcome that benefits the patient. This may seem obvious, but often patients do not consciously link behavior to outcome, and maladaptive defenses to difficult situations persist, whereas they might not if the new behavior is reinforced so that it becomes a more automatic response.

Maladaptive defenses tend to reinforce the intensity of the crisis. Examples include ego mechanisms that deny, falsify, or distort reality. Although a patient may need to do this initially to buffer the full effect of the crisis, maladaptive defenses in general provide a roadblock to resolving the crisis. This is illustrated in Case Example 13-8.

■ C A S E   E X A M P L E   1 3 – 8
■ Kevin's Story
■

Kevin Waller, age 16, has been arrested for selling cocaine in school. His mother is a single parent who works long hours, and she had been unaware that Kevin has been taking drugs, let alone selling them. She comes to the emergency department in crisis and distraught, but she is convinced that there must be some mistake. Her son is a good boy who would never be involved with something like this. She tells the nurse that she knows he has recently gotten mixed up with some bad friends, and they must have set Kevin up for this to avoid their own involvement. The nurse knows that there is considerable legal evidence to indicate that Kevin has been dealing drugs for some time.

The nurse's approach needs to be sensitive to the mother's need for denial at this time but not supportive of it or encouraging toward it. It is also important for the nurse to make the assessment, as well as the interventions, immediately therapeutic and relevant to the needs of the situation.

At this time, the nurse recognizes that Kevin's mother has limited ability to absorb the shock of her son's arrest. The nurse also recognizes that the mother has limited ability to imagine alternative explanations for either her son's involvement or the resolution of the crisis.

Because a realistic appraisal of the problem is essential to the development of appropriate interventions, the nurse knows that she must address the problem directly and quickly. As a first level of response, the nurse attempts to widen the mother's constricted view of the situation. To rebut the mother's denial, the nurse begins by acknowledging the mother's pain and reframing her current dilemma as a life problem in need of a solution.

"Mrs. Waller, I know this must be a terrible shock for you. It's not uncommon for parents to find out about their children's drug use in just this way. Our job will be to help you make some sense out of what has happened and to look at some ways that we might use this situation as a positive turning point in your family. You say that you know that Kevin has gotten involved recently with bad companions. What has this been like for you?" ■

Note that in the nurse's response, she does not refute Mrs. Waller's description. Instead, she implicitly broadens the implications of Mrs. Waller's findings by suggesting that her experience is not uncommon. Immediately following this suggestion, the nurse moves the discussion toward the ideas of intervention and finding meaning in the event for purposes of assessment and intervention.

The desired outcome in crisis intervention is behavioral change that allows the client to assume some sense of control over his or her life comparable to or exceeding precrisis functioning.

Reinforcement of behavior plays an important role in empowering patients to take charge of their lives. It takes many avenues. For example, it may include behavioral modeling or role playing. You can take the role of an employer or significant family member in helping patients make crucial requests or respond to difficult dialogues. This strategy is particularly helpful in situations in which the predicted responses are likely to be accusatory or rejecting. Direct interventions, such as anticipatory guidance, specific assertiveness training, or behavioral rehearsal, also support desired behaviors.

Basic exploration of the consequences to various choices proves helpful for many patients for two reasons: First, it provides a forum for discovering and resolving cognitive distortions, and second, it helps them problem solve possible objections and consider ways to resolve them. Strategic questions might include

What would happen if you decided to do this instead of . . . ?
What is the worst possible scenario if you decide to do . . . ?
How do you think your husband [wife, parent, friend, boss] will react if you do . . . ?

Depending on the situation, it may be advantageous to point out that change in one person always makes those around them a little uncomfortable, and even a desired change initially can breed objections. This strategy is particularly relevant to use in maturational crisis. Developing alternative strategies in case the first initiative does not work should be the norm rather than the exception in crisis intervention.

Acknowledging the patient's efforts can be as effective as noting successful achievement. It is a particularly important strategy when the expected outcome does not occur, as it frequently does not, the first time around. Efforts can be reworked into the necessary modifications more easily if the patient can see the relationship between the previous efforts and the next step. The nurse's statement in the following example acknowledges the patient's efforts and reframes her concern within the broader context of developing alternative options to resolving her problem.

Nora: "I did as you told me, I asked my husband to come into the crisis center for this appointment, but he refused to come. It's really pretty hopeless. There's no one who can help me at home."

Nurse: "Nora, I know that you would like to get his cooperation, and it took courage to ask him. But I wouldn't look at it as a failure. You may have 'seeded' the idea of help with him, and more important, you were able to say what you needed. That's a new behavior for you that you will need to resolve this situation. Now, let's look at some other options for getting you the help you need."

Termination Phase: Evaluation

Termination dates and goals to be accomplished are established within the first or second contact. Because crisis intervention is of limited duration, time frames should be honored. Crisis intervention strategies always entail a review process that is both self-reflective and planned. It is important for patients to see the significance of their efforts, to articulate sources of social support, and to identify, in closing, not only strategies to reduce stress but also those competencies needed to promote personal well-being. During the final session, you and the patient mutually assess goal accomplishment or lack of attainment. Reasons why certain outcomes occurred during the intervention process are discussed in detail. Particularly relevant are the mention of changes the patient has made in attitude and mastery of coping skills. This discussion fosters further consolidation and internalization of more effective coping strategies. Anticipatory guidance helps the patient foresee future situations that may become problematic.

As you review goal achievement with the patient, it is important to focus on what this event means to the patient and what has been learned from living through the stress. This learning may prove helpful to the patient in the future as other stressful situations are encountered. Included in the formative evaluation is the degree to which the patient seems to be handling feelings associated with the crisis as well as the concrete action steps taken to resolve the crisis. For example, has the patient achieved a reality-based perception and cognitive mastery over the crisis event and surrounding circumstances? Were there earlier unresolved issues that contributed to the development of the current crisis, and, if so, have they been addressed?

The summative evaluation criteria relate to these questions: "Is the patient's basic level of functioning at or above the precrisis state?" "Should this case be closed, or are there other agencies or referrals that should be contacted?" An evaluation of progress helps the patient place the whole sequence of events in a positive perspective and brings closure to an important period in the patient's life. Without attention to the evaluation phase of the nursing process, an excellent assessment and comprehensive, appropriate nursing interventions are rendered ineffective.

Not every crisis situation is resolved satisfactorily within the given time frame. Although the goal of crisis intervention is to enhance the coping skills, effectiveness, and competence of the patient in the short term, individuals may need assessment of potential in the long term to stabilize these adjustment skills. Three identifiable coping patterns usually suggest the need for further treatment.

First, some people seem to cope successfully with a difficult crisis-producing situation for some time and then fall apart. Emotional exhaustion ensues because the person runs out of energy. Or a person in the midst of a crisis develops a physical illness. Patients or family members who appear to be the rock of Gibraltar, able to weather and coordinate all aspects of a crisis situation, are particularly vulnerable to fallout once the crisis is under control.

Second, you might observe a person's attempting to cope with stress by becoming more and more involved with extraneous activities. These activities can become a trap with no exit because the reflective time needed for transformation and growth is missing.

Third, sometimes a person becomes so involved in a crisis situation that everything else in the person's life becomes connected with the crisis. Earlier conflicts resurface and are interwoven with the current circumstances without the person being able to distinguish between past and current history.

Crisis intervention, by definition, is short term, and it is not designed to deal with larger life issues. At the same time, it often pokes at the edges of a personal journey and permits access to a more detailed portrait of self with unbelievable vividness. In the face of crisis, emotional barriers are lifted, and feelings previously denied emerge spontaneously into view. Travel to emotional health and well-being, although still not easy, at least becomes more understandable. Because crisis often offers an opportunity to delve into previously unavailable personal accounts of a journey, you can use it as the springboard for engaging the patient traveler in a deeper search for personal truth. You need to "seize the moment" to provide information that otherwise might fall on deaf ears or to suggest further referral for a more careful review of underlying personality dynamics. Because a relationship between you and the patient now exists, it is easier within the context of the crisis intervention to propose further intervention. An example of a useful way to propose follow-up treatment is as follows: "John, you know we have done some really good work together in getting you stabilized about your wife's decision to get a divorce. But this is a very hard situation for you to deal with, and you probably will continue to have feelings that will come in potentially overwhelming waves at times when you least expect it. I'd like to suggest that you consider making an appointment with _____ for follow-up continuation of your care related to these issues and what to expect as you work through this difficult time in your life."

Establishing the link between the good work accomplished to date and future opportunities for personal growth helps facilitate compliance. If the patient is not interested in follow-up care at this time, you still can furnish written information about resources should the need for further treatment arise.

In most communities, there are social service and legal agencies or services specifically designed to aid the traveler in crisis—and beyond. Community agencies and professionals frequently used as referral resources include private and public social services, police officers, lawyers, physicians, clergy members, school personnel, self-help groups (e.g., Shanti, for AIDS victims; Alzheimer's and related disorders support groups for family members, and financial resource agencies such as Social Security. Giving patients information about resources empowers them and provides them with more leverage in difficult interpersonal situations.

Making referrals is an art. It begins with your knowledge of relevant referral sources and the best ways to access them. By calling different service agencies in the community, you can learn about fees, accessibility, means of contact, and services offered. Giving a phone number to a patient is usually not sufficient. It is not always as easy as it looks to access important referral resources even when your coping skills are intact. For the patient emerging from a crisis, trying to access social services through the general information number and being either put on hold or directed through a maze of different departments is frustrating. A quick call from you can ensure contact when the patient's coping skills are deficient. When more than one agency or professional is involved in the care of the patient, coordination of efforts and frequent contact become essential. Otherwise, the interventions may work at cross purposes or duplicate efforts, which is confusing to the patient and ultimately frustrating for the professionals or agencies involved. Table 13–5 summarizes the do's and don'ts of psychological first aid.

TABLE 13–5 Do's and Don'ts of Psychological First Aid

DO'S	DON'TS
Contact	
Listen carefully	Ignore either facts or feelings
Reflect feelings and facts	Judge or take sides
Communicate acceptance	
Dimensions of the Problem	
Ask open-ended questions	Rely on yes/no questions
Ask person to be concrete	Allow continued abstractions
Assess lethality	Ignore "danger" signs of lethality, violence, or physical emergency
Possible Solutions	
Encourage brainstorming	Allow tunnel vision
Deal directly with blocks	Leave obstacles unexplored
Set priorities	Tolerate a jumble of needs
Concrete Action	
Take one step at a time	Attempt to solve it all now
Set specific short-term goals	Make binding long-term decisions
Confront when necessary	Be timid
Be directive, if and only if you must	Retreat from taking responsibility when necessary
Follow-Up	
Make a contract for recontact	Leave details up in the air, or assume that client will follow through on plan on his or her own
Evaluate actions steps	Leave evaluation to someone else

From Slaikeu, K. (1984). *Crisis intervention: A handbook for practice and research.* ©1984 by Allyn and Bacon. Reprinted by permission.

Although recordkeeping is always important, it is critical that it be accurate and complete as it relates to crisis intervention treatment. The patient record should contain the date and time of admission, interview notes with a precise description of the patient, an initial treatment plan, behavioral notes, treatment, and behavioral responses. Notations regarding physician and family notifications should be made with name, date, time, and response included. A rationale for exceptions to regular protocols should be entered in the documentation. For example, if the patient is not allowed to see his or her family because of impending violence, this reason for postponing the visitation should be written in the nursing notes.

When individuals or families are in crisis, they frequently act irrationally. It is not uncommon for a patient who clearly needs crisis intervention to refuse treatment or to decide he or she wants to leave the treatment center, emergency department, or psychiatric unit before being fully evaluated or against medical advice. Unless the patient is a danger to self or others, he or she must be allowed to leave. It is important, however, not only to discuss with the patient the risks of taking this action but also to record in the patient's chart the nature of the discussion, the patient's response, behaviors noted, and the time and date of departure. Recorded information also should include the names of the physician, social worker, and family members who were notified; the times and date; and their responses. Clearly state that the patient left against medical advice, what instructions were given, if any, and further treatment or referrals suggested.

*W**hat do you think?** What are your personal strengths that help you deal with difficult situations?*

➤ *Check Your Reading*
37. How might the nurse use a patient's strengths in crisis intervention?
38. What is meant by normalizing feelings?
39. What should be included in a nursing documentation for a patient in crisis?

Generic Crisis Intervention in Disasters

Crisis intervention in disaster situations requires a generic rather than individual approach. Generic support as a crisis intervention strategy is based on a public health model and is designed to reach large numbers of individuals in as short a time as possible. Obviously, it is most effective in large-scale disasters and community crisis situations. *Generic support* interventions focus on facilitating needed connections with appropriate agencies, provisions, and basic supplies such as food, water, and shelter to sustain the individual temporarily until more permanent arrangements can be made. Treatment goals emphasize relief for groups rather than individuals.

Providing immediate, tangible relief and training large groups of people to understand the meaning of the crisis and the tasks needed for return to equilibrium are central goals. By contrast with the directive role you assume in individual crisis situations, crisis intervention in large-scale disasters supports the sense of participation by the local citizens. Generic crisis intervention strategies generally are used in disasters in which large numbers of people have experienced loss and disruption. Case Example 13–9 illustrates this approach.

■ **CASE EXAMPLE 13–9**
■ **The Story of a Virginia Flood**

On November 4, 1985, the city of Roanoke, Virginia, experienced a flood that resulted in the deaths of 10 people, left hundreds homeless, and caused an estimated $750 million worth of damage. After this disaster, Mental Health Services of the Roanoke Valley launched a plan to facilitate recovery. The agency immediately distributed educational materials to explain the normal emotional reactions to such a catastrophe. They encouraged people to come and seek help at the Mental Health Center. A program for flood victims and for rescue and medical personnel was organized by a team of specially trained counselors. ■

After the immediate impact of the crisis, when interventions focused on providing basic food, water, and shelter to the caregiver group, your role shifts to strengthening the individual coping strategies of the person or people involved. Young children and the elderly are populations particularly vulnerable to long-standing emotional strain as a result of a disaster. Parents may need particular attention so that they can resume their parental responsibilities as soon as possible. Encouraging children to express their feelings through words, images, or the use of play therapy helps mitigate their anxiety and stimulates their sense of mastery over an incomprehensible situation. Children are particularly susceptible to misinterpretation of events. They may not appear upset, but they are absorbing all of the data surrounding the hazardous event without necessarily being able to understand or integrate it. For example, a 9-year-old girl witnessed the sudden and precipitous death of a favorite grandmother as she went with her in the ambulance to the emergency department. Everyone assumed she was old enough to understand what had happened and undervalued the meaning of the experience for her. Twenty years later, this young woman is unable to enter an emergency department or hospital.

Psychiatric Emergency Services

Psychiatric emergency services often take a proactive community-based approach in the form of mobile crisis teams. These teams are composed of interdisciplinary, specially trained crisis intervention workers. The mobile crisis service functions as an outreach mechanism for people who might not seek treatment under their own initiative. This evaluative emergency psychiatric service provides the initial point of entry into the larger mental health system for patients in psychiatric crisis. Operating around the clock, the mobile crisis team responds to calls in the community and conducts preliminary assessments and first-order interventions in the field for people in crisis with concurrent probable mental illness or situational crisis. Patients served might include a frail elderly patient who refuses to eat, an agoraphobic patient, or a confused schizophrenic patient living in the community.

Usually, it is the family rather than the patient who initiates the request for treatment because either they are unable to provide the required care or the patient is unwilling to consider hospital-based services. Frequently, the person or family requesting the service, in addition to the patient, is in a state of acute crisis. By providing immediate support, reinforcing family strategies, and referring to the appropriate support services, an acute crisis can be reduced and it may be possible to avert the need for rehospitalization of a chronically ill mental patient. Acutely suicidal, homicidal, or intoxicated patients are not treated by the team. This form of alternative mental health services for the patient in crisis is particularly effective for treating transitory psychiatric crisis in the deinstitutionalized mentally ill.

Caring for Yourself

Working with acute crisis situations is emotionally and spiritually draining. For many crisis situations, there are no authoritative or definitive answers to serious life questions. The human carnage and destruction of all that is important to a person's sense of self and well-being, often occurring in a matter of moments, affects the caregiver as well as the victim. There remain existential questions that continue to haunt the crisis worker about their own contributions, the meaning of life, their place in it, and sometimes God's place in it. Careful retrospective analysis of a crisis situation and one's role in helping patients resolve it can reveal its truth and transform its meaning, thereby putting it in perspective.

Nurses actively engaged in crisis work need a formalized mechanism for understanding their reactions to catastrophic events beyond their control. Providing consistent, caring support to people in acute states of emotional disequilibrium demands a steadiness and a balance that simultaneously require understanding and backing from the caregiver. If the crisis affects the individual worker personally as well as professionally, the problem is more complex. For example, a disaster, such as a hurricane or earthquake, can create a role conflict for nurses who are torn between attending to their personal family needs and their professional responsibility to those of the larger community (Stanley, 1990).

Critical Incident Debriefing

With every crisis situation, professional caregivers have fears and discomforts that cannot be addressed in the critical moments of crisis intervention. These feelings need to find their voice once the immediate crisis subsides. Usually, this is best accomplished with a group format. It is important for nurses working with crisis situations to understand that they are not alone with their reactions. What nurses find during postcrisis group recall is that other workers' experiences parallel and echo their own, and this can be reassuring to the individual nurse. There is common recognition that one's own sense of discomfort is embedded in the context of an unfamiliar world in which previously learned coping strategies did not hold up. Although talking about it may not fully resolve a personal ache, the level of discomfort generally is lessened following a **critical incident debriefing.** Talking, expressing feelings, and exploring ways to deal with the feelings are all positive ways to cope with stress and to put it in perspective. The balancing factor of having a designated time and place to talk about the fears and discomforts of working with people in terrible circumstances helps to mitigate the tension and resolve a personal sense of feeling out of control. Moreover, shared experiences and actions broaden nurses' professional framework for understanding and coping with potentially awkward, confusing, and untenable feelings.

A critical incident stress debriefing approach to stress reduction is used with personnel in high-stress settings. This technique was first used informally to reduce the impact of psychological stress casualties among emergency service personnel dealing with war casualties and has been broadly applied across a wide variety of clinical settings. Debriefing after major or cumulative crisis circumstances, such as an unusual number of deaths on a critical care unit, mass casualties, or environmental devastation, is an effective and essential way to reduce collective stress among nursing personnel. The concept can also be used with any group of nurses routinely working with patients to resolve crisis situations in psychiatric and medical settings, for example, with case management, in which crisis situations are compounded by limited resources.

The goals of the debriefing process relate to helping the individual understand what happened from a big picture perspective. The process provides the nurse with a safe place to air feelings, assists the nurse with differentiating between the things that can and cannot be controlled related to resource allocation, reduces the nurse's tension to a workable level, and restores the nurse to precrisis functioning.

Critical incident stress debriefing includes a five-phase format:

1. Fact
2. Thought
3. Reaction
4. Teaching
5. Reentry

In the *fact phase*, each participant is invited to share his or her perception of the incident. As the group members describe the incident, new information and pieces of information are integrated into a more understandable whole.

The *thought phase* builds on this information by asking participants to reflect on the incident and to share what they were feeling personally during different parts of the crisis.

In the *reaction phase*, participants are asked to evaluate the impact of the emotional aspects of the incident (e.g., "What was the worst part of the incident for you?"). Previously undiscussed and less acceptable feelings are allowed to emerge in a safe environment. Knowing that other people experience the same feelings as you do and that those feelings are normal behavioral responses to abnormal circumstances is often a relief to people who work with intense stress and have no place to share their feelings and concerns. Participants discuss stress-related symptoms they had during the incident or are experiencing currently.

The *teaching phase* focuses on specific cognitive, emotional, and spiritual strategies to reduce stress and ways to enhance group support of each other.

In the final *reentry phase*, the facilitator encourages questions designed to put closure on the incident and provides a summary of the process. Individual referrals for further counseling, if needed, are provided at this time (Rubin, 1990).

Conclusions

The role of the psychiatric nurse is a broad one and is not limited to "just talking" to patients and families. The interventions available to the nurse include all the somatic interventions used in traditional medical-surgical units, excellent biopsychosocial and spiritual assessment skills, teaching of "book knowledge," understanding and acceptance of mental illness, skills to manage the illness and restore the individual or family to wholeness, advocacy efforts, case management skills, and discharge planning.

Education about psychiatric illness and how to manage it is one of the most helpful strategies that we can offer patients and families. By increasing their knowledge, we make a direct and lasting impact on their journey; we provide them with the tools and information to make informed decisions, to handle symptoms, to understand their rights and responsibilities, and to journey with a bit more control and choice. By sharing knowledge, we affirm the collaborative and partnership roles we have with patients and families. We are not in charge of the patient's journey; we are more like coaches. We run alongside. We encourage. We challenge, and we support. We affirm, and we stimulate hope.

Because behavioral therapy is based on learning principles, behavioral management techniques are important to the role of the psychiatric nurse as teacher. Psychiatric nurses have roles teaching behaviorist principles to educators, parents, and managers in a great range of fields. For those working within the constraints of today's health care settings, behaviorism can offer short-term interventions for those unable to undergo long-term therapy. For patients who seek techniques for self-management, behavioral strategies can improve the quality of their lives. By focusing on observable actions, health care professionals—and their patients—can achieve measurable results.

Finally, the psychiatric–mental health nurse draws on teaching and other skills in crisis intervention, whether the crisis be a psychiatric emergency involving a drug overdose, a community crisis such as a flood, or a disaster such as a plane crash. In the initial stages of crisis, the psychiatric nurse's role is to stabilize the person, family, or community whose journey is in crisis. Part of the stabilization involves a "coaching" role in discovering effective solutions to the crisis. Later, after stabilization, the psychiatric nurse helps patients in crisis integrate the meaning of the crisis into the story of their life's journey.

Key Points to Remember

- Basic psychiatric interventions include much more than just talking. The psychiatric nurse's repertoire includes many skills: relationship building and supportive interventions; health status assessment and somatic interventions; teaching of self-care knowledge (book knowledge about the illness, medications, and other items) and self-care skills, including coping and problem-solving strategies; strategies to staying spiritually well; behavioral modification techniques; crisis situation interventions; advocacy efforts; case management; and discharge planning.
- The mentally ill person and his or her family need to fully understand the scope of the individual's illness.
- Patient education is an integral part of quality and cost-effective care, and it is the process of deliberately creating cognitive, affective, behavioral, and psychomotor changes.
- The function of education is to develop organized bodies of knowledge and generic problem-solving skills.
- Learning is a dynamic process that incorporates readiness to learn, motivation, acquisition of new knowledge, attitudes and skills, and the resulting ability to change behavior.
- Learning takes place in both formal and informal contexts.
- Principles of learning guide you in carrying out the phases of the educational endeavor.
- Principles of adult learning guide you in developing learning programs that take into account the attributes of the adult learner.
- The educational process involves the following phases: assessment, diagnosis, outcome identification, planning, implementation, and evaluation.
- The educational process begins with a thorough assessment of the learner's needs, learning style, and any obstacles to learning.
- On the basis of assessed information, educational planning proceeds with the identification of the overall goal and long-term outcomes.
- After the overall goal and long-term outcomes are identified, behavioral objectives, which are specific, measurable, and patient centered, are delineated to guide the learning process and set the parameters for the implementation and evaluation phases.
- Succinct activities are set forth to meet the learning behavioral objectives.
- Implementing the plan involves either an individual or a group approach to the learning endeavors.
- Learning activities may include lectures, discussions, question and answer sessions, demonstrations and return demonstrations, self-study programs, workbook assignments, role play, and games. The teaching activity chosen must be best suited for each patient's learning needs, style of learning, and behavioral objectives.
- The last phase of the process is evaluation of how well criteria were met, both for each learning objective and for the overall educational endeavor.
- Retention of information and understanding can be evaluated through direct discussion, observation, or testing.
- Educating patients about mental illness incorporates all of the information about general patient education, taking into account that serious mental illness is debilitating to the patient and the family.
- The mentally ill person may not be capable of making relevant, competent decisions or carrying out problem-solving activities as other patients can.
- The necessary information incorporated into teaching patients about mental illness flows from expressed major concerns.
- The biopsychosocial-spiritual model provides one of the broadest frameworks from which to teach about the many facets of living with mental illness.
- The most relevant content of the biopsychosocial-spiritual model includes information about the nature of mental illness, information about different diagnoses, associated symptoms, probable causes, treatment options, medications, prognosis, coping, and managing stress.
- Behavioral therapy provides a systematic way to examine and change human behavior through manipulation of its antecedents and consequences.
- Target behaviors need to be defined operationally as discrete behavioral actions.
- The Premack principle postulates that a high-frequency behavior (preferred activity) can be especially effective as a reinforcer for a low-frequency behavior (a less preferred activity).
- Reinforcers can be positive or negative, tangible or social. Secondary reinforcers are most effective because they are attached to a number of reinforcers from which the patient can choose.
- Shaping is a technique used by the therapist to reward behaviors that are approximations of the desired behavior and gradually to increase expectations as the patient masters smaller approximations until the goal is met.

- People learn from observation of others as well as from direct behavioral strategies.
- Relaxation strategies, biofeedback, and flooding are important self-management strategies that can be used whenever needed and at relatively low cost.
- Crisis is a time of decision.
- Elements of a crisis include a critical stressor, a vulnerable state, failure of normal problem-solving methods, lack of social supports, and intolerable tension.
- Balancing factors, such as social support, redefining the goals, and a realistic appraisal of the crisis situation, can avert a crisis state.

- A crisis state is not a pathological state.
- A crisis is categorized as situational or maturational.
- Evaluation of lethality is a first-order consideration in assessment in crisis intervention.
- Assessment and intervention strategies are closely linked in crisis intervention.
- Interventions are based on the problem-solving mode, with attention focused on the immediate situation.
- Referral is an important part of crisis intervention.
- A critical incident stress debriefing format provides a formalized opportunity for nurses to gain new understanding and personal awareness of reactions to difficult crisis situations.

Learning Activities

1. Review the detailed content outline in Appendix I. Develop a sample teaching plan for one topic that you would like to present to a patient with whom you are working.
2. What teaching strategies are most effective in facilitating your learning? Why?
3. What is your learning style? On what do you base your conclusion? How would you determine the learning style of a patient with whom you were working?
4. What is your preferred method of accessing information? How do you know this about yourself? How would you assess a patient's preferred method of accessing information?
5. Think back to a time when you confronted a potential crisis. Perhaps it involved the death or illness of a family member, friend, or pet; the suicide of a classmate; the loss of a first love; or a move to a new area. Or perhaps it was an experience that was personally significant to you because it was a first experience. Perhaps it was your 1st day of clinical as a nursing student or maybe your first semester away from home. Next, identify the factors that made the crisis potentially overwhelming and those that helped reduce the sense of crisis. How did you cope? Were you able to talk with sympathetic friends, student support services, or family members who could console and support you?

   Next, share your experience with your classmates and develop a list of the defining characteristics of the crisis and the most successful coping strategies that you discovered. Discuss how these experiences can be used to shape your responses to patients in crisis.
6. Consider the following scenario:
   a. Mr. Terrera has brought his wife to the emergency department because he is worried about her. Their son committed suicide about 3 weeks ago. According to Mr. Terrera, Mrs. Terrera has not been able to sleep and refuses to eat. She says, over and over again, "Why did it have to happen this way?" She cries all the time since her son's death. The couple is Spanish, and Mrs. Terrera does not speak English fluently. Using the strategies presented in this chapter, role play the initial interview in groups of four students. One student should act as observer and provide feedback to the "nurse interviewer."
7. Analyze these scenarios and identify the following for each:
   - Central or immediate problem
   - Contributing factors
   - Obstacles to problem-solving
   - Desired outcomes

   Then, on your own, develop a nursing strategy, including prioritized nursing actions, for each case. Discuss your results in small groups. Come to a consensus as to how you would approach each of the patients, what considerations would be most important, and who should be involved in the treatment process.
   a. Joan Ferrenz is 24 years old. Her mother drove her to the emergency department after Joan told her she had swallowed a significant number of Tylenol pills and drank a fifth of whiskey.
   b. John Taylor was brought by the police to the emergency department. He seems easily distracted and very angry.
   c. Carol Moore is a borderline schizophrenic patient who is well-known to the emergency department staff members. She has just cut her wrists with a knife and appears quite distressed.
   d. Tim Jackson's girlfriend told him she didn't want to see him anymore. He doesn't know how he will live without her and has come to the emergency department complaining of shortness of breath, profuse sweating, and heart palpitations.
8. Identify a behavior that you would like to change. Develop an operational definition of the behavior, and count the number of times you do it in 2 weeks. For example, snacking may be a problem. Keep a journal for 2 weeks and count the number of times a day you snack. Note the times and what you are doing just before you have the urge to snack. Identify what happens after you snack and the consequences of your snacking.
9. Select a complex behavioral outcome, for example, conducting an election for class office, planning a

party, cleaning the house, planning Thanksgiving dinner, or completing an assignment. Specify all of the behavioral components incorporated in the final outcome and order them sequentially as subsets to achieving the goal.

10. Plan a behavioral program to change the specific behavior of a friend, colleague, relative, or yourself.

Specify your observational method and justify its selection. Collect the baseline data over a predetermined period. Identify the desired outcome. Describe the reinforcers and reasons for selection. Consider any negative implications or unexpected consequences. Use behavioral strategies to teach a child a skill.

Critical Thinking Exercises

1. The community health nurse, Ms. Peabody, was making a 10-day follow-up visit to Mrs. Alverez after her abdominal surgery. As Ms. Peabody entered the house, Mrs. Alverez's daughter, Maria, met her at the door stating, "My brother has been shot by a gang member and my mother is dying. Please help us."
   1. What assumptions is Maria making about Ms. Peabody?
   2. What assumptions can Ms. Peabody make about what has happened?
   3. What other information is needed to assess the crisis level accurately?

   Recognizing a crisis situation, Ms. Peabody makes an assessment of everyone's coping behaviors. She notes that Maria is crying hysterically, Mrs. Alverez is lying in bed in a fetal position, and the son who was shot is sitting in his room watching MTV. He does not appear to be hurt.
   4. What conclusions can be drawn about this scene?
   5. How would Ms. Peabody check out her assumptions about this crisis situation?
   6. What alternative interpretation could explain the characters' behavior?

2. Sabrina, a student in her 1st week of the psychiatric clinical, was assigned to Ms. Kim Kenny, a depressed 28-year-old woman. Sabrina noticed in the patient's chart that she had a history of asthma, had smoked for 15 years, and was a waitress in a gambling casino. She decided to do some health teaching with Ms. Kenny. Because this was her third meeting with her, Sabrina felt comfortable approaching her, stating, "Kim, I think you need to stop smoking. I have a lot of good pamphlets that tell you why smoking is bad for you. You, of all people, should know that smoking will only make your asthma worse." Ms. Kenny sat listening as she was told about how bad smoking was. At the end of the talk, Ms. Kenny said, "I know I should stop, but where I work everybody smokes."
   1. Under what assumptions is the student operating in this interaction?
   2. What could she have assumed instead?
   3. Why do you think she made these assumptions?

The next day, Sabrina had a meeting scheduled with Ms. Kenny at 11:00 AM. At 11:30, Ms. Kenny ran up to Sabrina, apologizing for being late. It seems that one of the other patients was showing her how to make an ashtray in ceramics class.
   4. Make sense out of the data.
   5. What conclusions can you draw about Ms. Kenny's readiness to stop smoking?
   6. Suggest other approaches. Might they have had a different result?

3. Ms. Trudy Henry, a student nurse, has just learned about behavioral conditioning therapy in her psychiatric nursing class. Two days earlier, Trudy found a young kitten in the parking lot of her apartment building that was very thin and looked as though it had not eaten for days. When she offered it food, the cat attempted to bite her. She managed to feed the animal and gave it shelter in her home without getting bitten. She noticed that any time that she attempted to touch the cat (which she named Nipper) for any reason, it used a biting movement with its jaw but did not inflict harm. She wondered if biting was Nipper's means of relating. Armed with her new knowledge about behavioral conditioning, Trudy set out to test her hypothesis and to make a plan to decrease the biting.
   1. What assumptions is Trudy making about Nipper's behavior?
   2. What assumptions is Trudy making about behavioral conditioning?
   3. What are possible ways that she could test her assumptions?

Trudy's plan was this: "Each time Nipper attempts to bite, I will hold and stroke his back, gently touch his nose, and say to him in a soft quiet tone, 'you're such a beautiful kitty cat.'" Trudy decided against spanking him on the tail with a newspaper each time he attempted to bite.
   4. What evidence does the reader have to determine Trudy's understanding of behavioral conditioning?
   5. What alternative approaches, using behavioral conditioning concepts, could be considered?
   6. What conclusions can the reader draw from the above data?

Additional Resources

Basics of Cognitive Therapy

http://mindstreet.com/cbt.html

*The Beck Institute for Cognitive Therapy
and Research*

http://www.beckinstitute.org/

Crisis, Grief, and Healing

http://www.webhealing.com

*Midwest Center for the Treatment of Stress
and Anxiety*

106 North Church Street
Suite 200
P.O. Box 205
Oak Harbor, OH 43449
800-944-9428 (information)
800-944-9496 (customer information)
800-515-1133 (support services)
http://www.attackinganxiety.com

Offers *Attacking Anxiety and Depression: A Self-
Help, Self-Awareness Program.*

References

Aguilera, D. (1994). *Crisis intervention: Theory and methodology* (7th ed.). St. Louis, MO: Mosby-Year Book.

Aguilera, D. C., & Messick, J. M. (1974). *Crisis intervention: Theory and methodology.* St. Louis, MO: C. V. Mosby.

American Nurses Association. (1994). *Standards of psychiatric mental health clinical nursing practice.* Washington, DC: American Nurses Association Press.

Arnold, E. (1999). Health teaching in the nurse-client relationship. In E. Arnold & K. Boggs (Eds.), *Interpersonal relationships: Communication skills for nurses* (3rd ed.). Philadelphia: W. B. Saunders.

Bandura, A. (1971). *Social learning theory.* New York: General Learning Press.

Bandura, A. (1986). *Social foundations of thought and action.* Englewood Cliffs, NJ: Prentice-Hall.

Bassett, L. (1997). *Attacking anxiety and depression: A self-help, self-awareness program for stress, anxiety & depression.* Oak Harbor, OH: Midwest Center for Stress and Anxiety.

Beckingham, A., & Baumann, A. (1990). The aging family in crisis: Assessment and decision making models. *Journal of Advanced Nursing, 15,* 782-787.

Bisbee, C. (1991). *Educating patients and families about mental illness: A practical guide.* Rockville, MD: Aspen.

Bloom, B., & Krawnthol, D. (1984). Taxonomy of educational objectives: The classification of educational goals. In *Cognitive domain* (Handbook I). New York: Longman.

Caplan, G. (1964). *Principles of preventive psychiatry.* New York: Basic Books.

Caplan, G. (1974). *Support systems and community mental health: Lectures on concept development.* New York: Behavioral Publications.

Cardell, R., & Horton-Deutsch, S. (1994). A model for assessment of inpatient suicide potential. *Archives of Psychiatric Nursing, 8,* 366-372.

Carrieri-Kohlman, V., Douglas, M. K., Gormley, J. M., & Stulbarg, M. S. (1993). Desensitization and guided mastery: Treatment approaches for the management of dyspnea. *Heart & Lung, 22,* 226-234.

Daley, D., Bowler, K., & Cahalane, H. (1992). Approaches to patient and family education with affective disorders. *Patient Education and Counseling, 19,* 163-174.

DeCoux, V. (1990). Kolb's Learning Style Inventory: A review of its applications in nursing research. *Journal of Nursing Education, 29,* 202-207.

Erikson, E. H. (1963). *Childhood and society.* New York: Norton.

Erikson, E. H. (1968). *Identity, youth, and crisis.* New York: Norton.

Hillard, J. (1990). *Manual of clinical emergency psychiatry.* Washington, DC: American Psychiatric Press.

Holmes, T. H., & Rahe, R. H. (1967). The social readjustment rating scale. *Journal of Psychosomatic Research, 11,* 213-218.

Jacobson, E. (1938). *Progressive relaxation.* Chicago: University of Chicago Press.

Kleeman, K. (1989). Families in crisis due to multiple trauma. *Critical Care Nursing Clinics of North America, 1*(1), 25.

Lazarus, A. (1976). *In the mind's eye.* New York: Rawson.

Lindemann, E. (1944). Symptomatology and management of acute grief. *American Journal of Psychiatry, 101,* 151-158.

Melick, M., Logue, J., & Frederick, C. (1982). Stress and disaster. In L. Goldberger & S. Breznitz (Eds.), *Handbook of stress: Theoretical and clinical aspects.* New York: Free Press.

Miller, W., & C'deBaca, J. (1994). Quantum change: Toward a psychology of transformation. In T. Heatherton & J. Weinberger (Eds.), *Can personality change?* Washington, DC: American Psychological Association.

Moller, M. D., & Murphy, M. F. (1997). The three r's rehabilitation program: A prevention approach for the management of relapse symptoms associated with psychiatric diagnosis. *Psychiatric Rehabilitation Journal, 20*(3), 42-48.

Moller, M. D., & Murphy, M. F. (1998). *Recovering from psychosis: A wellness approach.* Nine Mile Falls: Psychiatric Rehabilitation Nurses.

Ost, L. G., Westling, B. E., & Hellstrom, K. (1993). Applied relaxation, exposure in vivo and cognitive methods in the treatment of panic disorder with agoraphobia. *Behavioral Research Therapy, 31,* 383-394.

Premack, D. (1965). Reinforcement theory. In D. Levine (Ed.), *Nebraska symposium on motivation* (pp. 123-180). Lincoln, NE: University of Nebraska Press.

Redman, B. (1993). *The process of patient education* (7th ed.). St. Louis, MO: C. V. Mosby.

Scholing, A., & Emmelkamp, P. M. G. (1993). Cognitive and behavioural treatments of fear of blushing, sweating or trembling. *Behavioral Research Therapy, 31,* 155-170.

Silber, K. P., & Haynes, C. E. (1992). Treating nailbiting: A comparative analysis of mild aversion and competing response therapies. *Behavioral Research Therapy, 30*(1), 15-22.

Skinner, B. F. (1953). *Science and human behavior.* New York: Macmillan.

Slaikeu, K. (1984). Crisis intervention: A handbook for practice and research. Boston: Allyn and Bacon.

Stanley, S. (1990). When the disaster is over: Helping the healers to mend. *Journal of Psychosocial Nursing and Mental Health Services, 28*(5), 12-16.

Thorndike, E. (1913). *Educational psychology: The Psychology of Learning.* New York: Teachers College Press.

Travelbee, J. (1969). *Intervention in psychiatric nursing: Process in the one-to one relationship.* Philadelphia: F. A. Davis.

Tyhurst, J. (1957). The role of transition states—including disasters—in mental illness. In *Symposium on preventive and social psychiatry.* Washington, DC: Walter Reed Army Institute of Research.

Uomoto, J. M., & Brockway, J. A. (1992). Anger management training for brain injured patients and their family members. *Archives of Physical Medicine and Rehabilitation, 73,* 674-679.

Vanderhorst, K., & Carson, V. B. (1998). Outcomes in psychiatric home care for children and adolescents. *The Journal of Care Management, 4*(4), 54, 57-60.

Williamson, J. (1990, Summer/Fall). Reaching children at greatest risk. *Child World, 35,* 65-69.

Suggested Readings

Moller, M. D., & Murphy, M. F. (1997). The three r's rehabilitation program: a prevention approach for the management of relapse symptoms associated with psychiatric diagnosis. *Psychiatric Rehabilitation Journal, 20*(3), 42-48.

Moller, M. D., & Murphy, M. F. (1998). *Recovering from psychosis: A wellness approach.* Nine Mile Falls: Psychiatric Rehabilitation Nurses.

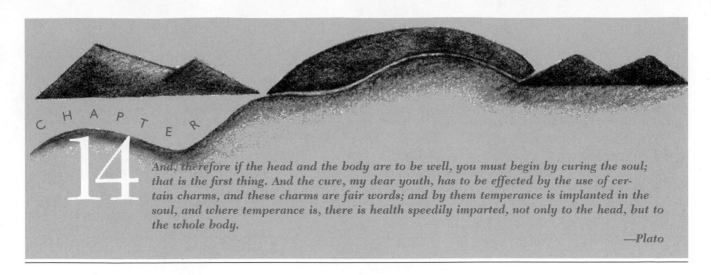

Advanced Therapeutic Interventions

Learning Objectives

After studying this chapter, you should be able to:

1. Compare and contrast brief and long-term approaches to individual therapy.
2. Describe the major components of brief psychotherapy.
3. Identify the primary tenets of cognitive behavioral psychotherapy.
4. Define the essential components of two family frameworks.
5. Describe the family therapy process.
6. Specify the use and components of the genogram as a tool in family therapy.
7. Identify the stages of group development.
8. Characterize leader and co-leadership functions.
9. Contrast inpatient and outpatient group psychotherapy.
10. Describe the essential elements of psychodrama.

Key Terminology

Adjourning phase
Anxiety
Automatic thinking schema
Boundaries
Brief psychotherapy
Catharsis
Cognitive behavioral psycho-
    therapy
Cognitive distortions
Core beliefs

Differentiation of self
Emotional cut-off
Emotional reactivity
Equifinality
Family
Family projection process
Forming phase
Genogram
Group dynamics
Group process

Group-specific norms
Heterogeneous groups
Homeostasis
Homogeneous groups
Insight
Multigenerational transmis-
    sion
Norming phase
Norms
Performing phase

Psychodrama
Psychotherapy
Self-differentiation
Self-understanding
Sibling position
Storming phase
Subsystems
System
Triangles
Universality

Portions of this chapter were adapted from chapters from the last edition contributed by Marcia Cooley, PhD, RN, CS-P, and Suzanne Sayle Jimerson, MS, RN, CS-P.

Advanced practice psychiatric nursing continues the journey and builds on the basic interpersonal theory and skills described in the 1950s by Hildegard Peplau. Rooted in the latest knowledge of professional nursing, neurobiology, psychopharmacology, and human development across the life span, advanced nursing interventions are designed to help mentally ill patients and their families cope more effectively with difficult emotional problems. This chapter focuses on specific specialized treatment modalities that the psychiatric nurse with an advanced degree and extensive clinical experience in the specialty uses in a variety of clinical settings.

Advanced practice nursing requires the clinician to be a registered nurse, to hold a master's degree, and to have significant work experience in the nursing clinical specialty. To practice in psychiatric nursing as a clinical specialist, the advanced practice nurse must meet specific practice requirements, have additional post-master's supervision, and pass a national certification examination in adult or in child and adolescent psychiatric mental health nursing prepared by the American Nurses Credentialing Center (ANCC).

As mental health care moves into the community, psychiatric nurses may consider expanded options in integrated primary health care as psychiatric primary care nurse practitioners (NPs). Psychiatric primary care NPs are educationally and experientially equipped to meet the complex primary and specialized care needs of mentally ill patients. Advanced practice nurses have the unique opportunity to provide a continuum of mental health services through dual pathways: the psychiatric primary care NP and the clinical specialist in psychiatric mental health nursing.

Although national certification is required for third-party reimbursement of psychiatric mental health services, each state, through legal statute and the state board of nursing, determines the scope of practice for advanced practice nurses in their state. Depending on specific state regulations, the advanced practice nurse in psychiatric nursing may be licensed as an NP or as a clinical specialist. For example, an advanced practice nurse in Maryland is licensed as a clinical specialist without prescriptive privileges. In Washington, D.C., only a few miles away, the same nurse is licensed as an NP with prescriptive privileges. Many states grant advanced practice psychiatric nurses authority to prescribe psychotropic drugs.

Advanced practice nurses licensed as clinical specialists function as independent practitioners. NPs in psychiatric nursing practice collaboratively with a physician with a legal written agreement. Both psychiatric primary NPs and clinical specialists can provide psychotherapy, typically in one or more of three formats: brief individual, family, or group therapy. The advanced practice nurse functions as a therapist within one or more of the therapeutic modalities presented in this chapter.

PSYCHOTHERAPY

Psychotherapy is often called the "talking cure" because of its dependence on verbal interaction. Talking about difficult emotional situations with a competent and understanding therapist has helped many patients and families develop a better understanding of their symptoms and more effective coping mechanisms. Psychotherapy was originally developed by Freud and his colleagues in the 19th century as a long-term intervention to correct early psychological trauma and facilitate personality change; however, trends in psychiatry have forced psychotherapy into a time-limited structure. The goals of **brief psychotherapy** are to help patients overcome or modify feelings, behaviors, and thoughts that are interfering with their meeting personal goals. Brief psychotherapy models narrow the goal of personality change to focus on specific behavioral conflicts or issues that can be treated successfully in a short period. Case Example 14–1 is about Peggy, who came to a clinical nurse specialist hoping for relief from her pain and suffering.

■ **CASE EXAMPLE 14–1**
■ **Peggy's Story**

For months, Peggy had been struggling with a kind of drowning feeling mixed with anxiety that made her feel irritable and mean, a view shared by her peers who found her behavior difficult. During these months, there were times when she couldn't get out of bed in the morning to attend her college classes. She wasn't doing well in most of her subjects and found it difficult to concentrate. Peggy was the first in her family to go to college, and she really wanted to succeed. Oh, she could just hear her mother yelling at her, "Who do you think you are anyway? Good enough to go to college—huh." Peggy found it difficult to be interested in much of anything in college and didn't even want to play tennis, which was something she used to like very much. Over the past few months, she had gained a significant amount of weight, and she felt that she looked ugly with the added weight. She had begun to abuse alcohol.

Peggy wasn't sure what this appointment could do for her except make her more anxious and irritable. She had to wait 2 weeks between the phone call and the appointment. Her roommates made her call because they said she was unbearable; they were tired of it and were considering asking her to move somewhere else. She had punched a wall once, and she stayed in her room a lot lately, often drinking beer, smoking cigarettes, and not wanting anything to do with her roommates. Peggy wondered what talking to someone would help—she couldn't possibly tell this nurse everything! If she did, the nurse wouldn't want anything to do with her anyway. Besides, she herself didn't even know what everything was. What if the nurse laughed at her? ■

HISTORY OF PSYCHOTHERAPY

As the quote that opens this chapter indicates, ancient scholars recognized that talking could bring about psychological healing. Early theorists thought that the emotions were controlled by the lunar cycles (thus, the term *lunacy* to describe mental illness). Individuals were reluctant to recognize and take responsibility for their personal feelings. As civilization progressed, blame for mental illness went from celestial bodies to magical fluids such as black bile, to spirits, and to the devil. Mental illness was often considered a permanent affliction, and those who suffered were often condemned to die or imprisoned in dungeons for life. Some were hanged for practicing witchcraft or burned for sorcery or committing acts directed by the devil (Brigham, 1994). An initial paradigm shift (moving from one thought system to another) about the origins of emotions came from St. Augustine, an early leader of the Christian church. He believed psychological self-understanding was a pathway to changing behaviors by first changing inner values (Alexander & Selesnick, 1968).

Toward the end of the 19th century, Freud changed the landscape of theoretical thinking about mental illness by attributing its origin to faulty relationships from early in life that continued to plague a person. According to Freud, it was important to systematically explore a person's early life experiences—a process that was expensive and could take several years of daily or three times a week visits—for full memory recall of childhood experience. The causes of mental illness were still considered to be external, the faulty relationships the child was exposed to early in life. The role of the physician was to observe these memories and to guide the patient toward understanding his or her influence on present behavior. Because the therapist did not react the way an early dysfunctional caretaker did, the patient was free to respond in a different manner. The therapist guided the patient, through careful observations and questions, to an understanding, called **insight,** into how his or her early childhood experiences were influencing present difficulties. With these insights, the patient was able to "unhook" himself or herself from these past defense mechanisms and was able to begin exploration of more satisfying ways of relating to others. The relationship with the therapist—a neutral, caring, sounding board—was considered healing in and of itself (Strachey, 1958).

We know that the etiology of mental illness is multifactorial—a combination of biological factors, multiple life stressors, social factors, and spiritual distress that encourage the development of dysfunctional behavioral symptoms. The discovery that biological factors are implicated in the development of mental illness forced a reappraisal of the value of psychotherapy as a primary treatment modality. This, with the observation that new and effective psychotropic drugs with fewer side effects seemed to have a favorable effect on emotional and mental symptoms, encouraged a revised understanding of mental illness as having a biological rather than a psychological origin. For a short time, it seemed the decade of the brain's biological and pharmaceutical focus would eclipse psychotherapy as the treatment of choice for mental illness. There was little question that medication shortened treatment, but it became clear that the patients who most successfully modified psychological symptoms combined psychotherapy with medication. It also became clear, with the success of shorter time frames for psychotherapy, that biological interventions facilitated the success of brief therapeutic interventions, resulting in impressive positive clinical outcomes.

Then came managed care, in which a third party (the insurance company) outside the therapist-patient relationship became an overseer of the treatment process. Payment for therapy, including initial evaluation, became subject to this third-party approval. The evolution of brief psychotherapy occurred as much from economic constraints as from clinical issues. As Puskar (1996) observed, "psychiatric nursing does not have the luxury of providing long-term therapy to patients whose insurance only covers 20 sessions" (p. 6).

Other sociopolitical factors affecting the delivery of mental health care include the deinstitutionalization of the mentally ill; the movement of health care, in general, toward short-term community-based interventions; and the preventive focus of intervention. Combined, these factors have led to a significant paradigm shift in the treatment of mental illness and significant implications for advanced practice psychiatric nursing.

Patients must be in a severe psychiatric crisis to gain admission to an inpatient setting. They move rapidly through assessment, stabilization, and discharge planning—sometimes within hours or days. Stabilization of the acute symptoms rather than the psychodynamic issues underlying the acute symptoms becomes the focus of the hospital stay. Symptoms that indicate the patient is harmful to self or others are aggressively treated; behavioral issues are identified in the inpatient setting and treated superficially by teaching patients coping skills and by carefully planning for follow-up.

Leibenluft and Goldberg (1993) presented guidelines for short-term inpatient therapies. They viewed hospitalization as only the beginning stage of recovery and envisioned more in-depth work as taking place in outpatient therapy. Discharge planning for short-term inpatient therapy takes on a high priority and focuses on four areas (McGihon, 1994):

1. Medication compliance
2. Symptom recognition and management
3. Relapse prevention
4. Follow-up treatment plan

Knowing how to move a patient through a community-based psychiatric care continuum is also important. Table 14–1 displays some of the differences between long-term and short-term psychotherapy.

What do you think? Should managed care companies dictate therapeutic interventions? Defend your answer.

► *Check Your Reading*

1. What qualifications does the psychiatric advanced practice nurse need to practice?
2. Why is psychotherapy called the talking cure?
3. What was Freud's role in the development of psychotherapy?

TABLE 14–1 Comparison of Short-Term and Long-Term Therapy	
SHORT-TERM THERAPY	**LONG-TERM THERAPY**
Patient seeks change in the presenting problem.	Patient seeks major personality change.
Therapist sees the patient as healthy.	Therapist sees the patient as ill.
Therapy reinforces strengths and teaches new behaviors.	Therapy is the most important part of the person's life.
Therapy is helpful during specific times of life.	Therapy is ongoing over a long period.
Patient works toward goals outside therapy sessions.	Patient brings memories to the session to work through during sessions.
Therapist is active and presents ideas.	Therapist is a listener, reflector, and questioner.
Goals of therapy are mutually defined.	Goal of therapy is determined by the therapist.
Termination time is known.	Termination time is unknown.

Adapted from Budman, S., & Gurman, A. (1988). *Theory and practice of brief therapy.* New York: Guilford Press.

4. What factors influence the development of brief therapy models?
5. Name the priority areas in discharge planning.

BRIEF INDIVIDUAL PSYCHOTHERAPY

Individual brief psychotherapy models are designed as action-oriented, present-focused, structured, time-limited interventions. Although the specific emphasis varies, these models use solution-focused techniques to help patients resolve core conflicts; the goal is for the patients to return to their premorbid state of functioning in a short period. Strategies are designed to help patients gain insight quickly and take concrete action to resolve targeted issues (Mann, 1973). Therapy draws from more than the relationship between therapist and patient. It can include joint sessions with significant others and use of time outside the therapy session for homework assignments. Other strategies incorporate role playing, recognizing and promoting patient strengths, and expecting patients to assume primary roles in their therapy. Therapists often ask patients to learn more about their problems outside their sessions through reading assignments and by attending community support groups and classes on themes such as stress management and assertiveness.

Brief therapy models use the patient's strengths and existing resources to facilitate change and alleviate the presenting problems. The therapist views the patient as basically well but at a point in life's journey at which new behaviors need to be learned. The therapeutic approach underscores the positive attributes a patient brings to therapy; facilitates development of a working partnership between the nurse and the patient; helps the patient develop future-oriented, positively worded goals; and identifies actions necessary for reaching those goals (Mason, 1994). The advanced practice nurse functions as the patient's professional partner, bringing to the therapeutic situation a theory-based knowledge of psychology and nursing. With this knowledge, the therapist often teaches the patient about the nature of his or her mental illness and offers suggestions about new ways of handling symptoms. With knowledge of the patient's history and current problem, the therapist defines, along with the patient, the goals for treatment and the approximate length of time needed to reach these goals. The therapist actively presents ideas for change and expects the patient to be motivated and to use these ideas outside the therapy session. Brief therapy models offer the therapist the flexibility to try different ideas and therapeutic techniques and the opportunity to plan therapy sessions for times when the sessions most benefit the patient. For example, the therapist might schedule sessions at progressively lengthened times.

Process

Assessment

Initial contact with the patient sets the stage for what will happen throughout the therapy process. In the first session, the therapist identifies and clarifies with the patient a central issue or core conflict that they can focus on in therapy. The therapist listens to the patient tell his or her story and what he or she has used to date to cope with the issue or conflict. The therapist conceptualizes the patient's difficulty compassionately in terms of the emotional pain it creates for the patient. At the same time, the therapist emphasizes the patient's *being* in the world versus *being* in therapy. Brief therapy models are task oriented in that they require the patient to *do* something to cope more effectively with the central issue or core conflict.

As a therapist, knowledge about health care from biological, psychological, social, cultural, and spiritual domains allows him or her to consider the patient from a unique holistic perspective. The wholeness of that view empowers both the patient and the nurse to reach for higher levels of wellness. The nurse brings to the initial interview a high degree of respect for human potential, recognizing that each encounter with a patient is an opportunity for growth for the patient as well as for the nurse.

Identifying the central issue is extremely important in the first session. The therapist listens to the presenting problem with utmost care and concern using integrated open-ended questions such as the following:

Has this problem ever occurred before?
Does this problem feel familiar to you?
What have you tried to do to make this better?

What has worked for you in the past when you have been faced with a difficult issue?

After listening to the patient's presenting problem and gathering a preliminary patient history, the therapist follows with a short explanation of the expected roles of the therapist and patient in the therapy process. The therapist explains that he or she will help the patient understand problems and come up with ideas to alleviate them but that it will be up to the patient to take an active part in the therapy process in order to make it work.

■ PEGGY'S STORY CONTINUES

When Peggy left her first session with the nurse therapist, she was amazed at how different this nurse was from what she expected. The nurse said that therapy would involve a lot of planning between them, and she asked Peggy to prioritize her problems. Peggy decided that not being able to get out of bed several times a month was highest on the list. Then she said that she wanted to work on her relationship with men because there was one guy at her part-time job whom she thought she might like. She also said that she would like to feel friendlier toward her family.

With these problems outlined, she and the nurse established goals. Together, they decided one goal would be that Peggy could choose to stay in bed 1 weekend day per month, with the understanding that she would get up on all other days at a prescribed time. To reach that goal, Peggy needed to do several things. First, she needed to establish consistent bedtime rituals and not have any caffeine after noon. Then she needed to start exercising every other day. The nurse gave Peggy some articles on exercise, caffeine, and sleep. The nurse told her how sleep deprivation affects mental health. The nurse said that if these ideas did not help, she might be able to temporarily prescribe some medication to help Peggy sleep. All of that happened in the first session. The nurse invited her to call if anything came up and said that they would work on making goals for her other high-priority problems in future sessions. She suggested they meet every other week so that Peggy would have time between sessions to work on her goals. ■

Outcome Identification

Outcome identification takes place in the first session. Once the core conflict is clear to both patient and therapist, the next step is to ask the patient what he or she wishes would happen to solve the problem. Referred to as the "miracle question"—What would happen if you woke up tomorrow and no longer had this problem?—the answer to this question gives the therapist an idea of how realistic the perceived solution is likely to be. It also can reveal how powerless the patient feels about the problem and what strengths the patient can bring toward alleviating the problem. This information gives the therapist an idea of how the patient views

a therapeutic partnership as well as how severe or chronic the patient's problem is.

Together, the therapist and the patient plan goals for therapy. To establish realistic outcomes, the therapist and patient need to think of specific behaviors that the patient will recognize if the goal is met. For example, if Peggy indicates that her goal is to get rid of her anxiety, the therapist might help her to recast her goal into behavioral terms:

• Be able to stay focused on and finish one school report before starting another rather than having six uncompleted reports.
• Be able to sleep through the night.

Throughout the therapy process, the therapist and patient evaluate whether these treatment goals are being met or need to be revised.

Once the goals of therapy are decided, the patient and therapist can work on the patient's central issue. The therapist may ask the patient to prioritize which elements should be addressed first. Concentrating on the central issue helps the patient keep focused and raises his or her awareness of the complex conflicts embedded in the central issue. The patient must be aware that making this kind of a change may require additional work outside the therapy session and that such work may be hard and emotionally painful.

During the first session, the therapist discusses the endpoint for therapy and what can be achieved regarding the patient's central issue within the time-limited nature of managed care treatment. The practical side of the therapy needs to be discussed, such as telephone calls, session lengths, lateness, billing procedures, missed appointments, and vacations. Also, the patients need to be told what they should do if they cannot reach the psychotherapist in an urgent or emergency situation. These issues need to be addressed in family and group therapy as well.

Planning and Intervention

To use a brief therapy model effectively, the therapist must be able to fully engage the patient as a partner throughout the healing process. Often, an analogy about a commonly understood medical problem, such as diabetes, helps guide the patient toward understanding his or her role. For example, after patients are diagnosed with diabetes, they are taught about the disease, how to monitor some aspects of life, and how diabetes affects the body. Most notably, patients may need to check their blood sugar levels throughout the day and respond to abnormal levels with dietary changes. The dietary changes are individualized and necessary to achieve normal blood sugar levels. If blood sugar levels do not return to normal, medication may be indicated.

The homework patients do throughout the therapeutic journey is analogous to monitoring blood sugar levels but involves monitoring moods and modifying behaviors to promote the return of the patient's mental health to normal. If a patient's mental health problems are severe due to internal chemical imbalances or do not respond to the patient's attempts to change, psychopharmacology may be indicated. Again, the analogy with the diabetic patient can be helpful, explaining that sometimes the only way for blood sugar levels to remain within normal limits is through chemical intervention.

During each session, the therapist checks in with the patient regarding homework completion and plans for the next step. Homework tasks related to coping more effectively with the core conflict or central issue help maintain continuity between sessions and reinforce the idea that working on problems in the context of the world is more important than simply working on them in the therapy session.

If homework is not completed, the therapist explores why. Sometimes, the assigned homework is not appropriate but the patient agreed to it to win the approval of the therapist. Other times, the patient does not perceive the assignment as relevant or may not really be ready to make the needed change. Talking about what went wrong and making needed modifications are essential. The therapist-patient relationship should change the patient's life in positive ways that both participants can identify.

One key to short-term therapy is the personal and interpersonal strengths that patients use to help them meet their own needs and live a satisfactory life (de Shazer et al., 1986). Noting strengths helps the therapist choose the most appropriate ways to meet treatment goals; the therapist analyzes which brief therapy techniques the patient would view as helpful and in what ways they would build on the patient's strengths. For example, Peggy's awareness that something is wrong and her motivation to seek therapy are personal strengths. Because Peggy is engaging in the therapeutic process even though she fears it makes the therapist realize that Peggy is willing to take interpersonal risks.

The therapist treating Peggy in brief therapy might supplement the sessions by having Peggy read about anxiety, teaching her relaxation techniques, or encouraging her to take a class on stress management. Written exercises designed to help Peggy observe herself and the anxiety-producing environments are helpful. As the therapist thinks of ways to help the patient in the journey toward the goals, the duration and frequency of sessions become more infrequent. Often, the initial two or three visits are weekly. Later, the visits may become biweekly and then monthly. The longer time between sessions coincides with the patient's learning what must be done outside the sessions to promote mental health.

Pharmacologic Intervention

Peggy's mood disorder may be severe enough that there is a chemical imbalance that medication can help to bring within normal limits. Some states allow an advanced practice nurse in psychiatric nursing to prescribe psychotropic medications. Prescription writing has allowed these nurse therapists to provide holistic rather than fragmented care under a written collaborative agreement with a physician. Helping the patient choose psychopharmacology, decide the right dosage, and mon-

itor side effects, if any, all are part of the helping relationship between the advanced practice nurse and the patient. Often, the ability to prescribe helps the patient on a short-term basis and is necessary to understand the patient better. For instance, if a patient comes in complaining of sleep deprivation as a presenting problem, it is difficult to obtain an adequate history and mental status because sleep deprivation itself causes lack of focus, irritability, decreased concentration, hypervigilance, and sometimes confusion. If the therapist can help the patient sleep with 2 or 3 nights of psychopharmacology, a much more accurate assessment can then be done.

Termination

Termination of brief therapy is predetermined—usually, there are no more than 20 sessions. Termination can occur before this predetermined time if the mutually defined goals are reached, and it sometimes occurs because the insurance company mandates a shortened time frame. Often, work on the presenting problem has a positive effect on other areas of the patient's life. Termination is an opportunity to review acquired behaviors and to plan with the patient how these behaviors can be used in the future to enhance the patient's overall health. There is understanding between the therapist and the patient that there may be other points in the patient's life, such as periods of high stress or times of developmental transitions, when the patient may need a mental health consultant to maximize health potential. The patient is welcome to return. Because the door is left open for the patient to return and because the relationship with the therapist is one of mutuality, termination often does not bring up strong feelings of loss and abandonment as it may in long-term therapy.

There is little question from personal anecdotes that patients find brief individual therapy helpful, but more evidence-based clinical outcome research studies are needed to validate this methodology in the treatment of mentally ill individuals (Crits-Christoph, 1992).

■ PEGGY'S STORY ENTERS A NEW ■ CHAPTER

As Peggy continued to define her goals and, with the nurse's help, to find ways to meet them, she became more self-confident and better able to see how she could have control over many things in her life. With her new boyfriend, for instance, her goal was to move slowly in the relationship and to avoid using alcohol as a crutch to help her feel more comfortable. With the nurse, she was able to role play to tell her boyfriend about herself without needing alcohol to calm her anxiety. When the time came, although she was nervous, she did it. She found herself hanging out less and less with her old buddies who drank. She discovered that what she really wanted to do was help disadvantaged kids like herself who do not feel loved while growing up. She switched her major at school to emphasize child health. As a part-time job, she worked in a home for emotionally disturbed children.

Peggy was now meeting with the nurse only once a month. They had a total of 12 sessions (plus a few phone calls). The nurse felt that Peggy had good solutions to her problems if she would give herself time to problem solve and continue to identify and define her personal needs. At the last session, the nurse suggested that perhaps a break in therapy would be appropriate—that Peggy needed to take her new life skills and practice them so that they became a part of her. At the last session, the nurse and Peggy summarized everything that Peggy had learned and then made a list of the important things for Peggy to remember when taking care of herself. The nurse suggested she tape that list where she could see it daily. Finally, the nurse said that Peggy might need to return for therapy at other times in her life, and that would be just fine. ■

What do you think? Is the patient being shortchanged in therapy by not focusing on the psychodynamic issues underlying the problem?

➤ *Check Your Reading*
6. What is the focus during a first interview?
7. Describe the process for developing patient outcomes.

Cognitive Behavioral Psychotherapy

Cognitive behavioral psychotherapy is a form of brief psychotherapy based on the premise that the way people *perceive* an event, rather than the event itself, determines its relevance and a person's emotional response. A. Beck (1976) at the University of Pennsylvania believed that people develop early beliefs **(core beliefs)** about themselves that later in life become activated, stimulating automatic cognitive interpretations. These personalized interpretations, if negative and self-critical, can lead to depression. These core beliefs are pervasive, overgeneralized, and rigid.

To maintain the validity of these core beliefs, people develop intermediate beliefs (rules, attitudes, assumptions) that support the core belief (J. Beck, 1995). For example, Peggy's core belief that she is basically incompetent can lead her to the erroneous assumption that she will not be successful academically no matter how hard she studies. In turn, she feels sad and experiences the "drowning feeling" that causes her to not sleep at night and then to be too exhausted to attend her college classes. Her core beliefs lead to generalized thoughts and feelings of anxiety and depression that prevent full attention to her studies and bring about a self-fulfilling prophecy of academic inadequacy.

Beck (1976) postulated that negative thoughts and cognitive distortions contribute to and perpetuate the patient's emotional difficulties and moods that, in turn, prevent goal achievement. Examples of **cognitive distortions** include the following:

- *Arbitrary inference:* Drawing a conclusion about an event without any evidence
- *Selective abstraction:* Drawing a conclusion on the basis of one fact rather than considering all facts
- *Overgeneralization:* Drawing a conclusion about oneself on the basis of a single fact or event
- *Magnification and minimization:* Drawing a conclusion through exaggeration or underestimation
- *Inexact labeling:* Drawing a conclusion on the basis of emotional response rather than facts

The goal of cognitive behavioral psychotherapy is to train patients to recognize their automatic thoughts and cognitive distortions. During the initial interview, the therapist assesses for cognitive distortions in the patient's responses. The therapist then explains the theory of cognitive distortions and educates the patient about how problems are perpetuated by these distortions. This is further explored by having the patient review his or her thoughts each day or write thoughts about a specific ongoing negative situation, such as the patient's relationship with his or her boss. The patient is asked to keep a journal, or log, of this work, which is then brought to therapy and explored in the session. Box 14-1 provides a format for questioning automatic thoughts.

After several instances of distorted thinking have been explored, a theme, or **automatic thinking schema,** may begin to emerge. These schemata are different from cognitive distortions in that they are usually well hidden from the patient's consciousness. They are basic attitudes about self, such as being stupid or unworthy, that have been learned in childhood and later fueled and

Box 14-1 ■ ■ ■ ■ ■
Questioning Automatic Thoughts

1. What is the evidence?
   What is the evidence that supports this idea?
   What is the evidence against this idea?
2. Is there an alternative explanation?
3. What is the worst that could happen? Could I live through it?
   What is the best that could happen?
   What is the most realistic outcome?
4. What is the effect of my believing the automatic thought?
   What could be the effect of changing my thinking?
5. What should I do about it?
6. What would I tell ____ (a friend) if he or she were in the same situation?

From Beck, J. (1995). *Cognitive therapy: Basics and beyond.* Questioning automatic thoughts in cognitive therapy. New York: Guilford Press, p. 109. © Copyright 1993 by Judith S. Beck, PhD. Reprinted with permission.

supported by the cognitive distortions needed to maintain the schema. These schemata are revealed as the therapist helps the patient formulate more healthy perceptions and thoughts.

To benefit from cognitive behavioral psychotherapy, the patient must be willing to do the homework (for example, keeping the journal) and be able to tolerate exploring his or her thoughts. The patient must also be from a social, family, and community environment that supports change. Cognitive psychotherapy is usually short-term, anywhere from 8 to 20 sessions. It is goal oriented. Therapist and patient must agree to work toward alleviating specifically identified problems. Insurance companies generally pay for cognitive psychotherapy because a well-defined goal can be accomplished within the number of sessions authorized by the insurance company.

■ CASE EXAMPLE 14-2
■ Janet's Story

Boy was I a wreck when I went into that therapy session today! I sure dumped a lot of stuff on that nurse therapist. As I was telling her my history, I realized how negative I am in so many ways in my life. She said she would like to learn more about that and began telling me about how automatic thoughts sometimes get in the way of being able to evaluate situations appropriately. She said that sometimes these negative thoughts come so easily because they are based on deeply and long-held thoughts about ourselves. She asked me what my first thought was in the morning and I told her that it was wondering what would go wrong today. She asked what it would be like if I woke up pondering what I would handle well today? While it seemed like a relief to think that, I quickly knew better.

She then said it would be worthwhile to explore these negative thoughts and gave me some interesting homework. I am supposed to keep a chart and describe a situation, my automatic thoughts about it, and then rewrite the situation in a way that comes out better for me. If I was having trouble with rewriting, she suggested I call some friends and get their ideas. She said there are usually different ways to respond to situations and the charting would help me see that. She said with practice, the goal of all this charting is to interrupt automatic negative responses and replace them with responses that are more positive. We did a sample one during the session. ■

What do you think? Some have said that therapy used to focus on healing, but now focuses on treatment of symptoms. How would you respond to that statement?

➤ *Check Your Reading*
   8. Describe two techniques often used in cognitive behavioral therapy.
   9. What are cognitive distortions?

FAMILY THERAPY

Family therapy is a second specialty treatment modality, practiced by a nurse with a master's degree and specialized training in family therapy. This family therapist treats the family as a unit or assists an individual in coping more effectively with family issues. Families are important to nurses because families are the context in which individuals live, and they are units to be analyzed as "patients." Demographic trends in family life are found in Box 14-2.

Sometimes, gathering data on the family situation is necessary to support the individual patient fully. At other times, the family as a unit needs treatment, and the

Box 14-2 ■ ■ ■ ■ ■
Demographic Trends in Family Forms

Smaller Families: Decreased family size results in stronger emotional bonds and more investment in each child.

Increase in Empty Nest Time: Longer life spans result in a longer empty nest stage and possibly relate to increased divorce rates.

Increase in Number of Dependent Elderly: Longer life spans increase the number of elderly who may be dependent on others.

Increase in Number of Older Women Living Alone: The increased chance of survival for women has lengthened the period of widowhood.

Increase in Number of Never-Married Adults: More and more people postpone marriage or decide not to marry at all.

Older First-Time Mothers: Marriage postponement and dual-career families result in older first-time mothers and children spaced farther apart.

Separation of Children From Biological Parents: Increased divorce rates result in greater numbers of children living with single-parent or blended families.

Increase in Number of Children Born Outside Legal Marriage: New technologies, changes in societal values, and increasing teenage pregnancy rate result in more children being born into alternative family forms.

Unavailability of Family to Care for Dependent Members: The increased number of women in the work force removes family members to care for young, elderly, and ill members.

Adapted from Glick, P. C. (1988). Fifty years of family demography: A record of social change. *Journal of Marriage and the Family, 50,* 861-873.

entire family becomes the "patient." Family therapy is particularly useful in the following situations:

1. When an individual is struggling with family as well as personal issues

2. When a family needs professional assistance in understanding the patient's perspective or coping with difficult feelings

3. When the family unit is the focus of treatment, for example, in a divorce situation

Box 14–3 ■ ■ ■ ■ ■
Definition of Family Forms

Nuclear: A father, mother, and at least one child living together but apart from both sets of their parents

Extended: Three or more generations including married brothers and sisters and their families

Three Generational: Any combination of first-, second-, and third-generation members living within a household

Dyad: Any two members, typically husband and wife, living alone without children

Single Parent: Divorced, never-married, separated, or widowed man or woman and at least one child; most single-parent families are headed by women

Step-Parent: One or both spouses divorced or widowed and remarried into a family with at least one child

Blended or Reconstituted: A combination of two families with children from one or both families and sometimes children of the newly married couple

Single Adult Living Alone: An increasingly common occurrence for the never-married, divorced, or widowed

Cohabiting: An unmarried couple living together

No-Kin: A group of at least two people who have no legalized or blood ties but who share a relationship and exchange support

Compound: One man (or woman) with several spouses

Gay: A homosexual couple living together with or without children

Commune: More than one monogamous couple sharing financial and social resources

Group Marriage: All individuals married to each other and considered parents of all the children

Family therapists believe that although personality traits are present at birth, people do not develop their personality in a vacuum. They develop it within a uniquely formed group—the family unit. Families are part of the emotional context that structures our personality development. It is within the family unit that a child grows, develops, establishes self-worth, and learns lifelong patterns and beliefs about life. Family relationships continue to influence our lives whether we see other family members frequently or not at all. Families can be a significant resource to help people maintain their health and to provide support when illness strikes. Or they can create unnecessary ongoing emotional pain. Dysfunctional family relationships can contribute to the development of abnormal behaviors within a particular family member socially labeled as deviant or suggestive of mental illness. Within the original family context, the behavior serves a function, but the same behaviors are destructive either to the individual or to the larger community system. Family therapy helps family members map information about dysfunctional patterns surrounding a presenting problem. The therapist and family members begin to examine assumptions or beliefs that prevent family members from altering their roles in maintaining problems. Together, they develop strategies to develop new behavioral patterns and constructive belief systems that support more satisfying relationships (Carr, 1998).

Families are defined in many different ways (Box 14–3). Basic to most definitions is that the **family** is a natural social group or **system** with a coordinated power structure, rules, and ascribed membership roles that have developed over time. The individuals comprising the family unit are connected emotionally with one another in persistent open and covert ways that enhance or compromise individual functioning.

Although *family* is defined as a social group, families differ from other social groups in that membership is automatic and continuous. The specific group composition is predetermined by virtue of birth, adoption, marriage, or long-term close association. Few social groups span the time frames that family does . . . from womb to tomb . . . and beyond. Families create patterns, identities, and expectations across generations, many of which are unspoken and not fully understood.

■ **CASE EXAMPLE 14–3**
■ **The Brannigan's Story**

Marian and Ben Brannigan have decided to try family therapy as a last resort before Ben, who recently asked Marian for a divorce, takes the steps to file for it. Marian does not want the divorce but agrees that the marriage is not satisfying. Although opposed in principle to the idea of divorce, Ben is convinced that what started out as a union that both partners valued has deteriorated into bitter strangers living in the same house. In his mind, this is no longer a marriage, and he no longer has faith that things can be different.

Things have gotten progressively more difficult in this family. Ben is a physician and spends long hours at the hospital, which Marian resents. Marian is a full-time housewife, inclined to angering quickly and harboring grudges. Not only is their marriage "on the rocks" but also their 12-year-old daughter Margie's grades have slipped dramatically and she seems withdrawn. The school psychologist has recommended family treatment.

This recent turn of events is not the first time this family has experienced emotional difficulty. Shortly after Marian and Ben married, Marian's father had an affair, and she has always suspected her husband of infidelity even when there was no reason to support her belief. This created dissension in the marriage, particularly because Ben's father had left his family when Ben was 3 years old, and commitment to marriage is something Ben feels strongly about. Marian and Ben's first child, Brent, drowned in the family swimming pool while Ben's mother was watching him. Following the accident, Ben has had little contact with his mother. Neither Ben nor Marian ever really got over Brent's death, nor have they really processed its meaning in their marriage. Over the years, they began to distance from one another without really realizing that it was happening. When Margie was born, Marian became totally absorbed in her care; her child, rather than her husband, became her top priority.

Ben feels that Marian blames him, in some way, for Brent's death, although she repeatedly said she knew it was an accident. Ben loves Margie but feels he can't get close to her except when Marian is not around. As the years have passed, Ben has become extremely critical of Marian regarding her obsession with Margie. He withdraws when she becomes angry, and he feels that he can never measure up to her expectations. Marian looks to Ben for financial support but little else. She experiences his time at the hospital as abandonment and thinks it is deliberate avoidance of his home responsibilities. She is no longer interested in him sexually and, although she finds him a handy support for social gatherings, she spends as little time as possible with him otherwise. For Ben this is not enough. He wants to throw in the towel and start again with a woman who can value him for who he is, and he wants a different relationship with his daughter, which he feels is impossible if he remains in the home. ■

This family would benefit from family therapy. It would help them understand how each of their behaviors influences the family as a whole and its individual members. Each family member is hurting in a different way, but their hurts, their problems, and the ultimate solutions are highly interrelated. Viewing their situation from a family perspective offers each person the opportunity to change his or her automatic pathological reactions to each other. As the family members begin to understand how their interactive patterns with each other perpetuate the problems and affect each family member's behavior, they can begin to learn different ways to communicate that favor true relationships and more effective coping mechanisms.

Historical Perspective

Family therapy as a treatment modality began in the 1950s and blossomed over the next 2 decades into a primary treatment modality. Early family theorists used biologically based natural systems theory to inform and guide their treatment of patients and their families. They compared the family system to the human body; system failure in one part of the body affects other body systems.

Systems analysis began as an engineering concept (cybernetics) designed to help engineers arrange complex data into a meaningful whole. Family therapy provides a similar cohesive organizing framework for understanding and treating complex family issues. When a therapist encounters a family clinically, the amount of information they provide is overwhelming and often conflicting. A systems model observes the family as a unit, studying patterns of conflict as the focus of diagnosis and intervention. The therapist considers relational patterns as they contribute to the functioning of the whole and does not focus on the individual symptoms. This format allows for a many-sided analysis and a deeper understanding of the ways in which individual parts contribute to an understanding of the whole (Simon, 1998).

Family theorists do not deny the existence of personal problems or intrapsychic pathologies. Nor do family therapists think that the family causes the pathology in a patient. The problem itself is reframed as a process question in need of a solution answer to which all family members can contribute. Family therapists focus their attention on the strong influence of family rules that support dysfunctional behavior and try to help family members change those rules and behaviors that do not work. They look at the role that the family plays in enabling dysfunctional behaviors and they help the family or individual seeking treatment for family issues rediscover the hidden strengths residing within the family that can be used to solve difficult relational issues. General principles of natural systems theory include the following:

- Every subsystem is a part of a larger system. Individuals are part of a larger family system and families are part of a larger community system influenced by its culture, politics, and environmental changes.
- The system is more than the sum of its parts. The whole can be understood only by looking at the pattern of relationships within the system rather than looking at individual parts in isolation.
- Living systems demonstrate **equifinality**—the ability to achieve the same final goal in a variety of ways.
- Systems strive for **homeostasis**—the tendency of systems to be self-regulating. Through a variety of mechanisms, systems maintain coherence within the system when challenges arise from the environment.
- Systems have feedback loops defined as "the process by which a system gets the information necessary to self-correct in its effort to maintain a steady state

or move toward a pre-programmed goal" (Nichols & Schwartz, 1998, p. 116).

- The way the system interprets events influences the way individuals within the system respond to them.

The validity of family therapy as a powerful intervention tool for the advanced psychiatric nurse is well evidenced in the resiliency of its main principles a half century later (Walsh, 1998). Two theories that are particularly useful in thinking about family therapy are Bowen's (1978) family system theory, which helps the therapist describe levels of dysfunction and the manner in which they occur, and Minuchin's (1974) structural theory, which examines the family system through the lens of its organizational boundaries.

Bowen's Family Systems Model

Bowen (1978) believed that chronic anxiety accompanying faulty family relationships was the basis of psychopathology. He suggested that the emotional disorders he observed in an individual patient were an individualized expression of disturbed relationships that occurred within the family across generations. Although we now know that the role of biological factors is basic to understanding major mental disorders, family relationships can provide either support or additional stress that contribute to symptoms or their resolution.

Bowen offered that the family contains opposing forces toward fusion and undifferentiation or toward self-differentiation and maturity. Healthy families demonstrate higher levels of **self-differentiation**—described as individual members recognizing and acknowledging their position on issues within the family without fear of reprisal. Dysfunctional families exhibit fusion in an undifferentiated ego mass in which individual family members do not think or feel for themselves.

Kerr and Bowen (1988) developed eight principles and later added a ninth—spirituality—which they never fully developed. Bowen viewed the basic forces shaping family functional behavior as

1. Multigenerational transmission process
2. Differentiation of self
3. Triangles
4. Nuclear family emotional system
5. Family projection process
6. Emotional cut-off
7. Sibling position
8. Societal regression
9. Spirituality

Bowen's family systems theory conceptualizes the family as an emotional unit composed of a complex network of interlocking relationships that can be analyzed through a multigeneration historical study of family patterns. He proposed that the interlocking and counterbalancing relationships that occur in family systems are similar to those found in all natural systems.

Bowen described a *nuclear family* as a relational unit consisting of those living in the same household, embedded in an extended family unit. The *extended family*, also referred to as the family of origin, consists of grandparents, aunts, uncles, and cousins. When people marry or choose to live together as a family unit, they leave an established family unit (extended family) to create their own nuclear family unit. Each person brings his or her own set of perceptions and expectations about the family that they wish to create together. Their union represents a blend of the family values, emotional reactivity, and ways of doing things from both family units. In second marriage blended families, the relationships are even more complicated than in biological families. The degree to which differences are respected and worked through openly helps determine the mental health of the family unit.

The nuclear family emotional system, applied to the Brannigan family, consists of Ben, Marian, Brent, and Margie. Brent continues his family membership even in death and has his own unique contributions to the behaviors of the family system. The extended family consists of both sets of parents, including Marian's absent father and Marian and Ben's cousins, aunts, uncles, and grandparents. What happens to the nuclear emotional system in this family is determined, in part, by the expectations and values that each member brings to the union. What happens also reflects the unique situational events that this family will experience during the course of its life together—for example, Ben's work demands, Brent's death, and the family's subsequent cut-off from Ben's mother.

Two of the most important concepts in Bowen's theory, anxiety and differentiation of self, are interrelated; they target the difference between thinking and feeling. **Anxiety** is viewed as the arousal of the organism on perceiving a real or imagined threat (Papero, 1990). The higher the level of chronic anxiety in the family, the more each individual life course becomes determined by reactive mechanisms rather than thought. **Differentiation of self** refers to the degree to which an individual can separate thought from feeling. Bowen defined this concept as "an instinctually rooted life force that propels each human to become an emotionally separate person with the ability to think, feel and act for self" (Kerr & Bowen, 1988, p. 95). An individual with a high degree of differentiation of self reacts with a high degree of thought and low degree of emotional reactivity.

Emotional reactivity is a tendency to react automatically to a situation without being able to separate thoughts from feelings. Undifferentiated family systems are fused or emotionally stuck together and tend to function automatically even with low anxiety levels. Family members retain emotional attachments to their family of origin and give in to the dominant emotions and patterns of dysfunctional family members even when these emotions and patterns do not make sense. They have unconsciously sacrificed their own individual needs to secure acceptance from others.

As individual family members become aware of the emotional processes in their family, they can reclaim the possibility of defining a personal self that represents their true beliefs within the family system. Their awareness of family patterns passed from previous generations to the present enables them to choose to transcend repetitive patterns of social behavior through deliberate action. Adult children can begin to understand that their parents were the product of their own set of parenting patterns and unable to break them. This understanding can lead to forgiveness that would not be possible without knowledge of the larger family context.

According to Bowen, a person's level of differentiation reflects his or her emotional independence from and within the family as an emotionally separate person, and he suggested that people at lower levels of differentiation experience psychological problems. Gavazzi (1993) tested, in adolescents, the assumption that level of self-differentiation is related to increased life problems. He found level of differentiation, or the family's tolerance for individuality and intimacy, to be significantly correlated with presenting problems of adolescents in a clinical setting. Other emotionally laden problems such as being depressed, using drugs and alcohol, running away, having few or no friends, and experiencing academic difficulties were associated with lower levels of differentiation.

The process of self-differentiation requires that people develop an "I" position within the family and allow other family members similar emotional space to have their own "I" position. While remaining respectful of other family members' opinions, the differentiated family member is able to define what is important to him or her within the family unit and to make choices that move beyond an automatic predetermined emotional response to anxiety-producing situations.

Becoming self-differentiated requires courage because the family system tries to force a person back into more comfortable, instinctual ways of relating. Although it is impossible to ever become fully self-differentiated or impervious to the emotional influence of the family unit, it is possible to become better differentiated within even the most impossible family situation. The process of redefining what a person needs from someone else and what position that person wants to take in the family also creates bridges to stronger relationships in many broad aspects of life. With the Brannigan family, the therapist would be concerned with helping Ben and Marian recognize that their problems lie in the way they communicate with each other and that the next step is to explore ways they can make their situation better.

Bowen introduced the concept of triangle as the "building block of the immature family" unit. He proposed that individuals use **triangles,** defined as an emotional device in which a person unconsciously focuses attention on a different object, person, or situation, even an illness, to defuse anxiety and emotional discomfort within the family system. In any two individuals, most noted in a marriage, tension lies in the struggle between togetherness and separateness. It is difficult to sustain a close twosome for too long. Typically, the twosome attempts to manage this tension by "triangling" in a third person, object, or even a problem. In any triangle, there is a close side, a distant side, and a side where tension or conflict occurs between the two people.

Any mother who has invited children to visit knows what a triangle is. Two children who usually play well together suddenly explode into trouble when a third is added. "Mommy, he won't play with me!" is a familiar refrain as one child sides with another and the third is left out in the cold. In times of calm, being in the most distant position is uncomfortable. People struggle to regain closeness. When the situation is tense, however, the most distant position is usually the most comfortable. People in the triangle maneuver to claim that outside position.

Because triangles are used by family members to reduce anxiety, it stands to reason that the greater the anxiety, the larger and more complex the number of triangles. Bowen referred to multiple triangles existing simultaneously within the family as interlocking triangles. For example, a child's failure in school may in part reflect anxiety about what is going on between his or her parents, but the parents seek treatment to resolve their child's poor school performance without looking at their own behavior with each other. Each parent blames the other or the child for the problem grades. This is not to say that the triangled person, event, or object causes the problem, only that the triangled one increases the emotional reactivity in the family by diverting attention from anxiety within a two-person system to an outside circumstance. Repetitive patterns of behavior, for example, mother always siding with daughter against father, one family member always in the spotlight for either good or bad behavior and another in the opposite position, suggest a triangle. Alcohol, extramarital affairs, even a midlife crisis can represent a triangle in a family threatened by anxiety.

In the Brannigan family, there are several triangles. One is Ben with his concentrated relationship with work and a distant relationship with Marian and Margie. Marian has Margie in an overly intense relationship to protect herself against the pain of a distant relationship with Ben. As Ben and Marian focus on Margie's failing grades, they can ignore their own serious marital problems. Ben draws attention to Marian's obsession with her daughter instead of telling her directly of his own feelings of being shut out. Marian uses her relationship with Margie as a substitute for the intimacy she craves from Ben.

The key to managing triangles is not to avoid them—an impossibility—but to learn to manage and retain a self within them. "Detriangling" requires thinking one's way out of the reactivity. It requires remaining connected with all the people while defining a self or stating an "I" position. The natural tendency is to desire approval or to seek distance to escape the tension.

Bowen claimed that all individuals belong to a larger emotional system with common systemic behavioral characteristics that, like biological characteristics, are transmitted across generations (Innes, 1996). Behaviors such as chronic alcoholism, divorce, multiple marriages, and abuse tend to repeat as behavioral patterns in successive generations. Bowen called this basic family therapy principle **multigenerational transmission.** In the Brannigan family, the fathers of both Ben and Marian failed to keep their commitments to marriage in their families of origin for different reasons. Ben appears to be repeating this pattern with Marian's strong but unconscious support. The therapist would help Ben and Marian understand how their early family history intersects with the present and a familiar expectation that father will be absent. Through recognition of historical patterns in their families of origin, Ben and Marian could learn to make different choices that would challenge their beliefs about the father's role in parenting, thereby enhancing their relationship.

Bowen believed that the interactive patterns the therapist observes with marital partners may, in part, be explained by their **sibling position** in their family of origin. Birth order helps determine ways of relating to others in relationships. For example, the oldest or only child is more likely to be overly responsible and serious, the middle child is likely to be somewhat of a maverick, and the youngest is more likely to be fun loving and disinclined to make decisions. Although not cast in stone, these personality characteristics develop on the basis of birth order and become familiar patterns of behavior. The more closely the functional position of the marriage partners resembles the original sibling position in childhood, the more successful the union; for example, two oldest children who marry will probably have trouble with competition, whereas two youngest children are likely to experience difficulty with decision-making.

Bowen's concept of the **family projection process** occurs when the family focuses on a particular family member as having all of the positive attributes in the family or all of the pathology—often, the latter is the most vulnerable because of a situational, physical, or mental handicap. The intense focus on this child or the child's behavior helps divert focus from the real family issues. This child is used unconsciously to stabilize the system. As long as the family projection process continues, the entire family is crippled. In the Brannigan family, Margie has become the recipient of the family projection process, with each parent critical of the other's handling of her. Her grades have become an issue, but little attention is paid to her perception of the family dynamics. Margie shows her pain by behaviors, the only way she can communicate without incurring the wrath of either parent.

One way family members handle the family projection process is through the concept of **emotional cut-off.** This is manifested by an adult family member attempting to cut-off from painful relationships by avoiding them. The purpose of the cut-off is to isolate the pain by breaking off all contact, for example, with geographic distance or by not talking to certain or all family members. Cut-offs, like other forms of dysfunctional behavior, tend to appear with regularity in subsequent generations. Ben was emotionally cut-off from his father at an early age, and later he emotionally cut-off from his mother following Brent's death. A Bowen therapist would explain the role of emotional cut-offs in family system dynamics and would suggest that Ben probably carries strong feelings about his mother with him even though he has not seen her in years. Encouraging Ben to reconnect with his mother and to talk through Brent's death with her would be a useful therapeutic intervention.

Treatment

Bowen family therapists view themselves as coaches to the family. The role of the therapist is to help the family decrease its anxiety, gain a broader perspective on problems, and become aware of the ways emotional reactivity influences individual and family functioning. Coaching people to define self, that is, to develop a more solid self in the face of forces to fuse with others, is one of the main strategies.

Starting with a genogram (Figure 14–1), a Bowen family therapist gathers information that helps the family members look at relationships between family processes and events, track multigenerational patterns, and connect with important relationships. Education, questioning, analogies, and observations are techniques the coach uses to attempt to maintain a neutral position, manage anxiety, and define self to the family. In this school of thought, the therapist considers it essential that each patient continue to work on her or his own level of differentiation while concurrently participating in family therapy.

Bowen advocated looking at what goes on between people rather than what goes on within them as the focus of treatment. The patient or family seeking family therapy is viewed as a partner in the process of looking at the family unit and in assuming full responsibility for his or her feelings. A Bowen therapist educates individual family members about triangles and coaches them to talk directly with each other rather than triangling in another family member to defuse their anxiety. The therapist would suggest that Margie's psychological development can be crippled by her mother's overprotection and her father's absence in her life and would coach both parents to develop a more realistic, evenhanded approach to her development. Simultaneously, the therapist would ask the couple to spend time with each other as a homework assignment to strengthen their relationship as a couple.

By teaching people to become aware of their own emotional process within the family and to use "I think" responses based on fact and their personal "I" position, rather than "I feel" responses based on emotional reactivity, the therapist helps people to become self-differentiated. Relevant homework assignments address both working on aspects of the problem and the interpersonal conditions supporting it.

What do you think? What happens when you take "I" stands in your own family? What would you like to happen? What triangles exist within your family? How do you interact within those triangles?

► *Check Your Reading*

10. Identify two principles associated with a systems framework of family therapy.
11. What does the term *differentiation of self* mean?
12. Describe a triangle. What purpose does a triangle serve?
13. What is the role of the therapist using a Bowen framework?

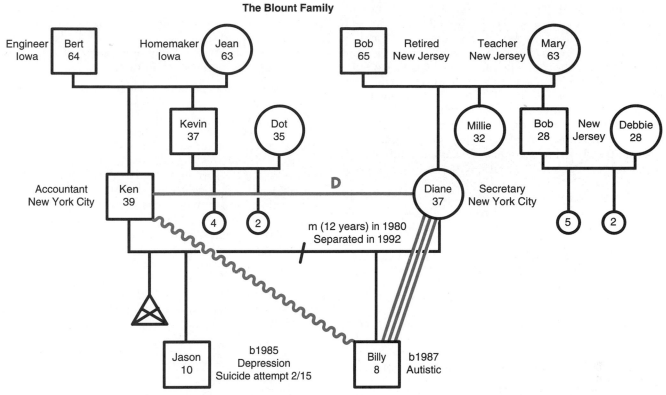

Figure 14–1
A sample genogram.

Minuchin's Structural Theory

Salvador Minuchin's (1974) structural theory of family looks at three essential elements of family organization: structure, subsystems, and boundaries. According to Minuchin, *structure* refers to how the family is organized and the interdependent functioning of its subsystems as the major determinants of individual behaviors. A structural approach examines and describes expected family transactions that have developed into unrelenting automatic behavioral expectations and patterns with dysfunctional unspoken rules that do not always fit a change in situation. Minuchin maintained that the structure of a family is not explained by its composition as a blended, single-parent, or traditional family unit. Structure describes the way relationships are played out in the family unit and the way in which family members interact with each other. The Brannigan family, for example, is an intact traditional family with mother, father, and child having problems. The structural relationships within this family, however, would be described differently—as an intense overinvolvement between mother and daughter, a conflictual distant relationship between husband and wife, and a disengaged relationship between father and daughter.

With a structural framework, the therapist looks at the family unit from the perspective of hierarchical subsystems for the purpose of description and the basis for intervention. **Subsystems** are defined subgroups of people within the family who connect with each other to perform different family functions. Subsystems include siblings, parents, or coalitions of like-minded family members. The spousal unit constitutes one subsystem, parents are viewed as a second subsystem, parent-child as a third subsystem, and siblings as a fourth subsystem. Other family subsystems are organized according to gender, common interests, functional ability, or family function. Within each subgroup, a person may act quite differently, play different roles, and demonstrate different skills. For example, the behaviors of a married man with his children, his wife, and his parents are likely to be different in focus, process, and content.

Family systems have **boundaries** or imaginary walls, both around them and between their subsystems. These boundaries are invisible emotional limits that regulate the amount and intensity of interpersonal contact. Boundaries that are permeable and clear, allowing information to flow in and out, lead to open, healthier systems. Boundaries that are impermeable shut the system off from information, resources, and sources of support. Clear boundaries between subsystems help maintain individual integrity while reinforcing the con nectivity of family members to the larger family unit.

In the Brannigan family, the spousal subsystem is in chaos. The boundaries in the parent-child subsystem have been violated because of the close coalition of Marian with Margie, with Ben in the odd man out position. Diffuse boundaries create issues with personal privacy. Boundaries that are too rigid preclude the necessary nurturance and personal involvement all family members need to grow and develop. Minuchin contended that the boundaries of most families fall within a continuum ranging from *enmeshment* (diffuse boundaries) to *disengagement* (rigid boundaries). An enmeshed family has no boundaries and consequently remains in chaos because its anxiety runs wild and unchecked. By contrast, the disengaged family has such rigid boundaries that it is unable to relax them or to accept the emotional support from family members that might be forthcoming if the boundaries could be loosened enough to allow input. Minuchin would describe the Brannigan family as enmeshed because the boundaries are not clear and family members are highly reactive to the emotional needs and challenges of each other.

With a structural approach, the therapist's role is an active one. The therapist actively challenges the maladaptive reactive transactional patterns to help the family system explore and develop a different level of homeostasis, one in which boundaries are reasonable, consistent, and open to emotional input from others without being compromised. The goals of treatment (Goldenberg & Goldenberg, 1996) are

1. To help families develop clearly defined generational boundaries

2. To establish a common front on important family issues, such as discipline, and realistic behavioral standards for family members

3. To help open communication pathways and to redefine pathological coalitions that exclude interdependency among all family members

A structural therapist would help Ben to take a more active role with Margie and would coach Marian to allow more emotional space for this to occur. The therapist might suggest homework assignments for Ben to take time with Margie alone. Another strategy would be to work out, with both parents, a united front in parenting Margie and time together, apart from Margie, to rebuild their spousal subsystem.

> **W**hat do you think? How would you define the boundaries within your own family?

> ► *Check Your Reading*
> 14. What would a structural therapist look for in describing family structure?
> 15. What is the role of boundaries in a structural family therapy approach?

Psychoeducation, a Prevention Tool

Psychoeducation is a family therapy tool that is becoming increasingly popular as a strategy to reduce risk factors associated with the development of behavioral symptoms. Examples of situations in which this would be appropriate include

1. Information and training about a specific area of family life, such as communication skills training or parent effectiveness training

2. Information and support to families dealing with a specific stress or crisis, such as a family support group for Alzheimer's disease

3. Prevention and enrichment, such as premarital counseling, for families not in crisis

Research supports the effectiveness of psychoeducation in a variety of ways. For example, the improvement of communication skills enhances the marital relationship and parent-child relations (Hawkins & Roberts, 1992). Parent effectiveness training (Gordon, 1980) improves parent-child openness and empathy (Grando & Ginsberg, 1976) and provides help for families of people with severe mental illness (Pollido, 1998). Roosa, Gensheimer, Short, Ayers, and Shell (1989) developed a program directed at preventive intervention for children in alcoholic families, which resulted in less depression and acting out and more positive coping for children who participated in this 8-week program. And North (1998) described a psychoeducational model for family caregivers of schizophrenic patients. Psychoeducational programs are relatively inexpensive and often effective in influencing family life.

■ CASE EXAMPLE 14–4
■ The Thomas's Story

The Thomas family is having a difficult time as the teenage children grow up. Josh, the 15-year-old child, is skipping school and receiving bad grades. Josh frequently stays out beyond his 11:00 PM curfew, and he refuses to do his chores. He is constantly argumentative, and family members find themselves frequently involved in fights that end in Josh's storming out of the house. Sometimes Luann, a single parent, becomes so frustrated that she will slap Josh across the face. When this happens, her mother, Dorothy, and her 13-year-old daughter, Julie, retreat to their rooms.

Josh complains that he does not have the freedom he deserves as a 15 year old. He believes his life and his school performance are his own business and that his mother should stay out of the picture. Luann is very worried about Josh's educational success. Luann interprets Josh's behavior to mean that he is likely to have trouble adapting to a difficult world. Her behavior is fueled by worry. Luann believes that she is struggling to help Josh learn to be a functional adult. This family is able to tolerate individual differences but is struggling to allow Josh some autonomy.

Luann happens to see an advertisement for parent effectiveness training for parents of adolescents. The series of classes runs for 12 weeks and is open to anyone in the community as a service of the community mental health clinic. The series is run by a nurse in the clinic and is attended by a group of 17 parents, who meet weekly for the 12 weeks. The class consists of a 30-minute educational session followed by a group discussion. Luann learns some effective techniques to help her set limits on Josh's behavior. She also learns information about adolescence and the importance of providing freedom, when possible. By listening to other families' experiences, she begins to see how her problems with Josh are universal and to form ideas about how to deal with them.

At every session, reading and homework are assigned. In the third session, every parent maps out a plan for dealing with the behavior of the adolescent and providing realistic consequences. Luann sits down with Josh, explains carefully what his limits are, and takes an "I" position that states what she is going to do. Support from the group helps her maintain her objective plan and decreases her tendency to react to Josh automatically. At first, Josh acts out even more, but when he realizes that she is not going to back down, he begins to obey the family rules. Luann, however, has to work to keep her mother from interfering with her discipline. Dorothy thinks the punishments are too harsh and feels sorry for Josh. A triangle develops in which Josh runs to Grandma for protection when he is in conflict with Mom.

Luann begins to realize the techniques she learned would also be helpful with Julie, even though Julie reacts to her in different ways. Eventually, Luann becomes a peer counselor who helps run the classes. Josh stays in school and graduates. He is now attending a community college. ■

Process

The therapeutic process can begin the moment a family member picks up the telephone to call for an appointment. An experienced therapist learns a great deal about the family's perception of the problem and how family members are managing tension by assessing how the family members present the problem on the telephone, whom they single out as the sick or problem individual, and whom they expect to attend the therapy. Most professionals are careful to structure even beginning contacts with families to maximize obtaining such information. See What Families Need to Know: Common Questions When Beginning Therapy.

The first interview can take place in a hospital, a psychiatric assessment center, a clinic, a mental health center, or the home. The first interview sets the stage for the family to begin to see a family problem rather than an individual concern. Neutrality, honesty, and careful statement of the boundaries or the limits both of the therapy and the therapist are important in the first encounters. The initial interview has many purposes. Information about family dynamics and family history must be obtained. Practical concerns such as phone numbers, health insurance information, and other health care sources are addressed. The family may come to the session wanting to talk about the problem and expecting that one session will even determine a solution. Most often, the therapist must help family members broaden perception to include the whole family.

At times, family members are anxious or angry, and this first session is used to help them become calmer. The therapist's challenge is to remain neutral and yet connect with each family member. Ask each member for a perception of the problem and indicate that all family members are important. As the therapist gathers information about the family, some relevant questions might include the following:

Why has the family come for help now?
How do family members describe the problem?
Do family members describe the problem as a family or an individual issue?
Is there a dual medical or psychiatric diagnosis that must be considered?

It is important to discuss the history of the problem, noteworthy events surrounding its onset, and previous attempts to correct it. The therapist is curious about dysfunctional communication patterns and interpersonal conditions supporting the problem. Integrated with a hypothesis about what the family is doing to perpetuate their presenting problem is the challenge to family members to see and take responsibility for their own role in the process.

In the initial session, the therapist makes contact with each family member and listens carefully to his or her perspective on the problem. The therapist assesses individual family members' constructions of family problems (Heatherington, 1998). For example, the therapist would want to know (Cierpka, 1998)

How much anxiety is the family experiencing now?
How much have family members experienced in the past?
What are the current indicators of social, emotional, and physical health or dysfunction?
Historically, what has the level of functioning been for each member individually and the family as a unit?
Is this a family that typically functions well but is now under stress? Or is this a family that consistently functions with a high level of anxiety?
Is this a crisis related to a long-standing pattern of dysfunctional relating?

As the issues become clearer, the therapist helps the family summarize an agreed on perception of the problem as the basis for discussing what sorts of interventions might be attempted. Before the family leaves the session, an initial contract is formulated that describes the expected encounters; the time, frequency, and duration of sessions; and the responsibilities of nurse and family members. The family should emerge from the session with a calmer and clearer view of the problem and some hope that family life can be strengthened by the contact.

Genogram, an Assessment Tool

A **genogram** is a format for drawing a family tree that records information about family members and their relationships for at least three generations (McGoldrick & Gerson, 1985). An assessment tool useful throughout the contact with the family, a genogram makes it easier for a therapist to think about the family members, patterns, and significant events that are important in the family's care. A genogram also may be used as a therapeutic tool to help individuals see family processes more clearly because it provides a basis for helping people

WHAT PATIENTS NEED TO KNOW

Common Questions When Beginning Therapy

How do I decide if our problems could be helped with family therapy?

Family therapy can be useful for problems, such as marital conflict, that are clearly identified as family problems. It is also often useful when the issue involves disturbances in family relationships such as those that occur between parent and child, caregiver and care receiver, or siblings. Waiting until the problem is out of hand is like waiting until one's blood pressure is too high. Often, therapy can be useful in a preventive way to help people work on their relationships before they are in serious trouble. Many therapists use family systems concepts with individuals who are interested in working on their own functioning. Some therapists see only one person in the family.

How do I know the theoretical orientation of the therapist, and does it matter?

When the call is made to set up the first appointment, you can ask the therapist to explain his or her theoretical orientation. The style in which a therapist works will become clearer after you are actually in therapy. Although some would disagree, the theory used may not be as important as the fit between the particular therapist and the patients. Gender should also be considered. Will someone in the family be uncomfortable or feel as if sides are being taken if the therapist is a man or a woman? Once therapy begins, if the style of the therapist is not helpful, you can always ask for a referral to someone else.

Is therapy covered under my insurance, and how much will it cost?

Treatment of emotional problems that are clearly identified as psychiatric illnesses in the *Diagnostic and Statistical Manual, Fourth Edition* is often more likely to be reimbursed than family therapy. However, health care plans differ as to what they cover. The best advice is to call your insurance representative and ask if the therapy is covered. Often, there is a deductible or copayment. Therapists also differ in the ways they manage their billing. In some cases, one family member is identified as the patient and other family members join the treatment sessions under that billing.

What can I expect to happen during the first session?

For some therapists, the therapeutic process begins with the first telephone call. The therapist may want to discuss the problem on the telephone or develop some sense of what the family is like before the family comes to the office. The therapist may set some rules; for example, a therapist might insist that all family members come to the appointment. Sometimes, homework is given for the family to complete before the first appointment. The first session is usually an information-gathering session. The therapist attempts to gain some understanding of the problem and help the family reframe the problem. Although patients may experience some relief, it often takes several sessions before anything is "resolved."

How long will therapy take?

Time varies according to the problem and many other factors. The therapist sets mutual goals and discusses the expected time with the family early in the encounter.

examine how ingrained assumptions and beliefs influence the way they choose to conduct their lives (Halevy, 1998). Although the therapist may think he or she knows what the family should do, interpretations that come from family members themselves are usually more accurate and useful for change. The picture of the family that is presented on the genogram helps the observer think about the family systemically and over time. Sometimes, when a larger picture is presented, connections among events and relationships become clearer and are viewed in a more objective way (see Figure 14-1).

Genograms serve several functions. Collecting and recording information for the genogram are ways for the interviewer and family to connect in personal but emotionally safe ways. A genogram also provides the interviewer with information about how the members of the family think about the family problems and interact with other members. Beginning to record information on a genogram can defuse issues or reduce anxiety about family problems. During the process of describing family relationships, people are required to think, organize, and present facts. The therapist joins with the family and helps to normalize and reframe problems so that they are viewed in a larger context. This type of interaction helps individual family members step back and think about an issue in a calmer way.

Typically, the genogram is constructed in the beginning of therapy and revised as new information becomes available. Three parts to genogram construction must be considered:

1. Mapping family structure
2. Recording family information
3. Delineating family relationships

First, the therapist and family completing the assessment fill in the facts about the family. Later, they return to describe the process of family interaction. A diagram of family members placed in each generation is drawn using horizontal and vertical lines. Symbols are used to represent pregnancies, miscarriages, marriages, and deaths (see Figure 14-1). Males are placed on the left of the horizontal line, females on the right. Placing the oldest sibling on the far left and progressing toward the right represents birth order. In the case of multiple marriages, the earliest is placed on the left, with the most recent on the right.

Helpful family information includes ages, birth dates, death dates, geographical locations, occupations, and educational levels. Critical family events such as moves, marriages, divorces, losses, and successes are recorded. Family members' physical, emotional, or social problems or illnesses are identified. A chronology or time line of family events often helps people see relationships between events and behavior changes. Observing and describing family relationships are the most crucial elements, and it is often the most helpful to the family. Complex relationship patterns can be inferred from observations and from family members' comments and analyses (Friedlander, 1998). Triangles are present in every family. Attempting to map the primary or most influential triangles in the family is a part of describing the family relationships. Helpful questions to gain a full perspective might include

What do you remember about discipline in your family?
What happened if your parents disagreed about something?
How did your parents show love?
How did you know the rules in your family?

Last, the family genogram should include any history of mental illness, substance use, or trauma. Reviewing this history provides an opportunity to educate the patient about familial tendencies of many mental health disorders. Once assessment data are complete, the therapist's attention turns to

- Determination of needs or areas of concern
- Assessment of family functioning
- Determination of patterns of family interaction
- Identification of components or targets of care
- Priority setting of identified needs

Outcome Identification

Treatment goals must be specific, communicated to involved family members, and agreed on. They should include long-term and short-term outcomes. The outcomes should take into consideration its potential effect on the individual, other family members, and the family as a whole. Specify goals in the form of measurable outcomes. For example, knowing that a family member wants to be a more effective parent is not the same as noting how often the parent interacts with the child without anger. Short-term goals progress, with modification, toward long-term goals as the family and therapist learn what works and make adjustments to new information.

Intervention

Interventions are directed by principle rather than by rote. Basically, the therapist helps the family see its own patterns of operation in a different way. Once the family can become thoughtful about its own operation, family members begin to think themselves out of the problem. Watching family members rediscover their own potential in developing creative solutions is one of the most rewarding aspects of family therapy. The family creates solutions that are likely to work. The therapist uses a variety of strategies to help families develop more effective ways of interacting with each other and take "I" positions within the family system, including role playing, helping them anticipate consequences, and providing constructive encouragement.

Families tend to resist change. Even when the change is most likely beneficial to the family, family members prefer to remain as they are. It is easier to keep what is known than to exert energy to move into the unknown. Recognize the importance of sequencing steps in the process or timing in suggesting options for change. For instance, families have difficulty changing during times of crisis or stress, yet that is often the best time to change because the family then sees the need for change. Change is most likely to occur after perceptions of the situation begin to change. Working on the family members' thinking about the problem is the first step to intervention. Helping them modify feelings and behavior comes next. Family therapy interventions are outlined in Box 14-4.

Box 14-4 ■ ■ ■ ■ ■
Family Therapy Interventions

- Teach the family members to decrease anxiety by focusing on thinking rather than feeling.
- Broaden the family members' perspectives by mapping the multigenerational family system, gathering facts, and reframing individual interpretations.
- Manage your own self by monitoring your anxiety.
- Identify the primary triangles and teach the family members to manage themselves within them.
- Track the family emotional process.
- Teach the family to explore connecting to others and healing cut-offs.
- Coach the family toward identifying possible solutions that come from family members.
- Help family members monitor and become more aware of individual reactions to emotional triggers.
- Increase awareness by teaching the family concepts of family functioning.
- Coach family members toward defining self.
- Maintain neutrality.
- Define an "I" position for yourself as therapist.

A change in even one person within the system always affects the entire system, although the effects may be subtle and not immediate, because what we do and the way we react have an impact on others. The changes may or may not be positive. For example, suppose a family coping with a chronic illness depends mostly on the caregiving of a 40-year-old sister. If the sister changes her behavior and starts claiming some time for herself, the care for the ill member might deteriorate; other family members pulled in to assist may experience more stress; and the family dynamics change. The sister's choice is not necessarily an incorrect one for either herself or other family members. It simply points out how interconnected individual family members' behaviors are with the functioning of the entire family system. Anticipating consequences is an important dimension of making changes.

The more important a family member is to family functioning, the more impact a change in that member has on the family. Not all family members change equally or have equal capacity to change. Identifying the family member most likely to be able to change is a good strategy when you are helping the family to modify its functioning. The member who is healthy—and in many cases more upset with the situation—is more likely to be able to effect change within the family than the member who is dysfunctional and satisfied with the status quo.

Family members' strengths are important to use in helping them resolve problems. For example, at times, Harry is lazy and irresponsible. Is it also possible that Harry adds humor and genuineness to a restricted family environment? Can the problem be reframed and seen as an asset?

A family's capacity to change is related to its level of functioning. The family has probably operated at a certain level of health for a long time before the family therapist appears on the scene. Having realistic ideas about what can be accomplished for each family member is necessary. If family members can begin to think about their issues in ways that lead to small improvements or maintenance of boundaries, this can be described as a positive outcome.

System boundaries regulate information to and around that system. Families that are closed (i.e., families with boundaries that are not permeable) often like to try to deal with problems themselves. Helping them accept help from extended family, the community, or professionals may involve exploring their beliefs and offering help while acknowledging the family's preferred style. Other families may have had past experiences with resources that turned out to be ineffective or inadequate. Making sure that resources are reliable and that family members have realistic expectations of what the resource can provide is a way to circumvent a repeat of earlier experiences.

Two-person systems are unstable. Triangles, coalitions, and alliances between family members are facts of family life. A relationship with only one part of a family activates triangles and decreases the effectiveness of intervention. The therapist needs to relate to the entire family system in a neutral way by maintaining connections with everyone. High levels of anxiety decrease a person's ability to think and increase automatic behaviors. The therapist tempers the amount of anxiety by being calm and in touch with the family system. This requires the therapist to carefully monitor his or her own anxiety and to pay close attention to remaining a nonanxious presence in the situation.

Termination

Ending a meaningful relationship always elicits feelings for both family and therapist. In any relationship that is defined as potentially therapeutic, attention must be paid to the termination process. Termination is a time when everyone involved must deal with personal feelings about separation. The therapist engages the family in a discussion of goal accomplishment, satisfaction with the process, and plans for continuation of health maintenance. The therapist tries to find a way to frame the outcomes of the visits to indicate success for the family, even if the original goals were not met. In almost every contact, the therapist and the family learned something or grew in some way that could be presented as success.

If referrals or transfers are needed, the therapist arranges these during the termination process. It also is important to establish criteria that will let the family know when to seek health care again. For example, the reappearance of the signs and symptoms of a chronic mental illness would be a signal for the family to contact the clinic. A crisis situation such as a death, birth, job loss, physical illness, or divorce also might trigger a need for therapy.

What do you think? Develop a genogram for your own family. What patterns are you able to see?

▶ *Check Your Reading*
16. What is a genogram?
17. What are the functions of a genogram?
18. Identify at least three of the principles of family intervention.

GROUP PSYCHOTHERAPY

Group psychotherapy is a third practice framework that advanced practice nurses use in psychiatric settings. Therapists view group therapy as a social microcosm in which patients can examine their behavior and reactions to others in a safe environment. Foulkes (1975) referred to group therapy as a "hall of mirrors" in which people can see themselves reflected in others. Group therapy is a powerful therapeutic tool to help patients correct maladaptive personal behaviors and to enhance a patient's ability to function as a contributing member of the community. The experience of being in a group does not deny the uniqueness of each person. Rather, it allows people to directly experience their talents and possibilities through the eyes and personal experience of others.

History

The value of group formats in promoting healing and fostering behavioral change was acknowledged in early tribal rituals and medieval morality plays. Ceremonial rituals specifically identified people as valid members of their community or religious group, thereby symbolizing their "belonging" to something larger. Medieval morality plays used human dilemmas and direct audience participation to encourage the audience to share vicariously with the actors. The plays often showed successful solutions to difficult life problems.

Group psychotherapy, as a recognized form of psychological treatment, traces its origins to the early 1900s. In 1907, Joseph Pratt, an internist in Boston, developed a psychoeducational method for teaching patients with tuberculosis about their disease and improving their morale. He used a combination of lecture and informal group discussion. Pratt (1992) described the informal group discussion meeting as

the most important feature of the class system. It is held every Friday in a large, cheerful room at Massachusetts General Hospital. The class meeting is a pleasant social hour for the members. One confided to the friendly visitor that the meeting was her weekly picnic. Made up as our membership is of widely different races and different sects, they have a common bond in a common disease. (p. 29)

The success of his group treatment approach inspired Pratt and others to use a group format to treat other chronic diseases such as diabetes. Later, Pratt expanded its use to the treatment of neurotic disorders. The idea of sharing a "common bond in a common disease," which Pratt advocated at the turn of the century, serves as the basis for many contemporary support and mutual help groups. The notion of combining psychoeducation with informal group discussion is used increasingly with patients and families because of the benefit of combining didactic information with individuals' experiences (North, 1998).

Samuel R. Slavson, considered the Father of Group Psychotherapy in America, worked with inner-city children and adolescents. He found that a group format using a combination of games, tools, and food to engage children in actively communicating with each other encouraged cooperative behavior among children who otherwise might not talk to each other (MacKenzie, 1992). This work laid the groundwork for group activity therapy, in which arts and crafts help children experience and direct their energies in productive ways. Today, Slavson's principles of group treatment are found in short-term psychoeducation programs in elementary schools and in focus groups related to parental divorce, drug abuse, and social skills training (Scheidlinger, 1994).

An experiential form of group psychotherapy, called *psychodrama,* originated from Moreno's earlier work in Vienna with the "theatre of spontaneity," in which he used role-playing techniques to help people reenact emotionally difficult situations experientially. Moreno is credited with introducing the phrase *here and now* to

psychotherapy (Kaplan & Sadock, 1993), which means that the focus is on how these situations might be experienced currently rather than as something that has no application to the present. Psychodrama bridges reality and fantasy by creating a stage that provides the patient with a "space for living" (an experiential space). Moreno pioneered techniques that are the basis for other forms of psychiatric treatment, such as role playing, role reversals, mirroring, and the empty chair technique used in gestalt therapy.

Group psychotherapy as a primary form of treatment for people with emotional problems achieved widespread recognition during World War II when, due to the limited number of available therapists, psychiatric casualties from the war were treated in small groups rather than individually. The success of this intervention in the military became its strongest marketing tool, and therapists outside the military began to consider group therapy a primary treatment modality. Today, patients of all ages with varied medical and psychiatric diagnoses appear to benefit from group therapy. In fact, contemporary estimates are that more than half of "all psychiatric inpatient settings in the U.S. currently employ group treatment modalities" (Scheidlinger, 1994, p. 223). As managed care increasingly oversees mental health care delivery, group therapy as a treatment modality is likely to emerge as a major form of mental health treatment.

> **W***hat do you think?* Think about groups of which you are a member. What roles do you play?

► *Check Your Reading*
19. What role did World War II play in the development of group psychotherapy?
20. What role does group therapy play in helping people bring about behavioral change?

Characteristics

The characteristics of effective and ineffective groups are presented in Table 14–2. Nurses with basic training in group dynamics can lead psychoeducation and resocialization or reminiscence groups, but specialized advanced training at the masters level is required for leading a psychotherapy group. *Group psychotherapy* is defined as a structured, regular, predetermined meeting between two or more patients for the purpose of achieving identified health-related goals. Group therapy uses peer relationships as well as the professional relationship between the therapist and patients in the group in a collaborative, structured, time-limited format to provide symptom relief, resolution of interpersonal problems, and personal growth. Patients can directly experience their pain and interpersonal problems through talking about them and receive helpful feedback from other patients that allows them to respond to their personal circumstances differently within a safe, healing interpersonal environment (Alonso & Swiller, 1992). Each group

TABLE 14–2 Characteristics of Effective and Ineffective Groups

EFFECTIVE GROUPS	INEFFECTIVE GROUPS
Goals are clearly identified and collaboratively developed.	Goals are vague or imposed on the group without discussion.
Open, goal-directed communication of feelings and ideas is encouraged.	Communication is guarded: feelings are not always given attention.
Power is equally shared and rotates among members, depending on ability and group needs.	Power resides in the leader or is delegated with little regard to member needs. It is not shared.
Decision-making is flexible and adapted to group needs.	Decision-making occurs with little or no consultation.
Controversy is viewed as healthy because it builds member involvement and creates stronger solutions.	Consensus is expected rather than negotiated based on data. Controversy and open conflict are not tolerated.
A healthy balance exists between task and maintenance role functioning.	One-sided focus on task or maintenance role functions excluding reciprocal function.
Individual contributions are acknowledged and respected.	Individual resources are not utilized. Conformity, the "company man or woman," is rewarded.
Diversity is encouraged. Interpersonal effectiveness, innovation, and problem-solving adequacy are evident.	Diversity is not respected. Problem-solving abilities, morale, and interpersonal effectiveness are low and undervalued.

From Arnold, E., & Boggs, K. (1999). *Interpersonal relationships: Communication skills for nurses* (3rd ed., p. 273). Philadelphia: W. B. Saunders.

is made up of individuals, and the character of the group is formed by the combination of each patient's interpretation of reality, values, communication, and experiences. Within the psychotherapy group, each patient influences group dynamics and in turn is affected by the group as a whole. A healthy group personality has a direct effect on each patient's task accomplishment and satisfaction with outcomes.

Purpose

The purpose of a therapy group varies with the needs of its patients and the expertise of the therapist. For example, the psychoeducational purpose of some therapeutic groups is to help patients and families better understand the disease process, treatment, or modifiable risk factors (Pollido, 1998). Other groups are designed to help patients understand and modify maladaptive patterns of relating to others. Their goal is to strengthen healthy patterns of behavior and to help patients learn new, better ways of relating. Self-help and mutual aid groups frequently do not have a professional leader. Their purpose is to provide patients and families having similar health concerns a place to share their experiences, derive comfort, share information, and exchange practical advice. The purpose and related goals of a therapy group should reflect the desired outcomes of patients' treatment plans and the characteristics of the milieu. The purpose and related goals should be achievable, personally meaningful, and appropriate to the setting (Table 14–3).

Curative Factors

Yalom (1995) identified 11 curative factors found in effective groups:

1. Catharsis
2. Universality
3. Self-understanding
4. Recapitulation of the primary family
5. Cohesion
6. Altruism
7. Instillation of hope
8. Identification
9. Interpersonal learning
10. Guidance
11. Existential factors

TABLE 14–3 Different Types of Groups

TYPE OF GROUP	OPPORTUNITIES PROVIDED BY GROUP CATEGORY
Therapy groups	Reality testing Encouraging personal growth Inspiring hope Strengthening personal resources Developing interpersonal skills
Support groups	Giving and receiving practical information and advice Supporting coping skills Promoting self-esteem Enhancing problem-solving skills Encouraging client autonomy Strengthening hope and resiliency
Activity groups	Getting people in touch with their bodies Releasing energy Enhancing self-esteem Encouraging cooperation Stimulating spontaneous interaction Supporting creativity
Education groups	Learning new knowledge Promoting skill development Providing support and feedback Supporting development of competency Promoting discussion of important health-related issues

From Arnold, E., & Boggs, K. (1999). *Interpersonal relationships: Communication skills for nurses* (3rd ed., p. 266). Philadelphia: W. B. Saunders.

Yalom believed that the therapy group offers a complex social microcosm of the real world in which people can explore different ways of communicating in a safe environment guided by a professional. **Catharsis** refers to the expression of emotion, which Yalom maintained is a major value of group psychotherapy. The group offers patients an opportunity to identify and distinguish their feelings, to express feelings honestly and openly in a socially acceptable manner, and to become the master rather than the victim of their emotions. This may be the first opportunity for some patients to do this.

Other important curative factors are those of **universality** and **self-understanding.** A major benefit of group therapy is that it helps patients realize that they are not alone and that other people have had similar life experiences—and survived them. Being in a group tends to stir up feelings from the first group most people had membership in—namely, their families. Yalom refers to this as *recapitulation of the primary family.* Patients in the group can become aware of how they are reacting to others in the group "as if" they are family members and can experiment with different ways of understanding and responding to previously painful events in their lives.

In a therapy group, the therapeutic alliance is referred to as *cohesion.* Yalom (1995) described group cohesion as the "we-ness" of the group, the sense that the group is important to the group members. Cohesion is composed of all the factors that make the group attractive for a member. In a cohesive group, the members like and respect one another, strongly desire to achieve identified group goals, and are willing to lend their efforts to make it happen. Cohesion contains the same dimensions as one-to-one relationships: unconditional acceptance, genuineness, empathy, and valuing of the members as unique (MacKenzie, 1990).

Yalom believed that *altruism,* or the personalized help that one group member extends to another, is another curative factor. The group experience offers hope to individuals who have trouble feeling that their problems can have healthy resolutions (Gunther, 1998). From there, *hope* develops, as people listen to each other's stories and draw from the experiences of others *(identification)* in understanding their behaviors and what is happening to them. Group sessions are powerful, special encounters that would not occur spontaneously for most people. Group sessions lead to *interpersonal learning* about more effective ways to relate to others. Group members provide guidance and practical suggestions to each other.

Yalom proposed that group therapy offers patients an opportunity to find new meaning in their lives by enlarging their perspectives by drawing attention to *existential factors* such as spirituality and questions about the meaning of life. In an age of technology, more group theorists are incorporating spiritual and religious themes as a focus of inquiry in group psychotherapy (Jacques, 1998).

Two definitions useful in the study of group psychotherapy are group dynamics and group process. **Group dynamics** refers to verbal and nonverbal behaviors that occur among group members. **Group process** refers to the natural developmental sequence of the group's activity. Both are concepts useful in understanding small group behavior. Following are some of the factors that the psychiatric advanced practice nurse considers in starting, maintaining, and terminating a psychotherapy group. Structural factors contributing to behavioral dynamics in therapeutic groups include member selection, group size, time frame, setting, and therapist competence.

Concepts in Group Dynamics

Patient Selection

Member selection is based on a patient's treatment need and capacity to contribute to group goals. Group members do not know each other before entering the group, and it is best not to include people in the same group who socialize with each other. It is not possible to have full control over patient selection, particularly in inpatient or partial hospitalization settings, but the therapist should carefully consider the rationale for including patients who are actively psychotic, uncontrolled manic, paranoid, or hostile (even in inpatient settings). These individuals cannot benefit from the group when their symptoms are intense, and they disrupt the group even with the most skilled leadership.

Functional Similarity

Yalom (1995) suggested that group members have enough in common with each other to feel interpersonally comfortable in the group and refers to this capacity as *functional similarity.* By this he meant that group members should have sufficient levels of functional ability and social recognizability to allow them to engage in meaningful conversation. Significant differences in educational level, life experiences, or developmental level can be barriers to full participation. When group members feel uncomfortable, they are not as likely to talk with each other. The leader should avoid including members who are the only ones with permanent characteristics such as different race, gender, education, or age than the other members.

MacKenzie (1992) referred to this as the "Noah's Ark" phenomenon. That is, a therapy group ideally should have at least two members with similar characteristics. Pairing members in this way precludes the creation of a group social isolate. For example, it would not be appropriate to place a single adolescent girl in a group of adolescent boys. When one therapist made this error and the girl's mother told the therapist her daughter was uncomfortable as the only girl, the therapist's response was that they were all adolescents and had similar issues. Not so! The adolescent girl continued for a few more sessions and then dropped out, feeling like a failure. Had one other female been in the group or had this young girl been placed in a different adolescent group of a mixed membership or of only girls, the outcome might have been different. Being one of a kind is a common experience for women and minorities in Alcoholics

Anonymous, which is often predominantly white and male. In making a referral to a self-help group, encourage a person to try several and find the one that best fits her or his needs. On the other hand, Yalom stressed the need for the group to be composed of members with different diagnostic elements so that members have opportunities to learn how to relate comfortably to people with opposing ideas and ways of responding.

Capacity to Contribute

Group members must be able to both contribute to group goals and derive benefit from this treatment modality. Usually, patients with more than mild cognitive disorders, antisocial behaviors, strong hostility, or paranoid symptoms do not profit from group intervention. First, their symptoms disrupt the group functioning. Second, their pathologies interfere with their own ability to derive benefit because their symptoms preclude the necessary cooperation with other members. They should be included only after their symptoms are under sufficient control that they gain some benefit from group membership. All group members need to be able to contribute in a meaningful way to the functioning of the group as a whole.

Matching Individual Need With Membership

Another factor to consider with group composition is the issue of a homogeneous compared with heterogeneous group membership. **Homogeneous groups** include patients with similar diagnoses, similar age group, or same gender. They are particularly effective when treating disorders in which denial plays a role, for example, addiction or eating disorders. Single-gender consciousness-raising groups can empower the participants in ways that might not be possible in a mixed group. **Heterogeneous groups** draw their membership from a variety of diagnoses. These groups are composed of men and women, rather than being single gender, and prospective members can run the age gamut of adulthood. The advantage of a heterogeneous group is that the rich complexity of its membership can provide several different ways of approaching interpersonal relationships. The format works well with patients experiencing relationship difficulties.

Choosing Open or Closed Groups

Another decision is whether to have open or closed membership. *Open groups* are those in which group membership changes frequently. This type of group is found in inpatient settings that depend on member residency and in many mutual help and support groups. *Closed groups* are those in which group membership does not change for the life of the group or only for a clearly understood reason. Members often must meet certain criteria for acceptance, such as a diagnosis or a particular therapeutic issue. For example, Alcoholics Anonymous is open only to people with a drug problem.

People need the assurance of full understanding of a particular diagnosis by others in the group to speak frankly. Psychotherapy groups can share characteristics of both open and closed membership. They are open in that as one member leaves the group, another fills the empty slot, but they have a closed membership in that members cannot arbitrarily enter the group simply because they have similar interests or problems.

Group Size

The size of the group influences group dynamics. Usually, a larger group limits the opportunity to share personal material. However, a larger group offers a cost-effective way to deliver educational information. Psychoeducational groups can consist of 10 to 15 members. In psychoeducational groups, the members discuss a particular topic such as medication, prevention, or symptom management of a mental disorder, but the process does not allow individuals to address personal psychological issues unrelated to the discussion topic.

Most insight-oriented therapy groups limit membership to six to eight. This size not only allows for a variety of interpretations but also permits sufficient interpersonal space for intimate sharing. Therapy groups need to have at least five members. With fewer than five members, the group is likely to produce an emotional intensity or to form subgroups, both of which are difficult to regulate.

Time Boundaries

Time boundaries in group therapy are extremely important. Most group therapy sessions last 75 to 90 minutes. Therapy sessions should begin and end on time. Attention to time boundaries respects the need of individuals to have lives outside the group and firmly integrates the group as a set pattern in the patient's life. The group space becomes a special agreed on time for self-exploration. Nothing interferes with it, and members can then plan activities in their lives to include their commitment to the group. Most individuals begin to depend on it and block out the time as their group time. Rescheduling meetings without having a definite rationale communicates to group members that the leader does not consider the group space to be important.

The time frame for group psychotherapy, if known, should be discussed in the pregroup interview and reinforced during the first session. Some groups are open-ended, but most have built-in time frames of 6 to 20 sessions in managed care outpatient settings and significantly fewer sessions in inpatient settings. I recommend setting a defined time frame for group therapy, even in outpatient settings, given managed care constraints. A new contract may be renegotiated with members if they achieve the original goals or the time period elapses. Making the assumption that the group should continue without further negotiation can be a mistake. Members can construe this assumption as a "bait and switch" that will affect further group participation. A more straightforward approach is to review members' progress and to solicit input as to how each group member would like to proceed. Individual decisions to leave the group at this point should be honored without any undue pressure to continue.

Inpatient Versus Outpatient Groups

Inpatient groups differ from outpatient groups in several ways. Group membership in inpatient groups depends on the particular patient population. Because of short stays, the focus of the group may be on spotting maladaptive behaviors that can be worked on in outpatient therapy and stabilizing symptoms enough to permit discharge. The content and process of inpatient psychotherapy is more superficial than in outpatient settings. With inpatient therapy, the therapist takes a much more active role, clarifies more often, and directs the process of establishing appropriate norms.

Because most inpatient treatment groups tend to be integral parts of a larger therapeutic protocol, the therapist needs to establish, in the initial session, that he or she will be sharing information from group sessions with other health team members. This disclosure is an explicit group norm because the leader must have the freedom to share information that could affect group treatment (Kibel, 1993). For example, members are bound to report any clandestine activities, such as members having intimate relationships with each other, smoking marijuana, or drinking alcohol. To withhold this kind of information can damage trust in group sharing and in treatment goals.

Socialization among members of both inpatient and outpatient groups is an issue. In the inpatient setting, activities that promote socialization receive support. The leader encourages members to continue the dialogue outside the therapy group that was begun in the group. The work of the outpatient group depends on limited social contact outside the group because members need to experience the full impact of intimate self-disclosure *within* the group. Consequently, regular socialization outside the group usually is discouraged. Confidentiality for group members is an expected norm but not one that the leader can enforce, legally. However, the leader can strengthen this norm by stressing its importance in keeping the group a safe place to reveal oneself. Lymberis (1993) noted that the "competence of the group leader is the best defense against member-to-member exploitation" (p. 352).

> *What do you think?* Reflect on groups to which you belong. How do these groups differ from therapeutic groups?

> ### ➤ *Check Your Reading*
> 21. How does the size of the group affect interaction?
> 22. Why are time boundaries important in group psychotherapy?
> 23. What is the meaning of universality in the group context?

Process

Phases of Group Development

Groups go through phases of development just as individuals do in one-to-one therapeutic relationships. The phases are sequential and overlapping, beginning with planning, which takes place before the group starts, and ending with termination and referrals, if needed. Tuckman (1965) described the phases of group development as forming, storming, norming, performing, and adjourning.

PREINTERACTION PHASE
The leader's first task is to establish a suitable foundation for the group by selecting an appropriate time and place for the group sessions and clearing these arrangements with other staff members. Psychotherapy groups must take place in a quiet, well-ventilated room where the group is not disturbed, and the chairs should be arranged so that all group members face each other.

The initial assessment interview takes place as an individual session before the first group session. Assessment interviews provide the therapist with an important opportunity to evaluate motivation and personal commitment. A potential member can be diagnostically suitable for the group and likely to benefit from the experience but, for a variety of reasons, lack the necessary commitment for group membership. Unless the person can be encouraged to find a reason for joining the group or is able to see the possible benefit, postponing membership or selecting a different treatment format is better. Potential group members who cannot make the time commitments, for example, someone who has to travel as part of the job, are not good candidates. Their "in and out" attendance pattern can be disruptive and is usually not tolerated well by other group members.

Another important goal of the pregroup assessment interview is to make entry into the group easier. People may have preconceptions about group therapy that the therapist can dispel. During this initial discussion, the patient begins to experience the "person" of the leader. Experiencing the group leader as a human being and a consistent member of the group beforehand often reduces patient anxiety about joining the group (Piper & Perrault, 1989). During the pregroup assessment interview, the therapist can provide necessary information about the group purpose, format, and expectations, and the patient can ask questions that may make the difference between whether he or she accepts or rejects group membership.

FORMING PHASE
The **forming phase** of group therapy is similar to the orientation phase in individual therapy in which group members begin to know each other. The therapist can begin the group with a self-introduction and ask members to say their names and tell the group something about themselves. The manner in which individuals express themselves and the type of information they choose to share provide important data that can be used later, in the working phase. However, the therapist

needs to make sure that members do not prematurely disclose lengthy intimate details about themselves because premature sharing can lead to intense discomfort when the sharer reflects on it, resulting in unanticipated termination. Preventing premature sharing can be accomplished by simply stating that the patient may want to bring up the topic later, when the group members know more about each other. Yalom (1995) also suggested letting members know from the start that the content for group discussion should be in the "here and now"; prolonged discussion of past events is not the focus. The group offers its members the unique opportunity to react to each other in the present, where other members can offer support or constructive feedback.

Acceptance, inclusion, and trust are primary values held by members in beginning group meetings. Initially, group communication tends to be tentative, polite, and guarded, as members explore their values and ideas with each other. They need to know that other group members, including the leader, will respect their contributions and will not make them look foolish to their peers. Finding that other members have had similar experiences and related feelings helps strengthen initial emotional bonding among group members. The group leader encourages the development of universality by linking member contributions together, pointing out similarities, and stressing the importance of group members as therapists for each other.

When the group begins to meet, the leader plays an active role in establishing the group structure. A standard first meeting format is to (1) identify the group's purpose and goal; (2) name fundamental structural norms such as expected attendance, confidentiality, and what to do in case of absence; and (3) explain how the group will function. A general statement about the nature of the work (i.e., that the group provides a place where members can discuss serious personal issues and receive feedback from each other) establishes the task of the group as serious. If members have never been in group therapy before, the therapist briefly educates them as to their roles as members. One way to introduce this is to make a simple statement about group goals and help members clarify the meaning of the goals. Letting members ask questions consistent with their personally held values tends to encourage greater commitment. Sufficient time to review and respond to individual concerns helps members feel heard and saves later frustration from unclear expectations.

Group Contract. The group contract spells out the boundaries of the relationship, issues of confidentiality, behaviors expected of the patients, and behaviors expected of the group therapist. In most psychotherapy groups, contracts are spoken rather than written. The contract represents the working agreement among individual members and the group leader and contains rules about absences, time and place of contact, relationships outside the group, and confidentiality. The group contract keeps the leader and members on track and focused on the reasons for the group's existence and its established therapeutic goals.

Ending Sessions. Toward the end of each meeting, even the first one, members are asked to summarize their reactions to the discussion. This process helps provide closure to issues. A strong summary statement also allows a concentrated glimpse at possible misperceptions or important feelings that have not emerged into full view and otherwise might go unaddressed. Here the therapist might say, "This would be a good topic for us to start with next time." After each session, record-keeping is completed on each group member related to the patient's response. A clinical summary is made related to progression toward desired outcomes.

STORMING PHASE

The transition stage of group of development consists of two interrelated phases, the storming phase and the norming phase. The **storming phase** of group development signals movement beyond the initial hesitancy and fear about being in the group. It can appear as a subtle questioning of appropriateness of time or group objectives. This opens the door to exploration of stronger feelings, hidden agendas, and open conflicts as members struggle with issues of power and control. Although uncomfortable, this phase of group development is absolutely essential because it sets the foundation for the development of the group-specific norms that will guide the group in the working phase. Fortunately, this phase usually does not last long. Establishing trust remains a central task for this phase of group development.

During the storming phase, the therapist acts as the gatekeeper by helping individual group members identify but move beyond their personal agendas and engage in group dialogue. During this phase, group members begin to engage with each other at a deeper level and to reveal more of their issues while asking for a similar commitment from others. Most significant for the group's development is the therapist's ability to act as a nonanxious presence in helping members maintain a positive attitude and commitment during the storming phase. This task is not easy, particularly if the therapist comes under attack. Group members look to the therapist to take the lead in modeling appropriate group behaviors. How the therapist conducts the sessions—listening and responding nondefensively to individual members and modeling respect for people's right to differ while maintaining the interest and boundaries of group members—is critical to successful resolution of this phase.

During the transition phase, the therapist becomes an "affirmer of standards," reflecting a basic respect for each person's contribution. This attitude encourages patients to take risks in communicating by making the interpersonal environment safe for each group member. As members work through their differences, the stage is set for the **norming phase,** in which the group, as a whole, develops the specific behavioral standards it needs to work through difficult issues.

NORMING PHASE

During the norming phase, the group develops *norms*—behavioral standards and basic operating procedures—that provide structural boundaries and guidelines for behaviors that will or will not be tolerated. Some behaviors are classified as universal **norms** because they are standards found in all psychotherapy groups. These are predetermined norms, voiced during the opening session, that include regular attendance, confidentiality, and the expectation of verbal contributions. Other standards are **group-specific norms,** which emerge from the needs of group members to facilitate goal achievement. For example, group-specific norms for a chronic schizophrenic therapy group might include specific basic group behaviors such as talking one at a time, not leaving the room during the session, refraining from violent behavior toward other group members, and refraining from obscene language. Specific norms in a drug abuse group would be to remain drug-free during the group sessions.

The more ownership individual members take in developing realistic norms, the more effective the group is likely to become. Group pressure on members who do not conform to expected norms helps reinforce bonding. Because norm violations by one group member affect the entire group, the leader must always address norm violations as being significant. When confronting a group member, the leader or group members need to understand why they are confronting and to deliver the feedback about specific observable behaviors. Confrontations should not be judgmental; they should be delivered from an "I" position and should focus on the effect of the behavior on other group members rather than labeling the member as "bad." Confrontations may need to occur more than once during the life of the group. Sometimes, a group-specific violation occurs when the group is facing a particularly difficult issue. Corey and Corey (1997) suggested that "the quality of the confrontations that occur in a group is an index of how effective the group is" (p. 89).

PERFORMING (WORKING) PHASE

Once the ground rules for operating the group are in place, members actively engage in working on group-determined agendas. The **performing phase** is characterized by cohesion and productivity, and the most in-depth work of the group takes place during this phase. Without the preliminary phases of forming, storming, and norming, however, the work could not be accomplished because the necessary trust and cooperation would not be present. Self-disclosure is more spontaneous and honest in the performing phase. Members know what to expect from each other. In the process of working through differences, a genuine respect for other members has developed, members trust the comments of others, and the sense of belonging is at its highest peak. Here, group members experience the altruism of helping others, interpersonal learning, self-understanding, and recapitulation of the family that Yalom (1995) identified as curative factors.

Throughout the performing phase, the therapist's primary function is to facilitate movement toward the group goals by providing an accepting interpersonal environment in which group members feel supported in exploring difficult issues. Group members take more responsibility for leadership activities and, in essence, become therapists for each other, although the group therapist retains overall accountability for maintaining group structure and ensuring progression toward group goals. The therapist needs to redirect group discussion when it becomes lost in detail or stuck in superficial discussion by asking relevant open-ended and focused questions. These interventions help the group explore problem areas in greater depth.

Using a variety of strategies to broaden the expressiveness of members helps deepen their connections. Neutral probes may encourage further details. The therapist consistently tries to engage the group as a whole in the problem-solving mode, so that all can learn from the shared experience. Seeking solutions consistent with treatment goals is an important function of group process. Often, group involvement with one member's dilemma mirrors other group members' difficulties with similar issues, and the therapist is in an excellent position to draw attention to this connection.

ADJOURNING (TERMINATION) PHASE

Good endings are as important as good beginnings in group life. The **adjourning phase** of group relationships occurs in a variety of ways: members leave, the group disbands, or a member is asked not to return for violating the group contract. Most often, individual group members leave a psychotherapy group because their work is finished or because they are discharged from the hospital or treatment program. Preparation for voluntary endings in an outpatient group can begin with a norm established in the first meeting or during the initial interview when the therapist asks each group member to tell the group of impending departure 1 week and to return the next to say goodbye.

Terminations are important both for the group as a whole and for the patient. Sufficient time for a fitting goodbye should be provided during each patient's last session. Ask the patient to tell the group what has been helpful and to say something to each group member. Another strategy is to ask each group member to share perceptions of the exiting patient with him or her. Generally, the therapist saves his or her remarks for last, to emphasize or neutralize other patient comments, if necessary. Sometimes, when a group member has been important to the group, the group is angry about the departure, and the words are not particularly supportive. The therapist may have to suggest, gently, that the group is having trouble giving up a valued member. If done with tact, this intervention can help members get in touch with their feelings. When eliciting feelings from other group members, Buchanan (1980) advised "keep it simple. Ask the group members how they feel and they will usually respond with short and direct statements" (p. 52). Recommendations for further referral usually are done individually and not as an explicit part of the group's termination process.

If the group as a whole is ending, the therapist can help the group summarize goal achievement and gain closure on any unresolved issues. Providing feedback about positive goal achievement individually and collectively is important to individual members and the group as a whole. In contrast to the performing (working) phase, the task of the adjourning phase is not to open new business. Rather, the intent is to gain closure on the experience. For many, the ending in one group frequently serves as an important element in considering membership in another therapy group.

Leadership Functions

The role of the leader in group treatment is not one simply of neutral observer or facilitator of the action. Rather it is one of *conductor* and *artist*. As conductor, the therapist takes primary responsibility for ensuring that the boundaries of the group are intact, that individual group members are not too vulnerable in the group, and that the group is moving toward achievement of group goals. The artistry of leadership is reflected in the therapist's ability to promote a spontaneous, interpersonal flow of communication among group members. It involves knowing when to confront and when to use a more laid-back approach, when to comfort and when to take a stern stand about an issue, when to help the group put closure on a topic and when to pursue a topic in more depth. Part of the healing process involves members' getting to know the therapist as a real person, not only as compassionate, trustworthy, and competent but also as capable of making mistakes. Effective leaders are sensitive to their own feelings and concerns as they emerge within the context of the group. Self-awareness allows the therapist the necessary objectivity to consistently act as an objective participant-observer.

The leader observes and comments on common themes expressed among members and the nature of members' interactions with each other. Feedback between patient and therapist takes place but is not the primary focus. Instead of answering the member directly, the leader redirects the question back to the group for discussion or broadens its application beyond that of the individual member. The continued presence of a caring, competent leader who is an active participant and who reinforces member feedback equips patients to become primary therapists for each other.

Co-leadership

Co-leadership refers to an equal peer relationship in which two mental health professionals assume shared leadership responsibility for the conduct of the group. There are many advantages to co-leadership, but one of the most important is having someone available to process the group, that is, talk about what happened, after each session. An equally informed and competent member who has shared in the same experience can be extremely valuable. The opportunity to share insights about the group process is an important source of clarification and support.

One co-leader often picks up on issues and feelings that the other may have missed. A co-leader can bring an issue forward directly or can nonverbally cue the other co-leader to its presence. If one co-leader makes a mistake in processing, the other can correct it and model for group members that differences in opinion and personal reactions need not be destructive. Patients sometimes split the co-leaders into polarities—nurturing versus harsh, bumbling versus competent. Although the co-leader under attack cannot always respond directly without appearing defensive, the other can redirect the transference focus without incurring the rage of the patient. This can be done with a statement such as, "It seems as though you are having a great deal of conflict with your feelings about Joan [group co-leader]. Any ideas what that is about?"

Co-leadership can be a growth experience for the therapists involved, as well as for the group. As the two co-leaders learn from each other, the experience becomes one of peer supervision. It also is hard work because it demands a high level of trust between the co-leaders. Therapists who choose to work together should be in agreement philosophically, although their basic communication style may differ. Ideally, their individual communication styles complement rather than mirror or conflict with each other. Essential to effective co-leadership is the need to establish norms of openness, honesty, and respect for each other's opinions, even when they disagree about how something should be handled. The co-leadership relationship will develop over time and, like other relationships, functions best when communication is harmonious and collaborative (Mackenzie, 1997).

Psychodrama

Psychodrama is a specific type of action-oriented group therapy sometimes conducted by advanced practice nurses with specialized training. According to Moreno (1964), the goal of this treatment approach "is not to analyze the patient, but to help him dream again." Moreno thought that traditional methods of group psychotherapy did not allow patients to really get in touch with their feelings, which they described but did not re-experience. With psychodrama, the patient (protagonist) is brought directly into the situation as an active participant. The director coordinates the process so that the group and the protagonist receive maximal benefit. Other group members act as auxiliary egos or play the roles of significant others with whom relationships are being explored. The action takes place as if it is unfolding in the present, even if the incident took place many years ago. The primary advantage of psychodrama is its direct access to reenacting painful situations so that the painful emotions associated with it can be reworked with the potential for spontaneously learning new responses in a safe therapeutic environment.

Warm-Up

Setting the scene for the psychodrama is part of the warm-up. This allows the protagonist time to become acquainted with the format and others who are taking part in the psychodrama. The same rules about confidentiality that apply to other therapeutic relationships and explanations of what will be placed in the patient's chart apply to psychodrama.

A double is used when the protagonist has difficulty expressing feelings about all or part of the situation. The double mimics the protagonist's body posture and gestures and puts into words the feelings suggested in the protagonist's nonverbal portrayal. The individual playing the double can be a group member, a staff member, or the group leader. By reinforcing appropriate feelings or strengthening the focus on an issue, the protagonist can deepen the meaning or develop new understandings of a situation.

For example, Sacks (1993) suggested the following sequencing of a scenario. The *protagonist* might say, "My mother went to the A&P and bought those stupid kiwis for a dollar each. Then she came back and paid the mortgage 3 weeks before it was even due. Then she bought this big stupid thing that . . . ." The double might respond, "She *always* throws her money away, and it drives me crazy" (p. 217). Psychodrama is an intense form of group psychotherapy for the protagonist. Periodically asking the protagonist how he or she is doing is essential. This brief questioning allows the patient to reflect on what is happening and to make necessary corrections if the process is too intense.

Achieving Closure

A critical dimension of the psychodrama process is achieving closure. Because of the powerful feelings that emerge from a psychodrama session, you have an ethical and therapeutic responsibility to allow enough time for closure and to provide for follow-up support with unit personnel, if warranted. Otherwise, an individual can have a powerful experience but little opportunity to integrate it into other parts of life or to consider the meaning of uncomfortable feelings associated with the psychodrama encounter.

ETHICAL AND LEGAL ISSUES

The advanced practice nurse in psychiatric nursing has moral and legal obligations to the patient, to the profession, and to himself or herself. These include

1. Having the requisite knowledge and skills necessary for effectively working with patients and their families in a variety of clinical settings and restricting scope of practice to these patient populations

2. Abiding by agency policies and legal guidelines for practice

3. Having self-awareness of potential biases, differences in values, beliefs, and attitudes that can affect therapeutic work and seeking consultation or referral when this occurs

4. Being sensitive to cultural, gender, religious, and political issues that influence therapeutic work

5. Avoiding personal or business relationships with patients or their families that are not part of the therapy process

6. Consulting with professional colleagues or qualified supervisors whenever there is a professional, ethical, or legal concern (the AACN requires that nurses in advanced practice seek peer supervision and have a consultative-referral relationship with a qualified physician)

7. Developing written informed consent procedures that are presented to the patient during the first session and as the need arises

8. Discussing payment and other business practices up front and following through with them

9. Introducing therapeutic strategies that respect the patient's autonomy and right to self-determination

10. Being careful with recordkeeping

11. Being aware of situations in which he or she must legally break confidentiality (e.g., to notify the authorities in cases of abuse or to warn someone of potential harm)

Conclusions

This chapter provides an overview of individual, family, and group therapy—treatment modalities that the advanced practice nurse in psychiatric nursing can use with patients and families. Advanced practice psychiatric nursing is a creative, skilled practice discipline dedicated to helping people resolve important psychological issues and achieve maximal mental health and well-being.

Individual brief therapy models are designed as action-oriented, present-focused, structured, time-limited interventions. Therapist and patient determine a core conflict or focal issue that will become the focus of treatment. Treatment can be a single session or may extend over 6 to 20 sessions. The termination date is predetermined and agreed on in the first session. Cognitive therapy is a specialized form of brief therapy based on the premise that the way people perceive an event rather than the event itself determines its relevance and a person's emo-

tional response. Therapeutic interventions are directed toward helping individuals resolve focal conflicts or target issues and correct the dysfunctional thinking that supports them.

Family therapy is based on natural systems theory. *Family* is defined as a natural social group or system with a coordinated power structure, rules, and ascribed roles of membership that have developed over time. Families come in many forms, ranging from single parent to traditional, with mother, father, and children. The family genogram is an assessment tool the nurse can use to track significant family events and relationships. The family therapist works to help family members understand family dynamics and take positions within the family unit consistent with their personal beliefs and values.

Group therapy is a third therapy form used by advanced practice nurses in psychiatric nursing. Group psychotherapy is defined as a structured, regular, predetermined meeting between two or more people for the purpose of achieving identified health-related goals. Group therapy uses peer relationships as well as the professional relationship between the therapist and patients in a collaborative, structured, time-limited format to provide relief of symptoms, resolution of interpersonal problems, and personal growth.

There is general agreement that treatment of mental illness combining psychotherapy and pharmacology is more effective than either one alone. Nurse therapists need to devise outcome studies for various psychotherapies practiced by nurses and to define that practice as unique to advanced practice psychiatric nursing. With such studies, nurses could advocate for patients with data showing that mental health care is an important aspect of patients' overall health.

Key Points to Remember

- Advanced practice nursing interventions require a master's degree and certification as an adult or child and adolescent clinical specialist or an NP in psychiatric mental health nursing.
- Psychotherapy is frequently referred to as the talking cure.
- The evolvement of brief psychotherapy occurred in response to advances in biological understandings of mental illness, economics, and sociopolitical factors influencing mental health care delivery.
- Brief individual psychotherapy is an action-oriented, present-focused, structured, and time-limited form of therapy.
- The role of the therapist in brief psychotherapy is an active one.
- The therapist and patient form a partnership to help the patient develop new, more effective ways of coping.
- During the first session, the therapist and patient select a core conflict or central issue to focus on for the duration of therapy.
- Homework is an important component of brief psychotherapy.
- Termination is predetermined.
- Cognitive behavioral psychotherapy is a form of brief psychotherapy focused on correcting the cognitive distortions that maladaptively influence the patient's behavior and feelings.
- Family therapy is based on natural systems theory.
- Families are systems in which the whole is viewed as greater than and different from the individual parts.
- Family patterns of interaction tend to extend over generations (multigenerational transmission).
- Self-differentiation allows a person to separate thinking from feeling with greater freedom to act in his or her best interests.
- A Bowen therapist acts as a coach to families in distress by helping them develop different ways of interacting with each other.
- According to Bowen, the two important variables in human functioning are level of differentiation and anxiety.
- The triangle is a three-person emotional system that shapes most human interaction.

- A structural family therapy framework actively challenges the maladaptive reactive transactional patterns to help the family system explore and develop a different level of homeostasis.
- An effective family assessment tool is the genogram, which is used to describe family facts and relationships.
- Evaluating the effectiveness of family therapy includes an examination of the effects on different members and subsystems as well as on the entire family unit.
- The goal of group psychotherapy is to assist patients to resolve behavioral symptoms and to develop higher levels of functioning in interpersonal relationships.
- The dynamics of group psychotherapy are influenced by member selection, time frameworks, and leader expertise.
- The sequential development of group therapy follows the pattern of forming, storming, norming, performing, and adjourning.
- Yalom identified 11 curative factors found in effective psychotherapy groups: catharsis, universality, self-understanding, recapitulation of the primary family, cohesion, altruism, instillation of hope, identification, interpersonal learning, guidance, and existential factors.
- Most psychotherapy groups are composed of six to eight patients. This group size permits greater emotional sharing than a larger group would allow.
- Group members usually do not know each other before entering the group. It is best not to include in the same group people who socialize with each other.
- Universal group norms include issues of confidentiality, attendance, and absences.
- Group members generally have some say in setting group goals and establishing group-specific norms that are comfortable for all group members.
- The content of most psychotherapy groups relates to emotional sharing in a here-and-now context.
- Psychodrama is action-oriented group psychotherapy in which participants reenact past experiences in the present.

Learning Activities

1. Interview a nurse psychotherapist to discover the types of patients who are coming for psychotherapy. Some of the questions you might ask include the following: What are your greatest challenges as a therapist? What are your greatest frustrations as a therapist? How has managed care affected your clinical practice?

2. Many movies and books depict the therapy process. Watch or read one and identify the techniques. Some suggestions include the movies *Good Will Hunting* and *What About Bob?* and the book *I Never Promised You a Rose Garden.*

3. During a meeting with one of your psychiatric patients, construct a time line that indicates all the important or nodal events or family stressors that have occurred for the patient during the past 10 years. Include both normal developmental and unexpected crises. Does the patient see any relationship between these events and personal health?

4. Make a list of all the possible behaviors a family can use to help members cope with a serious illness. See if your classmates can add to it. Which of these behaviors does your own family use? How difficult would it be for your family to try some new ones?

5. Construct a genogram with one of your patients. Try to collect data about at least three generations. Be sure to include both facts and emotional relationships. Does the genogram help the patient see any connections he or she has not seen before? Do you think the patient is generally objective or generally blaming in describing the family?

6. Pick a concept of interest to psychiatric nurses such as caring, empowerment, or belonging. Imagine an incident related to the topic and write a description of nurses employing the concept. Include participants, set the scene, and explain the incident's meaning to you. Share your story with a small group of students. As each student shares a story, identify underlying themes. Have one student act as scribe and record the underlying themes. Define the concept by identifying themes discussed in small groups with the whole class. Develop a common definition for the concept.

7. Identify a support group in your community and arrange to talk with the contact person or to attend the group. (Usually, community support groups are listed in the community newspaper with time, place, and contact person.) Ask about the group's purpose, format, session times, fees, and any other information you can glean about the group. Share this information with your clinical or student group.

Critical Thinking Exercises

Nurse Sweeney recently attended a course about cognitive psychotherapy. She plans to incorporate the concepts into her practice as a nurse psychotherapist. To formulate her nursing interventions using Beck's concepts, she presented the following patient to the course instructor. Mrs. Kennal, a 60-year-old schoolteacher, recently had surgery for breast cancer. She was unable to return to teaching because she did not want to touch anyone or anything. She believed that she would contaminate others and give them cancer. Because she feared being alone and helpless, Mrs. Kennal refused to drive to her doctor's appointments.

1. What assumptions can Nurse Sweeney make about Mrs. Kennal's behaviors?

2. What evidence supports these assumptions?

3. What cognitive distortions might Mrs. Kennal be making about her physical health?

Nurse Sweeney determined that Mrs. Kennal had used distorted thinking when she believed the cancer had contaminated her and in turn she would contaminate others. She also used it in her belief that the stress of teaching and controlling children in the classroom caused her to get cancer.

1. How would Nurse Sweeney test her conclusions?

2. Suggest other alternatives to those stated.

Susie had planned to attend junior college 10 miles away from the family home after graduation, but about a month after she declared this decision, she announced to her parents at dinner that she was going away to a private college. She stated that her basketball coach could get her financial help and she could get a 50% scholarship. She failed to tell her parents that her boyfriend would also be going to this school.

1. What would Bowen say about triangles in this family?

2. What assumptions might Susie be making or reacting to?

3. Consider possible reactions that her parents might have to Susie's announcement.

Susan and Ron are senior nursing students going through their psychiatric nursing practicum. Their assignment was to organize a medication teaching group for the patients on the general psychiatric unit. They recruited five patients: Mrs. G, a 45-year-old school bus driver admitted because of a recent accidental medication overdose; Mr. Z, a 22-year-old college student recently admitted with a delusion that the devil was stealing his mind and soul; Mr. S, a 40-year-old depressed secretary ready for discharge; Mr. J, a 42-year-old paranoid computer operator; and Ms. B, a 33-year-old phobic telephone operator. Everyone met in the conference room sitting in chairs around a long table.

1. What assumptions can you make about Susan and Ron's knowledge of groups?

2. What evidence do you have to support your assumptions?

3. Give an alternative explanation as to why this group might have been chosen.

At the beginning of group, Ron and Susan asked patients to introduce themselves and identify which medications they were taking. When Mrs. G began to talk about the sadness she felt and how the paroxetine HCl (Paxil) she was taking helped her, Mr. Z stood up and announced that she should read the Bible more and then she would not be sad. At this time, Ms. B covered her ears, started to cry, and said, "I want to leave."

1. Put yourself in each patient's place and identify her or his point of view.

2. Make sense out of what might be happening.

3. How might the leader respond effectively in this situation?

Additional Resources

American Academy of Child and Adolescent Psychiatry (AACAP)

3615 Wisconsin Avenue, NW
Washington, DC 20016-3007
202-966-7300
http://www.aacap.org

Campaign for Our Children

120 West Fayette Street
Suite 1200
Baltimore, MD 21201
410-576-9015
http://www.cfoc.org

References

Alexander, F., & Selesnick, S. (1968). *The history of psychiatry.* New York: New American Library.

Alonso, A., & Swiller, H. (1992). *Group therapy in clinical practice.* Washington, DC: American Psychiatric Press.

Arnold, E., & Boggs, K. (1999). *Interpersonal relationships: Professional communication skills for nurses* (3rd ed.). Philadelphia: W. B. Saunders.

Beck, A. (1976). *Cognitive theory and emotional disorders.* New York: International University Press.

Beck, J. (1995). *Cognitive therapy: Basics and beyond.* New York: Guilford Press.

Bowen, M. (1978). *Family therapy in clinical practice.* New York: Aronson.

Brigham, A. (1994). The moral treatment of insanity (July, 1847). *American Journal of Psychiatry, 151*(6), 11–16.

Buchanan, D. (1980). The central concern model, a framework for structuring psychodramatic production. *Group Psychotherapy, Psychodrama and Sociometry, 33,* 25–32.

Budman, S., & Gurman, A. (1988). *Theory and practice of brief therapy.* New York: Guilford Press.

Carr, A. (1998). Positive practice in family therapy. *Journal of Marital and Family Therapy, 23,* 271–293.

Cierpka, M. (1998). Stereotypical relationship patterns and psychopathology. *Psychotherapeutic Psychosomatics, 67,* 241–248.

Corey, G., & Corey, M. (1997). *Groups: Process and practice* (5th ed.). Monterey, CA: Brooks/Cole.

Crits-Christoph, P. (1992). The efficacy of brief dynamic psychotherapy: A meta-analysis. *American Journal of Psychiatry, 149,* 151–158.

de Shazer, S., Berg, I., Lipchik, E., Nunnally, E., Molnar, A., Gingerich, W., Weiner-Davis, M. (1986). Brief therapy: Focused solution development. *Family Process, 25,* 207–221.

Foulkes, S. H. (1975). *Group analytic psychotherapy: Method and principles.* London: Gordon & Breach.

Friedlander, M. (1998). Assessing clients' constructions of their problems in family therapy discourse. *Journal of Marital Family Therapy, 24,* 289–303.

Gavazzi, S. (1993). The relation between family differentiation levels in families with adolescents and the severity of presenting problems. *Family Relations, 42,* 463–468.

Glick, P. C. (1988). Fifty years of family demography: A record of social change. *Journal of Marriage and the Family, 50,* 861–873.

Goldenberg, I., & Goldenberg, H. (1996). *Family therapy: An overview* (4th ed.). Pacific Grove, CA: Brooks/Cole.

Gordon, T. (1980). Parent effectiveness training: A preventative program and its effect on families. In M. J. Fine (Ed.), *Handbook on parent education.* New York: Academic Press.

Grando, R., & Ginsberg, B. G. (1976). Communication in the father-son relationship: The parent-adolescent relationship development program. *The Family Coordinator, 25,* 465–473.

Gunther, M. (1998). A place called HOPE: Group psychotherapy for adolescents of parents with HIV/AIDS. *Child Welfare, 77,* 251–271.

Halevy, J. (1998). A genogram with an attitude. *Journal of Marital and Family Therapy, 24,* 233–242.

Hawkins, A. J., & Roberts, T. A. (1992). Designing a primary intervention to help dual-earner couples share housework and child care. *Family Relations, 41,* 169–171.

Heatherington, L. (1998). Assessing individual family members' constructions of family problems. *Family Process, 37,* 167–187.

Innes, M. (1996). Connecting Bowen theory with its human origins. *Family Process, 35,* 487–500.

Jacques, J. (1998). Working with spiritual and religions themes in group therapy. *International Journal of Group Psychotherapy, 48,* 69–83.

Kaplan, H., & Sadock, B. (1993). *Comprehensive group psychotherapy.* Baltimore: Williams & Wilkins.

Kerr, M., & Bowen, M. (1988). *Family evaluation.* New York: Norton.

Kibel, H. (1993). Inpatient group psychotherapy. In A. Alonso & H. Swiller (Eds.), *Group therapy in clinical practice* (pp. 93–111). Washington, DC: American Psychiatric Press.

Leibenluft, E., & Goldberg, R. (1993). Guidelines for short-term inpatient psychotherapies. *American Journal of Psychiatry, 143,* 1507–1517.

Lymberis, M. (1993). Ethical and legal issues in group psychotherapy. In A. Alonso & H. Swiller (Eds.), *Group therapy in clinical practice* (pp. 343–356). Washington, DC: American Psychiatric Press.

MacKenzie, K. R. (1997). *Time-managed group psychotherapy: Effective clinical applications.* Washington, DC: American Psychiatric Press.

MacKenzie, K. R. (1990). *Introduction to brief group psychotherapy.* New York: Harper & Row.

MacKenzie, K. R. (1992). *Classics in group psychotherapy.* New York: Guilford Press.

Mann, J. (1973). *Time-limited psychotherapy.* Cambridge, MA: Harvard University Press.

Mason, W. (1994). Solution-focused therapy and inpatient psychiatric nursing. *Journal of Psychosocial Nursing, 32*(10), 46-49.

McGihon, N. (1994). Health care reform: Clinical implications for inpatient psychiatric nursing. *Journal of Psychosocial Nursing, 32*(11), 31-33.

McGoldrick, M., & Gerson, R. (1985). *Genograms in family assessment.* New York: Norton.

Minuchin, S. (1974). *Families and family therapy.* Cambridge, MA: Harvard University Press.

Moreno, J. L. (1964). *Psychodrama* (Vol. 1). New York: Beacon House.

Nichols, P., & Schwartz, R. (1998). *Family therapy: Concepts and methods* (4th ed.). Needham Heights, MA: Allyn & Bacon.

North, C. (1998). The family as caregiver: A group psychoeducation model for schizophrenia. *American Journal of Orthopsychiatry, 68*(1), 39-46.

Papero, D. (1990). *Bowen family systems therapy.* Boston: Allyn & Bacon.

Piper, W. E., & Perrault, E. (1989). Pretherapy preparation for group members. *International Journal of Group Psychotherapy, 38,* 17-34.

Plato. (1952). *The dialogues of Plato.* Chicago: William Benton.

Pollido, D. (1998). Content and curriculum in psychoeducation groups for families of persons with severe mental illness. *Psychiatric Services, 49,* 816-822.

Pratt, J. (1992). The class method of treating consumption in the homes of the poor. In K. R. MacKenzie (Ed.), *Classics in group psychotherapy* (pp. 25-30). New York: Guilford Press.

Puskar, K. (1996, July 15). The nurse practitioner role in psychiatric nursing: Expanding advanced practice through the NP role. *Online Journal of Issues in Nursing.* (Available at http://www.nursingworld/ojin/tpc1/tpc1_E2.htm)

Roosa, M., Gensheimer, L., Short, J., Ayers, T., & Shell, R. (1989). A preventive intervention for children in alcoholic families: Results of a pilot study. *Family Relations, 38,* 295-300.

Sacks, J. (1993). Psychodrama. In H. Kaplan & B. Sadock (Eds.), *Comprehensive group psychotherapy* (3rd ed.). Baltimore: Williams & Wilkins.

Scheidlinger, S. (1994). An overview of nine decades of group psychotherapy. *Hospital and Community Psychiatry, 45,* 217-224.

Simon, F. (1998). Beyond bipolar thinking: Patterns of conflict as a focus for diagnosis and intervention. *Family Process, 371,* 215-232.

Strachey, J. (Ed.). (1958). *Standard edition of the complete psychological works of Sigmund Freud* (Vol. 12). London: Hogarth Press.

Tuckman, B. (1965). Developmental sequence in small groups. *Psychological Bulletin, 63,* 384-399.

Walsh, F. (1998). The resilience of the field of family therapy. *Journal of Marital Family Therapy, 24,* 269-271.

Yalom, I. D. (1995). *The theory and practice of group psychotherapy* (4th ed.). New York: Basic Books.

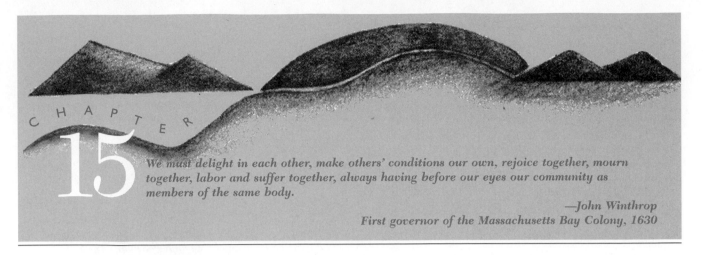

The Continuum of Care

Learning Objectives

After studying this chapter, you should be able to:

1. Discuss at least three events that influenced the development of community mental health (CMH) care.

2. Describe the group of chronically mentally ill served by CMH care.

3. Define the terms *institutionalization, deinstitutionalization, revolving door cycle,* and *catchment area.*

4. Define the acute, transitional, and follow-up phases of the psychiatric continuum.

5. Define milieu therapy and name contemporary settings in which it is used.

6. List the components of milieu therapy.

7. Define and give examples of primary, secondary, and tertiary prevention.

8. Describe how psychiatric home care is a bridge to community care.

9. Discuss Bay Area Health Care's model of psychiatric home care.

10. Discuss at least three of the housing options available to the chronically mentally ill.

11. Apply the nursing process in cases in which the focus of care is on the community.

Key Terminology

Adult foster care
Catchment area
Chronically mentally ill
Clinical case management
Community mental health center (CMHC)
Congregate housing
Continuum of psychiatric treatment
Crisis unit

Day treatment
Deinstitutionalization
Holding environment
Homebound
Independent housing
Institutionalization
Intermittent supervised residential setting
Milieu

Milieu therapy
Mobile treatment
Outpatient therapy
Primary prevention
Psychiatric home care
Psychosocial rehabilitation program
Residential therapeutic community

Revolving door cycle
Seriously and persistently mentally ill
Secondary prevention
Sheltered housing
Tertiary prevention
Therapeutic community
24-Hour supervised residential setting

In order for you to function effectively to meet the mental health needs of your patients, you must have a clear understanding of the full continuum of psychiatric care. Whether or not you specialize in psychiatric nursing, you need to know about the range of services available to treat mental illness and to promote mental health. Due to the nature of mental illness, the concept of a treatment continuum is especially important. Patients who experience mental illness during their life journey often require help for extended periods in several different settings.

The psychiatric treatment continuum may be viewed as having three phases: acute, transitional, and follow-up (Segal, Hazan, & Kotler, 1990) (Figure 15–1). Patients use acute care for crisis intervention under high-risk circumstances. When patients make the transition from acute care, they may move to follow-up care or remain in transitional care for an extended period, depending on their needs for support. Transitional care may also be used after follow-up care in an attempt to prevent acute care. And some patients may access follow-up care merely for short-term stressful life situations.

There are several contemporary issues dramatically affecting the delivery of mental health services (LeCuyer, 1992; Watson, 1992):

1. Decreased length of stay across all treatment settings
2. Maintenance of seriously mentally ill patients in the least restrictive settings
3. Advances in biomedical treatment
4. Cost-containment efforts
5. Aging population

These factors present many challenges to the psychiatric nurse who must establish therapeutic relationships more quickly than in years past while preparing comprehensive discharge recommendations for the patient's next level of care.

The purpose of this chapter is to introduce you to the various settings for psychiatric treatment. Significant concepts underlying community mental health (CMH)

are discussed. You meet one young patient and follow him through his journey in the mental health system. After a brief historical perspective, each level of care in the continuum is defined. Finally, the steps of the nursing process are applied to a community example to differentiate these steps from those taken in other examples of individual patients presented in this book.

Peter's Story

Peter is in the outpatient clinic this morning for an emergency evaluation. He is met by Marianne, a psychiatric nurse. Peter is accompanied by Kim, his case manager, who is concerned about Peter's behavior during the past 24 hours. Kim reports to Marianne, "I got a call early today from the residential program director who said that Peter has been more irritable and argumentative. He has been verbalizing threatening statements that have something to do with someone's trying to get him kicked out of town. Peter has not been sleeping well lately—in fact, the past 2 nights he slept only 1 to 2 hours. I'm worried about him. Until today I have never been afraid of him, but today he threatened to hurt me if I didn't get him out of town."

Peter's History

Marianne reviews Peter's history and finds that he has been out of a state hospital for only 1 month. There he received treatment for 6 months, but before entering the state hospital, Peter had been in another hospital close to his parents' home, which had closed its units and relocated Peter. Peter's history includes three psychiatric admissions and placements in several residential settings in his home county, from which he ran away many times, often back to the state hospital. Peter has been threatening to staff members in the past, but he has never harmed himself or others while

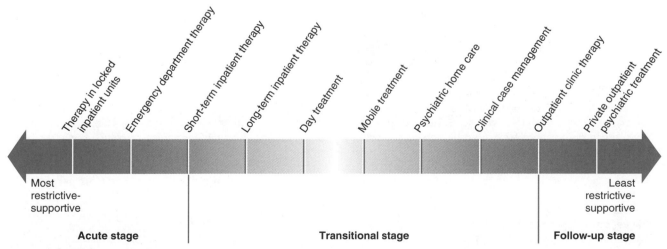

Figure 15–1
The psychiatric treatment continuum.

hospitalized. He assaulted his father and a police officer several years ago. Peter has demonstrated impaired judgment by running away without money or resources in cold weather, and he has been consistently unable to manage his resources when in the community. In addition to the residential placements, Peter has lived at the YMCA and a group home, but he always ran out of money and ran away from these settings.

Peter's Current Condition

In the waiting room, Peter sits several seats away from Kim. He appears restless. He scans his environment, mumbles, smiles, and giggles to himself. Abruptly Peter stands up and yells, "I have to see the doctor now . . . or somebody's gonna be sorry!"

Marianne observes Peter's distress and sees him promptly. Peter appears a little more comfortable in Marianne's office, away from the busy waiting room. Marianne asks Peter to tell her what is happening with him. Peter states, "There are forces that want me out of this town; if I can't get help, I might have to hurt somebody. I have been hearing voices . . . they say they will kill me. Can you help me?" Marianne responds, "You are in a safe place, Peter. We will help you. You will not be alone, and we will not let anything harm you." Marianne documents evidence of auditory hallucinations, delusional thoughts, and high anxiety and feelings of being unsafe. Peter appears calmer and agrees to remain in Marianne's office with Kim while he waits to see the psychiatrist. Marianne uses another office to make calls to determine the available resources that may be needed to help Peter remain safe. She finds that a bed is available in the local hospital's acute psychiatric unit, and a direct admission is possible with the treatment team's referral.

Peter is seen by the psychiatrist, and the treatment team refers Peter to the acute care setting for stabilization of his schizophrenia. Marianne meets with Peter to tell him of the recommendation for inpatient care. Peter seems relieved and agrees to enter the hospital as a voluntary patient.

Inpatient Setting

Peter is admitted to a locked inpatient unit where he remains for 5 days. Medication is adjusted, Peter benefits from a low-stress environment, and an attempt to identify stressors is made.

Peter is accompanied to the hospital by Kim. Because Marianne has arranged for a direct admission to the psychiatric unit, Peter does not go to the emergency department before admission to the psychiatric unit. Before admission, Peter was pacing and talking about people who want to run him out of this town. Now, however, Peter seems to be familiar with hospital routines and appears less agitated.

Miguel, a psychiatric nurse, is Peter's primary nurse. Miguel's initial assessment of Peter includes psychiatric and medical history, presenting problem, medications, psychosocial history, and mental status. Miguel reviews patient rights with Peter and provides him a copy. When Peter is calm, Miguel gives Peter a tour of the unit and introduces him to other patients and to staff members. The unit routine is discussed.

Peter's medication is adjusted, and Miguel documents Peter's responses and assesses him for side effects. Miguel remains in contact with Kim (Peter's case manager) and Marianne (Peter's outpatient clinic nurse) regarding discharge plans. Peter's symptoms stabilize within 4 days. He no longer refers to being run out of town. He reports a decrease in auditory hallucinations and is less frequently heard mumbling to himself. During the hospitalization, no contributing stressors were identified that explained Peter's increased symptoms. Peter does admit that he does not have any friends and is away from his family.

For support, the inpatient unit refers Peter to the crisis unit, with a plan for him to return to residential housing in about 1 week. But before Peter leaves the hospital for the crisis unit, Miguel schedules him an appointment at the clinic with Marianne, the clinic nurse, to monitor his medication.

Outpatient Clinic

Peter sees Marianne, who is an advanced practice clinician (i.e., clinical specialist), in the outpatient clinic before he goes to the crisis unit. Marianne monitors Peter's medication, mental status, and community adjustment. She provides psychoeducation to Peter, his family, and his care providers at the residential program. Peter arranges individual therapy with her.

Within the nurse-patient therapeutic relationship, Peter expresses to Marianne his distress with his diagnosis, his despair at his loss of potential, and his questioning of religious beliefs related to having a chronic illness. Peter and his family have a strong religious faith, and Peter's illness has been perceived by his family as a loss of faith. Additionally, he is in a community that is no longer near his church. He expresses guilt that he has not attended religious services, as was his practice when he lived in his home community.

Over the course of his lifetime, most of his treatment will be provided in this setting. The outpatient clinic, or community mental health center (CMHC), provides evaluation, medication, emergency evaluation, and case management. The clinic is the hub of Peter's treatment.

Case Management

In the meantime, Kim, Peter's case manager, works to link him with needed medical services. For example, Kim arranges for Peter to have some dental work done by a dentist who donates services to disabled people. She also helps Peter contact his pastor and arrange for a visit.

Residential Therapeutic Community

The purpose of Peter's stay in the crisis unit is to enable him to return to his day program while there are staff members available at night. When Peter returns to his day program, it is discovered that there are irreconcilable differences between Peter and the two men who share his apartment.

The two men had played a couple of jokes on Peter and had been doing pranks to make him react. Peter had difficulty coping with being the brunt of the jokes because he was new to the apartment, and his illness makes environmental stress difficult to handle. A team meeting is called, including Peter, Marianne, Kim, and residential and crisis unit staff members. Now less symptomatic, Peter is able to ask for a different residential arrangement. Another apartment is found with one other male patient. Peter agrees to a 2-week trial of living in the new apartment. Until he demonstrates that he is comfortable, Peter will have increased staff member support in his residential setting.

Peter's story illustrates the appropriate use of resources across the **continuum of psychiatric treatment** (see Figure 15-1). He was able to access acute care without an emergency department evaluation because he had a case manager to coordinate his community services. He was already under care in the transitional stage, depending on a day treatment program and case management to help him function at his optimal level of independence. (He also had the support of supervised residential housing, which is described later.) His actual psychiatric treatment at the follow-up level of care was in the outpatient clinic.

As a young adult with schizophrenia, Peter is a member of the population called **chronically mentally ill** or **seriously and persistently mentally ill.** This group is defined as "Those individuals who are, have been, or might have been but for the deinstitutionalization movement on the rolls of the long-term mental institutions, especially state hospitals" (Bachrach, 1979, p. 387). (See Chapter 24 for further discussion of nursing care for the schizophrenic patient.)

WHO ARE THE CHRONICALLY MENTALLY ILL?

The chronically mentally ill are a diverse group with a variety of diagnoses, including schizophrenia; major affective disorders; and organic disorders secondary to trauma, disease, or substance abuse. They include the chronically mentally ill elderly, who may reside independently with supportive family nearby or with a supportive network of caring people who might include landlord, mail carrier, local grocer, and others who look out for the individual's welfare (Buckwalter & Light, 1989). Some of the chronically mentally ill elderly live with family and friends; some live in supervised housing, such as foster care or nursing homes (Richter, 1990).

Chronically mentally ill patients may hold jobs in the community during periods when symptoms are in remission; those with residual symptoms that interfere with their functional capacity may rely on disability checks and sporadic employment. They may reside in foster or group homes. Some seek shelter in decrepit urban hotels, whereas others take to the street and end up in shelters for the homeless. Some of those with severe mental illness reside, inappropriately, in prisons. Many have complicating patterns of substance abuse.

For some, substance abuse is a primary problem. For others, substance abuse may be an attempt to self-medicate to ease the pain of a difficult life (Bostelman et al., 1994; Conway, Melzer, & Hale, 1994).

The group of chronically mentally ill range in age from the young, who have never experienced long-term institutionalization, to the old, who suffer from deinstitutionalization. All experience problems of being emotionally and mentally disabled and must live with the stigma of mental illness. Sheets, Prevost, and Reihman (1982) identified three subgroups among the young (from 18 to 30 years of age) chronically mentally ill: a subgroup that is high-functioning, a subgroup that is passively accepting (low energy, low demand), and a subgroup that actively denies they have mental illness (high energy, high demand). Those who aggressively deny the reality of their illness have the most difficulty accepting any help, including supervised housing. They prefer the independence of hotels and the streets. Those who choose to live with limited interpersonal contact may withdraw, may neglect themselves, and may stop taking their medications, and they are especially vulnerable to exploitation by others. There has been reported success, however, in working with these patients to persuade them to accept help within the CMH care system and to accept residential living arrangements (Cutler, 1986).

What do you think? Compare the continuum of psychiatric services with what you know is available for other diseases such as diabetes or congestive heart disease. Is there a difference? If so, why?

► *Check Your Reading*

1. Why is the continuum of services important for psychiatric patients?
2. What are the three phases of the psychiatric treatment continuum?
3. Name three issues currently affecting delivery of mental health services.
4. What is the general definition for the population called "chronically mentally ill" or "seriously and persistently mentally ill"?

HISTORICAL PERSPECTIVE

In order for you to appreciate the current structure of mental health services, with its strengths and its weaknesses, you need to understand significant points of history. Policy and funding decisions by the federal government have had a profound effect on the health care system (Buerhaus, 1998). Before 1963, CMH care was nonexistent in the United States. Severely impaired patients were admitted to psychiatric hospitals, where they frequently remained the rest of their lives. Admission to a psychiatric hospital was viewed as the end of the road, the last stop for dealing with chronic, seemingly intractable problems.

When the phenothiazine drugs (e.g., chlorpromazine [Thorazine]) were produced in the 1950s, it caused a revolution in treatment (Buerhaus, 1998). With the elimination of the most bizarre psychiatric symptoms, patients were able to be discharged back into the community. But new obstacles were encountered: many patients did not have a family to welcome them back home and they needed new living arrangements; some patients still showed symptoms that interfered with normal social behavior; other patients suffered from signs of **institutionalization,** a condition characterized by dependency with impaired social interactions, decision-making, and independent living skills resulting from long-term care in an institutional setting.

In 1955, Congress created the Joint Commission on Mental Illness and Health to analyze the needs and resources of the mentally ill and to make recommendations for national policy (Krauss & Slavinsky, 1982). In 1961, the Commission published its report recommending that treatment be moved from the state hospital to the community setting, which is known as **deinstitutionalization.** The goals were as follows, as quoted by the Commission (Joint Commission on Mental Illness and Health, 1961):

The objective of modern treatment of persons with mental illness is to enable the patient to maintain himself in the community in a normal manner. To do so, it is necessary (1) to save the patient from debilitating effects of institutionalization, (2) to return to home and community life as soon as possible, and (3) thereafter, to maintain him in the community as long as possible. Therefore, aftercare and rehabilitation are essential parts of all services to mental patients, and the various methods of achieving rehabilitation should be integrated in all forms of services, among them day hospitals, night hospitals, aftercare clinics, public health nursing centers, foster family care, convalescent nursing homes, rehabilitation centers, work services and ex-patient groups. (p. 16)

In 1963, Congress passed the Community Mental Health Act, which established the comprehensive **community mental health center (CMHC)** (Bachrach, 1979). Each CMHC was to provide five services:

1. Inpatient care
2. Outpatient care
3. Partial hospitalization
4. Emergency care
5. Consultation and education

It was expected that federal funds would not be needed in the long term; instead, services would eventually be funded by state and local governments and by fees for service. In 1965, Medicare and Medicaid legislation was passed that provided health insurance for the elderly and the poor, including payment for mental health care.

Before the new community system had a chance to become firmly established, state hospitals began to discharge large numbers of patients to reduce costs. Communities were not prepared with the necessary supports to receive these patients. Housing and treatment facilities were scarce and the community attitude was inhospitable; patients were mocked, feared, and stigmatized for conditions over which they had no control. Largely unwelcomed and rebuffed, many patients found that life outside the hospital was too stressful to tolerate. Their symptoms worsened and they sought readmission to the hospital, starting a **revolving door cycle:** short inpatient stays, rapid discharge, and eventual relapse with repeated admissions.

In the 1970s, federal funds continued to cover CMHCs, and additional requirements were set: specialized services were mandated for children, the elderly, transitional housing, drug abuse, and alcohol abuse. In 1979, psychiatric home care was added to Medicare benefits for home health services. It was becoming clear that state and local governments were not able to match federal funds, and that rural and poor areas would not be self-sufficient with fees.

During the 1960s and 1970s, length of stay in inpatient and outpatient treatment was based mainly on physicians' clinical judgment and paid as fee for service. Although all insurance plans, including Medicare and Medicaid, had an annual or lifetime limit for mental health care coverage, there was no external control on the patient's use of the benefit. A hospital stay might extend from 1 to 6 months; outpatient treatment continued as long as the patient was making progress. Discharge goals in each setting were based on resolution of all problems. The cost of medical care, both general and psychiatric, increased significantly.

Throughout the 1980s, the federal government significantly altered its support to mental health services. There was increased attention to the rising costs of health care and concern about the national budget deficit. The Omnibus Budget Reconciliation Act (OBRA) of 1982 shifted the administration of mental health programs to the individual states, and each state received a block grant to cover services. The Community Mental Health Systems Act of 1980, with the goal of improving coordination between CMHCs and hospitals, was repealed. As of 1984, all federal funding for CMHCs was terminated and centers were mandated to return to the core five services again.

As the 1980s and 1990s unfolded, the focus on controlling health care costs intensified, leading to the rising dominance of managed care (Grob, 1994). It became clear that federal funding would not increase and future Medicare policy would reflect the same issues as the private sector: to emphasize preventive services, to constrain provider payments, and to shift more care out of acute care settings and into the community and home arena (Buerhaus, 1998). States began to privatize the payment system for Medicaid patients, and the Medicare population was bombarded by managed care invitations to switch their benefits. In every setting, clinical staff members were being urged to do more with less. Drolen (1990) warned that this aggressive emphasis on efficiency would have a demoralizing effect on human service workers.

Another major innovation of the 1990s was the increased involvement of recipients of services in the planning efforts (Chamberlin & Rogers, 1990). Former-patient groups and self-help groups began organizing in the 1970s and gradually gained a voice in public policy. Public Law 99-660 required the participation of various constituencies including ex-patients in planning for community-based mental health care. Managed care organizations were increasingly interested in evaluating quality of services, seeking consumer feedback as a significant element (Chisholm et al., 1997).

> **W**hat do you think? What role should former and current patients play in designing a more effective mental health delivery system?

> ➤ *Check Your Reading*
>
> 5. Describe psychiatric treatment for patients before 1963.
> 6. What skills do patients lose during institutionalization?
> 7. Name the three goals of the deinstitutionalization movement in 1961.
> 8. What are the five services provided by CMHCs?
> 9. Explain the meaning of revolving door cycle.
> 10. Describe three clinical consequences of managed care.

EVOLVING CONCEPT OF MILIEU TREATMENT

As you may realize, many aspects of treatment have been affected by these major policy changes. New treatment modalities have emerged and traditional concepts have had to evolve. The psychiatric treatment continuum as we know it developed. But one aspect of treatment that stretches across the whole continuum is the use of the environment as a therapeutic factor, called milieu therapy.

When we talk about the environment in psychiatry, we refer to the **milieu,** defined as "the surroundings, especially of a social or cultural nature" (Flexner, 1993, p. 1220). We all have experienced environments that make us feel good—where we can be ourselves and know that we are accepted, and where we feel comfortable and at ease. Recognizing the significance of the environment led to the treatment approach called **milieu therapy,** which is the management of the environment to create or facilitate a healing context for the patient (Mosher, Kresky-Wolff, Matthews, & Menn, 1986).

Milieu therapy takes naturally occurring events from the environment and uses them as rich learning opportunities for patients. These naturally occurring events include interactions and the daily ebb and flow of routine activities, also known as therapeutic milieu (Rubin, 1991). Historically, milieu therapy was consid-

ered an inpatient modality; it began in the United States in the 1960s. It was based on a psychoanalytical theory, with the physician making a diagnosis and a prescription for a controlled environment including staff members' behavior (LeCuyer, 1992).

At the same time, the concept of **therapeutic community** was also proliferating. Originally defined by Dr. Maxwell Jones when he was treating soldiers returning from World War II in England, this inpatient approach stressed democratic decision-making by patients and staff members. Instead of a physician-prescribed environment, decisions about daily life activities were made by the group (Almond, 1974).

The psychiatric nurse has always had a central role in maintaining the therapeutic milieu. As noted in Chapter 4, the American Nurses Association standards include milieu therapy as one of the core nursing interventions. Although it was once considered only an inpatient modality, today you need to view milieu issues as part of the treatment continuum, as patients move more rapidly across settings.

The curative nature of the milieu is based on four assumptions:

1. A therapeutic relationship that is characterized by respect, support, and genuine interest is healing and may be a prototype for other relationships.
2. Personalities in the milieu are heterogeneous and the patient has opportunities to interact with patients and staff members in multiple roles.
3. Patient ego strengths can be used and supported as each patient participates in treatment in the group setting.
4. Group processes provide learning opportunities for patients and allow staff members to observe multiple social behaviors, which helps to determine the best treatment plan for each patient.

Gunderson's Components of Milieu Therapy

Gunderson (1983) identified five components of milieu therapy. The interaction of the components promotes change by providing a safe environment that allows for intrapsychic growth (Gunderson, 1983; Walker, 1994). Illustrated in Figure 15–2, these components are solid for the inpatient milieu and permeable for the community setting. Figure 15–2 demonstrates that the components of milieu therapy can constrict or expand like a lens, depending on the patient's needs.

Structure

The goal of having a structured environment is to provide opportunities for interactions at both individual and group levels (Gunderson, 1983). These interactions may be both formal and informal. A structured and orderly environment assists the patient to feel secure and allows the patient to choose from available activities as much as possible.

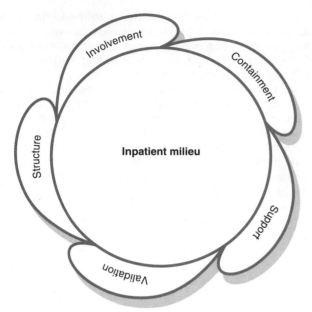

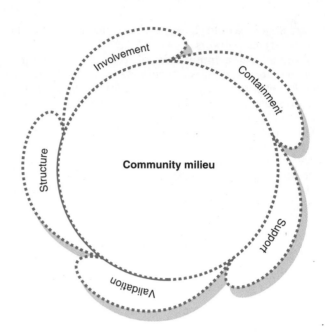

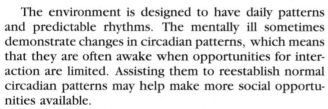

Figure 15–2
Gunderson's components of milieu therapy.

The environment is designed to have daily patterns and predictable rhythms. The mentally ill sometimes demonstrate changes in circadian patterns, which means that they are often awake when opportunities for interaction are limited. Assisting them to reestablish normal circadian patterns may help make more social opportunities available.

Level systems (patient privilege systems) may be used as a form of structure in the inpatient setting (Walker, 1994). Such systems allow patients to earn privileges by meeting behavioral expectations. For example, on admission, all patients begin at the lowest level with the fewest privileges. As patients demonstrate behavioral control, compliance with treatment, and symptom control, the privileges increase. Changes in the level usually require a written physician's order. The privileges may include permission to leave the unit, permission to leave the hospital, inclusion in special activities, and use of specific facilities.

Involvement

Interacting with others provides an opportunity to increase ego strength and modify one's personality (Gunderson, 1983; Walker, 1994). The milieu promotes interpersonal and interactional skills. The level of involvement is matched with the abilities of the individual. For example, people with symptomatic thought disorders tolerate interaction less well than other patients and may require low stress involvement.

The settings for interactions vary greatly. In inpatient settings, one-to-one relating groups, community meetings, and free social time provide opportunities for involvement. In the community, partial hospitalization programs, psychosocial programs, outpatient therapy groups, individual therapy, volunteer work, support groups, and employment are just a few of the settings for involvement.

Containment

Containment involves assisting the patient to be safe and to learn to discharge unaccepted burdens in an acceptable manner (Gunderson, 1983). Teaching appropriate expression is done in one-to-one interactions as well as through group activities. Patients are given the opportunity to learn that if they cannot contain themselves, then society has mechanisms to assist. The inpatient setting provides one-to-one verbal interventions, time outs, seclusion, as-needed medications, and restraints, whereas the community uses police officers, courts, and emergency mental health workers.

Support

Safety, support, and control are important milieu factors (Gunderson, 1983). Patients need protection from themselves if they are suicidal, homicidal, or self-mutilating. This protection takes the form of periodic observation at needed intervals, ranging from constant one-to-one supervision to every 15 minutes to monthly monitoring in the community.

The milieu provides a holding environment that is supportive without excessive demands. Such an environment is often required for patients with chronic or serious mental illnesses. Winnicott (1960) described a **holding environment** as one that provides consistency, caring, and object constancy, thereby facilitating growth, intimacy, and possibly use of higher defenses.

Validation

Validation is affirmation of individual worth. It involves reassuring patients that what they are experiencing is within the realm of human experience (Gunderson, 1983; Walker, 1994). The staff members' demonstrations of care and concern serve to substantiate a patient's self-worth. The milieu provides an opportunity to have symptoms validated and taken seriously. This information can teach patients how to cope with symptoms and life experiences.

Validation and human connectedness belong to the dimension of caring for the spiritual being. In connecting with each other in a safe relationship, both patient and nurse have an opportunity to experience the spirituality of reflective relating.

> **W**hat do you think? Think about milieus with which you are involved. What makes some supportive environments and others not?

➤ *Check Your Reading*
11. What is the definition of milieu therapy?
12. How is the therapeutic community model different from the original model for milieu therapy?
13. Describe three assumptions about the curative effect of the milieu.
14. What are Gunderson's five components of milieu therapy?

FOCUS ON PREVENTION

A second significant concept that relates to various settings in CMH is the public health definition of prevention. The principles of primary, secondary, and tertiary prevention provide direction for nursing interventions.

In **primary prevention,** the nurse focuses on preventing new occurrences of mental illness. The nurse develops interventions and programs to eliminate stresses that lead to or aggravate existing mental disorders. Examples include teaching parenting classes for new parents; offering support to self-help groups; and advocating within the political arena for the rights of the mentally ill.

Secondary prevention involves treating a diagnosed disorder within a given individual and making referrals to decrease the incidence of mental disorders. Examples of nursing interventions include providing nursing care in the acute setting, crisis or hotline services, and psychotherapy (advanced practice nurse).

Tertiary prevention involves providing rehabilitation services to patients who have been diagnosed with a mental disorder. Nursing interventions include discharge planning and referring to aftercare, teaching patients to manage their medications, and helping patients to adjust to a new residence away from home.

OVERVIEW OF TREATMENT SETTINGS

Acute Stage

Short-Term Inpatient, Locked Unit

The most restrictive and supportive level of treatment in the acute stage of the continuum is the short-term inpatient unit. Hospitalization is designed to provide containment and structure to patients who are at risk for harming themselves or others. Remember Peter's story: he had persistent symptoms in the community and required several transitional services, but he was a candidate for admission to a hospital only when he threatened his case manager.

The short-term unit may be locked to contain involuntary and voluntary patients while they are undergoing comprehensive assessments. The hospital milieu is powerful and requires attention and management to remain a therapeutic force (Frank & Frank, 1991). Otherwise, the collective emotional and behavioral problems of patients lead, by default, to a negative milieu.

The nurse provides 24-hour care and observation and participates in the multidisciplinary treatment plan. Significant aspects of the nurses' role include

1. Orienting patients to the environment as frequently as necessary
2. Assessing the physical needs of patients and staff members for safety
3. Teaching and role modeling effective communication
4. Teaching health-related issues to patients and families
5. Monitoring the effectiveness of medications
6. Setting limits as needed, including using time outs, seclusion, and restraint appropriately

All patients are on some kind of observation status, and close observation is actually a form of restraint, which must be used carefully (Dennis, 1997).

In the era of hospital stays of less than 1 week, the nurse (and the treatment team) must focus on specific goals and measurable outcomes (Vaughn, Webster, Orahood, & Young, 1995). Often, the unit specializes in one type of psychiatric disorder (e.g., affective disorders). Nursing interventions must be well-defined and tied to specific patient outcomes (Delaney, 1997). The nurse may lead groups that begin on admission and may continue after discharge (Delaney, Ulsafer-Van Lanen, Pitula, & Johnson, 1995). Any special physical needs of patients must also be addressed. For example, if a patient has chronic fatigue syndrome, he or she should not be expected to do all of the usual activities in the milieu (Anderson & Jayner, 1995).

Once the patient has a comprehensive assessment and diagnosis, and the appropriate treatment plan is initiated, linkage is made with aftercare services, and discharge is possible to the next level of care (Hughes & Ashby, 1996). The goal is to create a successful treatment plan for the patient in his or her community (Mindich & Hart, 1995). For Peter, it took only 5 days to adjust his medication and to reduce his verbal threats. He was discharged to his day program, case manager, and outpatient clinic follow-up, with a referral to a temporary, more supervised residence.

> **W**hat do you think? Compare and contrast the nurse's role on an inpatient psychiatric unit with that of a nurse on a medical unit.

➤ *Check Your Reading*
15. What is the meaning of primary prevention?
16. Give an example of a nursing intervention for secondary prevention.
17. What are the criteria for admission to an inpatient unit?
18. What are the discharge criteria for inpatient treatment?

Emergency Department

The other setting for the acute stage of treatment is the hospital emergency department. Weissberg (1991) called this setting "the new asylum for the poor" (p. 317) because some patients have no other resources for emergency or follow-up care. The emergency department may provide primary care for the seriously mentally ill and mentally ill chemical abusers (Oldham, Lin, & Breslin, 1990). Also, patients may be brought in by police officers or family members in a crisis situation.

The nurse, with the support of the emergency department physician and the on-call psychiatrist, makes a thorough assessment and a referral for inpatient or community treatment. Significant nursing responsibilities include assessing the patient for suicidal and violent potential; providing the patient with an environment to decrease stimuli; providing crisis intervention for the patient and family or care provider; treating the patient with neuroleptic medication; and teaching the patient and family about illness and treatment resources. If there is a risk that the patient might lose control, restrictive measures, including seclusion and restraint, may be used.

The therapeutic potential of the psychiatric emergency department is best realized when it is connected to the larger mental health system of the community. In order to make the most appropriate referral, the nurse needs to be aware of the full continuum of services in that community. If the nurse determines that the patient poses a risk to self or others, the referral is for hospitalization. However, all other problems receive referrals for some level of community care, which takes place during the transitional or follow-up stage of the treatment continuum.

Transitional Stage

Long-Term Inpatient Facilities

The patients served in long-term facilities include those who have not stabilized in short-term settings, have been involuntarily committed (including in forensic units), or are chronically ill and unable to maintain themselves safely in the community. Although these units are less common today compared with the 1960s, the patients are younger, sicker, and more violent. Most treatment teams would prefer a less restrictive setting for the patient, but it is difficult to predict violence in this population (Sclafani, 1986). Patients referred through the legal system may be confined for up to 6 months at a time before reevaluation and for much longer periods if they are found to be not criminally responsible for a crime.

Long-term facilities often have a shortage of professional staff members, including registered nurses, and supervising nonprofessional staff members is a significant part of the nurse's responsibility. Nurses must be creative in developing a therapeutic milieu with limited resources. Studies in long-term units that employed milieu therapy showed reduced use of multiple drugs, decreased overall neuroleptic usage, and fewer negative interpersonal interactions (Kurg-Cringle, Blake, Dunham, Miller, & Annecillo, 1994; Uys, Mhlaluka, & Piper, 1996).

Just as in the short-term setting, restrictive interventions must be used when necessary, including seclusion, restraint, and one-to-one observation. Discharge planning for this population is a continuing challenge. With the advances in antipsychotic medication and the development of more intensive residential supervision, many of these patients will someday return to the community. Barker, Davison, Turner, & Park (1997) described an intensive residential therapeutic service for chronic psychotic patients as one example of innovative community support.

Peter's story illustrates the potential level of independence for the seriously and persistently mentally ill. Peter had been in state hospitals for longer than 6 months before his release to his team of caregivers. With a history of assault to his father and the police and his multiple failed attempts at community living, Peter could have been considered hopeless for community treatment. But his hospital treatment team developed an intensive support system for him, including the day program, case management, outpatient therapy, and supervised residence. Although he may continue to need brief hospitalizations for crises, his quality of life in his community is much higher than if he were permanently confined to an institution.

What do you think? When you think about working in a transitional unit, what thoughts and feelings do you have?

➤ *Check Your Reading*
19. In what stage of the treatment continuum is the emergency department situated?
20. Describe three types of patients who may be in long-term units.
21. Why is milieu treatment important for long-term units?

Day Treatment

Day treatment or partial hospitalization programs are intensive outpatient treatments that use all the modalities of the acute hospital without evening and overnight components. They are appropriate for patients who need acute treatment but do not require 24-hour nursing care because they have adequate support to maintain them at home. All admissions are voluntary.

The admission criteria are clear-cut just as they are for acute hospitalization:

1a. Treatment is needed to prevent hospitalization for a patient in crisis.

or

1b. Treatment allows a patient to be discharged earlier from a hospital to day treatment; it thus serves as a step-down level of care.

and

2. There is a responsible relative or caregiver who can ensure the patient's safety overnight.

The nurse works with the multidisciplinary team to develop a treatment plan based on recommendations from the hospital or the outpatient referral source. Group therapy, psychopharmacology, family therapy, activity therapy, educational groups, and case management are the main treatment modalities. The therapeutic milieu is significant because patients interact in a structured setting with a variety of social roles. Just as in a hospital, safety is a primary concern, and staff members are trained to cope with behavioral emergencies. But if a patient requires seclusion or restraint for risk behavior, this community setting calls emergency assistance to refer the patient to an emergency department.

The trend for decreased length of stay applies to day treatment also. Once based on an average of 30 days, now a stay may last only 1 to 2 weeks. Many day programs have created their own continuum of services. Full-time day treatment, consisting of several group treatments per day for 5 days a week, is tapered to intensive outpatient treatment of fewer than 5 days a week or partial days. The goal for discharge is to stabilize the current symptoms, to educate the patient and family about the problem and treatment, and to make appropriate referrals for community follow-up in less restrictive (and less costly) settings.

With the seriously and persistently mentally ill, the patient may be referred to a long-term **psychosocial rehabilitation program** as part of the discharge plan. These programs are based on a rehabilitation model instead of a medical model. Instead of a focus on treating illness, the focus is on social and vocational training and pretraining, if necessary. The goal is to help the patient become as economically self-sufficient as possible. Case management is often included in this setting, but no psychiatric treatment is provided. Nurses need to be aware of rehabilitation principles and actively seek this specialized resource whenever appropriate, and they should keep in mind rehabilitation's potential to provide supported education opportunities (Palmer-Erbs, 1996, 1997).

Mobile Treatment

Mobile treatment refers to an outreach approach in which teams of professionals go into the community to treat the patient in the home or in the neighborhood. Patients referred to mobile treatment are often unable to comply with outpatient appointments or medication.

Often called treatment resistant, they may be young, uneducated, unemployed, homeless adults. They are diagnosed with serious and persistent mental illness, personality disorder, posttraumatic stress disorder, or substance abuse. Without treatment, they tend to overuse emergency departments and experience recurrent contacts with the legal system (Guy, 1997).

As a member of the team, you go to the patient's residence or favorite neighborhood haunt. You must become familiar with the patient's usual patterns of behavior and must be flexible about the treatment setting. Treatments provided include administration of intramuscular medications, crisis intervention, and supportive case management to help the patient to access needed social and economic resources. Some program team members actually drive patients to outpatient appointments, and some outreach may be done by day treatment staff members.

Funding of these programs is often connected to local government grants or demonstration projects and thus can be tenuous. Length of stay is unpredictable because the discharge plan is often unacceptable to the patient. Although patients may develop some trust in their own milieu with these caregivers, they often are unwilling to return to the more structured outpatient setting.

Clinical Case Management

Clinical case management is a treatment modality in which the case manager performs the following functions:

1. Assesses patient needs
2. Develops a plan for service
3. Links the patient with needed services
4. Monitors the effectiveness of services
5. Advocates for the chronically mentally ill, as appropriate

Case management may be provided as one of the comprehensive services in other community-based programs. Or there may be specific local government funding for a target population. Clearly, one group that desperately needs case management is the chronically mentally ill. The presence of one familiar, long-term relationship helps these patients to access the multitude of community services that they need, in a manner that preserves their dignity. (See Chapter 13 for more discussion about case management.)

In Peter's story, this episode of his problem began with a disagreement with his roommates. Unable to clearly verbalize his distress, his psychotic symptoms worsened. When the case manager was called by Peter's residential staff member, she recognized Peter's potential for loss of control and smoothly moved him to an inpatient setting via the emergency evaluation at the clinic. Consider the alternative scenario. Peter could have assaulted someone at the house; he could have been arrested by the police and taken to jail or to the emergency department in handcuffs. In the emergency department, Peter could have been subjected to a lengthy evaluation in a frightening environment, finally entering a hospital in a much worse condition than he was in when he was actually admitted. He could have lost his housing because of his dangerousness and then would have been transferred to a long-term institution until new housing could be found. ■

What do you think? Compare and contrast the continuum of psychiatric services with what is available for medical patients.

➤ *Check Your Reading*

22. What is the main difference between inpatient treatment and a partial hospital program?
23. What is the purpose of a psychosocial rehabilitation program?
24. Why are patients referred to mobile treatment?
25. List three functions of a clinical case manager.

Psychiatric Home Care

The last treatment in the transitional stage of the continuum is psychiatric home care. **Psychiatric home care** was defined in 1979 according to Medicare guidelines that require

1. The patient to be certified by a physician as homebound
2. The patient to have a psychiatric diagnosis
3. The patient to need the skills of a psychiatric nurse
4. The plan of care to be under the direction of a physician

Homebound status means that patients have a condition, either physical or emotional, that generally precludes them from leaving home without significant assistance from another person; therefore, the patients rarely leave home (Eggland, 1987; Carson, 1994a, 1998). Examples of conditions that support homebound status are shown in Box 15-1.

The patient's diagnoses must include a recognized psychiatric diagnosis from *Diagnostic and Statistical Manual of Mental Disorders, Fourth Edition* such as Depression or Anxiety Disorder or a dual diagnosis of mental disorder and substance abuse. The majority of patients treated in psychiatric home care are older than 65 years of age and generally have multiple physical diagnoses as well.

A skilled psychiatric nurse is defined, as follows, by Medicare guidelines (Independence Blue Cross and Blue Shield, 1993): a nurse with a master's degree in psychiatric nursing or community health nursing; a bachelor's degree in nursing, with 1 year of adult or geriatric psychiatric experience; or a diploma or associate degree

in nursing, with 2 years of adult or geriatric psychiatric experience.

The written plan of care must be established and reviewed by a physician; in other words, the nurse is working at all times under a physician's orders. Initially, Medicare required the physician to be a psychiatrist, but that condition was changed in response to national pressure about the needs of many elderly patients who could not or would not go to a psychiatrist.

Patients with acute care needs are referred to psychiatric home care, either to facilitate a more rapid discharge from a higher level of care, such as a hospital or a partial hospital program, or to prevent hospitalization and excessive use of emergency departments. Medicare and Medicaid insist on homebound status in order to reimburse for home care. But other third-party payers use *home care* even when patients are ambulatory in the community. The goal of psychiatric home care is to link the patient to less restrictive follow-up care in the community.

Psychotherapy is not the main treatment modality in psychiatric home care. As evidenced by the variety of the nurses' educational backgrounds, psychiatric home care usually involves interventions at the basic level of psychiatric nursing practice. Rarely, a managed care payer may request individual psychotherapy, which does require an advanced practice nurse.

After a thorough assessment of the patient, the home environment, and the support system, the main nursing interventions (Carson, 1994a, 1994c, 1994d, 1994e, 1995, 1998; Davis, 1987; Minnesota Community Health Services, 1981; Newton & Brauer, 1989; Pelletier, 1988; Thobaben, 1989) used include the following:

Box 15-1 ■ ■ ■ ■ ■
Examples of Patient Conditions That Might Be Grounds for Considering a Person Psychiatrically Homebound

- Confusion, disorientation, and poor judgment
- Psychomotor retardation caused by severe depression
- Altered perception or cognition
- Altered thought processes
- Risk for self-harm
- Vulnerability in the community
- Poor impulse control
- Requirement of 24-hour supervision
- Impairment in social interactions
- Excessive fear or anxiety
- Agoraphobia
- Need for assistive devices (e.g., cane, walker, wheelchair) for mobility
- Inability to leave home independently
- Inability to leave home without taxing effort
- Dependence on assistance from others for leaving home

1. Instruction for patients and families
2. Case management
3. Provision of respite to families
4. Assistance to patients to achieve spiritual wellbeing

Box 15-2 lists the most common interventions used in psychiatric home care.

In addition, the nurse collaborates as necessary with members of the multidisciplinary team from the home care agency—social worker, home health aide, occupational therapist, physical therapist, speech therapist—to promote the patient's maximal rehabilitation.

One major influence on the development of psychiatric home care across the United States during the 1990s was the Bay Area Health Care model (Carson, 1994a) (Figure 15-3). The symbol of a home is used to conceptualize the model. The foundation of the house is a moral and spiritual one, indicating that the nurse approaches patients with an attitude of respect. The nurse must be resolute in standing by patients, recognizing them as people of worth and dignity who have strengths as well as disabilities. This includes promoting health by sustaining the patient's physical, emotional, and spiritual life (Carson, 1994b, 1998). Note that this holistic approach is not a reimbursable skill but arises from the individual nurse's professional dedication.

The walls of the house are made up of assessment skills and relationship building. These walls provide the necessary supports to all other therapeutic interventions. A comprehensive nursing assessment evaluates mental status, using standardized rating scales; activities of daily living (ADLs); medication issues; psychiatric follow-up issues; social support; and spiritual issues. Relationship building demands verbal and nonverbal communication techniques. These techniques convey to

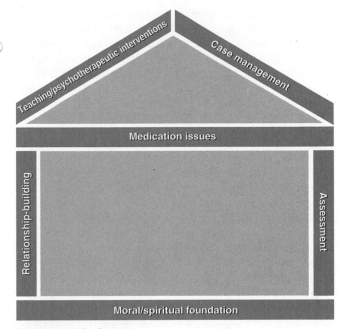

Figure 15-3
The symbol of a home is used to conceptualize the Bay Area Health Care's psychiatric home care model. (Redrawn from Carson, V. B., Jacik, M., & Platman, S. [1994]. *Psychiatric home care manual*. Baltimore: Bay Area Health Care.)

the patient genuine interest, which assists in therapeutic changes.

The second floor of the house (see Figure 15-3) is made up of issues surrounding medications. Many psychiatric patients have difficulty complying with long-term medication regimens. There are many reasons why patients resist taking their medication: disliking side effects, forgetting dosage schedules, exceeding financial

---

Box 15-2 ■ ■ ■ ■ ■
Nursing Interventions Commonly Used in Psychiatric Home Care

Continual Assessment of

- Medication compliance
- Medication side effects
- Mental status
- Nutrition and hydration
- Sleep pattern

Teaching About

- New medication regimens
- Coping patterns related to whatever issues the patient is confronting
- Activities of daily living to meet basic needs
- Communication skills
- Signs and symptoms of exacerbations of illness
- Access to medical follow-up

Application of Psychotherapeutic Skills to

- Improve self-concept
- Decrease fear
- Decrease anxiety
- Decrease hopelessness
- Increase motivation
- Increase spiritual well-being
- Decrease eating pattern disturbances
- Decrease sleep pattern disturbances
- Increase social interaction
- Increase diversional activities

Case Mangement to

- Manage and evaluate care on a regular basis
- Coordinate unskilled services
- Coordinate skilled services
- Coordinate community resources

limits, and denying illness. Finding solutions to these concerns must be tailored to each individual. Just teaching about the main effects and side effects of medications can powerfully influence some patients. For other patients, establishing compliance kits (a container for holding medicine with designated days and times), rearranging medication time schedules, or advocating with physicians for modified dosages can be beneficial (Brown, Wright, & Christensen, 1987; Collins-Colon, 1990; Davidhizar & McBride, 1985; Witt, 1981).

The two sides of the roof (see Figure 15–3) are teaching and psychotherapeutic interventions and case management. In order to clarify interventions and goals in behavioral language in ways that third-party payers can understand, almost all therapy issues are translated into teaching terms. Teaching is concrete with results described in measurable outcomes. For example, when nurses teach about depression, components include causes; physical, cognitive, interpersonal, and spiritual effects; guilt; and cognitive coping strategies. Case management is essential to link the patient to community resources that can support health and independence and prevent rehospitalization. As noted earlier, the nurse case manages other disciplines from the home health agency and makes community referrals (e.g., to an outpatient clinic, to a psychosocial center, to a senior center, or even to a transportation system to access these services).

Follow-Up Stage

The final stage of the treatment continuum is the follow-up stage, which is the least restrictive level of care. **Outpatient therapy** in a clinic or with a private therapist represents the most independent level of functioning for the patient. Patients are responsible for scheduling their own appointments with the therapist and for following through on treatment recommendations for medication and behavioral change. CMHCs were originally designed to serve a defined population of 75,000 to 200,000 residents, called a **catchment area.** Geographical limitations may become obsolete as managed care systems expand.

As described earlier in this chapter, patients may be referred to outpatient therapy from an acute or transitional treatment facility after their crisis symptoms have stabilized and they are able to return to living in the community. Or patients may access this level of care strictly as outpatients seeking counseling to cope with stressful events along their life's journeys, such as family conflict, divorce, or death of a loved one.

The milieu in these settings is not well recognized but encompasses the physical environment, including support staff members and issues about access. Waiting rooms and treatment rooms need to be comfortable and safe. Secretaries, receptionists, and other paraprofessionals need to be trained to observe the waiting areas and to recognize acute patient problems requiring immediate clinical attention. The intake process needs to be timely, friendly, and free of barriers such as a high

fee without a sliding scale or lack of public transportation.

Outpatient clinics are staffed by a variety of mental health professionals. The role of the nurse depends on the nurse's educational background. The basic level nurse provides medication administration and monitoring, teaching, case management, and crisis intervention. The advanced practice nurse provides individual, group, and family therapy.

Length of treatment is based on the patient's and the therapist's evaluations of improvement in the identified problems, within the limits of the third-party payer system or self-payment. Some patients receive brief therapy of four to eight sessions with or without medication, and then they are discharged completely. Other patients, including the seriously and persistently mentally ill, may continue in outpatient treatment for years in order to prevent relapse and rehospitalization.

W*hat do you think?* Do you think psychiatric home care should require an advanced practice psychiatric nurse?

➤ *Check Your Reading*

26. What are the four Medicare requirements for psychiatric home care?
27. What part of the treatment continuum contains home care?
28. Is psychotherapy the goal of psychiatric home care?
29. What does the symbol of the house mean in the Bay Area Health Care model of home care?
30. What treatment environments are used in the follow-up stage of the continuum?
31. What is the catchment area?

Continuum of the Residential Therapeutic Community

Just as psychiatric treatment meets the needs of patients across a continuum, so also there is a continuum of residential services that provide a range of support from most restrictive to least restrictive (Figure 15–4). Sommers (1987, p. 170) stated, "the character of a psychiatric patient's residential surroundings and social milieu can influence the success she/he experiences in attempting to adjust to life in the community." These settings are generally organized by psychosocial rehabilitation agencies that provide, in addition to job training, the development and maintenance of social networks and supports (Stroul, 1989).

The concept of a **residential therapeutic community** is based on 3 decades of research into CMH services. Studies repeatedly showed that there are patients with a tenuous adjustment to community life: they have limited coping skills, show powerful dependency needs, and tend to develop severe psychiatric symptoms in response to mild to moderate degrees of

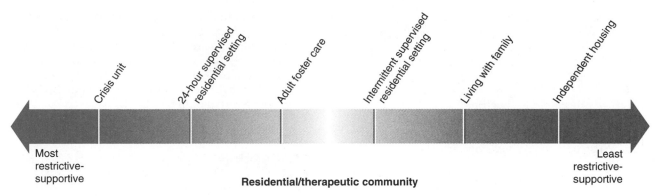

Figure 15–4
The continuum of the residential therapeutic community.

stress (Stein & Test, 1980). When offered a 24-hour support program, including housing, medication monitoring, transportation to clinic appointments, and even guardianship to monitor finances, these patients made better social and work adjustments (Test, Knoedler, & Allness, 1985).

There is a relationship between the residential continuum and the treatment continuum. Patients do not need an equal level of intensity in both systems. That is, a patient may receive one level of treatment services and a different level of residential support. Generally, a patient in a highly supportive residential arrangement may use a lower level of treatment over the long term. For example, a paranoid schizophrenic patient living in a 24-hour supervised residence would probably use less crisis intervention and more outpatient care. Conversely, the more outpatient treatment that is provided, the lower the level of residential support that is needed.

The **crisis unit** offers the most restrictive support level of the residential continuum. There is 24-hour staff coverage provided by paraprofessionals to produce a supportive, low-stress environment. The patients are voluntary and must agree to follow treatment recommendations from the referring clinician in the emergency department or the outpatient setting. The service is usually limited to 2 weeks or less and the goal is to prevent hospitalization. In Peter's story, he was referred to the crisis unit on discharge from the hospital in order for staff members to evaluate him closely for 1 week before allowing him to return to his less supervised housing.

The next less restrictive level is the **24-hour supervised residential setting.** At this level, the patient lives in a group setting for a longer period, with 24-hour supervision from paraprofessional staff members to assist with and teach ADLs. There may be house meetings and democratic house rules reflecting elements of the inpatient therapeutic community approach. Treatment is usually provided off-site in some type of day program and communication between house staff members and clinical staff members is essential. As you recall, it was a call from a house staff member that first identified Peter's relapse and alerted the clinical staff members to take action.

Another setting with 24-hour supervision is **adult foster care.** In this arrangement, the patient lives in a family home for support and assistance with ADLs. This service may be provided by the Department of Social Services (DSS). The DSS caseworker coordinates communication between the family and the treatment team. This level of care is well suited to the elderly patient who has had a long hospital stay but is not intended for any patients with a potential for violent behavior.

Less restrictive than 24-hour settings is the **intermittent supervised residential setting.** The patient still lives in a group residence, but staff supervision may be only a few hours per week. The patient may live alone or with one or two roommates in an apartment and may still attend a structured day program off-site. Supervised residences are also called **sheltered housing** or **congregate housing.**

The next less restrictive step along the housing continuum is living with family. For patients who have family and still need help to monitor medications and assist with transportation to appointments, this level provides for their maximal independence in the community. The patient may be receiving treatment at the outpatient level or still require ongoing day treatment. Actually, the majority of patients are discharged from emergency departments or hospitals directly back to their families, underscoring the need to provide family education in every treatment plan across the continuum (Yamashita & McNally, 1998). Another important need of families caring for the long-term mentally ill is linkage to caregiver support groups (Hunt, 1996).

The final and least restrictive level of residence is **independent housing.** Living in independent housing is the goal for many patients. This level of independence is usually attained when patients become employed or have financial assistance in the form of government-subsidized housing. Patients may require ongoing outpatient treatment or may be discharged completely after all appropriate community referrals are made.

What do you think? Should housing be provided for the seriously and persistently mentally ill as part of their insurance coverage?

➤ *Check Your Reading*

32. In general, what agencies support supervised residences for psychiatric patients?
33. Name three examples of supports in the residential therapeutic community.
34. What is the difference between a crisis unit and a 24-hour supervised setting?
35. What population is well suited to adult foster care?
36. What level of supervision do patients receive in sheltered housing?
37. Name two significant needs of families who care for the mentally ill.

Other Professional and Informal Helpers

Despite the best efforts of treatment staff and housing staff members, it is still not possible for them to meet all the diverse needs of patients living in the community. As you know, in your own life you interact with a variety of people on a regular basis, all of whom create your natural social network. For patients who may be unable to establish their own support system, often it is the psychiatric nurse who seeks out formal and informal helpers.

Examples of sources of formal professional helpers include public welfare agencies, courts, schools, churches, charitable organizations, child day care centers, social services organizations, Meals-on-Wheels, local pharmacies, and crisis services agencies. The nurse provides the patient with contact people or actual referrals to these services, as needed.

The potential informal helpers are identified by learning about the patient in his or her unique environment. For every patient who arrives in the emergency department or hospital and is called "homeless" or "without family," there is someone whom the patient considers significant. A careful social history or home visit can reveal this contact and make it possible to reestablish a linkage on discharge. The list of informal helpers may include family members not living with the patient, friends, neighbors, members of neighborhood organizations, self-help group members, church members, teachers, police officers, landlords, or even mail carriers.

NURSING PROCESS: COMMUNITY AS PATIENT

In CMH care, as in other areas of nursing, you rely on the nursing process to gain an understanding of the patient, to diagnose the patient's needs, to determine appropriate outcomes, to plan effective and appropriate interventions, and to evaluate the results of the interventions. The one area that sets CMH care apart is that sometimes the patient is an individual or family, and sometimes the patient is the community. This discussion leads you through the application of the nursing process in the community setting.

Assessment

You may focus a community assessment in a number of different ways. For instance, you might be interested in gauging community acceptance of a mental health initiative. The following questions are appropriate to this type of assessment:

- Do you believe that former patients of mental hospitals are able to function well in your community?
- Would you have any objections if an organization that you belonged to accepted a former mental patient as a member?
- What would your feelings be if a former mental patient moved next door to you?
- Do you think you could ever become friends with a former mental patient?

Diagnosis

The analysis of these answers leads to nursing diagnoses for the community, such as

- Knowledge Deficit related to lack of understanding of the characteristics of the chronically mentally ill
- Anxiety related to misinformation about the chronically mentally ill
- Ineffective Community Coping related to the high stress level associated with perceptions of the chronically mentally ill

Outcome Identification

The expected outcomes for a community might be

- After presentation of educational talks and materials, a random posttest of the community will show significantly greater understanding of the characteristics of the chronically mentally ill.
- The response to the posttest questions measuring affective and attitudinal issues will show a significant change toward greater acceptance of and more positive feelings toward the mentally ill.

- Plans for the development and enhancement of existing resources and programs to meet the needs of the chronically mentally ill will come from the community.

Planning

The plan that is developed to achieve these expected outcomes might rely heavily on education. The nurse, as program coordinator, might target public forums such as schools, clinics, churches, neighborhood recreation centers, and health fairs as sites to begin educating the community. Possible short-term goals and interventions for such a plan might include the following.

Expected Outcome

After presentation of educational talks and materials, a random posttest of the community will show significantly greater understanding of the characteristics of the chronically mentally ill.

Short-Term Goal

Community members will participate in a variety of educational programs offered throughout the community.

Expected Outcome

The response to the posttest questions measuring affective and attitudinal issues will show a significant change toward greater acceptance and more positive feelings.

Short-Term Goal

Community members will take a pretest and a posttest to measure their attitudes toward the chronically mentally ill.

Expected Outcome

Plans for developing and enhancing existing resources and programs to meet the needs of the chronically mentally ill will come from the community.

Short-Term Goal

Community members will participate in small focus groups to identify existing resources, plan what re-sources are needed, and plan how to develop needed resources to support the chronically mentally ill.

Implementation

The interventions to support this plan might include

- Develop a brochure outlining the achievements of many who are chronically mentally ill.
- Develop a slide and lecture presentation depicting the mentally ill in productive occupations contributing to the health of the community.
- Focus on the spiritual benefits of caring for and being tolerant of those who are less fortunate than ourselves.
- Explain the economic benefits that a community receives when it cares for its own and does not send the mentally ill to a state institution.

The interventions are limited only by the creativity and resources of those presenting such an educational program.

Evaluation

A project of this magnitude requires ongoing or formative evaluation. Issues that must be evaluated include but are not limited to the following:

- Is the community assessment comprehensive enough? Are there areas that have not been explored?
- Is the planned teaching approach at an appropriate level for the community?
- Are the teaching materials effective?
- Are facilities available to offer the programs?
- Are community members adequately informed regarding the upcoming educational programs?

The summative evaluation of this particular approach is specified in the objectives. There are other ways, however, to gauge effectiveness of a program. For instance, if a halfway house opened in a particular neighborhood, observations about how former patients were treated when they went for walks and frequented stores and other neighborhood establishments would be subjective data to support or refute the success of a community-based intervention.

> ➤ *Check Your Reading*

38. Give three examples of professional helpers in the community.
39. How do you, as the nurse, identify the patient's informal helper?
40. Name one method used to assess a community as the patient.
41. What nursing diagnosis is likely to occur in every community project?
42. What approach can be used to measure outcomes for a community?
43. What is the primary nursing intervention used to treat a community?

FUTURE DIRECTIONS

As we look to the future of nursing in the psychiatric treatment continuum, it seems that we are still struggling to meet the goals of the 1961 report from the Joint Commission on Mental Illness and Health. That is, can we help create a system that is truly integrated to help the psychiatric patient to function at the highest possible level in the community?

Nurses are in a strategic position to influence the future development of mental health care. Traditionally, we have demonstrated a holistic approach to patients and their families, with respect for the patient's autonomy to encourage self-direction. This view provides nurses with a vantage point to advocate for change within the health care system and within the community. Such advocacy could influence reform within the system and lessen community responses that stigmatize people with psychiatric histories. History proves, both here and abroad, that public policy does not always support effective programs, but political pressures can result in revised policy (Murdock, 1995; Sullivan, 1997).

The psychiatric mental health nurse, with a biopsychosocial and spiritual orientation, is uniquely qualified to deliver care to patients across the therapeutic continuum. Krauss (1989) argued that of all disciplines involved in CMH care, the nurse was the best prepared to offer to the chronically mentally ill the three "Cs": care, comprehensiveness, and continuity. She asserted that nurses are prepared "through the power of privileged intimacy and with the authority of our roles as clinician, teacher, advocate, and reformer of the health care system" (p. 59). (See Chapter 39 for more discussion about future trends.)

Conclusions

The concept of CMH care is an important force in psychiatric care; it is alive and still struggling for the best method of implementation. In the 1960s, state hospitals cared for more than 50% of all psychiatric patients. Thirty years later, with more than 2.5 million severely mentally ill in the United States, only about 10% were cared for in state hospitals. The pattern of psychiatric care in the 1990s was brief hospitalization during the acute phase of an illness and rapid return to community living. Usually, only the most dysfunctional people and those who pose a serious threat to themselves and others reside in long-term psychiatric facilities.

The therapeutic milieu exists on a continuum of treatment settings. Milieu therapy includes a treatment component, and nurses often provide that treatment component.

To ensure that the milieu is positive, psychiatric and mental health care providers are responsible for managing socioenvironmental factors. Mentally ill individuals need nurses to develop programs, monitor progress, provide consultation, and maintain the therapeutic milieu in both inpatient and community treatment settings.

Psychiatric home care is a fairly new approach to treating psychiatric patients. This is a promising treatment modality that recognizes that patients frequently do better when they remain within the comforts of their own homes. It also recognizes that psychiatric home care is effective as a cost-containment measure. Psychiatric home care is likely to become increasingly more important as a primary treatment approach for the chronically mentally ill in a cost-cutting, resource-driven health care system.

Key Points to Remember

- Before 1963, CMH care was nonexistent. Institutionalization refers to the process of becoming dependent on an institution for care and decision-making.
- Deinstitutionalization refers to the process of preparing patients who have spent a great deal of time within institutions for life in the world.
- CMH care serves the needs of the chronically mentally ill, also referred to as the seriously and persistently mentally ill.
- The chronically mentally ill are a diverse group made up of people of all ages with many different psychiatric diagnoses.

- CMH care focuses on the community, the individual, and the family.
- A catchment area is a city or several rural communities with a total population ranging from 75,000 to 200,000 residents.
- The services offered by CMH care include CMHCs; a variety of living arrangements, including single-room occupancy and sheltered or congregate housing; support groups; day treatment centers; mobile treatment teams; and community services.
- Nurses focus on primary, secondary, and tertiary prevention in the community setting.

- The nursing process can be applied to a community as a whole or to an individual or family within the community.
- The interventions used by the CMH nurse include teaching, case managing, consulting, providing therapy, networking, crossing boundaries to forge linkages, and advocating.
- Gunderson's (1983) components of milieu therapy include structure, involvement, containment, support, and validation.
- Contemporary settings for milieu therapy include the following inpatient settings: locked inpatient units, emergency departments, short-term psychiatric units, and longer-term psychiatric units. Community milieu settings include day treatment, mobile treatment, psychiatric home care, and outpatient clinics. Nurses may provide direct care and consultation in residential and psychosocial program settings.
- Psychiatric home care is growing because of increased consumer demand, growth of the population needing the service, and pressures toward cost containment.
- The overall goals of psychiatric home care are to improve quality of life, to prevent unnecessary hospitalizations, and to maximize patients' potential to live in their own homes.
- Bay Area Health Care's model of psychiatric home care has six components: the foundation is a moral and spiritual one; the walls are made up of assessment and relationship-building skills; the second floor is made up of medication issues; and the roof is constructed of teaching and psychotherapeutic interventions and case management.

Learning Activities

1. Conduct an informal survey in your community. Ask your family and neighbors how they would react to having a halfway house for the chronically mentally ill established in their community.
2. Find out where the nearest CMHC is in your area. Call to find out what services are offered to patients.
3. Call the mental health association in your community. Ask if there are any self-help groups in your area. If there are, what services do they provide?
4. What milieu therapy settings have you seen in clinical environments or while visiting or working in health care settings? What are the positive features? What aspects are negative?
5. As you participate in your psychiatric nursing experiences, take note of the discharge planning that is going on for each patient. Is anyone referred for psychiatric home care? Could any patient benefit from psychiatric home care services?

Critical Thinking Exercises

Penny Johnson, a 27-year-old former drug abuser, attends a women's group led by the psychiatric nurse specialist Mrs. Hargood every Monday and Thursday in the partial hospitalization program. During group, she expresses great concern that her 4-year-old daughter's father has just been released from jail and wants to live with her. She thinks he is still taking drugs.

1. What assumptions do you think Penny is operating under?
2. How could Mrs. Hargood check these assumptions out by some simple inquiry?
3. Suggest a response to Penny's concerns.

Jerome, an elderly patient who walks Penny home every day, tells the group that he has a gun and would shoot "this guy" if he ever comes around to bother Penny.

1. What assumptions might Jerome have about his relationship with Penny?
2. Consider the nurse's legal responsibility to report this threat.
3. What other evidence is needed to draw a conclusion about the situation?

References

Almond, R. (1974). *The healing community: Dynamics of the therapeutic milieu.* New York: Jason Aronson.

Anderson, J. S., & Jayner, D. (1995). Milieu issues in the treatment of a person with chronic fatigue syndrome on an inpatient unit. *Journal of American Psychiatric Nurses Association, 1*(1), 12-15.

Bachrach, L. L. (1979). Planning mental health services for the chronically ill patient. *Hospital and Community Psychiatry, 30,* 387-392.

Barker, P., Davison, M., Turner, J., & Park, B. (1997). Intensive care for people with serious mental illness. *Nursing Standard, 11*(34), 40-42.

Bostelman, S., Callan, M., Rolincik, L. C., Gantt, M., Herink, M., King, J., Massey, M. K., Morehouse, D., Sopata, T., & Turner, J. (1994). *Public Health Report, 109,* 153-157.

Brown, C. S., Wright, R. G., & Christensen, D. B. (1987). Association between type of medication, instruction, and patient's knowledge, side effects, and compliance. *Hospital and Community Psychiatry, 38*(1), 55-60.

Buckwalter, K. C., & Light, E. (1989). New directions of psychiatric mental health nurses: The chronically mentally ill elderly. *Archives of Psychiatric Nursing, 3*(1), 53-54.

Buerhaus, P. I. (1998). Financing, demographic, and political problems confronting Medicare in the U.S. *Image: Journal of Nursing Scholarship, 30,* 117-123.

Carson, V. B., Jacik, M., Platman, S. (1994a). *Psychiatric home care manual.* Baltimore: Bay Area Health Care.

Carson, V. B. (1994b). Caring: The rediscovery of our nursing roots. *Perspectives in Psychiatric Care, 30*(2), 46.

Carson, V. B. (1994c). Doing psych, but talking med-surg language. *Caring, 13*(6), 32-41.

Carson, V. B. (1994d). Spiritual care of Evelyn. *Caring, 13*(12), 27-29.

Carson, V. B. (1994e, January). Spirituality and depression: An important relationship. *Smooth Sailing: DRADA Newsletter,* 34.

Carson, V. B. (1995). Bay Area Health Care model of psychiatric home care. *Home Healthcare Nurse, 13*(4), 26-32.

Carson, V. B. (1998). Designing an effective psychiatric home care program. *Home Healthcare Consultant, 5*(4), 16-21.

Chamberlin, J., & Rogers, J. A. (1990). Planning a community-based mental health system. *American Psychologist, 45,* 1241-1244.

Cutler, D. L. (1986). Community residential options for the chronically mentally ill. *Community Mental Health Journal, 22*(1), 61-72.

Chisholm, M., Howard, P. B., Boyd, M. A., Clement, J. A., Hendrix, M. J., & Reiss-Brennan, B. (1997). Quality indicators for primary mental health within managed care: A public health focus. *Archives of Psychiatric Nursing, 11,* 167-181.

Collins-Colon, T. (1990). Do it yourself medication management for community based clients. *Journal of Psychosocial Nursing and Mental Health Services, 28*(6), 25-27.

Conway, A. S., Melzer, D., & Hale, A. S. (1994). The outcome of targeting community mental health services: Evidence from the West Lambeth schizophrenia cohort. *British Medical Journal, 308,* 627-630.

Davidhizar, R. E., & McBride, A. B. (1985). Teaching the client with schizophrenia about medication. *Patient Education and Counseling, 7,* 233-255.

Davis, E. J. (1987). Home care: What is needed? *Public Health Nursing, 4*(2), 82-83.

Delaney, K. R. (1997). Milieu therapy: A therapeutic loophole. *Perspectives in Psychiatric Care, 33*(2), 19-28.

Delaney, K., Ulsafer-Van Lanen, J., Pitula, C. R., & Johnson, M. E. (1995). Seven days and counting: How inpatient nurses might adjust their practice to brief hospitalization. *Journal of Psychosocial Nursing and Mental Health Services, 33*(8), 36-40.

Dennis, S. (1997). Close observation: How to improve assessments. *Nursing Times, 93*(24), 54-56.

Drolen, C. S. (1990). Current community mental health center operations: Entrepreneurship or business as usual? *Community Mental Health Journal, 26,* 547-558.

Eggland, E. T. (1987). Home health care. *Nursing 87, 10,* 75-80.

Flexner, S. B. (Ed). (1993). *Random house unabridged dictionary* (2nd ed.). New York: Random House.

Frank, J. D., & Frank, J. B. (1991). Psychotherapy in a controlled environment. In J. D. Frank & J. B. Frank (Eds.), *Persuasion and healing* (pp. 274-294). Baltimore: Johns Hopkins University.

Grob, G. N. (1994). Government and mental health policy: A structural analysis. *Milbank Quarterly, 72*(3), 471-500.

Gunderson, J. G. (1983). An overview of modern milieu therapy. In J. G. Gunderson, O. A. Wills, Jr., & L. R. Mosher (Eds.), *Principles and practice of milieu therapy* (pp. 1-13). New York: Jason Aronson.

Guy, S. (1997). Assertive community treatment of the long-term mentally ill. *Journal of the American Psychiatric Nurses Association, 3,* 185-190.

Hughes, K. H., & Ashby, C. (1996). Essential components of the short-term psychiatric unit. *Perspectives in Psychiatric Care, 32*(1), 20-25.

Hunt, U. (1996). Care study. Shared experience: Running a carers' support group. *Mental Health Nursing, 16*(4), 24-27.

Independence Blue Cross and Blue Shield, Medicare Intermediary [Transmittal letter]. (1993).

Joint Commission on Mental Illness and Health. (1961). *Action for mental health* (pp. 16-19). New York: Basic Books.

Krauss, J. (1989). The three Cs and the chronically mentally ill. *Archives of Psychiatric Nursing, 3*(2), 59-60.

Krauss, J., & Slavinsky, A. (1982). *The chronically ill psychiatric patient and the community* (pp. 76, 78). Boston: Blackwell.

Kurg-Cringle, R., Blake, L. A., Dunham, D., Miller, M. J., & Annecillo, C. (1994). A nurse-managed inpatient program for patients with chronic mental disorders. *Archives of Psychiatric Nursing, 8*(1), 14-21.

LeCuyer, E. A. (1992). Milieu therapy for short stay units: A transformed practice theory. *Archives of Psychiatric Nursing, 6,* 108-116.

Mindich, D. S., & Hart, B. (1995). Linking hospital and community. *Journal of Psychosocial Nursing and Mental Health Services, 33*(1), 25-28.

Minnesota Community Health Services, Office of Community Development. (1981). *Home care guidelines.* Minneapolis, MN: Minnesota Department of Health.

Mosher, L. R., Kresky-Wolff, M., Matthews, S., & Menn, A. (1986). Milieu therapy in the 1980's: A comparison of two residential alternatives to hospitals. *Bulletin of the Menninger Clinic, 50,* 257-268.

Murdock, D. (1995). Redefining the targets for mental illness. *Nursing Standard, 9*(49), 28-30.

Newton, N. A., & Brauer, W. F. (1989). In-home mental health services. *Caring, 8*(6), 16-19.

Oldham, J. M., Lin, A., & Breslin, L. (1990). Comprehensive psychiatric emergency services. *Psychiatric Quarterly, 61,* 57-67.

Palmer-Erbs, V. (1996). Psychosocial rehabilitation: A breath of fresh air in a turbulent health care environment. *Journal of Psychosocial Nursing and Mental Health Services, 34*(9), 16-21.

Palmer-Erbs, V. K., & Unger, K. V. (1997). An innovation in psychosocial rehabilitation programming: Supported education. *Journal of Psychosocial Nursing and Mental Health Services, 35*(1), 16-21.

Pelletier, L. R. (1988). Psychiatric home care. *Journal of Psychosocial Nursing and Mental Health Services, 26*(3), 22-27.

Richter, J. M. (1990). Social support: The chronically mentally ill institutionalized elderly. *Journal of Gerontological Nursing, 16*(8), 32-35.

Rubin, R. L. (1991). Child psychiatric nursing. In G. W. Stuart & S. J. Sundeen (Eds.), *Principles and practice of psychiatric nursing* (pp. 852-877). Washington, DC: C. V. Mosby.

Sclafani, M. (1986). Violence and behavior control. *Journal of Psychosocial Nursing, 24,* 9-13.

Segal, S. P., Hazan, A. P., & Kotler, P. L. (1990). Characteristics of sheltered care facility operators in California in 1973 and 1985. *Hospital and Community Psychiatry, 41,* 1245-1248.

Sheets, J. L., Prevost, J. A., & Reihman, J. (1982). Young adult chronically mentally ill patients: Three hypothesized subgroups. *Hospital and Community Psychiatry, 33,* 197-203.

Sommers, I. (1987). Tolerance of deviance and community adjustment of the mentally ill. *Community Mental Health Journal, 23,* 159-171.

Stein, L. I., & Test, M. A. (1980). An alternative to mental hospital treatment: Conceptual model, treatment program and clinical evaluation. *Archives of General Psychiatry, 37,* 392-397.

Stroul, B. A. (1989). Community support systems for persons with long-term mental illness: A conceptual framework. *Psychosocial Rehabilitation Journal, 12,* 9-26.

Sullivan, P. (1997). Mental health nursing. The care program approach: A nursing perspective. *British Journal of Nursing, 6,* 208.

Test, M. A., Knoedler, W. H., & Allness, D. J. (1985). The long-term treatment of young schizophrenics in a community support program. In *The training in community living model: A decade of experience. New Directions for Mental Health Services.* No. 26. San Francisco: Jossey-Bass.

Thobaben, M. (1989). Developing a psychiatric nursing home health service. *Caring, 8*(6), 10-14.

Uys, L. R., Mhlaluka, N. G., & Piper, S. E. (1996). An evaluation of the effect of program changes in an acute psychiatric care unit. *Curationis: South African Journal of Nursing, 19*(3), 21-27.

Vaughn, K., Webster, D. C., Orahood, S., & Young, B. C. (1995). Brief inpatient psychiatric treatment: Finding solutions. *Issues in Mental Health Nursing, 16,* 519-531.

Walker, M. (1994). Principles of a therapeutic milieu: An overview. *Perspectives in Psychiatric Care, 30*(3), 5-8.

Watson, J. (1992). Maintenance of therapeutic community principles in an age of biopharmacology and economic restraints. *Archives of Psychiatric Nursing, 6,* 183-188.

Weissberg, M. (1991). Chained in the emergency department: The new asylum for the poor. *Hospital and Community Psychiatry, 42,* 317-318.

Winnicott, D. W. (1960). The theory of the patient-infant interaction. *International Journal of Psycho-analysis, 41,* 585-595.

Witt, R. (1981). Medication compliance among discharged psychiatric patients. *Issues in Mental Health Nursing, 3,* 305-317.

Yamashita, M., & Forsyth, D. M. (1998). Family coping with mental illness: An aggregate from studies in Canada and U.S. *Journal of the American Psychiatric Nurses Association, 4*(1), 1-8.

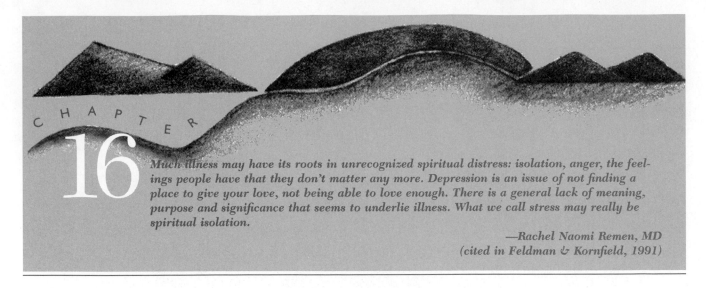

16

Much illness may have its roots in unrecognized spiritual distress: isolation, anger, the feelings people have that they don't matter any more. Depression is an issue of not finding a place to give your love, not being able to love enough. There is a general lack of meaning, purpose and significance that seems to underlie illness. What we call stress may really be spiritual isolation.

—Rachel Naomi Remen, MD
(cited in Feldman & Kornfield, 1991)

Alternative Therapies

Learning Objectives

After studying this chapter, you should be able to:

1. Describe traditional Chinese medicine.
2. Define life force.
3. Define acupuncture and discuss its use.
4. Discuss two conditions for which herbal therapy is used.
5. Define imagery and discuss its use.
6. Define therapeutic touch and discuss its use.
7. Define therapeutic massage and discuss its use.
8. Discuss the concept of energy transformation.
9. Define bioenergetics and discuss its use.
10. Define biofeedback and discuss its use.
11. Identify Western mind-body-spirit therapies including electroconvulsive therapy, hydrotherapy, phototherapy, sleep deprivation, psychotropic medications, nutritional and exercise interventions, religious practices, prayer, meditation, and "doing good works."

Key Terminology

Bioenergetics	Imagery	Prayer	Therapeutic massage
Biofeedback	Life force	Psychotropic medications	Therapeutic touch
Ch'i	Meditation	Qi'gong	Traditional acupuncture
Electroconvulsive therapy	Nutrition	Relaxation	Traditional Chinese medicine
Exercise	Orthomolecular therapy	Religious practices	Transcendental meditation
Hydrotherapy	Phototherapy	Sleep deprivation therapy	Yin and yang

In Chapter 1, we introduced the idea of a world view and said that this textbook is based on a theistic world view, which holds that God exists, and that He is all powerful, personal, and intimately involved in our everyday lives. Yet even those who share a theistic world view—and certainly those who hold other world views—have different beliefs about the role of alternative therapies in mental illness.

Each nurse and each patient must make an informed choice about these therapies. See Snapshot: Nursing Interventions Specific to Mind-Body-Spirit Therapies. To make such a choice, you and your patient need to understand the basis for these therapies. You need to be able to compare and contrast your own world views with the beliefs on which these therapies are based, and you need to decide whether these therapies are consistent with your world views.

Two principal types of alternative therapies for mental illness exist: those stemming from an Eastern tradition and those stemming from a Western tradition. In this chapter, we present a brief overview of the alternative therapies stemming from both traditions. As you read and study this material, we encourage you to think critically about the alternative therapies. Consider how they fit with your own world view. Consider how they fit with a theistic world view. Consider the degree to which these therapies find support in objective research.

Millie's Story

Millie is 52 years old, very much overweight, depressed, and about ready to give up. She tells her story to an acupuncturist.

"I've seen them all—doctors, therapists, even nutritionists—and not one of them has been able to provide me with any relief. I'm broke and still sick. Life is so difficult. I decided you were my last shot. I'm always in the dumps; I feel nauseated most of the time. I am so sensitive to foods and lots of other things around me. I have a spastic colon, chest problems, abdominal gas, and dizziness, and I'm fat. I'm so tired I can barely get started each day. I know my thyroid is slow. I suffer from migraine headaches; I also have sugar problems, but I crave chocolates.

"I wish I could have made something of myself. I had the ability, I just didn't have any motivation. The closest I ever came to success was when I owned my own flower shop. I had to sell it about 4 years ago—the allergies became too much for me. Sure I had allergy tests, but I didn't believe the results. The tests showed that I had no allergies. Why would I want to cut myself off from something that I was good at? I used to treat projects in the flower shop as people. I

SNAPSHOT

Nursing Interventions Specific to Mind-Body-Spirit Therapies

What do you need to do to develop a relationship with a patient who uses mind-body-spirit therapies?
- Listen to the patient and his or her explanation of the signs and symptoms of his or her problems.
- Maintain an open mind regarding other methods of treatment.
- Allow the patient to express his or her feelings about frustrations with traditional therapies.
- Explore strategies, successes, and failures of different complementary therapies and their effectiveness and other alternatives.

What do you need to assess regarding the patient's health status?
- Assess the patient using a mind-body-spirit model to evaluate the effectiveness of alternative therapies on all levels of functioning.

What do you need to teach the patient or the patient's caregiver?
- Provide information on alternative and complementary therapies.
- Explore possible strategies and investigate new models.
- Evaluate the effectiveness of alternative and complementary therapies and impart that information to the patient, the patient's family, or the patient's caregiver.
- Teach coping skills, relaxation techniques, and other methods to reduce stress and anxiety.
- Investigate community referral sources that provide complementary services and provide the patient with information about access.

What skills will you want the patient or caregiver to demonstrate?
- Ability to try and practice new strategies, allowing you the opportunity to provide feedback on technique and redirection, when necessary.
- Ability to express feelings and thoughts about the strategies' effectiveness.
- Ability to evaluate when strategies are effective.
- Establish a caring, understanding environment that allows the patient to believe in the treatment.
- Provide a safe and therapeutic environment that allows the patient to explore alternative strategies.

could make flowers blend from being nothing to being beautiful in an arrangement. This is something I have never been able to do with myself.

"I have always been weird, and I have never belonged anywhere. When I was a little girl I hated school. That's when I started to have stomach pains and would throw up. I just wanted to stay home with my mother.

"No, my mom was not affectionate, but somehow I felt safe with her. She didn't talk much either. It's funny—I remember her telling me that I was an accident and that I wasn't wanted, but I still felt good being with her. I didn't have any friends. In fact, I tried to stay away from other kids. I even quit high school because I didn't like to be around other kids. I worked for a while and then decided that I ought to go back to night school and get my high school diploma. After that, I went to college. I did well and graduated with a degree in early childhood education. And you know what? I do not like children or understand them. I don't have a clue why I did that.

"I got married for the first time in 1965. I knew almost immediately that I had made a mistake. My life went downhill fast; I developed more physical problems, and I started to see a psychiatrist. Finally, in 1971, my husband came home, packed his bags, and just left.

"In 1974 I married again. The marriage is okay. Am I happy? No, but it's better than being alone. Sometimes, my husband gets on my case for being fat. He never says anything positive about me. We don't talk much either.

"I think I believe in God or at least in a higher power. I pray to Him to take care of me, but He doesn't seem to listen. I guess there are others with more important problems than mine. I think maybe some of my problems are related to my karma—you know, I need to work out my bad deeds from a former life.

"I take Nardil [phenelzine sulfate] every day, Synthroid [levothyroxine sodium], Phenergan [promethazine HCl], and lots of herbs and megavitamins."

Millie's journey is clearly a complicated tapestry. Millie has many problems, and she has found no lasting solutions in traditional medical, psychiatric therapy, and spiritual care. She has now turned to an alternative therapist.

EASTERN MIND-BODY-SPIRIT THERAPIES

Historical Development

Taoism

Taoism came into being as a guiding philosophy around 2500 BC—perhaps even earlier. Taoism teaches

- We comprise the reality of existence.

- If we live within the natural rhythms of the universe, we will be whole.
- We are one with all that is around us.
- Paying attention to nature and all her changes (endless birth, growth, death, and renewal) allows us to sense that we are no different from what we see around us.
- We must respect the life force of nature.
- We are essentially divine. We ourselves, therefore, possess the creative energy or life force to change. This energy is called the **Ch'i,** or **yin and yang.**

According to Taoists, this **life force** is a two-part force, with each part complementary to the other and neither part more important than the other. Good and evil, birth and death, action and inaction, flexibility and inflexibility, and love and fear are but a few facets of this two-part force. Health, according to Taoism, is the balance between these parts.

Taoism, therefore, focuses on understanding imbalances. According to Taoism, health involves being balanced in our natural rhythms, and illness emanates from imbalances. For example, human beings are by nature diurnal beings, awake and active during the day and asleep and inactive during the night. If we adopt a nocturnal pattern, we are out of balance with our nature. Taoism teaches that this imbalance may harm our well-being, because fighting our natural rhythms consumes a great deal of energy (Chia, 1983; Cleary, 1992).

Taoists believe that staying in tune with the natural rhythms is what we are to do to complete our life journey. In Taoism, the goal of life is transformation, which means returning to and being reabsorbed into the life force. Taoists also believe that nature gives us guidance in our quest for balance.

A practitioner operating from a Taoist perspective therefore teaches patients to remain balanced between the two parts. The premise is that it is better to maintain order than to spend time correcting disorder (Chopra, 1991a, 1991b; Dreher, 1990).

What do you think? How would you incorporate the notion of maintaining balance into your own views about a healthy lifestyle? Do you think imbalance is a factor in serious mental illnesses?

➤ *Check Your Reading*
1. What is Taoism?
2. What is the Ch'i, or life force?
3. What does Taoism say about the role of balance in achieving healing of mind, body, and spirit?

Traditional Chinese Medicine

Traditional Chinese medicine is based on Taoist natural philosophy. The goal of traditional Chinese medicine is to promote harmony (health) or order out of chaos (illness) (Schatz, Larre, & Rochat de la Vallée, 1986).

Traditional Chinese medicine is a vast system of medicine based on a constellation of concepts, theories, laws, and principles of energy movement within the body. Specific modes of therapy in traditional Chinese medicine include acupuncture, diet therapy, exercises, herbal therapy, and manipulation of the musculoskeletal system. These modes of therapy are aimed at addressing the patient's illness in relation to the complex interaction of mind, body, and spirit. Adherents of traditional Chinese medicine say that it addresses not only symptoms but also what they call *cosmological* events—events that relate to the dynamics of the universe.

According to traditional Chinese medicine, the Ch'i, or life force, circulates throughout the universe and in our bodies in precise channels called meridians. (These meridians become significant in the practice of acupuncture.)

Traditional Chinese medicine incorporates a five-element theory that is a concrete expression of the Taoist concept of Ch'i, yin and yang, or life force. In this five-element theory, every substance, including the elements of the body, is classified as one of five primordial elements: wood, fire, earth, metal, and water (Figure 16-1). For instance, a practitioner of traditional Chinese medicine would say that the spleen and stomach "are of the realm of earth." The lungs and large intestines, on the other hand, "belong to metal."

These elements are said to act on one another as part of a dynamic system. For example, a practitioner of traditional Chinese medicine would say that fire animates earth, that earth produces metal, that metal enriches water, that water produces wood, and that wood gives rise, in turn, to fire. In this system, the transition of the five elements reflects the human condition of transformation, and transformation, in this system, is the essence of healing (Feng & English, 1973; Kaptchuk, 1983).

According to traditional Chinese medicine, the relationships among the elements can be both nurturing and destructive. Thus, they illustrate the delicate interaction between yin and yang and the need to maintain balance.

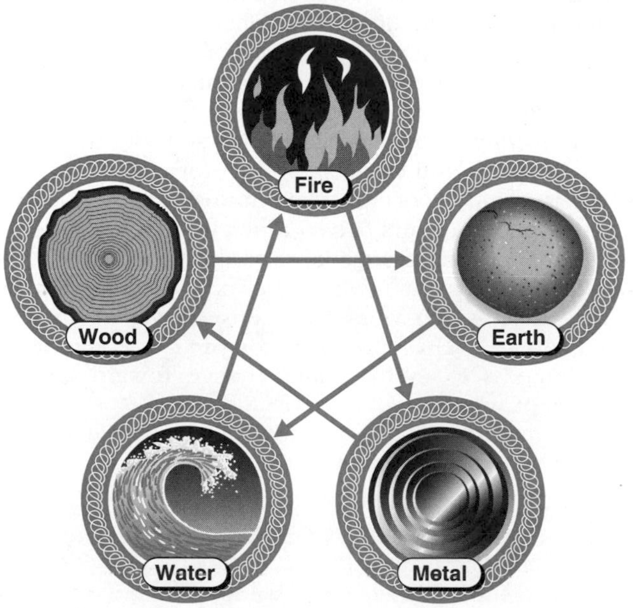

Within this view, health depends not only on the web of relationships within the five-element energy system but also on the relationships within the patient's environment, including

- Relationships with individuals, families, and communities
- Relationships with seasons, climates, and other physical phenomena
- Relationships with emotional, mental, and spiritual influences

Just as any other health care practitioner would, a practitioner of traditional Chinese medicine assesses the patient through a thorough history and physical examination. However, the practitioner of traditional Chinese medicine uses the history and physical examination to gain an understanding of the imbalances of mind, body, and spirit that have caused the patient's illness. Diagnosis, in traditional Chinese medicine, involves not only questioning the patient but also observing his or her body structure, skin color, breath, body odors, nail condition, voice, gestures, mood, and pulse.

Practitioners of traditional Chinese medicine say that *pulse diagnosis* is an art requiring years of practice. The practitioner identifies six pulses in each wrist, using both a light and a firm touch. She or he then describes the qualities of the pulses, using terms such as *fast, slow, weak, slippery, astringent, stretched,* and *tardy.* This information is used to identify the patient's current health status and health history as well as to make a prognosis for future health (Connelly, 1987).

As Millie's story continues, her problems are assessed by an acupuncturist, a practitioner of traditional Chinese medicine.

Figure 16-1
The ancient Chinese five-element model of energy transformation.

"Millie, based on my assessment, I believe that you are stuck in transformation from early in life. You are unfulfilled in what we call your earth nature. First of all, I believe that you have what we call a disturbance in earth as your center. You see, earth is our center, our soul, where our sense of self resides. Earth flourishes in our late summer, when the spring's birth comes to fruition. It is our ripening stage. It is the element within us that has to do with bonding and nourishment. The digestive organs (where we 'rot and ripen' our foods) are the targets of illness in our earth nature.

"From birth, you did not seem to bond spiritually with your mother and perhaps not even physically. Your mother fed you from a bottle rather than from her breasts. Not surprisingly, you developed a milk allergy early on. From earliest infancy, you could not digest and assimilate all that was around you—not only foods but also, metaphorically, your family and others.

"Also, Millie, your ripening, or maturity, is yet to come. Transformations are difficult for you. Your organs of birth (your ovaries and uterus) have been targets of disease. You have never been able to conceive and bear children. Indeed, your reproductive abilities floundered before they began.

"Earth is our 'mother,' from whom we derive all nourishment. Your history of disease in your uterus (including irregular and troublesome periods, fibroids, endometriosis, and early menopause) reflects this unfulfillment in your earth nature. Your organs of fruition failed. Your sense of career never germinated. You were not able to give birth, so to speak, to your life's ambitions. Consequently, you have had no ambitions. You have not been able to nourish yourself, let alone others. All of these problems deal with nourishment or lack of nourishment in mind, body, and spirit.

"Second, I believe that you have a disturbance in earth as your protector. Earth is not only our center but also our protector, where we live and thrive. If our earth within is imbalanced, we develop problems with nourishment and our immune systems. Conceiving anything, including children and ideas, and bringing projects to fulfillment, become difficult, if not impossible. Life is stuck in incompleteness, with no forward movement.

"Third, I believe that you have a disturbance in earth as your rootedness. You see, our earth is our rootedness. If we are not properly rooted, we cease to be grounded and balanced. Our self-esteem then becomes vulnerable to forces outside ourselves, as does our sense of purpose. Because earth normally provides our stability, instability is a sign of imbalance in our earth nature. Thus, your life has been characterized by wandering—nothing that you have ventured has come to fruition. Your only identity is manifested in symptoms to be addressed and cured. Your symptoms give you substance. Weight or body fat is protective. With excessive body fat, your earth nature is expressing imbalance by establishing a protective wall of insulation from life.

"In addition to disturbances in your earth nature, I believe that you also have some disturbance in what we call your fire nature. Fire nourishes earth. Warmth and caring (the fire of life) allow the fruits of the earth to grow. Millie, you never experienced this vital essence. How could you thrive? You never experienced a sense of belonging, a sense of being held in the bosom of the earth mother or in the bosom of your family. You never experienced touch, which is essential for grounding the human spirit and connects us all to one another. Without the ultimate communicator 'touch' in your life, you have never felt connected with anyone.

"What I would like to do now is to work with you on a treatment plan that will address these disturbances in your earth nature and fire nature."

What do you think? The above assessment is very different from what you have experienced within Western medicine. What are your thoughts about this approach? If you were conducting a nursing assessment of Millie, what would you assess?

➤ *Check Your Reading*
4. What is traditional Chinese medicine?
5. What are the five elements in traditional Chinese medicine?
6. What are yin and yang?
7. How is healing defined in traditional Chinese medicine?

An Eastern View of Healing

To understand healing from an Eastern world view, we must examine the goals, principles, and stages involved in healing. The goals of healing are

- Be in harmony with one's environment and all of creation in mind, body, and spirit.
- Reawaken the spirit to its possibilities.
- Reconnect with life's meaning.

According to this world view, the principles of healing are

- All nature (i.e., all living systems) tends toward order and harmony.
- All living systems are interdependent.
- Illness, or "dis-ease," is a pattern or patterns in the healing continuum of life.
- Healing is transformational and evolutional.
- All healing is manifested as a simultaneous, yin and yang reflection of the whole being in a state of transition.
- All healing is engendered through love and compassion. Love is the "author" of all healing.
- All healing is spirit centered.

Finally, in an Eastern world view, the stages of healing are

- *Awakening* represents a time—often triggered by crisis or illness—in which the person is said to sense a need for change, a feeling of diminution in the quality of life.
- *Intentionality and focus* occur when the person desires to change his or her consciousness from patterns of "disharmony" to patterns of healthy behaviors and seeks to ease the pain of spiritual discomfort and to obtain help.
- *Commitment* occurs when the person forges healing relationships and establishes goals for change.
- *Transformation* occurs when mutual, creative, active participation occurs between practitioner and patient toward ongoing change in mind, body, and spirit.
- *Attainment* occurs when the patient incorporates new, healthy behaviors, has a sense of well-being, and accepts new challenges for growth. He or she has a willingness to evaluate and change toward greater levels of wholeness.
- *Empowerment* occurs when the person feels a sense of stability and harmony.

What do you think? How do these stages of healing fit in with your view of healing? Are there comparable concepts within Western medicine?

8. List two of the goals of healing from an Eastern world view.
9. Identify two of the principles of healing from an Eastern world view.
10. Identify the stages of healing from an Eastern world view.

Specific Therapies

Some specific body-mind-spirit therapies stemming from an Eastern world view are listed:

- Acupuncture
- Qi'gong
- Imagery
- Therapeutic touch
- Therapeutic massage
- Relaxation
- Bioenergetics
- Transcendental meditation
- Biofeedback

This list of therapies, each of which we discuss in more detail in the next sections, is not all-inclusive. However, it is representative of the more common approaches used by practitioners of the therapies stemming from an Eastern world view.

ACUPUNCTURE

Traditional acupuncture is a system of health care and treatment based on the concept of *energetics.* According to Seem (1987), in his book *Body Mind Energetics,*

[T]his view of functional energetic systems and their interrelation portrays the body as a microcosm of the forces of the universe, with man situated between heaven (the sun and moon and the cosmos) and Earth. A dynamic series of energetic fluctuations, working on the human organism from above and below, constitutes the body of a living system. (p. 1107)

As we noted previously when we discussed traditional Chinese medicine, practitioners of acupuncture believe that energy courses through human beings in precise meridians. They believe that this energy is flowing, dynamic, observable, and measurable, and that its transition affects the balance of health. A practitioner of acupuncture identifies this balance by examining the ways in which people respond to problems. The practitioner then uses the technique of acupuncture to address the promotion of health and the prevention of illness (Requena, 1986). Today, acupuncture is used to treat a wide variety of illnesses, including sciatica, varicose veins, premenstrual syndrome, infertility, breast lumps, irritable bowel syndrome, arthritis, substance abuse, weight loss, and more (http://acupuncture.com/Acup/AcuInd.htm, 1999). In fact, the National Acupuncture Detoxification Association advocates widespread use of acupuncture detoxification using the principles of Chinese medicine (http://acupuncture.com/Acup/NadaPg1.htm, 1999).

The practitioner first performs an in-depth assessment of the patient's history. She or he then performs a thorough Eastern physical examination, in which she or he assesses the patient's energy balance by several means. For example, she or he might employ pulse diagnosis; temperature-taking; examination of the facial features (called *physiognomy*); examination of the dynamics of the patient's structure and functioning; and observation of the patient's skin color, voice, and emotions.

Based on the collected data, the practitioner identifies the pattern of disruption of the patient's energy. She or he states the diagnosis in terms of the five-element system of traditional Chinese medicine and the networks of the acupuncture meridians (see Figure 16-1). The practitioner identifies these disruptions as energy blockages manifested in mind, body, and spirit.

The practitioner then develops a comprehensive treatment plan unique to the particular patient. Where the practitioner has identified energy blockages, she or he inserts long needles, which look rather like small knitting needles, into specific points along the imbalanced meridians. Acupuncturists have identified at least 722 such acupuncture points, although only about 40 to 50 are in common use. By inserting these needles, practitioners believe that they can manipulate, disperse, or reactivate energy.

Acupuncturists also practice the less well known but related procedure known as *moxibustion*. In this procedure, the practitioner burns a substance called *moxi,* which is derived from the plant *Artemista vulgaris,* a member of the chrysanthemum family. This burning produces heat over the patient's energy points. This heat penetrates the skin and, practitioners believe, alters the flow of Ch'i, or energy (Chow, 1984).

Similar to moxibustion is a practice known as *cupping*. Instead of burning leaves, cupping uses suction above the body part that requires treatment. Air inside a cup is warmed and the cup is turned upside down over the body at particular points. The vacuum created by the heat is said to expel dryness from the body, warm the Ch'i, and reduce swelling (Cassileth, 1998).

Acupuncturists evaluate the impact of their interventions both by how the patient feels in mind, body, and spirit and by what the practitioner observes. Interestingly, an acupuncturist considers all change positive. An acupuncturist considers the absence of change "energy stagnation."

A unique aspect of acupuncture is that the practitioner provides hands-on patient care 100% of the time during acupuncture therapy. Another benefit, according to practitioners, is that because the acupuncture needles actually penetrate the patient's energy field, the energy of the practitioner is always joined with that of the patient.

Focus and intent of both the patient and the practitioner are said to be essential to the process of acupuncture. The practitioner focuses entirely on the patient and teaches the patient to focus inward to try to feel the energy flowing or not flowing. When the patient experiences a sensation that might indicate energy blockage, the practitioner asks him or her to focus on the meaning of that blockage. Practitioners view this process of focusing as essential for achieving balance. For example, if the patient experiences a "knot" in the stomach, the acupuncturist might ask him or her to focus on what he or she is not able to digest in life.

Acupuncturists also use herbs, nutrition, and exercise to promote health. According to acupuncturists, herbs promote healing by influencing the energy field internally by altering ingestion and assimilation, much as the needles would act externally. Likewise, they say that diet and exercise keep energy flowing through nourishment and movement. Table 16–1 lists some herbal remedies commonly used in acupuncture (http://acupuncture.com/Herbology/CaHerb.htm, 1999).

Let's return now to Millie, to see how her acupuncturist addressed her problems.

Millie's acupuncturist determined that Millie's healing required that she enter into what she called "a journey of transcendence—a rising above your symptoms and an opening of the window to your truth." Her practitioner therefore chose counseling, teaching, and traditional acupuncture as primary interventions. She also interspersed other therapies to complement and enhance these primary modes of treatment. These secondary interventions included imagery, therapeutic massage, and simple exercise. She also focused on proper nutrition.

The practitioner stated her goal for Millie's acupuncture as follows: "By the end of the first acupuncture treatment, Millie will experience changes in the sound of her voice, her emotions, and her general well-being." The practitioner tried to meet this goal by administering three acupuncture treatments to help Millie "open her energy fields," thereby allowing Millie to unblock behavioral patterns and create change.

What do you think? Do you think you have energy fields that can be manipulated by a practitioner? Does being in the presence of a very

depressed individual or a very anxious individual affect your own energy? If so, how do you explain this phenomenon?

▶ *Check Your Reading*
11. To what does the term *energetics* refer?
12. Describe the process of acupuncture.
13. What is unique about the process of acupuncture?

QI'GONG

Qi'gong is used as a gentle technique to calm the mind and improve stamina. Qi'gong exercises involve concentrated, controlled breathing with simple, repetitive motions, similar to tai chi. Qi'gong is both internal and external. Internal qi'gong is practiced alone by the individual and promotes self-healing and health maintenance. It is performed with little to no movement and requires intense concentration focused on moving Ch'i throughout the body. External qi'gong is a special skill developed by master therapists that emits their own Ch'i and influences the health of others, similar to therapeutic touch or psychic healing. The force is both invisible and unmeasurable.

Qi'gong lowers the heart rate, lowers blood pressure (BP), improves relaxation, lowers the stress level, reduces anxiety, and provides a feeling of increased well-being and peace of mind. Although studies of qi'gong have resulted in extensive writings in China, they are anecdotal and do not meet Western standards for validity (Cassileth, 1998).

IMAGERY

Imagery, simply put, is "the mind thinking in pictures" (Epstein, 1989, p. 59). The idea of using imagery as an intervention is to visualize not only what is real but also what one wants to *become* real. The idea is that our mental pictures actually change reality. In some situations, imagery does indeed seem to change reality; why that happens, however, is the subject of controversy.

From an Eastern perspective, the spiritual basis of using imagery as an intervention is the belief that the only reality is *Brahman,* the universal energy. By creating an image, we can thus change reality and move toward healing.

The science of psychoneuroimmunology offers an alternative explanation for the success of imagery. Psychoneuroimmunology does not suggest that cancer, pain, or any disease process is unreal. Instead, it suggests that as human beings we are created in such a way that when we think positive thoughts (the process of thinking being in itself biochemical), we generate a health-enhancing effect in our immune systems. Conversely, when we are besieged by stress and we perceive our situation to be hopeless, we produce a different type of biochemical process, resulting in a depletion of our immune systems (Carson, 1993).

As used in health care, imagery is the imagination of health. As Thomas Moore (1992) wrote in his popular book, *Care of the Soul,* "a poetic reading of the body

TABLE 16–1 Herbal Remedies

Detoxifying Herbs	**Antibiotics**
Red clover	Goldenseal
Alfalfa	Echinacea
Passion flower	Myrrh
Dandelion	Garlic
Elderberry	
Catnip	**Digestive Herbs**
	Licorice
Nerve Tonics	Peppermint
Valerian	Ginger
Skullcap	Slippery elm
Hops	Chamomile
Passion flower	
Antifungal Herbs	
Pau d'arco	
Aloe vera	
Tea tree oil	

as it expresses itself in an illness calls for a new appreciation for the laws of imagination . . . ." (p. 159). Imagery is often used in treating patients with medical disorders that are resistant to traditional approaches: patients with AIDS, patients in hospice care, patients with chronic pain, and patients with cancer. Case Example 16–1 illustrates the successful use of imagery in a 13-year-old with advanced cancer.

■ CASE EXAMPLE 16–1
■ C.R.'s Story

C.R., aged 13, was admitted to our center with the diagnosis of Ewing's sarcoma Stage IV with bilateral lung metastasis. Cyclic chemotherapy was initiated during the 4-day hospitalization. We were asked to see the patient on the last day because of pain. In the initial conversation with the parents they expressed great interest in having their son learn imagery exercises for pain control and sleeping and also asked if the patient could use this "to fight cancer."

Patient was in bed on the initial visit. He was irritable, tense, and complaining of pain in his back at the intravenous site. When asked if he wanted to move via wheel chair to our office, he declined. The initial practice was conducted in a four-bed room where we made a tape of the initial exercise. Patient indicated that he could not visualize switches and preferred to focus on the perception of numbness in the areas of discomfort. He relaxed very well using favorite place imagery, which included imagining that he was playing with his cat. The patient was given the option of deciding when to practice although we recommended B.I.D. practice. It was suggested that he induce numbness for gradually increasing periods of time. It was suggested that, although he could use the tape when he wished, at least half the practice should be without assistance of the tape. The patient quickly demonstrated improvement in pain control and decrease in requirements for pain medications. After discharge he was followed on an ambulatory basis with three individual practice sessions and group practice sessions. He spoke frequently about his imagery to combat cancer. The Acterberg-Lawlis interview concerning cancer imagery was filled out by him as follows:

He said that his cancer cells looked like black knights lined up for attack. He perceives them being "not strong enough to beat the white knights" who are the white blood cells. He sees the white blood cells charging all over the place and sees more of them than the black knights. The cancer cells are smaller than a white cell. The white knights fight the black knights by "piercing them, chopping them up with their daggers, they always do their job." The drugs are vicious beasts that go along with the white knights and eat up what's left. To the question, "How well does your treatment work to kill off disease," he answers, "The white knights and vicious beasts always win they don't have much to do now." He stated that he thinks about his imagery treatment on and off every day. ■

Abstracted from Olness, K. (1981). Imagery (self hypnosis) as adjunct care in childhood cancer: Clinical experience with 25 patients. *American Journal of Pediatric Hematology/Oncology, 3,* 313.

Millie's practitioner initiated the use of therapeutic imagery after three acupuncture treatments so that Millie could begin to visualize a more balanced body functioning as it should without allergies and illness. According to her practitioner, "Body image was an ongoing issue of malfunction and helplessness for Millie."

The practitioner stated the goal of imagery for Millie as follows: "Millie will state that she can imagine living her life allergy-free and with a healthy body."

The practitioner helped Millie meet this goal by teaching Millie how to practice imagery and encouraging her to do so on a regular basis. The rationale for this intervention was that the use of imagery could help Millie to change her image of her self and her health and, subsequently, lead to change in the reality of her health as well.

W*hat do you think?* How do you use imagery in your own life? Many athletes report that before competition they "rehearse" their performance in their minds. Is this a form of imagery?

► *Check Your Reading*
14. Define the term *imagery*.
15. What is the purpose of imagery?

THERAPEUTIC TOUCH

Dolores Krieger (1981), a pioneer in **therapeutic touch,** described the technique as "a conscious intentional therapy" (pp. 62-63). It is a spiritual intervention without a basis in established religion. On the surface, it appears to be similar to the Christian practice of "laying on of hands," but in reality it is worlds—and world views—apart.

According to Macrae (1991),

The practice of therapeutic touch involves the use of oneself (that is, one's own localized energy field) as an instrument to help whatever areas within the patient's field that have become obstructed and disordered by disease. (p. 18)

Essential to the practice of therapeutic touch are the beliefs that we are all healers and that a life force that we can manipulate is present in all of us. This universal energy is said to seek balance on all levels of mind, body, and spirit.

According to practitioners of therapeutic touch, the practitioner places his or her hands over a person, intentionally intervening in that person's energy field. The practitioner moves the person's life force to areas of depletion and clears blockages in the energy field to allow a free and ordered flow of energy and to promote healing (Hamilton, 1991; Heidt, 1991).

The practice of therapeutic touch involves five steps (Kreiger, 1979):

1. The practitioner centers himself or herself by

focusing on his or her own thoughts, clearing the mind to communicate with the person's energy field.

2. The practitioner assesses the patient's energy field by passing his or her hands, held 2 to 6 inches above the person's body, looking for blockages in energy flow.

3. The practitioner unruffles the patient's energy field by sweeping his or her hand in a downward motion past the person's toes and out of the body.

4. The practitioner directs and modulates the energy field.

5. The practitioner stops the therapy when he or she can no longer recognize bilateral differences in the patient's energy field.

To assess the patient's energy field, the practitioner sweeps his or her hands over the patient's body. During this sweep, he or she is said to feel a number of sensations, which are described as follows (Macrae, 1991):

Healthy energy flow: Evenly distributed and unbroken
Loose congestion: A cloud or wave of heat or heaviness
Light congestion: Coldness, or no response to the vibrations
Deficit: A hollowness, or depletion of vibration
Imbalance: An area's vibrations not flowing in harmony with the whole

Practitioners of therapeutic touch say that their assessment involves total interaction with the patient's energy field; they listen, observe, and *feel* in such a way as to gain an in-depth understanding of the patient's energy balance. The practitioner intuits the patient's vibrations, so to speak.

The aspect of therapeutic touch aimed at healing involves a second sweep across the patient's body. This time, the practitioner focuses on trying to manipulate energy imbalances and on transferring energy from himself or herself to the patient in an effort to create balance (Hanley, 1991; Hover-Kramer, 1991).

A good deal of research on therapeutic touch has been conducted, some of it funded by the Office of Alternative Medicine of the National Institutes of Health. Grad's 1963 and 1969 studies of therapeutic touch are particularly noteworthy, and Krieger cited them as foundational to her own work. Interestingly, Clark and Clark (1984) reviewed Grad's work, as well as the work of other nurse researchers on therapeutic touch, and concluded that research on therapeutic touch showed transient benefits, no significant benefits, or a need for replication of the research.

Janet Quinn (1989), a nurse researcher whose work was funded by the National Institutes of Health, tested the theories of intentionality and energy exchange, both of which are central to the practice of therapeutic touch. Quinn hypothesized that patients who were treated with therapeutic touch would experience a decrease in anxiety, as measured by decreased BP, decreased heart rate, and reduced anxiety scores, compared with patients who were treated with a technique that mimicked therapeutic touch. In her studies, Quinn found that the benefits of therapeutic touch were not significantly different from the effects of the technique that mimicked therapeutic touch.

Rosa, Rosa, Sarner, and Barrett (1998) studied 16 therapeutic touch practitioners to see if they could perceive a human energy field in a blind study. Results showed that of trials with 280 practitioners, only 123 correctly identified the field (44%). The conclusion of this study leaves doubt that therapeutic touch is statistically significant and that statements of feeling the human energy field were not different than would have been achieved through chance.

Nevertheless, many nurses who use therapeutic touch cite anecdotal evidence of the technique's effectiveness in calming patients and instilling a sense of peace. It seems reasonable to ask, therefore, whether the effects of therapeutic touch observed by nurses are related to the technique of therapeutic touch or whether they are related to the bestowing of kindness, a gentle touch, and focused attention.

What do you think? If a technique cannot be validated by the scientific method, should it be used with patients?

► *Check Your Reading*
16. Define the term *therapeutic touch.*
17. What is the purpose of therapeutic touch?
18. What is the spiritual basis of therapeutic touch?

THERAPEUTIC MASSAGE

Therapeutic massage is an alternative approach to healing that employs a "systematic manipulation of soft body tissue by such movements as rubbing, kneading, pressing, rolling, slapping and tapping" (Beck, 1988, p. 12). Therapeutic massage, which includes such variations as shiatsu, acupressure, *tui na,* Swedish massage, Rolfing, and polarity therapy, derives from Japanese, Chinese, European, and North American traditions.

Therapeutic massage has been reported as effective in calming infants and has been used to improve immune function in people infected with HIV.

Depending on the provider's point of view, the purposes of therapeutic massage may include opening energy channels, releasing a blocked life force, and promoting relaxation. Therapeutic massage is said to have a systemic effect, in that it promotes better circulation in the blood vessels and lymphatics, leading to metabolic balance. Additionally, practitioners say that it enhances detoxification and excretion of built-up waste products from both muscles and organs.

The practitioner assesses the patient through a brief history and physical examination. Depending on her or his perspective, the practitioner may look for areas of blocked energy by examining the patient's musculoskeletal structures and soft tissues, as well as by observing the patient's gait, posture, and expressions. The practitioner may attempt to reestablish the patient's energy flow by manipulation and what is called healing intent. The practitioner may also try to help the patient to release pain or blocked emotions in the process of relaxation.

According to experienced practitioners with an Eastern world view, the massage practitioner becomes attuned to the life force as he or she reads the symptoms of imbalance (e.g., muscle spasms, fatigue, and depression) and validates with the patient the changes resulting from therapy.

From a secular as well as a theistic perspective, therapeutic massage works because a patient who receives the massage interprets the actions of the practitioner as loving and caring. Biochemical changes result, leading to feelings of calm and peacefulness.

Millie's acupuncturist determined that it would be appropriate to use therapeutic massage to alleviate Millie's "stuckness" in circulation and her issues of "bound-up muscular tension" and "holding onto" emotional tension. The practitioner selected therapeutic massage in particular to address these problems because she felt that Millie needed a hands-on therapy to ground her through human contact.

The practitioner stated the goal of therapeutic massage with Millie in this way: "Millie will verbalize greater connectedness with others after 1 month of therapeutic massage sessions."

What do you think? What place do you think that therapeutic massage might have in the care of the seriously mentally ill?

► *Check Your Reading*

19. Define the term *therapeutic massage*.
20. What is the purpose of therapeutic massage?
21. What is the Eastern spiritual explanation of the effectiveness of therapeutic massage?
22. What is a Western spiritual-biochemical explanation of the effectiveness of therapeutic massage?

RELAXATION

Relaxation is a technique that combines imagery with progressive tensing and relaxing of muscle groups throughout the body. It is an intervention that can be interpreted through either an Eastern pantheistic or a Western theistic perspective. From an Eastern pantheistic perspective, relaxation is therapeutic because it enables a person to achieve harmony with the universal energy force. From a Western theistic perspective, relaxation is therapeutic because it activates God-given biochemical mechanisms for healing.

BIOENERGETICS

According to practitioners of **bioenergetics**, *bioenergy* (another name for the life force, or Ch'i) is a force that can be manifested in physical or emotional planes. If a person experiences distress in the physical plane, say

these practitioners, it is also manifest in the emotional plane. Healthy people are said to experience a free flow of bioenergy; they are emotionally responsive and physically relaxed. Unhealthy people, they say, often block the expression of feelings. According to practitioners of bioenergetics, this blockage is transformed into rigid musculature. Healing is said to come about through the release of physical tensions, which allows the expression of repressed feelings and eventual resolution of conflict.

The practitioner of bioenergetics is in direct contact with the patient. The practitioner helps the patient to complete exercises that result in the stretching of muscles and the highlighting of areas of tension. The practitioner then participates with the patient in the acting out of emotional responses; he or she encourages the open expression of feelings, which in turn is said to result in freer flow of bioenergy and healing.

TRANSCENDENTAL MEDITATION

Transcendental meditation is a process whereby a person strives to experience *pure consciousness,* or oneness with the universal energy force. Transcendental meditation was introduced into the United States by the Maharishi Mahesh Yogi in the late 1950s and 1960s. The Maharishi Mahesh Yogi said that his purpose in spreading the technique of transcendental meditation was to encourage people to focus less on the material world (which he viewed as unreal) and more on the immaterial energy force (which he viewed as real). He said that as we focused less on the material world and more on the spiritual world, social problems would be eliminated. The Maharishi Mahesh Yogi did not propose that meditation led to good works or social action but that meditation itself changes reality.

Meditation has a long history within the theistic world view. Throughout history, individuals have meditated to move away from the distractions of the world and to be able to hear the voice of God. Meditation provides the benefits of relaxation and stress reduction, which in turn lowers the levels of stress hormones, improves immune functioning, diminishes chronic pain, and improves mood. It allows the body to promote self-healing (Cassileth, 1998).

Transcendental meditation is a technique that must be taught and requires a number of steps:

1. A teacher initiates the person into transcendental meditation with an initial instructional presentation covering the benefits of the practice.

2. In a second presentation, the teacher presents the steps of transcendental meditation.

3. The teacher interviews the person.

4. The teacher provides individual instruction.

5. The teacher gives the student a unique *mantra,* frequently a word with spiritual significance, which the student is to focus on and repeat hypnotically.

6. The individual practices transcendental meditation independently but returns at least three times for monitoring by a mentor who ascertains the student's progress and answers questions.

➤ *Check Your Reading*
23. What is bioenergy?
24. Define the term *transcendental meditation*.
25. What is the purpose of transcendental meditation?
26. What is the purpose of bioenergetics?
27. What did the Maharishi Mahesh Yogi say that transcendental meditation would accomplish?

BIOFEEDBACK

Like relaxation, **biofeedback** is an effective technique that we can explain through both an Eastern pantheistic perspective and a Western theistic perspective. From an Eastern pantheistic perspective, biofeedback is therapeutic because the body is basically an energy field that needs to be rebalanced and brought into harmony with the universe. From a Western theistic perspective, biofeedback is therapeutic because it taps into a God-given biochemical healing mechanism.

Biofeedback teaches the patient to bring under conscious control such functions as respiratory rate, heart rate, BP, and skin temperature. The goal of bringing these functions under voluntary control is to relieve such physiological problems as migraine headaches, stuttering, insomnia, chronic pain, and anxiety.

Biofeedback training involves several steps:

1. Becoming aware of the functioning associated with the targeted symptom (e.g., noting the changes that occur preceding and during a migraine headache)
2. Learning to recognize internal changes associated with the targeted symptom
3. Learning to voluntarily alter those internal changes
4. Becoming motivated to learn this control

Practitioners of biofeedback facilitate the process of acquiring sensitivity to internal changes through the use of electronic equipment. This equipment measures biochemical changes in the body and signals the patient of these changes. The equipment includes

- An EEG to monitor changes in brain waves (alpha, delta, and theta waves). This device is used for patients with anxiety and general tension, stuttering, insomnia, and chronic pain.
- A thermistor to measure skin temperature. This device is used to help patients with migraines learn to shift blood volume from central to peripheral sites, such as the hands.
- An electromyograph to measure muscle relaxation. This device is used in patients with *bruxism* (grinding of the teeth) and spasticity.
- A galvanometer, to measure galvanic skin response. This device is used to help patients recognize unconscious emotional states.

➤ *Check Your Reading*
28. What is biofeedback?
29. Identify at least four conditions in which biofeedback could be used.
30. Identify at least two of the electronic instruments used in biofeedback.
31. What are the four steps used in the process of biofeedback?

WESTERN MIND-BODY-SPIRIT THERAPIES

In addition to the Eastern mind-body-spirit therapies explored in this chapter, Western mind-body-spirit therapies are used in the treatment of psychiatric patients. These include **electroconvulsive therapy, phototherapy, sleep deprivation therapy** (covered in depth in Chapter 25), **psychotropic medications** (covered in Chapter 17), hydrotherapy, nutrition, exercise, prayer, meditation, religious practices, and "good works."

Hydrotherapy

Hydrotherapy involves the use of water in the treatment of mental illness. Traditionally, it called for the patient to be wrapped in wet packs or cold sheets. This technique resulted in subduing and quieting the patient. Historically, the practice was often associated with the early insane asylums, where the treatment was punitive. However, this technique, which may sound punitive and primitive, is less restrictive than medication and is effective in calming patients who are out of control. Alternative therapists recommend soaking in hot water to restore proper circulation, relax the body, and reduce stress (Cassileth, 1998).

Nutrition

Nutrition is an essential consideration when working with a patient who has a mental illness. Because psychiatric illnesses affect the whole person, it is not surprising that patients with mental illnesses frequently have inadequate diets. Often, either their diets are deficient in the proper nutrients, or they eat too much or too little. Research demonstrates the intimate connection between nutrition and behavioral issues. For instance, anemia, which is the most common deficiency disease, often causes depression. Scientists at the University of California, Davis, reported that omitting breakfast can interfere with cognition and learning in the classroom (Pollett, Cueto, & Jacoby, 1998). As you conduct patient assessments, be sure to assess the patient's nutrition, and be prepared to address this area in health teaching.

Medications and Food

One important area of nutrition to consider is the interaction of foods and medications. For instance, some medications, such as antidepressants classified as monoamine oxidase inhibitors (MAOIs), involve dietary restrictions. Patients taking MAOIs are instructed to avoid eating foods that contain a substance called tyramine. These foods, taken with MAOIs, could cause a hypertensive crisis, in which the patient's BP soars to dangerous levels (see Chapter 17).

Millie takes Nardil [phenelzine sulfate], an MAOI, yet she continues to eat chocolate, which contains tyramine. Consequently, she becomes very ill. ■

Caffeine and Other Stimulants

Another important area of nutrition to consider is the ingestion of foods or substances that produce or exacerbate psychiatric symptoms. For instance, patients with anxiety disorders should avoid stimulants, such as those found in over-the-counter diet and cold preparations, as well as caffeine. These substances can intensify anxiety in patients already struggling with anxiety disorders.

For instance, caffeine triggers increased activity of the sympathetic nervous system, which causes the fight-or-flight physiological response typical of an anxiety attack. It is helpful to advise patients to cut down caffeine intake slowly over a period of months, for example, first substituting decaffeinated coffee and then herbal teas for regular coffee. In fact, many herbal teas, such as chamomile, hops, and peppermint, actually have a relaxing effect on the body (Communication Channels, 1994; Danton, Altrocchi, Antonuccio, & Basta, 1994; Hunt, 1989). Table 16–2 lists caffeine withdrawal symptoms.

Foods High in Sugar

Another important area of nutrition to consider is the ingestion of large quantities of refined simple sugars. Refined simple sugars can affect mental health by causing a "roller coaster effect" in energy levels, leading to

TABLE 16–2 Caffeine Withdrawal Symptoms	
Anxiety	Headache
Apathy	Inability to concentrate
Constipation	Insomnia
Cramps	Irritability
Craving	Nausea
Depression	Nervousness
Dizziness	Runny nose
Drowsiness	Tachycardia
Fatigue	Tinnitus
Feeling hot and cold	Vomiting

anxiety and depression. Foods such as cookies, candies, cakes, pies, soft drinks, ice cream, and other sweet foods quickly break down into glucose in the digestive tract. Glucose then moves rapidly into the bloodstream and is taken up by the cells of the body to satisfy their energy needs.

To handle this overload of glucose, the pancreas releases large amounts of insulin, an important protein that helps transport glucose from the blood into the cells of the body. Frequently, however, the pancreas "overshoots" and releases too much insulin. This results in a rapid fall in blood glucose, producing the roller coaster effect typically felt by a person with hypoglycemia or premenstrual syndrome.

To correct this situation, the adrenal glands release cortisol and other hormones. These substances cause the liver to release stored glucose to return blood glucose levels to normal. Unfortunately, as the adrenal glands are at work boosting blood glucose levels, they are simultaneously heightening alertness and producing symptoms of anxiety.

Eating complex carbohydrates is better for our physical and emotional well-being than eating refined sugars. Our bodies must work harder to break down complex carbohydrates into glucose than they work to process simple sugars. The sugars in complex carbohydrates, therefore, enter our bloodstream at a more even rate than do simple sugars. Fruit-based desserts and fruit salads can be satisfactory substitutes for foods high in simple sugars. Fruits also contain fiber, which delays the rate at which sugars are absorbed into the bloodstream (Lark, 1994).

Alcohol

People with moderate to severe anxiety and mood swings should avoid alcohol entirely or limit its use to occasional small amounts. Alcohol is a simple sugar, which is rapidly absorbed by the body. Like other simple sugars, alcohol worsens the symptoms of hypoglycemia, causing an increase in anxiety and mood swings. Additionally, the use of alcohol is contraindicated with most psychotropic medications (Lark, 1994; Seligman, 1994) (http://www.greentree.com/article.html?num=299, 1999).

Food Additives

Some people are sensitive to food additives, which can produce anxiety-like symptoms including rapid heartbeat, shallow breathing, headaches, "spaciness," and dizziness. Aspartame (Nutrasweet) and monosodium glutamate (MSG) are two of the most popular additives that have been repeatedly implicated in the production of unpleasant physical and psychological reactions.

Dairy Products

For some people, eating dairy products worsens symptoms of depression and fatigue. To ensure adequate intake of calcium and protein, counsel such patients to substitute beans, peas, soybeans, sesame seeds, and green leafy vegetables for dairy products. Soy milk, potato milk, and nut milk, which are available at natural food stores, are excellent substitutes for cow's milk (Lark, 1994).

Wheat and Other Gluten-Containing Grains

In anxious and depressed people who are sensitive to some foods, the ingestion of wheat may worsen the anxiety and depression. The causative component of wheat appears to be gluten, a protein derivative that gives dough its tough, elastic character. People suffering from severe anxiety should eliminate wheat from their diets for at least 1–3 months. Oats, barley, and rye, which also contain gluten, should be eliminated initially. For some people, even corn and rice can increase symptoms of anxiety, fatigue, and depression.

Buckwheat, on the other hand, is easily digested by most people who are sensitive to gluten. It comes from a different plant family than wheat and other gluten-rich grains. Quinoa and amaranth are other good choices; all are available at natural food stores. Buckwheat, quinoa, and amaranth are also excellent sources of the B vitamins, vitamin E, many essential minerals, complex carbohydrates, essential fatty acids, and fiber. For people sensitive to wheat and other gluten-containing foods, a good meal might consist of beans and buckwheat bread with vegetables, or corn bread and split pea soup (Lark, 1994).

Vegetables and Fruits

Swiss cheese, chard, broccoli, beet greens, mustard greens, kale, raisins, blackberries, and bananas are rich in calcium, magnesium, and potassium, which are important minerals that help improve endurance, stamina, and vitality. Brussels sprouts, parsley, peas, tomatoes, potatoes, berries, and melons supply a good dose of vitamin C, which is essential for the production of adrenal hormones (Lark, 1994).

Seeds and Nuts

Raw flax seeds and pumpkin seeds are excellent sources of two essential fatty acids: linoleic acid and linolenic acid. Adequate levels of essential fatty acids are important in preventing both the emotional and physical symptoms of premenstrual syndrome, menopause, emotional upsets, and allergies. Sesame and sunflower seeds are excellent sources of linoleic acid (Communication Channels, 1994; Danton et al., 1994; Hunt, 1989).

Vitamins, Minerals, and Amino Acids

Certain vitamins are essential to good mental health. For instance, vitamin B_1 (thiamine) is used by the brain to change glucose into fuel. A lack of thiamine can lead to depression, anxiety, and memory loss. Vitamin B_6 (pyridoxine) also seems connected to depression. The body needs vitamin B_6 to manufacture serotonin, one of the substances implicated in mood regulation. Folate (folic acid) helps in the production of neurotransmitters, and a deficiency of folate is implicated in depression. Vitamin C (ascorbic acid) is essential to a healthy immune system, and a healthy immune system is essential to warding off depression. Stress, smoking, and pregnancy deplete the body of vitamin C, leaving the individual vulnerable to bouts of depression (http://www. greentree.com/article.html?num=299, 1999).

The use of specific vitamins, minerals, and amino acids in tablet, capsule, or powder form to balance a person's nutritional needs is called **orthomolecular therapy.** Orthomolecular therapy is not synonymous with megavitamin therapy. In *megavitamin therapy,* a person consumes massive quantities of vitamins, far exceeding recommended daily allowances, in an attempt to achieve overall health. In orthomolecular therapy, the person consumes specific vitamins, minerals, and amino acids (sometimes in large quantities, when a deficiency is severe) to correct a specific imbalance thought to underlie a specific problem.

A number of conditions appear to respond to orthomolecular therapy. For instance, brewer's yeast (500 mg three times a day with meals) along with B-complex vitamins (including niacin) (50 mg three times a day with meals) has been effective in treating anxiety and exhaustion. Rheumatoid arthritis, a severe, crippling form of arthritis, sometimes responds to treatment with pantothenic acid (500 mg four times a day). Likewise, phenylalanine seems to increase the body's pain tolerance, and senility and senile dementia may respond to L-glutamine (1 g daily, progressing to 2 g by the end of 1 month). Similarly, antioxidants (vitamin C, vitamin E, selenium, zinc, and β-carotene) may bind with pesticide residues on fruits and vegetables and protect us from the harmful effects of these chemicals (Salaman, 1989). Niacin and foods high in fiber also seem to act as detoxifiers.

Herbal Supplements

ST. JOHN'S WORT

St. John's wort *(Hypericum perforatum)* is a yellow flowering plant that grows wild in Europe and the United States. It seems to affect the brain and control mood swings. It has been used to control pain and to treat stress and anxiety for centuries in traditional, native, and folk healing. Hypericin, the main ingredient, has few side effects, and it is not known how it works. Although St. John's wort is effective, its administration is not an accurate science, dosages may vary by patient and herbal formula, and there is little regulation for production and sales. St. John's wort is not regulated by the Food and Drug Administration, and it is considered a nutritional supplement and not a prescription medication.

DeSantis and Nolan (1996) reviewed 23 clinical studies that measured the effectiveness of St. John's wort. Studies showed that patients were less depressed when taking the herbal preparation than when taking a placebo. Further studies need to be completed that compare the effects of St. John's wort to those of selective serotonin reuptake inhibitor antidepressants to determine a safe and effective dose and formula that further evaluate the placebo effect.

St. John's wort seems to have certain advantages over prescription antidepressants, including

- There have been no reports of sexual dysfunction.
- It helps with insomnia, actually increasing deep sleep, whereas prescription antidepressants decrease deep sleep.

The most commonly reported side effects of St. John's wort include sensitivity to sunlight, fatigue, and upset stomach (http://www.greentree.com/article.html?num=149). The use of St. John's wort is not appropriate if

- The individual is pregnant.
- The individual is taking a prescription antidepressant.
- The individual has a history of seizure disorders.
- The individual has an estrogen-dependent cancer (the herb contains a mild phystoestrogen).
- It is causing feelings of confusion, severe headaches, a sudden rise in BP, pupil dilation, and heart palpitations.

KAVA

Kava is a member of the pepper family and was used for centuries in the South Pacific. Kava is widely prescribed in Europe for anxiety and insomnia. Kava's popularity rests on its nonaddictive characteristics and the fact that it does not produce the morning after "hangover" frequently associated with prescription anxiolytics such as diazepam (Valium). In a double-blind study of individuals' reactions to everyday stress, the group taking kava displayed a significant decrease in stress levels, whereas the placebo group showed no reduction. Anecdotal evidence suggests that kava produces more relaxed, less aggressive, and more social behavior. It provides menopausal women relief from anxiety and nervousness. At very high dosages and over a prolonged period, kava may cause the skin to become dry and scaly. Kava may worsen the condition of people with Parkinson's disease.

VALERIAN

Another popular remedy in Europe, valerian is used to treat restlessness and sleep disorders. Valerian acts like a minor tranquilizer and may be taken as a tea or an extract. Its mechanism of action is unknown, and it seems to produce no side effects.

Exercise

Exercise is as important for the psychiatric patient as it is for any other patient and should be a part of your care of people with mental health problems. Some psychiatric illnesses and some psychotropic medications produce lethargy and listlessness. Patients may become sedentary and may therefore benefit from health teaching, encouragement, and concrete suggestions about ways to increase physical activity in their lives.

Additionally, physical exercise, particularly aerobic exercise, discharges the fight-or-flight energy associated with anxiety. Exercising results in increased oxygenation and blood circulation and revitalizes organ systems. The removal of waste products such as carbon dioxide, lactic acid, and other products of metabolism is more efficient with increased exercise.

Exercise results in the release of hormones called β-endorphins, substances thought to be responsible for the "runner's high" experienced by runners. Running, bicycling, walking, and swimming can increase β-endorphin levels significantly and should be included in the treatment plan of all patients with mental illness (Communication Channels, 1994; Danton et al., 1994; Hunt, 1989).

According to an Ohio State Univerity Study, exercise may reduce anxiety and depression in patients with chronic obstructive pulmonary disease (COPD). Charles Emery, coauthor of the study, believed the results to be especially important because patients with COPD often limit their physical activity. In a 10-week study that included 79 COPD patients older than the age of 50 years, the patients were randomly assigned to three groups. One group participated in regular exercise, an educational class about COPD, and a stress management class. The second group had the educational and stress management classes but no exercise. The third group was put on a waiting list with no treatment during the course of the study. Those who participated in exercise showed decreases in anxiety and depression, but those who participated in the educational programs only did not (http://www.greentree.com/article.html?num=102).

Religious Practices

Religious practices, including prayer (discussed separately), attendance at worship services, and reading of Scripture and other spiritually related materials, have been shown to be protective behaviors against a wide range of medical illnesses, including mental illness. There is ample research to demonstrate that religiosity is inversely related to psychopathology, particularly depression; social isolation; suicide; death anxiety; substance abuse; and support of euthanasia and physician-assisted suicide. Conversely, religiosity is positively correlated with improved functioning and overall healthier lives (Alvarado, Templar, Bressler, & Thomas-Dobson, 1995; Bachman, Aloser, Doukas, Lichtenstein, Corning, & Brody, 1996; Baume, O'Malley, & Bauman, 1995; Brown, Ndubuisi, & Gary, 1990; Ellison, 1995; Gartner, Larson, & Allen, 1991; Idler & Kasl, 1992; Koenig, 1995; Koenig, George, Meador, Blazer, & Dyck, 1994; Levin & Vanderpool, 1987; Matthews, 1997, 1998a, 1998b; Paykel, Myers, Lindenthal, & Tanner, 1974).

Prayer

Prayer, simply stated, is "talking to God." In a theistic world view, prayer is one of the main spiritual tools for seeking God's help. People with a theistic world view pour out their hearts to God, believing that He understands their struggles, accepts them as they are, sustains them in their sorrows, celebrates with them in their joys, and strengthens them in their journeys.

Prayer is a powerful form of communication. It allows a person to feel connected to a being who not only is greater and more powerful but also loves unconditionally (Poloma, 1993). People have few other (if any) resources to which to turn for such communion. However, prayer recognizes that God is the creator, and that the person praying is the *created*. Although many people view prayer as a means of manipulating God, the authors of this book believe that the person who is praying *cannot* manipulate God, because we see God as sovereign—as exercising absolute authority over the universe (Carson, 1989, 1993; Carson & Green, 1992). Nevertheless, we believe that through prayer we sometimes receive authentic healing from our pain (Dossey, 1996; Kaufman, 1997; Matthews, 1997).

Studies have shown that Americans are a praying people (Gallup & Jones, 1989; Poloma, 1993). In fact, 4 decades of Gallup polls have consistently demonstrated that 9 of 10 Americans pray, on occasion (Gallup & Jones, 1989).

In a study by Poloma (1993), prayer was associated with mental health. A positive relationship existed between prayer and three out of four indicators of quality of life: life satisfaction, general happiness, and existential well-being. Poloma also found that prayer contributes as much as a comfortable income and contributes more than gender, education, or age to one's sense of being satisfied with life. What is it about prayer that makes this difference? It is not the frequency or type of prayer that contributes to well-being; it is the extent and depth of intimacy with God that most contributes to such well-being.

In two other studies, one by Carson and Green (1992) and one by Carson (1993), participants who tested positive for HIV who were spiritually well and hardy indicated that the most important behavior in which they engaged was prayer.

Meditation

Meditation, when viewed from a theistic perspective, is quite different from transcendental meditation and other Eastern forms of meditation. From a theistic world view, the purpose of meditation is "to be still and know that God is God" (Poloma, 1993, p. 49). The focus is not on overcoming self-identity so as to be one with an impersonal, universal energy force but rather on communing in deep relationship with the Almighty. The 1989 Gallup poll (Gallup & Jones, 1989) found that people who engaged in meditative prayer stated that they spent time "quietly thinking about God," "feeling the presence of God," "trying to listen to God speaking," and "worshipping and adoring God" (p. 45). The focus of meditation or meditative prayer is on God—not on one's own needs or problems. This focus on God, with its interior stillness, allows for an inner response. People who engage in this type of prayer experience a positive effect on measures of mental health and well-being.

Doing "Good Works"

In his book *Man's Search for Meaning,* concentration camp survivor Viktor Frankl (1965) said that two factors determined whether a prisoner of a World War II concentration camp survived. The first factor was the good fortune of not being selected for extermination in the gas chambers. The second factor was the prisoner's level of spiritual well-being—his ability to find meaning in the most bestial of conditions. Frankl noted that many of the prisoners who survived were the first to share a piece of bread with another who seemed more in need, managed to keep a sense of humor, focused on others at their own expense, encouraged others when circumstances seemed bleak, and led others in prayer or song to raise hope.

Doing such good works and helping others even when our own circumstances would have us act selfishly and shun others somehow exerts a transforming power on us. In reaching beyond ourselves and our own difficulties, we somehow ultimately bring good on ourselves. Doing good works is love in action, and love in action is a strong tool for promoting physical, mental, and spiritual health in others, and, ultimately, in ourselves.

Conclusions

Sometimes patients do not find relief from their mental illnesses through traditional methods of Western medicine. Consequently, they may turn to alternative mind-body-spirit therapies.

Many of these therapies, such as acupuncture, imagery, therapeutic touch, therapeutic massage, relaxation, bioenergetics, transcendental meditation, and biofeedback, are rooted in the spiritual world view of Eastern pantheism. Other alternative therapies are rooted in Western medicine or in a Western theistic world view. These therapies include electroconvulsive therapy, psychotropic medications, hydrotherapy, nutrition, exercise, and religious practices such as prayer, meditation, and doing good works.

We encourage you to think critically about these alternative mind-body-spirit therapies. Keep abreast of the research being conducted on these therapies. Think about the degree to which they are consistent with your own world view. Think about the implications of these therapies when dealing with patients and other health care professionals who hold different world views.

Key Points to Remember

- Taoism teaches that reality is energy and that our goal is to live in unity with all that surrounds us.

- According to pantheism, the Ch'i (life force or yin and yang) is the divine energy within and outside of us.

- Traditional Chinese medicine is the foundation of the current mind-body-spirit therapies rooted in pantheism. Traditional Chinese medicine focuses on our unity with nature and on maintaining balance in our energy systems and relies on a five-element energy system.
- Acupuncture deals with moving energy through the meridians of the body to restore energy balance.
- Imagery is a technique that focuses on changing reality by creating a different mental image. From a pantheistic view, the basis for this practice is the belief that the only reality is the divine energy; all else is illusion.
- Therapeutic touch attempts to manipulate energy through the practitioner's use of her or his hands to move energy from one area of the patient's body to another and to direct energy from the practitioner to the patient for the purpose of enhanced healing.
- From the viewpoint of pantheism, therapeutic massage unblocks energy flow and connects patient and practitioner through human touch.
- Relaxation is a technique that combines imagery with progressive tensing and relaxing of muscle groups throughout the body.

- Bioenergetics is concerned with removing blockages to promote the flow of bioenergy, or Ch'i.
- Transcendental meditation focuses on getting beyond the self and becoming one with the universal energy force.
- Hydrotherapy, which has traditionally involved wrapping patients with wet packs, is a Western mind-body-spirit therapy used to calm agitated patients.
- Nutrition is an important consideration in mental health.
- Exercise is beneficial to mental health because it decreases anxiety and depression and increases a sense of well-being.
- Prayer, especially meditative prayer, is associated with mental health and well-being.
- Religious practices, including attendance at religious services, reading religious works, and participating in activities sponsored by religious groups, are all positively related to measures of mental health and well-being.
- Doing good works contributes to a sense of spiritual well-being and is a powerful tool for promoting physical, mental, and spiritual health.

Learning Activities

1. Examine your own world view. Does your world view allow for the use of any of the alternative therapies discussed in this chapter? If so, which ones? On what basis do you draw your conclusions?
2. Imagine that a patient for whom you are caring tells you that she is also seeing an acupuncturist. What would your reaction be? What would you say to your patient?
3. Interview two other health professionals. Ask them to define the concept of world view. Ask them if they understand the world views undergirding the alternative therapies rooted in Eastern medicine. What is your reaction to their responses?
4. Investigate what types of alternative therapies are practiced in your area. Call two of these practitioners, and ask what types of patients seek help from them. Ask them to explain their world view or the belief system undergirding their practice.

Critical Thinking Exercise

Mrs. Robinson, a 36-year-old woman, had been admitted to the inpatient psychiatric unit with a diagnosis of depression. During her 7-day inpatient treatment, Mrs. Robinson complained about frequent low back pain. When Nurse Chelo approached her room to discuss discharge plans, Mrs. Robinson asked what Nurse Chelo thought about her getting acupuncture for her low back pain. When Nurse Chelo asked the patient if she had discussed it with her physician, Mrs. Robinson stated, "I asked him about it once and he just laughed. He told me that as soon as my depression disappeared, my back pain would also disappear."

1. What is Mrs. Robinson's physician's point of view regarding acupuncture?
2. What assumptions can you draw about Mrs. Robinson's point of view?

3. What other evidence would you need to support your assumptions about Mrs. Robinson's physician's point of view?

Nurse Chelo had just read about acupuncture in her new psychiatry textbook and decided to give Mrs. Robinson some information about the treatment.

1. What could happen as a result of Nurse Chelo's giving information?
2. If Nurse Chelo's response had been different, what else might have happened?
3. What conclusions (if any) can you make about the decision that Mrs. Robinson will make about acupuncture?

Additional Resources

Alternative Medicine Home Page

http://www.pitt.edu/~cbw/altm.html

ITM Online: Chinese, Tibetan, Ayurvedic, Native American, and Thai Medicine

http://www.europa.com/itm/

National Center for Complementary and Alternative Medicine

http://nccam.nih.gov
Part of National Institutes of Health, Washington, D.C.

National Institute for Healthcare Research

800-580-NIHR
http://www.nihr.org
nihr@nihr.org (e-mail)

Nutrition and Mental Illness: Sampling of the Current Scientific Literature Part 2

http://www.thorne.com/townsend/nov/null.html

References

Alvarado, K. A., Templar, D. I., Bressler, C., & Thomas-Dobson, S. (1995). The relationship of religious variables to death depression and death anxiety. *Journal of Clinical Psychology, 51,* 202-204.

Bachman, J. G., Aloser, K. H., Doukas, D. J., Lichtenstein, R. L., Corning, A. D., & Brody, H. (1996). Attitudes of Michigan physicians and the public toward legalizing physician assisted suicide and voluntary euthanasia. *New England Journal of Medicine, 334,* 303-309.

Baume, P., O'Malley, E., & Bauman, A. (1995). Professed religious affiliation and the practice of euthanasia. *Journal of Medical Ethics, 21,* 49-54.

Beck, M. (1988). *The theory and practice of therapeutic massage.* New York: Milady.

Brown, D. R., Ndubuisi, S. C., & Gary, L. E. (1990). Religiosity and psychological distress among blacks. *Journal of Religion and Health, 29*(1), 55-68.

Carson, V. B. (1989). *Spiritual dimensions of nursing practice.* Philadelphia: W. B. Saunders.

Carson, V. B. (1993). Prayer, meditation, exercise, and vitamin use: Behaviors of the hardy individual who is HIV+, diagnosed with ARC or AIDS. *Journal of the Association of Nurses in AIDS Care, 4*(3), 18-28.

Carson, V. B., & Green, H. (1992). Spiritual well-being: A predictor of hardiness in the AIDS patient. *Journal of Professional Nursing, 8,* 209-220.

Cassileth, B. R. (1998). *The alternative medicine handbook: The complete guide to alternative and complementary therapies.* New York: Norton.

Chia, M. (1983). *Awaken healing energy through the Tao.* New York: Aurora Press.

Chopra, D. (1991a). *Creating health.* Boston: Houghton Mifflin.

Chopra, D. (1991b). *Perfect health: The complete mind/body guide.* New York: Harmony Books.

Chow, E. P. Y. (1984). *Traditional Chinese medicine: A holistic approach.* Diamond Bar, CA: Quest.

Clark, P., & Clark, M. J. (1984). Therapeutic touch: Is there a scientific basis for practice? *Nursing Research, 33*(1), 37-40.

Cleary, T. (1992). *I ching: The book of change.* Boston: Shambala.

Communication Channels, Inc. (1994). Supplements can help some anxiety disorders. *Better Nutrition for Today's Living, 56*(6), 20-21.

Connelly, D. M. (1987). *Traditional acupuncture: The law of the five elements.* Columbia, MD: The Centre for Traditional Acupuncture.

Danton, W. G., Altrocchi, J., Antonuccio, D., & Basta, R. (1994). Nondrug treatment of anxiety. *American Family Physician, 49,* 161-177.

DeSantis, P. A. G. M., & Nolan, W. A. (1996). St. John's wort as an antidepressant. *British Medical Journal, 313,* 241-242.

Dossey, L. (1996). *Prayer is good medicine.* New York: Harper.

Dreher, D. (1990). *The Tao of inner peace.* New York: Harper-Collins.

Ellison, C. G. (1995). Race, religious involvement, and depressive symptomatology in a Southeastern U. S. community. *Social Science and Medicine, 40,* 1561-1572.

Epstein, G. (1989). *Healing visualizations: Creating health through imagery.* New York: Bantam Books.

Feldman, C., & Kornfield, J. (Eds.). (1991). *Stories of the spirit, stories of the heart: Parables of the spiritual path from around the world.* San Francisco: Harper.

Feng, G., & English, J. (1973). *Tao te ching. A new translation of Lao Tsu.* London: Wildwood House.

Frankl, V. E. (1965). *Man's search for meaning.* New York: Washington Square Press.

Gallup, G., & Jones, S. (1989). *100 questions and answers: Religion in America.* Princeton, NJ: Princeton Religion Research.

Gartner, J., Larson, D., & Allen, G. (1991). Religious commitment and mental health: A review of the empirical literature. *Journal of Psychology and Theology, 19,* 6-25.

Grad, B. (1963). A telekinetic effect on plant growth. *International Journal of Parapsychology, 5,* 117-133.

Grad, B. (1969). Some biological effects of the laying-on-of-hands: A review of experiments with animals and plants. *Journal of the American Society for Psychical Research, 59,* 96-127.

Hamilton, D. (1991). Vital energy: The antebellum health movement. *Journal of Holistic Nursing, 9*(3), 10-18.

Hanley, M. A. (1991, Winter). Therapeutic touch: The art of improvisation. *Journal of Holistic Nursing, 9*(3), 26-31.

Heidt, P. R. (1991). Therapeutic touch: The caring environment. *Journal of Holistic Nursing, 9*(3), 19-25.

Hover-Kramer, D. (1991). Energy fields: Implications for the science of human caring. *Journal of Holistic Nursing, 9*(3), 59.

Hunt, D. (1989). *No more fears.* New York: Warner Books.

Idler, E. L., & Kasl, S. V. (1992). Religion, disability, depression, and timing of death. *American Journal of Sociology, 97,* 1052-1079.

Kaptchuk, T. (1983). *The web that has no weaver: Understanding Chinese medicine.* New York: Congdon and Weed.

Kaufman, D. (1997, Fall). Interview with C. Everett Koop, M. D. *Faith & Medicine Connection, 2*(1), 4.

Koenig, H. G. (1995). Use of acute hospital services and mortality among religious and non-religious copers with medical illness. *Journal of Religious Gerontology, 9*(3), 1-21.

Koenig, H. G., George, L. K, Meador, K. G., Blazer, D. G., & Dyck, P. B. (1994). Religious affiliation and psychiatric disorder among Protestant baby boomers. *Hospital and Community Psychiatry, 45,* 586-596.

Krieger, D. (1979). *The therapeutic touch: How to use your hands to help or to heal* (pp. 62, 63). Englewood Cliffs, NJ: Prentice-Hall.

Kreiger, D. (1981). *Foundations for holistic health nursing practices: The Renaissance nurse.* Philadelphia: J. B. Lippincott.

Lark, S. M. (1994). Strike back at high anxiety: Natural ways to stay calm in stressful times. *Vegetarian Times,* (198), 90-93.

Levin, J. S., & Vanderpool, H. Y. (1987). Is frequent religious attendance really conducive to better health? Toward an epidemiology of religion. *Social Science and Medicine, 24,* 589-600.

Macrae, J. (1991). *Therapeutic touch.* New York: Alfred A. Knopf.

Matthews, D. (1997). Flexing spiritual muscles can prevent illness. *Faith and Medicine Connection, 2*(1), 1.

Matthews, D. (1998a). Religious commitment and depression. *Faith & Medicine Connection, 2*(2), 3.

Matthews, D. (1998b). Spirituality: A new prescription for depression. *Faith & Medicine Connection, 2*(2), 1.

Moore, T. (1992). *Care of the soul.* New York: HarperCollins.

Olness, K. (1981). Imagery (self hypnosis) as adjunct care in childhood cancer: Clinical experience with 25 patients. *American Journal of Pediatric Hematology/Oncology, 3,* 313.

Paykel, E. S., Myers, J. K., Lindenthal, J. J., & Tanner, J. (1974). Suicidal feelings in the general population: A prevalence study. *British Journal of Psychiatry, 124,* 460-469.

Pollitt, E., Cueto, S., & Jacoby, E. R. (1998). Fasting and cognition in well- and undernourished schoolchildren: A review of three experimental studies. *American Journal of Clinical Nutrition, 67*(Suppl. 4), 779S-784S.

Poloma, M. (1993). The effects of prayer on mental well-being. *Second Opinion, 18*(3), 37-51.

Quinn, J. (1989). Therapeutic touch as energy exchange: Replication and extension. *Nursing Science Quarterly, 2*(2), 79-87.

Requena, Y. (1986). *Terrains and pathology in acupuncture.* Brookline, MA: Paradigm.

Rosa, L., Rosa, E., Sarner, L., & Barrett, S. (1998). A close look at therapeutic touch. *Journal of the American Medical Association, 279,* 1005-1010.

Salaman, M. (1989). Super nutrition for super health. *Bestways, 17*(4), 38-42.

Schatz, J., Larre, J., & Rochat de la Vallée, E. (1986). *Survey of traditional Chinese medicine.* Columbia, MD: Traditional Acupuncture Institute.

Seem, M. (1987). *Body mind energetics.* Rochester, VT: Thorsons.

Seligman, M. E. P. (1994). What you can change and what you cannot change. *Psychology Today, 27*(3), 34-47.

Suggested Readings

Bratman, S. (1997). *The alternative medicine sourcebook: A realistic evaluation of alternative healing methods.* Los Angeles: Lowell House.

Carson, V. B. (1993). Prayer, meditation, exercise, and vitamin use: Behaviors of the hardy individual who is HIV+, diagnosed with ARC or AIDS. *Journal of the Association of Nurses in AIDS Care, 4*(3), 18-28.

Clark, P., & Clark, M. J. (1984). Therapeutic touch: Is there a scientific basis for practice? *Nursing Research, 33*(1), 37-40.

Hanley, M. A. (1991, Winter). Therapeutic touch: The art of improvisation. *Journal of Holistic Nursing, 9*(3), 26-31.

Hunt, D. (1989). *No more fears.* New York: Warner Books.

Lark, S. M. (1994). Strike back at high anxiety: Natural ways to stay calm in stressful times. *Vegetarian Times,* (198), 90-93.

Marti, J. E. (1998). *The alternative health and medicine encyclopedia.* Detroit, MI: Visible Ink Press.

Oliveira, A., & Crowe, R. (1995). Complementary therapies. In P. Kelly, S. Holman, R. Rothenberg, & S. P. Holzemer (Eds.), *Primary care of women and children with HIV infection.* Boston: Jones & Bartlett.

Poloma, M. (1993). The effects of prayer on mental well-being. *Second Opinion, 18*(3), 37-51.

Quinn, J. (1989). Therapeutic touch as energy exchange: Replication and extension. *Nursing Science Quarterly, 2*(2), 79-87.

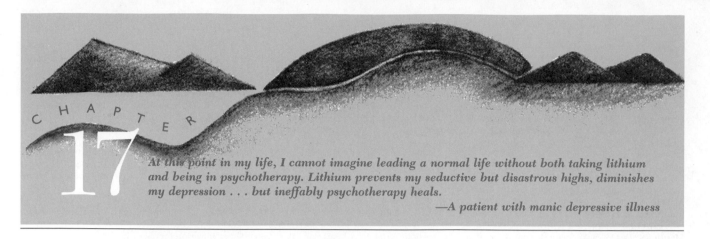

At this point in my life, I cannot imagine leading a normal life without both taking lithium and being in psychotherapy. Lithium prevents my seductive but disastrous highs, diminishes my depression . . . but ineffably psychotherapy heals.

—A patient with manic depressive illness

Psychotropic Drugs

Learning Objectives

After studying this chapter, you should be able to:

1. State the mechanism of action of each family of psychotherapeutic drugs.
2. State the principal uses of each family of psychotherapeutic drugs.
3. State the major adverse effects, side effects, and related nursing interventions of each family of psychotherapeutic drugs.
4. State the major drug interactions of each family of psychotherapeutic drugs.
5. Apply the nursing process to a patient requiring psychotherapeutic drugs.
6. Identify the spiritual implications of taking psychotherapeutic drugs.

Key Terminology

Acute dystonia
Agranulocytosis
Akathisia
Antianxiety agents
Anxiolytics
Antidepressants
Antipsychotic agents
Atypical agents
Benzodiazepines
Butyrophenones
Carbamazepine

Chlorpromazine
Clozapine
Extrapyramidal reactions
Haloperidol
High potency
Lithium
Low potency
Monoamine hypothesis of depression
Monoamine oxidase inhibitors
Negative symptoms

Neuroleptic malignant syndrome
Neuroleptics
Olanzapine
Parkinsonism
Phenothiazines
Positive symptoms
Psychotherapeutic drugs
Quetiapine fumarate
Receptors
Reuptake

Selective serotonin reuptake inhibitors
Serotonin syndrome
Synaptic transmission
Tardive dyskinesia
Transmitter
Tricyclic antidepressants
Valproic acid
Ziprasidone

Our topic for this chapter is **psychotherapeutic drugs**—drugs used to treat psychiatric disorders. This group of drugs has four major divisions: (1) antipsychotic agents (used primarily for schizophrenia), (2) antidepressants, (3) lithium and other drugs for bipolar disorder (manic-depressive illness), and (4) anxiolytics (used to relieve anxiety). None of the psychotherapeutic agents is curative; these drugs offer only symptomatic relief. Furthermore, no one drug represents ideal therapy by itself; rather, all of these agents are best used in conjunction with some form of psychotherapy. Unfortunately, not all patients receive ideal treatment; many are left to rely on drug therapy alone. Conversely,

This chapter, including Figures 17–1 and 17–2 and Tables 17–1 through 17–12, is adapted from Chapters 11 and 24 through 27 of Lehne, R. A. (1994). *Pharmacology for nursing care* (2nd ed.). Philadelphia: W. B. Saunders.

patients who could benefit from drug therapy (along with psychotherapy) may fail to receive the medication that they need—thus needlessly prolonging discomfort (Abramowicz, 1994).

Nursing's role is critical in the use of psychopharmacology. Nurses are frequently in a position to assist the patient in making informed choices regarding the place of medications in the whole scheme of therapy. Nurses' assessment skills provide invaluable information regarding the effectiveness of medications, the interactions of medications, and the side effects experienced by particular patients. Furthermore, nurses are frequently involved in direct administration of medications, teaching about the effects of safe use of medications, and following up medication effectiveness in the long term. Additionally, nurses are increasingly in positions of not only monitoring medications prescribed by others but also actually prescribing the medications themselves (Bailey, 1996). Thus, it is critical for nurses in psychiatry to understand the actions of medications.

The journey of Dr. Royce Opara illustrates the consequences of failing to prescribe psychotherapeutic drugs for the patients who need them.

 ### Dr. Royce Opara's Story

Dr. Royce Opara, a 37-year-old physician, was admitted to a private psychiatric hospital in early January 1979. He was a board-certified internist and was also a subspecialist in nephrology. He had been married three times and had three children, one with his current wife and two with his second wife.

Dr. Opara had a history of brief periods of anxiety and depression that had been treated on an outpatient basis. Although he had received treatment during periods of difficulty during his prior marriages, before this admission he had been suffering from anxious and depressive symptoms for approximately 2 years. Since 1977, he had been treated as an outpatient with a combination of individual psychotherapy and tricyclic antidepressant medication. He did not maintain the recommended dose of antidepressant medication, and his condition deteriorated as problems with his wife increased over conflict about her desire for another child. Because of strong cultural biases, he resisted the suggestion of family therapy. Hospitalization was recommended when he became suicidal and increased his consumption of cocaine from occasional to daily use.

On admission to the facility, the admitting psychiatrist found him verbally abusive, obstinate, and agitated. He was diagnosed as suffering from a narcissistic personality disorder and manic-depressive illness, depressed type. He was hospitalized for several months. He was often unpleasant, aggressive, and noncompliant. During this time, he continued to be treated with individual psychotherapy four times a week but with no psychotherapeutic medications. He lost a considerable amount of weight, experienced severe insomnia, and had marked psychomotor agitation. His agitation, manifested by incessant pacing, was so extreme that his feet became swollen and blistered, requiring medical attention. His progress was minimal, forcing the family to become increasingly concerned.

Finally, a brother, who was a cardiologist, convinced the family to seek a second opinion from a psychiatrist who lived in a nearby metropolitan area. In response to his inquiry, the clinical staff at the hospital held a clinical case conference to review the patient's treatment. They decided to make no major changes and specifically decided not to institute any medication regimen. Dr. Opara's condition did not improve. Later, in an unpublished diary, he described his hospitalization as a living hell. After several months, his relatives convinced him to leave the hospital. He was subsequently transferred to a private psychiatric facility in another state. His discharge diagnosis was manic-depressive illness, depressed type. At the new facility, he was diagnosed as having a psychotic depression, agitated type, and treatment with a combination of phenothiazines and tricyclic antidepressants was initiated. Within 3 weeks his condition had improved, and within 3 months, he was discharged (with a final diagnosis of manic-depressive illness, depressed type with psychotic features). He resumed his professional work, and as of 1990, he continued to function well without rehospitalization.

He subsequently initiated a lawsuit against the first facility, claiming that as a result of negligence in not administering drug treatment—to which he had responded favorably in the past—he lost his standing in the professional community and custody of his children. He was awarded financial damages by an arbitration panel in an amount agreed on by both parties, thus averting a jury trial.

Although Dr. Opara may have received some benefit from treatment with antidepressant medications in past episodes of illness, for the first 7 months of hospitalization on this admission, pharmacological agents were withheld in favor of a treatment approach based on psychodynamic formulations of the etiology of anxiety and depression. Thus, the influence of possible endogenous genetic and biological dysfunction was ignored.

MECHANISMS BY WHICH CENTRAL NERVOUS SYSTEM DRUGS ACT

All of the psychopharmacological drugs produce their therapeutic effects by altering communication among neurons within the central nervous system (CNS). In all cases, this is accomplished by influencing synaptic transmission (rather than by axonal conduction). Accordingly, in order to understand how these drugs act, we need to know the ways in which they can alter communication between neurons at synapses. To establish this understanding, we first review the steps in **synaptic transmission,** after which we discuss the ways in which drugs can affect each step (Lehne, 1994c).

Steps in Synaptic Transmission

Synaptic transmission takes place in five basic steps. These are depicted in Figure 17–1 and discussed in this section.

Step 1: Synthesis

For synaptic transmission to take place, molecules of **transmitter** must be present within the nerve terminal. Hence, we can look on synthesis of transmitter as being the first step in transmission.

Step 2: Storage

Once the transmitter is synthesized, it must be stored until the time of its release. Storage of transmitter molecules takes place within vesicles, which are tiny packets present in the axon terminal. Each nerve terminal contains a large number of transmitter-filled vesicles.

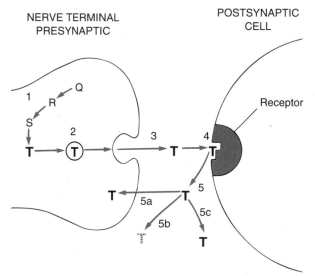

Figure 17–1
Steps in synaptic transmission. *Step 1,* Synthesis of transmitter (T) from precursor molecules (Q, R, S). *Step 2,* Storage of transmitter in vesicles. *Step 3,* Release of transmitter. In response to an action potential, vesicles fuse with the terminal membrane and discharge their contents into the synaptic gap. *Step 4,* Action at receptor. Transmitter binds (reversibly) to its receptor on the postsynaptic neuron, causing a response in that cell. *Step 5,* Termination of transmission. Transmitter dissociates from its receptor and is then removed from the synaptic gap by (a) reuptake into the presynaptic neuron, (b) enzymatic degradation, or (c) diffusion away from the synaptic gap.

Step 3: Release

Release of transmitter is triggered by the arrival of an action potential at the axon terminal. The action potential initiates a process in which vesicles undergo fusion with the terminal membrane, causing release of vesicular contents into the synaptic gap. With each action potential, only a small fraction of all vesicles present in the nerve terminal are caused to discharge their contents.

Step 4: Receptor Binding

After their release, transmitter molecules diffuse across the synaptic gap and then undergo reversible binding to receptors on the postsynaptic neuron. This binding initiates a series of events that result in either excitation or inhibition of the postsynaptic neuron. Thus, binding of transmitter can either increase or decrease the chances that the postsynaptic neuron will fire an action potential of its own.

Step 5: Termination

Transmission is terminated by dissociation of transmitter from its receptors, followed by removal of free transmitter from the synaptic gap. Transmitter can be cleared from the synaptic gap by three processes:

1. **Reuptake** into the presynaptic neuron
2. Enzymatic degradation
3. Diffusion

In those synapses in which transmission is terminated by reuptake, axon terminals contain "pumps" for the active transport of transmitter molecules back into the neuron (see Figure 17–1, step 5a). After reuptake, molecules of transmitter may be degraded, or they may be repackaged in vesicles for reuse. In synapses in which transmitter is cleared by enzymatic degradation (see Figure 17–1, step 5b), the synapse contains large quantities of transmitter-inactivating enzymes. Although simple diffusion away from the synaptic gap (see Figure 17–1, step 5c) is a potential means of terminating transmitter action, this process is slow and generally of little significance.

Effects of Drugs on Synaptic Transmission

In this section, we look at the specific ways in which drugs can alter the steps of synaptic transmission. By way of encouragement, although this information may appear complex, it is not. In fact, most of it is self-evident.

Transmitter Synthesis

Drugs can either increase or decrease transmitter synthesis. A drug that increases synthesis increases the amount of transmitter stored in presynaptic vesicles. As a result, when an action potential reaches the axon terminal, more transmitter is released; therefore, more transmitter is available to **receptors** on the postsynaptic cell, thus intensifying transmission at that site. Conversely, a drug that decreases transmitter synthesis causes the transmitter content of vesicles to decline, resulting in reduced transmitter release and suppression of synaptic transmission.

Transmitter Storage

Drugs that interfere with transmitter storage reduce synaptic transmission. This occurs because disruption of storage depletes vesicles of their transmitter content, thus decreasing the amount of transmitter available for release.

Transmitter Release

Drugs can have one of two effects on transmitter release: they can promote release or they can inhibit release. Drugs that promote release intensify transmission; conversely, drugs that inhibit release suppress transmission.

Receptor Binding

Many neuropharmacological drugs act directly at receptors. Drugs in this category are known to act one of three ways:

1. Bind to receptors and cause receptor activation
2. Bind to receptors and prevent receptor activation by the natural transmitter at that site (or by other drugs that bind to that receptor)
3. Bind to the receptors and enhance the actions of the natural transmitter at that site

Drugs that directly activate receptors are called agonists. Conversely, drugs that prevent receptor activation are called antagonists. Receptor agonists and antagonists constitute the largest and most important groups of neuropharmacological drugs.

Termination of Transmitter Action

Drugs can interfere with the termination of transmitter action by two mechanisms: blockade of transmitter reuptake or inhibition of transmitter degradation. Drugs that act by either mechanism cause the concentration of transmitter in the synaptic gap to rise, thus intensifying transmission.

What do you think? With what we know about the biological basis for psychiatric illnesses, could what happened to Dr. Opara happen today?

► Check Your Reading
1. How are neurotransmitters stored in the nerve terminal?
2. What are the two possible outcomes when a transmitter binds to its receptor on a postsynaptic neuron?
3. What is the general term for a drug that causes receptor activation when it binds to a receptor? What is the term for a drug that prevents receptor activation as a result of receptor binding?
4. What is the effect of a drug that blocks transmitter reuptake?

ANTIPSYCHOTIC AGENTS

The **antipsychotic agents** are a chemically diverse group of compounds that are used to treat a broad spectrum of psychotic disorders. Specific indications include schizophrenia, delusional disorders, acute mania, depressive psychoses, and drug-induced psychoses.

Antipsychotic agents catalyzed revolutionary change in the management of psychotic illnesses when they were introduced in the early 1950s. Before these drugs became available, persistent psychoses were largely untreatable, and patients were fated to a life of institutionalization. With the advent of antipsychotic medications, many patients with schizophrenia and other severe psychiatric disorders have been able to leave psychiatric hospitals and return to the community. Others have been spared hospitalization entirely. For those who must remain institutionalized, antipsychotic drugs have at least been able to reduce suffering.

The antipsychotic drugs fall into two major groups: traditional antipsychotics and atypical antipsychotics. All of the traditional agents block receptors for dopamine in the CNS, and they all can cause serious movement disorders, referred to as extrapyramidal reactions (Blair & Dounce, 1993). Although the **atypical agents** also block dopamine receptors, the pattern of blockade differs from that of the traditional agents. The atypical agents have a greater selectivity for specific dopamine receptors. As a result, the risk of extrapyramidal reactions with the atypical agents is low (Boxes 17–1 and 17–2).

Traditional Antipsychotic Agents

In this section, we discuss pharmacological properties shared by all of the traditional agents. Much of our attention focuses on adverse effects. Of these, the extrapyramidal reactions are of particular concern. Because of these neurological side effects caused by dopamine blockade, the traditional antipsychotics are known alternatively as **neuroleptics.** The word *neuroleptic,* which is derived from Greek, literally means "clasp the neuron."

B o x 1 7 – 1 ■ ■ ■ ■ ■
Antipsychotic Drugs

It is important for nurses to understand the difference between typical and atypical antipsychotics.

Box 17-2 ■ ■ ■ ■ ■
Atypical Antipsychotic Medications

- Effectively treat positive and negative symptoms
- Work on multiple receptor sites
- Lower risk of tardive dyskinesia and extrapyramidal symptoms
- Have lower prolocatin levels than traditional antipsychotic medications
- May increase compliance due to fewer side effects
- Enhance quality of life

Classification

The traditional antipsychotics can be classified according to potency or chemical structure. From a clinical viewpoint, classification by potency is more informative.

POTENCY

Traditional antipsychotic agents can be classified as **low potency,** medium potency, or **high potency** (Table 17–1). The low-potency drugs, represented by chlorpromazine (Thorazine), and the high-potency drugs, represented by haloperidol (Haldol), are of particular interest.

Although the neuroleptics differ from one another in potency, all of these drugs are essentially equal in their ability to relieve symptoms of psychoses. In pharmacology, the term *potency* refers only to the size of the dose needed to elicit a given response; potency implies nothing about the maximal effect that a drug can produce. Hence, when we say that haloperidol has a higher potency than chlorpromazine, we mean only that the dose of haloperidol required to relieve psychotic symptoms is smaller than the required dose of chlorpromazine; we do not mean that haloperidol can produce greater effects. When administered in therapeutically equivalent doses, both drugs elicit an equivalent antipsychotic response.

If the low-potency and high-potency neuroleptics possess the same therapeutic ability, why should we distinguish between them? The answer is that although these agents produce similar antipsychotic effects, they differ significantly in their side effects. Hence, by knowing the potency category to which a particular neuroleptic belongs, we can better predict that drug's undesired effects. This knowledge is useful in drug selection and patient care and education.

CHEMICAL STRUCTURE

The traditional antipsychotic agents can be placed into five major groups based on their chemical structures (Table 17–2). One of these groups, the phenothiazines, has three subdivisions. Drugs in all groups are equivalent with respect to antipsychotic actions.

Two chemical categories—the **phenothiazines** and the **butyrophenones**—deserve special attention. The phenothiazines were the first of the modern antipsychotic agents. **Chlorpromazine,** the prototype of the low-potency neuroleptics, is a member of the phenothiazine family. The butyrophenones stand out because they are the family to which haloperidol belongs. **Haloperidol** is the prototype of the high-potency antipsychotics.

Mechanism of Action

The traditional antipsychotic drugs block a variety of receptors within and outside the CNS. To varying degrees, these drugs produce blockade at receptors for dopamine, acetylcholine, histamine, and norepinephrine. There is little question that blockade at these receptors is responsible for the major adverse effects of the antipsychotics. However, because the etiology of psychotic illness is unknown, the relationship of receptor blockade to therapeutic effects can only be guessed. One theory suggests that neuroleptics suppress symptoms of psychosis by blocking specific subtypes of dopamine receptors in the mesolimbic and mesocortical areas of the brain, regions thought to be involved in the expression of positive and negative symptoms, respectively. In support of this theory is the observation that all of the traditional antipsychotics produce dopamine receptor blockade.

Therapeutic Uses

SCHIZOPHRENIA

Schizophrenia and schizoaffective disorder are the most common indications for antipsychotic drugs. These agents effectively ameliorate symptoms during acute psychotic episodes, and, when taken consistently, can greatly decrease the risk of relapse. Initial effects are seen in 1 to 7 days, but full effects develop gradually over 6 to 8 weeks. So-called **positive symptoms** (e.g., agitation, delusions, hallucinations) generally respond better than do the **negative symptoms** (e.g., social withdrawal, blunted affect, motor retardation). Although individual patients may respond better to one drug than to another, all of the traditional antipsychotic agents are equally effective. Consequently, selection among these drugs is based primarily on their side-effect profiles, rather than on their therapeutic effects. Because the high-potency agents generally cause fewer side effects than do the low-potency agents, many clinicians select a high-potency agent for initial treatment.

Please note that antipsychotic drugs do not alter the underlying pathology of schizophrenia. Treatment, therefore, is not curative—it offers only symptomatic relief.

BIPOLAR DISORDER (MANIC-DEPRESSIVE ILLNESS)

Most patients with bipolar disorder are managed with either lithium (for years, the drug of choice) or valproic acid. Neuroleptics, such as clozapine, may be used in acute cases (in combination with lithium or valproic acid) to help manage patients who are going through a severe manic phase or who are resistant to standard treatment (Mahmood, Devlin, & Silverson, 1998). Drugs for bipolar disorder are discussed later in the chapter.

TABLE 17-1 **Traditional Antipsychotic Drugs: Relative Potency and Major Side Effects**

		EQUIVALENT ORAL DOSE (mg)*	INCIDENCE† OF MAJOR SIDE EFFECTS			
POTENCY CLASS	DRUG		Sedation	Orthostatic Hypotension	Anticholinergic Effects	Extrapyramidal Effects
Low	Chlorpromazine (Thorazine)	100	High	High	Medium	Low
	Thioridazine (Mellaril)	100	High	High	High	Low
	Mesoridazine (Serentil)	50	High	Medium	Medium	Low
	Acetophenazine (Tindal‡)	20	Medium	Low	Low	Medium
	Loxapine (Loxitane)	10	Medium	Medium	Medium	High
	Molindone (Moban)	10	Medium	Low	Medium	Medium
Medium	Perphenazine (Trilafon)	8	Low	Low	Low	High
	Trifluoperazine (Stelazine)	5	Low	Low	Low	High
	Thiothixene (Navane‡)	4	Low	Low	Low	High
	Fluphenazine (Prolixin)	2	Low	Low	Low	High
High	Haloperidol (Haldol)	12	Low	Low	Low	High
	Pimozide (Orap)	1	Low	Low	Low	High

*Doses listed are the therapeutic equivalent of 100 mg of oral chlorpromazine.
†Incidence refers to early extrapyramidal reactions (acute dystonia, parkinsonism, akathisia). Incidence of late reactions (tardive dyskinesia) is the same for all of these drugs.
‡Discontinued.

TABLE 17-2 Traditional Antipsychotic Drugs: Chemical Classification, Routes, and Dosages

CHEMICAL CLASS AND GENERIC NAME	TRADE NAME	ROUTE	DOSAGE RANGE (mg/d)
Phenothiazine: Aliphatic			
Chlorpromazine HCl	Thorazine, Ormazine	PO, IM, R, L	30–500
Triflupromazine HCl	Vesprin	IM	30–90
Phenothiazine: Piperidine			
Mesoridazine besylate	Serentil	PO, IM, L	30–400
Thioridazine	Mellaril	PO, L	150–800
Phenothiazine: Piperazine			
Acetophenazine	Tindal	PO	60–120
Fluphenazine HCl	Prolixin, Permitil	PO, IM, L, D (q 2–4 wk)	2–40
Perphenazine	Trilafon	PO, IM, L	16–64
Trifluoperazine HCl	Stelazine	PO, IM, L	2–4
Thioxanthene			
Thiothixene	Navane	PO, IM, L	5–60
Butyrophenone			
Haloperidol	Haldol	PO, IM, L, D (q 4 wk)	2–100
Dihydroindolone			
Molindone HCl	Moban	PO, L	10–225
Dibenzoxazepine			
Loxapine succinate	Loxitane	PO, IM, L	30–250

D, depot-longacting injection; IM, intramuscular; L, liquid; PO, oral; R, rectal (suppository).

TOURETTE'S SYNDROME

This rare, inherited disorder is characterized by severe motor tics, barking cries, grunts, and outbursts of obscene language, all of which are spontaneous and beyond the control of the patient. At least two antipsychotic drugs, haloperidol and pimozide, can help to relieve symptoms.

OTHER USES

Neuroleptics can be used to treat delusional disorders and dementia and other *organic mental syndromes,* which are psychiatric syndromes resulting from organic causes such as infection, metabolic disorders, poisoning, and structural injury to the brain. In addition, these agents can partially ameliorate symptoms of Huntington's disease.

Adverse Effects

Although antipsychotic agents produce a variety of undesired effects, these drugs are generally safe; death by overdose is rare. Of the many side effects that these drugs can produce, the most troubling are the extrapyramidal reactions—especially **tardive dyskinesia.** It is important to note that the adverse effect profile of the low-potency agents differs from that of the high-potency agents. Specifically, the low-potency agents are associated with a higher incidence of sedation, hypotension, and anticholinergic effects, whereas the high-potency agents are associated with a higher incidence of early extrapyramidal reactions (see Table 17-1).

Extrapyramidal reactions are movement disorders resulting from effects of antipsychotic drugs on the extrapyramidal motor system. The extrapyramidal system is the same neuronal network that, when it malfunctions, is responsible for the movement disorders of Parkinson's disease.

Four types of extrapyramidal reactions occur. They differ from one another with respect to time of onset and management. Three of these reactions—**acute dystonia, parkinsonism,** and **akathisia**—occur early in therapy and can be managed with a variety of drugs. The fourth reaction—tardive dyskinesia—occurs late in therapy and has no satisfactory treatment. Characteristics and management of the four extrapyramidal reactions are summarized in Table 17-3.

The early reactions occur less frequently with low-potency agents (e.g., chlorpromazine) than with high-potency agents (e.g., haloperidol). In contrast, the risk of tardive dyskinesia is equal with all antipsychotics.

ACUTE DYSTONIA

Acute dystonia develops within the first few days of therapy—frequently, only hours after the first dose. The reaction can be both disturbing and dangerous. Typically, the patient develops severe spasm of the muscles of the tongue, face, neck, or back. *Oculogyric crisis* (involuntary upward deviation of the eyes) and *opisthotonos* (tetanic spasm of the back muscles causing the trunk to arch forward while the head and lower limbs are thrust backward) may also occur. Severe cramping can cause joint dislocation. Laryngeal dystonia can impair respiration. The cause of acute dystonia is unknown.

This acute and intense dystonia (neurotransmitter involvement is explained in Box 17-3) constitutes a crisis that requires rapid intervention—it is painful and traumatic to the patient. Initial treatment consists of anticholinergic medication (e.g., benztropine and diphenhydramine) administered intramuscularly (IM) or intravenously (IV). As a rule, symptoms resolve within 5 minutes of IV administration and within 15 to 20 minutes of IM administration.

It is important to differentiate between acute dystonia and psychotic hysteria. Misdiagnosis of acute dystonia as hysteria could result in escalation of antipsychotic dosage, thus causing the acute dystonia to become even worse.

PARKINSONISM

Antipsychotic-induced parkinsonism is characterized by bradykinesia, mask-like facies, drooling, tremor, rigidity, shuffling gait, *cogwheeling* (ratchet-like movements), and stooped posture. Symptoms usually develop several weeks after starting antipsychotic medications and are indistinguishable from those of idiopathic Parkinson's disease.

Neuroleptics cause parkinsonism by blocking dopamine receptors in the striatum. Because idiopathic Parkinson's disease is also due to reduced activation of striatal dopamine receptors, it is no wonder that Parkinson's disease and neuroleptic-induced parkinsonism share the same symptoms.

Neuroleptic-induced parkinsonism is treated with some (but not all) of the drugs used to treat Parkinson's disease. Specifically, centrally acting anticholinergic drugs (e.g., benztropine mesylate [Cogentin], diphenhydramine HCl [Benadryl], and amantadine HCl [Symmetrel]) may be employed. Levodopa, however, should be avoided, because this drug promotes activation of dopamine receptors and might therefore counteract the beneficial effects of antipsychotic treatment.

Use of antiparkinsonian drugs does not continue indefinitely. Antipsychotic-induced parkinsonism tends to resolve spontaneously, usually within a few months after its onset. Hence, antiparkinsonian drugs should be withdrawn by tapering after a few months to determine if they are still required.

AKATHISIA

Akathisia is characterized by pacing and squirming brought on by an uncontrollable need to be in motion. This profound sense of restlessness can be disturbing. The syndrome may occur almost immediately after a single dose and may persist for weeks after medications have been discontinued. The cause is unknown. Like other early extrapyramidal reactions, akathisia occurs most frequently with high-potency antipsychotics.

Three types of drugs have been used to diminish symptoms: (1) anticholinergic agents, (2) β-adrenergic blockers, and (3) **benzodiazepines.** Although drugs can be helpful, reducing antipsychotic dosage or switching to a low-potency agent may be more effective.

It is important to differentiate akathisia from worsening of psychotic symptoms. If akathisia were to be confused with anxiety or psychotic agitation, it is likely that antipsychotic dosage would be increased, thus making akathisia more intense, and this increased dosage may cause the patient to behave in a way that results in the

Box 17–3 ◼ ◼ ◼ ◼ ◼
What Happens in Dystonic Reactions

1. Dopamine and acetylcholine exist in a balance to enhance smooth muscle contraction.
2. When too much dopamine is blocked, it allows for increased amounts of acetylcholine, thereby disrupting the balance.
3. When this happens, muscles become rigid, as in dystonic reactions.
4. To restore the balance, an anticholinergic agent is given.

TABLE 17–3 Extrapyramidal Reactions to Antipsychotic Drugs

TYPE OF REACTION	TIME OF ONSET	FEATURES	MANAGEMENT
Early Reactions			
Acute dystonia	1–5 d	Spasm of muscles of tongue, face, neck, eyes (ocologyric crisis) and back (opisthotonus)	Anticholinergic drugs (e.g., benzotropine) IM or IV
Parkinsonism	5–30 d	Bradykinesia, mask-like facies, tremor, rigidity, shuffling gait, drooling, cogwheeling, stooped posture	Anticholinergics (e.g., benzotropine, diphenhydramine), amantadine, or both
Akathisia	5–60 d	Compulsive, restless movement; symptoms of anxiety, agitation; subjective reports from patients, "Feels like I'm going to jump out of my skin."	Reduce dosage or switch to a low-potency antipsychotic. Anticholinergic drugs, beta-blockers, and benzodiazepines may help.
Late Reaction			
Tardive dyskinesia	Months to years	Orofacial dyskinesias, choreoathetoid movements	Best approach is prevention; no reliable treatment. Trial with clozapine may help.

IM, Intramuscular; IV, intravenous.

use of seclusion or restraints (Box 17–4). Additionally, akathisia has been associated with suicide attempts.

TARDIVE DYSKINESIA

Tardive dyskinesia develops in 20% to 40% of patients during long-term therapy and is the most troubling of the extrapyramidal reactions. The risk increases with longer treatment and higher dosage. For many patients, symptoms are irreversible (Kane, Woerner, Pollack, Safferman, & Lieberman, 1993).

Tardive dyskinesia is characterized by involuntary *choreoathetoid* (twisting, writhing, worm-like) movements of the tongue, face, and extremities. Patients may also present with lip-smacking movements, and their tongues may flick out in a fly-catching motion. One of the earliest manifestations is the appearance of slow, worm-like movements of the tongue. Involuntary movements that involve the tongue and mouth can interfere with chewing, swallowing, and speaking. Eating difficulties can result in malnutrition and weight loss. There is also an increased risk for choking. Over time, involuntary movements of the limbs, toes, fingers, and trunk can lead to an increased potential for falls, especially in the geriatric population. For some patients, symptoms decline after a dosage reduction or drug withdrawal; for others, tardive dyskinesia is irreversible.

The cause of tardive dyskinesia is complex and is not completely understood. One theory suggests that symptoms result from excessive activation of dopamine receptors. It is postulated that, in response to chronic receptor blockade, dopamine receptors of the extrapyramidal

system undergo a functional change such that their sensitivity to activation is increased. Stimulation of these "supersensitive" receptors produces an imbalance in favor of dopamine and thus produces abnormal movement. In support of this theory is the observation that symptoms of tardive dyskinesia can be reduced (temporarily) by increasing antipsychotic drug dosage, which causes greater receptor blockade. Because symptoms eventually return even though antipsychotic dosage is kept at an elevated level, dosage elevation cannot be used to manage tardive dyskinesia.

Tardive dyskinesia has no reliable means of treatment; hence, prevention is the best approach. Antipsychotic drugs should be used in the lowest effective dosage for the shortest time required. After 12 months, the need for continued therapy should be assessed. If drug use must continue, a neurological evaluation should be done at least every 3 to 6 months to detect early signs of tardive dyskinesia. The Abnormal Involuntary Movement Scale (AIMS) is commonly used to evaluate involuntary movements of patients who take neuroleptic medications (Box 17–5). For patients with chronic schizophrenia, dosage should be tapered periodically to determine the need for continued treatment.

If signs of tardive dyskinesia appear but the patient requires continued antipsychotic therapy, what should be done? Unfortunately, this question has no easy answer. If drug use continues, tardive dyskinesia may become progressively worse; thus, discontinuation would seem desirable. If treatment ceases, however, relapse of psychosis may occur; hence, discontinuation may well be harmful. In the face of this dilemma, the clinician should discuss the options with the patient and a family member so that the patient can make an informed decision regarding continued treatment. It has been noted that symptoms of tardive dyskinesia have abated in some patients after substitution of an atypical antipsychotic agent (e.g., clozapine) for a traditional antipsychotic agent (Shriqui, 1998). Accordingly, a trial with an atypical agent may be a reasonable choice for the patient who cannot simply discontinue antipsychotic treatment (Kane, 1998). Box 17–6 lists nursing insights about tardive dyskinesia.

NEUROLEPTIC MALIGNANT SYNDROME

Neuroleptic malignant syndrome (NMS) is an idiosyncratic hypersensitivity to antipsychotics that is believed to affect the thermoregulatory mechanism of the body. It is a rare but serious reaction that carries a 4% risk of mortality (decreased from 20% in the late 1980s because of early recognition and treatment). Primary symptoms are "lead pipe" rigidity; fever (temperature may exceed 41°C); sweating; and autonomic instability, manifested as dysrhythmia and fluctuations in blood pressure (BP). Frequent laboratory findings include an elevated *creatine kinase,* which is a muscle enzyme, and an elevation in the white blood cell count (WBC). The patient's level of consciousness may rise and fall, he or she may appear confused or mute, and he or she may develop seizures or go into a coma. Death can result from respiratory failure, cardiovascular collapse, dysrhythmias, and other causes. NMS is more likely to occur with high-potency agents than with low-potency agents

---

Box 17–4 ■ ■ ■ ■ ■
Nursing Thoughts About Extrapyramidal Symptoms

- Dystonic reactions are distressing to patients and lead to noncompliance.
- Dystonic reactions involving the laryngeal muscles produce laryngospasm, which is life-threatening.
- Patients with drug-induced parkinsonism are prone to injury by falls and food aspiration due to swallowing difficulties.
- Patients with bradykinesia due to drug-induced parkinsonism may be misdiagnosed as being depressed and receive another medication, which may cause additional side effects.
- Akathisia is experienced as the most discomforting side effect from antipsychotic medications; this discomfort can lead to noncompliance, which is associated with suicide attempts.
- Drug-induced akathisia may precipitate violent behavior in patients and may appear to worsen patient's psychosis. This may lead to increased dosage or use of seclusion and restraint.
- Anticholinergic drugs can produce euphoria and have an abuse potential in susceptible individuals.

Box 17–5 ■ ■ ■ ■ ■
Abnormal Involuntary Movement Scale

Patient identification _____ Date _____

Rated by _____

Either before or after completing the examination procedure, observe the patient unobtrusively at rest (e.g., in waiting room).

The chair to be used in this examination should be a hard, firm one without arms.

After observing the patient, he/she may be rated on a scale of 0 (none), 1 (minimal), 2 (mild), 3 (moderate), and 4 (severe) according to the severity of symptoms.

Ask the patient whether there is anything in his/her mouth (i.e., gum, candy, etc) and if there is to remove it.

Ask patient about the *current* condition of his/her teeth. Ask patient if he/she wears dentures. Do teeth or dentures bother patient *now?*

Ask patient whether he/she notices any movement in mouth, face, hands or feet. If yes, ask patient to describe and to what extent they *currently* bother patient or interfere with his/her activities.

| 0 | 1 | 2 | 3 | 4 | Have patient sit in chair with hands on knees, legs slightly apart, and feet flat on floor. (Look at entire body for movements while in this position.) |

| 0 | 1 | 2 | 3 | 4 | Ask patient to sit with hands hanging unsupported. If male, between legs, if female and wearing a dress, hanging over knees. (Observe hands and other body areas.) |

| 0 | 1 | 2 | 3 | 4 | Ask patient to open mouth. (Observe tongue at rest within mouth.) Do this twice. |

| 0 | 1 | 2 | 3 | 4 | Ask patient to protrude tongue. (Observe abnormalities of tongue movement.) Do this twice. |

| 0 | 1 | 2 | 3 | 4 | Ask patient to tap thumb with each finger as rapidly as possible for 10–15 seconds; separately with right hand, then with left hand. (Observe facial and leg movements.) |

| 0 | 1 | 2 | 3 | 4 | Flex and extend patient's left and right arms. (One at a time.) |

| 0 | 1 | 2 | 3 | 4 | Ask patient to stand up. (Observe in profile. Observe all body areas again, hips included.) |

| 0 | 1 | 2 | 3 | 4 | Ask patient to extend both arms outstretched in front with palms down. (Observe trunk, legs, and mouth.)* |

| 0 | 1 | 2 | 3 | 4 | Have patient walk a few paces, turn, and walk back to chair. (Observe hands and gait.) Do this twice.* |

*Activated movements.

From National Institute of Mental Health. (1976). Abnormal involuntary movement scale. In Guci, W. (Ed.), *The ECDEU assessment manual* (pp. 534-537). Rockville, MD: U.S. Department of Health, Education and Welfare.

(Addonizio, 1991; Byrd, 1993; Caroff & Mann, 1991; Keck, Pope, Cohen, & McElroy, 1991).

Treatment consists of supportive measures, drug therapy, and immediate withdrawal of antipsychotic medication. Hyperthermia should be controlled with antipyretics and cooling blankets. Hydration should be maintained with IV fluids. Two drugs—dantrolene and bromocriptine—are helpful. *Dantrolene,* which is a direct-acting muscle relaxant, reduces rigidity and hyperthermia. *Bromocriptine,* which is a dopamine receptor agonist, helps to relieve CNS toxicity.

Resumption of antipsychotic therapy after an episode of NMS carries a significant risk that NMS will reoccur. Because NMS has a high rate of morbidity and mortality, the decision to resume treatment must be made with great care. If continued treatment with an antipsychotic is clearly required, the lowest effective dosage should be employed, and high-potency agents should be avoided.

ANTICHOLINERGIC EFFECTS

Antipsychotic drugs produce varying degrees of muscarinic cholinergic blockade (see Table 17–1). By blocking muscarinic receptors, these drugs can elicit a full spectrum of anticholinergic responses (e.g., dry mouth,

Box 17-6 ■ ■ ■ ■ ■
Nursing Insights About Tardive Dyskinesia

- Persistent use of traditional antipsychotics may result in TD in 20% to 60% of patients at a rate of 4% to 5% of exposure to traditional antipsychotics.
- TD can lead to life-threatening respiratory and GI complications.
- TD may decrease life expectancy.

GI, gastrointestinal; TD, tardive dyskinesia.

blurred vision, photophobia, urinary hesitancy, constipation, and tachycardia). Patients should be informed about these responses and taught how to minimize danger and discomfort. As indicated in Table 17-1, anticholinergic effects are more likely with low-potency agents than with high-potency agents.

ORTHOSTATIC HYPOTENSION
Antipsychotic drugs promote orthostatic hypotension by blocking α-adrenergic receptors on blood vessels. α-Adrenergic blockade prevents compensatory vasoconstriction when the patient stands; thus, BP falls. Patients should be informed about signs of hypotension (e.g., lightheadedness and dizziness) and be advised to sit or lie down if these signs occur. In addition, patients should be informed that hypotension can be minimized by moving slowly when standing up. With hospitalized patients, BP and pulses should be checked before and 1 hour after drug administration. Measurements should be made while the patient is lying down and again after he or she has been sitting or standing for 1 to 2 minutes. If BP is low and pulse rate is high, the drug should be withheld and the physician consulted. Hypotension is more likely with low-potency antipsychotics than with high-potency drugs (see Table 17-1). Tolerance to hypotension develops in 2 to 3 months.

SEDATION
Sedation is common early in treatment but often subsides within 1 week of beginning treatment. Neuroleptic-induced sedation is thought to result from blockade of histamine receptors in the CNS. Daytime sedation can be minimized by administering the entire daily dose at bedtime. Patients should be warned against participation in hazardous activities until sedative effects diminish.

SEIZURES
Antipsychotic drugs can reduce seizure threshold, thus increasing the risk of seizure activity. The risk of seizures is greatest in patients with epilepsy and other seizure disorders. These patients should be monitored. If loss of seizure control occurs, the dosage of their antipsychotic medication may need to be decreased or the dosage of their antiseizure medication may need to be increased.

SEXUAL DYSFUNCTION
Antipsychotics can cause sexual dysfunction in women and men. In women, these drugs can suppress libido

and impair the ability to achieve orgasm. Additional research is ongoing to determine what other gender-specific drug reactions women experience (Kulkarni, 1997). In men, neuroleptics can suppress libido and cause erectile and ejaculatory dysfunction; the incidence of these effects is 25% to 60%.

Drug-induced sexual dysfunction can make treatment unacceptable to sexually active patients, thus leading to poor compliance. A reduction in dosage or switching to a high-potency antipsychotic may reduce effects on sexual function. Patients should be counseled about possible sexual dysfunction and encouraged to report problems.

DERMATOLOGIC EFFECTS
Drugs in the phenothiazine class can sensitize the skin to ultraviolet light, thus increasing the risk of severe sunburn. Patients should be warned against excessive exposure to sunlight and advised to apply a sunscreen or wear protective clothing. Phenothiazines can also produce pigmentary deposits in the skin, cornea, and lens of the eye.

Handling antipsychotics can cause contact dermatitis in patients and health care personnel. Dermatitis can be prevented by avoiding direct contact with these drugs. Health care personnel can wear latex gloves; patients can do the same or use tweezers to take the medication.

NEUROENDOCRINE EFFECTS
Antipsychotics increase levels of circulating prolactin by blocking the inhibitory action of dopamine on prolactin release. Elevation of prolactin levels promotes *gynecomastia* (breast growth) and *galactorrhea* (excessive, sometimes spontaneous, milk flow) in up to 57% of women. Up to 97% experience menstrual irregularities. Gynecomastia and galactorrhea can also occur in men. Because prolactin can promote growth of prolactin-dependent carcinoma of the breast, neuroleptics should be avoided in patients with this form of cancer. Note that although antipsychotic drugs can promote the growth of cancers that already exist, there is no evidence that antipsychotic drugs actually cause cancer.

AGRANULOCYTOSIS
Agranulocytosis (a significant suppression in white cell count, which can be life threatening) is a rare but serious reaction. Among the traditional antipsychotics, the risk is highest with chlorpromazine and certain other phenothiazines. Because agranulocytosis severely compromises the ability to fight infection, WBCs should be obtained whenever signs of infection (e.g., fever, sore throat) appear. If agranulocytosis is diagnosed, the neuroleptic should be withdrawn. Agranulocytosis reverses when treatment is discontinued.

OPHTHALMOLOGIC EFFECTS
Antipsychotics can cause white, brown, or gray lenticular opacities that may result in loss of visual acuity and, in severe cases, blindness. Seen with use of chlorpromazine and thioridazine, these opacities can be detected by slit lamp examination. These drugs can also cause a type of retinopathy in which a brown discoloration of sight is due to an interaction with melanin.

PHYSICAL AND PSYCHOLOGICAL DEPENDENCE

Development of physical and psychological dependence is rare. Patients should be reassured that addiction and dependence are not likely to occur. Although physical dependence is minimal, abrupt withdrawal of antipsychotics can precipitate a mild abstinence syndrome. Symptoms result from chronic cholinergic blockade and include restlessness, insomnia, headache, gastric distress, and sweating. Abstinence syndrome can be avoided by withdrawing antipsychotic medication gradually.

Drug Interactions

Drugs with anticholinergic properties intensify anticholinergic responses to neuroleptics. Patients should be advised to avoid all drugs with anticholinergic actions, including antihistamines and specific over-the-counter sleeping aids.

CENTRAL NERVOUS SYSTEM DEPRESSANTS

Neuroleptics can intensify CNS depression caused by other drugs. Patients should be warned against using alcohol and all other drugs with CNS-depressant actions (e.g., antihistamines, opioids, and barbiturates).

LEVODOPA

Levodopa is a drug used to treat Parkinson's disease, and this drug may counteract the antipsychotic effects of neuroleptics. Conversely, neuroleptics may counteract the therapeutic effects of levodopa. These interactions occur because levodopa and neuroleptics have opposing effects on receptors for dopamine: levodopa activates these receptors, whereas neuroleptics cause blockade. Thus, levodopa is not used in patients treated with antipsychotic drugs.

Safety Profile

The traditional antipsychotic drugs are safe; death by overdose is extremely rare. With chlorpromazine, for example, the therapeutic index is about 200; that is, the lethal dose of this drug is 200 times greater than the therapeutic dose.

Overdosage produces hypotension, CNS depression, and extrapyramidal reactions. Extrapyramidal reactions can be treated with antiparkinsonian drugs. Hypotension can be treated with IV fluids plus an α-adrenergic agonist such as phenylephrine. There is no specific antidote for CNS depression. Excess drug should be removed from the stomach by gastric lavage. Emetics cannot be used because their effects are blocked by the antiemetic action of the neuroleptic.

Depot Preparations

The depot antipsychotics are long-acting, injectable preparations used to treat patients with persistent schizophrenia. The objective is to prevent relapse and maintain the highest possible level of functioning. The rate of relapse is lower with depot therapy than with oral therapy. Depot preparations are valuable not only for all patients who need long-term treatment but also for those who have difficulty with compliance. There is no evidence that depot preparations pose an increased risk of side effects, including NMS (Huttunen et al., 1996).

Three depot preparations are available: haloperidol decanoate (Haldol Decanoate), fluphenazine decanoate (Prolixin Decanoate), and fluphenazine enanthate (Prolixin Enanthate). After IM or subcutaneous injection, active drug (fluphenazine or haloperidol) is slowly absorbed into the blood. Because of this slow, steady absorption, plasma drug levels remain relatively constant between injections. The dosing interval is once every 2 to 4 weeks. Typical maintenance dosages are presented in Table 17–4.

Atypical Antipsychotic Agents

Atypical antipsychotic agents differ from traditional agents in that they cause few or no extrapyramidal symptoms (EPSs), including tardive dyskinesia. In fact, tardive dyskinesia may actually remit when patients are switched from a traditional antipsychotic drug to an atypical one (Gallbofer, 1998; Shriqui, 1998). This may be due to a greater selectivity for dopamine receptor subtypes and activity at other transmitter systems. Several others are being tested in clinical trials.

Clozapine

Clozapine (Clozaril), approved for use in the United States in 1989, is the first of the atypical antipsychotic drugs that is indicated for patients with schizophrenia who have not responded to traditional agents or who cannot tolerate their extrapyramidal effects. The drug's major adverse effect is agranulocytosis, and a few deaths have occurred despite weekly hematologic monitoring. Clozapine is considered the "gold standard" in the treatment of refractory schizophrenia (Chouinard et al., 1993; Jann, 1991; Jaretz, Flowers, & Millsap, 1992; Lehne, 1994a; Meltzer, Burnett, Bastani, & Ramirez, 1992). Gelenberg (1998b) reported that in a number of studies, the clinical efficacy of clozapine is so outstanding that even though the drug costs more than most of the

TABLE 17–4 Depot Antipsychotic Preparations		
GENERIC NAME (TRADE NAME)	**ROUTE**	**TYPICAL MAINTENANCE DOSAGE**
Haloperidol decanoate (Haldol Decanoate)	IM	50–100 mg every 4 wk
Fluphenazine decanoate (Prolixin Decanoate)	IM, SC	2.5–25 mg every 2 wk
Fluphenazine enanthate (Prolixin Enanthate)	IM, SC	2.5–25 mg every 2 wk

IM, intramuscular; SC, subcutaneous.

older antipsychotics, in the long run, it is more cost effective.

MECHANISM OF ACTION

Like traditional antipsychotic agents, clozapine blocks receptors for dopamine. However, the pattern of blockade is unique compared with that of traditional agents: clozapine produces relatively strong blockade of dopamine$_1$ receptors and relatively weak blockade of dopamine$_2$ receptors. This pattern of selective receptor blockade may explain the drug's relative lack of extrapyramidal effects and, together with its high degree of serotonin blockade, may also underlie its therapeutic effects. In addition to blocking receptors for dopamine, clozapine blocks receptors for serotonin, norepinephrine, histamine, and acetylcholine.

THERAPEUTIC USES

Because of the risk of fatal **agranulocytosis,** clozapine is generally reserved for *refractory patients*—those patients with persistent schizophrenia or schizoaffective disorders who have not responded to traditional antipsychotic drugs. In this treatment-resistant group, clozapine has had a 40% to 60% success rate. Not only do patients respond but also the quality of the response is often superior to that seen with traditional drugs. Patients are more animated, behavior is more socially acceptable, and rates of rehospitalization are lower. Because the incidence of extrapyramidal effects with clozapine is low, the drug is well suited for patients who have experienced severe EPSs with traditional antipsychotic drugs.

ADVERSE EFFECTS

In contrast to traditional antipsychotics, clozapine carries a low risk of extrapyramidal effects. Tardive dyskinesia has not been reported. In fact, tardive dyskinesia may improve when patients switch to clozapine from a traditional agent. Neuroendocrine effects (e.g., galactorrhea, gynecomastia, and amenorrhea) and interference with sexual function are minimal.

Agranulocytosis

Clozapine produces agranulocytosis in 1% to 2% of patients. The overall risk of death is about 1 in 5000; the usual cause is related to gram-negative septicemia. Agranulocytosis typically occurs during the first 6 months of treatment. Its cause is not known.

Because of the risk of fatal agranulocytosis, weekly hematologic monitoring is mandatory during the first 6 months; after 6 months, monitoring is biweekly. If the total WBC falls below 3000/mm^3 or if the granulocyte count falls below 1500/mm^3, treatment should be interrupted. When subsequent daily monitoring indicates that counts have risen above these values, clozapine can be resumed. If the total WBC falls below 2000/mm^3 or if the granulocyte count falls below 1000/mm^3, clozapine should be permanently discontinued. WBC should be monitored weekly for 4 weeks after drug withdrawal.

Patients must be informed about the risk of agranulocytosis and told that clozapine will not be dispensed if the weekly or biweekly blood test is not done. Also, patients should be given information about early signs of infection (e.g., fever, sore throat, fatigue, and mucous membrane ulceration) and instructed to report these signs immediately.

Seizures

Generalized tonic-clonic convulsions occur in 3% of patients taking clozapine. The risk of seizures is dose related, with a higher incidence occurring in patients receiving doses greater than 600 mg. Patients who have experienced a seizure should be warned not to drive or to participate in other potentially hazardous activities while on this medication.

OTHER ADVERSE EFFECTS

The most common side effects of clozapine are drowsiness and sedation (40%), dizziness (20%), hypersalivation (30%), tachycardia (25%), and constipation (14%). Additional effects include postural hypotension (9%) and elevation of body temperature (5%). The made-for-television movie, *Out of Darkness,* starring Diana Ross as a patient with paranoid schizophrenia, dramatically depicts a patient's transformative response to the use of clozapine.

DRUG INTERACTIONS

Because of its ability to cause agranulocytosis, clozapine is contraindicated for patients taking other drugs that can suppress bone marrow function (e.g., carbamazepine [Tegretol] and many anticancer drugs). Cimetidine and erythromycin can increase levels of clozapine. Smoking, carbamazepine, and phenytoin can decrease levels of clozapine. Increased levels of clozapine can lead to toxicity, whereas decreased levels may diminish its efficacy.

DOSAGE AND ADMINISTRATION

To minimize clozapine's side effects, treatment should begin with a 12.5-mg dose, followed by 25 mg once or twice daily. Dosage is then increased by 25 mg/day until it reaches 300 to 450 mg/day. Further increases can be made once or twice weekly, in increments no larger than 100 mg. The usual maintenance dosage is 300 to 600 mg/day in two or three divided doses. Maximal dosage is 900 mg/day. However, dosage may be lower for the elderly.

Risperidone

Risperidone (Risperdal), approved for use in 1993, produces strong blockade at serotonin$_2$ receptors and weaker blockade at dopamine$_2$ receptors. Antipsychotic effects are equivalent to those of haloperidol and may have a more rapid onset. Both positive and negative symptoms are improved. Interestingly, low doses of risperidone (less than 10 mg/d) are more effective than high doses. Like clozapine, risperidone causes fewer EPSs than do the traditional agents (Borison, Diamond, Pathiraja, & Meibach, 1992; Land & Salzman, 1994; Marder & Meibach, 1994). In comparison with clozapine, risperidone does not cause agranulocytosis. Volavka (1988) reported that risperidone was studied for its antiaggressive effects in 139 patients with schizophrenia. On the Brief Psychiatric Rating Scale, a more significant decrease in hostility was demonstrated with risperidone than with haloperidol or placebo (Volavka, 1998).

MECHANISM OF ACTION

Risperidone, a benzisoxazole, is a serotonin-dopamine antagonist. Risperidone has a high affinity for dopamine$_2$ receptors and is correlated with the control of positive symptoms; however, that same action is ineffective in the treatment of the negative symptoms. Risperidone also has a high affinity for 5-hydroxytryptamine (5-HT$_2$) receptors, and this blockade is associated with the amelioration of negative symptoms.

THERAPEUTIC USES

Risperidone has demonstrated equal efficacy in the treatment of schizophrenia when compared with haloperidol. It is a reasonable choice to use when patients have experienced EPSs, have not been able to tolerate the traditional antipsychotic side effects, have not responded to other agents, or have significant negative symptoms. In spring 1997, Janssen Pharmaceuticals, which manufactures Risperdal [risperidone], announced a project to link people with schizophrenia to local and national resources to help them stay with their treatment plans (see Additional Resources; Enos, 1997).

ADVERSE EFFECTS

Extrapyramidal side effects of risperidone have been noted in doses greater than 10 mg/day. Other reported side effects are insomnia (26%), agitation (22%), anxiety (12%), constipation (7%), nausea (5%), dyspepsia and vomiting (5%), dizziness (4%), and sedation (3%).

DRUG INTERACTIONS

Risperidone is metabolized in the liver by the cytochrome P-450 2D6 enzyme. What this means is that certain drugs could change risperidone metabolism, such that higher or lower doses would be necessary to achieve therapeutic efficacy. Significant interactions have not been reported; however, the potential for drug interactions exists if the patient is taking other medications that are metabolized by this cytochrome.

DOSAGE AND ADMINISTRATION

The initial dosage of risperidone is 0.5 mg twice a day. The dosage is then titrated up (slowly in elderly) for 2 to 3 days, then at weekly intervals to 4 mg to 8 mg where efficacy is observed. Remember, in doses greater than 10 mg/day the risk of EPS increases.

Other Drugs

Since the success of clozapine, which was the first antipsychotic drug approved by the Food and Drug Administration (FDA) after 1975, there has been a renewed scientific, social, political, and economic interest in the drugs used to treat the schizophrenias. As discussed earlier, risperidone was approved in 1993, and there are now several other atypical antipsychotic drugs available.

OLANZAPINE

Olanzapine (Zyprexa) received FDA approval in November 1996 after short-term (6-week) controlled trials involving more than 3200 schizophrenic inpatients. Compared with the placebo group, patients treated with olanzapine 10 to 15 mg/day had superior scores on several important psychiatric scales including Positive and Negative Symptoms, Brief Psychiatric Rating Scale (psychosis cluster) and Clinical Global Impressions (severity scale) (Antipsychotic olanzapine approved, 1996). Olanzapine structurally resembles clozapine, and like quetiapine fumarate (Seroquel), it is an antagonist at the dopamine and serotonin receptors. Both olanzapine and quetiapine fumarate are regionally selective for neurons in the limbic and frontal cortex but not for dopamine neurons in the striatum. Because of this there is a decrease in motor side effects, lowering the incidence of EPS. These agents have demonstrated efficacy in reducing the positive and negative symptoms of schizophrenia.

Dosing for olanzapine is interesting because the recommended starting dose is also the recommended therapeutic dose of 10 mg/day. For elderly patients or for patients predisposed to hypotension, the initial dose should be 2.5 to 5 mg/day. Depending on targeted symptoms and tolerance of the drug, it may not be necessary to titrate to 20 mg/day, which is the maximal recommended dose.

Reported side effects are headache (17%), insomnia (20%), constipation (9%), weight gain (6%), akathisia (5%), and tremor (4%). There is also a transient elevation in liver transaminase (alanine aminotransferase, previously serum glutamic-pyruvic transaminase) and prolactin levels that usually subside after the 1st month of treatment. A low potential for drug interaction is reported. Olanzapine is being considered for newly diagnosed patients, refractory patients, and patients in acute exacerbation of psychosis (Littrell, 1997).

QUETIAPINE FUMARATE

Quetiapine fumarate, approved in November 1997 by the FDA for management of psychotic disorders, has a higher affinity for 5-HT$_2$ receptors compared with dopamine$_2$ receptors (*Medical Sciences Bulletin,* 1997). The dosage initially is 25 mg twice a day, increasing in increments of 25 to 50 mg twice or three times a day starting the 2nd or 3rd day until it reaches the dose range of 300 to 400 mg (for average dose efficacy). The maximal dose is 800 mg/day. Side effects reported for quetiapine fumarate are headache (19%), somnolence (18%), constipation (9%), and weight gain (2%) (Arvanitis & Miller, 1997; Small, Hirsch, Arvanitis, Miller, & Link, 1997).

ZIPRASIDONE

Ziprasidone (Zeldox) is under development and is chemically unrelated to any other antipsychotic drug. The mean dose used in clinical trials was 80 mg twice a day (dose range, 80 to 160 mg), and it has been reported to have efficacy comparable to that of haloperidol; In addition, improvement in negative symptoms has been observed. There appears to be an absence of significant weight gain with ziprasidone, which is an undesirable side effect of all other previous atypical antipsychotics (Brook, Swift, & Harrigan, 1997).

Ziprasidone is the only atypical antipsychotic that has a parenteral (IM) form. Clinical studies found ziprasidone to be rapidly effective (beneficial effects up to 4 h) and well-tolerated. Doses of 2 and 20 mg were used and produced no EPS or akathisia. Mild to moderate somnolence, nausea, and postural hypotension were the most common side effects reported. Table 17–5 provides a comparison of atypical antipsychotics.

Using Antipsychotic Drugs to Treat Schizophrenia

Characteristics of Schizophrenia

Although we have discussed and profiled many antipsychotic agents, we need to review the characteristics of schizophrenia itself and additional considerations regarding drug therapy. For a more complete discussion of the illness, see Chapter 24.

Schizophrenia is a chronic psychotic illness characterized by disordered thinking, feeling, and perception. Secondary to the disorder is a reduced ability to comprehend reality. Symptoms usually emerge during adolescence or early adulthood.

ACUTE EPISODES

During an acute psychotic episode, delusions and hallucinations are frequently prominent. Delusions are typically religious, grandiose, or persecutory. Auditory hallucinations, which are more common than visual hallucinations, may consist of voices arguing or commenting on one's behavior. The patient may feel that he or she is under the control of external influences. Disordered thinking and loose association may render rational conversation impossible. Affect may be blunted or labile. Misperception of reality may result in hostility and uncooperativeness. Impaired self-care skills may leave the patient disheveled and dirty. Patterns of sleeping and eating are usually disrupted.

RESIDUAL SYMPTOMS

After florid symptoms (e.g., hallucinations and delusions) of an acute episode remit, less vivid symptoms may remain. These include suspiciousness; poor anxiety management; and diminished judgment, insight, motivation, and capacity for self-care. As a result, patients frequently find it difficult to establish close relationships, maintain employment, and function independently in society. Suspiciousness and poor management of anxiety contribute to social withdrawal. An inability to appreciate the need for continued drug therapy may cause noncompliance, resulting in relapse and possibly hospital readmission.

TABLE 17–5 Comparison of Atypical Antipsychotics

ADVANTAGES AND DISADVANTAGES	CLOZAPINE	RISPERIDONE	OLANZAPINE	QUETIAPINE	ZIPRASIDONE
Advantages					
Efficacy in treatment for positive and negative symptoms	X	X	X	X	X
May improve cognition	X	X	X	X	X
EPS	X	Dose related	Rare	X	Rare
Low incidence of tardive dyskinesia	X	Unknown	Unknown	Unknown	Unknown
No effect on prolactin levels	X	Dose related	X	X	X
Injectible form					X
Disadvantages					
Agranulocytosis	X				
Weekly or biweekly blood draw	X				
Weight gain	X	X	X	Unknown	Minimal
Long titration period	X			X	
Sedation	X	Some	Some	X	Some
Galactorrhea or amenorrhea		Dose related			Unknown
Akathisia	Minimal	Dose related	Minimal	Minimal	Dose related

LONG-TERM COURSE

The long-term course of schizophrenia is characterized by episodic acute exacerbations separated by intervals of partial remission. As the years pass, some patients experience progressive decline in mental status and social functioning, whereas others may stabilize. Maintenance therapy with antipsychotic drugs reduces the risk of acute relapse but may not prevent long-term deterioration, depression, and suicide.

POSITIVE VERSUS NEGATIVE SYMPTOMS

The symptoms of schizophrenia can be divided into two major groups: positive symptoms and negative symptoms. *Positive symptoms* can be viewed as an exaggeration or distortion of normal function, whereas *negative symptoms* can be viewed as a loss or diminution of normal function. Positive symptoms include hallucinations, delusions, agitation, tension, and paranoia. Negative symptoms include lack of motivation, poverty of speech, blunted affect, poor self-care, and social withdrawal.

In general, traditional antipsychotic drugs have a greater impact on positive symptoms than on negative symptoms. The atypical antipsychotic drugs are equally efficacious in the treatment of the positive and negative symptoms, which enhances the patient's quality of life.

Drug Therapy for Symptoms of Schizophrenia

Drug therapy for schizophrenia has three major objectives:

1. Suppression of acute episodes
2. Prevention of acute exacerbations
3. Maintenance of the highest possible level of functioning, thus returning control to the patient

This section presents a discussion of measures to achieve these objectives.

PREADMINISTRATION ASSESSMENT

Before treatment, patients should undergo a thorough mental status examination and a physical examination to determine whether the psychotic episode is due to an immune disorder or a thyroid disorder or is drug-induced. It is important to find out if there is a family history of mental illness. It is also important to determine if the patient has a history of taking medication for schizophrenia and if so, what medication; an important factor in predicting positive outcomes for schizophrenic patients is previous response to treatment. The patient should be observed for overt behavior (e.g., gait, pacing, restlessness, and volatile outbursts), emotional state (e.g., depression, agitation, and mania), intellectual function (e.g., stream of thought, coherence, hallucinations, and delusions), and responsiveness to the environment.

Patients who must avoid specific antipsychotics or use them with caution must be identified. Traditional antipsychotic agents are contraindicated for patients who are comatose or severely depressed and for patients with Parkinson's disease, prolactin-dependent carci-

noma of the breast, bone marrow depression, and severe hypotension or hypertension. These drugs should be used cautiously in patients with glaucoma, adynamic ileus, prostatic hypertrophy, cardiovascular disease, hepatic or renal dysfunction, or seizure disorders. Clozapine is contraindicated for patients with a history of clozapine-induced agranulocytosis, those with bone marrow suppression, and those taking myelosuppressive drugs, which include many anticancer drugs.

DRUG TREATMENT

Treatment is usually initiated with one of the traditional antipsychotic agents. Although all of the traditional agents produce equivalent therapeutic effects, some patients may respond better to one agent than to another. Accordingly, if treatment with one traditional agent is unsuccessful, a trial with a drug from a different chemical class should be undertaken.

Selection among the traditional antipsychotic drugs is based largely on side effects. The patient should not be given a drug that, because of its side-effect profile, is especially likely to cause discomfort, inconvenience, or harm. For example, certain patients (e.g., those with prostatic hypertrophy or glaucoma) are especially sensitive to anticholinergic drugs. Accordingly, these patients should not be treated with low-potency neuroleptics. By similar logic, if the patient has a history of extrapyramidal reactions, high-potency agents should be avoided. By properly matching patients and drugs, side effects can be minimized, comfort can be maximized, and compliance can be promoted. Table 17–6 indicates the traditional antipsychotic agents that should be avoided in the presence of certain predisposing factors.

In the United States, there are several atypical antipsychotics that may be rational alternatives to the traditional antipsychotic agents. Because these drugs are associated with a low incidence of extrapyramidal reactions, they are especially well suited for patients who have experienced severe extrapyramidal reactions to traditional agents. Also, because of their superior ability to relieve negative symptoms, these drugs may be beneficial for patients whose negative symptoms have not responded to traditional agents. Because clozapine can produce fatal agranulocytosis, it is not considered a drug of first choice; rather, clozapine should be reserved for patients who have not responded to trials with at least two other agents.

DOSING

Dosing with neuroleptics is highly individualized. Unresponsive patients may need doses that are 10 to 20 times greater than those used for highly responsive patients. Elderly patients require relatively small doses—typically 30% to 50% of those taken by younger patients.

Dosage size and timing are likely to change over the course of therapy. During the early phase of treatment, antipsychotics should be administered in divided daily doses. Once an effective dosage has been determined, the entire daily dose may be given at bedtime for many antipsychotic agents. Because antipsychotics cause sedation, this practice can promote sleep and decrease

TABLE 17-6 Antipsychotics That Should Be Avoided in the Presence of Certain Predisposing Factors	
PREDISPOSING FACTOR	**ANTIPSYCHOTIC AGENTS TO AVOID**
Glaucoma, prostatism, adynamic ileus, urinary hesitance	Low-potency agents (anticholinergic actions can exacerbate these disorders)
Use of anticholinergic drugs (e.g., tricyclic antidepressants)	Low-potency agents (anticholinergic effects will intensify muscarinic blockade)
Old age	Low-potency agents (the elderly are especially sensitive to the anticholinergic and sedative effects of these drugs)
Active lifestyle	Low-potency agents (sedative effects can interfere with function)
Delirium	Low-potency agents (anticholinergic action can exacerbate delirium)
Cardiovascular disorders	Low-potency agents (anticholinergic and hypotensive actions can exacerbate these disorders)
History of extrapyramidal reactions	High-potency agents (disruption of extrapyramidal function is greatest with these drugs)
Active sex life in males	Thioridazine (this agent may inhibit ejaculation)

drowsiness during the day. During long-term therapy, the dosage should start low and titrate slowly to achieve the lowest effective amount to reduce targeted symptoms and achieve optimal functioning of the patient.

ROUTES OF ADMINISTRATION

Antipsychotic drugs are administered orally, IM, subcutaneously, IV, and by rectal suppository. Routes for individual agents are summarized in Tables 17-2 and 17-4.

Oral

Oral administration is preferred for most patients. Antipsychotics are available in tablets, capsules, and liquids for oral use. The liquid formulations require special handling. These preparations are concentrated and must be diluted before use. Dilution may be performed with a variety of fluids, including fruit juices, milk, and carbonated beverages. The oral liquids are sensitive to light and must be stored in amber or opaque containers. Liquid formulations of phenothiazines can cause contact dermatitis; nurses and patients should take care to avoid skin contact with these preparations. If a spill occurs, the affected area should be flushed.

Intramuscular

IM injection is generally reserved for patients with severe, acute schizophrenia and for long-term maintenance therapy. Injections should be made into the deltoid or gluteal muscle, and the site should be rotated. The Z-track method is preferred because it is less painful (decreases skin irritation) and facilitates slow, steady absorption. Depot preparations are given every 2 to 4 weeks (Davis, Metalon, Wantabe, & Blare, 1994) (see Table 17-4).

INITIAL THERAPY

With adequate dosing, symptoms begin to resolve within 1 to 7 days. However, the full therapeutic response develops gradually over 6 to 8 weeks.

Some symptoms resolve sooner than others. During the 1st week, the goal is to reduce agitation, hostility, anxiety, and tension and to normalize sleeping and eating patterns. During the next 6 to 8 weeks, symptoms should continue to steadily improve. The goals over this interval are increased socialization, improved self-care and mood, and improved formal thought processes. Of the patients who have not responded within 6 weeks, 50% are likely to respond by the end of 12 weeks.

It is important to note that not all symptoms respond equally. As discussed earlier, positive symptoms generally respond better than do negative symptoms.

MAINTENANCE THERAPY

Schizophrenia is usually persistent and requires prolonged treatment. The purpose of long-term therapy is to reduce the recurrence of acute florid episodes and to maintain the highest possible level of functioning. Unfortunately, although long-term treatment can be effective, it also carries a risk of adverse effects, especially tardive dyskinesia.

After control of an acute episode, antipsychotic therapy should continue for at least 12 months. Withdrawal of medication prior to this time is associated with a 55% incidence of relapse, compared with only 20% in patients who continue drug use. Accordingly, patients must be educated and "buy into" the benefit of continued therapy for the entire 12-month course, even though they may be symptom-free and consider themselves "cured."

After 12 months, an attempt should be made to discontinue drug use, provided that symptoms are absent. About 25% of patients do not need drugs beyond this time. To avoid adverse reactions to drug withdrawal, dosage should be reduced gradually. It is important that medication not be withdrawn at a time of stress (e.g., when the patient is being discharged from the hospital). If a relapse occurs in response to withdrawal, drug treatment should be reinstituted. For many patients, resumption of treatment diminishes symptoms and prevents further relapse.

When long-term therapy is conducted, dosage should be adjusted with care. To reduce the risk of tardive dyskinesia and other adverse effects, a minimal effective dosage should be established. Annual attempts should be made to lower the dosage or to discontinue treatment entirely.

Long-acting (depot) antipsychotics are especially well suited for long-term therapy. Depot therapy has three major advantages over oral therapy:

1. Relapse rate is lower with depot therapy.
2. Depot therapy maintains steady drug levels between doses.
3. Total dose per unit time is lower with depot therapy, thus reducing the risk of side effects.

There is no evidence that depot preparations carry a higher risk of tardive dyskinesia or NMS. In the United States, only 10% of patients receive depot therapy. This low rate of use is based in part on the widely held (but incorrect) perception that depot therapy is for "losers"—patients who suffer recurrent relapse because of persistent noncompliance with oral therapy.

PROMOTING COMPLIANCE

Poor compliance is a common cause of therapeutic failure and is responsible for a substantial number of hospital readmissions. Compliance can be difficult to achieve because treatment is prolonged, patients may fail to value the need for therapy, or patients may be unwilling or unable to take medicine as prescribed. In addition, side effects can discourage compliance.

Compliance can be enhanced by

- Ensuring that medication given to a hospitalized patient is actually swallowed and not *cheeked* (hidden in the patient's mouth)
- Educating family members regarding medications, signs and symptoms of relapse, and the importance of keeping outpatient appointments
- Providing the patient with written and verbal instructions on dosage size and timing and encouraging him or her to take the medicine exactly as prescribed
- Informing the patient and family members that antipsychotics must be taken regularly to be effective and thus cannot be used on an as needed basis
- Informing the patient about side effects of treatment and teaching him or her how to minimize undesired responses
- Assuring the patient that antipsychotic drugs do not cause addiction
- Establishing a good therapeutic relationship with the patient and his or her family members
- Using a depot preparation (e.g., fluphenazine decanoate, haloperidol decanoate) for long-term therapy

B o x 1 7 – 7 ▪ ▪ ▪ ▪ ▪
Medication Noncompliance

Estimated rate of noncompliance = 50% to 80%

Noncompliance includes early discontinuation

Discontinuance may be due to
- Side effects
- Knowledge deficit about medications
- Economic issues
- Stigma of mental illness

(Box 17–7 lists some reasons for medication noncompliance.)

***W**hat do you think?* What are your thoughts about the compliance issues related to psychotropic medications? Lack of compliance with medications costs the health care system millions of dollars in rehospitalizations. Should patients have the right to refuse psychotropic medications, even if that refusal results in extremely high treatment costs? How would you work with a patient and his or her family to ensure better compliance? What techniques would you use?

▶ *Check Your Reading*

5. What is the major indication for antipsychotic drugs?
6. How are antipsychotic drugs thought to act?
7. What are the early extrapyramidal reactions, and how are they treated?
8. What is tardive dyskinesia, and how is it treated?
9. What are the signs and symptoms of NMS?
10. What is the significance of clozapine-induced agranulocytosis?
11. What are the features of an atypical antipsychotic medication?

ANTIDEPRESSANTS

As their name suggests, **antidepressants** are drugs used to treat depression. These agents fall into four groups:

1. Tricyclic antidepressants
2. **Monoamine oxidase inhibitors** (MAOIs)
3. **Selective serotonin reuptake inhibitors** (SSRIs)
4. Miscellaneous antidepressants

The principal indication for these drugs is major depression, although there are a host of other uses (e.g., chronic pain, enuresis, obsessive-compulsive disorder [OCD], premenstrual symptoms) (Gelenberg, 1998e). As a rule, antidepressants are not indicated for uncomplicated bereavement. It should be noted that antidepressants are not merely general psychic stimulants; rather, these drugs act selectively to alleviate symptoms of depression (Brasfield, 1991; Cohn et al., 1990; Ereshefsky, 1995; Lehne, 1994b).

Major Depression: Characteristics, Pathogenesis, and Overview of Treatment

Characteristics

Before discussing the antidepressant drugs, it is helpful to briefly review the characteristics of depression. For a more complete discussion of depression, refer to Chapter 25.

The principal symptoms of depression are (1) depressed mood and (2) loss of pleasure or interest in all or nearly all of one's usual activities and pastimes. Associated symptoms include insomnia (or sometimes hypersomnia); anorexia and weight loss (or sometimes hyperphagia and weight gain); mental slowing and loss of concentration; feelings of guilt, worthlessness, and helplessness; thoughts of death and suicide; and overt suicidal behavior. For a diagnosis to be made, symptoms must be present most of the day, nearly every day, for at least 2 weeks.

Major depression is a frustrating illness because symptoms may not correspond with external events. That is, rather than occurring in response to life's tragedies, symptoms of major depression may descend "out of the blue"; otherwise healthy individuals—unexpectedly and without apparent cause—find themselves feeling profoundly depressed.

It is important to distinguish between major depression and normal grief or sadness. Whereas major depression is an illness, grief or sadness is not. Rather, grief and sadness are appropriate reactions to a major life stressor (e.g., death of a loved one, loss of a job). In most cases, grief and sadness resolve spontaneously over several weeks and do not require medical intervention. If, however, symptoms are unusually intense, and if they fail to abate within an appropriate time, a major depressive episode may have been superimposed. In these cases, treatment is indicated.

Pathogenesis

The etiology of major depression is undoubtedly complex and not yet known. Because depressive episodes can be triggered by stressful life events in some people but not in others, it would appear that, for some people, a predisposition to depression exists. Social, developmental, and biological factors, including genetic heritage, may all contribute to that predisposition.

The Greeks were the first to introduce the term, *melancholia*. They believed that depression was caused by excessive amounts of black bile (melancholia literally means "black bile"). Accounts and treatment of depression were written about in biblical times—King Saul suffered from depression and David played his harp for him, which temporarily lifted Saul's spirits. The theory that depression is biologically based is not a well-known concept. There exist public misconceptions that depression is not a biological malady.

Current theory states that depression is associated with regional brain dysfunction. Research is directed to correlating observed symptoms and behaviors with disturbed chemistry. This can be seen by using technology such as PET and single photon emission computed tomography (SPECT) scans.

Two neurotransmitters are correlated with depression: serotonin and norepinephrine (monoamines). The first, serotonin, which originates in the dorsal and median raphe nuclei of the brain stem, is widely distributed in the forebrain. The function of this system is thermoregulation, feeding, and regulation of mood and emotion. It is also involved in control of sleep, wakefulness, and sexual behavior. (So one may conclude that when serotonin is involved, one is either awake, sleeping, or having sex!) It is also hypothesized that affective disorders and OCD are related to a dysfunction of serotonin.

The norepinephrine or noradrenergic pathway arises from the locus coeruleus, and cells are scattered throughout the ventral and lateral tegmental region of the medulla, and the fibers are distributed throughout the neocortex and involve the hypothalamus. Its function is rather famous for it has sympathetic nervous system control that includes regulation of BP and, of course, the fight-or-flight syndrome. Norepinephrine, as serotonin, is involved in sleep and wakefulness as well as the hypothalamic function of thermoregulation, thirst, and hunger. This is why when people are depressed, they complain of decreased or increased appetite and weight loss or gain.

Clinical observations made in the 1960s led to formulation of the **monoamine hypothesis of depression,** which asserts that depression is caused by a functional insufficiency of monoamine neurotransmitters (norepinephrine, serotonin, or both) in the brain. This hypothesis is based mainly on two observations: (1) depression can be induced with reserpine, a drug that depletes monoamines from the brain, and (2) the drugs used to treat depression intensify monoamine-mediated neurotransmission. Although these observations do indeed support the monoamine hypothesis, it is likely that this somewhat simplistic theory will need refinement as our understanding of the brain deepens. However, despite its shortcomings, the monoamine hypothesis does provide a useful conceptual framework for understanding the antidepressant drugs.

Treatment

Depression can be treated with three modalities: (1) drugs, (2) electroconvulsive therapy (ECT), and (3) psychotherapy. Each modality has a legitimate role.

Drugs are the primary therapy for major depression. Currently available antidepressants are listed in Table 17-7.

For many patients, the **tricyclic antidepressants** are drugs of first choice. These agents are effective and relatively safe and can be administered easily. The SSRIs are as effective as the tricyclics, have a better safety profile, and are better tolerated. As a result, fluoxetine HCl (Prozac), the prototype of the family, has achieved widespread popularity. MAOIs are generally reserved for patients who have not responded to tricyclics or to one of the SSRIs. However, for patients with atypical depression, MAOIs are the drugs of choice. Antianxiety agents (e.g., diazepam [Valium]) can be employed in depression, but their use is not routine. As a rule, CNS stimulants (e.g., amphetamines, methylphenidate) are without benefit in depression. As discussed later, patients with bipolar depression can be treated prophylactically with lithium or valproic acid.

ECT is a valuable tool for treating depression. This procedure is effective, and beneficial responses develop more rapidly than with drugs. Accordingly, ECT is indicated when speed is critical (i.e., in severely depressed, suicidal patients) or when a patient has failed to respond to antidepressants. There is also literature that suggests positive outcomes for use of ECT with the elderly and for

TABLE 17–7 Antidepressants: Adverse Effects and Effects on Neurotransmitters

	TRANSMITTER REUPTAKE ANTAGONISM		ANTICHOLINERGIC ACTIVITY	SEDATION	HYPOTENSION	SEIZURE RISK	CARDIAC TOXICITY	OTHER SIDE EFFECTS
	NE	5-HT						
Tricyclic Antidepressants								
Amitriptyline	++	+++	++++	+++	+++	+++	+++	
Desipramine	++++	+	++	++	+++	+++	+++	
Doxepin	++	++	+++	+++	+++	+++	++	
Imipramine	+++	+++	+++	+++	+++	+++	++++	
Nortriptyline	+++	++	++	++	+	+++	+++	
Protriptyline	+++	+	+++	+	++	+++	++++	
Trimipramine	+	+	+++	+++	+++	+++	+++	
MAOIs								
Isocarboxazid	*	*	0	+	+++	0	0	Hypertensive crisis from tyramine in food
Phenelzine	*	*	0	+	+++	0	0	
Tranylcypromine	*	*	0	†	++	0	0	
Selective Serotonin Reuptake Blockers								
Fluoxetine	0	++++	0	†	0	+	0	Skin rash
Fluvoxamine	0	++++	0					
Paroxetine	0	++++	0	0	0		0	
Sertraline	0	++++	0	†	0	+	0	
Miscellaneous Antidepressants								
Amoxapine	+++‡	++‡	+++	++	+	+++	+	Parkinsonism
Bupropion	§	§	++	†	++	++++	+	Seizures
Maprotiline	+++	+	+++	+++	+++	+++	+++	Seizures
Trazodone	0	++	0	+++	+++	+	+	Priapism
Nefazodone	0	+++	+	++	+	+	0	Visual trails on initiation (resolves); Minimal sexual side effects
Venlafaxine	+++	+++	+	+	++	+	+	Dose-regulated hypertension
Mirtazapine	0	++	++	+++	+	+	0	Rare neutropenia

*MAOIs do not block transmitter reuptake. Rather, they increase intraneuronal stores at NE, 5-HT, and DA.

†Produces moderate stimulation, not sedation.

‡In addition to blocking NE and 5-HT reuptake, amoxapine blocks receptors for DA.

§Bupropion primarily inhibits reuptake of DA rather than NE or 5-HT.

0, no effect; +, minimal effect; ++, mild effect; +++, moderate effect; ++++, strong effect; DA, dopamine; 5-HT, 5-hydroxytryptamine (serotonin); MAOI, monoamine oxidase inhibitor; NE, norepinephrine.

treatment for those diagnosed with psychotic depression.

The role of psychotherapy in major depression is largely supportive; symptoms do not respond nearly as well to psychotherapy alone as they do to medication. However, although of less direct benefit than drugs, psychotherapy can help to relieve suffering by providing insight, reassurance, and caring. Research has demonstrated that by combining both psychotherapy and pharmacotherapy, there are better outcomes in relapse rates (Box 17–8).

TRICYCLIC ANTIDEPRESSANTS

The first tricyclic agent—imipramine HCl (Tofranil)—was introduced to psychiatry in the late 1950s. Since then, the ability of the tricyclics to relieve depressive symptoms has been firmly established. The most common adverse effects of the tricyclics are sedation, orthostatic hypotension, and anticholinergic effects. The most hazardous adverse effect is cardiac toxicity.

Mechanism of Action

The tricyclic drugs are blockers of monoamine (norepinephrine and serotonin) reuptake. By blocking reuptake, the tricyclics can increase the amount of these transmitters available for receptor binding, thereby intensifying their effects. Such a mechanism would be consistent with the monoamine hypothesis of depression. The monoamine hypothesis, which asserts that depression stems from a deficiency in monoamine-mediated neurotransmission, predicts that drugs capable of increasing the effects of monoamines reduce symptoms of depression. This prediction is fulfilled by the tricyclic drugs. The relative abilities of individual tricyclics to block reuptake of norepinephrine and serotonin are summarized in Table 17–7.

We should note that blockade of reuptake, by itself, cannot fully account for the therapeutic effects of the tricyclics. This statement is based on the observation that clinical responses to the tricyclics (relief of depressive symptoms) and the biochemical effects of the tricyclics (blockade of transmitter uptake) do not occur in the same time frame. That is, whereas the tricyclic drugs block transmitter uptake within hours of administration, relief of depression takes several weeks to develop. Hence, it would appear that in the interval between the onset of uptake blockade and the onset of a therapeutic response, intermediary neurochemical events must be taking place. Just what these events might be is unknown.

Box 17–8 ■ ■ ■ ■ ■
Positive Patient Outcomes

Positive patient outcomes are enhanced by using a combination of pharmacological treatments and nonpharmacological treatments.

Pharmacokinetics

Tricyclic antidepressants have half-lives that are long and variable. Because their half-lives are long, the tricyclic antidepressants can usually be administered in a single daily dose. However, because their half-lives are variable, the tricyclic drugs require individualization of dosage.

Therapeutic Uses

Depression. *Tricyclic antidepressants* (so named because of their chemical structure of three hydrocarbon rings) are useful drugs for treatment of major depression. These drugs relieve symptoms of depression by elevating mood, decreasing morbid preoccupation, improving appetite, and restoring normal sleep patterns.

It is important to note that the tricyclic agents, and all other antidepressants, do not relieve symptoms immediately. Initial responses take from 1 to 3 weeks to develop. One or 2 months may be needed before a maximal response is achieved. Because therapeutic effects are delayed, tricyclic antidepressants cannot be used on an as needed basis. Furthermore, because responses are delayed, a therapeutic trial should not be considered a failure until medication has been administered for at least 1 month without success.

Suicide is always a concern during the treatment of depression because the patient may be so despondent that he or she perceives suicide as the only means of relieving his or her suffering. To reduce the chances of suicide, several precautions can be taken. First, because antidepressants take several weeks to alleviate symptoms, hospitalization should be considered for the patient in acute distress presenting with suicidal tendencies. Hospitalization provides immediate safety while aftercare plans are being formulated. In addition, because the antidepressants themselves can be vehicles for suicide, the patient should not be given access to a large supply of these drugs. Accordingly, you should ensure that each dose is actually swallowed and not cheeked. This precaution prevents the patient from accumulating multiple doses that might be taken with suicidal intent.

Bipolar Disorder. *Bipolar disorder* (manic-depressive illness) is characterized by alternating episodes of mania and depression (see Chapter 25). Tricyclic antidepressants can be helpful during the depressive phase of this illness.

Panic Disorder. Panic disorder is characterized by spontaneous panic attacks. Primary associated symptoms are anticipatory anxiety and phobic avoidance (e.g., agoraphobia). Tricyclic antidepressants can eliminate panic attacks in approximately 75% of those treated. The associated symptoms (anticipatory anxiety and phobic avoidance) are not affected.

Adverse Effects

The most common undesired responses to tricyclics are orthostatic hypotension, sedation, and anticholinergic effects. The most serious adverse effect is cardiac toxicity. Adverse effects of individual tricyclics are summarized in Table 17–7.

Orthostatic Hypotension. Orthostatic hypotension is the most serious of the common adverse responses to treatment. Hypotension is caused mainly by blockade of α-adrenergic receptors on blood vessels. The patient should be informed that orthostatic hypotension can be minimized by moving slowly when assuming an upright posture. Also, the patient should be instructed to sit or lie down if symptoms of hypotension (dizziness, lightheadedness) occur. For the hospitalized patient, BP and pulse rate should be monitored on a regular schedule (e.g., four times daily). These measurements should be taken while the patient is lying down and again after the patient has been sitting or standing for 1 to 2 minutes. If BP is low and pulse rate is high, medication should be withheld and the physician should be notified.

Anticholinergic Effects. The tricyclic antidepressants can block muscarinic-cholinergic receptors, thus causing an array of anticholinergic effects (e.g., dry mouth, blurred vision, photophobia, constipation, urinary hesitancy, and tachycardia). The patient should be informed about possible anticholinergic responses and instructed in ways to minimize discomfort (e.g., eating sugarless candies, increasing fiber intake).

Diaphoresis. Despite their anticholinergic properties, tricyclic antidepressants often cause *diaphoresis* (sweating). The mechanism of this paradoxical effect is unknown.

Sedation. Sedation is a common response to the tricyclic drugs. This response is probably due to blockade of histamine receptors in the CNS. The patient should be advised to avoid hazardous activities if prominent sedation occurs. Sometimes, taking medications before bedtime reduces this effect.

Cardiac Toxicity. Tricyclics can adversely affect cardiac function; however, in the absence of overdosage or preexisting cardiac impairment, serious cardiotoxicity is rare. These drugs affect the heart by decreasing vagal influence on the heart (secondary to muscarinic blockade) and by acting directly on the bundle of His to slow conduction. Both effects increase the risk of dysrhythmia. To minimize adverse cardiac effects, patients older than 40 years of age and those with heart disease should undergo an EEG evaluation before treatment and periodically thereafter.

Seizures. Tricyclic antidepressants lower the seizure threshold. Caution must be exercised in patients with epilepsy and other seizure disorders.

Hypomania. Occasionally, the tricyclics produce too much of a good thing, elevating mood from depression all the way to *hypomania* (mild mania). If hypomania develops, the patient should be evaluated to determine whether elation is drug induced or symptomatic of manic-depressive illness.

Drug Interactions

Monoamine Oxidase Inhibitors. The combination of a tricyclic antidepressant and an MAOI can lead to severe hypertension from excessive adrenergic stimulation of the heart and blood vessels. Excessive adrenergic stimulation occurs because (1) inhibition of MAO causes accumulation of norepinephrine in adrenergic neurons and (2) blockade of norepinephrine reuptake by the tricyclics decreases norepinephrine inactivation. Because of the potential for hypertensive crisis, combined therapy with tricyclic antidepressants and MAOIs is generally avoided.

Direct-Acting Sympathomimetic Drugs. Tricyclic antidepressants potentiate responses to *direct-acting sympathomimetics* (i.e., drugs such as epinephrine and norepinephrine that produce their effects by direct interaction with adrenergic receptors). Stimulation by these drugs is increased because tricyclics block their uptake into adrenergic terminals, thus prolonging their presence in the synaptic space.

Indirect-Acting Sympathomimetic Drugs. Tricyclic antidepressants decrease responses to *indirect-acting sympathomimetics* (i.e., drugs such as ephedrine and amphetamine that produce their effects by promoting release of transmitter from adrenergic nerves). Effects of indirect-acting sympathomimetics are reduced because tricyclics block uptake of these agents into adrenergic nerves, thereby preventing them from reaching their site of action within the nerve terminal.

Anticholinergic Agents. Because the tricyclic antidepressants exert anticholinergic actions of their own, these drugs intensify the effects of other medications that exert anticholinergic actions. Consequently, patients receiving tricyclic agents should be advised to avoid all other drugs with anticholinergic properties, including antihistamines and certain over-the-counter sleeping aids. Additionally, these drugs may cause delirium (from the French *delirare*, "to be crazy"), especially in the elderly population.

Central Nervous System Depressants. Depression of the CNS caused by the tricyclics increases when using other drugs that have CNS-depressant properties. Accordingly, the patient should be warned against taking other CNS depressants, such as alcohol, antihistamines, opioids, and barbiturates.

Toxicity. Overdosage with tricyclic antidepressants is often life threatening. (The lethal dose is only eight times the average daily dose.) To minimize the risk of death by suicide, the acutely depressed patient should be given no more than a 1-week supply of medication at one time.

Clinical Manifestations. Symptoms of tricyclic overdose result primarily from anticholinergic and cardiotoxic actions. The combination of cholinergic blockade and direct cardiotoxicity can produce dysrhythmia, including tachycardia, intraventricular block, complete atrioventricular block, ventricular tachycardia, and ventricular fibrillation. Responses to peripheral muscarinic blockade include hyperthermia, flushing, dry mouth, and dilation of the pupils.

CNS symptoms are prominent. Early responses are confusion, agitation, and hallucinations. Seizures and coma may follow.

Treatment. Absorption of ingested drug can be reduced with gastric lavage followed by administration of activated charcoal. Physostigmine (a cholinesterase inhibitor) is given to counteract anticholinergic actions. Propranolol, lidocaine, or phenytoin can be given to control dysrhythmia. Dysrhythmia should not be treated with procainamide or quinidine because these drugs aggravate cardiac depression.

Dosage and Administration

Dosages for individual tricyclics are summarized in Table 17–8. General guidelines on dosing follow.

Initial doses of tricyclic antidepressants should be kept low (e.g., 50 mg of imipramine/d for the adult outpatient). Low initial doses minimize adverse reactions and, as a result, help to promote compliance. High initial doses are both undesirable and unnecessary. They are undesirable because they pose an increased risk of adverse reactions. They are unnecessary in that onset of therapeutic effects is delayed regardless of dosage, and therefore aggressive initial dosing offers no benefit.

Because of interpatient variability in metabolism of tricyclics, dosing is highly individualized. As a rule, dosage is adjusted on the basis of clinical response. However, in the absence of a therapeutic response, plasma drug levels can be used as a guide for dosage determination. Levels of imipramine, for example, must be above 150 ng/ml for antidepressant effects to occur. If a patient has not responded to imipramine, measurements should be made to ensure that plasma drug levels are greater than 150 ng/ml. If drug levels are below this value, the dosage should be increased.

Once an effective dosage has been established, most patients can take their entire daily dose at bedtime because the long half-lives of the tricyclic antidepressants make divided daily doses unnecessary. Once-daily dosing at bedtime has several advantages: (1) it is simple to perform and thus facilitates compliance, (2) it promotes sleep by causing maximal sedation at night, and (3) it reduces the intensity of side effects during the day. Although once-daily dosing is generally desirable, not all patients can use this schedule. The elderly, for example, can be especially sensitive to the cardiotoxic actions of the tricyclics. As a result, if the entire daily dose is taken at one time, effects on the heart might be intolerable.

Once remission has been produced, therapy should continue for at least 6 months. Failure to take medication for this period is likely to result in relapse. Patients should be encouraged to continue drug therapy even if they are symptom-free and feel that further medication is not needed.

All of the tricyclic agents can be administered by mouth, the usual route for these drugs. Two agents—amitriptyline HCl [Elavil] and imipramine—may also be given by IM injection. IV administration is not used. Because effects take weeks to develop, there would be no advantage to this route.

T A B L E 1 7 – 8 Adult Dosages for Antidepressants

GENERIC NAME	TRADE NAME	INITIAL DOSE*† (mg/d)	DOSE AFTER 4–8 WEEKS* (mg/d)	MAXIMAL DOSE‡ (mg/d)
Tricyclic Antidepressants				
Amitriptyline	Elavil, Enovil	30–100	100–200	300
Desipramine	Norpramin	75	150–200	300
Doxepin	Adapin, Sinequan	30–150	100–200	300
Imipramine	Tofranil	75–100	100–200	300
Nortriptyline	Aventyl, Pamelor	75–100	75–150	150
Protriptyline	Vivactil	15–60	15–60	60
Trimipramine	Surmontil	50–150	50–150	200
Monoamine Oxidase Inhibitors				
Isocarboxazid	Marplan	20–30	20–30	30
Phenelzine	Nardil	45	60–90	90
Tranylcypromine	Parnate	20	20–60	60
Selective Serotonin Reuptake Inhibitors				
Fluoxetine	Prozac	20	20–40	80
Fluvoxamine	Luvox	50	100–300	300
Paroxetine	Paxil	20	20–60	60
Sertraline	Zoloft	50	50–200	200
Miscellaneous Antidepressants				
Amoxapine	Asendin	50–75	200–300	300
Bupropion	Wellbutrin, Zyban	200	300	450
Maprotiline	Ludiomil	75	150–225	225
Trazodone	Desyrel	150	100–150	600

*Doses listed are total daily doses. Depending on the drug and the patient, the total dose may be given in a single dose or in divided doses.
†Initial doses are employed for 4–8 weeks, the time required for most symptoms to respond. The smaller dose within the range listed is used initially. Dosage is gradually increased as required.
‡Doses higher than these may be needed for some patients with severe depression.

Drug Selection

In the United States, seven tricyclic antidepressants are available (see Tables 17-7 and 17-8). When administered in adequate doses, all seven agents are equally effective at reducing symptoms of depression and panic disorder. Principal differences among these agents concern side effects (see Table 17-7).

Selection among tricyclic agents is made on the basis of side effects. For example, if the patient has been experiencing insomnia, a drug with prominent sedative properties (e.g., doxepin) might be selected. Conversely, if daytime sedation is undesirable, a weak sedative agent (e.g., desipramine) might be preferred. Elderly patients with glaucoma or constipation and males with prostatic hypertrophy can be especially sensitive to anticholinergic effects; for these patients, a drug with weak anticholinergic properties (e.g., desipramine) would be appropriate.

MONOAMINE OXIDASE INHIBITORS

The MAOIs are second-choice or third-choice antidepressants for most patients. Although these drugs are as effective as the tricyclics, they are more dangerous. Of particular concern is the risk of hypertensive crisis in response to ingestion of certain foods and drugs (Gelenberg, 1998b). With the advent of newer alternatives to the tricyclic antidepressants, indications for the MAOIs continue to decline.

Only two MAOIs are approved for use in the United States (see Tables 17-7 and 17-8). One of these drugs—isocarboxazid—was previously available, but it has been withdrawn from the market in the United States. Hence, only two MAOIs—phenelzine and tranylcypromine—are prescribed.

Mechanism of Action

Before discussing the MAOIs, we need to discuss MAO itself. MAO is an enzyme present in the liver, the intestinal wall, and the terminals of adrenergic nerves. The function of MAO in nerve terminals is to convert monoamine transmitters (norepinephrine, epinephrine, serotonin) into inactive products. In the liver and intestine, MAO serves to inactivate biogenic amines present in food; in addition, these enzymes can inactivate biogenic amines administered as drugs.

Antidepressant effects of the MAOIs appear to result from inhibition of MAO within nerve terminals (Figure 17-2). By inhibiting intraneuronal MAO, these drugs increase the amount of norepinephrine and serotonin available for release from neurons of the CNS. The intensified transmission that occurs when these transmitters are released in supranormal amounts is thought to be responsible for relief of depression.

The MAOIs can act on MAO in two ways: reversibly and irreversibly. Phenelzine produces irreversible inhibition. Tranylcypromine produces reversible inhibition. Recovery from irreversible inhibition requires synthesis of new enzyme, a somewhat slow process. Hence, the effects of the irreversible inhibitors persist for about 2 weeks after drug withdrawal. Recovery from reversible inhibition is more rapid, occurring in 3 to 5 days.

Antidepressant effects of the MAOIs cannot be fully accounted for by MAO inhibition alone. This statement is based on the fact that the biochemical action of these drugs (inhibition of MAO) takes place rapidly, whereas the clinical response (relief of depression) takes weeks to develop. Hence, it would appear that in the interval between initial inhibition of MAO and alleviation of depression, additional neurochemical events must be taking place. It is these as yet unknown events that are ultimately responsible for the beneficial response to treatment.

Therapeutic Uses

Depression. The MAOIs are as effective as the tricyclic agents for relieving depression. However, because their use can be hazardous, MAOIs are generally reserved for patients who have not responded to tricyclics or the newer antidepressants. For one group of patients—those with atypical depression—MAOIs are drugs of first choice. As with the tricyclic agents, beneficial effects take a week or more to develop.

Other Uses. MAOIs have been used with some success in the treatment of bulimia, OCD, and panic disorder. Like the tricyclics, MAOIs can eliminate spontaneous panic attacks in patients with panic disorder.

Adverse Effects

Central Nervous System Stimulation. Unlike the tricyclic agents, MAOIs cause direct CNS stimulation (in addition to acting as antidepressants). Excessive stimulation can produce anxiety, agitation, hypomania, and even mania.

Orthostatic Hypotension. Despite their ability to increase the norepinephrine content of peripheral sympathetic nerves, the MAOIs reduce BP when administered in usual therapeutic doses. The patient should be informed about signs of hypotension (dizziness, lightheadedness) and advised to sit or lie down if these occur. Also, the patient should be informed that hypotension can be minimized by moving slowly when assuming an erect posture. For the hospitalized patient, BP and pulse rate should be monitored regularly (e.g., three or four times daily). These measurements should be taken while the patient is lying down and after the patient has been sitting or standing for 1 to 2 minutes.

Hypertensive Crisis From Dietary Tyramine. Although the MAOIs normally produce hypotension, these drugs can be the cause of severe hypertension if the patient should ingest foods that contain *tyramine,* a substance that promotes the release of norepinephrine from sympathetic nerves. Hypertensive crisis is characterized by headache, tachycardia, hypertension, nausea, and vomiting.

Before considering the mechanism by which hypertensive crisis is produced, let us consider the effect of tyramine under drug-free conditions. In the absence of MAO inhibition, dietary tyramine does not represent a threat. Much of the tyramine in food is metabolized by MAO in the intestinal wall. Furthermore, any dietary tyramine that is not absorbed passes directly to the liver via the hepatic portal circulation. Once in the liver,

A Neurotransmission
without MAOIs

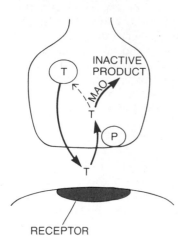

B Neurotransmission
with MAOIs

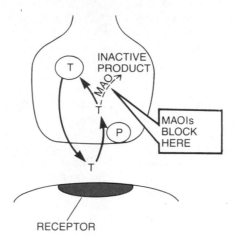

Figure 17–2
Mechanism of action of monoamine oxidase inhibitors (MAOIs). *A*, Under drug-free conditions, much of the norepinephrine or serotonin that undergoes reuptake into nerve terminals becomes inactivated by MAO present within the terminal. This inactivation process helps maintain an appropriate concentration of transmitter within the terminal. *B*, MAOIs prevent inactivation of norepinephrine and serotonin, thereby increasing the amount of transmitter available for release. Release of supranormal amounts of transmitter intensifies transmission. MAO, monoamine oxidase; P, uptake pump; T, transmitter (norepinephrine or serotonin).

tyramine is immediately inactivated by MAO. Hence, as long as hepatic MAO is functioning, dietary tyramine is prevented from reaching the general circulation and, therefore, is devoid of adverse effects.

In the presence of MAOIs, the picture is different. Dietary tyramine can produce a life-threatening hypertensive crisis. The mechanism of this reaction has three components. First, inhibition of neuronal MAO augments norepinephrine levels within the terminals of sympathetic neurons that regulate cardiac function and vascular tone. Second, inhibition of hepatic MAO allows dietary tyramine to pass directly through the liver and enter the systemic circulation intact. Third, on reaching peripheral sympathetic nerves, tyramine stimulates the release of the accumulated norepinephrine, thus causing massive vasoconstriction and excessive stimulation of the heart; hypertensive crisis results. There is a potential risk with the excessive hypertension that due to the sudden increase in BP, small vessels in the brain may hemorrhage.

To reduce the risk of tyramine-induced hypertensive crisis, the following precautions must be taken:

- MAOIs must not be dispensed to patients who are considered incapable of rigid adherence to dietary restrictions.
- Before an MAOI is dispensed, the patient must be fully informed about the hazard of ingesting tyramine-rich foods.
- The patient must be provided with a list of specific foods and beverages to avoid. These foods, which include most cheeses, yeast extracts, fermented sausages (e.g., salami, pepperoni, bologna), and aged fish or meat, are listed in Table 17–9.
- The patient should be instructed to avoid all drugs that are not specifically approved by the physician.

The patient should be informed about the symptoms of hypertensive crisis (headache, tachycardia, palpitations, nausea, vomiting) and instructed to notify the physician immediately if these develop. If the physician is unavailable, the patient should go directly to an emergency department.

In addition to tyramine, several other dietary constituents (e.g., caffeine, phenylethylamine) can precipitate hypertension if ingested by patients taking MAOIs. Foods that contain these compounds are listed in Table 17–9. The patient should be instructed to avoid them.

Drug Interactions

The MAOIs can interact with many drugs to cause potentially disastrous results. Accordingly, the patient should be instructed to avoid all medications—prescription agents and over-the-counter drugs—that have not been specifically approved by the physician. It is also wise to suggest that your patient wear a Medic Alert bracelet should an emergency situation arise in which the patient could not give information. This would alert medical personnel so that caution could be observed should there be a need for medications.

Indirect-Acting Sympathomimetic Agents. Indirect-acting sympathomimetics (e.g., ephedrine, amphetamine) are drugs that promote the release of norepinephrine from sympathetic nerves. Use of these agents by patients taking MAOIs can result in hypertensive crisis. The mechanism of this interaction is the same as that described for tyramine. The patient should be instructed to avoid all sympathomimetic drugs, including ephedrine, methylphenidate, amphetamines, and cocaine. Sympathomimetic agents may be present in cold remedies, nasal decongestants, and asthma medications; all of these preparations should be avoided unless approved by the physician.

Interactions Secondary to Inhibition of Hepatic Monoamine Oxidase. Inhibition of MAO in the liver can decrease the metabolism of several drugs, including epinephrine, norepinephrine, and dopamine. These drugs must be used with caution because their effects are intensified and prolonged.

Tricyclic Antidepressants and Selective Serotonin Reuptake Inhibitors. The combination of tricyclic antidepressants with MAOIs may produce hypertensive episodes or hypertensive crisis. As a result, this combination is not employed routinely. However, although potentially dangerous, the combination can benefit certain patients. If this combination is employed, caution must be exercised. SSRIs should not be used with MAOIs.

Antihypertensive Drugs. Combined use of MAOIs and antihypertensive agents may result in excessive lowering of BP. This response should be no surprise considering that MAOIs, by themselves, can cause hypotension.

Meperidine. Meperidine HCl (Demerol HCl) can cause *hyperpyrexia* (excessive elevation of temperature) in patients receiving MAOIs. Accordingly, if a strong analgesic is required, an agent other than meperidine should be chosen. Furthermore, the analgesic should be administered in its lowest effective dosage.

SELECTIVE SEROTONIN REUPTAKE INHIBITORS

Drugs that produce selective blockade of serotonin reuptake are now available (see Tables 17–7 and 17–8). These drugs are as effective as the tricyclic antidepressants and are safer, because of a better side effect profile and decreased risk of death by overdose. Fluoxetine, the most popular of these drugs, can be considered the prototype for the group. Accordingly, we focus our discussion on this agent.

Fluoxetine

Since its introduction, fluoxetine has become the most widely prescribed antidepressant in the United States. The drug is as effective as the tricyclic agents, causes fewer side effects, and is less dangerous when taken in overdosage.

Mechanism of Action. Fluoxetine causes selective inhibition of serotonin reuptake. This action is thought to underlie its antidepressant effects. The drug has no effect on dopamine or norepinephrine. In contrast with the tricyclic agents, fluoxetine does not block cholinergic, histaminergic, or α-adrenergic receptors. Furthermore, fluoxetine more commonly produces CNS excitation rather than sedation.

Pharmacokinetics. Fluoxetine is well absorbed after oral administration, even in the presence of food. The drug is widely distributed throughout the body and is highly bound (94%) to plasma proteins. Fluoxetine undergoes extensive hepatic conversion to norfluoxetine, a metabolite with pharmacological actions like those of fluoxetine itself. Norfluoxetine is eventually converted to inactive metabolites that are excreted in

---

TABLE 17–9 Foods That Can Interact With Monoamine Oxidase Inhibitors

FOODS THAT CONTAIN TYRAMINE

Category	Unsafe Foods (High Tyramine Content)	Safe Foods (Little or No Tyramine)
Vegetables	Avocados, especially if overripe; fermented bean curd; fermented soybean; soybean paste	Most vegetables
Fruits	Figs, especially if overripe; bananas, in large amounts	Most fruits
Meats	Meats that are fermented, smoked, or otherwise aged; spoiled meats; liver, unless *very* fresh	Meats that are known to be fresh (exercise caution in restaurants; meat may not be fresh)
Sausages	Fermented varieties: bologna, pepperoni, salami, others	Nonfermented varieties
Fish	Dried or cured fish; fish that is fermented, smoked, or otherwise aged; spoiled fish	Fish that is known to be fresh; vacuum-packed fish, if eaten promptly or refrigerated only briefly after opening
Milk, milk products	Practically all cheeses	Milk, yogurt, cottage cheese, cream cheese
Foods with yeast	Yeast extract (e.g., Marmite, Bovril)	Baked goods that contain yeast
Beer, wine	Some imported beers, Chianti wine	Major domestic brands of beer, most wines
Other foods	Protein dietary supplements, soups (may contain protein extract), shrimp paste, soy sauce	

FOODS THAT CONTAIN OTHER VASOPRESSORS

Food	Comments
Chocolate	Contains phenylethylamine, a pressor agent; large amounts can cause a reaction.
Fava beans	Contain dopamine, a pressor agent; reactions are most likely with overripe beans.
Ginseng	Headache, tremulousness, and manic-like reactions have occurred.
Caffeinated beverages	Caffeine is a weak pressor agent; large amounts may cause a reaction.

the urine. Because the drug has a long half-life (approximately 7 days), elimination of the drug may last weeks, especially in elders. The long half-life also allows for once-daily dosing. Steady-state plasma drug levels are reached after about 4 weeks.

Therapeutic Uses. Fluoxetine is used primarily to treat major depression. Antidepressant effects begin in 1 to 3 weeks and are equivalent to those produced by the tricyclics. The drug is also approved for OCDs and has been used to treat bulimia (DeVane, 1992; Grimseley & Jann, 1992; Jenike, Baer, & Greist, 1990).

Adverse Effects. The most common reactions to fluoxetine are nausea (21%), headache (20%), and manifestations of CNS stimulation including nervousness (15%), insomnia (14%), anxiety (10%), agitation and akathisia. Anorgasmia, delayed ejaculation, and other sexual dysfunctions occur frequently. Fluoxetine can cause dizziness and fatigue; patients should be warned against participation in hazardous activities (e.g., driving). Rash, which can be severe, has occurred in less than 4% of patients; in most cases, rashes readily respond to drug therapy (e.g., antihistamines, glucocorticoids) or to withdrawal of fluoxetine. Other common reactions include diarrhea (12%), excessive sweating (8%), and anorexia with associated weight loss (11%).

In contrast with the tricyclic agents, fluoxetine produces little or no cardiotoxicity, hypotension, or muscarinic blockade. Overdosage causes nausea, vomiting, and signs of CNS stimulation (e.g., agitation, restlessness, hypomania, seizures). Because fluoxetine is not cardiotoxic, overdosage is less dangerous than with the tricyclics and not likely to be fatal as a single agent overdose.

Drug Interactions. Fluoxetine should not be combined with MAOIs, because severe adverse effects have been reported. MAOIs should be withdrawn at least 14 days before starting fluoxetine. When fluoxetine is discontinued, at least 5 weeks should elapse before an MAOI is given due to its prolonged half-life by the metabolite norfluoxetine. **Serotonin syndrome,** a potentially life-threatening event, can occur from interaction with an MAOI. Symptoms include anxiety, diaphoresis, rigidity, hyperthermia, autonomic hyperactivity, and coma (Ciraulo & Shader, 1990a, 1990b; Sternbach, 1991). Gelenberg (1998d) suggested that any patient taking an antidepressant be warned about the possibility of withdrawal symptoms. He suggested using the mnemonic FINISH developed by Berber:

F = flu-like symptoms
I = insomnia
N = nausea
I = imbalance
S = sensory disturbances
H = hyperarousal (anxiety)

Fluoxetine inhibits a liver enzyme system (the cytochrome P-450 system) that is responsible for metabolizing many other drugs, including the tricyclic antidepressants. As a result, concentrations of these other drugs may increase, possibly to dangerous levels. Accordingly, caution should be exercised if these combinations are used.

Dosage and Administration. Fluoxetine may be taken with or without food. The initial dosage recommended by the manufacturer is 20 mg/day. Many patients, especially the elderly, are sensitive to the 20 mg/day dose and experience anxiety, agitation, and insomnia. In view of the many reports, the manufacturer began to distribute 10-mg capsules. This should be a consideration for the elderly and for patients who are known to be drug sensitive. If needed, the dosage may be increased gradually to a maximum of 80 mg/day; however, doses greater than 20 mg/day may increase toxicity more than they increase beneficial effects. If daily doses above 20 mg are used, they should be divided. Elderly patients and patients with impaired liver function should take lower doses.

Other Selective Serotonin Reuptake Inhibitors

In addition to fluoxetine, three other SSRIs are available: fluvoxamine maleate (Luvox), sertraline HCl (Zoloft), and paroxetine HCl (Paxil). All three drugs have properties similar to those of fluoxetine. They all produce selective blockade of serotonin reuptake, relieve symptoms of major depression, and cause CNS stimulation rather than sedation. Like fluoxetine, these drugs cause fewer anticholinergic effects than the tricyclics and less orthostatic hypotension. In addition, they are much safer than the tricyclics when taken in overdose. Common side effects include nausea, headache, nervousness, diarrhea, and insomnia. As with fluoxetine, the incidence of sexual dysfunction (especially anorgasmia) is high (Chouinard, Goodman, Greist, Jenike, & Rasmussen, 1990). A discussion regarding potential drug to drug interactions follows the sections Dual Mechanism Drugs and Other Novel Antidepressants.

Dual Mechanism Drugs

Venlafaxine (Effexor) and nefazodone HCl (Serzone) are the "dual mechanism" drugs. Venlafaxine inhibits both norepinephrine and serotonin uptake, providing a dual mechanism of action. There is minimal interaction with α-adrengergic, muscarinic, serotoninergic, histaminic, or opioid receptors. Recommended initial dosing is 75 mg/day in divided doses with increases every 4 days. Drug efficacy is reported in doses of 225 mg with a maximal dose of 375 mg/day.

Common side effects are nausea, somnolence, dizziness, dry mouth, and sweating. Of note and an important consideration is that venlafaxine causes an increase in BP (mean increase, <7.2 mmHg in diastolic pressure) (Product Monograph) in doses greater than 200 mg/day. BP monitoring is essential. Clinically significant elevations of BP warrant discontinuance of venlafaxine.

Nefazodone is structurally related to trazodone HCl (Desyrel) and was approved for treatment of major depression in December 1994. Studies have also found it to be efficacious in reducing the anxiety and sleep disturbances seen in depression and improving symptoms of premenstrual syndrome. Nefazodone, a phenylpiperazine, has a potent serotonin blocking effect and serotonin reuptake inhibition.

Drug efficacy is reported at doses between 300 and 600 mg/day. Dose initiation should begin at 100 mg twice a day and titrated every 4 to 7 days as tolerated until symptoms being to resolve. Elderly patients or those with concomitant medical problems should be started at 50 mg twice a day and titrated weekly, as tolerated. Side effects reported are headache, dry mouth, nausea, somnolence, and dizziness. These side effects, as with the other antidepressant medications, usually subside as the drug is tolerated. Nefazodone produces minimal sexual side effects.

OTHER NOVEL ANTIDEPRESSANTS

Mirtazapine is a piperazinoazepine and is a *tetracyclic* (four carbon rings). The neurochemical action includes antagonism of α_2-adrenergic receptors, which causes an increase in norepinephrine levels; serotonin$_2$ and serotonin$_3$ antagonism; and antihistaminergic properties. The main side effects include sleepiness and weight gain. Dosing for mirtazepine begins with 15 mg/day at intervals of 1 to 2 weeks to a maximal 45 mg/day. It is the first α_2 antagonist available for the treatment of depression in the United States.

Drug to Drug Interactions

All antidepressants have the potential for drug interactions. Antidepressant drugs differ in their protein-binding potential, which can affect their propensity for drug interactions. In general, all SSRIs are highly protein bound, increasing the risk for drug interactions. This potential can be of clinical importance especially when drugs such as digoxin and warfarin sodium (Coumadin) (often taken by the elderly) are prescribed because they have a narrow therapeutic window (as levels rise so does risk for toxicity).

Many drug interactions with antidepressants occur because of their effects on the cytochrome P-450 isoenzyme system. These enzymes are important because (1) enzymes catalyze chemical reactions and (2) many medications are metabolized by these enzymes. Thirty isoenzymes of P-450 have been identified and four families of these isoenzymes are recognized as being involved in drug metabolism. Drug labeling often includes what isoenzyme is used in metabolization to indicate possible drug interactions.

Inhibition of enzymes can lead to elevations in drug plasma levels with subsequent toxicity. Also, drug inhibitions can be associated with inefficacy of drug if that isoenzyme is needed to convert an inactive parent drug to the therapeutic active metabolite. One example is fluvoxamine, which contains a warning for potential theophylline toxicity. Fluoxetine and fluvoxamine inhibit the 2D6 isoenzyme, and they interact with tertiary amines (amitriptyline and imipramine). Because of this, both SSRIs can triple the concentration of imipramine. Nefazodone is a potent inhibitor of P-450 3A4. Also, a warning on the labeling includes the information that triazolam (Halcion) and alprazolam (Xanax) doses should be reduced by 50% to 75%, and astemizole (Hismanal) can be fatal if the drug is used coadministered with nefazodone.

When giving an antidepressant, be aware of drug interactions when there is coadministration of that drug and others as antihypertensives, anti–blood-clotting agents, and medications for allergies and sinusitis.

MISCELLANEOUS ANTIDEPRESSANTS

Trazodone

Trazodone blocks serotonin reuptake and may also stimulate serotonin receptors directly. Antidepressant effects take several weeks to develop and are equivalent to those of the tricyclic agents.

Common side effects are sedation, orthostatic hypotension, nausea, and vomiting. In contrast with the tricyclic agents, trazodone lacks anticholinergic actions and is not cardiotoxic. Accordingly, trazodone may be preferred for elderly patients and other persons for whom the cardiac and anticholinergic effects of the tricyclics may be intolerable.

Trazodone can cause *priapism* (prolonged, painful erection of the penis). In some cases, surgical intervention has been required. Priapism itself or the procedures required for relief can result in permanent impotence. Patients should be instructed to notify the physician or to go to an emergency department if persistent erection occurs. (Prolonged clitoral erection is exceedingly rare.)

Overdosage with trazodone is considered safer than with tricyclic agents or MAOIs. Death from overdosage with trazodone alone has not been reported, although death has occurred after overdosage with trazodone plus other CNS depressants.

Amoxapine

Amoxapine (Asendin) has both antidepressant and neuroleptic properties. Antidepressant effects are equivalent to those of the tricyclics.

Amoxapine has relatively weak anticholinergic and sedative properties. After overdosage, the risk of seizures with this drug is greater than with the tricyclics. Caution should be exercised in patients with epilepsy.

Like the antipsychotics, amoxapine can block receptors for dopamine. As a result, the drug can cause extrapyramidal side effects (e.g., parkinsonism, akathisia). Because of the risk of tardive dyskinesia (an extrapyramidal effect that develops with prolonged use of dopamine antagonists), long-term use of amoxapine should be avoided.

Bupropion

Bupropion HCl (Wellbutrin) is a unique antidepressant similar in structure to the amphetamines. Like the amphetamines, this agent has stimulant properties and suppresses appetite. Bupropion is devoid of the anticholinergic, antiadrenergic, and cardiotoxic effects associated with the tricyclic agents. Antidepressant effects begin in 1 to 3 weeks and are equivalent to those of the tricyclics. The mechanism by which depression is relieved is probably related to norepinephrine reuptake blockade via an active metabolite; however, it remains unknown.

Bupropion is generally well tolerated. The most common adverse effects are weight loss, dry mouth, and dizziness. Other undesired responses include tremor, agitation, and insomnia.

At doses greater than 450 mg/day, bupropion produces seizures in about 0.4% of patients. The risk of seizures is greatly increased in patients with predisposing factors, such as head trauma, preexisting seizure disorder, CNS tumor, and use of other drugs that lower seizure threshold.

Dosing must be done carefully to minimize the risk of seizures (risk is dose and serum level related). Dosage escalation must be done slowly. The initial dosage is 100 mg twice a day. After 4 days, the dosage can be increased to 100 mg three times a day. If necessary, the dosage can be increased to a maximal 150 mg three times a day.

Maprotiline

Although maprotiline HCl (Ludiomil) is structurally different from the tricyclic antidepressants (maprotiline has four rings rather than three), this drug is similar to the tricyclics with respect to therapeutic effects and side effects. The principal difference between these drugs is that maprotiline is more likely to cause seizures, even when used in moderate doses; after overdosage, about 30% of patients experience seizures. Because of the risk of seizures, maprotiline should not be taken by patients with a history of seizure disorders. The drug's side effect profile is summarized in Table 17-7. Usual dosages are shown in Table 17-8.

> **What do you think?** If a patient said to you, "I am scared to take Prozac, I hear it makes you suicidal," how would you respond?

➤ *Check Your Reading*

12. What is the usual time course for developing a therapeutic response to antidepressant drugs?
13. What are the most common adverse effects of the tricyclic antidepressants?
14. What is the most serious adverse effect of the tricyclic antidepressants?
15. Why are tyramine-containing foods dangerous for patients taking MAOIs?
16. What is the principal advantage of SSRIs over tricyclic antidepressants?

LITHIUM AND OTHER DRUGS FOR BIPOLAR DISORDER

Our topic in this section is drug therapy of bipolar disorder, also known as manic-depressive illness. For years, the mainstay of pharmacological therapy was lithium, and in 1996, valproic acid received the FDA approval for its use in the treatment of bipolar disorder. Let us examine an overview of bipolar disorder.

Clinical Manifestations

Before considering drug therapy, it is helpful to briefly review the characteristics of bipolar disorder. A more complete discussion of this illness can be found in Chapter 25.

Manic-depressive illness is a cyclic disorder characterized by recurrent fluctuations in mood. Typically, patients experience alternating episodes of mania and depression separated by periods in which mood is normal. The characteristics of depressive episodes are described in the preceding section and are not repeated here.

Manic episodes are characterized by heightened mood (euphoria), hyperactivity, excessive enthusiasm, and flight of ideas. Manic individuals display overactivity at work and at play and have a reduced need for sleep. Mania produces excessive sociability and talkativeness. Extreme self-confidence, grandiose ideas, and delusions of importance are common. Manic individuals frequently indulge in high-risk activities (e.g., questionable business deals, reckless driving, gambling, sexual indiscretions), giving no forethought to the consequences. Symptoms in the late stages of a manic episode may resemble those of paranoid schizophrenia (hallucinations, delusions, bizarre behavior).

As noted, most individuals with bipolar disorder go through alternating episodes of mania and depression. Untreated episodes of mania or depression generally last from 4 to 13 months. For the majority (approximately 70%) of patients, periods of normal mood separate the episodes of mania and depression. As time passes, manic and depressive episodes tend to occur more frequently.

Overview of Drug Therapy

Drug Selection

Drug therapy for bipolar disorder is summarized in Table 17-10. As indicated, the mainstay of therapy was lithium. In 1995, another drug, **valproic acid** (Depakene or Depakote) was approved by the FDA for use in the treatment of bipolar disorder. Lithium and valproic acid can provide symptomatic control during both the manic phase and the depressed phase. In addition, when taken prophylactically, both can reduce the frequency and severity of recurrent manic and depressive episodes. When used to control acute mania, lithium is often combined with a benzodiazepine (if symptoms are mild) or with an antipsychotic agent plus a benzodiazepine (if symptoms are severe). When used during the depressed phase, lithium is usually combined with an antidepressant. However, there is a risk that the antidepressant will transport the patient from depression into mania.

Many antiseizure drugs—**carbamazepine**, lamotrigine (Lamictal), and gabapentin (Neurontin)—have been used on an investigational basis to treat manic-depressive illness. These drugs can control symptoms during manic and depressive episodes and can provide prophylaxis against recurrent mania and depression. These agents represent an alternative to lithium for patients who fail to respond to lithium or who find its

TABLE 17-10 Drug Therapy for Bipolar Disorder	
ILLNESS PHASE	**DRUGS**
Manic phase	
Moderate symptoms	Lithium* + a benzodiazepine
Severe symptoms	Lithium* + an antipsychotic agent + a benzodiazepine
Depressive phase	Lithium + a tricyclic antidepressant or bupropion
Normalized phase	Lithium (for prophylaxis against recurrence of mania or depression)

*For lithium nonresponders, addition or substitution of carbamazepine or valproic acid may be helpful.

side cffccts intolerable (Semenchuk & Labiner, 1997; Gelenberg, 1998c).

Promoting Compliance

Poor patient compliance can frustrate attempts to treat acute manic episodes. Patients may resist treatment because they fail to see anything wrong with their thinking or behavior. Furthermore, the manic experience is not necessarily unpleasant. In fact, individuals going through a manic episode may well enjoy it. As a result, in order to ensure adequate treatment, hospitalization is often needed. To achieve this, collaboration with the patient's family may be required. Because hospitalization per se will not guarantee compliance, lithium administration should be observed to ensure that each dose is actually taken.

After an acute manic episode has been controlled, long-term prophylactic therapy is indicated, making compliance an ongoing concern. To promote compliance, the patient and family should be educated about the nature of manic-depressive illness and the importance of taking medication as prescribed. Family members can help to ensure compliance by overseeing medication use and by urging the patient to visit a physician or psychiatric clinic if a pattern of noncompliance develops.

Lithium

Lithium can provide symptomatic control in patients with manic-depressive illness. Beneficial effects were first described by John Cade, an Australian, in 1949. However, because of concerns about toxicity—lithium has a low therapeutic index—lithium was not approved for use in the United States until 1970. Because significant injury can occur when plasma drug levels are only slightly greater than the therapeutic level, monitoring of lithium levels is mandatory.

Lithium is a simple inorganic ion that carries a single positive charge. In the periodic table of elements, lithium falls within the same group as potassium and sodium. Accordingly, lithium has properties in common with these two elements. Trace amounts of lithium occur

naturally in animal tissues but has no known physiologic function.

PHARMACOKINETICS
Absorption and Distribution
Lithium is well absorbed after oral administration. The drug distributes evenly to all tissues and body fluids.

Excretion
Lithium has a short half-life, owing to rapid renal excretion. Because of its short half-life and high toxicity, the drug is usually administered in divided daily doses; large, single daily doses greater than 1500 mg are generally avoided. Because lithium is excreted by the kidneys, it must be used with great care in patients with renal impairment.

Sodium depletion decreases renal excretion of lithium, causing the drug to accumulate. Toxicity may result. Accordingly, it is important that sodium levels remain normal. Patients should be instructed to maintain normal sodium intake; a sodium-free diet cannot be used. Because diuretics promote lithium accumulation, these agents must be employed with caution. Sodium loss secondary to diarrhea causes renal sodium and lithium retention and can be sufficient to cause lithium accumulation leading to toxicity. Thus, the patient should be forewarned of this possibility.

Plasma Lithium Levels
Measurement of plasma lithium levels is an essential feature of treatment. Lithium levels must be kept below 1.5 mEq/L; levels greater than this can produce significant toxicity. For initial therapy of a manic episode, lithium levels should range from 0.8 to 1.2 mEq/L. Once the desired therapeutic effect has been achieved, the dosage should be reduced to produce maintenance drug levels of 0.4 to 1.0 mEq/L. Blood for lithium determinations should be drawn in the morning, 12 hours after the evening dose (Gerner & Stanton, 1992; Lehne, 1994b).

To keep lithium levels within the therapeutic range, plasma drug levels should be monitored routinely. Levels should be measured every 2 to 3 days at the beginning of treatment and every 1 to 3 months during maintenance therapy.

THERAPEUTIC USES
Manic-Depressive Illness
Lithium is a first-line drug of choice for controlling manic episodes in patients with manic-depressive illness and for long-term prophylaxis against recurrent mania and depression in these patients.

In manic patients, lithium reduces euphoria, hyperactivity, and other symptoms but does not cause sedation. Antimanic effects begin 5 to 7 days after the onset of treatment. However, full effects may not be seen until 2 to 3 weeks after therapy begins. For many patients, adjunctive therapy with a benzodiazepine or an antipsychotic agent can be helpful. Benzodiazepines (e.g., lorazepam [Ativan] and clonidine [Klonopin]) are used to provide sedation in patients with relatively mild symptoms of mania. Antipsychotics (e.g., haloperidol) may be required to provide rapid control in patients with severe symptoms.

Prophylaxis with lithium may not prevent episodes of depression. If depression occurs, adjunctive therapy with an antidepressant is indicated.

Other Uses

Although approved only for treatment of manic-depressive illness, lithium has been used with varying degrees of success in other psychiatric disorders, including alcoholism, bulimia, schizophrenia, and glucocorticoid-induced psychosis. Nonpsychiatric uses include hyperthyroidism, cluster headache, migraine, and syndrome of inappropriate secretion of antidiuretic hormone. In addition, lithium can raise neutrophil counts in children with chronic neutropenia and in patients receiving anticancer drugs or zidovudine (AZT).

MECHANISM OF ACTION

We do not know the underlying cause of manic-depressive illness, nor do we know how lithium stabilizes mood. Lithium has multiple effects on the nervous system. The drug can alter the synthesis, storage, release, and reuptake of neurotransmitters (norepinephrine, serotonin, dopamine, acetylcholine, γ-aminobutyric acid [GABA]). Also, lithium can alter the distribution of neuronally important ions (calcium, sodium, and magnesium). In addition, lithium can influence the function of second-messenger systems. Which, if any, of these actions underlies lithium's therapeutic effects is unknown.

ADVERSE EFFECTS

Adverse effects of lithium can be divided into two categories: (1) effects that occur at excessive drug levels and (2) effects that occur at therapeutic drug levels. In the discussion that follows, adverse effects produced at excessive lithium levels are considered as a group. Effects produced at therapeutic levels are considered individually.

Adverse Effects When Lithium Levels Are Excessive

Certain toxicities are closely correlated with the concentration of lithium in plasma. As indicated in Table 17–11, mild responses (e.g., fine hand tremor, gastrointestinal upset, thirst, muscle weakness) can develop at lithium levels that are still within the therapeutic range (i.e., below 1.5 mEq/L). When plasma levels exceed 1.5 mEq/L, more serious toxicities begin to appear. At drug levels above 2.5 mEq/L, death has resulted. Patients should be informed about early signs of toxicity and instructed to interrupt lithium use if these appear. The most common cause of lithium accumulation in compliant patients is sodium depletion.

Treatment of acute overdosage is primarily supportive; there is no specific antidote to lithium toxicity. The severely intoxicated patient should be hospitalized. Hemodialysis is an effective means of lithium removal and should be considered whenever drug levels exceed 2.5 mEq/L.

TABLE 17–11	Toxicities Associated With Excessive Plasma Levels of Lithium
PLASMA LITHIUM LEVEL (mEq/L)	**SIGNS OF TOXICITY**
<1.5	Nausea, vomiting, diarrhea, thirst, polyuria, lethargy, slurred speech, muscle weakness, fine hand tremor
1.5–2.0	Persistent GI upset, coarse hand tremor, confusion, hyperirritability of muscles, ECG changes, sedation, incoordination
2.0–2.5	Ataxia, giddiness, high output of dilute urine, serious ECG changes, fasciculations, tinnitus, blurred vision, clonic movements, seizures, stupor, severe hypotension, coma, death (usually secondary to pulmonary complications)
>2.5	Symptoms may progress rapidly to generalized convulsions, oliguria, and death

ECG, electrocardiogram; GI, gastrointestinal.

Adverse Effects When Lithium Is at Therapeutic Levels

Tremor. Patients may develop a fine hand tremor, especially in the fingers, that can interfere with writing and other motor skills. Lithium-induced tremor can be augmented by stress, fatigue, and certain drugs (e.g., antidepressants, antipsychotics, caffeine). Tremor can be reduced with a β-adrenergic blocking agent (e.g., propranolol HCl [Inderal]) and by measures that reduce peak levels of lithium (i.e., reduction of dosage, use of divided doses, or use of a sustained-release formulation).

Renal Toxicity. Long-term administration of lithium has occasionally been associated with degenerative changes in the kidney. The risk of renal injury can be reduced by keeping the serum levels in the therapeutic range. Kidney function should be assessed before treatment and once a year thereafter.

Goiter. Long-term use of lithium can cause *goiter* (enlargement of the thyroid gland). Although usually benign, lithium-induced goiter is sometimes associated with hypothyroidism. Treatment with thyroid hormone or withdrawal of lithium reverses thyroid hypertrophy. Measurement of thyroid hormones (T_3 and T_4) and thyroid-stimulating hormone should be obtained before treatment and annually thereafter.

Teratogenesis. Use of lithium during the 1st trimester of pregnancy is associated with a low incidence of birth defects (usually malformations of the heart). Accordingly, lithium is contraindicated during the 1st trimester of pregnancy. Furthermore, unless the benefits of therapy clearly outweigh the potential risk to the fetus, lithium should be avoided during the remainder of pregnancy as well. Women of childbearing age should be counseled about the importance of avoiding pregnancy while taking lithium.

Adverse Effects During Lactation. Lithium readily enters breast milk and can achieve concentrations that are potentially harmful to the nursing infant. Consequently, breast-feeding during lithium therapy should be discouraged.

Polyuria. Polyuria occurs in 50% to 70% of patients taking lithium chronically. In some patients, daily urine output may exceed 3 L. Lithium promotes polyuria by antagonizing the effects of antidiuretic hormone. To maintain adequate hydration, patients should be instructed to drink 8 to 12 glasses of fluids daily. Polyuria, nocturia, and excessive thirst can discourage patients from complying with the prescribed regimen.

Lithium-induced polyuria can be reduced with a thiazide diuretic. The mechanism of this paradoxical effect is not known. Unfortunately, thiazides can increase plasma levels of lithium. Accordingly, a reduction in lithium dosage is required.

DRUG INTERACTIONS
Diuretics
Diuretics promote sodium loss and can thereby increase the risk of lithium toxicity. Toxicity can occur because, in the presence of low sodium, renal excretion of lithium is reduced, causing lithium levels to rise.

Anticholinergic Drugs
Anticholinergic drugs can cause urinary hesitancy. Combined with lithium-induced polyuria, this effect can result in considerable discomfort. Unfortunately, the combination of lithium plus an anticholinergic drug cannot always be avoided. Patients frequently require concurrent therapy with agents that have prominent anticholinergic properties (e.g., antipsychotics, tricyclic antidepressants).

PREPARATIONS AND DOSAGE
Lithium is available as two salts: lithium carbonate and lithium citrate. With either salt, administration is oral. Lithium formulations and trade names are summarized in Table 17-12. Cautions pertaining to lithium are listed in Box 17-9.

Lithium can cause gastric upset. This can be reduced by administering lithium with meals or with milk.

Dosing with lithium is highly individualized. Dosage adjustments are based on plasma drug levels and clinical response.

Plasma drug levels should be kept within the therapeutic range. Levels between 0.8 and 1.2 mEq/L are generally appropriate for acute therapy of manic episodes. For maintenance therapy, lithium levels should range from 0.4 to 1.0 mEq/L. (Levels of 0.6 to 0.8 mEq/L are effective for most patients.) To avoid serious toxicity, lithium levels should not exceed 1.5 mEq/L.

Knowledge of plasma drug levels is not the only guide to lithium dosing; consideration of the clinical response is at least as important. When evaluating the appropriateness of a lithium dosage, we must not forget to look at the patient. Laboratory tests are all well and good, but they are not a substitute for clinical assessment. If, for example, blood levels of lithium appear proper, but clinical evaluation indicates toxicity, there is no question as to the action that should be taken; the dosage should be reduced, despite the apparent acceptability of the dosage as reflected by plasma drug levels.

Carbamazepine and Valproic Acid

Carbamazepine and valproic acid were originally developed and marketed for treatment of seizure disorders. Since then, these drugs have been used with success to treat patients with bipolar disorder. At this time, carbamazepine is reserved for patients who have failed to respond to lithium or who cannot tolerate the side effects of lithium (McElroy, Keck, Pope, & Hudson, 1992).

Carbamazepine was the first drug to be widely studied as an alternative to lithium for patients with manic-depressive illness. Like lithium, carbamazepine reduces symptoms during manic episodes and depressed episodes. In addition, the drug appears to provide effective prophylaxis against recurrence of mania and depression. For patients with severe mania and for those who *cycle,* that is, move rapidly between depression and mania,

TABLE 17–12 Lithium Preparations			
LITHIUM SALT	**FORMULATION**	**LITHIUM CONTENT***	**TRADE NAME**
Lithium carbonate (Li_2CO_3)	Capsules	4.06 mEq lithium (150 mg Li_2CO_3) 8.12 mEq lithium (300 mg Li_2CO_3) 16.24 mEq lithium (600 mg Li_2CO_3)	Eskalith, Lithonate
	Tablets	8.12 mEq lithium (300 mg Li_2CO_3)	Eskalith, Lithane, Lithotabs
	Tablets: slow release	8.12 mEq lithium (300 mg Li_2CO_3)	Lithobid
	Tablets: controlled release	12.18 mEq lithium (450 mg Li_2CO_3)	Eskalith CR
Lithium citrate	Syrup	8 mEq lithium/5 ml (equivalent to 300 mg Li_2CO_3)	Cibalith-S

*Lithium content is expressed in two ways: (1) milliequivalent (mEq) of lithium ion and (2) milligrams (mg) of the particular lithium salt of which the preparation is composed.

carbamazepine may be superior to lithium. When given to manic patients who have failed to respond to lithium, carbamazepine has had a success rate of about 60%. For treatment of acute manic episodes, the dosage should be low initially (200 to 400 mg/d) and then gradually increased to as much as 1.6 to 2.4 g/day. Lower doses should be employed when carbamazepine is used together with lithium, valproic acid, or an antipsychotic drug. The mechanism by which carbamazepine stabilizes mood is unknown.

Valproic acid, indicated for use in bipolar disorder, is also used as a first-line agent. Clinical studies indicate that valproic acid can control symptoms of acute manic episodes and can provide prophylaxis against recurrent episodes of mania and depression. Like carbamazepine, valproic acid appears especially useful for patients with rapid-cycling bipolar disorder. Dosing should be initiated at 10 to 15 mg/kg/day in one to three divided doses, increased by 5 to 10 mg/kg/day at weekly intervals until therapeutic levels are achieved. Valproic acid alters GABA-mediated neurotransmission, and this action may underlie the drug's mood-stabilizing effects. Valproic acid serum levels of at least 50 ng/ml are required for therapeutic efficacy.

Side effects include anorexia, nausea, vomiting, drowsiness (most common), and tremor. There also have been reported elevations in serum transaminases and hepatotoxicity, which is rare.

Gabapentin and lamotrigine are two anticonvulsant agents that appear to have mood-stabilizing properties. Until additional controlled studies have been performed, these agents should be reserved for the treatment of patients who do not respond to or who are unable to tolerate the standard treatments.

> **W**hat do you think? Imagine you are working with a patient diagnosed with bipolar disorder. After taking lithium for several months, the patient says to you, "If this is what feeling normal is like, you can have it. I prefer the highs of mania." How would you respond?

➤ *Check Your Reading*
17. What is the role of lithium in the treatment of bipolar disorder?
18. What is the reason for monitoring lithium blood levels?
19. What blood level of lithium should not be exceeded?
20. What is the relationship of sodium intake and sodium levels to lithium toxicity?
21. Which drugs are used as alternatives to lithium in treating bipolar disorder?

ANTIANXIETY AGENTS

Anxiety is a common complaint, and the drugs employed for treatment are prescribed widely. Drugs used to relieve anxiety are called **antianxiety agents** or **anxiolytics;** an older term for these drugs is *tranquilizers.*

Before the benzodiazepines became available, anxiety was treated with barbiturates and other general CNS depressants—drugs with multiple undesirable qualities. First, these drugs are potent respiratory depressants that can readily prove fatal in overdosage. As a result, they are "drugs of choice" for suicide. Second, because they produce subjective effects that many people find desirable, general CNS depressants have a high potential for abuse. Third, with prolonged use, most general CNS depressants produce significant tolerance and physical dependence. Fourth, barbiturates and certain other CNS depressants stimulate synthesis of hepatic drug-metabolizing enzymes and can thereby decrease responses to other drugs. Because benzodiazepines are just as effective as the general CNS depressants but do not share their undesirable properties, benzodiazepines have largely replaced the general CNS depressants for managing anxiety and insomnia.

Benzodiazepines

Benzodiazepines are drugs of first choice for treating anxiety. In addition, these agents are used to promote sleep, induce general anesthesia, and manage seizure disorders, muscle spasm, panic disorder, and withdrawal from alcohol (Lehne, 1994a). Benzodiazepines were introduced in the early 1960s and are among the most widely prescribed drugs in the United States. Perhaps the most familiar member of the benzodiazepine family is diazepam. The most frequently prescribed members are lorazepam and alprazolam.

The popularity of benzodiazepines stems from their clear superiority over the alternatives: barbiturates and other general CNS depressants. Benzodiazepines are safer than the general CNS depressants and have a lower potential for abuse. In addition, benzodiazepines produce less tolerance and physical dependence and are subject to fewer drug interactions.

Because all of the benzodiazepines produce similar effects, we consider the family as a group, rather than focusing on individual agents.

Overview of Pharmacological Effects

Practically all responses to benzodiazepines result from actions in the CNS. Benzodiazepines have few direct actions outside the CNS. All of the benzodiazepines produce a similar spectrum of responses. However, because of pharmacokinetic and potency differences, individual benzodiazepines may differ in their clinical applications.

CENTRAL NERVOUS SYSTEM

All beneficial effects of benzodiazepines and most adverse effects result from depressant actions in the CNS. With increasing dosage, effects progress from anxiolysis to sedation to hypnosis to stupor.

Benzodiazepines depress neuronal function at multiple sites throughout the CNS. These drugs reduce anxiety through effects on the limbic system, a neuronal network associated with emotionality. They promote sleep through effects on cortical areas and on the sleep-wake cycle. They induce muscle relaxation through effects on supraspinal motor areas, including the cerebellum. Two important side effects—confusion–cognitive dulling and amnesia—result from effects on the hippocampus and cerebral cortex.

CARDIOVASCULAR SYSTEM

When taken orally, benzodiazepines have negligible effects on the heart and blood vessels. In contrast, when administered IV—even in therapeutic doses—benzodiazepines can produce profound hypotension and cardiac arrest.

RESPIRATORY SYSTEM

Compared with the barbiturates, the benzodiazepines are weak respiratory depressants. When taken alone in therapeutic doses, these drugs produce little or no depression of respiration; with toxic doses, respiratory depression is moderate, at most. With oral therapy, clinically significant respiratory depression occurs only when benzodiazepines are combined with other CNS depressants (e.g., opioids, barbiturates, alcohol).

Mechanism of Action

Benzodiazepines potentiate the actions of GABA, the primary inhibitory neurotransmitter found throughout the CNS. These drugs enhance the actions of GABA by binding to specific receptors in a supramolecular structure known as the GABA receptor-chloride ion channel complex. Benzodiazepines do not act as direct GABA agonists.

Because benzodiazepines act by amplifying the actions of endogenous GABA, rather than by directly mimicking GABA, there is a limit to how much CNS depression these drugs can produce. This explains why benzodiazepines are so much safer than the barbiturates—drugs that can directly mimic GABA. Because benzodiazepines simply potentiate the inhibitory effects of endogenous GABA and because the amount of GABA in the CNS is finite, there is a built-in limit to the depth of CNS depression that the benzodiazepines can produce. In contrast, because the barbiturates are direct-acting CNS depressants, maximal effects are limited only by the amount of barbiturate administered.

Pharmacokinetics

ABSORPTION AND DISTRIBUTION

Most benzodiazepines are well absorbed after oral administration. Because of their high lipid solubility, benzodiazepines readily cross the blood-brain barrier to reach sites within the CNS.

METABOLISM

Most benzodiazepines undergo extensive metabolic alterations. With few exceptions, the metabolites are pharmacologically active. As a result, responses produced by administering a particular benzodiazepine often persist long after the parent drug has disappeared from the plasma. Hence, there may be a poor correlation between the plasma half-life of the parent drug and the duration of pharmacological effects. Flurazepam, for example, whose plasma half-life is only 2 to 3 hours, is converted into an active metabolite with a half-life of 50 hours. Hence, administration of flurazepam produces long-lasting effects, despite the fact that within 8 to 12 hours of its administration, flurazepam itself can no longer be detected in the blood. Diazepam has a similar long-acting metabolite, desmethyl-diazepam.

In patients with liver disease, metabolism of benzodiazepines can decline, thereby prolonging and intensifying responses. Because certain benzodiazepines (oxazepam, temazepam, and lorazepam) undergo little metabolic alteration, these agents may be preferred for patients with hepatic impairment.

TIME COURSE OF ACTION

Benzodiazepines differ significantly from one another with regard to time course of action. These agents differ in onset of action, duration of action, and tendency to accumulate with repeated dosing.

Because all of the benzodiazepines have essentially equivalent pharmacological actions, selection among these drugs is based, in large part, on differences in time course. For example, if a patient needs medication to accelerate falling asleep, a benzodiazepine with a rapid onset of action (e.g., triazolam) would be indicated. However, if medication is needed to prevent waking later in the night, a benzodiazepine with a slower onset (e.g., estazolam) would be preferred. For treatment of anxiety, a drug with an intermediate duration of action is desirable. For treatment of any benzodiazepine-responsive condition in the elderly, a drug such as lorazepam, which is not likely to accumulate with repeated dosing, is generally preferred.

Therapeutic Uses

The benzodiazepines have three principal indications: (1) anxiety, (2) insomnia, and (3) seizure disorders. In addition, these drugs are employed as preoperative medication and to manage muscle spasm, panic disorder, and withdrawal from alcohol. Although all benzodiazepines share the same pharmacological properties and therefore might be equally effective for all of these applications, not every benzodiazepine is actually employed for all potential uses. The principal factors that determine the actual applications of a particular benzodiazepine are the pharmacokinetic properties of the drug itself and the research and marketing decisions of pharmaceutical companies.

ANXIETY

Benzodiazepines are drugs of first choice for treating anxiety. Although all benzodiazepines have anxiolytic properties, only eight are marketed for this indication (Table 17-13). Anxiolytic effects result from depressing neurotransmission in the limbic system and cortical areas. Guidelines for managing anxiety with benzodiazepines are presented later in the chapter.

INSOMNIA

Benzodiazepines are drugs of first choice for treating insomnia. These drugs decrease latency time to falling asleep, reduce awakenings, and increase total sleeping time. Although all benzodiazepines can relieve insomnia, only a few are actually marketed for this use.

PANIC ATTACKS

Alprazolam, in high doses, provides effective treatment of panic disorder. Although several other medications, including SSRIs (e.g., fluoxetine), imipramine (a tricyclic antidepressant), and phenelzine (an MAOI) are also effective, only alprazolam and fluoxetine are actually approved by the FDA for this indication.

Adverse Effects

Benzodiazepines are generally well tolerated, and serious adverse reactions are rare. Compared with the barbiturates and other general CNS depressants, the benzodiazepines are remarkably safe drugs.

CENTRAL NERVOUS SYSTEM DEPRESSION

When taken in sleep-inducing doses, benzodiazepines cause drowsiness, lightheadedness, incoordination, and difficulty in concentrating. When these effects occur at bedtime, they are generally inconsequential. However, if sedation and other manifestations of CNS depression persist beyond waking, interference with daytime activities can occur.

PARADOXICAL PSYCHOLOGICAL EFFECTS

When employed to treat anxiety, benzodiazepines sometimes cause paradoxical responses, including insomnia, excitation, euphoria, heightened anxiety, and rage. If these reactions occur, benzodiazepines should be withdrawn. These reactions are more likely to occur in children, the elderly, and the developmentally disabled.

ANTEROGRADE AMNESIA

Benzodiazepines can cause *anterograde amnesia* (impaired recall of events that take place after commencement of treatment). Anterograde amnesia has been especially troublesome with triazolam. If patients complain of forgetfulness, the possibility of drug-induced amnesia should be evaluated.

RESPIRATORY DEPRESSION

Benzodiazepines are only weak respiratory depressants. Death from overdosage with oral benzodiazepines alone has never been documented. Hence, in contrast to the barbiturates, benzodiazepines present little risk as vehicles for suicide. It must be emphasized, however, that although respiratory depression with oral therapy is rare, benzodiazepines can cause severe respiratory depression when administered IV. In addition, substantial respiratory depression can result from combining oral benzodiazepines with other CNS depressants (e.g., alcohol, barbiturates, opioids).

TABLE 17-13 Major Drugs for Anxiety

GENERIC NAME	TRADE NAME	USUAL ADULT DOSAGE RANGE (mg/day)
Benzodiazepines		
Alprazolam	Xanax	.5–4
Chlordiazepoxide	Librium, others	15–100
Clorazepate dipotassium	Tranxene, Gen-Xene	7.5–60
Diazepam	Valium, others	2–40
Halazepam	Paxipam	80–60
Lorazepam	Ativan	2–4
Oxazepam	Serax	15–90
Prazepam	Centrax	10–60
Nonbenzodiazepine		
Buspirone HCl	BuSpar	10–40

Potential for Abuse

The abuse potential of the benzodiazepines is lower than that of the barbiturates and most other general CNS depressants. The behavior pattern that constitutes "addiction" is uncommon among patients who take benzodiazepines for therapeutic purposes. When asked about drug-use patterns, people who regularly abuse drugs rarely indicate a preference for benzodiazepines over barbiturates. Because their potential for abuse is low, benzodiazepines are classified under Schedule IV of the Controlled Substances Act. This contrasts with the barbiturates, most of which are classified under Schedule II or III.

Adverse Effects During Pregnancy and Lactation

Benzodiazepines are highly lipid soluble and can readily cross the placental barrier. Reports based on benzodiazepine use during the 1st trimester of pregnancy suggest an increased risk of congenital malformations, such as cleft lip, inguinal hernia, and cardiac anomalies. Use near term can cause CNS depression in the neonate. Because they present a risk to the fetus, most benzodiazepines are classified in FDA Pregnancy Category D (i.e., there is a proven risk of fetal harm, but, depending on the patient, the potential benefits of use during pregnancy may justify the risk). Four of these drugs—estazolam, quazepam, temazepam, and triazolam—are classified in Category X (i.e., the risks of use during pregnancy clearly outweigh any possible benefits). Women of child-bearing age should be warned about the potential for fetal harm and instructed to discontinue benzodiazepines if pregnancy occurs.

Benzodiazepines enter breast milk with ease and may accumulate to toxic levels in the breast-fed infant. Accordingly, these drugs should be avoided by nursing mothers.

Tolerance and Physical Dependence

With prolonged use of benzodiazepines, tolerance develops to some effects—but not to others. No tolerance develops to anxiolytic effects, and tolerance to hypnotic effects is generally low. In contrast, significant tolerance develops to antiseizure effects. Patients who are tolerant to barbiturates, alcohol, and other general CNS depressants show some cross-tolerance to benzodiazepines.

Benzodiazepines can cause physical dependence, but the incidence of substantial dependence is low. When benzodiazepines are discontinued after short-term use at therapeutic doses, the resultant withdrawal syndrome is generally mild and often goes unrecognized. Symptoms include anxiety, insomnia, sweating, tremors, and dizziness. Withdrawal from long-term high-dose therapy can elicit more serious reactions, such as panic, paranoia, delirium, hypertension, muscle twitches, and outright convulsions. Symptoms of withdrawal are usually more intense with benzodiazepines that have a short duration of action. With one agent—alprazolam—dependence may be a greater problem than with other benzodiazepines. Because benzodiazepine withdrawal syndrome can resemble an anxiety disorder, care must be taken to differentiate withdrawal from the return of original symptoms.

The intensity of withdrawal symptoms can be minimized by discontinuing treatment gradually. Doses should be tapered over several weeks. Substituting a benzodiazepine with a long half-life for one with a short half-life is also helpful. Patients should be warned against abrupt cessation of treatment. After discontinuation of treatment, patients should be monitored for 3 weeks for indications of withdrawal or recurrence of original symptoms.

Drug Interactions

Benzodiazepines undergo few important interactions with other drugs. Unlike barbiturates, benzodiazepines do not induce hepatic drug-metabolizing enzymes. Benzodiazepines therefore do not accelerate the metabolism of other drugs. Triazolam and alprazolam are metabolized by cytochrome P-450 3A4, and the levels can significantly increase when given with other drugs metabolized by this enzyme (e.g., nefazodone).

CENTRAL NERVOUS SYSTEM DEPRESSANTS

The CNS-depressant actions of benzodiazepines combine with those of other CNS depressants (e.g., alcohol, barbiturates, opioids). Although benzodiazepines are safe when used alone, these drugs can be extremely hazardous in combination with other depressants. Combined overdosage with a benzodiazepine plus another CNS depressant can cause profound respiratory depression, coma, and death. Patients should be warned against use of alcohol and all other CNS depressants.

Dosage and Administration

All benzodiazepines can be administered orally. In addition, three agents—diazepam, chlordiazepoxide, and lorazepam—may be administered parenterally (IM and IV). When used for sedation or induction of sleep, benzodiazepines are almost always administered by mouth. IM and IV administrations are reserved for acute management of alcohol withdrawal (chlordiazepoxide—IM), severe anxiety (lorazepam—IM), status epilepticus (diazepam—IV), and other emergencies. Dosages for anxiety are summarized in Table 17–13.

ORAL

Patients should be advised to take oral benzodiazepines with food if gastric upset occurs. Also, they should be instructed to swallow sustained-release formulations intact, without crushing or chewing. Patients should be warned not to increase the dosage or discontinue therapy without consulting the physician.

For treatment of uncomplicated insomnia, benzodiazepines should be given on an intermittent schedule (e.g., 3 or 4 d/wk) in the lowest effective dosage for the shortest duration required. This minimizes physical dependence and associated drug-dependency insomnia.

INTRAVENOUS

IV administration, rare in psychiatric practice, is hazardous and must be performed with care. Life-threatening reactions (e.g., severe hypotension, respiratory arrest, cardiac arrest) have occurred with diazepam. In addition, IV administration carries a risk of venous thrombosis, phlebitis, and vascular impairment.

To reduce complications from IV administration, the following precautions should be taken:

1. Inject the drug slowly.
2. Take care to avoid intraarterial injection and extravasation.
3. If direct venous injection is impossible, make the injection into infusion tubing as close to the vein as possible.
4. Follow the manufacturer's instructions regarding suitable diluents for preparing solutions.
5. Have facilities for resuscitation available.

Acute Toxicity

ORAL OVERDOSAGE

When administered in excessive dosage by mouth, benzodiazepines rarely cause serious toxicity. Symptoms include drowsiness, lethargy, confusion, and ataxia. Life-threatening cardiovascular and respiratory effects are uncommon. If an individual known to have taken an overdose of benzodiazepines does exhibit signs of serious toxicity, it is probable that another drug was taken as well.

INTRAVENOUS TOXICITY

When injected IV, even in therapeutic doses, benzodiazepines can cause severe adverse effects. Life-threatening reactions (e.g., profound hypotension, respiratory arrest, cardiac arrest) occur in approximately 2% of patients.

TREATMENT
General Treatment Measures

Benzodiazepine-induced toxicity is managed in the same fashion as toxicity from barbiturates and other general CNS depressants. Oral benzodiazepines can be removed from the body with gastric lavage followed by ingestion of activated charcoal and a saline cathartic; dialysis may be helpful if symptoms are especially severe. Respiration should be monitored, and the airway should be kept patent. Support of BP with IV fluids and norepinephrine may be required.

Treatment With Flumazenil

Flumazenil (Romazicon) is a competitive benzodiazepine-receptor antagonist. The drug can reverse the sedative effects of benzodiazepines but may not reverse benzodiazepine-induced respiratory depression. Flumazenil is approved for treating benzodiazepine overdosage and for reversing the effects of benzodiazepines following general anesthesia. The principal adverse effect is precipitation of convulsions. This effect is most likely in patients taking benzodiazepines to treat epilepsy and in patients who are physically dependent on benzodiazepines.

Buspirone

Buspirone HCl (BuSpar) is a relatively new and different antianxiety medication. The drug has minimal CNS-depressant actions and does not enhance the depressant effects of alcohol, barbiturates, and other general CNS depressants. Buspirone is said to reduce anxiety while producing even less sedation than benzodiazepines. The drug is devoid of hypnotic, muscle relaxant, and anticonvulsant actions.

Mechanism of Action

The mechanism by which buspirone acts has not been established. The drug binds with high affinity to receptors for serotonin type 1A and with lower affinity to receptors for dopamine. Buspirone does not bind to receptors for GABA or benzodiazepines.

Therapeutic Uses

Buspirone is labeled for short-term treatment of anxiety; however, when taken for as long as 1 year, the drug showed no reduction in antianxiety actions. For treatment of anxiety, the drug appears to be as effective as benzodiazepines. Buspirone lacks sedative effects and is not indicated for insomnia. Patients may feel that buspirone is not working because of a delayed onset of action and want to stop taking the medication. Onset of efficacy is usually reported at about a week, whereas with benzodiazepines, relief from anxiety is reported almost immediately. Use of buspirone is discussed further in the section Management of Anxiety later in the chapter.

Adverse Effects and Drug Interactions

Buspirone is generally well tolerated. The most common reactions are dizziness, nausea, headache, nervousness, lightheadedness, and excitement. The drug is nonsedative and does not interfere with daytime activities. Furthermore, the drug poses little or no risk of suicide; huge doses (375 mg/d) have been given to healthy volunteers with only moderate effects (e.g., nausea, vomiting, dizziness, drowsiness, miosis). Buspirone does not enhance the depressant effects of alcohol, barbiturates, and other general CNS depressants.

Tolerance, Dependence, and Abuse

Buspirone has been used for up to 1 year without evidence of tolerance, physical dependence, or psychological dependence. No withdrawal symptoms have been observed on termination of treatment. There is no cross-tolerance between buspirone and benzodiazepines, barbiturates, or other sedative-hypnotics.

To date, there is no evidence that buspirone has a liability for abuse. Accordingly, the drug is not regulated under the Controlled Substances Act.

Management of Anxiety

Anxiety is a nearly universal experience that often serves an adaptive function. When anxiety is moderate and situationally appropriate, drug therapy may not be needed or even desirable. In contrast, for patients with generalized anxiety disorder (GAD), symptoms are prolonged and potentially disabling; hence, anxiolytic therapy is frequently required.

Situational Anxiety Versus Generalized Anxiety Disorder

SITUATIONAL ANXIETY
Situational anxiety is a normal response to a stressful situation (e.g., family problems, school, test-taking, financial difficulties). Although symptoms may be intense, they are also temporary. If necessary, drugs can be used to provide relief, but treatment should be short-term. Situational anxiety is common among patients with medical illnesses and those anticipating surgery.

GENERALIZED ANXIETY DISORDER
The hallmark of GAD is unrealistic or excessive anxiety about two or more life circumstances that lasts for 6 months or longer. Other psychological manifestations include vigilance, tension, apprehension, poor concentration, and difficulty falling or staying asleep. Somatic manifestations include trembling, muscle tension, restlessness, and signs of autonomic hyperactivity (e.g., palpitations, tachycardia, sweating, clammy hands).

Treatment of GAD consists of psychotherapy and anxiolytic drugs. Psychotherapy provides support and encouragement and can improve coping abilities in anxiety-provoking situations. For some patients, this therapy may be all that is needed. However, if symptoms are intensely uncomfortable or disabling, antianxiety drugs are indicated. In most cases, benzodiazepines are preferred. Along with psychotherapy and drugs, the treatment program can include relaxation therapy (e.g., meditation, relaxation exercises, biofeedback) to reduce tension.

Drug Therapy of Anxiety

BENZODIAZEPINES
Benzodiazepines are drugs of first choice for anxiety. These widely used agents have rendered older anxiolytics obsolete. Because all benzodiazepines have similar CNS effects, selection among these drugs is largely a matter of prescriber's preference. Dosages for anxiety are summarized in Table 17–13.

Since the introduction of benzodiazepines in the 1960s, attitudes toward these drugs have changed. When they first became available, benzodiazepines were used somewhat indiscriminately. In all probability, many people who did not really need these drugs were receiving them. Because of the freedom with which benzodiazepines had been dispensed, physicians were sometimes accused of poor medical practice. Furthermore, the frequent use of benzodiazepines led to public concerns about addiction. In response to these developments, two changes took place: (1) physicians restricted their prescribing of benzodiazepines and (2) patients tended to self-administer less medication than had been prescribed. The unfortunate result is that overtreatment was to some extent replaced with undertreatment.

The current consensus is that benzodiazepines have a completely legitimate role in the therapy of severe anxiety and that these drugs, like all others, must simply be used with discretion. When they are clearly indicated, benzodiazepines should be prescribed in a sufficient dosage and for a sufficient duration to achieve their objective: relief of symptoms and improvement of overall function. To help ensure that benzodiazepines are taken as prescribed, patients should be made to feel that their use of an anxiolytic is appropriate and that they should not be ashamed of their legitimate medical need.

It is difficult to predict how long anxiolytic drugs should be taken. To determine the need for continued therapy, patients should be reevaluated on a regular basis. In some cases, use of an "on-off" dosing schedule may be helpful. In such a regimen, treatment is interrupted periodically (e.g., every 6 to 8 wk). If anxiety returns, treatment can resume.

BUSPIRONE
Buspirone is an alternative to benzodiazepines for treating anxiety. This drug differs from benzodiazepines in four important ways:

1. It does not cause sedation.
2. It has no abuse potential.
3. It does not potentiate other CNS depressants.
4. Its antianxiety effects take 1 week to begin and several weeks to reach their peak.

Because therapeutic effects are delayed, buspirone is not suitable for patients who need immediate relief, nor is it suitable for use on an as needed basis. Because buspirone has no abuse potential, the drug may be especially appropriate for patients known to abuse alcohol and other drugs. Because it lacks depressant properties, buspirone is an attractive alternative to benzodiazepines in patients who require long-term therapy but who cannot tolerate benzodiazepine-induced sedation and psychomotor slowing. Buspirone does not display cross-dependence with benzodiazepines. Hence, when patients are switched from benzodiazepines to buspirone, the benzodiazepine should be tapered off while initiating buspirone (to prevent a withdrawal syndrome). Patients who have taken benzodiazepines should be told that buspirone does not produce sedation and that its effects take 1 week or more to develop; this information allows expectations to be realistic.

BETA-BLOCKERS
β-Adrenergic blocking agents (e.g., propranolol) can relieve symptoms caused by autonomic hyperactivity

(tachycardia). These drugs may be most valuable as an aid to coping with situational anxiety, such as that experienced by individuals who are overly apprehensive about public speaking.

➤ *Check Your Reading*

22. Why are benzodiazepines preferred to barbiturates and other general CNS depressants for treating anxiety?
23. What are physical dependence and withdrawal concerns with benzodiazepine therapy?
24. What are the principal differences between benzodiazepines and buspirone?
25. How long should antianxiety therapy last?

NURSING PROCESS

In the past, initiation of psychopharmacological intervention was the prerogative of the treating psychiatrist, but more than 40 states have granted prescriptive authority to Certified Specialists in Psychiatric and Mental Health Nursing. Regardless of whether the prescriber is a psychiatrist or an advanced practice nurse, the decision about which medication to use is based on several factors, including the patient's preference and responsiveness to particular drugs in the past; a family member's treatment response; the drug's side effect profile; and the clinician's own observations about efficacy. Often, however, the decision to change to another medication is based on the observations and documentation of nurses regarding the patient's responsiveness or lack of responsiveness to a medication. Therefore, it is imperative that you understand not only the goals of treatment but also the effects of medications. The application of the nursing process to the patient receiving psychopharmacologic therapy depends on the specific patient and the specific disorder being treated. However, to give an example of the application of the nursing process to the patient receiving psychopharmacologic therapy, we consider the psychopharmacologic treatment of schizophrenia. To begin, let us take a look at Case Example 17–1 to understand the importance of medication issues to the schizophrenic patient.

■ CASE EXAMPLE 17–1
■ Loren's Story

Loren Evans was a 35-year-old woman who was separated from her husband. The couple had been married for 15 years and were parents of two boys, ages 8 and 11, who were in the custody of their father. Loren had a diagnosis of schizophrenia, chronic undifferentiated type. The onset of her illness occurred when she was an 18-year-old sophomore in college, majoring in nursing. She reported several inpatient admissions and was being treated on an outpatient basis at a research center. She attended weekly group therapy sessions. Over the past 3 years, Loren participated in several drug treatment protocols and was

now in a study designed to determine the lowest possible dose of a neuroleptic required to control psychotic symptoms. The protocol required that Loren go on a drug-free trial period from the medication regimen of fluphenazine 10 mg three times a day.

To observe for signs and symptoms of recurring illness, she had been referred to a home health agency. A request was made for a psychiatric certified specialist to perform weekly assessments to monitor mental status as Loren was titrated off medication and to perform health teaching about the earliest prodromal symptoms signaling impending acute recurrence. Loren has been medication-free for the past 3 months. During that time, she experienced three major stressors: (1) the break-up of a relationship with an older man; (2) an allergic reaction to penicillin, which was treated with prednisone; and (3) refusal by her estranged husband to allow Loren unsupervised visits with her children. Over the past 2 weeks, Loren has exhibited mild anxiety and difficulty sleeping. She also has expressed dissatisfaction with her outpatient treatment and has expressed an intent to withdraw from the program. The certified specialist was concerned that Loren was beginning to exhibit subtle signs and symptoms of impending illness and reported her observations to the treatment team at Loren's outpatient program. Two days after the last home visit, Loren presented at her therapy session in an acutely agitated state and was subsequently admitted to an inpatient unit with a diagnosis of acute exacerbation of schizophrenia, chronic undifferentiated type. She was again started on an antipsychotic medication, and 2 weeks after the admission was discharged to an outpatient program. She exercised her right to refuse treatment at the research center and opted instead for a day treatment program, which combined pharmacological interventions with a psychosocial component.

Initial Phase of Illness

Assessment

During the initial phase of the patient's illness, you assess the presence of psychotic behavior. Questions you might ask include the following:

Are there any true drug allergies?
Is the patient willing to take the medication? If so, by what route?
Is the patient likely to cheek or hide pills in her mouth?
Is she more likely to swallow a liquid preparation?
Will the patient require IM administration of medication?
Is the patient aggressively acting out? If so, will you need help in administering medication?
Does the patient understand the need for medication?
Does the patient exhibit movement disorders from use of neuroleptic medication? You will administer the AIMS to assess for this (see Box 17–5).

Diagnosis

The nursing diagnosis during the initial phase of treatment might be Ineffective Individual Coping related to auditory hallucinations as evidenced by agitation, pacing, insomnia, and threatening gestures.

Outcome Identification

The expected outcome of the initial phase of treatment is normalization of behavior and is expressed as follows. The patient's behavior will return to normal as evidenced by cessation of agitation, pacing, and threatening gestures and by sleeping 7 to 8 hours per night at the end of 1 week of receiving antipsychotic medication.

Planning and Implementation

Because the patient is in a state of acute psychosis and may be uncooperative to the point of refusing medication (particularly pills, which are easily cheeked), you need to plan "how" medication will be administered. For instance, in the case of a patient who is a threat to others, you might obtain an order to administer the medication IM. You must know which medications are available in IM and in liquid forms and which are not. You can change the form of medication (pill to liquid) without the physician's order, but you cannot change the route of administration (oral to IM) without a specific written order. Indeed, in an acutely ill patient a liquid preparation has a more rapid onset of action than the pill form. You are exercising clinical judgment in determining the form of medication to readily achieve the aim of bringing behavior under control.

Evaluation

In the first phase of treatment, successful medication management is demonstrated by a decrease in the level of agitation, hostility, combativeness, and aggressiveness displayed by the patient. Also, usual patterns of sleeping and eating begin to return.

Second Phase of Illness

Assessment

The second phase of the patient's illness is characterized by stabilization. This phase extends from 1 to 3 weeks and is characterized by the gradual reduction in the medication dosage. During the phase of stabilization, you monitor the patient's behavior for any signs and symptoms of recurring illness. It is during this phase that you assess for improvement in socialization, mood, and self-care activities. Because the patient may no longer be acutely psychotic and may be amenable to health teaching, you assess the patient's level of knowledge about the illness and the medications.

Diagnosis

The nursing diagnosis during the phase of stabilization might be Knowledge Deficit about the effects and side effects of antipsychotic medications related to unfamiliarity with the illness and treatment as evidenced by patient's verbalization of incomplete or inaccurate information.

Outcome Identification

The expected outcome of the stabilization phase is as follows. The patient and family will be able to state the positive effects and side effects of the prescribed antipsychotic medication and will verbalize willingness to adhere to medication schedule.

Planning and Implementation

Plan, based on assessment of willingness to learn, intellectual functioning capabilities, and barriers to learning (e.g., language), how to teach the patient and the patient's family about the illness as well as the medications that the patient is taking. Teaching focuses on identifying prodromal signs and symptoms and on encouraging the patient's active cooperation in self-reporting symptoms. The patient can be taught to be aware of even the slightest feelings of tension, anxiety, and unusual thoughts. Medication teaching focuses on knowing what the medication does, what side effects it produces, how to cope with side effects, and any adverse effects that the patient needs to monitor (Box 17-10).

Figures 17-3 through 17-5 show sample medication teaching tools that are appropriate to use in patient and family education for patients with schizophrenia. Figures 17-6 through 17-8 show similar teaching tools for use in patient and family education for patients with depression, mania, or anxiety.

Evaluation

Evaluation of the teaching plan can be done by verbal return demonstration to show that the patient understands the teaching, or a written test can be used to evaluate the level of learning that has taken place. Another technique is to have the patient pick out the medications they will take and state the prescribed time. Figure 17-9 shows a sample medication pretest and posttest used in evaluation.

Box 17-10 ■ ■ ■ ■ ■
Patient Education

- Do not give too much information at one time.
- Use reinforcement.
- Give written and oral information.
- Involve family or significant others.

Text continued on page 455

Patient: _____

Provider: _____

Date: _____

THORAZINE FACT SHEET

Trade Name: Thorazine

Generic Name: chlorpromazine

Purpose: To relieve the symptoms of your illness, including voices, visions, bothersome thoughts that you can't control, excessive fearfulness, believing people are saying bad things about you, thinking you have special powers, etc.

Warnings:
- Notify your doctor if pregnant or planning a pregnancy.
- Do not drive or operate machinery until you know how you will react to this medicine.
- Avoid drinking alcohol while taking this medicine.
- If your skin or the whites of your eyes get yellow or you get unexplainable sore throat, fever, and weakness, call your doctor *IMMEDIATELY.*
- Can cause tardive dyskinesia (TD). *IF* this occurs, it is slowly progressive, potentially irreversible involuntary movements of mouth, lips, and extremities. Your doctor will monitor and discuss continuing this medication with you.
- Always tell your doctor *all* medicines you are taking.
- Do not stop taking your medicine without your doctor's approval. The dosage should be slowly decreased. Stopping all at once may cause withdrawal symptoms.
- Do not give this medication to other people.
- If you need an antacid, take it two hours before or after this medication.
- During summer when it is hot and you are sweating more, increase fluids.
- If you have a seizure disorder, the frequency or severity of seizures may increase. Tell your doctor right away.

Common Side Effects	What To Do
Shakiness, restlessness, stiffness, thick tongue, neck twisting, eyes rolling up	Take your _____ as prescribed. This medication is used to treat these symptoms. If you have no medication to treat these symptoms, call your doctor or go to Emergency Room.
Dizziness	Drink fluids, change position slowly.
Blurred vision	Should clear up in 2–3 weeks.
Sensitivity to the sun	Wear a sun block outside. Wear protective clothing.
Constipation	Eat bulk foods, drink fluids, drink prune juice, exercise.
Dry mouth	Suck on sugarless hard candy or chew gum. Practice meticulous dental care.

- You are taking _____ mg _____ times a day. Do not stop taking without your doctor's supervision as your symptoms may occur.
- If you miss a dose and remember within 2–3 hours, take it. Otherwise, skip it and take remaining doses as scheduled. DO NOT double up.

Figure 17–3
Medication teaching tool for chlorpromazine (Thorazine). (From Carson, V. B. [1994]. *Bay area psychiatric home care manual.* Baltimore: Bay Area Health Care. Copyright © 1994, Bay Area Health Care.)

Patient: _____

Provider: _____

Date: _____

CLOZARIL FACT SHEET

Trade Name: Clozaril

Generic Name: clozapine

Purpose: To relieve the symptoms of your illness, including voices, visions, bothersome thoughts that you can't control, excessive fearfulness, believing people are saying bad things about you, thinking you have special powers, etc.

Warnings:
- This drug can cause your white blood cell count to fall very low (agranulocytosis) and reduce your ability to fight infection. Weekly blood tests are essential. Your prescription cannot be filled without proof of weekly blood tests.
- Do not drive or operate machinery until you know how you will react to this medicine.
- Avoid drinking alcohol while taking this medicine.
- Always tell your doctor *all* medicines you are taking.
- Do not stop taking your medicine without your doctor's approval. The dosage should be slowly decreased. Stopping all at once may cause withdrawal symptoms.
- Do not give this medication to other people.
- If you need an antacid, take it two hours before or after this medication.
- During summer when it is hot and you are sweating more, increase fluids.
- Keep all appointments with your doctor and the laboratory so that your response to this drug can be evaluated. Your dose may need to be adjusted, especially during the first few weeks.

Common Side Effects	What To Do
Flu-like symptoms, sore throat, weakness, fever, mouth sores, any sign of infection	Stop taking clozapine and contact your prescriber immediately.
Seizures, tremor	Stop taking clozapine and contact your prescriber immediately.
Fast or irregular heart beat, difficulty breathing	Stop taking clozapine and contact your prescriber immediately.

- You are taking _____ mg _____ times a day. Do not stop taking without your doctor's supervision as your symptoms may occur.
- If you miss a dose and remember within 2–3 hours, take it. Otherwise, skip it and take remaining doses as scheduled. DO NOT double up.

Figure 17–4
Medication teaching tool for clozapine (Clozaril). (Modified from Carson, V. B. [1994]. *Bay area psychiatric home care manual.* Baltimore: Bay Area Health Care. Copyright © 1994, Bay Area Health Care.)

Patient: _____

Provider: _____

Date: _____

PROLIXIN FACT SHEET

Trade Name: Prolixin

Generic Name: fluphenazine

Purpose: To relieve the symptoms of your illness, including voices, visions, bothersome thoughts that you can't control, excessive fearfulness, believing people are saying bad things about you, thinking you have special powers, etc.

Warnings:
- Notify your doctor if pregnant or planning a pregnancy.
- Do not drive or operate machinery until you know how you will react to this medicine.
- Avoid drinking alcohol while taking this medicine.
- If your skin or the whites of your eyes get yellow or you get unexplainable sore throat, fever and weakness, call your doctor *IMMEDIATELY.*
- Can cause tardive dyskinesia (TD). *IF* this occurs, it is slowly progressive, irreversible involuntary movements of mouth, lips and extremities. Your doctor will monitor and discuss continuing this medication with you.
- Always tell your doctor *all* medicines you are taking.
- Do not stop taking your medicine without your doctor's approval. The dosage should be slowly decreased. Stopping all at once may cause withdrawal symptoms.
- Do not give this medication to other people.
- If you need an antacid, take it two hours before or after this medication.
- During summer when it is hot and you are sweating more, increase fluids.
- If you are allergic to aspirin or yellow dye (present in some foods and medications), tell your doctor.
- If you have ever had a bad reaction to insulin, shock therapy or any other tranquilizer, notify your doctor immediately.
- Before *any type* of surgery with a general anesthetic, tell the doctor you are taking prolixin.

Common Side Effects	What To Do
Shakiness, restlessness, stiffness, thick tongue, neck twisting, eyes rolling up	Take your _____ as prescribed. This medication is used to treat these symptoms. If you have no medication to treat these symptoms, call your doctor or go to Emergency Room.
Dizziness	Drink fluids, change position slowly.
Blurred vision	Should clear up in 2–3 weeks.
Sensitivity to the sun	Wear a sun block outside. Wear protective clothing.
Constipation	Eat bulk foods, drink fluids, drink prune juice, exercise.
Dry mouth	Suck on sugarless hard candy or chew gum. Practice meticulous dental care.

- You are taking _____ mg _____ times a day. Do not stop taking without your doctor's supervision as your symptoms may occur.
- If you miss a dose and remember within 2–3 hours, take it. Otherwise, skip it and take remaining doses as scheduled. DO NOT double up.

Figure 17–5
Medication teaching tool for fluphenazine (Prolixin). (From Carson, V. B. [1994]. *Bay area psychiatric home care manual.* Baltimore: Bay Area Health Care. Copyright © 1994, Bay Area Health Care.)

Patient: _____

Provider: _____

Date: _____

PAMELOR FACT SHEET

Trade Name: Pamelor

Generic Name: nortriptyline

Purpose: This drug is used to treat depression.

Warnings:
- This drug can take 2–3 weeks to work.
- Do not drive or operate machinery until you know how you'll react to this medication.
- Always tell your doctor *all* medicines you are taking.
- See your doctor regularly for check-ups.
- Ask your doctor for advice about drinking alcoholic beverages.
- Women who are pregnant, plan to become pregnant, or are breast-feeding should inform their doctor.
- Do not allow anyone else to take this medication.
- Before surgery, inform your doctor you are taking this drug.
- This drug can cause an irregular heart beat.

Common Side Effects	What To Do
Drowsiness, weakness, tiredness, excitement, insomnia, blurred vision, difficulty urinating	Take this drug at bedtime if it causes drowsiness. Take this drug in the morning if it causes insomnia. If you take the drug more than once a day, ask your doctor if you can take it all at once. These symptoms should decrease over time. If they do not, contact your doctor.
Dizziness, lightheadedness, faintness when getting up from a sitting or lying position	Get up slowly.
Persistent fine tremor; shuffling walk; slow speech; difficulty swallowing; drooling; slow, jerky movements; jaw, neck, and back muscle spasms; inability to sit still; sore throat; fever; skin rash; yellowing of skin or eyes; irregular heart beat	Contact your doctor.
Sensitivity to the sun	Wear protective clothing and sunscreen when out in the sun.
Constipation, difficulty urinating, blurred vision	Contact your doctor if these symptoms are severe or persist.

- You are taking _____ mg _____ times a day. Your schedule is _____ .
- If you miss a dose and remember within 2–3 hours, take it. Otherwise, skip it and take the remaining doses as scheduled. DO NOT double up.

Figure 17–6

Medication teaching tool for nortriptyline (Pamelor). (Modified from Carson, V. B. [1994]. *Bay area psychiatric home care manual.* Baltimore: Bay Area Health Care. Copyright © 1994, Bay Area Health Care.)

Patient: _____

Provider: _____

Date: _____

NARDIL FACT SHEET

Trade Name: Nardil

Generic Name: phenelzine

Purpose: This drug is a monoamine oxidase inhibitor (MAOI) and is used to treat depression and anxiety.

Warnings:
- Avoid foods and beverages containing tyramine while taking medication and for two weeks after stopping medication. These foods and beverages include avocados (especially if overripe); fermented bean curd; fermented soybean; soybean paste; figs (especially if overripe); bananas (in large amounts); meats that are fermented, smoked, or otherwise aged; spoiled meats; liver (unless *very* fresh); fermented sausages such as bologna, pepperoni, and salami; dried or cured fish; fish that is fermented, smoked, or otherwise aged; spoiled fish; practically all cheeses; yeast extract (e.g., Marmite, Bovril); imported beers; Chianti wine; protein dietary supplements; soups (may contain protein extract); shrimp paste; and soy sauce. Also avoid chocolate, fava beans, ginseng, and caffeinated beverages.

- If you experience a severe headache, neck stiffness or soreness, nausea or vomiting, sweating (with fever or cold, clammy skin), dilated (large) pupils and increases sensitivity to light, and rapid or slow heart beat with chest pain, stop taking the medication and call your doctor immediately. These may be signs of an extreme rise in blood pressure.

- Do not drive or operate machinery until you know how you will react to this medication.

- Always tell your doctor *all* medicines you are taking and never take any medicines or drugs without asking your doctor first.

- See your doctor regularly for check-ups.

- Do not stop taking this medication without talking to your doctor.

- Ask your doctor for advice about drinking alcoholic beverages.

- Women who are pregnant, plan to become pregnant, or are breast-feeding should inform their doctor.

Common Side Effects	**What To Do**
Dizziness; lightheadedness; faintness when getting up from a sitting or lying position.	Get up slowly.
Dry mouth.	Suck sugarless hard candy or chew sugarless gum.
Restlessness; difficulty sleeping; constipation; difficulty urinating; loss of appetite; drowsiness; weakness; fatigue; rash; swelling of feet, ankles or lower legs; blurred vision; decreased sexual ability.	Contact your doctor if these symptoms persist or are severe.

- You are taking _____ mg nardil _____ times a day. Your schedule is _____

- If you miss a dose and remember within 2–3 hours, take it. Otherwise, skip it and take remaining doses as scheduled. DO NOT double up.

Figure 17-7
Medication teaching tool for phenelzine (Nardil). (Modified from Carson, V. B. [1994]. *Bay area psychiatric home care manual.* Baltimore: Bay Area Health Care. Copyright © 1994, Bay Area Health Care.)

Patient: _____

Provider: _____

Date: _____

LITHIUM FACT SHEET

Trade Names: Cibalith-S, Eskalith, Eskalith CR, Lithane, Lithobid, Lithonate, Lithotabs

Generic Name: lithium

Purpose: This drug stabilizes the mood of people with manic-depressive illness (extreme mood changes from depression or anger to elation). It is also used investigatively to treat other mental conditions and illnesses.

Warnings:

- Lithium can decrease alertness and coordination. Do not drive a car or operate dangerous machinery until you know how this drug affects you.

- Keep all appointments with your doctor and the laboratory. You probably will have blood tests periodically to monitor the amount of lithium in your blood and also urine tests, especially if you experience side effects. Your dose may need to be adjusted occasionally.

- Drink 12 full glasses of water or other beverages each day (unless your doctor tells you otherwise) and use a moderate amount of salt on your food. However, if your doctor puts you on a low-salt or low-sodium diet, follow it.

- Avoid beverages with sugar because sugar causes cavities in your teeth and caffeine increases urination, which may alter the effect of lithium.

- If you are pregnant, may become pregnant, or are breast-feeding, tell your doctor before taking lithium. If you become pregnant, notify your doctor promptly.

- Many drugs can alter the effect of lithium. Before you take lithium, tell your doctor what prescription and nonprescription drugs you are taking. All of your doctors and dentists should know that you take lithium so that they can avoid prescribing drugs, especially ibuprofen (Advil, Motrin, or Nuprin) and sodium bicarbonate and other antacids containing sodium without consulting your doctor.

- If you are allergic to aspirin or tartrazine (yellow dye present in some processed foods and medications, including lithium) or have thyroid, kidney, heart or blood vessel disease, tell your doctor before taking lithium.

- Do not allow anyone else to take this medication.

Common Side Effects	What To Do
Nausea; loss of appetite; stomach bloating; abdominal pain.	Take lithium with meals. If these effects persist, contact your doctor.
Fine tremor of the hands.	Avoid beverages that contain caffeine (coffee, tea and cola). If the tremor worsens, spreads to other parts of the body, or is bothersome, call your doctor.
Headache; mild loss of memory; confusion; acne.	If these problems are bothersome, contact your doctor.
Dry, coarse skin; hair loss; mental dullness; sensitivity to cold; fatigue; sleepiness; slow reflexes; weight gain.	Contact your doctor.

Figure 17-8

Medication teaching tool for lithium. (From Carson, V. B. [1994]. *Bay area psychiatric home care manual.* Baltimore: Bay Area Health Care. Copyright © 1994, Bay Area Health Care.)

Illustration continued on following page

<table>
<tr><th>Common Side Effects</th><th>What To Do</th></tr>
<tr><td>Dry mouth; thirst; increased urination.</td><td>Drink plenty of water (or other beverages), especially if you have vomiting, diarrhea or a fever. Contact your doctor if you have increased urination or prolonged vomiting, diarrhea or a fever.</td></tr>
<tr><td>Lithium intoxication: shaking of the hands; muscle twitching; weakness or incoordination; vomiting; diarrhea; drowsiness.</td><td>Stop taking the medication and contact your doctor immediately.</td></tr>
</table>

- You are taking _____ mg nardil _____ times a day. Your schedule is _____

_____ .

- If you miss a dose and remember within 2–3 hours, take it. Otherwise, skip it and take remaining doses as scheduled. DO NOT double up.

LITHIUM TOXICITY

Symptoms: Feels like you are drunk (slurred speech, staggering walk, bad shakes, confused) and with the "flu" (nausea, vomiting, diarrhea).

If you have these symptoms, it may mean you have too much lithium in your blood. DO NOT TAKE THE NEXT DOSE OF LITHIUM. CALL YOUR DOCTOR OR GO TO EMERGENCY ROOM TO HAVE SOME BLOOD DRAWN FOR A LITHIUM LEVEL.

How to prevent this from happening:

1. Take lithium *exactly* as prescribed by your doctor.
2. Get lab work done as soon as doctor requests it.
3. DO NOT change the amount of salt or fluids you are taking in.
4. Tell your doctor if you are sick with the flu—vomiting or diarrhea—or if you have a kidney infection.
5. Tell your doctor if you get put on "water pills."
6. Drink a bit more fluid when it's hot and you are sweating.
7. Let your doctor know if you go on any special diet for weight, blood pressure, etc.

Figure 17–8 *Continued*

MEDICATION PRE-POST TEST

PATIENT: _____

NURSE: _____

DATE: _____ SCORE: _____

1. I am taking (name medication[s]).

2. I am taking _____ mg _____ times per day.

3. My schedule is _____ .

4. My medication helps me:
   a. Feel less sad.
   b. Feel less nervous.
   c. Feel less bothered by bad thoughts I can't control.
   d. Other (list any other benefits).

5. If I miss a dose of my medicine, I should:
   a. Double up on the next dose.
   b. If I remember to take it close to the regularly scheduled time, I should take it and stay with my normal schedule.
   c. If it is several hours from when I should have taken it, I will forget the missed dose and get right back on my normal schedule with the next dose.

6. My medication may make me feel drowsy and even clumsy. When I first begin taking the medicine it is a good idea to:
   a. Stay at home all the time until I feel more alert and sharper in my thinking.
   b. Avoid driving a car or operating machinery until I know how I will react to this medicine.
   c. Avoid taking the medicine right before I need to be alert in my actions and thinking.
   d. Tell my doctor I want another medication.

7. If I am going to have surgery, even dental surgery, I should:
   a. Stop taking medication the day before the surgery.
   b. Tell my surgeon all the medications I am taking.
   c. Take more of my medication right before surgery to put me in a better state of mind.

8. Before drinking any alcohol, whether in beer, wine, whiskey, wine coolers, or over-the-counter medications, I should:
   a. Stop taking my medication.
   b. Talk to my doctor about whether it is safe or not to mix alcohol with this medicine.
   c. Read the label on the bottle or package containing the alcohol to see what I should do.

9. If I am taking this medicine, there are certain things that I should tell my doctor. Please check off at least three things from the following list:
   ____ a. I have a history of an eating disorder.
   ____ b. I have a history of seizures.
   ____ c. I am pregnant or want to become pregnant.
   ____ d. I am breast-feeding.
   ____ e. I am taking other medications.
   ____ f. I have certain allergies.
   ____ g. I have a history of heart problems or high blood pressure or have had a recent heart attack.
   ____ h. I have a history of kidney disease.
   ____ i. I am a diabetic.

10. A friend asks me for a dose of my medicine to help him/her feel better. I should:
    a. Refuse and explain that the medicine may make him/her sick.
    b. Give one dose away just so the friend can see if it helps or not.
    c. Freely share my medicine with other people who have the same symptoms as I.

If you are taking a medication to make you feel less sad, please answer the next four questions.

11. My medication can produce some side effects that are bothersome but not serious. These include (please choose at least two from the following list):
    ____ a. Drowsiness, feeling tired, weak.
    ____ b. Excitement, insomnia, blurred vision.
    ____ c. Lightheadedness when I get up too quickly from lying down or sitting to a standing position.
    ____ d. Sensitive to sunlight.
    ____ e. Dry mouth.
    ____ f. Constipation, blurred vision, difficulty urinating.

Figure 17–9

Medication pretest and posttest. (From Carson, V. B. [1994]. *Bay area psychiatric home care manual*. Baltimore: Bay Area Health Care. Copyright © 1994, Bay Area Health Care.)

Illustration continued on following page

12. My medication does not make me feel better right away. It may take as long as:
   a. Two to three weeks.
   b. Three to four weeks.
   c. Five to six weeks.

13. Most of the side effects that my medication produces can be dealt with easily. Column A lists the side effects and Column B lists the common remedies. Please match the remedy with the side effect.

Column A	Column B
____ a. Drowsiness	____ 1. Take medicine with meals
____ b. Excitement, insomnia	____ 2. Wear sunblock and hat
____ c. Sensitive to sunlight	____ 3. Chew sugarless gum and suck on sugarless hard candy.
____ d. Dry mouth	____ 4. Eat more bulk foods, drink more water.
____ e. Constipation	____ 5. Take medicine at bedtime.
____ f. Nausea	____ 6. Take medicine in morning.

14. There are some side effects that I should immediately tell my doctor about. Which of the following fall into that category (check all that apply)?
   ____ a. High fever, chills, sore throat.
   ____ b. Change in skin color.
   ____ c. Any unusual bleeding.
   ____ d. Swelling of feet and lower legs.
   ____ e. Headache.
   ____ f. Diarrhea.

If you are taking medicine to make you feel less nervous, please answer the next three questions.

15. My medication can be habit forming. I should:
   a. Take the medication exactly as my doctor tells me to.
   b. Only take the medication when I feel desperate.
   c. Stop taking the medication as soon as I feel better.

16. When I feel better, I should:
   a. Stop taking the medication.
   b. Work with my doctor on a schedule to wean me off the medication.

17. Stopping the medication abruptly can cause me to:
   a. Have a heart attack and other coronary complications.
   b. Have seizures and experience withdrawal.
   c. Need more of the medication.

If you are taking a medicine to help you feel less bothered by troublesome thoughts you cannot control, please answer the following four questions.

18. My medicine can cause some unpleasant side effects that involve unusual movements. If I notice that I can't sit still (I have dancing feet) and I feel jittery inside, or I am experiencing spasms of my muscles in my face or other places in my body, I probably need to take some Cogentin, Benadryl, Artane, or amantadine as ordered by my doctor. If I do not have any of these medicines available, I should:
   a. Stop taking my medicine.
   b. Call my doctor immediately or go to an emergency department.
   c. Take a double dose of my medication.

19. My medication can cause tardive dyskinesia, a more serious movement disorder with jerky movements of the face and extremities. If this happens to me, my doctor will probably:
   a. Increase the dose of my medicine.
   b. Decrease the dose of my medicine.
   c. Stop my medication immediately.

20. Because of the side effects of my medicine, my doctor may have also placed me on another medication, such as Benadryl, Cogentin, Artane, Kemadrin, Akineton, or amantadine. These medications are used to control:
   a. The movement problems that come with my medicine.
   b. The dry mouth and constipation that come with my medicine.
   c. The blurred vision that comes with my medicine.

Figure 17–9 *Continued*

21. These additional drugs also have side effects. These include:
    a. Dry mouth, blurred vision, constipation.
    b. Fast heart beat.
    c. Seizures.
    d. Parkinson's disease.

If you are taking Tegretol or Dilantin please answer the following question.

22. Sometimes the dose of my medicine must be adjusted. Because of this it is important that I:
    a. Get my blood drawn so that my doctor can monitor how much of the medicine is in my system.
    b. Eat a balanced diet with 8 full glasses of water a day.
    c. Collect my urine for 24 hours to see that I am urinating the right amount.

Figure 17–9 *Continued*

Third Phase of Illness

Assessment

The third stage is the maintenance phase of treatment. The goal of maintenance is to maintain the patient on the lowest possible dose of medication. At this stage, the patient is probably being treated as an outpatient. Those who have experienced a first episode may not require prolonged treatment and may be gradually withdrawn from medications over a period of 3 to 6 months. During the third phase of the patient's illness, assess for

- Stress in the patient's life (beginning employment, returning to school)
- Level of knowledge and compliance with medication
- Emotional issues such as powerlessness
- Spiritual issues such as the patient's belief that he or she is lacking in faith if he or she relies on medication; that he or she must not be good enough for God to heal him or her; that the illness is a punishment from God; therefore, he or she should not take medication

Diagnoses

The nursing diagnoses during the maintenance phase focus on coping with stress, increasing knowledge, enhancing compliance, decreasing feelings of powerlessness, and relieving spiritual distress in the patient. Appropriate nursing diagnoses might include

- Ineffective Individual Coping related to multiple stressors as evidenced by verbalizations of nervousness and decreased ability to concentrate
- Knowledge Deficit related to medication action as evidenced by patient's inability to state reason for taking medication
- Noncompliance related to discomfort of side effects of antipsychotic medication as evidenced by increasing disorganization in thoughts and verbalizations regarding the negative effects of medication

- Powerlessness related to inability to control illness as evidenced by verbalizations that medication is a crutch and that patient is weak
- Spiritual Distress related to patient's disappointment that God does not heal him or her as evidenced by verbalizations such as, "I must not be good enough, or God would cure me without medications"

Outcome Identification

The expected outcome of the maintenance stage is reducing the patient's medication to the lowest level that maintains stable behavior. Stable behavior could be expressed in the following manner:

- The patient's behavior will remain stable, oriented to reality, and nonaggressive while a low dose of antipsychotic medication is used.
- The patient will exhibit effective coping strategies.
- The patient will verbalize an understanding of medication purpose, side effects, and schedule.
- The patient will verbalize that control over illness exists in decisions to understand and take medications.
- The patient will discuss feelings toward God and recognize that God uses multiple avenues for healing, including medications.

Planning and Implementation

Nursing interventions include the following:

- Teach the patient coping abilities to deal with stress.
- Reinforce medication and other health-related teaching with emphasis on acknowledging the role of stress in precipitating acute exacerbations of illness.
- Negotiate with the patient ways to increase compliance, such as changing the time the medication is taken or the form of medication or using medication boxes to assist patient in remembering when to take it.
- Acknowledge the patient's feelings of powerlessness over the illness and the inability to control symptoms without medications.

- Emphasize the areas of life where the patient retains control.
- Empathize with the spiritual distress that frequently accompanies chronic illnesses where medication usage is a fact of life.
- Discuss spiritual beliefs that impact on medication use and offer an alternative view on the use of medication as a healing tool of God.

Patients whose illness is chronic (two or more episodes) may be maintained on a single dose of medication that can be administered at bedtime. Nighttime administration helps to minimize the sedative effect of many of the antipsychotics. This sedative effect during the daytime may interfere with social participation as well as participation in nonpharmacological treatments, which are also of value in returning the patient to an optimal state of functioning. Chronically mentally ill patients may display persistent symptoms that are not responsive to traditional medication management, such as fixed systematized delusions, impaired insight, and inappropriate affect. These patients may be excellent candidates for the use of clozapine, risperidone, olanzapine, or quetiapine fumarate (see the Snapshot of Nursing Interventions Specific to Psychotropic Medications).

Evaluation

Evaluation includes reviewing whether the patient's symptom profile is improved, whether he or she is compliant with the medication regimen, and whether he or she is knowledgeable about the prescribed medication.

SNAPSHOT

Nursing Interventions Specific to Psychotropic Medications

Why you need to develop a therapeutic alliance with the patient taking psychotropic medications
- Nurses who are able to give accurate information in a clear, concise manner decrease patient anxiety.
- Increases the likelihood that patients will accept medication.
- Assists the patient in making an informed decision.

Assessment of health care status
- Potential for suicide (Statistics reflect that 20% of patients diagnosed with schizophrenia attempt suicide and 10% successfully complete the suicide.)
- Concurrent medical conditions
- History of medication compliance and history of admissions.
- Persistent side effects
- Knowledge level, willingness to learn (Remember that persistent positive symptoms of mental illness may impair cognition. Additionally, if internal stimuli are decreased, the patient's ability to focus and receive information is enhanced.)
- Social supports and community resources available to the patient
- Cultural beliefs and value system

What you need to communicate
- Importance of taking medications even though the patient feels good
- Mental illness is a disease as are hypertension, asthma, and diabetes. Medications help to lessen symptoms, not cure the disease.

What you need to teach the patient and/or the patient's caregiver
- Generic and trade names of medication (Have the patient identify the medication, state the time and the dose of the medication as he or she is selecting it out of a drawer or box.)
- Potential side effects and drug-food interactions of medication (Also, instruct the patient to report any side effects to the clinician who is monitoring the medication regimen.)
- Positive outcome (benefit) of taking medication
- Resources available for additional information

Other health professionals who might need to be a part of this plan of care
- Physician—to obtain informed consent (risk and benefits) and evaluate efficacy of medications
- Pharmacist—to monitor for potential interactions, ensure that accurate dose is dispensed, and provide information
- Social worker—to coordinate benefits (pharmacy) and outpatient therapy
- Occupational therapist—to assist with the patient's reintegration into the community, for example, to reach recreational activities to decrease stress
- Health aide or technician—to observe and report behavioral responses that may be related to medication, for example, sleeping thoughout the night may demonstrate the medication is decreasing a former symptom that exacerbated the illness

- Traditional antipsychotic drugs and atypical antipsychotic drugs differ in two principal ways: atypical antipsychotics are less likely to cause extrapyramidal reactions (including tardive dyskinesia) and atypical agents are more effective than traditional agents at relieving negative symptoms of schizophrenia.
- The major adverse effect of clozapine is agranulocytosis. Because of this potentially fatal effect, weekly blood tests are mandatory (during the first 6 months), and then the blood tests are bimonthly.
- As with the antipsychotics, therapeutic responses to antidepressants develop slowly (over a month or more).
- The most common adverse effects of the tricyclic antidepressants are sedation, orthostatic hypotension, and anticholinergic effects.
- The most serious adverse effect of the tricyclic antidepressants is cardiotoxicity, which can be fatal.
- Patients taking MAOIs must be warned against eating foods that contain tyramine because tyramine can cause a fatal hypertensive crisis in these people. Stimulant medications and SSRIs should also be avoided.
- The principal advantages of SSRIs over tricyclic antidepressants are that SSRIs cause fewer side effects (they do not cause hypotension, sedation, anticholinergic effects), and SSRIs are not cardiotoxic, which makes them much less dangerous when taken in overdose.
- Lithium and valproic acid are the principal treatments for bipolar disorder.
- To minimize the risk of toxicity, blood levels of lithium must be kept below 1.5 mEq/L. Monitoring of blood levels is essential.
- A reduction in sodium intake reduces lithium excretion, which causes lithium levels to rise, possibly to toxic concentrations. Patients must maintain normal sodium intake and sodium levels.
- Anticonvulsants, carbamazepine, lamotrigine, and gabapentin are alternatives to lithium for treating bipolar disorder.
- Benzodiazepines are preferred to barbiturates and other general CNS depressants for treating anxiety because benzodiazepines are much safer and cause fewer side effects.
- Although benzodiazepines can cause physical dependence, the withdrawal syndrome associated with these drugs is usually mild (although it can be intense with some patients).
- Four principal differences exist between buspirone and the benzodiazepines: buspirone lacks CNS-depressant actions; buspirone does not intensify the CNS-depressant effects of other drugs; antianxiety effects of benzodiazepines develop immediately, whereas therapeutic effects of buspirone may take a week to begin and a month or more to reach their peak; and buspirone has even less potential for abuse than the benzodiazepines.
- When patients are taking any type of medication, you are responsible for assessing mental status, effectiveness of medications, presence of side effects, degree of compliance, and the patient's and family's level of knowledge about the medication and the illness that the medication is being used to treat.
- One of the most common nursing diagnoses for patients taking psychotropic medication is Knowledge Deficit regarding medication use and side effects.
- The expected outcomes for patients taking any type of psychotropic medication focus on improvement in the patient's symptoms and functioning, increased knowledge regarding the illness and the medication, and appropriate levels of compliance with the medication regimen.
- Appropriate nursing interventions for patients taking any type of psychotropic medication include education of the patient and family regarding the illness and the medications and exploration of ways to improve compliance.
- Evaluation of the nursing care focuses on whether the patient's psychiatric symptoms decrease, whether the patient experiences side effects and how effectiv these side effects are controlled, whether the pati level of functioning improves, and whether the is compliant with taking the medication.

Learning Activities

1. Write in your journal your own reactions to the idea that you would have to take medication most of your life. Would it be difficult on you? What impact would this have on your self-concept? Your spirituality?
2. Interview two other people and ask the following questions:
   a. What is your attitude about taking medications?
   b. Do you have trouble remembering to take medications as they are prescribed?
   c. Would/Does taking medications on a regular basis affect your sense of well-being?

3. Begin to develop a medica 3-inch by 5-inch index c medication that your patie purpose of the medicati range, what dose your works, and any pre while taking the d the medication effects does yc side effects k

Conclusions

As with drug therapy of somatic disorders, drug therapy of mental illnesses has made a lot of progress but still has a long way to go. Since the 1950s, we have developed powerful drugs that can provide symptomatic relief for many patients. Unfortunately, for many others, treatment remains largely ineffective. Much of the difficulty resides with our incomplete understanding of mental illness. If we do not really understand the disorders we are trying to treat (and we do not), we have no rational basis for developing new drugs to treat them. Fortunately, with the rapid advances being made in psychiatry and neuroscience, there is reason to hope that safer and more effective psychotherapeutic agents are forthcoming.

Does the availability of psychotherapeutic drugs relieve you of your responsibility to provide good nursing care? Obviously not. In fact, with the advent of these drugs, nursing responsibilities have actually increased. If treatment is to be optimal, the nurse must evaluate the patient for a therapeutic response. Armed with this information, the prescriber is in a better position to make dosage adjustments or to decide to switch to another drug (if your evaluation shows that the current selection is not working). In addition to helping optimize therapeutic effects, it is your responsibility to help minimize adverse effects. This is done by observing the patient for adverse effects and intervening, as needed. Of equal importance, you must educate patients and their families about possible adverse effects along with measures to minimize discomfort or harm. Clearly, by providing informed and conscientious nursing care and patient education, you can greatly increase the chances of achieving the therapeutic goal—maximal benefit with minimal harm. Conversely, if the care and education that you offer are inadequate . . . well, we know that will not happen.

Key Points to Remember

- When a neurotransmitter binds to its receptor on a postsynaptic neuron, it can either increase or decrease the chances that the postsynaptic neuron will initiate an action potential of its own.
- Two major mechanisms can terminate neurotransmission: enzymatic degradation of neurotransmitter and reuptake of transmitter back into the presynaptic nerve terminal.
- A drug that blocks reuptake of a neurotransmitter intensifies synaptic transmission by that transmitter.
- The major indication for antipsychotic medications is schizophrenia.
- Traditional antipsychotic drugs are thought to produce their therapeutic effects by blocking receptors for dopamine.
- Responses to antipsychotic drugs develop slowly, requiring a month or more to produce a full effect. Antipsychotic drugs cause three types of early extra-

pyramidal reactions: acute dystonia, parkinsonism, and akathisia. Acute dystonia and parkinsonism can be treated with anticholinergic drugs (e.g., benztropine). Akathisia, although more difficult to treat, may respond to anticholinergic drugs, benzodiazepines, or beta-blockers. Also consider lowering the amount of drug or switching to another medication.
- Tardive dyskinesia is a late extrapyramidal reaction and has no reliable treatment.
- NMS, a life-threatening reaction to antipsychotic drugs, is characterized by muscular rigidity, high fever, and autonomic instability.
- Low-potency antipsychotics and high-potency antipsychotics produce equal therapeutic effects. These drugs differ, in that low-potency agents cause more anticholinergic effects, sedation, and orthostatic hypotension, whereas high-potency agents cause more early extrapyramidal reactions. Tardive dyskinesia is equal with both groups.

- Traditional antipsychotic drugs and atypical antipsychotic drugs differ in two principal ways: atypical antipsychotics are less likely to cause extrapyramidal reactions (including tardive dyskinesia) and atypical agents are more effective than traditional agents at relieving negative symptoms of schizophrenia.
- The major adverse effect of clozapine is agranulocytosis. Because of this potentially fatal effect, weekly blood tests are mandatory (during the first 6 months), and then the blood tests are bimonthly.
- As with the antipsychotics, therapeutic responses to antidepressants develop slowly (over a month or more).
- The most common adverse effects of the tricyclic antidepressants are sedation, orthostatic hypotension, and anticholinergic effects.
- The most serious adverse effect of the tricyclic antidepressants is cardiotoxicity, which can be fatal.
- Patients taking MAOIs must be warned against eating foods that contain tyramine because tyramine can cause a fatal hypertensive crisis in these people. Stimulant medications and SSRIs should also be avoided.
- The principal advantages of SSRIs over tricyclic antidepressants are that SSRIs cause fewer side effects (they do not cause hypotension, sedation, anticholinergic effects), and SSRIs are not cardiotoxic, which makes them much less dangerous when taken in overdose.
- Lithium and valproic acid are the principal treatments for bipolar disorder.
- To minimize the risk of toxicity, blood levels of lithium must be kept below 1.5 mEq/L. Monitoring of blood levels is essential.
- A reduction in sodium intake reduces lithium excretion, which causes lithium levels to rise, possibly to toxic concentrations. Patients must maintain normal sodium intake and sodium levels.
- Anticonvulsants, carbamazepine, lamotrigine, and gabapentin are alternatives to lithium for treating bipolar disorder.
- Benzodiazepines are preferred to barbiturates and other general CNS depressants for treating anxiety because benzodiazepines are much safer and cause fewer side effects.
- Although benzodiazepines can cause physical dependence, the withdrawal syndrome associated with these drugs is usually mild (although it can be intense with some patients).
- Four principal differences exist between buspirone and the benzodiazepines: buspirone lacks CNS-depressant actions; buspirone does not intensify the CNS-depressant effects of other drugs; antianxiety effects of benzodiazepines develop immediately, whereas therapeutic effects of buspirone may take a week to begin and a month or more to reach their peak; and buspirone has even less potential for abuse than the benzodiazepines.
- When patients are taking any type of medication, you are responsible for assessing mental status, effectiveness of medications, presence of side effects, degree of compliance, and the patient's and family's level of knowledge about the medication and the illness that the medication is being used to treat.
- One of the most common nursing diagnoses for patients taking psychotropic medication is Knowledge Deficit regarding medication use and side effects.
- The expected outcomes for patients taking any type of psychotropic medication focus on improvement in the patient's symptoms and functioning, increased knowledge regarding the illness and the medication, and appropriate levels of compliance with the medication regimen.
- Appropriate nursing interventions for patients taking any type of psychotropic medication include education of the patient and family regarding the illness and the medications and exploration of ways to improve compliance.
- Evaluation of the nursing care focuses on whether the patient's psychiatric symptoms decrease, whether the patient experiences side effects and how effectively these side effects are controlled, whether the patient's level of functioning improves, and whether the patient is compliant with taking the medication.

Learning Activities

1. Write in your journal your own reactions to the idea that you would have to take medication most of your life. Would it be difficult on you? What impact would this have on your self-concept? Your spirituality?

2. Interview two other people and ask the following questions:
   a. What is your attitude about taking medications?
   b. Do you have trouble remembering to take medications as they are prescribed?
   c. Would/Does taking medications on a regular basis affect your sense of well-being?

3. Begin to develop a medication file box. Write on 3-inch by 5-inch index cards the names of every medication that your patients are taking. Describe the purpose of the medication, the side effects, the dosage range, what dose your patient is taking, how the drug works, and any precautions that must be observed while taking the drug. Summarize the ways in which the medication benefits your patient. What side effects does your patient experience? How are these side effects handled?

Conclusions

As with drug therapy of somatic disorders, drug therapy of mental illnesses has made a lot of progress but still has a long way to go. Since the 1950s, we have developed powerful drugs that can provide symptomatic relief for many patients. Unfortunately, for many others, treatment remains largely ineffective. Much of the difficulty resides with our incomplete understanding of mental illness. If we do not really understand the disorders we are trying to treat (and we do not), we have no rational basis for developing new drugs to treat them. Fortunately, with the rapid advances being made in psychiatry and neuroscience, there is reason to hope that safer and more effective psychotherapeutic agents are forthcoming.

Does the availability of psychotherapeutic drugs relieve you of your responsibility to provide good nursing care? Obviously not. In fact, with the advent of these drugs, nursing responsibilities have actually increased. If treatment is to be optimal, the nurse must evaluate the patient for a therapeutic response. Armed with this information, the prescriber is in a better position to make dosage adjustments or to decide to switch to another drug (if your evaluation shows that the current selection is not working). In addition to helping optimize therapeutic effects, it is your responsibility to help minimize adverse effects. This is done by observing the patient for adverse effects and intervening, as needed. Of equal importance, you must educate patients and their families about possible adverse effects along with measures to minimize discomfort or harm. Clearly, by providing informed and conscientious nursing care and patient education, you can greatly increase the chances of achieving the therapeutic goal—maximal benefit with minimal harm. Conversely, if the care and education that you offer are inadequate . . . well, we know that will not happen.

Key Points to Remember

- When a neurotransmitter binds to its receptor on a postsynaptic neuron, it can either increase or decrease the chances that the postsynaptic neuron will initiate an action potential of its own.
- Two major mechanisms can terminate neurotransmission: enzymatic degradation of neurotransmitter and reuptake of transmitter back into the presynaptic nerve terminal.
- A drug that blocks reuptake of a neurotransmitter intensifies synaptic transmission by that transmitter.
- The major indication for antipsychotic medications is schizophrenia.
- Traditional antipsychotic drugs are thought to produce their therapeutic effects by blocking receptors for dopamine.
- Responses to antipsychotic drugs develop slowly, requiring a month or more to produce a full effect.
- Antipsychotic drugs cause three types of early extra-pyramidal reactions: acute dystonia, parkinsonism, and akathisia. Acute dystonia and parkinsonism can be treated with anticholinergic drugs (e.g., benztropine). Akathisia, although more difficult to treat, may respond to anticholinergic drugs, benzodiazepines, or beta-blockers. Also consider lowering the amount of drug or switching to another medication.
- Tardive dyskinesia is a late extrapyramidal reaction and has no reliable treatment.
- NMS, a life-threatening reaction to antipsychotic drugs, is characterized by muscular rigidity, high fever, and autonomic instability.
- Low-potency antipsychotics and high-potency antipsychotics produce equal therapeutic effects. These drugs differ, in that low-potency agents cause more anticholinergic effects, sedation, and orthostatic hypotension, whereas high-potency agents cause more early extrapyramidal reactions. Tardive dyskinesia is equal with both groups.

Critical Thinking Exercises

Lillian, a 40-year-old schoolteacher, was admitted to the inpatient unit for depression. She was overwhelmed with conflicts at work and with an impending divorce at home. Part of her treatment involved group counseling. Another part of her treatment involved the medication fluoxetine. Before discharge, the nurse provided Lillian with educational information about her newly prescribed drug, fluoxetine.

1. What information would you give to Lillian about fluoxetine?

2. What assumptions can the nurse make about Lillian's use of the drug?

3. What evidence would convince the nurse that the patient understood her information about the drug?

Lillian was discharged to the outpatient clinic. Two weeks later, when she arrived for her first appointment, she carried the *New York Times* bestseller *Listening to Prozac* (Kramer, 1993). Lillian seemed concerned about the stories that she heard from her friends about fluoxetine causing suicidal or homicidal tendencies.

1. What assessment and information does the nurse need to provide about what Lillian is telling her?

2. What are alternative explanations why Lillian might have expressed such concerns to the nurse?

3. What conclusions (if any) can be drawn about Lillian's comments to the nurse?

Additional Resources

Janssen Pharmaceutical's Person-to-Person Project

800-376-8282 (patient support)

This project offers educational, vocational, and community support to patients and families who are dealing with schizophrenia.

Promedica Research Center

3758 Lavista Road
Suite 100
Tucker, GA 30084-5648
404-982-0330

Promedica@aol.com (e-mail)
http://members.aol.com/promedica/promedica.html

The center publishes the newsletter *Probe*, which contains current information on drug research; the newsletter is available at no charge to nurses. Additionally, they have developed a number of excellent audiotape and booklet programs available for nurses and other mental health professionals. All of these audiotape programs are approved by the Georgia Nurses Association for continuing educational unit contact hours.

Psychopharmacology and Drug References on the Mental Health Net

http://www.cmhcsys.com/guide/pro22.htm#A

Psychopharmacology and Substance Abuse (American Psychological Association Division 28)

http://www.apa.org/about/division/div28.html

References

Abramowicz, M. (Ed.). (1994). Drugs for psychiatric disorders. *The Medical Letter on Drugs and Therapeutics, 36,* 89-96.

Addonizio, G. (1991). The pharmacologic basis of neuroleptic malignant syndrome. *Psychiatric Annals, 21,* 154-157.

Antipsychotic olanzapine approved. (1996). *Medical Sciences Bulletin: The Internet-Enhanced Journal of Pharmacology and Therapeutics. 19*(3), 2.

Arvanitis, L. S., & Miller, B. G. (1997). Multiple fixed doses of "Seroquel" (quetiapine) in patients with acute exacerbation of schizophrenia: A comparison with haloperidol and placebo. The Seroquel Trial 13 Study Group. *Biological Psychiatry, 15,* 233-246.

Bailey, K. P. (1996). Preparing for prescriptive practice: Advanced practice psychiatric nursing and psychopharmacology. *Journal of Psychosocial Nursing, 34*(1), 16-20.

Blair, D. T., & Dounce, A. (1993). Nonneuroleptic etiologies of extrapyramidal symptoms. *Clinical Nurse Specialist, 7,* 225-231.

Borison, R. L., Diamond, B. I., Pathiraja, A., & Meibach, R. C. (1992). Clinical overview of risperidone (pp. 173-179). In H. Y. Meltzer (Ed.), *Novel antipsychotic drugs.* New York: Raven Press.

Brasfield, K. H. (1991). Practical psychopharmacologic considerations in depression. *Nursing Clinics of North America, 26,* 651-663.

Brook, S., Swift, R., & Harrigan, E. P. (1997). The tolerability efficacy of intramuscular ziprasidone. *European Neuropsychopharmacology, 7*(Suppl.), S215-225.

Byrd, C. (1993). Neuroleptic malignant syndrome A dangerous complication of neuroleptic therapy. *Journal of Neuroscience Nursing, 215*(1), 62-65.

Caroff, S. N., Mann, S., et al. (1991). Neuroleptic malignant syndrome: Diagnostic issues. *Psychiatric Annals, 21,* 130-147.

Chouinard, G., Goodman, W., Greist, J., Jenike, M., & Rasmussen, S. (1990). Results of a double-blind placebo controlled trial of a new serotonin uptake inhibitor, sertraline, in the treatment of obsessive-compulsive disorder. *Psychopharmacology Bulletin, 26,* 279-284.

Chouinard, G., Jones, B., Remington, G., Bloom, D., Addington, D., MacEwan, G. W., Labelle, A., Beauclair, L., & Arnott, W. (1993). A Canadian multicenter placebo-controlled study of fixed doses of risperidone and haloperidol in the treatment of chronic schizophrenic patients. *Journal of Clinical Psychopharmacology, 13,* 25-40.

Ciraulo, D. A., & Shader, R. I. (1990a). Fluoxetine drug-drug interactions. I. Antidepressants and antipsychotics. *Journal of Clinical Psychopharmacology, 10,* 48-50.

Ciraulo, D. A., & Shader, R. I. (1990b). Fluoxetine drug-drug interactions. II. *Journal of Clinical Psychopharmacology, 10,* 213-217.

Cohn, C. K., Shrivastava, R., Mendels, J., Cohn, J. B., Fabre, L. F., Claghorn, J. L., Dessain, E. C., Itil, T. M., & Lautin, A. (1990). Double-blind, multicenter comparison of sertraline and amitriptyline in elderly depressed patients. *Journal of Clinical Psychiatry, 51,* 28-33.

Davis, J. M., Metalon, L., Wantabe, M. D., & Blare, L. (1994). Depot antipsychiatric drugs: Place in therapy. *Drugs, 47,* 741-773.

DeVane, C. L. (1992). Pharmacokinetics of the selective serotonin reuptake inhibitors. *Journal of Clinical Psychiatry, 53,* 13-20.

Enos, G. A. (1997). Pharmaceutical company launches schizophrenia support line. *Mental Health Weekly, 7*(17), 3-4.

Ereshefsky, L. (1995). Antidepressants: A pharmacologic rationale for treatment and product selection. *Formulary, 30*(1), 10-19.

Gelenberg, A. (1998a). Cost effectiveness of clozapine: Spend more, save more? *Biological Therapies in Psychiatry Newsletter, 21*(3), 1-2.

Gelenberg, A. (1998b). SRI withdrawal reactions. *Biological Therapies in Psychiatry Newsletter, 21*(6), 1-2.

Gelenberg, A. (1998c). SSRIs for PMDD. *Biological Therapies in Psychiatry Newsletter, 21*(4), 1-2.

Gerner, R. H., & Stanton, A. (1992). Algorithm for patient management of acute manic states: Lithium, valproate or carbamazepine. *Journal of Clinical Psychopharmacology, 12*(Suppl. 1), 575-635.

Grimseley, S. R., & Jann, M. W. (1992). Paroxetine, sertraline, and fluvoxamine: New selective serotonin reuptake inhibitors. *Clinical Pharmacy, 11*, 930-957.

Huttunen, M. O., Tuhkanen, H. Haavisto, E., Nyholm, R., Pitkanen, M., Raitasua, V., & Romanov, V. (1996). Low and standard dose depot haloperidol combined with targeted oral neuroleptics. *Psychiatric Services, 47*(1), 83-85.

Jann, M. W. (1991). Clozapine. *Pharmacotherapy, 11*, 179-195.

Jaretz, N., Flowers, E., & Millsap, L. (1992). Clozapine: Nursing care considerations. *Perspectives in Psychiatric Care, 28*(3), 19-26.

Jenike, M. A., Baer, L., & Greist, J. H. (1990). Clomipramine versus fluoxetine in obsessive-compulsive disorder: A retrospective comparison of side effects and efficacy. *Journal of Clinical Psychopharmacol, 10*, 122-124.

Kane, J. M., Woerner, M. G., Pollack, S., Safferman, A. Z., & Lieberman, J. A. (1993). Does clozapine cause tardive dyskinesia? *Journal of Clinical Psychiatry, 54*, 327-330.

Kane, J. M. (1998, May). Choosing an optimal antipsychotic agent, conventional or atypical. *Current Approaches to Psychoses Diagnosis and Management, 7*, 4-5.

Keck, P. E., Pope, H. G., Cohen, B. M., & McElroy, S. (1991). Risk factors for neuroleptic malignant syndrome. *Archives of General Psychiatry, 46*, 914-918.

Kramer, P. (1993). Listening to Prozac. New York: Penguin Books.

Kulkarni, J. (1997). Women and schizophrenia: A review. *Probe, 2*(5), 1-3.

Land, W., & Salzman, C. (1994). Risperidone A model antipsychotic medication. *Hospital and Community Psychiatry, 45*, 434-435.

Lehne, R. A. (1994a). Basic principles of neuropharmacology. In R. A. Lehne, *Pharmacology for nursing care* (2nd ed., pp. 101-108). Philadelphia: W. B. Saunders.

Lehne, R. A. (1994b). Drugs for bipolar disorder. In R. A. Lehne, *Pharmacology for nursing care* (2nd ed., pp. 295-302). Philadelphia: W. B. Saunders.

Littrell, K. H. (1997). Choosing an antipsychotic in the treatment of schizophrenia: Conversion to olanzapine. *Probe, 2*(3), 1-4.

Mahmood, T., Devlin, M., & Silverson, T. (1998). Clozapine in the management of bipolar and schizoaffective manic episodes resistant to standard treatment. *Probe, 3*(2), 1-3.

Marder, J. R., & Meibach, R. C. (1994). Risperidone in the treatment of schizophrenia. *American Journal of Psychiatry, 151*, 825-835.

McElroy, S. L., Keck, P. G., Pope, H. G., & Hudson, J. I. (1992). Valproate in the treatment of bipolar disorder: Literature review and clinical guidelines. *Journal of Clinical Psychopharmacology, 12*(Suppl.), 425-525.

Medical Sciences Bulletin: The Internet-Enhanced Journal of Pharmacology and Therapeutics. (1997, November). (241), 1-3.

Meltzer, H., Burnett, S., Bastani, B., & Ramirez, L. (1992). Effects of six months of clozapine treatment on the quality of life of chronic schizophrenic patients. *Hospital and Community Psychiatry, 41*, 892-897.

Semenchuk, M., & Labiner, D. (1997). Gabapentin and lamotrigine: Prescribing guidelines for psychiatry. *Journal of Practicing Psychiatry and Behavioral Health, 11*, 334-342.

Shriqui, C. L. (1998, May). Tardive dyskinesia in geriatric patients with psychoses. *Current Approaches to Psychoses Diagnosis and Management, 7*, 12-14.

Small, J. C., Hirsch, S. R., Arvanitis, L. A., Miller, B. G., Link, C. G. G. (1997). Quetiapine in patients with schizophrenia. A high- and low-dose double-blind comparison with placebo. Seroquel Study Group. *Archives of General Psychiatry, 54*, 549-557.

Sternbach, H. (1991). The serotonin syndrome. *American Journal of Psychiatry, 148*, 705-713.

Volavka, J. (1998, May). Violence and aggression in psychoses Are newer antipsychotic drugs effective? *Current Approaches to Psychoses Diagnosis and Management, 7*, 2-3.

Weiden, P. J. (1996, July). Prevention for extrapyramidal side effects. *Journal of Practicing Psychiatry and Behavioral Health*, pp. 240-253.

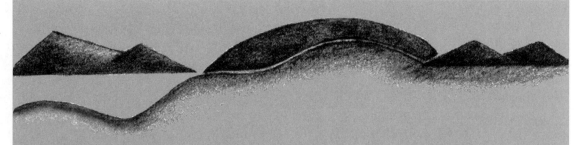

IV Travelers Across the Life Span

Traveler's Log

I have always enjoyed working with children. But it wasn't until I had two boys of my own and spent time as a classroom aide that I realized I was most intrigued by the inner lives of children. I read about play therapy and knew I wanted to learn more. I chose to study nursing because I believe nurses have a uniquely holistic approach to health care. I was lucky to find a job right after graduation from nursing school, working in a new psychiatric inpatient unit for children ages 3 to 15.

Children open up like flowers when given loving attention. I came to know my patients and their families well. They taught me what I needed to build on my theoretical education. I had to be open, to pay attention, and to learn from them by being present in the midst of their suffering and confusion. Here there could be creativity, playfulness, and even laughter. Going on with my studies, I learned to move treatment outside the hospital walls—outpatient assessments, group and individual therapy, parent-child therapy—and to build teams to provide home-based care. Much depends on parents coming to understand their child's strengths and vulnerabilities and developing a way to communicate this understanding. Parents must be the child's best advocate.

It has been an amazing journey. Along the way, I have learned much about resiliency, about hope, and about being a person. I have forged extraordinary friendships with colleagues . . . friendships that sustain and delight me. And I know that my encounters with children have enriched the course of both their paths and mine.

—Sarah Lechner

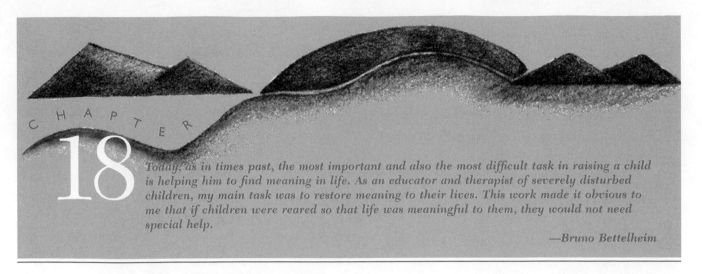

Today, as in times past, the most important and also the most difficult task in raising a child is helping him to find meaning in life. As an educator and therapist of severely disturbed children, my main task was to restore meaning to their lives. This work made it obvious to me that if children were reared so that life was meaningful to them, they would not need special help.

—Bruno Bettelheim

The Child

Learning Objectives

After studying this chapter, you should be able to:

1. Outline the stages of normal child development according to the major theorists.
2. Describe various coping strategies and their appropriateness to each developmental level.
3. Describe the risk factors associated with emotional disturbance in children.
4. Outline the salient features of the physical and mental status examinations for this population.
5. List specific areas of assessment and features to be observed within each area.
6. Identify the broad categories of childhood diagnoses according to the *Diagnostic and Statistical Manual of Mental Disorders, Fourth Edition* (DSM-IV).
7. Suggest one nursing diagnosis appropriate to each disorder.
8. Apply the nursing process to a patient situation.
9. Describe the various treatment modalities and the settings in which these are used.
10. List the principles of medication use in children.

Key Terminology

Anal phase	Goodness of fit	Oral phase
Attachment	Latency phase	Protective factors
Genital phase	Oedipal phase	Risk factors

In getting to know a troubled child, you need to come to the encounter with your whole self-memories, knowledge, hopefulness, earnestness, and also playfulness. Young people, whether eagerly or reluctantly, entrust themselves to a caring nurse. This trust can be seen as an act of courage and of hope.

To recognize this courage, to offer help, and to participate in hoping with a child are acts of love for the nurse. In the words of Bettelheim (1950), however, "love alone is not enough" (p. 4). Neither is intuition, nor empathy—"a corrective experience is not enough" (Winnicott, 1965, p. 258). These attributes are important, but you must also have a special kind of understanding guided by a basic knowledge of child development—physical, social, and psychological—and by a capacity to enjoy the intellectual challenge of learning about psychopathology. Understanding is informed by a deep interest in the inner lives of others and a willingness to examine yourself honestly and continually. With understanding, both nurse and child can learn and change.

Jordi's Story

It rained that morning. He liked the lightning, and the thunder was rumbly and warm. It was the rain that scared him. Every time it came, the same thought was there—rain forest—and it would repeat over and over again—rain forest, rain forest—and the same picture popped into his head—only lately he was more and more in the picture.

The trees were raining down. They weren't the tall, nice ones. They were short, fat, heavy, and stubby. They had giant roots that spread all over. And they came down from the sky to look for him, and one day one would come—the one that hated him most. It would crush him into the dirt. The roots would strangle him. He would be buried deeper and deeper.

They led him out of the house into the bus. It was different from the trains and their routes that he knew so well. Then they went out of the familiar neighborhood.

He was afraid to sit, and nobody objected to his standing the whole way. He felt very small. It made him feel a little bit bigger to stand. He kept his fist clenched tightly on the seat, and his body became more rigid. As familiar surroundings disappeared, he clenched the seat even tighter, feeling that this would keep him from disappearing too.

He felt that if he held himself tightly and didn't budge, he would not come apart. It took immense concentration to hold himself together. Each bump and jolt threatened to make him scatter into little pieces. A private battle was taking place between him and the lurching of the bus.

The attendant talked to him. He didn't answer. He couldn't hear her. Keeping himself in one part absorbed him totally. All of his senses were concentrated on the terrible effort.

Reprinted with the permission of Macmillan Publishing Company from *Jordi* (p. 6) by Theodore Isaac Rubin, MD. Copyright © 1960 by Theodore Isaac Rubin.

THE BEGINNING OF THE JOURNEY: CONSIDERATIONS IN WORKING WITH CHILDREN

Child as Sojourner

One reason people give for choosing to work with children is a liking for childhood spontaneity and

creativity. Although there are certainly elements of these qualities in child psychiatric nursing, disturbed children often experience themselves as out of control and terrified, or inhibited and joyless. Such children can only be helped by adults who can tolerate terror and unhappiness.

"What's wrong, Jordi? What? Tell me."

He hit himself with his closed fist again and again. "Hold my hand, Sally. Help me—hold me."

She held his hands between hers as he moaned, "Oh, oh." Then she managed to get him on her lap. She bent over him, held her arms around him, and hugged him tightly.

He felt warm and safe.

Reprinted with the permission of Macmillan Publishing Company from *Jordi* (p. 46) by Theodore Isaac Rubin, MD. Copyright © 1960 by Theodore Isaac Rubin.

Normal Development

Several theories of child development have flowered over the past century. Psychoanalytic theorists have each proposed a number of discrete phases that correspond to the individual's mastery of physical, environmental, and—primarily—emotional tasks. Freud (1938) described these phases as follows:

1. The **oral phase,** from birth to 18 months of age, so named because of the central role of the mouth in satisfying needs, experiencing intimacy, exploring the world, and expressing distress and satisfaction.

2. The **anal phase,** from 18 to 36 months of age, referring to the important role that control of the urethral and anal sphincters *(toilet training)* plays in the young child's life. Control involves both the regulation of pleasurable sensations and the assertion of autonomy.

3. The **Oedipal phase,** from the ages of 4 to 6 years, named, of course, for the Greek myth. This term describes the child's wish for exclusive possession of the parent of the opposite gender. In this phase, children are believed to develop a capacity for *triadic* relationships. The child can now appreciate the parents' relationship with one another as well as their joint relationship with the child.

4. The **latency phase,** roughly the period between the ages of 6 or 7 and 10 or 11 years. During this period, according to Freud, the urgent striving for a romantic attachment to the opposite-sex parent becomes *latent* (dormant).

5. The **genital phase,** from the ages of 12 to 20 years, the hallmark of which is a reworking of the original oedipal conflict. Its successful completion results in the young adult's forming an emotional and sexual attachment to an appropriate person outside of the family.

Building on her father's work but focusing more on the child's adaptation, Anna Freud (1936) described several *lines of development* in different spheres of functioning, such as in care of the body and all of its needs and in relationships, both intimate and social. Erikson (1963) proposed that maturation involves the mastery of a series of basic developmental crises across the life span. In Erikson's view, successful resolution of each crisis allows the individual to move ahead in a satisfactory manner. Failure to negotiate the crisis at any of these phases, however, results in a diminished sense of self and a lack of readiness to face the next challenge. Piaget (1932/1965) concentrated on the child's cognitive development, labeling styles of intellectual reasoning that move from simple to complex and from concrete to abstract. Each of these theorists is represented in Table 18-1.

CHILDHOOD

Childhood is a time of growth, increasingly complex socialization and sophisticated learning about all aspects of a particular culture, and a gradual movement from the personal productivity of play to the societal productivity of work. Each stage of development is complete in itself, so that the child is not merely an incomplete adult. Each stage along the journey has its own unique appeal and infuses the world with its own unique energy. Play, often called both the language and the business of childhood, can serve as a window into the child's life.

Understanding the Individual Journey

A solid grounding in child development is essential for *anyone* working with children. Reading original works by the major theorists is useful. Reading fictional and autobiographical accounts—particularly accounts from different racial or cultural perspectives—and watching movies that explore the child's experience can be helpful too.

As always, however, going directly to the source is most helpful. Children themselves can be the best teachers. You might begin by arranging to observe in a day care center, on a playground, or in a school. Ask the children you meet straightforwardly about their lives. They are often glad to be listened to and taken seriously.

Any understanding of a child's own journey, no matter how deep or rich, is incomplete without a sense of the child's place in the family. Chess and Thomas (1986) proposed the paradigm of **"goodness of fit"** as a way of approaching the parent-child relationship. This deceptively simple idea is important: It "is best if the children are valued for their unique and idiosyncratic traits, temperaments, skills, and weaknesses" (Pruett, 1996, p. 236).

What do you think? Do Freud's ideas have any relevance today?

▶ *Check Your Reading*
1. Name Freud's developmental stages and the ages to which they refer.

TABLE 18-1 Models of Child Development

THEORIST AND ORIENTATION	AGE AND DEVELOPMENTAL PHASE																		
	0	1	2	3	4	5	6	7	8	9	10	11	12	13	14	15	16	17	18
Freud— Psychosexual		Oral		Anal		Phallic– Oedipal			Latency					Genital				
Erikson— Social-emotional		Trust vs. mistrust		Autonomy vs. shame and doubt			Initiative vs. guilt		Industry vs. inferiority				Identity vs. role confusion			
Piaget— Cognitive		Sensorimotor			Preoperational					Concrete operational					Formal operational				
Anna Freud— Lines of Development		Dependency Suckling Weaning Wetting and soiling Body as a toy Irresponsibility in body management Egocentricity Dual unity			Part object Self-feeding Food fads Play Companionship			Family romance Rational eating Bladder and bowel control Work Responsibility in body management				Ambivalence			Adult object relationships			

2. Why is play important?

3. What did Erikson contribute regarding understanding child development?

Journey as It Touches the Family

"I was with strangers the whole Saturday and Sunday—the whole weekend."

"But you were home, Jordi."

"Home, home with the public—with strangers."

"Your mother and father were home, Jordi."

"They were public also—they were all away from me . . . ."

Reprinted with the permission of Macmillan Publishing Company from *Jordi* (p. 49) by Theodore Isaac Rubin, MD. Copyright © 1960 by Theodore Isaac Rubin.

The modern family is in peril. All too often, a family exists in isolation from any real sense of community. Within the family, individuals may feel isolated too. This sense of anomie appears to pervade all levels of American life. Kendall (1989) wrote of her work as a child psychiatric nurse consultant in a poor urban hospital setting:

Frequently, inner-city children from socially deprived environments are discharged home where the pressures of poverty, violence, overcrowding, separation (if placed in a foster home), apathy, and a myriad of additional problems again jeopardize the child's development, potentiating further crises and disturbances. (p. 145)

Describing the stereotype of a stable, middle-class, American nuclear family as unrepresentative of the human species, Konner (1982) stated that "subtly, deeply, persistently, it continues to serve as a yardstick for us, and this has to stop" (p. 287).

Regardless of social status or the constellation of family members, families of disturbed children often report that life at home holds little pleasure. So much time and energy are expended in efforts to manage the child's behavior, whether oppositional, withdrawing, or compulsive, that none is left for having fun. Siblings frequently feel cheated of a "regular life." A common cycle occurs as follows:

1. A child's minor disobedience turns into a crisis as everyone's anxiety level rises.

2. The parents react by yelling, hitting, or imposing a severe punishment.

3. Everyone ends up feeling terrible, and the parents try to undo the severity of the punishment by overindulging the disobedient child.

4. The child gets in the habit of pushing every difficulty to this conclusion and a pattern is established.

Nurses often work with young children in an unusually close and intimate manner, acting at times as *parent surrogates*. It is a difficult challenge in these circumstances to resist the temptation to become a better mother or father than the child's own—or perhaps even a better mother or father than the *nurse's* own. Becoming a better parent can be quite gratifying (for both nurse and child) but only for a short while. Becoming a parent surrogate poses risks, as competition may result in the angry withdrawal of the child's real parents. Other parents may depend on the nurse to maintain a high level of involvement, beyond what is reasonable or possible. Both of these risks touch on the nature of therapeutic work, on the difference between gratifying immediate needs and offering the possibility of long-term change. This dilemma might be summed up here by quoting a proverb: "Give a man a fish and you feed him for a day. Show him how to fish and you feed him for a lifetime."

Nurses are in a position to teach parents the skills they need both to care for their children and to anticipate developmental challenges, using available resources for support.

Broadening the Path: The Outside World

School

You need only reflect on your own childhood memories to know that school is an extremely important part of a child's life. A good school not only educates a child but also can enhance a child's social skills, self-esteem, and preparedness to meet many different kinds of challenges adaptively.

The good school experience depends, in part, on the following characteristics (Combrinck-Graham, 1996; Comer, 1996; Linney & Seidman, 1989):

1. Reasonable school size

2. Collaborative relationships between school personnel and parents

3. Strong administrative leadership

4. High degree of teacher autonomy

5. Orderly structure that involves students rather than oppressing them

6. Staff and parents maintaining high expectations for children

For disturbed and learning-disabled children, the good school experience also depends heavily on the school's ability to recognize and provide for these special needs, regardless of the child's age.

Friends

Traditional models of personality development have given little attention to "the influence of children upon children" (McDermott, 1996, p. 412). Yet from toddlerhood on, a child's interactions with other children are crucial for learning empathy, reciprocity, self-assertion, self-regulation, and intimacy. The peer group takes on increasing importance until eventually—by adolescence—it overshadows the family in the child's involvement and allegiance. "[S]elf-evaluation and evaluation of others, attachment and loyalty, and attribution of qualities evolve primarily through the peer culture" (Combrinck-Graham, 1996).

One of the most frequent complaints of disturbed children and their parents is that these children have great difficulty establishing and sustaining friendships. Hyperactive children are frequently unpopular and may play only with children younger than themselves. Depressed or anxious children often withdraw from social contact. Impulsive and aggressive children tend to alienate peers by their actions. Developmentally delayed children may lack the skills needed to engage in reciprocal social exchanges. Psychotic children may appear bizarre or frightening to others. Such children need direct help negotiating more satisfactory relationships. The plan of treatment should address this need.

Community

A fortunate child's community may include a neighborhood; a church, a synagogue, or a mosque; a circle of family friends and acquaintances; and familiar people encountered day to day in local shops, libraries, health clubs, or museums. An African saying, popularized in the title of a book (Clinton, 1996), captures this concept: "It takes a village to raise a child."

Yet many children do not grow up with a real sense of community. They may live with danger, homelessness, or isolation. They may attend a school far from home and have no friends nearby. The more you know about resources within the child's community, the more helpful you can be to parents who themselves may feel disconnected and alone. (See Chapter 15 for a further discussion about the place of the community in addressing the mental health needs of families.)

What do you think? Was there a special person in your life who strongly influenced your development?

> ➤ *Check Your Reading*
> 4. Name one significant consideration in understanding each of the following: child, family, and community.
> 5. Why do nurses need to consider models other than the middle-class nuclear family when evaluating family functioning?
> 6. What tasks are facilitated through friendships?
> 7. Why do nurses need to be aware of community resources?

Racial, Ethnic, and Cultural Differences

Nurses who have an opportunity to work with children and families from markedly different backgrounds are immeasurably enriched by what they learn. Both patient and nurse are part of a larger ecological system; each comes to an encounter with a lifetime of cultural experiences (see Chapter 12). Nurses from majority groups may be blind to their own assumptions because "cultural influences are woven into the personality like a tapestry" (McDermott, 1996, p. 411).

The best way to understand what a child and family experience, value, and believe is to learn directly from the child and other family members. Two general principles can guide your approach:

- Child-rearing practices do differ from culture to culture and among subgroups within the larger culture as well. These differences in practice have a strong effect on personality development in children (Caudill & Schooler, 1973; McDermott, 1996; Whiting & Edwards, 1988).
- Minority status is intrinsically neither a risk factor nor a protective factor but carries the potential to become one or the other. The influence of minority status depends on the pervasiveness of societal discrimination against the minority group; the fit between majority and minority beliefs, norms, and values; and the availability of strong adult role models and community support.

JOINING THE JOURNEY: THE THERAPEUTIC RELATIONSHIP

Wherever he went, she was there. Whatever he did, she was there. For a long time they said nothing to each other and never even touched each other. But—no matter what—there she was, close to him.

After a long time, a change took place.... He no longer felt that she was separate from him . . .

And then they began to talk.

Reprinted with the permission of Macmillan Publishing Company from *Jordi* (p. 18) by Theodore Isaac Rubin, MD. Copyright © 1960 by Theodore Isaac Rubin.

The therapeutic relationship is at the heart of child treatment, regardless of the modality or the setting. The phrase *continuity of care* has been stretched beyond recognition in this cost-conscious era to include institutions and entire service systems, but true continuity is provided by an ongoing relationship with an individual person. You need not do all of the work alone; you can advocate for a consistent care team. This team involves a partnership not only among professionals but also with the child and family. Take into account that a child, regardless of age, is a complete human being embedded in a family and community. In developing goals for treatment, incorporate these interlocking spheres. In the words of Winnicott (1957), include *The Child, the Family and the Outside World*.

Frequently, a disturbed child has become stuck in a cycle of maladaptive behaviors that draw forth unhelpful responses from those in the family and community who have also become stuck in responding a certain way. Thus, weaknesses and problems appear in both the child and others. Your challenge is to recognize ways in which these three spheres can become sources of strength. As Rutter (1987) found in his studies of resilience in children, each of these areas has the potential to become **protective factors.**

Transference

The psychoanalytic concept of transference is complicated in child treatment. As Anna Freud (1946) pointed out, because children are generally still living with their parents and are still in the midst of a primary relationship with them, transference in the strictest sense of the word cannot occur. In addition, the more closely and intimately a nurse must interact with a child—for example on an inpatient ward for young children—the more their relationship is an immediate and *real* one for both nurse and child. Yet elements of this relationship are transferential. Chethik (1989) called this displacement of ongoing issues from the family onto the nurse or therapist a "transference of current relationships." Thus, "dealing with the child's projected feelings is inevitable when working with children" (Critchley, 1985, p. 245).

Countertransference

Feelings of countertransference are similarly inevitable when working with children. Your goal is not to do away with or avoid such feelings but to make use of them for a deeper understanding. By examining these feelings, which involve unconscious communications, you can further the work of bringing hidden material to consciousness. This should be done with the help of a clinical supervisor.

Certain kinds of behavior are especially likely to evoke strong feelings in a caregiver (Lewis, 1996). Among these are expressions of hostility, destructiveness, aggression, extreme excitement, and seductive or sexualized behavior. Also, in conflicts between a child and a parent, you may overidentify with one or the other. Some common signals of countertransference can alert you:

1. Noticeable increase in anxiety
2. Sudden rush of any strong emotion
3. Persistent feeling of dislike for a child or parent
4. Boredom or sleepiness in the absence of real fatigue
5. Urge to argue with a child or parent
6. Wish to elicit gratitude from a child or parent

Equipment for the Journey: Coping Mechanisms

Anna Freud, in her 1936 monograph *The Ego and the Mechanisms of Defense,* outlined a developmental progression of unconscious mental processes that people use to mediate their experiences of both the inner world and the disappointments and dangers of external reality. Table 18-2 lists common unconscious

TABLE 18-2 Common Coping Mechanisms Grouped by Developmental Appropriateness	
AGE (y)	**COPING MECHANISMS**
0–5	Delusional projection
	Denial
	Distortion
3–15	Projection
	Fantasy
	Somatization
	Acting out
	Passive-aggressive behavior
3–adulthood	Intellectualization
	Repression
	Displacement
	Reaction formation
	Dissociation
12–adulthood	Altruism
	Humor
	Suppression
	Anticipation
	Sublimation

Adapted from Valliant, G. E. (1971). Theoretical hierarchy of adaptive ego mechanisms. *Archives of General Psychiatry, 25,* 107–118. Copyright 1971, American Medical Association.

strategies and the age groups in which they are typically seen. Such strategies are not inherently negative or positive. They cause trouble only when they interfere with satisfactory living. The most primitive are useful for young children; older children who rely only on these early defenses have a hard time adapting successfully to the demands of life.

What do you think? Can you think of a clinical experience in which you were fairly sure transference and countertransference were involved?

► *Check Your Reading*

8. Name one feature of transference unique to children.
9. What is countertransference?
10. Describe at least three manifestations of countertransference.
11. Give four examples of coping mechanisms and the developmental phase(s) to which each is appropriate.

Stumbling Blocks Along the Path: Epidemiology and Risk Factors

In a summary of 30 years of worldwide studies including more than 123,000 children, Verhulst and Koot (1992) reported that an average of 13% had a psychiatric disturbance of some kind. Five more recent studies cited by the same authors show an even higher range, between 17% and 26%. Overall, boys tend to have more problems with disruptive activity (also called *externalizing behaviors*).

In a nation and a world beset by a host of social ills, children are especially vulnerable. Nurses must remain at the forefront of efforts to reverse this trend. At the very least, you must be alert to certain **risk factors** as you look for ways to prevent or ameliorate mental illness in children. In the words of Solnit (cited in Provence & Naylor, 1983):

A high-risk environment is one which tends to complicate rather than facilitate a healthy development; it is one that uncovers and magnifies the [child's] and parents' vulnerabilities rather than providing the built-in support that will enable them to overcome weaknesses or deficits. (p. viii)

Poverty

The single most prevalent risk factor among children with behavior problems is a low socioeconomic status (Verhulst & Koot, 1992). Obviously, simply being poor does not cause difficulties. Children from extremely poor families can do extraordinarily well. As Winnicott (1971) put it, there is even "the possibility that for a baby or a small child a slum family may be more secure and 'good' as a facilitating environment than a family in a lovely house" (p. 142).

Poverty makes it far more likely, however, that a child will be deprived of optimal nutrition and stimulation, exposed to environmental dangers, given inadequate health care, poorly educated, and in many ways cut off from a rich cultural heritage and opportunities for creative expression. The effects of poverty on families—particularly on children—are at the root of an enormous social policy dilemma often portrayed as a burden on the middle classes. Instead, poverty really represents a tragic loss of human potential. Children and families in the mainstream of society are also terribly deprived, although in different ways, by this stratification of human activities.

Poor children, especially poor minority children, are more likely to be channeled through the juvenile justice system than are middle-class and white children displaying the same behavioral symptoms (Children's Defense Fund, 1989). A study led by Kazdin (cited in Rierden, 1993) found that 80% of children with chronic conduct problems grow up to become adults with similar chronic problems, such as unemployment, criminal behavior, failed marriages, alcoholism, substance abuse, and psychiatric disorders. "This is," Kazdin remarked, "probably the most costly mental health problem we face in the United States. Not only in terms of dollars but also in terms of human suffering" (cited in Rierden, 1993, p. 1).

Neglect and Abuse

In all states, nurses are mandated to report suspected child abuse. However, neglect and abuse are rarely as obvious as the well-publicized cases suggest. The reality is that defining neglect and abuse is difficult and controversial (Korbin, 1987). The American Humane Association (1981) described *neglect* as the "deprivation of necessities," such as "food, clothes, shelter, health care, education and responsible supervision." Yet, as Helfer (1987) pointed out, there is no consensus on the point at which a relative deprivation of any of these becomes clearly definable as neglect.

Abuse is an easily misunderstood word. It may broadly include severe emotional maltreatment or describe a serious physical injury or, far more frequently, repeated episodes of minor injuries (Wolfe, 1987). Therefore, try to be as specific as possible about the actual events and any physical evidence. Don't rely on vague terminology.

The short-term effects of parental violence include physical, developmental, and psychiatric symptoms (Kashani, Daniel, Dandoy, & Holcomb, 1992). Children who have suffered maltreatment are more likely to have difficulties in security of attachment (Main & Solomon, 1990), control of aggression (Scarpa, 1997), mood (Kazdin, Moser, Colbus, & Bell, 1985), self-esteem and social competence (Kazdin et al., 1985; Salzinger, Feldman, Hammer & Rosario, 1993), academic performance (Hoffman-Plotkin & Twentyman, 1984), and juvenile crime (Tarter, Hegedus, Winsten, & Atterman, 1984). They are also more likely to become abusing parents, although the great majority of abused children do *not* grow up to commit abuses (Wolfe, 1987). The National Research Council (1998) lists attributes that have been correlated with abuse, including poverty, social isolation, young parental age, and drug or alcohol use.

The importance of specifying what actually happened is equally true in sexual abuse, a phrase that can refer to a broad range of behaviors, from flashing, to fondling, to rape. Estimates suggest that as many as 38% of all girls are exposed to some form of inappropriate sexual contact during childhood (Russell, 1986), and this figure is likely to be even higher for girls in impoverished conditions (Wyatt, Newcomb, & Rierderle, 1993). The sexual maltreatment of boys is less commonly reported than that of girls. Effects of sexual abuse include fearfulness, a sense of being "damaged goods," depression, impaired peer relations, and a drop in academic performance (Sgroi, 1982). Frequently, such children become preoccupied by sexual matters and may become highly stimulated by the intimacy of a therapeutic relationship.

The degree and nature of harm are related, in part, to the age and temperament of the child. Other factors are the child's relationship with the person committing the offense, that person's age, the type and duration of the abuse, whether it involved affection and "specialness" or coercion and pain, and how the child's disclosure is handled.

Take care not to approach a discussion of sexual abuse with any assumptions about its meaning for a child. Children tend to be acutely sensitive to what an adult wants to hear about such matters—or does *not* want to hear. Sometimes a child is experiencing a great deal of conflict between negative and positive feelings related to the event and may be overwhelmed with guilt on disclosure.

Exposure to Violence

The average American child watches about 3 hours of television a day and by age 12 "has witnessed eight thousand murders and more than a hundred thousand other acts of violence, according to the American Psychological Association" (Auletta, 1993, p. 45). Fortunately, the average American child normally appears to be able to maintain a sense of all of this as make-believe, although studies suggest that exposure to media violence can increase the likelihood of aggressive behavior (Centerwall, 1992; Lagerspetz, 1989). Anecdotal evidence leads one to conclude that under extreme stress or in the presence of a thought disorder, a child has far more difficulty separating fiction from reality. Instances of violent action have been linked to the perpetrator's identification with a fictional aggressor. Incidents such as the killings of several youths in street fights immediately after showings of violent movies such as *The Warriors* in 1979 and *New Jack City* in 1991 are hard to ignore (Auletta, 1993).

Another layer of exposure to violence is the relentless reporting of news about real-life beatings, murders, war, and other disturbing events. Still closer to home is the violence urban children witness in their own neighborhoods. Many disadvantaged young people, especially poor black boys, express a sense of hopelessness about the future based on a belief that they are more likely to die in neighborhood violence than to reach adulthood (Garbarino, 1992).

By far the most immediate ill effects of exposure to violence are accrued by children from violent households. Children who are the targets of such violence may experience fear, anger, sadness, and depression (Brown & Finkelhor, 1986). Even when children are merely witnesses, they grow up with role models who are violent and who victimize others, and they are more likely to engage in violent behavior themselves (Farrington, 1978; Kashani et al., 1992) or to be repeatedly victimized in future relationships (Russell, 1986). In addition, the availability of firearms in the United States is epidemic; "one third of all 8-year-olds nationwide have access to a gun" (Garbarino, 1998, p. 107).

Parental Psychopathology

Conduct Disorder in Either Parent

Conduct disorder or criminal behaviors in either parent or in both parents have been associated with psychiatric disturbance in children (Kazdin, 1992; Rutter & Quinton, 1984). Whether this effect is due to inadequate parenting, modeling, or parental maltreatment—or to some combination of factors—remains unclear.

Depression in Mother

The other characteristic most strongly correlated with childhood psychopathology is maternal depression (Rutter, 1986). Although genetic factors are likely to be involved in this association, parental availability and the quality of caretaking are also important variables. Children of depressed mothers are more likely to have mood disorders and also are vulnerable to a range of other difficulties, including anxiety, poor self-esteem, and academic and conduct problems (Beck, 1998; Postnatal Depression, 1998).

Medical Illness and Disability

A number of authors have studied the relationship between psychiatric disturbances and medical illness (Graham & Turk, 1996; Lambert & Lambert, 1987) or disability (Breslau, 1985; Rose & Thomas, 1987; Sacks, 1988). According to Mrazek (1996), "Serious physical illness should be conceptualized as one of the most important early risk factors for emotional disturbance" (p. 1058). In a nursing study of behavioral disturbances in medically hospitalized children, McClowry (1991) pointed out that although the hospitalization may in itself be a stressor, other causes may underlie both the need for hospitalization *and* the emotional problems. Socioeconomic disadvantage is once again implicated as a contributing factor.

Nurses are often in a position to be especially helpful to children with medical illnesses or disabilities, whether they encounter such children in a medical, educational, or psychiatric setting. It is especially important that you understand that illness and disability have a *meaning* to a child and family. As stated by Kleinman (1988), health care providers have an "existential commitment to be with the sick person and to facilitate his or her building of an illness narrative that will make sense of and give value to the experience" (p. 54). With the help of a committed nurse, an illness or a disability can even provide a child and family with an opportunity for mastery and growth.

Medical illness or disability in the parent is also a risk factor for a child (Rutter, 1966). A significant number of children, especially in poor, urban areas, are affected by HIV and AIDS in family members. Michaels and Levine (1992) estimated that by the year 2000, between 80,000 and 110,000 children and teens will have been orphaned by maternal AIDS deaths.

Divorce

The divorce rate in the United States climbed sharply in the second half of the century, leveling off at approximately 50% (Hernandez, 1988). Children of divorce represent a disproportionate percentage of child psychiatric patients. In inpatient settings, this figure approaches 100% (Wallerstein & Corbin, 1996).

Divorce has an immediate, often obvious impact on children's lives. It is related to family conflict, disruption, loss, diminished parenting, diminished financial support, and at times increased dependence of the parent on the child (Peterson, Leigh, & Day, 1984; Wallerstein & Corbin, 1996). Although the initial impact can be addressed immediately and may be mitigated by time, social support, and treatment, divorce has also been found to have profound long-term effects on development (Kalter, 1987; Wallerstein & Blakeslee, 1989).

Longitudinal studies have indicated a complex blending of factors that contribute to postdivorce adjustment. These include individual resilience and the availability of encouragement either within or outside of the family. Wallerstein (1983) formulated six *psychological tasks* for the child of divorce:

1. Acknowledging the reality of the marital rupture
2. Disengaging from parental conflict and distress and resuming customary pursuits
3. Resolving losses
4. Resolving anger and self-blame
5. Accepting the permanence of divorce
6. Achieving realistic hope regarding relationships

What do you think? Is it harder to be a child now than it was when you were growing up?

➤ *Check Your Reading*

12. Up to what percentage of children are believed to have a psychiatric disturbance?
13. List six risk factors associated with mental illness in children.
14. Which of these risk factors is most strongly correlated?
15. Identify three of the six psychological tasks facing a child after parental divorce.
16. What effect does living in a violent household have on a child?
17. Why is poverty a risk factor for children?
18. Define neglect.

NURSING PROCESS

Assessment

Jordi was observed for hours. There were rooms with one-way mirrors and interviews and tests of all kinds. He played with blocks, ink blots, and little statues of children and adults.

Reprinted with the permission of Macmillan Publishing Company from *Jordi* (p. 12) by Theodore Isaac Rubin, MD. Copyright © 1960 by Theodore Isaac Rubin.

You will apply the same observational skills you learned in assessing a child's physical condition to assessing a child's psychiatric condition. The cornerstone of your assessment is a carefully gathered history that includes the child's motor, cognitive, and social development;

past illnesses and injuries; daily living skills; school performance; and course of symptoms. Box 18–1 provides a way of organizing a psychiatric nursing assessment. Figure 18–1 is a sample child-family assessment tool.

Physical Examination

A physical examination should be thorough and performed with sensitivity to the child's feelings. Obvious findings, such as abnormal head circumference, bruises, or abdominal distention, should be noted. *Any* unusual observation should also be recorded, because some rare neurodegenerative and neuromuscular disorders may be mistaken for primarily psychiatric illnesses.

Pay special attention to the neurological examination. Asymmetries, delays in coordination or speech, mixed or delayed "handedness," poor right-left discrimination, and visual difficulties suggest organic dysfunction. When mild, these have been referred to as *soft signs.* This is a vague term, poorly correlated with *specific* disorders, but evidence suggests that "soft signs on the neurological examination do reflect brain dysfunction in most cases and are influenced by heredity" (Pincus, 1996).

Mental Status Examination

Although questionnaires and structured interviews have been developed to ascertain the presence of psychiatric symptoms in children, the Mental Status Examination

Box 18–1 ■ ■ ■ ■ ■

Important Aspects of a Psychiatric Nursing Assessment

History
  Developmental milestones
  Socialization
  School performance and behaviors
  Eating, sleeping, and elimination patterns
  Medical illnesses or injuries
Physical examinaion
  Neurological examination
  Frank central nervous system anomalies
  Presence of "soft signs"
Mental status examination
  Appearance
  Anxiety level
  Attention span
  Relatedness
  Orientation
  Mood
  Thought processes
  Memory
  Presence of suicidal or homicidal ideation
  Coping mechanisms
  Quality and content of play

Child's Name: _____ Date: _____

Nurse's Name: _____

Goals for Visit: _____

Vital Signs (If Appropriate): T_____ P_____ R_____ B/P_____

Allergies NKA: _____ Drugs: _____ Food:_____ Other: _____

Reason for Referral (Need for Control; Safety; Behavioral Interventions; Family Support): _____

_____

_____

Family History (Genogram; Any Recent Stress; Who Resided in Home; Child's Relationship with Family Members; Patterns of Communication; Disciplinary Practices): _____

_____

_____

_____

_____

Developmental History (Child's Growth; Developmental Milestones; Current Level of Functioning; Parental Expectations): _____

_____

_____

_____

History of Previous Treatment (When? With Whom? Where? Outcomes?): _____

_____

_____

_____

History of Medical/Physical Problems: _____

_____

_____

Current Medical/Physical Problems: _____

_____

_____

Current Drug Therapy: Yes_____ No_____

    If yes, what medications does child take?_____

    Dose _____ Frequency_____

Nutrition and Sleep:

    Appetite Change Yes_____ No_____

    Weight Gain: Yes_____ No_____

    Weight Loss: Yes_____ No_____

    Eating Problems: _____

    Diet Restrictions: _____

    Caffeinated Beverage Intake: _____

    Food Allergies: _____

Overall Physical Appearance: Well Nourished _____ Obese_____ Poorly Nourished _____

    Frail _____ Run Down_____ Other_____

Regular Hours of Sleep: Yes_____ No_____

Difficulty Falling Asleep: Yes_____ No_____ Restlessness: Yes_____ No_____

Early A.M. Awakening: Yes_____ No_____ Nightmares: Yes_____ No_____

Dr. Verna Benner Carson
Psychiatric Home Care Manual

Figure 18-1
A sample child-adolescent-family assessment tool. (From Carson, V. B. [1994]. Psychiatric home care manual. Baltimore: Bay Area Health Care. Copyright © Bay Area Health Care, 1994.)

remains the primary tool of assessment. However, the interviewer conducting such an examination with a child must be more flexible and informal than with adults, providing both structured and unstructured opportunities for interaction.

A nurse may be conducting the Mental Status Examination alone or assisting another clinician. The interview should take place in a private space with play items, such as paper and crayons, clay, dolls, animal figures (dinosaurs are particularly appealing to young children), toy telephones, and a toy medical kit. The inclusion of toy guns is a personal choice and a controversial question with no "right" answer. Be prepared for the child to express aggression regardless of the toys provided. For preadolescents, you may want to have a small selection of card or board games you also enjoy playing.

Pay special attention to the beginning of the encounter, even before entering the playroom. The manner in which the child greets (or doesn't greet) you is significant, as is the way the child parts from the parent. Also valuable are comments made while *approaching* the interview room; such comments are often unguarded and can be extremely revealing. The ending of the interview may be similarly rich.

During the interview, which unfolds as a kind of conversation, note the child's appearance, coordination, tolerance of separation from the accompanying parent, mood, range of emotion, relatedness, and understanding of the reason for the interview. Questions can determine the child's orientation, general comprehension, and memory (e.g., make a game of listing three unrelated items and ask the child to recall them after 5 minutes). As the play or talking progresses, be attentive to the child's thinking—its content, speed, and order of flow. At some point, you must ask directly about hallucinations, suicidal thoughts and plans, sexual experience, and (depending on the age of the child) alcohol and drug use. Ask these questions in an empathic, straightforward, and low-key manner.

You should be developing working hypotheses about the DSM-IV differential diagnoses as well as tentative nursing diagnoses that will be solidified in planning treatment with the family. Throughout both evaluation and treatment, remember that much of a child's communication happens indirectly, sometimes without any words at all. Pay careful attention both to what children say and to what they do. Watch how they relate to the people around them, how they show they are anxious, and what comforts them. Consider your own feelings and associations and ask yourself what these might mean. While keeping a child company, try to imagine what it is like to *be* that particular child.

Specific Areas of Assessment

Play

It is in playing and only in playing that the individual child or adult is able to be creative and to use the whole personality, and it is only in being creative that the individual discovers the self (Winnicott, 1971, p. 54).

For a child, play means many things. It has been called "the vehicle by which the child masters the environment and his own impulses and increases his adaptive behavior" (Critchley, 1985). Play is also a young child's main form of communication, and you need to observe and respond to it with this in mind. Box 18-2 outlines some important features of a child's play.

> "He took the doorknob attached to a long string and ran past her out of the house. He had his jiggler now and was truly safe. He let his jiggler hang down in front of him and waited. Soon it would tell his feet where to go. . . . He walked and walked."
>
> Reprinted with the permission of Macmillan Publishing Company from *Jordi* (p. 5) by Theodore Isaac Rubin, MD. Copyright © 1960 by Theodore Isaac Rubin.

Jordi's early play behavior was solitary, repetitive, and lacking in imagination and narrative line. Jordi could not use play to explore or master his fears because he was unable to distinguish between fantasy and reality.

Box 18–2 ■ ■ ■ ■ ■
Important Aspects of Play

- *Content:* Themes such as aggression or nurturing may appear repeatedly, or play may involve a wide range of thematic material.
- *Anxiety:* Play may involve a manageable—even pleasurable—level of tension, or the child may be overwhelmed by anxiety and interrupt the play.
- *Imagination:* Imagination can range from simple manipulation of objects to richly elaborated fantasy play.
- *Discrimination between make-believe and reality:* Some children get lost in the play; others may assure the nurse "it's just pretend."
- *Narrative line:* Actions may be repeated endlessly, may jump from one to another, or may flow smoothly with a sense of a beginning and an ending.
- *Persistence:* One child may be easily frustrated and another may stick to a task such as building a tower until it is completed.
- *Reciprocity:* Some children ignore an onlooker completely; others invite the nurse to participate actively, seeking a shared experience.
- *Adherence to rules:* Blatant cheating is seen in young children and sometimes in older children with poor self-esteem; obsessional children may become so preoccupied by the rules that the point of the game is obscured.

> The monkey bars, crisscrossing up and down, forward and backward intrigued him.... He walked over cautiously and touched the closest bar. It was cold. A sinister chill ran through him.... It looked like a wonderful toy to climb over and swing from. And it looked like an awful monster that could tangle you up, crush you, and kill you. Her voice, soft and smooth, said, "Try it. It's fun, Jordi—fun—a toy. I'll show you."

Reprinted with the permission of Macmillan Publishing Company from *Jordi* (p. 39) by Theodore Isaac Rubin, MD. Copyright © 1960 by Theodore Isaac Rubin.

> Over the course of his treatment, Jordi gradually learned turn-taking in play, the usefulness of rules, and the pleasure of mastery. Finally, he was able to take part in school-age games with other children.

Reprinted with the permission of Macmillan Publishing Company from *Jordi* (pp. 51–52) by Theodore Isaac Rubin, MD. Copyright © 1960 by Theodore Isaac Rubin.

ATTACHMENT AND SEPARATION

In the narrowest sense of the word, **attachment** refers to the reciprocal relationship between a mother and an infant during the first months of the child's life. Long regarded as a critical aspect of human development, attachment became the focus of much scientific concern and interest during the 1940s and 1950s (Harlow & Harlow, 1962; Robertson, 1970; Spitz, 1945).

Two decades later, researchers began to study this relationship in a systematic way (Bowlby, 1969). The phrase *secure attachment* (Ainsworth, Blehar, Waters, & Wall, 1973) described an infant's sense of basic trust in the reliability of a supportive caretaker, or "good-enough mother" (Winnicott, 1971, p. 11). Secure attachment contrasted with *insecure attachment*, which has since been further broken down into three categories: insecure-avoidant, insecure-resistant, and insecure-disorganized-disoriented (Main & Cassidy, 1988). These are believed to grow out of the infant's experiences of not being comforted by a parent. Studies have suggested that a secure attachment is correlated with greater adaptive functioning in childhood, although this may not be an enduring effect (Thompson, 1996). Similarly, the infant's role has not been as well described as that of the mother (Stern, 1985).

In a broader sense, attachment also includes the capacity to form meaningful relationships with others throughout life. It is possible for a child, in the absence of a secure attachment in infancy, to develop better attachments later in life. Numerous authors have cited this capacity to form attachments as an important *source of resistance to risk* (Garmezy, 1987) or a *protective factor* (Rutter, 1987). To assess this capacity, observe the child's interactions with others and gauge the quality of the growing therapeutic relationship.

SEXUALITY

> The bath felt very nice. It was warm, and he was alone. He pushed the piece of wood around the tub and watched it skim over his knees and then back again over his belly. Then he held it down on the bottom of the tub and let it go suddenly, watching it shoot to the surface. Then he thought of his penis. First he squeezed it; then he rubbed it up and down. It felt nice, and it was good to be alone. When his penis stood up, he stared at it a while and wondered how this magic took place.

Reprinted with the permission of Macmillan Publishing Company from *Jordi* (pp. 51–52) by Theodore Isaac Rubin, MD. Copyright © 1960 by Theodore Isaac Rubin.

One of Freud's most revolutionary concepts was that of infantile sexuality. Although the concept came as a disagreeable shock to turn-of-the-century Vienna, for most of recorded human history and prehistory, not only was infantile and childhood sexuality universally accepted but also children were exposed to a full range of adult sexual expression, from birth onward, with no concern for their "corruption."

Children explore their bodies and find pleasure in exploration. Modern parents have become slightly more tolerant of this process, although tolerance often depends on the child's gender. For example, boys are now more frequently given the correct words for *penis, testicles,* and *scrotum,* whereas girls are often taught a substitute word or only the word *vagina,* not *vulva, labia,* or—particularly—*clitoris.* Boys, however, are more likely than girls to be discouraged from affectionate physical contact with others.

Despite relatively minor changes, parents continue to be at a loss in providing for their children's sexual development and safety. For the most part, they avoid sexual topics and redirect children's curiosity. Some clinicians have expressed worry that, in a climate of pervasive concerns about sexual molestation, the trend toward fathers' greater involvement in all aspects of child care may be hindered by fears of accusation (Levenkron, 1993). This would be especially unfortunate because fathers who are closely involved in caring for their infants are *less* likely to engage in sexual behavior with any children (Parker & Parker, 1984).

Worldwide studies of sexual mores place the United States among the most restrictive cultures in terms of child-rearing practices. As Konner (1982) put it,

[T]he Western family, including that of the United States at mid-century as well as that of Freud's Vienna, afforded children much less experience and information regarding sex, playful or serious, than did the average non-industrial society (p. 287).

Further,

[E]verything we know about higher primates points to a crucial role for experience in the growth of normal

behavior, and this is no less true of sexual than of other forms of behavior (p. 285).

One unfortunate outcome of these limitations is that while children are strongly discouraged from learning about sexual pleasure and eroticism, the media bombard everyone with contradictory cultural messages. This discrepancy appears to contribute to an extraordinarily high rate of sexual dysfunction—approaching 50%—in both men and women (Yates, 1996). Another contributing factor to adult sexual dysfunction is a history of sexual molestation as a child (Groth, 1979). Although most children who have been molested do not repeat this pattern in adulthood, some sexual dysfunctions in men *are* associated with pedophilia, and sexual problems between married couples are positively correlated with father-daughter incest (Groth, 1982).

During an assessment, ask the parents about what the child has been taught regarding sex and any other information that might be relevant. A good starting point is to invite the parents to speak about any concerns or questions they might have regarding their child's sexuality. Without an invitation, parents may hesitate to bring up this topic. In counseling parents, keep the following points in mind:

1. You can model an approach to the subject that is direct, unembarrassed, and sensible, using language appropriate to the parents' background and educational level.

2. Ask parents to clarify their attitudes and wishes about their child's sexuality by talking openly in a supportive environment.

3. If frank discussion reveals major conflict or sexual difficulties between parents, they should be encouraged to take this up in separate couples' treatment.

4. Your objective is to see that the child is protected as far as possible from *any* activity or event that is frightening, painful, overstimulating, or coercive.

Also observe the child for either overly inhibited or hypersexual behavior. Frank preoccupation with explicit sexual themes or knowledge of detail not explained by the parents' account should lead you to wonder about the possibility of molestation or exposure to adult sexual activities. Ask the child a question, such as "Have you ever been touched, or been asked to touch someone, in a way that made you feel excited, worried, or uncomfortable?"

Although Freud's term *latency* delineates the years (roughly between the ages of 6 or 7 and 10 or 11 years) when the child's hormone levels are stable and the oedipal preoccupation with the parents goes temporarily underground, experience tells us that latency-age children certainly continue to be interested in sex. They are, however, enlarging their repertoire of adaptive defense mechanisms and tend to become more modest and private about all bodily functions (although not in their humor!).

MORAL DEVELOPMENT

The development of moral decision-making skills has been relatively little studied. Yet, as Wolf (1996) pointed out, "The psychopathology of moral development is

likely to be as important for child psychiatry as that of attachment behavior" (p. 219). Philosophers, early psychoanalytic theorists, and behaviorists have based speculations about moral development largely on self-reflection and studies of adults. Piaget (1965) observed children's behavior and reasoning in normative settings and plotted time lines of moral reasoning that correspond with cognitive phases.

Kohlberg (1981) took this stage theory a step further, proposing a sequence of six stages of moral development grouped in three levels: the premoral level, the level of conventional role conformity, and the level of self-accepted moral principles. Kohlberg's conclusions have been widely criticized. Gilligan (1982) pointed out that the 25-year longitudinal study on which Kohlberg's work was based included only boys and men. She proposed a three-level theory of moral development for girls: concern for the self, caring for others in need, and concern and caring for all people (Gilligan, 1985). Gilligan argued that basing moral decisions on the primacy of caring relationships (for Kohlberg, a stage 3 characteristic) is a higher value than basing moral decisions on universal ethical principles (for Kohlberg, stage 6). Similarly, Hoffman (1984) proposed four levels in the development of empathy: global empathy, egocentric empathy, empathy for another's feelings, and empathy for another's general condition. Coles (1986) conducted phenomenological research with children who have maintained a highly evolved moral stance despite adverse social circumstances. Kagan and Lamb (1987) collected essays from studies in anthropology, philosophy, and developmental psychology in an attempt to answer four long-standing questions:

1. Is morality innate or learned?
2. How do standards for moral judgment develop as children grow older?

Dear God,
I do not think anybody could be a better God. Well I just want you to know but I am not just saying that because you are God. Charles

From Hample, S., & Marshall, E. (Eds.) (1991). *Children's letters to God: The new collection.* New York: Workman.

3. Are there universal standards that all children acquire?

4. Do gender and cultural differences have any bearing on moral development?

Faced with such questions, you may be wondering how parents can best meet their children's needs in this regard. The answer is probably disarmingly simple: When parents whose lives reflect their own values raise their children lovingly, the children are likely to grow up with similar values. "Moral education follows naturally on the arrival of morality in the child by the natural developmental processes that good care facilitates" (Winnicott, 1965, p. 100). During assessment, try to get a preliminary sense of the child's social judgment and capacity for empathy, the level of excitement evoked by cruelty or identification with an aggressor, and any expression of remorse for transgressions.

SPIRITUAL DEVELOPMENT

Perhaps even less well studied than moral development is the spiritual development of children and adolescents. Yet, as Coles (1990) reminded us,

[The] child's house "has many mansions"—including a spiritual life that grows, changes, responds constantly to the other lives that, in their sum, make up the individual we call by a name and know by a story that is all his, all hers. (p. 308)

Carson (1989) proposed spiritual development as a *two-directional process.* The horizontal dimension is concerned with spiritual values in day-to-day living, the vertical with an individual's relationship to a higher power. Carson distinguished between spirituality and religiosity, because many people abide by religious traditions without experiencing spiritual awakening, just as people without religious affiliation may espouse an essential spirituality.

Building on these stages of the development of faith put forward by Fowler (1984), by Aden (1976), and by Westerhoff (1976), Carson wove in Erikson's (1961, 1963) belief in the importance of hope, as shown in Table 18–3. As Carson pointed out, these theories have

Dear God It is great the way you always get the stars in the right places.

Jeff

From Hample, S., & Marshall, E. (Eds.) (1991). *Children's letters to God: The new collection.* New York: Workman.

been formulated in the context of Western cultures and Judeo-Christian values. One of the most striking differences between industrialized nations and the rest of the people of the world is that, in many indigenous cultures, spiritual teaching is part of daily life and childhood education. Children's heritage is inseparable from their responsibility to safeguard the tenets and practices of their creed. For example, writing of the Australian

TABLE 18-3 Spiritual Development

DEVELOPMENTAL STAGE	ERIKSON	ADEN	FOWLER	WESTERHOFF
Infancy	Hope	Faith as trust	Stage 0: undifferentiated	
Early childhood	Will	Faith as courage	Stage I: intuitive-projective	Experienced faith
Preschool	Purpose	Faith as obedience		
School age	Skill	Faith as assent	Stage II: mythical-literal	
Adolescence	Fidelity	Faith as identity	Stage III: synthetic-conventional	Affiliative faith
Young adulthood	Love	Faith as surrender	Stage IV: individuality, reflexive	Searching faith
Adulthood	Care	Faith as unconditional surrender	Stage V: polar-dialectical	
Maturity	Wisdom	Faith as unconditional acceptance	Stage VI: universalizing	Owned faith

Aborigines, Lawlor (1991) stated that for them, "childhood emerges out of the depths of the spirit of the natural world and is inseparable from that world" (p. 170).

Hollander (1981) emphasized the parents' role in assisting children to develop a spiritual awareness, particularly in families cut off from communal practices, by giving the child a context to support spirituality in daily activities. Sometimes, catastrophic events can bring a child face to face with a spiritual crisis. Sometimes, with help, the child can make good use of such a crisis to develop a profound inner strength.

Not part of any model of spiritual development, however, is the view that the child is *innately* religious, inhabiting a world suffused with undifferentiated godliness. This idea has run like a thread through Western mystical thought for thousands of years. From this perspective, promoting spiritual growth consists of protecting the child's inborn spiritual capacities from the negative influences of the material world. This belief can be traced as far back as Socrates, who expressed a conviction that each person is born endowed with complete knowledge and that this knowledge can be brought to consciousness by careful questioning. It appears in the words of Jesus to his disciples: "Except ye be converted, and become as little children, ye shall not enter the kingdom of heaven" (Matthew 18:3). And it appears nearly 2000 years later, in Wordsworth's poem, "Ode on Intimations of Immortality":

> *But trailing clouds of glory do we come*
> *   From God, who is our home:*
> *Heaven lies about us in our infancy!*

When considering a child's spiritual development, question both parents and child about spiritual faith, religious practices, and their importance to the family. Understanding another's values is an important part of empathy. As Carson (1989) reminded us, "[S]pirituality is not something to be judged but rather to be assessed and accepted."

SUICIDALITY

No statistics are kept of suicides among children under 5 years of age, but records show that it is the fifth leading cause of death in children between the ages of 5 and 14 (Pfeffer, 1997). The most prevalent methods of suicide in young children involve impulsive actions such as jumping from a height or running in front of a car, so separating possible suicides from the high number of accidental deaths in this age group is difficult.

The most immediate risk factor is *current suicidal ideation,* particularly in the presence of a lethal plan. Never dismiss this as a bid for attention. The best way to determine whether the child has a plan is to ask directly. Approach the topic naturally in the context of the mental status examination, but even with a gentle approach, make your questions clear and unambiguous: "Have you ever thought of hurting yourself or killing yourself? How would you do this? Are you feeling this way now?" A child at high risk for committing suicide must be kept safe and should be hospitalized, if necessary.

W*hat do you think?* Do any of these areas of child development make you uncomfortable?

► *Check Your Reading*

19. What do you assess as part of the physical examination?
20. Give an example to illustrate each of five features of a play assessment.
21. Name at least four specific areas of a child's psychiatric assessment.
22. What is the most immediate risk factor for a suicidal child?
23. Give one reason why a spiritual assessment is included in the overall assessment of children.

Diagnosis

Naming a psychiatric disorder does not mean that it exists the way objects or physical illnesses exist. This ambiguity may be especially true of many psychiatric diagnoses given to children, which (although they may be related to a neurological problem) are based on a cluster of attributes or behaviors and are not diseases. Also keep in mind that these attributes and behaviors are almost always just exaggerated versions of characteristics that all people share. The diagnosis is "not an end in itself, but a strategic doorway to treatment" (Nurcombe & Fitzhenry-Coor, 1987).

As Chapter 3 explains, you need to be familiar with the currently used psychiatric nosology, or classification system. The *Diagnostic and Statistical Manual of Mental Disorders, Fourth Edition* (DSM-IV) begins with a section addressing disorders "usually first diagnosed in infancy, childhood, or adolescence" (p. 37). These psychiatric diagnoses in turn suggest related nursing diagnoses.

For Jordi, the overriding nursing diagnosis is social isolation related to profound developmental delays, poor reality testing, and anxiety, as evidenced by lack of social skills and immature and bizarre behaviors.

Assessment data that support this finding might be stated as follows:

1. Jordi's parents state "He has no friends."
2. Jordi makes poor eye contact and rarely interacts with others.
3. Jordi displays several unusual sensitivities and fears.
4. Jordi appears to be responding to internal stimuli at times.

W*hat do you think?* Is it helpful to give a child a psychiatric diagnosis or not?

► *Check Your Reading*

24. Explain why most children's psychiatric disorders are different from a medical disease, such as diabetes.

Attention Deficit and Disruptive Behavior Disorders

ATTENTION-DEFICIT HYPERACTIVITY DISORDER

A DSM-IV diagnosis of Attention-Deficit Hyperactivity Disorder (ADHD) is based on symptoms that occur before age 7 years and have lasted at least 6 months. This diagnosis is further codified by the predominating symptoms—that is, whether the child is mainly inattentive, mainly hyperactive, or both.

In any classroom in the United States you may see a child with these symptoms. He is in constant motion: running when others walk, fidgeting as he waits in line, jumping up out of his seat, making mistake after mistake on his worksheets, not paying attention, or blurting out answers without waiting to be called on.

A large epidemiological study found that ADHD is the most common psychiatric diagnosis given to children between the ages of 4 and 11 years (Szatmari, Offord, & Boyle, 1989). In a representative sample of 1617 children, 9% of boys and 3.3% of girls were found to have ADHD. Other studies show that genetic factors explain about 50% of the variance (Weiss, 1996).

The first line of treatment for ADHD is often a stimulant medication such as methylphenidate or dextroamphetamine. Because the vast majority of children with ADHD show situational differences in hyperactivity (Weiss, 1996), however, the child's environment clearly plays a key role and must be taken into account.

Although Conduct Disorder occurs in children, it is more frequently seen in adolescents and is discussed in Chapter 19.

OPPOSITIONAL DEFIANT DISORDER

Oppositional defiant disorder is another diagnosis given to children who are often more readily perceived as troubling than troubled. Similarly, this diagnosis requires a minimum of four out of eight designated behaviors to be present for at least 6 months, including temper tantrums, arguing with adults, actively defying adult requests, provocative behavior, blaming others, and being easily angered. Again, because these behaviors are common, they must occur far more frequently than in others of the same mental age. As Rey (1993) pointed out:

Symptoms of oppositional defiant disorder may be the final common pathway of many etiological factors, alone or in combination, including genetic, constitutional, social, and psychological mechanisms. (p. 1775)

Nevertheless, an oppositional, defiant child is relatively rare in households in which parents agree on consistent, loving methods of providing structure and discipline. Oppositional children often have low self-esteem and may actually find their own behavior quite frightening. Nevertheless, they may also be frightened of giving up their defiance. It probably serves several functions, including distraction from fearfulness, sadness, and anxiety. The object of socializing such children is not to break them. As Cotton (1993) wrote:

Our patients are the discontented, sad and angry lions in the playing fields and classrooms of childhood. We want them to keep their lion strength, passion, and aggression, within the treatment settings and strategies we create for them. We don't want them to abandon the inner lion, but to befriend and tame it. (p. 2)

A combination of externally imposed limits, cognitive teaching of problem solving skills, and insight-oriented therapy can address both behaviors and feelings.

> **W**hat do you think? Should classrooms be changed to meet the needs of ADHD children?

➤ *Check Your Reading*

25. Name at least two characteristics of a child with ADHD.
26. Suggest two nursing diagnoses for a child with a disruptive behavior disorder.

ANXIETY DISORDERS

The anxiety disorders of childhood and adolescence include both specific and general disturbances. Anxiety, fear, and impaired social interaction are potentially useful nursing diagnoses in these disorders. Of the anxiety disorders, only separation anxiety disorder is listed in DSM-IV as a childhood disorder. It is most commonly seen in early childhood and in preadolescence. It is characterized by at least a 4-week duration of excessive and unrealistic worry about separation from the child's major attachment figures (usually, but not always, parents). Anxiety may be manifested by such things as persistent worries about possible harm to the parents and reluctance or refusal to be separated from them, for example, to attend school or to go to bed. These children often complain of a wide variety of physical symptoms as well.

Separation anxiety in the child is often seen concurrently with a similar anxiety in the parent, lending support to the theory of a genetic contribution to the disorder. In this instance, both child and parent can be helped by the experience of surviving separations.

Overanxious disorder of childhood, included in the category of generalized anxiety disorder, is diagnosed based on symptoms present for 6 months or more. Symptoms include excessive or unrealistic worries about several events or activities, past or future; irritability; difficulty concentrating; and difficulty falling asleep. A problem in offering comprehensive treatment for any of these disorders is that antianxiety medications, such as the benzodiazepines, which are traditionally used to help anxious adults, have not been found to be particularly effective or helpful in children. Somewhat more helpful are antidepressants, such as bupropion or nortriptyline.

Obsessive-compulsive disorder (OCD), now generally believed to be a neurophysiologically based illness with a genetic component, has also been noted to occur at a higher rate in relatives of people with Tourette's disorder (Pauls, 1996). Although a single specific mechanism has

DSM-IV Diagnosis: Attention-Deficit Hyperactivity Disorder

Diagnostic Criteria

A. Either (1) or (2):

(1) Six (or more) of the following symptoms of *inattention* have persisted for at least six months to a degree that is maladaptive and inconsistent with developmental level:

Inattention

(a) Often fails to give close attention to details or makes careless mistakes in schoolwork, work, or other activities.

(b) Often has difficulty sustaining attention in tasks or play activities.

(c) Often does not seem to listen when spoken to directly.

(d) Often does not follow through on instructions and fails to finish schoolwork, chores, or duties in the workplace (not due to oppositional behavior or failure to understand instructions).

(e) Often has difficulty organizing tasks and activities.

(f) Often avoids, dislikes, or is reluctant to engage in tasks that require sustained mental effort (such as schoolwork or homework).

(g) Often loses things necessary for tasks or activities (e.g., toys, school assignments, pencils, books, or tools).

(h) Is often easily distracted by extraneous stimuli.

(i) Is often forgetful in daily activities.

(2) Six (or more) of the following symptoms of *hyperactivity-impulsivity* have persisted for at least six months to a degree that is maladaptive and inconsistent with developmental level:

Hyperactivity

(a) Often fidgets with hands or feet or squirms in seat.

(b) Often leaves seat in classroom or in other situations in which remaining seated is expected.

(c) Often runs about or climbs excessively in situations in which it is inappropriate (in adolescents or adults, may be limited to subjective feelings of restlessness).

(d) Often has difficulty playing or engaging in leisure activities quietly.

(e) Is often "on the go" or often acts as if "driven by a motor."

(f) Often talks excessively.

Impulsivity

(g) Often blurts out answers before questions have been completed.

(h) Often has difficulty awaiting turn.

(i) Often interrupts or intrudes on others (e.g., butts into conversations or games).

B. Some hyperactive-impulsive or inattentive symptoms that caused impairment were present before age 7 years.

C. Some impairment from the symptoms is present in two or more settings (e.g., at school [or work] and at home).

D. There must be clear evidence of clinically significant impairment in social, academic, or occupational functioning.

E. The symptoms do not occur exclusively during the course of a Pervasive Developmental Disorder, Schizophrenia, or other Psychotic Disorder and are not better accounted for by another mental disorder (e.g., Mood Disorder, Anxiety Disorder, Dissociative Disorder, or a Personality Disorder).

Code based on type:

314.01 Attention-Deficit/Hyperactivity Disorder, Combined Type: If both Criteria A1 and A2 are met for the past six months.

314.00 Attention-Deficit/Hyperactivity Disorder, Predominantly Inattentive Type: If Criterion A1 is met but Criterion A2 is not met for the past six months.

314.01 Attention-Deficit/Hyperactivity Disorder, Predominantly Hyperactive-Impulsive Type: If Criterion A2 is met but Criterion A1 is not met for the past six months.

Coding note: For individuals (especially adolescents and adults) who currently have symptoms that no longer meet full criteria, "In Partial Remission" should be specified.

DSM-IV Diagnosis: Oppositional Defiant Disorder

Diagnostic Criteria

A. A pattern of negativistic, hostile, and defiant behavior lasting at least six months, during which four (or more) of the following are present:

(1) Often loses temper.

(2) Often argues with adults.

(3) Often actively defies or refuses to comply with adults' requests or rules.

(4) Often deliberately annoys people.

(5) Often blames others for his or her mistakes or misbehavior.

(6) Is often touchy or easily annoyed by others.

(7) Is often angry and resentful.

(8) Is often spiteful or vindictive.

Note: Consider a criterion met only if the behavior occurs more frequently than is typically observed in individuals of comparable age and developmental level.

Based on information from the *Diagnostic and Statistical Manual of Mental Disorders. Fourth Edition.* Copyright 1994 American Psychiatric Association.

MEDICAL DIAGNOSES AND RELATED NURSING DIAGNOSES

Attention-Deficit and Disruptive Behavior Disorders *Continued*

B. The disturbance in behavior causes clinically significant impairment in social, academic, or occupational functioning.

C. The behaviors do not occur exclusively during the course of a Psychotic or Mood Disorder.

D. Criteria are not met for Conduct Disorder, and, if the individual is age 18 years or older, criteria are not met for Antisocial Personality Disorder.

Related Nursing Diagnosis

Ineffective Family Coping: Compromised

Definition

A usually supportive primary person (family member or close friend) is providing insufficient, ineffective, or compromised support, comfort, assistance, or encouragement that may be needed by the client to manage or master adaptive tasks related to his or her health challenge.

Example

Ineffective Family Coping related to oppositional defiant disorder as evidenced by cycle of harsh punishment followed by overindulgent compensation.

---

yet to be demonstrated, studies suggest the involvement of the serotoninergic system of the brain (Scahill, Walker, Lechner, & Tynan, 1993).

The defining characteristics of OCD are obsessions (recurring, distressing thoughts or images), compulsions (repetitive, driven behaviors performed in response to obsessions), or both. In talking about these with young children you might call them "worries" and "habits." Treatment has focused on the use of medications (e.g., clomipramine or fluoxetine) that block the reuptake of the neurotransmitter serotonin to support behavioral approaches. Typically, parents of a child with this disorder find themselves gradually accommodating increasingly outlandish demands in a well-meaning but futile effort to help the child function. Learning to set limits supportively and to work with the child on treatment interventions, such as *exposure* (intentionally confronting the child with provocative stimuli) and *response prevention* (not allowing the compulsion) are important for both parents and nurses (March & Mulle, 1998).

Posttraumatic stress disorder is now recognized in children as well as in adults. Either posttraumatic stress disorder or acute stress disorder may follow a child's experiencing or witnessing a terrifying event in which threat of harm or death or actual harm or death occurs.

The difference between the two disorders is largely a matter of time of onset and duration of symptoms, both involving recurrent recollections of the event, disturbing dreams, increased anxiety, and avoidance of anything likely to remind the child of the event. Some symptoms may respond to antidepressant medication (Table 18–4). Children who have had such experiences tend to recreate them repeatedly in play; it is possible for a helping adult to guide this repetition into a sense of mastery.

What do you think? Can you remember having any distressing (to yourself) childhood worries or habits?

➤ *Check Your Reading*

27. Give an example of an unrealistic worry one might see in an overanxious child.
28. What is meant by *exposure* and *response prevention* in the treatment of obsessive-compulsive disorder?
29. Name two symptoms of posttraumatic stress disorder in children.

FEEDING AND EATING DISORDERS

Feeding and eating disorders, listed in DSM-IV in both the childhood section and a later, separate section, include a number of potentially serious problems in infants, children, and adolescents. Although anorexia and bulimia occur increasingly in grade-school children, these are discussed fully in Chapters 19 and 30.

Pica is defined as the ingestion of nonnutritive substances over a period of 1 month or more. Pica occurs primarily in mentally retarded children, young children in deprived environments, and in children whose mothers also had pica (Chatoor, 1997). In each of these instances, the pica should be addressed by a behavior management plan, while the related condition must also be considered and included in a broader plan of care.

Rumination disorder, a rare, poorly understood phenomenon, has been linked to serious difficulties in the parent-child relationship. It describes a pattern of regurgitating, rechewing, and swallowing food, although it is not due to a medical condition. At times, this disorder may occur in a biologically well-endowed infant because of maternal inadequacy, but it is more often seen in children with serious developmental delays.

Obesity, although not included in the DSM-IV as an eating disorder, is important to consider because it represents a serious, potentially life-threatening condition with psychological correlates; "at least 11% and possibly as many as 25% of US children . . . are overweight" (Hill & Trowbridge, 1998, p. 571). Essential to working with an obese child is the participation of a nutritionist, good medical management, an exercise

MEDICAL DIAGNOSES AND RELATED NURSING DIAGNOSES

Anxiety Disorders

DSM-IV Diagnosis: Separation Anxiety Disorder

Diagnostic Criteria

A. Developmentally inappropriate and excessive anxiety concerning separation from home or from those to whom the individual is attached, as evidenced by three (or more) of the following:

(1) Recurrent excessive distress when separation from home or major attachment figures occurs or is anticipated.

(2) Persistent and excessive worry about losing, or about possible harm befalling, major attachment figures.

(3) Persistent and excessive worry that an untoward event will lead to separation from a major attachment figure (e.g., getting lost or being kidnapped).

(4) Persistent reluctance or refusal to go to school or elsewhere because of fear of separation.

(5) Persistently and excessively fearful or reluctant to be alone or without major attachment figures at home or without significant adults in other settings.

(6) Persistent reluctance or refusal to go to sleep without being near a major attachment figure or to sleep away from home.

(7) Repeated nightmares involving the theme of separation.

(8) Repeated complaints of physical symptoms (such as headaches, stomach aches, nausea, or vomiting) when separation from major attachment figures occurs or is anticipated.

B. The duration of the disturbance is at least four weeks.

C. The onset is before age 18 years.

D. The disturbance causes clinically significant distress or impairment in social, academic (occupational), or other important areas of functioning.

E. The disturbance does not occur exclusively during the course of a Pervasive Developmental Disorder, Schizophrenia, or other Psychotic Disorder and, in adolescents and adults, is not better accounted for by Panic Disorder With Agoraphobia.

Specify if:

Early Onset: If onset occurs before age 6 years.

DSM-IV Diagnosis: Generalized Anxiety Disorder (includes Overanxious Disorder of Childhood)

DSM-IV Diagnosis: Obsessive-Compulsive Disorder

DSM-IV Diagnosis: Posttraumatic Stress Disorder

Related Nursing Diagnoses

Anxiety
Spiritual Distress

Definition

A vague, uneasy feeling whose source is often nonspecific or unknown to the individual.

Disruption in the life principle that pervades a person's entire being and that integrates and transcends one's biological and psychosocial nature.

Example

Anxiety related to separations, as evidenced by rapid heart beat, clinging, and inconsolable crying.

Spiritual Distress related to witnessing mother's murder, as evidenced by preoccupation with death, expressions of hopelessness.

Based on information from the *Diagnostic and Statistical Manual of Mental Disorders. Fourth Edition.* Copyright 1994 American Psychiatric Association.

---

program, and vigorous treatment of any underlying depression or anxiety. Without the child's interest and motivation and the active participation of the family, the child has little chance for successful weight reduction. If the child is still growing, attempting weight stabilization may be more realistic. (See Chapter 30 for more information on eating disorders.)

GENDER IDENTITY DISORDERS

Gender identity disorders should be clearly distinguished from homosexuality, which is a sexual orientation *not* a disorder. Homosexual people often recognize quite early that they are romantically and sexually interested in same-sex individuals. It is generally difficult for these children to find someone to talk to about their concerns, and clinicians should not respond to such a disclosure as if it were an indication of pathology.

Gender identity disorder in children is characterized by a persistent wish to be or a belief that one is of the opposite gender. Typically, symptoms such as persistent cross-dressing appear in the toddler and preschool years. Nursing diagnoses to consider are personal identity disturbance and social isolation.

TABLE 18-4 Commonly Used Medications in Child Psychiatry

MEDICATIONS	COMMON USES	RECOMMENDED DOSAGES	ADVERSE EFFECTS	NURSING CONSIDERATIONS
Stimulants				
Methylphenidate (Ritalin)	ADHD	10–30 mg/d in divided doses; not approved for children <6 y		Observe for a rebound effect in the late afternoon, with return or increase of the original behaviors.
Dextroamphetamine sulfate (Dexedrine)	ADHD	2.5–30 mg/d in divided doses; not approved for children <3 y	Decreased appetite, insomnia, growth delays, irritability, tachycardia	Be aware that stimulants may increase or "unmask" tics in children. Similarly, stimulants can make compulsive behaviors more marked. Monitor for lowering of the seizure threshold. Note any changes in mental status. Stimulants may, in rare cases, precipitate psychotic episodes.
Tricyclic antidepressants	Depression		Dry mouth, visual disturbances, sedation or insomnia; worsening psychoses, seizures; blood dyscrasias, cardiovascular changes, including rare *fatal* cardiac dysrhythmias	Insist on close monitoring for any ECG changes. Educate patients about reporting and alleviating uncomfortable side effects. Be aware that medication must be tapered to discontinue; abrupt withdrawal can cause extreme discomfort.
Nortriptyline (Pamelor)	Depression	30–50 mg/d; not recommended for children <12 y		Be alert to danger of overdoses, which may be fatal.
Desipramine (Norpramin)	Depression, ADHD	25–100 mg/d, not to exceed 150 mg/d; not recommended for children <12 y		
Amitriptyline (Elavil)	Depression	50 mg/d; not recommended for children <12 y		
Imipramine (Tofranil)	Depression, enuresis	Up to 100 mg/d, not to exceed 2.5 mg/kg for treatment of enuresis; not recommended for children <12 y except for treatment of enuresis (in children ≥6 y)		
Clomipramine (Anafranil)	OCD	Up to 3 mg/kg/d; not recommended for children <10 y		
MAOIs			Orthostatic hypotension; headache; sleep disturbances; gastrointestinal upset.	Be aware that combining MAOIs with tricyclics can cause severe seizures or hypertensive crises. A hypertensive crisis can also be induced by interaction with foods containing tyramine (cheese, beer, wine) as well as with amphetamines, cocaine, and caffeine. Because normal developmental issues make it unlikely that children can safely monitor their own use of such medications, the nurse should advocate an alternative.

Table continued on following page

TABLE 18-4 Commonly Used Medications in Child Psychiatry *Continued*

MEDICATIONS	COMMON USES	RECOMMENDED DOSAGES	ADVERSE EFFECTS	NURSING CONSIDERATIONS
MAOIs *Continued*				
Phenelzine sulfate (Nardil)		Not approved for use in children under 16 (but may still be prescribed)		
Tranylcypromine sulfate (Parnate)		Not approved for use in children (but may still be prescribed)		
Other Antidepressants				
Paroxetine HCl (Paxil) Fluoxetine HCl (Prozac) Sertraline HCl (Zoloft)	Depression	Safety and efficacy not established, but these drugs are increasingly prescribed for children.	Nausea, nervousness, sleep disturbances	Fluoxetine in particular may rarely be activating. Monitor children for increased agitation, aggression, or self-injurious behavior. None of these drugs should be given in conjunction with an MAOI (at least 5 wk should intervene between medications). These drugs are presumed to work by inhibiting reuptake of the neurotransmitter serotonin. Because of a potential interaction, parents should be warned not to give the nutritional supplement tryptophan (sometimes used to promote sleep).
Bupropion HCl (Wellbutrin)	Depression, ADHD	Not approved for use in children. If prescribed, likely dosage is 100–250 mg/d	Lowering of seizure threshold, dry mouth, sleep disturbances, gastrointestinal symptoms, tremor, rash or other allergic reactions	Never administer to children with seizure disorders, anorexia, or bulimia. Never give in conjunction with an MAOI (at least 2 wk should intervene between medications). Doses should be divided and single dose should never exceed 2 mg/kg.
Antihistamines				
Diphenhydramine (Benadryl)	ADHD, anxiety, bedtime sedation	Not approved for behavior disorders but used in child psychiatry for decades	Dry mouth, sedation or dullness, overexcitement	Be aware that parents may be using diphenhydramine without any medical supervision (the drug is readily available). Warn parents that overdoses may be dangerous or fatal, as can use of this drug in infants (including ingestion through breast milk). Asthma may be aggravated by use of diphenhydramine.
Hormones				
Desmopressin acetate (DDAVP)	Enuresis	0.1–0.4 ml intranasally at bedtime	Nasal congestion, headache, gastrointestinal symptoms, hyponatremia	Because of the rare fatalities with imipramine use, DDAVP is increasingly common. Severe hyponatremia can cause seizures.
Anticonvulsants	Seizures			Administer regularly and accurately. Decrease gastrointestinal upset by administering with food or liquid. Observe and report any and all seizure activity.
Carbamazepine (Tegretol)	Seizures, mood and behavioral disorders	15–30 mg/kg/d	Blurred vision, lethargy	

TABLE 18–4 Commonly Used Medications in Child Psychiatry *Continued*

MEDICATIONS	COMMON USES	RECOMMENDED DOSAGES	ADVERSE EFFECTS	NURSING CONSIDERATIONS
Anticonvulsants Continued				
Valproic acid (Depakene)	Seizures	15–60 mg/kg/d	Tremors, gastrointestinal symptoms	Single dose should not exceed 250 mg.
Phenytoin (Dilantin)	Seizures	4–8 mg/kg/d	Rash, hyperplasia of the gums, hirsutism	Nurse, patient, and parents must pay special attention to oral hygiene.
Phenobarbital	Seizures	3–6 mg/kg/d	Lethargy, hyperactivity	
Clonazepam (Klonopin)	Seizures	0.02–0.2 mg/kg/d	Lethargy, excessive salivation	Divide into 3 equal doses.
Diazepam (Valium)	Status epilepticus	IM: 2–5 mg in single dose IV: 5–10 mg at 1 mg/2–5 min		
Antipsychotics				
Neuroleptics	Schizophrenia and other psychotic disorders		Sedation, hypotension, extrapyramidal reactions	Because of their serious and wide-ranging adverse effects, neuroleptics should be used with extreme caution in children. Each drug has a unique combination of beneficial and adverse effects. Research each prescribed medication and educate parents about expected responses and reportable reactions. A low-dose anticholinergic such as biperiden hydrochloride (Akineton) or benztropine mesylate (Cogentin) may be used to mitigate extrapyramidal effects of some neuroleptics.
Phenothiazines				
Chlorpromazine (Thorazine)	Psychotic disorders	1–3 mg/kg/d in divided doses		
Thioridazine (Mellaril)	Psychotic disorders	1–3 mg/kg/d in divided doses		
Perphenazine (Trilafon)	Psychotic disorders	Pediatric doses not established; most often prescribed at 0.1–0.4 mg/kg/d in divided doses		
Butyrophenones				
Haloperidol (Haldol)	Psychotic disorders	0.05–0.15 mg/kg/d (up to 6 mg)		
Thioxanthines				
Thiothixene (Navane)	Psychotic disorders	6–10 mg/d in divided doses; not recommended for children <12 y		
Dibenzodiazepines				
Clozapine (Clozaril)	Refractory schizophrenia in adults and some adolescents	Pediatric dosages not established		Because clozapine can cause life-threatening agranulocytosis, it must be used according to the guidelines of the Clozaril National Registry.
Benzisoxazole Derivative				
Risperidone (Risperdal)	Psychotic disorders	Pediatric dosages not established		

Table continued on following page

TABLE 18-4 Commonly Used Medications in Child Psychiatry Continued

MEDICATIONS	COMMON USES	RECOMMENDED DOSAGES	ADVERSE EFFECTS	NURSING CONSIDERATIONS
Antimanic Agents Lithium carbonate (Eskalith) Lithium carbonate time release (Lithobid)	Bipolar disorders	900–1200 mg/d in divided doses; not recommended for use in children <12 y but may still be prescribed	Gastrointestinal symptoms, weight gain, tremors, polyuria and polydipsia, fatigue	In both children and adolescents, dosage must be titrated carefully, according to serum lithium levels. Therapeutic levels range between 0.6 and 1.2 mEq/L. Levels even slightly above this range can be toxic, and sensitive individuals may experience toxicity at lower ranges. Nurse, patient, and family should be alert for signs of toxicity. These include worsening of expected adverse effects, dizziness, ataxia, slurring of speech, and blurred vision.
Antihypertensive Agents Clonidine (Catapres)	Tourette's disorder, ADHD, opiate withdrawal	0.2–0.6 mg/d; not recommended for children <12 y but may still be prescribed	Dry mouth, drowsiness, gastrointestinal symptoms, orthostatic hypotension	Check orthostatic blood pressure before administering each dose. Be aware that clonidine should not be stopped abruptly; dosage should be tapered over 3–4 d before discontinuing, to prevent rebound hypertension.

ADHD, attention-deficit hyperactivity disorder; ECG, electrocardiographic; IM, intramuscular; IV, intravenous; MAOIs, monoamine oxidase inhibitors; OCD, obsessive-compulsive disorder.

TIC DISORDERS

Tic disorders include transient tic disorder, chronic motor or vocal tic disorder, and Tourette's disorder. A tic is defined as "a sudden, rapid recurrent, nonrhythmic, stereotyped motor movement or vocalization" (DSM-IV, 1994, p. 100). A significant percentage of all children, particularly school-age boys, are affected by tics at one time or another (Leckman & Cohen, 1999). Most of these tics, whether motor or vocal, disappear spontaneously within a few weeks or months. If tics persist for more than a year, the disorder is classified as chronic. If both motor and vocal tics persist, the child is given the diagnosis of Tourette's disorder.

"The first step in management of children with Tourette's syndrome is understanding them and their world" (Silver, 1988, p. 204). An upsurge of public interest and knowledge about Tourette's syndrome has been helpful for these children. A child with Tourette's is now more likely to be offered treatment rather than punished or ostracized. Still, adults are often at a loss at setting limits or holding the child responsible for the behavior. Keep in mind that tics *can* be suppressed; one of the goals of treatment is to find ways of strengthening the child's ability to suppress tics. These methods can include social sanctions, behavioral reinforcers, and medication. The child can also be taught to identify the urge to tic and develop alternative strategies for handling this feeling.

What do you think? Should preschool children be allowed to cross-dress?

> ➤ *Check Your Reading*
> 30. What is pica?
> 31. What is rumination disorder?
> 32. What is the difference between sexual orientation and a gender identity disorder?
> 33. Give a short definition of Tourette's disorder.

ELIMINATION DISORDERS

Functional *enuresis* is involuntary wetting not caused by an identifiable physiological condition such as urinary tract infections, which should be carefully ruled out. Enuresis can occur diurnally but is far more frequent at night. No single cause has been universally accepted, but most studies are now focusing on sleep and arousal patterns. Untreated, it resolves spontaneously in most cases by age 13 years or so. The condition is usually a source of considerable embarrassment and even shame for a child, however, and may interfere with such important social activities as sleepovers and camp attendance.

Although numerous approaches, such as establishing fluid restrictions, awakening schedules, and aversive consequences, have historically been tried, the most effective methods have been shown to be medication (imipramine or vasopressin [DDAVP]) and the bell-and-pad system (Mikkelsen, 1996). The bell-and-pad system uses an alarm triggered by the child during voiding. It is most successful if the parents participate by waking the child at the first sound of the alarm, supervising clean-up, and rewarding progress. If the child and family are motivated and willing to work at it, the bell-and-pad method offers the decided advantages of a sense of pride and mastery as well as an absence of potential adverse reactions.

Functional *encopresis,* or fecal incontinence, is far more rare than enuresis. Three categories of encopretic children have been proposed by Hersov (1985):

1. Children who volitionally soil
2. Children who have inadequate bowel control
3. Children who soil by leakage

This last category includes children who have frequent diarrhea as well as those who experience retention with overflow. In all cases, medical causes must be ruled out. Treatment should take the category into account, although aspects of the treatment may be similar. For example, children who retain feces probably need a bowel-cleaning regimen followed by daily laxatives, whereas children with loose stools may need a daily bulking agent. Education about bodily signals is helpful, as is a plan for sitting on the toilet for 10 or 15 minutes following meals. The child who has been deliberately

soiling as a means of communication can be helped toward self-expression through other means. If words are too difficult, art activities may be more satisfying.

> **W***hat do you think?* Have you known someone who wet the bed as a child?

➤ *Check Your Reading*
34. Suggest a treatment plan for nocturnal enuresis.
35. Define functional encopresis.

DEVELOPMENTAL DISORDERS

The developmental disorders are listed in the DSM-IV as Mental Retardation, Learning Disorder, Motor Skills Disorder, Communication Disorder, and Pervasive Developmental Disorder.

Mental retardation is defined by the American Psychiatric Association (1994, p. 39) as including both

---

MEDICAL DIAGNOSES AND RELATED NURSING DIAGNOSES

Feeding and Eating Disorders

DSM-IV Diagnosis: Anorexia Nervosa
See Chapter 30 for details.

DSM-IV Diagnosis: Bulimia Nervosa
See Chapter 30 for details.

DSM-IV Diagnosis: Pica

Diagnostic Criteria
A. Persistent eating of nonnutritive substances for a period of at least one month.
B. The eating of nonnutritive substances is inappropriate to the developmental level.
C. The eating behavior is not part of a culturally sanctioned practice.
D. If the eating behavior occurs exclusively during the course of another mental disorder (e.g., Mental Retardation, Pervasive Developmental Disorder, Schizophrenia), it is sufficiently severe to warrant independent clinical attention.

DSM-IV Diagnosis: Rumination Disorder

Diagnostic Criteria
A. Repeated regurgitation and rechewing of food for a period of at least one month following a period of normal functioning.
B. The behavior is not due to an associated gastrointestinal or other general medical condition (e.g., esophageal reflux).

C. The behavior does not occur exclusively during the course of anorexia nervosa or bulimia nervosa. If the symptoms occur exclusively during the course of Mental Retardation or a Pervasive Developmental Disorder, they are sufficiently severe to warrant independent clinical attention.

Medical Diagnosis: Obesity

Definition
The condition of weighing more than 120% of one's ideal body weight.

Related Nursing Diagnoses

Altered Nutrition: More Than Body Requirements
Risk for Injury

Definition
The state in which an individual is experiencing an intake of nutrients that exceeds metabolic needs.

A state in which the individual is at risk for injury as a result of environmental conditions interacting with the individual's adaptive and defensive resources.

Example
Alteration in Nutrition related to excessive caloric intake, as evidenced by weight of 325 lb.

Risk for Injury related to ingestion of objects, as evidenced by history of swallowing toy parts or paint chips.

Based on information from the *Diagnostic and Statistical Manual of Mental Disorders. Fourth Edition.* Copyright 1994 American Psychiatric Association.

MEDICAL DIAGNOSES AND RELATED NURSING DIAGNOSES

Tic Disorders

DSM-IV Diagnosis: Tourette's Disorder

Diagnostic Criteria

A. Both multiple motor and one or more vocal tics have been present at some time during the illness, although not necessarily concurrently. (A *tic* is a sudden, rapid, recurrent, nonrhythmic, stereotyped motor movement or vocalization.)

B. The tics occur many times a day (usually in bouts) nearly every day or intermittently throughout a period of more than one year, and during this period there was never a tic-free period of more than three consecutive months.

C. The disturbance causes marked distress or significant impairment in social, occupational, or other important areas of functioning.

D. The onset is before age 18 years.

E. The disturbance is not due to the direct physiological effects of a substance (e.g., stimulants) or a general medical condition (e.g., Huntington's disease or postviral encephalitis).

DSM-IV Diagnosis: Chronic Motor or Vocal Tic Disorder

Diagnostic Criteria

A. Single or multiple motor or vocal tics (i.e., sudden, rapid, recurrent, nonrhythmic, stereotyped motor movements or vocalizations), but not both, have been present at some time during the illness.

B. The tics occur many times a day nearly every day or intermittently throughout a period of more than one year, and during this period there was never a tic-free period of more than three consecutive months.

C. The disturbance causes marked distress or significant impairment in social, occupational, or other important areas of functioning.

D. The onset is before age 18 years.

E. The disturbance is not due to the direct physiological effects of a substance (e.g., stimulants) or a general medical condition (e.g., Huntington's disease or postviral encephalitis).

F. Criteria have never been met for Tourette's Disorder.

DSM-IV Diagnosis: Transient Tic Disorder

Diagnostic Criteria

A. Single or multiple motor or vocal tics (i.e., sudden, rapid, recurrent, nonrhythmic, stereotyped motor movements or vocalizations).

B. The tics occur many times a day, nearly every day for at least four weeks, but for no longer than 12 consecutive months.

C. The disturbance causes marked distress or significant impairment in social, occupational, or other important areas of functioning.

D. The onset is before age 18 years.

E. The disturbance is not due to the direct physiological effects of a substance (e.g., stimulants) or a general medical condition (e.g., Huntington's disease or postviral encephalitis).

F. Criteria have never been met for Tourette's Disorder or Chronic Motor or Vocal Tic Disorder.

Specify if:
Single Episode or *Recurrent*

DSM-IV Diagnosis: Tic Disorder, Not Otherwise Specified

Related Nursing Diagnosis

Knowledge Deficit

Definition

Absence or deficiency of cognitive information related to specific topic.

Example

Knowledge Deficit related to Tourette's Disorder, as evidenced by self-blame and uncontrolled rage.

Based on information from the *Diagnostic and Statistical Manual of Mental Disorders. Fourth Edition.* Copyright 1994 American Psychiatric Association.

"significantly subaverage functioning" and limitations in adaptive skills. Cognitive functioning is usually measured by a standardized test such as the Stanford-Binet Intelligence Quotient Test or the Wechsler Intelligence Scales for Children, Revised (WISC-R). Adaptive functioning may also be assessed by a standardized formal interview such as the Vineland Adaptive Behavior Scales (Sparrow, Balla, & Cicchetti, 1984), or it may be described informally by the child's parents.

In practice, far more weight is given to a child's score on cognitive tests. These intelligence quotient (IQ) tests measure a particular set of skills and "may not tell us much about *intelligence*" (Tanguay & Russell, 1996, p. 503). What they do provide is a delineating boundary for the diagnosis of mental retardation, which the DSM-IV specifies as an IQ score of 70 or below. Remember that the vast majority of retarded children have an IQ score of at least 55 (Tanguay & Russell, 1996) and the potential to enjoy a productive, loving, and fulfilling life. Psychiatric disorders do, however, occur at a disproportionately high rate among mentally retarded children (Rutter, Graham, & Yule, 1970).

Clinicians sometimes hesitate to use the phrase *mental retardation* when talking to parents, but it is extremely important for parents to understand their child's cognitive limitations as well as strengths. When parents have an inaccurate idea of their child, their expectations will not match the child's capacities, and they may be unable to provide appropriate support to enable their child to reach full potential. Parents also need help advocating for their child's special needs, both present and future.

The *pervasive developmental disorders* include autistic disorder, Rett's disorder, childhood disintegrative disorder, Asperger's disorder, and pervasive developmental disorder, not otherwise specified.

Autism may be viewed as the extreme end of a spectrum of deficits in the areas of relatedness, communication, and imaginative play. It is characterized by a lack of awareness of other people or the use of people as if they were things, abnormal verbal and nonverbal communication, and a preoccupation with repetition and sameness. Autistic children frequently display a number of distinctive movements called *stereotypies,* such as hand-flapping or rocking.

Autism is a poignant and thus far poorly understood disorder that has kindled a spark in popular interest in part because of high functioning in some autistic children with such skills as advanced reading abilities or savant qualities. Autism has been the subject of a number of books and movies, some autobiographical, which have unfortunately contributed to the misperception of most autistic individuals as normal or even quite brilliant—awaiting a magic cure to awaken them

MEDICAL DIAGNOSES AND RELATED NURSING DIAGNOSES

Elimination Disorders

DSM-IV Diagnosis: Enuresis

Diagnostic Criteria

A. Repeated voiding of urine into bed or clothes (whether involuntary or intentional).
B. The behavior is clinically significant as manifested by either a frequency of twice a week for at least three consecutive months or the presence of clinically significant distress or impairment in social, academic (occupational), or other important areas of functioning.
C. Chronological age is at least 5 years (or equivalent developmental level).
D. The behavior is not due exclusively to the direct physiological effect of a substance (e.g., a diuretic) or a general medical condition (e.g., diabetes, spina bifida, a seizure disorder).

Specify type:
Nocturnal Only
Diurnal Only
Nocturnal and Diurnal

DSM-IV Diagnosis: Encopresis

Diagnostic Criteria

A. Repeated passage of feces into inappropriate places (e.g., clothing or floor) whether involuntary or intentional.
B. At least one such event a month for at least three months.
C. Chronological age is at least 4 years (or equivalent developmental level).

D. The behavior is not due exclusively to the direct physiological effects of a substance (e.g., laxatives) or a general medical condition except through a mechanism involving constipation.
Code as follows:
787.6 With Constipation and Overflow Incontinence
307.7 Without Constipation and Overflow Incontinence

Related Nursing Diagnoses

Functional Incontinence

Self Esteem Disturbance

Definition

The state in which an individual experiences an involuntary, unpredictable passage of urine.

Negative self-evaluation/feelings about self or self capabilities that may be directly or indirectly expressed.

Example

Functional Incontinence related to enuresis, as evidenced by daily soiling of bedding.

Self Esteem Disturbance related to encopresis, as evidenced by embarrassment, shame, and secretiveness.

(Grandin & Scaviano, 1986; Greenfeld, 1986; Kaufman, 1976; Maurice, 1993).

Work with autistic children must rely heavily on concrete behavioral interventions, but "this is not to imply that psychodynamics are unimportant. On the contrary, all children are influenced by psychodynamics, and interactions with caretakers and environment have a deleterious, benign or beneficial effect on autistic children" (Campbell, Perry, & Green, 1984, p. 103).

Both Rett's disorder and childhood disintegrative disorder involve periods of normal development followed by the loss of previously acquired skills in several areas of development. Asperger's disorder was first described by Asperger (1944) as involving generally higher cognitive functioning than in most autistic children, along with difficulties with reciprocal relationships and characteristic preoccupations with such things as mechanical objects, telephone numbers, or bus schedules.

Pervasive developmental disorder, not otherwise specified (PDD-NOS), remains a sort of catch-all diagnosis whose broad application will probably be further categorized in the years to come. Globally, children considered to have PDD-NOS are those who have some autistic features but do not meet the criteria for autism or the other three pervasive developmental disorders. Although PDD-NOS is statistically far more prevalent than autism in children, little research has been done on this disorder. Nurses may encounter undiagnosed young children with peculiarities of speech, poor social skills, and restricted play behaviors (Cascio & Kilmon, 1997).

Specific developmental disorders include the following:

- *Learning disorders:* Reading disorder, mathematics disorder, disorder of written expression
- *Motor skills disorders:* Developmental coordination disorder
- *Communication disorders:* Expressive language disorder, mixed receptive expressive language disorder, phonological disorder, stuttering

Although the prevalence of learning disabilities has not been firmly established, it is believed to be somewhere between 5% and 10% of the general population (Centers for Disease Control and Prevention, 1987). Among psychiatrically disturbed children, however, the proportion is far higher because many learning disabled children also have emotional, social, and family problems. These may reflect a "dysfunctional nervous system" or may be a consequence of the frustration of being disabled (Silver, 1996, p. 521). Kazdin (1992) identifies learning disabilities as one of four major risk factors in developing serious behavior problems. A sad fact is that as many as one third of adolescent boys who end up in juvenile detention are learning disabled (Lewis & Balla, 1980; Robbins, Beck, Preis, Jacobs, & Smith, 1983).

Learning disabilities have also been correlated with diagnoses of conduct disorder and borderline personality disorder in adolescents (Hunt & Cohen, 1984). Regarding the communication disorders, Scahill proposed in a 1989 nursing research study that "children

with speech and language delays are at risk for accruing additional problems—including emotional and behavioral disturbances" (p. 3).

State educational systems generally specify diagnostic criteria for the provision of special education services. Nurses should be alert for any signs that a child has problems with perception, memory, understanding, verbal expression, abstraction, reading, writing, or problem solving. A nurse may recommend that a battery of psychoeducational tests be ordered to identify specific developmental disorders. Testing can be critical not only for the creation of a good educational plan but also to guide nursing treatment. Parents and children should be sensitively informed of learning strengths and weaknesses.

What do you think? Do you know what *your* learning strengths and weaknesses are?

▶ *Check Your Reading*

36. List the five broad categories of developmental disorders.
37. Make a statement about the association of learning disorders to other childhood and adolescent adversities.

DISORDERS NOT SPECIFIC TO CHILDREN

Several other categories in the DSM-IV are not specific to children but do occur in this population. Foremost among these are mood disorders. Depressive disorders do present in children with the classic signs of sadness, irritability, changes in appetite, and sleep disturbances. Another common symptom is a series of somatic complaints. At times, though, depression can be obscured by a child's inability to verbalize, by a high level of motor activity or impulsivity, and even by a veneer of cheerfulness.

Both major depressive disorder and the more chronic dysthymic disorder can be treated with a combination of psychotherapy and an antidepressant agent, such as one of the tricyclics or a newer medication, such as fluoxetine. Nursing diagnoses include impaired adjustment, sleep pattern disturbance, social isolation, hopelessness, spiritual distress, and potential for self-directed violence. (See Chapter 25 for more complete discussion of mood disorders.)

Bipolar disorders have only relatively recently been diagnosed in children and are often difficult to differentiate from other illnesses. Although rare, they should be considered for symptoms such as lability of mood, pressured speech, sleeplessness, tangentiality, paranoia, and bizarre behavior, especially when the onset is sudden and in the presence of a positive family history. It is essential to rule out alcohol-induced or drug-induced changes, even in children.

Similarly rare, schizophrenia has been diagnosed in children as young as 5 years of age. Onset is usually gradual, with auditory hallucinations, delusions, and thought disorders the most common manifestations. Positive family history is a risk factor. As in adult schizophrenia, useful nursing diagnoses include alter-ation in thought process, potential for injury, and self-care deficit. Treatment includes the use of neuroleptics.

Substance-related disorders are often overlooked by child mental health clinicians, but they are commonly seen not only in adolescents but also increasingly among younger children. Macdonald (cited in Bailey, 1992) called substance abuse "the most commonly missed pediatric diagnosis" (p. 1016). Be alert to the ease of availability of alcohol and drugs in the child's community. Attending local Al-Anon, Nar-Anon, or Families Anony-mous meetings help raise your awareness. Substance abuse can impede normal development, impair judg-ment, exacerbate emotional problems, and cause irre-versible physical harm. It may even be fatal.

What do you think? Do you know a child you think may be depressed?

➤ *Check Your Reading*
38. Name four possible signs of depression in children.
39. What has been referred to as "the most com-monly missed pediatric diagnosis"?
    Nursing Process

Outcome Identification

Identifying the outcome(s) of care for a child depends on the diagnoses, both DSM-IV as well as nursing. In Jordi's case, for example, expected outcomes might be

- The patient will demonstrate improved social skills.
- The patient will employ more adaptive coping skills when frightened, upset, or angry.
- The patient will begin to seek adult help and reassurance when confused by thoughts and percep-tions.

Planning

Once you have, with the help of the child and parents, identified the central problems and the available re-sources and strengths, you need to develop a plan of care or treatment. A nursing care plan is one way to organize and plan care. Including a brief paragraph can enable others involved in carrying out the plan to have a better understanding of the child's strengths, weak-nesses, and inner life.

Jordi is a boy with fundamental defi-cits in relatedness whose isolation has been made worse by a thought disorder. These problems, along with a high degree of anxiety, have resulted in a profound delay in acquiring skills of social interaction.

Strengths for Jordi are his tentative wish for interper-sonal contact and his ability to use the structure of a well-known environment for support.

The plan specifies expected outcomes and the short-term goals likely to lead to these outcomes. Although objectives are written from the child's per-spective, interventions are described from the nursing perspective.

Expected Outcome 1
The patient will demonstrate improved social skills.
Short-Term Goals. (1) The patient will successfully interact in a play situation with a trusted adult, and (2) the patient will begin to develop greater comfort and facility as he increases his contacts with other children.

Expected Outcome 2
The patient will employ more adaptive coping skills when frightened, upset, or angry.
Short-Term Goals. (1) The patient will decrease unsafe outbursts from several times a week to fewer than once a month, and (2) the patient will use words to describe his thoughts and feelings.

Expected Outcome 3
The patient will begin to seek adult help and reassurance when confused by thoughts and percep-tions.
Short-Term Goal. The patient will remain in verbal or physical contact with a trusted adult during episodes of disorganization.

What do you think? Should a nurse humor a patient by temporarily going along with a delusion?

➤ *Check Your Reading*
40. Identify two expected outcomes for Jordi.
41. State a goal for each of these outcomes.
    Nursing Process

Implementation

Individual Therapy

Psychotherapy takes place in the overlap between two areas of playing, that of the patient and that of the therapist. Psychotherapy has to do with two people playing together. The corollary of this is that where playing is not possible then the work done by the therapist is directed towards bringing the patient from a state of not being able to play into a state of being able to play. (Winnicott, 1971, p. 38)

The same basic principles that apply to adult therapy also apply to child therapy, although the means of communication, especially for younger children, are rather different. As Axline (1982) pointed out, there are some general rules that should apply to *all* interactions with children, both in therapy and in day-to-day life. These include respecting and accepting children as they are, maintaining sufficient limits to provide a sense of reassurance and security, encouraging the expression of feelings, letting them take their time, providing opportunities for creativity and spontaneity, and recognizing that immaturity is a phase of development and not a deficit.

In most settings, a nurse is required to have a master's degree to provide individual psychotherapy. At times, the nurse-psychotherapist plays along with the child; at other times, the nurse maintains a reflective stance. In either case, a balance between permissiveness and structure must be sought. Helping children express their fantasies—however messy and frightening—is necessary, but letting children actually destroy toys or hurt themselves (or the therapist) is likely to disrupt treatment seriously:

For a pretend or imaginary attack is one thing. It can ultimately be countered by the knowledge that the attack was not real. But as soon as an attack is made on a physical level, it acquires the possibility of actual hurt . . . of taking away the person who is struck. It can terrify the child. (Baruch, 1952, p. 85)

Generally it is best to meet at a consistent time, in a consistent place, making the same toys and materials available each session and confining the therapeutic work to the playroom. Interpretations should be used sparingly and in the initial phase of treatment should be made in the language of the play itself. That is, if a child is playing out a parent-child scenario, the therapist can comment on the interaction in the third person rather than abruptly (and intrusively) shifting to a direct reference to the child and parent. Children use metaphors naturally. Children also do astonishingly well making their own interpretations when they are engaged in therapeutic work.

Facility in verbalizing what a child is unable to express is an invaluable gift. When the time is opportune for making an important observation, the nurse-therapist should not hold back. Gently the nurse can create a vocabulary that is incorporated both in the play and in the child's growing self-understanding. A skilled therapist can engage in this delicate balancing act intuitively, making it appear effortless, but this level of expertise requires years of training and experience to achieve.

1. Build Jordi's capacity for reciprocal interactions; for example, practice turn-taking and other elements of conjoint play with him. Your relationship with the patient can function as a bridge to other relationships of trust.

2. Introduce Jordi to other children in a safe, familiar setting, allowing him to watch them for extended periods without interaction. You can minimize the patient's anxiety by maintaining sameness and allowing for gradual accommodation.

3. Gradually encourage Jordi to play alongside another child. Support Jordi in brief, structured interactions such as familiar turn-taking activities with other children. Help the patient increase a sense of control through mastery of each successive step before going on to the next one.

4. Maintain neutrality while keeping Jordi safe during outbursts. Avoid reinforcing behavior. High expressed emotion, either negative or positive, can become a reinforcer for maladaptive behavior.

5. Initially, use a safe holding technique during outbursts; gradually increase the expectation that Jordi will regain self-control without physical intervention. The nurse provides containment until the patient learns to take over that function for himself.

6. Help Jordi practice alternative expressions of upset and anger, including words. Having satisfactory experiences with more adaptive forms of self-expression can be self-reinforcing.

7. Assist Jordi to recognize cues to his own increasing agitation and positively reinforce adaptive coping techniques. Your aim is to help the patient learn a skill that can be built over the life span. Self-awareness is an important therapeutic tool.

8. During calm moments, help Jordi come up with words and phrases to represent his delusional ideas and his feelings. Use examples from stories or from other people if this is less threatening. Appeal to the patient's strengths to help him understand his own illness in simple, concrete, benign terms.

9. Verbalize your understanding of Jordi's feeling-states when he appears disorganized. Help the patient to shift focus from the unreality of his disordered thinking to the reality of his feelings.

10. Reassure Jordi of his safety; describe the real context he is in. Be careful not to collude with the patient's distorted perceptions.

FAMILY THERAPY

Family work has a special significance in child treatment because, as Critchley (1985) stated, "Most child therapists agree that, to achieve any long-term therapeutic gains, the child's family must be involved in the treatment process" (p. 247). This work may be approached through various means, including family sessions, parent support groups, or direct modeling and education (see Chapters 13 and 14). You can offer invaluable help because it is difficult to proceed further until the home situation is stabilized.

A few essential principles of behavior management can be taught: the parents are responsible for making decisions, including decisions about what choices the children can make.

1. The family should agree on a simple set of rules based on safety and respect for one another.

2. The family should agree on a set of consequences for breaking rules—these must be firm but reasonable.

3. The family should agree on a set of rewards that will be available for following the rules—preferably ones that rely heavily on family members doing enjoyable things together rather than on material objects.

4. The parents must keep in mind that all behavior is a form of communication: the goal is to help the child recognize this and find acceptable ways of expressing feelings.

When difficulties arise, the parents should be encouraged to let the child's struggle be against the rule, not against the parents. In that way, they may even allow themselves to feel frustrated along with the child instead of feeling frustrated by the child. Behavior management works to change the behaviors of the child by first changing the behaviors of the managers.

A special type of treatment for infants and very young children works with the mother-child dyad. Called *watch, wait and wonder,* this technique employs a number of sessions in which the parent is instructed to get on the floor and follow the child's lead for a period of time. The parent and therapist then talk about the play session, as the parent comes to recognize the reverberations of his or her own childhood in the relationship (Muir, 1992).

GROUP THERAPY

The first children's therapeutic play groups were organized in 1934 by Slavson (Critchley, 1985). These were structured by the therapist, both in the selection of membership and in the nature of the play, to provide corrective life experiences. Most groups for children since then have focused on socialization, self-disclosure, or particular activities with the intention of preparing them for similar situations in daily life. In the 1980s and 1990s, clinicians have explored the usefulness of the British group-as-a-whole theory for these age groups (Moss & Rakusin, 1990). This theory holds that the group itself must be seen as the patient, as an entity greater than the sum of its individual parts. The same defensive group behaviors and responses to therapy seen in adult groups can also be recognized and brought to awareness in groups of children as young as 3 years of age.

What do you think? Which of the modalities described do you think you would most enjoy?

► *Check Your Reading*

42. Which level of educational preparation is generally required to do individual psychotherapy?
43. Give one reason why it is important not to allow a child to hurt the therapist.
44. Why is it important for a child's family to be involved in treatment?
45. List four basic principles of behavior management techniques.

TREATMENT SETTINGS

Because some children require more intensive treatment and greater containment than can be provided by outpatient services, individual, family, and group therapy can also be offered as part of a comprehensive inpatient, day treatment, or residential program.

Inpatient Hospitalization. Inpatient hospitalization is the most restrictive modality and is generally reserved for comprehensive evaluation and treatment of the most seriously disturbed children. It is extremely expensive, not only in money but also in the emotional investment and time commitment required of the entire family. When successful, however, it can act as a catalyst for permanent changes in the child, family, and community and can dramatically improve the trajectory of a child's life.

As in adult psychiatry, the therapeutic milieu is one of the most powerful components of inpatient treatment. A well-functioning milieu provides containment, structure, support, involvement, and validation (Delaney, 1992). Figure 18–2 shows a schedule from a children's inpatient unit. The participation of the family in the milieu work can make the difference between temporary gains and permanent growth.

Residential treatment programs are neither as restrictive nor as intensive as inpatient wards. They provide structured living and education to children who have been unable, for whatever reason, to function adaptively at home. The availability of such programs varies from region to region, as does the quality of the facilities themselves. At their best, they offer stability and ongoing treatment while a family continues to work toward returning the child home. At worst, they may function as a sort of temporary orphanage, a way station between a terrible beginning and an uncertain future.

Partial hospitalization and—still less restrictive—day treatment programs generally follow a daily structure similar to the inpatient milieu, although usually with less stringent rules and with higher behavioral expectations for children. These patients can maintain sufficient self-control to live at home. Whether a child is being seen in outpatient therapy or in a day program, there is frequently an unmet need for home-based services. More and more agencies are establishing programs to meet this need. Sometimes a parent aide works with the child and family for several hours a week, sometimes a visiting nurse meets with the family to continue therapeutic work begun earlier. The potential for change with a home-based model of care is enormous.

Fragmentation of treatment delivery is perhaps the single greatest weakness in the system of mental health care available to children in the United States. Many advanced practice nurses looking toward children's future psychiatric needs advocate nursing case management as most effective in meeting those needs. A nursing case manager not only provides direct care and supervises an in-home aide but also functions as coordinator of various mental health services a child might need throughout development.

	MONDAY	TUESDAY	WEDNESDAY	THURSDAY	FRIDAY	SATURDAY	SUNDAY
			CHILDREN'S SCHEDULE				
7:30–8:00	Wake-up/room inspection	Wake-up/room inspection	Wake-up/room inspection	Wake-up/room inspection	Wake-up/room inspection		
8:00–8:30	BREAKFAST	BREAKFAST	BREAKFAST	BREAKFAST	BREAKFAST	Wake-up	Wake-up
8:30–9:00	Community meeting	Community meeting	Community meeting	Community meeting	Community meeting	BREAKFAST	BREAKFAST
9:00–10:00	School	School	School	School	School	Community meeting	Community meeting
10:00–12:00	Testing Appointments	Testing Appointments	Testing Appointments	Testing Appointments	Testing Appointments	Super clean-up Fun time	Clean-up Room inspection Fun time
12:00–12:30	LUNCH	LUNCH	LUNCH	LUNCH	LUNCH	LUNCH	LUNCH
12:30–1:00	Quiet time	Quiet time	Quiet time	Quiet time	Quiet time	Personal time	Personal time
1:00–2:00	Group therapy	Life skills activity group	Video club/ fitness fun	Group therapy	Fitness fun/ success club	Family activity (1:00–2:30)	Family activity (1:00–2:30)
2:00–3:00	Physical education	Free play outside	Library Read-aloud	Creative expression	Physical education	Personal time (2:30–3:00)	Personal time (2:30–3:00)
3:00–3:30	Snack	Snack	Snack	Snack	Snack	Snack	Snack
3:30–5:00	Game time/ individual therapy	Game time/ individual therapy	Game time/ individual therapy	Game time/ individual therapy	Game time/ individual therapy	Game time/ individual therapy	
5:00–5:30	Community meeting	Community meeting	Community meeting	Community meeting	Community meeting	Visiting (3:30–5:00)	Visiting (3:30–5:00)
5:30–6:00	DINNER	DINNER	DINNER	DINNER	DINNER	Community meeting DINNER	Community meeting DINNER
6:00–6:30	Rewards	Rewards	Rewards	Family night		Special activity	Rewards
6:30–7:15	Physical therapy/baths	Personal time	Personal time	Support groups	Personal time	Personal time	Personal time
7:15–8:00	Snack Bedtimes begin	Snack	Snack	Snack	Movie night	Snack	Snack Goodbye party

Figure 18–2
A sample schedule from an inpatient psychiatric unit for children.

► *Check Your Reading*

46. Briefly describe the characteristics of the different settings in which child psychiatric treatment is provided.
47. List the five descriptors of the well-functioning therapeutic milieu.

PSYCHOPHARMACOLOGY

Some experts decry the use of psychopharmacology under any circumstances; they point to the long-term adverse effects of neuroleptic medications and the common occurrence of stimulants prescribed by pediatricians without adequate monitoring (Breggin, 1994). Psychopharmacological agents do carry dangerous potential for unnecessary and even harmful use, and medication should never be a substitute for needed environmental changes. Clinical experience suggests, however, that some children benefit enormously from a carefully controlled, judicious use of medication and that to deny those children such a benefit is inhumane. Box 18–3 lists some basic principles of medication use in children.

Be sensitive to the family members' feelings about medication and about any previous experiences with either prescription or nonprescription drugs. It takes time and patience to discuss this important matter thoroughly. Often, even in the presence of strong ambivalence, the family's "expectations of pharmacotherapy's effects may be unrealistically high and attended by anxious hopes" (Munir, 1989, p. 113).

You also need to be familiar with the most commonly used psychiatric medications. Parents and children need education and support to make the best use of this intervention. Table 18-4 gives uses, dosages, adverse effects, and nursing considerations.

Evaluation

> "I can climb the bars now, Sally."
> "What was that, Jordi? I didn't hear you."
> "The bars, the monkey bars—now I can climb on them and play."
> "Yes, you sure can."
> "Sally, it's the bars and things, other things too."
> "Yes, there's been much, Jordi—many things."

Box 18-3 ■ ■ ■ ■ ■
Principles of Medication Use in Children

- Inclusion of parents and child in any decision regarding use of medication; any medication should be presented and used in the context of a comprehensive plan of treatment
- Completion of a thorough assessment, including an accurate diagnosis, before considering a medication trial
- Weighing of risks and benefits associated with each agent, paying special attention to developmental concerns
- Completion of requisite baseline measures, such as blood counts, vital signs, weight, electrocardioram
- Clear identification of target symptoms and selection of an objective means to evaluate the efficacy of the medication
- Awareness that children frequently show different responses from those of adults with similar symptoms
- Use of extreme caution; the least dangerous agent should be tried first, begun slowly and tapered if stopped unless immediate discontinuation is indicated by an adverse reaction
- Completion of an adequate trial and thorough documentation to prevent subjecting the child to unnecessary risk in the future
- Continued careful monitoring of both beneficial and adverse effects, with the active participation of parents and child
- Avoidance of polypharmacy

> And there were things, many things. There was incident after incident. There were bars, many bars—bars to cross, bars to climb, bars to knock down—and they did it. And it was hard work. But they struggled, and the bars came down.

Reprinted with the permission of Macmillan Publishing Company from *Jordi* (p. 62) by Theodore Isaac Rubin, MD. Copyright © 1960 by Theodore Isaac Rubin.

When the initial treatment goals and objectives are established, the nurse, the child, and the child's family should plan to review their progress periodically at reasonable intervals and to revise goals as may be appropriate. As with Jordi's care plan, it can be extremely helpful to include some measures of progress easily recognized by everyone. Losing sight of a child's gradual improvement causes family and child to become discouraged. Also, identify what should be accomplished to bring treatment to a successful conclusion.

The trend in child psychiatric treatment has been moving steadily away from long-term, exploratory work toward shorter-term, specific, identifiable behavioral achievements. Although short-term goals help focus treatment, limited time frames sometimes have the effect of replacing the forest with a succession of trees. As goals are attained, reviewed, and revised, keep a perspective on the longer view of this journey. Hold onto hope for the child so that goals achieved truly do become steps toward a richer, more fulfilling life. As feelingly expressed by Herskowitz (1989),

To be totally alive with one's senses, fully perceptive, emotionally unrestricted, to have a mind free to explore and make new connections, and a strong, agile body, is to live in a state of grace. (p. 68)

Termination

> Then he ran out of the room and out of the building. . . . He rode all over New York and cried most of the time. Then he thought about Sally and the times gone by. Then he thought about their talks of the last six months.
>   When he got back, it was six o'clock, but everybody was still there. . . .
>   He looked at her and said, "I came back, I came back. Sally, I came back to leave." ■

Reprinted with the permission of Macmillan Publishing Company from *Jordi* (p. 73) by Theodore Isaac Rubin, MD. Copyright © 1960 by Theodore Isaac Rubin.

Whether one works with a child for a brief time or for many years, the moment of ending the relationship is important and must be acknowledged as such. It is a time for reviewing the child's accomplishments, for expressing both the sadness of loss and

SNAPSHOT

Nursing Interventions Specific to Childhood Psychiatric Illness

What do you need to do to develop a relationship with a child suffering with a psychiatric illness?
- Respect and accept the child as he or she is.
- Maintain sufficient limits to provide a sense of reassurance and security.
- Encourage expression of feelings.
- Allow the child to take his or her time in talking.
- Provide opportunities for creativity and spontaneity.
- Be consistent in time and place of meetings.
- Verbalize what the child is unable to express.
- Maintain neutrality when the child shows intense feelings or has an outburst.

What do you need to assess regarding the patient's health status?
- Suicidal risk or self-destructive thoughts
- Neurological status—asymmetries, delays in coordination or speech, mixed or delayed "handedness," poor right-left discrimination and visual difficulties suggesting organic dysfunction
- Appearance, coordination, tolerance of separation from parent
- General orientation, comprehension and memory, presence of hallucinations and/or delusions
- Substance abuse
- Nutrition and sleep patterns
- Developmental history
- Family history with genogram
- Vital signs
- Weight, especially if the patient is experiencing changes in appetite
- Quality and content of play
- School performance and behaviors
- History of abuse or neglect
- Concurrent medical conditions

What do you need to teach the patient and/or the patient's caregiver?
- Medication issues—reason for taking; side effects and how to deal with them; untoward effects; warnings; importance of adhering to medication schedule
- The disease process and how it is expressed in the child
- Nutrition issues
- Emergency measures
- Importance of appropriate communication support
- Maintaining safety
- Importance of emotional support
- Importance of consistency

What skills will you want the patient and/or caregiver to demonstrate?
- Ability to enter into a no-harm contract and remain safe
- Ability to follow medication and treatment plan
- Ability to follow a behavioral plan
- Ability to perform personal care
- Ability to identify and express feelings
- Coping skills
- Relaxation techniques
- Ability to form friendships, to share, to show empathy
- Ability to discipline appropriately

What other health professionals might need to be a part of this plan of care?
- Physician—psychiatrist and/or primary care physician—who is usually in charge of the overall treatment plan including medication management
- Social worker—to assist with access to community supports; insurance issues; access to entitlements; connection with community-based treatments
- School personnel—to ensure that educational process meets needs of child

---

the security of knowing that the relationship has created a new strength within the child that will never be lost. Don't overidentify with a child or take an expression of anger personally. Right up to the last instant of departure, your focus is on the meaning of this event to the child and the child's need to master a separation.

Because the work of ending will have been done in the days or weeks leading up to it, the actual moment of "goodbye" may seem surprisingly anticlimactic. If all has gone well, the child is now ready to move ahead, despite a sense of loss and sadness. The child will be looking forward, toward the journey to come.

NURSING PROCESS APPLICATION

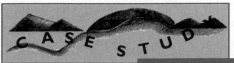

Betsy

Betsy is the 11-year-old daughter of Margaret, a 29-year-old single parent. Margaret brought Betsy to the clinic because she was "depressed" and not doing well in school. Two months ago, Margaret was hospitalized for 2 weeks because she was suicidal. While in the hospital, she began to resolve issues related to childhood sexual abuse by her father. She is currently being treated for depression with outpatient therapy and fluoxetine (Prozac). Margaret has full custody of both Betsy and Betsy's younger sister, Amy.

During the initial session, Betsy would not answer specific questions but did participate in drawing on the blackboard. Margaret stated that Betsy and Amy fight a lot and that they have no specific rules about bedtimes or mealtimes. Betsy cries frequently in the evening because she misses her father and grandparents. She is currently not doing well in school and spent the past 2 days in the nurse's office, too upset to be in class.

ASSESSMENT	• Child and mother anxious and upset • Mother describes feeling "overwhelmed" • Poor grades • Poor parenting skills • Lack of structure in home • Ambiguity regarding child and parent roles

DIAGNOSIS	**DSM-IV Diagnoses:** Separation Anxiety Disorder Generalized Anxiety Disorder **Nursing Diagnoses** • Altered Parenting related to inadequate role identity evidenced by description of feeling overwhelmed by task of parenting two children and maintaining full-time employment while recovering from depression, having an inadequate support system, and having a lack of appropriate role models • Altered Growth and Development related to inadequate maternal and paternal caretaking evidenced by poor performance in school, inability to concentrate in class, absences from class, and verbalizations of hopelessness and depression

OUTCOME IDENTIFICATION, PLANNING, AND IMPLEMENTATION

> **Expected Outcome 1:** By _____ the parent and child will interact in a positive manner.

Short-Term Goals	Nursing Interventions	Rationales
The child will remain psychologically safe.	1. Assess the parent's awareness of the child's needs. 2. Determine the parent's ability to nurture both child and self.	1–2. Ability to provide safety and nurturing is a basic function of parenting. The child may need to be removed from the home if she cannot perceive minimal psychological security at home.
By _____ the mother will begin to verbalize the child's need for nurturing.	1. Encourage the mother to verbalize the differences between ideal and actual parenting behaviors. 2. Encourage the mother to verbalize the need for self-nurturing as well as nurturing the child. 3. Provide opportunities for the mother to explore role identity through counseling (group or individual).	1–3. Parenting is a learned behavior. Often, parents rely on how they were parented. The fact that the mother sought help for her child is one indication of her desire to learn different ways to parent.

Expected Outcome 2: By _____ the parent and child will demonstrate decreased anxiety.

Short-Term Goals	Nursing Interventions	Rationales
By _____ mother and child will describe at least two ways they have learned to cope with anxiety in a positive manner.	1. Assess coping behaviors for dealing with anxiety. 2. Focus on positive behaviors and individual and collective strengths. 3. Teach mother and child positive ways of coping with anxious feelings, such as relaxation, drawing, painting, and affirmations.	1–2. Behavioral methods assist in the desensitization process. Gradual time away helps the child to learn to trust. 1–3. Assist the mother and child in cognitive awareness of ways to decrease anxiety and of the relationship between anxiety and behavior. Empower the mother and child to manage their own care eventually.
By _____ the child will be able to spend at least 2 hours away from the mother without increasing signs of anxiety.	1. Arrange for gradually increasing times for the child to be away from the mother. 2. Monitor for evidence of increased anxiety, such as increased vital signs, restlessness, apprehension, or increase in somatic complaints. 3. Encourage the child either to verbalize feelings or to express feelings through play or drawing.	3. Enable the child to work through fearful situations without somatization.

Expected Outcome 3: By _____ the parent and child will demonstrate clear role identities.

Short-Term Goals	Nursing Interventions	Rationales
By _____ the mother will verbalize expectations for self and child.	1. Encourage the mother to express her expectations freely. 2. Encourage the mother to determine how expectations were derived.	1. Parents may have unrealistic expectations of their ability to parent. 2. Expectations may reflect cultural or family of origin values. Increasing the mother's awareness may help her to be more realistic.
By _____ the mother will verbalize areas of failure to meet expectations.	1. Listen attentively. 2. Show empathy and understanding.	1–2. Failure to meet expectations leads to anger and frustration. The mother needs your unconditional acceptance.
By _____ the parent will develop parenting strategies that more clearly define the role of parent and child.	1. Help the parent develop more realistic expectations of an 11-year-old child. 2. Teach the mother appropriate growth and development for an 11-year-old child. 3. Assist the mother with limit-setting strategies and age-appropriate disciplinary measures.	1–3. Based on the way she has parented, the mother may be unaware of the norms for growth and development. Based on the history of abuse in her family, the mother may rely on ineffective ways of discipline and may be unaware of any other alternatives.

Expected Outcome 4: By _____ the child will perform at an age-appropriate level in school and at home.

Short-Term Goals	Nursing Interventions	Rationales
By _____ the child will express a willingness to attend school.	1. Explore with the child all possible reasons for not wanting to attend school. 2. Discuss the potential benefits of attending school. 3. Devise a behavioral chart that allows for rewards for days of school attended.	1–2. An 11-year-old child is old enough to reason. Exploring benefits of an education is beneficial. 3. The use of positive reinforcement is valuable when attempting to change behavior.

| By _____ the family will be able to use appropriate support services. | 1. Make appropriate referrals to parenting classes, social worker, and school counselor.
2. Monitor family progress.
3. Collaborate with involved health professionals. | 1–3. This family has multiple needs and will require the use of various health care professionals. Collaborating is an essential part of planning, maintaining, and evaluating care. |
| By _____ the parent will be able to set appropriate guidelines for bedtime and meals within 1 week. | 1. Assess current routines at home.
2. Assist the mother in defining routines that are compatible with adequate time for daily routines for the family and allow for adequate amounts of sleep and recreation.
3. Develop a chart for the family to use for the following week.
4. Monitor progress.
5. Offer praise as indicated. | 1. It is important to begin where the family is in regard to routine. If you change routines too quickly or severely, noncompliance can be expected.
2–3. Behavior modification is useful when providing structure for a family.
4–5. Positive reinforcement of efforts on a regular basis strengthens desired behavior. |

Expected Outcome 5: By _____ the mother and child will verbalize hopefulness and meaning in life.

Short-Term Goals	Nursing Interventions	Rationales
By _____ the mother will express hope for her own well-being as well as the well-being of her daughters.	1. Assess for suicidal ideation. 2. If suicidal ideation is present, determine the level of suicidality and initiate a plan of care for a suicidal patient. If suicidal ideation is not present at this time, encourage the client to explore resources such as significant others, a higher power, or God. 3. Encourage the mother to talk about her hope for the future. 4. Emphasize strengths and positive statements. 5. Assist to develop short-term goals.	1–2. Assessing for suicidality is always a priority intervention from an ethical and legal standpoint and may require immediate intervention. 3–5. These interventions aid in restoring esteem and confidence in self.
By _____ the daughter will express feelings of hope for her future.	1. Assess for suicidal ideation. 2. If suicidal ideation is present, determine the level of suicidality and initiate a plan of care for a suicidal patient. 3. Encourage the child to identify her losses. 4. Use a variety of modalities such as art, play, music, and drama to help the child work through the identified losses.	1–2. Asessing for suicidality is always a priority intervention from an ethical and legal standpoint and may require immediate intervention. 3–4. Unidentified, unresolved grief often leads to loss of hope.

EVALUATION   **Formative Evaluation:** The nurse observed that Betsy and her mother met each of the short-term goals in the time frames allotted. As her mother developed confidence in their ability to identify and respond to Betsy's needs, Betsy could tolerate longer periods away from her without increased signs of anxiety.

Summative Evaluation: Betsy was able to meet all of the expected outcomes with the help of the nurse and Margaret's referral to the local family mental health clinic for treatment of her depression. Over a 6-month period, Betsy's grades improved dramatically. Betsy looked forward to going to school and being with her friends. Both mother and child expressed satisfaction with their relationship.

Conclusions

Even with many similarities between the adult journey and the pediatric journey, children also present important differences. Most childhood psychiatric disorders refer to a number of attributes and behaviors that can be modified through a combination of treatment approaches. Mere recognition of these disorders does not tell us of the child's experience or allow us into the child's inner world.

The story of Jordi is the tale of a child whose development is placed in jeopardy by his own constitutional vulnerability and by a poor fit with his family and community. Fortunately, it is also the story of a child protected by his intelligence, by his parents' unselfish love for him, and most of all by the dedication and skill of a woman who learned to accompany Jordi on his journey, to share a vision of the world with him.

The practice of child psychiatric nursing is a rare experience, involving the nurse in work that is extraordinarily complex: it is at once beautiful and horrifying, intellectually challenging, emotionally demanding, and deeply fulfilling. It requires dedication to a kind of professionalism that does not distance you from a patient but makes you even more immediately available. If you choose this journey in nursing, you must have a solid knowledge of physical, cognitive, social, spiritual, and psychological development. You must enjoy and respect children. You must be prepared for serious self-examination. In return, you will be welcomed into the lives and hearts of children and their parents in a unique way: as a fellow sojourner, as a guide who is at the same time being guided, as a fully alive human being connecting with others in that momentary state of grace.

Key Points to Remember

- Child psychiatric nurses must have a basic knowledge of normal child and adolescent development.
- Psychiatrically disturbed children may experience themselves as out of control, terrified, inhibited, and without joy or hope.
- Each stage of child development should be thought of as complete in itself, with characteristic challenges and tasks appropriate to the child in each stage.
- Any understanding of a child's individual journey is incomplete without a sense of the child's place in the family.
- The nurse need not compete with the child's parents but rather should support and teach them.
- The nurse should have an understanding of and an appreciation for the community in which a child lives.
- Minority status is in itself neither a risk factor nor a protective factor but has the potential to become either one.
- The therapeutic relationship is at the heart of child treatment.
- Transference and countertransference are important concepts in child psychiatric nursing.
- Coping mechanisms are unconscious strategies for managing conflicts. They are not good or bad but can be either useful or troublesome depending on the person and the situation.
- A nurse should be alert to the presence of risk factors, such as poverty, neglect and abuse, exposure to violence, parental psychopathology, divorce, and medical illness or disability.
- The nurse draws on the same observational skills used for physical assessments to assess a child's psychiatric status.

- The cornerstone of a thorough psychiatric assessment is a carefully gathered history.
- Particular attention must be paid to the neurological examination.
- The nurse should attend to all areas of a child's life, such as play; attachments; sexual, moral, and spiritual development; and the presence of suicidal ideation.
- The nurse should be familiar with the DSM-IV nomenclature. The nurse should also be aware that most psychiatric diagnoses of childhood and adolescence describe a cluster of attributes or behaviors that are an exaggeration of normal characteristics.
- Nurses and other mental health professionals frequently miss substance abuse not only in adolescents but also in younger children.
- The child psychiatric nursing formulation provides an opportunity to convey a sense of who a child is.
- A nursing care plan should specify expected outcomes and short-term goals.
- Treatment modalities with children include individual therapy, group therapy, and family therapy. Treatment settings include outpatient clinics, inpatient and partial hospitalization programs, day treatment, and residential centers.
- Parents and children should be involved in making decisions about medication. Any medication should be used as part of a comprehensive plan of treatment.
- The nurse, the child, and the child's parents should plan to review their progress periodically.
- Regardless of how long a therapeutic relationship has lasted, the process of ending it is important and must be given attention.

Learning Activities

1. Take an informal survey of your friends and family members. Ask them to tell you about what helped them through any difficult time as they were growing up.
2. Arrange to observe for an hour at a school or a day care center. Write a process recording of an interaction there.
3. Call your local reference librarian or Chamber of Commerce and ask for statistics on the number of children in your area living below the poverty level.

Call the local court and ask for statistics on the number of children involved in the criminal justice system annually. Call the local child welfare department and find out what mental health services for children are in place in your area.

4. Find out if your place of worship offers any programs that would be helpful to troubled children and their families.

Critical Thinking Exercise

Nurse Hadden was approached by the second-grade teacher, Mrs. Lane, to discuss her concerns about one of her students, Timmy. Mrs. Lane reported that since Timmy started second grade, she noticed that he never stopped moving. He could not sit still to finish the reading assignment, he was always asking to go to the bathroom, he never seemed to listen when she told the children their directions, he blurted out words at unexpected times, and he recently started to push other children at recess.

1. What assumptions can you make about Timmy's behavior?

2. What evidence suggests that your assumptions are accurate or faulty?

3. If you are the nurse, what other evidence do you need to draw a conclusion about Timmy's behavior?

Two months later, Timmy's mother called the nurse to inform her that Timmy was taking methylphenidate (Ritalin). She requested that the nurse help monitor Timmy's medication.

1. What conclusions, if any, can be drawn about the outcome of the nurse-teacher discussion?

2. Suggest possible alternate explanations about Timmy's condition.

3. Assuming an alternate explanation, would the results be the same?

Additional Resources

The ARC Home Page
http://thearc.org/welcome.html

Family Village
http://www.familyvillage.wisc.edu

Speech-Language Pathology Website
http://www.ica.net/pages/fred

Autism Society of America
http://www.autism-society.org

International Rett Syndrome Association
http://www.rettsyndrome.org

Asperger's Disorder Homepage
http://www.ummed.edu/pub/o/ozbayrak/asperger.htm

ADD/ADHD Information Library
http://www.newideas.net/index.htm

Conduct Disorder in Children and Adolescents Fact Sheet
http://www.mentalhealth.org/publications/allpubs/ca-0010/conduct.htm

Guide to the Diagnosis and Treatment of Tourette Syndrome
http://www.mentalhealth.com/book/p40-gtor.html

National Association for Continence
http://www.nafc.org

References

Aden, L. (1976). Faith and the developmental cycle. *Pastoral Psychology, 24,* 215–230.
Ainsworth, M. D. S., Blehar, M. C., Waters, E., & Wall, S. (1978). *Patterns of attachment.* Hillsdale, NJ: Erlbaum.
Alsobrook, J. P., Grice, D., & Pauls, D. L. (1996). Genetic influences on child psychiatric conditions. In M. Lewis (Ed.), *Child and adolescent psychiatry* (2nd ed., pp. 351–363). Baltimore: Williams & Wilkins.

American Humane Association (1981). *National Analysis of Child Neglect and Abuse Reporting, 1979.* Washington, DC: US Department of Health and Human Services.

American Psychiatric Association (1994). *Diagnostic and statistical manual of mental disorders* (4th ed.). Washington, DC: American Psychiatric Association.

Asperger, H. (1944). Die "autischen psychopathen" im kindersalter. *Archive für Psychiatrie und Nervenkrankheiten, 117,* 76-136.

Auletta, K. (1993, May 17). What won't they do? *The New Yorker,* 45-53.

Axline, V. (1982). Entering the child's world via play experiences. In G. L. Landreth (Ed.), *Play therapy: The dynamics of the process of counseling* (pp. 47-57). Springfield, Il: Charles C Thomas.

Bailey, G. W. (1992). Children, adolescents and substance abuse [Special section]. *Journal of the American Academy of Child Psychiatry, 31,* 1015-1017.

Baruch, D. (1952). *One little boy.* New York: Julian Press.

Beck, C. T. (1998). The effects of postpartum depression on child development: A meta-analysis. *Archives of Psychiatric Nursing, 12*(1), 12-20.

Bettelheim, B. (1950). *Love is not enough.* Glencoe, IL: Free Press.

Bettelheim, B. (1975). *The uses of enchantment.* New York: Random House.

Bowlby, J. (1969). *Attachment and loss.* Vol. I: Attachment. New York: Basic Books.

Breggin, P. R. (1994). Toxic psychiatry. Why therapy, empathy and love must replace the drugs, electroshock and biochemical theories of the "new psychiatry." New York: St. Martin's Press.

Breslau, N. (1985). Psychiatric disorders in children with physical disabilities. *Journal of the American Academy of Child Psychiatry, 24*(1), 87-94.

Brown, A., & Finkelhor, D. (1986). Impact of child sexual abuse: A review of the research. *Psychology Bulletin, 99,* 66-77.

Campbell, M., Perry, R., Green, W. H. (1984). Use of lithium in children and adolescents. *Psychosomatics, 25*(2), 95-106.

Carson, V. B. (1989). *Spiritual dimensions of nursing practice.* Philadelphia: W. B. Saunders.

Cascio, R. S., & Kilmon, C. A. (1997). Pervasive developmental disorder, not otherwise specified: Primary care perspectives. *Nurse Practitioner: American Journal of Primary Health Care, 22*(7), 11, 15-16, 18.

Caudill, W., & Schooler, C. (1973). Child behavior and child rearing in Japan and the United States: An interim report. *Journal of Nervous and Mental Disorders, 157,* 323-338.

Centers for Disease Control and Prevention (1987). Assessment of the number and characteristics of persons affected by learning disabilities. In Interagency Committee on Learning Disabilities: *Learning disabilities: A report to the U.S. Congress.* Washington, DC: U.S. Department of Health and Human Services.

Centerwall, B. S. (1992). Television and violence: The scale of the problem and where to go from here. *Journal of the American Medical Association, 267,* 3059-3063.

Chatoor, I. (1997). Eating and nutritional disorders of infancy and early childhood. In J. Weiner (Ed.), *Textbook of child and adolescent psychiatry.* Washington, DC: American Psychiatric Press.

Chess, S., & Thomas, A. (1986). *Temperament in clinical practice.* New York: Guilford Press.

Chethik, M. (1989). *Techniques of child therapy: Psychodynamic strategies.* New York: Guilford Press.

Children's Defense Fund (1989). *A vision for America's future.* Washington, DC: Author.

Clinton, H. R. (1996). *It takes a village.* New York: Simon and Schuster.

Cohen, D. J., Bruun, R. D., & Leckman, J. F. (1988). *Tourette's syndrome and tic disorders.* New York: John Wiley.

Coles, R. (1986). *The moral life of children.* Boston: Atlantic Monthly Press.

Coles, R. (1990). *The spiritual life of children.* Boston: Houghton Mifflin.

Combrinck-Graham, L. (1996). Development of school-age children. In M. Lewis (Ed.), *Child and adolescent psychiatry* (2nd ed.). Baltimore: Williams & Wilkins.

Comer, J. (1996). Improving psychoeducational outcomes for African-American children. In M. Lewis (Ed.), *Child and adolescent psychiatry* (2nd ed.). Baltimore: Williams & Wilkins.

Cotton, N. (1993). *Lessons from the lion's den.* San Francisco, CA: Jossey-Bass.

Critchley, D. L. (1985). Individual and play group therapy. In D. L. Critchley & J. T. Maurin (Eds.), *The clinical specialist in psychiatric mental health nursing* (pp. 229-257). New York: John Wiley.

Delaney, K. R. (1992). Nursing in child psychiatric milieus. Part I: What nurses do. *Journal of Child Psychiatric Nursing, 5,* 10-14.

Erikson, E. H. (1961). In J. Huxley (Ed.), *The humanist frame.* London: Allen & Unwin.

Erikson, E. H. (1963). *Childhood and society.* New York: Norton.

Farrington, D. P. (1978). The family backgrounds of aggressive youths. In L. Hersov, & M. Rutter (Eds.), *Aggression and antisocial behavior in childhood and adolescence.* Oxford: Pergamon Press.

Fowler, J. W. (1984). Toward a developmental perspective on faith. *Religious Education, 69*(2), 207-219.

Freud, A. (1936). *The ego and the mechanisms of defense.* London: Hogarth.

Freud, A. (1946). *The psycho-analytic treatment of children.* London: Imago.

Freud, S. (1938). *The basic writings of Sigmund Freud* (A. A. Brill, Ed. and Trans.). New York: Modern Library.

Garbarino, J. (1992). The meaning of poverty in the world of children. [Special issue: The impact of poverty on children]. *American Behavioral Scientist, 35,* 220-237.

Garbarino, J. (1998, April 13). Interview by Linda Kramer. *People,* 107.

Garmezy, N. (1987). Stress, competence and development. *American Journal of Orthopsychiatry, 57,* 159-173.

Gilligan, C. (1982). *In a different voice: Psychological theory and women's development.* Cambridge, MA: Harvard University Press.

Gilligan, C. (1985). *Remapping development.* Paper presented at the biennial meeting of the Society for Research in Child Development, Toronto, Ontario, Canada.

Graham, P., & Turk, J. (1996). Psychiatric aspects of pediatric disorders. In M. Lewis (Ed.), *Child and adolescent psychiatry* (2nd ed., pp. 989-1005). Baltimore: Williams & Wilkins.

Grandin, T., & Scaviano, M. M. (1986). *Emergence: Labeled autistic.* New York: Warner Books.

Greenfeld, J. (1986). *A client called Noah: A family journey continued.* Washington, DC: Henry Holt.

Groth, A. N. (1979). Sexual trauma in the life histories of rapists and child molesters. *Victimology, 4,* 10-16.

Groth, A. N. (1982). The incest offender. In S. Sgroi (Ed.), *Handbook of clinical intervention in childhood sexual abuse.* Lexington, MA: Lexington Books.

Harlow, H. F., & Harlow, M. K. (1962). Social deprivation in monkeys. *Scientific American, 207,* 136-146.

Helfer, R.E. (1987). The litany of the smoldering neglect of children. In R. E. Helfer & R. S. Kempe (Eds.), *The battered child* (4th ed., pp. 301-311). Chicago: University of Chicago Press.

Hernandez, D. J. (1988). Demographic trends and the living arrangements of children. In E. M. Hetherington & J. D. Arsteh (Eds.), *Impact of divorce, single-parenting and stepparenting on children.* Hillsdale, NJ: Erlbaum.

Herskowitz, M. (1989). The nature of human nature. *Annals of the Institute for Orgonamic Science, 6,* 60-68.

Hersov, L. (1985). Faecal soiling. In M. Rutter & L. Hersov (Eds.), *Child and adolescent psychiatry: Modern approaches* (pp. 482-489). London: Blackwell Scientific.

Hill, J. O., & Trowbridge, F. L. (1998). Childhood obesity: Future directions and research priorities. *Pediatrics, 101* (Suppl. 3, Part 2), 570-574.

Hoffman, M. L. (1984). Moral development. In M. H. Bornstein & M. E. Lamb (Eds.), *Developmental psychology: An advanced textbook.* Hillsdale, NJ: Erlbaum.

Hoffman-Plotkin, D., & Twentyman, C. T. (1984). A multimodal assessment of behavioral and cognitive deficits in abused and neglected preschoolers. *Child Development, 55,* 794-802.

Hollander, A. (1981). *How to help your child have a spiritual life.* New York: Bantam.

Hunt, R. D., & Cohen, D. J. (1984). Psychiatric aspects of learning difficulties. *Pediatric Clinics of North America, 31,* 471-497.

Kagan, J., & Lamb, S. (1987). *The emergence of morality in young children.* Chicago: University of Chicago Press.

Kalter, N. (1987). The long term effects of divorce on children: A developmental vulnerability model. *American Journal of Orthopsychiatry, 57,* 587-600.

Kashani, J. H., Daniel, A. E., Dandoy, A. C., & Holcomb, W. R. (1992). Family violence: Impact on children. *Journal of the American Academy of Child and Adolescent Psychiatry, 31,* 181-189.

Kaufman, B. (1976). *Son-rise.* New York: Harper & Row.

Kazdin, A. E. (1992). Overt and covert antisocial behavior: Child and family characteristics among psychiatric inpatient children. *Journal of Child and Family Studies, 1,* 3-20.

Kazdin, A. E., Moser, J., Colbus, D., & Bell, R. (1985). Depressive symptoms among physically abused and psychiatrically disturbed children. *Journal of Abnormal Psychology, 94,* 298-307.

Kendall, J. (1989). Child psychiatric nursing and the family: A critical theory perspective. *Journal of Child and Adolescent Psychiatric and Mental Health Nursing, 2,* 145-153.

Kleinman, A. (1988). *The illness narratives.* New York: Basic Books.

Kohlberg, L. (1981). *The philosophy of moral development: Moral stages and the idea of justice: Vol. 1. Essays on moral development.* San Francisco, CA: Harper & Row.

Konner, M. (1982). *The tangled wing: Biological constraints on the human spirit.* New York: Henry Holt.

Korbin, J. E. (1987). Child abuse and neglect: The cultural context. In R. E. Helfer & R. S. Kempe (Eds.), *The battered child* (4th ed.). Chicago: University of Chicago Press.

Lagerspetz, K. (1989). Media and the social environment. In J. Groebel & R. A. Hinde (Eds.), *Aggression and war: Their biological and social bases.* Cambridge, England: Cambridge University Press.

Lambert, C. E., Jr., & Lambert, V. A. (1987). Psychosocial impacts created by chronic illness. *Nursing Clinics of North America, 22,* 527-533.

Lawlor, R. (1991). *Voices of the first days: Awakening in the aboriginal dreamtime.* Rochester, VT: Inner Traditions.

Leckman, J. F., King, R. A., & Cohen, D. J. (1999). Tics and tic disorders. In J. F. Leckman & D. J. Cohen (Eds.), *Tourette's syndrome: Tics, obsessions, compulsions.* New York: J. Wiley & Sons.

Levenkron, S. (1993, April). Addictions treatment with the eating disorders patient. Paper presented at Greenwich Hospital, Greenwich, CT.

Lewis, D., & Balla, D. (1980). Psychiatric correlates of severe reading disabilities in an incarcerated delinquent population. *Journal of the American Academy of Child Psychiatry, 19,* 611-622.

Lewis, M. (1996). Psychiatric assessment of infants, children, and adolescents. In M. Lewis (Ed.), *Child and adolescent psychiatry* (2nd ed., pp. 447-463). Baltimore: Williams & Wilkins.

Linney, J. A., & Seidman, E. (1989). The future of schooling. *American Psychologist, 44,* 336-340.

Main, M., & Cassidy, J. (1988). Categories of response to reunion with the parent at age 6: Predictable from infant classifications and stable over a 1-month period. *Developmental Psychology, 18,* 415-426.

Main, M., & Solomon, J. (1990). Procedures for identifying infants as disorganized/disoriented during the Ainsworth Strange Situation. In M. T. Greenberg & D. Ciechetti (Eds.), *Attachment in the preschool years: Theory, research and intervention* (pp. 121-160}. Chicago: University of Chicago Press.

March, J. S., & Mulle, K. (1998). *OCD in children and adolescents: A cognitive-behavioral treatment manual.* New York: Guilford Press.

Maurice, C. (1993). *Let me hear your voice: A family's triumph over autism.* New York: Fawcett Columbine.

McClowry, S. (1991). Behavioral disturbances among medically hospitalized school-age children. *Journal of Child and Adolescent Psychiatric and Mental Health Nursing, 4,* 62-67.

McDermott, J. F., Jr. (1996). The effects of ethnicity on child and adolescent development. In M. Lewis (Ed.), *Child and adolescent psychiatry* (2nd ed., pp. 411-415). Baltimore: Williams & Wilkins.

Michaels, D., & Levine, C. (1992). Estimates of the number of motherless youth orphaned by AIDS in the United States. *Journal of the American Medical Association, 268,* 3456-3461.

Mikkelsen, E. J. (1996). Modern approaches to enuresis and encopresis. In M. Lewis (Ed.), *Child and adolescent psychiatry* (2nd ed., pp. 583-591). Baltimore: Williams & Wilkins.

Moss, N., & Rakusin, G. (1990, January). *The application of British group-as-a-whole theory to group therapy with young children.* Paper presented at the Interdepartmental Conference at the Yale Child Study Center, New Haven, CT.

Mrazek, D. A. (1996). Chronic pediatric illness and multiple hospitalizations. In M. Lewis (Ed.), *Child and adolescent psychiatry* (2nd ed., pp. 1058-1066). Baltimore: Williams & Wilkins.

Muir, E. (1992). Watching, waiting, and wondering: Applying psychoanalytic principles to mother-infant intervention. *Infant Mental Health Journal, 13,* 319-328.

Munir, K. (1989). Child and adolescent psychopharmacology comes of age. In J. Ellison (Ed.), *Psychotherapist's guide to pharmacotherapy.* Chicago: Year Book.

National Research Council (1998). Chalk, R., & King, P. A. (Eds.). *Violence in families: Assessing, prevention and treatment programs.* Washington, DC: National Academy Press.

Nurcombe, B., & Fitzhenry-Coor, I. (1987). *Diagnostic reasoning and treatment planning: I. Diagnosis.* Paper presented at the Robinson Memorial Lecture, Perth, Australia.

Parker, H., & Parker, S. (1984). Cultural roles, ritual and behavior regulation. *American Anthropologist, 86,* 584-600.

Peterson, G. W., Leigh, G. K., & Day, R. D. (1984). Family stress theory and the impact of divorce on children. *Journal of Divorce, 7,* 1-20.

Pfeffer, C. R. (1997). Suicide and suicidality. In J. Weiner (Ed.), *Textbook of child and adolescent psychiatry.* Washington, DC: American Psychiatric Press.

Piaget, J. (1965). *The moral judgment of the child.* New York: Free Press.

Pincus, J. H. (1996). The neurological meaning of soft signs. In M. Lewis (Ed.), *Child and adolescent psychiatry* (2nd ed., pp. 479-484). Baltimore: Williams & Wilkins.

Postnatal depression linked to child behavioural problems. (1998). *Community Nurse, 4*(1), 8.

Provence, S., & Naylor, A. (1983). *Working with disadvantaged parents and their children.* New Haven: Yale University Press.

Pruett, K. D. (1996). Family development and the roles of mother and father in child rearing. In M. Lewis (Ed.), *Child and adolescent psychiatry* (2nd ed., pp. 215-221). Baltimore: Williams & Wilkins.

Rey, J. M. (1993). Oppositional defiant disorder. *American Journal of Psychiatry, 150,* 1769-1775.

Rierden, A. (1993, March 21). Ties that bind poverty's children. *The New York Times,* p. 1.

Robbins, D. M., Beck, J. C., Preis, R., Jacobs, D., & Smith, C. (1983). Learning disability and neuropsychological impairment in adjudicated, unincarcerated male delinquents. *Journal of the American Academy of Child Psychiatry, 22,* 40-46.

Robertson, J. (1970). *Young children in hospital* (2nd ed.). London: Tavistock.

Rose, M., & Thomas, R. (1987). *Children with chronic conditions: Nursing in a family and community context.* New York: Grune & Stratton.

Rubin, T. I. (1960). *Jordi.* New York: Macmillan.

Russell, D. E. H. (1986). *The secret trauma: Incest in the lives of girls and women.* New York: Basic Books.

Rutter, M. (1966). *Children of sick parents: An environmental and psychiatric study* (Institute of Psychiatry Maudsley Monographs, no. 16). London: Oxford University Press.

Rutter, M. (1986). The developmental psychopathology of depression: Issues and perspectives. In M. Rutter, C. E. Izard, & P. B. Read (Eds.), *Depression in young people: Developmental and clinical perspectives.* New York: Guilford Press.

Rutter, M. (1987). Psychosocial resilience and protective mechanisms. *American Journal of Orthopsychiatry, 57,* 316-331.

Rutter, M., Graham, P., & Yule, W. (1970). *A neuropsychiatric study in childhood.* London: Heinemann.

Rutter, M., & Quinton, D. (1984). Parental psychiatric disorder: Effects on children. *Psychological Medicine, 14,* 8-53.

Sacks, O. (1988). *Seeing voices: A journey into the world of the deaf.* Berkeley, CA: University of California Press.

Salzinger, S., Feldman, R. S., Hammer, M., & Rosario, M. (1993). The effects of physical abuse on children's social relationships. *Child Development, 64,* 169-187.

Scahill, L. (1989). *Detecting communication disorders in child psychiatric inpatients.* Unpublished master's thesis, Yale University, New Haven, CT.

Scahill, L., Walker, R. D., Lechner, S. N., & Tynan, K. T. (1993). Inpatient treatment of obsessive compulsive disorder in childhood: A case study. *Journal of Child Psychiatric Nursing, 6,* 5-14.

Scarpa, A. (1997). Aggression in physically abused children: The interactive role of emotional regulation. In A. Raine & P. A. Brennan (Eds.), *Biosocial bases of violence*. NATO ASI series: Series A: Life Sciences, 292 (pp. 341-343). New York: Plenum Press.

Sgroi, S. (1982). *Handbook of clinical intervention in childhood sexual abuse*. Lexington, MA: Lexington Books.

Silver, A. A. (1988). Intrapsychic processes and adjustment in Tourette's syndrome. In D. J. Cohen, R. D. Bruun, & J. F. Leckman (Eds.), *Tourette's syndrome and tic disorders*. New York: John Wiley.

Silver, L. B. (1996). Developmental learning disorders. In M. Lewis (Ed.), *Child and adolescent psychiatry* (2nd ed., pp. 522-528). Baltimore: Williams & Wilkins.

Sparrow, S., Balla, D., & Cicchetti, D. (1984). *The Vineland adaptive behavior scales* (Interview ed., expanded form). Circle Pines, MN: American Guidance Service.

Spitz, R. A. (1945). Hospitalism: An inquiry into the genesis of psychiatric conditions in early childhood. *Psychoanalytic Study of the Child, 1,* 53-74.

Stern, D. (1985). *The interpersonal world of the infant*. New York: Basic Books.

Szatmari, P., Offord, D. R., & Boyle, M. H. (1989). Ontario Child Health Study: Prevalence of attention deficit disorder with hyperactivity. *Journal of Child Psychology and Psychiatry, 30,* 219-230.

Tanguay, P. E., & Russell, A. T. (1996). Mental retardation. In M. Lewis (Ed.), *Child and adolescent psychiatry* (2nd ed., pp. 508-516). Baltimore: Williams & Wilkins.

Tarter, R. E., Hegedus, A. E., Winsten, N. E., & Alterman, A. I. (1984). Neuropsychological, personality and family characteristics of physically abused delinquents. *Journal of the American Academy of Child Psychiatry, 23,* 668-674.

Thompson, R. A. (1996). Attachment theory and research. In M. Lewis (Ed.), *Child and adolescent psychiatry* (2nd ed., pp. 100-108). Baltimore: Williams & Wilkins.

Verhulst, F. C., & Koot, H. M. (1992). *Child psychiatric epidemiology: Concepts and findings*. (Developmental clinical psychology and psychiatry, Vol. 23). Newbury Park, CA: Russell Sage.

Volkmar, F. R. (1996). Autism and the pervasive developmental disorders. In M. Lewis (Ed.), *Child and adolescent psychiatry* (2nd ed., pp. 499-508). Baltimore: Williams & Wilkins.

Wallerstein, J. S. (1983). Children of divorce: The psychological tasks of the child. *American Journal of Orthopsychiatry, 53,* 230-243.

Wallerstein, J. S., & Blakeslee, S. (1989). *Second chances: Men, women and children a decade after divorce*. New York: Ticknor & Fields.

Wallerstein, J. S., & Corbin, S. B. (1996). The child and the vicissitudes of divorce. In M. Lewis (Ed.), *Child and adolescent psychiatry* (2nd ed., pp. 1118-1127). Baltimore: Williams & Wilkins.

Weiss, G. (1996). Attention deficit hyperactivity disorder. In M. Lewis (Ed.), *Child and adolescent psychiatry* (2nd ed., pp. 847-853). Baltimore: Williams & Wilkins.

Westerhoff, J. (1976). Will our children have faith? (pp. 79-103). New York: Seabury Press.

Whiting, B., & Edwards, C. (1988). *Children of different worlds: The formation of social behavior*. Cambridge, MA: Harvard University Press.

Winnicott, D. W. (1957). *The child, the family, and the outside world*. London: Tavistock.

Winnicott, D. W. (1965). *The maturational processes and the facilitating environment: Studies in the theory of emotional development*. New York: International Universities Press.

Winnicott, D. W. (1971). *Playing and reality*. London: Tavistock.

Wolfe, D. A. (1987). *Child abuse: Implications for child development and psychopathology* (Developmental clinical psychology and psychiatry, Vol. 10). Newbury Park, CA: Russell Sage.

Wolff, S. (1996). Moral development. In M. Lewis (Ed.), *Child and adolescent psychiatry* (2nd ed., pp. 187-194). Baltimore: Williams & Wilkins.

Wyatt, G. E., Newcomb, M., & Rierderle, M. (1993). *Sexual abuse and consensual sex: Women's developmental patterns and outcomes*. Newbury Park, CA: Russell Sage.

Yates, A. (1996). Childhood sexuality. In M. Lewis (Ed.), *Child and adolescent psychiatry* (2nd ed., pp. 221-235). Baltimore: Williams & Wilkins.

Suggested Readings

Kendall, J. (1989). Child psychiatric nursing and the family: A critical theory perspective. *Journal of Child and Adolescent Psychiatric and Mental Health Nursing, 2,* 145-153.

Rubin, T. I. (1960). *Jordi*. New York: Macmillan.

Rutter, M. (1987). Psychosocial resilience and protective mechanisms. *American Journal of Orthopsychiatry, 57,* 316-331.

Winnicott, D. W. (1971). *Playing and reality*. London: Tavistock.

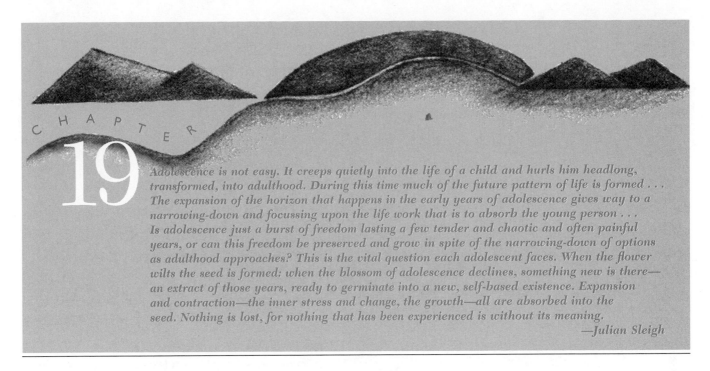

Adolescence is not easy. It creeps quietly into the life of a child and hurls him headlong, transformed, into adulthood. During this time much of the future pattern of life is formed . . . The expansion of the horizon that happens in the early years of adolescence gives way to a narrowing-down and focussing upon the life work that is to absorb the young person . . . Is adolescence just a burst of freedom lasting a few tender and chaotic and often painful years, or can this freedom be preserved and grow in spite of the narrowing-down of options as adulthood approaches? This is the vital question each adolescent faces. When the flower wilts the seed is formed; when the blossom of adolescence declines, something new is there— an extract of those years, ready to germinate into a new, self-based existence. Expansion and contraction—the inner stress and change, the growth—all are absorbed into the seed. Nothing is lost, for nothing that has been experienced is without its meaning.

—Julian Sleigh

The Adolescent

Learning Objectives

After studying this chapter, you should be able to:

1. Name and describe the three phases of adolescence.
2. Describe the adolescent in the context of family, school, peers, and community.
3. Discuss the symptoms of suicidality and violence in adolescents.
4. Discuss some aspects of adolescent sexuality.
5. Describe anorexia and bulimia in the adolescent patient.
6. Name several other body issues of adolescents.
7. Discuss adolescent spirituality.
8. Discuss the special considerations of establishing a therapeutic relationship with an adolescent.
9. Assist an adolescent in writing a treatment contract.
10. Describe some features of individual and group therapy with adolescents.

Key Terminology

Conduct disorder

Early adolescence

Imaginary audience

Late adolescence

Middle adolescence

Personal fable

505

In this chapter, we will look at the ways in which, in the culture of North America, adolescence is seen and experienced as a separate state, an extended transition between childhood and adulthood. Keep in mind what you learned in the last chapter: still pertinent are all the risk factors, coping mechanisms, areas of assessment, principles of medication use, and many of the diagnoses that we looked at in children. In the pages that follow, we will look briefly at some of the ways adolescents differ from children. We will consider some particular problematic behaviors, and look closely at some diagnoses you may encounter when working with disturbed youth.

We pour ourselves into the mold they
Made for us, and yet they say it's all wrong—
That we should ignore what we've learned
And learn what we've ignored
That life is not a joyful rollercoaster ride
But a bulldozer—miserably pushing its way
   Toward extinction! ■
                              —Charity Clemmer, 17

Charity's Story

Another generation, a place to start, a face to blame
For all mistakes inflicted upon the small
Form and bright eyes of the young.
To do as they say and not as they do...
Watching them with a longing for the truth
That is not found in clothes, sex, drugs, violence.
But we'll look anywhere.
Anywhere the bright lights lead us—
The lights of artificial skies and women
So thin and pale that ghosts can see
Right through them.
A path ends at the platform shoes
And cigarettes behind the school,
Away from the disgusted stare of the
Creators for their creations.
Placing fault on where they went wrong.
They say we're lost, mislead, polluted.
They call us slackers, losers, bad seeds...
Planted by the very hands that slap us.
They think that we're not listening,
Not understanding, because we don't agree
That the meaning of life is to do what
You're told and work hard for something
That you can never have: peace.
We are blamed for seeing what they
Are blind to. That this is not working.
That life is not a bulldozer driving
Toward extinction. That flowers should
Be picked and nature should not be
Pushed aside to make way for a new world
Where feeling is not important
And purpose is buried under misery.
So we pull, pull away from this bleak world,
Grappling for another, but not finding one
Except the metaphor they made for us:
The generation X, made to want and need
The things that turn the money over.
The generation that bends and molds
And tears its form to reflect the
Images of the hollow girl or shallow boy,
Lit up in our faces wherever we go.

CONTINUING THE JOURNEY: CONSIDERATIONS IN WORKING WITH ADOLESCENTS

Normal Adolescent Development

Adolescence in North America is generally considered to be a turbulent and stormy time. Nevertheless, the vast majority of adolescents do weather the storm of changing bodies, changing feelings, and the search for identity. A series of studies over three decades and across populations both in the United States and worldwide has found that approximately 80% of all adolescents "do not experience turmoil or psychological disturbance" (Offer, Schonert-Reichl, & Boxer, 1996, p. 279). This still means, however, that about 20% of teenagers are in a significant degree of distress. To understand the magnitude of this distress and how to help alleviate it, it will be helpful first to look at an overall picture of adolescent development.

Adolescence has been broken down into three general phases: early, middle, and late. **Early adolescence** corresponds to the beginning of puberty, that is, physical maturation and the development of primary and secondary sex characteristics. It is considered roughly to cover the ages of 11 through 13 in girls and 12 through 14 in boys. The tasks of early adolescence include acceptance of these enormous bodily changes and belonging to a (usually same gender) peer group. The changes of puberty tend to follow a predictable course. For girls, the beginning of breast development is followed by the appearance of pubic hair and a growth spurt. The onset of menarche comes later. For boys, pubic hair and penis growth usually precedes voice lowering and facial hair. The timing of puberty varies widely, however; it can occur several years earlier or later than the average. (The average itself has changed over the past 100 years, as we will discuss later.) The timing of puberty can have important effects on psychological development as well as on growth. Most young adolescents find bodily changes easier to accept if they happen in sync with the peer group. In addition, late developers often grow taller and longer-limbed, which can increase self-consciousness and dissatisfaction early on, although it may enhance peer admiration and self-acceptance later.

Middle adolescence, approximately 14 through 16 years in girls and 15 through 17 years in boys, is marked by the well-known struggle for independence, which often involves some degree of defiance and limit-testing. It is during this phase that the parent's role is perhaps most difficult but potentially most rewarding. In the words of Offer Schonert-Reichl, and Boxer (1996)

a good experience with parents will go a long way toward helping the adolescent's confidence in his or her self. The idea that one's parent can let go, still love the adolescent and allow him or her to experiment with different relationships is most important for healthy development. (p. 286)

Cognitive abilities increase, and many adolescents take great pleasure in their newfound facility in abstract thinking. Tasks include continued participation in a peer group, clarification of sexual orientation, exploration of intimacy, and development of a greater capacity for introspection and empathy.

During **late adolescence,** generally considered to end at the end of the 19th year, relative stability is generally attained in peer relationships, academic and leisure interests, and financial responsibility. Included in the tasks of this phase are the resolution of remaining dependency issues, commitment to a set of principles, crystallization of one's sex role, and choosing a vocation or career.

> **W***hat do you think?* Does adolescence really exist or is it a modern social construct?

➤ *Check Your Reading*
   1. What are the three phases of adolescence?
   2. Name one characteristic of each phase.
   3. Give an example of a task appropriate to each phase.

Understanding the Individual Journey

Each adolescent is unique. Yet each adolescent shares many of the same feelings, ambitions, fears, and concerns. It is a challenge to balance these two realizations in working with an adolescent patient. Elkind (1967) identified forms of normal egocentrism linked to Piaget's stages of cognitive development (see Chapter 18). The egocentrism of adolescence, Elkind argued, is brought about by the "conquest of thought." That is, the adolescent is now conceptually able to take into account the thought of others, but does not differentiate between those thoughts and his or her own preoccupations. Thus, the adolescent believes that others are as concerned about his or her appearance and behavior as he or she is. Anticipating others' reactions, the adolescent develops an internalized **imaginary audience** and gears his or her clothing, speech, and mannerisms to this admiring or critical phantom. But at the same time, a complementary belief in the adolescent's uniqueness

and consequent immortality arises. "It is as if the adolescent experiences the world with a unique sensory quality that is not shared by others: 'Nobody ever felt the way I do'" (Blos, 1962, p. 93). Out of this stance is constructed a **personal fable.** Lapsley (1993) emphasized that this phase is not pathological, but is a normal part of completing the second and final stage of the individuation process. The adolescent also may now establish "an I-Thou relationship with God as a personal confidant," looking for guidance and support (Elkind, 1967, p. 1031).

Similarly, Sleigh (1980) called this state of being a kind of "self-consciousness," embedded in the newly changing body. With this emerging identity, and an increasing estrangement from one's parents, comes a sense of isolation:

It is not easy to hand over to another person the power to gaze into one's feelings of emptiness and loss. Also it is not easy to put into words what is happening. The loneliness goes down to a level that can rarely be reached by another person. (p. 10)

Sleigh expressed a concern that so many distractions are provided by our culture that the adolescent is diverted from facing this loneliness and coming to terms with it. He encouraged those who would be helpful to allow the adolescent to "traverse the valley of aloneness" offering the reassurance that it is a threshold, not an end (p. 11). Sleigh referred us to Nouwen (1975) who taught

To live a spiritual life we must first find the courage to enter into the desert of our loneliness and to change it by gentle and persistent efforts into a garden of solitude. (p. 35)

The Journey as It Touches the Family

For the parents of an adolescent, the main task of this potentially stormy period is to survive. This does not mean passively waiting for the clouds to pass. It is a tremendously active process; it means examining the very values the adolescent may now be questioning or challenging, and reaffirming them. It means communicating directly and openly. It means growing along with the adolescent while remaining the adult. Most parents experience this challenge as a serious one: Psychoanalytically, adolescence is a time for reworking the family rivalries that characterize toddlerhood. Only now, as Winnicott (1971) put it, "growing up means taking the parent's place. *It really does*"(p. 144). Many cultures have incorporated formalized rituals that structure and contain this rite of passage. The mainstream culture of North America seems to lack such rituals, although in their absence some groups of young people develop their own maladaptive initiations. In the United States, even in the smoothest of transitions, normal adolescents pass through a phase of asking parents to leave them alone and to take care of them at the same time.

Divorce can have a particularly strong impact at this time, especially as adolescents take on the tasks of young adulthood and face a prospect of repeating patterns of failure in intimate relationships. An adolescent may also become preoccupied with the moral issues involved in a divorce and may side strongly with one parent against the other on that basis. The occurrence of divorce has been correlated with a higher rate of substance abuse in adolescents (Neher & Short, 1998) as well as poor health and nutrition, anxiety, depression, increased aggression, low self-esteem, and smoking (Thomson, 1998).

THE ADOLESCENT AND THE OUTSIDE WORLD

School

"The school, like the family, is charged with preparing the young to become successful adult workers, members of families, and citizens" (Comer, 1992, p. 2). In considering factors influencing adolescent development, school often tends to be overshadowed, even overlooked. Just the fact that in our culture the term *leaving school-age* is synonymous with *entering adolescence* is significant. However, both junior high and high school can be enormously powerful spheres of influence for the adolescent. Traditionally, school provides the basic setting for adolescents' social contacts. For youth involved in school sports teams, the experience can become a focal point of their lives over a period of years. In school, adolescents come in contact with adults—teachers, coaches, counselors, and administrators—who provide role models and important mentoring relationships. Such relationships can have profoundly positive effects on the trajectory of a young person's life. Also, increasingly, adolescents hone in on vocational and career interests in school, culminating in application to a chosen college, or graduating directly to the workforce.

Still, school for the adolescent is by no means a universally positive experience. For many, school is associated with academic failure, social rejection, and humiliation. For a tiny minority who have a disproportionately great effect on entire schools and towns, school becomes the setting in which the adolescent acts out a drama of revenge and retribution, causing damage and even taking lives. Although the incidence of violence has remained relatively stable, the nature of the violence in schools has become an enormous problem: one of every five U.S. high schools has at least one full-time police officer stationed through the school year. In a 1997 national survey by the Centers for Disease Control and Prevention (CDC) (Results of 1997 Youth Risk Behavior Study, 1998), at least 20% of all high school students carried weapons in school. A statewide survey in North Carolina found that 47% of males and 13% of females had carried a weapon to school in the past 30 days (Valois & McKeown, 1998). The solution would seem to lie not so much in the rush to enhance security in our schools with more metal detectors and guards but rather in simpler, more humane approaches. Projects that enhance community involvement in the schools, small class sizes, teachers who actually know their students, introduction of a violence-prevention curriculum, and integration of the emotional, social, and spiritual lives of people into the school discourse all would seem wiser ways of using scarce resources. In the words of Garbarino (1995), "big high schools are the single greatest threat the adolescent community faces" (p. 94). An adolescent needs to experience his or her participation and leadership truly making a difference.

Berg (1996) pointed out that "it has been shown that a sizable proportion of children at school show a considerable dislike of it and show a reluctance to attend" (p. 1105). There are certain specific problems that occur in relation to school attendance that may bring an adolescent into the mental health or legal system, or both. The first of these school phobia is most prevalent in the early adolescent years. *School phobia* is defined by the following characteristics: the child experiences emotional upset at the idea of attending school; the child's parents know the child is staying home and have made some attempt to encourage the child to go to school; serious antisocial behavior is not present. The onset is usually gradual, although it may be sudden. It may be related to a change in school setting or an increase in school demands and tends to be worst following vacations and on Monday mornings. It is most important that a concerted effort is made, with professionals, family, and school personnel working together, to ensure that the young adolescent attend consistently. Usually, once at school the child sheds her fear and behaves normally. If allowed to persist, however, school absence becomes entrenched, and the child typically becomes increasingly socially isolated and depressed (Berg, 1996).

Truancy is distinguished from school phobia in that the adolescent does not experience fear of going to school and usually tries to conceal his or her absence from parents. It is correlated with poverty, poor academic achievement, and an increased rate of delinquent behavior. Truancy can be carried to the extreme of permanent nonattendance, or "dropping out." Some schools, particular in poor, urban settings, have a staggeringly high truancy rate.

Friends

"There is an adolescent phase which has value in itself, and which makes adolescents want to club together in a mixture of *defiance* and *dependence*" (Winnicott, 1996, p. 138). The hallmark of adolescence is membership in a peer group. The quality of friendships undergoes a transformation in the adolescent years. No longer are friendships based mainly on day-to-day play and sharing of toys. Now, more abstract attributes become important: loyalty, empathy, self-disclosure (Offer et al., 1996). Friendships are forged that supplant the family as the primary source of intimacy and self-esteem. Such friendships may last a lifetime. Even gang membership may be seen for its positive attributes: an expression of the need for teenagers to establish a sense of identity and efficacy by affiliation with a group (Rodriguez, 1994). Some gangs, in recruiting youngsters, deliberately deemphasize dangerous or illegal activities and stress the advantages of family-like organizations that provide protection and opportunities for recognition and advancement.

"Compared to the family," wrote Csikszentmihalyi and Larson (1984), "friends have everything going for them, at least from the point of view of the adolescent" (p. 156). Teens choose their friends freely and can expect their approval and admiration. They do not have to negotiate the typical conflicts of home life, do not have to answer to friends, do not have to explain certain commonalities of adolescent life. If a conflict does arise, a friendship can be ended and another begun. In the typical American family, almost the only thing family members do together is watch television; teenagers spend most of their time together talking and engaging in activities. Adolescents spend more time with friends than does any other age group.

Inevitably, peers become the major influence in adolescence. Many adolescents bridle at the suggestion that peer pressure influences their decisions. In their experience, they feel free to do or not to do whatever their friends are doing. In fact, the power of a group to influence an individual's choices has been well-documented and is perhaps never more pervasive than during the teen years. Thus the adolescent's choice of a peer group is crucial. Association with deviant peers makes it likely that an adolescent will engage in deviant behavior. As Prothrow-Stith and Weissman (1991) put it, "The peer group is a refuge providing approval, warmth, friendship, sustenance and fun, but the refuge can become an unsafe haven" (p. 53). Csikszentmihalyi and Larson (1984) defined the ideal friendship as "one that contributes to order both at the personal and social levels in the short run, and at the same time helps a person find a meaningful place in the world over the years" (p. 157).

Community

The status and role of the adolescent in the community have shifted from time to time and from place to place. For example, in times of war, adolescents are viewed as a resource for the military. Even theoretical writings in such eras reflect a view of adolescents as mature and competent. When unemployment levels are high, teens tend to be viewed as immature and are encouraged by societal pressures to stay in school longer (Offer et al., 1996). In agricultural communities, the adolescent has historically been a valued asset, a source of strong labor and limitless energy. There has been work for teens to do, and elders to teach them how to do it; the difficulty lies only in convincing them to stay put when they dream of broader horizons.

In the blighted neighborhoods of the inner cities, on the other hand, teenagers are often seen as a menace to be controlled. In Brazil and Colombia, "clean-up crews," including off-duty police officers, have been responsible for the murders of thousands of street children. In the United States, a key speaker at the 1992 Republican convention urged military involvement to take back "our" cities, as if the impoverished young people living and dying in them were not also our children. And yet, the United States has not had the political will to control the number of guns that end up in the hands of children and teenagers. In the words of Venkatesh (1997), "Neither the structure nor the practice of the street gang can be understood apart from the social organizational context of the larger community it inhabits" (p. 82).

Many communities lack appropriate places for young people to gather. Groups cluster on street corners in the inner cities, congregate in parking lots in the suburbs, or make their way to the malls. As Finnegan (1998) commented, "As a hangout for teenagers, there could hardly be a worse place than the mall; they are in a universe in which consumption is the only value" (p. 35). In some neighborhoods, residents put pressure on the police department to enforce curfew laws.

Racial, Ethnic, and Cultural Differences

As we have seen in Chapter 12, culture, ethnicity, and race have a deep influence on the development and lifeways of each of us. Child-rearing practices differ widely, and even temperament has been shown to be subject to cultural influence. These differences become most relevant at the points where cultures intersect. For example, Native American and Asian children are raised to *accept* natural occurrences rather than to attempt to control them. Competition is not highly prized, since the emphasis is on sharing and loyalty to family and group. Modesty, interdependence, respect for elders, and emotional self-control are valued. Adaptive as these traits are within Native American and Asian communities, they can clash with the values of the dominant culture in the United States, putting the adolescent in a difficult position as he or she moves into a larger sphere of social interactions (McDermott, 1996). For African-American students, Comer (1996) said,

by mid-adolescence . . . social class and race-related expectations and occupational and career possibilities begin to greatly influence school performance . . . many capable young people go on a sharp psychosocial downhill course at this point, leading to school dropouts, teenage pregnancy, delinquency and crime. (p. 1100)

On the other hand, there are strong maturational influences at work in adolescence, frequently running counter to the culture of origin. Thus, often to the distress of parents and grandparents, teenagers tend to conform to the larger society's gender norms, regardless of upbringing (McDermott, 1996). The emphasis on youth, on the individual, on independence and freedom of choice, on open expressions of anger and sexuality can be extremely disruptive within the families of many minority adolescents, particularly in families who have immigrated or who live in relatively isolated communities. Figure 19–1 illustrates the many factors that have an impact on the developing adolescent.

> **W**hat do you think? Which played the biggest part in your adolescence, family, school, friends, or community?

➤ **Check Your Reading**
4. What is the imaginary audience?
5. Why is divorce especially hard on an adolescent?
6. Name one risk and one opportunity related to high school life.
7. Give an example of a clash of cultural values for adolescents.

RISKS OF ADOLESCENCE

Injurious Behaviors

According to statistics compiled by the CDC (1998), 72% of deaths between the ages of 5 and 24 years are caused by motor vehicle accidents, homicides, suicides, and accidental injuries. A contributing factor in these deaths is the adolescent egocentrism discussed earlier. A teenager who believes he or she is unique and immortal is not likely to refrain from reckless behavior despite evidence that this has been dangerous to others. Similarly, an adolescent convinced that no one else could feel as he or she does may be more liable to attempt suicide when filled with despair.

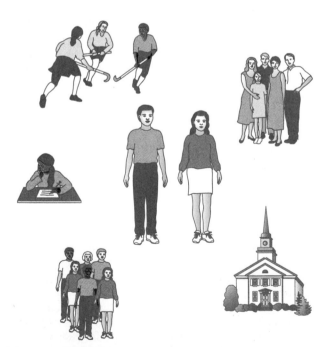

Figure 19–1
Forces that have an impact on an adolescent.

Suicidality

The management of suicidal behavior is "probably the most difficult issue in child psychiatric outpatient treatment and causes the most sleepless nights" (Lewandowski, personal communication, 1990). Risk factors include

- History of suicide attempt
- Mood disorder, disruptive disorder, substance abuse disorder, anxiety disorder, or schizophrenia
- Recent significant loss
- Death of a friend or family member by suicide, especially if recent
- Perception of isolation
- Family conflict
- Parental divorce and remarriage

Adolescent girls have a higher rate of suicidal gestures, most often by means of overdose; boys have a slightly higher rate of completion, with hanging and firearm use the most common methods. As many as 60% of adolescents have considered suicide (McKeown, Garrison, Cuff, Waller, Jackson, & Addy, 1998). The suicide rate among white male adolescents jumped 22% in the 1980s but stabilized over the 1990s, whereas the rate among black male adolescents continues to climb, more than doubling from the late 1970s to the late 1990s (CDC, 1998). Black middle-class youth appear to be at particular risk. A number of suicide assessment instruments exist, among them Beck's Scale for Suicide Ideation, Linehan's Reasons for Living Inventory (RLI), and a self-administered adaptation of the RLI by Coles called the Suicidal Behaviors Questionnaire (cited in Range & Knott, 1997).

Nurses should know that asking about suicidal thoughts does not increase risk for suicide, it lessens it. Nurses can play an important part in suicide prevention, not only by directly developing a relationship with and a care plan for the suicidal adolescent (Foote, 1997) but also through educating families about risk factors, warning signs, and protective factors. Parents should seek treatment for adolescents who show signs of depression. An adolescent who makes statements of hopelessness and self-hatred, or who gives away valued possessions, must be taken seriously. Parents should make an effort to encourage positive friendships and, by talking issues through with their teens, promote good judgment and problem-solving. Also, the negative stress of divorce and remarriage can be mitigated by an adolescent's experience of family cohesiveness (Rubenstein et al., 1998). Families can be helped to develop more positive patterns of communication and to involve adolescents in fun, productive activities without impinging on the growing need for independence. A sense of acceptance, engagement, purposefulness, and spiritual fulfillment makes suicidality unlikely.

Violence

Contributions to the development of violent behaviors are numerous. Being young, male, and raised in adverse circumstances is linked universally with increased rates of violence. Androgens are undoubtedly related to aggression, but hormones do not explain everything. In an earlier-mentioned North Carolina study, roughly half of all adolescent boys surveyed reported having had at least one physical fight in the preceding year; however, nearly one third of adolescent girls reported the same (Valois & McKeown, 1998). In Chapter 18, we looked at the effect of the media on behavior. The Center for Media and Public Affairs in Washington, D.C., tallied all violent acts on television over an 18-hour period in April, 1994. It recorded 2065 instances of violence (Kolbert, 1994). Video games have become increasingly violent and future games promise to be more violent still. One game depicts a man shooting unarmed bystanders in public places; another encourages players to torture their enemies.

Evidence exists that over half of all violent crimes are committed under the influence of alcohol (Pihl & Peterson, 1993). Gang membership also contributes to crime in several ways. Initiation rites and promotions frequently depend on the commission of assaults on rival gang members. Gangs involved in drug trafficking promote violent crime in users who have to find money to support their habits. Also, participation in group activities can have a disinhibiting effect on individuals, so that collectively they may commit offenses they would not carry through alone. Tolleson (1997) discussed the adaptive role violence can play in the lives of fearful, "mortally vulnerable" young gang members, an enactment of identification with the aggressor that transforms passivity into mastery. Only by making their world safer can we lessen their perceived need for a violent response.

Armstrong and Gurke (1997) pointed out that gangs have begun to "infiltrate all socioeconomic levels of most towns, cities and metropolitan areas" (p. 6) and stress the need for school nurses to get involved in intervention strategies. Similar arguments were made by Mondragon (1995) regarding nurses in primary care settings, and Prothrow-Stith and Weissman (1991) about emergency department personnel. Agreeing, Czerwinski and Moloney-Harmon (1997) called gun-related violence an epidemic and stated that "nurses must make a commitment to tackle this overwhelming, but solvable problem" (p. 209). In places where church groups and other volunteer organizations have taken strong stands, programs have been developed as gang alternatives where young people can put their creative energy, enthusiasm, and idealism to wonderful uses.

The psychiatric diagnosis most often associated with violence is **conduct disorder.** Conduct disorder is a label for disturbances of behavior contradictory to accepted social norms. These behaviors usually involve harming others or violating a trust. At least 3 of 15 criteria must have been present for 6 months or more, including stealing, running away, lying, fire-setting, truancy, and cruelty to animals (see Medical Diagnosis and Related Nursing Diagnosis: Disruptive Behavior Disorders).

A conduct disorder represents a description of a group of behaviors—such as impulsivity and violence—frequently clustered together. A number of investigators have begun studying the possible neurochemical contributions to such behaviors, most notably decreased noradrenergic and serotoninergic functioning (Eichelman, 1992; Quay, 1993). As always, however, you must also look beyond the behavior, or within it, to the communicative function it serves. The outside observer can easily recognize anger in a conduct-disordered adolescent, but the adolescent may be less clear about anger and less clear still about the other feelings underlying the actions. As Winnicott (1958) suggested, "there is a direct relationship between the antisocial tendency and deprivation," and, further, *"the antisocial tendency implies hope"* (p. 309).

Your first response as a nurse is to help provide what the adolescent is missing: that is, not some material thing but the safety of being contained and prevented from doing harm. With containment (which can be provided in a home or an institution), you can begin to link behaviors with feelings in a way that becomes comprehensible for an adolescent.

What do you think? What do you believe accounts for the increased seriousness of adolescent crime?

▶ *Check Your Reading*
 8. Give three risk factors for suicide.
 9. Name three contributing factors to adolescent violence.
10. List three symptoms of conduct disorder.

Alcohol and Substance Abuse

By the age of 18, in the United States, most young people have used drugs to "get high" (Cambor & Millman, 1996). There has been some discussion about the distinction between the terms *use* and *abuse,* with some arguing that because all unprescribed substance use is illegal for teens, it is ipso facto abuse. We will assume that some mild, recreational experimentation is normative, because it is engaged in by the vast majority of adolescents and since the majority of adolescents mature out of this phase. We will look briefly instead at adolescent abuse of or dependence on various substances including alcohol, marijuana, inhalants, cocaine, heroine, prescription drugs, "designer" drugs, steroids, and tobacco. (See Chapter 26 for an in-depth discussion of substance abuse, including the Diagnostic and Statistical Manual of Mental Disorders, Fourth Edition (DSM-IV) diagnostic criteria for Substance-Related Disorders.)

The DSM-IV defines *abuse* as use that is maladaptive and persists for at least a month. The epidemiology of adolescent substance abuse is difficult to determine. Surveys such as the Youth Risk Behavior Survey may miss the most chronic abusers, who are less likely to attend school consistently. Teens may not be truthful answering questions about illegal activities. Symptoms of substance abuse may be missed, in part, because they can resemble some of the normal behavioral changes of

MEDICAL DIAGNOSIS AND RELATED NURSING DIAGNOSIS

Disruptive Behavior Disorders

DSM-IV Diagnosis: Conduct Disorder

Diagnostic Criteria

A. A repetitive and persistent pattern of behavior in which the basic rights of others or major age-appropriate societal norms or rules are violated, as manifested by the presence of three (or more) of the following criteria in the past 12 months, with at least one criterion present in the past 6 months:

Aggression to people and animals

1. Often bullies, threatens, or intimidates others.
2. Often initiates physical fights.
3. Has used a weapon that can cause serious physical harm to others (e.g., a bat, brick, broken bottle, knife, gun).
4. Has been physically cruel to people.
5. Has been physically cruel to animals.
6. Has stolen while confronting a victim (e.g., mugging, purse snatching, extortion, armed robbery).
7. Has forced someone into sexual activity.

Destruction of property

8. Has deliberately engaged in fire-setting with the intention of causing serious damage.
9. Has deliberately destroyed others' property (other than by fire-setting).

Deceitfulness or theft

10. Has broken into someone else's house, building, or car.
11. Often lies to obtain goods or favors or to avoid obligations (i.e., "cons" others).
12. Has stolen items of nontrivial value without confronting a victim (e.g., shoplifting, but without breaking and entering; forgery).

Serious violations of rules

13. Often stays out at night despite parental prohibitions, beginning before age 13 years.
14. Has run away from home overnight at least twice while living in parental or parental surrogate home (or once without returning for a lengthy period).
15. Is often truant from school, beginning before age 13 years.

B. The disturbance in behavior causes clinically significant impairment in social, academic, or occupational functioning.

C. If the individual is age 18 years or older, criteria are not met for Antisocial Personality Disorder.

Specify type based on age at onset:

Childhood-Onset Type: Onset of at least one criterion characteristic of Conduct Disorder before age 10 years.

Adolescent-Onset Type: Absence of any criteria characteristic of Conduct Disorder before age 10 years.

Specify severity:

Mild: Few if any conduct problems in excess of those required to make the diagnosis and conduct problems cause only minor harm to others.

Moderate: Number of conduct problems and effect on others intermediate between mild and severe.

Severe: Many conduct problems in excess of those required to make the diagnosis or conduct problems cause considerable harm to others.

Related Nursing Diagnosis: Risk for Violence

Definition

A state in which an individual exhibits behaviors that can be physically harmful to the self or others.

Example

Potential for Violence related to Conduct Disorder as evidenced by Intermittent aggressive outburst.

Based on information from the *Diagnostic and Statistical Manual of Mental Disorders. Fourth Edition.* Copyright 1994 American Psychiatric Association. Nursing diagnoses and definitions from North American Nursing Diagnosis Association. (1999). *NANDA nursing diagnoses: Definitions and classification, 1999-2000.* Philadelphia: NANDA.

adolescence. In addition, substance abuse frequently occurs in young people with other psychiatric disorders, such as depression, anxiety, and conduct problems, further obscuring the picture (Stowell & Estroff, 1992). Keep in mind that there is a tendency for some adolescents to turn psychoactive substances in a misguided attempt to medicate themselves for their underlying anxiety and depression. Unrecognized and untreated, however, substance abuse undermines the most earnest therapeutic efforts. Figure 19–2 provides an Adolescent Substance Abuse Interview and Assessment Tool.

ALCOHOL

The most common psychoactive substance in use among adolescents is alcohol, and the trend has been toward earlier and earlier use. Most commonly, young people establish patterns of intermittent drinking, usually on weekends. Most drinking is done in group settings, originating perhaps in a wish to feel less awkward but culminating often in drinking to the point of illness or unconsciousness. At this stage, the adolescent's impaired judgment represents an enormous health risk. The greatest danger lies in risky behaviors engaged in while intoxicated, particularly driving and fighting. Another risk is the combined use of alcohol and sedatives, which can be fatal. Also, a young person under stress or with a genetic predisposition to alcoholism may become dependent and develop a pattern of compulsive drinking, impairing day-to-day functioning and jeopardizing his or her health.

Adolescent Chemical History Assessment

Patient's Name:_____ Date:_____

Nurse's Name:_____

The questions that follow are not definitive; they can be reduced in number, altered, expanded, or rearranged. This is a data-gathering, educational, diagnostic, and awareness-building tool.

1. What do you or have you used (including inhalants)?

2. How long have you used (beginning from experimentation)?

3. Do your parents know you use? What happened when they found out (if they did)? How did you feel about that?

4. How often are you high in a week (or significant period of time)? Drunk? What do "high" and "drunk" mean to you?

5. How many of your friends use? Acquaintances?

6. Are you close to someone you are convinced has a chemical problem? Have you told them about your concern, if you are concerned?

7. Are you taking medication?

8. Do you owe money for chemicals? How much?

9. How much do you spend for chemicals in a month (if you were to pay for all your chemicals)?

Figure 19–2

Adolescent chemical history assessment. DWI, driving while intoxicated. (From Hazelden Foundation, Center City, Minnesota.)

Illustration continued on following page

CANNABIS

Cannabis or marijuana, made from dried leaves and flowers of the hemp plant, *Cannabis sativa*, is also widely used among teenagers. Marijuana has myriad nicknames, among them "weed," "O.J." and "chronic." Most often smoked in a hand-rolled cigarette known as a "joint," marijuana is also used to replace the tobacco in a small cigar called a "blunt." Hashish, a less common, stronger substance also derived from cannabis, is normally smoked in a pipe. Marijuana and hashish may also be eaten. The effects of cannabis include heightened and altered perceptions and thought patterns, increased appetite, drowsiness, mood changes, and motor coordi-nation impairment. Acute paranoia may occur. Habitual use may lead to a decline in social and academic functioning and general apathy. This has been called the *amotivational syndrome* (Winger, Hofmann, & Woods, 1992). Bronchitis is seen in marijuana smokers. The reproductive system may be affected. Also, daily mari-juana use has an association with eventual abuse of other drugs such as cocaine and heroin.

INHALANTS

Following alcohol and marijuana, inhalants are probably the next substances probably most frequently abused by young adolescents. Inhalants include a wide variety of

10.   Who provides, if you are broke?

11.   Have you received any negative feedback about your use? How did it make you feel?

12.   Have you ever lost a friend because of your use? Boyfriends/girlfriends? What happened? How did you feel?

13.   Have you lost a job because of your use? What happened? How did you feel?

14.   Have you ever been "busted" (police, school, home, DWIs)? What happened? How did you feel?

15.   What time of day do you use?

16.   Do you use on the job or in school (during school)?

17.   How is school going for you? Grades, skips, fails, absences? How do you feel about that?

18.   Does it take more, less, or about the same amount to get high?

19.   Have you ever "shot up"? With what? Where on your body?

20.   What is a blackout? Ever had one? Did you ever pass out? What happened? How did it make you feel?

21.   Are you sexually active?

Figure 19–2 *Continued*

materials in everyday household use, such as glue, paint thinner, lighter fluid, spray paint, and gasoline, easily accessible to youngsters without money or transportation. A rag is typically saturated with the substance and held in the mouth (huffing) or put in a plastic bag that is placed over the face (sniffing). There is a real danger of suffocation from the plastic bag. Repeated use can cause lung and brain damage. Native American and Hispanic youth appear to be at the highest risk for inhalant abuse.

DEPRESSANTS

Another commonly abused class of drugs is depressants. Adolescents, especially younger adolescents, may obtain illegal prescription sedatives, including anxiolytics (e.g., diazepam, lorazepam), hypnotics (e.g., flunitrazepam [Rohypnol]), and barbituates (e.g., pentobarbital, secobarbitol), for recreational use. Habitual users tend to combine drugs and to develop tolerance, requiring high daily doses to obtain the desired effects, which include diminished anxiety and behavioral disinhibition. Withdrawal from continuous use of sedatives can cause severe central nervous system (CNS) and cardiovascular system dysregulation; it may even be fatal. If you suspect an adolescent is experiencing early sedative withdrawal, seek appropriate help at once. Accidental or deliberate sedative overdoses also cause many teenage deaths.

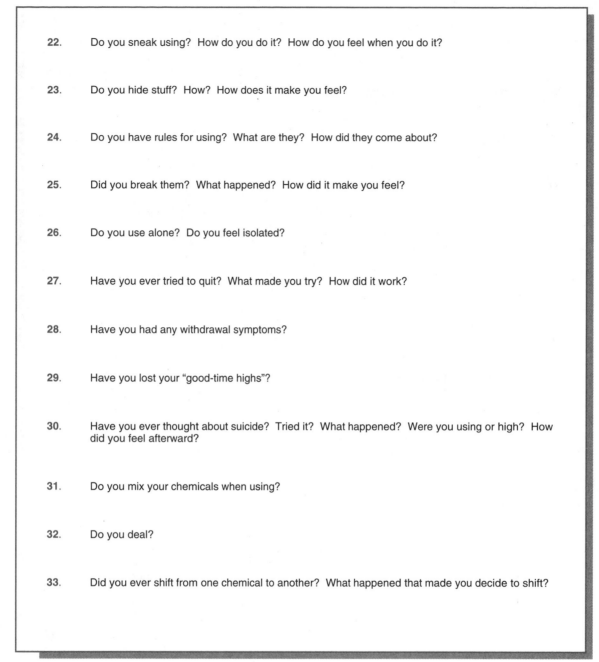

22.   Do you sneak using? How do you do it? How do you feel when you do it?

23.   Do you hide stuff? How? How does it make you feel?

24.   Do you have rules for using? What are they? How did they come about?

25.   Did you break them? What happened? How did it make you feel?

26.   Do you use alone? Do you feel isolated?

27.   Have you ever tried to quit? What made you try? How did it work?

28.   Have you had any withdrawal symptoms?

29.   Have you lost your "good-time highs"?

30.   Have you ever thought about suicide? Tried it? What happened? Were you using or high? How did you feel afterward?

31.   Do you mix your chemicals when using?

32.   Do you deal?

33.   Did you ever shift from one chemical to another? What happened that made you decide to shift?

Figure 19–2 *Continued*

Illustration continued on following page

Another sedative that has become a problem is flunitrazepam (Rohypnol). Called "rochas" or "roofies" and used by some young teens to reduce anxiety (similar to methaqualone), these are the pills known as the "date rape drug." One or two dissolved in an alcoholic beverage can render a young person unconscious within minutes; the victim generally has no memory of what occurs over the next several hours.

STIMULANTS

Amphetamines and ephedrine derivatives as well as cocaine are included among the stimulant class of drugs.

A small number of teens abuse stimulants in pill form; among these are chronic dieters. More commonly, a powdered form is inhaled nasally, or occasionally taken by intravenous (IV) injection. More potent, more dangerous, smokeable forms of cocaine ("crack") and methamphetamine ("ice") have tended to appear in epidemic proportions among impoverished youth populations, causing havoc in already vulnerable communities. Adverse effects, apart from disrupting daily life and emotional development, include CNS and cardiovascular system complications. Pregnant teens who abuse stimulants endanger their already compromised fetuses.

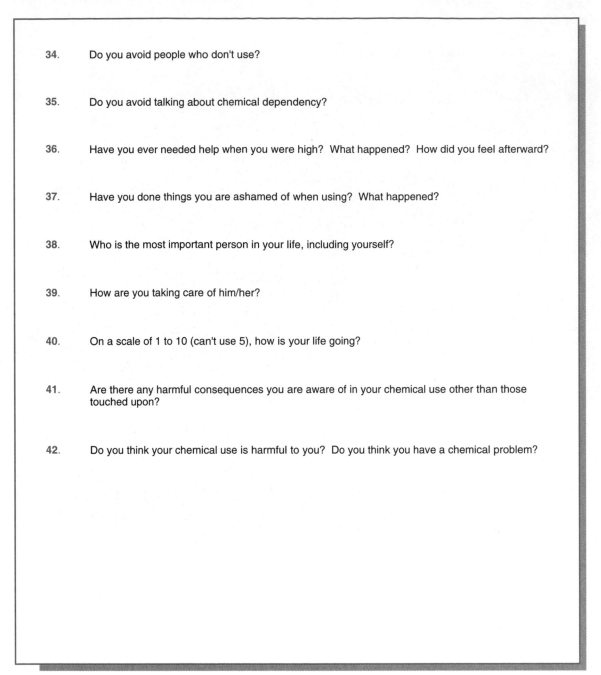

34.   Do you avoid people who don't use?

35.   Do you avoid talking about chemical dependency?

36.   Have you ever needed help when you were high? What happened? How did you feel afterward?

37.   Have you done things you are ashamed of when using? What happened?

38.   Who is the most important person in your life, including yourself?

39.   How are you taking care of him/her?

40.   On a scale of 1 to 10 (can't use 5), how is your life going?

41.   Are there any harmful consequences you are aware of in your chemical use other than those touched upon?

42.   Do you think your chemical use is harmful to you? Do you think you have a chemical problem?

Figure 19-2 *Continued*

OPIATES

Abuse of opiates includes the illegal use of drugs such as morphine, codeine, and synthetic opioids like Darvon and Percodan. The most commonly abused opiate, however, is heroin. Like the powdered stimulants, heroin is usually inhaled at first. It is described as bestowing a brief, compelling sensation of well-being and of freedom from anxiety. Highly addictive, it must be taken in increasingly large quantities, which often leads to intradermal and IV use. A 1986 study by the National Institute for Drug Abuse found that 1% of all high school seniors had injected heroin IV.

IV heroin users are at high risk for contracting such life-threatening illnesses as hepatitis and AIDS. Like crack and ice, heroin tends to make an appearance in an epidemic-like pattern, concentrating in the poorer inner cities and spreading to the more affluent surrounding communities and college towns. Its initial cheapness and availability contributes to dependence and the need for increasingly large purchases to support the habit, in turn contributing to an enormous increase in youth crime in affected areas. Heroin-addicted girls frequently turn to prostitution as a means of raising the necessary funds.

HALLUCINOGENS

For centuries, hallucinogens have been used by indigenous peoples in the context of religious rituals, to enhance the experience of a transcendent, collective consciousness. The best known hallucinogen is perhaps lysergic acid diethylamide (LSD), which became popular in the late 1960s. But more commonly used now are the so-called designer drugs, like MDMA ("Ecstasy"). Synthesized in private laboratories, these drugs inhabit a gray area of the law, outside the purview of the Food and Drug Administration (FDA). Acting on the serotonergic system, they affect mood and have relatively few physical side effects.

Their use is primarily in group settings like "mosh pits" at rock concerts or at "raves," parties where young people dance for hours, to the point of exhaustion. It is likely that these youths are seeking the same ancient sense of shared consciousness but, without a spiritual foundation, achieve instead a fleeting illusion of escaping reality. Other far more dangerous hallucinogens include phencyclidine (PCP) and ketamine—both developed as anesthetic agents. PCP, also known as "angel dust" and "illy," may be sprinkled on marijuana, mixed with other powdered drugs, or used to dip cigarettes into. It causes a state of depersonalization, paranoia, even delirium, resembling an acute schizophrenic episode. It has been associated with extremely violent outbursts and, in high doses, coma and death. Ketamine, called "special K," is similarly toxic.

STEROIDS
Although steroids are not listed in the DSM-IV and used for largely different reasons than the above-mentioned substances, they are a matter of concern for the nurse who works with adolescents. Taken primarily by boys involved in competitive sports or concerned about their developing physique, anabolic (muscle-building) steroid abuse can cause infertility, liver damage, and heart disease. As many as 11% of high school–aged boys take steroids, and a small percentage of female athletes do as well. Apart from a rapid increase in muscle bulk, noticeable effects of steroid use include worsening acne, mood swings, increased aggression, and increased libido.

TOBACCO
Nicotiana tabacum, or tobacco, was used for hundreds of years by indigenous peoples in the Western Hemisphere for medicinal purposes. Recently, in fact, with pressure on the tobacco industry to take responsibility for the dire consequences of its products, there is research being done into the potentially beneficial uses of its numerous component chemicals. One of these, the stimulant nicotine, has long been known to be a highly addictive substance. According to the Department of Education, the younger the smoker, the more likely severe levels of nicotine addiction will develop (Levant, 1998). Thirty-five percent of all high school students smoke (CDC, 1998).

In 1996, the FDA classified nicotine as a drug and banned all advertising aimed at minors. However, the tobacco industry still sponsors sporting events, maintains Web sites, and promotes movies featuring charismatic actors smoking cigarettes. Easily obtained despite laws banning sales to minors, tobacco has been shown to be a "gateway" drug (Lindsay & Rainey, 1997). Although not all teen smokers go on to become users of illicit substances, among those who do, the majority begin with cigarettes.

Assessing whether a young person is involved in substance abuse can be difficult. Substance abuse should be suspected in all instances of accidental injury and in any adolescent brought by parents to a hospital or clinic for evaluation. Some clinics and hospitals have policies of routine drug screens, making it possible to detect a percentage of users. If you are assisting with a physical examination, you can look for elevated vital signs, irregular heart rate, dilated or constricted pupils, lesions of the nasal mucosa, injection marks or skin abscesses, jaundice and abdominal tenderness. There are also questionnaires that can be administered, such as the Drug and Alcohol Problem (DAP) Quick Screen (Schwartz & Wirzt, 1990). But the therapeutic relationship is the context in which an adolescent is likely to begin to talk honestly about the problem and to come to terms with it. Because drug-abusing adolescents tend to associate with others like them, initiating a discussion regarding concerns they may have about friends can be an opener.

It helps to keep in mind that there are many reasons why adolescents begin abusing substances. Temperamentally, sensation seeking individuals are more likely to take risks with substance experimentation and other dangerous activities. Peer pressure has an enormous influence on adolescent behavior. As mentioned earlier, many young people with mental health problems attempt to alleviate these problems through a kind of self-medication. But do not underestimate the effect on the average teenager of anxieties caused by all the issues we have touched on. We are all looking for meaning in our lives.

Nancy Reagan was wrong to advise children that they can just say no. A hunger rises. It is not exactly a longing for drugs but for refreshment on the highest level: a new personality, a new world. . . . (Humphreys, 1987, p. 14)

We all have stress-reducing habits, ranging from secretive nail biting to shopping splurges. Mature individuals with adequate social support may have the self-discipline to seek out such life-enhancing practices as prayer, artistic expression, or meditation. But teens with low self-esteem, few credible role models, and little patience, bombarded by media promotions of instant gratification and subject to pressure from peers, can easily stumble into substance use that initially seems helpful. Your ability to accept the adolescent nonjudgmentally, while not endorsing self-harmful behavior, can be the beginning of disavowing these dangerous habits.

Identifying which individuals will "mature out" of using substances and which will go on to become chronic users is probably not possible, although certainly some adolescents can be seen to have more risk factors for addiction. These include adolescents who are low achievers and have low self-esteem, who take risks and are drawn to others with deviant behaviors, who are impulsive and aggressive, and who are experiencing intrapsychic distress (Brooks et al., 1995). School-based programs designed to prevent cigarette, alcohol, and drug use have not been shown to be especially successful thus far. Such programs "tend to increase alcohol and drug knowledge without decreasing or delaying the onset of use" (Houston & Weiner, 1997, p. 649). Family-based programs have had better success.

For the substance-dependent adolescent, treatment is difficult, particularly in a cost-constrained health care environment. The ideal setting is probably a therapeutic residential community, designed for adolescents as distinct from adults. Staffed by a team of professionals and recovering addicts, such a community takes into account that addiction and its sequelae have the effect of interrupting adolescent development. In this setting, abstinence is monitored. Individual and group therapy can be provided, and a pattern of attendance at Alcoholics Anonymous (AA) or Narcotics Anonymous (NA) meetings established. Noshpitz (1994) described the treatment resistance of young people who harbor a negative ideal:

In the drug-treatment setting . . . it is common to encounter adolescents who protest that they only have an addiction problem; once they break the habit, they would need no further help." (p. 348)

However, these young people have a strong inner belief that they are unworthy and bound to fail and will sabotage their own success because it is intolerable to them. The key is to forge a treatment alliance and gradually call the adolescent's attention to the process of self-destructiveness as it plays out in the context of the therapeutic community.

> **W**hat do you think? How do you feel about the movement to legalize drugs?

> ► *Check Your Reading*
> 11. What is the most commonly abused substance in adolescence?
> 12. Name some household products used as inhalants.
> 13. Give three signs of steroid use.
> 14. What is the ideal treatment setting for substance-dependent adolescents?

Self-Mutilation

A phenomenon seen primarily among adolescent girls, self-mutilation, also called "cutting," has a high correlation with depression and borderline personality disorder. The girl who cuts herself is "often emotionally inarticulate and emotionally imperceptive" (Levenkron, 1998, p. 49). She tends to be insecure in herself and to mistrust the solidity of her relationships with others.

The practice of cutting usually begins when the adolescent feels overwhelmed by a strong feeling of rage, anxiety, or sadness that she cannot express. Out of frustration she hurts herself in some way: cuts a hand on glass, scratches or burns herself, or bangs her head against a wall. The physical pain and subsequent endorphin release act as a distraction from the emotional pain, and the adolescent believes she has discovered a "cure." Levenkron (1998) quoted a young woman who stated "'It was like medicine for my fears'" (p. 32). Some

adolescents encourage one another to cut—even sharing cutting instruments and thus the risk of blood-borne diseases. Disgusted or nurturing responses of caretaking adults can also reinforce this habit.

Look for scars on the physical examination; ask about what kinds of things upset the adolescent and what techniques she uses to calm herself when feeling upset. By demystifying this disturbing behavior you can lay the groundwork for developing a plan to replace it with more adaptive coping skills.

Depression

Depression can be a contributing factor in all of the dangerous behaviors we see in adolescents. Chapter 25 gives a complete picture of major depressive disorder (MDD) and provides the DSM-IV diagnostic criteria as well as nursing diagnoses and interventions. For the adolescent, you should keep in mind that depression may manifest itself in various ways. The teen may lack energy and motivation, may show changes in appetite and sleep patterns, may seem sad and hopeless, but may also be primarily irritable or angry. He or she might engage in self-destructive acts due to depression and can have another diagnosis whose symptoms may mask the depression. In conduct disordered or anorexic adolescents, for example, depression may be missed as attention is focused on more immediately obvious issues. The use of an interview such as the KSADS (Chambers et al., 1985) can be helpful.

SEXUALITY

One cannot attempt to study any problem of adolescence without recognizing the basis of the new instinctual drive, which is biological . . . Puberty forces on each child a new orientation to the world. This new thing is the more difficult because the child does not see far ahead, and does not want to look. . . . (Winnicott 1996, p. 138)

A striking increase in erotic preoccupation is a hallmark of adolescent development, along with physical maturation. The body is flooded with gonadal hormones. "The boy is growing a new shape to his physical genitality, and a new excitability; the girl is experiencing menstruation, and a new uprush of feeling in personal relationships" (Winnicott, 1996, p. 138). Most girls begin puberty approximately 2 years before most boys and reach maturity more quickly once puberty begins. Tanner staging tracks the emergence of secondary sex characteristics (Tanner, 1974): you can obtain this information from a physical examination. Ask adolescents directly about sexual activity, keeping in mind that only when they trust you will they be candid.

Masturbation

Adolescent masturbation . . . becomes the regulator of tension and the bearer of fantasies which accompany, in their shifting content and pattern, the various phases of adolescent development. (Blos, 1962, p. 159)

Although there are cultural and gender differences, as well as differences between individuals and in the same individual over time, masturbation is a nearly universal phenomenon. The nurse's concern with masturbation regards the impact it may have on an adolescent's life. Many adolescents worry about their bodies, including their genitals—whether they are normal in size, in shape, and in function. They may have concerns or misperceptions about their erotic experiences, dreams, nocturnal emissions, and sexual fantasies. If you are doing a physical examination or assisting in one, it is helpful to tell an adolescent his or her body is normal without expecting to be asked. If you let an adolescent know you can talk about such concerns easily and reassuringly, you open the door for further discussion and questions that he or she has never dared ask anyone.

Masturbation is a normal and expectable part of growing up. But if an adolescent's functioning is being impaired in some way related to their masturbatory activities, they may need more specific help. For example, an adolescent may develop a *paraphilia;* that is, an item, sexual object, or situation that becomes a focus of sexual fantasy and a requirement for sexual arousal. If this involves culturally prohibited activities, the adolescent might be consumed with shame. If it involves other people unwilling—or legally and morally unable—to consent, the adolescent is at risk for endangering self and others. Repetitive fantasies of violent rape or of child molestation are a signal of sexuality gone awry. If an adolescent has a place to talk about these issues, there is a chance to avert harm being done.

Pregnancy

Fisher (1992), a Darwinian anthropologist, suggested that teenagers in hunter-gatherer societies have traditionally enjoyed many years of learning about and trying out sexual relationships without fear of pregnancy because of the late menarche of slim, physically active girls. The average age of menarche in the developed world has dropped rapidly from age 17.5 years in the early part of the 20th century to 12.2 years for white and 11.5 years for black girls (Lauton & Freese, 1981).

Now, of course, apart from the risk of pregnancy, all sexually active adolescents face the risk of contracting serious sexually transmitted diseases, including HIV. You can assess the need for appropriate guidance or health care. Do answer any questions in a direct and factual way: "A new need for factual truth appears at the onset of puberty" (Winnicott, 1996, p. 138). Adolescents will not accept adult advice or education that does not take into account the reality of "desire and the pleasurable aspects of sex" (Offer et al., 1996, p. 283).

Despite declining teen birth rates, the United States has the highest adolescent pregnancy rate in the developed world. Each year, 1 million American girls—4 out of 10—become pregnant. Ninety-five percent of these pregnancies are unwanted; one third end in abortion.

Some of the risk factors associated with teen pregnancy are having an early-onset psychiatric disorder, early menarche, having a mother who gave birth as a teen, engaging in substance abuse, experiencing early sexual abuse, having low parental monitoring, and not being involved in religious activities (Bardone et al., 1998, Kessler et al., 1997). The majority of adolescent girls who become sexually active do not plan their first episode of sexual intercourse. In addition, there appears to be a connection between low self-esteem and lack of the assertiveness needed to say "no" or to insist on protection.

Adolescent girls who maintain the pregnancy are at risk for dropping out of school—about 60% do so—and facing years of poverty. And such a teenage mother puts her child at risk for developing both physical and mental health problems, as we have seen in Chapter 18. Programs that teach either abstinence or contraceptive methods have been only moderately successful; more helpful are programs that also include exploration of future ambitions and goal-setting. Zwingle (1998) put it this way: "Hope is the most important method of birth control" (p. 49).

All too often, however, pregnancy is seen solely as an adolescent girl's issue. Obviously, it takes two people to create a baby. In an alphabetical list of things that can be done to make our culture less socially toxic for children, Garbarino (1995) stated "Men must change" (p. 169). By this he meant that men must spend more time actively engaged with their children. This change has to begin before children are conceived: we all, young men included, must start thinking of fathers as equally responsible. A recent study of adolescents' strategies to promote sexual encounters found significant gender differences. Among boys, plans included far more coercive strategies, including pressuring, raping, lying, and using substances to get a partner intoxicated or high (Eyre, Read, & Millstein, 1997).

Teenage boys need counseling about sex that includes respect for oneself and others: caring for body, feelings, and spirit. Young men facing the birth of an unplanned child also need "culturally specific . . . guidance within the web of legal, family and personal issues surrounding teenage fatherhood" (Kiselica, 1995, p. 1). They may need help negotiating a complex relationship with the child's mother, and coping with feelings about their own father's role in their lives.

Sexual Orientation

There have always been homosexual teenagers—approximately 6% to 10% of any given population—who have lived for the most part with a deeply distressing secret, often in shame, confusion, and self-hatred. The existence of a significant cohort of adolescents who identify themselves as gay, lesbian, or bisexual is a relatively new phenomenon. It has been historically accepted that many adolescents pass through periods of attraction to same-gender individuals and often experiment sexually. This is still the case: same-gender play usually takes place between under-15-year-olds, more often between boys than girls. But the common wisdom was that they would all "outgrow" it or that only in adulthood was one's ultimate orientation fixed. Only since the late 1980s or so has the mean age of self-identification dropped from early adulthood to mid-adolescence (Boxer, 1988). In one study of 194 homosexual adolescents, the average age of self-awareness was 10 years; the average age of self-labeling, 14; and the average age of first disclosure to another, 16 (D'Augelli, Hershberger, & Pilkington, 1998).

Although social stigmatization lessened somewhat in the 1990s, gay young people still face many barriers to acceptance. These young people face ridicule, ostracism, verbal abuse, and physical assault and are at risk for running away and becoming homeless. Most worrisome, they are also at high risk for suicide: studies have found rates of about 40% of homosexual adolescents with a history of attempted suicide (D'Augelli et al., 1998; Procter & Groze, 1994). Of completed suicides, gay youth account for nearly one third (Yates, 1996). Teens who disclose to their own families may be rejected, berated, or even assaulted by parents and siblings (D'Augelli et al., 1998). The brutal murder of a gay college student in Wyoming in October 1998 illustrated the extent to which gay youth are victimized.

To work with troubled gay adolescents, a nurse must first be aware of his or her own biases. Familiarize yourself with the barriers that exist in schools and even in health care settings and with issues surrounding "coming out" (Fontaine & Hammond, 1996; Nelson, 1997; Radkowsky & Seigel, 1997). Conveying an attitude of respect and inclusion enables the work to begin. Lock and Kleis (1998) urged, "It is of paramount importance that we who work with children and adolescents assist in changing homophobic attitudes" (p. 672).

> **W**hat do you think? What is your attitude toward adolescent homosexuality?

➤ *Check Your Reading*
15. How does "cutting" often begin?
16. How many teen pregnancies occur yearly in the United States?
17. Name three risk factors for teen pregnancy.

DIETARY BEHAVIORS

Adolescents have notoriously poor eating habits: skipping meals, snacking, eating on the run, gorging on fast foods. Largely because of the high proportions of calories, protein, and calcium in the typical American child's diet, teenagers in the United States today are more likely to reach their genetic potential in terms of height and weight. However, few teens eat the recommended number of servings of fruit and vegetables, and most far exceed the recommended limits on saturated fats. A diet of high calorie, high fat, and highly refined and processed foods, combined with inactivity, can cause immediate health problems for adolescents by contributing to overweight. Beyond that, lifelong habits are established

which lead to diabetes, heart disease, cancer, and strokes.

Adolescent girls tend to be acutely sensitive to body image. With social pressure to be thin, most girls respond to the normal weight gains of puberty with distress. Girls learn early on to ignore normal cues of hunger and satiety, attending instead to self-perceptions of fatness or thinness. The majority of all adolescent girls go on a weight-reducing diet at some point. Black girls used to be less diet-prone, but this is rapidly changing. A recent population-based study of 17,159 adolescent girls found that "ethnic subculture does not appear to protect against the broader sociocultural factors that foster body dissatisfaction" (French et al., 1997, p. 320). For a minority of girls, ignoring bodily cues and dieting develop into full-blown eating disorders.

Eating Disorders

Although not classified as eating disorders, overweight and obesity are increasingly prevalent in children and adolescents. A combination of high carbohydrate snack foods and a decrease in energy expenditure put adolescents—girls in particular—at risk for unhealthy overweight. (Obesity and binge eating are discussed more fully in Chapter 30.)

The eating disorders most prevalent in adolescence are anorexia nervosa and bulimia nervosa (see Chapter 30 for DSM-IV diagnostic criteria). The diagnosis of anorexia nervosa is based on four major identifying features: (1) a refusal to maintain minimal weight normal for height and age; (2) an intense fear of becoming fat; (3) a distorted body image; and (4) in females, the absence of at least three consecutive, postmenarchal menstrual cycles. Extremely rare in boys and in prepubertal children, anorexia is primarily an illness of adolescent girls.

Recognized as a psychiatric disturbance more than 100 years ago, anorexia has been the subject of intensified interest since the 1960s. It is extremely difficult to treat and potentially fatal. With more public awareness and earlier recognition, however, more girls may receive treatment early, when they have the best chance for recovery. One reason for the difficulty of treatment is that girls affected by this illness generally do not wish to be "cured," that is, to gain weight. The further the illness progresses, the more deeply entrenched is their resistance (Levenkron, 1993). Anorexia is frequently seen comorbidly with depression, anxiety disorders, and characterological disorders, such as borderline and dependent personality disorders (Hoffman & Halmi, 1993).

Wachsmuth and Garfinkel (1993) reviewed four basic goals of treatment:

1. Establishing and maintaining an ongoing treatment alliance
2. Weight restoration and reversal of the associated physical signs and symptoms of starvation
3. Improvement in eating behavior
4. Improvement in social functioning

They also noted that a wide range of types of therapy has been recommended, including, either singly or combined, family therapy, individual psychotherapy, psychoanalysis, group therapy, and behavioral therapy. These recommendations have been based largely on clinical experience rather than on controlled outcome studies. One study by Russell and colleagues (cited in Wachsmuth & Garfinkel, 1993) compared the effectiveness of individual to family treatment on an outpatient basis. This study found that for adolescents under 18 years of age and for patients with illness lasting fewer than 3 years, family therapy was significantly more effective. Although most anorexic adolescents do improve or recover, the illness is associated with a significant mortality rate of between 2% (Hall, Slim, & Hawker, 1984) and 18% (Theander, 1985). When the child's weight loss is extreme enough to warrant hospitalization, treatment may include tube feedings and strict behavioral contracts based on daily weights, with increasing privileges and autonomy in response to continued weight gain.

Garrett (1997) made the argument that although much emphasis is placed on the origins of anorexia, little is known about the recovery process. She decried the absence of "positive outcome indicators" in the research literature—that is, what actually helps people give up their obsession with food and weight. Garrett believed that the patients' stories about what caused their anorexia, and about their process of recovery, are most important. She suggested the following measures (p. 270):

1. Making recovery stories available to recovering anorectics.

2. Encouraging the retelling and rewriting of personal narratives as stories of overcoming and transformation; *not into static perfection, but of continuing spiritual search* [emphasis added].

3. Encouraging physical practices that deepen bodily awareness.

4. Taking seriously the spiritual lives of clients.

Bulimia nervosa, defined as episodes of binge eating alternating with extreme weight loss measures (such as self-induced vomiting or use of laxatives), is seen most frequently in high school-aged and college-aged young women. The subjective experience is typically reported to involve a feeling of being out of control and of being anxious about bodily appearances. Although this disorder is often associated with anorexia, bulimic individuals may range in weight from thin to obese and may keep their bulimia secret for many years before seeking help (Wozniak & Herzog, 1993). Bulimia can lead to significant medical problems ranging from erosion of tooth enamel to serious, even fatal, electrolyte imbalances. A promising treatment approach combines an exploration of interpersonal dynamics and behavioral interventions.

OTHER ISSUES RELATED TO THE BODY

Physical Activity or Inactivity

Teenagers have the potential to be at the peak of their physical development and to establish patterns of healthy activity that will serve them well for life. Predictably, however, an adolescent's focus is on the here and now. Problems related to this area range from obsessive over-exercise to an alarming lack of physical activity. Adolescents involved in sports may be under tremendous pressure to gain or lose weight; young men may increase intake of unhealthy foods and may begin using steroids, as we have seen. Those adolescent girls who engage in highly competitive sports, especially those in which weight affects performance such as gymnastics are at high risk for eating disorders. Young women may develop *exercise bulimia,* a pattern of excessive exercise for the purpose of weight loss.

Inactivity is increasingly common, however. According to the CDC (1998), 75% of high school students do not attend physical education classes. This is especially sad because for those young people who do engage in sports in an unpressured, enjoyable way, athletic activities provide opportunities for socialization, protection from trouble, and a peer-acceptable reason to refuse drugs and alcohol, as well as fitness, self-confidence, and satisfaction.

Sleep

After puberty, adolescents appear to need more sleep, in particular stage 4, nonrapid eye movement sleep, which occurs in the first third of the sleep period (Anders, 1997). Unfortunately, this occurs just as the adolescent is establishing a pattern of staying up later and later. This, added to the fact that many high schools begin classes very early in the morning, can lead to significant sleep deficits. Teens typically sleep late on weekends and may also fall asleep at home in the afternoon, or even on their desks at school. If the sleep cycle gets sufficiently disturbed, the body clock resets itself and the adolescent may develop a *circadian rhythm sleep disorder,* defined by the DSM-IV as follows:

A persistent and or recurrent pattern of sleep disruption leading to excessive sleepiness or insomnia that is due to a mismatch between the sleep-wake schedule required by a person's environment and his or her circadian sleep-wake pattern. (p. 573)

Treatment is through promoting 8 hours of sleep each night, a difficult achievement. If the pattern is too distorted, the circadian rhythm can be reset by advancing the hour of sleep, as for jet lag. Interesting the adolescent in the biology of the problem may help.

Clothing

Early adolescents in particular tend to be extremely attentive to appearance. Remembering the self-consciousness of adolescent egotism, this is not surprising. To be sure of fitting in and being acceptable to one's peers, most young people create and follow clothing fads. The "uniform" of any given adolescent group makes a statement that serves at least two functions: to distinguish the teen as *distinct from* others (little kids, parents, noncool people) and to distinguish the teen as like others (slightly older adolescents, friends, idols). Styles may also be calculated to shock. Subgroups among adolescents are identifiable by a "look" that is often adopted by the larger culture, with or without the accompanying behaviors. Thus the "grunge" movement that began in Seattle ended up ultimately being associated with the discredited "heroin-chic" of top designers appealing to teens. Similarly, the beltless, baggy, stocking cap fashion that began among prison populations became ubiquitous. As older generations seeking to retain their youth copy the look of the young, adolescents move on to a new style, while Madison Avenue rushes to keep up.

Fad clothing items can be very expensive. Sports heroes promote athletic shoes that cost well over $100. A certain watch, a pair of boots or sunglasses, a shearling lamb coat—these things can come to seem like necessities to an adolescent with fragile self-esteem. This can put impoverished adolescents at a disadvantage, or serve as an incentive to get involved in criminal activities to obtain the coveted items. There have been incidents of people being robbed, even killed, for jackets and shoes. Likewise, in every youth gang there are symbols, colors, and clothing mannerisms that signal gang membership. Many high schools have prohibited the wearing of any of these; a growing number of schools are adopting uniforms as an answer to some of these problems. In most therapeutic communities for substance abuse treatment, rules prohibit wearing clothing items associated with the drug culture.

Hair

Similarly, adolescents have, for several generations, used hair as a means of expression and cultural identification. It is difficult now to imagine how dangerously provocative the simple gesture of growing one's hair long could be for a young man in the 1960s. At the turn of the millenium, it takes quite an unusual hair color and style to turn heads, even in small towns and rural areas. Hair can make a statement about one's racial or ethnic identification. It can serve as a social bond between friends who braid or style one another's hair. When a young person enters the military, the hair is shaved in part as a symbol of transformation and humility.

In general, adolescents as a group have successfully asserted their right to wear their hair as they please. In general, too, adolescents have adopted an attitude of acceptance and playfulness toward their own and others' hair, although some teenagers suffer great unhappiness due to dissatisfaction with its texture, thickness, curl, or lack of curl. Failure to shampoo and care for one's hair can be a sign of serious depression. An unexpected, drastic change in cut or style may be an indication of a degree of impulsivity that should be watched.

Piercings and Tattoos

It seems that every adolescent cohort has to take bodily expression one step further to disconcert the parental generation. In the 1990s, tattoos and body piercing became extremely popular among adolescents. But beyond their shock value, piercings and tattoos can be seen as part of the adolescent need to establish an identity. They echo worldwide tribal body painting and scarification rituals at puberty. The tattoos themselves may tell parts of the *personal fable*. Also, the pain caused by tattooing evokes an endorphin response reminiscent of that seen in cutting. This paradoxical high is known as *ink fever.*

You may be called on to mediate a conflict over body "ownership" between parent and child. It is difficult, perhaps impossible, to convince an adolescent that he or she may have a change of heart and regret a body-altering decision. But parents may need support to set age-appropriate limits, and adolescents need education about piercing or tattooing procedures they intend to undergo. Both can entail real risks of infection, ranging from mild bacterial inflammation to serious diseases like hepatitis and even HIV.

SPIRITUALITY

So the young person can search for another source of inner strength. His emerging individualness is a sign that there is a central core in him which is like a tap-root, and to explore this tap-root is a valid quest, for it is vital to him and part of him and not a prop from outside. (Sleigh, 1980, p. 28)

As we have seen, our society has "remarkably few rites of passage that mark the stages of life" (Prothrow-Stith & Weissman, 1991, p. 52). Adolescents hunger for this: for the means of self-transformation, for symbols of maturity, for validation of one's place on earth. But even beneath the absence of such rites, "spirituality is at an ebb in the more advanced technological societies" (Csikszentmihalyi, 1993, p. 238). Compare these two passages about the spiritual climate facing the young people of this century. The first, from a 1909 book by Brierly, might have been written yesterday rather than at the start of the 20th century:

Men having lost the peace which the life of the spirit brings are trying to fill themselves with substitutes. Civilization is a scene of enormous activities at its circumference, with a desolating emptiness at its centre. Our science is bankrupt of spiritual satisfaction. Its only revelation is of its powerlessness to help us. The foaming activities of society and fashion are emptier still. (p. 8)

The second, written in 1993, continues as if in the same breath:

While religions have lost much of their power, science and technology have not been able to generate convincing value systems to replace them . . . The United States, in the midst of unprecedented material affluence, is suffering from symptoms of increasing individual and societal entropy: rising rates of suicide, violent crime, sexually transmitted disease, unwanted pregnancy—not to mention a growing economic instability fueled by the irresponsibly selfish behavior of many politicians and businessmen. (Csikszentmihalyi, 1993, p. 238)

What then must we do?

Parents who are members of a church or temple can be encouraged to attend services regularly and to take their children with them. Eron (1980), in a series of studies of the persistence of aggression in children, looked for attributes that later kept aggressive children out of trouble with the law. He found that church-going was a significant protective factor. Nurses who belong to formal religions can have the courage to let their lives and work be seen as a manifestation of their faith. Praying *with* an adolescent who welcomes it can be a powerful healing experience. Praying silently *for* an adolescent who rejects it can guide one's helping efforts. Without forcing one's beliefs on an adolescent, it is possible to encourage the flowering of his own beliefs. Remembering the true meeting Sleigh (1980) spoke of, we can see that

Greatness of soul is called up in a person who meets an adolescent and allows himself to be met in return. The memory of a true meeting can last and sustain a person through many times of doubt and self-deprecation. In such dark times one can say to oneself, "I know there is one who regards me." (p. 16)

Especially with support, every teenager has the potential to become a valued member of a spiritual community, even a spiritual leader.

For those who have no religious faith, it is still essential to believe in the future and to pass this belief along to the next generation. Csikszentmihalyi (1993) argued that even the most rational scientist must have "faith in evolution" (p. 291), including consciously directed cultural and moral evolution. He believed that people, in the absence of traditional belief systems, can and should still aspire to having spiritual skills and wisdom. He proposed these four axioms to guide a "fellowship of the future" (p. 289):

1. You are part of everything around you: the air, the earth, and the sea; the past and the future.
2. You shall not deny your uniqueness.
3. You are responsible for your actions.
4. You shall be more than what you are.

What do you think? Do you feel you can be open about your religious beliefs or doubts and at the same time respect another's absolutely?

▶ *Check Your Reading*
18. Name three of the goals of treatment for anorexia.
19. What percentage of high school students does not attend physical education classes?
20. In what ways could clothing cause serious problems for an adolescent?
21. How might a nonreligious person promote spiritual values for an adolescent?

JOINING THE JOURNEY: THE THERAPEUTIC RELATIONSHIP

Once he has come to accept his inner space, the adolescent is ready for his next formative experience, that of "meet-

ing" . . . This can be a rare event in life: we seldom really meet one another . . . And yet, for the adolescent, to be met is so necessary if the feeling of selfhood is to be confirmed . . . Meeting is not an invading or possessing or in any way an intruding: it is positive and unconditional . . . It is a corresponding, a sensitive relating, that says, "I see you as you are. I accept what I see, and I also see behind it much that will become." (Sleigh, 1980, pp. 14–15)

Building a therapeutic relationship with an adolescent demands confidence and a strong sense of one's own identity, a sense of comfort with one's memories of the teenage years. Erikson (1968) referred to *fidelity* as a virtue of the adolescent ego—that is, taking a philosophical stand and keeping faith with oneself. This does not imply a rigid belief in ideologies, for the adolescent is still searching. But the adolescent is striving to identify a unique and continuous *self*, striving to discover the meaning in life. And a helping professional "must stand for something and make his or her stand known" (Rachman & Ceccoli, 1996, p. 158). The constraints of time in a managed-care environment offer an additional challenge. Yet, if we keep in mind Sleigh's (1980) concept of meeting, we know that the fundamental nature of the encounter can transcend its brief duration. "The moment of recognition may be for an instant, but this instant has eternity in it, and the young person is affirmed" (p. 15).

Transference and Countertransference

Some nurses find working with adolescents to be especially challenging because of the potential for stirring up unresolved issues from their own adolescence. It is essential to be a close observer of one's feelings and responses. A nurse may feel a pull toward wishing the adolescent to live out his or her old fantasies or ambitions. Other nurses, particularly nurses who are parents of teenage children themselves, find it hard not to over-identify defensively with the adolescent's parents.

Teenagers also project feelings onto a caregiver. In their search for identity, adolescents are especially susceptible to idealizing or devaluing important adults. They may reexperience strong dependency needs and fantasize that the nurse will become a parent figure. They may identify a primary nurse or therapist as being too much like a restrictive parent and rebel. Or they may attempt to persuade this person to regress, to ally with them in revolt against a restrictive parent. Just as in working with children, recognizing the feelings that are stirred up is essential, not only as a way of preventing harm to the relationship. These feelings will also tell you much about the adolescent's inner experience. If you pay attention, the adolescent can teach you, on a feeling level, what it is to be in his or her place.

NURSING PROCESS

Assessment and Diagnosis

In 1988, the CDC established a Division of Adolescent and School Health (DASH). Its mission is to identify and monitor health risks among adolescents and to establish and evaluate national risk-prevention programs. The CDC (1998) contended that most serious problems that affect the entire population of the United States stem from six types of behaviors that "usually are established during youth; persist into adulthood; are interrelated; and are preventable" (p. 1):

1. Behaviors resulting in intentional or unintentional injury
2. Alcohol and drug use
3. Sexual behaviors
4. Tobacco use
5. Dietary behaviors
6. Physical inactivity

In considering nursing assessments and diagnoses, we will keep in mind the fact the behaviors adolescents engage in, both negative and positive, are likely to have repercussions throughout a lifetime.

In a review of the issues of some of the special considerations of adolescent life, we have examined both dangers and opportunities, both risk and protective factors. Some of what gives adolescence its greatness are its opportunities for idealism, creativity, mastery, self-discovery, autonomy, and intimacy.

Care Planning, Treatment, and Evaluation

In Chapter 11 you learned a great deal about nursing diagnoses and care planning; you also had, in Betsy's case, examples of nursing diagnoses and care planning in a child's journey toward health. In work with an adolescent, whenever possible, you will want to mutually arrive at realistic, attainable goals, using the adolescent's own words in creating the plan. Evaluation parameters should be built right into the plan. It might take the form of a contract, especially if dangerous behaviors are involved, such as substance abuse, cutting, or suicidal gestures. A sample contract is shown in Box 19-1.

Individual Therapy

Conducting individual therapy with an adolescent has some of the qualities of parenting referred to earlier. Playfulness and creativity are still central, although the quality of therapeutic sessions will be different. For an early adolescent, play therapy may take the form of a structured game that becomes the underpinning of a conversation. It may involve creating something during

---

Box 19-1 ■ ■ ■ ■ ■
Stephen's Contract

The Things I Am Working on Are

Being honest
Respecting myself and others
Staying clean and sober
Being safe

The Rules in My House That Go for Everybody Are

No hitting or yelling
Do chores on time
Tell other people what your plans are
Kids get a vote but parents make the final decision

The Rules That Go for Me Are

Don't take without asking
Get homework done before going out
Be home by 10 unless I have permission to be out later
No phone calls after 11:00 PM

My Privileges Are

Allowance
TV in my room
Using the car with permission
Having friends over

My Responsibilities Are

Load and run dishwasher
Take trash out
Keep my room clean
One big chore every weekend

- I will keep my counseling appointments.
- I will go to group every week.
- I will tell my parents the truth.
- I will agree to be drug-tested once a month.
- I will not do unsafe things.
- I will check in with my dad if I am feeling unsafe or like using.
- Every Saturday, at our family meeting, we'll go over how I've been doing during the week.
- If I stick to the contract, I will get 20 points toward getting my own telephone (200 points).
- Every little rule I break I lose 5 points.
- If I break a big rule I get no points and get grounded for a week.
- Once I earn the phone, we'll meet to work on a new contract.
- If I start using again I know I will have to go back into treatment.

SNAPSHOT

Nursing Interventions Specific to Adolescent Crisis

What do you need to do to develop a relationship with an adolescent?

- Need to "meet" the adolescent—offer unconditional acceptance and positive attitude and gentle encouragement for what the adolescent can become
- A strong sense of self and one's own identity
- A sense of comfort with one's memories of teenage years
- Honesty
- Awareness of transference and countertransference issues
- Sense of humor
- Encourage patient to identify and discuss feelings

What do you need to assess regarding the patient's health status?

- Suicidal risk or self-destructive thoughts
- Affective responses, including anger, anxiety, apathy, bitterness, denial of feelings; guilt, despondency; irritability; helplessness, hopelessness (may be evaluated and quantified using a standardized depression inventory such as the Beck, the Zung or the Hamilton Depression Inventory)
- Participation in dangerous behaviors; e.g. self mutilation, drug use, violence, gang-related activities
- Status of relationships with family and friends
- Diet: healthy? adequate? presence of eating disorder?
- Sleep: quantity? Does the adolescent get enough rest?
- Sexuality: Is teen sexually active? Is teen knowledgeable about "safer sex" practices? Sexual orientation?
- Response to and compliance with medication regimen and reasons behind noncompliance; delayed effectiveness
- School performance and adjustment
- Community stressors; e.g. violence in neighborhood
- Spiritual issues

What do you need to teach the patient and the patient's caregiver?

- Medication issues, reason for taking, side effects and how to deal with them, untoward effects, warnings, importance of adhering to medication schedule
- Disease process, causes, course, and treatments
- Nutrition issues
- Emergency measures
- Need for physical activity, healthy diet
- Importance of both friends and family to healthy adolescent
- Maintaining safety
- Lifestyle and compliance issues such as benefits of exercise, stress management, safer sex practices
- Importance of talking about feelings
- Importance of achieving spiritual well-being

What skills will you want the patient and caregiver to demonstrate?

- Ability to enter into a No-Harm Contract and remain safe
- Ability to follow medication and treatment plan
- Ability to share thoughts and feelings
- Ability to identify and express feelings
- Coping skills
- Stress management skills; e.g., physical exercise
- Planning a healthy diet
- Appropriate limit setting

What other health professionals might need to be a part of this plan of care?

- Physician-psychiatrist and/or primary care physician who is usually in charge of the overall treatment plan, including medication management
- Social worker to assist with access to community supports, insurance issues, access to entitlements, connection with community-based treatments

---

a session and talking about how the experience relates to the adolescent's life. If a game is the focus of a session, one must pay careful attention to both the adolescent's and one's own response to a competitive situation. Even a structured game can become a vehicle for exploring dynamic issues in a displaced manner, as long the goal of the session is kept in sight (Beiser, 1979). For a middle or late adolescent, therapy will largely consist of talk, with its risk of intimacy, its humor, and the building of a shared vocabulary. Some therapists choose to work with adolescents outside the office: taking a walk, even engaging in an activity such as shooting baskets. In working with an adolescent, a therapist may at times be more self-disclosing, as long as it serves the patient's interest to do so, rather than the therapist's needs. One should also be attentive to authenticity—the use of the adolescent's full self.

Group Therapy

Group therapy is an extremely useful mode of treatment for adolescents. Many therapists find this age group too difficult to work with in a group context, but they miss a valuable opportunity. In all stages of life, people are social beings, and in no stage more so than in adolescence. As Kymissis (1996) put it, "In the group, the peer affiliation becomes the major developmental force" (p. 28). With the support of the therapeutic structure, group members "find out who they are, where they belong, and where they want to go."

Use of appropriate structure and technique is essential for the group experience to be a positive one for members and leaders alike. It is sensible to group adolescents roughly by age, early-to-middle, and middle-to-late, depending upon developmental issues at stake. Groups may be gender-segregated or mixed, depending on the intended focus of the group. Groups should not exceed 8 to 10 members and should always be headed by a pair of coleaders. Kraft (1996) listed attributes necessary to working with this population of young people: "flexibility, perceptiveness, activity, warmth, creativity, understanding, empathy, self-awareness, and responsiveness" (p. 8). Rules are established to provide a sense of safety, and leaders aim to keep anxiety at manageable levels, freeing adolescents to express themselves in an atmosphere of acceptance. In the words of Kymissis (1996), "Some of the goals of adolescent groups are to enable adolescents to develop skills to cope with anxiety and to find security in themselves" (p. 29). Group therapy is particularly useful for adolescents dealing with substance abuse, eating disorders, grief and loss, suicidality, divorce, and AIDS in a family member.

Facing the constraints of shortened treatment parameters, there is a special need for accuracy in assessments, for concision of diagnoses, for efficiency of planning, with integration of evaluative criteria. Most especially, there is a need for sufficiency in treatment.

That is, although treatment may be brief, it must provide as much help as is necessary to achieve positive change.

Use of Medication

Generally, the same principles cited in the previous chapter still apply here. The same medications are used for teens, as well as others more commonly used for adults (see Chapter 17). There are, however, some special considerations in prescribing medications for adolescent patients. One of these involves being clear in one's thinking about the difference between drug abuse and medication use, and clarifying this distinction for the adolescent.

Adolescents are often given responsibility for managing their own medication. This practice must be reviewed carefully on a case-by-case basis. One danger is the very real risk of overdose in a depressed or impulsive adolescent. Another is the common problem of noncompliance. Some adolescents, even those who willingly inhale, ingest, or inject illicit substances, are reluctant to take medication. Many teens voice a fear of being somehow changed. Just at the moment when they are trying so hard to find themselves, they shun the possibility of being modified in a way beyond their control.

> **What do you think?** How do you feel about working with teenagers?

▶ **Check Your Reading**

22. Why must a health care provider "stand for something"?
23. How can countertransference be useful?
24. In what ways might an adolescent's treatment plan look different from a traditional care plan?
25. Describe some features of an adolescent therapy group.

Conclusion

Adolescence is a dynamic time: a period of growth, change, risk, and opportunity. A nurse working with an adolescent has a chance to make a positive difference not simply to the life of a developing young person, but also to the long life of the adult person the teenager will become. To do this, the nurse needs to understand normal adolescent development. The nurse must be aware of the areas in which any given adolescent is at particular risk, and be developing ideas about how these might be turned to the adolescent's advantage. As Garbarino

(1995) put it, "Risk accumulates; opportunity ameliorates" (p. 151).

Further, the nurse has to be confident and secure, prepared truly to "meet" an adolescent and to accept him or her without judgment. Belief in the future, and in an adolescent's potential, can be the foundation of a very meaningful encounter. This is a point in the child's journey where a helping adult can offer invaluable support and guidance, lighting the way along a path toward health, joy, and fulfillment.

Key Points to Remember

- Adolescence has been broken down into three phases: early, middle, and late.

- Early adolescence corresponds to the beginning of puberty.

- Middle adolescence is marked by the well-known struggle for independence.
- Late adolescence is generally considered to end at the end of the 19th year; relative stability is generally attained in peer relationships, academic and leisure interests, and financial responsibility.
- Each adolescent is unique.
- The adolescent's journey has a profound impact on the family.
- School is a powerful sphere for the adolescent.
- School phobia is most prevalent in the early adolescent years.
- Truancy is correlated with poverty, poor academic achievement, and an increased rate of delinquent behavior.
- Friends are one of the major influences during adolescence.
- Community environment, racial, ethnic, and cultural influences can affect adolescents positively or negatively.
- Adolescence is a time of risks and opportunities.
- The risks of adolescence includes engaging in injurious behaviors such as suicidality, violence, drug use, and self-mutilation.
- Depression is a factor that influences the adolescent's engagement in risky behaviors.
- Sexuality is a major focus of the developing adolescent.

- Masturbation is a common behavior of adolescence.
- Pregnancy is risk for sexually active adolescents—4 out of 10 American adolescents become pregnant.
- Dietary behaviors are frequently a risk factor for adolescents, who many times have notorious eating habits.
- Eating disorders, including anorexia nervosa and bulimia nervosa, along with obesity, are increasingly more prevalent in children and adolescents.
- Inactivity is increasingly a problem with adolescents.
- Adolescents need more sleep but they establish a pattern of staying up late, leading to significant sleep deficits.
- Clothing and hair styles are very important as ways of establishing a unique identity for adolescents.
- Spirituality is part of the adolescent's journey, but they need support to become a member of spiritual community.
- The therapeutic relationship with an adolescent has similarities with parenting.
- Transference and countertransference are major issues confronting the nurse in a therapeutic relationship with an adolescent.
- Individual and group therapies are appropriate interventions for adolescents.
- Medication use carries with it special considerations regarding the adolescent's compliance with medication.

Critical Thinking Exercise

Johnny's mother is concerned about certain behaviors that she observes and calls the school nurse for advice. Lately, Johnny has been quiet and barely communicative; he spends a great deal of time in his room away from the family. Last week she received a call from school informing her that Johnny had been truant three times in the past 2 weeks. Johnny has never been a problem child and this is very different behavior from his norm.

1. Based on this limited information, what are some initial possible explanations for Johnny's behavior?

2. If you were the school nurse, what additional information would you want from Johnny's mother regarding family dynamics? Peers? Johnny's physical health?

3. What information would you want from Johnny?

4. Based on the additional information you collect, what nursing diagnoses are you trying to rule out?

5. What advice would you give Johnny's mother?

Additional Resources

References

American Psychiatric Association. (1994). *Diagnostic and statistical manual of mental disorders* (4th ed., rev.). Washington, DC: Author.

Anders, T. F. (1997). Sleep disorders: Infancy through adolescence. In J. M. Weiner (Ed.), *Textbook of child and adolescent psychiatry* (2nd ed.). Washington, DC: American Psychiatric Press.

Armstrong, M. L., & Gurke, B. (1997). Gang membership and student behavior: Nursing's involvement with prevention, intervention, and suppression. *Journal of School Nursing, 13*(2), 6-12.

Bardone, A. M., Moffitt, T. E., Caspi, A., Dickson, N., Stanton, W. R., & Silva, P. A. (1998). Adult physical health outcomes of adolescent girls with conduct disorder, depression, and anxiety. *Journal of the American Academy of Child and Adolescent Psychiatry, 37,* 594-601.

Beiser, H. R. (1979). Formal games in diagnosis and therapy. *Journal of the American Academy of Child Psychiatry, 18,* 480-491.

Berg, I. (1996). School avoidance, school phobia, and truancy. In M. Lewis (Ed.), *Child and adolescent psychiatry: A comprehensive textbook* (2nd ed.). Baltimore: Williams & Wilkins.

Blos, P. (1962). *On adolescence.* New York: Free Press.

Boxer, A. M. (1988, March 27). *Betwixt and between: Developmental discontinuities among gay and lesbian youth.* Paper presented at the meeting of the Society for Research on of Adolescence, Alexandria, VA.

Brierly, J. (1909). *Aspects of the spiritual.* New York: Whittaker.

Brooks, J. S., Whiteman, M., Cohen, P., Shapiro, J., Balka, E. (1995). Longitudinally predicting late adolescent and young adult drug use: Childhood and adolescent precursors. *Journal of the American Academy of Child and Adolescent Psychiatry, 34,* 1230-1238.

Cambor, R. L., & Millman, R. B. (1996). Alcohol and drug abuse in adolescents. In M. Lewis (Ed.), *Child and adolescent psychiatry: A comprehensive textbook* (2nd ed.). Baltimore: Williams & Wilkins.

Centers for Disease Control and Prevention. What is Dash? Web site. Available at: http://www.cdc.gov/nccdphp/dash/what.htm. Accessed June 18, 1999.

Chambers. W. J., Puig-Antich, J., Hirsch, M., Paez, P., Ambrosini, P. J., Tabrizi, M. A., & Davies, M. (1985). The assessment of affective disorders in children and adolescents by semistructured interview. *Archives of General Psychiatry, 42,* 696-702.

Comer, J. (1992). School consultation. In R. Michels, A. M. Cooper, S. B. Guze, & P. Wilner, *Psychiatry* (vol. 2). Philadelphia: J. B. Lippincott.

Comer, J. (1996). Improving psychoeducational outcomes for African-American Children. In M. Lewis (Ed.), *Child and adolescent psychiatry* (2nd ed.). Baltimore: Williams & Wilkins.

Csikszentmihalyi, M., Larson, R. (1984). *Being adolescent.* New York: Basic Books.

Csikszentmihalyi, M. (1993). *The evolving self.* New York: Harper Collins.

Czerwinski, S. J., & Moloney-Harmon, P. A. (1997). Caught in the crossfire. Children, guns, and trauma: An update. *Critical Care Nursing Clinics of North America, 9,* 201-210.

D'Augelli, A. R., Hershberger, S. L., & Pilkington, N. W. (1998). Lesbian, gay, and bisexual youth and their families: Disclosure of sexual orientation and its consequences. *American Journal of Orthopsychiatry, 68,* 361-371.

Eichelman, B. (1992). Aggressive behavior: From laboratory to clinic. *Archives of General Psychiatry, 49,* 488-492.

Elkind, D. (1967). Egocentrism in adolescence. *Child Development, 38,* 1025-1034.

Erikson, E. (1968). *Youth and crisis.* New York: W. W. Norton.

Eron, L. D. (1980). Prescription for reduction of aggression. *American Psychologist, 35,* 244-252.

Eyre, S. L., Read, N. W., & Millstein, S. G. (1997). Adolescent sexual strategies. *Journal of Adolescent Health, 20,* 286-293.

Finnegan, W. (1998). *Cold new world.* New York: Random House.

Fisher, H. E. (1992). *The anatomy of love: The natural history of monogamy, adultery and divorce.* New York: Norton.

Fontaine, J. H., & Hammond, N. L. (1996). Counseling issues with gay and lesbian adolescents. *Adolescence, 31,* 817-830.

Foote, J. (1997). Practice. Teenage suicide attempts. *Nursing Times, 93*(22), 46-48.

French, S.A., Story, M., Neumark-Sztainer, D., Downes, B., Resnick, M., & Blum, R. (1997). Ethnic differences in psychosocial and health behavioral correlates of dieting, purging and binge eating in a population-based sample of adolescent females. *International Journal of Eating Disorders, 22,* 315-322.

Garbarino, J. (1995). *Raising children in a socially toxic environment.* San Francisco: Jossey-Bass.

Garrett, C. (1997). Recovery from anorexia nervosa: A sociological perspective. *International Journal of Eating Disorders, 21,* 261-272.

Hall, A., Slim, E., & Hawker, F. (1984). Anorexia nervosa: Long term outcome in 50 female patients. *British Journal of Psychiatry, 145,* 407-413.

Hoffman, L., & Halmi, K. (1993). Comorbidity and course of anorexia nervosa. *Child and Adolescent Psychiatric Clinics of North America, 2,* 129-144.

Houston, M., & Weiner. J. M. (1997). Substance-related disorders. In J. M. Weiner (Ed.), *Textbook of child and adolescent psychiatry* (2nd ed.). Washington, DC: American Psychiatric Press.

Humphreys, J. (1987). *Rich in love.* New York: Viking Penguin.

Kessler, R. C., Berglund, P. A., Foster, C. L., Saunders, W. B., Stang, P. E., Walters, E. E. (1997). Social consequences of psychiatric disorders, II: Teenage parenthood. *American Journal of Psychiatry, 154,* 1405-1411.

Kiselica, M. S. (1995). *Multicultural counseling with teenage fathers: A practical guide.* Thousand Oaks, CA: Sage.

Kolbert, E. (1994, December 14). Television gets closer look as a factor in real violence. *The New York Times,* p. A1.

Kraft, I. A. (1996). History. In P. Kymissis & D. A. Halperin (Eds.), *Group therapy with children and adolescents.* Washington, DC: American Psychiatric Press.

Kymissis, P. (1996). Developmental approach to socialization and group formation. In P. Kymissis & D. A. Halperin (Eds.), *Group therapy with children and adolescents.* Washington, DC: American Psychiatric Press.

Lapsley, D. K. (1993). Toward an integrated theory of adolescent ego development: The "new look" at adolescent egocentrism. *American Journal of Orthopsychiatry, 63,* 562-571.

Lauton, B., & Freese, A. S. (1981). *The healthy adolescent: A parents' manual.* New York: Scribner's.

Levant, G. (1998). *Keeping kids drug free.* San Diego, CA: Laurel Glen.

Levenkron, S. (1993, April). *Addictions treatment with the eating disorders patient.* Presented at a meeting at Special Lecture Series, Greenwich Hospital, Greenwich, CT.

Levenkron, S. (1998) *Cutting: Understanding and overcoming self-mutilation.* New York: W. W. Norton.

Lindsay, G. B., & Rainey, J. (1997). Psychosocial and pharmacological explanations of nicotine's "gateway drug" function. *Journal of School Health, 67*(4), 123-126.

Lock, J., & Kleis, B. N. (1998). A primer on homophobia for the child and adolescent psychiatrist. *Journal of the American Academy of Child and Adolescent Psychiatry, 37,* 671-673.

McDermott, J. F. Jr. (1996). The effects of ethnicity on child and adolescent development. In M. Lewis (Ed.), *Child and adolescent psychiatry* (2nd ed.). Baltimore: Williams & Wilkins.

McKeown, R. E., Garrison, C. Z., Cuffe, S. P., Waller, J. L., Jackson K. L., & Addy, C. L. (1998). Incidence and predictors of suicidal behavior in a longitudinal sample of young adolescents. *Journal of the American Academy of Child and Adolescent Psychiatry, 37,* 612-619.

Mondragon, D. (1995). Clinical assessment of gang violence risk through history and physical exam. *Journal of Health Care for the Poor and Underserved, 6,* 209-216.

Neher, L. S., & Short, J. L. (1998). Risk and protective factors for children's substance use and antisocial behavior following parental divorce. *American Journal of Orthopsychiatry, 68,* 154-161.

Nelson, J. A. (1997). Gay, lesbian, and bisexual adolescents: Providing esteem-enhancing care to a battered population. *Nurse Practitioner: American Journal of Primary Health Care, 22*(2), 94, 99, 103.

Noshpitz, J. D. (1994). Self-destructiveness in adolescence: Psychotherapeutic issues. *American Journal of Psychotherapy, 48,* 347-362.

Nouwen, H. J. M. (1975). *Reaching out—The three movements of spiritual life.* New York: Doubleday.

Offer, D., Schonert-Reichl, K. A., & Boxer, A. M. (1996). Normal adolescent development: Empirical research findings. In M. Lewis (Ed.), *Child and adolescent psychiatry: A comprehensive textbook* (2nd ed.). Baltimore: Williams & Wilkins.

Pihl, R. O., & Peterson, J. B. (1993). Alcohol/drug use and aggressive behavior. In S. Hodgins (Ed.), *Mental disorders and crime.* Newbury Park, CA: Sage.

Procter, C. D., & Groze, V. K. (1994). Risk factors for suicide among gay, lesbian, and bisexual youths. *Social Work, 39,* 504–513.

Prothrow-Stith, D., & Weissman, M. (1991). *Deadly consequences: How violence is destroying our teenage population and a plan to begin solving the problem.* New York: HarperCollins.

Quay, H. C. (1993). The psychobiology of undersocialized aggressive conduct disorder: A theoretical perspective. *Development and Psychopathology, 5,* 165–180.

Rachmann, A. W., & Ceccoli, V. C. (1996). Analyst self-disclosure in adolescent groups. In P. Kymissis & D. A. Halperin (Eds.), *Group therapy with children and adolescents.* Washington, DC: American Psychiatric Press.

Radkowsky, M., & Siegel, L. J. (1997). The gay adolescent: Stressors, adaptations, and psychosocial interventions. *Clinical Psychology Review, 17,* 191–216.

Range, L. M., & Knott, E. C. (1997). Twenty suicide assessment instruments: Evaluation and recommendations. *Death Studies, 21,* 25–58.

Results of 1997 youth risk behavior survey (YRBS). 1 in 5 teen-agers is armed, a survey (1998, August 14). *The New York Times,* p. A19.

Rodriquez, L. J. (1994). Gangs are part of the solution. *The Utne Reader, 64,* 58–59.

Rubenstein, J. L., Halton, A., Kasten, L., Rubin, C., & Stechler, G. (1998). Suicidal behavior in adolescents: Stress and protection in different family contexts. *American Journal of Orthopsychiatry, 68,* 274–284.

Schwartz, R. H., & Wirtz, P. W. (1990). Potential substance abuse: Detection among adolescent patients. *Clinical Pediatrics, 29*(1), 38–43.

Sleigh, J. (1980). *Thirteen to nineteen: Growing free.* London: Floris Books.

Stowell, R. J. A., & Estroff, T. W. (1992). Psychiatric disorders in substance-abusing adolescent inpatients: A pilot study. *Journal of the American Academy of Child and Adolescent Psychiatry, 31,* 1036–1040.

Tanner, J. M. (1974). Sequence and tempo in the somatic changes in puberty. In M. M. Grumbach, G. D. Grave, & F. E. Meyer (Eds.), *Control of the onset of puberty.* New York: John Wiley.

Theander, S. (1985). Outcome and prognosis in anorexia nervosa and bulimia: Some results of previous investigations, compared with those of a Swedish long-term study. *Journal of Psychiatric Research, 19,* 493–508.

Thompson, P. (1998). Adolescents from families of divorce: Vulnerability to physiological and psychological disturbances. *Journal of Psychosocial Nursing and Mental Health Services, 36*(3), 34–41.

Tolleson, J. (1997). Death and transformation: The reparative power of violence in the lives of Black inner-city gang members. *Smith College Studies in Social Work, 67,* 415–431.

Valois, R. F., & McKeown, R. E. (1998). Frequency and correlates of fighting and carrying weapons among public school adolescents. *American Journal of Health Behavior, 22*(1), 8–17.

Venkatesh, S. A. (1997). The social organization of street gang activity in an urban ghetto. *American Journal of Sociology, 103*(1), 82–111.

Wachsmuth, J. R., & Garfinkel, P. E. (1993). The treatment of anorexia nervosa in young adolescents. *Child and Adolescent Psychiatric Clinics of North America, 2,* 145–160.

Winnicott, D. W. (1958). *Collected papers.* London: Tavistock.

Winnicott, D. W. (1971). *Playing and reality.* London: Tavistock.

Winnicott, D. W. (1996). *Thinking about children.* Reading, MA: Addison-Wesley.

Wozniak, J., & Herzog, D. B. (1993). The course and outcome of bulimia nervosa. *Child and Adolescent Psychiatric Clinics of North America, 2,* 109–128.

Yates, A. (1996). Childhood sexuality. In M. Lewis (Ed.), *Child and adolescent psychiatry: A comprehensive textbook* (2nd ed.). Baltimore: Williams & Wilkins.

Zwingle, E. (1998, October). Women and population: The millennium series. *National Geographic,* 36–55.

Recommended Readings

Brown, C. (1965). *Manchild in the promised land.* New York: Macmillan.

Frank, A. (1993). *The diary of a young girl.* New York: Bantam.

Prothrow-Stith, D., & Weissman, M. (1991). *Deadly consequences: How violence is destroying our teenage population and a plan to begin solving the problem.* New York: HarperCollins.

Sleigh, J. (1980). *Thirteen to nineteen: Growing free.* London: Floris Books.

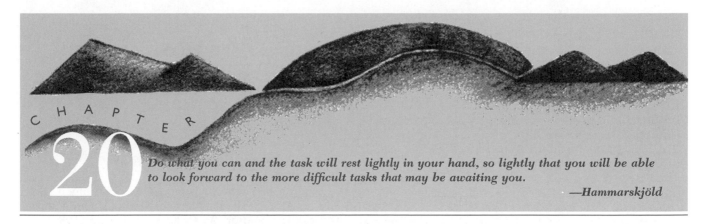

Do what you can and the task will rest lightly in your hand, so lightly that you will be able to look forward to the more difficult tasks that may be awaiting you.

—*Hammarskjöld*

The Adult

Learning Objectives

After studying this chapter, you should be able to:

1. Identify theories of adult development.
2. Describe developmental tasks in early and middle adulthood.
3. Describe mental health issues commonly faced by the traveler in early and middle adulthood.
4. Identify nursing interventions to promote mental health in the adult traveler.

Key Terminology

Adult	Dual-career families	Midlife crisis	Transitional period
Adult development	Horizontal stressors	Novice adulthood	Vertical stressors
Developmental eras	Menopause	Organismic	

Adulthood is the segment of the life journey that typically begins to unfold in the 20s (early adulthood) and extends through middle adulthood (age 35 to 55) and into late middle adulthood (age 55 to 64). The word **adult** derives from the Latin *adultus,* meaning to grow up. Adulthood is defined as being fully developed and mature. Another definition is a person who has reached a certain age (e.g., 21) as specified by law. What do we really mean, though, by *adulthood?* Is adulthood best described as a dynamic process or a stage of human development, or is it better characterized as a state distinguished by responsibility, love, and commitment? Is the experience of adulthood different for men and women and, if so, in what ways? What are the critical mental health issues particular to adulthood? What do nurses need to know to facilitate the human development and psychological well-being of adults in the 21st century?

Normal early and middle adult development may be a seamless narrative from the individual traveler's perspective, but the prologue actually begins in childhood. Before adulthood, a person's perspectives and identity evolve in relation to the groups to which a person belongs, all of which influence ideas, emotions, and behavior in different ways. The foundation for understanding the journey first rests with the past as the individual experienced it: parenting, life experiences, role models, education, articles or books read, movies seen, and so on. These factors have an intimate bearing on how the present is perceived and interpreted. The way people interact is a little different, even if they have been exposed to the same set of circumstances, because each person beholds reality differently. Reality is always shaped by the "I" of the beholder.

Adulthood offers each person a second chance to rewrite life's story. It provides an extended opportunity to shape a creative identity, this time with personal meanings reflective of personal choices. No matter how traumatic or disapproving childhood was, adulthood offers another possibility for personal fulfillment and satisfaction. Thus, the adult journey is distinctly and personally human, uniquely fitted to that person's travels, similar to but unlike any other.

In a sequential pattern experienced as a dynamic growth process, healthy adult travelers typically develop and refine their life stories, make necessary corrections, and embrace modes of behavior increasingly more consistent with their sense of self as a holistic being. For a significant number of adult travelers, the human meaning of the journey is compromised by serious physical or mental deficits or is cut short by death in early or middle adulthood. Consequently, exploring the possibilities for each day in the life of the adult is as important as considering developmental potential over the life span.

The story of early and middle adulthood is also about roles and relationships that can either support or contradict adult development, thereby enhancing or diminishing the skill of the traveler in negotiating the next step of the journey. Adulthood argues for responsibility, love, commitment, and balance as the defining characteristics of the journey to wholeness and maturity. In the final analysis, the quality of each adult traveler's journey is judged "by the content of their character" (King, 1963). Whether an individual is white or a person of color, rich or poor, handsome or ugly, too thin or too fat, educated or illiterate no longer matters. The manner in which each traveler has conducted the adult years is viewed as the only measure of success.

The Story of a Committed Young Man

A young man is adamant in His committed life. The one who was nearest Him relates how, on the last evening, He arose from supper, laid aside His garments, and washed the feet of His friends and disciples, an adamant young man, alone as He confronted His final destiny. . . .

He had assented to a possibility in His being, of which He had had His first inkling when He returned from the desert. If God required anything of Him, He would not fail. Only recently, He thought, had He begun to see more clearly, and to realize that the road to possibility might lead to the cross. He knew, though, that He had to follow it, still uncertain as to whether He was indeed the "One who shall bring it to pass," but certain that the answer could only be learned by following the road to the end. The end might be a death without significance as well as being the end of the road of possibility. . . . ■

From Hammerskjöld, D. (1964). *Markings* (L. Sjöberg & W. H. Auden, Trans.). (pp. 68–69). New York: Knopf.

BASIC ASSUMPTIONS ABOUT ADULTHOOD

Box 20-1 describes five basic assumptions about adult development.

First Assumption Discussion

Adulthood presents the opportunity for a much richer and longer experiential story, of which the individual is the primary author. As Costa and McCrae (1994) suggested, "personality cannot be grasped at a single cross section; it is necessary to see how it unfolds over a lifetime."

Second Assumption Discussion

Kelly and Rasey (1952) described the role of experience as follows:

Experience, then, is the process of undergoing the contact with the concrete, the working out of projected circumstances. It is built into structure, and man is made out of it. The organism is henceforth different, and if it were possible to repeat an experience, the outcomes would be different, since the repeated experience would really be encountered the second time by a different individual. (pp. 34–35)

The role of experience in shaping personal identity parallels the ideas of nursing theorists Rogers (1970) and Parse (1981). They asserted that it is impossible to experience the same phenomena in exactly the same

Box 20-1 ■ ■ ■ ■ ■
Five Basic Assumptions About Adulthood

1. The development in adulthood is much more complex than that of infant and child development.
2. Adulthood is a continuous, dynamic process of human development and adjustment, developed interactively through experience and education.
3. Adulthood cannot be measured by a steady, orderly progression through life.
4. Adult development is always contextually bound.
5. The experience of adulthood is different for women than it is for men.

Data from Costa & McCrae (1994); Gilligan (1982); Hayes (1994); Kelly & Rasey (1952); Lerner & Hood (1986); Parse (1981); and Rogers (1970).

way because of intervening life experience. Thus, motherhood can be repeated several times, but the experience of pregnancy and birth is slightly different with each child. Moreover, no two individuals ever experience the same phenomena in exactly the same way because each person brings different life expectancies and tools of experience to each situation. For example, the experience of giving birth is different for the first-time mother who gives birth in her 30s and one who gives birth at age 21.

Education influences human development by bringing new experiences and different ways of thinking. Education links culture, theory, and practical applications together and encourages the student to enter into dialogue about its meaning. Atchley (1991, p. 119) suggested that "the adult develops life principles—a philosophy of life—through an interaction between what is known, what is experienced, and his or her personality." Thus, for each person, the journey is a little different because the philosophy of life that directs it is uniquely tailored to the individual traveler.

Third Assumption Discussion

Adulthood can be described in general themes characterizing different developmental seasons. Although this information aids the nurse in helping patients understand their journeys and anticipate the next steps, adulthood is a living process, and each person embraces it differently (Lerner & Hood, 1986). **Adult development** is not about linear progression to an ideal state but about *being* an adult person. Tournier (1957, p. 230) noted that maturity is more than simply, "an accumulation of knowledge and experience, as if it were stones placed one upon another to form a monument." Adulthood therefore needs to be conceptualized as a condition of human *being*. "The flowering of the person is not a state at which we arrive, it is the movement that results from our incompleteness. . . . " Accordingly, "the concept of person belongs to the realm of quality, not quantity." The lived experience of adult development can be as passionate and varied as each person chooses to make it.

Fourth Assumption Discussion

To understand each adult's journey, you need to consider the landscape that enables and maintains its progression. An informative data assessment always contains information about the interplay between the human organism and the environment in normal circumstances. An effective treatment plan respects and actively incorporates the integration between the patient and current circumstances in his or her environment. Understanding a person's context helps ensure interventions that are personally meaningful because they acknowledge the patient's world as a significant part of the story. As Hayes (1994, p. 72) noted, "the client's history is not so much a record of one's life experience as it is a living representation of one's experience of life, of one *experiencing* life."

Fifth Assumption Discussion

There is growing recognition that the psychological make-ups of men and women may be as different as their physical differences, and these psychological differences may be complementary in developing a holistic, realistic knowledge of a situation. We have moved in the professional and popular literature from narrowed thinking that "anatomy is destiny," as Freud suggested, to equally fallacious reasoning that there are no real gender differences other than those that can be explained by social learning factors, to a conclusion that there are recognizable complementary differences that complete adulthood as a portrait of wholeness. Popular nonfiction presents differences in communication and psychosocial approaches to situations that appear to be gender-related. These books top the bestseller lists, finding avid readers trying to understand both themselves and their gender opposites.

There are two essential findings: (1) real differences are evident in the ways men and women seek and respond to their social world and (2) these differences need to be understood and appreciated as necessary to the larger purposes of our society. These realizations do not mean that only men have certain psychological characteristics or that women are the exclusive repository of others. The narrow attribution of characteristics as solely male or female is inaccurate. Also inappropriate is defining some traits as better or less effective and efficient in coping with life tasks. As both men and women recognize the value and uniqueness of each person, psychological differences begin to have the same potential for completion of wholeness as do physical differences.

THEORETICAL PERSPECTIVES ON ADULT DEVELOPMENT

In 1890, William James wrote that "[f]or most of us, by the age of thirty, the character has set like plaster, and will never soften again" (James, 1981, p. 126). Early psychologists, including Freud, asserted that personality characteristics were firmly established in early childhood and that modifying them in adult life was difficult, if not impossible. Few would disagree that an adult's response to life is deeply affected by innate temperament characteristics, position in family, and early childhood experiences. Each person establishes a continuity of self and personality, in which "changes can be incorporated into a whole that others still recognize as the same unique individual" (Atchley, 1991, p. 260).

In more recent times, developmental theorists such as Erikson (1978, 1980, 1982), Jung (1969), and Maslow (1969) argued that personality is *not* fixed in adulthood. They believed adulthood is a describable dynamic phase

Box 20–2 ■ ■ ■ ■ ■

Carl Jung's Theory of Adult Development

1. Personality development is a lifelong process with distinct changes occurring in midlife.
2. Young adults strive for mastery over the external world, experienced in work and relationships.
3. Societal dictates form the framework for development, with emphasis on competence in the work world and the development of ego-enhancing relationships.
4. Both men and women desire approval of others.
5. Men and women have complementary differences and similarities between them.
6. Advocated the broadening of social roles suggests that adult development limited to traditional gender roles can lead to one-sidedness in personality development.
7. Adults turn inward for sources of meaning in the second half of the life journey.
8. Adults at 35–40 undergo a transitional stage of development, characterized by emotional turmoil and individuals begin to question what they are doing.

Data from Jung, C. G. (1969). The stages of life. In H. Read, M. Fordham, & G. Adler (Eds.), *The collected works of C. G. Jung* (R. F. C. Hull, Trans.) (pp. 749–765). Princeton, NJ: Bollingen.

of human development in which men and women continue to develop psychologically into more complete human beings. Research into adult male development, for example, has characterized dynamic changes in middle-class men from young adulthood through middle age. Most significant changes are related to intimacy, career, and development of personal meaning (Levinson, Darrow, Klein, Levinson, & McKee, 1978; Vaillant, 1977).

Current theories of adult development are drawn from the work of Jung (1969), Erikson (1982), and Levinson and colleagues (1978). Their approach was **organismic** in that they believed that human development occurs as a natural qualitative maturation of personality. To a classic-stage theorist:

Each stage is a more differentiated, comprehensive, and integrated structure than is the one before it. Each succeeding stage represents the capacity to make sense of a greater variety of experiences in a more adequate way. (Hayes, 1994, p. 263)

Each sequential stage brings the potential for greater adaptation and differentiation, as adults qualitatively reorganize their lives psychologically and socially to meet current demands (Commons, Sinnott, Richards, & Armon, 1989). Common to classic-stage theories is the belief that young adults in their 20s are concerned with establishing themselves in a suitable occupation, selecting a life mate, and choosing a lifestyle with meaning. In

their 30s, these same adults focus on stabilizing their career choices and maximizing family commitments. Adults in their 40s are occupied with making contributions to society. In the 50s and early 60s, they reassess life's meaning, and many redirect their energies. Finally, in old age, adults look back on their lives with either pride or regret; the final ending is determined by all the events leading up to it. Although modern thinking challenges the idea that adult development is stage-related, stage theory continues to provide a relevant organizing framework that nurses can use with adult patients.

In describing Jung's midlife crisis, Staube (1981, p. 62) suggested that the "essence and goal of individuation became clear to him at midlife through his personal experience and his artistic elaboration of images that came to him from the depths of the creative psyche." The period of self-questioning can last over a significant time span—sometimes years.

Erik Erikson: Model of Personality Development

Erikson's (1980, 1982) seminal work on personality development (see Chapter 6) is particularly important in considering adulthood. He argued convincingly that all people, whether famous or unknown, continue to develop during their adult years in similar ways. Erikson (1958, 1969) based his accounts on the study of adult development observed in the life stories of successful adults across diverse cultures. He researched major historical figures such as Luther and Gandhi.

The cornerstone of Erikson's theory is identity. The first four stages of human development begin the process by arranging the building blocks of childhood to form the edifice of personal identity. The psychosocial crisis of identity versus identity diffusion reaches its ascendancy in late adolescence. The adolescent then prepares to assume the mantle of adulthood. As an adult, identity is first chosen in work and love and later expanded to include generative efforts for the benefit of the larger society. Erickson's extension of development through adulthood and old age established the field of life course development (Douvan, 1997).

Box 20-3 describes Erickson's partial model of personality development for three adult stages.

Box 20–3 ■ ■ ■ ■ ■

Erikson's Partial Model of Personality Development—Three Adult Stages

Young adulthood—Intimacy vs. isolation
Middle adulthood—Generativity vs. stagnation
Late adulthood/maturity—Ego integrity vs. despair

From ADULTHOOD by Erik H. Erikson, editor. Copyright © 1978, 1976 by the American Academy of Arts and Sciences. Reprinted by permission of W. W. Norton & Company, Inc.

For those who have successfully mastered psychosocial tasks during earlier phases of adult development, their identity is evident in their ego integrity. As mature adults reflect on the meaning of their lives, they achieve a wisdom that can only be acquired through fully lived experience. Although growing maturity brings with it an awareness of the finitude of life, fear of the unknown is significantly reduced when accompanied by feelings of a life well-lived with few regrets. This understanding makes it easier for a person to face the inevitability of death. A sense of despair emerges for those who feel they have not led a meaningful life and are unsure of their place in the greater scheme of life. Attention to making the early and middle adult years meaningful helps prevent despair in old age.

Daniel Levinson: A Theory of Adult Male Development

A theory of adult male development was described in the best-selling book, *The Seasons of a Man's Life,* published in 1978 by Levinson and colleagues. Their descriptions of milestones in adult development were based on a longitudinal series of interviews with 40 men who were between 35 and 45 years of age when first interviewed. The subjects represented a wide range in socioeconomic status, religious preference, and educational level. Five of the subjects were men of color. Adulthood, stated Levinson, is characterized by a series of negotiations between self and society. Figure 20–1 is a diagram of his theoretical model.

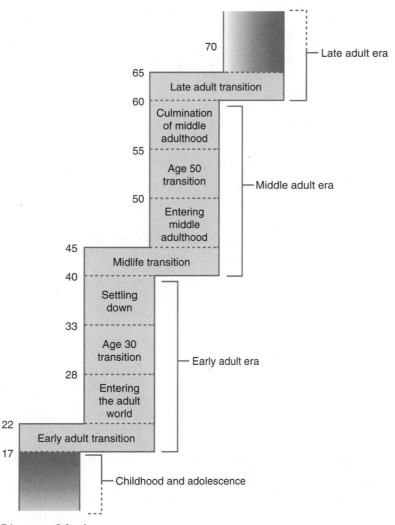

Figure 20–1
Levinson's theory of adult male development. (From *THE SEASONS OF A MAN'S LIFE* by Daniel J Levinson, et al. Copyright © 1978 by Daniel J Levinson. Reprinted by permission of Alfred A. Knopf Inc.)

Levinson and associates emphasized developmental life structures considered to represent the underlying pattern of each man's life. Their findings suggest a distinctive sequence in a man's life patterns. The pattern consists of "a series of alternating stable structure-building periods" (1978, p. 49), with intervening transition periods. During the life cycle, therefore, each man goes through long periods (eras) of relative stability in which developmental tasks are pursued within an existing life structure.

Levinson and colleagues (1978) referred to the sequential structure-building periods as **developmental eras.** Accordingly, he staged his theory of human development as four developmental eras ranging from birth to death: childhood and adolescence (0 through age 22), early adulthood (age 17 through 45), middle adulthood (age 40 through 65), and late adulthood (age 60 through 85). Each era spans approximately 20 to 25 years. Levinson and colleagues mention the first era—childhood and adolescence—and the last era—late adulthood—as phases of human development, but they are not explored in the depth he accords to early and middle adulthood.

Marking movement into each era of adult development is a **transitional period,** in which people question previous life structures, consider new possibilities, and make crucial new choices. The transitional periods overlap the era left behind and the next era, extending over a 5-year period. Transitions occur because the person no longer has confidence in the previous life structure and must consider new choices. Transitional periods typically are experienced as a personal crisis in which the past is integrated into the new future. Much of what has occurred before must be discarded or reworked in a new way. Each transition involves exit from past ideas about life; these ideas are not lost but are necessarily reworked for a new beginning. Entitled "Graceful Exit," an anonymous passage describes transition to the next life stage:

There's a trick to a graceful exit. It begins with the vision to recognize when a job, a life stage, a relationship is over—and to let go. It means leaving what's over without denying its validity in our lives. It involves a sense of future, a belief that every exit line is an entry, that we are moving on, rather than out.

The trick of changing well may be the trick of living well. It's hard to recognize that life isn't a holding pattern but a process. It's hard to learn that we don't leave the best parts of ourselves behind. We own what we learned back there. The experiences and the growth are grafted into our lives. And when we exit, we can take ourselves along— quite gracefully.

Although individuals differ in their precise movements through transitional stages created by biological, psychological, spiritual, and social circumstances, Levinson contended that his theory is applicable transculturally. The concept of transition is particularly useful in thinking about adulthood because it emphasizes the dynamic nature of life experience. Nurses can help healthy adults understand transitions as being uncomfortable but necessary steps in their adult journey.

Carol Gilligan: A Model of Women's Development

Gilligan (1982) proposed a model of women's development based on the notion that there are distinctive differences in the ways women physically, emotionally, and spiritually approach their adult years. Her work suggests that differences in the experience of adulthood are both individual and gender-related. Gilligan developed her theory in response to Kohlberg's research proposing that women display less moral maturity than men of the same age. Gilligan argued that the instrumentation used in Kohlberg's study put women at a disadvantage because it failed to account for values held by women in making their moral decisions.

Gilligan argued that women speak with a different voice, "a voice of 'care and connection' as opposed to the male voice of 'rights and justice,' and that this different moral voice arises out of a different sense of self" (Kitzinger, 1992, p. 241). Her model proposed that women's adult development occurs within the context of an embedded self. According to Gilligan, women strive to develop a sense of connectedness, whereas men struggle for autonomy. Self-realization for women comes from an involvement in meaningful relationships, that is, "networks . . . sustained by activities of caregiving and response" (Gilligan, 1982, p. 40). Although her work has been criticized for lack of empirical support, it has raised serious questions about adult development in women and has firmly established the validity of equal but different gender-linked approaches to major life events.

ADULT TRAVELER IN EARLY AND MIDDLE ADULTHOOD

Variation in Psychological Maturity

Physically, most people (except those with malnutrition or disease) have attained their full height by age 21 (Bogin, 1988). Legally, a person becomes an adult at age 18. Adulthood, as defined by age and physical maturity, generally occurs in a predictable and similar fashion whether the person is mentally healthy or mentally ill. People experience much variation, however, in their psychological maturity.

Normal adults of the same chronological age do not necessarily have comparable interests, nor are they working on similar developmental tasks. Life experience in adulthood is influenced by energy level, physical appearance, differences in health, self-management, and other social or organic factors that affect maturity. Unexpected twists to a life pattern and personal crises also affect the experience of adulthood. These factors help account for the wide range of interests, developmental tasks, and adjustment patterns found in adults. They are critical elements in the way individual adults perceive themselves, develop, and implement their life goals.

The call to assume the mantle of adulthood is one that people respond to differently for a variety of reasons. Some people never assume adult roles because of serious physical or emotional deficits, such as autism, active psychosis, head trauma, or profound mental retardation. Others discard adult roles as too confining and instead live their adult lives with the variations of personality disorders. This choice is often outside of insight and awareness. Still others assume adulthood with a vengeance that stifles creativity and precludes giving time to the child that lives within. This narrowed, distorted adulthood takes the form of neurosis. Biological and social factors impede or facilitate a person's experience of the journey in adulthood.

What do you think? As you look at the adults in your life, what makes a "good adult"? Where do you stand in your analysis of a "good adult"?

Adult Travelers in Their 20s: Novice Adulthood

A healthy transition from adolescence into adulthood is marked by excitement, confusion, and fear by most emerging young adults. They enter adulthood with a strong dose of idealistic thinking, filled with hope and dreams for the future, determined to make a difference. In early adulthood, life beckons with the promise of unlimited possibilities, and as Sheehey (1976, p. 85) noted, "the tasks of this period are as enormous as they are exhilarating."

Levinson wrote of the early to mid-20s as **novice adulthood.** Age 17 to 22 is considered a transitional period. Extending from 22 to 33 years of age, the novice faces four developmental tasks as represented in Box 20–4.

Levinson believed that those who are most successful in their careers have benefitted from a mentor relationship with a more experienced adult willing to share knowledge and to be a guide through the difficult paths of career and life. A number of studies have found that both men and women profit in their job advancement and satisfaction from mentor relationships (Burke & McKeen, 1990; Noe, 1988).

Society judges maturity by the individual's ability to assume adult roles. In the 20s, adult maturity is associated with the ability to establish financial and emotional independence from the family of origin. Using an element of choice, typically young adults choose to leave their family home, become self-supporting, choose a mate, and begin a meaningful career, although each person's journey continues to reflect rituals, beliefs, and values that symbolize that individual's role within the family and community. Adults in their 20s are intensely involved in and focused on their careers, or if they have not yet selected one, they are confused about which way to turn. As they progress through their 20s, decision making about the choice of a life's work becomes clearer. By age 30, most young adults have established their life's work. Delayed marriages and decisions to have no children or to delay having them become critical issues. Comparing their lives to those of others in the same age bracket is significant to adults in their 20s. Consequently, social norms and expectations become measures of success for young adults.

What do you think? As you look at yourself, how did you navigate or are you navigating your 20s?

Box 20–4 ■ ■ ■ ■ ■
Levinson's Developmental Tasks of the Novice Adult

1. Constructing an occupation
2. Gaining a marriage and family
3. Procuring a mentor relationship
4. Developing a dream that generates excitement and vitality such that career identity is personally meaningful and satisfying

From THE SEASONS OF A MAN'S LIFE by Daniel J Levinson, et al. Copyright © 1978 by Daniel J Levinson. Reprinted by permission of Alfred A Knopf Inc.

■ C A S E   E X A M P L E   2 0 – 1
■ Ashley's Story

Ashley Bennett is 24 years old. She graduated from college 2 years ago with a degree in interior design. Although her mother would have preferred that she stay in the area, Ashley was determined to start a life of her own. She selected Atlanta because it was a "young people's town," and the weather appealed to her. So she set out to seek her fortune.

Ashley found a job with a small interior design firm and began working as a design assistant. The pay was minimal, and like most young adults, Ashley found a gap between her current salary and what she would like to be earning. Nevertheless, she liked what she was doing, so she learned to budget her money and scaled her needs down to match her pocketbook. It was lonely away from home and school at first, with several crises of confidence. Ashley, however, was determined to make it on her own. Deciding to buy her first car was scary, but Ashley decided to go ahead anyway. She had to work at a second job to make her car payments and still feel comfortable financially, but it was worth it to her because she felt safe in her new car. She moved into a smaller apartment with two other roommates and took great pride in decorating it just as she wanted it. By the end of the 1st year, Ashley had successfully negotiated the transition from home and school to her own personally chosen living environment, from the security of family to an inner security based on her own accomplishments. ■

Case Example 20-1 illustrates the decision making common to young adults. In making the transition from adolescence to adulthood, Ashley learned many valuable lessons about money, friends, and negotiating her life circumstances. Has it been worth it? Yes. Can she expect to negotiate or relate to the future solely with what she has learned in her 1st year as an independent adult? No. But she is off to an excellent start in taking responsibility for her own actions and building a life that has meaning to her.

Adult Travelers in Their 30s: The Blending of Dreams Versus Reality

During their 30s, men and women further refine their life structures in ways that mature and stabilize their lives. Levinson and colleagues (1978) suggested that blending the lofty aspirations of the 20s with purposeful goals based in reality is the task of the 30s. Adults must become aware that a fruitful life requires concerted care and effort. Consequently, developmental efforts in the 30s are characterized by finding career and role relationships that are life-affirming, morally worthwhile, and personally satisfying. People learn that they can influence the world in their own way by what they choose to do and how they do it. In contrast with those in their 20s, adults in their 30s are ready to expand their energies in ways that allow them to change and grow as responsible adults. They want to make a difference by extending their talents to others. As Case Example 20-2 shows, finding a congenial social group often becomes the means to achieving adult social and civic responsibility in the community.

■ C A S E E X A M P L E 2 0 – 2
■ **Marian and Dave's Story**
■
■ Marian and Dave are in their early 30s. They have been married for 6 years and are expecting their first child. For the first few years of their marriage, they rented an apartment, but they recently moved into their first home. Both work full-time. They have recently joined a church and make genuine efforts to meet their neighbors because they want to become an active part of the community in which they hope to raise their child. Expenditures are now more carefully planned, more likely spent for the home or the birth of the baby rather than on spontaneous activities. Although work commitments remain important, Marian is considering changing jobs, working for a company closer to home. Dave clearly has deepened his professional commitment to his firm and works long hours not only for the paycheck but also for the satisfaction his work brings. Both Marian and Dave are aware that they have to make quality time for themselves a priority if they want their marriage commitment to continue to grow and develop. ■

A New Combination of Life Goals: Developing Comfort With Imperfections

Caring associated with generativity allows people to experience more humanized values and deeper interests in community with others. Although relationships remain significant, they become more reality-based. Important changes include a decreasing emphasis on appearances and developing comfort with imperfections, as this woman reveals:

The biggest difference for me is that I don't take myself so seriously. The other day I had some friends over for lunch. Just before they were set to arrive, I took a homemade quiche out of the oven, and it slipped out of my hands onto the floor. My beautiful quiche was completely destroyed. Had I been in my 20s, I would have thrown it out, gone quickly to the store to buy something else, or cried and taken my friends out to lunch. Instead I scooped the quiche back into the pan, served it with the explanation of what happened and we all had a good laugh. I realized they had come to see me, and that was the most important thing. I didn't have to be as perfect as I felt I needed to be in my 20s, and that is such a relief. (Arnold, 1994)

Toward the end of the 30s, Vaillant (1977) suggested, a phase of career consolidation between intimacy and generativity takes place. People seriously and methodically begin to examine life commitments and to evaluate their worth. Levinson's (1978) study reported similar findings. This transitional period sets the stage for a midlife crisis, which has typically affected men in their 40s. (Changes in work in the 21st century, however, may make the 30s a time of change rather than consolidation.)

Midlife Crisis: Questioning the Meaning of One's Life

The pace and rhythm of adulthood change dramatically with the midlife crisis, a transitional period beginning anywhere from age 35 to 50 (Kotre & Hall, 1990). Often, midlife is associated with changes and losses including declining health status, retirement, caregiving for aging parents, and unexpected responsibility for adult children and grandchildren (Samuels, 1997). Aging adults who have engaged in early-adulthood multiple roles will have a better chance at resolving midlife crises with a sense of well-being because of their practiced adaptability (Vandewater, Ostrove, & Steward, 1997).

A **midlife crisis** is an internal questioning of the meaning of one's life thus far—a turning point. Most people find that excessive reliance on the opinions of others gives way to a deeper understanding of what has true inner meaning for the person. The desired outcome of a midlife crisis is a realigning of attitudes and behaviors needed to complete the life cycle in a meaningful way.

Midlife crisis is forced on people by physical, social, and psychological factors needing attention in midlife. Initially, the crisis can be experienced as loss (Kalish, 1989). In midlife, body contours change; facial appearance and hair color sometimes show marked differences; and energy levels shift. Physical changes occur graphically in midlife, signaling for many the passage of years in ways not easily avoided. Although a gradual decline in physical capacity occurs in midlife, most people can do many of the activities they performed in earlier life but at a slower pace. Most important for reframing the midlife experience is a strong correlation among physical well-being, full engagement with life, and mental health. Nurses can help patients cope with the stress, anxiety, and depression often associated with this transitional period of life (Samuels, 1997).

RELATIONSHIPS

Psychological concerns in midlife typically focus on professional or personal relationships (or both) and on self-definition. Critical reevaluations of professional and personal relationships and their relevance for future growth can be quite unsettling, as this traveler in midlife reveals:

I experienced a significant change in thinking about myself, signaled first by a period of intense disequilibrium about the meaning of my life. I noticed with some shock that things of importance and concern to me for many years, for example, meeting the expectations of others, status, and recognition, were no longer critical issues, but I had nothing to take its place. (Arnold, 1994)

Divorce and remarriage are common outcomes of midlife evaluations. These changes may represent a creative life solution for those in long-term relationships that clearly have been destructive. For those whose personal needs transcend their long-term commitments, however, the outcome is clothed in irresponsibility and self-absorption. These people make choices for the wrong reason, as a way of retaining declining youth. The transitional midlife crisis, for some men and to a lesser extent, for some women, can include turning to another person as the source of intimacy. Such a turning provides the middle-aged adult with feelings of renewed youthful vigor and freedom from thoughts of aging (Staube, 1981). The financial havoc and emotional carnage of such decisions, however, can be serious costs for families and adult children. For many middle-aged adults who choose divorce, any self-absorbed peace is marred by ongoing problems.

Nurses can help patients sort out the meanings of relationships and can coach patients in reworking relationships that have become stale or unworkable. Therapeutic strategies can enhance the ability to reflect on life with responsibility and compassion. Adults often need help in mastering the difficult ordering of relationships and their meaning for the second half of life.

What do you think? Think of someone you know who has been through a divorce. What impact did this have on the person? On his or her family?

OPPORTUNITY FOR SELF-DEFINITION THROUGH MIDLIFE CRISIS

Many travelers speak of the midlife crisis as a rebirth—a freedom to be and to cherish—and a turning point of great significance in their life journey. Painful choices and inevitable shifts in self-concept form the foundation in the midlife journey toward wholeness. As Jung suggests, the journey necessarily entails an integration of all parts of self—inner strivings and outer accomplishments. It also is a time, however, when care of the human spirit becomes an important, exhilarating task (Lane, 1987). In Case Example 20-3, a woman speaks of her personal midlife crisis as a pivotal point in her journey. The crisis allowed her to make choices that were painful but significant to the completion of her life journey.

■ CASE EXAMPLE 20-3
■ Patricia's Story

Patricia grew up in a small town and became a nun in her late teens. For more than 19 years, she lived the vowed religious life. Always a positive person, Patricia accepted that her life was unfolding as it should until her mother became gravely ill, and Patricia as her only child received permission to care for her at home. She viewed this time as a period of reflection in which she experienced a profound midlife crisis, brought to the forefront of her mind by her current crisis. The role reversal of parent care and an awareness that something was missing from her life led her to question what was truly important to her. Patricia made the decision to leave the religious life, the wisdom of which she felt was reaffirmed in many ways during the ensuing years. She described the changes she experienced during her midlife crisis as shifting from doing what others expected to a realization that she had choices in life, that she was in charge of her own destiny. In the process of developing a lifestyle based on choice rather than expectation, Patricia experienced a new peacefulness, a "freedom to be," which she characterized as being able to enjoy herself and her life in fresh ways that brought renewal and exhilaration to her human existence. Patricia's crisis of meaning in her 40s contained many of the characteristics common to a midlife crisis:

- A life stressor (her mother's illness) requiring a different set of coping strategies
- Awareness of significant physical changes in herself and in her mother
- Realization of life's finiteness and that if changes are to occur, they must occur now
- A quest for meaning that arises as a powerful inner force in midlife ■

Adult Travelers in Their 40s: Discovering the Important Things in Life

Healthy adults in their 40s are much more complex human beings than they were in their 20s. They have gone forward and established careers and families, developed ideas about what is important to them, and contributed to their communities in meaningful ways. Life continues to change for travelers in their 40s, however, and adults find it necessary to break with the past, to test and experiment with new lifestyles, to explore new modes of creativity and generativity, and to rediscover what is meaningful in life.

Generational Responsibilities: Balancing Caregiver Roles With Reevaluation of the Direction of Later Life

Because both men and women are living longer, adults in their 40s may be caregivers for elderly parents and simultaneously be parents of late adolescent or adult children. As their adult children extend their education, parents often provide financial assistance for a much longer period than previously was the case (Kingson, Hirshorn, & Cornman, 1986). These demands create additional stress on adults already beginning to contemplate diminished income in their declining years. Adults in their 40s are more realistic and more sensitive to potential physical vulnerability in themselves (Buhler & Goldenberg, 1968; Gould, 1975). They pay more attention to their health.

In their 40s, healthy adults streamline their assets both figuratively and objectively (Thurnher, 1983). Although the process of consolidation takes place toward the end of the 30s, it reaches ascendancy in the early to mid-40s. Career reevaluation and significant career changes are common in the 40s, as individuals discover that their sense of self is in conflict with their chosen career. Even if the career has significant meaning, men and women at midlife generally are at the peak of their careers—and they know it. Moreover, current economic uncertainties have intensified the sense of midlife crisis for many, as middle management and senior-level workers in their 40s and 50s are often first cut in the downsizing of many companies and government jobs.

Typically, the impetus to develop a meaningful path to fulfillment and to plan the direction of later life takes on greater energy. At the same time, the midlife adult senses the need to balance commitments, to go with the flow of life.

Menopause: A Natural Life Process in the 40s and 50s

Menopause typically occurs as a natural life process during the 40s or 50s, presenting the female traveler with significant hormonal symptoms and cessation of menses. Menopause definitively marks the end of the reproductive years, and hormonal fluctuations associated with menopause frequently create mood changes that require psychiatric intervention (Mercer, Nichols, & Doyle, 1989). Strategies that reframe menopause as a natural process, occurring as an unavoidable interval in the story of adult women, but one that need not become a defining characteristic, are important nursing interventions. Especially useful is psychoeducation regarding the benefits and risks of hormonal therapy, anticipatory guidance about what to expect, and creative ways to negotiate life in the postmenopausal years.

A deliberate reframing of a natural physical process is particularly important because many research studies of perimenopausal and postmenopausal women speak of this time in a woman's life as one of physical loss and depletion, to be corrected with estrogen therapy. Psychological issues raised in research include perceived diminished sexual attractiveness and functioning. Absent are studies related to postmenopause as a time of positive transition, with potential for greater self-awareness, personal growth, and fulfillment, yet many women experience their postmenopausal years as positive. Once again, the popular literature takes the lead in addressing women's adult development (Sheehey, 1993), much as Levinson's work did for men in the 1970s.

Adult Travelers in Their 50s: Growth and Renewed Vitality

Referred to as *late middle adulthood,* the 50s typically offer a window of opportunity to integrate much of what has gone before into a fuller life story, and many unimportant details are discarded as irrelevant. Sheehey (1981) captured the essence of development in the second half of life with a quote from Schopenhauer:

The first 40 years of life furnish the text, while the remaining 30 supply the commentary; without the commentary we are unable to understand aright the true sense and coherence of the text, together with the moral it contains. (p. 289)

The renewed research interest in the period between 50 and 65 is partly a result of a dearth of information about this segment of adult development. Most studies of women in late midlife address this decade solely in relation to menopause or skip to the broader category of the older woman, as if this term equally described the psychological concerns of women in their 50s and women in their 70s. Studies of men in their 50s simply are not available. Part of the reason for fewer life scripts that cast men and women in their 50s in roles of renewal is that in the early part of this century, men and women reaching this age were considered old. Most could expect fewer than 19 more years of life, typically spent in retirement and ill health. Midlife men and women today can expect another 30 to 40 years during which the old rules about later adulthood no longer apply.

Healthy adults in their 50s are able to let go of the need to control what is happening and are better able to go with the flow of life as it presents itself. Relationships with significant others have the potential for deepening, partially because people have more time and maturity to devote to their nurturance. Adults in their 50s have the health and energy to devote to the relationships that are important to them. At the same time, adults in their 50s are more aware of time limitations in which to live a healthy and active lifestyle. They now recognize the need to use time well and that whatever they wish to do with the rest of their lives needs to be done now (Arnold, 1994). As health becomes more of an issue in the 50s, Fiske and Chiriboga (1990) noted

Health problems are not only major stressors in and of themselves, but they tend to precipitate a chain of secondary stressors. The onset of a serious health problem, especially during the later years, leaves a characteristic

signature: the loss of a sense of personal security, a heightened sense of vulnerability, acceleration of the psychological processes of aging. (p. 284)

Nurses need to consider the 50s an important segment in the life journey. During this time, a person's life story can be enhanced by helping the older midlife adult get in touch with the creative aspects of later life. It is becoming more and more the norm that late middle life offers adults an opportunity to become reenergized, moved by a clear sense of direction, and empowered by their maturity to engage with life in a new and innovative manner.

What do you think? Where are you in your life's journey? If you were to write your own story, what would the theme be?

➤ *Check Your Reading*
1. How would you describe the differences between adults in their 20s and those in their 50s?
2. What is meant by *midlife crisis,* and what factors influence its development?
3. What are the developmental tasks of the novice adult?

MENTAL HEALTH ISSUES IN NORMAL ADULTHOOD

In thinking about mental health issues facing the traveler in early and middle adulthood, first review the characteristics associated with emotional maturity (Box 20–5). No one is perfect and, consequently, people strive for but do not fully attain healthy maturity in all areas of

Box 20–5 ■ ■ ■ ■ ■
Suggested Measures of Maturity

1. Openness to being personally challenged
2. Dedication to the truth (reality principle)
3. Having multiple perspectives (being able to see that it is possible to look at a situation from several different and equally valid viewpoints)
4. Willingness to take responsibility for one's own actions
5. Being able to let go of impossible expectations and situations
6. Equal comfort in the company of others and in solitude
7. Capacity to establish loving but not binding bonds with others
8. Ability to make and keep commitments
9. Capacity to delay gratification for a greater good
10. Ability to admit when one is wrong and to make amends

their lives. Perhaps this is why people typically write their memoirs in their later years.

Self-Actualization: Realizing the Possibilities Life Has to Offer

Maslow (1969) and other humanist psychologists point to self-actualization as a natural force in normal personality development (see Chapter 6). Mastery of developmental tasks required for self-actualization in adulthood is contingent on the sense of being needed, meaningful interaction with peers, and increasing skill in handling complex problems and decisions about difficult life issues. For the traveler, self-actualization brings an ever-present sense of freshness and excitement about possibilities. The adult develops an experiential awareness and delight that life makes a difference. Knowledge that one's efforts have meaning and are the best one can offer fosters serenity and satisfaction. Life remains full of possibility for the self-actualizing adult, but it is coupled with the realization that one must go with the flow and rhythms of the journey, accepting and working with all that life presents. Self-actualized travelers are able to make significant contributions to the community, simply through their presence. Reed (1994, p. 64) referred to this self-transcendence as "a characteristic of developmental maturity whereby there is an expansion of self-boundaries and an orientation toward broadened life perspectives and purposes."

Vertical and Horizontal Stressors

Personal growth does not take place in a vacuum, and adult development closely interacts with a person's environmental context (Mercer et al., 1989). Vertical and horizontal stressors (Figure 20–2) are directly related to mental health issues in early and middle adulthood. They can prime the development of mental symptoms or lay the groundwork for personal growth.

Vertical stressors are carried from generation to generation in the form of beliefs, values, and modes of conduct. Inherent in one's culture, social community, and family background, vertical stressors contribute to or raise questions about each individual's unique experience of adulthood. For example, the type of social support a person received as a child can later influence the adult's ability to use social support effectively in adult relationships. Box 20-6 describes three adult modes of maladaptive support-seeking patterns of behavior stemming from inappropriate parenting.

Horizontal stressors occur as normative, expected, or unexpected life events. Neugarten (1977) proposed that life events serve as symbols of transitions during the course of each person's life trajectory. Normative life events typically occur more gradually than situational stressors, which are abrupt changes in the conduct of a person's life. Typical horizontal stressors during early adulthood can include starting a job, getting married, and having a first child. Later in life, these stressors can

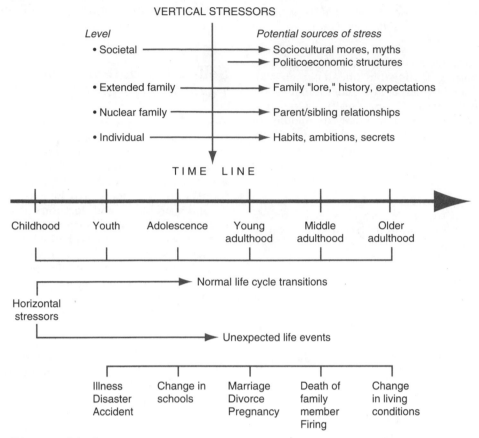

Figure 20–2
Vertical and horizontal stressors directly related to mental health in early and middle adulthood. (From Arnold, E., & Boggs, K. [1995]. *Interpersonal relationships: Communication skills for nurses* [2nd ed.]. Philadelphia: W. B. Saunders.)

include a last child leaving home, retirement, or birth of the first grandchild. The stressor can be pleasant or unpleasant, desired or undesired. Illness is an unexpected stressor that dramatically serves as a turning point in many adult journeys, as Case Example 20–4 illustrates.

■ **CASE EXAMPLE 20–4**
■ **Edward's Story**

Edward, a vigorous athlete and active man who swore he would never work behind a desk, was injured in an accident that left him completely paralyzed from the neck down. As he was being taken into the emergency room (15 years ago), he reported, "I felt as if God were speaking to me: 'You take control of the physical circumstances, I'll cover everything else.' I had a special feeling of warmth and security in my body." His fast-paced, perfectionistic life was suddenly changed. One week after the accident, he had an experience "that was like starting my life all over, being born again. I had to throw out everything I knew before starting all over again from scratch." Among the major changes he reported were a more compassionate and trusting sense of others, an appreciation of beauty

in the world, and "a deeper more enhanced dependence on God in controlling things we don't understand." ■

From Miller, W. & C'deBaca, J. (1994). *Quantum change: Toward a psychology of transformation*. In T. Heatherton & J. Weinberger (Eds.), *Can personality change?* (p. 269). Washington, DC: American Psychological Association.

Here a young adult chose to cope with his unfortunate circumstances in a positive manner. Health professionals play an important role in helping patients reframe critical stressors that occur naturally or as unexpected crises in ways that continue to promote self-actualization in adulthood (Clayton & Birren, 1980).

NURSING DIAGNOSES APPROPRIATE TO NORMAL ADULTHOOD

Appropriate nursing diagnoses provide defining characteristics and name causes of vertical stressors in adulthood. Typically, nursing interventions for healthy adults correspond to one or more of the nursing diagnoses summarized in Box 20–7.

Box 20-6 ■■■■■
Three Adult Modes of Maladaptive Support-Seeking Patterns of Behavior Stemming From Inappropriate Parenting

1. The *compulsively self-reliant person* has difficulty forming attachments, resulting from parental rejections of the child's attempt to form attachments.
2. The *compulsive caregiver* is often the result of having had a disabled or depressed mother who was unable to take care of the child and instead created a context in which the child took care of the mother. This person develops many relationships but always is a caregiver. Being cared for is uncomfortable, so that the individual avoids being placed in such a position.
3. The *compulsive support seeker* develops many relationships but is constantly in need of support. This distortion of attachment arises when too much support has been given to a child, who then never develops self-efficacy, or when an individual so deprived consistently seeks in adulthood what was unavailable as a child.

From Bowlby, J. (1977). The making and breaking of affectional bonds. Part I: Aetiology and psychopathology in the light of attachment theory. *British Journal of Psychiatry, 130*, 191-210.

Box 20-7 ■■■■■
Nursing Diagnoses Related to Adult Mental Health

1. Spiritual Distress
2. Body Image Disturbance
3. Compromised Ineffective Family Coping
4. Ineffective Individual Coping
5. Altered Family Processes
6. Sexual Dysfunction
7. Parental Role Conflict
8. Risk for Altered Parenting
9. Powerlessness
10. Knowledge Deficit
11. Self Esteem Disturbance

There are many possible reasons for the development of symptoms warranting a general diagnosis. Therefore, carefully inquire about possible causes related to one or more of the following: lack of knowledge regarding developmental milestones, recent moves, unrealistic expectations related to parenting or a job, dysfunctional marital relationships, or role reversals.

A comparison of normal developmental patterns with the patient's presenting symptoms provides the data necessary to arrive at appropriate nursing judgments for each adult patient. Specific nursing interventions should relate to the particular phenomena of concern, the desired outcome, and underlying dynamics of the situation. Primary prevention strategies should reduce risk factors and strengthen protective factors. Psychoeducation and social support also help improve the self-esteem and restart a productive self-concept in adult travelers.

ACCOMMODATING TO SOCIAL CHANGES: IMPLICATIONS FOR ADULT DEVELOPMENT

Chronological adult development based on stage theories does not take into full account social changes affecting women who juggle career concerns with family obligations or the relatively recent phenomenon of competent, hard-working adults laid off because of corporate restructuring or downsizing (MacKinnon-Slaney, 1994). Dramatic social changes since the mid-1960s have altered and will continue profoundly to affect our understanding of adult human development. The role of women has changed dramatically. Because these shifts affect family and work life, corresponding roles for men have undergone significant transformation (Carlsen, 1988). In most cultures, work roles for women for centuries have been gender-linked, with a strong emphasis on homemaking and child-rearing. The euphemism "keep them barefoot and pregnant" described what most women could look forward to as their career. If they worked, the cultural milieu traditionally confined women to a narrow range of occupational roles—nurse, teacher, social worker, or secretary. Only in cases of extreme emergency were women permitted to assume work roles traditionally reserved for men. For example, during World War II, women were allowed to become military pilots and to assume traditional male jobs in private industry. Once the war ended, however, this window of opportunity evaporated as if it had never existed.

In the 1990s, greater flexibility of social roles allowed both men and women a broader sense of identity and existential space to find their own truths. Men and women seek careers traditionally reserved for the opposite sex. For example, men become nurses; women become physicians and steam fitters; fire and police departments recruit women; traditionally male-only military colleges have been ordered to admit women to their ranks. These changes have also benefitted men, who now feel freer to develop closer relationships with their children and to share some of the burden for maintaining the family's financial resources with a spouse. The term *househusband* is now a legitimate phrase to describe men who choose to be homemakers whose wives are primary breadwinners.

Only since the 1960s have women been able to legitimately to expand their personal horizons beyond the home and to join men as equals in life and work (Baruch, Barnett, & Rivers, 1983; Josselson, 1987). Salary discrepancies still exist, however, and men statistically hold an advantage. In many companies, a "glass ceiling" limits promotion of women to the highest ranks. This means that even though women may have abilities equal to men, they face male bias in terms of moving up the career ladder. Even so, the lot of women in the workplace has improved dramatically. Women now have consistent roles in most employment areas, and a great range of occupational choices is open to the imagination and talents of women. In providing culturally specific health care, however, you need to realize that in many cultures, the role of women remains limited to subservient homemaker and childbearer.

Dual-Career Families

Since the late 1960s, there has been a dramatic change in the structure of the family and a broadening of social role expectations. Family units in which the father goes to work and the mother stays at home with the children are becoming increasingly uncommon. **Dual-career families,** those in which one partner works full-time and the other is employed at least 19 hours a week, are the rule rather than the exception. Yet women continue to consider home and work responsibilities in making career decisions (Paludi, 1991).

Research shows that greater flexibility of social roles for men and women are sources of satisfaction and benefit for children. Hoffman (1989) suggested that the cognitive, social, and emotional development of school-age children with working mothers parallels or is better than that of children with mothers at home. Employed mothers in Hoffman's study expressed satisfaction with their combined role and their relationship with their children. Moreover, their school-age children held less stereotyped views of male and female roles than the children of mothers who did not work. Gottfried, Gottfried, and Bathurst (1988) also found strong indications that paternal involvement enhanced their children's cognitive and psychosocial development. Still, many women experience deep personal satisfaction as full-time homemakers and mothers and select this option.

Changes in Family Structures

In addition to major changes in social roles occurring within the family unit, the definition of a family is much more diverse than it was 20 years ago. The traditional model of a married couple as mother and father and children who live with their biological parents still exists but is no longer the only acceptable option. The divorce rate has risen significantly, and more marriages terminate in divorce than in death. Households headed by a female single parent number more than one in five. For every three marriages that succeed, another two will be dissolved through separation and divorce (National Center for Health Statistics [NCHS], 1994).

Joint custody and parental visiting rights are facts of life for many families, with more than 1 million marriages ending in divorce each year (NCHS, 1994). Yet although many children grow up in single-parent or blended stepfamilies, Golombok and Fivush (1994) noted that the diversity of family form does not necessarily have an adverse impact on children. Rather, it is the quality of the parent-child relationships and alternative child-care arrangements that account for differences in child development. (See Chapter 18 for issues and interventions related to families.)

In the 1990s, many men and women chose to remain single. No longer was single life a sign of failure when a woman or man made a deliberate choice. Cohabitation between consenting adults, with or without children, also became a common long-term alternative to marriage. It also is much more acceptable for homosexual couples to raise children and to live together openly as couples (Patterson, 1992). Divergent lifestyles for men and women are more acceptable, and having a homosexual orientation is viewed as a sexual preference rather than the consequence of faulty parenting or a symptom of mental illness.

Women's patterns of marriage, childbearing, and caregiving have also changed considerably. Just a few decades ago, the childbearing decades were culturally limited to the early 20s through early 30s. Should a woman conceive a child in her late 30s or early 40s, the child was deemed a *change of life baby,* with the implication that conception was unplanned, an irregularity of nature associated with the beginning of menopause. Today, there is a blurring of life periods (Neugarten & Neugarten, 1986) as women postpone having children until they are older. Many adults approach marriage and childbirth as options rather than expectations of mature adulthood, and many more women have their first child in their late 30s and 40s. New reproductive technologies also allow women at older ages, women without partners, and lesbian couples to have children of their own.

The decision to postpone childbirth does not seem to carry adverse effects. In a comparative study of first children born in their parents' early 20s, 30s, and 40s, Daniels and Weingarten (1982) reported that age variation did not significantly affect accomplishment of parenting tasks. Becoming a parent at a later age required more initial adjustment, but these parents also reported greater ultimate satisfaction with their parenting than they believed they would have experienced with a first child at an earlier age.

Infertility

Having children still establishes a sense of continued identity for women. Childbearing is a normal life process, a recognized symbol of adult status and feminine identity (Phoenix, Woollett, & Lloyd, 1991). Women in the age group 15 to 44 with impaired ability to have children number 6.1 million (NCHS, 1995). *Infertility* is defined as the inability to have children for biological reasons. Causes of infertility are many and can occur in one or both partners. Infertility is not simply a biological crisis. It carries great potential for an identity crisis, particularly if the role of mother is central to a woman's identity or is viewed by the husband as important to the relationship. As one woman explained:

I think we've all grown up with the idea that pregnancy is what a woman does, it's the most natural thing, and we have a whole 2000 years of literature and culture that have always pointed in that direction. So there has been this tradition, and it's very hard at times to redefine oneself as a woman.

I figured I could sit in the backyard and make quilts and do handwork that I love to do, which in some ways I haven't done because now I see no purpose; it is more something to do if you're pregnant. There are some things I still haven't done, like fix up the patio with Astroturf, which would be nice for a child to play in. And some things I would do in the house that now really aren't needed since there are no kids. I had images and plans of things I would do. (Phoenix et al., 1991, p. 177)

Although typically considered a woman's issue, infertility in men is quite common and of considerable concern to the men involved. The procedures for assessing fertility are invasive and time-consuming. In vitro fertilization and adoption are possible solutions, but in vitro technology is expensive and not always successful. You can help patients work through the emotional aspects of infertility and can connect them with the appropriate medical services for explaining options or providing direct service. Note that people can be generative in many ways and that biological childbearing is only one of them. Helping men and women to see their reproductive capacity as something other than the defining characteristic of their masculinity or femininity is particularly important. (See Chapter 10 for communication and reframing strategies.)

Ending a Relationship

Achievement of intimacy is a significant psychosocial task of adulthood, so that the end of a relationship, whether in separation, divorce, or death, marks a turning point in the adult's journey. This process of loss applies to homosexual as well as heterosexual partners and can also apply to the end of a relationship with a dear friend, a meaningful job, or even a beloved pet.

Some of the factors affecting the intensity of the loss relates to the nature and length of the relationship, the level of conflict in or satisfaction with the relationship, and the amount of social support the person receives on an ongoing basis. Fiske and Chiriboga (1990) found that divorcing persons were more likely to experience both positive and negative changes in nearly all areas of their lives. One woman described some of the complications induced by a lost relationship:

In my 40s I was very involved in education, family, and community. It was exciting and fulfilling. The change at age 54 to a single lifestyle was traumatic. I had always felt that being married had given me the freedom to explore and engage in new activities with home and husband as always an emotional and financial safety net. Now it seems tiresome to make all decisions—and do all thinking—alone. In the past six years, I've also had to come to terms with the basic fact that there are many things over which we have absolutely no control. (Arnold, 1994)

In divorce, "burying" the partner is often harder than the separation when a partner dies. Frequently, divorced parents face continued involvement. Opportunities for despair as well as for personal growth accompany the process of working through either the voluntary or the involuntary ending of a relationship.

Becoming widowed in early and middle stages of adulthood is particularly traumatic because these widowed women have few peers who understand or can respond to their pain. At a time when their contemporaries are walking through life with a partner, widows are at a distinct disadvantage. Atchley (1991, p. 200) suggested that "the social disruption widowhood causes depends largely on the number of role relationships affected by the spouse's death." Fiske and Chiriboga (1990) observed that loss of a spouse was more devastating for men than for women. They postulated that women are more likely to have close relationships with a number of people, whereas many men have close relationships only with their wives. For many people, however, loss is poignant, as this woman describes:

At age 52, my husband of almost 33 years died. He was just 54 and had a brain tumor. This event so changed my life, my outlook, my future, my lifestyle that I have trouble thinking beyond it. His death is so all-consuming that age, stage, and outlook seem to be a result of that event. (Arnold, 1994)

Although this woman had many friends, the loss was still devastating. When tragedy strikes, a person's developmental world stops—at least for a time. Some life issues are not particularly age-related or more gracefully handled during one age period than another. Nor are the usual remedies useful, as another woman, an introvert by nature, states:

Social support is not a substitute for inner strength. Movies and dinner do not complete a sleepless night. I am a solitary person in most of life's crises and do not count on others to fill my needs or wipe my tears—a function of a miserable, bleak, and unsupported childhood. I have always worked at finding serenity and staying alive. I am no less in the world but embrace it more fully. (Arnold, 1994)

We often equate maturity, mental health, and the ability to resolve grief with the level of social support a person receives or seeks. Yet, as this woman's testimony shows, social support is critical for some, but the route others must take is different. You, therefore, need to be aware and supportive of personal choices.

The Not-So-Empty Nest

In past decades, the *empty nest* was identified as the basis for depression in midlife women. Contrary to popular belief, a number of researchers (Cooper & Gutmann, 1987; Neugarten, 1970) reported that the last child leaving home does not create depression for most women but that the empty nest actually liberates parents. Both working parents and home-oriented women experienced greater freedom, more free time, greater privacy, and more opportunities. This woman's statement captures her sense of personal growth:

My family has grown and gone, and the hectic pace of the 40s, which tore me between being a wife, mother, and caretaker for aging parents, has ended. Perhaps the very fact that the 40s were so full of obligations makes the 50s appear idyllic early on. I now have the time and means to work and play as I like. I am able to fulfill obligations because I want to, and not because I have to. I have passed the "have to" years and entered the "want to" years. (Arnold, 1994)

Lowenthal and Chiriboga (1972) reported exceptions to these findings in women with long-standing emotional problems whose lives revolved around their children. For these women, therapy can help them reestablish a stronger sense of self.

The empty nest is not an abrupt change for many adults today. Changing social and economic realities have created different mental health issues for both parents and adult children. Many young adults in their 20s are choosing to return home and to live with their parents for longer periods. For these young adults, building a solid career identity is threatened by economic uncertainty, and the comforts of home are far more appealing than the substandard housing arrangements they typically can afford. Consequently, some young adults are postponing major life commitments, including marriage, children, and home ownership, because of declining job opportunities and rising costs of housing and education. Additionally, the time required to earn a college degree can be more than 4 years, as evidenced in the T-shirt proclamation: "ECU, the best 5 or 6 years of my life."

For today's young adult, exercising the necessary self-discipline required for financial independence clearly is not easy. A generation ago, people bought only what they could afford because there were no financial structures to support other alternatives. Today's easy credit for purchases adults cannot really afford is creating a negative balance and significant debt, the magnitude of which is only beginning to be appreciated. The financial shortfall often is absorbed by parents, causing stress, anger, anxiety, and frustration for all concerned. Circumstances may warrant psychiatric intervention.

The Sandwich Generation

As more people live longer, adult children increasingly are called on to provide financial and other assistance to aging parents (Aldwin, Spiro, Levenson, & Bosse, 1989; Kingson et al., 1986). Actual physical care of the frail elderly creates an ongoing concern for those who cannot put an infirm parent in a nursing home for either financial or emotional reasons. At the same time, these adults have teenagers to parent. This social phenomenon has created the *sandwich generation,* in which adults age 53 to 65 have multiple caregiving responsibilities.

Women still remain the major caregivers to the elderly. Caught between two generations, both of which require care, many adults in midlife find it difficult to balance caregiving responsibilities. Teenagers require a different kind of parenting, and the frail elderly typically require the type of physical care accorded their children at an earlier age. Caregiving therefore requires a constant switching of gears. Moreover, caring for elderly parents is more difficult, first because the investment brings further dependence as the older adult becomes more frail and second because parenting the frail older adult necessarily entails role reversals.

Unemployment

The pervasive fear of job loss—affecting blue-collar and white-collar workers alike—is becoming a powerful

Box 20-8 ■ ■ ■ ■ ■
Empty

The empty nest
Quiet solitude
Time to read
Time to think
Time to write
of times gone by
Precious memories preserved
for coming generations.

The empty house
Quiet solitude
Time to clean
Time to organize
Time to buy new things
get rid of the old
Everything sparkling clean
for possible visitors

The empty life
Quiet solitude
Time to be alone
Time to contemplate
Time to enjoy life
and start anew
the slate wiped clean
Now what will I do?

By Lorraine Beldo. Copyright Lorraine Beldo, www.queenbee publishing.com.

force. For U.S. workers, the 1990s became the age of job insecurity. Each year, close to 2 million Americans permanently lose their jobs as companies downsize to remain competitive. Many of those who lose their jobs will be out of work for an extended period. Midlife layoffs in previously stable work situations create serious assaults on self-identity. Some people emerge stronger, but others are irreparably scarred. Being laid off invariably is experienced as a personal crisis of identity requiring significant attention to reframing one's sense of self in addition to the actual job search. From unskilled workers to corporate executives, employees increasingly are asking the same questions: will the current wave of corporate restructuring that is shaping the economy affect me, and how will I cope if I lose my job?

Adding to the anxiety is the structural shift in the work force from permanent positions to a contingent work force that includes many employees who are not part of the core establishment. Contingent work is defined in terms of whether the employment arrangement is expected to last longer than a year. The 1998 U.S. Bureau of Labor Statistics estimated that between 2.2% and 4.9% of the work force is contingent.

New jobs often are temporary positions with little or no job security, and they often carry no benefits such as health insurance, pensions, and paid vacations. Temporary and contingent workers now make up more than 18.6% of the work force; total temporary employment grew by 1.8 million from 1980 to 1995 (National Alliance of Business, 1996). These temporary workers are part-time, independent contractors, or self-employed.

In the past, hard work and loyalty paid off (Morrow & McElroy, 1987). Economic security was based on constancy, seniority, and dedicated work. This work ethic is fast becoming a relic of the past, replaced by structural changes in the work force that favor a temporary, or contingent, model. The use of consultants who are paid higher salaries but are not given benefits is becoming more and more prevalent. Companies choose to pay a little more for expertise in the short run, to be able to dismiss workers easily when company demands shift. The loyalty of the "company man" is evaporating, and work commitment is harder to sustain, as employees lose faith in their employer's ability to provide a caring, supportive work environment that rewards commitment.

Review of the literature reveals a higher incidence of mental health disruptions in the form of depression, loss of self-esteem, marital and family problems, and even suicide as correlates of job loss (Dooley & Catalano, 1991; Love & Torrence, 1989). Yet little is written about concrete preventive mental health strategies designed to help people cope with job loss in a world in which old paradigms about job search strategies no longer apply. A college degree no longer guarantees employment success, and career opportunities are far more competitive because of corporate restructuring, downsizing, and the automation of many skilled tasks once performed by human workers. Most companies are trying to do more with less, so that getting a job, regardless of age, is harder than it was even 5 years ago.

Getting another job becomes more difficult as one gets older. The U.S. Department of Labor identifies a *mature worker* as any employee age 40 or older. With the current restructuring of employment patterns, older workers report having a great deal of difficulty obtaining other jobs. Despite laws against discrimination of all types, age discrimination is a reality in today's job market. In 1989, the U.S. Senate Special Committee on Aging reported that more than a third of employers studied believed that age discrimination occurred on a regular basis. Older workers typically are stereotyped as being less creative or willing to find innovative solutions to challenging problems. They are viewed as less able to make quick decisions under pressure, as less interested in learning new technologies, and, in some instances, as untrainable. Many have made excellent salaries and earned management titles. Companies are hesitant to hire them because younger workers do not require the same salaries or entitlements and are willing to do the same jobs. Older workers report interview comments from potential employers such as, "You are overqualified for this job, and I don't think you would be really happy here" or "You have a lot of skills, but what we are looking for is someone who has this technical skill, which you don't seem to have." Issues such as retirement and health benefits also affect decisions about hiring the older worker because benefits most often are used by this age group and cost the company money without a commensurate return on investment. Characteristics associated with the successful older worker such as loyalty, expertise, and a record of steady performance are overlooked in today's unstable job market.

Many communities today are providing support for dislocated workers to learn the skills that will make them more competitive in the job market. Privately funded and volunteer organizations, such as Forty Plus, help the older worker find the necessary support and practical advice needed to negotiate today's uncertain job opportunities.

Adults as Lifelong Learners

Although adults now constitute approximately 50% of students in higher education (MacKinnon-Slaney, 1994), current theories to explain development in the adult learner pose more questions than provide answers. Adult learners come with a wide variety of life skills. Most are self-supporting. Most are looking for an educational experience that will build on their life experience and enhance the quality of their lives (Mezirow, 1990).

The characteristics and learning needs of the adult learner typically are much more diverse than they are for traditional college students in late adolescence and early adulthood (Bauer & Mott, 1990). Because of major differences in life experience, adults present a wider variation in their skill development and self-efficacy. The adult learner may have mastered life skills that will make learning tasks easier as the educational experience develops, but basic study skills and ability to organize content quickly typically benefit from having initial structural expectations and guidelines set forth by the instructor. Adult learners who have been out of school for a long time often lack confidence in their abilities to compete effectively in the classroom with younger students. Because adult learners are older and typically more experienced and self-motivated, their need for initial structure is often overlooked by instructors and frequently by the student as well. Additionally, experience with adult learners has shown that the essential components of learning and their application indicate that it is more important for the learner than for the teacher to determine what, when, and how to learn (Regan-Smith, 1998). Basic assumptions relevant to the process of learning in adulthood are presented in Box 20–9.

What do you think? Should individuals be prepared for adulthood in a structured way? Should our educational system prepare individuals for adulthood? If so, how should that be done?

The Future of Adult Development

In *A Tale of Two Cities,* the scene of an important social revolution several centuries ago, Charles Dickens began with the line: "It was the best of times, it was the worst of times." As we embark on the 21st century, we are arriving on the crest of unprecedented technological and sociological changes that will have important consequences for adult development. The technological revolution may indeed equal that of other social revolutions in its power. The potential for human development at the beginning of the 21st century to reach the best of times or the worst of times in large measure depends on

Box 20–9 ■■■■■
Educating the Adult Learner

1. We cannot teach another person directly; we can only facilitate his or her learning.
2. A person learns significantly only those things that he or she perceives as being involved in the maintenance of, or enhancement of, the structure of self.
3. Experience that is perceived as inconsistent with self can be assimilated only if the current organization of self is relaxed and expanded to include it.
4. The educational situation that most effectively promotes significant learning is one in which the threat to the self of the learner is reduced to a minimum.

the judgments of its adult population. Maturity and level of mental health affect important decisions.

New Theories Linked to Social Changes

Some developmental theorists link adult development more to maturational responses to life events and social relationships than to chronological age. These criteria may become more definitive ways to conceptualize developmental responses in a world of rapid social change, increasing focus on technology, and much less time for reflection. For example, genome therapy may dramatically improve the human life span, with projections that people could live to be 140 years old in the 21st century. How will this affect the staging of adult development? What will the quality of life be like? What are the implications for career development and personal relationships if the projection becomes a reality in the 21st century? Longevity is only one of the many changes tomorrow's adult can expect.

The process and outcome of change greatly affects our understanding of self and other adults. From a practical perspective, negotiating adulthood in the 21st century is a little like white water rafting. The waters are swift, rapidly changing, and exciting, but potentially dangerous. Careful preparation for the trip helps ensure its success. People need to draw the map, develop perspectives on how to navigate the rapids, and identify the specific strengths and values they need to bring as baggage on the kayak. Moreover, the white water rafter needs an experienced guide to direct the project and to warn of potential dangers.

Adult travelers need to act as guides and mentors for the next generation of adults by linking together the past, present, and future in a meaningful way. Descriptions of human development in adulthood that blend the best of past traditions with the realities of the present and the trends of the future need to be carefully interwoven into the fabric of community life. Those adults who will enhance and even shape our lives in the future need new explanations. The story of the adult traveler in the 19th century was of individualism and self-actualization, but as Keen (1991) suggested:

... [R]ecently it has begun to look as if individualism is rapidly leading us into anarchy. What was once our strength is now tearing us apart. We are losing our moral consensus, our sense of community, our willingness to sacrifice for a shared ideal of the future, our understanding of what it is that gives dignity to the life of a man or woman. (p. 145)

The 21st century offers an opportunity to blend strong community values with those of individuals, to uphold and affirm the values of individualism as necessary and valid to full participation in the community. Perhaps then, the story of adulthood in the 21st century could be of community and of building a "just and loving society" (Bellah, 1985, p. 83).

Havighurst (1953, 1973) suggested a number of problem areas that warrant research on personality through the life span. Among the areas of study are career changes in relation to personality, age, and sex, and the ways normal adults perceive the aging process as individuals, as family members, and as members of the wider community. Exploration of personality changes associated with alterations in physical vigor or health, the influence of leisure activities on adult personality development, documentation of human development in the 50s and 60s, attitudes toward death, and variables associated with development of dementia also are fruitful areas for inquiry into normal adult development.

Human Development as a Moral Imperative

Many of the decisions that technology and cost containment in health care have spawned will create moral dilemmas that focus on choice and responsibility. Human responses to these questions and the decisions made will reside in the hands and souls of adults. In an expanding concept of the meaning of adulthood, Tournier (1965) noted,

> . . . [T]o speak of the person, and of respect for the person, is to speak, not of that man which is physical, psychological or intellectual, but of what is spiritual in him, his moral conscience, his sense of responsibility, his freedom of choice. (p. 49)

Choice and responsibility are key to strategies for promoting adult mental health in this new century. Preventive psychiatry that is focused on reducing risk factors and strengthening protective factors is of primary importance. To exercise their response-ability appropriately, adults need to integrate biological, ethical, and social concerns as the building blocks of adult development in a new holistic paradigm. The means for this integration are education, values clarification, and social support to meet the challenge.

> **W**hat do you think? As you look at your own life, is this the "best of times" or "the worst of times" for you? Defend your answer.

> ➤ *Check Your Reading*
> 4. What are the differences between vertical and horizontal stressors in adult development?
> 5. What is meant by the sandwich generation?
> 6. What are the negative factors that can work against adult learning?

PROMOTING THE MENTAL HEALTH OF THE ADULT TRAVELER

Bellah (1985, p. 82) suggested that "if it is to provide any richness of meaning, the idea of a life course must be set in a larger generational, historical, and probably, religious context." In the early 20th century, Freud identified intrinsic personal fulfillment achieved through productive work and satisfying intimate relationships as the benchmark of adult mental health. These are likely

to remain contemporary standards of adult maturity. Telling the current story of adulthood, however, is an art that needs to be firmly anchored in both objective and subjective definitions of roles and social institutions of the past and present and integrated with those needed to achieve the visions of this millennium. An awesome undertaking, the story begins with this generation of adults. As Whitehead (1929) in his landmark book on education advised:

> The mind is never passive: it is a perpetual activity, delicate, receptive, responsive to stimulus. You cannot postpone its life until you have sharpened it. Whatever interest attaches to your subject matter must be evoked here and now; whatever powers you are strengthening in the pupil must be exercised here and now; whatever possibilities of mental life your teaching should impart, must be exhibited here and now. That is the golden rule of education, and a very difficult one to follow. (p. 18)

Human Character Development

Human character development is becoming increasingly important, primarily because of the crucial role contemporary adult travelers will play at every stage of their psychological growth in shaping the new world. Adults in the 21st century will be called on to consider important ethical questions: end-of-life decisions, fetal tissue research, prophylactic surgery on well children and adults with genetic predispositions to cancer, access to care in a cost-containment health care environment, subsidized care and housing for migrant workers, and other social dilemmas. None of these issues has clear-cut answers. Yet all of them are being woven into the social fabric of the 21st century.

Ladner (1995) suggested that the solution to these problems lies in education:

> Higher educational institutions are particularly suited to provide the leadership because they can link theory with practice and teach principle-centered leadership to today's college students. It doesn't matter whether one is a Republican, Democrat or independent: all students need to be guided by ethical imperatives if they are to be engaged in solving the problems of their generation. (p. C2)

Thus, broad-based education for adult learners is based on a strong moral imperative. Creating practical strategies to cope successfully with a world they did not create becomes a vital force in preventive adult mental health.

More than ever, tomorrow's adult will be a "tentative character type shaped by inherited values on the one hand and the challenges of the expanding frontier on the other" (Bellah, 1985, p. 39). For those dedicated to enhancing adult potential, the task is to preserve and integrate traditional values of responsibility, dedication to truth, and commitment as the cornerstone of adult maturity. Definitive educational strategies can support the learning needs of an increasingly diverse student population. At the same time, "There must be new flowerings, new prophets, new adventures, always new adventures—if the heart of man, albeit in fits and starts, is to go on beating" (Tournier, 1965, p. 39).

Education in Preventive Mental Health

Education is becoming increasingly important as a means of both shaping and telling the story of adulthood. Education acts as the gatekeeper, the first line of defense in reducing risk behaviors associated with mental illness and in promoting protective factors to enhance emotional health and well-being. Relevant curricula, however, need to support primary prevention. The current educational system also needs to reflect technical, social, and economic changes in society and to support purposeful character development. Formal and informal teaching methods related to health education should focus on the development of creative *processes* necessary to create a social environment, in particular, critical thinking and respect for diversity. Values clarification to improve the critical thinking and ethical decision-making abilities of adult travelers, combined with empowerment strategies, is a basic foundation for primary prevention mental health strategies in the 1990s and beyond. Broad-based curricula that integrate interventions supporting physical and emotional health can help alleviate many risk factors.

The restructuring of higher education also needs to account for the requirements of adult learners. Education should enhance personal development, thereby reducing unnecessary stress and frustration. Today's adult student population is much more diverse, with a tremendous range of interests, life experiences, maturity, and learning needs. Such diversity naturally affects students' approaches to learning tasks and requires a broader educational mix of teaching strategies to support significant differences in student learning requirements. Granting course credit for comparable life experiences makes the curriculum more flexible and tailored to individual student needs. Redesigning courses that build on rather than repeat student experience makes the concept of the university as a community of scholars accessible to more students. Recognizing the complexity of student learning needs while balancing them with realistic expectations of academic performance are key elements in the restructuring of curriculum models to enhance student learning.

Values Clarification

We need to ensure that humanistic society does not fall victim to the economic or technological tenor of the time. Thus, values clarification is becoming increasingly important as a preventive mental health strategy. Young and middle-aged adults need to achieve a solid and recognizable identity as members of a humanistic community, embracing the notion of a shared, personal participation in life and attention to values and the moral domain. They need to engage thoughtfully and compassionately in a continuous process of exploration, questioning and reflecting on critical matters, such as abortion, end-of-life decisions, access to health care, and care of the poor.

Young and middle-aged adult travelers need to make difficult ethical decisions related to the goals and purposes of technological advances. Values clarification can help them sort criteria and look closely at relevant data from a more holistic perspective. Sharing common concerns and discussing differences become simpler when issues are named and more than one voice is heard. The process of inquiry should be personal and should include the spiritual, social, affective (emotional), and intellectual self in the full cognitive (mental) engagement of the individual. Respect for ideas presented by people with different backgrounds and beliefs and dissimilar ways of thinking is essential.

Technology in Preventive Mental Health

Technology is important in preventive mental health because of the possibilities technology offers for early diagnosis and health education and because of the problems it generates in using it wisely. Technological change is as dramatic as the development of books during the Renaissance. In fact, the computer is likely to become the textbook of the future. The Internet has created an information superhighway, enabling people, students included, to access vast amounts of information in a wide spectrum of formats. The classroom as we know it today has broadened, as the world shrinks through the creative use of technology. Today, the instructor may be many miles away, as teaching is provided in virtual classrooms or at home, without a student ever having to put a foot in the classroom. Even surgery may be performed through interactive television.

Electronic interactive formats present an interesting and informative way to enhance student learning. Interactive video presents material within a situational or interpersonal context. This format helps a student recognize that facts are embedded in larger situations. They can see and hear how people evaluate and respond effectively to complex situations. Computer-generated simulations can provide practical applications for problem solving and allow more flexibility with differences in the time patterns some students need to learn. Yet it is critical that technology support but not replace the spontaneous, reasoned human element in health education. Facts need a context and tone for a collective meaning. Human beings are meaning makers, and no matter how sophisticated a decision-making software package, it can never replace human dialogue. Consequently, modeling behavior, developing social skills, and relating ideas to others must continue to be significant dimensions of health education.

The process of developing creativity is greater than the sum of its parts. The instructor must be able to understand and convey the social skills necessary to deal with the nuances, emotional sensitivities, and values of others in real-life situations. Personal encounters with the student about these matters are as important as mastering content. Fostering awareness of the human values and richness of shared discovery can occur only through ongoing conversations about meaning.

Empowerment Strategies

Most mentally healthy adults can generate their own answers and resolve their own problems in life with just a little support and guidance. Mentorship, particularly in novice adulthood, is an important element of preventive psychiatry (Levinson et al., 1978; Noe, 1988). Nurses can assist the adult traveler in learning assertive communication, negotiation, and conflict management strategies both spontaneously and in formal continuing education classes. Providing adults with information about the normal process of adult development and assisting them in developing parenting skills, caring for aging parents, or surviving loss of a relationship or job in times of distress can reframe a crisis into a challenging possibility. Informal health teaching that assists adult travelers to find meaning in their current situations and plan for the future is a preventive strategy, easily accomplished without significant financial outlay. During times of transition, nurses can help adult travelers reclaim a sense of self-mastery through simple open-ended questions, such as

- How are you adjusting to (identify the life transition: your job loss, having to care for your parents, the death of your spouse, your return to school)? Framing the question in this way suggests that the period of transition is one of temporary adjustment with a projected outcome that can be successful.
- What coping skills have you used in the past that have helped you? This question helps individuals identify productive coping skills that they may have forgotten, which can be used to negotiate the current transition successfully.

Social Support

Social support offers the adult opportunities to correct knowledge deficits, to develop networks that help enhance self-esteem, and to consider options for coping with difficult life problems. Primary prevention strategies in the form of stress management and coping skills, use of community resources, referral to appropriate support groups, and reading of material on parenting are simple interventions. Crisis intervention (see Chapter 13) should be offered to those individuals and families presenting with inadequate coping skills, insufficient support systems, and perceived powerlessness to direct their lives. A related intervention is to provide sufficient time for personal reflection and subsequent human dialogue. As Wicks (1985, p. 142) suggested, "Use any technique necessary to slow yourself down so that you don't rush to the grave missing the scenery in your life along the way."

Support groups are an invaluable form of social support. As a primary therapeutic intervention or as an adjunct to other therapies, they provide emotional respite and direction for adult travelers. Nurses can help individuals and families find new meaning in uncertain times through referral to the many support groups serving the community for adults in crisis.

One example of a support group is New Hope, a community-based job search group designed for people who have lost a job for any reason. The group has the collective purpose of helping the job seeker cope emotionally while looking for a new job, providing practical help and support with all aspects of the job search process and offering an opportunity for networking among job seekers. Explicit norms include confidentiality, mutual respect, and commitment to the job search process. The clientele using the services of the group is mixed, with a heavier concentration of white-collar, male, and older workers displaced from the work force after many years of service.

New Hope's interactive process is based on an *empowerment framework,* defined as "the interpersonal process of providing the resources, tools and environment to develop, build and increase the ability and effectiveness of others to set and reach goals for individual and social ends" (Hawkes, 1992, p. 609). To replace traditional paradigms of work efficacy and job security based on education, successful performance, and rational progression, the group has developed a different paradigm for the job search.

An explicit assumption is that workers face a new labor force paradigm of uncertainty and ambiguity in the workplace that applies to everyone, regardless of credentials and experience. Acknowledging this reality and developing initiatives to meet the challenge is an important group focus. Empowerment of self through personal responsibility is viewed as a primary strategy of effective job searching. Interventions are designed to help people identify their strengths and recognize their value as individuals apart from their jobs. Clients are encouraged to accept ambiguity in work and to develop competencies related to versatility and networking in a time of turbulent economic change. Specific techniques include developing professional networks and cooperative human relationships, learning to accept feelings, sharing job leads, acting through knowledge, and developing the tools needed to understand and respond effectively in a rapidly changing job market.

People enter New Hope not knowing what to expect, usually experiencing diminished self-esteem and identity, anticipating changes in lifestyle, and feeling vulnerable about the future. Members of the group have identified the following factors as helpful:

1. Having a place to talk
2. Finding that you are not alone
3. Networking
4. Maintaining motivation
5. Developing concrete strategies in the job search
6. Learning about resources
7. Gaining support from the other members

Participants in the group report the following outcomes as the result of group membership:

1. Networking skills
2. Résumé writing skills
3. Interviewing skills
4. Confidence building skills

New Hope offers a preventive mental health strategy to reduce anxiety, emotional pain, and loss while empowering people to negotiate a job search creatively. Similar support groups might promote empowerment and follow a similar format while helping individuals cope with divorce, death, illness, and many other vertical stressors that appear on the landscape of the adult journey.

What do you think? What sources of empowerment exist in your life? Are they social, spiritual, or psychological? How do these sources empower you to move forward on your journey?

➤ *Check Your Reading*

7. In what ways can education be considered a primary means of preventive psychiatry?
8. How are support groups used as a tool to promote mental health?
9. What do you think will be some of the major ethical issues facing adults in this century?

The case study about Dorothy presents a normal, predictable life crisis in the human journey of the adult traveler and suggests appropriate nursing interventions. For psychiatric conditions affecting adults, see Unit V.

NURSING PROCESS APPLICATION

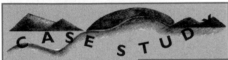

Dorothy

Dorothy is a 49-year-old executive secretary who lives in the Southwest. Her mother was diagnosed with lung cancer 6 months ago and is currently in the terminal stages. Her mother had a bilateral mastectomy 4 years ago for breast cancer. Two months ago, Dorothy divorced her husband of 20 years and is living alone in an apartment. Her two children are living on their own; one is in college, and one is married with two children. Her only sister lives on the West Coast and also works full time. As of now, Dorothy's only social outlet is an occasional evening out with her friends from church.

Dorothy's mother asked Dorothy to promise her that she would not put her in a nursing home. Every evening after work Dorothy drives to her mother's home to check on her. Having Dorothy move in is not an option because her mother lives in a one-bedroom apartment. When Dorothy comes to the doctor's office for a check-up, she tells you she is "exhausted, on edge, and frustrated and can't sleep through the night." She says that her mother is a strong person and she wants to abide by her wishes, but she isn't sure about what to do. When her father died several years ago, Dorothy was not there and still feels guilty. She also tells you that she is concerned that her mother's small savings will be gone soon.

ASSESSMENT

Assessment data are as follows:
- Insomnia
- Fatigue
- Anxiety
- Multiple personal stressors (divorce, multiple role changes)
- Financial concerns
- Perceived lack of support

DIAGNOSIS

DSM-IV Diagnosis: Adjustment Disorder, With Anxiety

Nursing Diagnosis: Caregiver Role Strain related to terminal illness of mother, financial concerns, and perceived lack of support evidenced by anxiety, insomnia, and feeling of extreme fatigue

OUTCOME IDENTIFICATION, PLANNING, AND IMPLEMENTATION

Expected Outcome I: By _____ the patient will obtain assistance with the demands of caring for her mother.

Short-Term Goals	Nursing Interventions	Rationales
By _____ the patient will verbalize tasks that could be delegated.	1. Assist the patient in developing a list of the tasks necessary to care for her mother. 2. Have the patient compile a list, and review it with her. 3. Help the patient decide which items on the list could be delegated and which items she needs to complete.	1–2. A structured activity will help the patient focus on and complete a specific task. 3. The patient will want to retain some tasks to remain a part of her mother's care, but delegating other tasks will enable the mother to remain at home, which is what she asked of her daughter.
By _____ the patient will identify resource persons, both inside and outside the family, that could assist with her mother's care.	1. Identify possible caregiver resources for the patient. 2. Develop possibilities for delegation of tasks that are within budgetary constraints. 3. Discuss the concept of respite care with the patient. 4. Assist the patient and caregiver to develop a daily schedule of direct care activities.	1. The patient may be unaware of all the resources that are available. 2. Planning without considering finances is not time-efficient. 3. The patient may be unaware of the concept of respite care. 4. A specific daily schedule will assist the patient in delegating activities.

Expected Outcome 2: By _____ the patient will develop a support system with neighbors, family, and friends.

Short-Term Goals	Nursing Interventions	Rationales
By _____ the patient will identify potential caregivers who could assist her.	1. Ask the patient to compile a list of potential caregivers from her neighbors, family, and friends. 2. Help the patient to identify the type and source of support or care that would be most beneficial.	1–2. Actually putting the list on paper will assist the patient in completing the task.
By _____ the patient will ask a neighbor or church member to sit with her mother while the patient attends a church service on the following Sunday.	1. Further assess the patient's spiritual needs and previous attendance at a church. 2. Asking for the help of a church member will assure the patient that others are willing to help her during this time.	1–2. The spiritual comfort found in attending a church service will be particularly helpful to the patient at this time.
By _____ the patient will invite a former friend over for lunch or dinner.	1. Encourage the patient to socialize and build up a support network. 2. Continue to encourage the patient to make contact with former friends.	1–2. Friends and family are often willing to help, but do not know what would be helpful.

Expected Outcome 3: By _____ the patient will verbalize the importance of self-care in maintaining the stamina needed to care for her mother.

Short-Term Goals	Nursing Interventions	Rationales
By _____ the patient will develop and implement a plan for daily regular exercise.	1. Assist the patient in maintaining a daily log of exercise and sleep patterns. 2. Teach the patient about the correlation of sleep and exercise.	1–2. Regular exercise is a stress reducer and sleep enhancer.
By _____ the patient will develop and implement a plan for healthy eating.	1. Encourage the patient to keep a daily diary of food intake. 2. Teach the patient about the pyramid plan for healthy nutrition on a daily basis. 3. Assist the patient to begin a nutritional plan that will be based on her likes and dislikes.	1. It is important to assess both areas of dietary intake that are healthy and those that need improvement. 2. The patient may be unaware of what entails healthy nutritional status. 3. Compliance in changing behavior is more likely if the patient does not have to make radical changes, particularly during times of other personal stress.

By _____ the patient will make and keep an appointment for a yearly physical examination.	1. Assist the patient in arranging for a time when she can see her physician that fits into her schedule. 2. Remind the patient that maintaining her own health is of the utmost importance right now.	1–2. Multiple life stressors can lead to a breakdown in the immune system and ultimately cause illness. Regular monitoring of health status is important at this time.

Nursing Diagnosis: Altered Role Performance related to change in marital status and role reversal with mother evidenced by inability to accept new role or to ask for help from others

---

OUTCOME IDENTIFICATION, PLANNING, AND IMPLEMENTATION

> **Expected Outcome 1:** By _____ the patient will be able to function comfortably in her new role.

Short-Term Goals	Nursing Interventions	Rationales
By _____ the patient will specify behaviors to meet new role expectations.	1. Ask the patient to make a list of necessary behaviors to accomplish her new role. 2. Offer suggestions such as assertiveness training. 3. Have the patient practice new behaviors with you in a role-play setting.	1–2. The patient may have some ideas in mind that would be helpful, but she may be so emotionally stressed that she is having difficulty generating new ideas for herself. 3. Initiating new behaviors is a difficult process. Practicing with someone who is accepting and encouraging fosters success.
By _____ the patient will discuss role performance with her sister and children and significant friends.	1. Have the patient delineate specific time frames for the change. 2. Assist the patient to express in behavioral terms what she expects from her sister and children.	1–2. Being specific in time frames and behavior will aid the patient in getting her needs met and is part of being an assertive person.
By _____ the patient will express satisfaction and acceptance with new role parameters.	1. Ask the patient to make a list of the pros and cons of her new role changes. 2. Encourage the patient to talk openly about any negative feelings she continues to have with her change in behavior with her sister, children, and friends.	1. Actually writing down the changes will help the patient to quantify any difficult areas. 2. Negative feelings usually indicate a form of resistance to change and may reveal some guilt about the change. Talking about these feelings to an accepting person may help alleviate the guilt.

> **Expected Outcome 2:** By _____ the patient will be able to express ambivalent feelings of anger, guilt, fear, and sadness over the role changes that are necessary at this time in her life.

Short-Term Goals	Nursing Interventions	Rationales
By _____ the patient will discuss a wide variety of feelings honestly and openly.	1. Ask the patient to keep track of feelings that occur in a 24-hour period. Provide her with a chart that describes feelings and feeling words. 2. Encourage the patient to make connections between strong negative feelings and bodily expressions. 3. Ask the patient to describe what bodily reaction she feels when she is angry or fearful. 4. Ask the patient to describe one or two things she feels hopeful about in the future.	1. The patient is probably being flooded with feelings and may be having difficulty distinguishing among them. 2–3. If the patient is unaccustomed to talking about or identifying feelings, making a connection with what is going on with her body will be helpful. 4. It is important to focus not only on negative feelings but also on positive ones.
By _____ the patient will seek the help of clergy or a therapist to help her with the grieving process.	1. Make the patient aware of all the grief she has experienced in the past year in regard to her divorce, her children leaving home, and her mother's history of poor health and impending death.	1. Often, patients are aware that they are experiencing a difficult time but do not have the necessary vocabulary to describe it. Labeling this process as the grief process and normalizing it for the patient may be helpful.

2.   Provide the patient with the names and phone numbers of nurse therapists or pastoral counselors who specialize in the grief process.

3.   Encourage the patient to make the appointment within 1 week.

2–3.   This patient has had considerable grief experiences in the past year, and working with a specialist in this area may prevent a delayed bereavement process.

EVALUATION

Formative Evaluation: Dorothy was able to meet each of the short-term goals in the time frames allotted. She developed strategies to provide respite from the constant care of her mother. Each week she appeared better able to ask for help and support from her friends and sister. She saw her physician and has taken steps to develop a more healthy lifestyle.

Summative Evaluation: Dorothy was able to meet all of the expected outcomes with the help and support of the nurse. She contacted a hospice and now has the support she needs to care for her mother. Dorothy states she feels she has regained balance in her life and no longer feels that her mother's care is a burden. In talking with her friends and reconnecting with her church, Dorothy has developed a strong support system that sustains her during this difficult time.

See the Snapshot Box of Nursing Interventions Specific to Facilitating a Patient's Journey Through the Crises of Adulthood.

SNAPSHOT

Nursing Interventions Specific to Crisis of Adulthood

What do you need to develop in a relationship with an adult who needs nursing care?

- Evaluate on which developmental level the adult is functioning, primarily to be able to communicate in a manner that fosters trust and a therapeutic relationship (i.e., level of maturity of the individual).
- Assess the adult's environment, which may be affecting the individual's ability to learn new behaviors.
- Note that communication between a man and a woman may require different strategies (e.g., a man may have difficulty accepting information from a female nurse clinician; a woman may need some self-disclosure by the nurse clinician before revealing personal information).
- Be caring, honest, empathetic, and professional.
- Provide information for further interventions and on the need for supportive others.

What do you need to assess related to the adult patient's health status?

- Observe for signs and symptoms of physical and psychiatric disorders gleaned by patient report and observation, for example, depression, anxiety, or paranoid thinking.
- Assess for risk of suicide or self-destructive thoughts.
- Perform complete physical and mental status examinations per protocols and assessment tools.

What do you need to teach the patient, the family, or the caregiver?

- Medication management for symptoms of physical or mental illness
- Stages of adult development and the common stressors found in each one
- Coping strategies to increase skills in dealing with stressors (e.g., relaxation exercises in anxiety-arousing situations, saying "no")

What skills do you want the patient or caregiver to demonstrate?

- Maturity appropriate to the developmental era of the adult traveler
- Positive coping skills
- Relaxation techniques and thoughts to reduce stress and anxiety
- Ability to express emotions and feelings without self-destructive behaviors
- Establish caring, long-lasting relationships with others
- Ability to secure and maintain work without major personal or professional difficulties
- Project positive self-esteem about body image as the adult traveler progresses through the life stages

What other health professionals might need to be a part of this plan?

- Physicians, nurse clinicians, caregivers, family, friends

Conclusions

Adulthood encompasses a long stretch of the developmental journey. The story of human life is about a journey toward wholeness. We see the journey physically begin with conception and end with death. In between, life offers each individual multiple opportunities through their personalized attitudes and actions of integrity, courage, justice, and compassion to make meaningful contributions to life and to experience tremendous satisfaction from the effort and outcome. Although childhood and adolescence are significant periods in providing the foundation for adulthood, this next life stage is even more significant because in every society, the adults become the critics, architects, and change agents of their generation.

Sufficient raw data suggest that adult development in the 21st century will be quite different and that today's adults will play a critical role in shaping a new reality. The current generation of young adults will be called to solve complex social, economic, and moral problems that simply did not exist even a few decades ago. Ladner (1995) submitted that youth are faced with a combination of such unprecedented social problems as teen pregnancy, violence, intergenerational poverty, and drugs. Although none of these problems is new, their combined prevalence among some groups and the extent of their impact are new phenomena. To these must be added the lack of access to health care (particularly for mental health), a graying population, dilemmas about end-of-life decisions, and high crime rates in virtually every segment of society. These external forces present mental health issues that require themes of exploration, risk-taking, and human character development combined in a completely different story of adult development. Successful negotiation of early and middle adulthood in the 1990s and beyond is both an awesome responsibility and a true adventure marked by personal challenge and opportunities for growth.

The tale of adulthood is experienced as an adventure in time and space. It typically begins when the traveler is ready to explore uncharted territory as an independent agent, with values as the compass, personal strengths as the tools, and mentors as guides along the way. Obstacles and detours emerge periodically in the landscape as unexpected crises, illness, and normative life events. The relevance of these crises is different for each traveler. Chance encounters also provide interruptions that affect the direction and meaning of the journey.

Atchley (1991, p. 115) noted that "like a road map, the abstract concept of the life course in reality is composed of a great many alternative routes to alternative destinations." The adult traveler may take many possible paths and must choose among them. The choices determine in part whether or not the traveler reaches a worthy goal. Each decision influences normal career and relationship cycles related to various life stages. The excursion through this part of the life journey is a special but limited period accorded to each traveler in which to discover a deeper sense of self and to establish one's place in the larger scheme of life.

Key Points to Remember

- Adult development is a dynamic life process characterized by responsibility and commitment.
- The experience of adulthood is different for men and women.
- In early adulthood, the focus is turned outward, toward meeting society's expectations. In midlife, the focus changes to an inward direction for meaning.
- Adults in their 20s are concerned with establishing a career, choosing a life mate, and selecting a mentor.
- Adults in their 30s consolidate and refine the commitments they made in their 20s.
- Physical, social, and emotional factors create a reevaluation of meaning in the 40s.
- A midlife crisis is a normal psychosocial event characterized by emotional upheaval but often resulting in a life that has more personal meaning.
- Adults in their 50s frequently experience a sense of renewal.

Learning Activities

1. In a relaxed position, close your eyes. Think about what it means to be your gender in society. What do you like best about being the gender that you are? How does your gender affect what you are doing? Now, think what it would be like to be a member of the opposite sex and ask yourself the same questions. What are you missing by being a member of the opposite sex? Share your thoughts with your classmates, and discuss the implications of your choices.

2. Adulthood offers each person an opportunity to shape a creative identity with personal meanings reflective of personal choices. This exercise asks you to consider what essential values are needed in charting a direction for the future. Look over the following list and rank the words in order of importance, with the most important first. When you are finished, share your answers with a partner and discuss how you came to your decisions.

Physical appearance	Choice
Comfort	Autonomy
Money	Equality
Working conditions	Articulateness
Living conditions	Innovation
Standard of living	Feelings

Honesty　　　　　Teaching
Caring　　　　　Learning
Flexibility　　　　Music and other arts
Motivation　　　　Religion
Freedom　　　　　Politics

3. Reflect over the past 10 years and identify the ways in which you have changed in your ideas, your outlook, and your feelings. Write a paragraph about how you see yourself today and another about how you were 10 years ago. Ask someone who knew you then how they would have expected to see you today. Share your observations with your small group and get their feedback.

4. Write a paragraph about how you see yourself in 5 years. What do you think might be different? What might stay the same? Share your observations with your small group and get their feedback.

Critical Thinking Exercise

Kathy, a wife and mother of two college students and a teenager, has decided to return to college to finish nursing school. Her husband recently had surgery that kept him out of work for 6 weeks. Her husband has always been a good provider. Although their savings are adequate, his income is directly affected by his ability to work. When she informed her husband of her decision, he commented, "You don't have to do that, I'll be all right."

1. Under what assumptions do you think Kathy is operating in this story?

2. What do you think is her husband's point of view?

3. How would you check these assumptions by some simple inquiry?

Six months later, Kathy was talking to Danielle, a fellow nursing student with two grown children. Kathy told Danielle that since her husband had returned to work, he has been given a work assignment in France and wants her to travel with him. The work assignment would be for 2 months in the early spring.

1. Make sense of this discussion.

2. Give a possible alternative interpretation of the situation that fits the facts.

3. What conclusions can you draw about Kathy's husband's point of view?

Additional Resources

Self-Help Sourcebook Online
http://www.cmhc.com/selfhelp/

References

Aldwin, C., Spiro, A., Levenson, M., & Bosse, R. (1989). Longitudinal findings from the normative aging study: Does mental health change with age? *Psychology and Aging, 4,* 295-306.

Arnold, E. (1994). *Portrait of change: Women in the second half of life.* Paper presented at the American Psychological Association Conference on Psychosocial and Behavioral Factors in Women's Health: Creating an Agenda for the 21st Century, Washington, DC.

Atchley, R. (1991). *Social forces and aging* (6th ed.). Belmont, CA: Wadsworth.

Baruch, G., Barnett, R., & Rivers, C. (1983). *Life prints: New patterns of love and work for today's women.* New York: McGraw-Hill.

Bauer, D., & Mott, D. (1990). Life themes and motivations of re-entry students. *Journal of Counseling and Development, 68,* 555-560.

Bellah, R. (1985). *Habits of the heart: Individualism and commitment in American life.* New York: Harper & Row.

Bogin, B. (1988). *Patterns of human growth.* New York: Cambridge University Press.

Bowlby, J. (1977). The making and breaking of affectional bonds. Part I: Aetiology and psychopathology in the light of attachment theory. *British Journal of Psychiatry, 130,* 191-210.

Buhler, C., & Goldenberg, H. (1968). Structural aspects of an individual's history. In C. Buhler & F. Massarik (Eds.), *The course of human life: A study of goals in the humanistic perspective* (pp. 54-63). New York: Springer.

Burke, R., & McKeen, C. (1990). Mentoring in organizations: Implications for women. *Journal of Business Ethics, 9,* 317-332.

Carlsen, M. (1988). *Meaning-making: Therapeutic process in adult development.* New York: Norton.

Clayton, V., & Birren, J. (1980). The development of wisdom across the life span: A reexamination of an ancient topic. In P. B. Baltes & O. G. Brim, Jr. (Eds.), *Life-span development and behavior* (Vol. 3). New York: Academic Press.

Commons, M., Sinnott, J., Richards, F., & Armon, C. (1989). Adult development: Comparisons and applications of developmental models (Vol. 1). New York: Praeger.

Cooper, K., & Gutmann, D. (1987). Gender identity and ego mastery style in middle-aged, pre and postempty nest women. *Gerontologist, 27,* 347-352.

Costa, P., & McCrae, R. (1994). Set like plaster? Evidence for the stability of adult personality. In T. Heatherton & J. Weinberger (Eds.). (1997). *Can personality change?* (pp. 21-40). Washington, DC: American Psychological Association.

Daniels, P., & Weingarten, K. (1982). *Sooner or later: The timing of parenthood in adult lives.* New York: Norton.

Dooley, D., & Catalano, R. (1991). Unemployment as a stressor: Findings and implications of a recent study. *WHO Region Publications European Series, 37,* 313-339.

Douvan, E. (1997). Erik Erikson: Critical times, critical theory. *Child Human Development, 28*(1), 15-21.

Erikson, E. H. (1958). *Young man Luther: A study in psychoanalysis and history.* New York: Norton.

Erikson, E. H. (1969). *Gandhi's truth.* New York: Norton.

Erikson, E. H. (Ed.). (1978). *Adulthood.* New York: Norton.

Erikson, E. H. (1980). *Identity and the life cycle.* New York: Norton.

Erikson, E. H. (1982). *The life cycle completed.* New York: Norton.

Fiske, M., & Chiriboga, D. A. (1990). The interweave of societal and personal change in adulthood. In J. Munnichs, P. Mussen, M. Fiske, & D. Chiriboga (Eds.), *Change and continuity in adult life.* San Francisco, CA: Jossey-Bass.

Gilligan, C. (1982). *In a different voice.* Cambridge, MA: Harvard University Press.

Golombok, S., & Fivush, R. (1994). *Gender development.* New York: Cambridge University Press.

Gottfried, A., Gottfried, A. W., & Bathurst, K. (1988). Maternal employment, family environment and children's development: Infancy through the school years. In A. E. Gottfried & A. W. Gottfried (Eds.), *Maternal employment and children's development: Longitudinal research.* New York: Plenum.

Gould, R. (1975). Adult life stages: Growth towards self-tolerance. *Psychology Today, 8,* 74-78.

Hammerskjöld, D. (1964). *Markings.* (L. Sjöberg & W. H. Auden, Trans.). New York: Knopf.

Havighurst, R. (1953). *Developmental tasks and education.* New York: David McKay.

Havighurst, R. (1973). History of developmental psychology. In P. Baltes & K. Schaie (Eds.), *Life span developmental psychology: Personality and socialization.* New York: Academic Press.

Hawkes, H. (1992). Empowerment in nursing education: Concept analysis and application to philosophy, education and instruction. *Journal of Advanced Nursing, 17,* 609-618.

Hayes, R. (1994). The legacy of Lawrence Kohlberg: Implications for counseling and human development. *Journal of Counseling and Development, 72,* 261-267.

Hoffman, L. (1989). Effects of maternal employment in the two-parent family. *American Psychologist, 44,* 283-292.

James, W. (1981). *The principles of psychology* (Vol. 1). Cambridge, MA: Harvard University Press.

Josselson, R. (1987). *Finding herself: Pathways to identity development in women.* San Francisco, CA: Jossey-Bass.

Jung, C. G. (1969). The stages of life. In H. Read, M. Fordham, & G. Adler (Eds.), *The collected works of C. G. Jung* (R. F. C. Hull, Trans.) (pp. 749-795). Princeton, NJ: Bollingen.

Kalish, R. (1989). *Midlife loss.* Newbury Park, CA: Sage Publications.

Keen, S. (1991). *Fire in the belly: On being a man.* New York: Bantam Books.

Kelly, E., & Rasey, M. (1952). *Education and the nature of man.* New York: Harper.

King, M. L., Jr. (1963, August 23). *I have a dream* [Speech]. Washington, DC.

Kingson, E., Hirshorn, B., & Cornman, J. (Eds.) (1986). *Ties that bind: The interdependence of generations.* Washington, DC: Seven Locks Press.

Kitzinger, C. (1992). The individuated self concept: A critical analysis of social constructionist writing on individualism. In G. Breakwell (Ed.), *Social psychology of identity and the self concept.* London: Surrey University Press.

Kotre, J., & Hall, E. (1990). *Seasons of life.* Boston: Little, Brown.

Ladner, T. (1995, January 15). Generation without a dream: What college students need to know about Martin Luther King, Jr. [Outlook section]. *Washington Post,* p. C-2.

Lane, J. (1987). The care of the human spirit. *Journal of Professional Nursing, 3,* 332-337.

Lerner, R., & Hood, K. (1986). Plasticity in development: Concepts and issues for intervention. *Journal of Applied Developmental Psychology, 7,* 139-152.

Levinson, D., Darrow, C., Klein, E., Levinson, M., & McKee, B. (1978). *The seasons of a man's life.* New York: Knopf.

Love, D., & Torrence W. D. (1989). The impact of worker age on unemployment and earnings after plant closings. *Journal of Gerontology, 44,* 190-195.

Lowenthal, M., & Chiriboga, D. (1972). Transition to the empty nest: Crisis, challenge, or relief? *Archives of General Psychology, 26,* 8-14.

MacKinnon-Slaney, F. (1994). The adult persistence in learning model: A road map to counseling services for adult learners. *Journal of Counseling and Development, 72,* 268-275.

Maslow, A. (1969). Various meanings of transcendence. *Journal of Transpersonal Psychology,* 56-66.

Mercer, R., Nichols, E., & Doyle, G. (1989). *Transitions in a woman's life: Major life events in developmental context.* New York: Springer.

Mezirow, J. (1990). *Fostering critical reflection in adulthood: A guide to transformative and emancipatory education.* San Francisco, CA: Jossey-Bass.

Miller, W., & C'deBaca, J. (1994). Quantum change: Toward a psychology of transformation. In T. Heatherton & J. Weinberger (Eds.), *Can personality change?* Washington, DC: American Psychological Association.

Morrow, R., & McElroy, J. (1987). Work commitment and job satisfaction over three career stages. *Journal of Vocational Behavior, 30,* 330-346.

National Alliance of Business (1996, June). *Workforce Economics Newsletter.*

National Center for Health Statistics (1987). Advance report of final marriage statistics. *Monthly Vital Statistics Report, 36,* 2.

National Center for Health Statistics (1994) and (1995). *Monthly Vital Statistics Report, 23,* 19.

Neugarten, B. (1970). Adaptation and the life cycle. *Journal of Geriatric Psychiatry, 4,* 71-87.

Neugarten, B. (1977). *Middle age and aging.* Chicago: University of Chicago Press.

Neugarten, B., & Neugarten, D. (1986). Age in an aging society. *Daedalus, 115,* 31-49.

Noe, R. (1988). Women and mentoring: A review and research agenda. *Academy of Management Review, 13,* 65-78.

Paludi, M. (1991). Sociophysiological and structural factors related to women's vocational development. *Annals of the New York Academy of Sciences,* 157-168.

Parse, R. R. (1981). *Man-living-health: A theory of nursing.* New York: John Wiley.

Patterson, C. (1992). Children of lesbian and gay parents. *Child Development, 63,* 1020-1042.

Phoenix, A., Woollett, A., & Lloyd, E. (Eds.). (1991). *Motherhood: Meanings, practices and ideologies.* London: Sage Publications.

Reed, P. (1994). Toward a nursing theory of self-transcendence: Deductive reformulation using developmental theories. In P. Chinn (Ed.), *Developing substance: Mid-range theory in nursing.* Gaithersburg, MD: Aspen. (Reprinted from *Advances in Nursing Science,* 64-77.)

Regan-Smith, M. G. (1998). Teachers' experiential learning about learning. *International Journal of Psychiatry in Medicine, 28*(1), 11-19.

Rogers, M. (1970). *An introduction to the theoretical basis of nursing.* Philadelphia: F. A. Davis.

Samuels, S. C. (1997). Midlife crisis: Helping patients cope with stress, anxiety and depression. *Geriatrics, 52*(7), 55-56.

Sheehey, G. (1976). *Passages: Predictable crises of adult life.* New York: Dutton.

Sheehey, G. (1981). *Pathfinders.* New York: Dutton.

Sheehey, G. (1993). *The silent passage: Menopause.* New York: Dutton.

Staube, J. (1981). *The adult development of C. G. Jung.* Boston: Routledge & Kegan Paul.

Thurnher, M. (1983). Turning points and developmental change: Subjective and "objective" assessments. *American Journal of Orthopsychiatry, 53,* 52-60.

Tournier, P. (1957). *The meaning of persons.* London: SCM Publishers.

Tournier, P. (1965). *The adventure of living.* New York: Harper & Row.

U.S. Senate Special Committee on Aging (1989).

Vaillant, G. (1977). *Adaptation to life.* Boston: Little, Brown.

Vandewater, E. A., Ostrove, J. M., & Steward, A. J. (1997). Predicting women's well-being in midlife: The importance of personality development and social role involvements. *Journal of Personality and Social Psychology, 72*(5), 1147–1160.

Whitehead, A. N. (1929). *The aims of education.* New York: Macmillan.

Wicks, R. J. (1985). *Touching the holy: Ordinariness, self-esteem, and friendship.* Notre Dame, IN: Ave Maria Press.

Suggested Readings

Bellah, R. (1985). *Habits of the heart: Individualism and commitment in American life.* New York: Harper & Row.

Gilligan, C. (1982). *In a different voice.* Cambridge, MA: Harvard University Press.

Levinson, D., Darrow, C., Klein, E., Levinson, M., & McKee, B. (1978). *The seasons of a man's life.* New York: Knopf.

Sheehey, G. (1976). *Passages: Predictable crises of adult life.* New York: Dutton.

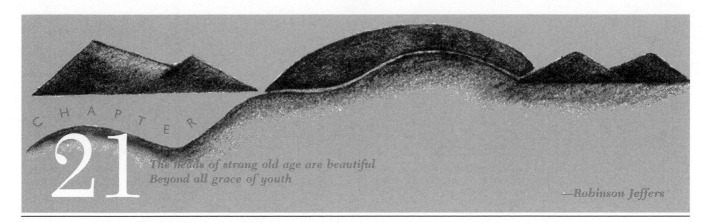

C H A P T E R

21

The heads of strong old age are beautiful
Beyond all grace of youth

—*Robinson Jeffers*

The Older Adult

Learning Objectives

After studying this chapter, you should be able to:

1. Describe facts about the aging population.
2. Describe normal mental health in late life.
3. List age-related changes.
4. Recognize factors that affect mental health assessment of the elderly.
5. Discuss developmental tasks of late life.
6. Identify risks and signs associated with depression in the elderly.
7. Discuss the symptoms, causes, and differentiation of delirium and dementia.
8. Describe unique features of anxiety and schizophrenia in older patients.
9. List basic measures to promote mental health in late life.
10. Apply the nursing process to a patient experiencing normal changes associated with the aging process.

Key Terminology

Ageism	Dementia	Old-old	Vigilance performance
Crystallized intelligence	Developmental tasks	Reminiscence	Young-old
Delirium	Fluid intelligence	Sundown syndrome	

More than 31 million Americans are older than 65 years of age, and most can be found living relatively normal lives in the community. They shop, maintain their households, pay their bills, and face the same stresses of daily life as adults of any age. They also face, to a greater degree than younger people, added stresses such as loss of loved ones, reduced income, forfeited roles, impaired function, and chronic illness. The road traveled in late life indeed can be a rocky one to navigate. The roads already journeyed, however, do give older travelers the added skill and strength required to face these challenges. Let us take a look at Mary Baxter's story for a glimpse of an elderly woman successfully navigating this part of life's journey.

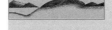 Mary's Story

Mary Baxter enjoys the warmth of the sun as she leisurely carries her groceries to the parking lot of the shopping center. She realizes that she once again has forgotten where she parked her car and wonders if this is a sign of a failing memory. "Well, I can't blame that on being 72," she chuckles to herself. "I've always had trouble remembering where I left the car."

Grocery shopping was particularly enjoyable today because she bought the food for the Sunday dinner she would prepare for her children and grandchildren. She has appreciated that her son and daughter live in communities that border the apartment complex in which she lives and that they feel free to drop in frequently. She has been equally glad to have her own space and to be able to spend time with her very active grandchildren on her own terms.

As she packs the groceries into her trunk, she notices a very impatient driver waiting for her parking space. Mary feels pressured and embarrassed that her lack of speed is causing inconvenience to another person. She nervously backs her car from the space at a faster pace than she would normally drive and is reminded of how she dislikes driving. Before her husband's death 4 years ago, she was always the pampered passenger. Her husband used to preheat the car before she entered it, open and close her door, chauffeur her to the front door of her destination . . . the little niceties that she misses. They now serve as daily reminders of the caring relationship she and her husband shared. She is getting on with her life and adequately taking care of herself, but the little things that are no longer shared with her husband remind her of the void that no amount of bus trips or bridge games can fill.

Mary reflects on that "horrible year of existence," her 1st year of widowhood. Her husband's sudden death left her unprepared for the adjustments she would need to make after devoting 47 years to being a wife and mother. She recalls the emptiness in her heart that she was unable to express to anyone. The seemingly pointless act of preparing a meal for one person caused her to skip meals and lose weight; rolling over in her sleep to find an empty space caused her to awaken and spend the remainder of the night watching television. Her physician saw the fatigue and weight loss and was quick to prescribe vitamins and sleeping pills, but the gnawing sadness and feeling that her life was in limbo did not leave her for more than a year. She thinks of her 90-year-old mother, now living in a nursing home, who was widowed at age 45, and wonders how she coped. "Time heals all," she thinks.

Mary feels fortunate that except for a little arthritis and farsightedness, she has good health and can take care of herself. She wonders about her own death, weighing the benefits of a sudden death like her husband's to dying gradually over a long period as she observes her mother doing. She prays that God will spare her the agony of a long life filled with pain and dependency and allow her to leave this world with dignity and some control over her circumstances. In the interim, she faces life 1 day at a time. ■

FACTS ABOUT THE OLDER POPULATION

Mary Baxter is hardly an unusual example of today's older adult; however, today's elderly are a diverse group. No longer do general descriptions about the "old popu-

lation" apply. The old can encompass healthy, active people like Mary Baxter and frail, dependent individuals, such as Mary's mother. In fact, the older population is now divided into subpopulations: the **young-old,** who are younger than age 75, and the **old-old,** who are age 75 and older. Each of these populations presents unique needs. For instance, the young-old may seek nursing assistance for guidance with health maintenance, retirement counseling, exercise programs, parent care, sexual adjustments, and selection of cosmetic surgeons. The old-old may desire assistance with administering medications, using assistive devices, selecting alternative housing, and thinking through advance directives (living will, document expressing individual's desires for care at a later time). (Of course, as every good nurse understands, individual differences within each subgroup reinforce the importance of astute assessment.) The age 75 and older population has been the fastest growing segment of the population, and this trend will continue, causing us to see more old-old people in society. The increasing prevalence of some mental illnesses accompanying age speaks to the increased need for geropsychiatric nursing services in the future.

Although the average life expectancy is 75.7 years for the total population, differences do exist between the genders and races. As Table 21–1 shows, women outlive men, resulting in a decrease in the ratio of males to females over the years. And although life expectancy has shown a steady increase for the white population, recent years have shown a decrease in life expectancy for black men and, to a lesser extent, a decrease for black women also.

Like Mary Baxter, most older women are widowed, whereas most older men have surviving spouses. The death of a spouse—and the emotional, financial, social, and sexual issues that result—offers opportunities for nursing intervention.

Women are more likely than men to be living alone, and a greater percentage of both genders are living alone than with their children (Table 21–2). About half of the elderly live within 25 miles of their children and have weekly contact with them. For both the elderly and their offspring, the arrangement of separate but close homes is preferable. Children do assist their elder parents with a variety of chores, and in turn they receive financial aid, child-rearing assistance, and emotional support.

Because of the "graying of America," more families are involved with caregiving of an elderly relative than ever before in history. An estimated 13.5 million, slightly more than 7% of the adult population, have disabled elderly parents or spouses at home or in an institution. Family members, not formal agencies, provide most care

TABLE 21–1 Life Expectancy in Years		
	MALE	**FEMALE**
White	73.0	79.1
Black	65.6	74.3

From U.S. Department of Commerce. (1993). *Statistical abstract of the United States* (113th ed., p. 85). Washington, DC: Bureau of the Census.

TABLE 21–2 Living Arrangements of Adults Age 65 Years and Older

	TOTAL (%)	MEN (%)	WOMEN (%)
Living alone	31.1	16.2	40.6
Living with spouse	54.5	75.1	39.9
Living with other relative	12.8	6.7	17.2
Living with nonrelative	2.3	2.1	2.4

From U.S. Department of Commerce. (1993). *Statistical abstract of the United States* (113th ed., p. 45). Washington, DC: Bureau of the Census.

to the elderly. In every clinical setting, nurses are involved with families of elders and must be prepared to offer interventions to promote the health of the entire family. (See Chapters 13 and 14 for more information on working with families.)

Although the rates for infections and injuries decline through the adult years, the rates of chronic illnesses significantly increase. In addition to the physical symptoms and caregiving demands imposed by these disorders, chronic illnesses can threaten mental health. For instance, the frustration of living with an incurable illness can cause depression. Uncertainty about the impact of the condition on roles, function, and life expectancy can produce anxiety. Furthermore, physiological disturbances caused by the illness can threaten homeostasis, resulting in delirium. The mind-body relationship is a significant concern for the chronically ill elderly. Psychiatric nurses must distinguish between common and pathological changes that occur with age (Table 21–3). You also need to identify unique

TABLE 21–3 Common Aging Changes

BODY SYSTEM	MANIFESTATIONS
Cardiovascular	Thickening and rigidity of heart valves Rise in aortic volume and systolic blood pressure Reduced cardiac output and efficiency Increased peripheral resistance Thickening and fragility of capillary walls
Pulmonary	Increased rigidity of lungs Decreased vital capacity and maximum breathing capacity Reduction in number and elasticity of alveoli Decreased ciliary activity Weaker thoracic muscles
Gastrointestinal	Increased prevalence of periodontal disease Reduced saliva production Increase in taste threshold, primarily affecting sweet and salty flavors Weaker gag reflex Reduced hunger contractions Decreased peristalsis
Genitourinary	Reduction in renal mass, glomerular filtration rate, renal blood flow, tubular function Decreased bladder capacity Hypertrophy of prostate gland Decreased testosterone production, sperm count, size of testes Decreased estrogen production, breast tissue, size of uterus Drier, more fragile vaginal canal
Musculoskeletal	Decreased muscle mass, strength, movement Increased brittleness of bones Deterioration of cartilage surface of joints
Neurological-Sensory	Decreased nerve cells, nerve conduction velocity, kinesthetic sense Presbyopia, narrowing of visual field, smaller pupil size, opacity and yellowing of lens Reduced lacrimal secretions Presbycusis Increased threshold for pain and touch Decreased olfaction
Integumentary	Reduced elasticity and moisture of skin Thinning of scalp, pubic, and axillary hair Slower growth of fingernails

symptoms (Box 21–1) and responses to treatment for physical health problems in the elderly.

> **W**hat do you think? Reflect on your experience with the elderly. How would you describe the elderly you know? Are they vibrant, healthy, and fully engaged in living? Are they confused, dependent, and physically debilitated? Do they represent a mix of both extremes? How would you describe your attitudes toward the elderly?

➤ *Check Your Reading*
   1. Why is it significant to subcategorize the elderly population?
   2. What differences in life expectancy exist between the genders and races?

DEVELOPMENTAL TASKS OF AGING

The path to old age is filled with unexpected twists and turns. Some parts of this adventure are filled with delightful new experiences, such as becoming a grandparent and exploring creative interests. The journey also includes obstacles and rocky roads, however, such as losing loved ones and adjusting to chronic illnesses. The challenges faced and adjustments made to achieve a sense of psychological and social well-being in late life are referred to as **developmental tasks.** Developmental tasks are part of an adult's continued growth through the life span and include (Eliopoulos, 1991)

   1. *Coping with losses and changes:* Development of health problems, meeting demands of chronic illness, retirement, decreased income, death of loved ones, change in residence

Box 21–1 ■ ■ ■ ■ ■
Differences in Presentation of Physical Illness in Late Life

Fever: Lower basal metabolic rate causes lower normal body temperature; febrile conditions are apparent at lower temperature levels than would occur with younger adults.

Pain: Altered pain sensations can result in little correlation between severity of problem and pain experienced; pain can be referred.

Cough: Reduced cough efficiency can result in significant accumulation of secretions in lungs without productive cough.

Confusion: Older adults are more likely to have impaired cognition as a result of many physical illnesses.

   2. *Establishing meaningful roles:* Redefining parent-child roles, entering a health care institution, grandparenting
   3. *Exercising independence and control:* Maximizing capabilities in light of disabilities, making decisions regarding self, dependent loved ones, lifestyle, and plans for the future
   4. *Finding meaning in life:* Balancing current limitations against a full life lived, reflecting on past accomplishments, leaving a legacy, connecting with others, growing spiritually

An outline of several theorists' views on development during aging is provided in Box 21–2.

You can facilitate good mental health in late life by assisting patients with the tasks of aging. Some basic measures include

   1. Making a sincere effort to learn about the patient, including family, background, work history, hobbies, and achievements.
   2. Listen with sincere interest.
   3. Encourage discussions of past events.
   4. Build on lifelong interests.
   5. Offer suggestions for meaningful family activities.
   6. Use humor therapeutically.
   7. Personalize the caregiving environment.
   8. Encourage maximum independence and decision-making.
   9. Emphasize capabilities and minimize limitations.

This act of recalling and reflecting on life experiences is a frequently observed behavior among older adults. Rather than an unhealthy process, reminiscing can be used therapeutically to help older adults achieve a sense of psychosocial and spiritual well-being. Box 21–3 includes a life review tool designed by Barbara Haight specifically to assist the elderly in the **reminiscence** process. You can help older people to

- Resolve unsettled issues.
- Appreciate the significance of their lives.
- Reaffirm their self-worth and identity.

Often, current stresses can be put into perspective and managed effectively when seen in the context of one's total life.

The regular, direct contact that nursing staff members have with older adults puts them in an ideal position to use reminiscence as a psychosocial intervention. Often, reminiscence can be an approach to interactions rather than a time-specific intervention. During routine interactions with patients, you can ask memory-evoking questions:

- What were styles like when you were young?
- What was it like for you to immigrate to America?
- What was the best holiday you can remember?

Show sincere interest and listen when patients talk about the past. Accept and validate feelings; for example, if someone like Mary Baxter becomes tearful discussing her husband's death, you might comment, "The loss of your husband must have been very painful for you." This statement could assist in triggering further

Box 21–2 ■ ■ ■ ■ ■
Major Developmental Theories of Aging

Erikson's Stages of Development

Erikson believed that individuals continue with the seven previous stages of psychological development as they age:
1. Trust versus mistrust
2. Autonomy versus shame
3. Initiative versus guilt
4. Industry versus inferiority
5. Identity versus identity confusion
6. Intimacy versus isolation
7. Generativity versus stagnation
8. The last stage, ego integrity versus despair, he viewed as the task in old age, in which the individual accepts his or her life as having been whole and satisfying to achieve ego integrity. Dissatisfaction and regrets with the life one has lived can lead to a sense of despair and disgust.

Peck's Tasks in Old Age

Peck identified three tasks faced in old age:
1. Ego differentiation versus work-role preoccupation: Developing satisfactions
2. Body transcendence versus body preoccupation: Finding psychological pleasures
3. Ego transcendence versus ego preoccupation: Feeling pleasure through reflecting on one's life rather than dwelling on the limited number of years left to live

Havighurst's Tasks of Aging

Havighurst described the following tasks of aging individuals:
1. Adjusting to decreased strength and health status
2. Maintaining involvement with friends and society
3. Establishing satisfactory living arrangements
4. Readjusting lifestyle to reduced income and retirement
5. Coping with the death of the spouse

Butler's Tasks of Late Life

Butler viewed the major tasks of late life as follows:
1. Adjusting to one's infirmities
2. Developing a sense of satisfaction with the life that has been lived
3. Preparing for death

Reprinted with permission from Eliopoulos, C. (1991). *Developmental tasks of aging (Long-term care educator,* Vol. 2, Lesson 6, p. 4). Glen Arm, MD: Health Education Network.

reflection. (See Chapter 10 for assistance with communication techniques to promote reminiscing.)

NORMAL MENTAL HEALTH IN LATE LIFE

Most people do not become child-like, rigid, cantankerous, or mentally incompetent as they age. Nor do they become wise, sedate, or more creative. Generally, under normal circumstances, their mental status is a reflection of the lifelong pattern: those who demonstrated high intellectual function in youth are likely to be the elders who find pleasure in the *New York Times* crossword puzzles. Those who were loners when young are unlikely to be gregarious club joiners during their senior years. The mental profile of older adults is diverse. General intellectual capacity does not decline with age, although some specific functions do demonstrate change. **Fluid intelligence,** which controls emotions, retention of nonintellectual information, creativity, spatial perceptions, and aesthetic appreciation, is thought to decline with age. **Crystallized intelligence,** involving the use of past learning and experiences for problem solving is maintained throughout adulthood.

Learning ability is maintained, although more time is needed for the early phases of the learning process. After a longer early phase, the elderly are able to learn at an equal pace with the young. **Vigilance performance,** the ability to retain information longer than 45 minutes, declines in old age. Older adults are more easily distracted by irrelevant information and stimuli and have a reduced ability to perform tasks that are complicated or demand simultaneous performance. Retrieval of information stored in long-term memory is slower. Mnemonic devices and other memory aids can improve some of this forgetfulness.

Drastic changes in personality are uncommon. If anything, people more openly express the personality they always had. Significant changes in personality can indicate a pathological process. Attitude, morals, and self-esteem tend to be stable through the life span.

The incidence of mental illness is higher among the old than the young. An estimated 25% of the elderly in the community and 50% of those in nursing homes have symptoms of mental illness (Eliopoulos, 1997). Almost 15% of the elderly have a problem with alcoholism. Approximately 65% of people admitted to nursing homes have Alzheimer's disease. Depression increases in prevalence with age, and suicide is considerably more common among older adults, particularly elderly white men, than other age groups.

W*hat do you think?* Have you ever listened to an elderly person reminisce? If so, what was your response to this person's walk down memory lane? Knowing what you know about the value of reminiscence, how can you use reminiscence to facilitate your journey with the patient? How is reminiscence a spiritual activity?

Box 21-3 ■■■■■■

Childhood

1. What is the very first thing you can remember in your life? Go back as far as you can.
2. What other things can you remember about when you were very young?
3. What was life like for you as a child?
4. What were your parents like? What were their weaknesses, strengths?
5. Did you have any brothers or sisters? Tell me what each was like.
6. Did someone close to you die when you were growing up?
7. Did someone important to you go away?
8. Do you ever remember being very sick?
9. Do you remember having an accident?
10. Do you remember being in a very dangerous situation?
11. Was there anything that was important to you that was lost or destroyed?
12. Was church a large part of your life?
13. Did you enjoy being a boy/girl?

Adolescence

1. When you think about yourself and your life as a teenager, what is the first thing you can remember about that time?
2. What other things stand out in your memory about being a teenager?
3. Who were the important people for you? Tell me about them. Parents, brothers, sisters, friends, teachers, those you were especially close to, those you admired, those you wanted to be like.
4. Did you attend church and youth groups?
5. Did you go to school? What was the meaning for you?
6. Did you work during these years?
7. Tell me of any hardships you experienced at this time.
8. Do you remember feeling that there wasn't enough food or necessities of life as a child or adolescent?
9. Do you remember feeling left alone, abandoned, not having enough love or care as a child or adolescent?
10. What were the pleasant things about your adolescence?
11. What was the most unpleasant thing about your adolescence?
12. All things considered, would you say you were happy or unhappy as a teenager?
13. Do you remember your first attraction to another person?
14. How did you feel about sexual activities and your own sexual identity?

Family and Home

1. How did your parents get along?
2. How did other people in your home get along?
3. What was the atmosphere in your home?
4. Were you punished as a child? For what? Who did the punishing? Who was "boss"?
5. When you wanted something from your parents, how did you go about getting it?
6. What kind of a person did your parents like the most? The least?
7. Who were you closest to in your family?
8. Who in your family were you most like? In what way?

Adulthood

1. What place did religion play in your life?
2. Now I'd like to talk to you about your life as an adult, starting when you were in your twenties up to today. Tell me of the most important events that happened in your adulthood.
3. What was life like for you in your twenties and thirties?
4. What kind of person were you? What did you enjoy?
5. Tell me about your work. Did you enjoy your work? Did you earn an adequate living? Did you work hard during those years? Were you appreciated?
6. Did you form significant relationships with other people?
7. Did you marry?
   (yes) What kind of person was your spouse?
   (no) Why not?
8. Do you think marriages get better or worse over time? Were you married more than once?
9. On the whole, would you say you had a happy or unhappy marriage?
10. Was sexual intimacy important to you?
11. What were some of the main difficulties you encountered during your adult years?
    a. Did someone close to you die? Go away?
    b. Were you ever sick? Have an accident?
    c. Did you move often? Change jobs?
    d. Did you ever feel alone? Abandoned?
    e. Did you ever feel need?

Summary

1. On the whole, what kind of life do you think you've had?
2. If everything were to be the same would you like to live your life over again?
3. If you were going to live your life over again, what would you change? Leave unchanged?
4. We've been talking about your life for quite some time now. Let's discuss your overall feelings and ideas about your life. What would you say the main satisfactions in your life have been? Try for three. Why were they satisfying?
5. Everyone has had disappointments. What have been the main disappointments in your life?

Box 21–3 ▪ ▪ ▪ ▪ ▪
Haight's Life Review and Experiencing Form *Continued*

6. What was the hardest thing you had to face in your life? Please describe it.
7. What was the happiest period of your life? What about it made it the happiest period? Why is your life less happy now?
8. What was the unhappiest period of your life? Why is your life more happy now?
9. What was the proudest moment in your life?
10. If you could stay the same age all your life, what age would you choose? Why?
11. How do you think you've made out in life? Better or worse than what you hoped for?

12. Let's talk a little about you as you are now. What are the best things about the age you are now?
13. What are the worst things about the age you are now?
14. What are the most important things to you in your life today?
15. What do you hope will happen to you as you grow older?
16. What do you fear will happen to you as you grow older?
17. Have you enjoyed participating in this review of your life?

Note: Questionnaire derived from new questions and two unpublished dissertations: Falk, J. (1969). *The organization of remembered life experience of older people: Its relation to anticipated stress, to subsequent adaptation and to age.* Unpublished doctoral dissertation, University of Chicago and Gorney, J. (1968). *Experiencing and age: Patterns of reminiscence among the elderly.* Unpublished doctoral dissertation, University of Chicago.
©1982 Barbara K. Haight, RNC, DrPH, Professor of Nursing, College of Nursing, Medical University of South Carolina, Charleston, SC 29425-2404. Used by permission.

► *Check Your Reading*
3. Describe the developmental tasks of late life.
4. What measures can you incorporate into routine nursing activities to facilitate reminiscence?
5. List major changes in mental function that occur with age.

PSYCHIATRIC DISORDERS IN THE ELDERLY

Depression

Depression increases in prevalence with age and is the most common psychiatric problem treated in the elderly. Obvious factors that cause the elderly to be at risk for depression are the multiple losses experienced with age (e.g., loved ones, income, roles, health, function, youthful appearance). Many chronic illnesses common among older persons are known to be accompanied by depression. These include cerebrovascular accident, chronic obstructive lung disease, Parkinson's disease, cancer, congestive heart failure, and multiple sclerosis. Drugs also may be a cause of depression. Depression may be associated with the age-related diminished production of mood-controlling neurotransmitters.

Signs of depression in the elderly are similar to those in younger adults (see Chapter 22 for discussion of loss and Chapter 25 for discussion of depression). However, poor grooming practices, slower movements, stooped posture, somatic complaints, reduced activity patterns, and other signs that would raise suspicion of depression in other age groups, may be overlooked in the elderly or attributed to physical health problems. Box 21–4 includes the Geriatric Depression Scale, a tool that eliminates somatic questions found on other depression inventories, the questions being designed with a yes-no response structure rather than a Likert scale to facilitate responses by the elderly.

You must look for even subtle clues of depression in the elderly and refer the patient for psychiatric evaluation in a timely manner. The basic care of the older depressed individual is similar to that for depressed adults of any age. Treatment includes psychotherapy and antidepressants. You should ensure that older depressed patients are afforded the full range of treatment options available. Support groups, financial assistance, and community resources can be especially helpful to patients with reactive depressions (those caused in response to situations such as change in income, death of loved one, relocation).

You can further assist older depressed patients by having frequent direct contact with them. Contact can be difficult because the behaviors of depressed patients—silence, slow response, pessimism, and irritability—can make caregivers uncomfortable. However, the need for human contact is important. Sitting in silence and using touch with depressed persons can be particularly important. You should encourage the open expression of feelings.

Monitoring the physical status of older depressed patients is particularly important because older people have a smaller margin of safety in the development of complications. Areas to observe include food and fluid intake, bowel elimination, and quality and quantity of sleep. Weight should be assessed frequently; weight changes of 5% or greater are significant for older adults. Pay attention to promoting a good physical state, which strengthens the patient's ability to work through depression.

Because suicide is a significant risk for the older depressed individual, be alert to clues to suicide. Note any sudden interest in putting affairs in order, giving away

B o x 2 1 – 4 ■ ■ ■ ■ ■
Geriatric Depression Scale

Choose the best answer for how you felt this past week.

° 1. Are you basically satisfied with your life? ....Yes No
2. Have you dropped many of your activities and interests? ....Yes No
3. Do you feel that your life is empty? ....Yes No
4. Do you often get bored? ....Yes No
° 5. Are you hopeful about the future? ....Yes No
6. Are you bothered by thoughts you can't get out of your head? ....Yes No
° 7. Are you in good spirits most of the time? ....Yes No
8. Are you afraid that something bad is going to happen to you? ....Yes No
° 9. Do you feel happy most of the time? ....Yes No
10. Do you often feel helpless? ....Yes No
11. Do you often get restless and fidgety? ....Yes No
12. Do you prefer to stay at home, rather than going out and doing new things? ....Yes No
13. Do you frequently worry about the future? ....Yes No
14. Do you feel you have more problems with memory than most? ....Yes No
° 15. Do you think it is wonderful to be alive now? ....Yes No

16. Do you feel downhearted and blue? ....Yes No
17. Do you feel pretty worthless the way you are now? ....Yes No
18. Do you worry a lot about the past? ....Yes No
° 19. Do you find life very exciting? ....Yes No
20. Is it hard for you to get started on new projects? ....Yes No
° 21. Do you feel full of energy? ....Yes No
22. Do you feel that your situation is hopeless? ....Yes No
23. Do you think that most people are better off than you are? ....Yes No
24. Do you frequently get upset over little things? ....Yes No
25. Do you frequently feel like crying? ....Yes No
26. Do you have trouble concentrating? ....Yes No
° 27. Do you enjoy getting up in the morning? ....Yes No
28. Do you prefer to avoid social gatherings? ....Yes No
° 29. Is it easy for you to make decisions? ....Yes No
° 30. Is your mind as clear as it used to be? ....Yes No

Score: _____ (Number of "depressed" answers)

Scoring key: The starred questions(*) should have a "yes" response. Count the number of "no's" from these. The remainder of the questions should be "no." Count the number of "yes" answers from these.
  Add the two scores together and interpret:
    Normal   0–10
    Mildly depressed   11–17
    Very depressed   >17
  From Yesavage, J. A., Brink, T. L., Rose, T. L., Lum, D., Huang, V., Adey, M., & Levier, V. O. (1982). Development and validation of a geriatric depression screening scale: A preliminary report agent. *Journal of Psychiatric Research,* *17*(1), 37–49.

possessions, self-neglect, hoarding medications, personality and behavioral changes, and comments alluding to ending one's life.

What do you think? What would you say to someone who described an elderly person as irritable, disheveled, hard to talk to, and sad and who concluded, "Well, what do you expect? He's 75."

➤ *Check Your Reading*
6. List subtle clues of depression that the older patient can exhibit.
7. Describe physical care considerations for the older depressed individual.

Delirium and Dementia

In the past, confusion in older individuals was not a cause for concern. Many practitioners considered a decline in intellectual function to be a normal outcome of aging and did nothing to evaluate or treat this finding. The result of this misunderstanding was that many older people with reversible confusional states did not receive the benefit of treatment and were unnecessarily subjected to serious complications, low levels of function, and poor quality of life. Fortunately, today's practitioners now recognize confusional states to be associated with pathological conditions and manage this finding more competently. (See Chapter 33 for a comprehensive discussion of cognitive disorders.)

A variety of conditions can lead to **delirium,** an acute cognitive impairment. Many of the potential causes of delirium, such as dehydration and infection, are common among the elderly. Thus, delirium is not a stranger to geriatric practice. In fact, altered cognition can be the first symptom apparent with pneumonia, dehydration, and other health problems in old age. Symptoms of delirium in the elderly typically appear abruptly and include

1. Disturbed intellectual function
2. Disorientation
3. Altered attention span
4. Poor memory
5. Labile mood
6. Meaningless chatter
7. Poor judgment
8. Altered level of consciousness

Shortness of breath, fatigue, and slower psychomotor activities are some of the physical signs that can accompany behavioral changes. Disturbances in sleep–wake cycles also can occur.

Identification and correction of the cause are essential to correcting the delirium. Acute confusion is reversible if treated promptly. The risk is that signs of confusion in older patients can be accepted as "normal," thereby delaying diagnosis and treatment. Confusion is particularly common in the acute care setting; some studies have indicated that nearly 7 in 10 elderly patients who become confused while hospitalized do not have their confusion identified by physicians and nurses (Foreman, 1990). The problem is compounded if the symptoms are treated rather than the cause (e.g., administering a tranquilizer to a patient who is hypervigilant as a result of the delirium rather than correcting the disturbance that caused the delirium).

A good history and evaluation of cognitive function are essential to recognizing the acute cognitive disorder of delirium. Failure to recognize the underlying cause not only allows altered mental function to continue but also risks ignoring a physical condition that could seriously threaten the elder patient.

Dementia is a serious chronic mental disorder. The nurse may play a significant role in ensuring that signs of confusion are recognized and evaluated in a timely manner. On first glance, patients with delirium and dementia appear to share similar symptoms. Both can demonstrate altered cognition and abnormal behaviors. Careful assessment, however, soon reveals the differences that separate these two conditions. The history of patients with delirium describes an abrupt onset of symptoms, whereas the history of patients with dementia indicates subtle, progressive development of symptoms over a long period. Even close family members may report having missed clues of dementia for extended periods because they may have blamed forgetfulness, inattention to self-care, and eccentric behaviors on advanced age. Also, assessment reveals some altered level of consciousness with delirium, whereas with dementia, the level of consciousness is unchanged.

Although the nursing care of dementia patients is covered in Chapter 33, some helpful tips are noted in this chapter for the care of the elderly with altered cognition (see Home Care Clinical Practice Guidelines—Dementia). Many age-related changes (e.g., changes in vision and hearing, slower responses) increase the risk for accidental injuries in the elderly. This problem is significantly compounded when the older adult has impaired cognition. Be attentive to protecting the patient by ensuring that hazardous or noningestible substances and medications are kept out of the patient's sight. Ensure that doors are alarmed to signal the patient's exit. Cap electrical outlets and designate a supervised, safe area for walking and wandering.

Pay special attention to the basic physical needs of the elderly who experience altered cognition. Patients who are restless and who wander require a higher caloric intake to meet needs. Encouragement at mealtimes, nutritional supplements, and easy-to-eat foods can promote intake. Monthly weights should be obtained; weight losses greater than 5% of total body weight are significant and warrant daily weight monitoring. Elimination patterns also should be monitored. Patients with altered cognition are likely to be unreliable historians of their bowel elimination patterns, and feces could become impacted if such patients are left to report their own constipation. Because these patients are less likely to notice and report rashes, lesions, masses, and other problems, inspect their entire skin surfaces regularly.

Promoting maximum independence is a desirable caregiving goal in all circumstances but can be particularly challenging when patients are cognitively impaired. Maximize existing function through basic nursing measures:

1. Affording ample time for the completion of tasks
2. Breaking tasks into simple steps
3. Guiding patients through activities by using one-stage commands
4. Giving clear, simple directions
5. Orienting patients to reality
6. Adhering to a consistent routine
7. Maintaining a stable environment

Some persons with impaired cognitive function display symptoms such as disorientation, agitation, and wandering as evening approaches, a condition referred to as **sundown syndrome** (because it manifests when the sun goes down). Although the cause is not fully understood, factors that contribute to sundown syndrome include recent relocation (e.g., admission to a health care facility), dehydration, sensory overload or deprivation, sleep disturbances, and change in circadian rhythms. Reducing a pronounced transition from day to night by keeping the room lighted can aid in preventing this syndrome. Also, keep familiar objects in the patient's view, make frequent contact, offer toileting assistance, and provide ample fluids.

Families need instruction in basic care techniques. Do not assume family caregivers understand how to feed, lift, or control inappropriate behaviors safely.

An altered state of cognition jeopardizes the patient's ability to make competent decisions. Even when confusion is time limited, as when delirium occurs secondary

Home Care Clinical Practice Guidelines–Dementia
THE ELDERLY ADULT (65+ YEARS)

Comprehensive Assessment Physical/Psychosocial/Spiritual
- Mental Status Assessment
- Depression Inventory
- Mini-Mental Status Assessment Tool
- Other Assessment Tools as Appropriate to Determine Delirium, Dementia (Alzheimer's), Depression (or Pseudo Depression)

Eligible
- Medical Clearance
- Suicidal–Passive Only
- With Support Person– Preferred

Admitted to Restore™ In-Home Mental Health Program

Referral to a Psychiatric Home Care Program

Pre-Admission Screening
- Physical Examination
- Psychiatric Hx

Ineligible
- Medical Complications
- Suicidal–Active

Establish Plan of Care

Standards of Practice are based on the ANA Standards for Psychiatric & Mental Health Nursing

Areas marked ☑ are mandatory for diagnosis

Health Status Assessment

Establish Measurable Outcomes

Assessment

Cardiovascular
- ○ ☑ Obtain complete set of vital signs, including sitting and standing blood pressure (hypotension)

Neurological/Psychological
Assess for:
- ○ ☑ Anxiety
- ○ ☑ Depressed mood (or pseudo depression)
- ○ ☑ Suicidal ideation
- ○ ☑ Orientation (person, place and time)
- ○ ☑ Psychosis (hallucination and delusions)
- ○ ☑ Somatization, i.e., headache, malaise, backaches
- ○ ☑ Sleep disturbance (notify nurse and/or physician if patient is awake all night)
- ○ ☑ Poor judgment, irritability, inappropriate behavior (particularly with dementia)
- ○ ☑ Major personality changes (dementia)

Neurologic
- ○ Loss of memory function (amnesia)
- ○ Loss of ability to understand the spoken/written word or inability to speak (aphasia)
- ○ Loss of ability to perform remembered motor tasks (apraxia)
- ○ Loss of ability to remember what things look like (agnosia)

Autonomic
- ○ Impaired or loss of motor tasks

Self Care Knowledge

Establish Measurable Outcomes

Patient/Caregiver Education

Medication Regimen
- ○ ☑ Response, side effects, compliance and schedule
- ○ ☑ Written materials provided

Caregiver/Social Support
- ○ ☑ Teach caregiver/family in appropriate level of patient care
- ○ ☑ Identify relative, friends and neighbors for support
- ○ ☑ Assist with location of support group to provide an outlet to express anger/ feelings of burden
- ○ ☑ Teach on the importance of structure for the patient's daily activities
- ○ ☑ Teach about effective communication and limit setting with patient

Emotional/Spiritual
As appropriate, encourage:
- ○ Expression of feelings
- ○ Supportive and non-judgmental approach
- ○ Spiritual interventions
- ○ Patient/family interactions
- ○ Empathetic approach
- ○ Validation of normalization of feelings
- ○ Written materials provided
- ○ Home management

Lifestyle and Compliance
- ○ Caregiver to communicate face to face with simple, direct statements
- ○ Maintain familiar objects in environment (calendars, clocks)
- ○ Caregiver to be taught about safety (night lights)
- ○ Caregiver to approach patient with a tolerant, calm, matter-of-fact attitude

Emergency Measures
- ○ Access 911/EMS
- ○ Access psychiatric nurse

Household Resources
- ○ Someone to stay with patient at all times

Home Safety
- ○ ☑ Remove safety risks in home for the prevention of falls
- ○ ☑ Remove any outdated drugs

(Continued on next page)

Home care clinical practice guidelines for the elderly adult with dementia. (From Staff Builders Home Health Care, Staff Builders, Inc, 1983 Marcus Avenue, Lake Success, NY 11042-7011.)

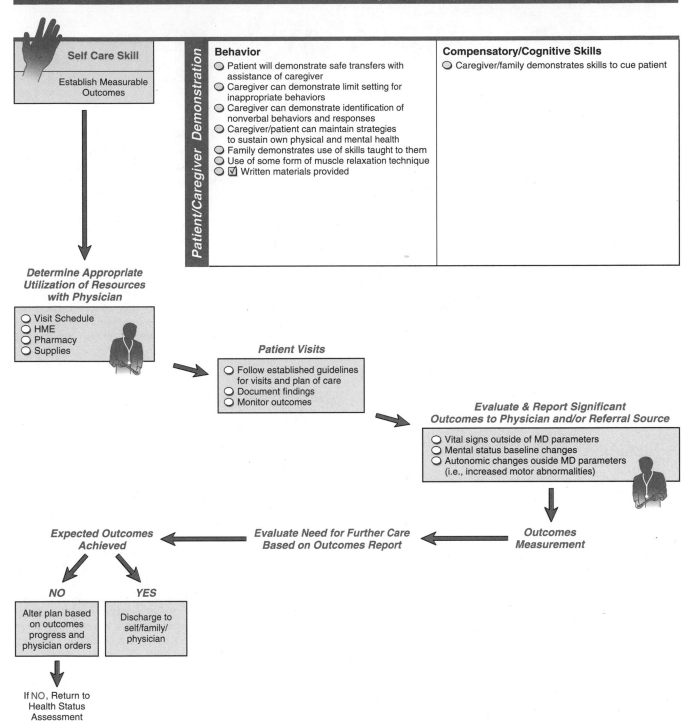

Home Care Clinical Practice Guidelines–Dementia
THE ELDERLY ADULT (65+ YEARS)

Self Care Skill

Establish Measurable Outcomes

Patient/Caregiver Demonstration

Behavior
- ○ Patient will demonstrate safe transfers with assistance of caregiver
- ○ Caregiver can demonstrate limit setting for inappropriate behaviors
- ○ Caregiver can demonstrate identification of nonverbal behaviors and responses
- ○ Caregiver/patient can maintain strategies to sustain own physical and mental health
- ○ Family demonstrates use of skills taught to them
- ○ Use of some form of muscle relaxation technique
- ○ ☑ Written materials provided

Compensatory/Cognitive Skills
- ○ Caregiver/family demonstrates skills to cue patient

Determine Appropriate Utilization of Resources with Physician
- ○ Visit Schedule
- ○ HME
- ○ Pharmacy
- ○ Supplies

Patient Visits
- ○ Follow established guidelines for visits and plan of care
- ○ Document findings
- ○ Monitor outcomes

Evaluate & Report Significant Outcomes to Physician and/or Referral Source
- ○ Vital signs outside of MD parameters
- ○ Mental status baseline changes
- ○ Autonomic changes ouside MD parameters (i.e., increased motor abnormalities)

Outcomes Measurement

Evaluate Need for Further Care Based on Outcomes Report

Expected Outcomes Achieved

NO

Alter plan based on outcomes progress and physician orders

If NO, Return to Health Status Assessment

YES

Discharge to self/family/ physician

---

to an adverse medication reaction, the patient is unable to fully comprehend and make rational decisions. Ensure that patients do not grant consent or otherwise make decisions that affect their person or their property. (See Chapter 33 regarding legal protection for the dementia victim's rights.)

What do you think? Is delirium a condition experienced only by the elderly? What could produce delirium in a young person? What techniques could you use to orient and maintain orientation in the elderly? What suggestions could you give to a family to ensure the environment was safe for their elderly loved one? What strategies could you advise them to incorporate into their daily routine to maintain orientation of their loved one?

➤ *Check Your Reading*
8. How does delirium differ from dementia?
9. What are the symptoms of sundown syndrome?

Anxiety

Despite its common occurrence, anxiety is often undetected, primarily because the elderly tend to present somatic complaints (e.g., upset stomach, insomnia, urinary frequency, fatigue) that confuse the diagnosis. A thorough evaluation can assist in identifying anxiety and causative factors. Because chronic illnesses are highly prevalent in the elderly, consider the role of the medical condition in causing symptoms of anxiety. Conditions related to anxiety include hyperthyroidism, malnutrition, hypoglycemia, and cardiopulmonary disease. Also, ingestion of sedatives, corticosteroids, over-the-counter cold and allergy medications, alcohol, and caffeine can cause symptoms of anxiety. Before treating anxiety as a psychiatric disorder, consider all other factors that could cause symptoms. (See Chapter 23 for generic information regarding care of the patient with anxiety.)

Schizophrenia

Schizophrenic elderly are few in number but pose caregiving challenges, partly because many older schizophrenics are in nursing homes. (The deinstitutionalization of these patients from mental hospitals a few decades ago has resulted in their reinstitutionalization in the nursing home setting.) Traditionally, nursing home staff have been ill-prepared to care for the mentally ill. In addition to the basic care afforded any patient with schizophrenia (see Chapter 24), older schizophrenics need particular attention paid to their physical health. These patients are less likely to seek and accept medical care, may not verbalize pain associated with physical illness, and can derive secondary gains by causing or complicating physical health problems—for example, through self-mutilation or picking at a wound. The close and regular contact of nursing staff with patients allows nurses to detect these problems and refer patients for treatment, as necessary.

Because knowledge regarding the effects of neuroleptics was scanty decades ago when many schizophrenic patients began using these drugs, tardive dyskinesia and other adverse reactions of neuroleptics are common findings among older schizophrenics. Even if these patients' use of neuroleptics has been recent, older patients are at greater risk for developing tardive dyskinesia and experiencing more problems, such as respiratory infections and malnutrition. Make sure that adequate precautions are taken when neuroleptics are used and that the physical health of these patients is closely monitored. (See Chapter 17 for an in-depth discussion of psychopharmacology.)

> **W**hat do you think? Because somatic concerns are frequent among the elderly what symptoms would you focus on if you were attempting to determine if an elderly person is depressed or anxious?

➤ *Check Your Reading*
10. Why is anxiety often undetected in older adults?
11. What are some reasons for older schizophrenics to avoid seeking medical care?

PROMOTING MENTAL HEALTH IN LATER LIFE

Positive mental health throughout the life span builds a strong foundation for good mental health in old age. The development of meaningful roles and interests, methods to manage stress effectively, good communication skills, and problem solving capabilities assists in promoting good mental health.

Identifying and Treating Physical Problems

The relationship of physical health to mental health is particularly significant in older patients. Cardiovascular disease, stroke, cancer, diabetes, and chronic obstructive pulmonary disease are among the chronic conditions highly prevalent among the elderly, which can cause symptoms of mental illness or impairment of mental function. Identify and treat physical health problems early to prevent complications. Also, consider the impact of a mental illness on physical health status because older patients have a smaller margin of safety to protect their physical health. For instance, a depressed older person who does not eat properly will become malnourished faster and easier than a younger adult. Patients are well equipped to heal following a mental illness if they are in optimal physical condition.

Dealing With Losses

The losses faced in old age are many and at times can be overwhelming. Nurses can guide older patients in using internal and external resources to cope with these losses. Listening to patients and encouraging reminiscence can help them to identify strategies that have been effective in adjusting to change and coping with misfortune. Information can be shared regarding community resources and support services that can assist with specific needs.

As losses are faced, feeling a sense of purpose can be difficult. Older people may be guided in identifying roles that have been valued and in developing ways to continue some degree of participation in these roles within any existing limitations. For instance, a recently retired schoolteacher who feels at a loss because of a lost work role can be encouraged to begin teaching a Sunday school class or to volunteer as a children's reading group leader at the local library. Hobbies and interests can be the source of new roles. For instance, the amateur toy train collector may find new opportunities in renting a table at a flea market to sell and trade collections or in giving lectures on collecting toy trains at the local community college. Of course, fulfillment and pleasure can be derived from exploring new interests and roles. A sense of integrity and productivity can be derived from purposeful activities.

The awareness of one's mortality is inescapable in old age. The frequently occurring death of loved ones and the development of serious illnesses themselves keep death a constant reminder. Cultural socialization and personal experience with death help determine the meaning that death holds for various individuals. For many people, spiritual beliefs provide an understanding of death and strength to accept the finiteness of life on earth. Great comfort can be obtained through the bond one possesses with a higher power. Older adults should be helped in obtaining spiritual support based on their personal belief systems. Be it attendance at a religious service, a bedside visit from clergy, or private time sitting in a garden, the need for nourishment of the soul must not be overlooked in care planning (Carson, 1999).

What do you think? If spirituality is helpful to the elderly person in dealing with loss, how can you support, strengthen, or facilitate the elderly person's spirituality?

➤ *Check Your Reading*
12. What are some basic measures to promote mental health in old age?

NURSING PROCESS

Assessment

Assessment in the elderly requires knowledge of both psychological and physiological changes that place older adults at risk for dysfunction.

Interviewing the Elderly

Adjustments to the interview process with older adults can facilitate data collection. Unlike today's younger generations who are accustomed to openly discussing their finances, sexual practices, family conflicts, and bodily functions, the elderly are part of a generation that viewed these topics as private, and, as a result, they may be uncomfortable discussing these personal matters.

You can respect these feelings while reviewing essential history by

1. Conducting the interview in a private area
2. Establishing rapport and putting the patient at ease
3. Explaining the type and purpose of the questions that will be asked and how this information will be used
4. Informing the patient of the right to refuse to answer questions

Common aging changes also require adjustments to the interview. Increased opacity of the lens with age results in a sensitivity to glare, such as bright sunlight shining through a window or fluorescent lights, that may not present a problem to younger eyes. A preoccupation with glare and missed visual cues could interfere with the older adult's participation in the interview. Normal body temperature is lower in many older adults, and older persons are more sensitive to cold environmental temperatures that are not bothersome to younger persons. (This problem can be compounded when the patient is clothed only in an examination gown while the caregiver is wearing layers of street clothes.) Make sure the environmental temperature is at least 75°F (23.8°C). Presbycusis is common in the elderly and interferes with the ability to adequately hear the interviewer's questions. Hearing competency should be evaluated before the interview and appropriate assistance (e.g., insertion of prescribed hearing aid, use of amplification device) provided to facilitate communication. The elderly patient's slower responses to stimuli can necessitate additional time for questions to be processed and responses formulated. Also consider the effects of illness and medications on such patients' abilities to participate in the interview.

Assessing Mental Status

Mental assessment in older adults involves some unique features. One important consideration is alteration in mental status as a result of physical illness. More likely than not, an acute confusional state or delirium is the mental manifestation of physiological disturbances. Fluid and electrolyte imbalances, fever, hyperglycemia, hypoglycemia, hypoxia, dehydration, hypotension, anemia, and adverse drug reactions are only some of the physical health problems that can lead to delirium. Depression can result from physical illnesses such as anemia, hypothyroidism, congestive heart failure, and stroke. The relationship of physical and mental health demands that a thorough physical evaluation accompany every mental health assessment.

A thorough health history is essential. Remember that new signs can develop as a result of changes in long-term health conditions. Be careful not to overlook obvious causes for an altered mental status. Laboratory tests can complement the physical examination and provide clues to potential disorders. Tests could include complete blood count, serum electrolytes, serological test for syphilis, blood urea nitrogen, blood glucose, bilirubin, blood vitamin level, sedimentation rate, and urinalysis. Electroencephalography, CT, MRI, and positron emission tomography are among the diagnostic tests that can be performed, depending on the suspected underlying cause.

Although an increasing number of practitioners are aware of the unique aspects of geriatric health problems, abnormal mental status in older adults still can be interpreted as a normal characteristic of old age. For instance, if Mary Baxter presented in an emergency department in a confused state, some staff members might view her as a "confused old lady" and miss or postpone diagnosing the cause of her symptoms. Delayed treatment and the development of complications could result. You must ensure that the stereotype of **ageism,** which characterizes the elderly as incompetent, does not influence assessment and treatment decisions. Advocate for competent evaluation and care of older adults.

> **W***hat do you think?* How have your attitudes toward the elderly been influenced by ageism?

Assessing Medication Issues

Because of the increased risk of drugs causing adverse reactions, many of which are manifested through altered mental status, a review of all prescription and nonprescription drugs used by the patient is essential. In addition, an assessment of factors that can affect drug administration, absorption, metabolism, and excretion is essential to ensure that medications result in greater benefits than risks to the older patient.

Advanced age can contribute to unique problems in drug therapy and warrant special nursing intervention. Tablets and capsules can stick to the oral mucosa and may not be swallowed as a result of drier mucous membranes of the oral cavity. If this occurs, not only are the drug's absorption benefits lost but the drug also can dissolve and cause irritation in the mouth or throat. Suppositories can take longer to melt because of a general lower body temperature and decreased circulation to the lower bowel and vagina. The risk is that suppositories can be expelled undissolved. Reduced muscle mass and inactivity can interfere with the absorption of intramuscular medications. Intravenous administration of drugs carries a risk of circulatory overload due to reduced cardiac efficiency with age.

The less acidic gastric environment common in old age can delay the absorption of drugs that require a low gastric pH. Reduced levels of serum albumin can create a problem when several protein-bound drugs (e.g., acetazolamide, amitriptyline, cefazolin, chlorpromazine, digitoxin, hydralazine, nortriptyline, phenytoin, salicylates, and warfarin) are administered together because less effective protein binding occurs. (This situation can be tricky in that if the serum albumin level is low, the patient can become toxic from protein-bound drugs despite having blood levels of the drugs within a normal or even low range.) Reduced numbers of functioning nephrons, decreased glomerular filtration rate, and less renal blood flow slow the filtration of drugs from the body and increase the ease with which drugs can reach toxic levels. Poor memory can interfere with the safe self-administration of drugs.

Special problems and risks associated with age-related changes should be considered and identified during the assessment and interventions planned accordingly.

Assessing Cognitive Function

A baseline evaluation of cognitive function should be performed on every older adult regardless of the clinical setting or specialty in which service is obtained. However, results of the initial test of cognitive function must be carefully interpreted. Although impaired cognition is not a normal characteristic of old age, it can result from the multiple stresses and stimuli during assessment. For example, a perfectly mentally competent older adult may test poorly immediately after admission to a health care facility because of the overwhelming number of activities he or she faces and anxiety about the situation. This same individual may score perfectly after having had several hours to adjust to the new environment. Labeling the person cognitively impaired on the basis of the intake assessment would be inappropriate and could risk biasing the care provided thereafter. When impaired cognition is observed during the initial assessment, repeated assessments are necessary.

Symptoms and observations noted during the assessment should be put in proper perspective before drawing conclusions about the older person's mental status. For instance

1. Inattention to self-care and grooming activities may be associated with arthritic fingers or fatigue secondary to anemia rather than a disturbance in mood or cognition.
2. Awakening from sleep at 3:00 AM every day could be caused by a sleep quota that has been fulfilled (about 5 to 7 hours of night sleep are adequate for most older adults) and may not be an indication of depression.
3. Grieving even though no loss of a significant person has occurred could be related to the loss of a beloved pet.
4. Suspiciousness about neighbors could be a valid perception of a crime risk rather than a manifestation of a paranoid disorder.

Family and social history are therefore important to understanding mental status.

> **W***hat do you think?* Medications are an important nursing concern when providing care for the elderly. What strategies could you devise to assist an elderly person who experiences impairment in sight, some forgetfulness, and arthritis in his or her hands to be compliant with a regimen of multiple daily medications?

SNAPSHOT

Nursing Interventions Specific to the Older Adult

What do you need to do to develop a relationship with an older patient suffering from a psychiatric disorder?
- Provide uninterrupted blocks of time to share with the patient.
- Ask patient for his or her preference for preferred name of address. Avoid using terms, such as "Pop," "Sweetie," or "Grandma," that could be offensive to the patient.
- Prevent environmental conditions that could be uncomfortable or distracting for older adults (e.g., glare from bright lights or direct sunlight coming through a window, background noise, room temperature below 70°F [21.1°C]).
- Be honest, empathetic, and compassionate.
- Explain and prepare the patient for activities.
- Pace communication to afford ample time for the patient to process, react, and respond. Although individuals differ, in general, more time is needed for older adults than for younger adults.
- Review the patient's life history and help the patient to identify accomplishments (e.g., raising a family, surviving the Great Depression, emigrating to a foreign country). Respect and preserve the patient's story.
- Encourage the patient to identify and discuss feelings.
- Involve family or significant others as desired by the patient.

What do you need to assess regarding the patient's health status?
- Impact of common aging changes on health status
- Self-care capacity
- Physiological responses, including appetite and weight changes, fatigue, sleep disturbances, immobility, constipation, headache, chest pain
- Cognitive responses, including confusion, slowed thinking, poor judgment
- Behavioral responses, including isolation; crying; agitation; pacing; substance abuse; slowed activity; poor personal hygiene; inability to perform instrumental activities of daily living (ADLs), such as cooking, balancing a checkbook, budgeting money, and structuring time
- Chronic conditions
- Weight, especially if the patient is experiencing changes in appetite
- Medications, including proper use, side effects, adverse effects, interactions, and effectiveness
- Family structure, availability, and relationships

- Caregiver availability and support; health and social agencies involved in care
- Knowledge level; ability and readiness to learn
- Housing
- Finances
- Psychological well-being, integrity
- Spiritual well-being; religious beliefs and values

What do you need to teach the patient or the patient's caregiver?
- Safe use of medications, including proper administration, management of side effects, recognition of adverse effects, precautions
- The disease process; its causes, course, and treatments
- Recognition of signs of change in condition, and complications
- Emergency measures
- Proper diet
- Emergency measures
- Importance of social support and strategies to obtain it
- Safety precautions related to disease and medications
- Stress management and other health practices
- Importance of emotional support

What skills will you want the patient and/or caregiver to demonstrate?
- Adequate self-care practices; ability to fulfill ADLs and instrumental activities of daily living (IADLs)
- Compliance with treatment plan
- Safe use of medications
- Ability to identify abnormalities that need to be brought to the attention of the provider
- Participation in leisure and social activities
- Ability to engage in interactions and activities that focus on significant loss, changing roles, clarification of values, spiritual well-being, and achievement of physiological integrity

What other health professionals might need to be a part of this plan of care?
- Physician, psychiatrist, or primary care physician—to take charge of the overall treatment plan including medication management
- Social worker—to assist with access to community supports, insurance issues, access to entitlements, connection with community-based treatments
- Psychiatric occupational therapist—to assist the patient with IADLs, such as time management, cooking, budgeting
- Nursing assistant or home health aide—to assist patient with personal hygiene and grooming, if necessary

➤ *Check Your Reading*

13. What are some precautions that you must take to ensure an accurate mental status assessment?
14. Describe factors that can influence the validity of data obtained during an interview with the older person.

Diagnosis

Analysis of the data leads you to determine appropriate nursing diagnoses for the elderly. The diagnoses depend on the data collected. For instance, a depressed elderly person might have the nursing diagnosis of hopelessness related to multiple losses evidenced by crying, sad affect, and expressions that life is not worth living. (See Chapters 23, 24, 25, and 33 for a comprehensive listing of nursing diagnoses for elderly adults experiencing stress and anxiety; schizophrenia; a mood disorder; or a cognitive disorder, such as Alzheimer's disease.)

Outcome Identification

The expected outcome depends on the diagnoses. For example, with a nursing diagnosis of hopelessness related to multiple losses, the expected outcome might be expressed as follows: the patient will experience less sadness and crying, express that life continues to be meaningful, and invest self in pleasurable diversional activities.

Planning

The nursing plan focuses on establishing short-term goals that lead to the accomplishment of expected outcome and on determining who will perform which nursing interventions. For example, the expected outcome might be supported by the following short-term goals:

1. The patient will discuss the multiple losses that have occurred.

2. The patient will discuss the impact of these losses.
3. The patient will express feelings of sadness.
4. The patient will identify activities that give meaning to life.
5. The patient will decide on one activity in which to invest self.
6. The patient will explore spiritual issues surrounding losses.

Accomplishing these goals might be delegated to the nurse as well as an activity therapist, an occupational therapist, a nursing assistant, and a representative of the patient's faith.

Implementation

Nursing interventions depend on the assessment, diagnoses, expected outcomes, and plan. See Snapshot: Nursing Interventions Specific to Major Depression. (See Chapters 23, 24, 25, and 33 for specific interventions related to stress and anxiety, schizophrenia, depression, and cognitive disorders.)

Evaluation

An evaluation includes a formative component, in which you evaluate the ongoing process, and a summative evaluation, in which you evaluate the overall effectiveness of the nursing care. Examine the comprehensiveness and accuracy of the assessment, the appropriateness of the nursing diagnoses and the expected outcome, and the specifics of the plan. Modifications are made throughout the entire process. The summative evaluation examines the achievement of the stated expected outcome. For example, if the patient experiences less crying and sadness, is able to see that life still has meaning, and is able to invest self in pleasurable activities, then the nursing care has been successful.

NURSING PROCESS APPLICATION

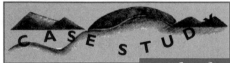

CASE STUDY

Richard

Richard is a 75-year-old retired mechanic who lives with his wife, Ruth. In July they celebrated 55 years of marriage. They have 5 children, 14 grandchildren, and 2 great-grandchildren. Richard is a devout practicing Catholic and has been able to find meaning in various life experiences. He is a healthy elder, and he and his wife enjoy traveling and spending time with their family. Working on the family genealogy on his home computer is one of his favorite hobbies.

Recently, he developed painful arthritis in both of his hands that prohibits him from any activity that requires movement of his hands and wrists. Richard has had several major health problems during his lifetime, such as loss of the sight in one eye, basal cell carcinoma, hypertension, and mild diabetes. Both chronic conditions are controlled with diet and medication. He tells the nurse in the physician's office that he cannot imagine continuing to live a productive life without the use of his hands and that he cannot tolerate the constant pain. The medication that the physician prescribed for the pain and inflammation is contraindicated because he is taking warfarin (Coumadin), which could cause hemorrhage. His wife tells you she is very worried about him.

ASSESSMENT	Assessment data are as follow: • Previously active elder • Devout religious practice • Ability to find solace in spiritual beliefs • Chronic arthritic pain associated with loss of function • Fear and apprehension • Increased pulse, respiration, and blood pressure • Insomnia • Good supportive network • History of ability to cope with grief associated with loss of a body function
DIAGNOSIS	**DSM-IV Diagnosis:** Rule Out Depression, Anxiety Disorder **Nursing Diagnosis:** Anxiety related to loss of control associated with inability to control pain, and loss of previous level of functioning manifested by excessive worry, insomnia, and increased vital signs.

OUTCOME IDENTIFICATION, PLANNING, AND IMPLEMENTATION

Expected Outcome 1: By _____ the patient will verbalize fear of loss of control associated with pain and decreased function.

Short-Term Goals	Nursing Interventions	Rationales
By _____ the patient will verbalize three specific fears that relate to loss of control.	1. Using therapeutic communication techniques, encourage the patient to verbalize subjective feelings, such as anger and sadness. 2. Ask the patient to locate these feelings in his body (e.g., shoulder, neck, stomach). 3. Encourage the patient to keep a record of feelings and associated fears. 4. Ask the patient to share his feelings and fears with his spouse or a health care professional.	1. These techniques will assist the patient in making the fear specific rather than general. This process will make the fear more manageable for the patient. 2. Identifying feelings is the first step in being able to work through them. Often, feelings are felt in the body, or somatized. 3–4. Recording fears and associated feelings is a therapeutic, effective way of working through them.
By _____ the patient will accurately describe current loss of function and how it has affected him.	1. Using therapeutic techniques, encourage the patient to describe in detail the current loss of function. 2. Ask the patient to describe specifically how the current loss of function is affecting him.	1–2. Having an empathic listener who will spend undivided time with the patient will aid in decreasing anxiety.
By _____ the patient will describe to the nurse a previous coping mechanism that worked for him when dealing with a fear associated with loss of function.	1. Ask the patient to describe a previous time in his life when he felt out of control. 2. Encourage the patient to describe his previous conquest over fear and anxiety regarding loss of function. 3. Validate the patient for being able to conquer this particular fear during his life journey.	1–3. Reminiscence empowers the patient to recognize previous coping mechanisms that work. The elderly have had many years of experience with loss, and these need to be validated.

Expected Outcome 2: By _____ the patient will demonstrate relaxation techniques.

Short-Term Goal	Nursing Interventions	Rationales
By _____ the patient will verbalize the rationale for and the components of a relaxation program.	1. Advise the patient regarding the relationship of anxiety, pain, and tension in the body. 2. Instruct the patient in deep breathing techniques. 3. Teach the patient to achieve progressive muscle relaxation, focusing on a specific muscle group or the entire body, beginning with the hands and feet and moving progressively upward. 4. Have the patient demonstrate to ensure that he understands and is achieving relaxation. 5. Inform the patient that repeated practice will enhance efficacy of this technique.	1–2. Persons with increased anxiety tend to be shallow breathers. 3–5. Return demonstration and practice will ensure that the technique will become an integral component of the patient's lifestyle.

Expected Outcome 3: By _____ the patient will experience reduced anxiety and improved sleep.

Short-Term Goals	Nursing Interventions	Rationales
By _____ pulse and respiration rates will return to normal.	1. Monitor vital signs for any physical signs of returning anxiety. 2. Encourage the patient to eliminate any additional life stressors in his home environment.	1. The neuroendocrine system is activated during fear and anxiety, and any increase may indicate that the patient is hiding his fear. 2. Structure and safety in his home environment will assist this patient in reducing tension and anxiety.
By _____ the patient will sleep for at least 4 hours without being awakened by pain. By _____ the patient will verbalize being refreshed or rested on awakening.	1. Have the patient avoid caffeine, alcohol, and strenuous activity 4 hours before sleep. 2. Promote relaxation at bedtime (e.g., with back massage, progressive relaxation techniques). 3. Encourage the patient to sleep in a comfortable environment that is conducive to sleep (e.g., with comfortable temperature, privacy, dimmed lights). 4. Provide sedation, if necessary, but inform the patient that this is a temporary solution.	1. All of these factors are known to interrupt normal sleep patterns rather than induce sleep. 2. Relaxation techniques are frequently helpful in attaining sleep. 3. External stimuli are known to interfere with normal sleep patterns. 4. This measure will assist the patient in achieving sleep until a normal pattern can be attained.

Expected Outcome 4: By _____ the patient will experience a decrease in pain and an increase in function.

Short-Term Goals	Nursing Interventions	Rationales
By _____ the patient will describe increased mobility of the affected joints.	1. Encourage the patient to keep a record of the amount of joint movement that he has on a daily basis. 2. Encourage the patient to expect a return of function that is reasonable considering the amount of dysfunction.	1–2. Empowers the patient to be an active participant in his own healing process, and helps the patient to be realistic in his recovery.

By _____ patient will verbalize a decrease in joint pain.	1. Provide the patient with a pain-rating scale and instruct him how to use it. 2. Ask the patient to keep a record of measures used to decrease pain. 3. Check with the patient's physician regarding the feasibility of adding an antidepressant medication such as amitriptyline to the patient's pain regimen.	1–2. Rating the pain empowers the patient to be an active participant in his own pain control and enables the nurse to monitor the effectiveness of all measures used. 3. Antidepressants used in small doses are effective analgesics and could assist the patient in improved sleep patterns.

Nursing Diagnosis: Potential for Enhanced Spiritual Well-Being related to the patient's previous ability to cope with loss and ability to find solace in spiritual beliefs.

OUTCOME IDENTIFICATION, PLANNING, AND IMPLEMENTATION

> **Expected Outcome 1:** By _____ the patient will verbalize this episode of illness as one of the many opportunities he has experienced in his life to find meaning and inner strength.

Short-Term Goals	Nursing Interventions	Rationales
By _____ the patient will make positive statements about his life and his relationship with God. By _____ the patient will verbalize that he is comfortable with his belief system.	1. Encourage and accept the patient's verbalizations about his belief system. 2. Provide spiritual counsel and reading material congruent with the patient's belief system. 3. Encourage the patient to discuss these statements with his wife and children.	1–2. A sense of integrity can result from being validated by caring professionals. 3. Relationship with significant others sustains a person's belief system during difficult times.

> **Expected Outcome 2:** By _____ the patient will verbalize a sense of hopefulness associated with his spiritual belief that pain and suffering are inevitable parts of the life cycle.

Short-Term Goals	Nursing Interventions	Rationales
By _____ the patient will state that his depression has abated. By _____ the patient will express a desire to continue to enjoy his family and friends.	1. Encourage the patient to articulate how this episode of chronic pain and discomfort was like others that he had in his lifetime. 2. Ask the patient to help you understand the specific measures that worked for him this time. 3. Encourage the patient to self-monitor for signs of returning depression. 1. Ask the patient what significant events are planned for his family (e.g., weddings, births, anniversaries). 2. Problem solve with the patient ways that he might be able to participate in these activities. 3. Encourage regular communication with his children and grandchildren.	1–2. These measures will enable the client to see how a strong belief system has helped him during his life. 3. Encourages the patient to be an active participant in his overall health care. 1–3. Hope often is associated with the desire to be a part of the future. The elderly often have to be reminded that they are an important part of the future for their family and friends.

In this case study, the expected outcomes represent the summative evaluation criteria, and the short-term goals represent formative evaluation standards.

Conclusions

The developmental theorist Erik Erikson believed that late adulthood is a time in which mental health requires a sense of integrity. For the elderly, integrity means pride in the past and contentment with the present. Without this sense of integrity, an elderly person may experience despair, "feeling that the time is now short, too short for the attempt to start another life and try out alternate roads to integrity" (Erikson, 1963, p. 228).

Nursing interventions can promote an elderly person's sense of integrity. Nurses need the time to spend with patients to help them validate their own experiences and belief systems. With integrity comes an ongoing commitment to life, however short the remaining time. For the elderly traveler, the last stage of the journey depends both on the road traveled and on a sense of self-worth, a belief that one's life will contribute to the future.

Key Points to Remember

- Most older adults live normal lives in a community setting.
- The elderly are a highly diverse group encompassing the young-old, who are younger than age 75, and the old-old, who are age 75 years or older.
- Caregiving of elders by families is on the rise. Approximately 7% of the adult population cares for a disabled spouse or parent at home.
- Chronic illnesses are highly prevalent in late life and can threaten mental health.
- Older adults face developmental tasks—challenges and adjustments in response to life experiences—that assist in achieving a sense of psychological and social well-being.
- Reminiscence can be used therapeutically to help the elderly resolve unfinished business, appreciate the significance of their lives, and reaffirm self-worth and identity.

- When assessing the mental health of older adults, consider the impact of physical health on mental status.
- Normal aging does not result in a decline in mental function; signs of mental impairment warrant a thorough evaluation.
- Although most symptoms of mental illnesses are similar in older adults to those in younger adults, the risk exists that these symptoms can be overlooked and attributed to growing old.
- Closely monitor the impact of mental illness on physical health. Older adults have a smaller margin of safety in developing complications.
- Nurses must take an active role in advocating that older adults receive timely intervention for mental health problems and that the rights of this vulnerable group are protected.

Learning Activities

1. Reminisce with a group of older adults and ask them to identify major stresses they faced in younger years. Ask them to discuss how these experiences helped them to cope with stresses they face currently.
2. Review the health histories of a group of patients. Identify physical conditions and medications that can cause or worsen mental health problems.
3. Examine several health care environments. Discuss

components of the environment that facilitate or interfere with optimal mental function of the elderly.
4. Review the care plans of older adults who have mental illnesses. Determine if adequate consideration is given to their physical health needs; revise the care plan as needed.
5. Think about components of your own life that will provide strength and meaning to you as you age.

Critical Thinking Exercise

Veronica, a nursing student, was assigned to Mrs. Donahue, a 70-year-old patient sitting in a geri-chair in the corner of the lounge on the inpatient psychiatric unit. While Veronica was doing a mini-mental status examination with Mrs. Donahue, she found out that she was a retired nurse who was going to be discharged to a nursing home. Mrs. Donahue complained about the loudness of the music on the unit and was sporting a black eye from a fall the night before when she attempted to walk to the dining room by herself.

1. What can you assume about Mrs. Donahue's condition?
2. What evidence supports your assumptions?
3. How could you find out if your assumptions are true?

As Veronica was talking to Mrs. Donahue, another patient approached Mrs. Donahue and began telling her about the medications she was taking. Mrs. Donahue promptly began to advise the other patient that she needed to take her medications with meals because they would upset her stomach. Mrs. Donahue also told the other patient to make sure that she reported any constipation.

1. Make sense of what might be happening.

2. What is the next thing you would say to Mrs. Donahue?

3. What is your purpose in responding in that way?

Additional Resources

American Association of Retired Persons (AARP)
601 East Street, NW
Washington, DC 20049

The American Association of Retired Persons is an advocacy group for the elderly; they also provide (for a reasonable fee) training materials associated with Reminiscence Therapy.

National Institute on Aging (NIA)

Public Information Office
Federal Building
Room 5C27, Building 3
9000 Rockville Parkway
Bethesda, MD 20892
http://www.nih.gov/nia

References

Carson, V. B. (1999). The grief experience: Life's losses and endings. In E. Arnold & K. Boggs (Eds.), *Interpersonal relationship skills for nurses* (pp. 169–172). Philadelphia: W. B. Saunders.

Eliopoulos, C. (1991). *Developmental tasks of aging (Long-term care educator,* Vol. 2, Lesson 6). Glen Arm, MD: Health Education Network.

Eliopoulos, C. (1997). *Gerontological nursing* (4th ed., p. 390). Philadelphia: J. B. Lippincott.

Erikson, E. (1963). *Childhood and society* (2nd ed., p. 228). New York: Norton.

Foreman, M. D. (1990). Complexities of acute confusion. *Geriatric Nursing, 11,* 136.

Suggested Readings

Bee, H. L. (1996). *The journey of adulthood* (3rd ed.). Upper Saddle River, NJ: Prentice-Hall.

Caprio-Prevette, M. D. (1996). *Memory enhancement program for older adults: A guide for practitioners.* Gaithersburg, MD: Aspen.

Eliopoulos, C. (1998). *Manual of gerontologic nursing* (2nd ed.). St. Louis, MO: C. V. Mosby.

Faran, C. J., Horton-Deutsch, S. L., Fiedler, R., & Scott, C. (1997). Psychiatric home care for the elderly. *Home Health Care Services Quarterly, 16*(1/2), 77–92.

Faran, C. J., Horton-Deutsch, S. L., Loukissa, D., & Johnson, L. (1998). Psychiatric home care of elderly persons with depression: Unmet caregiver needs. *Home Health Care Services Quarterly, 16*(4), 57–73.

Fidler, G. S. (1992). *Recapturing competence: A system's change for geropsychiatric care.* New York: Springer.

Lowenthal, D. T. (1990). Clinical pharmacology. In W. B. Abrams & R. Berkow (Eds.), *The Merck manual of geriatrics* (p. 181). Rahway, NJ: Merck Sharp and Dohme Research Laboratories.

Magai, C. (Ed.). (1996). *Handbook of emotion, adult development, and aging.* San Diego, CA: Academic Press.

Norman, I. J. (1997). *Mental health care for elderly people.* New York: Churchill Livingstone.

Rupp, J. (1996). *Dear heart, come home: The path of midlife spirituality.* New York: Crossroad.

Rybarczyk, B., & Bellig, A. (1997). *Listening to life stories: A new approach to stress intervention in health care.* New York: Springer.

Shepard, R. J. (1997). *Aging, physical activity, and health.* Champaign, IL: Human Kinetics.

Zarit, S. H., & Knight, B. G. (1996). *A guide to psychotherapy and aging: Effective clinical interventions in a life stage context.* Washington, DC: American Psychological Association.

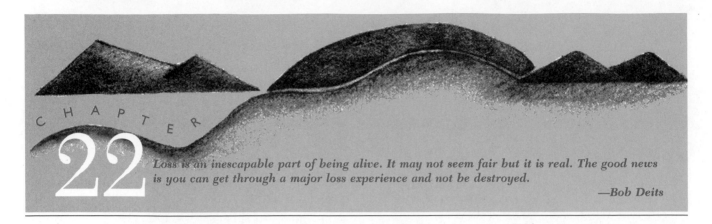

22

Loss is an inescapable part of being alive. It may not seem fair but it is real. The good news is you can get through a major loss experience and not be destroyed.

—*Bob Deits*

Loss

Learning Objectives

After studying this chapter, you should be able to:

1. Define loss and enumerate the types of losses people face in a lifetime.
2. Discuss the losses psychiatric patients face as a result of having mental health problems.
3. Name at least three people who have contributed to the work that has been done in the area of grief.
4. Describe the grief process: its length, stages, major tasks, and complications.
5. List several obstacles to grieving.
6. Describe the effects of loss and grieving on the person with mental illness.
7. Outline several strategies that people use to cope with significant losses.
8. Discuss how to assist a psychiatric patient to cope with loss using the nursing process.

Key Terminology

Complicated grieving	Grief	Grieving process	Loss
Disenfranchised grieving	Grieving patterns		

Loss is a pervading theme in the life journey that all people undertake. Although loss is usually considered to be something personal, the experience of loss is as universal as are the experiences of being born and dying. The life cycle is marked with advances, setbacks, changes, growth, and transitions, and amidst all of these is the experience of loss. People cope with their losses in individual ways. Loss can be an opportunity for growth and transformation or it can be considered a curse on one's life. Within this chapter, the student examines loss from a general perspective as well as from the perspective of the person who is battling mental illness; you explore the various ways that people cope with loss and how they choose to grieve their losses; and how you can help psychiatric patients to survive losses, grieve adequately, and grow through the experience. Using the nursing process, you journey with the psychiatric patient through her or his losses and help her or him discover ways of achieving a meaningful life, despite the losses faced. Let us take a look at Mary Ann's story to become acquainted with the experience of loss.

Mary Ann's Story

As Mary Ann sat in the warm sunshine, her heart was heavy and her thoughts confused. She had just written in her journal an account of the sad events that had occurred in her life within the recent past. She wished she could escape the memories and painful feelings she was experiencing, but they just would not go away.... Mary Ann had dreamed of a beautiful marriage and a commitment that would last a lifetime. In its place she had a broken dream and only the memory of what could have been. She had met her husband just 5 years ago. For 2 years they knew the excitement of being in love. They enjoyed each other, and love gave new meaning and direction to their lives. They shared, planned, and prepared. Finally, they entrusted their lives and love to each other in marriage. They moved to the mountains of Vermont to build the home of their dreams. They worked hard but did not seem to mind. They had a goal and a dream that they both shared.

One year passed, and conflict began to occur. Undiagnosed and untreated mental health problems in Mary Ann's husband, linked with the usual struggles of marital adjustment, soon brought the couple to a marriage counselor. The professional help was too little, and perhaps too late, to remedy the many problems that existed. Mary Ann's spouse feared change and the challenge of growth; thus, he resisted and blocked the counseling.

This couple had hardly begun their journey in married life when obstacles fell in their path. Mary Ann tried harder than ever to move around them and to look beyond them. She felt, however, that she was alone in this work. Then, as would any weary traveler, she stopped, retraced her steps, and sadly realized that her life was going nowhere. Her energies were being robbed as a result of the constant struggles. Her peace was threatened. Her spirits were down, and she had lost her zest for living. Life was a burden. Her journey was taking her in directions she had not chosen.

The choices had become clearer to her. She could give up the promises, the hopes, and the unrealized dreams, or remain in the struggle. If she remained, it would mean a struggle for survival that could cost her health, happiness, and well-being. She chose to let go of what was and to move in another direction. The new route was unclear and felt perilous at times. The pain, caused by the many losses incurred as a result of her choices, sometimes felt unbearable. She was leaving the marriage and abandoning her dreams. Mary Ann felt lonely and afraid, yet resolute and assured of the rightness of her decision. As she reflected on her lost marriage dream that day, she had a keen sense of all that she was losing. She was feeling the pain of letting go and the experience of grieving. ■

DEFINITION OF AND RESEARCH ON LOSS AND GRIEF

Loss Defined

In defining **loss** within a broad context, we might state that it is an event that involves the involuntary separation from something we have possessed and perhaps treasured. Loss requires that we give up that which is familiar, comfortable, and personal. In the introductory story, Mary Ann gave up her dream of a long happy marriage; she felt uncomfortable, in pain, and alone. She faced the challenge of adapting to a new set of circumstances and events in her life. Mary Ann's experiences with loss provide us a glimpse of how loss affects us all. Box 22–1 lists some general assumptions about loss.

Grief Defined

When someone you love has died, you face the difficult but important task of grieving or mourning. Grief involves the open expression of your thoughts and feelings regarding not only the death but also the person who has died. According to Wolfelt (1991a, pp. 11, 12), "You are beginning a journey that is often frightening, painful, overwhelming, and sometimes lonely."

Although grieving is most often linked with death experiences, it is a necessary process for all of the losses we face. The greater the commitment or investment we have in a person, object, project, or pursuit, the greater will be our sense of loss when it is gone. Significant losses are grieved intensely and for a longer period. Losses of lesser significance also are grieved but usually for a shorter time and with less sadness and pain. Sudden, unexpected losses are difficult to face and often are grieved for a longer period of time. This is because of the lack of preparation for their occurrence.

The terms *grieving, mourning,* and *experiencing bereavement* refer to the same process and are used interchangeably in this chapter. Gyulay (1989, p. 2) defined **grief** as "a journey toward healing and recovering from the pain of a significant loss." This definition contains two important goals that are a part of the grief process: healing oneself and recovering from the loss.

Box 22–1 ■ ■ ■ ■ ■
General Assumptions About Loss

- Loss is a universal experience among human beings.
- Loss is painful because it implies separation.
- Significant losses cause strong emotional responses.
- Loss requires adjustment to what is unfamiliar, uncertain, and often unchosen.
- The effects of a given loss can touch many lives.

Clinical Work and Studies Done on Loss and Grief

Freud's Contributions

Freud (1959) attempted to explore normal and complicated grieving reactions in his classic work *Mourning and Melancholia.* Although he is widely quoted, Freud really wrote little about mourning in comparison with the volumes he wrote on other topics. Freud suggested that mourning or grieving involves the task of detaching survivors from memories and hopes regarding the deceased.

Lindemann's Contributions

Eric Lindemann (1944) studied grief extensively during the 1940s. Through a series of interviews with grieving people, he was able to record basic patterns of acute grief, physical symptoms that accompany it, and mental changes in people who had suffered significant losses.

Engel's Contributions

George Engel (1964) built on the work of Lindemann. He identified the components of grief work to be

• Freeing oneself from an inordinate attachment to the deceased
• Readjustment to one's environment in which the deceased is no longer a part
• Undertaking new relationships and social interactions

Bowlby's Contributions

During the 1960s, John Bowlby's (1969) work focused on describing mourning as a process that has three overlapping stages:

• Numbness and disbelief
• Disorganization of the bereaved person's life and personality
• The reorganization process

Bowlby researched the "separation response syndrome" in the 1960s and 1970s as he did work in the area of grief and attachment.

Parkes' Contributions

Researchers focused strongly on grief in the 1970s, and this was paralleled with increased interest in death and dying. Among the noted authors and researchers in the areas of grief, death, and loss, was Collin Murray Parkes (1972). He conducted a series of bereavement studies in the 1960s and 1970s examining the effects of loss on the physical and mental health of people during the first 6 to 12 months of their bereavement period.

Rando's Contributions

Theresa Rando's (1984, 1993) extensive work in the 1980s and 1990s focused on the areas of grief and death.

She researched the course of the mourning process, the experiences of bereaved parents, and the increasing prevalence of complicated mourning. Complicated mourning can sometimes become a problem for a grieving person (Rando, 1993). Box 22–2 indicates some of the risk factors that could lead to this type of mourning.

Additional Contributions

A series of clinical studies addressing grief issues among parents who lost infants and young children were conducted in the late 1980s (Hutti, 1988). Margaret Shandor Miles and Alice Sterner Demi continued to do research in this area, focusing on dying children, parenting the child with a life-threatening illness, parental bereavement, survival guilt in bereaved parents and in those escaping natural disasters, and bereavement guilt after a suicide occurs (Miles & Demi, 1986, 1994).

With the increased numbers of traumatic and premature deaths in our contemporary society, it is not unusual for people to be faced with multiple deaths to mourn. This leads to what Kastenbaum (1991) termed *bereavement overload,* which requires professional care and supportive assistance to allow persons to grieve adequately. Posttraumatic stress reactions caused by accidents, natural disasters, war, suicide, and the increasing number of homicides in our society can complicate grieving significantly. Problems usually arise when a person focuses on grieving without paying attention to treating the posttraumatic stress.

During an interview conducted in 1991, Herman Fiefel, author of the book *The Meaning of Death* (1959), reflected on the stages of dying and phases of mourning outlined in literature and research. He warned about defining strict standards by which to plan care and provide support and instead advocated a focus on individual differences and personal needs and choices (Corless, Germino, & Pittman, 1994). This is in keeping with the trends of working with grieving people within support groups on a longer-term basis. Certainly, when we consider the grieving psychiatric patient, it is essential that support is provided in a time frame that ensures his or her safety and well-being. Table 22–1 shows the stages of grieving.

Box 22–2 ■ ■ ■ ■ ■
Risk for Complicated Mourning

1. There is sudden death that is traumatic, violent, or mutilating.
2. The death of a child has occurred.
3. An unhealthy relationship with the deceased (anger, ambivalence, dependence) has existed.
4. There is isolation or lack of an available social support system.
5. The mourner is burdened with significant stressors, ungrieved losses, or mental health/chemical dependency problems.

TABLE 22–1 The Stages of Grieving

STAGES	PREDOMINANT CHARACTERISTICS	DURATION
Stage I: Shock and Disbelief	Shock, numbness, disbelief, denial; inability to make decisions; difficulty in carrying on conversations; short attention span, high anxiety; physical symptoms such as nausea, vomiting, shortness of breath	Several hours, days, or weeks
Stage II: Attempts at Denial, Illusion of Normalcy	Seems anesthetized; sets about reestablishing order, stabilizing his or her life; appears that all is as before; makes decisions, greets friends, shops, tries to fill the void	A few weeks
Stage III: Feeling: Emotions, Loneliness, Emptiness	Begins the painful journey into the darkest areas of life; expresses strong emotions (intense anger, intense loneliness, guilt); negative themes emerge: "My life will never be the same." "It is impossible to ever be happy again." "Others do not understand me." Each person reacts differently. Some are stoic and logical; others feel the hurt deeply and show it; still others dwell on the loss, while some counterattack to dispel the anger (e.g., join Mothers Against Drunk Driving), and some actually become physically or psychologically ill.	Many months
Stage IV: New Awareness	A search for meaning begins; can find hopeful events once again. There is the belief that life can be happy, a view of self and the world is refashioned, there is a sense one will "make it."	Many months
Stage V: Acceptance	Accepting but not forgetting the loss, reinvestment in life's undertakings and social events, letting go and moving on.	A year or 2 (maybe longer)

Adapted from Veninga, R. L. (1985). *A gift of hope: How to survive our tragedies.* Philadelphia: Lippincott Williams & Wilkins.

What do you think? What losses have you experienced? How did you cope with the grief that followed those losses?

► *Check Your Reading*
1. Define loss.
2. Define grief, or the grieving process.
3. Identify three pioneers who did clinical work on loss and grieving.
4. What aspects of grief and mourning have been researched in the 1980s and 1990s?

LOSS

Loss and the Life Cycle

Loss is a common denominator throughout the life cycle. We each experienced our first loss when we were separated at birth from the warmth and safety of our mother's bodies and thrust into a world of noise, cold, brightness, and apparent confusion.

We come to know numerous losses that are inherent to the process of human growth and development. Perhaps the best example of these are the losses incurred because of the aging process. Life's circumstances and events cause us to face multiple losses as well. These can include the death of a family member, a friend, or a pet; losses incurred because of geographical moves; failure to obtain a given job, a promotion, a raise, a dream, or an *A* on an examination; financial losses or bankruptcy; and loss of health, a body part, self-image, or self-worth.

Westberg (1971) stated, in a practical manner, that

A list of losses would be inexhaustible. We can lose our health, our eyesight, our hearing. We can lose our home through fire or tornado or through financial ruin. In some families grief comes with the loss of a pet which has been a part of everything that has gone on in that household for ten years or more. Any of these things, and many more, sets in motion a cycle of grief. (p. 16)

Getting in Touch With Loss

We have a tendency to underestimate the impact of loss experiences on our lives. We try to move on with our lives as if the losses never occurred. We resist slowing down the pace of our rapidly moving lives to grieve our losses, or even to "count our blessings." The painful memories connected with loss are quickly repressed so that they do not interfere with our pursuits and undertakings. The tragedy of using repression is that the painful memories do not disappear. They are merely stored in the subconscious, to be dealt with at some later time. Stored grief and loss is cumulative and increases a person's vulnerability to experience a major grief reaction, triggered perhaps by a loss of lesser significance. The intensity of the grief reaction may lead the person to conclude that she or he has completely lost her or his emotional equilibrium. What the person fails to realize is that the personal grief encompasses not one loss but a series of losses. Some losses may be more significant than others, but all may have been repressed for some time.

The *Diagnostic and Statistical Manual of Mental Disorders, Fourth Edition* (DSM-IV) addresses the issue of grieving or bereavement by distinguishing symptoms related to "normal" bereavement from those of a major depressive disorder, exacerbated perhaps by a loss experience (see Medical Diagnoses and Related Nursing Diagnoses: Grieving).

In his book *Life After Loss,* Bob Deits (1988) wrote,

The only time you have to start working through your losses is today. Tomorrow will not be a better day to face up to the task. The only one who can make the journey through your grief is you. But as you make it, you will discover that you are equal to the challenge. (p. 82)

An excellent way to get in touch with losses experienced within your life is to use a personal survey or to prepare a loss inventory (Box 22–3). In doing this, you not only are able to recount loss events and their significance but also can recognize whether you adequately grieved these events.

Another exercise that is helpful in exploring issues of personal loss is to use a loss time line. To create a loss time line, randomly select a 5- or 10-year segment of your life, then plot losses chronologically. As the events take shape graphically on the time line, the proximity of the losses and the number of losses experienced become clear. Case Example 22–1 tells the story of one woman's losses, and Figure 22–1 demonstrates the use of a loss time line to illustrate her losses.

Although it is helpful to recognize one's losses, it is equally important to look at how a person like Susan

---

B o x   2 2 – 3 ■ ■ ■ ■ ■
A Personal Loss Inventory

1. The first significant loss I can remember in my life was _____
2. The circumstances were _____
3. My age was _____
4. The feelings I had at the time were _____ _____
5. The first death that made its impact on my life was _____
6. The thing I remember most about that experience was _____
7. I coped with the loss by _____
8. The most difficult death for me to face would be _____
9. My primary style of coping with loss is _____ _____
10. I know my grief over a loss is resolved when _____

Smith has dealt with each loss. In Susan's case, the losses were significant, and her ability to cope was certainly taxed. Did Susan take the time to grieve each loss? Did one grief period blend into another? Did Susan emerge from the period of loss well, whole, and healed?

MEDICAL DIAGNOSES AND RELATED NURSING DIAGNOSES

Grieving

DSM-IV Diagnosis: Bereavement

Diagnostic Criteria
This category can be used when the focus of clinical attention is a reaction to the death of a loved one. As part of their reaction to the loss, some grieving individuals present with symptoms characteristic of a Major Depressive Episode (e.g., feelings of sadness and associated symptoms such as insomnia, poor appetite, and weight loss). The bereaved individual typically regards the depressed mood as "normal," although the person may seek professional help for relief of associated symptoms such as insomnia or anorexia. The duration and expression of "normal" bereavement vary considerably among different cultural groups. The diagnosis of Major Depressive Disorder is generally not given unless the symptoms are still present 2 months after the loss. However, the presence of certain symptoms that are not characteristic of a "normal" grief reaction may be helpful in differentiating bereavement from a Major Depressive Episode. These include (1) guilt about things other

than actions taken or not taken by the survivor at the time of the death; (2) thoughts of death other than the survivor feeling that he or she would be better off dead or should have died with the deceased person; (3) morbid preoccupation with worthlessness; (4) marked psychomotor retardation; (5) prolonged and marked functional impairment; and (6) hallucinatory experiences other than thinking that he or she hears the voice of, or transiently sees the image of, the deceased person.

Related Nursing Diagnoses
Dysfunctional Grieving.

Definition
Extended, unsuccessful use of intellectual and emotional responses by which individuals attempt to work through the process of modifying self-concept based on the perception of the loss.

Example
Dysfunctional Grieving related to the loss of a child.

Diagnostic criteria reprinted with permission from the *Diagnostic and Statistical Manual of Mental Disorders, Fourth Edition.* Copyright 1994 American Psychiatric Association. Nursing diagnoses and definitions from North American Nursing Diagnosis Association. (1999). *NANDA nursing diagnoses: Definitions and classification 1999-2000.* Philadelphia: NANDA.

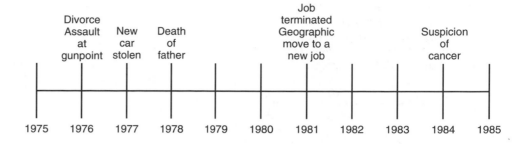

Figure 22-1
Example of a loss time line.

■ CASE EXAMPLE 22-1
■ Susan Smith's Story

Life was going well for 52-year-old Susan Smith. Although she had never had children, and although her marriage of 16 years had been rocky at times, she felt reasonably content with her lot in life. She had a well-paying job as an insurance executive, and she was in good health. Then, suddenly, her husband announced that he was leaving her. He wanted a divorce.

After the divorce in 1976, Susan moved to an upscale apartment in Baltimore. She had barely settled into her new home when, on her way home from work, she was robbed at gunpoint. Susan lost her purse, her credit cards, and her wallet, but otherwise escaped unharmed.

Susan purchased a new Oldsmobile after her divorce, and she felt proud of her ability, as a single woman, to afford such a prestigious car. However, in 1977, just 6 months after making her last payment on the car, local teens stole it and took it for a joyride, causing thousands of dollars of damage in the process.

Susan's life seemed to normalize in 1978, but by the end of that year, her father became gravely ill with pancreatic cancer and died.

After 3 years of uneventful living, Susan suddenly lost her job. Corporate reorganization and downsizing had left her with three options: take a major pay cut, take a lower-ranking position, or leave the company on severance pay. She chose the last option, and a long, tedious job search and a move to Colorado for a new job resulted.

Three-and-a-half years later, Susan received a call from her gynecologist after a routine mammogram. A suspicious shadow showed up on the film, and a biopsy was necessary "just to be safe." Despite her doctor's cautious optimism, Susan feared the worst: breast cancer. After a wait that seemed like an eternity, Susan underwent the biopsy. The reports, thankfully, were negative. Susan did not have breast cancer. ■

Loss and the Psychiatric Patient

Loss issues are a concern as you journey with a person who struggles with mental illness. Dealing with losses or going through a grief reaction can even precipitate a crisis or a psychotic episode in someone whose mental health is already fragile. The psychiatric patient is vulnerable to the same losses as the person who is emotionally sound. Additionally, the psychiatric patient experiences losses directly related to mental illness, including

1. Loss of job or career because of unstable mental health
2. Loss of financial well-being due to hospital bills or the inability to work
3. Loss of friends as a result of frequent hospitalizations or the inability to enter into meaningful relationships
4. Loss of rootedness and a place called "home" as a result of the tendency to disengage from reality and the flow of human life

Less obvious but just as significant are the losses of a more personal and spiritual nature, including

1. Loss of zest and joy for living when illness exacerbates
2. Loss of purpose and direction for life
3. Loss of existential meaning
4. Loss of health and wholeness
5. Loss of hope, especially during periods of psychosis or depression
6. Loss of grasp of what is real and true
7. Loss of physical and psychological stamina

When the psychiatric patient becomes trapped in his or her flight from reality or intense state of self-absorption, losses can be ignored easily. During periods of acute illness, losses cannot be fully perceived or grieved. The patient must experience emotional equilibrium before being able to process losses. During the time it takes for the psychiatric patient to regain emotional equilibrium, many losses may have occurred. Most significant of these losses are the deaths of parents, family members, close friends, or significant others. When mental health stabilizes, the person may be faced with many voids in her or his life, caused by the losses that have occurred. How, then, does she or he begin to grieve?

Similar is the plight of the person enmeshed in an addictive lifestyle. Years of events come and go without the addicted person being fully aware of his or her investment in these events. When the person begins a life of sobriety, he or she is faced with taking an inventory of all that has been missed, ignored, or avoided because of the addiction. Grieving these losses is a part of adjusting to a chemical-free lifestyle.

Your challenge as a psychiatric nurse involves helping the patient to reinvest in life once again through a recapturing of "what was" and a facing of "what is." Most certainly this process entails getting in touch with loss experiences that have occurred and discovering how they can be grieved. The work is slow and arduous.

Your interventions must be gentle, directive, and well paced so as not to overwhelm the patient. The goal is to journey with the psychiatric patient toward wellness and healing as he or she grieves. Let us turn our attention to the process of grieving.

> **W**hat do you think? How would you assist a psychiatric patient to deal with the many losses that accompany a psychiatric diagnosis?

> ➤ *Check Your Reading*
> 5. What are some typical losses faced in a lifetime?
> 6. What are some disadvantages of using repression as a means of coping with loss?
> 7. How does the DSM-IV differentiate a normal grief reaction from a Major Depressive Episode?
> 8. What are some of the losses that people with mental illness face?

GRIEF

The Length of the Grieving Process

One of the major concerns regarding the **grieving process** is how long it will last. Many of us would just as soon grieve for a few days or weeks and then have the process completed—quickly and easily. This does not happen, primarily because grieving is a process that takes time to unfold and be resolved.

Deits (1988) indicated that because grieving and recovery from grief are demanding, people often look for any way to get out of going through the process. To go through grief requires both stamina and an incredible amount of patience. This is especially true when one feels terribly sad, lost, lonely, angry, or all of these. To simply wait it out or endure it without any active participation in the process is counterproductive.

Experiencing the loss is the first step in letting go and moving beyond the loss experience (Carson, 1999). Lindemann (1944) indicated that experiencing the emotional pain of a loss is what many fear the most. This fear can block the grief process from happening at all.

People grieve in different ways and at different rates. The important factor is that they grieve as soon after the loss as they can rather than postponing this necessary process for long periods of time (Bouvard, 1988). People usually grieve most intensely during the first months following their loss. By the end of the 1st year, people who allowed the grieving to occur and who have had no complicating circumstances surrounding their grief process may be nearing some point of resolution (Caplan, 1974). We discuss the factors related to complicated grieving later in this chapter.

The length of the grief process is dependent on

- The significance of the lost object or person
- One's preparation for the separation
- The emotional strength and ability to cope possessed at the time of the loss

Mrs. Jackson's story (Case Example 22–2) demonstrates that grieving her significant loss, related to her husband's death, may be delayed until she has coped with more immediate problems or needs. These will certainly drain her emotional energy leaving her unable to mourn his loss until some later time.

■ CASE EXAMPLE 22–2
■ Mrs. Jackson's Story

Mrs. Jackson is 42 years old; she suffered with depressive episodes for 20 years of her life. She received some bad news from her 46-year-old husband one day. During his annual physical, something abnormal was seen on his chest radiograph. Mr. Jackson was the sole provider for his family of four, and he had to interrupt his work for an admission to the hospital. The couple live with their 16-year-old daughter and 17-year-old son in an apartment in the inner city, subsisting on a modest income.

Tests revealed that Mr. Jackson had inoperable lung cancer. Plans for treatment with chemotherapy were made. Despite the stress she felt regarding the failing health of her husband, Mrs. Jackson spent a period of time each day at the hospital, trying to emotionally support him as he faced his diagnosis and treatment.

On returning from the hospital one day, Mrs. Jackson was informed by her daughter, who also suffers from depression, that she was pregnant and did not know what to do. Mrs. Jackson needed to look at options and make decisions, but concern over her husband's condition seemed more immediate.

Treatment went poorly for Mr. Jackson—the tumor was not responsive to chemotherapy. His condition declined rapidly, and his wife was aware of this. While facing this dilemma, a call came from the school principal informing Mrs. Jackson that her son had been suspended from school for the possession and use of drugs. His admission back into school would be dependent on the completion of a drug rehabilitation program.

As the days passed, Mr. Jackson became weaker, and his death became more imminent. Mrs. Jackson kept news of problems at home from him. She was feeling more emotionally fragile as each day passed. She had always relied on her husband, and now he was no longer there for her.

Within days, Mr. Jackson died and his wife was faced with the loss of her husband, the funeral, loss of a source of income for the family, a son with a serious drug problem who was out of school, a daughter who was 2 months pregnant, her own failing mental health, the home, and financial affairs.

Mrs. Jackson will deal with the immediate needs first. Her grieving process will be delayed until the urgent issues are resolved. Her mental health will need attention before she is faced with another bout of major depression. Her financial problems and the needs of her son and daughter will be handled with the assistance of her sister. These issues, however, will take precedence. She will grieve the loss of her husband at a later time when she has the emotional energy to do so. ■

Let us reflect on the psychiatric patient who may be actively engaged in treatment for a psychotic episode or a progression of her or his particular form of mental illness. When a significant loss occurs during that period, varying reactions can be expected. If the person is not in touch with reality at the time of the loss, the loss event will come and go without the person facing it. He or she even may go through the motions of attending a wake and funeral. Grieving will occur at some later time when the acute manifestations of the mental illness have been controlled through treatment. News of a significant loss such as death, bankruptcy, or loss of a job can threaten an already weakened emotional state. This may result in a pathological grief reaction, a psychotic episode, or an acute depression with suicidal ideation. Mental illness, therefore, may complicate or delay the grief reaction and may extend the period of grieving.

Stages of Grieving

The stages of grieving have been outlined by many authors who have studied grief and loss. These include Engel (1964), Kübler-Ross (1969), Westberg (1971), and Veninga (1985), to name a few. Perhaps the best known of these are the stages of dying described by Dr. Elizabeth Kübler-Ross. The denial, anger, bargaining, depression, and acceptance that she discussed in her writings may easily be considered the stages of the grieving process. Table 22–1 clearly outlines the stages of grieving.

Major Tasks of Grieving

As shown in Box 22–4, a person faces major tasks in any grief process (Worden, 1982). Each of these tasks is ac-

Box 22–4 ■ ■ ■ ■ ■
Major Tasks of Grieving

1. *Accepting the reality of the loss*—believing the loss has really occurred, knowing the situation will not reverse itself
2. *Experiencing the emotional pain*—knowing the disappointment, the loneliness, the emptiness, the absence of what was, and feeling the emotions that accompany these realizations
3. *Adjusting to life without the "lost object"*—recognizing that one's life is not over or totally destroyed, knowing that one can go on
4. *Letting go and moving beyond*—reinvesting energies into new relationships and undertakings, discovering a new purpose and meaning for one's life

Adapted from Worden, W. (1982). *Grief counseling and grief therapy: A handbook for the mental health practitioner.* New York: Springer.

complished as the grief process unfolds. The reality of the loss is felt as acute pain, and energies are poured into coping with this reality. The person wonders whether he or she will ever feel better about the loss. As the months of grieving pass, the person begins to believe that he or she is adjusting to life without what was lost. However, the arrival and passing of a holiday or commemorative event may rekindle the pain and deep longing. The person questions whether any progress in grieving has been made. In time, more emotional energy is available for meeting responsibilities, facing challenges, and accepting new undertakings. All of this is a part of the adjustment to life without the lost object.

Patterns of Grieving

As mentioned, many people would prefer not to grieve at all because the process is long, difficult, and emotionally draining. We now look at normal **grieving patterns** and contrast them with those that are abnormal. Much has been written on the topic of abnormal grieving (Schneider, 1980). It also is called *complicated grief, morbid grief reactions, the pathological grief syndrome, distorted grief,* and *unresolved grief.*

Normal Grieving

If grieving were regarded as a readily accepted social process, people would find the freedom to share their grief with others. When assisted in their grief work by caring others, people grieve more quickly and easily. In U.S. society, overt expressions of grief are not always socially acceptable. As long as death, the ultimate loss experience, continues to be regarded as something tragic, catastrophic, and unnatural, so too will grieving be regarded as terribly painful and difficult and an intrusion on the American way of life. If a person cannot freely grieve the loss of a significant other, much less is she or he free to grieve other losses.

Table 22–2 outlines some of the characteristics of normal grief reactions. These are contrasted with complicated grief reactions.

Complicated Grieving

Grieving that is incapacitating and unusually long and involves some disorganized, depressed behaviors falls into the category of **complicated grieving.** Some persons are predisposed to this kind of grief reaction, as seen in those with a history of

1. Psychiatric problems involving recurring hospitalizations
2. Substance abuse, especially alcoholism
3. Death faced during childhood or adolescence
4. Conflicts with or marked dependency on the deceased
5. A death experience accompanied by a posttraumatic stress reaction
6. Depressive reactions to life's crises

TABLE 22–2 Characteristics of Normal and Complicated Grieving

CRITERIA	NORMAL GRIEF REACTIONS	COMPLICATED GRIEF REACTIONS
Feelings	A deep sadness; guilt and self-reproach for somehow being responsible; loneliness; listlessness; anger at others	Deep sadness that persists and easily turns into depression; episodes of self-reproach; guilt and worthlessness that may be accompanied by suicidal ideation; anger and blaming of those held responsible
Physical sensations	Hollowness in the stomach; tightness in the chest and shortness of breath; loss of appetite or tendency to overeat; lack of energy; fear of illness; insomnia or sleeping long hours to cope	Symptoms are similar to a normal grief reaction but persist much longer, leading to a disruption of one's daily routine; preoccupation with illness and pathology; acquiring symptoms experienced by the deceased
Thought patterns	Difficulty concentrating; inability to make decisions or choices; memory lapses; auditory or visual hallucinations in which one seems to connect with the "lost object"	Intense preoccupation with the "lost object" accompanied by a continuing hope of the object's return; cognitive processes may be disrupted over a longer period of time; auditory and visual hallucinations may become part of a psychotic episode; intellectual awareness of the loss devoid of feelings
Behavior	Absent-mindedness; social withdrawal or restless overactivity; crying; lack of libido; dreaming about the lost object	Persistent withdrawal from social contacts and activities leading to complete social isolation; dysfunctional living patterns related to poor decision-making; dreams that incorporate the lost object

Adapted from Schneider, J. (1980, Fourth Quarter). Clinically significant differences between grief, pathological grief, and depression. *Patient Counseling and Health Education*, 267–275.

Wolfelt (1991a, 1991b) described various categories of complicated grief.

Absent Grief. Absent grief entails prolonged denial, resulting from psychic numbing. This prevents a person from accepting the reality of a significant loss and from mourning that loss. The person experiencing absent grief is relatively unmoved and psychologically detached as he or she tells the story of the loss that has occurred. As mentioned earlier, persons actively pursuing an addictive lifestyle or caught in the throes of mental illness may exhibit absent grief, even when something or someone treasured is lost.

Delayed Grief. Delayed grief involves the postponement of grieving for weeks, months, or years. Delayed grief can be abruptly ended by subsequent losses that trigger grieving. Sometimes delays in grieving occur out of necessity, such as occurred in the case of Mrs. Jackson in Case Example 22–2. If a significant period passes after an actual loss experience, during which a person cannot or will not grieve, repression is the coping mechanism used.

Chronic Grief. Chronic grief is a persistent pattern of grieving that tends to be exaggerated and does not reach resolution. It creates disabling symptoms and dysfunctional people. Chronic grief is characterized by attempts to keep the deceased person alive, such as by maintaining his or her personal things intact and expecting that the deceased will reenter the mourner's life.

Distorted Grief. Distorted grief is that type of grief that Lindemann called a morbid grief reaction. Anger and guilt are the two emotional expressions that become distorted in this type of grieving. The person is caught up in a state of emotional upheaval that inhibits him or her from effectively carrying out personal responsibilities and activities.

Converted Grief. Converted grief can be referred to as a type of Somatization Disorder. It entails a preoccupation with physical or psychological symptoms that are not consciously linked by the person to his or her loss.

Depression is often seen as a component of both normal and complicated grief reactions. The helplessness and hopelessness of depression often rob the grieving person of the emotional energy needed to do grief work.

Grieving in Children

Children perceive loss and grieve differently than do adults. For instance, children under the age of 3 years do not have a clear concept of the finality of death. The reactions of young children to loss is greatly affected by the sadness and seriousness of the adults around them who are grieving a recent loss. They come to understand that death involves leaving and separation. However, because they do not comprehend the finality of death, they may look for and talk about the deceased person as if he or she were coming back.

Children 3 to 6 years of age have a keener sense of a loss experience. They know about separation from a parent and the anguish this causes. They also may know what it is like to lose a pet or friend. Fear of having caused a significant loss by unacceptable behavior is common. Trying to discuss ways of "undoing" a loss is also a preoccupation of the child.

As children reach the ages of 6 to 9 years, they begin to realize that death is permanent and nothing will reverse it. In this age range, children have a lot of questions that they expect will be answered. Adults struggle with being candid when it comes to providing children with information about loss, separation, and death.

As children reach the ages of 10 to 12, death becomes a more familiar experience to them, as does loss. They may have lost in games and sporting events, had friends move away, and perhaps experienced the death of a child they knew. They come to realize that death can come to anyone at any time.

Adolescents may vacillate between having a mature attitude and having a child-like attitude toward death. Adolescents have a tendency to want to defy death and to remain immune to it. They know about the losses one faces in life, but when it comes to accepting death as one of those losses, they show great resistance. Death to them is reserved for older people or for those who are ill.

Interventions that are useful for working with grieving children are outlined in Box 22-5.

Obstacles to Grieving

Many obstacles to grieving exist. Many people do not want to struggle with the pain of loss that grieving evokes. Grieving takes time, and some people do not want to put the time and energy into this process after a significant loss. Other factors may impede a person from expressing grief and from doing so in a timely manner. The following are some obstacles to grieving.

Living in a Modern Society

In 21st-century America, life is generally fast paced, success oriented, goal seeking, and proficiency prone. Little recognition is given to the importance of grief work, and sufficient time to complete it may not be allowed. In addition, our society is mobile. Many people find themselves without roots and a permanent place to call home because of their life's circumstances. When faced with a significant loss, many find that they are geographically distant from family and relatives. This leads to a sense of being disconnected from one's former support system while facing the loss. People may not yet have a community in the new place of residence in which to relate or from which to receive support. Thus, grieving is made more difficult.

Lack of Religious Rites and Rituals

Religious rituals and rites of passage, well supported and sanctioned by American society, can help people mourn and undertake their process of grieving. The funeral provides loved ones with an opportunity to publicly and reservedly display their grief. Through a ministry of prayer, consolation, and counseling, clergymen and clergywomen have supported countless people in their grief process. A strong faith and deep religious principles have sustained many grieving people during the long, hard months of grief. With the trend among younger Americans to withdraw from traditional church membership and participation, this vital source of strength and spiritual assistance can be lacking at a time when it could be beneficial.

In light of the benefits that a funeral ritual provides to the grieving, we might question what happens when a person is cremated? Cremation has become a more common practice in our society, and it is a choice that many dying people make. Cremation, without a memorial service to accompany it, can deprive grieving families and loved ones of the final act of separation from the deceased that funeral rites provide.

Social Norms for Grieving in Men

Men in our society have restrictions placed on them with regard to grieving. This prevents healthy expressions of grief and impedes the grief process. Wolfelt (1990) indicated that men are more likely to experience complicated grief processes, absent grief, delayed grief

---

Box 22-5 ■ ■ ■ ■ ■
Interventions to Use With Grieving Children

- Talk with children with openness and honesty; use "teachable moments," such as the death of a pet, changing seasons, or television programs to discuss death with children.
- Assure them of their safety and physical well-being.
- Assure them of being loved, despite difficult times.
- Explain and let them see feelings of grief. It is best to err on the side of too much disclosure of feelings than to deny them any exposure to grief.
- Assure them of the normalcy of their feelings. Let them know that loss brings intense feelings that must be dealt with.
- Include them in rituals of mourning.
- Recognize that mourning comes and goes for children (in part, as their denial or coping mechanism).
- Help the very young to remember the deceased through pictures, stories, and memories.
- Look for "magical thinking" about a return of the lost one back into their lives.
- Older children show resistance to accepting death as one of life's losses.
- Make sure that children are provided with honest answers to their questions about loss, separation, and death.
- Recognize that children are not born afraid of death—they learn to be afraid of it.
- Know that their grief will be expressed through play, artwork, and other behaviors rather than predominantly through verbalization.

Adapted from Rando, T. A. (1984). *Grief, dying, and death: Clinical interventions for caregivers.* Champaign, IL: Research Press.

reactions, or any manifestation of abnormal grieving as a result of socially dictated gender stereotypes. Several factors influence the manner in which men and boys grieve. These factors also affect their choice not to grieve (Table 22–3).

Unsanctioned Losses

Some losses are not validated or fully sanctioned by all of society (Doka, 1989). Among these unsanctioned losses are loss of a pregnancy through an abortion or a miscarriage; loss of a loved one by suicide; loss of someone with whom one had an extramarital affair, a homosexual relationship, or a nonmarital union; loss of financial stability through bankruptcy; and loss of one's job through dismissal with cause. Emotional, legal, and financial involvements related to these unsanctioned losses can compound the loss experience further. *Disenfranchisement* means being deprived of one's rights as a citizen. **Disenfranchised grieving** is a complicated form of grieving because it entails unsanctioned losses. Social stigma; difficulties with participation in mourning rites; delayed or private grieving; lack of social support systems; economic and legal problems; and the emotional burdens of guilt, shame, and blaming may exist. According to Pine (1972), disenfranchised grievers are an underclass of grievers. They are shunted out of the mainstream because their relationships may not be fully recognized (e.g., with abortions or miscarriages), illegitimate (e.g., with an extramarital affair or a nonmarital union), or unsanctioned (e.g., a gay partner). The losses may not fit the norm of being appropriate or have societal approval, such as with suicide, bankruptcy, or being dismissed with cause from one's job. Refer to What Patients and Families Need to Know: Grief for some common questions and answers.

Other Obstacles to Grieving

Other obstacles to grieving include

1. Inability to grieve because chemical dependence totally absorbs the person's life
2. An altered state of physical or mental health that warrants energy being placed on becoming physically or mentally well again
3. Facing multiple losses, as is the case in a fire or natural disaster in which possessions and loved ones are lost
4. Uncertainty about the loss because circumstances prevent confirmation of the certainty of the loss, as is the case with victims of war and war prisoners
5. Survivors find death from sudden illness (Sanders, 1982) more difficult to resolve

> **W**hat do you think? The average employee receives 3 days of paid leave following a significant loss. Is this adequate? If not, how long should the leave be? Is there anything else in addition to a paid leave that employers can provide to assist employees to deal with grief?

Grieving and the Psychiatric Patient

Having looked at how people not suffering from mental health problems face the major tasks of grieving, let us now explore how the psychiatric patient faces these tasks. The psychiatric patient grieves to the degree that she or he has the emotional energy and a grounding in reality to do so. In undertaking the first task of grieving—accepting the reality of the loss—the person may enter into denial as a means of coping. He or she may believe that what has been lost will be returned. Some patients may become psychotic or immersed in depression (Kutscher, 1968). These circumstances can inhibit any forward movement in accomplishing the tasks of grieving until they are resolved.

Psychiatric patients may avoid the second task of grieving—facing the pain of loss—by developing somatic symptoms that distract from grieving and result in a focus on physical illness. This may lead them to engage in an extensive diagnostic workup. Lindemann (1944) described this as symptom formation "by identification." Energies that could be spent on facing the pain of loss and adjusting to life without the lost object are spent on finding the cause of symptoms and controlling diseases that are thought to exist.

TABLE 22–3 Factors That Affect the Grieving of Men	
FACTOR	**EXPLANATION**
Social conditioning	Early lessons in life teach that boys and men do not cry; acceptable male feelings are fearlessness, aggressiveness, and defensiveness.
Reluctance to seek support	Grieving requires a reaching out to caring others and some dependence upon them; societal norms dictate that males be strong, independent, and self-sufficient.
Intolerance of slowing down to grieve	Grief work that terminates in growth and healing requires periods of quiet and time to process; masculinity is often equated with striving, accomplishing, and producing.
Inability to acknowledge pain	Men are influenced to believe that outwardly expressing the pain of loss is equated with weakness; since childhood they have learned that they must be strong, repressing what they feel.

Adapted from Wolfelt, A. (1990, Fall). Gender roles and grief: Why men's grief is naturally complicated. *Thanatos,* 20–24.

? WHAT PATIENTS AND FAMILIES NEED TO KNOW

Grief

Why do we grieve?

Grieving is our normal response to dealing with a loss. By working through the emotions of denial, anger, bargaining, depression, and acceptance, we are able to let go of the loss and focus on our life, our relationships, and our goals with renewed energy.

How do I know if I'm grieving?

You may experience a deep feeling of sadness and sorrow and sometimes guilt and anger about losing someone or something close to you. You may have physical symptoms such as muscle tension and weakness, a hollow feeling in the stomach, tightness in the chest, shortness of breath, or loss of appetite or overeating. In addition, you may have trouble sleeping and difficulty concentrating and making decisions. Sometimes you might feel you are going crazy because you dream about the lost person or imagine that he or she is still alive. You might think that you hear or see the lost person in a crowd. All of this is normal and will lessen with the grieving process.

When does grieving become abnormal?

When grief does not follow the typical pattern, becomes incapacitating, or is of unusually long duration, it can be considered abnormal. If you feel your grief is abnormal, seek professional help.

What can I do to help someone grieve?

It is important to be a good listener and allow the grieving person to "retell" their loss over and over. Do not tell the person not to cry. He or she needs to get his or her feelings out. Grief affects all members of a family, so do not forget the children. They, too, experience grief. Encourage the grieving person to seek solace and spiritual comfort within his or her religious traditions. Remember, grief is self-limiting and will resolve over time. Tell the person to be patient with himself or herself.

The third task of grieving—adjustment to life without the lost object—can be difficult for the psychiatric patient if the "lost object" is the person on whom she or he depended for support, care, and supervision. The reality of the loss can create feelings of panic revolving around survival issues. It is necessary to help the person to designate a substitute caregiver or a different support person. The challenge lies in helping the person to not feel totally destroyed or hopeless because of this loss.

The fourth task of grieving—letting go and moving beyond—can happen if the psychiatric patient is supported in her or his grieving over an adequate period of time. Assistance is given to help the patient process the significance of the loss. Letting go and moving on require bidding goodbyes and having reminiscences, coping with feelings of abandonment, and reaching out to others.

Significant losses may trigger intense feelings of shame, self-blame, and diminished worth and a more negative self-concept. When such feelings precipitate a dysfunctional existence, the major tasks of grieving cannot be accomplished without the assistance of psychiatric medications and counseling.

W*hat do you think?* If you were working with an adolescent with a diagnosed psychiatric problem, what interventions do you think might help that adolescent deal with a recent loss? Do you have

any experiences that might allow you to identify with such a patient? If so, what helped you?

➤ *Check Your Reading*

9. What factors affect the length of one's grieving process?
10. Describe what you consider to be two of the more difficult tasks of grieving.
11. What are some of the characteristics of normal grieving? Abnormal grieving?
12. How do children grieve differently than adults?
13. Identify three obstacles to grieving that exist within our society.
14. What problems does a psychiatric patient typically encounter as he or she tries to complete the tasks of grieving?

MOVING BEYOND LOSS AND GRIEF

In discussing some basic guidelines for doing grief work, Deits (1988) emphasized the importance of believing that grief has a purpose and that it will have an end. So many people, including the psychiatric patient, become caught in the process of trying to discover why the loss occurred. This need for a logical explanation is a natural response to any crisis or tragedy. Individuals look at what happened and want to discover who or what is to blame. In addition, they review how the loss happened to find meaning in what occurred. Tragedies somehow seem easier to face if a causative factor can be pinpointed. Yet, with some losses, the person cannot find clear reasons for the loss, people to blame, or particular circumstances to which the losses relate. The truth is that loss and grief occur in our lives because we are mortal human beings who live in an imperfect world with other human beings.

Coping with loss can become more difficult when the elements of retribution become enmeshed in the process. Grieving people easily can blame themselves, rightfully or erroneously, for a loss that has occurred. Self-recrimination and self-inflicted punishment in the form of guilt, shame, unforgiveness, or interminable sadness complicate grieving or slow it down significantly. The death of an infant or child from causes such as sudden infant death syndrome (SIDS), a spontaneous abortion or stillbirth, or an accident can provoke the distraught parents to blame each other. This can lead to marital strife, which makes coping with the loss much more difficult.

Guilt, shame, and self-recrimination also are seen in cases of suicide. It is difficult to face the haunting thought of being responsible for the death of a loved one. Sadness is mixed with feelings of negligence for being blind to or emotionally cut off from the person who just terminated his or her life. Grieving is painful and intense, and moving beyond the grief seems impossible.

Religious issues also may become a point of focus following loss. By nature, we are all spiritual beings. At our center is a yearning for association with and reliance on a presence greater than we are. We come to know that presence as God, a higher power, or some spiritual, bonding force. Some people believe that their loss represents God's punishment for past wrongdoings. Others feel betrayed or abandoned by God. It is not unusual to hear people cry out to God in dismay, "How could You do this to me?" "How could You let this happen?" Thus, God may be considered the direct cause of the loss. Some curse God as they curse their fate. Over time, many find comfort and solace in their relationship with their God and their church. A spiritual crisis (spiritual distress) precipitated by a painful loss can interfere with grieving.

Coping mechanisms are learned patterns of behavior that permit us to deal with stressful situations or crises. Their effectiveness is measured by their ability to bring some form of resolution to a stressful situation or by their ability to lower the feelings of distress being experienced. We learn to cope well or poorly, effectively or ineffectively. Our coping patterns can be changed or improved as necessity dictates. Box 22–6 provides a list of coping mechanisms classified into the categories of least effective, intermediately effective, and most effective. Some of these coping mechanisms provide short-term relief when used but do not lead to problem or crisis resolution. An example of this is a sense of humor. When situations are overwhelming,

---

B o x 2 2 – 6 ■ ■ ■ ■ ■
Coping Mechanisms

Least Effective

Suppression (not worrying, trying to forget)
Hypervigilance (expecting the worst, being unduly alert for "trouble")
Stoic submission (displaying unquestioning acceptance, being unmoved by the worst)
Passivity (thinking that others must help one, waiting to be directed or "saved")
Acting out (striking back, doing something . . . anything)
Blaming (faulting oneself, accusing others or circumstances)

Intermediately Effective

Humor (laughing it off, seeing the lighter side)
Tension reduction (eating, drinking, playing, working, smoking, or sleeping more)
Sharing responsibilities (delegating, relying on others)
Withdrawing (removing oneself for a while, stepping back to be objective)
Ventilating (unburdening periodically, discharging repressed emotions)

Most Effective

Confronting the issues (facing reality, problem solving) and seeking information (learning more, consulting the "experts")
Setting priorities (redirecting energies, focusing on important things)
Redefining goals (cultivating new dreams, rekindling hope)
Seeking support (sharing with friends, accepting encouragement and empathy)

---

being able to smile or to laugh lightens the intensity of the pain. This enables improved coping until some form of resolution of the situation is achieved.

You are invited to explore which coping mechanisms you use most. Being in touch with how you cope, as well as how you grieve your losses, helps you to become more effective as a helping professional, change agent, companion, and fellow traveler to the psychiatric patient. You assess coping patterns as you work with the grief-stricken mentally ill patient.

Deits (1988) wrote of the need to make a decision to go on with one's life after a major loss. If grieving people wait until they feel better before undertaking their grief work, precious time is lost. They can get trapped in their grieving. This leads to stagnation and fixation on their state of misery and pain. This is a real danger for the psychiatric patient who is prone to periods of depression and hopelessness. He or she may have a desire to regress to a safer way of being in which there is less chance of becoming involved with the pressures and responsibilities of life.

What do you think? How do your spiritual beliefs influence how you cope with loss and grief?

➤ *Check Your Reading*

15. What makes it more difficult for couples to cope with and grieve the loss of a child?
16. How is one's spirituality affected by a significant loss?
17. Define coping mechanisms.
18. Enumerate the coping mechanisms that you use most often in difficult times.

NURSING PROCESS

Let us return to the story of Susan Smith presented earlier in the chapter. When discussing loss as an experience of the human journey, it was suggested that a loss time line be used as a means of tracking loss experiences. An example was provided using a 10-year segment from Susan Smith's life (see Figure 22–1).

From 1975 to 1977, Susan faced three losses—a divorce, a physical assault and robbery, and the theft of her new automobile. The losses were close to each other in time. Strong emotional responses and some grieving occurred with each loss. The loss that was the most difficult for Susan to face, however, was the death of her father in 1978. She had been close to him. His diagnosis of pancreatic cancer came as a shock to the whole family. At the end of a 9-month period, this 72-year-old man, once vibrant and strong, had deteriorated physically and was in the terminal phase of his illness. Susan's father died in late October 1978. In December of that year, just 2 weeks before Christmas, Susan was admitted to the psychiatric unit of a large teaching hospital in her city. Her admitting diagnosis was Grief Reaction With Depressed Mood. The psychiatric nurse assigned to be the primary nurse for Susan met with her the day of her admission.

Assessment

Susan did not communicate much during the initial nursing assessment. The admission note of the attending physician indicated a history of chronic depression, as well as several short inpatient stays for treatment of the depression. Susan also had had 6 months of outpatient therapy following her divorce. The nurse performed a comprehensive assessment focusing on physical, emotional, social, and spiritual domains. Box 22–7 presents a summary of the assessment data obtained on Susan Smith.

Diagnosis

From the behaviors that Susan presented during the assessment, the psychiatric nurse identified the following nursing diagnosis: Dysfunctional Grieving related to a complicated grief reaction that is evidenced by withdrawal, seclusion, absence of friends and support persons, self-termination of employment, spiritual distress, and self-care deficits.

Outcome Identification

The expected outcomes for Susan's care include the following:
- Susan will resolve the issues surrounding her complicated grief reaction.
- Susan will display behaviors indicative of successful grieving, including returning to work, reengaging in life's activities, and resuming self-care activities; behaviors indicative of spiritual well-being; and evidence of reconnection with others.

Planning

Having assessed Susan's present status, the psychiatric team members developed a plan of care to assist Susan in dealing with her sadness and to help her to get in touch with her most recent loss experience and its impact on her life. The plan included a focus on improving patterns of self-care; resolving somatic symptoms such as anorexia, insomnia, and weight loss; establishing needed support systems; and promoting spiritual well-being. The short-term goals and expected outcomes, which represented a mutual effort by Susan and the staff members, were as follows.

Expected Outcome
Susan will resolve the issues surrounding her complicated grief reaction.

Short-Term Goals
- Susan will participate in daily sessions held with her therapist so that she can explore her recent significant loss.
- Susan will attend group therapy daily and be an active participant within the group.
- Susan will begin to express the emotions she has surrounding the loss of her father.
- Susan will report to her case manager, or to any nurse on duty, feelings of being out of control, hopeless, unable to go on, or intensely angry.

Expected Outcome
Susan will display behaviors indicative of successful grieving, including returning to work, reengaging in life's activities, and resuming self-care activities; she

Box 22-7 ■ ■ ■ ■ ■
A Summary of the Assessment Data on Susan Smith

Physical Status

The nurse observed a 52-year-old white woman with an appearance that bespoke neglect. Susan's clothes were soiled, her hair uncombed. She wore no cosmetics, looked older than her age, and sat stooped in her chair with eyes cast down. Susan looked pale and thin. She complained of weight loss, poor appetite, and indigestion when she did eat. Susan indicated that she had not been able to sleep for the past month or so.

Emotional Status

Susan spoke little and seemed quite withdrawn. Her responses to questions were one- or two-word answers, unless prompted to be more specific. She showed little emotion, especially when asked about her father's death. In a sad tone, she spoke of how special she had always been to him. They had always done so many things together. She could describe the details of her father's illness and death, but she offered factual information that was devoid of any feeling component. Susan was agitated at times, looking toward the door as if she were eager to leave. Most of the time she stared at the floor, finding it difficult to make eye contact.

Social Status

From the medical history, the nurse learned that Susan had become a recluse during the past 3 weeks. When Susan was asked about her job, she informed the nurse that she resigned 3 weeks ago because the pressures were too great to handle. She indicated that she liked being alone and enjoyed spending her free time in her apartment. When asked about her friends, she stated that her best friend, her father, had died.

Spiritual Status

Susan grew up attending church services in the Lutheran church. She stated that after her marriage ended so painfully, she stopped going to church. She thought God would save her father from dying so soon. "But He [God] failed to help me, just as He did when I was struggling in my bad marriage."

---

will exhibit behaviors indicative of spiritual well-being; and she will show evidence of reconnection with others.

Short-Term Goals
- Susan will bathe, comb her hair, and dress in her own clothing each day.
- Susan will be up and out of bed each day.
- Susan will eat four small meals each day and report any symptoms of discomfort that occur as a result of eating.
- Susan will use relaxation tapes at bedtime and report to the nurse each morning how well she slept.
- Susan will participate in the unit social activities.
- Susan will engage in interactions with others.
- Susan will discuss her feelings of abandonment and anger at God.
- Susan will plan for her return to work as soon as she is able to do so.

Implementation

Before looking at the interventions that the nurse chose to work with Susan, let us take a look at the Snapshot: Nursing Interventions Specific to Grief and Loss.

The general skills for adult patients guided the daily interactions between Susan and her psychiatric nurse and provided the foundation for a relationship of trust and respect. The mutual goals that had been established and identified as being feasible were reviewed daily. Thus, Susan was held accountable for her plan of care. Nursing interventions focused on present needs and the fulfillment of the mutual goals. The following nursing interventions were used in assisting Susan to deal with her bereavement:

- Encourage daily hygiene, grooming, and the wearing of personal clothing, as opposed to a hospital gown.
- Monitor food consumption at meal times.
- Provide a nutritious evening snack.
- Weigh the patient twice weekly.
- Teach Susan the basic concepts of relaxation therapy; provide a tape recorder and relaxation tapes at bedtime; monitor their effectiveness.
- Provide the medications prescribed for insomnia, depression, and gastric distress and note their effectiveness.
- Encourage social interaction and activities in the day room.
- Hold Susan responsible for participation in individual therapy sessions and group therapy.
- Engage the patient in conversation and encourage her to share how she is feeling at a given period of the day.

SNAPSHOT

Nursing Interventions Specific to Grief and Loss

What do you need to do to develop a relationship with a patient facing grief and loss?

- Be physically and emotionally present to the grieving person, despite his or her inability to easily relate.
- Let your genuine concern and caring show.
- Try to view the loss from the griever's unique perspective, as well as the perspective of his or her significant others.
- Allow crying, talking, a retelling of the loss event, and even periods of silence, without judgment or censure.
- Give the person encouragement to grieve but realize that you cannot take away the pain of loss being felt.
- Do not use false reassurances such as, "Feel better, your loved one is with God" or "You still have many years ahead in which to recuperate this loss." Reassurances don't help the actively grieving person to feel better.

What do you need to assess regarding the patient's status?

- Observe the grieving person for normal grieving patterns, exhibited within the expected time frame following the loss.
- Assess and teach the grieving person to assess for other significant losses that have never been mourned.
- Be attentive to the presence of obstacles to grieving in the person's personal life and life circumstances.
- Observe for complicated grief patterns (absent, delayed, chronic, distorted, or converted grief) and encourage professional help to work through them.
- Explore with the griever coping patterns used in the past, their effectiveness, and the need for new, more effective coping skills.
- Assess the need for medication and further psychiatric follow-up if grieving seems to be coupled with major depression.

What do you need to teach the patient and the patient's significant others about grief and loss?

- Grieving is a natural response to loss. If these feelings are repressed at the time of the loss, the grieving will occur at some later point in time.
- The grief process is much longer than a few days or weeks if a significant loss has occurred. Grieving follows various stages of progression until it is resolved.
- Each person grieves in his or her own unique way, but the tasks of moving through grief require one's full attention in order for the process to progress and resolve.
- New roles, strengths, and life skills can emerge as a result of seeing the grief process to its termination.
- There will be effects of grief on the body, mind, spirit, and relationships; thus there is the need for gentle care of self by the griever.
- There is importance in verbalizing feelings, no matter how strong they may be; maintaining good physical health while grieving; and having support people on whom one can depend.

What skills will you want the patient to demonstrate?

- Ability to verbalize feelings, needs, and the pain caused by the loss.
- Coping skills that bring about positive outcomes and reinforce internal strengths.
- Use of relaxation strategies, physical exercise, and good nutrition to promote physical and emotional well-being.
- Ability to use medications, counseling, and group support as a means of moving beyond grieving.
- Ability to obtain or regain spiritual strength and well-being.
- Ability to reinvest one's energies into new undertakings, new relationships, and a new tomorrow.

What other health professionals might need to be a part of this plan of care?

- Ongoing grief therapy, especially in the case of complicated grief reactions, requires the care and services of a psychiatrist, counselor, or social worker.
- A physician, whether a psychiatrist or primary doctor, may be needed to do any testing for physical illness or for the prescription of antidepressants or other medications.
- Social workers can assist the grieving person and his or her significant others to access financial services, community resources, and other entitlements.
- A grief support group, directed by a nurse or social worker, can facilitate grief work for self and others who have had similar experiences.

- Monitor for self-destructive tendencies.
- Observe the patient for changes in affect, statements of hopelessness or self-blame, increased depression or agitation, or threats of suicide.
- Explore feelings of abandonment expressed by the patient, and provide emotional support and availability.
- Encourage Susan to verbalize her feelings of abandonment by her father and by her God.
- Help Susan to explore her relationship with her father and the meaning of her life with and without him.
- Have Susan describe her spirituality and her present relationship to her God.
- Encourage Susan to write a farewell letter to her father in which she can express some of her feelings.
- Evaluate excuses for not being able to participate in therapy sessions.
- Monitor the effectiveness of Susan's mood-altering medications and communicate the need for dose adjustment.

Evaluation

The formative evaluation of Susan's care took place in weekly evaluations of treatment progress made by the case manager and other team members. A team conference was held during the 1st week of admission. Susan's treatment course and progress were discussed. Revisions were made in the plan of care as needed. The evaluations of each team member were based on whether progress was being made in decreasing Susan's depression; whether emotional, social, spiritual, and physical well-being were being established; and whether Susan was able to initiate grief work. Susan had em-

barked on the journey toward wellness, assisted by caring and supportive mental health professionals.

Once her condition stabilized and evident progress was made, Susan was discharged. The summative evaluation indicated that her mood was brighter and her affect more pleasant; she had gained 4 lb and reported sleeping much better. Susan had begun to express her feelings of loss regarding her father. She had spoken to the nurse about her feelings toward God; however, she was not willing to talk to a clergyperson and indicated that she still felt very angry toward God. The psychiatric team strongly advised Susan that although she had made tremendous progress, more work still needed to be accomplished. Susan was encouraged to join a support group designed for persons who have lost loved ones, as well as to continue to see an outpatient therapist.

What do you think? As you read about Susan, would you do anything different? If Susan had experienced a psychosis, how would you alter the plan of care?

➤ *Check Your Reading*
19. Identify at least one expected outcome in working with a patient with a nursing diagnosis of Dysfunctional Grieving.
20. Identify four interventions that you would use with a grieving adult.
21. Identify four general interventions that you would use with a grieving child.

Let's look at two additional case studies and apply the nursing process.

NURSING PROCESS APPLICATION

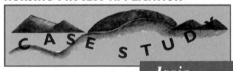

Josie

Josie is a 45-year-old nurse entrepreneur who has been feeling sad and guilty that she has been unable to spend time (due to a busy, traveling schedule) with her mother, who lives in another state and is dying of cancer. Two years ago, her mother, age 68, was diagnosed with adenocarcinoma of the colon. After Josie's mother recovered from the colon resection, she underwent weekly chemotherapy treatments for 18 months.

Although Josie was able to be with her mother for the surgery and visited her several times during the 18 months of chemotherapy, she tells her friends that over the past 2 years, she has felt helpless to assist her family because she lives out of state. Josie has experienced episodes of crying when driving her car and chokes up when she talks to friends about her mother. Recently, she has experienced a lack of interest in sex and increasing conflict with her spouse, who seems less than supportive, and she has lost interest in attending her exercise class and has stopped attending church. On her last visit with her mother, arrangements were made for her mother to enter a local hospice program.

ASSESSMENT   Assessment data are as follows:
- Guilt, sorrow, choked feelings, and altered libido

- Change in activity level—not attending exercise class
- Feelings of helplessness and spiritual distress noted in Josie's behavior

---

DIAGNOSIS   **DSM-IV Diagnosis:** Adjustment Disorder

Nursing Diagnosis: Anticipatory Grieving related to anticipated loss of mother (and spouse) as evidenced by feelings of guilt, sorrow, altered libido, change in activity level, "choked" feelings, and denial and minimization of situation by spouse

---

OUTCOME IDENTIFICATION, PLANNING, AND IMPLEMENTATION

> **Expected Outcome 1:** By _____ Josie will identify and express feelings appropriately about the anticipated loss of her mother.

Short-Term Goal	Nursing Interventions	Rationales
By _____ the patient will identify and express feelings to self and others.	1. Provide an open, accepting environment so that Josie feels free to discuss feelings and concerns. 2. Listen to Josie's perceptions of the situation by using therapeutic communication skills, active listening, silence, and acknowledgment.	1. Accept all grief behavior—the response is highly individual, as no two people experience or behave in the same way or at the same rate. 2. Any type of meaningful loss (e.g., loss of parent, body part, role, or functioning) will precipitate a reaction that will follow the general stages or patterns of the grief response.

> **Expected Outcome 2:** By _____ the patient will return to previous level of functioning.

Short-Term Goal	Nursing Interventions	Rationales
By _____ the patient will resume normal activity (within 3 weeks).	1. Encourage Josie to attend exercise class and discuss problems related to activity level, sexual desire, and role performance. 2. Assist in the use of creative visualization and relaxation skills for family members. 3. Provide teaching about common symptoms of grief, the strong emotional responses that can occur, and the importance of taking special care of herself during this period before and following a major loss. 4. Discuss control issues with family members; determine what is within the person's power to change and what is beyond her control.	1–2. During the grief process, changes may occur in self-care, appetite, and activity levels, which are normal and similar to anxiety responses. 3. The availability of support people facilitates the resolution of grief. Avoid reinforcing the belief that holding in feelings is a sign of emotional strength. 4. Feelings of control and ineffective coping skills contribute to a failure to resolve grief.

> **Expected Outcome 3:** By _____ the family will demonstrate acceptance of the need for counseling and hospice services support.

Short-Term Goal	Nursing Interventions	Rationales
By _____ the family will seek assistance during the grief process by participating in hospice care.	1. Encourage family members to use the services provided by hospice. 2. Refer to other resources such as clergy, religious affiliation, counseling, psychotherapy, and support groups as needed.	1–3. The availability of support persons facilitates the resolution of grief. A strong religious faith may assist family members in dealing with loss.

3. Incorporate family members in problem-solving, supporting, and assisting the mother to deal with the situation.

4. Encourage family members to become involved in activities unrelated to the anticipated loss

4. Rational thinking and involvement in everyday activities facilitate grief resolution. Cultural and social practices support individuals adjusting to separation and loss.

Nursing Diagnosis: Spiritual Distress related to anticipated loss of mother evidenced by feelings of helplessness and separation from church ties and support

---

OUTCOME IDENTIFICATION, PLANNING, AND IMPLEMENTATION

> **Expected Outcome 1:** By _____ the daughter will verbalize spiritual concerns and feelings about anticipated loss.

Short-Term Goal	Nursing Interventions	Rationales
By _____ the patient will verbalize feelings about spiritual crisis.	1. Encourage Josie to discuss what has triggered feelings of helplessness. Discuss differences among grief, guilt, and helplessness, and assist Josie to identify and deal with each.	1. Often feelings of helplessness may be triggered by false guilt. Grief occurs as a response to a loss. Guilt is about not doing something you feel you should have. Feeling helpless occurs as a response to feelings of powerlessness and loss of control over a situation.
	2. Focus on short-term, concrete goals that the patient can do now (being with her mother when she can, telephoning frequently, arranging business travel to stay over 1 or 2 days with her mother).	2. Patients may experience fewer feelings of hopelessness and helplessness if they can feel as though they are making progress in some small area.
	3. Incorporate family members in problem-solving, supporting, and assisting the mother to deal with the situation.	3. The availability of support people facilitates the resolution of grief. A strong religious faith may assist family members in dealing with loss.
	4. Encourage family members to become involved in activities unrelated to the anticipated loss.	4. Rational thinking and involvement in everyday activities facilitate grief resolution. Cultural and social practices support individuals adjusting to separation and loss.

EVALUATION

Formative Evaluation: Josie met all of her short-term goals. She had begun to share her feelings with one of her close girlfriends and her spouse. She stated that even though she did not feel like exercising, she was making the effort, and once she got to exercise class, she felt better. While visiting her mother, she accompanied her father to church, which made her feel better and supported her father.

Summative Evaluation: Josie met all of the expected outcomes. She was able to be with her mother when hospice care was initiated. She felt good about the hospice nurse who was to take care of her mother. As for dealing with her guilt about not spending "enough" time with her mother and not always being available to her, Josie stated, "I am aware of what is going on. I need to allow myself time to feel sad." It was suggested to Josie that she work with her business partner to have some time off in the next month and to not schedule any extra activities, as her mother's condition was deteriorating. Her ongoing plan of care was continued during this process.

NURSING PROCESS APPLICATION

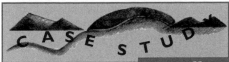

Camilla

Camilla is a 28-year-old mother who lost her 3-month-old son to SIDS 2 years ago. Since then, she has lost over 50 lb and is frail in appearance, with her current weight at 99 lb on her 5 ft 6 in. frame. She has lost total interest in work and has been on leave for the past 2 weeks because of constant crying spells, which have interfered with customer relations at her place of employment. Her husband reports that she has lost interest in sex and becomes agitated when he suggests they try to have another child.

ASSESSMENT	Assessment data are as follows: • Excessive crying, altered libido, lack of interest in work • Weight loss of 50 lb over past 2 years • Lack of resolution of normal grieving response
DIAGNOSIS	**DSM-IV Diagnosis:** Adjustment Disorder **Nursing Diagnosis:** Dysfunctional Grieving related to lack of resolution of unresolved issues of son's death 2 years ago as evidenced by excessive crying, weight loss, decreased libido, and lack of interest in normal work activities

OUTCOME IDENTIFICATION, PLANNING, AND IMPLEMENTATION

> **Expected Outcome 1:** By _____ the patient will have 2- to 3-lb weight gain.

Short-Term Goal	Nursing Interventions	Rationales
By _____ the patient will identify the weight loss as an issue related to the loss of her son and begin to gain weight by eating normally.	1. Discuss the symptom of weight loss and how it relates to the grieving process while motivating the patient to assume responsibility for self-care and well-being. 2. Explore with the patient fears associated with loss, particularly those related to loss of control.	1. Accept all grief behavior—the response is highly individual, as no two people experience or behave in the same way or at the same rate. 2. Any type of meaningful loss (e.g., loss of parent, body part, role, or functioning) will precipitate a reaction that follows the general stages or patterns of the grief response.

> **Expected Outcome 2:** By _____ the patient will work through the phases of grieving by expressing feelings about the loss of the infant to SIDS.

Short-Term Goal	Nursing Interventions	Rationales
By _____ the patient will verbalize behaviors associated with the normal stages of grief.	1. Identify which stage of grief the patient is stuck in or what is being expressed.	1. Often patients are fixed or stuck in the anger stage of the grieving process, in which the anger is directed inward and toward the self. An assessment of where the patient is in the grieving process is necessary to plan effective care.

2. Provide information about the normalcy of grieving and the typical feelings and actions associated with each of the stages of grief.

3. Encourage the patient to verbalize feelings and explore the reality of the loss and the means of resolution so that she can move on with her life.

4. Encourage the patient to review the loss in terms of the relationship and meaning it has in her life. When necessary, point out distortions and misinterpretations of the reality of the situation.

2. Knowledge of the stages of grieving may assist the patient in understanding the normal process of loss. The more significant the loss to the person, the more time is required for and the more severe the grief reaction.

3. Verbalizing feelings in a nonthreatening, supportive environment provides the basis for the patient to deal with the reality of the loss. This will assist the patient in recognizing her position within the grief process and help her come to terms with unresolved issues related to the loss.

4. Family members (especially mothers) who have lost a child to SIDS often have unresolved guilt issues—they feel they could have "done something" to prevent the death of their infant. Accurate information and identification of the reality of the situation and acknowledgment of the feelings of guilt may assist the patient to begin to resolve the grief.

Expected Outcome 3: By _____ the patient will participate in work activities and verbalize a sense of progress toward resolution of the grief and hope for the future.

Short-Term Goals	Nursing Interventions	Rationales
By _____ the patient will begin to resume normal activities and return to work.	1. Assist the patient with identifying methods for more adaptive coping with the loss of her son by focusing on assets and strengths. 2. Refer the patient to self-help groups for parents who have lost a child to SIDS (e.g., Compassionate Friends, SIDS Support Groups, National Sudden Infant Death Resource Center, SIDS Alliance).	1. Focusing on strengths and assets promotes self-esteem, encourages repetition of desirable behaviors, and aids in assisting the patient to cope with the situation. 2. Community outreach programs and groups are helpful in preventing prolonged grieving responses by providing immediate support and referral in the critical period after the death. Later, these self-help groups provide the opportunity for parents to draw support from other parents of SIDS infants.
By _____ the patient will begin to express feelings of hope for the future and a sense of control over her life situation.	1. Encourage the patient to find ways to experience pleasure as grief subsides and reinforce any experiences of pleasure. 2. Support and encourage the patient by reinforcing any creative efforts. 3. Encourage the use of self-affirmations.	1. Grief inhibits feelings of pleasure and joy in living. 2. Creative efforts can assist the patient in discovering a new purpose in life. 3. Self-affirmations enhance self-esteem.

EVALUATION

Formative Evaluation: Camilla met all of the short-term goals except the last one. She stated that it was hard for her to find joy in her life at this time; however, she did not feel as saddened and depressed over the situation.

Summative Evaluation: Camilla achieved all of her expected outcomes. By the end of a month, she had gained 10 lb and was able to go back to work. She stated, "I feel better knowing that I didn't do something to cause my son's death. I carried such a burden, thinking that I did something wrong. It feels much better to know that there was nothing I could have done to cause or prevent what occurred." To help her work on feeling more pleasure and joy in her life, the nurse encouraged her and her husband to identify those activities that they enjoyed doing when they first met. She expressed that she thought that she would feel more pleasure in time. The nurse modified her plan of care to give her additional time to integrate pleasurable activities and actions into her future.

Conclusions

In helping patients move beyond grief and loss, we help them realize that they are and can be stronger people for having faced the challenge of grieving. When helped to look back at how far they have come in the journey through grief, they realize that they have grown as they have moved forward. Building on newly found strength that comes as they pass through the grief process, they can dare to dream new dreams, set new goals, foster new relationships, and pursue new undertakings.

Sandra L. Bertman (1991), in her book *Facing Death*, writes about grieving and its effects:

Grief is not a disease. It is love not wanting to let go. It can be likened to a blow or a cut in which the wound gradually heals. For a while, one is acutely vulnerable, physically and emotionally. Though grief can be temporarily disabling, working through it ultimately brings strength. (p. 200)

How do you know when the psychiatric patient has completed the journey through grief and loss? The patient provides you with the information. She or he feels and looks better. Symptoms that seemed frightening early on are gone. Behavioral changes such as resocialization, energy expenditure in personal pursuits, a return to religious practices, and enthusiasm about be-

ing alive are observable. As you journey with the patient through grief, you will find that the process becomes more rewarding. You who have journeyed together through the dark times find light, as well as new direction, purpose, and meaning at the end of the process.

We end this chapter with the biblical text from the book of Ecclesiastes (3:1–8). The text fosters a sense of hope as it captures the journey of life:

There is an appointed time for everything, and a time for every affair under the heavens.
A time to be born, and a time to die; a time to plant and a time to uproot the plant.
A time to kill, and a time to heal; a time to tear down and a time to build.
A time to weep and a time to laugh; a time to mourn, and a time to dance.
A time to scatter stones, and a time to gather them; a time to embrace and a time to be far from embraces.
A time to seek, and a time to lose; a time to keep, and a time to cast away.
A time to rend, and a time to sew; a time to be silent, and a time to speak.
A time to love, and a time to hate; a time of war and a time of peace.

Key Points to Remember

- Loss accompanies all human beings in their life experiences from the moment of birth to death.
- Loss is an event within the life of a person that involves giving up that which is familiar, comfortable, and personal.
- Grief is a natural response to having lost something of significance in one's life. Grief involves feelings of sadness, emptiness, longing, pain, helplessness, and sometimes despair.
- Some people have a tendency to repress loss experiences rather than to face the emotional pain of grieving them.
- A way to get in touch with losses experienced in one's life is to do a loss inventory. A part of that process requires that one explore how losses were grieved after they happened.
- Psychiatric patients know the losses that come with their mental illness. These might include poor health, frequent hospitalizations, a meager support system because of the illness, inability to maintain steady em-

ployment, lack of purpose in life, and an inadequate grasp of what is real.
- According to cultural standards maintained in our American society, to grieve freely and openly is to demonstrate some degree of weakness.
- Eric Lindemann is a pioneer in the area of grief work. He did studies on grief and loss as early as the 1940s.
- John Bowlby described mourning as a process with three overlapping stages: numbness and disbelief, disorganization, and the reorganization of one's life and person.
- Theresa Rando did significant clinical work in the areas of grief and complicated grief during the 1980s and 1990s.
- People grieve in individual ways and for varying lengths of time. The grief process may extend from 12 to 24 months or even longer.
- Factors affecting a person's grief are the significance of what one has lost, the period of time it was possessed, the preparation one has had for the loss, and

the emotional strength or ability to cope possessed at the time of the loss.

- Significant losses for a psychiatric patient may precipitate a major grief reaction with depression or the exacerbation of the mental health problems already being treated.
- Major tasks of grieving include accepting the reality of the loss, experiencing the pain of the loss, adjusting to life without that which was lost, and reinvesting energy into going on with life.
- Normal grief reactions affect the feelings, behaviors, thought patterns, and physical well-being of a person. Symptoms lose their intensity as time passes.
- People predisposed to encounter an abnormal or complicated grief response are those chemically addicted; psychiatric patients; those facing sudden, violent, or mutilating deaths; victims of multiple, unresolved losses or multiple deaths; parents losing a child; and those with an unhealthy or dependent relationship to the deceased.
- Treating the grief of the psychiatric patient usually requires a period of hospitalization, the use of medications, and the use of psychotherapeutic interventions.

- Chronic grief can be characterized by attempts to keep the deceased alive by talking about him or her frequently, maintaining his or her personal things intact, or expecting that the deceased will reenter the mourner's life.
- Obstacles to grieving include societal norms about grieving patterns, gender roles and expectations, uncertainty about the loss, intolerance of slowing down to grieve, and unsanctioned losses.
- Unsanctioned losses are those losses related to situations that are not always socially acceptable, such as losses connected to abortion, suicide, divorce, nonmarital unions, homosexual unions, extramarital affairs, bankruptcy, and drug abuse.
- Tragedies and losses seem easier to cope with if a causative factor can be identified.
- Coping with loss can become more difficult if the elements of blame and retribution become enmeshed in the process.
- It is necessary to help psychiatric patients recognize that growth and new strength for living can be the positive outcome of grieving their losses adequately.
- Helping people say goodbye in some meaningful, creative manner helps them let go and move on.

Learning Activities

1. Prepare a loss time line covering the past 5 years of your life. Consider the kinds of losses you have experienced, how many you have had, and whether you took some time to grieve those losses.
2. Write in your journal about losing a special person in your life. Describe what impact this has had on you. What do you miss the most about that person? Are there some things you wish you would have said to him or her? Write about these things.
3. Read a book or some journal articles about the effects that the death of children, be they well children or sick children, have on their parents. How do the parents usually cope?

4. What are your personal thoughts about suicide? Read more about its occurrence among people your own age, those with mental health problems, and those who are chemically dependent. Talk with a friend about this topic.
5. Plan how you would help a patient deal with the losses in life faced because of mental health problems. Consider how mental illness has affected his or her life and well-being. Make your plan holistic.

Critical Thinking Exercise

Mrs. Naver, a 26-year-old mother of two children in her 3rd month of pregnancy, was admitted to the obstetrical unit with vaginal hemorrhaging at 1:00 AM. By 7:00 AM, it was clear that she was having a miscarriage. As Nurse Anders gently approached Mrs. Naver to assess her condition, the patient in a tearful, soft-spoken voice stated, "Why do those babies have to cry so loud, they kept me awake all night."

1. What assumptions can you make about Mrs. Naver?
2. How would you test these assumptions?
3. What inferences can you draw about the approach Nurse Anders should use?

As Nurse Anders is about to respond to Mrs. Naver's comment, Nurse Barr, a married nurse without children, comes into the room and tells the patient that she officially had a miscarriage and needs to have a surgical procedure to remove the remaining contents of her uterus. As the patient begins to sob loudly, Nurse Barr states, "At least you have two other children."

1. How do you think Mrs. Naver responded to Nurse Barr's comment?
2. What assumptions is Nurse Barr making?
3. How might she determine if her assumptions are faulty?

Additional Resources

Crisis, Grief, and Healing http://www.webhealing.com	*Grief and Loss Resource Centre* http://www.rockies.net/~spirit/grief/grief.html

References

American Psychiatric Association. (1994). *Diagnostic and statistical manual of mental disorders* (4th ed.). Washington, DC: Author.

Bertman, S. L. (1991). *Facing death.* New York: Taylor and Francis Publishers.

Bouvard, M. (1988). *The path through grief.* Wellesley, MN: Brewer Press.

Bowlby, J. (1969). *Attachment and loss* (Vol. I). New York: Basic Books.

Caplan, G. (1974). Forward. In I. Glick, R. Weiss, & C. M. Packer (Eds.), *The first year of bereavement.* New York: John Wiley.

Carson, V. (1999). The experience of grief. In E. Arnold & K. Bogg (Eds.), *Interpersonal relationships: Professional communication skills for nurses* (3rd ed.). Philadelphia: W. B. Saunders.

Catholic Biblical Association. (1983). *The new American Bible.* New York: Thomas Nelson.

Corless, I. B., Germino, B. B., & Pittman, A. (1994). Attitudes toward death: A personal perspective. In *Death, dying and bereavement.* Boston: Jones and Bartlett.

Deits, B. (1988). *Life after loss.* Tucson, AZ: Fisher Books.

Doka, K. (1989). *Disenfranchised grief—Recognizing hidden sorrow.* Washington, DC: Lexington Books.

Engel, G. (1964). Grief and grieving. *American Journal of Nursing, 64*(7), 93-96.

Fiefel, H. (1959). *The meaning of death.* New York: McGraw-Hill.

Freud, S. (1959). Mourning and melancholia. In *Collected Papers* (Vol. 4.). New York: Basic Books.

Gyulay, J. E. (1989). Grief responses. *Issues in Comprehensive Pediatric Nursing, 12,* 1-31.

Hutti, M. H. (1988). A quick reference table of interventions to assist families to cope with pregnancy loss or neonatal death. *Birth, 15*(1), 33-35.

Kastenbaum, R. (1991). *Death, society and human experience* (4th ed.). Columbus, OH: Charles E. Merrill.

Kübler-Ross, E. (1969). *On death and dying.* New York: Macmillan.

Kutscher, A. (1968). Psychiatric implications in bereavement. In *Death and Bereavement.* Springfield, IL: Charles C Thomas.

Lindemann, E. (1944). Symptomatology and management of acute grief. *American Journal of Psychiatry, 101,* 141-148.

Miles, H. S., & Demi, A. C. (1986). Guilt in bereaved parents. In T. Rando (Ed.), *Parental loss of a child: Clinical and research considerations.* Champaign, IL: Research Press.

Miles, M. S., & Demi, A. C. (1994). Bereavement guilt—a conceptual model with applications. In T. Corless, B. Germino, & M. Pittman (Eds.), *Death, dying, and bereavement.* Boston: Jones and Bartlett.

Parkes, C. M. (1964). Recent bereavement as a cause of mental illness. *British Journal of Psychiatry, 110,* 198-204.

Parkes, C. M. (1972). *Bereavement: Studies of grief in adult life.* New York: International Universities Press.

Pine, V. (1972). Social organization and death. *Omega, 3,* 149-153.

Rando, T. (1984). *Grief, dying and death: Clinical interventions for caregivers.* Champaign, IL: Research Press.

Rando, T. (1993). *Treatment of complicated mourning.* Champaign, IL: Research Press.

Sanders, C. (1982). Effects of sudden versus chronic illness death on bereavement outcome. *Omega, 13,* 227-241.

Schneider, J. (1980, Fourth Quarter). Clinically significant differences between grief, pathological grief, and depression. *Patient Counseling and Education,* 267-275.

Stearus, A. (1984). *Living through personal crisis.* Chicago: Thomas Moore Press.

Veninga, R. (1985). *The gift of hope: How we survive our tragedies.* New York: Little, Brown.

Westberg, G. (1971). *Good grief.* Philadelphia: Fortress Press.

Wolfelt, A. (1990, Fall). Gender roles and grief: Why men's grief is naturally complicated. *Thanatos,* 20-24.

Wolfelt, A. (1991a, Spring). Helping yourself heal when someone loved dies. *Thanatos,* 11, 12.

Wolfelt, A. (1991b, March/April). Toward an understanding of complicated grief: A comprehensive overview. *The American Journal of Hospice and Palliative Care,* 28-30.

Worden, W. (1982, 1990). *Grief counseling and grief therapy—a handbook for the mental health practitioner.* New York: Springer.

Suggested Readings

Deits, B. (1988, 1992). *Life after loss.* Tucson, AZ: Fisher Books.

Rando, T. (1993). *Treatment of complicated mourning.* Champaign, IL: Research Press.

Westberg, G. (1971). *Good grief.* Philadelphia: Fortress Press.

Worden, W. (1982). *Grief counseling and grief therapy—a handbook for the mental health practitioner.* New York: Springer.

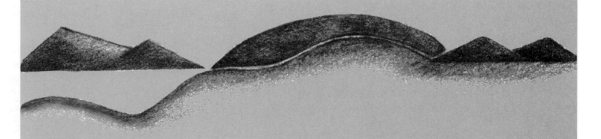

V The Wounded Traveler

Traveler's Log

I was working as a graduate student in a consultation-liaison role in a large medical center. Some of the work I performed included ongoing supportive psychotherapy with people on rehabilitation units. I stopped in to see Luke, a 17-year-old who had been in a car accident while fleeing police. Luke was paralyzed from the waist down. After a few minutes of catching up on events since I last saw him, he agreed to see me later in the day. The nurses working with Luke gave me an earful. He had been up to all kinds of trouble—at least from the perspective of those wanting a well-run unit. He was "noncompliant" at every opportunity, had "strange looking" visitors, played loud music, and had women visitors who were found on his bed with him. I tried not to smile as I imagined the situation from the perspective of a 17-year-old.

Later that day, Luke and I talked about what was important in his life, both before his injury and now. He described a pretty normal perspective for a 17-year-old in high school. His friends were important; he missed hanging out with them and felt he was out of touch with the direction his life was taking. He mentioned a girl he cared about. He feared that she was only staying with him because she felt sorry for him. He felt she should "just dump him" because he was "a loser" now. I asked about his sexuality and whether he had talked to anyone about the changes that had resulted from his paralysis. He started to cry. The subject had never been discussed. Through further discussion he realized that he could still be sexual. This opened the door to a discussion of his noncompliance and helped us to work together so that he could get his life back on track. Although this work was difficult, it was satisfying to realize that my skills had helped this young man to view his future more realistically.

—Joanne DeSanto Iennaco MS, RN,C

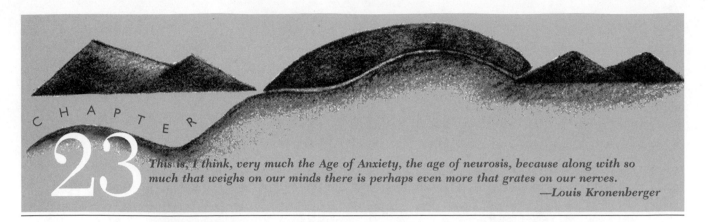

23

This is, I think, very much the Age of Anxiety, the age of neurosis, because along with so much that weighs on our minds there is perhaps even more that grates on our nerves.

—Louis Kronenberger

Stress and Anxiety Disorders

Learning Objectives

After studying this chapter, you should be able to:

1. Recognize signs and symptoms of anxiety.
2. Describe the stress response.
3. Identify key symptoms of the anxiety disorders.
4. Discuss psychobiological, psychodynamic, and behavioral theories about anxiety.
5. Define defense mechanisms.
6. Identify effective nursing interventions to decrease anxiety.
7. Discuss effective treatment for anxiety disorders including the role of the nurse.
8. Apply the nursing process to a patient with an anxiety disorder.

Key Terminology

Acute Stress Disorder
Agoraphobia
Anxiety
Anxiety disorder
Anxiety Disorder due to a General Medical Condition
Anxiety Disorder Not Otherwise Specified

Anxiolytic
Coping
Defense mechanisms
Generalized Anxiety Disorder
Immediate stress response
Intermediate stress response

Long-term stress response
Obsessive-Compulsive Disorder
Panic Disorder
Posttraumatic Stress Disorder

Social Phobia
Specific Phobias
Stress
Stress response
Substance-Induced Anxiety Disorder

Maturation is the task of a lifetime. It is known that growth and development do not begin at birth or end at a definitive age but that progressive unfolding is a journey traversing all the years of a person's life. In all lives, periods of contentment, sadness, and curiosity lead to growth, happiness, and sometimes despair. Life is sometimes in balance and sometimes not. During those parts of the journey that are not balanced, people tend to be more vulnerable to **anxiety,** an intense feeling of fear or dread with an uncertain cause.

Anxiety, in normal proportions, is a trigger that is helpful to growth. Normal anxiety is short-term and of low to moderate intensity. Mild to moderate feelings of vague unease are felt by almost everyone during periods of unrest throughout the life journey. Frequently, these periods precede significant changes, for example, going to school for the first time, leaving home for college, preparing for marriage, or the birth of a child.

But when anxiety is prolonged or excessive, a person may develop crippling physical or psychological symptoms. The anxiety disorders are a group of conditions characterized by symptoms of anxiety and behavioral efforts to avoid those symptoms. Acute anxiety is an unbearable feeling. It creates physical sensations of arousal (fight or flight); an emotional state of fear or panic; decreased cognitive problem-solving ability; and an altered spiritual state with hopelessness. Box 23–1 lists the range of signs and symptoms of anxiety. Anxiety is considered abnormal when reasons for it are not evident or when manifestations are excessive in intensity and duration (Brown, Barlow, & Liebowitz, 1994; Hoehn-Saric, 1979).

STRESS

It is impossible to discuss the concept of anxiety without also defining stress. According to Lazarus and Folkman

Box 23–1 ■ ■ ■ ■ ■
Physical, Emotional, Cognitive, and Spiritual Signs and Symptoms of Anxiety

Physical

Dry mouth
Elevated vital signs
Diarrhea
Increased urination
Nausea
Diaphoresis
Hyperventilation
Fatigue
Insomnia
Sexual dysfunction
Irritability
Tenseness

Emotional

Fear
Impending doom
Helplessness
Insecurity
Low self-confidence
Anger
Guilt

Cognitive

With mild anxiety, increased awareness and problem solving abilities

With anxiety increased above mild, narrowed perceptual field, missed details, diminished problem solving skills

Deteriorated logical thinking

Spiritual

Hopelessness
Feeling of being cut off from God
Anger at God for allowing the anxiety

(1984), psychological **stress** "is a particular relationship between the person and the environment that is appraised by the person as taxing and/or exceeding his or her resources and endangering his or her well being." There are universal stressors that would affect most people, for example, illness, accidents, and catastrophic events. However, because of individual interpretations of events, stressors are frequently person-specific. For example, one student may worry excessively about an examination, while a peer may not experience any associated distress.

Research shows that the **stress response** is a physiological reaction, which has been categorized into three phases that occur within 10 minutes of a stressful event. The first phase, or **immediate stress response,** occurs within 2 or 3 seconds of the onset of perceiving a threat: the sympathetic nervous system releases the catecholamines epinephrine and norepinephrine, and the individual shows perspiration, tremulousness, and rapid pulse and respiration.

The second phase, or **intermediate stress response,** occurs within 2 or 3 minutes of the stressor: the neurotransmitters have stimulated various organs and the liver triggers the release of glucose to provide the body with extra energy (Robinson, 1990).

The third phase, or **long-term stress response,** involves the endocrine system. The pituitary gland secretes adrenocorticotrophic hormone (ACTH), which stimulates the adrenal glands to produce cortisol, the stress hormone. This hormone produces multiple effects including elevating blood pressure and altering metabolism of fat and protein (Fitzgerald, 1997). For more discussion of brain physiology related to stress, see Chapter 7.

What do you think? When you look at your own stress response, are there situations that make you really "nervous" that other people would shrug off? Conversely, have you ever been surprised when someone becomes anxious in regard to a situation that doesn't bother you?

▶ *Check Your Reading*
1. What is the definition of anxiety?
2. What does it mean that stressors are "person-specific"?
3. Describe three physical symptoms of anxiety.
4. How does anxiety affect problem-solving and spirituality?
5. Describe the three phases of the stress response.

RELATIONSHIP BETWEEN ANXIETY AND STRESS

Anxiety is always part of the stress response, and in the healthy range, it alerts a person to take protective action in the face of potential danger. The range of intensity for anxiety is defined by four levels, from mild to panic. Table 23–1 contains an overview of the characteristics of

T A B L E 2 3 – 1 Characteristics of the Four Levels of Anxiety

LEVEL	PHYSIOLOGICAL	EMOTIONAL	COGNITIVE	SUBJECTIVE
Mild	Increase in pulse, B/P, and heart rate due to sympathetic arousal	Affect positive	Alert; aware; able to problem-solve	Attentive
Moderate	Muscle tension; diaphoresis; pupils dilated; increased pulse, B/P, and breathing rate; peripheral vasoconstriction	Tension, fear	Attention focused on issue of concern; able to shut out irrelevant data	Sense of helplessness; apprehensive expectation; sweating of palms; vigilance and irritability
Severe	"Fight or flight" responses; generalized sympathetic nervous system response; dry mouth; numbness of extremities	Distress, trembling	Sensory perception greatly reduced; person can focus only on small details; learning cannot occur	Dyspnea, dizziness; fear of going crazy; visual disturbances; motor tension with hyperactivity
Panic	Continued arousal	Emotionally overwhelmed; may regress to primitive coping behaviors	Responds only to internal distress	Feelings of impending doom or death; chest pain or discomfort

B/P, blood pressure.

each level. An example of mild anxiety is someone who overslept and is running to the bus stop to try to avoid being late to work. This person is excited but is able to concentrate and solve the problem. Moderate anxiety might occur after a narrow escape from a traffic accident. This person is aware of multiple physical symptoms including sweating, muscle tension, and dry mouth and is focused on the stressful event. Severe anxiety or panic may be precipitated by a life-threatening event. This person is focused solely on internal stimuli and is totally overwhelmed and unable to respond to external direction.

Normally, a person experiencing mild to moderate anxiety may use voluntary behaviors called **coping** skills to decrease the unpleasant feeling. Examples of coping behaviors are distraction, deliberate avoidance, and seeking information. Another common response to anxiety is the use of unconscious **defense mechanisms,** first described in the psychoanalytic literature by Freud. A person does not deliberately plan to use a defense mechanism; theoretically, the unconscious mind transforms the anxiety into a more tolerable symptom. Box 23-2 contains the definition of the most common defense mechanisms. For more in-depth discussion of psychoanalytic theory, see Chapter 6.

However, if stress continues at an unbearable level or a person lacks sufficient biological mechanisms for coping with anxiety, then a person is at risk to develop an **anxiety disorder.** According to the *Diagnostic and Statistical Manual of Mental Disorders, Fourth Edition* (DSM-IV), the anxiety disorders include eight major categories:

1. Generalized Anxiety Disorder
2. Panic Disorder
3. Phobias
4. Obsessive-Compulsive Disorder
5. Posttraumatic Stress Disorder
6. Acute Stress Disorder

7. Anxiety Disorder due to a General Medical Condition
8. Anxiety Disorder Not Otherwise Specified

These are the most common psychiatric disorders in America, affecting more than 23 million people, or 1 out of every 4 individuals, each year. In 1990, anxiety disorders cost the United States $46.6 billion with direct and indirect costs, almost one third of the national mental health bill of $148 billion (Brown & Lempa, 1996).

In this chapter, you are introduced to each type of anxiety disorder and to one patient, in particular, who suffered through a journey with Generalized Anxiety Disorder. We explore the symptoms, the possible causes, and the recommended treatments and nursing care of patients who suffer from these problems.

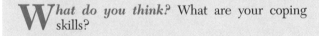

What do you think? What are your coping skills?

➤ *Check Your Reading*
6. Describe cognitive changes in the four levels of anxiety.
7. What is a person's subjective state at panic level anxiety?
8. Name three defense mechanisms and explain how they are different from coping skills.
9. Identify four different types of anxiety disorder.

 **Mrs. Anderson's Story**

Mrs. Anderson is a 66-year-old, married white woman who was referred to psychiatric home care by her internist because she is excessively

B o x   2 3 – 2 ■ ■ ■ ■ ■
Defense Mechanisms

Repression

This is the most basic of defense mechanisms. Components of it are present in many of the more complex defenses. In repression, whatever is a threat to the ego is banished from awareness. For instance, a person with multiple personalities is unaware of the alter egos because they are banished from awareness through repression.

Suppression

This mechanism is similar to "forgetting." The individual does not have recall for the threatening event but if cued is capable of remembering. Through suppression, threats to the ego are avoided.

Projection

The use of this mechanism causes threats to the ego to be disavowed by perceiving them to be outside of the self. Thus, the person who is angry assumes the object of the anger to be angry at him or her. This is a transformation of the anger, which is a threat to the ego.

Introjection

The process of taking in characteristics of others begins early in life. In its healthy form, children adopt morals and values from parents through this process. Introjection is related to three defenses: *identification, imitation,* and *incorporation.* Identification and imitation are more mature defenses, while incorporation is one that is primitive, (e.g., it develops in infancy and involves the taking in of whole aspects of the parent or other model).

Reaction Formation

This mechanism disguises the person's actual feeling, which is too threatening to experience. Thus, the person is aware of the opposite of his or her actual feeling, while the real, underlying feeling is repressed.

Undoing

With this mechanism, a thought or action is used to negate an anxiety-provoking experience. For instance, the person with obsessive-compulsive traits might keep several scheduling books to hold in check the impulse to be free of social restraints.

Displacement

This is a commonly used mechanism that alters the object of threatening feelings. For instance, a child might be angry at the teacher but instead picks a fight with a peer on the playground at recess.

Denial

Two forms of this mechanism exist: one is denial of a fact, and the other is denial of the significance of the fact. The first form is the more serious because it alters reality. The second alters one's response to that reality. As an example, denial is used when a patient does not accept that he or she has a drinking problem. An example of the less serious form of denial is seen when a person is persistently late for a scheduled class because that person is actually very fearful of the topic.

Regression

This mechanism makes it possible for the threatened person to move backward developmentally to a place where he or she is more secure. One who feels tense in social situations might physically lean on a partner and be quieter than usual. That person might also become uncharacteristically boisterous as in earlier adolescence. An example of regression in its most malignant form is when psychiatric patients who are acutely ill give up all social graces such as wearing clothes and using the toilet and eating, necessitating complete nursing care that mimics the parenting provided when the patient was an infant.

---

anxious. She had made four visits to the physician's office and two emergency department trips in the previous 4 months, with vague complaints of palpitations, constipation, and body aches. She has a history of hypertension, but her blood pressure has been controlled for some time with medication and diet. She also has a history of taking pain medications for various problems. The physician can find no significant physical cause for her complaints.

She lives with her 68-year-old husband, who suffered a heart attack 6 months earlier. He reported that he felt fully recuperated and was compliant with his treatment regimen. But he complained that his wife had changed in the past 6 months: she did not want him to leave her side and she worried constantly about his health.

The couple has been married 45 years, has no children, and lives in their own home in a quiet neighborhood. The husband is a retired salesman and she worked part-time at a local grocery store. They used to visit with neighbors, attend Methodist church regularly, and participate in church-related social events. But in the past 2 months, Mrs. Anderson has refused to go out of the house except for physician appointments. She insists that her husband stay home with her except for brief errands, such as grocery shopping.

Admission Status

On admission, Mrs. Anderson complains of insomnia, decreased appetite, constipation, backache, fatigue, and constant "worrying." "I've been a worrier all my life, but this is much worse," she says. She denies feeling anxious about anything except her physical problems. She has no history of suicidal ideation or gestures. She believes that the physician has missed the right diagnosis for her. She is angry that he refused to fill her prescription for propoxyphene (Darvon) and she refuses to fill her new prescription for alprazolam (Xanax)—"I don't want to get hooked on that dope." She recognizes that she has become socially isolated but blames it on her physical state. She is receptive to the home care psychiatric nurse once reassured that, indeed, she is a "real nurse."

Baseline Measurements

The nurse selects the Mini-Mental State Examination MMSE) and the Sheehan Patient Rated Anxiety Scale for baseline measurements of Mrs. Anderson's status (Figure 23–1). She scores 25 of 30 on the MMSE and 39 on the Sheehan scale, indicating short attention span and moderate anxiety. Also, she had lost 5 lb in the past 2 months, and her blood pressure is 130/85. The nurse consults with the physician and agrees that the patient shows symptoms of **Generalized Anxiety Disorder** (GAD).

Nursing Treatment

Over the next 8 weeks, the nurse assesses Mrs. Anderson's health status and provides education to improve her self-care, including new knowledge and new skills. After teaching that GAD is a treatable illness, she persuades the patient to try taking her new medicine. She focuses on nutrition and a healthy sleep pattern. She later teaches cognitive techniques to reframe negative thoughts, relaxation exercises, and coping skills. The nurse always includes Mr. Anderson in the teaching and encourages him to set reasonable limits on his wife's demands for his attention.

Discharge Status

At the end of the 8 weeks, Mrs. Anderson is retested on the same instruments: she scores 29 of 30 on the MMSE (improved attention span) and 4 on the Sheehan (within normal range). She reports that her sleep is back to normal and she no longer feels tired and worried all the time. She gained 3 lb and her blood pressure remains stable. She only uses acetaminophen (Tylenol) for an occasional headache. Her husband is pleased that she no longer wants him to stay at home all the time. They went back to church one time and plan to start attending the senior center weekly. She is compliant with her medication and her next checkup is scheduled with the physician in 3 months. ∎

GENERALIZED ANXIETY DISORDER

As illustrated in Mrs. Anderson's case history, the central feature of GAD is excessive, uncontrollable worrying over a period of at least 6 months. The patient is preoccupied with at least two life concerns, for example, finances, significant other's welfare, or health. Especially in the elderly, health (both one's own and that of a loved one), may be the predominant concern (Brawman-Mintzer et al., 1994). There is significant distress or impairment in social or occupational functioning.

Symptoms include motor tension, autonomic hyperactivity, and scanning behavior. Motor tension symptoms are trembling, shakiness, muscle tension, aches or soreness, and easy fatigability. Autonomic hyperactivity leads to shortness of breath, palpitations, sweating, dry mouth, dizziness, nausea or diarrhea, and frequent urination. Scanning behavior is evidenced by feeling on edge, having an exaggerated startle response, difficulty concentrating, sleep disturbance, and irritability.

The prevalence of GAD is about 3% to 4% of the U.S. population in a given year. Studies show that it primarily affects women, and there is a high likelihood of co-occurrence with panic disorder and major depression. Specifically, one epidemiologic study found that 58% to 65% of subjects who were diagnosed with GAD also had at least one other psychiatric disorder (Brown & Lempa, 1996). There is evidence of possible genetic influence for the disorder because first-degree relatives (mother, father, sibling, children) are 5.6 times more likely to have the same symptoms as compared with normal controls (Brown, 1995). One nursing research study suggested that adult children of alcoholics may be particularly vulnerable to severe anxiety disorders; stressors included divorce, separation, spousal abuse, and poor parental modeling (Haack & Alim, 1991).

Patients do not always seek psychiatric treatment for this problem and, indeed, may not initially admit to feeling anxiety. Instead, they may suffer for years until physical symptoms frighten them enough to seek medical attention, or they may self-medicate with alcohol, other substances, or prescription pain or sleeping medications. Nurses often find this problem while treating the patient for another complaint in the outpatient setting. Review What Patients and Families Need to Know: Anxiety Disorder for significant teaching issues for patients and families with GAD.

CP93-0327 (C1.VP)

	Project ID	Investigator ID	Today's Date			Visit	Patient ID	Birth Date				
			Month	Day	Year			Month	Day	Year	Form # 22.1	Page # 1 of 3

Investigator's Initials X

Patient's Initials X

SHEEHAN PATIENT RATED ANXIETY SCALE

INSTRUCTIONS: Below is a list of problems and complaints that people sometimes have. Part 1 asks about how you have felt during THE PAST WEEK; Part 2 asks about how you feel RIGHT NOW. Mark only one box for each problem, and do not skip any items.

PART 1--DURING THE PAST WEEK, HOW MUCH DID YOU SUFFER FROM . . .

	Not At All	A Little	Moderately	Markedly	Extremely
1. Difficulty in getting your breath, smothering, or overbreathing.	☐	☐	☐	☐	☐
2. Choking sensation or lump in throat.	☐	☐	☐	☐	☐
3. Skipping, racing, or pounding of your heart.	☐	☐	☐	☐	☐
4. Chest pain, pressure, or discomfort.	☐	☐	☐	☐	☐
5. Bouts of excessive sweating.	☐	☐	☐	☐	☐
6. Faintness, lightheadedness, or dizzy spells.	☐	☐	☐	☐	☐
7. Sensation of rubbery or "jelly" legs.	☐	☐	☐	☐	☐
8. Feeling off balance or unsteady like you might fall.	☐	☐	☐	☐	☐
9. Nausea or stomach problems.	☐	☐	☐	☐	☐
10. Feeling that things around you are strange, unreal, foggy, or detached from you.	☐	☐	☐	☐	☐
11. Feeling outside or detached from part or all of your body, or a floating feeling.	☐	☐	☐	☐	☐
12. Tingling or numbness in parts of your body.	☐	☐	☐	☐	☐
13. Hot flashes or cold chills.	☐	☐	☐	☐	☐
14. Shaking or trembling.	☐	☐	☐	☐	☐

Changes: date & initial in box at left in line with the change.

Layout and design © 1993 University of South Florida, Department of Psychiatry and Behavioral Medicine

CONTINUED ON BACK

Figure 23–1
The Sheehan Patient Rated Anxiety Scale. (Courtesy of David V. Sheehan, MD, University of South Florida, Institute for Research in Psychiatry, Tampa, Florida.)

Illustration continued on following page

Form # 22.1	Page # 2 of 3	DO NOT WRITE IN THIS AREA

SHEEHAN PATIENT RATED ANXIETY SCALE - Part 1 (Continued)

DURING THE PAST WEEK, HOW MUCH DID YOU SUFFER FROM . . .	Not At All	A Little	Moderately	Markedly	Extremely
15. Having a fear that you are dying or that something terrible is about to happen.	☐	☐	☐	☐	☐
16. Feeling you are losing control or going insane.	☐	☐	☐	☐	☐
17. SITUATIONAL ANXIETY ATTACK Sudden anxiety attacks with 4 or more of the symptoms listed previously that occur when you are in or about to go into a situation that is likely, from your experience, to bring on an attack.	☐	☐	☐	☐	☐
18. UNEXPECTED ANXIETY ATTACK Sudden unexpected anxiety attacks with 4 or more symptoms (listed previously) that occur with little or no provocation (i.e., when you are NOT in a situation that is likely, from your experience, to bring on an attack).	☐	☐	☐	☐	☐
19. UNEXPECTED LIMITED SYMPTOM ATTACK Sudden unexpected spells with only one or two symptoms (listed previously) that occur with little or no provocation (i.e., when you are NOT in a situation that is likely, from your experience, to bring on an attack).	☐	☐	☐	☐	☐
20. ANTICIPATORY ANXIETY EPISODE Anxiety episodes that build up as you anticipate doing something that is likely, from your experience, to bring on anxiety that is more intense than most people experience in such situations.	☐	☐	☐	☐	☐
21. Avoiding situations because they frighten you.	☐	☐	☐	☐	☐
22. Being dependent on others.	☐	☐	☐	☐	☐
23. Tension and inability to relax.	☐	☐	☐	☐	☐
24. Anxiety, nervousness, restlessness.	☐	☐	☐	☐	☐
25. Spells of increased sensitivity to sound, light, or touch.	☐	☐	☐	☐	☐
26. Attacks of diarrhea.	☐	☐	☐	☐	☐
27. Worrying about your health too much.	☐	☐	☐	☐	☐
28. Feeling tired, weak, and exhausted easily.	☐	☐	☐	☐	☐
29. Headaches or pains in neck or head.	☐	☐	☐	☐	☐
30. Difficulty in falling asleep.	☐	☐	☐	☐	☐
31. Waking in the middle of the night, or restless sleep.	☐	☐	☐	☐	☐

CONTINUED ON NEXT PAGE

Changes: date & initial in box at right in line with the change. ⟶

Figure 23–1 Continued

What do you think? Should every patient who sees a family practice or primary care physician be screened for anxiety? Defend your answer.

➤ *Check Your Reading*

10. What is the key symptom of GAD?
11. How does GAD interfere with social functioning?
12. What are genetic and social risk factors for GAD?

CP93-0327 Page 3 (C1.VP)

	Project ID	Investigator ID	Today's Date			Visit	Patient ID	Birth Date				
			Month	Day	Year			Month	Day	Year	Form # 22.1	Page # 3 of 3

Investigator's Initials: X

Patient's Initials: X

SHEEHAN PATIENT RATED ANXIETY SCALE - (cont'd.)

PART 1 (continued) --
DURING THE PAST WEEK . . .

	Not At All	A Little	Moderately	Markedly	Extremely
32. Unexpected waves of depression occuring with little or no provocation.	☐	☐	☐	☐	☐
33. Emotions and moods going up and down a lot in response to changes around you.	☐	☐	☐	☐	☐
34. Recurrent and persistent ideas, thoughts, impulses, or images that are intrusive, unwanted, senseless, or repugnant.	☐	☐	☐	☐	☐
35. Having to repeat the same action in a ritual, e.g., checking, washing, counting repeatedly, when it's not really necessary.	☐	☐	☐	☐	☐

PART 2 --
RIGHT NOW, AT THIS MOMENT . . .

	Not At All	A Little	Moderately	Markedly	Extremely
1. Mouth drier than usual.	☐	☐	☐	☐	☐
2. Worried, preoccupied.	☐	☐	☐	☐	☐
3. Nervous, jittery, anxious, restless.	☐	☐	☐	☐	☐
4. Afraid, fearful.	☐	☐	☐	☐	☐
5. Tense, "uptight."	☐	☐	☐	☐	☐
6. Shaky inside or out.	☐	☐	☐	☐	☐
7. Fluttery stomach.	☐	☐	☐	☐	☐
8. Warm all over.	☐	☐	☐	☐	☐
9. Sweaty palms.	☐	☐	☐	☐	☐
10. Rapid or heavy heart beat.	☐	☐	☐	☐	☐
11. Tremor of hands or legs.	☐	☐	☐	☐	☐

← Changes: date & initial in box at left in line with the change.

Figure 23-1 *Continued*

? WHAT PATIENTS AND FAMILIES NEED TO KNOW

Anxiety Disorder

What is anxiety disorder?

Anxiety is a diffuse response to a vague threat as compared to fear, which is an acute response to a clear-cut external threat. The physical symptoms of anxiety include an increase in blood pressure and heart rate. The palms become sweaty and the pupils dilate. The feelings that are involved are guilt, grief, and anger. Intellectual symptoms include an inability to concentrate, indecisiveness, inability to learn or reason, and worry. Social symptoms include talkativeness or extreme quietness, and apprehension with groups of people. Spiritual symptoms may include feelings of hopelessness and despair, fear of death or being a failure, and inability to find meaning in life.

Who is affected?

Women are more affected than men, and may have a relative who also feels symptoms. Some research shows that adult children of alcoholics may be especially vulnerable.

What is the prevalence?

The prevalence for Generalized Anxiety Disorder is 3% to 4% of the U.S. population in a given year. There is often co-occurrence with another psychiatric disorder such as Panic Disorder, Major Depression, or Substance Abuse.

What is the cause?

Research shows that there are definite brain structures and chemicals involved with anxiety. It is likely that an imbalance in brain chemicals leads to the experience of ongoing anxiety.

How is it treated?

Specific antianxiety or antidepressant medications are very helpful. Also supportive therapy is useful, including learning relaxation techniques, new ways of perceiving anxiety, and new behaviors to react to anxiety.

How can family and friends help?

Have patience and continue to believe that treatment will help. Encourage the patient to take medication as prescribed even if there is not immediate benefit. Also encourage the patient to participate in therapy and if possible, help with homework assignments.

PANIC DISORDERS

The distinctive feature of **Panic Disorder** is the experience of recurrent, unexpected panic attacks followed by at least 1 month of significant behavior change due to the attack (American Psychiatric Association, 1994). A panic attack usually lasts only for a few minutes, and begins suddenly with intense feelings of fear or impending doom. Symptoms include dizziness, faintness, choking, palpitations, trembling, nausea or abdominal distress, numbness, chest pain, and fear of dying or going crazy. There is no definable stimulus for the attack and after recurrent attacks, there is persistent worry about having another one.

After recurrent attacks, a person may avoid the location where an attack took place and the people involved. In some cases, the person develops **agoraphobia,** the fear of being in places or situations from which escape might be difficult or embarrassing in case of another attack. Frequent fears involve being outside the home alone, being in a crowd of people, standing in a waiting line, or traveling (Danton, Altrocchi, Antonuccio, & Basta, 1994; Hunt, 1988).

If untreated, this Panic Disorder significantly reduces one's productivity and quality of life. There is increased risk of alcohol and other drug abuse because of attempts to self-medicate. Marital and social relationships are altered to prevent or hide the attacks. There is also increased risk of suicide (Johnson, Weissman, & Klerman, 1990).

The prevalence of panic disorder is approximately 1% to 2% of the U.S. population, with women being twice as likely to develop symptoms. There is a high co-occurrence rate with other disorders: 25% of patients develop depression; 17% to 30% develop alcohol and drug abuse; 20% have a phobia; and 39% have a personality disorder (Brown & Lempa, 1996). It usually starts in a person's 20s and is rare after age 40 (Flint, 1994). There seems to be a genetic link because studies show that first-degree relatives have a 9.6 times higher risk for the disorder compared with normal controls (Brown, 1995).

Panic Disorder may present serious diagnostic difficulties because the symptoms mimic a variety of medical problems. Other conditions that need to be ruled out include coronary artery disease, irritable bowel syndrome, epilepsy, thyroid disease, mitral valve prolapse, hypoglycemia, pheochromocytoma, and multiple sclerosis (Brown & Lempa, 1996).

Patients often seek treatment for this terrifying disorder and the nurse finds these patients in the emergency department and inpatient and outpatient settings.

See What Patients and Families Need to Know: Panic Attacks for significant teaching issues for patients and their families.

> **What do you think?** Do you know anyone who suffers from panic attacks? Do you?

> ➤ *Check Your Reading*
> 13. Describe a panic attack.
> 14. How is agoraphobia associated with panic attacks?
> 15. Name three medical problems that could be confused with Panic Disorder.

PHOBIAS

The most widespread type of anxiety disorder is the Phobia, that is, a severe and persistent fear of a clearly identifiable object or situation despite the person's awareness that the fear is unreasonable. There are two broad categories for phobias: specific and social. **Specific Phobias** (once called simple phobias) are subdivided into five types: animals, natural environment (e.g., lightning or heights), blood-injection-injury type, situational (e.g., flying), and other (e.g., situations that could lead to choking or contracting an illness). **Social Phobia** (once called social anxiety disorder) relates to profound fear of social or performance situations in which embarrassment could occur. For example the person who fears eating out might accidentally overturn a water glass and others will stare; the singer will have stage fright; or the speaker will forget a portion of the speech (Seligman, 1994; Stein, Walker, & Forde, 1994).

The prevalence of phobias is approximately 13% to 15% of Americans in a given year. There appears to be a genetic influence because the first-degree relatives of a phobic person are 3.2 to 3.3 times more likely to also have a phobia compared with controls. Animal and natural environment phobias usually start in childhood, whereas situational phobias have onset in childhood or in the mid-20s.

Patients do not always seek treatment for a phobia, but they suffer great distress. They develop behaviors to avoid the phobic stimulus, for example, "I never drive over bridges." Or they anxiously anticipate and tolerate the stimulus, experiencing symptoms of a panic attack. They may show impairment in occupational, academic, or social functioning. Review What Patients and Families Need to Know: Phobias for teaching issues for patients and families.

> **What do you think?** Do you have any "unreasonable fears"? Do you know others who do? What impact can these fears have on life?

> ➤ *Check Your Reading*
> 16. Give two examples of a Specific Phobia.

WHAT PATIENTS AND FAMILIES NEED TO KNOW

Panic Attacks

What is a panic attack?

A panic attack is a specific period of intense fear or discomfort with at least four of the following symptoms: palpitations or pounding heart; sweating; trembling or shaking, sensations of smothering or difficulty breathing; feeling of choking; chest pain; nausea; feeling dizzy or faint; feeling of unreality or losing control; numbness; and chills or flushes. People often fear that they are having a heart attack or that they are going crazy.

Who is affected?

The symptoms usually start in young adulthood and affect women twice as often as men. There may be a genetic influence because relatives may also show the same symptoms.

What is the prevalence?

The prevalence in the U.S. population is approximately 1% to 2%. Many people also have symptoms of depression, substance abuse, or phobias.

What is the cause?

Current research indicates that an underlying chemical imbalance in the brain causes a panic attack. It is also thought that the tendency to experience panic attacks can be inherited.

How is it treated?

Antidepressant medications are very effective but may require several weeks of use before showing a benefit. Antianxiety medication may also be used during an acute attack. Therapy that teaches the person to relax and to recognize the symptoms as anxiety and not a heart attack is also helpful. It is very important to have a full physical examination to rule out any medical problem that could be confused with panic symptoms.

How can family and friends help?

Reassure the person that he or she is not dying during an attack. Stay calm and move the person to a quiet area. Encourage the person to take medication as ordered and to participate in treatment.

WHAT PATIENTS AND FAMILIES NEED TO KNOW

Phobias

What is a phobia?

A phobia is a severe and persistent fear of a specific object or situation despite the person's awareness that the fear is unreasonable. The feared object may be an animal or something in the environment, such as lightning. Or it may be a certain social situation, such as public speaking. The person will try to avoid the feared situation, and if it cannot be avoided, will experience intense anxiety and distress.

Who is affected?

Phobias about animals and natural environment events usually start in childhood, while situational phobias may start in the mid-20s. There seems to be a genetic influence because many times relatives also have a phobia. Many people hide a phobia because they are embarrassed about their reaction to a situation that most people consider to be ordinary.

What is the prevalence?

The prevalence is approximately 13% to 15% of the U.S. population in a given year. Phobias are the most common type of anxiety disorder even though many people never seek treatment.

What is the cause?

Like the other anxiety disorders, the exact cause is not known. It is possible that the person experienced an intense, frightening experience in childhood and then overreacts to a similar stimulus. Or, the object may symbolize something else frightening to the person. The panic symptoms may be due to a genetic susceptibility to overreact to fear.

How is it treated?

Behavioral therapy is very helpful for treating phobias. In a controlled environment with the therapist, the person is exposed to the feared object or imagery of the same and taught to alter his or her responses. Antianxiety medication may also be used to reduce the person's anxiety level.

How can family and friends help?

Do not ridicule the person about the fear. Encourage the person to take medication as ordered and to participate in therapy. If possible, help the person with homework assignments.

---

17. Describe Social Phobia.
18. What is the difference between a Phobia and Panic Disorder?

OBSESSIVE-COMPULSIVE DISORDER

In **Obsessive-Compulsive Disorder** (OCD), a person is preoccupied with recurrent, ritualistic thoughts or actions. Obsessions are persistent thoughts, ideas, impulses, or images that are intrusive and cause marked anxiety. Frequently, the content involves violence, contamination, and doubt about one's own performance. Compulsions are repetitive acts that follow an obsession, performed according to strict rules and aimed at decreasing the feeling of distress. The act is not realistically connected to the event or situation, but the person cannot resist the impulse to relieve the immediate anxiety. For example, common compulsive behaviors include hand-washing, counting, and checking something repeatedly.

The person usually recognizes or shows insight that the behavior is irrational and excessive. The rituals are time-consuming, taking up more than 1 hour a day. Efforts are made to ignore or suppress the impulses, which usually began in childhood. But the ongoing feeling of failure only increases the sense of shame, and many people keep their symptoms a secret. There is functional impairment in relationships as well as occupational or academic performance.

The lifetime prevalence of OCD is estimated at 2% to 3%, meaning that in the United States alone, there may be 5 to 7 million people suffering with symptoms. Some studies show that fewer than half of these people seek treatment, and a delay of 5 to 10 years before starting therapy is common. There is frequent co-occurrence with other psychiatric disorders (Brown, 1996). In one survey at an OCD clinic, patients also had major depression (66%), panic attacks (26%), and body dysmorphic disorder (23%). With childhood onset of OCD, there is frequent co-occurrence with tics, Tourette's disorder, or Sydenham's chorea. Another study of 100 patients with schizophrenia or schizoaffective disorder found OCD symptoms to be common and in need of treatment (Bermanzohn, 1997).

The nurse may encounter these patients in the outpatient or inpatient setting. As noted previously, the patient is often being treated for another disorder, possibly including alcohol or substance abuse. Significant teaching issues for these patients and their families are found in What Patients and Families Need to Know: Obsessive-Compulsive Disorder.

What do you think? Watch the movie *As Good As It Gets*. How would you describe the impact of OCD on Melvin Udall's (Jack Nicholson's) life?

► *Check Your Reading*

19. How are obsessions related to compulsions?
20. Does a patient know that the obsession is irrational?
21. Name three disorders that may co-occur with OCD.

POSTTRAUMATIC STRESS DISORDER

Posttraumatic Stress Disorder (PTSD) differs from the other anxiety disorders because the cause is a real and devastating event in the person's life. PTSD results from a pathological response to an overwhelming event that was beyond the individual's control, for example, a natural disaster such as an earthquake, a man-made disaster such as fire, or wartime horrors. Even medical professionals such as paramedics and nurses who repeatedly witness trauma, mutilation, and death are candidates for PTSD. Table 23–2 compares normal and abnormal responses to traumatic stress.

The primary feature of PTSD is that the victim continues to reexperience the event through intrusive thoughts or nightmares. Memories of the trauma occur at random times and the person struggles with obsessive thoughts about what was done and what was not done. Or symptoms may emerge when the person is exposed to situations that resemble or symbolize the original trauma. Fear and persistent states of arousal lead to difficulty falling asleep or remaining asleep. Hypervigilance with an exaggerated startle response may occur, and people have problems concentrating and completing tasks. The duration of the symptoms is at least 1 month, and the syndrome may emerge many months after the event. Some victims, however, have no memories of the trauma for a period. They may complain of feeling detached or separate from others and lose the ability to enjoy pleasurable events, reflecting psychic numbing.

In both cases, anger, sadness, rage, depression, or stoicism may be demonstrated. In the case of wartime veterans, in which the victim was actually a participant in violent acts, changes may occur related to aggression. Other victims show a reduced capacity to control affect, demonstrating unpredictable explosions of anger or an inability to express angry feelings.

WHAT PATIENTS AND FAMILIES NEED TO KNOW

Obsessive-Compulsive Disorder

What is obsessive-compulsive disorder?

Obsessions are intrusive, unwanted thoughts or impulses that repeatedly come to a person's mind. Compulsions are actions that are repeated related to obsessions. For example, a person has a disturbing thought and then acts it out, "My hands must be contaminated; I must wash them." On one level, the person knows that these thoughts are irrational. But on another level, he or she is afraid that the thought may be true. Trying to avoid the thought or the action leads to great anxiety.

Who is affected?

People of all ages, ethnic groups, and both sexes may be affected. Symptoms usually begin during teenage years or young adulthood. There is frequent co-occurrence with other psychiatric disorders including depression and panic attacks; in childhood, it may occur with tics or other neurological disorders.

What is the prevalence?

In the United States, the lifetime prevalence is estimated at 2% to 3%. Most people suffer symptoms for 5 to 10 years before seeking treatment because they feel ashamed of their lack of self-control.

What is the cause?

Similar to the other anxiety disorders, it is thought that symptoms result from an imbalance of chemicals in the brain. Multiple studies show that certain brain activities are altered by medications that decrease the symptoms.

How is it treated?

Medications including certain antidepressants are very helpful. Therapy is also beneficial with the goal of changing the person's behavior related to the obsession. Family members may be included in the therapy to role-play situations with the patient.

How can family and friends help?

Be patient and supportive. Do not make fun of the person and think that he or she can stop this behavior voluntarily. Encourage the person to take medication as ordered and to participate in therapy including homework assignments.

T A B L E 2 3 – 2 Phases of Normal and Pathological Responses to Traumatic Stress

NORMAL RESPONSE	PATHOLOGICAL RESPONSE
1. Outcry: Fear, sadness, rage	1. Being overwhelmed and disorganized by the reaction
2. Denial: Refusing to explore memories of the event	2. Panic or exhaustion secondary to the emotional reaction
3. Intrusion: Involuntary thoughts of the event	3. Extreme avoidance: Use of alcohol or other drugs and acting-out to deny distress
4. Working through: Exploration and integration of the traumatic event and its meaning	4. Flooding: Disturbing, persistent images and thoughts of the event
5. Completion: Reengagement and commitment to ongoing life	5. Psychosomatic responses: Bodily complaints developing in response to incomplete processing of the event
	6. Character distortions: Persistent changes in thoughts and behavior that evolve as defenses, causing chronic alterations in lifestyle

Modified from Horowitz, M. (1986). *Stress response syndromes* (2nd ed.). New York: Aronson.

The prevalence of PTSD is estimated around 7.8% of the U.S. population. This patient may seek treatment in an emergency department or the outpatient setting. Particularly in the emergency department PTSD may go untreated unless members of the nursing staff make a comprehensive assessment and initiate the appropriate referrals for treatment (Clark, 1997). Refer to What Patients and Families Need to Know: Posttraumatic Stress Disorder for a review of teaching material for this patient and his or her family.

What do you think? If trauma can produce long-term psychological effects in the form of PTSD, what should be done preventively when individuals have experienced trauma?

? WHAT PATIENTS AND FAMILIES NEED TO KNOW

Posttraumatic Stress Disorder

What is posttraumatic stress disorder?

Posttraumatic stress disorder is the development of certain specific symptoms following exposure to an extremely traumatic event. Symptoms include recurrent flashbacks and dreams of the event, and attempts to avoid thoughts, feelings, and activities associated with the event. The person often has difficulty sleeping and concentrating, and may feel numb or irritable.

Who is affected?

Anyone can be affected who is exposed to events such as military combat, violent personal assault, natural disaster, or any other life-threatening situation.

What is the prevalence?

In the general population, the incidence is approximately 7%, but in a high-risk population the percentage may be 50% (e.g., survivors of an earthquake).

What is the cause?

Several theories exist. Some researchers believe that it is not an illness, but rather, a maladaptive way of coping with severe stress. Others believe that the brain is actually altered by repeated exposure to trauma, and loses its control over the normal stress response.

How is it treated?

Medication and therapy are both used for treatment. Medicine may help with the anxiety and sleep symptoms. Therapy, especially group therapy, is needed for the person to work through the experience and to regain a sense of security.

How can family and friends help?

Be supportive and express hope that treatment will be effective over time. Encourage the patient to take medication regularly and to participate in therapy.

➤ *Check Your Reading*

22. Does PTSD occur immediately after the traumatic event?
23. Why are nurses at risk for PTSD?
24. Name three symptoms of PTSD.

OTHER ANXIETY DISORDERS

There are four more specific diagnoses included in the family of anxiety disorders. They are described briefly here so that you become acquainted with the terminology. The symptom pictures resemble the entities previously described.

First, a new category was added to the DSM-IV in 1994 to describe a close relative of PTSD called **Acute Stress Disorder.** Like PTSD, the problem begins with exposure to a traumatic event with a response of intense fear, helplessness, or horror. In addition, the person shows dissociative symptoms, that is, a subjective sense of numbing, feeling "in a daze," depersonalization, or amnesia and clearly tries to avoid stimuli that arouse recollection of the trauma. (For further information on dissociative behaviors, see Chapter 28.) But just like PTSD, the victim reexperiences the trauma and shows functional impairment in social, occupational, and problem-solving skills. The key difference is that this syndrome occurs within 4 weeks of the traumatic event and only lasts 2 days to 4 weeks.

The second diagnosis is **Anxiety Disorder due to a General Medical Condition.** The patient may exhibit severe anxiety, panic attacks, obsessions, or compulsions, but the cause is clearly related to a medical problem excluding delirium. The history, physical examination, and laboratory findings support a specific diagnosis, for example, hypoglycemia, pheochromocytoma, or thyroid disease.

Third, there is **Substance-Induced Anxiety Disorder.** Again, the patient may present with anxiety, panic attack, obsessions, compulsions, or a phobia. But the symptoms arise in the context of, or within 1 month of, Substance Intoxication or Withdrawal, for example, alcohol, amphetamines, or cocaine. Alternatively, the substance causing the symptoms may be a medication (e.g., a sedative or sleeping pill). The etiology is determined by a thorough history, physical examination, laboratory testing, and the recognition that the anxiety symptoms exceed the usual symptoms of intoxication or withdrawal. (For more information about substance abuse disorders, see Chapter 26.)

The fourth and final variation of anxiety disorders is **Anxiety Disorder Not Otherwise Specified.** This category describes patients with significant anxiety or phobic avoidance but without enough symptoms to meet the criteria for a particular anxiety or adjustment disorder diagnosis. The patient may show a mixed anxiety-depressive picture; demonstrate social phobic symptoms related to having another medical problem (e.g., Parkinson's disease); or present with insufficient data to rule out a general medical condition or substance use.

What *do you think?* If anxiety is commonly associated with medical conditions, how should the management of the anxiety be integrated into a primary care perspective?

➤ *Check Your Reading*

25. What is the difference between Acute Stress Disorder and PTSD?
26. How is the diagnosis confirmed for Anxiety Disorder due to a General Medical Condition?
27. Name four substances that may cause Substance-Induced Anxiety Disorder.
28. When is the diagnosis Anxiety Disorder Not Otherwise Specified used?

POSSIBLE CAUSES OF ANXIETY DISORDERS

Now that you have been introduced to the behavior patterns in anxiety disorders, we can explore some of the theoretical explanations for these phenomena. As with other forms of mental illness, there is no exact cause known at this time, and scientific studies are continuing. Three major approaches to understanding the causes for anxiety are psychobiological, psychodynamic, and behavioral.

Psychobiological Approaches

The psychobiological approach attempts to explain the symptoms of anxiety disorders as faulty operations of the multiple body systems involved in the normal stress response. Research has revealed a definite anatomical pathway, called the limbic system, underlying the experience of anxiety. The limbic system is composed of a group of structures that form a border separating the structures of the brain stem from the major sensory systems of the cortex. (See Chapter 7 for diagrams and discussion of brain structures.)

There are three limbic pathways. The first pathway includes the hypothalamus and the thalamus. The hypothalamus acts to regulate endocrine functions based on the input it receives from all limbic structures. The second pathway of the system contains the amygdala and hippocampus. These structures are involved with memory and evaluation of sensory information. Research suggests that new sensory input is combined in the hippocampus and amygdala with associations of prior experience before stimulating the hypothalamus. The third limbic pathway is the cingulate gyrus and septal circuit. Stimulation of this area elicits sexual functions and social behaviors. This area sends signals from the cortex to the lower limbic structures (Brown et al., 1994; Hill, 1991).

These anatomical pathways provide the structure for the electrical impulses that receive or send a response related to anxiety. In order for these neurons to communicate with each other, they release chemicals, or neurotransmitters, at each synapse. There are multiple neurotransmitters in the brain that regulate anxiety, including epinephrine, norepinephrine, dopamine, serotonin, and γ-aminobutyric acid (GABA). These neurotransmitters are involved in emotion, attention, and visceral regulation. Their receptors are found in blood vessels, heart, and lung tissue.

Norepinephrine seems to play a role in amplifying anxiety. GABA is the most abundant neurotransmitter (200 to 1000 times greater than norepinephrine or serotonin) and seems to be completely inhibitory; it reduces anxiety, lowers muscle tone, and modulates sleep (Hill, 1991). Evidence from drug studies suggests that the therapeutic effects of antianxiety medications come from decreasing serotonin or increasing GABA.

What do you think? If the cause of anxiety is biologically based, what is the role of "talking" therapy in the management of anxiety?

➤ *Check Your Reading*

29. What are the three pathways in the limbic system?
30. How is the neurotransmitter norepinephrine related to anxiety?
31. What is the role of the neurotransmitter GABA related to anxiety?

Obsessive-Compulsive Disorder. Research into the causes of OCD points to a dysregulation of serotonin levels. Drugs that can mimic serotonin can provoke obsessions and compulsions. But, at the same time, drugs that inhibit the reuptake of serotonin, making it more available, also show selective benefit for OCD symptoms. Further study is needed to clarify the exact mechanisms in the disruption (Glod & Cawley, 1997).

PET and MRI scans of the brains of OCD patients show an increase in brain activity in specific brain regions, namely, the orbital-frontal lobes and parts of the basal ganglia. The basal ganglia–frontal cortex and other systems form a connection to help inhibit thoughts and behaviors, acting like a "brake"; dysfunction in this pathway may be responsible for the persistent obsessive and compulsive behaviors. Notably, treatment, in the form of medication or psychotherapy, produces decreased blood flow and glucose metabolism in these regions (Glod & Cawley, 1997).

Panic Disorder. Research into the causes of panic disorder suggest that heredity and biological factors play a role (Brown & Lempa, 1996). The common symptom of hyperventilation led to the "suffocation alarm theory." This theory proposes that during a panic attack, the brain is falsely signaling a shortage of oxygen or an increase in carbon dioxide and setting off a suffocation alarm in a person with an inherently low threshold. Thus, a person who is sensitive to an imbalance of blood gases may be vulnerable to panic attacks.

Another physiological clue comes from the lactate sensitivity theory. The muscles of the body produce lactate (in the form of lactic acid) during vigorous exercise, showing the body straining to meet oxygen demands. Injections of sodium lactate precipitate panic attacks in four fifths of people with panic disorder but only produce panic symptoms in one fifth of the general population. Lactate sensitivity may be a genetic susceptibility for panic disorder.

Finally, for panic disorder, it was observed that stimulants that alter norepinephrine transmission can precipitate panic attacks (e.g., amphetamines, caffeine). Norepinephrine is normally released by the brain in emergencies. Possibly, hypersensitivity of receptors for norepinephrine or serotonin or GABA may contribute to the false signal that results in panic.

Posttraumatic Stress Disorder. Research into PTSD suggests biological changes in the hormones and cerebral cortex of animals and human beings exposed to aversive events. People exposed to stressful events showed an increased response with the sympathetic nervous system, including higher plasma catecholamine levels and higher urinary epinephrine and norepinephrine levels (Kolb, 1987). Perhaps people exposed to repeated stress, as in war, lose their physiological control of incoming stimuli, and cortical neurons become vulnerable to the neuroendocrine disturbance.

Another theory about PTSD involves the release of massive amounts of endorphins when a person is affected by a traumatic event. Endorphins produce an analgesic needed to survive the ordeal, and when the trauma ends, the endorphin levels decrease. It is thought that PTSD symptoms occur in response to the decrease in endogenous opioids such as endorphins (Van der Kolk, Boyd, & Krystal, 1984).

➤ *Check Your Reading*

32. What neurotransmitter imbalance seems to be related to OCD?
33. Name two genetic susceptibilities that may be related to Panic Disorder.
34. Describe how the brain could be altered by repeated traumatic events in PTSD.

Application to Mrs. Anderson

A psychobiological explanation for Mrs. Anderson's condition suggests the following. She was born biologically susceptible to anxiety due to genetic factors: she probably suffered from anxiety symptoms all of her life but did not seek help, using various pain medications to self-medicate during times of stress. There is no family history given, but on inquiry, one might find that there was a sibling or parent who would be described as "nervous." Especially in this generation, there would not be a free admission of emotional problems in the family because of the strong stigma related to mental illness.

When her husband was diagnosed with a life-threatening cardiac condition, she was severely stressed at the potential loss of her lifelong significant other. Instead of a self-limited stress response, her brain responded with a significant imbalance in the neurotransmitters. Her physical symptoms were directly related to the stress response (e.g., palpitations), or they were minor physical complaints (e.g., constipation, body aches) exaggerated by her preoccupation with finding something physically wrong.

Psychodynamic Approaches

Psychoanalytic theory developed by Sigmund Freud in the 19th century proposed that anxiety resulted from a failure to repress painful memories, impulses, or thoughts. He believed that the symptoms of anxiety disorders were actually these repressed thoughts breaking into consciousness in disguised forms. He developed the concept of unconscious defense mechanisms, which allow the person to avoid the painful feeling of anxiety by transforming it into a more tolerable symptom. (See Chapter 6 for more discussion of psychoanalytic concepts.)

Another psychological approach involves the theory of cognitive distortion, that is, the patient's problem is that he or she interprets reality in a negative way. Clark (1997) believed that panic disorder is not biological but instead represents a severe cognitive distortion. The patient misinterprets the symptoms of anxiety as symptoms of impending death, and it is the misinterpretation that leads to a full-blown panic attack (Seligman, 1994.)

A third psychological theory has been developed by Horowitz (1986) in research on PTSD. Horowitz viewed trauma as a stressor that affects a person's information-processing capacity. He noted that all people who survive a traumatic event have a "completion tendency," an unconscious tendency to think about the experience in an attempt to understand what has happened. The PTSD victim tries to integrate the feelings about the event and ruminates about the memories. The behavioral attempts at avoidance (e.g., repression of memories) are a defense against the avalanche of uncontrollable feelings. When a person cannot complete an understanding of the event, PTSD develops (see Table 23-2 to review normal versus pathological responses to trauma).

Application to Mrs. Anderson

A psychoanalytic explanation for Mrs. Anderson's symptoms might focus on her experiencing severe separation anxiety due to the fear of losing her husband through death. She repressed the real reason for her distress because it was too frightening to her conscious mind—remember that she never did admit that she was afraid of losing her husband and she barely acknowledged that she felt anxiety. She used her physical complaints as a means of seeking his constant attention and trying to prevent him from leaving her.

> ➤ *Check Your Reading*
> 35. What is the psychoanalytic explanation for anxiety symptoms?
> 36. How does cognitive distortion relate to panic attacks?

37. What is the completion tendency involved in PTSD?

Behavioral Approach

The behavioral theorists believe that anxiety is the outcome of conditioning; it is learned. Conditioning refers to the process of learning to react to a neutral stimulus the same way that one reacts to a stimulus that causes a natural response. For example, if someone made a loud noise to startle you every time you sat in a certain chair, soon you would begin to feel uncomfortable just looking at the chair, even without the noise. If a person experiences the physiological symptoms of anxiety in relation to an event, then that event will trigger the same reaction again. Review Chapter 6 for more discussion of behavioral theories.

Application to Mrs. Anderson

A behavioral approach to Mrs. Anderson's symptoms would focus on a particular behavior to change, for example, her reaction each time that her husband left the house. Each step in her behavior pattern would be identified. For example, does she start to pace, then look at the clock, then start to cry, and so on? Her positive behaviors would be reinforced and negative behaviors would be replaced with alternative actions through teaching.

What do you think? Could the cause of anxiety be an interplay among biological, psychodynamic, and behavioral factors? Explain your position.

OVERVIEW OF EFFECTIVE TREATMENTS

After learning about the range of patient symptoms and possible causes of anxiety disorders, you are ready to explore the successful treatment alternatives, including the role of the nurse. Pharmacotherapy and various forms of psychotherapy are indicated for all of these conditions. Blair (1996) pointed out that the nurse must use both biological and behavioral interventions to provide comprehensive care.

Medications

There are several classes of medications that specifically help to reduce the symptoms of these disorders. First, the benzodiazepines (e.g., alprazolam [Xanax], lorazepam [Ativan], and diazepam [Valium]) act directly to decrease anxiety by facilitating the action of the neurotransmitter GABA. Their effects are felt immediately. A second antianxiety drug, or **anxiolytic** is buspirone (BuSpar). It takes up to 4 to 6 weeks to show optimal effects, and its site of action is suspected to be serotonin receptors. Although it does not act as quickly as the benzodiazepines, it does have a lower potential for dependence and abuse (Porterfield, 1991).

The third class of medications is the antidepressants. Tricyclic antidepressants (e.g., imipramine [Tofranil], amitriptyline [Elavil], clomipramine [Anafranil]) block the reuptake of serotonin and norepinephrine. Therapeutic effects may take several weeks and cardiac side effects may be a disadvantage (e.g., dizziness or palpitations). The serotonin selective reuptake inhibitor (SSRI) antidepressants are also useful for anxiety (e.g., paroxetine [Paxil], sertraline [Zoloft], fluoxetine [Prozac]). They produce fewer cardiac side effects and less sedation than the tricyclics and do not have the risk of withdrawal symptoms of the benzodiazepines.

Other classes of drugs may also be used. The β-adrenergic blocking agents (propranolol, atenolol, metoprolol) may decrease symptoms of autonomic hyperactivity, such as tachycardia. Calcium channel blockers such as diltiazem (Cardizem) or verapamil (Calan) and anticonvulsants such as carbamazepine (Tegretol) have also shown some success (Brown & Lempa, 1996). Use of these medications, however, requires close medical monitoring because of the possible cardiac and respiratory side effects. For further discussion of psychopharmacology, refer to Chapter 17. Obviously, the nurse is actively involved in administering medication and educating both in the inpatient and community settings.

> ➤ *Check Your Reading*
> 38. What is the behavioral explanation for anxiety symptoms?
> 39. How do benzodiazepines act to decrease anxiety?
> 40. Name one advantage and one disadvantage to the use of buspirone.
> 41. What is a potentially serious side effect of tricyclic antidepressants?
> 42. Why do patients need close monitoring with atenolol?

Psychotherapy Approaches

Cognitive therapy and behavioral therapy that include a supportive focus on psychoeducation are the most effective therapeutic approaches to the anxiety disorders.

Cognitive Therapy

Cognitive therapy teaches patients about their thinking patterns so that they can change their reactions to the situations that cause anxiety. For example, a technique developed by Clark to treat panic attacks is surprisingly simple (Seligman, 1994). Patients are told that panic results when they mistake the normal symptoms of anxiety for symptoms of heart attack or dying. The physical reactions of anxiety are described so that the patient can recognize them as merely anxiety and not a life-threatening event. He or she practices dealing with the symptoms by breathing rapidly into a paper bag, which causes a build-up of carbon dioxide and shortness of breath, mimicking the sensations that provoke a panic

attack. The therapist points out that the symptoms are harmless and simply due to altered breathing. The patient learns to reinterpret the symptoms and no longer progresses to a full-blown panic attack.

In treating PTSD, Scurfield (1985) defined five aspects of treatment using a cognitive approach:

1. Developing trust within the therapeutic relationship
2. Educating the patient about the recovery process
3. Managing stress
4. Helping the patient to reexperience the trauma
5. Integrating the trauma experience

These patients often respond well to group therapy and must explore their spiritual values in order to find a new balance between themselves and the Supreme Being who allowed the trauma to take place.

Behavioral Therapy

Behavioral therapy tries to change the specific behaviors associated with a person's anxiety disorder. New behaviors are taught to reduce the sensations of anxiety, such as deep breathing or other relaxation exercises. Or the person with OCD or a phobia may be exposed to the stressor repeatedly in a controlled setting. This type of therapy, known as desensitization or exposure and response prevention, helps the patient modify or delay the automatic anxious response. Often, family members may be included for role playing to learn helpful interventions to support the patient with homework assignments and to monitor progress (Brown, 1996). To review more detail on behavioral therapy, see Chapter 13.

> ➤ *Check Your Reading*
> 43. What is the main goal of cognitive therapy?
> 44. Name two important aspects of treatment with PTSD patients.
> 45. What changes are patients expected to make in behavior therapy?

Role of the Nurse

As noted repeatedly, the nurse encounters patients with anxiety disorders in every possible treatment setting, including both psychiatric and medical units. The basic level psychiatric nurse is involved in treatment in the inpatient, partial hospital, or home care environments. The advanced practice psychiatric nurse works in all of those settings plus the outpatient mental health system. (See Chapter 15 for more discussion about the continuum of care.)

There are two important reasons why all nurses need to be knowledgeable about recognizing and treating anxiety. First, as described with PTSD, nurses are in a high-risk profession for developing stress-related problems. Also, as a predominantly female group, nurses are at a higher risk for most of the anxiety disorders. Even nursing students may experience more stress than their non-nursing counterparts, as reported in two studies of Hispanic student nurses (Huerta, 1997). Thus, every nurse, starting in nursing school, needs to be alert for

Box 23–3 ■ ■ ■ ■ ■
Nursing Strategies to Reduce Patient Anxiety

- Active listening to show acceptance
- Honesty; answering all questions at the client's level of understanding
- Clearly explaining procedures, surgery, and policies and giving appropriate reassurance based on data
- Acting in a calm, unhurried manner
- Speaking clearly, firmly (but not loudly)
- Giving information about laboratory tests, medications, treatments, rationale for restrictions on activity
- Setting reasonable limits and providing structure

- Encouraging patients to explore reasons for the anxiety
- Encouraging self-affirmation through positive statements, such as "I will," "I can"
- Using play therapy with dolls, puppets, games, drawing for young patients
- Using touch, giving warm baths, back rubs
- Initiating recreational activities, such as physical exercise, music, card games, board games, crafts, reading

Data from Gerrard, B., Boniface, W., & Love, B. (1980). *Interpersonal skills for health professionals.* Reston, VA: Reston Publishing.

signs of maladaptive responses to stress in herself or himself as well as in peers. Learning to practice stress management is essential for a successful nursing career (Jackson, 1997).

Second, all patients and families seeking attention for medical problems have one thing in common: they are anxious about the diagnosis and the treatment. Regardless of the severity of the problem from the medical point of view—a child with a nosebleed in an emergency department or an adult with a routine outpatient procedure—that patient and family are suffering some degree of anxiety. In order for the nurse to effectively perform the necessary procedures or teach, she or he must address the anxiety and try to reduce it to a mild level. Box 23–3 lists nursing interventions to decrease patients' anxiety in any nursing setting.

NURSING PROCESS

Now we can look specifically at the nursing process related to patients with anxiety disorders, using Mrs. Anderson's story as the primary example. All of these procedures pertain to the practice of the basic level psychiatric nurse.

Assessment

During the assessment interview, the nurse observes for behavior that shows the patient's usual coping pattern with anxiety. By definition, these patients never show the healthy response of learning new, positive, growth-producing behaviors to adapt. Instead, there are three maladaptive patterns that usually reflect an attempt to deny the original stressor: withdrawal and avoidance, acting out, or somatization.

For all patients with anxiety disorders, it is important to assess for suicidal ideation and level of social support. Approximately 20% of the people with Panic Disorder attempt suicide, which is even higher than those with depression (Brown & Lempa, 1996). Studies of people

undergoing stressful life events repeatedly show that social support is significant in helping them to cope better (Constantino & Bricker, 1997; Warren, 1997).

There are several standardized assessment tools used for anxiety disorders. They include Anxiety Disorders Interview Schedule–Revised (ADIS-R), Sheehan Patient Rated Anxiety Scale and the Modified Anxiety Scale, and Modified Spielberger State Anxiety Scale (Hoover & Parnell, 1984; Spielberger, 1984). These rating scales collect additional subjective data from the patient and help to provide a measurable baseline against which to monitor progress.

In the case of Mrs. Anderson, she was desperately trying to deny anxiety as the problem and became preoccupied with somatic complaints leading to social withdrawal. A comprehensive biopsychosocial and spiritual assessment showed these data.

Biological/Physical. Mrs. Anderson has decreased sleep, decreased appetite, constipation, backache, and high blood pressure.

Psychological/Emotional. She is anxious, has decreased concentration, is noncompliant with antianxiety medicine, has possibly abused pain medicines, and is self-imposed homebound.

Cognitive. Mrs. Anderson is alert, with rapid speech, and denial of suicidal ideation.

Sociological and Sociocultural. She is a 66-year-old white, married woman who is childless and retired with a history of social support with neighbors and church activities.

Spiritual. Mrs. Anderson is a Methodist, with a history of regular church attendance and involvement in group activities.

Mrs. Anderson scored 39 on the Sheehan Patient Rated Anxiety Scale, on which scores above 30 are considered abnormal and the goal is to bring the score below 10. The nurse also used the Mini-Mental State Examination to clarify cognitive functioning because the patient was elderly and could possibly have some deficits; her score of 25 out of 30 showed mild impairment in attention span. Based on the total data, the nurse formulated a discharge plan for Mrs. Anderson to return to her previous level of functioning in her marital and social relationships.

> **W**hat do you think? What skills have you developed to deal with your own anxiety? With the anxiety of others?

> ➤ **Check Your Reading**
> 46. Name two reasons why all nurses need to develop skills to treat anxiety.
> 47. What are three patterns that patients may use to avoid dealing with stress?
> 48. What is the primary safety factor to assess with all anxious patients?
> 49. What is the Sheehan scale?

Diagnosis

After analyzing the assessment data and conferring with the physician regarding the medical diagnosis, the nurse is ready to identify the relevant nursing diagnoses for the patient and family. Table 23–3 shows a comprehensive list of nursing diagnoses associated with stress and anxiety.

In reference to Mrs. Anderson, the nurse identified four nursing diagnoses related to anxiety:

Anxiety is related to her husband's health as evidenced by somatic complaints.

Ineffective Individual Coping is related to anxiety as evidenced by her excessive dependency on husband and misuse of pain medication.

Impaired Social Interaction is related to anxiety as evidenced by self-imposed homebound status and refusal of usual social contacts.

Ineffective Family Coping is compromised related to her anxiety as evidenced by her husband's inability to set realistic limits on her demands for attention.

The nurse also noted the patient's other problems, including alterations in sleep, nutrition, and knowledge deficit. In view of the patient's defensiveness about mental illness, the nurse prioritized the problem list to teach first about the illness and medication, second about the physical issues, and third about specific techniques to control anxiety. She shared her problem list with the patient and her husband, who agreed with the issues.

Outcome Identification

For each nursing diagnosis, there is a long-term goal or expected outcome. For anxious patients with multiple complaints, short-term goals are extremely important to demonstrate that progress is possible. Using Mrs. Anderson as an example, the following are some expected outcomes (long-term and short-term) for her episode of home care.

Problem
Anxiety

Long-Term Goal
By discharge, the patient will report significant decrease in anxiety.

Short-Term Goals
- By week 1, the patient will take alprazolam (Xanax) as ordered.
- By week 2, the patient will keep a daily log to record her anxiety level and activities.
- By week 3, the patient will demonstrate deep breathing.

Problem
Ineffective
Individual
Coping

Long-Term Goal
By 4 weeks, the patient will identify three coping alternatives.

Short-Term Goals
- By week 1, the patient will identify one past coping mechanism.
- By week 3, the patient will demonstrate progressive relaxation.

Problem
Ineffective
Family Coping
Compromised

Long-Term Goal
By 6 weeks, husband will leave patient at home alone for necessary outings.

Short-Term Goals
- By week 2, the patient will discuss feelings produced when husband leaves the house.
- By week 3, the patient and husband will both identify their feelings.
- By week 4, the patient will try thought-stopping techniques to block negative thoughts.

> ➤ **Check Your Reading**
> 50. Name four nursing diagnoses associated with anxious patients and their families.

Planning

To organize your plan of care for the anxious patient, you must consider three areas of concern. What physical and emotional health factors need ongoing monitoring, that is, how is the patient's health status? What information teaching does the patient (and family) need to increase his or her level of self-care? What skill teaching does the patient need to increase his or her level of self-care?

TABLE 23–3 Nursing Diagnoses Related to Stress and Anxiety

NURSING DIAGNOSIS	DEFINITION	EXAMPLE
Anxiety	A vague, uneasy feeling whose source is often nonspecific or unknown to the individual	Anxiety related to beginning new job
Impaired Verbal Communication	The state in which an individual experiences a decreased or absent ability to use or understand language in human interaction	Impaired Verbal Communication related to cultural differences
Decisional Conflict (specify)	The state of uncertainty about course of action to be taken when choice among competing actions involves risk, loss, or challenge to personal life values	Decisional conflict related to perceived threat to value system
Ineffective Family Coping: Compromised	A usually supportive primary person (family member or close friend) is providing insufficient, ineffective, or compromised support, comfort, assistance, or encouragement that may be needed by the client to manage or master adaptive tasks related to his or her health challenge	Ineffective Family Coping: Compromised related to multiple situational crises
Hopelessness	A subjective state in which an individual sees limited or no alternatives or personal choices available and is unable to mobilize energy on own behalf	Hopelessness related to long-term stress
Ineffective Individual Coping	Impairment of adaptive behaviors and problem-solving abilities of a person in meeting life's demands and roles	Ineffective Individual Coping related to recent unemployment
Parental Role Conflict	The state in which a parent experiences role confusion and conflict in response to crisis	Parental Role Conflict related to perceived inability to meet child's psychological needs
Altered Parenting	The state in which a nurturing figure(s) experiences an inability to create an environment that promotes the optimum growth and development of another human being	Altered Parenting related to chronic stress experienced by parents
Post-Trauma Response	The state of an individual experiencing a sustained painful response to an overwhelming traumatic event(s)	Post-Trauma Response related to terrorist attack
Powerlessness	Perception that one's own actions will not significantly affect an outcome; a perceived lack of control over a current situation or immediate happening	Powerlessness related to inability to deal with anxiety
Chronic Low Self-Esteem	Long-standing negative self-evaluation/feelings about self or own capabilities	Chronic Low Self-Esteem related to inability to problem-solve daily situations effectively
Impaired Social Interaction	The state in which an individual participates in an insufficient or excessive quantity or ineffective quality of social exchange	Impaired Social Interaction related to self-imposed isolation
Social Isolation	Aloneness experienced by the individual and perceived as imposed by others and as a negative or threatened state	Social Isolation related to inability to engage in satisfying personal relationships
Spiritual Distress (Distress of the Human Spirit)	Disruption in the life principle which pervades a person's entire being and which integrates and transcends one's biological and psychosocial nature	Spiritual Distress related to intense suffering
Risk for Violence: Self-Directed or Directed at Others	A state in which an individual experiences behaviors that can be physically harmful either to the self or to others	Risk for Violence: Self-Directed related to unrelenting course of anxiety disorder

Reprinted with permission from the *Diagnostic and Statistical Manual of Mental Disorders, Fourth Edition.* Copyright 1994 American Psychiatric Association. Nursing diagnoses and definitions from North American Nursing Diagnosis Association. (1999). *NANDA nursing diagnoses: Definitions and classification 1999–2000.* Philadelphia: NANDA.

For Mrs. Anderson, health problems requiring close monitoring included altered eating, sleeping, and elimination; pain and anxiety levels; and high blood pressure. Her knowledge deficits were related to her illness, Generalized Anxiety Disorder; her antianxiety medication, alprazolam (Xanax) and appropriate use of pain medication; and healthy habits to prevent relapse. The skill deficits identified for Mrs. Anderson involved cognitive skills to reframe negative thoughts; relaxation techniques and other coping skills; and communication skills for her and her husband to verbalize feelings and to set appropriate limits on behavior.

After you formulate your plan, you select the appropriate nursing interventions for your level of practice. As a basic level psychiatric nurse, you would plan to use counseling, psychobiological interventions, and health teaching for Mrs. Anderson.

Implementation

When implementing your care plan for the anxious patient, there are three specific features to remember. First, always address the patient's safety. Whether you are in the hospital or in the home, you must observe or teach the caregiver to observe the patient carefully. If there is any history of self-destructive behavior or substance abuse, precautions or contracting for safety may be necessary. Second, stay alert for any change in physical complaints that may signal new medical problems or exacerbations of known conditions. Third, recognize that anxious patients may be difficult to engage in treatment. Their attention span is short and they are fearful of change, especially if the nurse relates their physical symptoms to an emotional problem.

Psychobiological interventions include administering medication or teaching the patient to take medicine and observing for side effects and effectiveness. For Mrs. Anderson, her misunderstanding about her illness and psychotropic medication was a serious obstacle to medication compliance. In such cases, health teaching must precede the patient's acceptance of medication.

Counseling interventions include developing the therapeutic nurse-patient relationship and providing reassurance to the patient and family that treatment can be effective. Especially when medications take several weeks to show a beneficial effect, the patient's compliance often depends on his or her trust in the nurse.

Health teaching is important for anxious patients and their families. Knowledge about the illness and medications is usually new material for them and can help them overcome the stigma attached to emotional problems.

Teaching about physical exercise is also helpful. Aerobic exercise has the direct effect of discharging the "fight or flight" energy associated with anxiety. In addition, brisk exercise causes the body to release hormones called β-endorphins, which produce a feeling of well-being, or the "runner's high." Patients who suffer from significant muscle tightness and tension should include stretching exercises in their exercise program (Lark, 1994).

Likewise, nutrition teaching has specific benefits for anxious patients. They need to learn to avoid stimulants such as caffeine and diet pills and specific foods such as those high in refined sugar and alcohol. For some sensitive patients, dairy products, wheat, and gluten-containing grains may cause problems. On the other hand, specific foods may help reduce their anxiety, including vegetables and fruits, legumes, whole grains, seeds, and nuts (Communication Channels, Inc., 1994).

For Mrs. Anderson, teaching about her illness and medication helped her to accept treatment; she most likely would have remained noncompliant without the nurse's intervention. She also benefitted from learning about healthy eating, exercise, and sleeping habits.

In addition to knowledge teaching, skills teaching is pertinent for patients with anxiety. Various techniques to promote relaxation can be taught easily. Boxes 23-4 through 23-6 show directions to teach deep breathing and progressive relaxation. Other coping skills can be introduced, including some solitary activities and the use of social support. Improved communication skills are also needed to help patients and their families to identify and verbalize feelings more clearly.

Mrs. Anderson successfully learned deep breathing exercises and thought-stopping for her negative thoughts. She resumed her social contacts and returned to her previous social support system. She and her husband also learned to be more direct and honest in their communication with each other, thereby decreasing tension for both of them. See the Snapshot: Nursing Interventions Specific to Anxiety Disorder.

What do you think? As you read the interventions that were used to assist Mrs. Anderson, are there other interventions that you think should be offered? Would you consider investigating available community supports for patients and families dealing with anxiety? What benefits could such a service offer Mrs. Anderson and her husband?

► *Check Your Reading*
51. What are the three main principles to organize your care plan?
52. What is the main psychobiological intervention for the anxious patient?
53. Name two issues for knowledge teaching and two topics for skills teaching.

Evaluation

In evaluating the care plan for the anxious patient, the nurse does a formative evaluation throughout the course of treatment. That is, as you implement your planned interventions, you constantly compare the results to your expected outcomes. If the patient consistently succeeds with each short-term goal, you continue with the original plan. But if the short-term goal is not achieved or a new problem develops, you must go through each step of the nursing process to ask: Is there significant

Box 23–4 ■ ■ ■ ■ ■
Directions for Controlled Breathing

1. Lie flat on your back and pull your knees up. Keep your feet slightly apart and try to breathe in and out through your nose.
2. Inhale deeply. As you breathe in, allow your stomach to relax so the air flows into your abdomen. Your stomach should balloon out as you breathe in.
3. Visualize your lungs filling up with air so that your chest swells out.
4. Imagine that the air you breathe is filling your body with energy.
5. Exhale deeply. As you breathe out, let your stomach and chest relax. Imagine the air being pushed out, first from your stomach and then from your lungs.

Box 23–5 ■ ■ ■ ■ ■
Directions for Progressive Relaxation

When your muscles are tense, movement is limited and energy flow is constricted. Muscles receive decreased blood circulation and oxygenation while accumulating waste products such as lactic acid and carbon dioxide. The following exercise, performed with or without soothing music, facilitates relaxation:

- Lie in a comfortable position. Allow your arms to rest at your sides, palms down, and exhale slowly and deeply with your eyes closed.
- Become aware of your feet, ankles, and legs. Notice if these parts of your body have any muscle tension or tightness. If so, breathe deeply and concentrate on that part of your body until you feel it relax. Release any anxious feelings with your breathing, continuing until the feelings begin to decrease in intensity and fade.
- Next, move your awareness into your hips, pelvis, and lower back. Breathe deeply until you feel them relax. Release any negative emotions as you breathe in and out.
- Focus on your abdomen and chest. Notice any anxious feelings located in this area and let them drop away as you breathe in and out.
- Finally, focus on your neck, arms, and hands. Note any tension in this area and release it. With your breathing, release any negative feelings blocked in this area until you cannot feel them any more.
- When you have finished releasing tension throughout the body, continue breathing deeply and relaxing for another minute or two. At the end of this exercise, you should feel lighter, more energized, and in control. Your body is relaxed and calm, and more important, no longer primed for an anxiety attack.

Box 23–6 ■ ■ ■ ■ ■
Teaching Relaxation by Means of Guided Imagery

Place the patient in a quiet, calm environment that is free from other distractions such as noise, strong light, or extraneous conversation. You might choose to sit away from the direct gaze of the person and ask him or her to select a place that has been conducive to rest and peace in the past.

Then, ask the patient to close his or her eyes, if desired, and to imagine that peaceful place. Ask the patient to describe the place in terms of its appearance, its odors if appropriate, and other sensual characteristics such as its temperature. Use a quiet, subdued tone of voice to avoid interrupting the mood that is being established.

Should the patient identify a place such as the beach, you can prompt responses with such non-threatening questions as "What does the sky look like? What color is it? Is the air warm? How does the warm sand feel to your body? Are you alone on the beach?" You also could say "Tell me how the water feels to your foot. Tell me more about the things that you think and do at the beach."

All of these questions require that the patient focus on the place that is being described. Gradually, his or her focus on the stressful event is weakened, resulting in a temporary diminution of anxiety. Relaxation occurs as a result of associations with the nonthreatening and calming beach.

SNAPSHOT

Nursing Interventions Specific to Anxiety Disorder

What do you need to do to develop a relationship with a patient suffering with an anxiety disorder?
- Approach the patient with warmth, quiet demeanor, and acceptance.
- Present a calm and deliberate approach.
- Be honest, empathetic, and compassionate.
- Speak slowly and allow the patient time to respond.
- Address the patient by preferred name (do not assume it is okay to use the patient's first name until you ask the patient's preference). Talk with the patient and listen carefully to what the patient shares.
- Encourage the patient to identify and discuss feelings.

What do you need to assess regarding the patient's health status?
- Suicidal risk or self-destructive thoughts
- Affective responses, including anger, anxiety, irritability; helplessness (may be evaluated and quantified using a standardized anxiety inventory)
- Physiological responses, including dry mouth and gastrointestinal disturbances, appetite changes, diarrhea, increased urination, diaphoresis, fatigue, sexual disturbances, insomnia, hyperventilation, weight changes, and elevated vital signs
- Cognitive responses, including narrowed perceptual field with anxiety above the mild level, missed details, diminished problem solving skills, deteriorated logical thinking
- Behavioral responses, including "nervousness," irritability, tenseness, alcoholism, drug addiction, inability to relax, expressions of fear and impending doom, feelings of helplessness and insecurity, low self-confidence
- Spiritual responses, including hopelessness, feeling cut off from God, anger at God for allowing the anxiety
- Vital signs may be elevated
- Weight, especially if the patient is experiencing changes in appetite
- Response to and compliance with medication regimen and reasons behind noncompliance; delayed effectiveness of medication effect

- Degree of social support
- Knowledge level; ability and readiness to learn
- Concurrent medical conditions

What do you need to teach the patient and/or the patient's caregiver?
- Medication issues: reason for taking; side effects and how to deal with them; untoward effects; warnings; importance of adhering to medication schedule
- Disease process, causes of anxiety, course of disease, and treatments
- Nutrition issues, especially avoidance of caffeine
- Emergency measures
- Importance of social support and strategies to obtain it
- Maintaining safety
- Lifestyle and compliance issues, such as benefits of exercise and stress management
- Importance of emotional support
- Importance of achieving spiritual well-being

What skills will you want the patient and/or caregiver to demonstrate?
- Ability to enter into a no-harm contract and remain safe
- Ability to follow medication and treatment plan
- Ability to use thought-stopping techniques and other cognitive strategies to deal with distorted thinking patterns
- Ability to identify and express feelings
- Coping skills
- Relaxation techniques

What other health professionals might need to be a part of this plan of care?
- Physician—psychiatrist and/or primary care physician—is usually in charge of the overall treatment plan, including medication management
- Social worker—to assist with access to community supports; insurance issues; access to entitlements; connection with community-based treatments
- Psychiatric occupational therapist—to assist patient with instrumental activities of daily living such as time management, cooking, budgeting
- Nursing assistant or home health aide—to assist patient with personal hygiene and grooming, if necessary

assessment data missing? Is the nursing diagnosis correct? Is the expected outcome realistic and measurable? Is the intervention too weak (e.g., needs limit-setting instead of listening) or too strong (e.g., needs acceptance of the symptom rather than confrontation)? Based on your evaluation, revise the intervention or the timing of the plan appropriately.

For example, with Mrs. Anderson, the nurse originally planned on a primary focus on anxiety and thought that she would teach, in sequence, illness, medication, relaxation exercises, and thought-stopping. But the patient's insistence that her problems were physical cued the nurse to progress more slowly with teaching about anxiety. Instead, the nurse focused on more emotionally neutral subjects, such as nutrition and sleep tips, while she monitored the effects and side effects of the new medication. Only when the patient's anxiety was lessened could she listen and learn about relaxation and other coping skills to help herself.

The summative evaluation made at the end of treatment gives the overall comparison between the patient's status on admission and the changed status on discharge. Successful and unsuccessful outcomes are noted along with any new problems or issues identified. Again, with Mrs. Anderson, there was notable improvement in her scores on the standardized rating scales. She also reported subjective improvement with her alertness and level of worrying, backed up by her husband's report about her reduced dependence on him. The problem of misuse of pain medication never was addressed directly; once the patient began to take her alprazolam, her complaints about physical pains decreased and she stopped seeking prescription-strength medication.

In closing, it should be noted that Mrs. Anderson's response to treatment was more successful than many other patients with anxiety disorders. She had no suicidal risk, her substance abuse was not well-entrenched, she responded well to alprazolam, and she had a solid support system, including a physician who recognized her anxiety problem. For many patients, symptoms may be more severe and response to treatment may be less successful. Especially when patients require multiple medication trials before finding a suitable regimen, risk factors such as hopelessness and self-destructive behavior may increase. The role of the psychiatric nurse in providing ongoing support to the anxious patient is crucial to preserve the patient's hope in treatment and to reinforce his or her belief in self as a worthwhile human being.

Conclusions

Psychiatric nursing care of patients with anxiety disorders is challenging and ultimately satisfying. Anxiety disorders tend to be amenable to treatment with anxiolytic drugs, supportive psychotherapy, and behavioral and cognitive therapies. As you care for patients with anxiety, notice how readily anxiety is shifted to other patients and to the staff members. Take measures to prevent that process by identifying the source of the anxiety and to whom it belongs. It is also imperative that you correctly assess the patient's level of anxiety and that you take measures to bring distress to manageable levels. Finally, it is your responsibility to provide and maintain a safe environment for the patient, to determine when the patient may be at greater risk for self-injury or suicide, and to communicate those findings to the appropriate resources.

Key Points to Remember

- Anxiety is a feeling of alertness and concern that prepares a person to take action of some kind. Anxiety in normal proportions is a trigger that is helpful to growth. Normal anxiety is short-term and of low to moderate intensity.
- Anxiety disorders are characterized by symptoms of anxiety and efforts to avoid those symptoms.
- Anxiety affects the body, mind, spirit, and emotions.
- Anxiolytics are the drugs that usually are used to reduce anxiety.
- The etiology of anxiety is theorized in psychobiological, psychodynamic, and behavioral terms.
- Stress is the broader response of which anxiety is one dimension.

- Stress is examined in terms of its immediate, intermediate, and long-term responses.
- Anxiety occurs along a continuum ranging from mild to moderate to severe to panic.
- People cope with anxiety using either conscious coping mechanisms or preconscious or unconscious processes called defense mechanisms.
- GAD is characterized by unrealistic or excessive anxiety and worry about two or more life circumstances.
- GADs usually respond to benzodiazepines, as well as buspirone.
- Nursing implications for a patient diagnosed with GAD include medication teaching and monitoring.

- Panic Disorder is characterized by discrete periods of intense fear or discomfort that are recurrent.
- Panic Disorder may exist with or without agoraphobia.
- Patients experiencing panic attacks usually present in the emergency department.
- OCD is reflected in ritualistic behaviors that may occur in thought or action.
- Obsessions are persistent thoughts.
- Compulsions are repetitive behaviors that follow an obsession.
- PTSD is a maladaptive set of responses to an event that has been overwhelmingly distressing.
- PTSD presents with physiological as well as psychological symptoms.
- Both pharmacotherapy and psychotherapy are used in the treatment of PTSD.
- Phobias are irrational fears. Specific Phobia includes severe fear of clearly identifiable objects or situations; social Phobia is a profound and enduring fear of social or performance situations in which embarrassment could occur.
- Assessment of a patient with an anxiety disorder identifies the pattern used by the patient to cope with the anxiety.
- Assessment focuses on the defining characteristics of anxiety and its severity and the impact of the symptoms of anxiety on the patient's life.
- Nursing diagnoses for anxiety disorders include Anxiety, Fear, Social Isolation, Ineffective Individual Coping, High Risk for Self Directed Violence, and Post-Trauma Response.
- Expected outcomes include a decrease in the feelings of anxiety and increased coping abilities in dealing with anxiety.
- Nursing strategies vary depending on whether the patient is in residential or community-based treatment.
- Evaluation includes a formative and summative focus.

Learning Activities

1. Observe yourself the next time you are anxious. What behaviors are you exhibiting?
2. Write down the behaviors you use to cope with anxiety. Which are most effective?
3. Read *The Boy Who Couldn't Stop Washing* by Rappoport (1989). What impact do you think having OCD has on a patient's journey?
4. Observe your behavior with your peers, patients, and others. Are you able to calm others when they are anxious? If so, what behaviors are you using that are effective? If people become more "uptight" in your presence, examine what behaviors are causing them to escalate in their anxiety.
5. Observe someone who you think is effective with patients. What strategies do you observe the person using?

Critical Thinking Exercise

Mrs. Peterson, a 45-year-old patient on the psychiatry unit, approaches the nurse's station clutching her chest, gasping for air. Nurse A, a new nurse to the unit, does not know this patient's history. She asks the patient to sit down while she takes her vital signs. Nurse B, who knows that Mrs. Peterson has a history of anxiety attacks, tells Nurse A that the patient just wants attention and to ignore her hysteria.

1. What assumption is Nurse B making?
2. If Nurse A follows Nurse B's advice, what assumption is Nurse A making?
3. What other evidence is needed to determine the appropriate intervention?

Nurse A decides to consider an alternative approach. She notes that the patient's husband and a female visitor have just left the unit. She asks Mrs. Peterson about the intensity, duration, and severity of her pain. The patient reports that the pain started when her husband told her he has filed for divorce and does not want her to return to the house. When asked what would help her feel calmer, the patient states that diazepam (Valium) helps. Nurse A decides to give the patient diazepam and observe her frequently for the next hour.

1. What could have happened if Nurse A had not considered an alternative approach?
2. If Nurse B interacted with the patient, what else could have happened as a result?
3. What is an alternative to the above approaches?

Additional Resources

Anxiety Disorders Association of America (ADAA)

11900 Parklawn Drive
Suite 100
Rockville, MD 20852
301-231-9350
http://www.adaa.org

The Anxiety-Panic Internet Resource (LAPir)

http://www.algy.com/anxiety

Mosby's Psychiatric Nursing Video Series: Anxiety Disorders (Volume 1)

Mosby Year Book
11830 Westline Industrial Drive
St. Louis, MO 63146
800-426-4545
http://www.mosby.com

National Alliance for the Mentally Ill (NAMI)

200 North Glebe Road
Suite 1015
Arlington, VA 22203-3754
800-950-6264
http://www.nami.org

National Institute of Mental Health (NIMH) Panic Disorder Education Program

Room 7c-02
5600 Fishers Lane
Rockville, MD 20857
800-64-PANIC
http://www.nimh.gov/anxiety/anxiety/panic/index.htm

References

American Psychiatric Association. (1994). *Diagnostic and statistical manual of mental disorders* (4th ed.). Washington, DC: American Psychiatric Association.

Bermanzohn, P. (1997, Winter). Clinical chameleons: Obsessive-compulsive symptoms in schizophrenia. *NARSAD Research Newsletter,* 1-4.

Blair, D. T. (1996). Integration and synthesis: Cognitive behavioral therapies within the biological paradigm. *Journal of Psychosocial Nursing and Mental Health Services, 34*(12), 26.

Brawman-Mintzer, O., Lydiard, R. B., Crawford, M. M., Emmanuel, N., Payeur, R., Johnson, M., Knapp, R. G., & Ballenger, J. C. (1994). Somatic symptoms in generalized anxiety disorder with and without comorbid psychiatric disorders. *American Journal of Psychiatry, 151,* 930-933.

Brown, A. (1995, Fall). Advances in genetics of psychiatric disorders. *NARSAD Research Newsletter,* 9-15.

Brown, A. (1996, Spring). Searching for a better understanding of OCD. *NARSAD Research Newsletter,* 16-18.

Brown, A. & Lempa, M. (1996, Fall/Winter). Update on potential causes and new treatments for anxiety disorders. *NARSAD Research Newsletter,* 13-18.

Brown, T. A., Barlow, D. H., & Liebowitz, M. R. (1994). The empirical basis of generalized anxiety disorder. *American Journal of Psychiatry, 151,* 1271-1281.

Clark, C. C. (1997). Posttraumatic stress disorder: How to support healing. *American Journal of Nursing, 97*(8), 26-32.

Communication Channels, Inc. (1994). Fertility and anxiety affected by caffeine. *Better Nutrition for Today's Living, 56*(9), 22, 23.

Constantino, R., & Bricker, P. (1997). Social support, stress, and depression among battered women in the judicial setting. *Journal of the American Psychiatric Nurses Association, 3*(3), 81-87.

Danton, W. G., Altrocchi, J., Antonuccio, D., & Basta, R. (1994). Nondrug treatment of anxiety. *American Family Physician, 49*(1), 161-167.

Fitzgerald, L. (1997). Exploration along the stress axis. *NARSAD Research Newsletter, 9*(2), 1-3.

Flint, A. J. (1994). Epidemiology and comorbidity of anxiety disorders in the elderly. *American Journal of Psychiatry, 151,* 640-650.

Glod, C., & Cawley, D. (1997). The neurobiology of obsessive-compulsive disorder. *Journal of the American Psychiatric Nurses Association, 3*(4), 120-122.

Haack, M., & Alim, T. (1991). Anxiety and the adult child of an alcoholic: A co-morbid problem. *Family Community Health, 13*(4), 49-60.

Hill, L. (1991). The neurophysiology of acute anxiety: A review of the literature. *CRNA: The Clinical Forum for Nurse Anesthetists, 2*(2), 52-61.

Hoehn-Saric, R. (1979). Anxiety-normal and abnormal. *Psychiatric Annals, 9,* 447-449.

Hoover, R., & Parnell, P. (1984). An inpatient educational group on stress and coping. *Journal of Psychosocial Nursing, 22*(6), 17-22.

Horowitz, M. (1986). *Stress response syndromes* (2nd ed.). New York: Aronson.

Huerta, M. (1997). Stress and social support among Hispanic student nurses: Implications for academic achievement. *Journal of Cultural Diversity, 4*(1), 18.

Hunt, D. (1988). *No More Fears.* New York: Warner Books.

Jackson, I. (1997). Coping with stress. *Nursing Times, 93*(29), 31.

Johnson, J., Weissman, M., & Klerman, G. (1990). Panic disorder, comorbidity, and suicide attempts. *Archives of General Psychiatry, 47,* 805-808.

Kolb, L. (1987). Neuropsychological hypothesis explaining posttraumatic stress disorder. *American Journal of Psychiatry, 144,* 989-995.

Lark, S. M. (1994). Strike back at anxiety: Natural ways to stay calm in stressful times. *Vegetarian Times,* (198), 90-93.

Lazarus, R., & Folkman, S. (1984). *Stress: Appraisal and coping.* New York: Springer.

Porterfield, L. (1991, September/October). Update on anxiolytics. *Advancing Clinical Care, 14,* 15.

Robinson, L. (1990). Stress and anxiety. *Nursing Clinics of North America, 25,* 935-943.

Scurfield, R. (1985). Post-trauma stress assessment and treatment: Overview and formulations. In C. R. Figley (Ed.), *Trauma and its wake* (pp. 219-256). New York: Brunner/Mazel.

Seligman, M. E. P. (1994). What you can change and what you cannot change. *Psychology Today, 27*(3), 34-47.

Spielberger, C. (1984). *State trait anxiety inventory.* Palo Alto, CA: Consulting Psychologists Press.

Stein, M. B., Walker, J. R., & Forde, D. R. (1994). Setting diagnostic thresholds for social phobia: Considerations from a community survey of social anxiety. *American Journal of Psychiatry, 151,* 408-413.

Van der Kolk, B., Boyd, T., & Krystal, J. (1984). Posttraumatic stress disorder as a biologically based disorder: Implications of the animal mode of inescapable shock. In B. van der Kolk (Ed.), *Posttraumatic stress disorder: Psychological and biological sequelae.* Washington, DC: American Psychiatric Press.

Warren, B. J. (1997). Depression, stressful life events, social support, and self-esteem in middle class African American women. *Archives of Psychiatric Nursing, 11*(3), 107.

Suggested Readings

Lark, S. M. (1994). Strike back at anxiety: Natural ways to stay calm in stressful times. *Vegetarian Times,* (198), 90-93.

Rappoport, J. (1989). *The boy who couldn't stop washing.* New York: Dutton.

Robinson, L. (1990). Stress and anxiety. *Nursing Clinics of North America, 25,* 935-943.

Zetin, M., & Kramer, M. (1992). Obsessive-compulsive disorder. *Hospital and Community Psychiatry, 43,* 689-699.

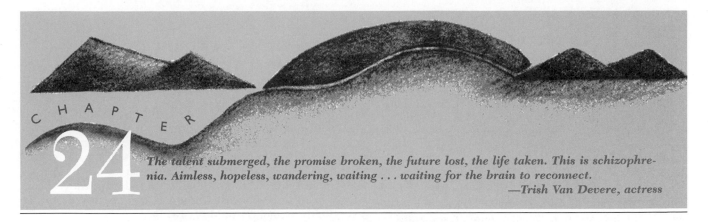

C H A P T E R

24

The talent submerged, the promise broken, the future lost, the life taken. This is schizophrenia. Aimless, hopeless, wandering, waiting . . . waiting for the brain to reconnect.
—*Trish Van Devere, actress*

Thought Disorders

Learning Objectives

After studying this chapter, you should be able to:

1. Describe the psychotic experiences that affect the journey of the patient with schizophrenia (e.g., delusions, hallucinations).
2. Define Bleuler's four "A's" of schizophrenia.
3. Describe first-rank and second-rank symptoms and positive, disorganized, and negative symptoms of an individual with schizophrenia.
4. Give examples of affective disturbance, disordered association of thought, autism, and ambivalence.
5. Discuss potential causes for the journey of schizophrenia.
6. Identify the role of psychotropic medications in the treatment of schizophrenia.
7. Describe the vulnerabilities of individuals with schizophrenia and strategies to prevent relapse.
8. Describe the vulnerabilities of individuals with schizophrenia for abusing substances and developing other medical illnesses and depression.
9. Describe the impact of the illness on the individual, family, and community.
10. Describe the nurse's role in facilitating the journey of the patient with schizophrenia and his or her family.
11. Identify assessment strategies for collecting data on a patient with schizophrenia.
12. Identify appropriate nursing diagnoses for a patient with schizophrenia.
13. Identify expected outcomes when working with a patient with schizophrenia.
14. Apply the nursing process to a patient with schizophrenia.

Key Terminology

Antipsychotic medication
Biological vulnerabilities
Delusions
Delusions of grandeur
Delusions of persecution
First-rank symptoms

Formal thought disorder
Hallucinations
Ideas of reference
Illusions
Loose association

Negative symptoms
Paranoid Personality Disorder
Personal vulnerabilities
Positive symptoms
Psychoeducation

Schizophrenia
Schizotypal-Personality
  Disorder
Second-rank symptoms
Word salad

The thought disorders are characterized by a disturbance in how an individual thinks, feels, relates to others and the environment, and perceives events that he or she experiences. The illness most frequently associated with thought disorders is schizophrenia. In his preface to the March 1998 issue of the *Psychiatric Clinics of North America,* devoted to the topic of schizophrenia, Dr. Peter Buckley observed, "Schizophrenia is still, arguably, the least understood and most ridiculed of all the major mental illnesses" (Buckley, 1998a, p. xiii). Andreasen and Carpenter (1993) observed that "the care and study of persons afflicted with schizophrenia is challenging, fascinating, and frustrating" (p. 26). These are the views of two prominent clinician-researchers who have devoted their careers to the study and treatment of schizophrenia. If this has been their experience, how much more confusing must it be to nurses who are just beginning their career journey and trying to learn the appropriate care for those who suffer from this illness. Perhaps a place to begin would be to hear the story of Ian Chovil.

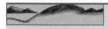

Ian's Story

Now in his 40s, Ian Chovil believes his illness started when he was 18 years old. His mother observed that he seemed to lose his ambition. He describes himself as "a strange kid, very anxious in any kind of social situation." While he was in graduate school he was hospitalized. He relapsed after his hospitalization and was not diagnosed; he went without treatment for the next 10 years. He further describes his life during these 10 years. "At first I believed I had dioxin poisoning. Then I believed I was a pawn in a war between people with supernatural powers, and then I thought aliens were putting me through a process that would result in my becoming an alien.... I really had to struggle just to survive, not knowing what was wrong. I was always below the poverty line, threatened by powerful enemies, eating at the missions when I was unemployed or going hungry." On his website Ian shares episodes of his life including experiences in jail, being homeless, and attempting suicide. He stated that he was "quite delusional and alone."

After a journey from Halifax to Victoria, he sought treatment for alcoholism. Although he acknowledges that he possibly will not experience what most of us take for granted, he describes himself as content. He states, "My life has a new purpose—to educate people about this devastating illness. And I can use my years of experience with schizophrenia for that." ■

Chovil, I. (1988). A mouse-guided tour of schizophrenia. *Living with schizophrenia, 2*(3), 8–10.

OUR UNDERSTANDING OF THOUGHT DISORDERS

Many identify schizophrenia as the most disabling of the major mental disorders. Most authorities on the subject believe schizophrenia is a major public health concern. An estimated 2 million Americans are afflicted with this serious mental illness. Based on these estimates schizophrenia is 5 times more common than multiple sclerosis, 6 times more common than insulin-dependent diabetes, and 60 times more common than muscular dystrophy (Keith, Reiger, & Judd, 1988).

An effort has been made to estimate the treatment costs for this disabling illness. One approach is to estimate the direct cost of treatment, while another approach seeks to determine indirect costs due to such factors as lost productivity (Rupp & Keith, 1993). In 1994, the cost of treating schizophrenia in the United States was estimated at $33 billion a year, with 25% of hospital beds occupied by patients with schizophrenia (*NAMI Advocate,* 1994). Jarboe and Kitts (1998) noted that some current estimates for direct and indirect costs may exceed $100 billion dollars annually.

> **W**hat do you think? As you begin to read this chapter, what are your thoughts about schizophrenia?

> ► *Check Your Reading*
> 1. What is a thought disorder?
> 2. Describe Ian's experience.
> 3. How many people are estimated as suffering from schizophrenia, and what is the probable cost of treatment for this illness?

It is now known that *schizophrenia* is a neurobiological disorder of the brain, and even though it is a severe mental illness, it is a treatable illness (Torrey, 1997). Sadly, however, up to 40% of persons with schizophrenia are not receiving treatment (Torrey, 1997).

The current understanding of this complex illness has taken many years of study and many dedicated persons. One of the early clinicians who sought to understand schizophrenia was Dr. Emil Kraepelin.

KRAEPELIN'S UNDERSTANDING OF SCHIZOPHRENIA

Emil Kraepelin, a European physician, named and attempted to identify the syndrome of dementia praecox (schizophrenia) in 1896. He classified psychoses into *dementia praecox* (a progressive intellectual deterioration with early onset) and manic-depressive psychosis, recognizing their similarities and lack of external causes. Kraepelin believed that dementia praecox was a sort of early senility with organic origin, was degenerative, and always ended in a state of disorganization after a chronic and deteriorating course. People afflicted with this illness, he assumed, never returned to their baseline level of functioning after becoming ill (Torrey, 1995). He also noted its occurrence in young, previously healthy persons.

BLEULER'S UNDERSTANDING OF SCHIZOPHRENIA

Dr. Eugen Bleuler, also a European physician, attempted to identify the behaviors typical of schizophrenia. In 1911, he renamed the illness schizophrenia rather than dementia praecox, deriving the name from the concept of "splitting," meaning that the patient is split off from reality, not that the person has a "split personality." This concept, however, is much misunderstood by the lay public and frequently misused. In this split from reality, thoughts and associations are fragmented and without meaning. The person's expressed emotions or facial expressions are not adequate or appropriate to the situation. Bleuler is best known for identifying the four "A's" associated with schizophrenia (Box 24–1), as follows:

1. The *affect* of the person with schizophrenia is disturbed, often blunted, resulting in a minimal change in facial expression and the consistent use of a monotonous tone of voice. Patients are typically described as having a flat affect, unable to joke or be engaged in conversation. Sometimes the person's affect is incongruous to the topic discussed; for example, the person describing some impulse to harm a family member may giggle. The person may become hostile when threatened.

2. *Association* between thoughts may be disrupted, providing the basis for describing this disturbance as a thought disorder. Sometimes thought blocking may occur, as evidenced by a person's difficulty in articulating a response to a question, or simply stopping in midsentence. The person may also lose track of a statement's meaning after starting a sentence, with resultant loose associations (e.g., "Look at my blue veins. I asked a Russian woman to make them red.") (Torrey, 1995, p. 45).

3. The person may appear to be *autistic*, preoccupied with self and inner experiences only, unable to relate to stimulation from the surrounding environment. It is not uncommon to see ill or nonstabilized patients with schizophrenia sitting on sofas or the floor of inpatient

recreation rooms, rocking, holding themselves, or appearing oblivious to the surrounding confusion and noise of the television and other patients arguing with one another.

4. The person demonstrates *ambivalence*, meaning that he or she simultaneously experiences strong positive and negative feelings, making it nearly impossible to make decisions. For instance, a person may be unable to decide to take medication, simultaneously believing the drug could be "poison" as well as a necessary treatment to relieve disturbing hallucinations (Kaplan & Sadock, 1995).

SCHNEIDER'S FIRST-RANK AND SECOND-RANK SYMPTOMS

Another description of symptoms, which some continue to use today, was developed by Dr. Kurt Schneider in 1959. He divided symptoms into **first-rank symptoms** and **second-rank symptoms.** Schneider emphasized that none of these behaviors is absolutely indicative of schizophrenia. The presence of several of these symptoms and the absence of any other identifiable pathological conditions, however, make the diagnosis of schizophrenia probable (Box 24–2).

Box 24–1 ■ ■ ■ ■ ■
Bleuler's "Four A's" of Schizophrenia

Affective disturbance
Disordered association of thought
Autism
Ambivalence

Box 24–2 ■ ■ ■ ■ ■
Schneider's First-Rank and Second-Rank Symptoms

First-Rank Symptoms

The hearing of one's thoughts spoken aloud
Auditory hallucinations that comment on the patient's behavior
Somatic hallucinations
The experience of having one's thoughts controlled (thought insertion)
The spreading of one's thoughts to others (thought broadcasting)
Delusions
The experience of having one's actions controlled or influenced from the outside (passivity experiences)

Second-Rank Symptoms

Other forms of hallucinations
Depression
Euphoria
Perplexity as disorders of affect and emotional blunting

Data from Kaplan, H., & Sadock, B. (1995). *Comprehensive textbook of psychiatry* (6th ed., p. 970). Baltimore: Williams & Wilkins.

W*hat do you think?* As you read Ian's story, what were your thoughts and feelings? Can you imagine how difficult just surviving was for him? Can you identify any of the four "A's or first- or second-rank symptoms in Ian?

➤ *Check Your Reading*
4. What was Kraepelin's contribution to our understanding of schizophrenia?
5. What are Bleuler's four "A's"?
6. What are first-rank symptoms?
7. What are second-rank symptoms?

Positive, Disorganized, and Negative Symptoms

Andreasen and Olsen (1982) recognized that schizophrenia is actually a group of heterogeneous disorders. In other words, it is probably more accurate to refer to the schizophrenias. They compared schizophrenia with collagen-vascular disease, observing that schizophrenia "is probably a group of related disorders that vary in their manifestations depending on the neurochemical or functional brain system being affected" (p. 789). Further, these researchers classified schizophrenia into three subtypes, which they conceptualized as positive (florid), negative (defect), and mixed. Thus, the symptoms of schizophrenia have been conceptualized into two broad categories, positive and negative (deficit) symptoms. A third category, disorganized, has been added because research has revealed that it is a dimension of the illness independent of the positive symptoms category (Box 24–3).

Liddle (1987) identified a separate syndrome, disorganization syndrome, in addition to positive and negative symptoms. He suggested that disorders of thought are major characteristics of the disorganized category, although he observed that other investigators assigned the symptoms of this syndrome to either positive or negative symptom groups. Because patients may have symptoms from more than one group of symptoms, he further attested that this phenomenon perhaps represents "discrete pathological processes occurring within a single disease" (p. 150). Docherty, DeRosa, and Andreasen (1996) reported findings they believed were consistent with other literature on schizophrenia, supporting "three relatively independent symptom dimensions: positive symptoms, negative symptoms, and disorganization symptoms" (p. 362).

Positive symptoms are present in the person with schizophrenia but absent in normal individuals. These symptoms generally respond well to medications. They include hallucinations and delusions. Disorganized symptoms include confused thinking and disorganized speech, disorganized behavior, and disorganized perceptions.

Negative symptoms are altered or defect emotional responses that respond less successfully to medication. These include apathy, social withdrawal, poverty of

Box 24–3 ■ ■ ■ ■ ■
Positive, Disorganized, and Negative Symptoms

Positive Symptoms

Delusions and hallucinations

Disorganized Symptoms

Confused thinking and disorganized speech
Disorganized behavior
Disorganized perceptions

Negative Symptoms

Flat or blunted emotions
Lack of motivation or energy
Lack of interest in things
Limited speech

Data from Frances, A., Docherty, J., & Kahn, D. The expert consensus treatment guidelines project for schizophrenia: A guide for patients and families. *The Journal of Clinical Psychiatry* Volume 57(Suppl. 12B), pp. 51-58, 1996. Copyright 1996, Physicians Postgraduate Press. Reprinted by permission.

thoughts, blunting of emotions, slow movement, and lack of drive. These negative symptoms can severely compromise a patient's ability to enter into a therapeutic relationship and also inhibit receptivity to compliance with prescribed medication regimens. These symptoms caused by the illness may inhibit a patient's ability to get well.

Crow (1980) argued that patients with predominantly positive symptoms (called type I, or florid) have less structural damage to the brain, a better response to antipsychotic drugs, and a better prognosis. Those with predominantly negative symptoms (type IIs, or defect) have more structural brain damage as seen on CT scans, a poorer response to drugs, and a worse prognosis (Andreasen, et al., 1986). Whether the two types represent two different causes of schizophrenia, however, is still unknown (Erlenmeyer-Kimling et al., 1993; Kay, 1990; Kay, Opler, & Lindenmayer, 1989; McGlashan & Fenton, 1993).

Crow (1980) speculated positive symptoms are primarily biochemical in origin and not related to structural abnormalities and tend to respond better to neuroleptic medication. These medications exert their therapeutic effect through blockage of dopamine transmission. As yet, PET studies (perhaps the most powerful techniques for studying the mechanisms that mediate abnormal mental phenomena) of persons with schizophrenia who have never been medicated have not shown any specific relationship between abnormal elevations in dopamine transmission as measured by $dopamine_2$ receptor density and prominent positive symptoms (Erlenmeyer-Kimling et al., 1993; Kay, 1990; Kay, Opler, & Lindenmayer, 1989; McGlashan & Fenton, 1993; Wong et al., 1986).

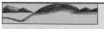 **Mark's Story**

In the 1970s, Mark Vonnegut, son of author Kurt Vonnegut, traveled toward a simpler life in Vancouver, British Columbia, leaving the staidness and conservatism of the East Coast. While in Vancouver, because of his own personal vulnerabilities, he became frankly psychotic. His first-person account, *The Eden Express,* is filled with descriptions from the ill person's perspective.

"By this time the voices had gotten very clear. At first I'd had to strain to understand them. They were soft and working with some pretty tricky codes. Snap-crackle-pop, the sound of the wind with blinking lights and horns for punctuation. I broke the code and somehow was able to internalize it to the point where it was just like hearing words. In the beginning it was mostly nonsense, but as things went along they made more and more sense. Once you hear the voices, you realize they've always been there. It's just a matter of being tuned in to them" (p. 106).

As Mark traveled with his friends and began homesteading with them in Vancouver, he began to experience more and more of the perceptual difficulties and misinterpretation of reality common to those experiencing their first psychotic break. Perhaps because he was living with such an antiestablishment group, the early clues to his psychotic disintegration were ignored or otherwise explained away. Eventually, though, even his tolerant group of friends recognized his need for psychiatric treatment. They could see that his bizarre behavior was causing him great distress and pain.

Subsequently, he was hospitalized on three occasions. After his recovery, Mark attended medical school at Harvard and has been successful practicing pediatrics in Boston (Vonnegut, 1975; Wyden, 1998). ■

Quotation from Vonnegut, M. (1975). *The Eden Express.* New York: Praeger.

DESCRIBING POSITIVE SYMPTOMS

Illusions and Hallucinations

Illusions occur when the patient misperceives or exaggerates stimuli in the environment. Persons with schizophrenia may see objects and people change their dimensions, their outline, and their brightness from minute to minute, as Mark Vonnegut so vividly described in *The Eden Express.* Sometimes these perceptual changes can signal the prodromal phase of schizophrenic illness. At other times, they can be part of the florid psychosis. At times, the patient may perceive a mirrored self-reflection change into a monster.

Hallucinations are sensory experiences of percep-

tions without corresponding stimuli in the environment (Table 24–1). They can occur in any sensory modality, but auditory hallucinations, or "hearing voices," are most commonly experienced by the individual with schizophrenia. The voices can be those of God, the devil, relatives, neighbors, or persons unknown to the patient. Auditory hallucinations often begin with friendly voices and progress to threatening, persecutory, and frightening messages and commands as the person decompensates. As the illness progresses, the patient is at risk to act on the voice commands. The voices are generally described as being "outside" and not merely thoughts spoken aloud. In Case Example 24–1 (see later under the role of nursing in the person with schizophrenia), Bill was at serious risk to harm himself in response to command hallucinations that told him to jump from the bridge.

Visual hallucinations occur less frequently in patients with schizophrenia, but they are not rare. When they occur in the absence of auditory hallucinations, they usually indicate a concurrent organic problem, such as alcohol withdrawal or drug toxicity.

Hallucinations must always be evaluated in their cultural context. In medieval times and today among some religious groups, visual hallucinations do not necessarily suggest mental illness. Arieti (1976) proposed the following criteria to distinguish religious hallucinations from the hallucinations experienced by individuals with schizophrenia:

- Religious hallucinations are usually visual.
- Religious hallucinations usually involve benevolent guides or advisors.
- Religious hallucinations are usually pleasant.

Tactile (touch), *olfactory* (smell), and *gustatory* (taste) hallucinations are less common. They are usually unpleasant.

TABLE 24–1 Types of Hallucinations	
HALLUCINATION	**EXAMPLE**
Auditory	Hearing choirs of angels inside one's head
Visual	Seeing a monstrous glowing face on the wall
Olfactory	Smelling acrid poison gas coming from a radiator
Gustatory	Tasting sharp lemon in absence of food
Tactile	Feeling small insects crawling under one's skin
Somatic	Sensing that a tunnel runs through one's head
Altered sense of self	Confusing one's own body with a doll or another person

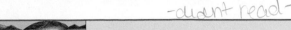

 **Lori's Story**

Lori was 17 years old, when as she describes, "uninvited and unannounced, the Voices took over my life" (p. 3). She was a camp counselor the summer before starting her senior year of high school. She describes it as "just an ordinary summer, and I was just an ordinary girl. Except that sometime during that summer things began to change" (p. 3). Two years before that fateful summer, Lori recalled memories of falling in love with an exchange student at the same camp. As she recalled the events of the summer before her senior year, her mood changed. She said it "began to turn black." One night, as she remembers, "a huge Voice boomed out through the darkness. 'You must die!' Other Voices joined in. 'You must die!' 'You will die!'" (p. 5–6).

In her own words, Lori continues, "Since that time, I have never been completely free of those Voices. At the beginning of the summer, I felt well, a happy healthy girl—I thought—with a normal head and heart. By summer's end, I was sick, without any clear idea of what was happening to me or why. And as the Voices evolved into a full-scale illness, one that only later I learned was called schizophrenia, it snatched from me my tranquility, sometimes my self-possession, and very nearly my life.

"Along the way I have lost many things: the career I might have pursued, the husband I might have married, the children I might have had. During the years when my friends were marrying, having their babies, and moving into the houses I once dreamed of living in, I have been behind locked doors, battling the Voices who took over my life without even asking permission.

"Sometimes these Voices have been dormant. Sometimes they have been overwhelming. At other times over the years they have nearly destroyed me. Many times over the years I was ready to give up, believing they had won" (p. 7).

While Lori was in college, she further describes her hallucinatory experiences. "Although the Voices still hovered around from time to time, fading in and out, disturbing my peace, they were much softer than they had been at camp, and in high school. They were more like chatterboxes in the back of my brain, talking to each other about me, narrating my every move. Most of the time I could retreat into sleep, and they wouldn't follow. If I couldn't sleep, I would close my eyes and take a series of deep breaths. I would chant to myself. 'You're not possessed by the devil.' Then I would silently address the Voices: 'Please,' I would beg, 'please leave me alone'" (p. 20).

"On the surface, things seemed great. Underneath, though, they were beginning to come apart. The Voices were coming louder and faster, startling me with their surprise visits to my brain. Only I didn't know they were in my brain. I heard them coming at me from the outside, as real as the sound of the telephone ringing.

"They popped up when I least expected them. Occasionally they were friendly, but mostly they re-

viled me, shouting in their hoarse, harsh tones: 'You must die, you bitch,' they shrieked. 'Die! Die! Die!' They filled me with anxiety. I'd turn around thinking somebody was in back of me, and no one would be there. On several occasions I tried beating through the bushes to flush out whatever or whoever it was that was taunting me. Of course, I was a bloody-fisted loser every time.

"I grew increasingly tense and nervous. I was always afraid I really was going to die, because that's what the Voices said would be my fate" (p. 21).

Eventually Lori required hospitalization as her symptoms intensified and became more incapacitating. She was actively suicidal as she became convinced that she was going to die, as the Voices continued to predict, and she determined it was her responsibility to bring about her own death. Again in her own words, she describes her hospital experience.

"All the time I was in the hospital they told me I was sick. They told me I was psychotic with hallucinations. I hated these two words. I knew they were not true. . . . Hallucinations meant that you were seeing something or hearing something that didn't really exist. But when I heard the Voices screaming at me, they were real. When the doctors and nursing staff told me that I was out of reality, and hallucinating, I hated them. What made me the psychotic one? What about all these judgmental people? What made them the experts? . . .

"My tormenters were real. I didn't want people telling me they were false or unreal. I wanted help in making them go away. That's what they should have been doing. But since they weren't, I just wanted to get out of there, and fast. I was twenty-four years old, and it was time I got on with my life" (p. 90).

During the course of her several hospitalizations, Lori received a variety of antipsychotic medications. None of them were completely effective in alleviating her symptoms. At one point she was treated with electroconvulsive therapy (ECT). In spite of energetic efforts to treat her illness, she experienced repeated hospitalizations, often following suicide attempts, during which she frequently required stays in the quiet room and sometimes was placed in cold wet-sheet packs. At one point, Lori experienced a particularly long stay in the hospital and continued to suffer great distress and hopelessness from her symptoms. Then she learned about a new medication that was being given experimentally to a few patients. She pleaded with her doctors to prescribe it for her. After careful review of her history and current situation, she was given the atypical antipsychotic medication, clozapine. As she began to feel better, she gained hope that she might be able to have a normal life. At first she missed the Voices and she felt a loneliness without their constant presence with her. The plans for Lori's discharge were made and she began to prepare for leaving the hospital.

After discharge she entered a halfway house, attended a day-treatment hospital, and regularly saw her therapist. She also spent time visiting her parents as well as developing the independence to live on her own. She now has her own apartment, works at a gift shop, and three times a month teaches classes about schizophrenia, clozapine, and how to stay well. ■

Delusions

Delusions are false fixed beliefs that cannot be corrected by reasoning. They may be simple and focused or detailed and involved. They are sometimes difficult to elicit on first encounter, although some patients have chronic fixed delusions and may describe them easily. The delusions of the individual with schizophrenia tend to be grotesque; loosely organized; and centered on themes of persecution, grandiosity, sex, bodily functioning, and control by others (Hagerty, 1984).

Delusions of persecution are most frequent and are the key symptom of paranoid schizophrenia. The ill person believes he or she is being persecuted by powerful agencies, such as the Federal Bureau of Investigation (FBI) or by specific people, such as a neighbor who can control him or her through walls and sometimes pipe in dangerous gases. Delusions of persecution may be more subtle. In Case Example 24-1 (see later in chapter), Bill's suspicion that the psychiatrist and nurse might be trying to harm him in their initial psychiatric interview was a delusion. The feeling of being controlled by some unseen mysterious force that exerts its power from afar occurs in most persons with schizophrenia at one time or another. Many individuals with schizophrenia believe their minds are controlled by telepathy or hypnotism. The person with schizophrenia today could be preoccupied by x-rays, spaceships, or atomic power that affects the mind and could take over the world. **Delusions of grandeur,** in which the patient assumes the identity of a famous individual such as Napoleon, Jesus Christ, or the president, are seen in schizophrenia as well as in mood disorders (see Chapter 25).

Ideas of reference are delusional ideas wherein people with schizophrenia believe that the actions of others are directed toward them. The patient may believe that the television announcer is referring to something the patient must do, or songs on the radio may have special significance. Some patients believe that others can read their thoughts or can put thoughts into their heads. One patient with schizophrenia showed the nurse a photograph of a pair of shoes leaning against a pillow. "Look, here is the evidence! The toes point toward the window where prostitutes walk up and down the street and call to my husband!"

W*hat do you think?* As you read Lori's story, what do you think it would be like living with "Voices"?

▶ *Check Your Reading*

8. What is a positive symptom? Give three examples.
9. What is a delusion?
10. What is the difference between an illusion and a hallucination?
11. What are ideas of reference?

DESCRIBING DISORGANIZED SYMPTOMS

Confused thinking and disorganized speech cause people with schizophrenia to have difficulty carrying on a conversation and in particular they find it difficult to communicate in coherent sentences.

Both the content of thought and the form of thought are disturbed in the person with schizophrenia. This **formal thought disorder** is different from the content disturbance in delusional thinking. The most common example of formal thought disorder is **loose association,** in which ideas shift from one subject to another, completely or only marginally related. The person appears unaware that the topics are disconnected. Statements having no meaningful relationship may be contained in the same expressed thought, or the person may shift from one frame of reference to another. When loosening of associations is severe, the person may become incoherent, with speech described aptly as **word salad.**

The person may experience thought blocking, in which thoughts and psychic activity unexpectedly cease. This can be a fleeting experience or can sometimes last for longer periods. Patients may appear perplexed and express the belief that someone has taken thoughts out of their heads.

The patient with schizophrenia has difficulty with concreteness and symbolism. Preoccupation with invisible forces, witchcraft, religion, and philosophy is common. The thinking of the person with schizophrenia is characterized by being overly symbolic as well as overly concrete.

The language of the person with schizophrenia may be difficult to understand. Because of the autistic nature of the illness, language becomes for the patient more a tool of self-expression than a tool of communication. Sometimes the person may create completely new words that are referred to as neologisms.

Slow movements and rhythmic gestures that are repetitious or ritualistic manifest disorganized behavior associated with this illness. For example, the patient may make a series of motions with the hands or feet before proceeding through a doorway.

Disorganized perceptions cause people with schizophrenia to distort everyday life experiences including feelings, sights, and sounds. The distortions of perception are such that even ordinary events or experiences are frightening and even distracting. They are abnormally sensitive to colors, noises, and shapes (Frances, Docherty, & Kahn, 1996). The person with schizophrenia tends to include many irrelevant items in thought and speech. Because of increased arousal level, people with schizophrenia show greater responsiveness to irrelevant stimuli and less responsiveness to relevant stimuli than normal persons. Consequently, irrelevant stimuli become incorporated into thought and speech.

DESCRIBING NEGATIVE SYMPTOMS

Part of the constellation of symptoms descriptive of schizophrenia are those labeled negative. These deficit symptoms can include affective flattening or blunting, poverty of speech or speech content, thought blocking, poor grooming, social withdrawal, lack of motivation, anhedonia (inability to take pleasure in activities or other people), and cognitive and attentional deficits.

When these symptoms occur during an initial breakdown, they often suggest the outcome of the disease and can be used as predictive factors. Catatonic symptoms (marked motor or psychomotor disturbance) and paranoid symptoms (suspicions) are often thought to be associated with better long-term outcomes. The predominance of negative symptoms, such as flattening of emotions and social withdrawal, is considered to be predictive of a poor outcome. Patients with negative symptoms tend to respond less well to medication and often have a history of poor adjustment before the onset of illness. They require an extensive support network to remain long-term in a community setting.

Social withdrawal, sloppiness about dress and hygiene, and loss of motivation and judgment are all common in schizophrenia. People with schizophrenia may sit silently while others converse, and families may express concern about the time a person spends alone. Sometimes, people with schizophrenia do nothing for extended periods, or they engage in pointless or repetitive activity. They may lose interest in their surroundings, become reclusive, lose all initiative, and even refuse to leave their own rooms. Researchers believe that this withdrawal may be a reaction to overstimulation, an adaptive response to a world the person experiences as too full of stimuli and too complex. Alternatively, withdrawal may be a response to understimulation. Close relationships may seem too frightening, and low self-esteem and feeling devalued by others add to the person's social withdrawal. Social withdrawal as a symptom of the illness has important implications in nursing treatment issues and family education.

> **W**hat do you think? How do you think you might communicate with a person who displayed loose associations?

➤ *Check Your Reading*

12. What is a disorganized symptom? Give three examples.
13. What is a negative symptom? Give two examples.
14. What are two different explanations for why persons with schizophrenia withdraw from social interactions?

INTERNATIONAL PILOT STUDY OF SCHIZOPHRENIA

Although there is evidence of variability of prevalence from one country to another (Torrey, 1995), schizophrenia occurs across all races around the world. When assessing the person with schizophrenia, nurses must be aware of the individual's cultural differences. Visual or auditory hallucinations with religious content may be a normal part of particular cultures' religious experiences. According to the *Diagnostic and Statistical Manual of Mental Disorders, Fourth Edition* (DSM-IV) (American Psychiatric Association [APA], 1994), there is evidence that supports a tendency to overdiagnose schizophrenia in some ethnic groups. In the United States, it has been reported that catatonic behavior is relatively uncommon in individuals with schizophrenia, but it is more common in non-Western countries. Individuals with the diagnosis of schizophrenia in developing nations seem to have a more acute course with a better outcome than do individuals in industrialized nations (APA, 1994).

In 1965, the World Health Organization initiated the International Pilot Study of Schizophrenia (IPSS) in an effort to obtain new knowledge about the epidemiology of the illness. One of the major objectives of IPSS was to develop and standardize diagnostic criteria that could be used in all nine countries in the study: Denmark, India, Colombia, Nigeria, England, the Soviet Union, Taiwan, the United States, and Czechoslovakia. A major problem in cross-cultural epidemiological studies has always been doubt that similar diagnostic criteria had been used to identify illness. For example, schizophrenia is diagnosed at much higher rates in the United States than in Great Britain and Europe.

A 12-point diagnostic system, shown in Box 24–4, was derived from the work of IPSS. The IPSS represented a major advance in the epidemiological study of mental illness, providing valuable information about the course of illness across nine cultures. One interesting conclusion from the study was that subjects who live in developing nations seemed to do better than those from more

Box 24–4 ■ ■ ■ ■ ■

Point Diagnostic System of the International Pilot Study of Schizophrenia

1. Restricted affect
2. Poor insight
3. Hearing one's thoughts spoken aloud
4. Absence of early waking
5. Poor rapport
6. Lack of depressed facial expression
7. Lack of elation
8. Widespread delusions
9. Incoherent speech
10. Unreliable information given
11. Bizarre delusions
12. Nihilistic delusions

highly developed societies. This determination followed a 2-year study of subjects who were interviewed a second time. This study laid the groundwork for future epidemiological research.

> ➤ *Check Your Reading*
> 15. What was the purpose of the IPSS?
> 16. Describe the 12-point diagnostic system derived from the work of the IPSS.

THE IMPACT OF THOUGHT DISORDERS ON THE JOURNEY

Age of Onset

As Mark's and Lori's stories indicate, onset of the illness is usually during adolescence or early adulthood. The disorder may, however, begin in middle or late adult life. Diagnosis of schizophrenia before age 10 or after age 50 is less common. The onset in males may be somewhat earlier than in females. The peak age of onset in men is between the ages of 15 and 25 and in women between ages 25 and 35.

Young Adults and Schizophrenia

The first "life break" or acute episode of the illness most frequently occurs in young adults or in those individuals just beginning to leave home and establish some sort of independence. Because of the dependence associated with any chronic illness, the timing of this "first break" may make the normal separation and individuation issues of late adolescence especially difficult to achieve. First signs are often gradual social withdrawal, loss of interest in school or work, unusual behavior, and angry outbursts.

People with schizophrenia are more likely to have a good outcome if they were considered relatively normal before becoming sick. Thus, if as children they were able to make friends with others, did not have major problems with delinquency, and achieved successfully in school according to their intelligence level, their outcome is likely to be good.

Torrey (1995) reflected that the young adult chronic population with schizophrenia so publicized today are simply more visible and not confined to institutions as they were years ago. He believes that 40 years ago, young adults with schizophrenia were hospitalized, usually for many years, during which time they were "socialized" to their disease. Most learned to expect little from life and to respect mental health personnel. When they were finally released into the community, these people were usually docile.

Young adults with schizophrenia today face much different circumstances. They are often hospitalized for 2 to 3 weeks at a time and are then followed up in community mental health clinics. By growing up around "normal" adolescents and young adults, they have different expectations—to be rid of their symptoms and lead a normal life. It is difficult to convince a young adult who sees an entire life stretching ahead that life will probably be a journey with chronic illness and that some sort of medication or at least monitoring will always be necessary. Because they are living in the community, these young people have access to alcohol and drugs, which they use just as their peers do (Nuechterlein et al., 1992).

Dealing with repeated episodes of schizophrenia and surviving the impact of the illness is a difficult struggle. Much energy is spent coping with the illness, severely reducing opportunities to accomplish normal developmental tasks that young adults face, such as finding a partner and raising a family. Some patients, even those with prolonged and episodic illnesses, however, do experience some recovery and may lead far richer, less chaotic, and more complex lives than was once imagined they could.

> **W***hat do you think?* What would be the most difficult struggle for a young person diagnosed with schizophrenia?

> ➤ *Check Your Reading*
> 17. What is the usual age of onset for schizophrenia?
> 18. How is life today different for the young person with schizophrenia than it was years ago?
> 19. Cite two factors that predict a good outcome for an individual diagnosed with schizophrenia.

First-Time Symptoms in the Elderly

It is estimated that around 10% of patients who are first admissions to a psychiatric hospital after age 60 exhibit symptoms of schizophrenia or are diagnosed with late-onset schizophrenia. The typical patient in this age group has a mixture of paranoid delusions and auditory hallucinations. Intellect and personality typically appear intact, in contrast with symptoms in young adults. Most studies indicate that women are more prone than men to develop late-onset schizophrenia (Castle & Murray, 1993). Several studies have indicated that patients with late-onset schizophrenia have a family history of psychoses rather than mood disorders. Grossberg (1997) noted the other 90% of patients past age 60 are those who experienced early-onset schizophrenia and now are entering their senior years.

A number of researchers have argued that sensory impairment, specifically deafness, may be a general risk factor for the development of hallucinations and delusions in later life. Deafness of many years' duration often precedes the development of symptoms of schizophrenia. Visual impairment has also been implicated by several authors as a risk factor. The mechanism by which sensory deficit leads to these symptoms is poorly understood but may be the "final straw" for a socially isolated and predisposed individual (Prager & Jeste, 1993).

The biochemistry of the mechanisms underlying late-onset schizophrenia might be a reversal of normal aging processes (i.e., increased dopamine). This process may produce an increased vulnerability to environmental stressors and sensory deficits that sometimes accompanies aging (Caligiuri, Lohr, Panton, & Braff, 1993; McDowd, Filion, Harris, & Braff, 1993).

Determining whether a person has schizophrenia rather than a dementing illness such as Alzheimer's disease, in which persecutory delusions also occur, is difficult. In fact, there are many causes for the development of hallucinations and delusions in the elderly population. Remember that schizophrenia is a possibility in the elderly. Hallucinations and delusions that occur in the elderly person reportedly have responded well to small doses of the newer atypical antipsychotic medications (e.g., risperidone) (Grossberg, 1997).

➤ *Check Your Reading*
20. What is the role of sensory deficits in developing late-onset schizophrenia?
21. Cite one diagnosis that occurs in the elderly that makes differential diagnosis for schizophrenia difficult.

THE TURBULENT JOURNEY FOR PATIENTS AND FAMILIES

Sylvia Geist called coping with schizophrenia, "a voyage through turbulence" (cited in Malloy, 1998, p. 495). This turbulence has been described by many patients and family members in a variety of references (Backlar, 1994; Bayley, 1996; Flynn, 1994; Malloy, 1998; Secunda, 1997; Simon, 1997; Willick, 1994; Wyden, 1998).

Many individuals with schizophrenia become chronic victims of the illness generally for their lifetime. The most disturbed of these individuals are tortured by voices and other personal "demons." Torrey (1995, pp. 131–134) reported a possible outcome of a 10-year disease course as

1. Twenty-five percent recover completely.
2. Twenty-five percent are much improved.
3. Twenty-five percent are modestly improved.
4. Fifteen percent remain unimproved.
5. Ten percent die. Most of these deaths are the result of suicide or accidents.

The stress of caring for these disturbed family members may strain a marriage, interfere with social life, and drain the family's resources. The cost of suffering to families cannot be estimated because the chronically ill person requires a lifetime commitment for care (Howard, 1994; Winter, 1990). Peter Wyden commented that mounting bills left him broke when insurance coverage ran out (Wyden, 1998). E. Fuller Torrey estimated that the costs for his sister's care for more than 35 years totaled over 1.5 million (Torrey, 1995).

The financial burden to both families and society is enormous, but the greater cost can never be approximated in economic terms. Torrey (1995) described these noneconomic costs as including

the effects of growing up normally until early adulthood, then being diagnosed with a brain disease that may last for the rest of your life. Hopes, plans, expectations, and dreams are abruptly put on hold. . . . There is no known

disease, . . . with non-economic costs so great as for schizophrenia. It is the costliest disease of all. (p. 18)

Arieti (1979), in discussing the impact of schizophrenia, concluded,

No war in history has produced so many victims, wounded so many people. No earthquake has exacted so high a toll; no other condition, that we know of has deprived so many young people of the promise of life. (p. 6)

All of us have experienced some glimpse of the agonies of families as well as the suffering of others involved in the tragic stories of John Hinkley, Ted Kaczynski, Michael Laudor, and Russell Weston. Following the shootings by Russell Weston, in the United States Capitol during spring 1998, Rosenfeld (1998), a journalist, reported stories of families affected and observed "having a mentally ill child or sibling changes your life forever" (p. B1). Writing from a parent's perspective, Dr. Martin S. Willick (1994) identified the experiencing of a son's illness as "mourning without end" (p. 5). Patricia Backlar (1994), a parent, described her own story as well as others and the multiple emotions and traumas experienced by them. Victoria Secunda (1997) also described her own story as a sibling of a mentally ill sister, as well as the story of 75 siblings and children, 12 parents, 15 spouses or partners, and 15 mental health consumers. Secunda described the life of a child of a mentally ill parent as a series of goodbyes and described the sibling's illness as "a kind of living death" (p. 82).

Clea Simon (1997) shared how alone she felt as a sibling of a brother and then a sister who became ill with schizophrenia. She asserted the commonality of aloneness in the many persons referred to in her story who also had a sibling ill because of schizophrenia. Robert Bayley (1996) described the illness's effect on his life as "constant pain and torment" (p. 727). He further recounted the misery he contends with from the voices and visions he experiences as well as the fatigue and isolation caused by the illness.

Dr. Nancy Andreasen (1984) knows schizophrenia firsthand as a clinician-researcher and has given a profound forecast on the potential of the future:

The psychiatrist who either discovers a definitive treatment for schizophrenia or identifies the major factors causing it will perhaps make the most important medical contribution of the twentieth century. When that happens, the impact on the lives of its victims and their relatives will be as great as when insulin was synthesized and used as a treatment for diabetes. (p. 53)

What do you think? What could you do to assist a family to cope with the news that their loved one has schizophrenia?

➤ *Check Your Reading*
22. What is the economic burden on family members of the illness of schizophrenia?
23. Describe the noneconomic burden on family members of schizophrenia?

CO-OCCURRENCE OF THOUGHT DISORDERS WITH OTHER DISORDERS

Becker's (1988) review of the literature led him to the following conclusions:

Depression is a frequent, not well understood complication of schizophrenia that may be associated with poor outcome features, including poor psychosocial functioning, relapse, and increased risk of suicide. (p. 1274)

Kane and Marder (1993) observed the "most common syndrome comorbid with schizophrenia is probably depression" (p. 121). They also noted the occurrence of depressive symptoms when patients were experiencing a worsening of their symptoms or when psychotic symptoms had become stabilized.

Black and Andreasen (1994) reported the occurrence of depressive symptoms in approximately 60% of patients with schizophrenia. Torrey (1995) emphasized that depression was the largest single contributor to the excess rate of death as a result of suicide among people suffering from schizophrenia. Estimates are that between 10% and 13% of people with schizophrenia die from suicide (Torrey, 1995). When suicide occurs it is generally during the first 10 years of the illness. Those at highest risk are men; persons with a remitting and relapsing course of illness; those who have a poor response to medications; those who are hopeless about the future; and persons whose current level of function is considerably lower than their earlier achievements in life. Persons who recognize the severity of their illness (have good insight) are also considered at high risk for suicide (Torrey, 1995).

Many individuals with schizophrenia have symptoms of coexisting medical conditions that are not reported by them or recognized by health care professionals. Jeste, Gladsjo, Lindamer, and Lacro (1996) have noted studies citing the underrecognition and underdiagnosis of medical comorbidity among psychiatric patients, especially those with schizophrenia. They further suggested patients with schizophrenia have a deficit in sensitivity to pain and this "combined with poor insight, may result in a lower rate of schizophrenia patients reporting physical problems to their physicians" (pp. 413–414). Dworkin (1994) reviewed the literature regarding pain insensitivity and concluded this situation is detrimental not only to the health of the patient with schizophrenia but could also be life-threatening. It is suggested that as many as 50% of coexisting medical conditions are not recognized and not diagnosed or treated. This has serious implications when the coexisting physical illness may exacerbate the symptoms of the psychiatric illness.

Substance abuse has been identified increasingly as a source of vulnerability and cause for relapse in patients with schizophrenia. Between 20% and 25% of psychiatric patients admitted with a diagnosis of schizophrenia report recent substance abuse (Norris & Naegle, 1990), and higher proportions of substance abuse can be uncovered if patients are laboratory tested. These patients are referred to as the dually diagnosed.

Use of illicit substances does not produce the mental illness of schizophrenia, as defined by DSM-IV criteria, although hallucinations, delusions, and paranoia can be a side effect of alcohol and cocaine abuse. Drug abuse of phencyclidine can trigger a drug-induced psychosis, indistinguishable in many ways from schizophrenia. Treating persons with schizophrenia and substance abuse problems requires an approach different from treating patients with strictly substance abuse problems. Substance abuse treatment programs, with their heavy emphasis on vigorous and dramatic confrontation, may produce too much anxiety for the individual recovering from schizophrenia. Most treatment centers do not usually wish to be burdened by the special needs of this population.

Patients with a primary diagnosis of substance abuse need to experience directly the devastation they are bringing on themselves so they can counteract the addiction. The interactions in these programs through peer group confrontation lead to extremely high levels of expressed emotion. One of the most significant findings in psychosocial investigations of the course of schizophrenia is that an environment with high expressed emotion (i.e., an environment rated high for criticism, intrusiveness, and hostility) is strongly associated with psychotic relapse (Koenigsberg & Handley, 1986).

> **What do you think?** Does the information on the impact of an environment with high expressed emotion suggest what a therapeutic milieu would be like?

➤ *Check Your Reading*

24. What is the most common syndrome occurring comorbidly with schizophrenia?
25. What is the frequency of unrecognized physical problems and the implications of not recognizing them when an individual has schizophrenia?
26. What is the impact of the use of illicit substances on the course of schizophrenia?
27. What can be the impact of traditional confrontational drug treatment programs on the patient who is dually diagnosed with both substance abuse and schizophrenia?

IMPLICATIONS OF THOUGHT DISORDERS

Among the many homeless people evident on the streets of our cities today are those with schizophrenia. These people who suffer the devastation of schizophrenia without treatment reflect some of the tragedy associated with schizophrenia. Torrey referred to this kind of situation as "a living hell" (1997, p. 19). Among this population there is a marked increase in death compared with the general population. Torrey also observed that public shelters are the only home many former state hospital patients, now in their 60s or 70s, have if they are not living on the street.

Although people with schizophrenia are generally considered harmless and not apt to harm others, there is an increase in violence attributed to mentally ill individuals, particularly those who are not taking medication. As a consequence of acts of violence, many of these ill persons are now among the imprisoned population rather than in a treatment setting in which proper diagnosis and appropriate medications could be prescribed. Homelessness, imprisonment, and other less than satisfactory living arrangements for the mentally ill have been attributed to the process of deinstitutionalization. Another phenomenon referred to as reinstitutionalization has subsequently occurred as jails, nursing homes, shelters, and the streets of our cities have replaced state-supported hospitals, in which so many patients formerly were found.

Violence toward family members is also being reported, although exact figures are not certain. Because many individuals are now living with parents or other family members, assaultive or violent behavior toward other family members (on the part of the mentally ill family member) can contribute to a frightening experience for all involved.

Still other people, although treated, remain chronically ill and disabled. They experience the associated wasting of productivity that they might have enjoyed if illness had not afflicted them. Recent evidence has suggested that delays in diagnosis and treatment contribute to irreversible damage to brain function (McGlashan & Johannessen, 1996).

Patients with schizophrenia often do not believe they are ill, thereby complicating their adherence to treatment. Cuesta and Peralta (1994) suggested lack of insight was a prominent symptom in schizophrenia and resulted from the illness itself. Fenton, Blyler, and Heinssen (1997) reported that symptom severity and lack of insight contributed to patients' nonadherence to their prescribed medications. It has also been recognized that the distress caused by the various side effects contributes to patient discontinuance of medication. Extrapyramidal symptoms (EPS) and weight gain, for example, can be influential in the process of ceasing to continue medications. In other instances, patients may feel better and see no need for continuing medication (Weiden, Raphin, Mott, & Frances, 1994).

The life expectancy of people with schizophrenia is shorter than that of the general population because of an increased suicide rate and death as a result of accidents and a variety of other causes. In the 1950s, when most patients were kept indefinitely on locked or unlocked hospital wards, suicide was not a significant problem.

The 5-year Schizophrenic Patient Outcomes Research Team (PORT) study, funded by the National Institute of Mental Health and the Agency for Health Care Policy and Research, sought to identify effective and appropriate treatment and determine the frequency with which these treatments were being used. The findings from the study exposed the inadequacy of prescribing treatments (e.g., pharmacotherapy, psychological treatment, family education and support, vocational rehabilitation, and service systems) that have been documented to be effective (Lehman, Steinwachs, & Coinvestigators, 1998).

There are a few reports of complete recovery from schizophrenia. The stories of Mark Vonnegut, Lori Schiller, and Frederick J. Frese, III, are encouraging and inspirational. In an autobiographical article, Frese (1994) described his life with schizophrenia. Dr. Frese is the Director of Psychology at a large state mental institution. In this position, he is involved in the care of many patients with chronic schizophrenia. He described his own 12 steps to recovery from schizophrenia (p. 24):

1. Denial is part of the illness and must be addressed early. Without acceptance that the person has a mental illness, there can be no healing.

2. Education about the illness is vitally important.

3. Medications are usually necessary to stabilize the biochemical imbalance in the brain, but street drugs and other chemicals serve only to destabilize a person with schizophrenia.

4. Delusional thinking can be seductive. Each individual needs to identify how delusions are patterned.

5. Circumstantiality, or the tendency to stray from a train of thought, is common. Patients need to teach themselves to stay on target in conversations.

6. Rehearsing in the form of talking to oneself is a common pattern. Patients need to learn to limit this activity to private times.

7. Immediate memory and decision-making abilities are often impaired. The person with schizophrenia needs to remember these limitations and be cautious when making decisions. Also important are developing coping strategies to augment problems with memory and letting others know that information processing occurs slowly.

8. Because the facial expressions of the person with schizophrenia tend to be delayed in responding to conversations with others, the other person may be uneasy. In close relationships, it is important for the person with schizophrenia to discuss this response pattern.

9. Stress-relieving hobbies such as playing, listening, or dancing to music; gardening; exercising; shopping; and reading are all essential to staying well.

10. Problems of stigma, discrimination, and ostracism are serious problems that need to be addressed carefully and systematically.

11. Making the decision to tell others about the schizophrenia is difficult. Explaining lost time spent in a hospital for crisis-oriented stabilization requires tremendous creativity.

12. Because loneliness is a serious problem for persons suffering with schizophrenia or other psychoses, networking with others who have similar problems is important. Organizations like the Alliance for the Mentally Ill and the National Mental Health Consumers' Association are wonderful resources.

What do you think? What personal qualities do you think are required to live fully with a chronic disease such as schizophrenia?

➤ *Check Your Reading*
28. What subgroup among persons with schizophrenia is at greatest risk for suicide?
29. Identify at least five of Frese's suggestions to individuals with schizophrenia for staying well.

DSM-IV DIAGNOSIS AND THE JOURNEY CURTAILED BY SCHIZOPHRENIA

Hall, Andrews, and Goldstein said that "schizophrenia is to psychiatry what cancer is to medicine: a sentence as well as a diagnosis" (cited in Torrey, 1995, p. 1).

Defining Thought Disorders

The APA (1994) has identified schizophrenia as a chronic disease that can be viewed from the perspective of three phases: (1) The acute phase occurs when the patient experiences psychotic symptoms. A prodromal phase is present prior to the acute phase. (2) The stabilization phase is associated with a decreasing severity of the symptoms. (3) The residual phase is present when the patient is without symptoms or the symptoms are experienced with less intensity.

Schizophrenia is a chronic disease that can be viewed from the perspective of four phases: (1) the prodromal phase occurs before the active phase; (2) the active phase occurs when the patient experiences psychotic symptoms; (3) the stabilization phase occurs when the

patient is in treatment but is still experiencing psychotic symptoms; and (4) the residual phase occurs after treatment when the patient is either without symptoms or the symptoms are experienced with much less intensity.

The DSM-IV identified five subcategories of schizophrenia, which include catatonic type, undifferentiated type, disorganized type, residual type, and paranoid type (APA, 1994). The characteristics of each of these types are described in Table 24–2.

Diagnostic Symptoms and Course of Illness

A diagnosis of schizophrenia requires that continuous signs of the illness have been present for at least 6 months. This period always includes an active phase with psychotic symptoms (e.g., hallucinations, delusions, formal thought disorder). The development of the active phase of schizophrenia is usually preceded by a prodromal phase that is marked by clear deterioration from the previous level of functioning. Prodromal symptoms include social withdrawal, poor hygiene, blunted affect, perceptual changes, and changes in usual interests and energy. The prodromal phase is extremely variable in length, and prognosis is especially poor when the person has had a slow downhill course for many years (APA, 1994).

During the active phase, psychotic symptoms are prominent. Such symptoms might include hallucinations, delusions, and formal thought disorder and must persist

TYPE OF SCHIZOPHRENIA	**CHARACTERISTICS**
Catatonic	Catatonic stupor (marked decrease in reactivity to the environment and/or reduction in spontaneous movements and activity) or mutism
	Catatonic negativism (an apparently motiveless resistance to all instructions or attempts to be moved)
	Catatonic rigidity (maintenance of a rigid posture against efforts to be moved)
	Catatonic excitement (excited motor activity, apparently purposeless and not influenced by external stimuli)
	Catatonic posturing (voluntary assumption of inappropriate or bizarre posture)
Undifferentiated	Prominent delusions
	Hallucinations
	Incoherence, or grossly disorganized behavior
	Lack of criteria for paranoid, catatonic, or disorganized type of disorder
Disorganized	Incoherence
	Marked loosening of associations, or grossly disorganized behavior
	Flat or grossly inappropriate affect
	Lack of criteria for catatonic type of disorder
Residual	Absence of prominent delusions, hallucinations, incoherence, or grossly disorganized behavior
	Continuing evidence of the disturbance, as indicated by two or more of the residual symptoms as listed in Table 24–3
Paranoid	Preoccupation with one or more systematized delusions or with frequent auditory hallucinations related to a single theme
	None of the following: Incoherence, marked loosening of associations, catatonic or grossly disorganized behavior

TABLE 24–2 Characteristics of Schizophrenia

Data from American Psychiatric Association. (1994). *Diagnostic and statistical manual of mental disorders. Fourth Edition.* Washington, DC: American Psychiatric Association.

for at least 1 week, unless they are successfully treated. The treatment phase is referred to as the stabilization phase. A residual phase usually follows stabilization of the illness. It is similar to the prodromal phase except that affective blunting and problems in role functioning are more prominent. The person may still experience hallucinations and delusions but is not so disturbed by them.

The person may return to his or her preillness level of functioning. The most common course is one of active illness episodes with some residual impairment between episodes. During the initial years of the disorder, the residual impairment often increases.

Under the diagnostic criteria of the DSM-IV, a diagnosis of Schizophrenia is made when strict criteria are fulfilled. These include the stipulation that the person must have exhibited symptoms for at least 6 months. In the past, failure to consider the 6-month duration of symptoms probably led to overdiagnosing of schizophrenia in the United States.

The DSM-IV described the essential features of schizophrenia as the presence of characteristic psychotic symptoms during the active phase of the illness with functioning below the highest level previously achieved lasting at least 6 months. The illness may include characteristic prodromal or residual symptoms (APA, 1994). At some phase, the illness always involves delusions, hallucinations, or certain characteristic disturbances, both in affect and in form of thought. An organic factor must not be responsible for the disorder, and these symptoms must not be due to a Mood Disorder or Schizoaffective Disorder. Schizoaffective Disorder is defined as one period of illness with symptoms of major depression or mania along with the symptoms of schizophrenia, including for some time delusions or hallucinations (APA, 1994). Table 24–3 describes differences in the course of schizophrenia.

Research has shown considerable differences in the long-term course of schizophrenia. The variations in course may be related to the different types of schizophrenia. In the period preceding the onset of frank psychosis, patients vary as to rapidity of onset, social withdrawal, and the presence or absence of perceptual changes. The active phase of hallucinations may be episodic or continuous and may or may not include negative symptoms. In late adult life, patients vary in the presence or absence of an improvement in psychosis and social capability (Carpenter & Kirkpatrick, 1988). Between episodes of illness, the extent of disability may range from none to disability so severe that institutional care is required.

➤ *Check Your Reading*
  30. How does the DSM-IV address the course of schizophrenia?
  31. How many types of schizophrenia does the DSM-IV identify?

Variations of Thought Disorders

Other variations of thought disorder that have been identified are Schizoaffective Disorder, Schizophreni-

form Disorder, and Delusional (Paranoid) Disorder. Schizoaffective Disorder is an illness that has symptoms with features of both schizophrenia and the mood disorders. Schizophreniform Disorder is an illness with a shorter onset and a shorter course. This diagnosis requires that both positive and negative symptoms be present for at least 1 month but less than 6 months. The current use of this diagnostic category is a protection for the premature diagnosis of schizophrenia (Andreasen & Black, 1995; Black & Andreasen, 1994).

Delusional (Paranoid) Disorder is manifested primarily through impaired thought processes in which the central focus is on distorted perceptions or paranoid (suspicious) thinking and behavior. The personality of the patient is basically intact, but nonbizarre delusions that are well systematized are present. The person's affect is congruent with the delusional thoughts he or she believes (Andreasen & Black, 1995; Black & Andreasen, 1994).

Personality disorders related to schizophrenia are the Schizotypal Personality Disorder and Paranoid Personality Disorder. **Schizotypal Personality Disorder** is a lifelong pattern of social detachment and inability to form relationships as well as cognitive or perceptual distortions and eccentricities in behavior (APA, 1994; Kety, 1985). The salient feature of **Paranoid Personality Disorder** is a lifelong suspiciousness of others that is

TABLE 24–3 Differences in the Course of Schizophrenia	
TYPE	**DESCRIPTION**
Subchronic	The time from the beginning of the illness, when the person first began to show signs of the disturbance (including prodromal, active, and residual phases) more or less continuously, is less than 2 years but at least 6 months.
Chronic	Same as above but more than 2 years.
Subchronic with acute exacerbation	Reemergence of prominent psychotic symptoms in a person with a subchronic course who has been in the residual phase of the disturbance
Chronic with acute exacerbation	Reemergence of prominent psychotic symptoms in a person with a chronic course who has been in the residual phase of the disturbance
In remission	The person is free of all signs of schizophrenia. Differentiating schizophrenia in remission from no mental disorder requires consideration of overall level of functioning, length of time since the last episode, total duration of the disturbance, and whether prophylactic medication is being given.
Unspecified	

unrelated to a full-blown schizophrenic disorder (APA, 1994).

Recognition of schizophrenia as a disease entity continues to be the subject of much confusion and debate. With considerable overlap among symptoms of different mental disorders, schizophrenia is probably more than one disease entity, with different types, subgroups, and brain dysfunctions. Psychotic symptoms also do not always indicate schizophrenia. Metabolic abnormalities as well as other neurological diseases can cause symptoms. For example, a person experiencing the sensation of bugs crawling over the skin could be suffering from a psychosis caused by alcohol withdrawal or even exposure to some toxic drug or chemical. People suffering from an acute episode of schizophrenic illness could also experience some of the same symptoms as a person experiencing drug withdrawal, usually accompanied by other symptoms, such as hearing voices.

Symptomatic definitions of mental states or disorders are imprecise, yet an accurate diagnosis is of utmost importance. The diagnosis determines the type of treatment. For instance, if the symptoms are a result of schizophrenia, antipsychotic medication is prescribed; if the symptoms result from drug withdrawal, benzodiazepines are the medication of choice.

➤ *Check Your Reading*

32. Why is it difficult to diagnose schizophrenia on the basis of psychotic symptoms alone?
33. Why is it important to differentiate schizophrenia from another disorder that might produce similar psychotic symptoms?

THE CAUSE OF SCHIZOPHRENIA

With the explosion of research in the neurosciences, knowledge about the cause of schizophrenia is continuing to expand (Carpenter, 1987). Yet scientists still do not know precisely what causes the diverse symptoms of schizophrenia; however, research results suggest a multifactorial etiology. It has long been debated whether schizophrenia is a neurodevelopmental or neuropathological disorder. The preponderance of research evidence suggests the hypothesis that schizophrenia is a neurodevelopmental brain disorder (Carpenter & Buchanan, 1995). Some established facts are shown in Box 24-5.

Although schizophrenia was once classified as a functional disorder (one with psychological origins), evidence supports the position that the brains of persons who have schizophrenia are different from those of persons who do not have this disease. The differences can be measured by gross pathology, by microscopic pathology, by neurochemistry, by cerebral blood flow and metabolism, electrically, neurologically, and neuropsychologically (Torrey, 1995).

➤ *Check Your Reading*

34. Describe the established facts of schizophrenia.
35. Why is schizophrenia no longer considered a functional disorder?

Box 24-5 ■ ■ ■ ■ ■
Established Facts About Schizophrenia

Schizophrenia is a <u>brain disease</u>. The brain does not appear to be functioning normally, but abnormalities in structure are debatable. Brain chemicals appear to be functioning abnormally.

The limbic system and its connections are primarily affected. Schizophrenia often runs in families. In the past, various types of family influences were proposed, such as deprivation or abnormalities in early mother-child relationships, but well-controlled studies have failed to identify any particular environmental factors. Stress does seem to have something to do with aggravating the illness in vulnerable individuals.

The brain damage may occur early in life. Factors such as inheritance, development before birth, and early trauma are thought to play a part in predisposing a person to schizophrenia.

Data from Torrey, E. F. (1995). *Surviving schizophrenia: A manual for families, consumers, and providers* (3rd ed.). New York: HarperCollins.

Genetic, Neuroimmunovirology, Birth and Pregnancy Complications

Hypotheses regarding the causation of schizophrenia include genetic, neuroimmunovirology, birth and pregnancy complications, neuroanatomical, and biochemical theories.

Genetic

There is general agreement by researchers that genetic predisposition plays a significant etiologic role in the development of schizophrenia (Kendler & Diehl, 1995). Schizophrenia occurs at an increased rate in first-degree relatives of patients with schizophrenia. These first-degree relatives have a 3% to 7% risk for developing schizophrenia. This increased risk is most evident in the study of twins with the monozygotic (identical) twin having a 40% to 50% rate for developing the disorder as compared with the 15% rate for the dizygotic (fraternal) twin (Jones & Cannon, 1998). Adoption studies have also supported the genetic relationship to schizophrenia, by establishing an increased risk in the absence of any contact with the biological relatives. Although these findings from family, twin, and adoptive studies suggest genetic factors rather than familial environment, we still do not know how the genetic transmission of schizophrenia takes place (Crow, 1993).

Infection

Researchers have long been interested in infection and the immune response as possible causative factors in schizophrenia. The advances in virology and immunology have enhanced the ability to test this hypothesis. This theory postulates that schizophrenia is caused by an infection (a virus) or by an autoimmune reaction against the central nervous system (CNS) tissue. This was supported by indirect evidence of possible geographical variance in the prevalence of the disorder, the season in which the birth occurred, and associations between the disorder and prenatal exposure to viral epidemics. There is no research evidence that irrefutably supports either the infectious or autoimmune theories as predominant etiological factors in schizophrenia. There are studies being conducted that are looking at the interactions between exposure to an infection or an autoimmune response in the early phases of brain development, specifically, the association between second-trimester influenza infections in mothers of schizophrenia patients (Jones & Cannon, 1998).

What do you think? A mother of a patient with schizophrenia tells you she feels guilty. She feels that she must have done something to cause this disease in her child. How would you respond to her?

➤ *Check Your Reading*

36. What do genetics suggest to us about schizophrenia?
37. What is the viral theory?

Birth or Pregnancy Complications

Individuals born to mothers who had pregnancy complications or born with a history of birth complications have a higher risk for developing schizophrenia as an adult. The cause of this increase in risk is not known. One theory is that fetal hypoxia (oxygen supply) may be the mechanism underlying the association between pregnancy and birth complications and the risk for development of the disorder. The oxygen-deprivation theory is interesting because many of the reported complications can be associated with temporary hypoxia. The hippocampus, a component of the limbic system, the cerebral cortex, and the basal ganglia are all brain regions frequently cited as deviant in schizophrenia and are the areas in the developing brain most sensitive to the adverse effects of hypoxia (Carpenter & Buchanan, 1995).

Neuroanatomical Theories

Many years have passed since researchers first demonstrated brain abnormalities on CT scans of individuals with schizophrenia (Gur & Pearlson, 1993). In the mid-1980s researchers shifted to the use of the more refined MRI technology for structural neuroimaging research in schizophrenia. These sophisticated structural brain imaging advances confirm that schizophrenia is a brain disease (Buckley, 1998b). Multiple research studies have consistently reported abnormalities of cerebral function and structure in all regions of the brain, specifically:

1. Enlargement of the lateral and third ventricles
2. Atrophy in the frontal lobe, cerebellum, and limbic structures
3. Increased size of sulci (fissures) on the surface of the brain
4. Decreased brain volume
5. Abnormalities in brain asymmetry

It is critical to consider two major factors in interpreting reported biological differences in schizophrenia:

1. The significance of the biological abnormality. A biological abnormality is, at most, a correlation and should not be assumed to be a causal factor.
2. Whether the abnormality is related to the disease process itself or to treatment, especially antipsychotic medication. This determination is often difficult.

In the studies reported, the brain changes are apparently not due to medication and are not limited to schizophrenia. They are also evident in patients with manic-depressive illness and other brain diseases (Andreasen et al., 1986; Breier et al., 1992; Pettegrew, Keshaven, & Minshaw, 1993; Utas & Cotman, 1993; Wolkin et al., 1992).

Suddath, Christison, Torrey, Casanova, and Weinberger (1990) studied brain structure in twins, one of whom had schizophrenia and one of whom did not. They found evidence of anatomical changes in the brains of twins with schizophrenia. The fact that the twins could be differentiated on the basis of structural differences probably meant that the cause of the underlying neuropathological process was not completely genetic.

➤ *Check Your Reading*

38. What have MRI and CT scans demonstrated about the brains of persons with schizophrenia?
39. What have twin studies demonstrated?
40. What are the two major cautions when interpreting brain studies?

The Limbic System

Another neuroanatomical theory is based on the knowledge of dopamine pathways in the brain and of brain behavior relations. This model is based on the premise that the brain is organized in neural circuits and that a structural or functional lesion somewhere in the circuit disrupts the entire circuit (Carpenter & Buchanan, 1995). Abnormalities in the limbic system in animals produce profound changes in emotion, inappropriate behavior, and an impairment in the animal's ability to screen out multiple visual stimuli. In humans, diseases of the limbic system are likely to produce schizophrenic-like symptoms. Many researchers have debated the location of the primary brain lesion that affects the development of schizophrenia. Many believe the site may be the limbic system (Torrey, 1995).

The identification of a lesion in one area of the brain, however, does not mean that the primary area of pathology has been defined. For example, identification of the limbic system as the site of pathology does not exclude that pathology could be caused by some type of hyperactive input from another region of the brain.

Also, a single pathological process in the brain can cause a wide range of phenomena in different patients, and a single specific abnormality in the brain can have many different causes. Parkinson's disease, for example, can have idiopathic, infectious, traumatic, or toxic causes (Kaplan & Sadock, 1995). The neuroanatomical theories attempt to account for the possible anatomical reason for the disturbed behaviors seen in people with the diagnosis of schizophrenia.

> ➤ *Check Your Reading*
> 41. Why is the limbic system important in understanding the symptoms of schizophrenia?
> 42. Why are researchers cautious about concluding that the limbic system is the primary site causing the disorder of schizophrenia?

Biochemical Theories

DOPAMINE THEORY

One of the most extensively studied theories related to the underlying biochemical basis of schizophrenia is that of the brain's use of dopamine. Dopamine is one of the brain's neurotransmitters that assists in the transmission of information between nerve cells. The drugs that reduce schizophrenic symptoms have been studied to determine their dopamine activity. The dopamine hypothesis of schizophrenia purports the illness may be related to overactive neuronal activity. There appears to be excessive dopamine levels in people with schizophrenia.

Pharmacological research demonstrates that drugs, such as amphetamines, that increase dopamine activity worsen schizophrenic symptoms, and drugs that decrease dopamine activity alleviate symptoms. Neuroleptic medications, such as the phenothiazines and the butyrophenones (e.g., haloperidol), have been extensively studied. Although these two classes of drugs are chemically quite different, they both block dopamine receptors and decrease schizophrenic symptoms. Speculation suggests that neuroleptic drugs act at the nerve synapse by binding dopamine receptor sites. The cause of excessive dopamine activity in people with schizophrenia is not known, and it is impossible to conclude that schizophrenia is caused by excessive dopamine. Symptoms could come from increased numbers of or activity of receptors.

More recent research studies suggest that there may also be a dopamine deficiency in patients with schizophrenia (Carpenter & Buchanan, 1995). This may call for a modification of the dopamine theory to incorporate the possibility of both dopamine excess and deficiency.

> ➤ *Check Your Reading*
> 43. What is the theoretical significance of dopamine to schizophrenia?

SEROTONIN THEORY

A serotonin deficiency in schizophrenia was proposed in the 1950s. This came about from the studies of the hallucinogen, lysergic acid diethylamide (LSD), which is chemically similar to serotonin and occupies serotonin receptor sites. Recently, the interest is on hypotheses that suggest a serotonin excess as causative of schizophrenia. Support for this theory is derived from the knowledge of brain behavior relations, the anatomy of neural transmitter systems, and drug mechanisms of action (Carpenter & Buchanan, 1995). There is speculation that even if serotonin does not play a major role in the neurochemistry of schizophrenia, serotoninergic agents may play a significant role in the treatment of psychosis (Wyatt, Kirch, & Egan, 1995).

Risk Factors for Schizophrenia

Karno and Norquist (1995) defined a risk factor as "an inherent or acquired characteristic or an external condition associated with an increased probability of developing schizophrenia" (p. 907). There are currently a number of epidemiological studies on schizophrenia that seek to determine the most important risk factors for this disorder. Risk factors can be described as demographic, such as age, sex, race, and social class. Precipitating factors are described as life events and migration. Predisposing factors are genes, perinatal complications, and infections. Risk for developing this disorder is increased if the person (APA, 1997, p. 6):

1. Is single
2. Is from an industrialized nation
3. Lives in a lower socioeconomic class
4. Is living in an urban center
5. Is a product of a difficult labor and delivery
6. Was born during the winter or recently experienced some stressful life event

Ethnicity and Racial, Age, and Sex Risk Factors

The research findings concerning differences in the prevalence and number of new cases in various ethnic and racial groups are not consistent. The mean age of onset for schizophrenia is below 45 years of age for both men and women. Late onset is not as uncommon as was once thought. This may be due to a failure to diagnose the disorder in the elderly because it has a different presentation. The lifetime risk is equal for males and females, with males having a younger age of onset and also a poorer outcome than females. Schizophrenia in males seems to have a more chronic and disabling course (Karno & Norquist, 1995).

Season and Birth Order Risk Factors

Individuals who develop schizophrenia show a slightly higher rate of being born in the winter and spring months above that which is found in the general population. Proposed explanations for this seasonal effect have been offered, which include environmental factors, a genetic factor, as well as more frequent sexual activity of parents of patients with schizophrenia. More research is needed on the seasonal hypothesis. Some early studies on the birth order of siblings have reported schizophrenia in the youngest children of large families and in first-born sons of small families. The value of these studies is still being debated, as results have not been consistent and as family size can affect the findings (Karno & Norquist, 1995).

> ➤ *Check Your Reading*
> 44. In what ways are people with schizophrenia exposed to a seasonal factor different from other people without schizophrenia?

Social Class Risk Factors

A number of studies have reported that schizophrenia is higher among members of lower social classes than upper social classes. Social causation is one explanation proposed, and social selection or drift theory is the other. Social causation factors are those that include more life event stressors, increased exposure to environmental and occupational hazards and infectious agents, poorer prenatal care, and fewer social supports if stressful events do occur. Social drift theory includes less upward mobility and a downward drift after the onset of symptoms. The disagreement over which explanation is the major factor continues, but recent research suggests that social drift processes are more important than social causation (Karno & Narquist, 1995).

Marital Status as a Risk Factor

Unmarried patients have shown higher rates of schizophrenia than married patients, which have led some to infer that single status contributes to the development of the disorder. Studies have not shown conclusively that marriage protects one against schizophrenia.

Urbanization and Industrialization as Risk Factors

Schizophrenia is reported to be higher in urban environments than in rural areas. Research data from the National Institute of Mental Health's (NIMH) Epidemiological Catchment Area (ECA) (1978 to 1984) study showed no difference in prevalence between urban and rural areas.

The Stress-Vulnerability Model

The stress-vulnerability model of schizophrenia identifies **biological,** environmental, and **personal vulnerabilities** that contribute to relapse or to minimizing symptoms of schizophrenia. The model also attempts initially to identify people who may be more vulnerable to developing the disorder. Earlier perspectives viewed schizophrenia as a chronic disorder attributable to a particular biological or environmental cause. This model emphasizes a permanent vulnerability to schizophrenia. Although some vulnerable individuals may never experience a psychotic episode, others have periodic episodes over many years (O'Connor, 1991). The stress-vulnerability model is complex and demands sophisticated research strategies to uncover factors associated with healthy and psychopathological development (Dworkin et al., 1993).

TREATMENT FOR SYMPTOMS OF THOUGHT DISORDER

The APA practice guidelines (1997) suggested conventional **antipsychotic medications** are indicated for almost all psychotic episodes in the acute phase as well as during the other phases. Psychotropic medications play an important part in the treatment of schizophrenia. Drugs do not cure but control symptoms—just as they do the symptoms of diabetes. These drugs are also called neuroleptics or major tranquilizers, but antipsychotic is the most descriptive name because their goal is not to produce tranquilization but to reduce and control psychotic symptoms. Chapter 17 provides an in-depth discussion of the medications used in treating schizophrenia.

The goals of antipsychotic therapy are

- To enable the patient to exert self-control (as contrasted with using the drug to control the patient)
- To relieve specific symptoms of psychosis
- To improve the patient's self-care ability

Until the late 1980s, clinicians reported that negative symptoms—apathy, withdrawal, loss of motivation, lack of social competence, blunted affect—responded poorly to medication (Gournay, 1993; Harris, 1988; Littrall & Magill, 1993; Marder & Meibach, 1994). However, the atypical serotonin-dopamine antagonist antipsychotic medications, for example clozapine and risperidone, have shown to have a favorable effect on negative symptoms (Möller, 1994).

Appropriate adjunctive medications may also be used, such as lithium, carbamazepine, or valproic acid. Antidepressants should be considered when depression is present. A benzodiazepine may be prescribed when panic, anxiety, and agitation are experienced by the patient.

Medications to treat EPS are also used. The antiparkinsonian drugs, or anticholinergics, include benztropine (Cogentin), biperiden (Akineton), and trihexyphenidyl (Artane). Because of the known ability of anticholinergics to block dystonic reactions, they have been used in conjunction with antipsychotic drugs since the antipsychotic drugs were introduced. They are also used to treat tremors and akathisia caused by antipsychotic drugs. The general practice today is to use them prophylactically, even before side effects appear, especially in patients who are younger or male, in whom dystonic symptoms are more common.

When pharmacologic treatments are not effective, ECT may be considered for the persistently psychotic patient. Although this treatment has been less frequently prescribed since the introduction of antipsychotic medication, there are indications for its use in selected instances.

Recommendations in the PORT study address the

above treatments as well as advocating psychosocial treatments such as assertive community treatment, vocational rehabilitation, and family education and support (Lehman & Steinwachs, 1998).

> **W**hat do you think? How would you respond to a patient who expressed concern over taking an antipsychotic medication?

> ➤ *Check Your Reading*
> 45. What are the purposes of antipsychotic treatment?
> 46. What are the antiparkinsonian drugs used to treat?

THE JOURNEY OF THE PERSON WITH SCHIZOPHRENIA AND THE ROLE OF NURSING

Patients with schizophrenia demand the best skills that nurses possess. Because of the difficulties these patients experience with communication and relatedness, nurses are challenged to reach out without being threatening, to be natural and honest while maintaining a professional role. Empathic understanding of the patient's experience is essential. To approach and develop a relationship with a person who may be misinterpreting the environment, the nurse must be sensitive to the psychotic person's difficulties. To employ the therapeutic use of self, the nurse must be aware of the process of a thought disorder while showing respect for the patient as a person. For example, it is helpful to assess the patient's perceptual differences by asking the patient about hallucinations and by observing behaviors that may indicate the patient is either responding or attending to internal stimuli. Next, ask the patient to describe experiences and note the degree to which this description differs from your perception of the environment. Case Example 24–1 describes the perception of reality of a person with schizophrenia.

> ➤ *Check Your Reading*
> 47. Why does the patient with schizophrenia pose a challenge to the psychiatric nurse?
> 48. How do you assess whether or not a person is experiencing hallucinations?

NURSING PROCESS

Nursing care for the person with schizophrenia requires an understanding of the patient's experience. The journey of the person with schizophrenia is marked by specific symptoms, which both diagnose the illness and describe the person's perceptions. Case Example 24–1 is one person's story of schizophrenia and supportive care.

■ **CASE EXAMPLE 24–1**
■ **Bill's Story**

—didnt read—

Bill is a 27-year-old single white man. He was brought into the psychiatric emergency department for evaluation by the police after he was observed standing and pacing near the railing of a bridge, muttering to himself. A bag of torn clothing and papers, a Bible, and half a bottle of haloperidol were found near him and brought to the emergency department. Initially, he was not cooperative with the questioning from the nurse and psychiatrist, and he accused them of trying to take thoughts from his head. The name of his therapist was on the bottle of pills, and he was contacted by phone.

The therapist told the health care personnel that he was concerned because Bill's mother had reported that Bill, concerned about side effects of haloperidol, had stopped taking his medication. Bill had left his mother's home to wander and had not been seen for several days. Bill did accept a dose of his regular medication, and he revealed some time later that he had been hearing voices inside his head telling him to jump from the bridge. He said in a soft voice over and over "I am what I am," and said that he saw the world with "deep eyes" and could feel the pain of others' poverty, hunger, and drug abuse. He felt pain in his body, "the pain of bullets," and expressed a desire to solve the world's problems. He believed he had a special gift, "mind throwing," through which he could control the thoughts of others. His repetition of the phrase "I am what I am" seemed related to his belief that he was the founder of a new religion.

When Bill accepted the haloperidol, he was also given a dose of benztropine (Cogentin) to prevent side effects from this neuroleptic medication. Routine blood tests included electrolytes and serum and urine toxicology tests. Toxicology studies were negative, and serum sodium was slightly elevated but not dangerously so, probably indicating that he had not been drinking enough fluids during the time he had been living on the street. He agreed to voluntary admission to the short-term psychiatric unit to prevent him from harming himself and to restabilize him on medications. ■

Assessment

Assessment of patients with schizophrenia occurs at the individual, family, and environmental levels. You must be aware of changes not only in the patient's physiological, psychological, and perceptual condition, but also in the patient's personal life. Factors to consider include living situation, family support, and stresses. You might assume that changes in any aspect of the patient's life could influence the potential for relapse (Savage, 1991).

Clinical Signs and Symptoms

Three key issues should be considered when assessing the symptoms of the patient with schizophrenia or a thought-disordered patient. The first is that no clinical sign or symptom is seen only in schizophrenia. Every sign or symptom can also be seen in other psychiatric and neurological disorders. To diagnose schizophrenia, a clinician must consider a mental status examination or examination of the person's presenting appearance as well as a history.

The second key issue is that the symptoms of the patient change over time. Symptoms depend on the course of illness and response to somatic therapy. The third issue is educational level. Intellectual ability and cultural background of the patient must be taken into consideration (Kaplan & Sadock, 1995).

Assessing Positive Symptoms

You might ask the patient (see Case Example 24-1) about voices and what he or she is experiencing, but you should expect that patients may not be forthcoming about their internal experiences. If the patient appears distracted, glances up at the ceiling for extended periods, appears to be talking to himself or herself yet denies hearing voices, record these observations. They may be evidence that the patient is hearing voices.

In identifying delusional thinking, the nurse should consider the method she or he uses to collect data. In Case Example 24-1, Bill did not trust the nurse or psychiatrist. This lack of trust interfered with Bill's ability to freely express his internal experiences. Therefore it is best to assess delusions by inquiring about their content while accepting the patient's perceptions: "You say people are following you. Who is following you? Do you have any thoughts about why they are following you?"

Initially, assess the delusional content to understand the patient's concerns. If you continue to focus attention on the delusion, however, you may inadvertently reinforce false beliefs. Be careful neither to argue with the patient over the delusions nor to condone them. Rather, listen to them, validate that you are correctly understanding the patient's perception of reality, and refocus the direction of the interview into reality. You can show understanding of the patient's perception and simultaneously introduce reality. For example, "I can see you are frightened and believe that the FBI is looking for you, but I have no reason to believe the FBI is after you."

Assessing Disorganized Symptoms

Interviewing a patient with a thought disorder is difficult. Keep the interview short. Focus on current issues. Patients think and reason on the basis of their own intricate private rules of reason. Thought processes do not lead to conclusions based on reality or universal logic. Thinking for the person with schizophrenia is said to be concrete, so that he or she may be unable to abstract when given a proverb to interpret. The expression "people in glass houses shouldn't throw stones," for example, might come to mean "people who live in houses made of glass might break windows if they threw stones out of them." The person with schizophrenia also may consider things to be identical merely because they share some properties. For example, "the Virgin Mary was a virgin. I'm a virgin; therefore I'm the Virgin Mary" (Arieti, 1979, p. 65). The patient thus loses the ability to generalize correctly.

Assessing Negative Symptoms

Observe the patient's behavior in respect to motivation, personal hygiene, emotional responsiveness, and ability to experience pleasure. The inability to experience pleasure (anhedonia) and interest in the surroundings, as well as poverty of speech or speech content, makes interactions difficult. Isolation and withdrawal are not uncommon.

Assessing for Safety Concerns

An important assessment area for the person with schizophrenia includes observation for evidence of depression, coexisting medical conditions, and abuse of substances. This includes assessing for the potential of harm to self or others. Suicidality and the possibility of aggressive or assaultive behavior are important factors to assess. The general health status of the patient should be determined and any abnormalities or symptoms of a coexisting medical condition need to be specified. It is also important to learn the patient's history of past and recent substance abuse.

Bill, in Case Example 24-1, is at high risk for suicide. Continual assessment of his suicidal ideation is important. Occasionally, people with schizophrenia commit suicide accidentally while in an acute stage of psychosis; they might, for example, not know they are unable to fly and may jump off a building.

Assessing for Response to Medications

The nurse needs to assess for the patient's responsiveness to medications prescribed in the past and currently. Nurses need to be diligent in observing for evidence of allergic reactions, extrapyramidal symptoms (EPS), abnormal involuntary movements (suggestive of tardive dyskinesia), and neuroleptic malignant syndrome. A medication assessment tool, the Simpson-Angus Rating Scale (for EPS), and the Abnormal Involuntary Movement Scale (AIMS) (assessing for the presence of tardive dyskinesia; see Chapter 17) as well as the nurse's observant eye can help in this assessment. See Box 24-6 for the Simpson-Angus Rating Scale.

Assessing for General Health

General health assessment includes the patient's diet, with the amount and types of fluid intake. The amount of sleep and quality of sleep should also be assessed. The type and frequency of exercise, as well as any types of repetitive activity, should be noted. The smoking habits of the patient including how much he or she smokes, should be determined. The patient's capability to attend to his or her personal hygiene including dental health needs is another significant area of concern.

Assessing Relationships

It is important to assess the social skills of the patient as well as the extent of interpersonal relationships present in his or her life, for example, the people with whom he

B o x 2 4 – 6 ■ ■ ■ ■ ■
Simpson-Angus Rating Scale

1. **Gait:** The patient is examined as he walks into the examining room; his gait, the swing of his arms, his general posture, all form the basis for an overall score for this item. This is rated as follows:
   0 Normal
   1 Diminution in swing while the patient is walking
   2 Marked diminution in swing with obvious rigidity in the arm
   3 Stiff gait with arms held rigidly before the abdomen
   4 Stooped shuffling gait with propulsion and retropulsion

2. **Arm dropping:** The patient and the examiner both raise their arms to shoulder height and let them fall to their sides. In a normal subject a stout slap is heard as the arms hit the sides. In the patient with extreme Parkinson's syndrome the arms fall very slowly.
   0 Normal, free fall with loud slap and rebound
   1 Fall slowed, slightly with less audible contact and little rebound
   2 Fall slowed, no rebound
   3 Marked slowing, no slap at all
   4 Arms fall as though against resistance; as though through glue

3. **Shoulder shaking:** The subject's arms are bent at a right angle at the elbow and are taken one at a time by the examiner who grasps one hand and also clasps the other around the patient's elbow. The subject's upper arm is pushed to and fro and the humerus is externally rotated. The degree of resistance from normal to extreme rigidity is scored as follows:
   0 Normal
   1 Slight stiffness and resistance
   2 Moderate stiffness and resistance
   3 Marked rigidity with difficulty in passive movement
   4 Extreme stiffness and rigidity with almost a frozen shoulder

4. **Elbow rigidity:** The elbow joints are separately bent at right angles and passively extended and flexed, with the subject's biceps observed and simultaneously palpated. The resistance to this procedure is rated. (The presence of cogwheel rigidity is noted separately.) Scoring is from 0 to 4, as in the Shoulder Shaking test.
   0 Normal
   1 Slight stiffness and resistance
   2 Moderate stiffness and resistance
   3 Marked rigidity with difficulty in passive movement
   4 Extreme stiffness and rigidity with almost a frozen shoulder

5. **Fixation of position or wrist rigidity:** The wrist is held in one hand and the fingers held by the examiner's other hand, with the wrist moved to extension flexion and both ulnar and radial deviation. The resistance to this procedure is rated as in Items 3 and 4.
   0 Normal
   1 Slight stiffness and resistance
   2 Moderate stiffness and resistance
   3 Marked rigidity with difficulty in passive movement
   4 Extreme stiffness and rigidity with almost a frozen shoulder

6. **Leg pendulousness:** The patient sits on a table with his legs hanging down and swinging free. The ankle is grasped by the examiner and raised until the knee is partially extended. It is then allowed to fall. The resistance to falling and the lack of swinging form the basis for the score on this item:
   0 The legs swing freely
   1 Slight diminution in the swing of the legs
   2 Moderate resistance to swing
   3 Marked resistance and damping of swing
   4 Complete absence of swing

7. **Head dropping:** The patient lies on a well-padded examining table and his head is raised by the examiner's hand. The hand is then withdrawn and the head allowed to drop. In the normal subject the head will fall upon the table. The movement is delayed in extrapyramidal system disorder, and in extreme Parkinsonism it is absent. The neck muscles are rigid and the head does not reach the examining table. Scoring is as follows:
   0 The head falls completely, with a good thump as it hits the table
   1 Slight slowing in fall, mainly noted by lack of slap as head meets the table
   2 Moderate slowing in the fall, quite noticeable to the eye
   3 Head falls stiffly and slowly
   4 Head does not reach examining table

8. **Glabella tap:** Subject is told to open his eyes wide and not to blink. The glabella region is tapped at a steady, rapid speed. The number of times patient blinks in succession is noted:
   0 0 to 5 blinks
   1 6 to 10 blinks
   2 11 to 15 blinks
   3 16 to 20 blinks
   4 21 or more blinks

Box continued on following page

B o x   2 4 – 6   ■ ■ ■ ■ ■
Simpson-Angus Rating Scale *Continued*

9. **Tremor:** Patient is observed walking into examining room and then is reexamined for this item:
  0 Normal
  1 Mild finger tremor, obvious to sight and touch
  2 Tremor of hand or arm occurring spasmodically
  3 Persistent tremor of one or more limbs
  4 Whole body tremor
10. **Salivation:** Patient is observed while talking and then asked to open his mouth and elevate his tongue. The following ratings are given:

0 Normal
1 Excess salivation to the extent that pooling takes place if the mouth is open and the tongue raised
2 When excess salivation is present and might occasionally result in difficulty in speaking
3 Speaking with difficulty because of excess salivation
4 Frank drooling

From Simpson G. M., Angus, J. W. S. (1970). A rating scale for extrapyramidal side effects. *Acta Psychiatrica Scandinavica Supplementum, 212,* 11-19.

or she interacts. The patient's tendency toward isolation, or extent of isolation behaviors, is also essential data for the nurse.

Assessing Spiritual and Religious Issues

Frequently, persons with schizophrenia experience delusions and hallucinations with religious content, and some health care providers tend to dismiss religious or spiritual verbalizations as psychotic murmurings. This response is unfortunate but may be changing; DSM-IV included religious and spiritual problems under additional conditions that may be a focus of clinical attention (APA, 1994). Studies have shown that individuals with schizophrenia who have a religious foundation and church participation have fewer exacerbations of the illness and spend less time hospitalized. Similar findings have been demonstrated when the caregiver of the person with schizophrenia is religious and views the caretaking role as a ministry and not as a burden (Larson & Larson, 1991; Larson, Milano, & Barry, 1996).

The nurse should ask about religious commitment, religious practices, and spiritual issues, such as the meaning of the illness to the person, the role of God, and sources of hope and support. These may be sources of great comfort to the patient and need to be encouraged, not denied (Carson, 1994; Larson & Larson, 1991). Leon, in Case Example 24-2, in the midst of active delusions of persecution, maintained his lifelong habit of reading Scripture every night.

■ CASE EXAMPLE 24-2
■ Leon's Story

"You asked me why I read the Bible every night. Well, I have done it as long as I can remember. My favorite passage is Psalm 23. I read that one every night before I go to bed. Even when I am really sick and hearing voices, I still read Psalm 23. I know that the Lord is not going to take away this schizophrenia . . . I wish He would . . . but He gives me strength . . . and I know that one day all my suffering will be over and I will be with Him. Reading the Bible reminds me that I am never alone." ■

Another individual with schizophrenia described his religious experience (Case Example 24-3).

■ CASE EXAMPLE 24-3
■ Story by an Anonymous Writer

"I am particularly indebted to Judaism, my religion, which helped me to overcome the very debilitating social effects of my illness. In becoming a devoted servant of God, I began sharing my religious experiences with other members of the Jewish community. In this way I began to socialize more and to make friends." ■

From Anonymous. (1996). First person account: Social, economic, and medical effects of schizophrenia. *Schizophrenia Bulletin, 22*(1), 183.

What do you think? How should religion and spirituality be assessed when the patient is experiencing religious delusions?

► Check Your Reading

49. What areas of assessment need to be of concern to the nurse?
50. What assessment tools may be of assistance in assessing a patient's response to psychopharmacological therapy?
51. What do you assess in regard to spiritual or religious issues?
52. State two findings that support the positive role of religion in the life of the individual with schizophrenia.

Assessing the Family Environment

The family environment and the family's ability to provide support have a powerful impact on the ability of the person with schizophrenia to function independently. Although no longer seen as the cause of mental illness, families are required to adapt to an immensely difficult situation. It is important to keep this focus in mind when assessing family functioning. Researchers have extended the scope of research beyond the husband-wife and parent-child relationships to encompass sibling relationships as well. The following findings may be useful in assessing sibling relationships. Gerace, Camilleri, and Ayers (1993) found that siblings identify their involvement in the care of a sibling with schizophrenia in three ways:

1. *Collaborative.* The sibling shared the caretaking responsibilities with the parents and other family members and was actively involved in collaboration with the health team.
2. *Crisis oriented.* The sibling's involvement was situation-specific with no carryover between crises. In these family situations, virtually no long-term planning decreased the incidence of crises.
3. *Detached concern.* The sibling is involved indirectly and attempts to create distance between self and the ill brother or sister and sometimes between self and the entire family.

The focus on siblings is significant because it directs attention to another area of potential support for the person with schizophrenia. It also increases sensitivity to the needs of families who daily care for a family member with schizophrenia.

The family assessment includes information on whether or not there are other family members with any history of mental illness, especially schizophrenia, mood disorders, or substance abuse. History of any of these disorders may indicate a genetic predisposition toward development of illness. Mental illness in other family members also directly affects the family's ability to provide long-term support to a family member with schizophrenia.

FAMILY COMMUNICATION PATTERNS

Although research on this issue is inconclusive, family communication patterns may determine the type of intervention needed. The family may need assistance in responding to the ill family member, who may be speaking in a thought-disordered way. Also, the family may need assistance in modifying an overstimulating or high-demand environment, which research has demonstrated to be particularly toxic for persons with schizophrenia (Lefley, 1992; Miklowitz, 1994).

THE ENVIRONMENT

To determine support and services available, it is essential to look beyond the patient and immediate family. Consideration should be given to community groups and organizations such as the National Alliance for the Mentally Ill (NAMI), a national family support system network with local chapters.

FAMILY STRESS AND COHESION

Chronic schizophrenia in a family member creates considerable psychological distress. Behaviors that families identify as stressful are gross deficits in task functioning, failure to take care of personal needs, difficulties in handling money, an inability to plan for the future, and episodic eruptions of deviant and sometimes threatening behavior (Hatfield & Lefley, 1987). It is essential to assess and document the patterns of family interaction and, in the inpatient setting, note the effects of family visits on the patient (Case Example 24–4).

Skipped

■ CASE EXAMPLE 24–4
■ Win's Story

We walk on stiff dry grass, bare trees motionless, pointing to a near-perfect blue sky. The only stir is the rustling of the dry leaves beneath our feet. I listen to her and think: Oh God, the pain. I had closed it off so well since the last time . . .

(Like Grendel, it crouches there on the fringe of my consciousness, waiting for precisely the right moment to slouch in and mar all the perfect blue domes and scorch the whole brown earth to black.)

"The staff is nice to us, very courteous and polite. The food's not bad." She kicks a stone in her path. "But they don't let us have seconds on meat or dessert. We get fresh fruit everyday, and with Christmas coming we'll get special things."

I glance sidelong at her, my sometime daughter, so beautiful, even in her sickness unto death. Surely you've made a mistake, God, not her . . .

I say nothing, merely look at my feet as I walk and wait for her to speak again. I pray her words won't come out chaotic and irrelevant. Sometimes, I want to grab what she says out of midair and shove it back in her mouth, demand that she retract what she's saying and tell her, "No, no! You don't mean that!" But when I think it, the darkness around her eyes reproaches me. *Stop,* they say, *You don't know what you're asking. I've been there, I know.*

"It's really not bad here. Marie and I are good friends. She gave me a martini last night. She mixed it in a shampoo bottle."

Outdoors, with night coming on, I'm grateful that here, at least, there is a semblance of order and predictability without the incoherent mumblings and uncoordinated movements and stares of non-recognition.

You've got it all wrong, God, she doesn't belong here! You've made a mistake! She's intelligent . . . she's artistic . . . she's got talent . . .

On Tuesdays, she paints ceramic ashtrays in the shape of hearts and stars . . .

With some animation, she tells me about her courses at the "University-Without-Walls." She is very tired, she says, because she was up late the past few nights studying and practicing chords on the piano, 156 of them. She has to be able to identify any one of them for her final exam. She expects to pass, even though she's never played the piano.

We trudge down the hill to the gardens. Amid the flowerless shrubs, standing tall, defiant against last week's freezing rain that bends them to the ground, is a quiescent waterfall and fish pond; the water runs empty except for soggy black leaves. "One of the patients here designed this park, but I think he's gone now." I notice her left foot dragging slightly. It does that when she gets tired. I suggest we start back to her unit.

Retracing our steps back up the hill, something comes to me, something I have denied for 9 years. Not the pain—no, no denying that—but the fact that she may not leave here this time. Before, I had known she would get better, and she did. But each time it has taken longer for her to recoup her losses—more medication, more effort—and this time, she seems not so fervent or angry or committed to her cause. She seems, in fact, quite content. Her hallucinations aren't nearly so bothersome as they once were; they're not all bad, she assures me, some quite pleasant, actually.

I reckon that now she has crossed over the line that once she drew between herself and "the dopies and the droolies and the druggies." I brood that maybe there is nothing in my world to draw her back. Heretofore, when the "real world" had become too much for her, she would "dip in and out of psychosis"—or so her therapist said. But now her stays in the never-never land seem to be growing longer and the drugs and psychotherapy less effective. Someday, I feel sure, she will slide irretrievably into the world of her own making and not come back—and what will I tell myself then? The time, the effort, the expertise that has gone into her care and keeping—it was all for naught?

She leads me to what she calls her favorite place, a slab of concrete with a dozen picnic tables stacked away for the season, echoes that there once was a summer. She stops to extract a cigarette from the pocket of her jacket, but she has no match. She stops a fellow patient passing by for a light.

Why does her madness repel me? Why do I ache at the thought of her slipping into an oblivion where I cannot follow? She functions well here. She has everything she needs: food, shelter, friends, caretakers. Why can't I let her go? She's better off here, without me. They can give her everything I can't . . . and more. They can give her what I and the world can't: permission to be crazy.

Clouds to the west mount as the sun hides just beyond the horizon. The air is as still and cold as the stone steps leading to the residence hall. She says something about the job she might get when she graduates to the halfway house. But there is no future in her voice. And as I have no future to offer her either, we turn toward the place from whence we came.

Here in the usually noisy and always smoke-filled C-2 recreation room, I deposit her, a fragment of my loss and helplessness, and then I walk to my car. I bury whatever grief I can in the night and the cold, knowing it will be resurrected the next time I come—just as surely as the picnic tables will be spread out in the spring and the waterfall will be turned on. ■

From Winship, W. (1993). First person account: How do I let go? *Schizophrenia Bulletin, 19*(4), 853–854.

W*hat do you think?* Reread Win's story. Is there any hope you could offer?

► *Check Your Reading*
53. What is included in a family assessment?
54. What are the issues that families have the most difficulty with in dealing with a family member with schizophrenia?

Diagnosis

Medical diagnoses are descriptive, so that a minimum number of symptoms meeting a minimal level of severity lead to a medical diagnosis. Symptoms listed in the DSM-IV form the constellation of medically relevant symptoms. Nursing diagnoses, in contrast, describe the quality, content, or context of the patient's health concern and its relationship to contributing factors.

Nurses do not wish to duplicate the medical diagnosis but must use the language of medicine to describe

TABLE 24–4 Nursing Diagnosis: Altered Thought Processes

TYPE OF THOUGHT	DEFINITION	EXAMPLE
Paranoid delusions	Belief that others are trying to harm the individual	A man notices a woman on the street and believes she is going to kill him.
Grandiose delusions	Belief that one has special powers or is a special person	A man believes he has the power to control the weather or is Jesus Christ.
Erotomania	Belief that another person is deeply in love with one (usually famous)	A woman believes she is engaged to Senator Edward (Ted) Kennedy, although they have never met.
Thought broadcasting	Belief that one's thoughts can be heard by others	A man believes his thoughts are broadcast over television.
Somatic delusions	Belief that one's body is altered from its normal structure or function	A woman believes that her bowels are filled with cement and refuses to eat.
Ideas of reference	False belief that public events are related to the individual	A man believes he has caused the bombing of Beirut.

symptoms. Thus both symptoms and their severity are included in the nursing diagnosis. Clear descriptions of psychiatric symptoms are essential to assess the effects of medication as well as the patient's potential for self-harm. Patients who are admitted to the hospital in an acute crisis, such as Bill in Case Example 24–1, are responding to vivid auditory hallucinations and require restabilization on higher-than-normal doses of medication. Therefore, in arriving at a nursing diagnosis, you must describe accurately what you observe as well as what the patient describes (Table 24–4).

Standardization of nursing actions and common terminology are an important foundation for the provision of nursing care and are provided through the nursing diagnosis, which is the basis for the nursing care plan. Certain nursing diagnoses are common to individuals with specific psychiatric disorders. See Medical and Nursing Diagnoses: Thought Disorder. Nursing diagnoses for people with schizophrenia focus on alterations in the pattern of activity, cognition, emotional processes, interpersonal processes, and perception.

► *Check Your Reading*
55. What do the nursing diagnoses provide that the medical diagnoses do not provide?
56. Cite two appropriate nursing diagnoses for a patient with schizophrenia.

Outcome Identification

As with any chronic illness, the nurse must be careful to set realistic outcomes for patients with schizophrenia. Unfortunately, deterioration in all aspects of functioning is part of the illness. The most troublesome areas of patient functioning should be the focus of expected outcomes, setting incremental, short-term outcomes that can set the stage for achieving more long-term outcomes. For example, you might expect a patient experiencing hallucinations to define and test reality at the time of discharge. For a patient exhibiting delusional thinking, you might expect the patient to distinguish between the delusions and reality.

Planning

As the nurse plans for the care of a person with schizophrenia, there are multiple considerations beyond that of initial stabilization. These considerations include discharge planning that focuses on community-living options and the availability of crisis-oriented inpatient treatment.

Role of the Nurse in Discharge Planning

From the moment of admission to the inpatient system, the nurse needs to assess factors related to the precipitating crisis and/or relapse with the purpose of formulating the discharge plan. Establishing a working relationship with the patient and family should lay a foundation for the entire process of treatment as early as possible during acute psychosis. A working alliance needs to be developed between the nurse and the patient and family

so that family strengths are maximized and resources identified. It is important not to focus on weaknesses and deficits. In the initial encounter, which lays the foundation for discharge planning, the nurse needs to gain an understanding of life experiences that might contribute to the stress level of a patient or other family members. Identify primary support people. A contract that establishes rules and expectations of treatment with specific, attainable, and mutually agreed-on goals helps target discharge criteria. Issues that contributed to the present hospitalization are explored. It is helpful to ask questions such as

- Are there factors in the patient's life that contributed to his or her inability to maintain health? If so, what can be done to eliminate or mediate those factors?
- Are there problems related to substance abuse that were not taken into account when the person was last in the hospital or last in contact with an outpatient therapist?
- Is there a change in social support that increased the patient's stress level?

Community-Living Options

Until the mid-1950s no one worried about community aftercare for psychiatric patients because almost no patients with schizophrenia left the mental hospital. The current trend in the treatment of the severely ill thought-disordered patient involves a variety of community-based treatment approaches. This trend has resulted in shorter periods of hospitalization, with inpatient care only for the acute phase of illness, and increased dependence on a wide assortment of aftercare and rehabilitation services. Community-based treatment has also resulted in large numbers of psychiatrically impaired persons returning to their families. Many live with their families throughout their adult lifetimes; in fact, a number of studies have reported that from 25% to 60% of deinstitutionalized patients return to their families (Torrey, 1995).

Crisis-Oriented Inpatient Treatment

Patients need to be hospitalized during the acute phase of illness, when they are no longer able to live in the community or with their loved ones. They may enter the health care system by seeing their regular outpatient therapist or a community outreach worker on a mobile treatment team, or the family may bring a patient into a hospital's emergency department for evaluation. Depending on local regulations, families dealing with an ill family member who appears to be losing control at home may seek an emergency petition requiring the police to bring the person to the local hospital for evaluation. If the person is not living with his or her family, a landlord or caretaker can petition the court to seek an evaluation. Patients can sometimes become violent, especially as they misperceive cues from others. In these instances, or in instances in which people may be at risk of imminently harming themselves, police can usually bring the person to a hospital for psychiatric evaluation.

MEDICAL DIAGNOSES AND RELATED NURSING DIAGNOSES

Thought Disorder

Medical Diagnoses (DSM-IV):

Schizophrenia: Paranoid type; catatonic type; disorganized type; undifferentiated type; and residual type

Nursing Diagnoses (NANDA)

Impaired Verbal Communication
Family Coping, Ineffective
Individual Coping, Ineffective
Personal Identity Disturbance
Altered Role Performance
Impaired Social Interaction
Self Care Deficit
Self Esteem Disturbance
Sensory/Perceptual Alteration
Social Isolation
Altered Thought Processes

DSM-IV Diagnosis:

Schizophrenia

Diagnostic Criteria

A. Characteristic symptoms: Two (or more) of the following, each present for a significant portion of time during a 1-month period (or less if successfully treated):
  (1) Delusions
  (2) Hallucinations
  (3) Disorganized speech (e.g., frequent derailment or incoherence)
  (4) Grossly disorganized or catatonic behavior
  (5) Negative symptoms, that is, affective flattening, alogia, or avolition

Note: Only one Criterion A symptom is required if delusions are bizarre or hallucinations consist of a voice keeping up a running commentary on the person's behavior or thoughts, or two or more voices conversing with each other.

B. Social/occupational dysfunction: For a significant portion of the time since the onset of the disturbance, one or more major areas of functioning such as work, interpersonal relations, or self-care are markedly below the level achieved before the onset (or when the onset is in childhood or adolescence, failure to achieve expected level of interpersonal, academic, or occupational achievement).

C. Duration: Continuous signs of the disturbance persist for at least 6 months. This 6-month period must include at least 1 month of symptoms (or less if successfully treated) that meet Criterion A (i.e., active-phase symptoms) and may include periods of prodromal or residual symptoms. During these prodromal or residual periods, the signs of the disturbance may be manifested by only negative symptoms or two or more symptoms listed in Criterion A present in an attenuated form (e.g., odd beliefs, unusual perceptual experiences).

D. Schizoaffective and Mood Disorder exclusion: Schizoaffective Disorder and Mood Disorder With Psychotic Features have been ruled out because either (1) no Major Depressive, Manic, or Mixed Episodes have occurred concurrently with the active-phase symptoms; or (2) if mood episodes have occurred during active-phase symptoms, their total duration has been brief relative to the duration of the active and residual periods.

E. Substance/general medical condition exclusion: The disturbance is not due to the direct physiological effects of a substance (e.g., a drug of abuse, a medication) or a general medical condition.

F. Relationship to a Pervasive Developmental Disorder: If there is a history of Autistic Disorder or another Pervasive Developmental Disorder, the additional diagnosis of Schizophrenia is made only if prominent delusions or hallucinations are also present for at least a month (or less if successfully treated).

Classification of longitudinal course (can be applied only after at least 1 year has elapsed since the initial onset of active-phase symptoms):
  Episodic With Interepisode Residual Symptoms (episodes are defined by the reemergence of prominent psychotic symptoms); also specify if: With Prominent Negative Symptoms
  Episodic With No Interepisode Residual Symptoms
  Continuous (prominent psychotic symptoms are present throughout the period of observation); also specify if: With Prominent Negative Symptoms
  Single Episode in Partial Remission; also specify if: With Prominent Negative Symptoms
  Single Episode in Full Remission
  Other or Unspecified Pattern

The early warning signs of relapse in people with schizophrenia have been identified only through a circuitous process unique to each patient (although with some commonalities), in contrast to most chronic illnesses, such as diabetes, in which systematic clinical observation has identified the early warning signs of the illness not being in control. The outcome of most studies of schizophrenia is that the illness is primarily one characterized by exacerbations and remissions. The most common outcome after an acute psychotic episode is a nonpsychotic deficit characterized by blunted affect, low energy levels, social withdrawal, and increased vulnerability to stress (Frese, 1994; Herz, Keith, & Docherty, 1990).

MEDICAL DIAGNOSES AND RELATED NURSING DIAGNOSES

Thought Disorder Continued

Related Nursing Diagnosis

Sensory/Perceptual Alteration: Auditory/Visual

Definition

Condition in which sensory stimuli are not experienced realistically or are misinterpreted

Example

Sensory/Perceptual Alteration: Auditory related to schizophrenia as evidenced by auditory hallucinations and subjective complaints about internal voices

Related Nursing Diagnosis

Altered Thought Processes

Definition

Condition in which an individual's thought processes are interrupted or not based in reality

Example

Altered Thought Processes related to schizophrenia as evidenced by delusional thinking; inability to concentrate; altered attention span; misinterpretations of reality; hypervigilance; impaired ability to make decisions, solve problems, reason, abstract, conceptualize, or calculate; inappropriate social behavior

Based on information from the *Diagnostic and Statistical Manual of Mental Disorders. Fourth Edition.* Copyright 1994 American Psychiatric Association. Nursing diagnoses and definitions from North American Nursing Diagnosis Association. (1999). *NANDA nursing diagnoses: Definitions and classification, 1999–2000.* Philadelphia: NANDA.

W*hat do you think?* What should society provide for the patient with schizophrenia in order for him or her to live a healthy, productive life?

➤ *Check Your Reading*

57. Identify two aspects of the nurse's role in discharge planning.
58. Why are community-living options an important consideration in discharge planning for the person with schizophrenia?

Implementation

Underlying all nursing interventions in the care of patients with a thought disorder is the establishing, maintaining, and terminating of the nurse-patient relationship. As mentioned earlier, a working alliance with the patient and family is necessary to establish the trust for achieving these ends. Specific interventions depend on both the medical and the nursing diagnoses. General guidelines are listed in Boxes 24–7 and 24–8.

Nurse as a Supportive Counselor

Patients with schizophrenia respond best to supportive counseling that focuses on strengths, increasing coping and problem-solving skills and offering affirmation, long-term concern, hopefulness, and commitment. Analytical insight-oriented therapy is too stressful for the person with schizophrenia and is inappropriate because the

illness is biologically based. Case Example 24–5 expresses the needs and the request of an individual with schizophrenia.

■ CASE EXAMPLE 24–5
■ A Poem by Vicki Lynn Bentley

I don't want your sympathy;
I want your acceptance!
I don't want your condemnation;
I want your compassion!
I don't want your patronage;
I want your support!
I don't want your indulgence;
I want an opportunity
    a chance to live
    a chance to serve
    a chance to die
knowing that I have lived up to my potential
as a human being. ■

From Bentley, V. L. (1994). Battling schizophrenia: My fight for dignity. *Journal of Psychosocial Nursing and Mental Health Services, 32*(3), 48.

➤ *Check Your Reading*

59. What are the functions of supportive counseling for the person with schizophrenia?
60. Why is insight-oriented counseling inappropriate for the person with schizophrenia?

Patients need the opportunity to express their concerns and struggles while learning to live with an illness

Box 24-7 ■ ■ ■ ■ ■

Interventions for a Patient With Altered Thought Processes

> Convey acceptance of patient, but do not confuse delusion with reality.
>
> Do not argue or deny the belief. Denial may impede the development of a trusting relationship.
>
> Reinforce and focus on reality in the here and now.
>
> Assist and support the patient in an attempt to verbalize feelings of anxiety, fear, and other emotions.

as complex as schizophrenia. The many psychosocial issues and concerns associated with daily living can be shared with an understanding caregiver in the counseling setting.

McGlashan (1994) advocated relationships with the person experiencing schizophrenia. He observed that "relationship treatments . . . are the oldest we have" and he emphasized the need "to reassess and reassert their relevance and worth" (p. 189).

Nurse as Teacher to Patient and Family

Persons with schizophrenia who receive neuroleptic medication and basic supportive care have been shown to relapse at the rate of 20% to 40% during the 1st year after hospitalization (O'Connor, 1991). Recognizing early signs of relapse can help reverse the pattern and decrease the suffering as well as the cost burden associated with relapse (Weiden & Olfson, 1995). According to the stress-vulnerability perspective, the onset of psychotic episodes results from interactions among four factors: basic vulnerabilities, environmental stress, per-

Box 24-8 ■ ■ ■ ■ ■

Interventions for a Patient With Auditory-Visual and Sensory-Perceptual Alterations

> Observe the patient for signs of hallucinations. Early intervention may prevent aggressive behavior as a result of misperception of stimuli or response to command hallucination.
>
> Avoid touching the patient. Touch may be perceived as threatening or could be sensorially painful.
>
> Do not validate the hallucination but accept that the patient is having the experience.
>
> Try to connect the occurrence of hallucinations with times of increased anxiety.
>
> Involve the patient in interpersonal activities that could provide distraction and bring him or her back to reality.
>
> Medicate with antipsychotic drugs as prescribed.

sonal factors, and environmental protectors (Goldstein, 1987). Because of the multiple factors involved in this dynamic system, the degree of change in stressors or protectors that begins the trend toward relapse cannot be predicted. See What Patients Need to Know: Schizophrenia and What Families Need to Know: Schizophrenia.

Becoming aware of early prodromal signs that signal the beginning of a relapse facilitates efforts to initiate restabilization. People with schizophrenia and their families typically are able to describe symptoms that are individual. Often, sleep changes, anxiety, and depression as well as general social withdrawal are the first signs the person or family notices. Although these signs can sometimes be subtle, helping the family and patient to identify the individual pattern and notify the outpatient therapist early can prevent relapse. Evidence indicates that most psychotic relapses are preceded by at least 2 weeks of prodromal symptom increases (O'Connor, 1991). The high rate of restabilization with early intervention suggests that if clinicians respond to all increases in early signs with increased surveillance and support, reduction of stimulation, and perhaps a temporary increase in medication, many relapses can be averted.

The goal of teaching is to identify target symptoms that are reliably associated with significant worsening of symptoms for a particular patient and not present at other times. Sometimes, early signs subside without deliberate intervention. By involving both patients and their families in the process of routine symptom monitoring, the burden can be lessened. It is important to develop an anticipatory plan that delineates the steps to be taken when family members identify symptomatic changes believed to signal exacerbation. It is also important that patients and families understand the relationship between stress and relapse. When stressful events occur or accustomed supports are lost, informed patients and families recognize the need for especially vigilant monitoring.

Psychiatric rehabilitation nurses Moller and Murphy (1998, pp. 10-12) identified six steps to prevent relapse. The patient and/or supportive caregiver should

1. Identify the problem symptoms.
2. Identify symptoms that signal relapse.
3. Identify and use symptom management techniques.
4. Identify symptom triggers.
5. Identify ways to cope with triggers.
6. Live a wellness lifestyle.

These authors have emphasized the necessity of maintaining a level of wellness to prevent relapse. They acknowledge the vulnerabilities that persons with chronic disorders have for exacerbation of symptoms. See Snapshot: Nursing Interventions Specific to Schizophrenia.

► **Check Your Reading**

61. What are the benefits of teaching patients and families to identify the early signs of illness exacerbation?
62. What interventions can be instituted to prevent relapse when prodromal signs are identified?

WHAT PATIENTS NEED TO KNOW

Schizophrenia

What causes schizophrenia?

The cause of schizophrenia is not precisely known, but the following are generally accepted facts: (1) the brain's chemicals appear to be functioning abnormally; (2) development before birth, early trauma, and inheritance are believed to be predisposing factors; and (3) relatives of people with schizophrenia have a greater chance of developing the disease than the general population.

Are there different types of schizophrenia?

There are five types of schizophrenia: paranoid (characterized by extreme suspiciousness, delusions of grandeur, and delusions of persecution); catatonic (characterized by a stuporous condition associated with rigidity, posturing, and waxy flexibility); disorganized (characterized by flatness of affect, silliness, incoherence); undifferentiated (characterized by symptoms found in more than one type); and residual (characterized by absence of delusions, hallucinations, or grossly disorganized behavior). Specific symptoms are diagnosed with each type. Symptoms must be present for at least 6 months to be labeled schizophrenia.

What happens if I don't take my medications?

It is important to take both the antipsychotic and the antiparkinsonian medications to control the symptoms. If the medications are stopped, a recurrence of the symptoms is likely.

What if the symptoms reappear?

Symptoms can recur, even with medication therapy and supportive care. Early recognition of signs such as social withdrawal, sleep changes, increased anxiety, and stress may be observed. It is important to understand the relationship between stress and relapse. Relying on family members and friends is important during a relapse.

Will I always have schizophrenia?

Yes, it is a disease process, one in which controlling the symptoms and living with the illness are important. There is no cure, but medications, community and family support, and therapy can be helpful.

To assist the patient experiencing the positive symptoms of hallucinations and delusions caregivers, family members, and the patient need to know how to manage such troublesome symptoms. When the nurse or family member can communicate with the patient in a genuine and accepting manner, mutual trust can be attained that facilitates the discussion of symptoms. Moller and Murphy (1998, pp. 7-13–7-15)

WHAT FAMILIES NEED TO KNOW

Schizophrenia

Will my family member ever be cured?

Schizophrenia is a chronic disease and similar to other chronic diseases, has early warning signs of being out of control. It is important to know that this illness is characterized by exacerbations and remissions. Often, when the symptoms of an acute episode subside, the person has blunted affect and a low energy level, and may withdraw from social and family situations.

What can I do to help my family member?

It is helpful for the family to become aware of the patient's pattern of activity to detect early signs of relapse. Learning how to identify these target symptoms and routine symptom monitoring by both patient and family can assist in restabilization with early intervention. Most of the time, a 1- to 2-week period with prodromal symptoms such as sleep changes, depression, anxiety, and social withdrawal precedes a period of exacerbation.

What resources are available?

Several programs are available to assist the family with support and educational information (see resources at the end of the chapter). Joining a support group with members who have the same experience as yourself can be helpful in providing social and emotional support in dealing with schizophrenic behavior. Education programs in both the community and the hospital can provide necessary important information on medication and side effects, communication techniques for dealing with negative feelings, and managing disruptive behavior.

SNAPSHOT

Nursing Interventions Specific to Schizophrenia

What do you need to do to develop a relationship with a patient suffering with schizophrenia?

- Approach the patient with a calm, honest, genuine, and accepting manner.
- Spend short periods of time with the patient even if he or she converses minimally and/or with difficulty.
- Demonstrate honest interest and concern in the patient's perceptions of their illness and situation.
- Speak distinctly and clearly with short sentences and with one thought per sentence.
- Address the patient by his or her preferred name (don't assume it is okay to use the patient's first name until you ask the patient's preference). As you talk with the patient, listen carefully and respectfully to what he or she shares. Also, avoid speaking of the patient by diagnosis, that is, the schizophrenic patient.
- Encourage the patient to identify and discuss feelings.
- Find ways to express hope without negating the struggle and suffering experienced by the patient.

What do you need to assess regarding the patient's health status?

- General health status assessment includes appetite, diet, weight changes, constipation, and sleep disturbance.
- Disturbance in the patient's thought processes, including presence of hallucinations and/or delusional thinking
- Disturbance in speech, such as poverty of speech or content
- Response to and adherence with medication regimen and reasons for nonadherence; assess for side effects; the presence and identification of side effects may be evaluated by using assessment tools such as the Simpson-Angus Rating Scale and the Abnormal Involuntary Movement Scale.
- Behavioral responses, including isolation and withdrawal, repetitious actions, poor personal hygiene, lack of motivation, decreased interest, and/or inability to experience pleasure
- Affect or emotional responsiveness, including blunted or flat affect
- Vital signs, including sitting and standing when patient is taking medication that may cause orthostatic hypotension
- Degree of social support and persons who provide it

- Capability for independent living, such as managing daily schedule, money, self-care of laundry and other housekeeping (e.g., cooking), work or vocational skills
- Potential for suicidal and/or assaultive behaviors

What do you need to teach the patient and/or the patient's caregiver?

- Disease process of schizophrenia, causes, course of illness, and treatment
- Medications prescribed, including the reason for taking, side effects (untoward as well as expected), and importance of adhering to the medication schedule
- Importance of maintaining a healthy lifestyle—diet, exercise, proper sleep, and opportunity for spiritual practices
- Signs of relapse, in particular, prodromal or trigger symptoms
- Importance of emotional and social support and where to obtain it
- Maintaining safety for the patient and self, including emergency measures

What skills will you want the patient and/or caregiver to demonstrate?

- Ability to perform personal care
- Ability to identify and express feelings
- Coping skills
- Ability to follow the medication plan
- Ability to handle an emergency situation and maintain safety

What other health professionals might need to be a part of this plan of care?

- The psychiatrist and/or primary care physician is usually in charge of the overall treatment plan including medication management.
- The psychiatric mental health nurse (generalist or clinical specialist), assists with assessment and management of the patient's treatment plan.
- The social worker can assist with access to community supports; insurance issues; access to entitlements; and connection with community-based treatments.
- The psychiatric occupational therapist assists the patient with instrumental activities of daily living, such as time management, cooking, and budgeting.
- The nursing assistant or home health aide assists the patient with personal hygiene and grooming, if necessary.
- The case manager can assist with the patient's treatment plan and help to coordinate the patient's access to all resources needed to remain independent in the community.

suggested the following guidelines for managing hallucinations as they occur:

- Establish a trusting interpersonal relationship.
- Assess for symptoms of a hallucination.
- Focus on the symptom and ask the person to describe what is happening.
- Identify if drugs and/or alcohol have been used.
- If asked, point out simply that you are not experiencing the same stimuli.
- Help the person describe and compare the present and previous hallucination.
- Encourage the person to observe and describe thoughts, feelings, and actions, both present and past, as they relate to the hallucination.
- Help the person describe needs that may be reflected in the content of the hallucination.
- Help the person identify if there is a correlation between the hallucination and the needs it may be reflecting.
- Suggest and reinforce the use of interpersonal relationships in meeting the need.
- Identify how other symptoms of psychosis have affected the person's ability to carry out activities of daily living.

The other positive symptom that may interfere with the ill person's life are delusions. Moller and Murphy (1998, pp. 8-15–8-16) made intervention suggestions for effectively managing these symptoms:

- Don't paraphrase the person's words and descriptions.
- Observe for evidence of concrete thinking.
- Observe for symptoms of Formal Thought Disorder.
- Observe for the ability to accurately use cause and effect reasoning.
- Distinguish between the description of the experience and the factual state of the situation—look for the kernel of truth.
- Identify if the delusion is falsifiable.
- Begin to carefully question, with sincerity, the facts as they are presented and the meaning to the patient.
- Assess the duration, frequency, and intensity of the delusion.
- Place the delusion in a time frame and identify triggers.
- Identify emotional components of the delusion.
- Promote distraction as a way to stop focusing on the delusion.
- Discuss consequences of the delusion when the person is ready.

Other areas of teaching that the nurse is ideally suited to provide are general health principles including proper diet, exercise, and general good health habits. In addition to understanding the management of symptoms, general knowledge regarding mental illness and its treatment (e.g., psychopharmacological treatment and the side effects of medications) is also useful information (Brooker, 1990; Moller & Murphy, 1997; Moller & Wer, 1989; Murphy & Moller, 1993).

Nurse as Protector From Self-Injurious Behavior

The nurse may be an important influence in assisting the individual who is suicidal from carrying out the actions that could be detrimental. In anticipating violent behavior the nurse's interventions protect not only the patient but also staff colleagues and other patients.

The nurse may need to mobilize other colleagues to assist in maintaining a watchful support with the patient until the suicidal or assaultive impulses have subsided. In the inpatient setting, the nurse may suggest the patient spend time in his or her room or use the quiet room until assaultive impulses have abated to the degree safety is ensured for all in the environment.

When the nurse intervenes to correct existing physical conditions, psychiatric symptoms may also be reduced. In addition, life-threatening consequences may be averted.

When a patient presents with both schizophrenia and a substance abuse problem, treatment must be directed toward both conditions. For instance, the patient may need to undergo detoxification from the abused substances before adequate, appropriate medication can be prescribed. Once the patient is receiving neuroleptic medications for schizophrenia, consideration must be given to appropriate and concurrent substance abuse treatment, including attendance at a 12-step program and a substance abuse education group. Treating only the schizophrenia and ignoring the substance abuse problem sets the patient up for failure. Both issues require treatment.

Programs that treat psychiatric patients often experience difficulty in treating patients with substance abuse problems because they may have little expertise with drug withdrawal protocols and do not have a well-planned psychosocial approach to the treatment of schizophrenia and substance abuse together. Because of the high rates of relapse of substance-abusing psychiatric patients and the common feeling that the patient is deliberately sabotaging treatment, health care providers and family may have a vehement negative response to the patient or feel hopeless and demoralized. It is important that this dual diagnosis problem is faced squarely with treatment programs for both problems to avoid countertherapeutic reactions.

The importance of a strong therapeutic alliance to successful outcomes of treatment cannot be overemphasized. You may need to function more as a coach to the patient in a nonjudgmental relationship, working to build adaptive behaviors and extinguish maladaptive ones, focusing on positive steps the patient has made. Patients should be encouraged and admired for their constructive alternative behaviors.

A group **psychoeducation** approach, with combined education and support about schizophrenia and the complications of substance abuse, may be useful. Group support can be helpful for a patient trying to make behavioral changes and may help reduce loneliness and provide concrete encouragement. It may also provide education and support for families and health care providers, who are the necessary psychosocial link to recovery for a person with schizophrenia.

> ➤ *Check Your Reading*
>   63. What is the importance of providing safety for the patient with suicidal or assaultive impulses?
>   64. What are the components of an effective treatment program for dually diagnosed patients?
>   65. What is the purpose of a psychoeducation group for the dually diagnosed patient?

Nurse as Collaborator With Patient and Family

Frese (1998) stressed the strength of the consumer's desire to be involved in the treatment program. Helping patients (who also often wish to be addressed as consumers and survivors) reenter society is a task Frese saw as a part of the role of those in the caring professions. The nurse can ideally become a central initiator of such a role in the nurse-patient relationship.

Reinhard (1994) recommended the nurse be involved as a family consultant. She advised a partnership with families to promote advocacy for obtaining better community resources for the mentally ill. She viewed this as "crucial" because many caregiving parents were aging and had concerns about the care of their children when they could no longer provide the needed care.

Rosalyn Carter (1998), former First Lady, long an advocate for better psychiatric care, regarded collaborative efforts with families as essential to help combat the stigma of mental illness. Nurses are welcome participants in advocacy organizations such as NAMI.

Nurse as Manager of Biological Interventions

The nurse has a significant role in administering prescribed medications as well as noting the patient's response to the medications. The nurse can also be mindful of the patient's diet and fluid intake, especially of drinks containing caffeine. It is known that caffeine as well as nicotine interfere with the absorption of antipsychotic medications (Moller, 1996; Moller & Murphy, 1998; Torrey, 1995).

The nurse can facilitate patient adherence to medications prescribed as she or he demonstrates interest and concern for the side effects the patient experiences. When the nurse listens carefully to the patient's responses to medication-taking, comfort measures such as chopped ice or sugar-free hard candy for dry mouth can be suggested. A distressing and frequent side effect of antipsychotic medications is weight gain. The nurse can provide dietary advisement and collaboration with a dietitian (Jackson & Haynes-Johnson, 1988). In addition, the nurse has frequent opportunities to provide information about the medications that patients are taking and instruct them about side effects. The nurse also has a significant responsibility to be vigilant regarding the most serious side effects and administer prescribed medications for them when indicated and report all undue responses to the prescribing psychiatrist.

Health teaching about the effects of cigarette smoking and caffeine on patient symptoms and the efficacy of medications is another important concern. A higher dose of antipsychotic medication may be required when high levels of caffeine and nicotine are ingested (Moller, 1996; Moller & Murphy, 1998; Torrey, 1995). Ingestion of high levels of sugar and chocolate may also increase a serotonin imbalance. It must also be kept in mind that chocolate and many soft drinks (colas) contain caffeine (Moller & Murphy, 1998).

> ➤ *Check Your Reading*
>   66. What collaborative role does Reinhard suggest for the nurse?
>   67. How can the nurse respond to the patient's reports of side effects?
>   68. What dietary teaching should the nurse give the patient related to medications?

Nurse as a Referral Source for Social Support

Krauss and Gourley (cited in Backlar, 1994) believed "the diagnosis of a serious and persistent mental disorder like schizophrenia launches a family into a world characterized by tumult, confusion, loss, grief, and conflict" (p. 153). These authors recognized both the family's and patient's need for information as well as a need to know where to find help.

The nurse has a crucial role in assisting families and patients to find the social supports that will enable the patient to adjust and cope in the community and help prevent relapse. One of the most effective organizations providing support to both patients and family members (consumers and survivors) is NAMI. A local chapter is available in almost every community. NAMI has also established support groups for siblings, who have often been neglected in the past. Other self-help groups may be available in a given community. Regional mental health centers can be a source of information for the location nearest the family and patient.

An increasing number of personal account books and articles are available chronicling the stories of many people who have experienced mental illness firsthand (Secunda, 1997; Simon, 1997; Wyden, 1998). Rosalyn Carter, with Susan Golant (1998), wrote an informative and supportive publication that may also be useful to families. These sources often help patients feel less alone with their problems and may also assist them in learning meaningful ways to cope with their own situations.

Leete (1987) attested to the value of peer-run groups in providing support, friendship, hope, and modeling. She also believed families and patients were entitled to education about illness, symptoms, course, and treatment.

FAMILY SUPPORT AND EDUCATION

Two types of clinical programs—psychoeducation and support groups—have been reported as strategies to help families cope with the problems posed by the symptoms of psychiatric illness. The support group consists of nonstructured discussions usually led by family members to provide social support. A psychoeducation group is usually conducted by mental health professionals. This type of group has an organized, structured format designed to educate families about mental illness and its treatment. The thrust of the family education and management strategy is to lower the emotional climate of the home while maintaining reasonable expectations for patient performance, that is, striking a balance between overstimulation and understimulation. The interventions attempt to

- Increase the stability and predictability of family life by decreasing the family's guilt and anxiety
- Increase self-confidence
- Provide a sense of cognitive mastery through the provision of information concerning both the nature and the course of schizophrenia as well as specific management strategies thought to be helpful in coping with schizophrenic symptoms on a day-to-day basis

When this family education process is effective, it decreases the intensity of interaction between the patient and family members and diminishes the possibility of patients being overstimulated by even the simplest elements of family life (Hogarty et al., 1990).

Both psychoeducational programs and support groups appear to be helpful to families, and it is unclear whether one modality is more helpful than the other (Wiedemann et al., 1994). The information provided by a psychoeducation group may make patient behavior more understandable and less bothersome to family members. In addition, because of the emphasis on communication and problem solving in the psychoeducation model, relationships with relatives and friends may improve, contributing to a feeling of increased social support (Kane, Dimartino, & Jimenez, 1990). Some find the organized structure of the psychoeducation group comforting, whereas those with a higher tolerance for ambiguity might favor the free-flowing discussions of the support group. Psychoeducation groups usually cover the following topics in four or more sessions:

1. Schizophrenia
2. Medication side effects and communication
3. Communicating negative feelings and problem solving
4. Reducing stress and managing disruptive behavior

Moller and Murphy (1997) developed a wellness-approach educational program for patients, families, and caregivers. They have demonstrated substantial cost savings in the prevention of relapse in patients who have participated in the program.

> ➤ *Check Your Reading*
> 69. What are two of the purposes of family education regarding schizophrenia?
> 70. Identify two topics covered in a psychoeducation group.

Nurse as Facilitator of Empowerment

Knowledge is a source of power. When patients and families are provided necessary knowledge about illness, symptom triggers, clues to relapse, and ways to care for themselves, they become empowered to live with an illness such as schizophrenia. When patients and families learn ways to prevent relapse of illness, to maintain recovery, and to facilitate important aspects of rehabilitation they can gain hope (Moller & Murphy, 1998).

Byrne and her colleagues (1994) believed hope is fostered through relationships. They concluded a belief in the patients' abilities could be a powerful influence in assisting patients and families while living with a chronic illness such as schizophrenia. Howard (1994) reported that hope as "a sustaining factor" provided purpose and encouragement for the continuation of caregiving (p. 112).

> ➤ *Check Your Reading*
> 71. What is the role of hope in facilitating empowerment?

Nurse as Facilitator of Spiritual Growth

Spiritual interventions are an essential component of care. This component focuses on the meaning of the illness to the patient as well as the patient's relationship with God. Sometimes the patient's behavior during exacerbation is so bizarre that health care providers forget that what is being observed are symptoms. The patient is not the symptoms, and the patient is not the illness. When a patient is viewed as the illness, any attempts to understand the suffering and the existential meaning of the illness generally cease. Likewise, efforts to focus on the patient's strengths and supports, including the patient's relationship with God, are ignored. Jean Vanier, founder of L'Arche movement in which mentally handicapped people, once institutionalized, are given homes in the community, emphasized the spiritual aspect of care (cited in Suska, 1991):

There are three gifts of growth: one is community, a network or covenanted relationships. You would not have chosen some of them. There's a mystery of community, a discovery of forgiveness. The community is to encourage growth, to confirm and challenge. But it can only challenge if it comforts and confirms.

There is no community without prayer. Prayer is to say Father, which says I trust. The first part of prayer is the cry, the cry of the wound. The second part of prayer is the prayer of rest, of bridegroom and lover. The cry leads to rest. Prayer finally leads to an offering. Prayer becomes the sacrament of the poor. (p. 328)

What do you think? How would you provide spiritual care to a patient with schizophrenia?

> ➤ *Check Your Reading*
> 72. Why is it essential to provide spiritual interventions in the care of the person with schizophrenia?

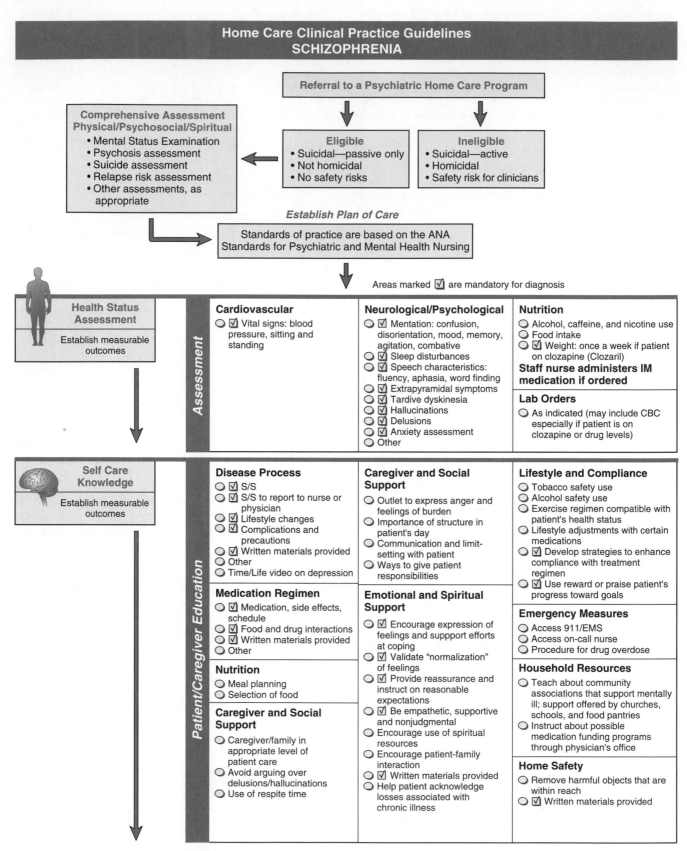

Home Care Clinical Practice Guidelines
SCHIZOPHRENIA

Referral to a Psychiatric Home Care Program

Comprehensive Assessment Physical/Psychosocial/Spiritual
- Mental Status Examination
- Psychosis assessment
- Suicide assessment
- Relapse risk assessment
- Other assessments, as appropriate

Eligible
- Suicidal—passive only
- Not homicidal
- No safety risks

Ineligible
- Suicidal—active
- Homicidal
- Safety risk for clinicians

Establish Plan of Care

Standards of practice are based on the ANA Standards for Psychiatric and Mental Health Nursing

Areas marked ☑ are mandatory for diagnosis

Assessment

Health Status Assessment

Establish measurable outcomes

Cardiovascular
- ○ ☑ Vital signs: blood pressure, sitting and standing

Neurological/Psychological
- ○ ☑ Mentation: confusion, disorientation, mood, memory, agitation, combative
- ○ ☑ Sleep disturbances
- ○ ☑ Speech characteristics: fluency, aphasia, word finding
- ○ ☑ Extrapyramidal symptoms
- ○ ☑ Tardive dyskinesia
- ○ ☑ Hallucinations
- ○ ☑ Delusions
- ○ ☑ Anxiety assessment
- ○ Other

Nutrition
- ○ Alcohol, caffeine, and nicotine use
- ○ Food intake
- ○ ☑ Weight: once a week if patient on clozapine (Clozaril)

Staff nurse administers IM medication if ordered

Lab Orders
- ○ As indicated (may include CBC especially if patient is on clozapine or drug levels)

Patient/Caregiver Education

Self Care Knowledge

Establish measurable outcomes

Disease Process
- ○ ☑ S/S
- ○ ☑ S/S to report to nurse or physician
- ○ ☑ Lifestyle changes
- ○ ☑ Complications and precautions
- ○ ☑ Written materials provided
- ○ Other
- ○ Time/Life video on depression

Medication Regimen
- ○ ☑ Medication, side effects, schedule
- ○ ☑ Food and drug interactions
- ○ ☑ Written materials provided
- ○ Other

Nutrition
- ○ Meal planning
- ○ Selection of food

Caregiver and Social Support
- ○ Caregiver/family in appropriate level of patient care
- ○ Avoid arguing over delusions/hallucinations
- ○ Use of respite time

Caregiver and Social Support
- ○ Outlet to express anger and feelings of burden
- ○ Importance of structure in patient's day
- ○ Communication and limit-setting with patient
- ○ Ways to give patient responsibilities

Emotional and Spiritual Support
- ○ ☑ Encourage expression of feelings and suppport efforts at coping
- ○ ☑ Validate "normalization" of feelings
- ○ ☑ Provide reassurance and instruct on reasonable expectations
- ○ ☑ Be empathetic, supportive and nonjudgmental
- ○ Encourage use of spiritual resources
- ○ Encourage patient-family interaction
- ○ ☑ Written materials provided
- ○ Help patient acknowledge losses associated with chronic illness

Lifestyle and Compliance
- ○ Tobacco safety use
- ○ Alcohol safety use
- ○ Exercise regimen compatible with patient's health status
- ○ Lifestyle adjustments with certain medications
- ○ ☑ Develop strategies to enhance compliance with treatment regimen
- ○ ☑ Use reward or praise patient's progress toward goals

Emergency Measures
- ○ Access 911/EMS
- ○ Access on-call nurse
- ○ Procedure for drug overdose

Household Resources
- ○ Teach about community associations that support mentally ill; support offered by churches, schools, and food pantries
- ○ Instruct about possible medication funding programs through physician's office

Home Safety
- ○ Remove harmful objects that are within reach
- ○ ☑ Written materials provided

Home care clinical practice guidelines for schizophrenia. (From Staff Builders Home Health Care, Staff Builders, Inc, 1983 Marcus Avenue, Lake Success, NY 11042–7011.)

Illustration continued on following page

Home Care Clinical Practice Guidelines
SCHIZOPHRENIA

Self Care Skill

Establish measurable outcomes

Patient/Caregiver Demonstration

Personal Care
- ○ Bathing and hygiene
- ○ Dressing

Behavior
- ○ Develop behavioral contract for _____
- ○ Thought-stopping techniques
- ○ Maintain boundaries
- ○ Limit setting for inappropriate behaviors
- ○ Participation in "no harm" contract
- ○ Socially appropriate behavior of _____
- ○ Appropriate expression of feelings
- ○ Impulse control
- ○ Identification of nonverbal behaviors and responses
- ○ Assertiveness techniques
- ○ Problem-solving tehniques
- ○ Other
- ○ ☑ Written materials provided

Coping Skills
- ○ ☑ Demonstrate health care maintenance strategies to sustain own physical and mental health
- ○ Efforts are made to adjust to illness
- ○ ☑ Participates in self-care or patient care
- ○ Family voices concerns, feelings, and questions and uses information taught to them
- ○ Use of some form of muscle relaxation technique
- ○ ☑ Written materials provided

Compensatory and Cognitive Skills
- ○ Reframe negative thought patterns
- ○ Demonstrates short-term recall through repetition
- ○ Visual lists or pictures to cue
- ○ Skill use of memory journal or calendar
- ○ Other
- ○ ☑ Written materials provided

Determine Appropriate Utilization of Resources With Physician
- ○ Visit schedule
- ○ HME
- ○ Pharmacy
- ○ Supplies

Patient Visits
- ○ Follow established guidelines for visits and plan of care
- ○ Document findings
- ○ Monitor outcomes

Evaluate and Report Significant Outcomes to Physician and/or Referral Source
- ○ Vital signs outside parameters
- ○ Mental status baseline changes
- ○ High risk for suicide, substance abuse, or self-destructive behaviors
- ○ Assessment tool scores indicate moderate to severe symptoms
- ○ Adverse side effects from medications (i.e., EPS, GI distress, excessive weight gain or loss, disturbed sleep patterns)
- ○ Labs outside of therapeutic range

Outcomes Measurement

Evaluate Need for Further Care Based on Outcomes Report

Expected Outcomes Achieved

NO

Alter plan based on outcomes progress and physician orders

If NO, Return to Health Status Assessment

YES

Discharge to self, family, or physician

Evaluation

To complete the nursing process, you evaluate changes in patient status and behavior in response to nursing interventions. Evaluation criteria are linked to nursing goals and an understanding of the limitations and vulnerabilities of the patient with schizophrenia based on a biopsychosocial and spiritual perspective.

The formative evaluation looks at the short-term goals identified for the patient and makes necessary adjustments as the patient's situation changes. The database is continually updated, the nursing diagnoses revised, and expected outcomes modified to meet changes in the patient's situation. For instance, the formative evaluation looks at the patient's immediate response to antipsychotic medication, response to the caregiver, increasing ability to manage personal care, and any changes in symptoms, such as hallucinations or delusions. The summative evaluation reviews the entire nursing process and draws conclusions about the effectiveness of nursing interventions in meeting the expected outcomes. Issues such as community placement, successful acclimation to a psychosocial program, long-term compliance with medications, and resolution of family concerns are addressed in the summative evaluation.

It is important when evaluating the effectiveness of care provided to the chronically ill patient, such as the person with schizophrenia, that an exacerbation of the illness is not viewed as a treatment failure. Chronic illnesses are episodic, with remissions and exacerbations. Individuals with schizophrenia need the freedom to "get sick" without the burden of being blamed as if they have failed the treatment team. Andreasen (1994) believed people with schizophrenia need to be allowed to have a "sick role." She asserted,

> *As brain diseases, mental illnesses are as legitimately physical as cancer or heart disease. As legitimate physical illnesses, the various mental illnesses must be given equal treatment by health care providers. People who suffer from these illnesses must be seen as genuinely ill, accorded the sick role, and provided with comprehensive and humane treatment.* (p. 34)

Andreasen (1984) suggested the person who "hears voices can hope that medication will drive away the voices and that he can return to a relatively normal life." She further observed that the person with schizophrenia with defect symptoms has lost the capacity to suffer and to hope—and at present, medicine has no good remedy to offer for this loss" (pp. 62–63). Fortunately, the advent of atypical antipsychotic medications during the 1990s has provided a new element of hope for those who experience negative or defect symptoms. The stories of Lori Schiller and Jeff Wyden represent two such hopeful outcomes (Schiller & Bennett, 1994; Wyden, 1998).

Another area of evaluation to be considered is the efficacy of nursing interventions. The nurse must evaluate the effectiveness of her or his own interventions. When another approach or intervention might be indicated, the nurse must have the courage to modify a previous intervention and try again.

➤ ***Check Your Reading***

73. How should recognition that schizophrenia is a chronic illness affect the evaluation process?

NURSING PROCESS APPLICATION

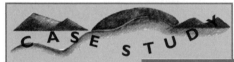

CASE STUDY

Ernie

Ernie is a 55-year-old white man who has been a salesman in the auto industry for the past 30 years. Over the past few months, Ernie's sales have declined significantly. Recently, his coworkers reported to their boss that Ernie has been behaving in a peculiar fashion. Each morning he arrives at his office, picks up his telephone, looks under it, and unscrews the face plate to check for a microphone. Ernie is sure that someone is tapping his telephone to sabotage his sales. Ernie's usual attire and appearance have also become increasingly untidy and unkempt. He has complained to coworkers about having difficulty sleeping.

During the nursing admission, Ernie states, "My coworkers are plotting against me." The nurse notes that Ernie is very cautious and anxious about signing the insurance and admission forms. During the entire process, he sits on the edge of his chair, answers questions evasively, and avoids direct eye contact with the nurse.

ASSESSMENT

Assessment data are as follows:

- Extreme anxious suspicion of coworkers and nurse
- Poor personal hygiene
- Hypervigilance and hyperalertness

DIAGNOSIS	DSM-IV Diagnosis:	Schizophrenia, paranoid type
	Nursing Diagnosis:	Altered Thought Processes related to delusional thinking as evidenced by verbalizations that coworkers are plotting against patient, extreme suspicion, and anxiety.

Expected Outcome 1: By _____ the patient will be able to distinguish between situations that arouse suspicion and delusional thinking and situations that reflect reality.

Short-Term Goal	Nursing Interventions	Rationales
By _____ the patient will have improved reality testing and decreased delusional thinking.	1. Accept the patient by letting him know you respect his feelings and point of view, even though you do not share them. 2. Do not deny or say directly that the patient's thinking or belief is wrong. 3. Assess the patient's delusions and ability to test reality daily. Do not dwell on delusions once the assessment is done; refocus on reality. 4. Reframe the patient's frightening delusional system of thinking. Assess for events that increase the patient's anxiety and determine what triggers delusions. 5. Assist the patient to affirm himself as a worthy human being who finds meaning in relatedness with others. 6. Administer antipsychotic medications.	1. This approach promotes an unconditional acceptance that will be helpful in developing basic trust with the patient. 2. This type of confrontation may escalate the patient's anxiety further because he may feel threatened, or confrontation may lead to counter-arguments with more delusional details. 3. Ongoing assessment provides data to determine if treatment (therapy, medication) is making any progress in alleviating the altered thinking processes. 4–5. Persecutory delusions can arise from spiritual distress associated with a negative, hopeless view of life. As the patient begins to value himself, he will convey a positive self-concept. 6. Medication therapy relieves target symptoms of psychosis (delusions). It does not cure but controls symptoms.

Expected Outcome 2: By _____ the patient will identify trusting characteristics in a relationship and begin to develop a relationship with at least one other person during hospitalization.

Short-Term Goals	Nursing Interventions	Rationales
By _____ the patient will develop a therapeutic relationship with the nurse.	1. Make short, frequent visits or contact with patient. 2. Avoid whispering around the patient and arguing. 3. Inform the patient of anticipated schedule changes. 4. Maintain a concerned but not overly concerned attitude toward the patient. 5. Understand that it is difficult for the patient to be self-aware and that self-disclosure is often uncomfortable.	1–4. This is a most helpful approach for establishing trust with a patient. 5. Pushing or pressuring the patient may cause an increase in anxiety. Allow the patient to set the pace in the relationship.
By _____ the patient will increase social skills.	1. Encourage the patient to participate in activities when he feels comfortable in doing so. 2. Provide feedback on behavior, reinforce strengths, and build on them.	1–2. Sharing experiences and participating in activities is a way for the patient to validate thoughts and feelings and receive feedback.

	Nursing Diagnosis:	Self Care Deficit related to altered thought processes and anxiety as evidenced by difficulty in dressing appropriately and maintaining personal hygiene.

> **Expected Outcome 3:** By _____ the patient will perform self-care at his highest level of functioning and ability.

Short-Term Goal	Nursing Interventions	Rationale
By _____ the patient will dress appropriately and maintain personal hygiene.	1. Provide a quiet, nonstimulating environment. 2. Give positive feedback for efforts to dress appropriately and maintain grooming.	1–2. Excessive anxiety and preoccupation with safety and delusions contribute to a lack of attention to personal hygiene and appearance. Positive feedback promotes self-esteem and a sense of control.

EVALUATION

Formative Evaluation: Ernie met each of his short-term goals. He immediately began to attend to appropriate personal hygiene practices, and his appearance during the first few days of treatment dramatically improved because of the therapeutic effect of antipsychotic medication. Ernie was able to establish a trusting relationship with the nurse but was not comfortable sharing his feelings in a group setting.

Summative Evaluation: Ernie achieved all of the expected outcomes except that he continued to have difficulty thinking about returning to work. Assisting Ernie to develop and increase his social skills required giving him additional time to meet this goal. Ernie was able to state how ashamed he felt about his behavior at work and did express a considerable amount of apprehension as to how his coworkers might view him. Ernie's ability to begin to share his feelings with the group was an initial step for him to begin to reestablish his relationships with his coworkers.

To continue to reinforce and strengthen Ernie's efforts to recognize his sense of self-worth, the treatment team made positive comments. Further therapy revealed that Ernie's father was authoritarian and critical, whereas his mother was domineering and argumentative. Ernie began to understand how this type of parenting style led to his forming a negative view of life with a general mistrust of others and lack of security while growing up.

NURSING PROCESS APPLICATION

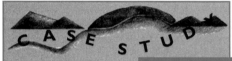

Cindy

Cindy, age 20, has been diagnosed with Schizophrenia, undifferentiated type. She has shared little of her family background with her college roommate, preferring instead to be alone rather than talk. For the past month, her roommate has noticed that Cindy seems to be off in her own world. She has noticed Cindy "talking to someone" even when there was no one in the room. During the admission interview, Cindy sat quietly and seemed to be listening and watching as if someone were talking to her. She was totally unaware of her surroundings and seemed preoccupied. Occasionally, she would laugh, look up at the ceiling, and nod her head as if in agreement.

ASSESSMENT

Assessment data are as follows:
- Acting as if she is listening to sounds—auditory hallucinations
- Looking up at ceiling and nodding head—visual hallucinations
- Unawareness of surroundings
- Laughing at inappropriate intervals

DIAGNOSIS

DSM-IV Diagnosis: Schizophrenia, undifferentiated type

Nursing Diagnosis: Sensory/Perceptual Alteration: Hallucinations, Auditory and Visual related to social withdrawal as evidenced by listening to sounds, looking up and nodding to the ceiling, and laughing at inappropriate intervals.

OUTCOME IDENTIFICATION, PLANNING, AND IMPLEMENTATION

> **Expected Outcome 1:** By _____ the patient will be able to define and test reality, eliminating the occurrence of hallucinations.

Short-Term Goals	Nursing Interventions	Rationale
By _____ the patient will have improved reality testing	1. Evaluate and observe for hallucinations. Redirect the patient back to reality by distracting her with conversation. 2. Avoid touching the patient. Reduce environmental stimuli.	1. Early assessment may prevent escalation of behavior into aggression. 2. Distortion of reality may lead to misinterpretation of a physical touch, and along with excessive environmental stimuli, can increase the patient's anxiety and precipitate a hallucination.
	3. Administer antipsychotic medications as ordered.	3. Antipsychotic (neuroleptic) agents reduce psychotic symptoms, such as hallucinations.
	4. Determine when anxiety increases. Stay with the patient to ensure safety.	4. Escalating anxiety often precedes hallucinations.
By _____ the patient will interact with others without hallucinating.	1. Assist the patient to increase social interaction gradually, starting first with one-to-one interaction and then progressing to small groups. 2. Be available in a consistent, no-demand supportive relationship.	1–2. Social isolation and lack of interpersonal relationships contribute to the use of hallucinations as a substitute for human interaction. A slow, gradual approach to interaction with others based on reality allows the opportunity for some desensitization because interpersonal contacts often precipitate anxiety.
By _____ the patient will be able to understand the hallucinatory experience and how it relates to stress and anxiety.	1. Investigate with the patient sources of stress and explain the relationship of anxiety and stress on the hallucinations. 2. Teach the patient to verbalize fears and methods to manage anxiety and stress constructively.	1. Hallucinations can be reduced by taking medications and reducing stress. 2. Verbalization of fears reduces anxiety. Alternative coping methods may help the patient manage anxiety.

EVALUATION

Formative Evaluation: Cindy met all of the short-term goals. Her hallucinations stopped after her medication was stabilized.

Summative Evaluation: Cindy achieved the expected outcome of being able to test reality. With time, she was able to refrain from responding to internal visions and voices. She understood the importance of taking her medication and was hopeful that it would control her symptoms. Her roommate remained supportive to her during the entire hospitalization process. Cindy learned not only to listen to her own feelings, fears, and concerns but also to share with her roommate (who had some of the same fears) some of her fears about college and "being on her own."

Conclusions

Andreasen (1994) speaks for anyone whose life has been touched by schizophrenia, when she describes this illness as a terrible disease. Keith, Rieger, and Judd (1988) summarized the result of schizophrenia as an assault on "virtually everything that is distinctly 'human'" (p. 1). These authors also believed no other illness of the 20th century combined the "frequency of occurrence, degree of disability, and squandered human potential that characterizes Schizophrenia" (p. 1). However, in the later years of the 1990s, rays of hope for new treatments and better understanding of the illness were emerging. Increasing sophistication in brain research is one of the hopeful advances of our lifetime. Although our understanding of the disease has increased, we still know little.

Present treatments are directed at controlling symptoms and somehow learning to live with the illness. No current treatment even hints at curing schizophrenia. Although we need to support continuing research directed at identifying specific causes and effective treatments, our attention must equally be directed to the caring aspect of treatment. Instead of stigmatizing and blaming the person with schizophrenia or their family, we need to develop programs that decrease family burden, to recognize the commitment to care made by families, and to reach out with compassion to the suffering individual. Krauss and Gourley (cited in Backlar, 1994) viewed the psychiatric nurse as "the bridge between diagnosis and treatment of the disease and recovery from the illness—between clinical management and day-to-day living" (p. 163). The psychiatric nurse, who frequently has extensive contact with patients and their families over a long period, knows these problems and needs to be a voice for improved care of the mentally ill.

Key Points to Remember

- Schizophrenia is to psychiatry what cancer is to medicine. The toll is tragic in patients, families, and society as a whole.
- Schizophrenia typically strikes in late adolescence or early adulthood.
- Most people with schizophrenia become chronic victims of the disease.
- In schizophrenia, normal perceptions of reality become distorted, resulting in auditory, visual, olfactory, or gustatory hallucinations; delusions; illusions; and a variety of other symptoms.
- A defect in the limbic system of the brain resulting in an inability to filter and select stimuli is suspected in many instances of schizophrenia.
- Schizophrenia is considered a formal thought disorder, although more than thoughts are involved in the illness.
- Because of their difficulty in communicating and relating, patients with schizophrenia pose a challenge to the psychiatric nurse.
- Kraepelin distinguished the symptoms of schizophrenia from manic-depressive psychosis.
- Bleuler identified the four "A's" of schizophrenia: affect, association, autism, and ambivalence.
- Schneider identified first-rank and second-rank symptoms of schizophrenia.
- Andreasen and her colleagues identified schizophrenia by the presence of positive, negative, and disorganized symptoms.
- The IPSS identified a 12-point diagnostic system that standardized diagnosis of schizophrenia across nine cultures.
- The DSM-IV identifies specific symptoms that must be met in diagnosing Schizophrenia and specifies that the symptoms must have been present for at least 6 months.
- The DSM-IV classifies Schizophrenia according to course and subtype.
- Current research into the cause of schizophrenia has focused on the structure and function of the brain and the role of the limbic system, genetic factors, dopamine, and viral transmission.
- Conventional and atypical antipsychotic medications are the first-line treatment of choice for the symptoms of schizophrenia.
- Assessment of the patient with schizophrenia involves assessing positive, disorganized, and negative symptoms; psychosocial and family support; spiritual and religious issues; and comorbidity with depression, a coexisting medical condition, and substance abuse.
- Nursing diagnoses use the symptom descriptions provided by medical diagnoses but expand those descriptions to include the patient's response to symptoms.
- Expected outcomes and short-term goals for a patient with schizophrenia must be realistic and allow for periods of exacerbation.
- Implementation includes medication issues, teaching the patient and family to identify and manage symptoms, supportive counseling, psychoeducation and support for families, managing a coexisting substance abuse problem, and spiritual interventions.
- Evaluation includes focusing on the immediate stabilization of the symptoms of the patient with schizophrenia in the midst of an acute exacerbation as well as the long-term adjustment of the patient.

Learning Activities

1. Read Mark Vonnegut's *The Eden Express* (1975), Lori Schiller's *The Quiet Room* (1994), or Peter Wyden's *Conquering Schizophrenia* (1998). What impressions do you get about schizophrenia? How does what you read challenge your stereotypes of schizophrenia?

2. Attend a NAMI meeting in your area. Observe the responses of the attendees to the illness of a family member or themselves. Compare their stories to those of Lori (*The Quiet Room*) and Jeff (*Conquering Schizophrenia*) and their families.

3. Research your community's resources. What is available for the long-term support of patients with schizophrenia and their families?
4. Ask five people what they know about schizophrenia. Compare what they tell you with the facts about schizophrenia. How does lack of knowledge contribute to stigma and discrimination?
5. View the videotape *Full of Sound and Fury* (may be available at a local library near you). Identify positive, disorganized, and negative symptoms observable in patients with schizophrenia who are featured in the film.
6. Invite some classmates to join you and visit Ian Chovil on his website (http://www.mgl.ca/~chovil). Discuss the information you have about schizophrenia and compare this with Ian's story. What contribution do

you perceive he is making and what is your impression of this resource for patients and their families? Would you use this resource as a referral?
7. Try to imagine yourself with a disease such as schizophrenia. Your brain no longer works the way that it used to or the way that it should, but you still have the same needs for love, companionship, friendship, and understanding. How do you think you would be treated? What do you think and feel about your own answer?
8. Reflect on the impact of advances in brain research into the causes of schizophrenia on stigma and discrimination. How might new knowledge change public perception of mental illness?
9. Identify something you can do in your community to reduce stigma. How might you implement this action?

Critical Thinking Exercise

Mr. Rhodes, a 39-year-old patient who was due to be discharged from the mental health unit in 2 days, watched the nurses discussing the flow of patient activity on the unit. About 20 minutes later, as he was approached by the nurse to plan for discharge, Mr. Rhodes said to the nurse, "You put thoughts into my head, didn't you?"

1. What assumption is the patient making?
2. What evidence suggests that the patient's conclusion may be faulty?
3. What inferences can the nurse draw from the patient's statement?

Based on her keen observational skills and her knowledge of patients with thought disorders, the nurse responded, "Mr. Rhodes, I did not put any thoughts in your head. It sounds like it is a very frightening experience for you. Tell me about it."

1. What conclusions has the nurse drawn about the patient's thought system?
2. What is the style of intervention?
3. What are alternative approaches that the nurse might use?

Additional Resources

Medic Alert Foundation

2323 Colorado Avenue
Turlock, CA 95382
800-432-5378
A Medic Alert bracelet or necklace is available with a 1-year membership, and there is a program for people who cannot afford the fees. It is a simple tool to ensure that people with schizophrenia receive proper care in an emergency department or to help family members find a loved one who has stopped taking medication and is experiencing behavioral problems in public.

The Mental Illness Education Project, Inc.

22-D Hollywood Avenue
Hohokus, NJ 07423
800-343-5540
201-652-1973 (fax)
New videotape for families and mental health professionals entitled, Families Coping with Mental Illness.

National Alliance for Research on Schizophrenia and Depression (NARSAD)

60 Cutter Mill Road
Suite 404
Great Neck, NY 11021
516-824-0091
516-487-6930 (fax)
NARSAD provides an informative newsletter.

National Alliance for the Mentally Ill (NAMI)

200 North Glebe Road
Suite 1015
Arlington, VA 22203-3754
800-950-6264 (helpline)
703-524-9094 (fax)
http://www.nami.org
NAMI support programs: contact your local NAMI chapter or the national office. Family to Family Education Program: a 12-session course for families of people with serious mental illnesses. Living With Schizophrenia: a 2-session program presented by consumers to other consumers.

Continued on following page

Additional Resources *Continued*

National Institute of Mental Health (NIMH)

Public Inquiries Branch
National Institute of Mental Health
Room 7C-02
5600 Fishers Lane
Rockville, MD 20857
Booklet prepared by the Schizophrenia Research Branch, NIMH, entitled, *Schizophrenia: Questions and Answers* (DHHS Publication No. ADM 90-1457), lists other organizations for family and patient support.

Person-to-Person

P.O. Box 21510
Boulder, CO 80308-4510
800-376-8282
http://www.mentalwellness.com
Provides free educational and support services for people taking risperidone (Risperdal). Developed by Janssen Pharmaceutica.

Schizophrenia Society of Canada

814-75 The Donway West
Don Mills
Ontario M3C 2E9
416-445-8204
416-445-2270 (fax)

Zyprexa Patient Assistance Program
P.O. Box 25768
Alexandria, VA 22313
800-488-2133
Designed to assist providers, patients, and patient caregivers through reimbursement support and through temporary provision of olanzepine (Zyprexa) at no charge to eligible patients.

References

American Psychiatric Association. (1994). *Diagnostic and statistical manual of mental disorders* (4th ed.). Washington, DC: Author.

American Psychiatric Association. (1997). Practice guideline for the treatment of patients with schizophrenia. *American Journal of Psychiatry, 154,* (Suppl.), 1-63.

Andreasen, N. (1984). *The broken brain: The biological revolution.* New York: Harper & Row.

Andreasen, N. (1994). Introduction. In P. Backlar, *The family face of schizophrenia: True stories of mental illness with practical advice from America's leading experts.* New York: Putnam's.

Andreasen, N., & Black, D. (1995). *Introductory textbook of psychiatry.* Washington, DC: American Psychiatric Press.

Andreasen, N., & Carpenter, W. (1993). Diagnosis and classification of schizophrenia. In D. Shore (Ed.), *Special report: Schizophrenia 1993* (pp. 25-40). Rockville, MD: National Institute of Mental Health.

Andreasen, N., Nasrallah, H., Dunn, V., Olson, S. C., Grove, W. M., Ehrhardt, J. C., Coffman, J. A., & Crossett, J. H. W. (1986). Structural abnormalities in the frontal system in schizophrenia. *Archives of General Psychiatry, 43,* 136-144.

Andreasen, N., & Olsen, S. (1982). Negative v. positive schizophrenia. *Archives of General Psychiatry, 39,* 789-794.

Anonymous. (1996). First person account: Social, economic, and medical effects of schizophrenia. *Schizophrenia Bulletin, 22,* 183-185.

Arieti, S. (1976). *Creativity: The magic synthesis.* New York: Harper Colophon.

Arieti, S. (1979). *Understanding and helping the schizophrenic: A guide for family and friends.* New York: Simon and Schuster.

Backlar, P. (1994). *The family face of schizophrenia: True stories of mental illness with practical advice from America's leading experts.* New York: Putnam's.

Bayley, R. (1996). First person account: Schizophrenia. *Schizophrenia Bulletin, 22,* 727-729.

Becker, R. E. (1988). Depression in schizophrenia. *Hospital and Community Psychiatry, 39,* 1269-1275.

Bentley, V. (1994). My fight for dignity. *Journal of Psychosocial Nursing and Mental Health Services, 32*(3), 48.

Black, D., & Andreasen, N. (1994). Schizophrenia, schizophreniform disorder, and delusional (paranoid) disorder. In R. Hales, S. Yudofsky, & J. Talbott (Eds.), *The American Psychiatric Press textbook of psychiatry* (2nd ed.). Washington, DC: American Psychiatric Press.

Breier, A., Buchanan, R. W., Elkashef, A., Munson, R. C., Kirkpatrick, B., Gellad, F. (1992). Brain morphology and schizophrenia. *Archives of General Psychiatry, 49,* 921-926.

Brooker, C. (1990). The health education needs of families caring for a schizophrenia relative and the potential role for community psychiatric nurses. *Journal of Advanced Nursing, 15,* 1092-1098.

Buckley, P. (1998a). (Guest Ed.) Preface. *Psychiatric Clinics of North America, 21,*(1) xiii-xv.

Buckley, P. (1998b). Structural brain imaging in schizophrenia. *Psychiatric Clinics of North America, 21*(1), 77-92.

Byrne, C. M., Woodside, H., Landeen, J., Kirkpatrick, H., Bernardo, A., & Pawlick, J. (1994). The importance of relationships in fostering hope. *Journal of Psychosocial Nursing, 32*(9), 31-34.

Caligiuri, M. P., Lohr, J. B., Panton, D., & Braff, D. L. (1993). Extrapyramidal motor abnormalities associated with late life psychosis. *Schizophrenia Bulletin, 19,* 747-754.

Carpenter, W. (1987). Approaches to knowledge and understanding of schizophrenia. *Schizophrenia Bulletin, 13,* 1-18.

Carpenter, W., & Buchanan, R. (1995). Schizophrenia: Introduction and overview. In H. Kaplan, & B. Sadock (Eds.), *Comprehensive textbook of psychiatry* (6th ed., pp. 889-901). Baltimore: Williams & Wilkins.

Carpenter, W., & Kirkpatrick, B. (1988). The heterogeneity of the long-term course of schizophrenia. *Schizophrenia Bulletin, 14,* 645-652.

Carson, V. B. (1994, January). Spiritual issues in the care of the mentally ill. *DRADA Newsletter, 2.*

Carter, R., & Golant, S. (1998). *Helping someone with mental illness: A compassionate guide for family, friends, and caregivers.* New York: Times Books.

Castle, D. J., & Murray, R. M. (1993). The epidemiology of late-onset schizophrenia. *Schizophrenia Bulletin, 19,* 691-700.

Chovil, I. (1988). A mouse-guided tour of schizophrenia. *Living with Schizophrenia, 2*(3), 8-10.

Crow, T. J. (1980). Molecular pathology of schizophrenia: More than one disease process? *British Medical Journal, 280,* 66-68.

Crow, T. J. (1993). Should contagion be resurrected?—A response to Butler and Stieglitz. *Schizophrenia Bulletin, 19,* 455-460.

Cuesta, M. J., & Peralta, V. (1994). Lack of insight in schizophrenia. *Schizophrenia Bulletin, 20*(2), 359-366.

Docherty, N. M., DeRosa, M., & Andreasen, N. (1996). Communication disturbances in schizophrenia and mania. *Archives of General Psychiatry, 53,* 358-364.

Dworkin, R. (1994). Pain insensitivity in schizophrenia: A neglected phenomenon and some implications. *Schizophrenia Bulletin, 20,* 235-248.

Dworkin, R. H., Cornblatt, B. A., Friedman, R., Kaplansky, L. M., Lewis, J. A., Rinaldi, A., Shilliday, C., & Erlenmeyer-Kimling, L. (1993). Childhood precursors of affective vs social deficits in adolescents at risk for schizophrenia. *Schizophrenia Bulletin, 19,* 563-578.

Erlenmeyer-Kimling, L., Cornblatt, B. A., Rock, D., Roberts, S., Bell, M., & West, A. (1993). The New York high-risk project: Anhedonia, attentional deviance, and psychopathology. *Schizophrenia Bulletin, 19,* 141-152.

Fenton, W. S., Blyler, C. R., & Heinssen, R. K. (1997). Determinants of medication compliance in schizophrenia: Empirical and clinical findings. *Schizophrenia Bulletin, 23,* 637-651.

Flynn, L. (1994). Schizophrenia from a family point of view: A social and economic perspective. In N. Andreasen (Ed.), *Schizophrenia from mind to molecule.* Washington, DC: American Psychiatric Press.

Frances, A., Docherty, J., & Kahn, D. (1996). The expert consensus treatment guidelines project for schizophrenia: A guide for patients and families. *Journal of Clinical Psychiatry, 57*(Suppl. 12B), 51-58.

Frese, F. J. III. (1998). Advocacy, recovery, and the challenges of consumerism for schizophrenia. *Psychiatric Clinics of North America, 21,* 233-249.

Frese, F. J. III. (1994). A calling. *Second Opinion, 19*(3), 11-25.

Gerace, L. M., Camilleri, D., & Ayers, L. (1993). Sibling perspectives on schizophrenia and the family. *Schizophrenia Bulletin, 19,* 637-648.

Goldstein, M. (1987). Psychosocial issues. *Schizophrenia Bulletin, 13,* 157-167.

Gournay, K. (1993). Trends in managing schizophrenia. *Nursing Standard, 7*(12), 31-36.

Grossberg, G. (1997). The older schizophrenic. *Treatment Today, 9*(2), 19, 23.

Gur, R. E., & Pearlson, G. D. (1993). Neuroimaging in schizophrenia research. *Schizophrenia Bulletin, 19,* 337-353.

Hagerty, B. (1984). *Psychiatric mental health assessment.* St. Louis: C. V. Mosby.

Harris, E. (1988). The antipsychotics. *American Journal of Nursing, 88,* 1508-1512.

Hatfield, A., & Lefley, H. (Eds.). (1987). *Families of the mentally ill: Coping and adaptation.* New York: Guilford Press.

Herz, M., Keith, S., & Docherty, J. (Eds.). (1990). *Psychosocial treatment of schizophrenia* (Vol. 4). Amsterdam: Elsevier.

Hogarty, G., Anderson, C., Russ, D., Korblith, S., Greenwald, D., & Javna, C. (1990). Family psychoeducation, social skills training and maintenance chemotherapy in the aftercare of schizophrenia. *Archives of General Psychiatry, 43,* 633-642.

Howard, P. (1994). Lifelong maternal caregiving for children with schizophrenia. *Archives of Psychiatric Nursing, 8*(2), 107-114.

Jackson, R. T., & Haynes-Johnson, V. (1988). Nutritional management of patients undergoing long-term antipsychotic and antidepressant therapies. *Archives of Psychiatric Nursing, 2*(3), 146-152.

Jarboe, K. S., & Kitts, C. D. (1988). Diagnosis, neurobiology and treatment of first-episode schizophrenia. The continuum of psychosis: Antipsychotic management. *Journal of the American Psychiatric Nurses Association, 4*(Suppl.), S2-S9.

Jeste, D., Gladsjo, J. A., Linfamer, L. A., & Lacro, J. P. (1996). Medical comorbidity in schizophrenia. *Schizophrenia Bulletin, 22,* 413-430.

Jones, P., & Cannon, M. (1998). The new epidemiology of schizophrenia. *Psychiatric Clinics of North America, 21*(1), 1-25.

Kane, C., Dimartino, E., & Jimenez, M. (1990). A comparison of short-term psychoeducational and support groups for relatives coping with chronic schizophrenia. *Archives of Psychiatric Nursing, 4,* 343-353.

Kane, J., & Marder, S. (1993). Psychopharmacologic treatment of schizophrenia. In D. Shore (Ed.) *Special report: Schizophrenia.* Rockville, MD: National Institute of Mental Health.

Kaplan, H., & Sadock, B. (1995). *Comprehensive textbook of psychiatry* (6th ed.). Baltimore: Williams & Wilkins.

Karno, M., & Norquist, G. (1995). Schizophrenia: Epidemiology. In H. Kaplan & B. Sadock (Eds.), *Comprehensive textbook of psychiatry* (6th ed., pp. 902-910). Baltimore: Williams & Wilkins.

Kay, S. R. (1990). Significance of the positive-negative distinction in schizophrenia. *Schizophrenia Bulletin, 16,* 635-652.

Kay, S. R., Opler, L. A., & Lindenmayer, J. P. (1989). The positive and negative syndrome scale (PANSS): Rationale and standardization. *British Journal of Psychiatry, 155*(Suppl. 7), 59-65.

Keith, S. J., Reiger, D. A., & Judd, L. J. (Eds.). (1988). Schizophrenia: The disorder and its scope. *A national plan for schizophrenia research: report of the National Advisory Mental Health Council* (pp. 1-2). Publ. No. (ADM) 88-1571. Rockville, MD: National Institute of Mental Health.

Kendler, K. S., & Diehl, S. R. (1995). Schizophrenia: Genetics. In H. Kaplan & B. Sadock (Eds.). *Comprehensive textbook of psychiatry* (6th ed., pp. 942-957). Baltimore: Williams & Wilkins.

Kcty, S. (1985). Schizotypal personality disorder: An operational definition of Bleuler's latent schizophrenia? *Schizophrenia Bulletin, 11*(4), 590-594.

Koenigsberg, H. W., & Handley, R. (1986). Expressed emotion: From predictive index to clinical construct. *American Journal of Psychiatry, 143,* 1361-1373.

Larson, D., Milano, M. G., & Barry, C. (1996). Religion: The forgotten factor in health care. *Electric Library,* 1-10.

Larson, D. B., & Larson, S. S. (1991). Religious commitment and health: Valuing the relationship. *Second Opinion, 17*(1), 26-40.

Leete, E. (1987). The treatment of schizophrenia: A patient's perspective. *Hospital and Community Psychiatry, 38*(5), 486-491.

Lefley, H. (1992). Expressed emotion: Conceptual, clinical, and social policy issues. *Hospital and Community Psychiatry, 43*(6), 591-598.

Lehman, A. F., Steinwachs, D. M., & Coinvestigators (1998). At issue: Translating research into practice: The schizophrenia patient outcomes research team (PORT) treatment recommendations. *Schizophrenia Bulletin, 24*(1), 1-32.

Liddle, P. (1987). Symptoms of chronic schizophrenia: A reexamination of positive-negative dichotomy. *British Journal of Psychiatry, 151* (8), 145-151.

Littrall, K., & Magill, A. M. (1993). The effect of clozapine on preexisting tardive dyskinesia. *Journal of Psychosocial Nursing and Mental Health Services, 31*(9), 14-18.

Malloy, Ruth. (1988). First person account: My voyage through turbulence. *Schizophrenia Bulletin, 24,* 495-497.

Marder, S., & Meibach, R. (1994). Risperidone in the treatment of schizophrenia. *American Journal of Psychiatry, 151,* 825-835.

McDowd, J. M., Filion, D. L., Harris, J., & Braff, D. L. (1993). Sensory gating and inhibitory function in late-life schizophrenia. *Schizophrenia Bulletin, 19,* 733-746.

McGlashan, T. H., & Fenton, W. S. (1993). The positive-negative distinction in schizophrenia. *Archives of General Psychiatry, 49*(1), 63-72.

McGlashan, T. H. (1994). Psychosocial treatment of schizophrenia: The potential of relationships. In N. Andreasen (Ed.), *Schizophrenia: From mind to molecule.* Washington, DC: American Psychiatric Association.

McGlashan, T. H., & Johannessen, J. O. (1996). Early detection and intervention with schizophrenia: Rationale. *Schizophrenia Bulletin, 22,* 201-222.

Miklowitz, D. (1994). Family risk indicators in schizophrenia. *Schizophrenia Bulletin, 20,* 137-146.

Möller, H. J. (1994). Pharmacotherapy for negative symptoms. *Interview for Current Approaches to Psychoses Diagnosis and Management* (Vol. 3, pp. 1, 3-4). Princeton, NJ: Excerpta Medica, Inc.

Moller, M. (1996, November/December). Practical points to enhance the effectiveness of medications: Part two. *NAMI Advocate,* 16-17.

Moller, M., & Wer, J. (1989). Simultaneous patient/family education regarding schizophrenia: The Nebraska model. *Archives of Psychiatric Nursing, 3,* 332-337.

Moller, M. D., & Murphy, M. F. (1997). The three R's rehabilitation program: A prevention approach for the management of relapse symptoms associated with psychiatric diagnosis. *Psychiatric Rehabilitation Journal, 20*(3), 42-48.

Moller, M. D., & Murphy, M. F. (1998). *Recovering from psychosis: A wellness approach.* Nine Mile Falls, WA: Psychiatric Rehabilitation Nurses, Inc.

Murphy, M. F., & Moller, M. (1993). Relapse management in neurobiological disorders: The Moller-Murphy management tool. *Archives of Psychiatric Nursing, 7,* 226-235.

NAMI Advocate, 15. (1994, January).

Norris, E., & Naegle, M. (1990). The complexities of treating the dually diagnosed substance abuser. *Addictions Nursing Network, 2*(4), 4-7.

Nuechterlein, K. H., Dawson, M. E., Ventura, J., Goldstein, M. J., Snyder, K. S., & Mintz, J. (1992). Developmental processes in schizophrenic disorders: Longitudinal studies of vulnerability and stress. *Schizophrenia Bulletin, 18,* 387-424.

O'Connor, F. (1991). Symptom monitoring for relapse prevention in schizophrenia. *Archives of Psychiatric Nursing, 5,* 193-201.

Pettegrew, J. W., Keshaven, M. S., & Minshaw, N. J. (1993). ^{31}P nuclear magnetic resonance spectroscopy: Neurodevelopment and schizophrenia. *Schizophrenia Bulletin, 19,* 35-53.

Prager, S., & Jeste, D. V. (1993). Sensory impairment in late-life schizophrenia. *Schizophrenia Bulletin, 19,* 755-772.

Reinhard, S. C. (1994). Perspectives on the family's caregiving experience in mental illness. *Image: Journal of Nursing Scholarship, 26*(1), 70-74.

Rupp, A., & Keith, S. J. (1993). The costs of schizophrenia assessing the burden. *Psychiatric Clinics of North America, 16,* 413-423.

Rosenfeld, M. (1998, July 31). Tears of blood for families of schizophrenia, a gunman's shots strike at their hearts. *The Washington Post,* p. B1.

Savage, P. (1991). Patient assessment in psychiatric nursing. *Journal of Advanced Nursing, 16,* 311-316.

Schiller, L., & Bennett, A. (1994). *The quiet room.* New York: Warner Books, Inc.

Secunda, V. (1997). *When madness comes home: Help and hope for children, siblings, and partners of the mentally ill.* New York: Hyperion.

Simon, C. (1997). *Mad house: Growing up in the shadow of mentally ill siblings.* New York: Doubleday.

Suddath, R., Christison, G., Torrey, E. F., Casanova, M. F., & Weinberger, D. R. (1990). Anatomical abnormalities in the brains of monozygotic twins discordant for schizophrenia. *New England Journal of Medicine, 322,* 789-794.

Suska, M. A. (1991). *Cry of the invisible.* Baltimore: Conservatory Press.

Torrey, E. F. (1995). *Surviving schizophrenia: A manual for families, consumers, and providers* (3rd ed.). New York: HarperCollins.

Torrey, E. F. (1997). *Out of the shadows: Confronting America's mental illness crisis.* New York: John Wiley.

TV Ontario in association with Mental Health Division of Health & Welfare of Canada and Association of General Hospitals Psychiatric Services. (Producer), & Magidson, D. (Director). *Full of sound and fury* [Film]. (Available from Filmakers Library, Inc., 124 East 40th Street, Suite 901, New York, NY 10016.)

Utas, J., & Cotman, C. W. (1993). Excitatory amino acid receptors in schizophrenia. *Schizophrenia Bulletin, 19,* 105-117.

Van Devere, T., quoted in *Schizophrenia: Youth's greatest disabler.* Richmond, British Columbia, Canada: British Columbia Schizophrenia Society.

Vonnegut, M. (1975). *The Eden express.* New York: Praeger.

Weiden, P. J., & Olfson, M. (1995). Cost of relapse in schizophrenia. *Schizophrenia Bulletin, 21,* 419-429.

Weiden, P., Raphin, B., Mott, M., & Frances, A. (1994). Rating of medication influences (ROMI) scale in schizophrenia. *Schizophrenia Bulletin, 20,* 247-310.

Wiedemann, G., Hahlweg, K., Hank, G., Feinstein, E., Muller, U., & Dose, M. (1994). Deliverability of psychoeducational family management. *Schizophrenia Bulletin, 20,* 547-556.

Willick, M. S. (1994). Schizophrenia: A parents' perspective—mourning without end. In N. Andreasen (Ed.), *Schizophrenia: From mind to molecule.* Washington, DC: American Psychiatric Press.

Winship, W. (1993). First person account: How do I let go? *Schizophrenia Bulletin, 19,* 853-854.

Winter, D. (1990). Questions and answers about schizophrenia. *Journal of Psychosocial Nursing, 28*(8), 7.

Wolkin, A., Sanfilipo, M., Wolf, A. P., Angrist, B., Brodie, J. D., & Rotrosen, J. (1992). Negative symptoms and hypofrontality in chronic schizophrenia. *Archives of General Psychiatry, 49,* 959-965.

Wong, D. F., Wagner, H. N., Tune, L. E., Dannals, R. F., Pearlson, G. D., Links, J. M., Tamminga, C. A., Broussolle, E. P., Ravert, H. T., Wilson, A. A., Toung, J. K. T., Malat, J., Williams, J. A., O'Tuama, L. A., Snyder, S. H., Kuhar, M. J., & Gjedde, A. (1986). Positron emission tomography reveals dopamine receptors in drug-naive schizophrenics. *Science, 234,* 1558-1563.

Wyatt, R., Kirch, D., & Egan, M. (1995). Schizophrenia: Neurochemical, viral and immunological studies. In H. Kaplan & B. Sadock (Eds.), *Comprehensive textbook of psychiatry* (6th ed.). Baltimore: Williams & Wilkins.

Wyden, P. (1998). *Conquering schizophrenia: A father, his son, and a medical breakthrough.* New York: Alfred A. Knopf.

Suggested Readings

Backlar, P. (1994). *The family face of schizophrenia: True stories of mental illness with practical advice from America's leading experts.* New York: Putnam's.

Frese, F. J. III. (1994). A calling. *Second Opinion, 19*(3), 11-25.

Schiller, L. & Bennett, A. (1994). *The quiet room.* New York: Warner Books.

Secunda, V. (1997). *When madness comes home: Help and hope for children, siblings and partners of the mentally ill.* New York: Hyperion.

Winter, D. (1990). Questions and answers about schizophrenia. *Journal of Psychosocial Nursing, 28* (8), p. 7.

Wyden, P. (1998). *Conquering schizophrenia: A father, his son and a medical breakthrough.* New York: Alfred A. Knopf.

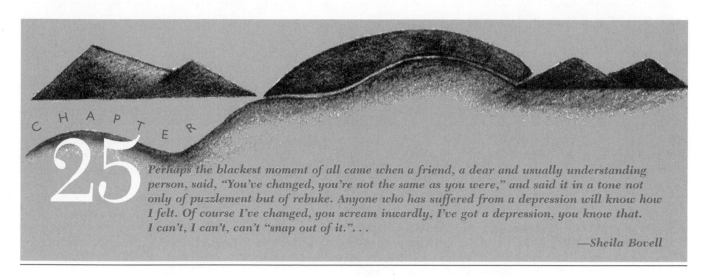

Perhaps the blackest moment of all came when a friend, a dear and usually understanding person, said, "You've changed, you're not the same as you were," and said it in a tone not only of puzzlement but of rebuke. Anyone who has suffered from a depression will know how I felt. Of course I've changed, you scream inwardly, I've got a depression, you know that. I can't, I can't, can't "snap out of it.". . .

—*Sheila Bovell*

Mood Disorders

Learning Objectives

After studying this chapter, you should be able to:

1. Define terms such as depression, mania, affective, bipolar, hypomania, dysthymia, and cyclothymia.

2. Discuss the current research related to pharmacological, neurochemical, endocrinological, and genetic causes of mood disorders.

3. Discuss the association of depression with other medical conditions.

4. Describe the importance of family involvement in the treatment of patients with mood disorders.

5. Describe the emotional, psychological, and spiritual components to consider throughout the nurse-patient journey characterized by mood disorders.

6. Identify expected outcomes for patients with depression and mania.

7. Discuss the treatment options available to patients experiencing mood disorders.

8. Describe the nursing role in each treatment option available to patients experiencing mood disorders.

9. Identify the nursing interventions for assisting families of patients with mood disorders.

10. Apply the nursing process to a patient diagnosed with depression and a patient diagnosed with bipolar disorder mania.

Key Terminology

Affect	Empowerment	Mixed episode	Rapid cycling
Bipolar disorder	Euthymia	Mood	Seasonal affective pattern
Cyclothymia	Hypomania	Postpartum depressive	Self-attitude
Depression	Longitudinal course specifiers	pattern	Vital sense
Dysthymia	Mania		

The mood disorders are characterized by disturbance in mood (profound sadness or apathy, irritability, or elation). This group of disorders is distinguished by two important facts: (1) they rank among the most serious health problems in the United States and (2) they are among the most poorly diagnosed and treated of the health problems in the United States.

No one is immune from mood disorders. They are common in men, women, adolescents, and children. Mood disorders affect the way people feel about themselves and the world in which they live. People with **depression** experience feelings of unbearable sadness or irritability, despair, and hopelessness. They frequently desire suicide. In addition, depression carries with it disturbances in emotional, cognitive, behavioral, somatic, and spiritual dimensions of the individual. People with **mania** experience feelings of excitement, elation, or extreme irritability. Mania also carries disturbances in emotional, cognitive, behavioral, somatic, and spiritual dimensions. Both depression and mania include the possibility of psychotic behavior. All of the mood episodes and mood disorders involve variations of or combinations of depression and mania.

Expenditures related to affective (or mood) disorders in the United States were an estimated $20.8 billion in 1985. By 1990, the total estimated costs had increased to $25.4 billion. The lifetime risk for major depression in men is 5% to 12% and in women, 10% to 25%. In the United States 5% of adults suffer from major depression in any given year. Fifteen percent of the patients with major depression will die by suicide (Hughes, 1997).

Clinical depression commonly co-occurs with general medical illnesses, although it often goes undetected and untreated. In fact, although the rate of major depression among persons in the community is estimated to be about 5%, among primary care patients, it is between 5% and 10%, and among medical inpatients, it is between 10% and 14% (Hays, Wells, Sherbourne, Rogers, & Spritzer, 1995). Research suggests that recognition and treatment of co-occurring depression may improve the outcome of the medical condition, enhance the quality of life, and reduce the degree of pain and disability experienced by the medical patient (Hays, Wells, Sherbourne, Rogers, & Spritzer, 1995).

Affective disorders represent 21% of the costs of all mental illnesses (Rice & Miller, 1995). Clinical depression is a common and highly treatable illness affecting over 17 million American adults—with or without a co-occurring condition—each year. Unfortunately, two thirds of them do not receive treatment, in part because the effects of depression are not understood to be symptoms of an illness. With proper treatment, nearly 80% of those with depressive illness can feel better, and most within a matter of weeks (D/ART, 1999).

About 25% of the first episodes of bipolar disorder occur before age 20. As many as half of the people who experience serious depression also have episodes of mania. About 1.5% of the U.S. population has bipolar disease. Ten percent to 15% of these bipolar patients commit suicide (Bowden, 1997). Hormonal factors may account for the greater rates of rapid cycling (meaning highs and lows in a short period of time) by women, but in general, women and men are equally affected with bipolar disorder (Bowden, 1997).

These illnesses are relapsing, episodic conditions, although their pattern varies with each individual. About 70% of patients who have suffered from depression can expect to face the illness again. The median number of recurrences during a lifetime is four. Women experience more depression than men between ages 18 and 44, and especially after age 25. For some reason, between 44 and 65 years of age, the difference is less pronounced, but after age 65, women are again far more likely to be depressed than men. Not only is depression more common in women but also it is often accompanied by other symptoms such as anxiety, sleep disorders, panic attacks, and eating disorders (Blehar & Oren, 1997).

Peter's Story

April 4, 1983, was a gorgeous spring day. The banners were waving in a balmy breeze, and short sleeves were the order of the day. I was excited and excitable, hopeful and expectant—certainly, a man at ease in his surroundings. In this setting my experience with manic-depressive illness began.

It was the opening-day game for the Baltimore Orioles, a team I have followed religiously for years. Better yet, "The Birds," as true fans call them, were ahead. Normally, I would have been overjoyed by a win in the home opener. But in the sixth inning, in the midst of celebrating with friends and my favorite sports team, I began to feel fuzzy, blurry-eyed, unsure of myself, afraid of the crowd, uneasy about the height of our seats over the field. I became very quiet.

My friends noticed the change in my mood on the way home: my short answers, the lack of life in my voice, my pregame excitement extinguished. I recall telling them that I felt that my mind was tired, but now I know that on that day I came face-to-face with my first biochemical depression.

Recognition of Illness

I was born and live today in a small town in West Virginia where I practice medicine. I am fortunate to have a loving, caring wife who is also my best friend. We have three children, ages 12, 6, and 4. The 6-year-old is a boy, surrounded by his sisters in age.

Looking at my family tree, I should not have been surprised to have psychiatric illness at some point in my life. My great-grandfather exhibited times of great activity and great melancholy, according to my grandmother's writings. She herself was diagnosed with manic-depressive illness, but she was never treated. My father was an alcoholic who died as a result of his drinking. His life included great business successes and failures, several divorces, and frequent depressions.

With what I suppose was an inherited predisposition, I met with several stresses during the months before the Orioles' opening day. My grandmother, with whom I enjoyed a very close relationship all my life, passed away. In the same month, my father died.

My wife and I were expecting a new baby at the end of April. My work weeks at my office climbed to 75 hours.

The low and fearful mood I experienced at the game was just the beginning. For weeks, I progressively lost more and more motivation, curiosity, and creativity. My appetite waned, and my sleep was disturbed. At first, I sought relief in my office and tried, literally, to work through it. I realized that this was not a solution when one morning I could not force myself to get out of bed and go to work.

Treatment

I saw a doctor and got medication, but it seemed to work too well; and I became manic. I became oblivious to reason and experienced extreme financial difficulties as a result of spending sprees. Delusions of grandeur, sexual indiscretions, and extreme irritability threatened my marriage.

For 5 months, I experienced cycles of mania and depression every 10 days. My doctor tried changing the dosage of my medication. My wife, Karen, and I both knew what was sure to follow with each new cycle, and the feeling was oppressive. We were unable to count on anything enjoyable in the future, knowing that I would be unreachably high, severely depressed and anxious, or in transition from one to the other.

When I look back on that period of several months, I wonder at the fact that my wife stayed with me. I am thankful that she was able to remember things about me when I was well that helped to carry her through this low point of our time together.

Still seeing no improvement, I became a research volunteer at the National Institute of Mental Health (NIMH) on September 14, 1983. As time passed, a more effective medication for my particular brand of bipolar disorder was found; the proper dosage was determined, and I improved immediately. While it was extremely difficult being away from my family and my work during my stay at the NIMH, I had many introspective moments to think about piecing my life back together.

Rehabilitation

Before I returned home, I began to carefully rebuild my marriage, faith, friendships, and business. My wife never wavered, nor, at its foundation, did my faith. Former friends looked askance, as if they could not believe that I was now "normal" after being on a "psych ward." Present friends were happy for my health and interested in the new genetic principles behind the biochemistry of my illness. I called each of my own patients to inform them of my renewed well-being and to assess their intentions. This was an incredibly difficult experience, but it was central to my plans to reestablish myself professionally.

Today, I continue to take only lithium carbonate. Minor mood swings still come and go with this medication but not of a severity near that which I experienced during 1983. I have not missed a day of work or of active living since March 26, 1984, when I first returned to the practice of dentistry. I complain at times about the increased appetite, some weight gain, and the occasional fatigue that I experience with the medication, but I continue to take it. Staying well is so important to me.

I went trout fishing recently—one of the few things I love more than the Orioles. When I returned home, Karen told me, as she often does, how happy she was to have me healthy. I was happy to hear that and to feel that. The baby I mentioned as an added stress in 1983 is a beautiful little girl named Erica Marcia.

I reflect often on the five years since her birth and am thankful we are all together. I don't know whether we need to be concerned about Erica or our other children having this illness. I hope and pray always that the researchers working on affective disorders have continued success. In the meantime, we all need to help educate Erica and others and give them hope for the future. There is a great deal more to be done in the world. ■

From DePaulo, J. R., Jr., & Ablow, K. R. (1998). *How to cope with depression: A complete guide for you and your family* (pp. 41–43). New York: McGraw-Hill. Reproduced with permission of The McGraw-Hill Companies.

OUR UNDERSTANDING OF MOOD DISORDERS

Almost 90 years ago, Emil Kraeplin best described manic and depressive conditions as two parts of a "single disease process." He also reported that he found nothing wrong in the brains of *affectively ill* (referring to mood disorders) patients who had died and that he could offer no truly effective treatments. As a result, there was doubt that these conditions were bodily diseases. The doubt about a physiological explanation gave greater credence to psychoanalytic theory as a treatment for the mentally ill. Before long, however, psychiatrists using psychoanalysis realized how ineffective it was with most severely depressed or manic patients. As a result, for many years the most seriously ill individuals were not treated. Recognition and treatment of depression is crucial, especially for medically ill patients. Depressive disorders may adversely affect survival, the length of a hospital stay, compliance with therapy, the ability to care for oneself, and the quality of life (Shelton, 1996).

Within the past 50 years, new medical treatments have evolved that are helpful and safe in the treatment of serious mood disorders. The development of these treatment tools supports the view that major forms of mental illness not only can be distinguished from each other but also respond to specific medical treatments. Often, the optimal benefits of treatment may require up to several months to become manifest. The risk for relapse is minimized for patients who respond to treatment and continue maintenance therapy at the same dosage for at least 2 years. Relapse rates are approximately 50% when a drug is discontinued after 2 years of remission during maintenance treatment (Friedman, Mitchell, & Kocsis, 1995).

Most of the research interest and funding have focused on discovering better psychopharmacological treatments for the disease. Little attention has been paid to the emotional, psychological, and spiritual aspects and origins of mood disorders.

The Impact of Mood Disorders on the Journey

Unfortunately, diagnosis of mood disorders is hampered by our inability to describe moods and changes in mood. This imprecision limits our ability to understand mood problems in a "medical sense." It is not an easy task to discuss basic but complex feelings the same way we talk about physical pain. We can usually describe physical pain by its location, intensity, and beginning.

Mood symptoms are generally more difficult to pinpoint. For instance, the word *depression* is often used to describe unpleasant feelings such as sadness, loss, or nostalgia, which are normal feelings of living. This usage complicates the process of distinguishing the disease of depression, which is a more fundamental and pervasive experience. Depression goes beyond sadness. It seriously affects an individual's feelings about the future and erodes the most basic attitudes about self. Sometimes this depression can deepen and widen to poison self-attitude and feelings about life, creating despair, hopelessness, and spiritual distress.

Mood refers to an individual's pervasive feeling state. A normal mood, also referred to as **euthymia,** refers to what is usual, common, or expected in a given situation (Figure 25-1). For example, when good things happen to us, we find ourselves in a good mood. When we have problems, disappointments, and setbacks, it is normal to be in a bad mood, or to experience **dysthymia.** Normal moods are reactive. Our moods respond and react to situations, to what happens to us, and to what is important to us. Normal mood will change in proportion to life situations. For example, the normal change in mood after the death of a loved one is usually severe and markedly different from the mood change following the loss of an inanimate object.

Historically, there has been considerable controversy about the relationship between long-standing depression and personality traits. The German psychiatrist Kurt Schneider described the concept of a "depressive personality" as an entity distinct from major mood disorders (Goldberg, 1997). Psychoanalytic investigators have linked the depressive personality with masochistic or self-defeating character disorder, distinct in theory from major affective illness (Kernberg, 1988).

Affect is a term closely related to mood. **Affect** refers to the feelings that are reflected on our faces, in our expressions, and by our demeanor. Affect is fleeting. The full range of affect indicates normal changes that occur in our facial reflection of feelings. Flat affect indicates no changes in our facial reflection of feelings.

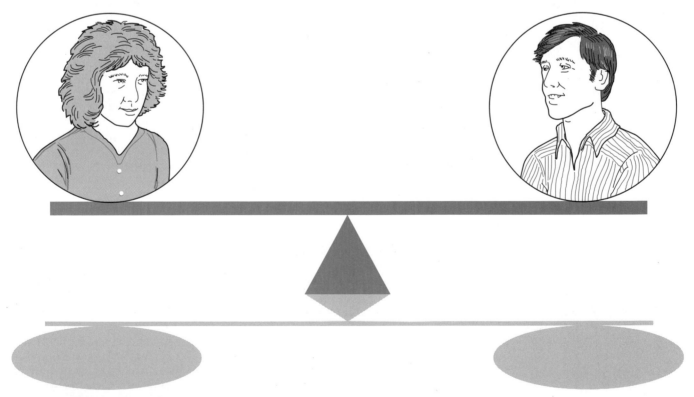

Figure 25-1
The term *euthymia* refers to a normal mood—what is usual, common, or expected in a given situation.

Blunted affect indicates minimal changes in our facial reflection of feelings.

Co-Occurrence of Mood Disorders With Other Disorders

Complicating the course of the mood disorders is a high rate of comorbidity (co-occurrence) with other psychiatric disorders. These include anxiety disorders, substance-related disorders, eating disorders, obsessive-compulsive disorder (OCD), somatization disorders, and personality disorders. In addition, mood disorders have a high rate of co-occurrence with other general medical conditions including stroke, dementia, diabetes, coronary artery disease, cancer, chronic fatigue syndrome, and fibromyalgia.

Co-Occurrence With Other Psychiatric Disorders

Severe forms of anxiety—phobias, panic attacks, obsessions, and compulsions—may occur alone or as a part of depression. People with panic attacks have been found to have a higher-than-expected number of relatives who suffer from a major depressive disorder. Data on eating disorders (anorexia nervosa and bulimia nervosa) suggest that depression is common in young women who suffer from dysregulation of food intake. Data also suggest that focus on the eating disorder, not the depression, is usually the most efficacious approach to treatment. From 80% to 100% of patients who are diagnosed with OCD also experience symptoms of depression. In these patients, the OCD is the focus of treatment. Patients who do not have OCD but present with severe depression often experience problems with obsessive thoughts. In these patients, the depression is the focus of treatment. Depressed patients often see their primary physicians with complaints of aches and pains. Primary physicians often focus entirely on the patient's somatic complaints to the exclusion of the depression. It is vital to recognize and assess somatic symptoms as possible indicators of depression.

Another classification of psychiatric disorders that occur with depression is personality disorders. Generally, when depression is complicated by a personality disorder, the course is more complicated, with increased rates of suicide attempts, self-harm, and treatment failure. In a multiple regression analysis, the only factors that remained significant were personality disorder prior to treatment failure, near delusional status, and younger age. Interestingly, persons with one or no predictors of poor response responded to treatment 91% of the time, whereas those with two or more predictors had only 25% response. This study indicates that there are specific clinical predictors of treatment failure and that combinations of factors exert a more powerful negative effect (Shelton, 1996).

Additional problems are created by the use of substances such as alcohol, nicotine, cocaine or other street drugs, and prescribed drugs. People appear to use these and other drugs to medicate depression or to induce the elevated moods associated with bipolar disorder. The relief provided by these substances is described by some patients as a "calming effect" or by others as "instant energy." Although these drugs may produce short-term relief of the symptoms of depression and mania, they lead to long-term problems of addiction. In his book *Darkness Visible: A Memoir of Madness,* William Styron described the advent of his most menacing forms of depression after he was forced to give up his alcohol addiction (Styron, 1990).

Co-Occurrence With Medical Conditions

At least 10% of major depression stems from a medical illness. Depression occurs in up to 50% of patients with Alzheimer's dementia and can cause worsening of cognitive deficits, particularly memory deficit. Both hypothyroidism and, more rarely, thyrotoxicosis have been shown to cause symptoms of depression. Over 40% of patients with parkinsonism develop depression, as do more than 25% of stroke victims, especially those with left hemispheric strokes (Hays et al., 1995). Depression has been reported with most malignancies and may be present several years before a tumor is diagnosed. In some groups of cancer patients, depression has been found to have an incidence of approximately 40%, suggesting an increased risk of developing depression with a diagnosis of cancer, as well as during treatment (Hays et al., 1995).

In addition, diabetes mellitus, myocardial infarction, head injury and normal-pressure hydrocephalus, central nervous system (CNS) tumors, chronic pain, and infections, especially those of viral origin, are considered contributory factors that are highly associated with the development of depression (Hays et al., 1995).

Patients with depression characteristically complain of fatigue and lack of energy. The complaint of chronic fatigue is not sufficient to meet the criteria for chronic fatigue syndrome. If both depression and chronic fatigue syndrome are present, however, the patient is treated for depression. Patients diagnosed with fibromyalgia have higher lifetime rates of major depressive disorder than do rheumatoid arthritis patients (Pagano, 1996). When fibromyalgia coexists with depression, the depression is treated. Other symptoms noted in the *Diagnostic and Statistical Manual of Mental Disorders, Fourth Edition* (DSM-IV) (American Psychiatric Association [APA] 1994) can include weight loss or gain, insomnia or hypersomnia, guilt, poor concentration, thoughts of death or suicide. Systematic signs and symptoms associated with rheumatoid arthritis include malaise, fatigue, unexpected weight loss, depression, and rheumatoid vasculitis (Pagano, 1996).

Implications of Mood Disorders

The journey toward wellness for individuals with mood disorders involves acceptance that the mood disorder is a medical illness requiring aggressive treatment. These illnesses bring untold misery, along with wasted days, months, and even years of impaired functioning at work and in personal life. Loss of productivity and its economic cost to society affect businesses in the billions of dollars (Hughes, 1997).

These diseases have a frightening mortality rate. Suicide is the most serious complication. In fact, suicide is one of the top 10 causes of death at all ages (Isacsson, Bergman, & Rich, 1996). An estimated 2000 teenagers per year commit suicide in the United States, making it the leading cause of death, after accidents and homicide (Brown, 1996). The most serious symptoms of depression are hopelessness, despair, and a sense of spiritual emptiness. Those who feel that life is meaningless and that God has abandoned them consider suicide a viable option.

As common and as potentially serious as the mood disorders are, one would expect physicians to be vigilant regarding the diagnostic possibility of a mood disorder. Yet these illnesses are misdiagnosed by physicians, misunderstood by the lay public, and too often ignored or considered a character weakness or a temporary difficulty that an individual can just "snap out of." The lack of acceptance by the medical community as well as by the general public increases the difficulty the patient experiences in accepting the illness. Yet acceptance of the illness is a prerequisite for the patient to benefit fully from all available treatment. Only through acceptance can the individual learn to exert control over the illness and to make responsible decisions related to coping with the illness on a daily basis.

Mood disorders are holistic. They affect physical, emotional, cognitive, social, occupational, and spiritual dimensions. Peter described his personal experience with **bipolar disorder** (a mood disorder characterized by extreme shifts in mood from sadness to either elation or irritability). Peter's story is a glimpse into the life of one person with a mood disorder.

What do you think? If Peter had chosen to deny his illness, how different do you think his outcome would have become? Explain. Do you believe that Peter should have discussed his illness with his patients? Give reasons why or why not?

> *Check Your Reading*
> 1. What are the symptoms of depression?
> 2. What are the symptoms of mania?

DEFINING MOOD DISORDERS

Included in mood disorders are mood episodes. These include major depressive, manic, mixed, and hypomanic episodes, which are not disorders in themselves but provide the building blocks for the major disorders. Mood disorders are further categorized into depressive

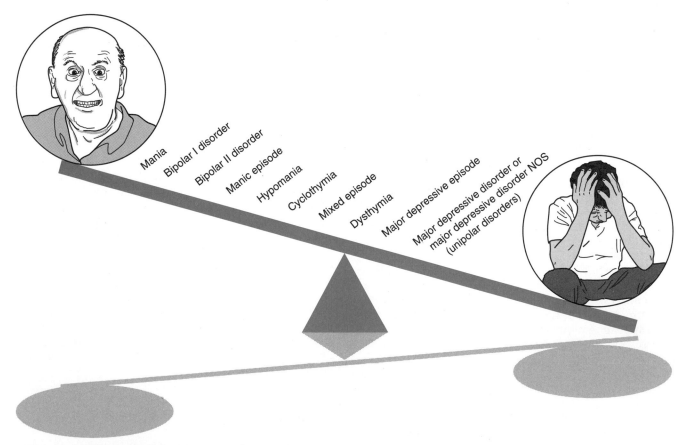

F i g u r e 2 5 – 2
The see-saw continuum of mood disorders.

TABLE 25–1 Definitions of Mood Episodes

Major Depressive Episode	Characterized by feelings of either depression or the loss of interest in nearly all activities. Symptoms must last at least 2 weeks. At least four other symptoms from the following list must be present: changes in appetite or weight, sleep, or psychomotor activity; feelings of worthlessness and guilt; difficulty concentrating or making decisions; recurrent thoughts of death or suicidal ideation, plans, or attempts
Manic Episode	Characterized by a period in which there is a dramatic change in mood; either elation and expansiveness or irritability is present. This change in mood must last at least 1 week (less if hospitalization is required). At least three other symptoms from the following list must be present: inflated self-esteem or grandiosity, decreased need for sleep, pressured speech, flight of ideas, distractibility, increased involvement in goal-directed activities or psychomotor agitation, and overinvolvement in pleasurable activities with potentially damaging consequences (e.g., hypersexuality, impulsive spending)
Mixed Episode	Characterized by rapidly changing, alternating moods (sadness, irritability, euphoria) accompanied by symptoms from both manic and depressive episodes lasting at least 1 week. Disturbance severely affects functioning, may require hospitalization, and may result in the emergence of psychotic behaviors
Hypomanic Episode	Characterized by at least 4 days of abnormally and persistently elevated, expansive, or irritable mood accompanied by at least three additional symptoms seen in a manic episode. Disorder is not severe enough to impair functioning seriously or to require hospitalization. Disorder does not involve psychotic behavior.

disorders (also referred to as unipolar disorders) and bipolar disorders. Depressive disorders include Major Depressive Disorder, Dysthymic Disorder, and Depressive disorder Not Otherwise Specified (APA, 1994). Bipolar disorders include Bipolar I Disorder and Bipolar II Disorder, Cyclothymic Disorder, and Bipolar Disorder Not Otherwise Specified (Figure 25-2). Tables 25-1 to 25-3 provide the definitions of the mood episodes, depressive disorders, and bipolar disorders. Note that some of these conditions involve milder symptoms than those seen in major depressive disorder or bipolar disorder. **Hypomania,** for example, is a manic state not severe enough to impair functioning. **Cyclothymia** involves relatively mild depressive symptoms.

Diagnostic Symptoms

A limitation of the DSM-IV or any other checklist of symptoms is that it does a better job of deciding who should be called depressed or manic than it does of describing the ill person's experience. Emphasis is on the patient's sadness, not on the potentially devastating effects of hopelessness and isolation (Rauch & Hyman, 1995). For instance, knowing that Peter was diagnosed with bipolar disorder provides no information regarding his suffering, the struggles that he experienced in his move toward stability, the personal trials and tribulations he endured, or the support that he received from his wife, Karen. Nursing diagnoses, in contrast, do more to describe the person's experiences.

In diagnosing a mood disorder, the clinician assesses presenting signs and symptoms, the patient's history and prior response to treatment, and the family's history. The central issues are whether the patient is experiencing a persistent change in mood, **self-attitude** (self-esteem or self-confidence), and **vital sense** (physical and bodily health). In Peter's story, all of these

symptoms were present. He described "feeling fuzzy, blurry-eyed, unsure of myself, afraid of the crowd, uneasy about the height of our seats over the field. I became very quiet" (DePaulo, 1989). Peter noted that he had a genetic background that made him vulnerable to developing a mood disorder. His story illustrates the dramatic swing between depression (the feelings that

TABLE 25–2 Definitions of Depressive Disorders

Major Depressive Disorder	A major mood disorder characterized by one (single) or more (recurrent) episodes of major depression, with or without full recovery between episodes
Dysthymic Disorder	A mood disorder characterized by depressed mood and loss of interest or pleasure in activities of life, with some additional signs and symptoms of depression present most of the time for at least 2 years. Many patients with dysthymia go on to develop major depressive episodes.
Depressive Disorder Not Otherwise Specified	A category of mood disorder characterized by specified depressive features that do not meet the criteria for Major Depressive Disorder, Dysthymic Disorder, Adjustment Disorder With Depressed Mood, or Adjustment Disorder With Mixed Anxiety and Depressed Mood

TABLE 25-3 Definitions of Bipolar Disorders

Bipolar I Disorder	A major mood disorder characterized by episodes of major depression and mania or hypomania. The diagnosis of Bipolar I Disorder requires one or more episodes of mania.
Bipolar II Disorder	A major mood disorder characterized by the occurrence of one or more Major Depressive Episodes accompanied by at least one Hypomanic Episode. The presence of a Manic Episode or a Mixed Episode excludes the diagnosis of Bipolar II Disorder.
Cyclothymic Disorder	A mood disorder of at least 2 years' duration characterized by numerous periods of mild depressive symptoms not sufficient in duration or severity to meet the criteria for Major Depressive Episode interspersed with periods of hypomania. Some view this as a mild form of bipolar disorder.
Bipolar Disorder Not Otherwise Specified	A mood disorder characterized by bipolar features that do not meet the criteria for any specific bipolar disorder.

began while watching the baseball game) and the severe symptoms of mania: "I became oblivious to reason and experienced extreme financial difficulties as a result of spending sprees. Delusions of grandeur, sexual indiscretions, and extreme irritability threatened my marriage" (DePaulo, 1989). The primary risk factors for depressive disorder are shown in Box 25-1.

Variations of Mood Disorders

As you can see in Tables 25-1 to 25-3, mood episodes and disorders are all characterized by a dysfunctional regulation of mood. For example, in the mixed affective disorder, or **Mixed Episode,** symptoms of depression

Box 25-1 ■ ■ ■ ■ ■
Risk Factors for Depression

- Prior episodes of depression
- Family history of depressive disorder
- Prior suicide attempts
- Female gender
- Age of onset under 40 years
- Postpartum period
- Medical comorbidity
- Lack of social support
- Stressful life situations
- Current alcohol or substance abuse

and mania occur together. The two most common mixed states are dysphoric (unhappy) mania and exalted depression. In dysphoric mania, individuals have high energy levels, racing thoughts, and pressured speech. Instead of being in an elated mood, however, they report feeling irritable, fearful, or unhappy. Exalted depression is also characterized by depressed mood but is accompanied by grandiose delusions.

In addition to the diagnoses seen in Tables 25-1 to 25-3, the DSM-IV specifies criteria for a patient's most recent mood episodes as

1. Mild, moderate, or severe without psychotic features; severe with psychotic features; in partial remission; or in full remission. These criteria apply to Major Depressive Episode, Manic Episode, and Mixed Episode.
2. With catatonic features
3. With melancholic features
4. With atypical features
5. With postpartum onset

DSM-IV also specifies the course of recurring episodes as

- Longitudinal course specifiers (with or without full interepisode recovery)
- With seasonal pattern
- With rapid cycling

Postpartum depressive pattern describes mood disturbance that can be applied to any of the mood disorders when the onset is within 4 weeks after the delivery of a child. For instance, a woman could be diagnosed with major depressive disorder with postpartum onset or bipolar disorder with postpartum onset. Symptoms of depression seem to be exacerbated in some women during times of dramatic hormonal changes, such as the plummeting levels of estrogen and progesterone during the premenstruum, post partum, and possibly at menopause. Although some women experience a major depressive disorder with postpartum onset, many others experience only transient mood changes. Women with histories of mood disorders before pregnancy are more likely to suffer more severely during the postpartum period and are also at greater risk of developing a mood disorder unrelated to childbirth later in life (Handal, 1998). On the positive side, however, pregnant women often have the lowest incidence of depression. Despite the seriousness of postpartum psychosis, it does not contribute greatly to the prevalence of major mood disorders in women (Blehar & Oren, 1997).

Beck's (1993) study of postpartum depressive pattern cited loss of control as the basic sociopsychological problem. One mother stated, "I had absolutely no control, and that was the scariest thing because I always had control." Women with postpartum depression lack control over their emotions, thought processes, and actions. As one mother described, "I just couldn't get out of the pain. It's like you hurt so bad, and you don't want to be that way, and yet you lose all control of everything." The major problem related to these disorders is delayed recognition and treatment, which affects not only the depressed mother but also her infant and the rest of her family. "When I was sick, I didn't want my baby. I didn't love my husband. I didn't want to work. I hated everything. When I got better, it all melted away" (Beck, 1993, p. 47).

Longitudinal course specifiers are used to characterize the course of illness in patients who experience recurrent Major Depressive Disorder, Bipolar I Disorder, or Bipolar II Disorder. These specifiers are applied to the period between the two most recent episodes. There are four longitudinal course patterns:

1. Recurrent, with full recovery between episodes and with no Dysthymic Disorder
2. Recurrent, without full recovery between episodes and with no Dysthymic Disorder
3. Recurrent, with full recovery between episodes, superimposed on Dysthymic Disorder
4. Recurrent, without full recovery between episodes, superimposed on Dysthmic Disorder

Seasonal affective pattern describes a variation of mood disorder typically characterized by depression occurring in the fall and winter and normal moods in the spring and summer. Less commonly reported are patients with recurrent summer episodes of depression. The disease has been referred to as seasonal affective disorder (SAD). Although the depression in SAD meets all the diagnostic criteria for major depression, several mood symptoms seem to be more common. As in any major depressive disorder, people with SAD have changes in appetite and sleep patterns. The SAD patient, however, almost always has an increase in sleep, complaints of chronic winter fatigue, an increase in appetite, and a craving for sweets and starch-rich foods. SADS patients also selectively eat sweets under emotionally difficult conditions (when depressed, anxious, or lonely) (Krauchi, Reich, & Wirz-Justice, 1997). Seasonal depressions tend to be of the atypical type but even those with an atypical type of depression appear different than SADS patients suggesting that SAD patients are a separate subtype of depression with an overlapping symptom picture (Tam, Lam, Robertson, Stewart, Yatham, & Zis, 1997).

Seasonal variations of mood are believed to be determined by the amount of time exposed to light rather than by temperature changes. Researchers have identified that seasonality of the affective state has been reported to vary indirectly in proportion to the latitude in temperate regions. The higher the latitude, the greater the risk of SAD (Suhail & Cochrane, 1997).

Because people with SAD have difficulty regulating serotonin levels during the winter, their craving for carbohydrates is a way of compensating. This theory explains why patients respond favorably to selective serotonin reuptake inhibitors (SSRIs) such as the antidepressants, fluoxetine (Prozac) and sertraline (Zoloft). However, the cornerstone of treatment is light therapy. Rosenthal (1994) stated that it is not the kind of light but the intensity that matters.

Another theory is focused on melatonin, a hormone produced by the pineal gland, which is strongly influenced by light exposure. Each night, like clockwork, the pineal gland releases melatonin into the bloodstream in minute quantities and continues to do so until dawn. Although it is unclear whether melatonin is instrumental in causing seasonal changes in human beings, the research in this area may prove critical in understanding and treating SAD.

Treatment of SAD with light is still being refined. Because it is not the kind of light but the intensity of light that is key, the following is a typical regimen: 4 to 6 hours of bright light each day seems necessary. The light must be 5 to 10 times brighter than ordinary room light, about the same brightness as can be seen looking out a window on a sunny spring day. Patients sit a few feet from the special fluorescent bulbs and read, sew, or do paperwork. They must keep their eyes open and are instructed to glance directly into the light for a few seconds every minute or so. The maintenance of light therapy–induced remission from depression in patients with SAD mood cycles seems to depend on the functional integrity of the brain serotonin system, which might be involved in the mechanism of action of light therapy (Neumeister et al., 1997; Beauchemin & Hay, 1997).

The characteristics of **rapid cycling** include four episodes of a mood disturbance occurring in the previous 12 months and meeting the criteria for Major Depressive Disorder, Manic Episode, Mixed Episode, or Hypomanic Episode. The episodes are delineated by either partial or full remission of at least 2 months or by a switch to an episode of the opposite mood (e.g., Major Depressive Episode switches to Manic Episode). Peter described rapid cycling of his bipolar illness.

What do you think? What is the difference between a seasonal depression and a major depression? Explain by giving examples of each.

➤ *Check Your Reading*
3. Define mood.
4. Define affect.
5. What are the central issues when diagnosing a mood disorder?
6. What is the difference between Bipolar I Disorder and Bipolar II Disorder?
7. What is a seasonal affective pattern?
8. What does rapid cycling mean?

CAUSE OF MOOD DISORDERS

There are many theories regarding the causation of depression. Research supports the influence of many factors.

Sleep and Its Effects

Research demonstrates a relationship between sleep and mood disorders. One of the hallmarks of major depression is sleep disturbance. Depressed individuals typically have EEGs with abnormalities in the duration and intensity of rapid eye movement (REM) sleep. These findings however, lack the consistency necessary to use the EEG as a diagnostic tool.

Deprivation of sleep in the latter part of the night, when more time is spent in REM sleep, correlates with improvement in patients' moods. Although the improvement lasts in a few patients, most have a relapse of their depressed mood as soon as they get some sleep. Research also demonstrates that sleep deprivation can precipitate manic episodes in patients with bipolar illness. This finding is important because it suggests that by observing regular bedtimes, bipolar patients may reduce their risk of an episode of mania. Patients must be alert to the symptoms of impending episodes such as altered sleep patterns that often precede, accompany, or precipitate mania (Bowden, 1997). Depression as well as drugs that have a (CNS) stimulant effect can also affect sleep patterns (Novak & Shapiro, 1997).

Pharmacological Factors

Scientists have observed that reserpine, the antihypertensive medication, causes symptoms of major depression, drowsiness, lethargy, and nightmares, but it is also recognized that this medication depletes the neurotransmitter norepinephrine in nerve cells. The tendency to trigger symptoms of major depression is shared by many drugs used to treat high blood pressure. Of particular interest is that the tricyclic antidepressants and the monoamine oxidase inhibitors (MAOIs) used to treat depression *increase* the availability of norepinephrine and have a positive effect in altering mood (Novak & Shapiro, 1997).

Steroids are a large group of medications that can cause mood changes in either direction, depression or mania. Oral contraceptives are related to steroids. These too cause depression. Sedatives and minor tranquilizers, used to treat anxiety symptoms and to induce sleep, frequently cause mood symptoms and are prone to abuse, thereby causing further complications. In addition, poisons such as lead at low levels of exposure can cause depression (Novak, 1997). Table 25–4 lists many classes of drugs that may induce depression.

Neuronal Factors

Abnormalities of the nervous system result from bodily disturbances that involve injury or malfunction of the brain. Huntington's disease, for example, is a rare genetic condition in which an adult experiences a decline in intellectual abilities and an inability to control movements. Interestingly, symptoms of bipolar illness often appear early in the course of Huntington's disease. Parkinson's disease is another, more common abnormality, in which movement disorders result from neuronal death of two connecting regions within the brain. These nerves use the neurotransmitter dopamine to communicate with one another. People with Parkinson's disease often suffer from depression. Their mood disturbances are treated with traditional antidepressant medications.

Another neuronal cause of depression is a cerebrovascular accident, or stroke, which is characterized by sudden interruption of the blood supply to the brain. Studies show that among patients who suffer strokes, about 25% develop major depression. Injury to the brain is thought to cause depression by destroying nerves that

TABLE 25–4 Drugs That May Induce Depression	
CLASSIFICATION	**DRUG NAME**
Analgesics and nonsteroidal antiinflammatory agents	Indomethacin
Antihypertensives	Reserpine Methyldopa (Aldomet) Clonidine Guanethidine Propranolol (Inderal) Hydralazine
Antimicrobials	Co-trimoxazole Sulfonamide Cycloserine Gram-negative agents
Antiparkinsonian drugs	L-Dopa Amantadine
Antipsychotic drugs	Enanthate/decanoate Haloperidol Fluphenazine
Cardiovascular agents	Digitalis Procainamide
Sedatives and antianxiety drugs	Benzodiazepines Barbiturates Chloral hydrate Ethanol
Steroids and hormones	Corticosteroids Estrogen Progesterone Oral contraceptives
Stimulants and appetite suppressants	Amphetamine Fenfluramine Phenmetrazine

Data from Frederick, P. (1989). Southwestern Internal Medicine Conference: Depression and medical illness. *American Journal of Medical Science, 298*, 64; and Derogatis, L. R., & Wise T. N. (1989). *Anxiety and depressive disorders in the medical patient* (p. 125). Washington, DC: American Psychiatric Press. From Neese, J. B. (1991). Depression in the general hospital. *Nursing Clinics of North America, 26*, 619.

use the catecholamine neurotransmitters. The location of the injury within the brain predicts both the likelihood and the severity of depression. A stroke in the left front quadrant of the brain carries a 60% chance that the individual will experience a major depressive disorder, a significantly greater chance than if the stroke is in any of the other quadrants of the brain (Shua-Haim, Sabo, Comsti, & Gross, 1997).

Ample evidence supports the role of neurotransmitters in the cause of depression (Franson, Renner, & Grossberg, 1994; Rauch & Hyman, 1995). Antidepressant medications actually target specific neurotransmitter systems. (For more about the role of neurotransmitters, see Chapter 7.)

Endocrinological Factors

The endocrine system is another physiological system linked with mood disorders. The endocrine system contains the body's network of glands that release hormones into the bloodstream affecting every organ of the body. The thyroid gland is a major part of the endocrine system. When too little thyroid hormone is released into the bloodstream, hypothyroidism results. In addition to causing muscle aching, hair loss, constipation, and diminished hearing, a deficiency in thyroid hormone also causes depression.

Cushing's disease, another endocrine abnormality, results from excessive stimulation of the adrenal glands by the pituitary gland. This overstimulation causes the adrenals to produce too much of the hormone cortisol. People suffering from Cushing's disease often have round, moonlike faces and rotund abdomens. Many suffer from diabetes and high blood pressure. Some of these patients also develop symptoms of mania and depression that are not always recognized and treated (Hirschfeld, 1997; McDonald & Nemeroff, 1998).

Genetic Factors

As Peter noted, his family tree should have prepared him for his mood disorder. Mood disorders do run in families, and patients are usually anxious about the chances of passing the disorder on to their offspring. People who have a first-degree relative (parent, sibling, or child) with a major depressive disorder are one and a half to three times as likely as the general population to have the same disorder. Up to 25% of those with a major depressive disorder have a relative with a mood disorder of some kind. The hereditary occurrence of bipolar illness is even more striking. Up to 50% of those with bipolar illness have a relative with some mood disorder, 10 to 20 times the rate in the general population. Working with families in which several members have bipolar disorder, a Johns Hopkins group found no evidence of linkages to chromosome 18 in families with apparent maternal transmission and solid evidence of linkage to chromosome 18 in families with apparent paternal transmission (DePaulo, 1996).

Studies of identical twins, whose genes are exactly the same, show that if one twin suffers from depression or bipolar illness, the chance that the other twin will develop the illness is 50% to 90%. If only one gene were involved and if there were no environmental contribution, we would expect a 100% concordance rate for these disorders in identical twins (DePaulo & Ablow, 1989). These findings, however, indicate that although there is a strong genetic influence in the development of mood disorders, other influences are important contributors. One important factor could be that the disorder in the affected twin is the result of a nongenetic cause, possibly neuronal, endocrinological, or pharmacological. A second explanation could be that only a vulnerability to the mood disorders is passed through the genes and that environmental factors may trigger a genetic predisposition in a person. Environmental factors could include difficult relationships, financial trouble, legal problems, and the medications and medical conditions related to mood disorders.

Adoption studies also support the view that depressive illnesses are inherited. Children of affectively ill parents who are adopted into families having no history of these illnesses still show three times as many depressive disorders as the biological children in the same families (DePaulo & Ablow, 1989).

The role of genetics versus environment is often debated among mental health professionals as well as the lay public. Rather than a competition between genetics versus environment or nature versus nurture, an interrelationship is likely. The relationship is probably nature *and* nurture. Genetic research should eventually identify environmental factors in the prevention and treatment of mania and depression.

The complexities surrounding the search for the genes responsible for depression and bipolar illness are enormous. Recent research findings indicate that there are genetic differences between Bipolar I Disorder and Bipolar II Disorder. In addition, people who have panic disorder as well as bipolar disorder appear to have an inherited gene located in a specific region of chromosome 18, designated 18q. Also implicated are chromosomes 4, 21, and perhaps the X chromosome. The determination of the different subtypes will lead to more specific treatment therapies and better responses (McMahon, 1997).

Research also indicates that it is highly unlikely that only one gene is involved, and even if the person carries the gene or genes, there is no guarantee that he or she will become ill. Minor gene interactions with the environment might precipitate the first manic or depressive episode (e.g., sleep reduction, drug or alcohol intake, childbirth). Other genes might either trigger or protect against the disease. Physical and psychological factors also clearly play an important (although currently unidentified) role in triggering and maintaining or protecting against an underlying genetic predisposition to these illnesses (McMahon, 1997). Spiritual factors may also play a role in promoting resiliency against mood disorders.

Psychodynamic Causes

A variety of psychodynamic theories address the causes of mood disorders. Psychoanalytic theory, developed by Freud, seeks to uncover unconscious conflicts that contribute to psychiatric symptoms. Freud emphasized the importance of unresolved trauma or difficulties in the cause of psychiatric illnesses. Depression, for example, is sometimes understood in psychoanalysis as anger turned inward after a real or perceived loss. Working in therapy to uncover the sources of the anger enables the person to face inner conflicts and early life experiences that created the symptoms (Freud, cited in Gaylin, 1968). Current thinking attributes psychotherapy as helping the psychosocial and interpersonal adjustment of the person, whereas drugs help with the physiologically based symptoms. Psychotherapy seems to help by improving the patient's willingness to continue with the medication treatment (Goldstein, 1998).

In bipolar illness, psychodynamic theories describe the patient's abnormal character development and inability to maintain good relationships. These features, coupled with an ongoing sense of impending loss of objects, produce a rageful stance toward these objects and their inability to gratify self-centered demands (Freud, cited in Gaylin, 1968). Fromm-Reichmann (1949) similarly described a "lack of subtlety," a "lack of any close interpersonal relatedness," and a tendency to exaggerate the intensity of interactions with other people as characteristics of patients with bipolar illness. Studies of families with a high incidence of bipolar illness have demonstrated the importance of rigid role conformity within the family system. Speculation suggests that the combination of a domineering parent and unrealistically high expectations led to a "walled-in existence" and deep hostility later manifested as depression or mania (Finley & Wilson, 1951).

Communication patterns between spouses have proved to be critical to child-rearing practices. Mayo (1979) found that many of the spouses of patients viewed manic or depressive episodes as willful acts of irresponsibility or manifestations of weakness of character and self-indulgence that had to be met with a firm display of power and control. The unspoken but powerfully communicated message to children is that mommy (or daddy) is "sick" through some personal fault. Such a message places children in a conflictual position between the parents. The child may view the "sick" parent as lovable but irresponsible and the well parent as responsible but feared. A pattern develops in which caretaking roles are vague, loyalties tenuous, and affection and approval dependent on a family member's degree of health and responsibility. This pattern disrupts unity and closeness of family members. In a recent study of marital functioning and depressive symptoms, results highlighted the cyclical course of dysphoria and stress among wives (Davila & Bradbury, 1997).

The cognitive model provides shorter-term therapy than the years of therapy so common to psychoanalysis. The most important cognitive theories relate to depression. These include Beck's cognitive model and Seligman's (1975) learned helplessness model.

The basic premise of Beck's cognitive model is that depressed persons think and process information in negative ways, even in the midst of contradictory evidence. This thinking develops over time as the person experiences stress in life. Early stress seems to shape the development of cognitive patterns in a negative self-referring manner. These negative patterns are believed to remain dormant until they are activated by stressful environmental experiences (Beck, Rush, & Shaw, 1979; Beck, 1996).

The learned helplessness theory postulates that depression occurs in people who perceive their own behavior out of control and feel helplessness (Seligman, 1975). Seligman's original theory was modified to include a cognitive dimension suggesting that the cognitive interpretation of what happens is critical. Therefore, attributions that people make about particular events and the degree of importance that they attach to these events are believed to be central to the development of depression (Abramson, Seligman, & Teasdale, 1978). More recent studies with dysphoric and nondepressed undergraduate students concluded that the inference of negative characteristics about the self from negative life events, coupled with the experience of negative life events, contributed to the development of depression through hopelessness (Kapci, 1998). This reinforces the earlier theories of Seligman and Abramson.

The interpersonal psychotherapeutic model explains depression (Klerman, Weissman, Rounsaville, & Chevron, 1984). Central to this model is the belief in a relationship between depression and current interpersonal functioning. Multiple interpersonal factors are important in the development of depression. These include unsatisfactory early interpersonal experiences, stresses in current interpersonal relationships, and lack of supportive relationships.

Interpersonal psychotherapy has been modified in the 1990s for different age groups and types of mood and nonmood disorders and for use as a long-term treatment. Having begun as a research intervention, interpersonal psychotherapy has yet to be well disseminated among clinicians. The publication of efficacy data, the recent appearance of two practice guidelines that include interpersonal psychotherapy among treatments for depression, and the interest in defined treatments for managed care have led to increasing requests for information and training. Additionally, despite overlaps and similarities, interpersonal psychotherapy is distinct from short-term psychodynamic psychotherapy (Markowitz, Svartberg, & Swartz, 1998; Weissman & Markowitz, 1994).

Given the need for integration of the medical condition and the understanding of the human response to the depressive experience, Calarco and Krone (1991) developed an integrated model of depressive behavior (Figure 25–3). This model reflects interaction among the variables of cognition, interpersonal response, and biological response. In addition, this interaction is affected by both acute and chronic stressors that affect a person's

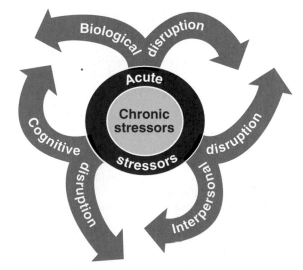

Figure 25–3
Calarco and Krone's integrated model of depressive behavior. (From Calarco, M., & Krone, K. [1991]. An integrated nursing model of depressive behavior in adults: Theory and implications for practice. *Nursing Clinics of North America, 26,* 573–583.)

thoughts about self, relationships with others, and biological integrity. The center of this model reflects the critical component of acute and chronic stressors that may influence depression and mania. The cognitive component of the model addresses the negative view of self and the future as well as the cognitive disruptions (i.e., decreased concentration, decreased decision-making and problem solving ability, and short-term memory deficits) seen in many who suffer from depression. The biological component reflects the physiological symptoms of depression, such as sleep disruption, appetite changes, and fatigue, as well as the biochemical changes in the brain and hormonal changes. The interpersonal component reflects the social withdrawal and isolation common in depression as well as the helplessness, frustration, and anger often generated in family and friends (Calarco & Krone, 1991; Mossey, Knott, Higgins, & Talerico, 1996).

> **W**hat do you think? What do you feel were the acute and chronic stressors that influenced Peter's mania? Explain.

➤ Check Your Reading

9. What is the relationship between sleep and mood?
10. Name three drugs that are implicated in causing depression.
11. According to psychoanalytic theory, what causes depression?
12. According to the cognitive model, what causes depression?
13. According to the interpersonal model, what causes depression?

NURSING PROCESS

Assessment

Because mood disorders are holistic, you are concerned with much more than just an assessment of mood. You are also concerned with an assessment of *self-attitude* (feelings of self-worth) and *vital sense* (sense of physical well-being). The typical physical signs of mood disorders include eating and sleep disturbances as well as changes in sexual interest and activity. Boxes 25-2 and 25-3 outline the areas of concern in assessing depression and mania. A number of effective scales are available to quantify the degree of both depression and mania, such as the Zung Self-Rating Depression Scale (Box 25-4) and the Young Mania Rating Scale (Box 25-5).

In addition to the areas of assessment listed in Boxes 25-2 and 25-3, you need to collect data concerning

- The patient's feelings, attitudes, and knowledge about the illness
- The degree and intensity of suicidal thinking and the potential risk for suicide
- The family's feelings, attitudes, and knowledge about the illness

- Issues of powerlessness
- Spiritual concerns such as hopelessness
- Social isolation

Patient's Feelings, Attitudes, and Knowledge

Patients with mood disorders express a wide variety of negative feelings. These include shame, humiliation, fear of reprisals if others find out, denial, anger, fear of experiencing a relapse, fear of passing the disorder onto their children, and fear of rejection by significant others. The feelings of shame and humiliation derive from the belief that the patient is to blame for the illness and somehow should have been able to control it. These feelings are compounded if the patient has experienced a psychotic episode. Recollections about inappropriate or bizarre behavior, embarrassing actions, or financial problems lead the patient to further shame. The self-blame and sense of personal inadequacy go beyond feeling responsible for the illness and extend to therapy itself. Some patients, believing if they just worked harder in therapy they would feel better, are hesitant to bring up their mood problems with their therapists. Admitting to feelings of depression or elation is like admitting that the therapy is a failure or that they themselves are a failure at therapy.

The fear of reprisal if others find out about the illness is a strong barrier effectively blocking both women and men from seeking treatment. People prefer suffering in isolation to the anticipated reactions of others' knowing that they are suffering with a mental illness. Fear of losing employment, employee benefits, and social stature are just a few of the concerns that patients with mood disorders confront.

Denial, another common response of the patient with a mood disorder, is normal when people are confronted with painful and destructive life events. Denial allows slow assimilation of thoughts and feelings that are initially overwhelming, even devastating, to accept (Hales, Rakel, & Rothschild, 1994; McDonald & Nemeroff, 1998). Denial was described by Endler (1990), a psychologist writing about his illness and the effect on those around him (Case Example 25-1).

Skipped

■ CASE EXAMPLE 25-1
■ Norman's Story

When I first started getting depressed, not only did I deny it to myself but so did my friends and colleagues. My gradual withdrawal from interaction, my lack of cheerfulness, and my quietness were interpreted by them as anger at something they had done wrong. My children said nothing to me. My colleagues said nothing to me, and the professionals that I worked with said nothing to me. I'm sure that some, if not most of them, must have noticed that something was wrong with me. ■

From Endler, N. (1990). *Holiday of darkness: A psychologist's personal journey out of his depression* (p. 148). Toronto, Ontario, Canada: Wall & Emerson.

B o x   2 5 – 2   ■ ■ ■ ■ ■

Indicators of Depression

Signs of Low Mood

- *Withdrawal:* A person suffering from depression may lose interest in activities that once gave him or her pleasure and may participate less in social interactions.
- *Negativism:* A person who is usually tolerant of many different viewpoints may become excessively skeptical when depressed. He or she may stubbornly resist the suggestions, orders, or instructions of others.
- *Unhappiness:* A depressed person may experience persistent sadness or frequent crying.

Signs of Lowered Self-Attitude

- *Self-deprecating, guilty, or self-blaming comments:* When depressed, a person may put himself or herself down with comments such as "I'm such a failure; I wonder how you stay with me." A depressed person may also accept blame for problems that do not exist or are clearly not his or her fault.
- *Expressions of hopelessness:* In depression, a person may experience unusually persistent pessimism and may express despair in suicidal statements or acts.

Signs of Decreased Vital Sense

- *Decreased attentiveness to oneself or to one's tasks:* A depressed person may neglect his or her appearance and let assignments at school, housework at home, or projects at work slide.

- *Decreased energy:* A person with depression may complain of fatigue and lack of energy or "motivation." He or she may have particular difficulty getting activities started, especially in the early morning hours.
- *Decreased ability to concentrate:* Depression often makes it difficult for a person to think through a problem and, thus, to initiate and complete a complex mental task. A usually avid reader may begin to read many books but may not finish them. A faithful correspondent may be unable to write.
- *Excessive indecisiveness:* A depressed person may vacillate between choices to an unusual degree and may defer decision-making to others. This may be true even for simple decisions that were previously made routinely.

Additional Signs

- *Change in weight or in eating patterns:* Decreased appetite leading to weight loss is a common symptom of depression. In some depressives (especially those whose depressions come during a particular season of the year), appetite and weight increase.
- *Change in sleep patterns:* Characteristically a depressed person's sleep is interrupted, especially in the early morning hours (2 to 6 AM), but in some depressives sleep is excessive and waking is difficult.
- *Change in sexual interest and activity:* Characteristically, sexual interest and performance are decreased in a depressed person.

From DePaulo, J. R. Jr., & Ablow, K. R. (1989). *How to cope with depression: A complete guide for you and your family.* New York: McGraw-Hill. Reproduced with permission of The McGraw-Hill Companies.

In manic-depressive illness, which often involves a psychotic diagnosis, an uncertain course, and a lifetime sentence of medication, anger is a common reaction. Although the anger is an understandable response, it often leads patients irrationally to reject an effective treatment or to vent their anger on the clinician.

Another issue for people recovering from mood disorders is fear of relapse or recurrence. A patient describes this feeling: "I think a person who's had a history of depression always fears that the bottom's going to fall out and they are going to get depressed again." The poet Robert Lowell (1977) wrote a similar description of depressed individuals: "If we see a light at the end of the tunnel, it's the light of an oncoming train" (p. 31). Several questions form the crux of patients' concerns. Will there be further episodes? How frequently? Will they be debilitating? Will I be able to work, earn a living, occupy myself, and fulfill my responsibilities? These questions reflect the long-term meaning of the illness to patients. Related to the fear of recurrence of illness, patients agonize over the possibility that their children will inherit the mood disorder.

The fear of rejection by significant others is of great consequence. Part of the symptom profile of the mood disorders is their ability to disrupt interpersonal relationships with coworkers, family, and friends. Widely varying reactions to the patient may include anger, concern, withdrawal, unrealistically low or high expectations, rejection, and denial of the illness (Mossey et al., 1996). Negative reactions of others affect the patient's already diminished sense of self.

A patient's information needs are another vital area to assess. For instance, distinguishing between normal and abnormal moods can be quite confusing for patients. The patient who is angry, irritable, a little down, or even feeling especially good may worry that these feelings are not part of the normal range of human emotion but are early symptoms of depression or hypomania. These overlapping emotions can be confusing and arouse anxiety in many patients who may then question their own

Box 25-3 ■ ■ ■ ■ ■
Indicators of Mania

Signs of Elevated or High Mood

- *Excessive cheerfulness:* A manic person may be unusually elated.
- *Irritability:* A person with mania may become irritable even over small matters, especially when one attempts to reason with him or her.
- *Anger beyond irritability:* When suffering from mania, a person may develop a haughty or superior stance that is not usual for him or her.

Signs of Increased Self-Attitude

- *Expressions and acts of unusual optimism:* These activities can evidence poor judgment. Unfortunately the overconfident, manic person's energy is often channeled into inappropriate, dangerous, or indiscreet behavior. A normally conservative person may undertake foolish or risky business ventures, may engage in sexual indiscretions, or may speak in overly critical or judgmental terms, often at inappropriate times and about sensitive subjects.

Signs of Increased Vital Sense

- *Increased energy:* A person with mania may appear tireless in the face of physical and mental efforts that would greatly tax an unaffected person. He or she may feel completely refreshed after just a few minutes or hours of sleep.
- *Increased activity:* The increased energy of mania often translates to a host of new projects at work, a seemingly insatiable desire to socialize, or greatly increased participation in sexual activities.
- *Excessive talking:* A person with mania may seem to talk endlessly, sometimes jumping haphazardly from idea to idea. Alternatively, a manic person may adopt an unusually abrupt and short or clipped manner of speaking to others.

Additional Signs

- *Change in eating patterns:* A manic person may have a voracious appetite or may be too busy to eat.
- *Change in sleep patterns:* When suffering from mania, a person feels less need for sleep, so sleep is usually decreased.
- *Change in sexual interest:* Sexual interest is often increased in a manic person.

From DePaulo, J. R. Jr., & Ablow, K. R. (1989). *How to cope with depression: A complete guide for you and your family.* New York: McGraw-Hill. Reproduced with permission of The McGraw-Hill Companies.

---

judgment and become unduly concerned about recurrences of their affective illness" (Harris, 1996). Patients need information about the following:

- The nature and causes of mood disorders
- Treatment options, including the value of psychotherapy used in conjunction with medications
- The actions and side effects of medications
- The importance of social support
- The need to take control of decisions related to the illness
- The importance of spiritual support
- The need to manage stress, which can be a precipitant of both mania and depression

The better an individual is able to manage life stress, the better the chance of leading a relatively stable life.

Suicidality

Suicide assessment is critical with depressed patients. Assess whether or not the patient is currently suicidal. Ask the patient, "Have you thought of hurting yourself? Are you presently considering hurting yourself? If you have been thinking about suicide, do you have a plan? What is the plan? Have you thought about what life would be like if you were no longer a part of it?" These questions are essential for identifying suicidal ideation and the lethality of any plan.

Consider a patient's prior history of suicide attempts and depression to be clear indicators that the patient is at high risk in the present for attempting suicide. A patient whose depression is lifting is at higher risk for suicide than a severely depressed individual. Increased energy occurs as the depression lifts. The energy is not enough to make the patient feel good or hopeful, but it is enough to carry out a suicidal plan. (Chapter 31 presents a comprehensive review of suicide.)

Family Feelings, Attitudes, and Knowledge

Include the reactions of family and friends in the assessment. Unfortunately, many of those closest to the patient mistakenly believe that depression is a self-induced illness. These people provide well-intentioned but inaccurate advice to the depressed person to "pull yourself up by the bootstraps," meaning "avoid giving in to the depression." Ironically, in depression it is the bootstraps that are defective, and no amount of effort can snap the individual out of the depression.

The illness affects the patient's working, playing, thinking, feeling, and communicating. Family members

Box 25–4　■ ■ ■ ■ ■
Zung Self-Rating Depression Scale

The Measurement of Depression
William W. K. Zung, MD

A self-rating depression scale (SDS) for the quantitative measurement of depression as an emotional disorder based upon an operational definition was first published in 1965 (Zung, 1965). This was followed by a series of reports that described its validity and reliability on the basis of investigations performed in the United States as well as in other countries throughout the world (Zung, 1958, 1972, 1989; Zung & Wonnacott, 1970).

Although devised for use in psychiatric research, the scale readily lends itself to use in the general practice of medicine in which most depressions are first encountered. The use of the SDS in a variety of patients with physical complaints with no apparent organic basis may uncover and measure depression in the so-called masked depressions. This saves valuable time for the doctor and the patient, since the unmasking of the patient's depression by the doctor is the first necessary step toward treatment.

How to Use the Self-Rating Depression Scale
Depression is defined operationally as a syndrome comprised of coexisting signs and symptoms that signify the presence of pathologic disturbances or changes in four areas: somatic, psychologic, psychomotor, and mood.

The SDS comprises a list of 20 items. Each item relates to a specific characteristic of depression. The 20 items together comprehensively delineate the depressive disorders as they are widely recognized. Opposite the statements are four columns headed: *None or a Little of the Time, Some of the Time, Good Part of the Time,* and *Most or All of the Time.*

For each item, the patient is asked to put a check mark in the box according to how it relates to his or her feelings within a specified time period: "during the past week." Although some depressed patients orally volunteer little information, most will readily cooperate when asked to check the scale if told that this will help the doctor know more about them.

To obtain the patient's depression rating, the completed scale is placed under the transparent overlay for scoring, and the indicated value for each item is written in the margin and totaled. This raw score is then converted to an SDS Index based on 100. The SDS Index is a total indication of "How depressed is this patient?" in terms of the operational definition and is expressed as a percentage. Thus, an SDS score of 65 may be interpreted to mean that the patient demonstrates 65% of the depression measurable by the scale.

Individual item scores tell us what specific sign or symptom the patient is manifesting, whereas aggregate scores of several items tell us in what area(s) the patient is having the most difficulty. For example, items 1 and 3 refer to affect; items 2 and 4 through 10 measure physiologic disturbances; items 12 and 13 measure psychomotor disturbance; and items 11 and 14 through 20 measure psychologic disturbances.

The statements in the scale are worded in the everyday language of the patient. Questions about how to complete the scale usually indicate the patient's desire to cooperate with the physician. For example, a patient may ask how to check item 5 because he or she is on a diet and therefore should not be eating as much. In this case, the patient is asked to answer as if he or she were not on a diet.

After the patient has filled out the scale, take a moment to check that all statements have been answered.

Interpretation of SDS Ratings in Depression and Other Emotional Disorders
"Depression" as a word can be used to describe: (1) an affect that is a subjective feeling tone of short duration, (2) a mood that is a state sustained over a longer period of time, (3) an emotion that comprises feeling tones along with objective indications, and (4) a disorder that has characteristic symptom clusters and complexes of signs and symptoms. The SDS is intended to rate depression as a disorder. However, the SDS is not intended to differentiate the different types of depression. It serves rather to quantitatively measure the intensity of depression, regardless of the diagnostic label used (Zung, 1973).

---

and friends may operate under the misconception that they have somehow caused the illness. The truth is that they could not have caused this kind of depression, and they cannot make it go away. Commonsense solutions such as logic, advice, reassurance, and sympathy all miss the mark in helping the person; family and friends begin to feel that they are failures. Feelings such as helplessness, anger, frustration, guilt, irritability, fearfulness, hopelessness, and being tired of hearing all of the depression problems are understandable reactions of the patient's loved ones (Davila & Bradbury, 1997).

In manic-depressive illness, in which psychosis is often a component of the symptoms, the patient is frequently hospitalized. The psychosis transforms the patient into a stranger whose bizarre behavior betrays the intimacies shared within the family. Often, the stranger is angry and does not respond to love or acceptance. It is not surprising that relatives react with withdrawal, denial, and an inability to comprehend what has happened.

In working with depressed patients, recognize that depression is an illness that can cause marked changes in

Box 25-4 ■ ■ ■ ■ ■
Zung Self-Rating Depression Scale *Continued*

Certain safeguards are incorporated in the construction of this rating scale. The patient is unable to discern a trend in answers because half of the statements are worded symptomatically positive and half are worded symptomatically negative. For example, item 1, "I feel downhearted, blue, and sad," is a positive statement. Item 2, "Morning is when I feel the best," is a negative statement reflecting the opposite of the way most depressed patients feel (worse in the morning). Negatively worded items are identified by asterisks on the transparent overlay, and the key words of the negative item appear in italics. In addition, an even rather than an odd number of columns is used to offset any possibility of a patient's checking middle columns in order to appear "average."

By combining results from several studies, the SDS Index can be interpreted as follows:

SDS INDEX	EQUIVALENT CLINICAL GLOBAL IMPRESSIONS
Below 50	Within normal range, no psychopathology
50–59	Presence of minimal to mild depression
60–69	Presence of moderate to marked depression
70 and over	Presence of severe to extreme depression

The above interpretations are based on data that compare depressed versus nondepressed patients as well as depressed patients versus normal subjects in the 20- to 64-year-old range. High scores are not in themselves diagnostic but indicate the presence of symptoms that may be of clinical significance.

Results from several studies have shown that there is usually some depressive symptomatology present in almost all of the psychiatric disorders. Patients may have several diagnoses: headache AND depression, schizophrenia AND depression, diabetes AND depression. Thus, a primary diagnosis other than depression does not eliminate the possibility that the patient is also depressed. If the SDS Index is above 50, the patient may need treatment for the depression in addition to treatment for the primary diagnosis.

Diagnostic Criteria for Depressive Disorders and Their Relation to SDS Items

The SDS items are not in the same order as in the SDS scale but are listed opposite corresponding symptoms of depression organized into (I) pervasive affective, (II) physiologic, (III) psychomotor, and (IV) psychologic disturbances.

In the items, words that appear in italics reflect the opposite of what most patients complain of. As stated earlier, these words have been converted from symptomatically positive to symptomatically negative statements to prevent the patient from discerning the pattern of his or her answers.

Excerpts from Zung, W. W. K. (1965). A self-rating depression scale. *Archives of General Psychiatry, 12,* 63–70, and Zung, W. W. K. (1973). From art to science: The diagnosis and treatment of depression. *Archives of General Psychiatry, 29,* 328–337.

a person's mood, thinking, bodily functions, and behaviors. Many people, including health care providers, associate only sadness or suicidal thinking with depression. It is important for you to assess the family's level or understanding about the mood disorder.

Norbeck, Chaftez, Skodol-Wilson, & Weiss, (1991) studied the needs of family caregivers in different age groups and found that the most frequently identified need by family members was for information about the illness, behavior management, coping, and making decisions. These needs probably stem from the ambiguous nature of mood disorders, which may develop insidiously and unpredictably, leaving families without the clear explanations or directives that they desire. The battle against depression starts with education. Erasing the myths and stigma that still surround the disease is particularly important for childhood depression (Fassler, 1997).

Issues of Powerlessness

As you get to know the patient, you also gather information about the patient's perceived sense of powerlessness. When illness develops, the sense of control over one's life may be threatened. People's responses to the stress of illness depend on personal characteristics and social resources. These responses significantly affect the person's health and well-being. Feelings of powerlessness stem from the unpredictability of the mood disorders as well as some of the treatment issues.

For instance, taking medications, feeling unsure about the prognosis of the disorder, and fearing the possibility of future exacerbations leave the person feeling totally vulnerable. Patients frequently express dissatisfaction over taking medications, particularly if the medications have annoying side effects. Complaints about medication may represent covert expressions of

B o x 2 5 – 5 ■ ■ ■ ■ ■
Young Mania Rating Scale

Guide for Scoring Items—The purpose of each item is to rate the severity of that abnormality in the patient. When several keys are given for a particular grade of severity, the presence of only one is required to qualify for that rating.

The keys provided are guides. One can ignore the keys if that is necessary to indicate severity, although this should be the exception rather than the rule.

Scoring between the points given (whole or half points) is possible and encouraged after experience with the scale is acquired. This is particularly useful when severity of a particular item in a patient does not follow the progression indicated by the keys.

1. *Elevated Mood*
   0. Absent
   1. Mildly or possibly increased on questioning
   2. Definite subjective elevation; optimistic, self-confident; cheerful; appropriate to content
   3. Elevated, inappropriate to content; humorous
   4. Euphoric; inappropriate laughter; singing
2. *Increased Motor Activity—Energy*
   0. Absent
   1. Subjectively increased
   2. Animated; gestures increased
   3. Excessive energy; hyperactive at times; restless (can be calmed)
   4. Motor excitement; continuous hyperactivity (cannot be calmed)
3. *Sexual Interest*
   0. Normal; not increased
   1. Mildly or possibly increased
   2. Definite subjective increase on questioning
   3. Spontaneous sexual content; elaborates on sexual matters; hypersexual by self-report
   4. Overt sexual acts (toward patients, staff, or interviewer)
4. *Sleep*
   0. Reports no decrease in sleep
   1. Sleeping less than normal amount by up to one hour
   2. Sleeping less than normal by more than one hour
   3. Reports decreased need for sleep
   4. Denies need for sleep
5. *Irritability*
   0. Absent
   2. Subjectively increased
   4. Irritable at times during interview; recent episodes of anger or annoyance on ward
   6. Frequently irritable during interview; short, curt throughout
   8. Hostile, uncooperative; interview impossible
6. *Speech (Rate and Amount)*
   0. No increase
   2. Feels talkative
   4. Increased rate or amount at times, verbose at times
   6. Push; consistently increased rate and amount; difficult to interrupt
   8. Pressured; uninterruptible, continuous speech
7. *Language-Thought Disorder*
   0. Absent
   1. Circumstantial; mild distractibility; quick thoughts
   2. Distractible; loses goal of thought; changes topics frequently; racing thoughts
   3. Flight of ideas; tangentiality; difficult to follow; rhyming, echolalia
   4. Incoherent; communication impossible
8. *Content*
   0. Normal
   2. Questionable plans, new interests
   4. Special projects; hyperreligious
   6. Grandiose or paranoid ideas; ideas of reference
   8. Delusions; hallucinations
9. *Disruptive-Aggressive Behavior*
   0. Absent, cooperative
   2. Sarcastic; loud at times, guarded
   4. Demanding; threats on ward
   6. Threatens interviewer; shouting; interview difficult
   8. Assaultive; destructive; interview impossible
10. *Appearance*
    0. Appropriate dress and grooming
    1. Minimally unkempt
    2. Poorly groomed; moderately disheveled; over-dressed
    3. Disheveled; partly clothed; garish make-up
    4. Completely unkempt; decorated; bizarre garb
11. *Insight*
    0. Present; admits illness; agrees with need for treatment
    1. Possibly ill
    2. Admits behavior change, but denies illness
    3. Admits possible change in behavior but denies illness
    4. Denies any behavior change

From Young, R. C., Biggs, J. T., Ziegler, V. E., & Meyer, D. A. (1978). A rating scale for mania: Reliability, validity and sensitivity. *British Journal of Psychiatry, 133*, 429–435.

powerlessness to control the illness and to prevent it from recurring. Some patients may feel that by taking the medical approach they have abdicated all control to others. These feelings can lead to rejection not only of medication but also of therapy. A comprehensive assessment identifies feelings of powerlessness and considers the resolution of these feelings in the plan of care.

Spiritual Issues

The many spiritual side effects of depressive illness warrant assessment. Experiences common to depressive illness, such as marital and family problems, divorce, and sudden unemployment, contribute to the downward spiral of negative self-reflections. The depressed person thinks in negative ways about self, the environment, and the future, resulting in a loss of faith in self, others, life, and ultimately God (Carson, 1994; Kerr, 1987-1988). The sense that God ceases to care and is removed is probably one of the most devastating symptoms of depression. Once this sense of separation has occurred, the person often considers suicide a viable option to end the pain of the illness. The sense of aloneness and abandonment in a hostile world is unbearable (Miller, 1987).

You need to inquire about spiritual issues. Ask questions, such as

What role has God played in your illness?
What role do you think God will play in your healing?
Of what significance are your religious beliefs and practices?
What are your sources of hope and comfort?
What is your God like?
What can I do to assist you in meeting your spiritual needs?

The answers to these questions allow you to address spiritual issues adequately in the plan of care.

Social Isolation

The amount of social support available to the patient is important. Individuals suffering with mood disorders frequently experience disruptions in their relationships with others. Depression causes loss of interest in activities that were formerly pleasurable and satisfying. The result is withdrawal from friends, family, and other sources of social support. In mania, the patient displays a superior sense of self and is irritable, argumentative, and rigid, thus creating a wall between self and others. Frequently, the patient's perception of isolation is painfully and objectively true.

What *do you think?* Why is a depressed person more at risk to commit suicide when he or she is feeling better? Explain.

▶ *Check Your Reading*

14. Identify at least five areas to assess in a patient with a mood disorder.
15. Identify at least three of the negative feelings expressed by patients suffering with mood disorders.
16. What do you assess in regard to suicide risk?
17. Why is powerlessness an important issue?

Diagnosis

Arriving at nursing diagnoses in mood disorders demands that you understand the complex interplay of concepts such as self-concept, anxiety, and hostility. The nursing diagnoses provide a way of attributing meaning to the information gained in the assessment. By linking behaviors, nursing diagnoses facilitate understanding of the patient's problems. For patients diagnosed with a mood disorder, the following are primary nursing diagnoses in establishing the plan of care:

- Anxiety
- Impaired Verbal Communication
- Ineffective Individual Coping
- Hopelessness
- Risk for Injury
- Altered Nutrition
- Powerlessness
- Self Care Deficit
- Self Esteem Disturbance
- Sexual Dysfunction
- Sleep Pattern Disturbance
- Social Isolation
- Spiritual Distress
- Altered Thought Processes
- Risk for Self Directed Violence

See Medical Diagnoses and Related Nursing Diagnoses: Depression and Mania.

Outcome Identification

The expected outcomes for a patient experiencing indicators of either depression or mania (see Boxes 25-2 and 25-3) are shown in Box 25-6. Remember that outcomes, like your assessment, need to include family members affected by the illness.

Planning

In addition to the expected outcomes, establish short-term goals with the patient. These goals vary according to whether the patient is being treated in an outpatient or an inpatient setting. Hospitalization implies that the illness is more serious. In general, whether the symptoms are depression or mania, the patient needs the structure provided by an inpatient setting. Review the expected outcomes. The short-term goals directly relate to these outcomes. Box 25-7 shows short-term goals appropriate for inpatient care.

What *do you think?* In today's managed care environment, how might you prioritize your patient's short-term goals in an inpatient setting? Explain.

▶ *Check Your Reading*

18. Identify at least five nursing diagnoses that might be appropriate for a depressed patient; at least five appropriate nursing diagnoses for a manic patient.
19. Identify three expected outcomes for a patient with depression; and three expected outcomes for a patient with mania.

MEDICAL DIAGNOSES AND RELATED NURSING DIAGNOSES

Depression

DSM-IV Diagnosis: Major Depressive Disorder, single episode

Diagnostic Criteria
A. Presence of a single Major Depressive Episode.
B. The Major Depressive Episode is not better accounted for by Schizoaffective Disorder and is not superimposed on Schizophrenia, Schizophreniform Disorder, Delusional Disorder, or Psychotic Disorder Not Otherwise Specified.
C. There has never been a Manic Episode, a Mixed Episode, or a Hypomanic Episode. *Note:* This exclusion does not apply if all of the manic-like, mixed-like, or hypomanic-like episodes are substance or treatment induced or are due to the direct physiological effects of a general medical condition.
   Specify (for current or most recent episode):
      Severity/Psychotic/Remission Specifiers
      Chronic
      With Catatonic Features
      With Melancholic Features
      With Atypical Features
      With Postpartum Onset

DMS-IV Diagnosis: Major Depressive Disorder, recurrent

Diagnostic Criteria
A. Presence of two or more Major Depressive Episodes. *Note:* To be considered separate episodes, there must be an interval of at least 2 consecutive months in which criteria are not met for a Major Depressive Episode.
B. The Major Depressive Episodes are not better accounted for by Schizoaffective Disorder and are not superimposed on Schizophrenia, Schizophreniform Disorder, Delusional Disorder, or Psychotic Disorder Not Otherwise Specified.
C. There has never been a Manic Episode, a Mixed Episode, or a Hypomanic Episode. *Note:* This exclusion does not apply if all of the manic-like, mixed-like, or hypomanic-like episodes are substance or treatment induced or are due to the direct physiological effects of a general medical condition.
   Specify (for current or most recent episode):
      Severity/Psychotic/Remission Specifiers
      Chronic
      With Catatonic Features
      With Melancholic Features
      With Atypical Features
      With Postpartum Onset
   Specify:
      Longitudinal Course Specifiers (With and Without Interepisode Recovery)
      With Seasonal Pattern

20. Identify three short-term goals for a patient with depression; and three short-term goals for a patient with mania.

Implementation

Nurse as a Counselor

Many of the feelings and attitudes that patients are confronted with are issues that you will deal with in your role as counselor. Therefore, your interpersonal and communication skills are essential when assisting the patient with a mood disorder. For instance, a generalist in psychiatric nursing

- Spends time with the patient to provide support and a reminder of reality.
- Approaches the patient using a moderate, level tone of voice, avoiding appearing overly cheerful.
- Uses active listening to indicate concern for the patient and to show that the patient is worthwhile.
- Communicates using simple, direct sentences, avoiding complex sentences or directions.

- Avoids asking too many questions or questions that are too probing.
- Encourages the patient to talk about feelings in whatever way that the patient is comfortable doing so.
- Establishes a contract with patient. If, for example, negativism dominates the patient's conversation, limit the focus on negativity to an agreed-on amount of time, after which the patient agrees to discuss other topics.
- Allows and encourages crying.
- Avoids cutting off the patient's conversation with false reassurance and platitudes.
- Provides positive feedback as the patient achieves goals of treatment. Explores the patient's strengths and coping responses.

Many patients diagnosed with mood disorders are also in therapy, which is conduced by psychiatrists, advanced practice certified psychiatric–mental health nurses, psychiatric social workers, or psychologists. Psychotherapy alone may treat mild and some moderate forms of depression. In patients with major depressive disorder or bipolar disorder, however, the combination

Related Nursing Diagnoses	Definition	Example
Risk for Self-Directed Violence	A state in which an individual experiences behaviors that can be physically harmful either to self or to others	High Risk for Self-Directed Violence related to depressed mood and feelings of worthlessness as evidenced by verbalization of suicidal ideation or pain or both
Self-Esteem Disturbance	Negative self-evaluation or feelings about self or self capabilities, which may be directly or indirectly expressed	Self-Esteem Disturbance related to negative view of self as evidenced by expressions of worthlessness
Powerlessness	Perception that one's own actions will not significantly affect an outcome; a perceived lack of control over a current situation or immediate happening	Powerlessness related to belief that agreeing to take medications or participating in therapy relinquishes control of illness to others as evidenced by refusal to participate in treatment program
Spiritual Distress	Disruption in the life principle that pervades a person's entire being and that integrates and transcends one's biological and psychosocial nature	Spiritual Distress related to sense of despair and feelings of abandonment by God as evidenced by inability to pray or practice other meaningful spiritual activities
Social Isolation	Aloneness experienced by the individual and perceived as imposed by others and as a negative or threatened state	Social Isolation related to feelings of inadequacy in social interactions as evidenced by withdrawal, problematic interactions with others, and seeking to be alone
Altered Thought Processes	A state in which an individual experiences a disruption in cognitive operations and activities	Altered Thought Processes related to neurobiological changes as evidenced by delusions, confusion, and impaired problem solving
Altered Nutrition: Less than Body Requirements	A state in which an individual experiences an intake of nutrients insufficient to meet metabolic needs	Altered Nutrition, Less than Body Requirements related to depressed mood, loss of appetite or lack of interest in food as evidenced by weight loss, weakness, poor muscle tone, and poor skin turgor
Sleep Pattern Disturbance	Disruption of sleep time causes discomfort or interferes with desired lifestyle	Sleep Pattern Disturbance related to depressed mood, anxiety, and fears as evidenced by difficulty falling asleep, early morning awakening, and complaints of feeling tired
Self Care Deficit	A state in which the individual experiences an impaired ability to perform self care activities	Self Care Deficit related to depressed mood as evidenced by disheveled clothing, offensive body odor, failure to brush teeth, and uncombed hair

Based on information from the *Diagnostic and Statistical Manual of Mental Disorders. Fourth Edition.* Copyright 1994 American Psychiatric Association. Nursing diagnoses and definitions from North American Nursing Diagnosis Association. (1999). *NANDA nursing diagnoses: Definitions and classification, 1999–2000.* Philadelphia: NANDA.

MEDICAL DIAGNOSES AND RELATED NURSING DIAGNOSES

Mania

DMS-IV Diagnosis: Bipolar I Disorder, single manic episode

Diagnostic Criteria

A. Presence of only one Manic Episode and no past Major Depressive Episodes. *Note:* Recurrence is defined as either a change in polarity from depression or an interval of at least 2 months without manic symptoms.

B. The Manic Episode is not better accounted for by Schizoaffective Disorder and is not superimposed on Schizophrenia, Schizophreniform Disorder, Delusional Disorder, or Psychotic Disorder Not Otherwise Specified.

> *Specify:*
>> Mixed: If symptoms meet criteria for a Mixed Episode
> *Specify* (for current or most recent episode):
>> Severity/Psychotic/Remission Specifiers
>> With Catatonic Features
>> With Postpartum Onset

DSM-IV Diagnosis: Bipolar I Disorder, most recent episodic mania

Diagnostic Criteria

A. Currently (or most recently) in a Manic Episode.

B. There has previously been at least one Major Depressive Episode, Manic Episode, or Mixed Episode.

C. The mood episodes in Criteria A and B are not better accounted for by Schizoaffective Disorder and are not superimposed on Schizophrenia, Schizophreniform Disorder, Delusional Disorder, or Psychotic Disorder Not Otherwise Specified.

> *Specify* (for current or most recent episode):
>> Severity/Psychotic/Remission Specifiers
>> With Catatonic Features
>> With Postpartum Onset
> *Specify:*
>> Longitudinal Course Specifiers (With and Without Interepisode Recovery)
>> With Seasonal Pattern (applies only to the pattern of Major Depressive Episodes)
>> With Rapid Cycling

---

of psychotherapy and medications has been proved to be more effective than either treatment alone. Current data suggest that if a depressed patient shows at least partial improvement after 6 to 8 weeks of treatment with relatively high medication doses, there is a reasonable likelihood that further improvement may occur. In contrast, if no signs of improvement are evident after at least 6 weeks of treatment, a medication change is warranted (Goldberg, 1997).

Psychotherapy serves a number of purposes. First, it teaches a person alternative ways to handle stresses. Second, it helps explore how the illness affects the person's life. Therapy helps patients in "learning to unravel what is normal personality from what the illness has superimposed upon it—turbulence, impulsiveness, lack of predictability, and depression" (Goodwin & Jamison, 1990, p. 732). Third, psychotherapy deals with denial. Denial is diminished by exploring the meaning of the illness with the patient. The natural course of the illness, its high relapse rate, and risks and benefits of medications are discussed. Fourth, psychotherapy provides a safe place to express feelings of anger and shame and have them accepted. Fifth, therapy allows for the conceptualization of mood disorders as fundamentally medical. This determination decreases stigma; provides effective, specific treatment; and minimizes family and patient responsibility as the cause of the illness. The therapist, however, needs to avoid focusing on the medical approach to the exclusion of all else. Such an approach might mean that significant life issues and problems

adjusting to the illness may be ignored. Research indicates that several forms of short-term psychotherapy, such as supportive, cognitive, and interpersonal, are effective in treating depression (Bachelor, 1996).

SUPPORTIVE PSYCHOTHERAPY

The objectives for supportive psychotherapy are the following (Bachelor, 1996; Bloch, 1979):

1. Promote the patient's best psychological and social functioning.

2. Bolster self-esteem and self-confidence.

3. Make the patient aware of what can and cannot be achieved, both personal limitations and the limitations of treatment.

4. Prevent undue dependence on professional support and unnecessary hospitalizations.

5. Promote the best use of available support from family and friends.

Supportive psychotherapy with medication treatment is most appropriate for patients with severe forms of depressive illness. For those whose abilities to understand the illness are impaired, the therapist provides concrete explanations about depression or mania. Therapists continually encourage patients and convey optimism about the future. Patients require frequent repetition of the message of optimism before they derive any benefit. Recovered patients often report that the persistent hopefulness of their therapist and others kept them from giving up before treatment worked or before the

MEDICAL DIAGNOSES AND RELATED NURSING DIAGNOSES

Mania Continued

Related Nursing Diagnoses	Definition	Example
Risk for Injury	A state in which an individual is at risk of injury as a result of environmental conditions interacting with the individual's adaptive and defensive resources	Risk for Injury related to extreme hyperactivity as evidenced by increased agitation and lack of control over behavior
Risk for Violence: Self-Directed or Directed at Others	A state in which an individual experiences behaviors that can be physically harmful to either self or others	Risk for Violence: Self-Directed or Directed at Others related to degree of manic excitement, delusional thinking, and hallucinations as evidenced by threats to self and others and impulsive and volatile behaviors
Altered Nutrition: Less than Body Requirements	The state in which an individual experiences an intake of nutrients insufficient to meet metabolic needs	Altered Nutrition: Less than Body Requirements related to inability to sit still long enough to eat as evidenced by weight loss
Sensory/Perceptual Alterations	A state in which an individual experiences a change in the amount or patterning of oncoming stimuli accompanied by a diminished, exaggerated, distorted, or impaired response to such stimuli	Sensory/Perceptual Alterations related to possible sleep deprivation as evidenced by auditory and visual hallucinations
Impaired Social Interaction	The state in which an individual participates in insufficient or excessive quantity or ineffective quality of social exchange	Impaired Social Interaction related to narcissistic behavior as evidenced by inability to sustain relationships
Sleep Pattern Disturbance	Disruption of sleep time causes discomfort or interferes with desired lifestyle	Sleep Pattern Disturbance related to excessive hyperactivity and agitation as evidenced by difficulty falling asleep and sleeping for only short periods

Based on information from the *Diagnostic and Statistical Manual of Mental Disorders. Fourth Edition.* Copyright 1994 American Psychiatric Association. Nursing diagnoses and definitions from North American Nursing Diagnosis Association. (1999). *NANDA nursing diagnoses: Definitions and classification, 1999–2000.* Philadelphia: NANDA.

illness remitted on its own. The truthful message to be communicated is that success is almost always the outcome of determined treatment. Even if the patient's disorder cannot be helped with current medical treatments, new treatments are always being developed.

Supportive psychotherapy for manic patients can be particularly difficult. Patients with mania usually have difficulty accepting that they suffer from a disease requiring immediate medical treatment. They may need supervision in spending their money or their time, and they cannot trust their confident and cheerful feelings to lead them to rational actions. Often, supportive therapy of a manic patient takes the form of finding any area of mutual understanding that allows a short-term agreement about treatment. These agreements can "carry" the patient, family, friends, and clinician until a more normal mood returns (DePaulo & Ablow, 1989).

COGNITIVE AND INTERPERSONAL PSYCHOTHERAPIES

Studies conducted by the National Institute of Mental Health show that in outpatients with mild and moderate depression, cognitive and interpersonal short-term psychotherapies are helpful. Both of these approaches can be used alone or in conjunction with pharmacological approaches.

The goal of cognitive psychotherapy is to correct negative thinking that determines feelings and behavior. For example, depressed patients frequently view life through gray-tinted glasses. They expect the worst from themselves, from others, and from the environment. They view the future as hopeless. They predict that these inadequacies and this current pain will continue indefinitely. "Everything I do turns out badly" is a characteristic self-evaluation of a depressed patient. The expectation of failure paralyzes the person from initiating new behaviors. The therapist, using verbal procedures and behavior modification techniques, works with the patient (Beck et al., 1996) to

- Teach the patient to recognize automatic negative thoughts and to change them.
- Identify distortions in the patient's self-image and view of the world.
- Identify and correct dysfunctional beliefs about events.

Interpersonal therapy focuses on the patient's relationships with others. The emphasis is on the "here and now" and on current problems. Interpersonal therapy differs from other psychotherapies in that it is time-limited and focuses primarily on both the patient's current symptoms of depression and the interpersonal context associated with the depression.

Nurse as Teacher to Patient and Family

An essential nursing role is that of a teacher. Many people lack understanding about the causes, characteristics, and appropriate treatments for the mood disorders. Because of this knowledge deficit, patients tend to blame themselves for their illness, and others do the same. When people understand all of the components of the mood disorders, they are less frightened and are more hopeful (McAllister & Ryan, 1997). Using brief supportive psychotherapy, lasting positive changes in interpersonal functioning occurred in subjects with this technique (Rosenthal, Muran, Pinsker, Hellerstein, & Winston, 1999). The teaching role is built into every nurse-patient interaction. Frequently, opportunities present themselves quite informally, so that you can speak to issues such as the biological basis for depression or mania or the importance of treatment. In Case Example 25–2, Joe benefitted from his sister-in-law's persistence, support, and encouragement. But most of all, her constant nonthreatening approach to teaching broke Joe's resistance and opened him to the possibilities of treatment. (See What Patients and Families Need to Know: Symptoms of Mania and What Society Needs to Know: Symptoms of Depression.)

Skipped

■ CASE EXAMPLE 25–2
■ Joe's Story

I had been feeling pretty bad for almost a year. Looking back on that time, I know that I was depressed. After a year, it wasn't getting better. In fact, there were mornings when I contemplated ways to end my life. I can hardly believe that I actually felt that despairing. One of the most

---

Box 25–6 ■ ■ ■ ■ ■
Expected Outcomes for Patients Experiencing Depression or Mania

Depression	Mania
The Patient Will	**The Patient Will**
· Remain free from self-inflicted harm	· Remain free from self-inflicted harm
· Be free of psychotic symptoms	· Be free of restlessness, hyperactivity, and agitation
· Demonstrate functional behavior in activities of daily living	· Be free of threatened aggression toward others
· Maintain balanced physiological functioning	· Demonstrate behaviors indicating feelings of self-worth
· Demonstrate an increased ability to deal with feelings of sadness, anxiety, or frustration	· Demonstrate appropriate appearance and behavior
· Demonstrate behaviors indicative of improved self-esteem	· Be free of psychotic symptoms
· Demonstrate increased spiritual well-being	· Demonstrate functional behavior in activities of daily living
· Demonstrate increased understanding of illness	· Maintain balanced physiological functioning
· Demonstrate increased understanding of treatment options	· Demonstrate increased spiritual well-being
· Identify a support system in the community	· Demonstrate increased understanding of illness
	· Demonstrate increased understanding of treatment options
The Family Will	· Identify a support system in the community
· Demonstrate increased understanding of depression and its symptoms	
· Verbalize the recognition that the family is not responsible for the cause or the healing of the depression	**The Family Will**
· Demonstrate increased understanding of the treatment issues in depression	· Demonstrate increased understanding of mania and its symptoms
· Identify a support system in the community	· Verbalize the recognition that the family is not responsible for the cause or the healing of the mania
· Demonstrate increased spiritual well-being	· Demonstrate increased understanding of the treatment issues in mania
	· Identify a support system in the community
	· Demonstrate increased spiritual well-being

Box 25-7 ■ ■ ■ ■ ■

Planning Short-Term Goals for Hospitalized Patients Who Are Depressed or Manic

Depression

The Patient Will

- Be free of self-inflicted harm
- Be oriented to person, place, and time
- Express feelings
- Communicate with congruent verbal and non-verbal messages
- Express anger or hostility outwardly in a safe manner
- Participate in activities
- Verbalize feelings of self-worth
- Verbalize hopefulness

Mania

The Patient Will

- Be free of self-inflicted harm
- Refrain from harming others
- Be oriented to person, place, and time
- Eat enough to maintain energy needs
- Restore balance in rest and activity
- Engage in therapeutic interactions

important factors in my seeking treatment was my sister-in-law's constant teaching and encouragement. She is a psychiatric nurse, and I guess it was pretty obvious to her that I was sick. She always asked me how I was doing, which reminded me that she cared.

But what really helped was her teaching. She would talk about a psychiatric patient she was working with in a general way, and then she would use this to lead into a discussion of depression, its symptoms, and the effectiveness of treatment. Then I remember her saying things like, "Some people feel that if they accept help, then that proves that they are weak. Can you believe what society has done to people suffering from psychiatric disorders? Somehow we convince them that it is their fault and deny them the very thing that would alleviate their suffering."

I know now that she was saying these things to me in the only way that I could hear them. Had she been direct with me I would have vigorously denied that I had a problem. One morning I cried like a baby; I just couldn't get out of bed. I knew I couldn't go on like this. My wife said, "Call Vickie; she'll know what to do." So I did. She gave me the name of a wonderful psychiatrist and a nurse psychotherapist. The doctor started me on fluoxetine (Prozac), which has worked wonders in my life. I feel better than ever! But the nurse is helping me to look at some negative thinking patterns that have always kept me from getting the most out of life. I am so grateful to Vickie. I think she may have saved my life. ■

You may also teach in formal ways, perhaps to groups of patients or families as well as to the community at large. Formal presentations provide the opportunity to educate a large number of people. Ideally, such presentations are followed by time for individual counseling. This allows people who are reticent to speak in a large group to have their questions answered and to seek advice, referrals, or support on a one-on-one basis. Formal presentations can effectively eliminate or reduce stigma by providing accurate information.

Included in the topics that you can address are medication issues along with other strategies to deal with stress and stay well. In addition, teach the patient about the importance of social support and the significance of spirituality to healing. Patient teaching also focuses on assisting the patient to communicate explicitly and honestly about needs. For example, the patient might say, "I know you mean well, but please don't do that." Another helpful thing for patients to recognize and be able to communicate to family members is that needs may change as the episode improves or worsens. The patient might say, "Something that isn't helpful to me today doesn't mean I might not want it tomorrow." The patient can learn to communicate gratitude even when the help offered is not what is needed. The patient in this situation might say, "I know you mean well by trying to talk to me, but I just can't talk right now." Clear feedback helps family members and others close to the patient remain long-term resources for the patient.

Nurse as Protector From Self-Injurious Behavior

Protecting patients from harming themselves or others is a priority in dealing with patients diagnosed with mood disorders. The nursing interventions include the following:

- Establish a written no-suicide contract with the patient.
- Make sure safety of the patient is ensured, whether the patient is experiencing suicidal ideation or also has intent and a plan. For a patient with ideation, intent, and plan, one-on-one contact with a staff member *at all times* (even when sleeping and in the bathroom) is necessary. The patient is restricted to the hospital unit and is permitted nothing that could cause self-harm (sharp objects, a belt). A patient who poses a less serious threat is assigned one-on-one contact with a staff member at all times but may go off the unit to attend activities while continuing one-on-one supervision. For a patient who expresses suicidal ideation and no plan, knowing the whereabouts of the patient at all times is sufficient. The patient may be accompanied by a staff member while off the unit, but one-on-one supervision is not required.
- Explain suicidal precautions to the patient.
- Be aware of potentially dangerous objects in the environment such as sharps, matches, lit cigarettes, and glass containers. These items should not be in the patient's possession.
- Check the environment to ensure that windows in the room are locked and are not accessible to the patient.

WHAT PATIENTS AND FAMILIES NEED TO KNOW

Symptoms of Mania

What is mania?

Mania is the term used to describe an elevated or "hyper" mood. Mania can range from mild symptoms to symptoms severe enough that the afflicted person requires hospitalization. Symptoms of mania include an exaggerated feeling of importance, increased activity, poor judgment, distractability, decreased need for sleep, and racing thoughts and speech.

Can some people have symptoms of both mania and depression?

A person can have both manic symptoms and depressive symptoms; this condition is termed bipolar disorder or mixed affective disorder. The symptoms range from mild to severe. Switching from manic symptoms to depressive symptoms can occur quickly or be independent of each other for a longer period.

What causes a person to become manic?

Considerable research on mania and depression over the past several years indicates that mania is the result of a chemical imbalance. It is also well known that a manic episode can be precipitated by a loss or a major stressor.

How is mania treated?

Because mania is biochemical, medications are effective in helping the symptoms subside. Lithium carbonate, a mineral, is one of the major drugs used. It works by stabilizing the extremes of low or high moods. Research has found several other mood stabilizers to be effective. Often, it may take a combination of two or more medications to stabilize the mood.

Will I need to be on medication for the rest of my life?

In many instances, people with symptoms of mania need to be on medications for the rest of their lives. Just as people who develop diabetes need to take insulin on a daily basis, people with bipolar disorder frequently need some type of medication to maintain a balance. When taking medications to treat mania, it is necessary to monitor blood levels and be under the supervision of a physician.

- Observe the patient, frequently observing behavior patterns. Note the patient's response to different activities on the unit, various staff members, and participation in tasks and activities.
- Be aware of relationships the patient may be forming on the unit. Be especially alert to relationships with other patients who may be manipulated into cooperating with the patient's suicide plan.
- As the patient takes medication, watch carefully to ensure that the patient is not cheeking and saving it.
- Observe any changes in the patient's mood.
- Encourage the patient to discuss feelings. Do not reinforce dwelling on previous suicide attempts or the details of such events.
- Communicate that the patient is a worthwhile human being and that there is always hope.
- Attempt to determine what keeps the patient "hanging on" and then reinforce that issue. For instance, if a patient says the only thing that keeps her from committing suicide is her children, reinforce how important it is for her to remain alive for them.
- Explore spiritual issues with the patient. Make a referral to clergy if necessary.
- Encourage the patient's expression of anger.
- Assist the patient to examine life, including the home environment and relationships outside of the hospital.

- Help the patient to identify situations and feelings that precipitate suicidal ideation. Assist the patient to plan how to deal with these feelings and situations to avert a disaster.

Nurse as Collaborator With Patient and Family

Your work in assisting family members to know how to help the patient is essential. When family members feel that they are partners in the health team, they can be useful in the present condition of the patient and also a long-term resource for him or her. To partner with a family, you need to assist family members to pull together. Your communication and interpersonal and counseling skills are essential. You affirm family efforts on behalf of the patient, make suggestions for continued well-being, provide information so that family members can be more effective, and invite them to collaborate in planning the patient's care. Such an approach presents a unified, supportive, and realistically hopeful environment in which the patient can begin the healing process.

In the "old" psychiatry, the relationship between the patient and physician or therapist was a privileged and confidential relationship. It was strictly forbidden that a

? WHAT SOCIETY NEEDS TO KNOW

Symptoms of Depression

How would I recognize depression in someone?

There are many indicators that a friend or family member may be suffering from depression. Often when a person is grieving a major loss, the term *depressed* is used to define normal sadness and pain. With the illness of depression, however, the sadness is overwhelming, and the person feels hopeless, helpless, and irritable. There is a noticeable change in eating habits and sleeping patterns, either sleeping too much or inability to feel rested after sleep. A person with depression loses energy and is unable to enjoy activities that previously brought pleasure. The person often cannot think or concentrate. A person who describes recurring thoughts of death or suicide needs to be seen by a physician immediately.

What are the major causes of depression?

There is no one single cause for depression. Researchers have found that depression tends to run in families. Also, some type of chemical imbalance frequently is present. Neurotransmitters are substances in the brain that allow brain cells to communicate with others. In depression, the deficiency in these chemicals causes insomnia, irritability, anxiety, fatigue, and lack of energy. Researchers do not know if these imbalances cause the disease or if the illness gives rise to the imbalances. It is not uncommon for major losses or stressors to precipitate a depressive illness.

How many people have depression?

Depression is the most common of all mental illnesses and often goes untreated because well-meaning family and friends advise the depressed person to "snap out of it." It is estimated that in any 6-month period, 9.4 million Americans suffer from depression. Depression is more common in women but does affect both genders and all age groups.

What can be done to treat depression?

Because a chemical imbalance is frequently the cause of depression, medications are typically indicated for treatment. These medications do not solve the stressors and problems that may have precipitated the symptoms, but they provide a person with the energy to deal with the issues. Antidepressants work by altering the brain's response to certain chemical reactions. Because these medications take about 4 to 6 weeks before they are fully effective, psychotherapy is usually recommended. Medications or psychotherapy, or a combination of both, usually relieves the symptoms of depression in weeks.

From American Psychiatric Association. (1994). *Let's talk about depression.* Washington, DC: American Psychiatric Association.

---

family member be informed about anything that was going on between the physician and patient. Fortunately that has changed. If collaboration with the family is permitted by the patient, more complete information is brought to the clinician and can greatly influence both the patient's diagnosis and the treatment. Most experienced clinicians recognize that a concerned family member can be the best support for both clinician and patient.

This partnership can be used to develop a plan to prevent relapses. Discuss the patient's symptoms and learn to recognize early warning signs of the illness as well as potential stressors that may precipitate an episode of illness. Sometimes the patient and family member can contract on the family member's role in helping the patient stay well. This supportive relationship, with the clinician as coach and facilitator, recognizes the family and patient as the vital motivators of maintaining wellness and support. This position is empowering for both the patient and the family and facilitates success.

You can teach the family the importance of decreasing the focus on the patient and trying as much as possible to "normalize" family routines. If the family is to remain intact, family members must avoid becoming dominated by the depressed person's needs. This is tremendously hard because even a depressed person who cannot speak or move and is immobilized by depression is a kind of magnetic focus for everyone in the family. Maintaining normal levels of socializing with family and friends is important. Obtaining support from others assists the family members to avoid feeling guilty and taking responsibility for the illness.

Nurse as Facilitator of Empowerment

The nurse can be of great assistance to the patient struggling for control and acceptance of the inevitable changes that come with illness. Using empowerment strategies, you can function in the role of facilitator and resource person, recognizing that self-awareness, self-growth, and resources are the tools that facilitate empowerment (Gibson, 1991; McAllister & Ryan, 1997).

Gibson (1991) defines **empowerment** as a social process of recognizing, promoting, and enhancing people's abilities to meet their own needs, solve their own problems, and mobilize necessary resources to take control of their own lives. In helping people assert control over their health, you are not only a resource person but also a mobilizer of resources. You need to facilitate access to both personal and environmental resources that foster a sense of control and self-efficacy and support health (Jones & Meleis, 1993).

Power, a component of the word *empowerment,* is synonymous with energy. Natural power is the capacity of acting or being active. Other synonyms are strength, efficacy, and effectiveness, implying "power to." Empowerment can occur when you and the patient are mutually active, respecting one another's needs and working together to achieve a result.

McKay, Forbes, and Bourner (1990) identified three components of mutual empowerment for patient and nurse: knowledge, confidence, and communication skills. The patient requires knowledge about the illness, and you need to be able to admit any knowledge deficits and find what the patient needs to know. The patient and nurse need to be able to listen and understand each other and effectively share information. The patient needs to experiment with information and advice given and confidently apply this knowledge to personal health care. You also need to be aware of the patient's understanding of the information provided and the extent of the patient's ability to cope through help and support rather than control and direction. Both you and the patient need confidence in each other to form a successful relationship. Figure 25–4 illustrates empowerment in nursing.

Nurse as Facilitator of Spiritual Growth

Nurses are in a unique position to understand the body, mind, and spirit relationship. The depressed person's spirit is oppressed. The mind is filled with thoughts of despair. The body is sluggish, dull, and unalive. Through understanding these factors, you can help the patient alter his or her perception of life. Through treatment,

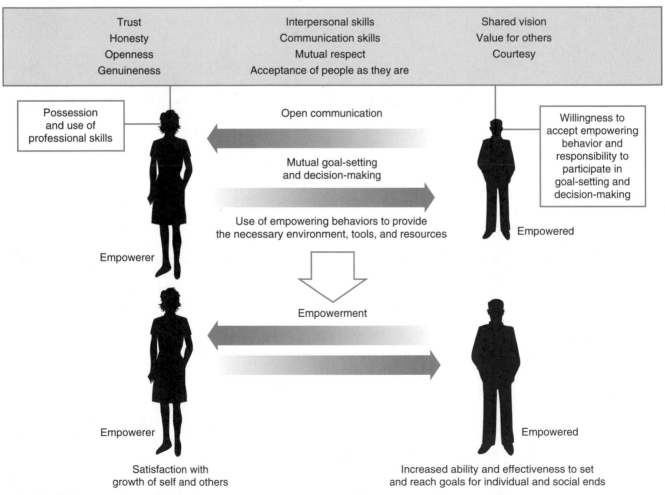

Figure 25–4

Empowerment in nursing. (From Hawks, J. [1992]. Empowerment in nursing education: Concept analysis and application to philosophy, learning and instruction. *Journal of Advanced Nursing, 17,* 613. Reprinted by permission of Blackwell Scientific Publications, Oxford, England.)

the person may achieve a higher level of wellness and understanding than before the illness began.

Continue to pursue treatment that works, but in the meantime, encourage and support a person's faith and convictions about life and God and, above all else, the will to live. The person may emerge from the painful experience having found knowledge and meaning and feels that this experience has been growth producing. Thurman provided a glimpse or such hope: "The roots are silently at work in the darkness of the earth against the time when there shall be new leaves, fresh blossoms, green fruit. Such is the growing edge" (cited in Miller, 1987).

The search for spirituality in our society is expressed individually as well as collectively through religious practices and convictions. Despite the erosion of the spirit during episodes of depressive illness, individuals are still drawn toward God and spiritual practices. Sometimes the spirituality and the beliefs of others serve to anchor a person in the present and provide hope that is so lacking internally. Although spirituality is a private affair, a matter of the heart, it is enhanced when intimacy and caring are part of a person's experience. The patient's spirituality may be bolstered by loved ones who continue to be faithful in their prayers, in their religious practices, and in the encouragement they offer the patient that things will get better (Carson, 1994). There is a strong connection among healthy, caring communities, healing, and spirituality (Wuthnow, 1994). Ralph Waldo Emerson described the spirit: "It is one of the most beautiful compensations of life that no man can seriously help another without helping himself." Figure 25-5 illustrates the Calarco and Krone (1991) model modified to include the spiritual dimension.

Nurse as a Referral Source for Social Support

In an effort to connect with one another in the search for spirituality, self-help or mutual support groups have developed as an important adjunct to treating patients with mood disorders and family members. Members come to meetings to share feelings and experiences with other people who have also experienced illness. They go away feeling satisfied that they may have helped another with their sharing. To qualify as a participant, the person has to have the illness and be willing to use the experience to help others. Meetings are run by and for members.

Although the term *self-help* is traditionally used in the literature, mutual help connotes the reality of these meetings as members struggle together to find solutions to problems related to illness. In mutual help groups, people experience the support and validation of others in similar situations. This process helps to decrease the social isolation so often experienced by both the patient and family members. William Styron (1990) wrote about his friend who had also experienced depression

His support was untiring and priceless. It was he who kept admonishing me that suicide was "unacceptable," and it was also he who made the prospect of going to the hospital

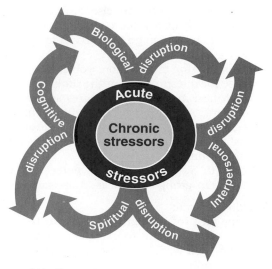

Figure 25–5
Calarco and Krone's integrated model of depressive behavior, modified to include the spiritual dimension. (Modified from Calarco, M., & Krone, K. [1991]. An integrated nursing model of depressive behavior in adults: Theory and implications for practice. *Nursing Clinics of North America, 26*, 573–583.)

less fearsomely intimidating. I still look back on his concern with immense gratitude. The help he gave me, my friend later said, had been a continuing therapy for him, thus demonstrating that, if nothing else, the disease engenders lasting fellowship. (p. 125)

Studies have shown that breast cancer patients who attended mutual help groups lived longer, regardless of the stage of their cancer or their treatment regimens. Support groups enhance the effectiveness of the medical treatment. Patients attending support groups are less depressed, fatigued, and confused and are actively coping better than those not in support groups. Apparently, sharing experiences, feelings, and fears with others reduces anxiety and promotes constructive behavior.

Skovhold (1974) summarized the benefits of this "helper therapy" principle. First, the effective helper often feels an increased level of interpersonal competence as a result of making an impact on another person's life. Second, the effective helper often feels a sense of equality in giving and taking. Third, the effective helper is often the recipient of valuable personalized learning acquired while working with someone in need. Finally, the effective helper often receives social approval from the people he or she helps. It has been hypothesized that all four factors, rather than any one, make helper therapy potent (Gartner & Reissman, 1984).

Members of a mutual help group for people with affective disorders reflect on their experience of belonging in a group facilitated not by professionals but by people who are affected by the illness themselves. "I wept when I first met Bob. I couldn't believe there was anyone else like me." Another group member described the experience, "It gives you a marker. If you see others worse than yourself, then you get some idea of how you are. It makes me feel I can't be that bad if I managed to do something for somebody else." Another member expressed the long-term value of the group: "I see the group as a safety net. I can go back to it if my depression returns."

Through supplying information, you can be an important resource for questions about the illness and dissemination of written material that ensures accuracy about mood disorders. As people with the illness and family members gain confidence in their knowledge and understanding of mood disorders, they will be less afraid to confront the stigma.

According to Silverman (1978), nurses collaborate with mutual help groups in at least four ways:

1. Making referrals
2. Serving on professional advisory boards
3. Serving as consultant to existing groups
4. Initiating and working on the development of new mutual help groups

Nurses can recruit patients, family members, and other mental health professionals into collaborative ventures such as mutual help groups. See the list of Additional Resources at the end of the chapter.

Nurse as Manager of Biological Interventions

MEDICATIONS

Although Chapter 17 provides a comprehensive review of the medications that are used in the treatment of mood disorders, there are still medication-related issues for the nurse to address. Research indicates that the most effective treatment for mood disorders includes both medication and psychotherapy. Not only does psychotherapy make it more likely that the patient will stay on medication, but also medication makes it more likely that the patient will continue in psychotherapy.

The medication-related issues to address are

- Establishing open and honest communication with the patient.
- Dealing with the stigma associated with taking medications.
- Providing accurate information about drugs, their actions, and side effects.
- Teaching the patient to address medication issues with the prescribing physician assertively.

The nurse needs to understand accurately what the patient is experiencing as a result of the medications. For instance, patients may withhold information about side effects they are experiencing, the lack of effectiveness of the medication, or the fact that they have stopped taking the medication. Factors that may precipitate the patient's noncompliance with antidepressant therapy include

- An attitude that the medication is a crutch
- Feelings or guilt and worthlessness
- Fears of drug dependency and addiction
- Lack of acceptance that a mood disorder is really a medical illness
- Feelings of shame, embarrassment, and stigma attached to mental illness and the idea of being "crazy"

Even when they are helped by medication, people may continue to believe they should have been able to handle the illness without medication. They may feel that if they tried a little harder or had done this or that differently, they would not have become ill. When faced with disagreement in their choice of treatment by their friends or family, the struggle is all the more difficult without a supportive therapist.

Adequate teaching cannot occur unless the nurse has established an environment in which the patient can honestly discuss feelings about medication. You must fully understand how the patient thinks and feels about medication. You must be cognizant of the patient's right to choose medications as part of treatment. Common nursing reactions to a patient's noncompliance are anger and frustration and a sense that the patient is rejecting interventions. You must guard against letting these feelings limit the exploration of a patient's choice to stop taking medications.

ELECTROCONVULSIVE THERAPY

Electroconvulsive therapy (ECT) induces a seizure by applying electric current. ECT provides the most rapid relief of any treatment for severe depression. Most of the severely ill patients who fail to respond to medication respond to ECT. This form of treatment should be considered when drug therapy has failed, when the patient is at high risk for suicide or starvation, or when depression is judged to be overwhelmingly severe. It is also particularly useful when the depressed person is troubled by delusions or hallucinations (DePaulo & Ablow, 1989).

ECT was discovered in the mid-1920s. At that time, it was the only treatment available and was frequently used and misused. In the mid-1960s, the use of general anesthesia and a muscle relaxant, most commonly succinylcholine, became a clinical standard for use with ECT. Since then, the frequency of adverse effects related to seizure have essentially become nonexistent (Abraham, Neese, & Westerman, 1991; Blazer & Cassel, 1994).

ECT treatments are given three times a week, with an average series involving 8 to 12 treatments and a duration of 2 to 4 weeks. How ECT works is still not clear. It appears to alter receptors for the catecholamine neurotransmitters in a way similar to that of the tricyclic antidepressants. The most common side effects are amnesia of events occurring near the period of the treatment and the potential for transient confusion as a result of the seizure and the barbiturate anesthetic.

Following a course of ECT, patients may have some memory deficits for the period before ECT was begun. These memory deficits tend to disappear with time, and in most cases patients suffer little long-term memory loss. Measuring the extent of memory loss is complicated because depression itself impairs concentration and memory. The memory deficits of which the patient complains may be the product not of the ECT but of the preexisting depression. Controversy still continues about whether any mild cognitive deficits remain after ECT (Blazer, 1994). Even with this controversy, ECT is the fastest-acting, most efficient form of therapy for depression and is considered safer than tricyclics in many cases. It is well tolerated and has a response rate of 70%

to 80%; however, the duration of the response may be as short as 1 month (Blazer, 1994).

Most patients who have had repeated episodes of depression are started on antidepressants after the course of ECT is completed. These act as an added precaution against the return of symptoms. A few patients do need a prolonged course of ECT. Those with a severe major depression that does not respond to medications may be prescribed continuation therapy called maintenance ECT (Sackheim, 1995). These patients receive a regular course of ECT and then continue their treatments on a reduced schedule, often on an outpatient basis, for several months. They may have one treatment a month or be treated less often. Table 25–5 outlines the nurse's responsibilities in monitoring the patient receiving ECT treatment. See Home Care Clinical Practice Guidelines: Depression.

***W**hat do you think?* How might you structure your nursing interventions with a patient who is in denial about his or her illness? Explain.

> *Check Your Reading*

21. In the role of counselor, identify five things that you would do.
22. Name two areas that you would teach the patient and family.
23. How do you collaborate with the patient and family?
24. What is empowerment?
25. Identify three ways that you can be a facilitator of empowerment for the patient.
26. How can you facilitate spiritual growth in the patient?
27. Identify at least two ways that nurses collaborate with support groups.
28. Name two things that you would teach a patient who was preparing to have ECT.

Evaluation

If you have established clear goals with the patient and the family, you can easily determine whether the plan needs to be modified or continued. The formative evaluation addresses such questions as the following:

- Has the patient remained safe? Has the patient made suicide attempts? If so, how does the plan need to be modified to ensure the patient's safety?
- Has the patient "connected" with a caring professional while in the hospital?
- Has the patient reestablished balance in eating, sleeping, and activity?
- Is the patient feeling better? Is there a noticeable improvement in mood, sociability, energy level, and interest in life?
- Has there been a significant improvement in the patient's score on the standardized depression inventory?
- Does the patient verbalize understanding of medication issues?
- Does the patient verbalize understanding of illness issues?
- Is the patient participating in therapy?
- Is the family involved in the patient's care?
- Has the patient begun to address the spiritual components of the illness?

The summative evaluation deals with issues such as discharge planning, referral to a support group, continuation of therapy, and the patient's ability to establish realistic goals.

***W**hat do you think?* In formulating discharge plans for your patient, why do you think it is important to facilitate a referral to a support group? Explain.

TABLE 25–5 Nursing Interventions for the Patient Receiving Electroconvulsive Therapy

BEFORE TREATMENT	DURING TREATMENT	AFTER TREATMENT
Provide teaching for the patient and family regarding the risks and benefits of ECT. Include the rationale for ECT, how ECT works, side effects of ECT, ECT procedures, activity after ECT, and ECT outcomes.	Before the procedure, check emergency equipment.	Reorient the patient.
	Keep NPO several hours before the treatment.	Be with the patient for comfort and support.
Offer handouts that might include a guide to ECT.	Remove potentially harmful objects, such as jewelry or dentures.	Assist family members to understand behavior associated with confusion or memory loss.
Make a videotape available that might outline the necessary information about ECT. Use this as a follow-up to your explanation to reinforce teaching or to stimulate questions and discussion.	Check vital signs.	Discuss with the patient and family how ECT has affected them and the effect it has on the patient's individual symptoms of depression.
	Maintain patent airway.	
	Position on side until alert.	
Whenever possible, encourage the exchange of information between patients and family members about their experiences with ECT.	Assist with ambulation.	
	Offer analgesic or antiemetic as needed.	

ECT, electroconvulsive therapy; NPO, nothing by mouth.

Home Care Clinical Practice Guidelines
DEPRESSION

Referral to a Psychiatric Home Care Program

Eligible
- Suicidal-passive only
- Not homicidal
- No safety risks

Ineligible
- Suicidal-active
- Homicidal
- Safety risk for clinicians

Comprehensive Assessment Physical/Psychosocial/Spiritual
- Mental Status Examination
- Depression Inventory
- Suicide Assessment
- Relapse Risk Assessment
- Other assessment tools as appropriate

Establish Plan of Care

Standards of Practice are based on the ANA Standards for Psychiatric & Mental Health Nursing

Areas marked ☑ are mandatory for diagnosis

Health Status Assessment
Establish Measurable Outcomes

Assessment

Cardiovascular
- ◯☑ Vital signs: blood pressure, sitting and standing

Gastrointestinal
- ◯ Anorexia
- ◯ Bowel movements including frequency, consistency, shape, odor, volume, color, continence
- ◯ Nausea and vomiting

Neurological/Psychological
- ◯☑ Mentation: confusion, disorientation, mood, memory, agitation, combative
- ◯☑ Sleep disturbances
- ◯☑ Speech characteristics: fluency, aphasia, word finding
- ◯☑ Extrapyramidal symptoms
- ◯☑ Hallucinations
- ◯☑ Delusions
- ◯ Other

Nutrition
- ◯ Alcohol, caffeine and nicotine use
- ◯ Food intake
- ◯ Weight

Lab Orders
- ◯ SN to draw blood for therapeutic drug levels (e.g. Lithium, Tegretol)

Self Care Knowledge
Establish Measurable Outcomes

Patient/Caregiver Education

Disease Process
- ◯☑ S/S
- ◯☑ S/S to report to Nurse/MD
- ◯☑ Lifestyle changes
- ◯☑ Complications/precautions
- ◯☑ Written materials provided
- ◯ Other
- ◯ Time/Life video on depression

Medication Regimen
- ◯☑ Medication, side effects, schedule
- ◯☑ Food and drug interactions
- ◯☑ Written materials provided
- ◯ Other

Nutrition
- ◯ Meal planning
- ◯ Selection of food

Caregiver/Social Support
- ◯ Caregiver/family in appropriate level of patient care
- ◯ Identify relative, friends and neighbors for support/ visitation
- ◯ Use of respite time
- ◯ Outlet to express anger/feelings of burden
- ◯ Importance of structure in patient's day
- ◯ Communication and limit setting with patient
- ◯ Ways to give patient responsibilities

Emotional/Spiritual
- ◯☑ Encourage expression of feelings and suppport efforts at coping
- ◯☑ Validate "normalization" of feelings
- ◯☑ Provide reassurance and instruct on reasonable expectations
- ◯☑ Be empathetic, supportive and non-judgmental
- ◯ Encourage use of spiritual resources
- ◯ Encourage patient/family interaction
- ◯☑ Written materials provided
- ◯ Help patient acknowledge losses associated with chronic illness

Lifestyle and Compliance
- ◯ Tobacco safty use
- ◯ Alcohol safty use
- ◯ Exercise regimen compatible with patient's health status
- ◯ Lifestyle adjustments with certain medications
- ◯☑ Develop strategies to enhance compliance with treatment regimen
- ◯☑ Use reward or praise patient's progress toward goals

Emergency Measures
- ◯ Access 911/EMS
- ◯ Access on-call nurse
- ◯ Procedure for drug overdose

Household Resources
- ◯ Teach about community associations that support mentally ill; support offered by churches, schools, food pantries
- ◯ Instruct about possible medication funding programs through physician's office

Home Safety
- ◯ Remove harmful objects that are within reach
- ◯☑ Written materials provided

Home care clinical practice guidelines for depression. (From Staff Builders Home Health Care, Staff Builders, Inc., 1983 Marcus Avenue, Lake Success, NY 11042-7011.)

Illustration continued on following page

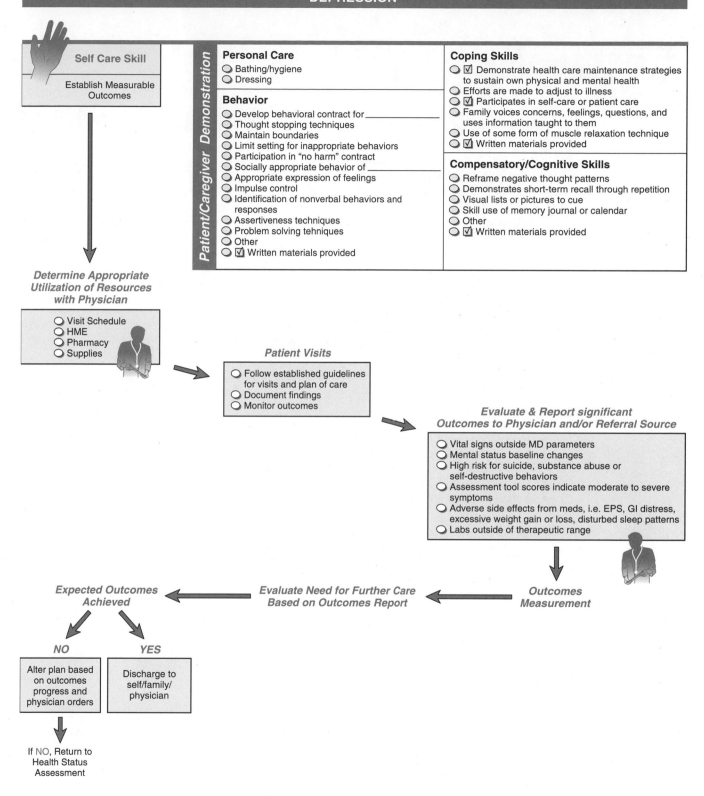

Home Care Clinical Practice Guidelines
DEPRESSION

Self Care Skill

Establish Measurable Outcomes

Patient/Caregiver Demonstration

Personal Care
○ Bathing/hygiene
○ Dressing

Behavior
○ Develop behavioral contract for _____
○ Thought stopping techniques
○ Maintain boundaries
○ Limit setting for inappropriate behaviors
○ Participation in "no harm" contract
○ Socially appropriate behavior of _____
○ Appropriate expression of feelings
○ Impulse control
○ Identification of nonverbal behaviors and responses
○ Assertiveness techniques
○ Problem solving tehniques
○ Other
○ ☑ Written materials provided

Coping Skills
○ ☑ Demonstrate health care maintenance strategies to sustain own physical and mental health
○ Efforts are made to adjust to illness
○ ☑ Participates in self-care or patient care
○ Family voices concerns, feelings, questions, and uses information taught to them
○ Use of some form of muscle relaxation technique
○ ☑ Written materials provided

Compensatory/Cognitive Skills
○ Reframe negative thought patterns
○ Demonstrates short-term recall through repetition
○ Visual lists or pictures to cue
○ Skill use of memory journal or calendar
○ Other
○ ☑ Written materials provided

Determine Appropriate Utilization of Resources with Physician

○ Visit Schedule
○ HME
○ Pharmacy
○ Supplies

Patient Visits

○ Follow established guidelines for visits and plan of care
○ Document findings
○ Monitor outcomes

Evaluate & Report significant Outcomes to Physician and/or Referral Source

○ Vital signs outside MD parameters
○ Mental status baseline changes
○ High risk for suicide, substance abuse or self-destructive behaviors
○ Assessment tool scores indicate moderate to severe symptoms
○ Adverse side effects from meds, i.e. EPS, GI distress, excessive weight gain or loss, disturbed sleep patterns
○ Labs outside of therapeutic range

Expected Outcomes Achieved

Evaluate Need for Further Care Based on Outcomes Report

Outcomes Measurement

NO   *YES*

Alter plan based on outcomes progress and physician orders

Discharge to self/family/ physician

If NO, Return to Health Status Assessment

➤ *Check Your Reading*
1. Identify at least five areas that you would review in a formative evaluation.

2. What would be important to consider in a summative evaluation?

NURSING PROCESS APPLICATION

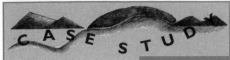

Wanda

Wanda is a 45-year-old woman who was admitted to the psychiatric hospital yesterday because she was no longer able to work or care for herself or her family. Her 25-year-old daughter, Laronda, became worried when she noticed that her mother was sleeping all the time, was not eating, and talked about "ending it all because life is just too difficult." Laronda is present with her mother during the admission process.

When you interview Wanda for the first time, you find that she is the single mother of three children. Laronda is also a single mother of two children and is attending community college, sharing the care of the two children with her mother. Wanda's son James is 23, works in a restaurant, and is also a part-time student. When Wanda speaks of her youngest son, Jesse, you notice that tears begin to well up in her eyes. She shares that Jesse, who is 20, became involved in drugs and gang activity several years ago and is currently serving a 10-year prison term for possession of drugs and armed robbery. He was incarcerated 6 months ago, and Laronda tells you her mother hasn't been the same since. Laronda is concerned because her mother has lost interest even in her grandchildren and going to church. Wanda tells you, "I know that God left me; I am such a bad person—nothing I do is right."

ASSESSMENT

The assessment data are as follows:
- Insomnia
- Sad affect
- Decreased appetite
- Verbalizations of despair: "Life is just too difficult."
- Loss of interest in previously enjoyable activities
- Verbalizations of shame and guilt: "I am a bad person."
- Verbalizations of abandonment by God: "I know God has left me."

DIAGNOSIS

DSM-IV Diagnosis: Major Depressive Disorder, single episode

Nursing Diagnosis: Hopelessness related to long-term stress and loss of belief in God, evidenced by vegetative symptoms of depression and verbalizations of despair and abandonment by God.

OUTCOME IDENTIFICATION, PLANNING, AND IMPLEMENTATION

Expected Outcome 1: By _____ the patient will be free of suicidal and depressive symptoms.

Short-Term Goals	Nursing Interventions	Rationale
By _____ the patient will sleep uninterrupted for at least 6 hours, and her appetite will return to normal.	1. Monitor and assess the patient's sleeping and eating patterns. 2. Administer medication as needed for sleep if the patient is unable to gain restful sleep. 3. Determine the patient's food preferences. 4. Encourage socialization while eating as the patient is ready.	1. Before intervention, it is important to establish a baseline. 2. If the patient's sleep has been disturbed for a long period, it may be necessary to intervene chemically initially. 3–4. Promote compliance and provide for decreased alienation.
By _____ the patient will report a mood change consistent with hopefulness.	1. Conduct a suicide assessment and initiate appropriate staff supervision depending on the level of risk.	1. Hospitalization for depression usually indicates that the patient is at high risk for suicide.

2. Administer antidepressant medications as ordered.

3. Teach the patient individually or in a group setting specifically how antidepressant medications alleviate the symptoms of depression.

2. To stabilize the mood and promote sleep, medications are often indicated when persons are hospitalized.
3. Teaching the patient about the physiological action of medications ensures compliance.

By _____ the patient will be able to verbalize feelings associated with depression.

1. In group therapy or individually, encourage the patient specifically to verbalize the feelings associated with hopelessness.
2. As trust is developed, encourage open expression of the patient's feelings about her son's incarceration.
3. Remain nonjudgmental and accepting.

1. Patients are often reluctant to talk about negative feelings because of the fear of overwhelming emotional pain.

2–3. There is shame associated with incarceration, and the patient may have been reluctant to share her feelings with anyone.

Expected Outcome 2: By _____ the patient will participate willingly in daily activities on the unit and engage in self-care behaviors.

Short-Term Goals	**Nursing Interventions**	**Rationale**
By _____ the patient will initiate self-grooming activities.	1. Offer genuine praise for the patient's efforts for goal setting, grooming, and other self-care activities.	1. Genuine, specific praise promotes continuance of positive behaviors. Patients tend to refute any praise that is general, such as "You look nice today."
By _____ the patient will willingly attend all unit functions.	1. Encourage the patient to participate in all activities that promote positive thoughts, feelings, and validation, such as recreational therapy, communication with her daughter, and perhaps a grief group.	1. These activities foster inclusion and decrease the alienation associated with hopelessness.

Expected Outcome 3: By _____ the patient will demonstrate hopefulness regarding her future life.

Short-Term Goals	**Nursing Interventions**	**Rationale**
By _____ the patient will (on three separate occasions) state something that she is hopeful about.	1. Encourage the patient to express negative feelings of hopelessness, despondency, and alienation. 2. Identify positive parts of the patient's existence, such as the loving support of her two older children and her grandchildren, her participation in a group, and something she has accomplished on the unit. 3. Help the patient identify behaviors that promote hopelessness, such as not attending group activities, eating alone, or ruminating about events over which she has little or no control. 4. Educate the patient about positive thinking and how to create a place of safety in her mind to combat hopelessness.	1. This process allows the patient an opportunity to ventilate feelings that have been pent up for a long time. 2. Helping the patient see positive people and situations promotes the expectation that hope is possible. 3. This process enables the patient to recognize experiences that precipitate feelings of hopelessness. 4. Feelings of hopelessness will inevitably reappear, and it is important that the patient is ready to deal with these feelings rather than perceive she has no control over them.

Expected Outcome 4: By _____ the patient will find hope and meaning in her relationship with God.

Short-Term Goals	**Nursing Interventions**	**Rationale**
By _____ the patient will make a positive statement about God.	1. Provide models of persons from literature or the Bible who have overcome misfortune.	1–3. Knowing that others have been able to overcome painful and shameful situations is often comforting.

By _____ the patient will verbalize how the events in her life, particularly her son's incarceration, have affected her on her life's journey.

2. Encourage the patient to discuss these situations and attempt to relate them to herself.

3. Ask the patient to think about how the situation relates to her situation and how they are alike.

4. Explain to the patient the importance of attempting to find meaning in all of life's events, even the most difficult ones.

5. Ask the patient if there are any spiritual resources that would be helpful to her at this time. Ask if there is something that you could do to respond to her distress.

4. Finding spiritual meaning in pain and trauma helps the process of grieving and acceptance.

5. Assisting the patient in rekindling her relationship with God is a loving and compassionate act because the patient is vulnerable and unable to do this for herself at this time.

Nursing Diagnosis: Chronic Low Self Esteem related to long-standing history of minimal accomplishments and losses, evidenced by self-negating verbalizations and feelings of shame, guilt, and despair.

Expected Outcome 1: By _____ the patient will demonstrate behavior consistent with increased self-esteem.

Short-Term Goals	Nursing Interventions	Rationale
By _____ the patient will verbalize feelings of self-worth.	1. Encourage the patient to engage in self-care grooming activities.	1. Attending to grooming is often an initial step in feeling better about oneself.
By _____ the patient will demonstrate absence of self-negating statements.	2. Honestly praise the patient for all observable accomplishments.	2. Patients with low self-esteem do not benefit from flattery or insincere praise. Honest, positive feedback enhances self-esteem.
By _____ the patient will actively engage in group therapy and activities on the unit.	3. Begin with simple recreational activities or art projects and proceed to more complex situations in a group context.	3. Initially the client may be too overwhelmed to engage in activities with more than one person.
	4. If the patient persists in negativism about self, place a limit on the length of time you will be able to listen to negativity. For example, agree to 10 minutes of negativity followed by 10 minutes of positive comments.	4. Time limits allow the client a safe time and place to ventilate negative feelings and demonstrate thought-stopping, the conscious interruption of negative thoughts.
	5. Explore with the patient her personal strengths and suggest making a written list to use as a reminder when negativity returns.	5. Having a written list to review can help the patient during difficult times after discharge, when the support of hospital staff is not there.

Expected Outcome 2: By _____ the patient will demonstrate understanding of the effect of negative self-talk and irrational belief systems.

Short-Term Goals	Nursing Interventions	Rationale
By _____ the patient will verbalize realistic statements about self and others.	1. Listen and accept the patient's irrational beliefs and feelings without judgment.	1–2. When the patient perceives your listening and confronting as a caring intervention, she will be better able to accept what you are intending her to hear.
By _____ the patient will accept praise from the staff without self-negating comments.	2. Respectfully confront persistent irrational beliefs, such as "I am a bad person," or all-or-nothing thinking.	
	3. Encourage thought-stopping and thought-substituting techniques.	3. This technique enables the patient to replace irrational thoughts with rational ones.

4.   Give the patient positive affirmation when she is able to accept praise verbally or nonverbally.

4.   Positive feedback encourages positive behavior.

By _____ the patient will practice suggestions for increasing self-esteem and will request support from the staff and peers.

1.   Encourage the patient to be proactive and assertive.
2.   Teach the necessary assertive skills and help the patient to distinguish between assertiveness and aggressiveness.
3.   Have the patient practice new behaviors with the staff and her peers.
4.   Encourage the patient to identify her own needs and to practice asking for what she needs.

1–3.   Becoming proactive and assertive is a skill and requires coaching.
2.   It is not unusual for people with passive personalities to become aggressive because they have allowed transgressions to occur for a long time.

4.   Part of being assertive is becoming aware of your own needs and asking for help when necessary.

Expected Outcome 3: By _____ the patient will verbalize a desire to live and develop realistic plans for the future.

Short-Term Goals	Nursing Interventions	Rationale
By _____ the patient will verbalize a desire to live by identifying daily goals and at least one long-term goal.	1. As the depression lifts, encourage the patient to set a daily goal and to put it in writing. An example is to call her daughter or write her son a letter. 2. Once daily goals are achieved and the patient has experienced some success, assist the patient in formulating long-term goals, such as a change in career, financial goals, interpersonal goals, or goals related to her health.	1–2. Writing both daily goals and long-term goals enables the patient to begin to believe in herself. Having a plan for the future is a proactive way of combating depression.

EVALUATION

Formative Evaluation: Wanda met all of her short-term goals. She said that she wasn't aware of how depressed she had become. She had always been a person with a strong drive and ambition, and this episode of depression took her by surprise. Wanda realized that the low self-esteem was not new but resolved to continue to work on feeling better about herself.

Summative Evaluation: Wanda also met all of the stated long-term goals. At the time of discharge, the staff told Wanda that they were concerned for her continued support. Wanda was a compliant patient and responded well to the structure provided by the hospitalization and the caring and concern of the treatment team. Wanda's typical role is to be a caretaker, and she was just beginning to learn to accept praise and genuine concern from others without negating it. The treatment team recommended that Wanda see a psychotherapist either individually or in a group for at least 6 months. See the Snapshot of Nursing Interventions Specific to Major Depression.

SNAPSHOT

Nursing Interventions Specific to Major Depression

What do you need to do to develop a relationship with a patient suffering with major depression?

- Approach the patient with warmth, quiet demeanor, and acceptance.
- Share time with the patient even if he or she talks little or not at all.
- Be honest, empathetic, and compassionate.
- Avoid lighthearted or too forceful an approach.
- Speak slowly and allow the patient time to respond.
- Address the patient by preferred name (don't assume it is okay to use the patient's first name until you ask the patient's preference); talk with the patient and listen carefully to what the patient shares.
- Find ways to express hope without negating the pain experienced by the patient.
- Encourage the patient to identify and discuss feelings.

What do you need to assess on the patient's health status?

- Suicidal risk or self-destructive thoughts
- Affective responses, including anger, anxiety, apathy, bitterness, denial of feelings; guilt, despondency; irritability; helplessness, hopelessness (may be evaluated and quantified using a standardized depression inventory such as the Beck, the Zung, or the Hamilton)
- Physiological responses, including gastrointestinal disturbances; appetite changes; constipation; fatigue; sexual disturbances; sleep disturbances; weight changes; headache, menstrual changes
- Cognitive responses, including confusion; slowed thinking; indecisiveness; problems with concentration; self-blame; pessimism
- Behavioral responses, including isolation and withdrawal; crying; agitation; alcoholism; drug addiction; slowed activity; poor personal hygiene; underachievement; inability to perform instrumental activities of daily living such as cooking, balancing a checkbook, budgeting money, and structuring time
- Vital signs, including sitting and standing blood pressure if patient is taking medication that leads to orthostatic hypotension
- Weight, especially if patient is experiencing changes in appetite

- Response to and compliance with medication regimen and reasons behind noncompliance; delayed effectiveness of medication
- Degree of social support
- Knowledge level; ability and readiness to learn
- Concurrent medical conditions

What do you need to teach the patient and/or the patient's caregiver?

- Medication issues; reason for taking; side effects and how to deal with them; untoward effects; warnings; importance of adhering to medication schedule
- Disease process; causes of depression; course of disease; and treatments
- Nutrition issues
- Emergency measures
- Importance of social support and strategies to obtain it
- Maintaining safety
- Lifestyle and compliance issues, such as benefits of exercise and stress management
- Importance of emotional support
- Importance of achieving spiritual well-being

What skills will you want the patient and/or caregiver to demonstrate?

- Ability to enter into a no-harm contract and remain safe
- Ability to follow medication and treatment plan
- Ability to use thought-stopping techniques and other cognitive strategies to deal with distorted thinking patterns
- Ability to perform personal care
- Ability to identify and express feelings
- Coping skills
- Relaxation techniques

What other health professionals might need to be a part of this plan of care?

- Physician (psychiatrist and/or primary care physician)—usually in charge of the overall treatment plan including medication management
- Social worker—to assist with access to community supports; insurance issues; access to entitlements; connection with community-based treatments
- Psychiatric occupational therapist—to assist patient with instrumental activities of daily living such as time management, cooking, and budgeting
- Nursing assistant or home health aide—to assist patient with personal hygiene and grooming, if necessary

Conclusions

Mood disorders are common and are frequently overlooked by some health professionals and misunderstood by others. The challenge for the nurse is to recognize the often misleading symptoms of depressive illnesses and assist the patient through diagnosis and treatment. Assessment of individual, family, spiritual, and environmental factors are important in planning for the patient's care. You need to address the impact of the illness on the patient's self-perception and sense of control over life. Through empowerment, you can encourage and develop a collaborative approach to helping, which is important to preventive health. With this approach, patients are assisted in taking responsibility and control of their own health care decisions. Additionally, family members need to be included as caregivers in the process. Provide them with the necessary preparation and support.

Both patients and family members need access to reliable written information and teaching about the illness. You need to be familiar with community resources that can help patients and families. You need to have a good working knowledge of the mutual help groups available and use them as referral sources. These groups assist patients to prevent or recover from illness and to attain their optimal level of health and independence. The stigma associated with mood disorders must be addressed through education and research efforts. Increased knowledge of the biological and genetic influences leads to a better understanding of how physical and psychosocial stressors may influence these illnesses. With more specific and accurate information to give people about depression and manic-depressive illnesses, fear and stigma can be reduced.

Mood disorders are treatable diseases. William Styron (1990) shared this message:

For those who have dwelt in depression's dark wood, and known its inexplicable agony, their return from the abyss is not unlike the ascent of the poet, trudging upward and upward out of hell's black depths and at last emerging into what he saw as "the shining world." There, whoever has been restored to health has almost always been restored to the capacity for serenity and joy, and this may be indemnity enough for having endured the despair beyond despair. (p. 84)

Key Points to Remember

- Mood disorders affect the way people feel about themselves. The impact of these disorders is holistic.
- Depressed people tend to be sad, irritable, despairing, hopeless, and suicidal.
- Manic people tend to be excited and elated or extremely irritable.
- All the mood disorders involve variations of, or combinations of, depression and mania.
- Mood disorders affect as many as 10% to 15% of Americans. They affect a person's most productive years. They are relapsing, episodic, and if left untreated, become more frequent and severe.
- Mood disorders have a high rate of co-occurrence with other disorders.
- Mood disorders have a high mortality rate. Suicide is the most common complication.
- Diagnosis of mood disorders is hampered by our inability to describe moods and changes in moods.
- Mood refers to a person's pervasive feeling state. A normal mood is euthymia; a bad mood is dysthymia; a high mood is elation.
- Affect refers to the fleeting feelings that show on our faces.
- Diagnosis of mood disorders looks at whether the patient is experiencing a persistent change in mood, self-attitude, and vital sense.

- The cause of mood disorders is most likely due to multiple factors, including sleep alterations; pharmacological interventions; and neuronal, endocrinological, genetic, and psychodynamic causes.
- Assessment of a patient with a mood disorder involves collecting data regarding the patient's mood, self-attitude, and vital sense. In addition, standardized depression inventories are frequently used. Information is collected about suicidal ideation, intent, and plan; the family's feelings, attitudes, and knowledge; issues of powerlessness spiritual concerns, and social isolation.
- There are many nursing diagnoses appropriate for the patient with a mood disorder.
- Expected outcomes focus on the patient's safety, normalization of mood, return of energy level to normal, and functional improvement.
- Implementation involves multiple roles, including counselor, teacher, protector, collaborator, facilitator of empowerment, facilitator of spiritual growth, referral source for social support, and manager of biological interventions.
- Evaluation examines the assessment data and the original short-term goals and expected outcomes. If the patient has made progress toward goal achievement, the plan is continued; if the progress has not been made, the plan is modified.

Learning Activities

1. Monitor your own moods for a week. How would you describe your mood changes? Is there wide variability in your moods? What affects your own mood changes? When you feel blue, what helps you to feel better?

2. Read William Styron's account of his depression. Write your reactions to his story in your journal.

3. People who suffer with mood disorders are afraid that if others know the diagnosis, they will be stigmatized. What do you think about people who have mood disorders? Would you want to work with a person who suffers with periodic depressions?

How do you think people who have mood disorders should be treated? Ask five other people (a mix of health professionals and nonhealth professionals) what they think about people with mood disorders. From these interviews and your own reactions, how real is the issue of stigma? How can stigma be countered?

Critical Thinking Exercises

Mrs. Buzzer, a 25-year-old woman, was brought to the crisis unit after she was found directing rush-hour traffic wearing red leotards, a see-through bathing suit top, and a bright green feather in her safari hat. When she spoke to the nurse on the unit, she stated, "I am the Amazon queen of all people." Mrs. Buzzer asked the nurse if she could call her sister to bring other clothes for her to wear. The nurse debated whether to allow this request.

1. What assumptions can be made about Mrs. Buzzer's behavior?

2. What evidence suggests that the nurse should deny or approve the request?

3. What might happen if she denies the request?

The following afternoon, Mrs. Buzzer's husband called the unit stating that he had received a call from a department store telling him that his wife had charged $500 on their credit card to buy shoes and dresses. She told the salesgirl that she was on her way to Africa to hunt baboons.

1. Make sense of the information.

2. What conclusion can be made about whether the nurse denied or approved the request?

3. What evidence leads you to draw this conclusion?

Additional Resources

Depression and Related Affective Disorders Association (DRADA)

Meyer 3–181
600 North Wolfe Street
Baltimore, MD 21287-7381
410-955-4647 (Baltimore)
202-955-5800 (Washington, DC)
drada-g@welchlink.welch.jhu.edu (e-mail)
This nonprofit organization is composed of individuals with mood disorders, family members, and mental health professionals. It offers information, education, referral, and support services to people nationwide. DRADA sponsors a nationally renowned training program for group leaders.

Depression Awareness, Recognition, and Treatment Program (D/ART)

5600 Fisher's Lane
Suite 10-85
Rockville, MD 20857
301-443-4140
301-443-4045 (fax)

National Self-Help Clearinghouse
Provides a list of resources throughout the United States that can help in networking and providing consultative assistance.

References

Abraham, I., Neese, J., & Westerman, P. (1991). Depression: Nursing implications of a clinical and social problem. *Nursing Clinics of North America, 26,* 527-535.

Abramson, L., Seligman, M., & Teasdale, J. (1978). Learned helplessness in humans: Critique and reformulation. *Journal of Abnormal Psychology, 87,* 49-74.

American Psychiatric Association. (1994). *Diagnostic and statistical manual of mental disorders* (4th ed.). Washington, DC: Author.

Bachelor, A. (1996). Cognitive and psychodynamic correlates of depressive symptomatology. *Psychological Report.*

Beauchemin, K. M., & Hay, P. (1997). Phototherapy is a useful adjunct in the treatment of depressed inpatients. *Acta Psychiatrica Scandinavica 5,* 424-427.

Beck, A., Rush, A., Shaw, B., (1979). *Cognitive theory of depression.* New York: Guilford Press.

Beck, C. (1993). Teetering on the edge: A substantive theory of postpartum depression. *Nursing Research, 42*(1), 42-47.

Beck, D. A. (1996). Minor depression: A review of the literature. *International Journal of Psychiatry Medicine, 26,* 177-209.

Blazer, D. G., & Cassel, C. F. (1994). Depression in the elderly. *Hospital Practice, 29,* 37-41.

Blehar, M. C., & Oren, D. A. (1997). Gender differences in depression. *Medscape Health, 2*(2),

Bloch, S. (1979). Supportive psychotherapy. In S. Bloch (Ed.), *An introduction to the psychotherapies* (pp. 196-220). New York: Oxford University Press.

Bowden, C. L. (1997). Treatment options in bipolar disorder: Mood stabilizers. *Medscape Mental Health, 2*(7),

Brown, A. (1996, Winter). Mood disorders in children and adolescents. *NARSAD Research Newsletter.*

Calarco, M., & Krone, K. (1991). An integrated nursing model of depressive behavior in adults: Theory and implications for practice. *Nursing Clinics of North America, 26,* 573-583.

Carson, V. B. (1994, January). Spirituality and depression. *Smooth Sailing: DRADA Newsletter,* 34.

D/ART (Depression/Awareness Recognition and Treatment). (1999). Depression co-occurring with general medical disorders. Available at: http://www.nimh.nih.gov/dart/index.htm.

Davila, J., & Bradbury, T. N. (1997). Marital functioning and depressive symptoms: Evidence for a stress generation model. *Journal of Personality Social Psychology, 73,* 849-861.

DePaulo, J. R., & Ablow, K. (1989). *How to cope with depression: A complete guide for you and your family.* New York: McGraw-Hill.

DePaulo, J. R. (1996, March). *Recent findings in the genetics of bipolar disorder.* Paper presented at the DRADA Symposium.

Derogatis, L. R., & Wise, T. N. (1989). *Anxiety and depressive disorders in the medical patient* (p. 125). Washington, DC: American Psychiatric Press.

Endler, N. (1990). *Holiday of darkness: A psychologist's personal journey out of his depression.* Toronto: Wall & Thompson.

Fassler, D. G. (1997). *Childhood depression: Early recognition leads to successful treatment.* Paper Presented at the American Academy of Child and Adolescent Psychiatry.

Finley, C., & Wilson, D. (1951). The relation of the family to manic-depressive psychosis. *Diseases of the Nervous System, 12,* 39-43.

Franson, K. L., Renner, J. A., & Grossberg, G. (1994). A practical guide to the use of antidepressants in the elderly. *Clinical Geriatrics, 2,* 39-49.

Frederick, P. (1989). Southwestern Internal Medicine Conference: Depression and medical illness. *American Journal of Medical Science, 298,* 64.

Friedman, R. A., Mitchell, J., & Kocsis, J. H. (1995). Retreatment for relapse following desipramine discontinuation in dysthymia. *American Journal of Psychiatry, 152,* 926-928.

Fromm-Reichmann, F. (1949). Intensive psychotherapy of manic-depressives: A preliminary report. *Confina Neurologica, 9,* 158-165.

Gartner, A., & Reissman, F. (1984). The self-help revolution. New York: Human Services Press.

Gaylin, W. (Ed.). (1968). *The meaning of despair: Psychoanalytic contributions to the understanding of depression.* New York: Science House.

Gibson, C. (1991). A concept analysis of empowerment. *Journal of Advanced Nursing, 16,* 354-361.

Goldberg, J. F. (1997). The treatment of chronic depression: Current strategies and future directions. *Medscape Mental Health, 2*(6), 18-22.

Goldstein, D. M. (1998, April 12). Pharmacological treatment of mood disorders. Presentation, Georgetown Medical Center, Depression and Related Affective Disorders Association (DRADA), Washington, DC.

Goodwin, F., & Jamison, K. (1990). *Manic-depressive illness.* New York: Oxford University Press.

Hales, R. E., Rakel, R. E., & Rothschild, S. (1994). Depression: Practical tips for detection and treatment. *Patient Care, 28,* 60.

Handal, K. (1998). Depression in women. Available at: http://thriveonline.aol.com/health/depression/depression.

Harris, M. F. (1996). Anxiety and depression in general practice patients: Prevalence and management. *Medical Journal of Australia, 164,* 526-529.

Hawks, J. (1992). Empowerment in nursing education: Concept analysis and application to philosophy, learning and instruction. *Journal of Advanced Nursing, 17,* 613.

Hays, R. D., Wells, K. B., Sherbourne, C. D., Rogers, W., & Spritzer, K. (1995). Functioning and well-being outcomes of patients with depression compared with chronic general medical illnesses. *Archives of General Psychiatry, 52*(1):11-19.

Hirschfeld, R. M. A., (1997). The National Depressive and Manic Depressive Association Consensus statement on the undertreatment of depression. *Journal of the American Medical Association, 277,* 333-340.

Hughes, D. (1997, January). The cost of depression in the elderly. Effects of drug therapy. *Drugs Aging,* 20.

Isacsson, G., Bergman, U., & Rich, C. L. (1996). Epidemiological data suggest antidepressants reduce suicide risk among depressives. *Journal of Affective Disorders, 41*(1), 1-8.

Jones, P., & Meleis, A. (1993). Health is empowerment. *Advances in Nursing Science, 15*(13), 113-118.

Kapci, E. G. (1998). Test of the hopelessness theory of depression: Drawing negative inference from negative life events. *Psychological Report, 82,* 355-363.

Kernberg, O. F. (1988). Clinical dimensions of masochism. *Journal of American Psychoanalytic Association, 36,* 1005-1029.

Kerr, N. (1987-1988). Signs and symptoms of depression and principles of nursing intervention. *Perspectives in Psychiatric Care, 14*(2), 48-63.

Klerman, G., Weissman, M., Rounsaville, B., & Chevron, E. (1984). *Interpersonal psychotherapy of depression.* New York: Basic Books.

Krauchi, K., Reich, S., & Wirz-Justice, A. (1997). Eating style in seasonal affective disorder: Who will gain weight in winter? *Comprehensive Psychiatry, 38*(2), 80-87.

Lowell, R. (1977). *Day by day.* New York: Farrar, Straus and Giroux.

Markowitz, J. C., Svartberg, M., & Swartz, H. A. (1998). Is IPT time-limited psychodynamic psychotherapy? *Journal of Psychotherapeutic Practice Research, 7,* 185-195.

Mayo, J. (1979). Families of manic-depressive patients: Effects of treatment. *American Journal of Psychiatry, 136,* 1535-1539.

McAllister, M., & Ryan, M. (1997). Generating ideas for teaching mental health. *Nursing Journal of Psychiatric Mental Health Nursing, 4*(2), 111-115.

McDonald, W. M., & Nemeroff, C. B. (1998). Practical guidelines for diagnosing and treating mania and bipolar disorder in the elderly. *Medscape Mental Health, 3*(2). Available at: http://psychiatry. medscape.com/medscape/psychiatry/journal.

McKay, B., Forbes, J., & Bourner, K. (1990, April). Empowerment in general practice: The trilogies of caring. *Australian Family Physician,* 513-520.

McMahon, F. J. (1997, April 18). Genetic advances: Addition by division. Paper presented at the Depression and Related Affective Disorders Association (DRADA) at Johns Hopkins Symposium, Baltimore, MD.

Miller, L. (1987, September 1 & 15). Spiritual aspects of depression. *Friends Journal,* 6-8.

Mossey, J. M., Knott, K. A., Higgins, M., & Talerico, K. (1996). Effectiveness of a psychosocial intervention, interpersonal counseling for subdysthymic depression in medically ill elderly. *Journal of Gerontology, Series A: Biological Sciences and Medical Sciences, 51*(4), 172-178.

Neese, J. B. (1991). Depression in the general hospital. *Nursing Clinics of North America, 26,* 613-622.

Neumeister, A., Praschak-Rieder, N., Hesselmann, B., Vitouch, O., Raub, M., Barocka, A., & Kasper, S. (1997). Rapid tryptophan depletion in drug-free depressed patients with seasonal affective disorder. *American Journal of Psychiatry, 154,* 1153-1155.

Norbeck, J., Chaftez, L., Skodol-Wilson, H., & Weiss, S. (1991). Social support needs of family caregivers of psychiatric patients from three age groups. *Nursing Research, 40,* 208-213.

Novak, M., & Shapiro, C. M. (1997). Drug-induced sleep disturbances: Focus on nonpsychotropic medications. *Drug Safety, 16*(2), 133-149.

Pagano, M. P. (1996). Rheumatoid arthritis: An update. *Clinical Reviews, 6*(8) 65-68, 71, 75-76, 78.

Rauch, S. L., & Hyman, S. E. (1995). Approach to the patient with depression. In A. H. Goroll, L. A. May, & A. G., Mulley, Jr. (Eds.), *Primary care medicine,* (3rd ed., pp 1033-1044.). Philadelphia:

Rice, D. P., & Miller, L. S. (1995). The economic burden of affective disorders. *British Journal of Psychiatry, 166* (Suppl.), 34-42.

Rosenthal, R. N. (1994, Fall). Seasonal affective disorder: Presentation to DRADA. *Smooth Sailing,* (2), 3-4.

Rosenthal, R. N., Muran, J. C., Pinsker, H., Hellerstein, D., & Winston, A. (1999). Interpersonal change in brief supportive psychotherapy. *Journal of Psychotherapeutic Practice Research, 8*(1), 55-63.

Sackheim, H. A. (1995). Continuation therapy following ECT: Directions for future research. *Psychopharmacology Bulletin, 25,* 501–521.

Seligman, M. (1975). *Helplessness.* San Francisco: Freeman Press.

Shelton, R. C. (1996). Treatment-resistant depression: Therapeutic approaches. *Medscape Mental Health, 1*(2).

Shua-Haim, J. R., Sabo, M. R., Comsti, E., & Gross, J. S. (1997). Depression in the elderly. *Hospital Medicine, 33*(7), 45–46, 48, 52, 55–56, 58.

Silverman, P. (1978). *Mutual help groups: A guide for mental health workers* (Publication ADM 78-646). Rockville, MD: National Institute of Mental Health.

Silverman, P., & Murrow, H. (1976). Mutual help during critical transitions. *Journal of Applied Behavioral Science, 12,* 411–418.

Skovhold, T. (1974). The client as a helper: A means to promote psychological growth. *Counseling Psychology, 4,* 58–64.

Styron, W. (1990). *Darkness visible: A memoir of madness.* New York: Random House.

Suhail, K., & Cochrane, R. (1997). *Seasonal changes in affective state in samples of Asian and white women. Social Psychiatric Epidemiology, 32,* 149–157.

Tam, E. M., Lam, R. W., Robertson, H. A., Stewart, J. N., Yatham, L. N., & Zis, A. P. (1997). Atypical depressive symptoms in seasonal and nonseasonal mood disorders. *Journal of Affective Disorders, 44*(1), 39–44.

Weissman, M. M., & Markowitz, J. C. (1994). Interpersonal psychotherapy: Current status. *Archives of General Psychiatry, 51,* 599–606.

Wuthnow, R. (1994). Sharing the journey: Support groups and America's quest for community. New York: Fall Press.

Suggested Readings

Abraham, I., Neese, J., & Westerman, P. (1991). Depression: Nursing implications of a clinical and social problem. *Nursing Clinics of North America, 26,* 527–535.

Beck, C. (1993). Teetering on the edge: A substantive theory of postpartum depression. *Nursing Research, 42*(1), 42–47.

Gibson, C. (1991). A concept analysis of empowerment. *Journal of Advanced Nursing, 16,* 354–361.

Jones, P., & Meleis, A. (1993). Health is empowerment. *Advances in Nursing Science, 15*(13), 1–13.

Story, M., & Anderson, G. (1992, June). Assessment and treatment strategies for depressive disorders commonly encountered in primary care settings. *Nurse Practitioner,* 25–36.

Books Selected by DRADA

DePaulo, J. Jr., & Ablow, K. R. (1989). *How to cope with depression.* New York: Ballantine Books.

Dowling, C. (1993). *You mean I don't have to feel this way?* New York: Bantam Books.

Duke, P., & Hochman, G. (1992). *A brilliant madness: Living with manic-depressive illness.* New York: Bantam Books.

Goodwin, F. K., & Jamison, K. R. (1990). *Manic-depressive illness.* New York: Oxford University Press.

Ingersoll, B. D., & Goldstein, S. (1995). *Lonely, sad and angry: A parent's guide to depression in children and adolescents.* New York: Doubleday.

Jamison, K. R. (1993). *Touched with fire: Manic-depressive illness and the artistic temperament.* New York: The Free Press.

Jamison, K. R. (1995). *An unquiet mind.* New York: Vintage Books.

Mondimore, F. (1993). *Depression: The mood disease* (Rev. ed.). Baltimore: Johns Hopkins University Press.

Papolos, D. F., & Papolos, J. (1997). *Overcoming depression* (Rev. ed.). New York: HarperCollins.

Resnick, W. M. (1988). *The manual for affective disorder support groups.* Baltimore: DRADA.

Rosenthal, N. E. (1993). *Winter blues: Seasonal affective disorder: What it is and how to overcome it.* New York: Guilford.

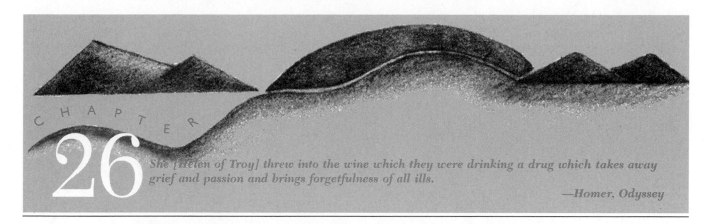

She [Helen of Troy] threw into the wine which they were drinking a drug which takes away grief and passion and brings forgetfulness of all ills.

—Homer, Odyssey

Psychoactive Substance Abuse Disorders

Learning Objectives

After studying this chapter, you should be able to:

1. Discuss the historical context of substance use disorders.
2. Define substance use disorders and related terminology.
3. Identify two theoretical perspectives on the cause of substance use disorders.
4. Discuss the four primary drug classifications.
5. Describe the nurse's role in the treatment of patients with substance use disorders.
6. Identify three populations with special needs.
7. Determine three changes in family dynamics that occur as a consequence of a family member's substance use disorder.

Key Terminology

Addiction	Dependence	Korsakoff's syndrome	Relapse prevention
Alcoholics Anonymous	Detoxification	Narcotic analgesic	Substance (drug or chemical)
Blackouts	Dual diagnosis	Physical dependence	abuse
Cocaine blues	Enabling behaviors	Polydrug dependence	Substance (chemical) depen-
Codependency	Flashback	Projection	dence
CNS stimulants	Halfway house	Psychoactive substances	Tolerance
Craving	Hallucinogens	Psychological dependence	Toxicity
Cross-tolerance	Hypnotic sedative	Rationalization	Wernicke's encephalopathy
Delirium tremens	Intoxication	Recovery	Withdrawal
Denial	Kindling effect	Reinforcing properties	

This chapter tells the story of the human journey anesthetized by the routine use of a psychoactive substance. A person's life journey, obscured from personal awareness by alcohol or other psychoactive substances, is a static one. The traveler and those closest to him or her are immobilized by the alcohol or drug use, unable to move forward or fully process what is happening around him because of his single-minded focus on substance use. As a result, the story of the journey stops midstream as if stuck in time and space, as a nonconsecutive chapter in the person's story because its author has lost his or her voice.

Substance use disorders are unlike any other, replete with paradoxes and social, moral, and legal overlays.

Although the disorder is self-inflicted, it develops without the full awareness or consent of its victims. This disorder directly affects the diagnosed patient as well as having equally devastating effects on family members who never ingest a psychoactive substance.

Additionally, society bears the economic burdens of this disorder. In a report published in May 1998, the government reiterated data from 1992, the most recent year for which sufficient data were available. That data indicated that alcohol and drug abuse cost $246 billion per year, which represents $965 for every man, woman, and child living in the United States in 1992 (Inteli-Health-Home, 1998). Substance abuse is classified as a medical disorder; however, many consider it a social, moral, and behavioral disorder. It is the only medical disorder for which one can be jailed rather than being treated medically. Understanding the complex interrelationships among the physical, psychological, spiritual, and social dimensions of substance use disorders is the first step in developing a comprehensive treatment plan applicable to the needs of affected patients and their families. Understanding these interrelationships can help you to assist those suffering with substance use disorders to consider the potential of leading a richer human existence without drugs or excessive use of alcohol. We begin with the story of Joe, a professional young man with a future who sees only the benefits of drug use and none of its disadvantages. To him, and many others, recreational drug use is harmless. This chapter argues that this assumption simply is not true for far too many people.

Joe's Story

I first tried hallucinogens in college after having smoked pot for a few years in high school. I guess it was both intense curiosity and part peer pressure from the guys in the dorm that led me to try mescaline and then LSD [lysergic acid diethylamic] later on. The first sensation is a temporary nausea and an extremely heightened sense of awareness, as if I have had many cups of coffee and things have sped up dramatically. Light is much brighter, colors are more vivid, and hearing is much keener, with music being especially pleasurable. All the senses are more intense and seem to blend together, mixing with thoughts and emotions. These thoughts, feelings, and perceptions sweep together and seem to drift and pull me away as if I am floating, so that I can literally get swept away in thoughts that seem to last forever. At times I can be talking a lot, laughing and then minutes later, I am anxious and scared. Sometimes I cry with overwhelming waves of emotion. The crying can be primal and hurting and healing all at once. The feelings of ecstasy have an "electric" quality, as if one were having sex with the brain. Sometimes, a feeling of being "at one with the universe" and with people around me is comforting and is very magical. It also is rather fleeting.

After many experiences with LSD, I would say that the environment and my underlying emotional state were key to how the trip would go! If I had already been elated or happy-go-lucky, it would be an overall intensely pleasurable experience. If I had any doubts about myself or if I was under a lot of pressure or turmoil, it was like experiencing a really bad nightmare, yet I was awake. I soon learned that I had to be careful when I chose to take LSD, the dosage was critical, and I had to try to steer myself toward a good mood if I decided I was going to trip.

I go back to it from time to time, especially if I am going to an intense jazz or rock concert. Although it is mostly uplifting and freeing to my spirit, it is still very mysterious to me. It is as if I am unlocking the door to my closet and seeing myself and people without masks—a little scary at times. Even if I go through an hour or so of hell with bad emotions, paranoia, and painful memories, it is so cathartic. I feel as if I have had an intense spiritual reawakening, as if being reborn. To be able to really understand suffering and the peace that follows that experience is very comforting and humbling. This, I think, is one of the attractions of LSD: to be able to be free, uninhibited, and even to cry like a baby and to comfort myself! Did I ever get enough consoling or relief as a child? This could be the real unanswered question here. ■

This story was written by Joe approximately 3 weeks after a bad "trip" on LSD, in which he was almost mugged and spent the night sleeping in a doorway. Although Joe was badly frightened by his experience and its potential to harm him, the draw of hallucinogenic drugs was just as strong 3 weeks later as it was before his bad experience with the voluntary use of LSD. It was almost as if the bad effects of his last trip were erased from memory.

Joe's selective memory and euphoric recall of the positive aspects of his drug experience, as well as his rationalization of the negative consequences, are not unusual. In large part, they derive from the substance's effects on the brain.

HISTORICAL PERSPECTIVE

A detailed historical perspective is beyond the purpose of this book. However, it is important to recognize that the journey to view substance abuse as a disorder has been influenced by religious, societal, and political views.

In 1956, alcoholism was officially labeled as a medical disease by the American Medical Society, and 4 years later, the classification of alcoholism as a treatable medical disease received further credibility with the publication of Jellinek's (1960) classic text, *Disease Concept of Alcoholism*. Jellinek argued that alcoholism should not be considered a uniform disorder, suggesting that the cause and effects of the disorder in a given individual are variable and multifactoral. This was a new concept that significantly changed the perception of the

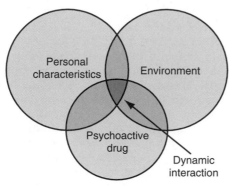

Figure 26–1
The polygenic model of transmission of substance use disorders.

disorder from a personal one to a highly interactive one with a polygenic mode of transmission affected by context and other personalized variables (Figure 26-1 and Box 26-1).

A narrowed focus on alcohol as primarily a sociobehavioral problem continued despite the more enlightened view of it as a medical disorder. This view had peaked during the early 1900s as society sought to deal with the issue by making psychoactive substance use a criminal activity (Kleber, 1990). In 1914, passage of the Harrison Narcotic Act mandated that narcotics be identified as controlled substances that could be dispensed only for medical reasons after stringent legal guidelines. The implications of this act automatically transformed an identified disease process into a criminal act on paper and also, more importantly, in the eyes of the society who voted it into law. The law provided a statute for prosecuting individuals for the possession and distribution of drugs, but so many people were jailed for drug-related offenses that they overflowed the prisons.

In addition to legal condemnation of psychoactive substance use, there were strong moral admonitions against alcohol use. Drug abuse was thought to be an offense against society; therefore, on January 6, 1919, the Eighteenth Amendment to the U.S. Constitution

Box 26–1 ■ ■ ■ ■ ■
The History of the Definition and Treatment of Alcoholism

- *Early 19th century.* In 1814 Benjamin Rush wrote a book on alcoholism as a disease called *An Inquiry into the Effects of Ardent Spirits Upon the Human Body and Mind,* which proposed that individuals who displayed repeated drunken behavior had an addiction to alcohol. He postulated that there may be a hereditary or a contagious factor to repeated use of alcohol (Rush, 1934).
- *Early 19th century.* The Protestant clergy joined physicians and urged temperance. The moral implications became part of the societal view of individuals who became intoxicated.
- *1851.* Maine enacted the Maine Liquor Law to control alcohol use through legislation.
- *1857.* The first treatment facility (inebriate asylum) was established by Joseph Turner in Binghamton, New York.
- *1870.* A physician group founded the American Association for the Cure of Inebriates.
- *1876.* The first periodical on alcoholism as a disease, the *Quarterly Journal of Inebriety,* was established.
- The American Association for the Study of Alcohol and Other Narcotics was formed with the merger of the Medical Temperance Association and the American Association for the Cure of Inebriates. This organization studied the physiological basis for the changes that occur with long-term use of drugs and alcohol. There was an attempt to formulate an understanding of the disease process of drug and alcohol abuse as well as to define terms, such as *chronic alcoholism, habitual, inebriety,* and *periodic drinking.*
- *1918.* The federal Prohibition Act deemed the use of alcohol illegal. This failed owing to the illegal

production and sale of alcoholic beverages. The act greatly influenced the study of alcoholism, and reinforced the belief that it is a moral condition as opposed to a disease state. Physicians were legally punished for prescribing medications to assist with withdrawal states. The study of alcoholism and drug addiction was removed from medical school curricula.
- Psychoanalytic schools of thought defined alcoholism as an internal psychological conflict resulting from fixation in the oral stage of development. Often, alcoholism was seen as a symptom of early traumatic childhood experiences that were not resolved because of an ineffectual ego state.
- *1956.* The American Medical Association encouraged hospitals to admit patients who had the diagnosis of alcoholism.
- *1935.* AA was founded by Bill Wilson and Bob Smith, MD.
- *1960.* E. M. Jellinek proposed that alcoholism is a progressive disorder. He identified stages of progression of alcoholism from psychological tolerance to physical tolerance and dependence on the substance (Jellinek, 1960).
- Current psychological schools of thought that are based on the analytical model attribute the abuse of drugs and alcohol as self-medication to deal with internal psychological conflicts.
- *Early 1980 to present.* Current exploration of the addiction process evaluates the long-term effects on the individual. Genetic studies; the effect of different substances on the brain and the fetus; and the physiological causes of withdrawal and the brain reward system are being studied.

specifically prohibited alcohol consumption in the United States. This began the Prohibition era. Passage of the law satisfied the many temperance and prohibition groups who hoped to eliminate the problem of alcoholism by making the selling or consumption of alcohol illegal. Initially, the law significantly reduced alcohol consumption, but within 10 years, alcohol consumption equaled pre-Prohibition levels. The Prohibition amendment was repealed in 1933, largely because it was ineffective. One positive effect was that it drew the nation's attention to the presence of a serious social problem and to the search for a more effective treatment approach. With the prisons overflowing with recalcitrant alcoholics, it was clear that incarceration was an insufficient deterrent to addictive behavior. As a result, two federal prison hospitals were specifically designated for the care and drug treatment of inmates. Patients were admitted voluntarily to these experimental treatment programs, one near Lexington, Kentucky, and the other in Fort Worth, Texas.

In 1970, again in response to a dramatic increase in drug-taking behaviors, Congress passed the Comprehensive Drug Abuse Prevention and Control Act, more commonly referred to as the Controlled Substances Act. This legislation assigned therapeutic use of psychoactive substances to one of five categories, reflecting a balance between medical use and potential for abuse (Table 26–1). Those drugs assigned to Schedule I are not available commercially even with a prescription. Written prescriptions are required for Schedule II drugs. Schedule III and IV drugs can be obtained with oral or written prescriptions, but there is a limit to how often the prescription can be refilled in a 6-month period without a new prescription. Schedule V drugs are easily obtainable, some in low quantities without a prescription. There are harsh legal penalties for dispensing drugs in violation of this act.

Synthetically Derived Psychoactive Substances

In 1903, the first barbiturate became available and thus began the history of sedative, hypnotic, and anxiolytic

TABLE 26–1 Controlled Substances Act Classification*

DRUG	CSA* SCHEDULE	MEDICAL USE
Narcotics		
Opium	II, III, IV	Analgesic, antidiarrheal
Morphine	II, III	Analgesic, antitussive
Codeine	II, III, V	Analgesic, antitussive
Heroin	I	None
Hydromorphone HCl (Dilaudid), meperidine HCl (Demerol HCl; Mepergan)	II	Analgesic
Depressants		
Chloral hydrate	IV	Hypnotic
Barbiturates	II, III, IV	Anesthetic, anticonvulsant, sedative
Benzodiazepines	IV	Antianxiety, anticonvulsant, sedative
Methaqualone (Quaalude)	I	Hypnotic sedative
Stimulant		
Cocaine	II	Local anesthetic
Amphetamines	II	Attention-deficit disorders, narcolepsy, weight control
Phenmetrazine (Preludin)	II	Weight control
Methylphenidate HCl (Ritalin)	II	Attention-deficit disorders, narcolepsy, weight control
Hallucinogens		
LSD	I	None
Mescaline and peyote	I	None
PCP (also called angel dust)	I	None
Marijuana	I	None
THC	I, II	Cancer chemotherapy antinauseant
Hashish	I	None
Hashish oil	I	None

*CSA criteria: Schedule I, no recognized medical use, high abuse potential; Schedule II, some medical use, high abuse potential; Schedule III, medical use, moderate to high abuse potential; Schedule IV, medical use, low abuse potential; Schedule V, medical use, very low abuse potential.

CSA, Controlled Substances Act; LSD, lysergic acid diethylamide; PCP, phencyclidine HCl; THC, tetrahydrocannabinol.

abuse as a source of psychoactive substance use disorders. Physical and psychological dependence on natural and synthetic hypnotics developed with alarming frequency as drug experimentation became commonplace with the recreational use of marijuana, cocaine, LSD, and phencyclidine (PCP). Recreational drug use rates peaked during the 1960s and 1970s, and declined in the 1980s (U.S. Department of Health and Human Services, 1990).

The benzodiazepines were developed in the 1960s as synthetic minor tranquilizers to replace the more dangerous barbiturates for reducing anxiety. Initially, these drugs were thought to be nonaddictive and were prescribed with impunity. They were added to the list of controlled drugs in the 1970s when their physically addictive properties became apparent.

Hallucinogenic drugs such as LSD also were introduced in the 1960s and achieved peak popularity in the 1970s. However, the bad trips, unpredictability of effects, and notoriety associated with people diving out of windows under the influence of a flashback shortened their popularity. PCP became the hallucinogenic drug of choice shortly afterward. A relatively cheap drug to synthesize, PCP also is one of the most dangerous, capable of producing irreversible neuropsychological damage. Cannabis (marijuana), a favorite with adolescents, has continued its strong status as the most frequently used illicit drug. In the 1980s, there was a decline in illicit drug use from the rates in the 1960s and 1970s, but it remains a major focus for treatment planning (U.S. Department of Health and Human Services, 1990).

Establishing a Treatment Focus

Establishing a realistic and compassionate treatment plan for substance use disorders received a strong boost from the efforts of Bill Wilson, a New York stockbroker, and Dr. Bob Smith, a surgeon from Akron, Ohio, the original cofounders of **Alcoholics Anonymous** (AA). In 1935, these two men developed a lay fellowship organization dedicated to providing support for recovering alcoholics who wished to become and remain sober. Bill Wilson had been under the care of Dr. William Silkworth, who detoxified thousands of alcoholics and believed that alcoholics have a sensitivity, an "allergy" for alcohol that causes the individual to drink in an uncontrollable manner. Following a relapse, Wilson had a spiritual experience while recovering at Towns Hospital. This spiritual experience came from the Oxford Group, which was a spiritual organization that encouraged alcoholics to join in order to recover from alcoholism.

The basic 12-step program developed by Wilson and Smith formed an important foundation for the therapeutic modification of alcoholism and associated **codependency** behaviors in family members. This model is used worldwide for the treatment not only of alcoholism but also of many other addictive behaviors. Basically, the 12-step program provides guidelines for healthy living. The first step is the belief that the alcoholic is powerless over alcohol and is derived from Dr. Silkworth's concept of the allergy to alcohol, which provides an understand-

ing for the compulsion to use the substance. The teachings of the Oxford Group and the spiritual exercises of St. Ignatius form the spiritual basis for AA (Miller & Chappel, 1991).

From the initial two founding members, AA has grown to have worldwide membership of more than 1.5 million recovering alcoholics. For the first time, alcoholics received respect for their efforts to remain sober as well as encouragement and hope from others who had successfully mastered their addictive behaviors, often on a daily basis. There is no direct cost to join, and members can receive lifelong support, if needed. Active and ongoing involvement with AA or Narcotics Anonymous still remains one of the most effective treatments and adjuncts to therapy for substance use disorders.

In 1970, the Hughes Act (P.L. 91-616) created the National Institute of Alcohol Abuse and Alcoholism as an independent institute within the National Institute of Mental Health. This act gave formal recognition to the importance of the issue as a public and social phenomenon, distinguishable from other mental illnesses. The institute was charged with developing comprehensive programs for the prevention and treatment of alcoholism. Major initiatives included the Employee Assistance Programs, which are state and federal programs for education about and treatment of drug abuse, primary prevention, and enhancement of third-party insurance plans for treatment coverage.

In the early 1980s, the American Nurses Association (ANA) established addictions as an independent area of specialized nursing practice. Since that time, the ANA, the Drug and Alcohol Nurses Association (DANA), and the National Nurses Society on Addictions (NNSA) have joined forces to develop standards of nursing practice and appropriate prevention strategies to address primary, secondary, and tertiary prevention of addictions (ANA, 1988; NNSA, DANA, ANA, 1987). The ANA Standards of Addictions Nursing Practice are shown in Box 26-2. The American Psychiatric Association (APA) developed a clinical practice guideline for the treatment of substance abuse and nicotine dependence (APA, 1995, 1996). The goals of these standards are to develop an understanding of patterns of abuse and addiction and to develop a comprehensive treatment approach to a complex mental health problem.

Recognizing the theoretical paradox of psychoactive substances being simultaneously useful as medicinal agents and highly destructive as recreational drugs is important because it helps the nurse understand the confusion that continues to exist about the most appropriate treatment for substance use disorders. Federal guidelines for the treatment of alcohol abuse have been passed into law and are meeting with some success. People with drug abuse problems can no longer be discriminated against in work and educational settings. Despite significant advances, there is more work to be done because a legalistic treatment approach to a medical disorder persists. Viewing substance use disorders as a weakness of character and addressing them as moral-legal issues remain a popular but single-minded approach to a complex problem. In fact, no other mental or physical disorder carries quite the same moral and

Box 26–2 ■ ■ ■ ■ ■

American Nurses Association Standards of Addictions Nursing Practice

Standard I: Theory: The nurse uses appropriate knowledge from nursing theory and related disciplines in the practice of addictions nursing.

Standard II: Data Collection: Data collection is continual and systematic and is communicated effectively to the treatment team throughout each phase of the nursing process.

Standard III: Diagnosis: The nurse uses nursing diagnoses congruent with accepted nursing and interprofessional classification systems of addictions and associated physiological and psychological disorders to express conclusions supported by data obtained through the nursing process.

Standard IV: Planning: The nurse establishes a plan of care for the patient that is based on nursing diagnoses, addresses specific goals, defines expected outcomes, and delineates nursing actions unique to each patients needs.

Standard V: Intervention: The nurse implements actions, independently and/or in collaboration with peers, members of other disciplines, and patients in prevention, intervention, and rehabilitation phases of the care of patient with health problems related to patterns of abuse and addiction.

   Standard Va: Intervention: Therapeutic alliance
   Standard Vb: Intervention: Education
   Standard Vc: Self help groups:
   Standard Vd: Pharmacological therapies:
   Standard Ve: Therapeutic environment:
   Standard Vf: Counseling:

Standard VI: Evaluation: The nurse evaluates the responses of the patient and revises nursing diagnoses, interventions, and treatment plan accordingly.

Standard VII: Ethical Care: The nurse's decisions and activities on behalf of patients are in keeping with personal and professional codes of ethics and in accord with legal statutes.

Standard VIII: Quality Assurance: The nurse participates in peer review and other staff evaluation and quality assurance processes to ensure that patients with abuse and addiction problems receive quality care.

Standard IX: Continuing Education: The nurse assumes responsibility for his or her own continuing education and professional development and contributes to the professional growth of others who work with or are learning about persons with abuse and addiction problems.

Standard X: Interdisciplinary Collaboration: The nurse collaborates with the interdisciplinary treatment team and consults with other health and evaluating programs and other activities related to addictions nursing.

Standard XI: Use of Community Health System: The nurse participates with other members of the community in assessing, planning, and implementing and evaluating community health services that attend to primary, secondary, and tertiary prevention of addictions.

Standard XII: Research: The nurse contributes to the nursing care of patients with addictions and to the addictions area of practice through innovations in theory and practice and participation in research, and communicates these contributions.

Reprinted with permisson from American Nurses Association, *Standards of Addictions: Nursing Practice with Selected Diagnoses and Criteria,* © 1988 American Nurses Publishing, American Nurses Foundation/American Nurses Association, Washington, DC.

legal stigma consistently associated with psychoactive substance use disorders.

The use of legal constraints is not without merit, but it complicates treatment in many cases. As a deterrent to drug abuse and a motivator for treatment, legal consequences for drug abuse play an important role in prevention and treatment. More often than not, it is to avoid or comply with legal consequences of drug abuse that the person with a substance use disorder first enters treatment. These same legal consequences, however, make pregnant women reluctant to admit to drug use and parents uneasy about reporting drug use among their sons and daughters. Equally detrimental to a therapeutic approach are the moralistic attitudes of health professionals and the general public regarding the role of willpower in the development of a substance use disorder.

With the emergence of a resource-driven health care delivery system, insurance companies are limiting third-party reimbursement for drug treatment and rehabilitation. There is irony in the paradox of mandating employers and schools to recognize substance use disorders as medical disabilities and to support treatment efforts for its sufferers while limiting treatment for a chronic disorder. In practical terms, the cost-containment measures for treatment of substance use disorders make it financially unavailable for a significant portion of the population who desperately need such services.

DEFINITION

Substance use disorder is a broad, generic diagnostic term used by the medical community to describe a predictable, composite set of physical symptoms and behavioral patterns associated with the voluntary ingestion of a psychoactive substance. The symptom pattern of the disorder is characterized by ongoing compulsive use of one or more psychoactive substances. Consumption continues as a compelling drive, despite increasingly negative life consequences and adverse social responses from significant others regarding drug-taking behaviors.

The term **psychoactive substances** refers to any mind-altering agents capable of modifying a person's behavior, mood, thinking, arousal level, state of consciousness, and perceptions. Changes in behavior occur because of the drug's effect on the normal synaptic transmission of internal messages in the brain, with special attention given to the role of acetylcholine, norepinephrine, dopamine, and serotonin (Leccese, 1991). Although virtually all medications are capable of producing neuropsychological effects, with many having the potential for creating abuse and dependence, substance use disorders are concerned primarily with the use of distinctly psychoactive substances voluntarily ingested for other than medical purposes. These substances, commonly referred to as drugs rather than medications, include a number of legally sanctioned drugs such as alcohol, benzodiazepines, narcotics, caffeine, and nicotine. The list of illegal drugs used recreationally includes hallucinogens, phencyclidine, cocaine, opiates, amphetamines, barbiturates, and volatile solvents.

Related Terminology

Terms used to describe the behaviors associated with substance use disorders include drug addiction, drug abuse, and chemical dependency. The World Health Organization (WHO) defined **addiction** as "a state of chronic intoxication produced by the repeated consumption of a drug (natural or synthetic)"; characteristics include (Kleber, 1990, p. 59):

1. Overpowering desire or need (compulsion) to continue taking the drug and to obtain it by any means
2. Tendency to increase the dose
3. Psychic (psychological) and, generally, a physical dependence on the effects of the drug
4. Detrimental effect on the individual and society

Substance (drug or chemical) abuse is another term frequently used to describe substance use disorders. The term refers to the nontherapeutic use of psychoactive agents or the illicit use of a prescribed drug on a regular, binge, or episodic basis. To meet *Diagnostic and Statistical Manual of Mental Disorders, Fourth Edition* (DSM-IV) criteria for substance abuse, the patient must have gone for at least a month, or frequently a longer period, without meeting the criteria for psychoactive substance dependence, which involves physical dependence and withdrawal symptoms.

Box 26–3 presents a broad glossary of terms related to substance use disorders. Distinctions among drug misuse, drug habituation, and drug abuse are also important in a discussion of drug-taking behaviors. *Substance misuse* embraces a wide spectrum of drug-taking behaviors. Examples include taking a legitimate drug prescription in a nonprescribed manner, obtaining it in an unlawful way or without a legitimate medical reason, and giving a prescribed medication to a friend. *Substance (drug) habituation* refers to regular use without developing physical dependence. This term is used by many substance users to describe the recreational use of marijuana or LSD. The distinction in many cases is one of semantics; the line between drug dependency and recreational use of drugs on a regular basis is a relatively thin one.

Substance (chemical) dependence is the pathological use of a psychoactive drug over a significant period of time with symptoms of physical and psychological addiction to the drug such that it interferes with physical, social, or occupational functioning. Evidence of sustained pathological use includes an inability to control use of the drug despite clear knowledge of the problems associated with its use and the development of craving and physical symptoms when the drug is withdrawn. A primary distinction between drug abuse and chemical dependency is that the former represents a voluntary behavior and the latter does not. With drug abuse, a person voluntarily ingests a psychoactive substance as a free and conscious act, whereas with chemical dependence, although the person voluntarily ingests the substance, his or her action is compulsive (Allen, 1998).

Difficulty in Establishing a Common Definition

Establishing a commonly held definition for substance use disorders has proved difficult for the medical community because it is such a complex disorder. The National Commission on Marijuana and Drug Use (1973) noted that "drug using behavior is described by such an array of non-specific, unscientific and judgmental terms that it is often difficult to ascertain who is being described and what behavior is being evaluated" (p. 73).

Although the official classification of substance use disorders is a medical one, if you were to seek a sample of definitions from the general public, you would be more likely to hear moral, social, and behavioral definitions. Many define it as a lack of willpower; a societal problem associated with poverty, deprivation, and homelessness; or a response to parental neglect or training. Some view it as a criminal problem in which young people are seduced into drug-taking behaviors by hardened criminals intent on making a fortune without actually working for it. All of these definitions fit some aspect of the meaning of a substance use disorder. Yet all are incomplete explanations.

Regardless of how it is defined, substance use disorders represent a multifactorial behavioral syndrome with physical, social, spiritual, and psychological consequences for the individual, family, and society. As Hughes (1989) suggested, "addiction is more than a toxic state, a criminal offense, a disease, a mental health problem, or an unhealthy habit. It also is a social problem that affects every aspect of life—physical,

Box 26-3 ■ ■ ■ ■ ■
A Glossary of Terms Related to Substance Use Disorders

Blackouts: Amnesia for events and conversations despite appearing normal and engaging in conversation of which there is no memory later

Cross-tolerance: Capacity of psychoactive drugs with similar pharmacological properties to produce the same adaptive changes as the original drug, making them interchangeable in effects on the brain

Detoxification: Medically supervised elimination of the drug from the body.

Drug addiction: Compulsive use of a drug that produces a state or period of chronic intoxication

Flashbacks: Reexperiencing of emotions and behavioral effects of drug without further drug intake and after the drug has cleared the body

Kindling effect: Reinforcing property of addictive drugs in which the brain's reward system in the basal forebrain becomes sensitive to the memory of pleasure exerted by the drug (this activates the addict's desire for the drug)

Overdose: Physical and potentially life-threatening symptoms directly related to drug ingestion

Physical dependence: Withdrawal syndrome of physical symptoms that occur when the drug is withdrawn and persist until system functioning readapts to the predrug state

Potentiation: Capacity of two psychoactive drugs to produce psychological and physical effects greater than the sum of two agents; also referred to as "synergistic" effects

Psychoactive Substance: Any mind-altering agent that alters a person's mood, behavior, perceptions, thinking, arousal level, or state of consciousness

Psychological dependence: Craving or insatiable hunger for a drug even after successful detoxification

Recovery: Sobriety; comfortable abstinence from drug

Reinforcing properties: Positive behavioral effects of drug taking and negative memories of withdrawal reactions

Relapse: Reemergence of symptoms associated with substance abuse disorders

Substance abuse: Nontherapeutic use of psychoactive drugs or illicit use of a prescribed drug

Substance use disorder: Mental disorder characterized by pathological use of a psychoactive drug over a significant period of time that interferes with physical stability, and emotional, social, or occupational functioning

Tolerance: Decreased sensitivity to drug with chronic use that allows a person to increase the dosage of a psychoactive drug without suffering toxic effects

Withdrawal: Physical symptoms directly related to the abrupt termination of the psychoactive drug

---

psychological and interpersonal" (p. 10). To this must be added the profound effect substance use disorders have on the spiritual life of the patient, family, and community. The diagnosis usually entails a person's serious loss of contact with his or her inner spirit, intrapersonally and interpersonally, leaving the perception of almost everything other than the drug use completely devoid of meaning. The loss of a loved one in a random alcohol-related accident and the human suffering this disorder causes others bring to mind the senselessness of drug-induced behaviors on innocent victims.

THEORETICAL MODELS

Theoretical models traditionally provide a way of making sense of a phenomenon and offer a map to understanding the relationship within it. Two of the more popular explanations of substance abuse disorders center on alcoholism as a prototype and describe a disease model and a model of faulty adaptation. There is persuasive evidence that there is a genetic predisposition to the development of alcoholism in some individuals (Stone & Gottesman, 1993). Among identical twins (monozygotic) the concordance rate for the development of alcoholism was much greater than for fraternal twins (dizygotic) in a number of research studies (Merekangas, 1990). Other studies of familial predisposition strongly implicate the role of genetics in the development of alcoholism, because having a first-degree blood relative with alcoholism increases the incidence of alcoholism to anywhere from two to four times the probability in the normal population (Milkman & Shaffer, 1985).

Several studies point to the possible role of dopamine in the reinforcing effects of several types of drug classifications, again suggesting a biological explanation for the development of chemical dependency (Stone & Gottesman, 1993). Most studies suggest that a genetic biochemical susceptibility combined with the learned behaviors developed through living in a dysfunctional family place the affected individual at high risk for developing chemical dependency. After an extensive review of the literature, Stone and Gottesman (1993) concluded that genetic factors contribute to the development of alcoholism, but their precise levels of influence differ related to gender, age of onset, and severity of the disorder. There is more evidence of genetic links with males, early onset, and severe drinking patterns. No single gene and no single biochemical or structural defect are likely to mediate the disorder. Instead there appears to be a multifactorial polygenic mode of transmission related to the development of alcoholism.

By contrast, the adaptive model suggests that substance use disorders occur as a socially caused phenomenon, the result of learned social coping strategies based on substance use. Proponents of this model cite addictive behaviors learned in the family of origin as primary etiological factors. Adaptive models fault sociocultural factors that allow children early access and show role modeling of drug behaviors by adults and peers as causative agents. These models suggest that for children who are exposed to drugs as a way of earning money, coping with stressful situations, and achieving acceptance in a social group, it is difficult to consider other alternative options. For children growing up in a drug culture—smoking pot, drinking alcohol, and using intravenous (IV) drugs—drug-taking behaviors are normal and living without the drug is intolerable. Mynatt (1996), in a study exploring the etiology of chemical dependency in nurses, identified three factors that are important influences to developing a substance abuse pattern of behavior. The nurses in this study reported that their family of origin was chaotic, often involving alcohol and substance abuse; there was victimization, such as verbal, emotional, physical, and sexual abuse; and they experienced low self-esteem.

Most theoretical explanations suggest a polygenic mode of transmission, which consists of the dynamic relationship among the individual's unique psychobiological make-up, genetic and environmental factors, and the effects of the particular psychoactive substance on that person's physical and emotional system. A multimodal framework helps explain why two individuals with similar genetic backgrounds may turn out quite differently and likewise why two individuals from very different family backgrounds can have similar problems with chemical dependence. Considering the context for drug-taking behaviors provides an explanation for the many different types of responses a single drug can have on a person.

> **W**hat do you think? How do you explain a substance abuse disorder? What is your theory? Do you believe it is an illness, a character weakness, a legal problem?

▶ *Check Your Reading*
1. In what ways do drug abuse and chemical dependency differ?
2. How does the historical context of substance use disorders contribute to our understanding of substance use disorders?
3. How would you describe the role of genetic factors in the development of alcoholism?

COMMON PROPERTIES OF PSYCHOACTIVE SUBSTANCES

A number of common properties associated with all psychoactive substances bear mention before discussing the individual drug classifications. These include

1. Acute and chronic structural and functional changes in the brain associated with drug intake
2. Variable effects on the person taking them
3. The concepts of dependence, tolerance, and reinforcing properties, which are unique characteristics of most psychoactive substances and are not found in other pharmacological classifications
4. The concepts of recovery and relapse prevention after cessation of drug intake

Changes in Brain Structure and Function

Psychoactive drugs act directly on one or more of the delicate electrochemical neurotransmitters in the brain that convey information and regulate mood. The area of the brain that is most affected by these substances is the chemical circuit that joins the ventral tegmental area and the nucleus accumbens, known as the medial forebrain bundle. The medial forebrain bundle is in the basal forebrain, which is responsible for judgment and problem-solving. This area also houses the amygdala, which is the structure where emotions, sex drive, appetite, and aggressive behaviors are formulated. The circuit sets priorities for the individual by mitigating behaviors that ensure the survival of the organism. Stimulation of the nucleus accumbens gives the individual pleasure and reinforces the behavioral pattern. This pattern may be repeated over time when the stimulation of the nucleus accumbens takes place, even if there are negative consequences.

Addictive drugs appeal to this reward system by sabotaging the normal functions of this area of the brain (Grinspoon, 1998). Their differential actions alter the normal electrochemical circuits in the brain and interfere with the normal biochemical balance of the body. Even single doses can dramatically disrupt the intricate internal biochemical processes in the brain that influence behavioral responses. Prolonged or chronic use can reset the body's internal biochemical response system in a new homeostatic but distinctly abnormal pattern. Paradoxically, over time, the drug abuser's behavior may appear more "normal" while on the drug and may look bizarre when the drug is withdrawn precipitously.

Moreover, chronic drug use affects not only the chemistry in the brain but also indirectly or directly, many critical body systems. Cardiovascular damage, coma, seizures, respiratory collapse, hepatic failure, renal failure, hemorrhagic disorders, transient psychosis, and nutritional deficiencies are serious secondary medical consequences of prolonged psychoactive drug abuse.

Psychoactive drugs lower resistance to infection and many are immunosuppressive. Unintentional suicides, automobile accidents, physical injuries, and homicides occur under the influence of psychoactive drugs.

Variable Effects

Substance use disorders are much more complicated to understand and treat than other mental disorders because they can have multiple and variable physical effects on different people and on the same person under different circumstances. Unlike other medications, psychoactive substances produce unexpected effects that vary with the dosage of the drug, the environmental context in which the drug is taken, and the person's mood at the time of ingestion. Alcohol, for example, produces an initial euphoria in which the affected person feels more socially competent and lighter in mood. At a higher dosage, however, sedation and central nervous system (CNS) depression occur. Cocaine has local anesthetic properties as well as powerful CNS stimulant action. Some alcoholics do not show any CNS changes on physical examination. Although they are in the minority, their testimony to the lack of ill effects associated with their disorder is unsettling because it encourages others to assume that excessive alcohol intake is not dangerous. Other factors, such as the person's body weight and musculature, rate of metabolism, food consumed before drug ingestion, mood at the time of ingestion, other drug use, tolerance variability, and mode of administration, also affect the way in which the brain responds to the presence of a psychoactive substance.

Dependence

In 1964, WHO identified dependence as the distinguishing characteristic of sustained abnormal drug use. **Dependence** is defined as "a state of psychic or physical dependence or both, on a drug, arising in a person following administration of that drug on a periodic or continuous basis. The characteristics of such a state vary with the agent involved" (p. 60).

Chemical dependence derives from structural and functional changes in the brain as the brain adapts to the chronic presence of a psychoactive substance such that the adaptation requires continued ingestion of the drug to prevent unpleasant withdrawal symptoms. There are two types of dependence, both of which are important to the understanding of substance use disorders: physical and psychological dependence. People who are considered to have a substance use dependency are sometimes referred to as being chemically dependent.

Physical Dependence

Physical dependence is described as a physical need for the psychoactive substance. The person suffers marked physiological symptoms when the drug is withdrawn and the physical need for the drug is directly related to the drug used or its interaction with other psychoactive substances. All of the sedative-hypnotic and narcotic-analgesic pharmacological classifications can create physical dependencies. Abrupt, unsupervised withdrawal from these drugs in heavy consumers can result in respiratory collapse and sudden death.

Intoxication

Intoxication occurs with clinically significant signs and symptoms associated with recent ingestion of a psychoactive substance not attributable to any other medical or psychological condition. A person can be intoxicated and not suffer the subsequent withdrawal effects that a person with a chronic condition would, or the intoxication can be superimposed on a drug dependency, resulting in acute symptoms.

Withdrawal

Withdrawal describes the spontaneous removal of the drug from the body system as either an unplanned event or a gradual tapering of the drug under medical supervision. Symptoms from unintended or unsupervised withdrawal can cause death as a result of cardiac arrest. Without a secure environment and medical supervision, withdrawal symptoms are so uncomfortable that they act as a reinforcement for further drug use.

Detoxification

Detoxification refers to a medically supervised withdrawal process over a prescribed time, ranging from 7 to 28 days. Observation and treatment of medical complications, short-term use of pharmacological agents to reduce patient discomfort, and intense motivational-educational therapeutic approaches are used to quickly reestablish a drug-free state in the chemically dependent patient.

Toxicity

Toxicity (overdose) refers to toxic physiological symptoms caused by taking too much of a drug or mixing drugs that *potentiate,* which means enhance the physical effects of each primary drug. People can become comatose, suffer cardiac arrhythmias or respiratory collapse, and die quickly from overdose. Overdoses can occur in first-time users who have not built up a tolerance to heavy doses of a drug. They can also occur in chronic drug abusers who ingest a purer form of a drug, which has not been cut, or who ingest more than one drug simultaneously. *Cut* refers to the process by which the drug is diluted by other substances for street consumption.

Psychological Dependence

Some psychoactive substances do not establish physical tolerance. Instead, they create a **psychological dependence** in which obsessive thinking about the drug causes the person to repeatedly seek drug relief despite the inevitable compromise of personal values, violation of conduct codes, and negative consequences of drug-taking behaviors. This compulsion to use the drug, despite negative consequences, is due to the reward system that takes place in the prefrontal cortex. Dopamine is released in the basal forebrain and the reward (experience of pleasure) is greater than expected by the nucleus accumbens. The dopamine is what is experienced as pleasurable by the individual, based on the way the brain releases dopamine. It is a signal for the obsessional thought about the drug to become the driven compulsive behavior to use the drug without considering any negative consequences (Grinspoon, 1998). This disturbance of the usual feedback and control in the system can cause changes in functioning over time. Drugs identified with a heavy incidence of psychological dependence among chronic abusers include cocaine, marijuana, and the hallucinogens. Because of its reinforcing properties, psychological dependence can be as debilitating as physical dependence in the persistence of a substance use disorder.

Tolerance

Tolerance is a common property of psychoactive substance disorders and a precursor of chemical dependence. Tolerance refers to the body's need for larger amounts of a psychoactive substance to achieve the same effects previously obtainable with less of the drug. Ingestion of increasingly greater amounts has no toxic effects as the neurotransmitters in the brain begin to adapt to biological alterations created by the presence of the drug. This increases the likelihood of greater drug use and eventual dependence.

Tolerance varies from individual to individual: not everyone who takes the same amount of a drug responds in a similar fashion. For example, some people can drink large amounts of alcohol without ill effects, whereas others can consume little and experience hangovers. In general, people with low tolerance to a drug are at lower risk for developing a substance use disorder than people with high tolerance because the effects are uncomfortable.

Cross-tolerance is the term used to describe

1. Capacity of other psychoactive substances in the same drug classification to enhance (potentiate) the effects of the primary abused drug
2. Ability of the primary drug to expand similar behavioral responses to other psychoactive substances after repeated exposure to a single drug

Because most people diagnosed as having a substance use disorder are, in reality, polydrug users, understanding the mechanisms of cross-tolerance is critical for effective nursing care.

Most CNS stimulants, hypnotic sedatives, and benzodiazepines potentiate or enhance the effects of each other and alcohol. The additive effects of the drug combinations can kill the drug user, whereas each drug taken individually would not have the same consequence. A popular combination of drugs with poten-

tially lethal effects for the user is excessive alcohol and benzodiazepines. Cross-tolerance also must be considered when medicating patients who require a narcotic analgesic for pain relief (e.g., surgical and hospice patients). Because of cross-tolerance, almost anyone with a history of or a current substance use disorder will require larger doses of narcotic-analgesics, even if they have not used drugs for many years.

Reinforcing Properties

Reinforcing properties refer to the positive or negative behavioral effects of self-administered psychoactive substances that serve to intensify desire or hunger for the drug. Psychological dependence is always associated with reinforcing properties, the most significant of which is **craving,** whereby the person experiences an insatiable compulsive desire for a particular psychoactive substance accompanied by vivid remembrances of either the good feelings the drug produces or the relief of anxiety and mood swings. Although exactly how it works is not fully understood (see Chapter 7 for physiological explanation), the **kindling effect** is a reinforcing property of addictive drugs in which the brain's reward system in the basal forebrain becomes sensitive to the memory of pleasure exerted by the drug. This activates the addict's desire for the drug (Du Pont & Gold, 1995). The euphoric recall of the drug experience by the reward system of the brain permits the substance abuser to selectively remember the feelings with no linkage to the potential self-destructive effects of the drug, much as Joe related earlier in his story.

Positive reinforcing properties consist of the initial mood elevation associated with effects of the drug on dopaminergic synapses, implicated in the brain reward circuitry. Activation of the natural brain reward system may provide immediate anxiety relief, temporary pain relief, natural euphoria, and increased energy. Negative reinforcing properties include the dysphoric or depressed mood that occurs in many substance users after the drug effects wear off. Usually, the unpleasant feelings create such emotional discomfort that quick relief from further ingestion of the drug is sought. Thus, painful memories of the withdrawal syndrome may provide the most powerful reinforcers for psychoactive substance addiction.

Recovery and Relapse Prevention

Two other common properties of substance use disorders relate to the treatment process involving concepts of recovery and relapse prevention. Because these disorders represent a chronic disease condition, the word "cure" is not used, even years after the last ingestion of a psychoactive drug. **Recovery** in substance use disorders is a psychologically comfortable abstinence from alcohol and other dependency-producing drugs. Recovery fe, and people in the rehabilitative phase identify themselves as recovering (not recovered) alcoholics and recovering (not recovered) addicts. This psychological reframing cues the person to remember that recovery requires a daily effort to remain abstinent.

The other concept deemed important in the understanding and treatment of drug dependencies is **relapse prevention.** Relapse occurs when the symptoms of a disease reappear after a period of improvement, and the person begins taking the drug again. Many substance users require more than one treatment episode because substance use disorders are chronic disorders. When the patient relapses, it is as if he or she had never stopped using drugs. Although discouraging, this fact does not preclude active intervention as quickly as possible.

Relapse prevention includes a wide variety of nursing strategies that help recovering addicts develop meaningful life goals that do not include the use of psychoactive drugs, find new support systems, and learn new coping strategies. Relapse prevention is particularly important during the first few months after intensive treatment and during stressful times. One way to guard against recidivism is to help the patient develop a written prevention plan and to work with others in the patient's life to empower them to assist the patient in achieving the goal of abstinence. Active involvement in AA, Cocaine Anonymous, or Narcotics Anonymous also can be lifesaving in helping the person with a substance use disorder maintain his or her resolve (see Case Example 26–2, later in this chapter).

TRAJECTORY OF THE JOURNEY INTO SUBSTANCE USE DISORDERS

Understanding the sequential pattern of behaviors associated with addiction provides the nurse with a firm knowledge base and credibility in helping patients constructively confront the magnitude of their problem. Clearly, there is a defined developmental path associated with substance use disorders that begins with social or medical use of a psychoactive substance and ends with the consistent presence of addictive behaviors. Usually, the road to chemical dependency begins innocently enough, and the point at which voluntary use becomes involuntary cannot be readily identified. Many factors such as drug availability, personality factors, genetic predisposition, exposure to stressful situations, and environmental support conspire to produce substance use disorders.

First-time use of a psychoactive substance typically occurs within the context of a young person's social and developmental peer group, as Joe related in his story. Alternatively, it can develop from the use of medically prescribed drugs to reduce anxiety, relieve physical pain, or promote sleep. The drugs help people feel better, and they begin to depend on the drugs for relief from minor emotional and physical discomfort. No one would identify the possibility of addiction as a consequence of regular ingestion of psychoactive substances. If you asked novice drug takers why they take drugs, use pot, drink alcohol, or snort cocaine, they would tell you "to relax," "as part of having a good time," "it makes me feel good," "it gets me more in touch with myself," or "simply out of curiosity because my friends use them."

Others would describe the "thrill-producing" effects of the drug experience. They would suggest that the drugs stimulate a sense of spontaneous awareness, oneness with the world, and self-confidence while diminishing boredom, tension, and meaninglessness.

The crossover from experimental, recreational use to habitual use is subtle. Solitary use, hiding the habit, and growing tolerance are definitive signs of growing dependence. Many people also have help in establishing habitual use in a drug supportive environment. The drugs are readily available and often are offered free or at low cost to the potential consumer. Once the drug habit has taken effect, full price is charged and the person has become enslaved in the drug-taking behavior.

As the habit increases, faith in the drug to relieve stress begins to replace trust in other interpersonal relationships. New friends interested in similar drug experimentation crowd out old relationships, and an extraordinary loyalty builds up among them, fueled by a secret that they all share and must protect: their use of psychoactive drugs (Case Example 26–1).

■ **C A S E   E X A M P L E   2 6 – 1**
■ **Dana's Story, Part 1**

I never grew up wanting to be a drug addict or an alcoholic. In fact, I was always taught in school and by my parents that drugs were bad and bad things could happen to you if you used them. So I really grew up afraid of them. I think the reason I picked up my first drink and later my first drug was, as for most people, because of peer pressure. I saw all my friends doing it and they weren't jumping off buildings or wanting to fly, and nobody was dying or freaking out. I didn't see any bad things happening to them. In fact, nothing but good things were happening. They were more popular than me; they were being invited on dates and I wasn't. I guess after a while, I wanted to do drugs so I could be like them.

Some people's theory about people on drugs or alcohol is that there is a void in their lives, a hole in their gut they can't seem to fill, or a lack of self-esteem. That was true with me. I didn't have enough self-esteem to stand on my own two feet and not "follow the crowd." I didn't know I was okay just the way I was. I needed acceptance from these people I thought were my friends. I didn't think I was pretty, I thought I was fat, and I just didn't think I was good enough. But when I was drinking or on drugs, well that's a different story. I was pretty, thin, funny, life of the party, cracking jokes. Everybody noticed me and liked me. If feeling like that meant that I had to drink, well so be it. I was having the time of my life.

That feeling lasted about 3 to 4 years. Then I started feeling not good enough again. I guess there were always periods of feeling like that when I was by myself, but now the feelings started coming back even when I was out with my friends, cracking jokes and being the life of the party. Everyone else still seemed to like me except me. So those awful feelings that drugs at one time suppressed came back even stronger. Because this time, the feelings were not only of not being good enough but also of fear that I was going to get caught soon if I kept it up, either by my parents or the police. I guess some people would call that paranoia. I also had feelings of guilt that I treated my family badly, that I wasn't there for them. It was more important for me to be out with my friends than to talk with them or help my mom out. At family functions, I would try to slip away to smoke a joint or make an excuse not to go so I could go out with people who didn't care about me. I guess I started realizing these people were not my friends when I started to see how they behaved not only toward me but toward other people. I saw them doing raunchy things to people, fighting and making fun of them because they were too drunk or messed up to do any better. The stealing, the lies, the manipulation, the schemes really bothered me. Of course at this point, I really didn't think any of this had to do with drugs. I blamed it on everyone and everything else. ■

Denial and rationalization provide structure and meaning to drug-taking behaviors (Crigger, 1998). In the patient's mind, personal reverses are associated with anything from a problem boss to the wife's nagging despite what everyone in close contact with the patient can observe: the problems exist in relation to the effects of a psychoactive substance. Physical evidence of organ system involvement appears in the form of physical disorders and neurological impairment. Frequently, those most intimately involved with the effects of dependency behaviors shake their heads in amazement that chemically dependent people cannot distance themselves from a chemical that literally is destroying them and everything that is important to them. Without treatment, substance dependence inevitably leads to personal, marital, financial, and job-related reverses directly attributable to the effects of the disorder. Death and impoverishment, the loss of everything that is meaningful, and often serious harm to others are potential outcomes.

DIAGNOSTIC CLASSIFICATIONS

DSM-IV General Classification

The DSM-IV distinguishes between psychoactive substance-induced organic mental disorders and those that clearly evidence abuse and dependency without definitive organic sequelae. The DSM-IV does not make generic distinctions related to the specific drug causing the disorder. **Polydrug Dependence** involves the regular use of three or more psychoactive substances over a period of at least 6 months.

The rationale for classifying psychoactive substance disorders within a generic category of substance use or substance dependence relates to commonalities in psychological behavioral patterns across drug classifications. Regardless of specific cause (which is important in treating toxicity and withdrawal), it is the outcome of psychoactive drug use, shared in common by all drug classifications, that is most likely to account for the problems associated with the disorder. With the exception of the acute withdrawal stage, the medical treatment and rehabilitation of any drug dependency are similar in approach and not dependent on a precise knowledge of the causative agent. Considering all psychoactive substance disorders collectively as a primary

medical phenomenon rather than focusing on the specific drug is useful in an age when most substance abusers use more than one psychoactive substance. The DSM-IV classification of substance abuse and substance dependence disorders is presented in the box Medical Diagnoses and Related Nursing Diagnoses: DSM-IV Criteria for Substance-Related Disorders.

Nursing Diagnoses

The nursing diagnoses for substance use disorders refer to the functional patterns a patient presents. Management of acute symptoms relates to the specific differential classification of the disorder. In the rehabilitative phase, however, the nurse sees similar functional patterns in need of nursing intervention across all pharmacological categories, a strong representative sample of which is provided in Box 26–4.

Differential Classification

In addition to making general diagnostic distinctions among substance intoxication, abuse, and dependence, the DSM-IV further categorizes psychoactive substance use disorders according to their general pharmacological effects on the brain and CNS. Four primary classifications cover most of the illicit drug use responsible for the diagnosis of substance use disorders:

1. Hypnotic sedatives
2. Hallucinogens
3. Narcotic analgesics
4. CNS stimulants

Two additional categories for over-the-counter drugs and volatile solvents are used (see Box 26–5).

Alcohol Use Disorders

Alcohol is a CNS depressant derived from the fermentation of sugar, starch, or other carbohydrates. The drug is rapidly metabolized, appearing in the bloodstream within 5 minutes and affecting the higher cortical functions in the brain almost immediately. Most people can metabolize approximately 1 oz per hour. Milk and fatty foods delay the absorption rate. With consistent use, alcoholics can metabolize liquor more quickly, leading to the assumption that they can handle their liquor better. What actually happens is that they develop greater tolerance for the substance.

Another common myth is that the percentage of alcohol accounts for drug dependency. Many people naively think that if they drink beer or wine they will not become alcoholics. Unfortunately, this simply is not true, and many alcoholics drink only beer or wine. The standard beverage equivalency is as follows:

- One beer equals 4 oz of whiskey.
- One glass of wine equals 1 to 1.5 oz of whiskey.

Alcohol has the unique distinction among abused psychoactive substances of being legally sanctioned,

MEDICAL DIAGNOSES AND RELATED NURSING DIAGNOSES

Substance-Related Disorders

Dependence and Abuse

Substance Dependence

A maladaptive pattern of substance use, leading to clinically significant impairment or distress, as manifested by three or more of the following occurring at any time in the same 12-month period:

1. Tolerance, as defined by either of the following:
   a. Need for markedly increased amounts of the substance to achieve intoxication or desired effect
   b. Markedly diminished effect with continued use of the same amount of the substance
2. Withdrawal, as manifested by either of the following:
   a. The characteristic withdrawal syndrome for the substance (refer to criteria A and B of the criteria sets for withdrawal from the specific substances)
   b. The same (or closely related) substance is taken to relieve or avoid withdrawal symptoms
3. The substance is often taken in larger amounts or over a longer period than was intended
4. A persistent desire or unsuccessful efforts to cut down or control substance use
5. A great deal of time is spent in activities necessary to obtain the substance (e.g., visiting multiple doctors or driving long distances), use the substance (e.g., chain smoking), or recover from its effects
6. Important social, occupational, or recreational activities given up or reduced because of substance use
7. Continued substance use despite knowledge of having had a persistent or recurrent physical or psychological problem that was likely to have been caused or exacerbated by the substance (e.g., current cocaine use despite recognition of cocaine-induced depression, or continued drinking despite recognition that an ulcer was made worse by alcohol consumption)

Specify if:

With Physiological Dependence: Evidence of tolerance or withdrawal (i.e., either item (1) or (2) is present).

Without Physiological Dependence: No evidence of tolerance or withdrawal (i.e., neither item (1) nor (2) is present).

There are modifiers that address the issue of course. First, it is most important to recognize that once a person has ever had a pattern of substance use that meets criteria for dependence, the person can no longer qualify for a diagnosis of abuse for that substance. However, the patient may meet criteria for early remission, full or partial, or sustained remission, full or partial. There is a modifier that applies to a patient who is on agonist therapy, such as methadone maintenance or nicotine replacement, when the agonist medication is not being abused. There is also a modifier that applies to a patient who is in a controlled environment for 1 month or longer where no criteria for dependence or abuse are met, but the person is in an environment where controlled substances are highly restricted, such as locked hospitals, therapeutic communities, or substance-free jails.

Substance Abuse

A. A maladaptive pattern of substance use leading to clinically significant impairment or distress, as manifested by one or more of the following occurring at any time during the same 12-month period:

1. Recurrent substance use resulting in a failure to fulfill major role obligations at work, school, or home (e.g., repeated absences or poor work performance related to substance use; substance-related absences, suspensions, or expulsions from school; neglect of children or household)
2. Recurrent substance use in situations in which it is physically hazardous (e.g., driving an automobile or operating a machine when impaired by substance use)
3. Recurrent substance-related legal problems (e.g., arrests for substance-related disorderly conduct)
4. Continued substance use despite having persistent or recurrent social or interpersonal problems caused or exacerbated by the effects of the substance (e.g., arguments with spouse about consequences of intoxication, physical fights).

B. Has never met the criteria for Substance Dependence for this class of substance.

Substance Intoxication and Substance Withdrawal

Substance Intoxication

The development of a reversible substance-specific syndrome due to recent ingestion of (or exposure to) a substance. (Note: different substances may produce similar or identical syndromes.)

Substance Withdrawal

The development of a substance-specific syndrome due to the cessation of, or reduction in, substance use that has been heavy and prolonged.

The substance-specific syndrome causes clinically significant distress or impairment in social, occupational, or other important areas of functioning.

Not due to a general medical condition and not better accounted for by another mental disorder.

MEDICAL DIAGNOSES AND RELATED NURSING DIAGNOSES

Substance-Related Disorders Continued

Related Nursing Diagnosis	Definition	Example
Ineffective Coping, Individual	The state in which an individual experiences or is at risk of experiencing an inability to manage internal or environmental stressors adequately because of inadequate resources (physical, psychological, behavioral)	Ineffective Coping, Individual related to substance use evidenced by using drugs to relieve anxiety
Ineffective Denial	The state in which an individual minimizes or disavows symptoms or a situation to his or her detriment of health	Ineffective Denial related to substance use evidenced in refusal to admit problem

Based on information from the *Diagnostic and Statistical Manual of Mental Disorders. Fourth Edition.* Copyright 1994 American Psychiatric Association. Nursing diagnoses and definitions from North American Nursing Diagnosis Association. (1999). *NANDA nursing diagnoses: Definitions and classification 1999-2000.* Philadelphia: NANDA.

easily obtainable at a relatively low cost, and actually promoted by advertising in the media (Gualtieri, 1990). Anyone 21 years or older can purchase alcohol legally over the counter, and even the most rural communities support a liquor store. Liquor stores are looked on as social gathering sites and reservoirs of information about the community in many urban settings, particularly in less affluent neighborhoods. In some communities, liquor stores are willing to cash paychecks, thus implicitly encouraging people to spend at least part of their paycheck on liquor.

Society actively supports the use of alcohol in moderation. Socially, it is not only acceptable to drink but, in many circles, expected. How many parties have you attended where alcohol was not served? If it was not served, you probably heard some derogatory comments about its absence. Often, there is a special table or area set aside for alcoholic beverages. Other party edibles do not enjoy a similar emphasis. There is little question that alcohol enlivens parties and social gatherings by producing a temporary state of light-heartedness and a reduction of self-consciousness, particularly in people who feel insecure about themselves. Taken in excess, alcohol inevitably leads to trouble, destroying the life of the party and in some instances taking the life of a partygoer through physical fights, overdose, or accident.

Television portrays social drinking as both normal and desirable. Only since the 1990s have drug prevention messages been shown with any regularity in television public service announcements. Interestingly, these advertisements target the adolescent. Drug problems among adults and the elderly usually are addressed in documentaries, but they are rarely addressed in preventive messages seen on television (McCracken, 1998).

The incidence and prevalence of alcohol use as a mind-altering drug provide staggering evidence of the magnitude of the problem. As the most frequently used and abused psychoactive substance in the United States, alcohol often is the first psychoactive drug used by potential polydrug abusers. Up to 20 million Americans could be diagnosed in any given year as having a major problem with alcohol, and approximately 40% of the population have lived some part of their lives in alcoholic families (Robertson, 1993).

Alcohol has been identified as both a cause and an effect of homelessness, placing the homeless individual at risk for infection, AIDS, tuberculosis, victimization, and hypothermia (U.S. Department of Health and Human Services, 1990). According to government studies, alcohol claims up to 100,000 lives per year. It is a factor in more than half of the reported automobile accidents and emergency department admissions, and it is an underlying dynamic in many medical conditions. Moreover, alcoholism accounts for up to 50% of the violence between spouses and is a contributing factor in one third of child molestation cases (Silverstein, 1990); the costs to the American public related to alcohol problems were estimated to exceed $70 billion per year.

Alcoholism is listed as the third leading cause of death, and cirrhosis, its most common sequelae, is the fifth leading cause of death in the United States. Because the range between a nontoxic dose of alcohol and a lethal dose is relatively narrow, death can occur with little warning and with no intent. The life span of the alcoholic is shortened considerably. Figure 26-2 provides some of the data related to the far-reaching social implications of alcohol abuse.

Physical Symptoms

Chronic alcoholism affects every organ in the body. Alcohol contains calories, but they are empty calories,

Box 26-4 ■ ■ ■ ■ ■
Nursing Diagnoses for Patients With Substance Use Disorders

Biological Responses

Sensory/Perceptual Alteration
Self Care Deficit
Injury, Potential for
Sexual Dysfunction
Infection, Potential for
Sleep Pattern Disturbance
Nutrition, Altered: Less than Body Requirements
Pain
Growth and Development, Altered

Cognitive Responses

Knowledge Deficit
Thought Processes, Altered
Noncompliance (specify)

Psychosocial Responses

Impaired Verbal Communication
Ineffective Individual Coping
Social Isolation
Anxiety
Family Processes, Altered
Parenting, Altered
Violence, Potential for
Growth and Development, Altered

Spiritual Responses

Spiritual Distress
Powerlessness
Hopelessness
Dysfunctional Grieving

Modified from American Nurses Association (1988). *Standards of addictions: Nursing practice with selected diagnoses and criteria.* Kansas City, MO: Author.

Box 26-5 ■ ■ ■ ■ ■
Classification of Commonly Abused Drugs

Central Nervous System Sedatives, Hypnotics, and Anxiolytics

· Barbiturates (phenobarbital sodium [Luminal Sodium], amobarbital sodium [Amytal Sodium], phentobarbital sodium [Nembutal Sodium], secobarbital sodium [Seconal Sodium], thiopental sodium [Pentothal])
· Alcohol
· Meprobamate (Miltown)
· Benzodiazepines (chlordiazepoxide HCl [Librium], diazepam [Valium], alprazolam [Xanax], triazolam [Halcion], flurazepam [Dalmane])

Stimulants

· Amphetamines (dextroamphetamine sulfate [Dexedrine])
· Cocaine
· Caffeine

Narcotic Analgesics

· Opium
· Heroin
· Morphine
· Codeine
· Methadone
· Other synthetic analgesics (hydromorphone HCl [Dilaudid], oxycodone HCl [Percodan], propoxyphene HCl [Darvon], pentazocine lactate [Talwin], meperidine HCl [Demerol HCl])

Hallucinogens

· LSD
· Canabis, marijuana, hashish
· Mescaline, peyote
· PCP (also called angel dust)

Over-the-Counter Drugs

Containing
· Atropine
· Scopolamine
· Antihistamines

Solvents

· Aerosol sprays
· Glue
· Gasoline
· Paint thinner
· Nail polish remover

LSD, lysergic acid diethylamide; PCP, phencyclidine HCl.

meaning that it is missing essential amino acids, vitamins, and minerals. A typical alcoholic who consumes up to 50% of his or her caloric intake in the form of alcohol develops a severe nutritional deficiency. Malnutrition and irritation of the intestinal mucosa create a lack of thiamine (vitamin B_1), leading to numbness, changes in gait, and pain in the extremities associated with peripheral neuritis.

Pancreatitis, cirrhosis of the liver, and diabetes occur with greater frequency in alcoholics than the general population and, untreated, can lead to death. Many alcoholics also demonstrate a low-grade hypertension. Some of the more common effects of chronic alcohol use on body systems were presented in Box 26-6.

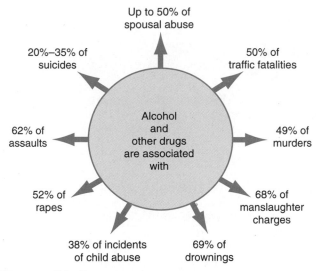

Figure 26–2
The social implications of alcohol abuse. (From The fact is ... OSAP responds to national crisis [MS400]).

Up to 50% of
spousal abuse

20%–35% of
suicides

50% of
traffic fatalities

62% of
assaults

Alcohol
and
other drugs
are associated
with

49% of
murders

52% of
rapes

68% of
manslaughter
charges

38% of incidents
of child abuse

69% of
drownings

Psychological Symptoms and Behavior Patterns

Psychological markers of alcoholism are overuse of defensive mental mechanisms to explain drug use, most prominently, denial, rationalization, and projection. **Denial** is apparent in the alcoholic's insistence that he or she does not have a problem despite concrete evidence of significant interference with normal life patterns directly attributable to his or her drug habit, such as missed days at work, traffic tickets for alcohol-related behaviors and automobile accidents, the obvious concerns of others, and related physical ailments. Statements such as, "I don't have a problem; it's your attitude that's a problem" or "I can stop any time I want to" are strong indicators of denial. **Rationalization** appears in the form of self-imposed rules that explain the person's drinking habits as legitimate. Sample statements include "I'm not an alcoholic because I just drink on weekends" or "I limit myself to beer; none of the hard stuff for

me." **Projection** is evidenced in the blaming of external forces (e.g., a nagging wife, an impossible boss, a stressful job) for stimulating the need to drink.

The alcoholic's use of these mental mechanisms is not a conscious effort to conceal the truth. Rather, it stems from an unconscious shield of self-deception that protects the individual emotionally and is the direct result of the reinforcing properties of the drug due to the brain reward circuit. **Blackouts** occur when there is neuronal irritability that erases the alcoholic's memory of self-destructive behaviors while under the influence. Breaking through this denial system is essential in supporting self-diagnosis, the cornerstone of successful rehabilitation in alcoholism. Assisting the patient to collect information about behavior that occurred during a blackout is one helpful way of knocking on the door of denial.

Establishing the Diagnosis

Major symptoms supportive of a diagnosis of alcohol dependency include the following:

1. Withdrawal symptoms and significant interference with psychosocial functioning in family and job relationships
2. Tolerance, as evidenced by the ability to consume the equivalent of a fifth of liquor or having a blood alcohol level of 100 dl or greater
3. Indiscriminate or regular drinking despite social or medical contraindications
4. Blackouts
5. Arrests for driving while under the influence of alcohol

In making a differential diagnosis of alcoholism, the nurse obtains a family history, history of drug use, and a description of the behavior patterns described previously, which usually can be ascertained in an assessment interview. It is important to ask questions about preexisting mental disorders, metabolic conditions, cardiac and gas exchange problems, prescribed medications, and head injuries, all of which have symptoms that sometimes mimic acute intoxication or withdrawal symptoms. Often, the nurse can smell alcohol on the patient's breath (Arthur, 1997; Brown, Pirmohamed, & Park, 1997; Markey & Stone, 1997; Tierney, 1997).

Two of the most common assessment tools used to establish a definitive diagnosis are the Michigan Alcoholism Screening Test (MAST) and the CAGE-AID questionnaire. The MAST consists of 23 questions that provide fairly reliable data about the drug habit (Box 26–7). The CAGE-AID questionnaire is shown in Box 26–8. Two or more positive answers suggest a diagnosis of substance use disorder and three or more confirm it. The CAGE instrument obviously is easier but slightly less reliable because it is more prone to answers reflecting social desirability. The homepage of the National Clearinghouse for Alcohol and Drug Information's Website (1998) has a questionnaire that asks the following questions:

Do you drink alone when you feel angry or sad?

Box 26–6 ■ ■ ■ ■ ■
Common Effects of Chronic Alcohol Use on Body Systems

- Polyneuropathy
- Chronic gastritis
- Cardiomyopathy
- Increased incidence of cancer (mouth, esophagus, pharynx, liver, larynx)
- Teratogenic fetal effects
- Cirrhosis
- Permanent brain damage
- Decreased immunity to infection

B o x   2 6 – 7   ■ ■ ■ ■ ■
The Michigan Alcoholism Screening Test (MAST)

Points		
2	(*1.)	Do you feel you are a normal drinker?
2	2.	Have you ever awakened the morning after some drinking the night before and found that you could not remember part of the evening before?
1	3.	Does your wife (or parents) ever worry or complain about your drinking?
2	*4.	Can you stop drinking without a struggle after one or two drinks?
1	5.	Do you ever feel bad about your drinking?
2	(*6.)	Do friends or relatives think you are a normal drinker?
0	7.	Do you ever try to limit your drinking to certain times of the day or to certain places?
2	*8.	Are you always able to stop drinking when you want to?
5	(9).	Have you ever attended a meeting of Alcoholics Anonymous (AA)?
1	10.	Have you gotten into fights when drinking?
2	11.	Has drinking ever created problems with you and your wife?
2	12.	Has your wife (or other family member) ever gone to anyone for help about your drinking?
2	(13.)	Have you ever lost friends or girlfriends/boyfriends because of your drinking?
2	(14.)	Have you ever gotten into trouble at work because of drinking?
2	15.	Have you ever lost a job because of drinking?
2	(16.)	Have you ever neglected your obligations, your family, or your work for two or more days in a row because you were drinking?
1	17.	Do you ever drink before noon?
2	18.	Have you ever been told you have liver trouble? Cirrhosis?
2	(19.)	Have you ever had delirium tremens (DTs), severe shaking, heard voices, or seen things that weren't really there after heavy drinking?
5	(20.)	Have you ever gone to anyone for help about your drinking?
5	(21.)	Have you ever been in a hospital because of your drinking?
2	22.	Have you ever been a patient in a psychiatric hospital or on a psychiatric ward of a general hospital where drinking was part of the problem?
2	23.	Have you ever been seen at a psychiatric or mental health clinic, or gone to a doctor, social worker, or clergyman for help with an emotional problem in which drinking has played a part?
2	24.	Have you ever been arrested, even for a few hours, because of drunk behavior?
2	(25.)	Have you ever been arrested for drunk driving or driving after drinking?

*Negative responses are alcoholic responses.
( ) Indicates questions included in the Brief MAST.
__ Indicates questions included in the SMAST (a shortened version of the MAST with good reliability).
Scoring: A score of three points or less is considered nonalcoholic; four points is suggestive of alcoholism; a score of five points or more indicates alcoholism.
Reprinted with permission from *Journal of Studies in Alcohol*, vol. 36, pp. 117–126, 1975. Copyright by Alcohol Research Documentation, Inc., Rutgers Center of Alcohol Studies, Piscataway, NJ 08855.

Does your drinking ever make you late for work?
Does your drinking worry your family?
Do you ever drink after telling yourself you won't?
Do you ever forget what you did while you were drinking?
Do you get headaches or have a hangover after you have been drinking?

The individual is instructed that any "yes" answers to these questions may indicate that she or he has a drinking problem. One therapeutic intervention aimed at assisting the patient to be able to evaluate her or his own drinking pattern and override the mechanism of denial is to ask the patient to complete more than one alcohol assessment tool and to discuss the results in an assessment interview.

Treatment for alcoholism is primarily psychosocial and educational, following the mandated general pattern presented later in this chapter for acute and rehabilitation phases of all substance use disorders. Disulfiram (Antabuse) is sometimes used in the treatment of alcoholism during the rehabilitation phase to reinforce the alcoholic's desire to stop drinking. The drug acts as an antagonist to alcohol by blocking its breakdown of acetaldehyde, which in turn results in the development of acute physical distress. When the person on disulfiram takes an alcoholic drink, within 5 to 10 minutes, systemic symptoms begin to appear known as the "acetaldehyde syndrome" (Leccese, 1991). Flushing, a throbbing headache, nausea, vomiting, muscular aches, weakness, difficulty breathing, and chest pains ensue. It usually takes 5 days for the body to clear the disulfiram out of the system, an important point to teach the patient to determine his or her level of understanding. Patients on disulfiram require close medical supervision and education about the danger of taking alcohol concurrently.

Zacharias, Rodriquez-Garcia, Hanz, and Hooper (1998) reported that as many as 40% of all patients in general hospitals are admitted because of complications related to alcohol. These researchers advocated a clinical pathway for alcohol withdrawal that provides consistency, coordination, and an interdisciplinary approach. Sander (1997) also identified the need for better intervention on medical units and developed a protocol that allows nurses to assess alcoholism with greater accuracy.

Toxicity

Physical signs and symptoms of alcohol toxicity with different blood levels are presented in Table 26-2. Combined with other hypnotic sedatives, the merged synergistic effects of alcohol and a benzodiazepine or barbiturate can prove fatal. Suicide and accidental death caused by overdose or lethal toxic combinations with other psychoactive drug substances make alcohol abuse dangerous.

Psychological symptoms associated with toxicity in-

clude marked alterations in sensory perceptions can resemble psychosis. The alcoholic present agitated state and experiences extrasensory strange voices, sounds, or shadows. Audito hallucinations usually are menacing, of form of rats or snakes. By contrast, with psychotic episode, the patient retains place, and time.

One of the most serious effect abuse is the development of irre Occurring in chronic alcoholics **Wernicke's encephalopath** early stage of the more ch brain dysfunction associated Symptoms of Wernicke's result of thiamine defic treatment in most cases ataxia, gaze disturban Alcohol abstinence c of thiamine has bee treatment of this disor serious organic disorder mar Essentially, brain cells have been hol. Memory is grossly impaired, espe memory, and the person exhibits confabulati disturbances. CT scan reveals profound brain a

Box 26-8 ■■■■■

CAGE-AID

Nurses are in a unique position to have an impact on addiction problems by using screening tools in clinical situations unrelated to addiction. Nurses are usually the first medical professional to access the individual for complaints offered. A 1991 study by Tolley and Rowland concluded that nurses were the preferred providers for developing and implementing addiction screening programs.

The NIAAA in 1990 defined screening as a process that identifies people at risk for the disease. There are two types of addiction screening most frequently used. The first is a self-reporting or interview-based questionnaire, and the second type is the clinical laboratory test. Screening can only detect the presence or absence of a substance use problem. Assessment and diagnostic procedures should follow in order to pinpoint the problem in detail and drive a referral for necessary care.

The screening process consists of a single event. It can be accomplished in a short time, 10 to 15 minutes, and is a statistically reliable procedure. Screening has broad applicability for the general public; the tools are easily answered and interpreted; minimal training is needed to administer the screening; and the cost of administering the tool is low. In order for the screening process to be effective, a procedure is necessary

for referring patients with positive results for further assessment.

The CAGE questionnaire is used to screen for problems with alcohol abuse and dependence. The CAGE-AID is the adapted tool to include other drugs. They are the most widely used screening tools due to their ease of use. The questionnaire consists of four questions. A score of one "yes" is indicative of further assessment. Studies have shown the CAGE correctly identifies 75% of alcoholics and 96% of nonalcoholics.

CAGE-AID Screening Tool

1. C—Have you ever felt you ought to cut down on your drinking (drug use)?
2. A—Have people annoyed you by criticizing your drinking (drug use)?
3. G—Have you ever felt bad or guilty about your drinking (drug use)?
4. E—Have you ever had a drink (used drugs) first thing in the morning—eye-opener—to steady your nerves or get rid of a hangover?

One positive answer indicates a possible problem; two positive answers indicate a probable problem.

Note: The CAGE questionnaire is complete to screen for problems with alcohol without the drug use substitution in the ( ). The addition of the ( ) is what changes the tool to the CAGE-AID (altered to include drugs).
Data from Fleming, M. F., & Barry, K. L. (1992). *Addictive disorders.* St. Louis, MO: C. V. Mosby; and Ewing, J. A. (1984). Detecting alcoholism: The CAGE questionnaire. *Journal of the American Medical Association, 252,* 1905-1907, Excerpts (modified) p. 1907, Copyright 1984, American Medical Association.

TABLE 26-2 Physical Signs and Symptoms of Alcohol Toxicity With Different Blood Levels*	
BLOOD ALCOHOL LEVEL	**PHYSICAL SIGNS AND SYMPTOMS**
20–99 mg/dL	Changes in mood, impaired judgment, muscle incoordination
100–199 mg/dL	Marked cognitive impairment, pronounced muscle incoordination, prolonged reaction time; should not be allowed to drive
200–299 mg/dL	All of the above plus marked ataxia, nausea, vomiting, slurred speech
300–399 mg/dL	Amnesia, hypothermia, tremors, severe dysarthria
400–700 mg/dL	Coma, respiratory failure, death

*A person is considered legally drunk with a blood alcohol level of >100 mg/dL.

and there is no treatment available to reverse the dementia with Korsakoff's syndrome.

Withdrawal

Withdrawal symptoms can include diaphoresis, mild disorientation, headaches, conjunctival injection, cardiac palpitations, hypertension, anorexia, insomnia, generalized weakness, tremors, nausea and vomiting, temporary hallucinations, decreased attention span, fear, suspiciousness, and heightened anxiety. The most serious form of withdrawal is known as **delirium tremens** (DTs), which occurs as a result of acute CNS irritability approximately 48 to 72 hours after the last drink. DTs are characterized by profound disorientation, coarse tremors, gross perceptual distortions, visual hallucinations, tachycardia, marked increase in blood pressure, grand mal seizures, and fever. Five percent of individuals who have DTs die even if medical treatment is instituted; death occurs from cardiac or respiratory failure, dehydration, and liver disease (Sullivan, 1995).

Dual Diagnosis

Alcoholism can occur concomitantly with a psychiatric disorder; many people self-medicate to reduce feelings of inferiority, depression, and anxiety. There are clinicians who believe that alcoholism is related to deep-seated psychopathology. Others insist that alcoholism must be considered as a primary disorder due to the research on the physical changes within the brain's reward circuitry system. These clinicians believe that the alcoholism must be treated as separate from any underlying personality dynamics. For the former, there is a natural tendency to look for underlying psychopathology as "causing" the need to take drugs. The latter belief leads the clinician to treat the alcoholism with medication, AA meetings, and psychoeducation. **Dual diagnosis** is a

major emerging problem, as evidenced by estimates suggesting that up to 60% of persons with substance use disorders also have a dual psychiatric diagnosis. Rosenberg and Drake (1998) developed the Dartmouth Assessment of Lifestyle Instrument (DALI) to assess substance abuse among the mentally ill. The researchers found that their instrument provided more accurate information than other more commonly used assessment tools.

Many patients use alcohol or other psychoactive drugs to forestall depressive symptoms, alleviate anxiety, stop frightening hallucinations, or express anger. The most common dually diagnosed psychiatric disorders are Schizophrenia, Major Depression, Panic Disorder, Antisocial Personality Disorder, and Eating Disorder. Developing knowledge about dual diagnosis suggests the need for a coordinated treatment approach with these patients (Gafoor & Rassool, 1998).

Most clinicians believe that it is important to treat alcoholism as a primary disease process while recognizing and handling the coexistence of other mental disorders in the rehabilitative phase. The rationale for treating the substance use disorder first is that the drug use typically interferes with an accurate assessment of the underlying psychiatric disorder. What looks like a serious personality disorder or depression can clear or improve when the alcohol or drug abuse is modified. The person under the influence of drugs cannot even begin to address the underlying psychological issues while the psychoactive properties of the drug are affecting thought processing and decision-making. There is an alteration of mood and thought process owing to changes in the availability of the principal neurotransmitters.

Treatment of the coexisting psychiatric disorder begins as soon as initial detoxification is complete. It is a critical component of aftercare because many patients use psychoactive substances instead of appropriate medication to self-medicate their anxiety and depressive symptoms (Claassen, et al., 1997). Using prescribed antipsychotic or antidepressant medication and developing different coping strategies through long-term supportive or insight psychotherapy may be crucial to the success of treatment for the substance dependency.

Sedative, Hypnotic, or Anxiolytic Use Disorders

Psychoactive drugs in this psychopharmacological classification include

- Benzodiazepines
- Barbiturates
- Minor tranquilizers, such as meprobamate (Equanil), diazepam (Valium), alprazolam (Xanax), and oxazepam (Serax)

These drugs act as CNS depressants and, in low doses, relieve anxiety and relax inhibitions. Psychological relief is obtained rapidly after ingestion because **hypnotic sedatives** produce a short-term sense of euphoria and well-being with few side effects at low doses. With high doses, however, hypnotic sedatives can depress vital CNS functions, particularly those involving respiratory centers. All of the hypnotic sedatives can be obtained legally, and they are all capable of producing psychological and physical dependence.

Benzodiazepine Use

The benzodiazepines are the most commonly prescribed anxiolytic (antianxiety) medications for treatment of insomnia, panic attacks, and mild tension states. Listed as Schedule IV drugs, they are highly effective as short-term treatment for anxiety related to situational circumstances. Diazepam, oxazepam, and chlordiazepoxide (Librium) also have an important medical use in treating the withdrawal symptoms of alcohol and other psychoactive substances that predispose an individual to violent behaviors. Usually, 50 to 100 mg is given intramuscularly and repeated every 4 to 6 hours until the acute effects are under control. Thereafter, the drug is given orally and tapered slowly. Beyond this period, these drugs should be given with great care, if at all, because of their addictive properties to reduce the anxiety of the recovering alcoholic. This pharmacological classification is more likely to be the drug of choice for older adults, who typically are not thought to have substance use disorders. Problems arise when benzodiazepines are prescribed but not monitored carefully.

Toxicity. The rationale for monitoring these drugs closely stems from the fact that, although moderate and long-acting benzodiazepines have a wider threshold of safety than other sedatives, they are potentially lethal in combination with other psychoactive drugs (Ghodse, 1994). Cross-tolerance to other hypnotic sedatives is high, and lethal overdoses occur when benzodiazepines are ingested with other psychoactive drugs. Oversedation or respiratory depression occurs in the elderly, and the benzodiazepines are a major contributing factor in psychiatric emergencies and unintentional death.

Withdrawal. Compared with the other drugs in this classification, the benzodiazepines have a relatively long half-life in the bloodstream. Consequently, onset of withdrawal to intermediate and long-acting benzodiazepines occurs within 3 to 5 days after cessation of the drug. Often the cause-and-effect relationship between drug withdrawal and emergence of symptoms is not always recognized because withdrawal symptoms are not abrupt (Mondanaro, 1990). Shorter-acting benzodiazepines such as triazolam (Halcion), alprazolam, lorazepam (Ativan), and oxazepam produce more severe withdrawal symptoms that begin soon after the drug is withdrawn. Treatment consists of gradual withdrawal of the drug, psychotherapy, and skill development of different, more effective coping strategies.

Barbiturate Abuse

Barbiturates derive from barbituric acid and produce pharmacological effects similar to those of alcohol. They are frequently the drug of choice among the middle class, who initially use them primarily as a prescribed drug from their physician to relieve insomnia or minor anxiety. Mode of administration is usually oral, with IV use by serious drug abusers. IV use of barbiturates is popular because it is financially easier to support than a heroin addiction.

Barbiturates also are used frequently in conjunction with other drugs to enhance euphoric effects or to help avoid the intensity of withdrawal symptoms. Barbiturate intoxication is associated with poor judgment, exaggeration of sexual and aggressive tendencies, sluggishness, and psychomotor impairment. It is frequently associated with unintentional overdose in children and is the drug classification most frequently implicated in adult attempted suicides. Barbiturates potentiate the effects of alcohol, and death occurs with a characteristic pattern of seizures and cardiorespiratory collapse. Withdrawal symptoms are severe and include agitation, tremors, delirium, and convulsions.

A major problem with barbiturate addiction is its legal availability through medical prescription. The addiction may go undiscovered because the abuser often can receive several prescriptions for the same drug from different physicians to support an undiagnosed habit.

Hallucinogen Use Disorders

The **hallucinogens** are a unique classification of psychoactive drugs for two reasons:

1. There are marked differences in the ways people experience them, ranging from no effect whatsoever to profound changes in perception, as described in Joe's story.

2. There are no distinct physical withdrawal effects.

Naturally occurring hallucinogens include mescaline and peyote taken from the cactus plant and psilocybin derived from mushrooms and marijuana. Synthetically derived hallucinogens include LSD and PCP, among others. The exact mechanism by which synthetic psychedelic drugs interact with the CNS is not readily identified, although LSD appears to interfere with the serotonin receptors of the neurons (Buskist & Gerbing, 1990). The blocking of important neuron receptors frees the neurons and gives rise to the out-of-body and intense emotional feelings experienced by the user, hence the typing as psychedelic drugs. The mode of administration is oral, usually as a tasteless powder that the person licks from a small blotter-type paper or swallows in pill form.

The hallucinogens involve sensory perceptual changes with a characteristic intense emotional experience and heightened awareness. When perceptual changes occur, the range can vary from having the experience of a freeing, pleasurable trip to greater perception to primary effects of an intensely dysphoric mood and paranoid ideation. They also vary from situation to situation so that the same person can experience good or bad trips from ingestion of the same drug at different times. **Flashbacks,** which represent a reexperiencing of the intense feelings associated with a previous drug-taking episode without further drug ingestion, can create a severe panic attack or psychotic behavior.

Flashbacks are sometimes activated with cannabis ingestion in the LSD user (Ghodse, 1995).

Phencyclidine Use

PCP, or angel dust, became popular in the late 1950s but lost its popularity 2 decades later because of its potential to cause psychosis and violence. This drug sometimes is classified as a hallucinogen because its pharmacological effects produce similar dramatic subjective effects and perceptions. PCP affects the opiate receptors associated with motivation and emotion (Buskist & Gerbing, 1990). The drug stimulates the release of dopamine and, taken in large doses, can precipitate a schizophrenic-like disorder. PCP stimulates paranoid ideation, auditory hallucinations, and a highly inconsistent pattern of behavior in users ranging from excitement to catatonic stupor.

Toxicity. PCP toxicity is most likely to present as a medical or psychiatric emergency in the form of an acute psychosis, and a person taking PCP is capable of sudden violent, impulsive behavior. Some report experiencing rageful delusions with a sense of having superhuman strength. During a bad trip, a person can experience panic attacks. Many former PCP users are found among the homeless or on chronic psychiatric units with a drug-induced psychosis.

Complications of Chronic Use. Chronic PCP use can result in permanent neurological and cognitive changes evidenced by loss of memory and impulse control, slowed thinking, dulled reflexes, and difficulty concentrating. Unfortunately, the strong feelings of invincibility, power, and strength are pleasurable enough that giving it up is difficult for most serious PCP abusers.

Cannabis Use Disorders

Of all the illicit drugs, cannabis is the most commonly used, especially by adolescents. Marijuana and its close cousins, hashish and tetrahydrocannabinol (THC), are derived from the Indian hemp plant, *Cannabis sativa.* The gummy resin covering the flowering tops and upper leaves contains the psychoactive agents responsible for the mind-altering properties of the drug. THC is the primary active ingredient in marijuana. Over the years, marijuana has been classified as a stimulant and, more recently, as a hallucinogen. Medically, THC has been used successfully in the treatment of glaucoma and in the relief of the nausea associated with cancer chemotherapy.

The most common route of administration for marijuana is inhalation into the lungs via smoking, which produces almost immediate effects. Some users ingest marijuana orally but because three times as much of the drug must be taken to achieve the same effects, this mode of administration is less favored. Drug effects are almost immediate. For most users, there is a sense of euphoria and a feeling of serenity. Time either is suspended or accelerated, depending on the overall mood of the user. There are marked perceptual changes in vision, hearing, taste, touch, and smell. With some people, visual and auditory perceptions are not pleasant; they are frightening and accompanied by a sense of depersonalization. A user described it as follows: "I felt as though I was going to die. My heart pounded and I could hear the clock ticking as though it was part of me. Everything was swimming around me and I thought someone was going to kill me." The drug remains in the body for up to 6 weeks after smoking it.

Relatively inexpensive and easily accessible, marijuana's initial euphoria and later the euphoric recall make it difficult for patients to give it up in favor of working through difficult problems without its support. One patient describes it as follows: "When things get really overwhelming, I can tune out with pot. It dulls the sensation and I think things are manageable again. I know it won't last, but for the moment, I can pretend, and I feel like I can cope. It doesn't help in the end, but I can't stand feeling that I have no control over what's happening to me."

Another reason for its popularity is the general belief that marijuana is not harmful. As one young man expressed it, "Give me one good reason why I shouldn't smoke it. It doesn't hurt me and it doesn't impact on anyone else like alcohol and other drugs do. Why shouldn't I use it?" There are several reasons why regular use of marijuana is harmful to the self as well as to others. The most commonly observed developmental pattern of drug abuse follows an ordered sequence of alcohol, cigarettes, and marijuana. There is slim but growing evidence of teratogenic effects on the fetus with prolonged marijuana use.

Marijuana clearly is a gateway drug in the typical progression to chronic use and IV administration of more addictive, opioid ("hard") drugs. Many people use the drug to self-medicate dysphoric mood and depressive symptoms. The quick high marijuana creates allows the person to feel in control again and to avoid painful emotional realities by slipping past them into the oblivion of the drug effects. Long-term use of the drug seems associated with a lack of motivation or initiative. Known as the "amotivational syndrome," individuals with a history of long-term marijuana use demonstrate a characteristic aimlessness and lack of realistic goal attainment. Sometimes, it is difficult to follow their conversations, and there is a tendency for the person to focus only on tangential parts of difficult reality circumstances.

In a few cases, a functional psychosis from chronic use can develop, lasting for a few hours or days and characterized by deep confusion, depersonalization, and hallucinations. The symptoms resolve quickly with antipsychotic medication but can reappear with resumption of marijuana use. Cannabis psychosis is more prevalent in countries with extremely heavy use (e.g., the West Indies and parts of Asia). Although marijuana toxicity can produce serious psychological symptoms and paranoia, the drug does not appear to have the fatal potential of overdose associated with other psychoactive substances.

Opioid Use Disorders

The **narcotic analgesics** are opioid agonists consisting of heroin, morphine, fentanyl, codeine, and methadone. With the exception of heroin, all of these drugs have significant medical value in regulated dosage for pain relief, and codeine is used as an active ingredient in medications for cough suppression. The opioids stimulate the neural activity of the opiate receptors and bind with various opioid receptors, thereby giving these narcotics their deserved reputation as effective pain killers. Reinforcing effects of this pharmacological drug classification appear to be related to their effect on dopaminergic pathways, particularly along the mesocorticolimbic circuits believed to be the reward and pleasure centers of the brain (Jaffe & Martin, 1990). In addition to providing physical relief from pain, the opioids suppress emotional tensions. Reduction of emotional pain and anxiety allows the heroin abuser to assume a passive adaptation to painful inner pressures.

Heroin, with no medical value, is a depressant drug and the most widely misused. Street names for heroin include "H," Harry, horse, or China white. High-grade heroin finds its way into this country from Southeast Asia, an area that includes Myanmar, Thailand, and Laos. Heroin is illegally transported in false-bottom suitcases, in passenger bags, and even in the stomachs of airline passengers who swallow rubber pouches filled with the drug; the incidence of heroin smuggling began to increase dramatically in the mid- to late 1990s.

Opiates usually are taken orally and through IV injection. Because IV injection produces the most intense and immediate effects, most serious narcotic addicts prefer "mainlining" as the mode of administration. The disadvantages of IV drug administration are related to infections and vein collapse with frequent use. Fever of unknown origin in any drug abuser should raise suspicion of endocarditis, or "cotton fever," a condition brought about by the direct IV injection of small particles or bacteria into the bloodstream. Novice narcotic abusers frequently use intramuscular or subcutaneous injections, referred to as "skin popping," before moving into IV modes of administration.

Complications of Chronic Use. Organ system complications associated with heroin abuse include endocarditis, pulmonary edema, and pulmonary fibrosis caused by the insoluble materials used to cut the drug for IV administration that collect in the lung. The most serious effects of heroin abuse are acute respiratory depression and pulmonary edema, which not infrequently result in cardiorespiratory arrest and the rather quick death of the victim.

Hepatitis is a frequent medical complication; IV drug use can account for up to 80% of hospitalizations for this disorder (Levine, et al., 1995). Septic conditions contribute to bacterial meningitis and skin lesions. Opiates create a state of chronic constipation, with the onset of diarrhea and abdominal cramping occurring symptomatically on withdrawal. There is a susceptibility to infection, and the development of hyperplastic nodes ("addicts' nodes") offers clear indication of the immunosuppressive qualities of heroin dependency. AIDs is a complication due to the sharing of needles and *works* (the equipment used to prepare the solution for injection).

Toxicity. Opiate overdose constitutes a medical emergency requiring immediate recognition and treatment. It is characterized by pinpoint pupils, depressed respiration, cardiac arrhythmias, convulsions, and coma. Death

can result from pulmonary edema (Schuckit, 1995). Treatment consists of administering an opioid antagonist (e.g., naltrexone [ReVia]) that can reverse the symptoms in a relatively short time. An adverse reaction can occur, however, in the form of withdrawal symptoms. Clonidine, alone and in combination with naltrexone, also has proved effective in detoxification protocols with heroin addicts.

Withdrawal. Although withdrawal symptoms do not constitute a medical emergency, they are extremely uncomfortable for the patient. Because of the discomfort involved, many patients seek immediate relief by using the drug again, and it is difficult for them to remain drug-free. Characteristic symptoms include delusional thinking, nightmares, severe tremors, diaphoresis, frequent yawning, abdominal pain, muscle spasm, and tearing. Withdrawal symptoms can be reversed with tapered doses of methadone. This drug acts as a heroin agonist, having analgesic effects without producing the high typically associated with heroin.

Methadone Treatment. Methadone was the first drug used for the treatment of heroin addiction. Although marked differences exist between the natural and synthetic chemical bases for the opiates, their effects on the neurotransmitter system in the brain are similar. Because of their close resemblance to each other, administering controlled doses of methadone to heroin addicts has received support from both the medical and legal communities as a safe, long-term treatment for heroin dependency. First prescribed in 1965, administration of the synthetically developed methadone seems to correct the unyielding chemical imbalance in brain metabolism related to chronic use of heroin. Heroin addicts receiving oral methadone in controlled dosages do not seem to experience the euphoria or withdrawal symptoms associated with heroin dependency or the damaging toxicological side effects associated with heroin consumption (Table 26–3).

In 1972, the Food and Drug Administration (FDA) reclassified methadone in a special drug category that would allow its medically supervised administration to addicts with chronic, intractable addictions to heroin. Drug addicts requiring detoxification are entitled to methadone treatment for up to 21 days. Federal guidelines for inclusion in a maintenance treatment protocol include a history of opiate dependency of more than 2 years and evidence of physical withdrawal symptoms associated with this drug classification. The only exception to this rule is the administration of methadone to a drug addict who is hospitalized for an illness other than drug dependency for more than 21 days. Methadone can be given to the patient until recovery from the illness is complete to curb withdrawal symptoms.

The expected outcomes of methadone maintenance are twofold (Gerstein & Harwood, 1990):

1. To reduce illicit use of heroin and the criminal behaviors used by heroin addicts to sustain their habit
2. To improve the psychological well-being and social productivity of the heroin addict

Clinical efficacy is demonstrated in the marked decrease in criminal activities and social rehabilitation attributable

TABLE 26-3 Using the Nursing Process in Detoxification With Methadone

STEP	DRUG ADMINISTRATION
Assessment	
1. Obtain complete assessment data regarding heroin use.	
2. Establish a diagnosis of opiate dependence based on IV use, urine screens, and naloxone testing.	
Planning	
1. Gain patient's cooperation.	
2. Provide information regarding methadone, mechanism of action, side effects, and so on.	
Implementation	
1. Administer medication.	10 mg
2. Observe for signs of opiate intoxication and withdrawal.	
3. Monitor vital signs.	
4. Establish methadone maintenance dosage once patient is stabilized (24–48 h).	20–30 mg/d
5. Reduce methadone dosage by 5 mg/d.	
6. Use supportive counseling and education during withdrawal.	Detoxification can be completed in 7–14 d
7. Reassure patient that withdrawal symptoms are normal even with methadone and will diminish.	

IV, intravenous.

to maintenance treatment programs for hard-core heroin addicts.

Sympathomimetic Use Disorders

Drugs pharmacologically classified as **CNS stimulants** (amphetamines, cocaine, nicotine, and caffeine) act on catecholamine neurotransmitters, serotonin, norepinephrine, and dopamine in the brain.

Amphetamine Use

The most commonly used amphetamines include dextroamphetamine (Dexedrine), methamphetamine, and methylphenidate (Ritalin). Amphetamines originally were used as appetite suppressants for weight loss.

Because of their energizing effects, this class of drugs also is used by athletes and long-distance truck drivers to increase energy and counteract fatigue. Medically, the drug classification is sometimes used in the treatment of depression, particularly when associated with narcolepsy. Methylphenidate is an effective medication used to offset the symptoms of attention-deficit hyperactivity disorder.

Cocaine Use

Cocaine has emerged as the signature drug of the CNS stimulants, and cocaine abuse increased with alarming frequency in the 1990s. Cocaine is a drug of choice among higher socioeconomic groups; the true incidence of cocaine use may be underreported.

Cocaine is derived from a plant, *Erythroxylon*. Cocaine alkaloid can be broken up into smaller pieces referred to as "crack," so named because of the crackling sound of the substance when heated. Compared with the cost of powdered cocaine, crack is cheap, purer, and more available in individual doses. Crack is *freebased*, a term used to describe taking the pure cocaine alkaloid and smoking it in a pipe or sprinkling it on a marijuana joint.

Like heroin, cocaine is smuggled into the United States and Canada from foreign sources, chiefly from Colombia, South America, where the plant grows well. Pharmacologically, cocaine affects the metabolism of dopamine, norepinephrine, acetylcholine, and serotonin. Of primary importance in understanding the action of cocaine on the brain is understanding its effects on the dopaminergic system. In the brain, this psychoactive substance blocks the reuptake mechanism of dopamine, thus prolonging the activity of the neurotransmitter in the synapse. This action may be responsible for cocaine's strong reinforcing effects. Cocaine has definite stimulant properties; it produces euphoria, increased energy, improved performance, loss of fatigue, and a sense of well-being and freedom from boredom.

Cocaine is a short-acting drug, particularly when injected or smoked as crack (APA, 1994). This makes it attractive as a mood-altering drug because it also produces a sense of power unparalleled in other psychoactive drugs. There is an almost instantaneous positive sense of well-being, heightened sense of competency, and increased sex drive. Although some consumers experience an initial nausea, it is transitory and usually does not detract from the enhanced sense of well-being and self-esteem that accompanies cocaine. The euphoric effects of the drug block out or "numb" uncomfortable emotional pain and counteract the boredom and emptiness of life.

Modes of administration vary:

- Insufflation (snorting or inhaling)
- IV injection (used with traditional cocaine powders)

With insufflation, the drug is inhaled into the lung and transported almost immediately to the brain via the circulatory system. Less frequently used methods include oral ingestion and chewing coca leaves much as one would chew tobacco. Cocaine also can be injected subcutaneously or intramuscularly.

The pattern of cocaine abuse is different from that of other psychoactive drugs in that abusers are "binge" rather than "maintenance" abusers, with binges lasting from several hours to several days. Nightclubs are fertile grounds for encouraging the habit, because the drugs are sold in these establishments. Between binges, the cocaine addict may be drug-free. Because it is a short-acting drug, physical tolerance does not develop in the same manner as with other psychoactive substances.

Complications of Chronic Use. The crack or cocaine abuser often presents in the emergency department as acutely anxious, possibly combative, and paranoid. Potentially violent behavior is always a possibility with a person under the influence of cocaine. The patient has a tendency to misinterpret the environment, which heightens the potential for violence. The cocaine addict responds best to a quiet and soothing environment with sufficient space and openness in communication and gestures.

Extensive use can produce nasal ulcerations, chronic cough or sore throat, malnutrition, and insomnia. Significant snorting can irrevocably affect the nasal mucosa, and chronic use can stimulate characteristic repetitive behaviors such as picking at the skin. Some patients experience psychotic symptoms such as auditory and tactile hallucinations (coke bugs) and paranoid ideation.

Although ingestion of cocaine produces euphoric effects that are intense and rapid, they are followed by an equally intense emotional low, and this may account for the strong psychological dependence on cocaine. The rapid, cycling bipolar effects of excitement and depression may be the result of the temporary dopamine increase noted with acute cocaine administration followed by a dramatic decrease in dopamine level found with repeated administration. The fact that the dysphoric symptoms can be corrected with subsequent cocaine administration increases the likelihood of persistent psychological dependence.

Of particular clinical concern is the development of **cocaine blues,** a sequela of drug cessation that consists of a dysphoric mood having clinical significance and suicidal ideation. The deep depression that often accompanies cocaine withdrawal makes the client a strong suicide risk and increases the desire for the drug to relieve the overwhelming dysphoric mood and associated feelings.

Typically, the cocaine addict is a polydrug user, which further complicates treatment initiatives. This may occur because cocaine produces such an uncomfortable level of stimulation that alcohol, marijuana, and other hypnotic sedatives are used to equalize the stimulating effects of the drug. A favored combination of many cocaine abusers is IV injection in combination with heroin, known as "chasing the dragon." Cocaine provides the high, and heroin helps to mellow the sharper stimulating effects of cocaine that can be troublesome. Cocaine also is used by heroin addicts to provide energy and sometimes the courage needed to perform criminal acts to sustain the heroin habit. This combination is referred to as "speedballing"; many heroin addicts list heroin as their primary drug and cocaine as secondary.

Toxicity. Cocaine toxicity was the second most frequent cause of death reported to the American Association of Poison Control Centers in 1988. Although chronic use can lead to toxic overdose, it is not necessary to be a long-time abuser to suffer significant side effects. Death can result in first-time users as well as in those severely addicted to cocaine. Toxicity and potential for overdose are greater with this particular drug than with other drugs because the purity of the drug can be as high as 90%; in addition, when it is free-based, it enters the brain with minimal alteration in drug concentration. Overdose can produce severe systemic responses, including respiratory collapse and sudden death. Thus, death can be instantaneous.

Other signs and symptoms of cocaine toxicity include acute anxiety, extreme agitation, seizures, cardiac arrhythmias, and pulmonary edema. Unfortunately, there are no drug antagonists to arrest the toxic effects of cocaine overdose. Naloxone is given to reduce the concurrent toxic effects of other drugs, namely narcotics, in the victim's body systems.

CNS stimulant toxicity in nonlethal situations usually is self-limited. Delusional symptoms are treated symptomatically with supportive measures. Antipsychotic medication is given when warranted, and a benzodiazepine such as diazepam or oxazepam is used in the first few days of treatment to reduce agitation. A peculiarity of cocaine is its natural sedative effect as it wears off; it is important not to oversedate the cocaine patient because this can heighten the possibility of respiratory depression with drug cessation.

Withdrawal. Patients experiencing withdrawal symptoms complain of headache, lethargy, craving, muscle pain, eating disturbance, alterations in sleep patterns, irritability, and paranoid or delusional thinking.

Treatment Considerations

Cocaine addiction is difficult to treat because of its rewarding or reinforcing properties. To neutralize the effects of craving, part of the treatment process for cocaine abusers is deliberate exploration of the positive effects of the drug with an eye to substitution.

Generally, a structured, intensive outpatient substance abuse program is needed to provide the setting required for drug abstinence and rehabilitation. More often than not, cocaine addictions coexist with other psychiatric disorders, the most common being major or bipolar depression, panic disorder, and attention-deficit hyperactivity disorder (Miller, Mahler, Belkin, & Gold, 1990). Thus, the underlying disorder must also be treated simultaneously. Antidepressants and lithium have been used with some success in reducing the craving and dysphoric mood associated with cocaine addiction withdrawal.

Caffeine and Nicotine Use

Caffeine and nicotine are not always thought of as drugs to be abused because they do not present the same destructive clinical impairment associated with substance abuse or dependence. Yet both are capable of producing tolerance and withdrawal symptoms with excessive, chronic use, and both are found in the

DSM-IV classification. Caffeine is found in a number of drinks, including coffee, tea, and soft drinks; in some analgesics; and in diet aids and cold medications. Toxicity is characterized by increased anxiety, irritability, psychomotor agitation, diaphoresis, and tinnitus. In a small number of cases, excessive caffeine can result in cardiac arrhythmias, grand mal seizures, and respiratory collapse. Caffeine is known to exacerbate peptic ulcers and circulatory failure. Women can sometimes decrease the symptoms of premenstrual syndrome by eliminating caffeine from their diet 2 weeks before the menses. Drowsiness, depression, headache, irritability, and dysphoric mood often are signs of caffeine withdrawal.

Nicotine typically does not create the social problems that other forms of dependence create. What it does generate is a serious health risk not only for smokers but also for those most intimately involved with them. Cancer of the lung, larynx, throat, and mouth; emphysema and other lung conditions; and cardiac and circulatory problems have been observed with heavy use of nicotine. Inhalation of passive smoke by nonsmokers can produce similar symptoms in people who have never smoked. Women who smoke frequently have low birth weight babies. For all of these reasons, habitual use of nicotine is a major health hazard.

Nicotine withdrawal occurs within 24 hours of cigarette stoppage. Symptoms include irritability, insomnia, tension, and decreased heart rate. Weight gain, emotional sensitivity, and irritability are characteristic of deliberate smoking cessation. The undesirable withdrawal symptoms and craving for cigarettes that remain long after cigarette smoking has stopped reduce the success rate. Those who wake up to a cigarette and who crave it when ill or who are willing to stand outside in the bitter cold to have a cigarette have the most difficulty giving it up. There is a high incidence of nicotine dependence among the mentally ill and those with other substance use disorders. Treatment for dependence consists of a variety of measures ranging from self-hypnosis, nicotine gum or patch, bupropion (Zyban), family support, and self-help groups (APA, 1996).

Volatile Solvent Use Disorders

During the 1990s, it became fashionable for adolescents to inhale volatile solvents such as glue, gasoline, paint thinners, and cleaners and other propellants for their stimulant effects. The substances are inhaled through the nose and mouth via a cloth or a plastic bag saturated with the substance or are sprayed directly from the can into the nose or mouth. The effects of the drug are immediate, and intoxication can result in a number of signs and symptoms, among them lethargy, psychomotor retardation, and generalized muscle weakness. Some propellants, in particular, can freeze the larynx or cause respiratory and cardiac depression. Toxicity can lead to cirrhosis or renal failure. The expected outcome of treatment, as in other dependencies, is complete abstinence. The same supports, however, are not available for the treatment of this dependence compared with other types of substance use disorders.

What do you think? What are your thoughts about free needle exchange as a response to the drug problem in our country?

➤ *Check Your Reading*

4. What are the distinguishing characteristics of substance dependence?
5. How does alcohol compromise a person's life journey?
6. What role does craving play in cocaine addiction?

NURSING PROCESS: ACUTE PHASE

Treatment of substance use disorders generally is broken down into two phases. The first is the acute phase, in which the nurse assesses and treats the medical, toxic, or withdrawal symptoms associated with the disorder. This phase typically lasts a short time and culminates in the medical stabilization of the patient's condition. This is followed by a much longer phase of treatment—rehabilitation—lasting months, years, or, with most people having this disorder, a lifetime.

The acute phase consists of all of the nursing interventions associated with the medical stabilization of the patient's symptoms. Patients demonstrating acute toxicity or withdrawal symptoms require immediate triage. The nurse elicits information related to amount and type of drug taken within the past 48 hours and routes of administration. This information is used to determine whether lavage is necessary and as a basis to administer drug antagonists, if appropriate. Relevant nursing diagnoses can include one or more of the following:

- Injury
- Potential for Altered Nutrition: Less than Body Requirements
- Sleep Pattern Disturbance
- Impaired Gas Exchange
- Fluid Volume Deficit
- Cardiac Output, Altered
- Self Care Deficit: Feeding, Hygiene, Toileting
- Thought Processes, Altered
- Sensory/Perceptual Alterations: Visual, Auditory, Tactile
- Violence, Potential for Self Directed or Directed at Others
- Breathing Pattern, Ineffective
- Communication, Impaired Verbal
- Self Concept, Disturbance in: Personal Identity

Expected treatment outcomes relate to the restoration and maintenance of physiological and psychological stability. Treatment is largely symptomatic and immediate. Depending on the nature and severity of the emergency situation, nursing interventions to meet any or all of the following treatment goals are appropriate:

- Prevention of cardiovascular collapse
- Support of the respiratory system

- Identification of psychoactive drugs and removal, if ingested orally
- Administration of narcotic antagonist, if appropriate
- Treatment of hypotension or hypertension
- Prevention of treatment of seizures
- Prevention of aspiration
- Treatment of hypothermia or hyperthermia
- Protection from self-inflicted or other-directed injury

Monitoring vital signs, establishing an adequate airway, administering oxygen if needed, and using IV fluids are first-priority nursing interventions. If the patient is an IV drug abuser, the likelihood of cotton fever, thrombophlebitis, endocarditis, hepatitis, AIDs, and bacteremia are considered. Look for needle marks over veins, indicative of recent injection, and signs of hyperthermia. Fever of unknown origin may be the only indicator of endocarditis, persisting even in the absence of positive test cultures. Look for other evidence of drug complications, such as electrolyte or nutritional deficiencies. These observations offer more precise data about the type of intervention needed. For example, recent oral ingestion of drugs can be reversed with proper administration of emetic medications. Routine measurement of intake and output and frequent vital signs is imperative because the patient's condition can change quickly. Urine and blood toxicology tests help determine drug toxicity levels, which are needed to make a differential diagnosis from psychosis and as the basis for choosing immediate treatment options. Most psychoactive drugs and their metabolites clear the body system within 48 hours unless the patient is a chronic abuser of the drug. Benzodiazepines take longer to clear the system, and the toxic effects of chlordiazepoxide do not peak until 5 to 7 days after ingestion (Haack, 1998).

While under the acute influence of drugs, the patient is likely to be a danger to self or others. Thus, assessing the patient's potential for violence or suicide related to sensory-perceptual deficits created by the drug toxicity is in order. If this potential is noted, the nurse needs to take appropriate measures to ensure patient and nursing personnel safety (see Chapter 33 for treatment of delirium).

Once the patient's immediate life-threatening needs are under control, the nurse turns his or her attention to simplifying the patient's environment. Placing the patient in a quiet, well-lit room, orienting the patient, and providing information about necessary procedures help decrease patient anxiety. Seizure precautions minimize chances of injury from seizure activity. Table 26–4 presents a minicare plan for the following common nursing diagnoses found in the acute phase of treatment of a substance use disorder:

Potential for Injury Related To substance abuse toxicity
Decreased Cardiac Output Related To effects of substance abuse toxicity
Altered Thought Processes Related To drug toxicity

NURSING PROCESS: REHABILITATION PHASE

The rehabilitative treatment of patients with substance use disorders requires an integrated psychopharmacological and behavioral psychiatric approach for successful outcome; family therapy also is appropriate when

---

TABLE 26–4 A Mini-Care Plan for the Acute Phase of Treatment of Substance Use Disorder

EXPECTED OUTCOME	NURSING ACTIONS
Long Term Patient will maintain psychological and physiological stability.	
Short Term Patient will maintain physical homeostasis.	1. Monitor vital signs every 15 min until stabilized. 2. Administer oxygen and other medications as needed. 3. Observe and report signs of impending seizure. 4. Monitor and report intake, output, and critical laboratory values. 5. Use IV therapy or oral fluids to correct nutritional deficiency.
Patient will verbalize orientation to person, place, and time.	1. Speak to the patient in a calm voice and use short sentences. 2. Orient patient to unit, and explain all procedures. 3. Administer antianxiety medications as ordered.
Patient will remain injury-free during detoxification.	1. Establish a calm environment with low lights and minimal stimuli. 2. If restraints are necessary, explain their use in simple terms and reassure the patient they will be removed when the patient is no longer a danger to self or others. 3. Stay with the patient if he or she is agitated or confused. 4. Institute seizure precautions, if needed.

IV, intravenous.

the family unit is intact. Schuster and Snyder (1990) noted,

just as insulin will not save a diabetic who cannot change his diet and life style, medications to treat drug addiction will not work by themselves. They must be part of a comprehensive treatment program that gives addicts the capabilities to achieve a life without drugs. (p. 72)

A critical part of the treatment process for chronic substance use disorders is the development of a new lifestyle completely devoid of old patterns and, in most cases, of past drug-using companions.

Assessment

The rehabilitative phase begins with education about the nature of addictive behaviors and a comprehensive personal assessment of past and present drug use. The information sought includes a history of the drinking or drug abuse pattern, social functioning, resources, and level of basic skill development. A complete history of the patient's drug abuse pattern includes age of onset, types of substances abused (including alcohol), mode of administration, usual conditions or situations in which drug-taking behaviors occur, previous treatment attempts, and medical treatments for secondary symptoms. Employment history, legal status, and family history provide an insight into the level of disruption in the chemically dependent person's life related to substance abuse. Mental status and questions about disturbances in mood elicit important information about associated psychiatric problems that may compound the drug abuse. Questions to include in a substance abuse history are presented in Figure 26–3.

Interviewing family members has two purposes:

1. It helps to verify the substance user's historical perspective, supplying missing details and modifying information in joint consultation with the patient.

2. It provides an opportunity to observe the interactions between the patient and family members.

The latter offers important clues about behaviors that may be reinforcing or enabling the disorder to continue without treatment. For example, the discovery that family members have been covering for the substance user so that he or she will not lose his or her job is an invaluable source of information about enabling behavior.

Although the primary diagnosis may be the substance use disorder, evidence of an underlying untreated psychiatric disorder may interfere with the patient's ability to engage fully in the rehabilitation process. Thought disturbances and tangential thinking may suggest a secondary problem with psychosis, whereas lack of anxiety and disregard for the rights of others may indicate an underlying personality disorder. When circumstantiality, perseveration, and disordered thinking are marked during the intake interview, an organic component should be considered. Evaluation of impulse control yields information about the patient's need for structure in planning treatment. Those with poor impulse control need a stronger treatment structure and more personalized support to remain with the treatment program.

Self-diagnosis and motivation for treatment form the cornerstone of successful treatment. Motivation to change is perhaps the most important aspect of a favorable prognosis, and self-diagnosis of the problems created by substance use allows the substance user to take responsibility for his or her actions. In addition to providing an accurate database, the assessment process forms an important bridge to engaging the patient in the treatment process and encouraging self-diagnosis.

When a patient lacks motivation for treatment, as many do initially, therapeutic confrontation is a strategy often used to break through denial of the disorder's impact on the chemically dependent person's life and those most important to him or her. The family, with the treatment team's help, presents the substance user with irrefutable evidence of behaviors related to chemical abuse or dependency with a firm call for treatment. This strategy is likely to have the greatest impact on patient readiness, particularly if coupled with realistic consequences for noncompliance. Another benefit is that it engages family cooperation from the outset of treatment.

Johnson (1990) defined a therapeutic confrontation as "meaningful people presenting reality to a person in a receivable way" (p. 3). Family members prepare for the confrontation in much the same way as a student would prepare for an important class presentation. Specific relevant data are presented in a logical and meaningful way so that the person receiving the information can easily comprehend it. The presented data include external problems (marital, social, occupational, financial) and personal problems, such as physical impairments, that are explicitly linked to specific substance use activities. Each person presents how the behavior he or she describes affects them personally. Factual information about the progression, treatment, and consequences of substance abuse is presented in a nonemotional, supportive manner. Attempts by the substance user to divert attention from the discussion or to make excuses without relating them to the problem of substance abuse are not accepted. Only the behaviors, and not the motivations, are up for consideration. Several pertinent behavioral examples are hard to refute even by the most hard-core chemically dependent person. Implementable consequences of noncompliance are identified, and the person is advised that the decision to seek treatment is no longer an option.

Arrangements for immediate detoxification are made before the confrontation, and, in many cases, a professional specially trained in therapeutic confrontations for addictive behaviors is present. The family must be willing to follow through on the consequences identified in the confrontation, and often the family needs a significant time beforehand to work through feelings about participating in it. Nevertheless, therapeutic confrontation is a powerful tool that has been used successfully as a motivator for treatment.

Wing (1991, 1993) has identified a model for alcoholic recovery that can be used within a nursing framework. She identified four stages of recovery:

1. *Denial:* The recovery behavior is the decision to remain abstinent.

Questions to Include in the Substance Abuse History

History of substance use	History of experimentation with any drugs in childhood. Any current recreational drug or alcohol use (obtain the following information for each drug used [e.g., nicotine, alcohol, cocaine] including drug of choice). Age of first use. Duration of use, method of (e.g., intravenous injection, snorting, smoking). Last use. Amount and cost of drug used per day or week. Patterns of binge use, amount used during a binge. Method used to support habit (e.g., stealing, prostitution, employment, Aid to Dependent Children checks). History of needle sharing (if intravenous drug user).
Presence of withdrawal symptoms	Alcohol—morning shakes, seizures (if pertinent, last seizure and type of seizure), hallucinations (visual, auditory, or tactile). Opioid—nausea, vomiting, abdominal pain or cramps, diarrhea, chills, runny nose and eyes, sweating, bone or muscle pain. Cocaine—depression, suicidal thoughts (if pregnant, contractions, hyperactive baby).
Substance-related illnesses	Hepatitis, pancreatitis, gastrointestinal bleeding, heart complications, frequent bronchitis or pneumonia, positive HIV test (date of last test), cellulitis, frequent sexually transmitted disease and treatment dates.
Treatment history	Attempts at self-detoxification and outcome, names of treatment programs and dates, length of stay, and drug-free period after each treatment. Longest drug-free period, activities during that time.
Past medical history	Admissions for liver disease, peptic ulcers, heart attack, surgical procedures, history of diabetes, hypertension.
Medications	Prescribed and over the counter—usual dose, amounts actually used.
Family history	History of substance abuse. (Go back at least two generations and include current close relatives.)
Childhood history	Problems growing up, history of physical/sexual/emotional abuse, family relationships.
Consequences of substance use	Losses (jobs, property, relationships, children, self-respect, health).
Legal history	Arrests, incarcerations, current status (e.g., parole, probation).
Psychiatric history	Admissions, any known diagnoses, medications, history of suicide attempts or thoughts.
Social history	Marital status, number of children, ages and whereabouts, living situation and source of support, level of education, and work history.
Sexual history	Sexual orientation, history of multiple partners, use of safe sex methods, history of rape, problems with impotence or other sexual dysfunction.
Gynecological history	Last menstrual period, irregularities, birth control method, gravidity, parity, abortions, miscarriages, ectopic, complications during pregnancy, source of prenatal care, history of drug use during pregnancy, health of newborns.
Review of systems	Evaluate present status, whether intoxicated or in withdrawal at time of visit.

F i g u r e 2 6 – 3
Questions to include in the substance abuse history. (From Caulker-Burnett, I. [1994]. Primary care screening for substance abuse. *Nurse Practitioner,* *1*9[6], 42–48.)

2. *Dependence:* The recovery behavior is the decision to make behavioral changes due to internal desires rather than others' wishes.

3. *Behavior change goals that are healthy:* The recovery behavior is to take responsibility for one's own actions and to develop a positive view of self.

4. *Life planning, emotional maturity, and long-term goal setting:* The recovery behavior is to set responsible goals for oneself in a mature manner that takes into consideration the needs of family members or individuals in the work environment.

Nursing diagnoses relevant to the rehabilitation phase may include one or more of the following:

- Ineffective Individual Coping
- Altered Family Processes
- Coping
- Ineffective Family Coping, Compromised, Dysfunctional
- Knowledge Deficit
- Social Isolation
- Spiritual Distress
- Self Care Deficit: Feeding, Bathing/Hygiene, Dressing/Grooming, Toileting
- Self Concept, Disturbance in: Self Esteem, Personal Identity, Role Performance
- Powerlessness

Outcome Identification

The expected outcomes of treatment are simple to identify and difficult to implement:

- The patient will remain drug-free.
- The patient will establish and maintain a productive and satisfying lifestyle.

Short-term goals consistent with the patient's nursing diagnoses are mutually defined so that they are acceptable to the chemically dependent person and the family. This helps promote ownership of treatment goals and motivation to achieve them. In most instances, goal achievement requires a total commitment and daily effort. Setting goals 1 day at a time that are action oriented, realistic, and achievable increases self-awareness and self-confidence.

Planning

Figure 26-4 presents the continuum of treatment options for drug abuse. Inpatient treatment of substance use disorders has been severely curtailed in a climate of restricted health benefits for mental disorders. Nevertheless, a variation on the Minnesota model, originally developed by three treatment centers in Minnesota—Pioneer House, Hazelden, and Wilmar—continues to be operative in the treatment of substance use disorders. The Minnesota model uses the 12 steps of AA (Box 26-9) as the foundation for treatment, and the staff usually consists of recovering addicts as well as health professionals specially trained in the treatment of addictive disorders. The treatment protocol involves admission to a residential treatment facility with a heavy emphasis on self-diagnosis, intensive group counseling, educational lectures, and mandatory AA attendance.

Table 26-5 provides suggested nursing actions for inpatient treatment or day treatment of substance use disorder. After discharge, the patient continues with an outpatient group for a few weeks or months, as needed.

The goal of this progressive treatment approach is to help the patient in the rehabilitative phase develop self-confidence and make needed connections in the community for continued aftercare.

Implementation

Nursing intervention strategies for the patient with a substance use disorder tend to be highly structured with an emphasis on self-diagnosis, limit-setting, group therapy, skill development, and family treatment.

Self-Diagnosis

Self-diagnosis forms the cornerstone of treatment, and it is not easy for someone locked in a rigid world in which

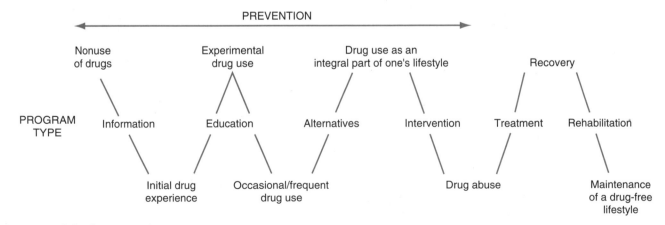

Figure 26-4

The continuum of treatment options for substance use disorders. (From French, J. F., & Kaufman, N. J. [1981]. *Handbook for prevention evaluation.* Rockville, MD: National Institute on Drug Abuse.)

emotional reactions, mental processes, and spiritual values were controlled by a psychoactive substance for a long time. As the initial euphoria about taking the first step toward abstinence subsides, there is an awareness of the radical lifestyle changes required to maintain it. Old routines and personal habits that activate alcoholic or drug-taking behaviors have to be replaced with new and productive patterns of behavior; long-standing angers and resentments need a different outlet and resolution. These changes go to the core of a person's self-concept, and the former substance user must now confront many painful attitudes and emotional responses. On a daily basis, the recovering addict must accept self and others as imperfect human beings living in an imperfect world, without the use of a psychoactive substance to dull the reality. There is the knowledge that in times of stress the person will be drawn once again to the landscape of substance use because this is familiar territory, whereas working through difficult life problems without alcohol or drugs is not as well known. There are many blanks in the patient's mental map that need to be filled in. The recovering addict must discover the precise details to fill in the puzzle of the past and develop a new set of puzzle pieces. The human context against which the map of the person's life is drawn must be fluid enough to provide meaningful choices and fixed enough to provide the structure necessary for survival.

Rehabilitative efforts begin with helping the patient self-diagnose situations and feelings likely to get in the way of developing a different drug-free self-identity. Breaking through the denial is a necessary first step in the recovery process for the patient and family members. This can be accomplished in a number of ways, and the process usually begins with education. Providing basic information about the nature and development of the disorder offers hope and help with the realization that substance use disorders are treatable. An educational format provides a nonthreatening way to deliver emotionally charged information about a disorder that is difficult to understand and accept. Providing opportunities for the patient to learn about the disease surprisingly provides information he or she has never heard before. Intensive group discussion of feelings expressed in the educational segment is an invaluable tool for breaking through the denial.

Group Therapy

Group therapy and self-help groups that are focused on abstinence and the behaviors needed to achieve it are the treatment of choice for alcoholics and drug abusers (Galanter, Castaneda, & Franco, 1991). This is true for several reasons. First, groups provide a social network for the patient. Many need this because without the bond of drinking or drug abuse, they have no friends. Other group members also provide consensual validation for the patient's experience and challenge any deceptions. They provide a powerful mechanism for breaking through the patient's denial because they have been there and know exactly how to get at the truth. At the same time, the group can support the patient's efforts to remain abstinent, and this is highly reinforcing. They provide an opportunity to share the pain, shame, and small triumphs with others who understand. Group confirmation of similar feelings and experiences allows maladaptive behaviors and feelings to be normalized rather than repressed or exaggerated. The patient practices reality testing by sharing with others having similar experiences and finding self-confidence in the confrontations and problem-solving strategies. The acceptance that comes from other group members who like you just the way you are and yet encourage you to become all that you are capable of is empowering.

TABLE 26-5 Suggested Nursing Actions for Inpatient Treatment or Day Treatment of Substance Use Disorder

EXPECTED OUTCOME	NURSING ACTIONS
1. Patient will verbalize that he or she is chemically dependent and is powerless over his or her drug habit.	1. Assess patient's current knowledge base. 2. Encourage expression of feelings related to substance abuse. 3. Describe natural progression of the disorder. 4. Identify resources for support and information. 5. Give positive reinforcement for self-diagnosis and assumption of personal responsibility for treatment 6. Encourage involvement of significant others in treatment.
2. Patient will participate in all treatment activities.	1. Assess patient's motivation to change. 2. Establish schedule with patient and hold patient accountable for attendance. 3. Enforce agreed-on contingencies for manipulative and acting-out behaviors. 4. Encourage and reinforce acceptance of responsibility. 5. Mutually identify problems in coping and help patient develop prevention plan. 6. Refer patient to community agencies and Alcoholics Anonymous or Narcotics Anonymous before discharge. 7. Arrange for aftercare and easy revisiting of therapeutic community for discharged patient.

Behavioral Therapy

Limit-setting is the behavioral component of the intervention and is designed to help patients respond constructively to the ongoing stresses of everyday life in a self-disciplined way. Part of the behavior pattern seen frequently in patients with substance use disorders is the avoidance of responsibility for common life tasks coupled with the making of excuses for dealing with unmet obligations. Correction of the attitudes and behaviors that support a lifestyle of denial and rationalization is difficult but necessary. Mixed with the behaviors are unresolved negative attitudes and feelings of alienation, anger, loneliness, and self-doubt that form the underpinnings of resumption of drug-taking behaviors. Patients have learned to repress feelings and bottle them up inside until they explode, often with disastrous results or until these feelings are acted out with the help of a psychoactive drug. Clear, consistent limits provide the external structure many patients need to internally respond effectively to their environment. Over time, these limits help the patient to internalize the process of setting limits on her or his own behavior in line with the needs of self and others. To be effective, the recovering substance user should participate actively in setting her or his own behavioral expectations. This helps ensure ownership of the behavior.

The steps in a behavioral approach to treatment follow:

1. Identify the rule, behavior, or emotion that is the focus of the intervention.

2. Ask the patient to express feelings about it and possible alternative solutions.

3. Agree on behavioral expectations.

4. Identify mutually defined natural and realistic consequences of noncompliance.

5. Explain in what ways consequences for rule violations will be applied and when.

6. Ask the patient for cooperation with protocol.

7. Use a written contingency contract, if needed.

8. Develop criteria for termination of the consequence.

9. Use agreed-on consequences immediately and without exception in a matter-of-fact but supportive way for infractions.

Following these steps often is difficult for the beginning practitioner who has established a relationship with the patient and wants to focus on a person's efforts as well as intervention outcomes. To apply a consequence when the patient slips seems unfair because the patient appears to be trying hard and reasons given for noncompliance are plausible. Remembering that the nature of the disease is built on excuses provides the basis for understanding that the patient must accept full responsibility for mistakes. It is critical to the treatment process that the patient acknowledge full accountability for the natural consequences of his or her behavior. Thus, all caregivers should remain firm in using agreed-on consequences for seemingly minor infractions that ordinarily would escape notice in other patients.

Developing Social Skills

Social skills development is a critical aspect of successful treatment. Skill development related to basic management of uncomfortable emotions (e.g., anger) and the ability to recognize the situations that provoke them occur in small group sessions. Identifying feelings of anger, fear, and vulnerability is frightening to people for whom emotions are not an acceptable part of life. Seeing others link behaviors to feelings as a norm of the group encourages the likelihood of similar effort on the patient's part. During this process, the patient learns to identify internal warning signs that could lead to potential relapse. Signs of increasing stress that require attention include

1. Increased desire for sugar or food binges
2. Inability to concentrate
3. Sleep disturbances
4. Mood swings
5. Increased stress

Patients are susceptible to the devitalizing effects of stress until they learn effective coping strategies to reduce it. A compassionate, goal-directed approach helps patients assume accountability for thoughts and feelings. Keeping patients on track and clarifying roles and expectations aid in building needed trust and self-confidence. Broad guidelines to help patients develop more effective coping patterns without drug use are presented in Box 26–10.

Another strategy in the early stages of supportive intervention is accomplished through cognitive restructuring (see Chapter 14). Cognitive restructuring involves becoming aware of faulty thinking patterns, validating perceptions and feelings with others, and practicing adaptive responses and behaviors. Restructured phrases remind the patient to "live and let live," to live "one day at a time," and that "easy does it," all slogans of AA. Living these platitudes provides a format for living in the present and taking responsibility for one's own needs as well as those of others. See Snapshot: Nursing Interventions Specific to Substance Disorder.

Providing Structural Supports

For those who need it, a drug-free therapeutic community in a hospital, day treatment setting, or halfway house offers a safe place where chemically dependent persons can develop skills needed in the larger community of life. The amount of help each person needs varies depending on their premorbid functioning, social support, and a host of other variables. Some patients can manage with little structure and a strong focus on developing adaptive skills in managing emotions. Others need a defined environmental or treatment structure for a period to resume responsibility and develop increased independence in conducting a life without drugs. With some, strict limit-setting, privilege systems, and an uncompromising program schedule provide the basic foundation for psychosocial skill development and gradual integration back into the community and family as a responsible, drug-free person.

Halfway houses are communal living situations that provide structure and support for those recovering addicts who lack family support and who cannot live on their own. Each halfway house has its own set of rules and expectations for those living in the house, with

regular group meetings to discuss relevant issues. Housed in the community, the recovering patient can attend school or work during the day and return to a supportive environment each evening for meals and emotional sustenance. Usually, the stay ranges from 1 to 4 months. Halfway houses provide an effective transitional bridge from the therapeutic inpatient community to the outside community, especially when coupled with outpatient treatment.

Aftercare

Patterns leading to substance use disorders are hard to erase, and recovering from a substance use disorder involves more than simply abstinence. Although it is easier for the patient in a detoxification program to feel confident about resisting the temptation to use drugs as a coping mechanism, this can lead to a false sense of confidence. Stresses are reduced, and the patient has a structure to his or her daily routine. The resolve may be there, but, once discharged, the stresses return and the old companions are available. Faulty thinking patterns

---

Box 26–10 ■ ■ ■ ■ ■

Guidelines to Help Patients Develop More Effective Social Patterns Without Drug Use or Alcohol

Phase I: Self-Diagnosis

Identifying problem situations
Identifying feelings associated with need for drugs
Linking feelings with problem situations

Phase II: Self-Awareness

Identifying fears and vulnerabilities
Linking behaviors and feelings
Identifying behaviors needing change
Developing insight into impact of behaviors on self and others

Phase III: Self-Change

Identifying alternative constructive changes
Expressing feelings and needs to others
Establishing realistic daily goals and meeting them
Making amends when appropriate
Managing difficult emotions productively
Anticipating difficult situations

Phase IV: Integrating Gains

Developing a written prevention plan
Identifying and contacting outside resource supports

Nursing Interventions Specific to Substance Disorder

What do you need to do to develop a relationship with a patient suffering with a substance abuse disorder?

- Approach the patient with warmth, quiet demeanor, and acceptance.
- Be honest, empathetic, and compassionate. Don't feed into the patient's denial about drug use.
- Be aware of manipulative behaviors.
- Set appropriate limits on manipulative behavior.
- Address the patient by his or her preferred name (don't assume it is okay to use the patient's first name until you ask the patient's preference); talk with the patient and listen carefully to what the patient shares.
- Encourage the patient that healing and recovery are possible.
- Encourage the patient to identify and discuss feelings.
- Encourage the patient to identify and discuss people, places, and situations that prompt drug use.
- Remain matter-of-fact and nonjudgmental in approach.

What do you need to assess concerning the patient's health status?

- Suicidal risk or self-destructive thoughts
- Affective responses, including anger, depression and anxiety. Use standardized instruments.
- Assess substance abuse with CAGE or MAST.
- Physiological responses, including gastrointestinal disturbances; appetite changes; sexual disturbances; sleep disturbances; weight changes.
- Cognitive responses, including confusion; slowed thinking; indecisiveness; problems with concentration; self-blame; pessimism
- Behavioral responses, including denial, blackouts; isolation and withdrawal; crying; agitation; alcoholism; drug addiction; slowed activity; poor personal hygiene; occupational difficulties; interpersonal difficulties; problems with the legal system
- Vital signs
- Weight, especially if the patient is experiencing changes in appetite
- Response to and compliance with medication regimen and reasons behind noncompliance; delayed effectiveness of drug

- Degree of social support
- Knowledge level; ability and readiness to learn
- Concurrent medical conditions
- Readiness to change lifestyle
- Readiness to use community resources

What do you need to teach the patient and/or the patient's caregiver?

- Medication issues; reason for taking; side effects and how to deal with them; untoward effects; warnings; importance of adhering to medication schedule
- Disease process; causes of substance abuse disorder; course of disease; treatment
- Withdrawal process—what to expect
- Nutrition issues
- Emergency measures
- Importance of social support and strategies to obtain it; importance of changing social support if that support promotes drug usage
- Maintaining safety
- Lifestyle and compliance issues, such as benefits of exercise and stress management
- Importance of emotional support
- Importance of achieving spiritual well-being
- Importance of group support for continued healing, that is, Alcoholics Anonymous (AA), Narcotics Anonymous (NA)

What skills will you want the patient and/or caregiver to demonstrate?

- Ability to enter into a no-harm contract and remain safe
- Ability to follow medication and treatment plan
- Ability to use thought-stopping techniques and other cognitive strategies to deal with situations, thoughts, and feelings that are associated with drug use
- Ability to identify and express feelings
- Coping skills
- Relaxation techniques

What other health professionals might need to be a part of this plan of care?

- Physician—psychiatrist and/or primary care physician—who is usually in charge of the overall treatment plan including medication management
- Social worker—assists with access to community supports, such as AA, NA, etc; insurance issues; access to entitlements; connection with community-based treatments

of relying on the drug rather than other people, of not asking for help, and of not sharing important feelings are well ingrained. Without ongoing external support and structure, the patient's coping mechanisms may be too fragile to withstand the chronic daily stresses that occur in everyone's life, particularly when drug availability presents itself as an easy out. Thus, ongoing aftercare is an essential part of the rehabilitative recovery process in the treatment of substance use disorders.

Aftercare takes a variety of forms. It often includes a structured plan for relapse prevention, active participation in continuing treatment and self-help groups, and access to the original professional treatment center as needed. Education and support are provided in equal proportion. Patients need to understand that the pathological physiology developed in their systems with chronic drug use will persist throughout their lifetime. This means they cannot use drugs again. If they do, the drug effects are reactivated as if they had never stopped taking drugs. Staying off drugs when this has been a way of life requires intense effort one day at a time, and for some, the craving will never disappear completely. See What Society Needs to Know: Alcoholism, Cocaine Addiction, and Heroin Addiction.

Developing Realistic Community Supports

For many patients, significant changes in their external world are needed because it is not unusual for some to have entered treatment with the loss or threat of loss of employment as the primary motivating factor. Returning to the workplace is frightening as well as a benchmark of recovery that can lead to a different and balanced sense of identity. Counseling and role playing related to explaining their recovery process, knowing how to respond to the discomfort of others who do not know how to react to them, and direction in handling the need to prove themselves in the workplace are practical interventions that should be taught to patients before they return to the workplace. Unfortunately, many times these issues do not receive the attention they should with the recovering patient.

Many businesses have state or federal Employee Assistance Programs and vocational rehabilitation for those who have difficulty returning to the work force. Helping the patient seek another career when the original one is not conducive to recovery or is no longer available is also an important aspect of the recovery plan.

WHAT SOCIETY NEEDS TO KNOW

Alcoholism, Cocaine Addiction, and Heroin Addiction

What is alcoholism?

Alcoholism is a term that applies to end stage of the continuum of nonuse versus addiction to alcohol. Addiction implies complete loss of control and drinking in spite of alcohol-related problems that involve social and occupational functioning. Alcoholism usually develops over many years of heavy drinking when the patient experiences a physiological and psychological dependence. With physical dependence tolerance develops (drinking more and more to achieve the same effect) and withdrawal (increased heart rate and blood pressure, irritability, and possible seizures). Psychological dependence involves compulsive use and craving.

What is cocaine addiction?

Cocaine is a naturally occurring stimulant extracted from the leaf of the coca bush. Cocaine affects the central nervous system and changes the way a person thinks, feels, and behaves. Dependence on this drug develops very quickly. The initial high (lasting 15 to 30 minutes) is followed by a deep depression. This reinforces the addictive nature of cocaine. Long-term chronic users have violent temper outbursts, disturbed thinking, and paranoia. Effects on the heart can lead to cardiac failure and death.

What is heroin addiction?

Heroin is an illegal street drug; therefore, addiction to heroin usually entails some type of antisocial or criminal behaviors. Heroin intoxication is manifested by constricted pupils, decreased breathing, drowsiness, lowered blood pressure, and slurred speech. There is often an initial euphoria and impaired memory and judgment. Withdrawal from heroin is similar to a bad case of influenza and is not life-threatening. To recover from heroin addiction, methadone substitution is often used along with counseling and job training.

What does recovery from these three conditions entail?

Abstinence from the mood-altering chemical is usually necessary along with the continued, sustained support of a 12-step program. Certainly, there must be a desire to change behavior. In some instances such as with heroin addiction, a therapeutic community is necessary to maintain abstinence. At one time it was believed that a person had to "hit bottom" to recover. Today, with the help of professionals, interventions for each of these addictions can occur at an earlier point in the progression of the illness.

Vocational and educational counseling, legal counseling, marital counseling, and development of realistic support systems in the community require a collaborative interdisciplinary approach to be successful.

Referral to Self-Help Groups

Referral to self-help groups in the community may be an important element of the rehabilitative process, particularly in a resource-driven health care system that no longer pays for the ongoing treatment many patients need. Groups such as AA, Cocaine Anonymous, and Narcotics Anonymous use a 12-step program to help those afflicted with substance use disorders develop a different lifestyle. The recovering addict typically is introduced to the group as a mandatory part of the treatment plan, or he or she goes because someone else thinks it is a good idea. Hearing the facts from those who have been there and who are willingly making the commitment to achieve a drug-free lifestyle is a particularly effective part of the chemically dependent person's education.

AA is the prototype for all support groups dedicated to the treatment of substance use disorders. It consists of "a fellowship of men and women who share their experience, strength and hope with each other that they may solve their common problem and help others to recover from alcoholism. The only requirement for membership is a desire to stop drinking" (AA, 1955, p. 564). Led by fellow alcoholics, the AA organization provides formal meetings and informal support to those alcoholics who wish to become and remain sober. There are both open and closed meetings. Open meetings generally have a few designated speakers who tell the group about how AA has benefitted them in their recovery process. In addition to these larger speaker meetings, there are smaller closed-group meetings with opportunities to discuss more personal issues with others and step meetings for more complete discussion of ways to meet the 12 steps needed for recovery. Groups for special needs (e.g., gays, women, minorities, professionals) are available in most larger urban communities. AA also provides an important informal network of support to those in need through its sponsorship component. Each new member who desires it is paired in a one-to-one relationship with a person who has been sober for some time. This person usually is of the same sex to forestall development of difficult intimate relationships. The sponsor is always available to the new member by telephone for encouragement, for clarification, and as a sounding board, particularly during the early stages of recovery. Vulnerable periods are the 1st month and after the first anniversary. Milestones are marked publically in the meeting with a token, speech, and sometimes refreshments. See What Patients and Families Need to Know: 12-Step Programs.

The effectiveness of the 12-step program and its influence in reducing the incidence of recidivism with substance use disorders are indisputable, as described in Case Example 26–2.

■ CASE EXAMPLE 26–2
■ Dana's Story, Part 2

Narcotics Anonymous really changed my life. I got into it in the following way. I was visiting my aunt in the hospital. My cousin was there, and we had partied together before. The subject of drugs came up, and she mentioned that she had quit and she did it through Narcotics Anonymous. Well, I thought that was great for her; she had finally gotten her life together; I was forgetting, of course, to look at my own life. She offered to take my sister and I to a meeting with her. My sister went, but I passed. A couple of weeks later, I decided to go, really, just out of curiosity. I didn't like my first meeting, I think, because I was so preoccupied with looking around to see if anyone was looking at me and just feeling very uncomfortable. It also wasn't exciting enough for me. I guess when you live in the fast lane long enough, sitting in a room with people and having everything that goes on be organized takes a little getting used to. I was real scared and couldn't wait to get out of there. I have no idea what made me do it, but I went to another meeting later that week. I felt more comfortable and met a lot of real good people, I guess because I wasn't in a race to get out the door. I started to go regularly and someone told me, "Just try it for 30 days and if you don't like it, the drugs aren't going anywhere." So that's what I did and I've been there ever since. That was 3 years ago.

I am now 21 years old and live in my own apartment that I share with a girl I met in the program. I'm taking risks, like moving out, buying a car, looking into college, and getting involved with different causes and movements I believe in. I'm doing things I wouldn't have done before, like sticking up for myself and not accepting unacceptable behavior. Narcotics Anonymous and the people in it taught me that I am someone, that I am pretty, and that I am important. They try to show you and to help you to live life on life's terms, which isn't always easy whether you use drugs or you don't. It wasn't hard for me to give up my old friends, because once I stopped getting high most of them really didn't want me around anyway. They told me in Narcotics Anonymous that if I missed my friends to just stick around and they would come back if they didn't die first. Now a lot of people I used to party with are with me in the rooms of Narcotics Anonymous. Narcotics Anonymous has definitely given me back respect for myself. They gave me back a chance at life and trying to be the best person I can be. ■

Evaluation

The evaluation criteria are directly linked to achievement of the patient outcomes identified earlier in the chapter. What the nurse should look for is evidence that the patient is taking steps to reduce risk factors for potential relapse. The recovering substance user should be able to verbalize and demonstrate lifestyle changes needed to achieve and maintain abstinence from psychoactive substances. Successful treatment results are seen in the patient's ability to cope with life situations in a

? WHAT PATIENTS AND FAMILIES NEED TO KNOW

12-Step Programs

What do you mean by a 12-step program?

A 12-step program is a fellowship of men and women who have a common problem (alcoholism, substance abuse, relationships, overeating, gambling, and so on). The only requirement for membership is the desire to stop a behavior that has become unmanageable. Twelve-step programs are not allied with any sect, denomination, political affiliation, religious institution, or organization. These programs will not endorse or oppose any causes and are completely based on voluntary membership and are totally self-supporting.

Where did 12-step programs originate?

In 1935 Bill W. and Dr. Bob founded the original 12-step support group for alcoholics. Shortly thereafter, Al-Anon was founded by Lois Wilson, the wife of Bill W. Since that time hundreds of 12-step support groups have begun that follow the model of Alcoholics Anonymous.

How are 12-step programs helpful?

Twelve-step programs provide an anonymous setting in which people with similar problems can share experience, strength, and hope. People who attend these meetings on a regular basis find a sense of community and are able to find acceptance and unconditional love and support. The 12 steps are "worked through" with the help of the members or a sponsor. The essence of the steps entails admitting that you have a problem, acknowledging that you are in need of a power greater than yourself to stop the behavior, admitting strengths and weaknesses, making amends to others you have offended as a result of the problem, and helping others through the same process. Twelve-step members do not actively solicit members but are always available when a potential member asks for help.

Isn't it necessary to have professional help When you have a substance abuse disorder?

To help an addicted person with the potentially harmful symptoms of withdrawal, medical attention is often necessary because death can be a complication of improperly managed withdrawal. In some cases in which there is a dual diagnosis (an addictive process and a mental illness) present, professional help is indicated. Otherwise, programs like Alcoholics Anonymous have helped millions of people worldwide.

---

realistic way without drug use. This person is able to acknowledge and work through difficult feelings and to seek support from people and God rather than drugs in times of distress. Specific examples of evaluation criteria are presented subsequently in the case study. Indicators of potential difficulty maintaining abstinence care include insomnia or hypersomnia, racing thoughts, increased irritability or agitation, social isolation, and withdrawal.

VULNERABLE POPULATIONS AND SUBSTANCE USE DISORDERS

Although substance use disorders cross all social and economic groups, certain populations are at higher risk for experiencing the disorder or present special needs associated with their substance use. For example, cultural differences in drinking patterns and whether or not the unfavorable behavioral effects of alcoholic behavior are tolerated by the society play a role (Helman, 1990). Ethnic cultures that support controlled drinking in moderation as a normal part of life while strongly disapproving of any forms of intoxication or deviant behavior associated with drinking are less likely to experience significant problems. Thus, Italians and Jews who incorporate moderate intake of alcohol into mealtimes and social-religious functions have significantly lower rates of alcoholism.

Extremes in attitudes about drinking seem to produce the negative drinking patterns likely to lead to alcoholism. In the Irish culture, there is no one dependable attitude toward drug consumption. Large quantities of alcohol consumption are encouraged at social functions, and yet alcohol consumption is strongly disapproved of as a regular part of life. The alcoholism rate among the Irish is higher than average. Other cultures that specifically condemn alcohol use on religious grounds—Mormons, certain Muslim cultures, and Baptists, for example—have a slightly higher than normal incidence of deviant drinking patterns.

Disadvantaged minority groups have a proportionately higher incidence of chemical dependency than the dominant culture for another social reason. They often become drug dealers because the instant money, lure of excitement, and comradery of seemingly self-made, confident individuals in control of life and the people around them are powerful seducers of the young and the poor living in substandard conditions with little promise of a better life. The power of such enhancements is hard to eradicate. Alcoholism is identified as one of the leading health problems in the African American ghetto community activated by informal structures of unemployment, availability of alcohol, peer pressure, and social norms that support drinking as an important part of life. Hispanics and Native Americans have similar issues of deprivation, availability, and social support of drug-taking behaviors that make them high risk for drug abuse. Among Native Americans, the second leading cause of death in young men is alcohol abuse, and it is estimated that "95% of American Indian families are affected either directly or indirectly by a family member's alcohol abuse" (U.S. Department of Health and Human Services, 1990, p. 39).

Women

Finnegan and Kandall (1992) estimated that women account for approximately 34% of those diagnosed with substance use disorders. Yet addiction in women is largely hidden because it carries an even greater stigma than for men. Social conditioning about the role of women, even in an era of women's liberation, does not allow for the same type of understanding accorded their male counterparts. Yet women typically experience symptoms of alcoholism at a faster rate than men do, and there is a stronger link between stress and development of symptoms (Quinby & Graham, 1993). Substance use disorders are often associated with secondary social problems for women, with a higher reported incidence of abuse, incest, and exploitation among women diagnosed as chemically dependent. Instead of turning to crimes like stealing to support their drug dependency, women are more likely to become prostitutes. This increases the risk of AIDS and other sexually transmitted diseases in this population.

Treatment issues for women also are more complicated because physicians tend to overlook substance use disorders as a primary diagnosis in women. They are more likely to treat women's signs and symptoms of alcoholism as secondary to their presenting psychological and medical symptoms or as reflecting self-medication for such symptoms. These women are more likely to be found in general mental health treatment centers being treated for a depressive disorder rather than in chemical dependency programs, where their substance use disorder could be addressed. Nurses can become strong advocates for these women, who frequently lack the judgment or skills to act in their own best interests.

Adolescents

Adolescence is a time of rapid transition of biological and psychological changes unparalleled in most other life stages. Adolescents are prone to explore different life experiences, among them experimentation with drugs. In fact, 47% of high school graduating seniors in the United States admitted to illicit drug use (Muramoto & Leshau, 1993).

For teenagers, the first drink or experiment with psychoactive drugs often signifies "risk-taking," doing what adults do. "Binge" drinking at parties and smoking pot with friends are tolerated without significant stigma attached. Peer pressure and a desire to appear successful with friends take precedence in activity choices without the reflective thinking that would look at the more adverse consequences of such risk-taking behavior.

Because drug abuse retards attainment of developmental milestones, the adolescent literally suffers from developmental arrest at the point that the chemical dependency begins. Thus, the 18-year-old adolescent who began drinking at age 12 years developmentally stopped maturing at age 12 years and frequently has the psychosocial skills of a beginning adolescent when chemical dependency is brought under control. The phenomenon of developmental arrest with psychoactive disorders is important in treatment and discharge planning. Otherwise, the recovering adolescent is thrown into social situations that chronologically he or she should be able to handle without much guidance but developmentally cannot without assistance and support. Dana's story describes a typical chain of events associated with substance use disorders in adolescence—a typical trajectory from simple recreational use to a full-blown addiction marked with denial, rationalization, and projection. Dana did not see that she was in trouble until it was almost too late. Dana was lucky because her story has a happy ending. She found Narcotics Anonymous and through this group eventually found herself.

Some adolescents are more at risk than others for the development of a substance use disorder. A number of studies have identified difficult family situations, interpersonal skill deficits, early delinquent behaviors, and exposure to psychoactive drugs as strong predictors of adolescent chemical dependency. Family discord in the form of bitter custody battles, inconsistent rules, splitting of child-rearing approaches that leave the child in the middle, and lack of supervision contribute to a higher incidence of substance abuse disorders in these adolescents. Adolescents introduced to drug use by their parents or significant others in the home are particularly at risk for the development of chemical dependency. So are adolescents who do not fit into their peer group because of differences in cognitive, attentional, behavioral control, or peer relations skills. Social and intellectual differences become more apparent during pubescence and with the added stress of moving from junior high to high school. The combination of easy availability of drugs and a need to belong is particularly dangerous for insecure adolescents. In many instances, boredom and low self-esteem heighten the prevalence of drug abuse among disenchanted adolescents. When life does not have much to offer and psychoactive drugs can transform that reality into a more pleasant one, drug-taking behaviors become commonplace. Other social factors that influence drug-taking behaviors revolve around the lifestyles of high school dropouts and unemployed youth who have easy access to drugs, higher levels of stress, and lower conformity to social norms. Chemical dependency in the adolescent progresses more rapidly than in adults. An adolescent can become an alcoholic with 6 months of heavy drinking.

The Unborn

All psychoactive drugs cross the placenta, and most are capable of causing serious teratogenic effects in the fetus. In the United States, it is estimated that 2.6 million infants born each year will have had significant exposure to alcohol through maternal abuse, and approximately 1 in 100 will demonstrate clinical teratogenic effects as a result (Finnegan & Kandall, 1992). Heavy drinking increases the risk of miscarriage and stillbirth. Excessive use of alcohol during pregnancy can lead to the development of fetal alcohol syndrome (FAS) in the newborn. Alcohol passes through the placenta from the mother to the fetus, and the amount of alcohol consumed by the fetus equals that consumed by the mother. Approximately 5000 infants are born each year with FAS (Streissguth, 1986, 1997).

The incidence of FAS is higher among specific ethnic groups. For example, it occurs 33 times more often in Native Americans and 6.7 times more often in the African American population than in whites. The probability of having a second FAS child increases for women who have one FAS infant.

FAS presents with a distinctive pattern of physical and mental defects. It is one of the three most prevalent causes of mental retardation in the newborn (Johnson, 1990). Infants born with this condition suffer gross structural malformations. They appear retarded with abnormally small heads and a higher incidence of microcephaly. There is a distinctive narrowing of the eyes and low nasal bridge. Almost half of the infants born with FAS have a heart defect, and many suffer defects in their joints and are of low birth weight. There is a correlation of severe mental deficiency in infants with noticeable physical defects. Such children are prone to behavioral problems and characteristically demonstrate short attention spans, nervousness, and poor coordination (Finnegan & Kandall, 1992). There is no treatment for FAS.

Cocaine dependency in the mother can cause serious problems in pregnancy. Women who consistently use cocaine are at risk for miscarriage and premature birth. There is evidence that regular cocaine use contributes to the development of abruptio placentae, a condition in which the placenta breaks away from the uterine wall, causing excessive bleeding and possible termination of the pregnancy. Newborns subjected to the cocaine dependence of their mothers demonstrate withdrawal symptoms after birth. Frequently, they are jittery, irritable, and difficult to comfort (Finnegan & Kandall, 1992). Because of their drug-related personality characteristics and the drug dependency of the mother, children of cocaine addicts are at increased risk for child abuse.

Opiates are appetite suppressants, often compromising the birth weight of the infant as well as the mother. Prenatal sedative and opiate dependence can endanger the birth process and create serious problems for the newborn. Passive heroin addiction can be fatal for the newborn cut off from the maternal supply at birth when the umbilical cord is cut. Withdrawal symptoms include high-pitched cry, CNS excitability, poorly coordinated sucking-swallowing reflex, muscle hypertonicity, and hyperirritability. If the mother has an opiate dependency, there is a 60% chance that the infant will suffer withdrawal symptoms once the cord is cut.

The problem of passive drug addiction in the newborn is further complicated by associated sociomedical complications (e.g., polydrug use, poor nutrition, heavy smoking, and inadequate prenatal care). Hospitals are experiencing a marked increase in the number of seriously ill and "boarder" infants associated with maternal substance abuse. The expanding population of passively addicted boarder infants, abandoned by mothers incapable of caring for them, creates a unique health care challenge and suggests the need for nontraditional models of intervention and innovative ways to engage and treat substance-abusing adolescents in the community. Allowing grandparents to assume custody for the infant can be a faulty solution because problems with drug abuse and dysfunctional family patterns often are prevalent in the grandparents' household as well. Even after successful detoxification, children exposed to psychoactive drugs in utero experience a higher incidence of developmental delays and significant behavioral problems in childhood and adolescence. Table 26–6 summarizes the teratogenic effects of psychoactive substances.

The Elderly

Substance use disorders in the elderly have been called the "hidden addiction" because one does not usually think of the elderly as having drug problems. The problem becomes increasingly more prevalent as more people are living longer. Psychoactive drug use in the elderly is most likely to involve alcohol or benzodiazepines prescribed for mild tension or sleeplessness. In general, psychoactive drugs, as are most other drugs administered to the elderly, are metabolized much more slowly than they are at an earlier stage of life, and individual responsiveness to drug actions is more variable in the elderly than at any other stage of life. As a result, the effects of the drug occur with greater intensity and last longer. Prescriptions to relieve sleeping problems that are actually caused by undiagnosed depression in the elderly may actually intensify rather than treat the underlying problem.

Treatment of the elderly follows therapeutic approaches similar to those used for other chemically dependent populations with regard to detoxification, family interventions, and the need for long-term follow-up. Additionally, lack of family and occupational supports, lost as the person ages, may require a greater emphasis on social, financial, and medical support services in the community as part of the treatment plan.

People With Acquired Immunodeficiency Syndrome

IV drug abuse has played a major role in the spread of the AIDS virus; IV drug abusers form the second largest primary risk group for development of the disorder. Secondary victims include newborn infants and nonabusing heterosexual or homosexual partners. According to the Centers for Disease Control and Prevention

T A B L E 2 6 – 6 Teratogenic Effects of Psychoactive Substances

PSYCHOACTIVE SUBSTANCE	MEDICAL USE	TERATOGENIC EFFECTS
Alcohol	Formerly used to stop contractions in premature labor	Weak to strong teratogenic effects FAS Low birth weight Central nervous system dysfunction Learning disabilities Decreased maternal folate levels Retardation
Benzodiazepines	Short-term treatment of alcohol withdrawal; anxiolytic	Transient fetal tachycardia Neonatal withdrawal effects First trimester—cleft palate
Barbiturates	Seizure control in epilepsy	May decrease fetal movement resulting in malpresentation during birth Anomalies similar to FAS Neonatal toxicity: poor sucking reflex and hypotonia Neonatal withdrawal: restlessness, irritability, hyperreflexes, and disturbed sleep patterns
Cocaine	None	Constricts placental and umbilical blood vessels Fetal hypoxia Intrauterine growth retardation Premature labor Neonatal withdrawal: irritability, hypertonicity, and tremor Increased incidence of childhood behavior problems, ADD
Opiates	None	Spontaneous miscarriage Higher incidence of stillbirth Intrauterine growth retardation Higher incidence of toxemia Low birth weight Neonatal withdrawal: impaired sucking, hyperactivity, hypertonicity, vomiting, sleep disturbances, diarrhea, and tremors Childhood behavior problems

ADD, attention-deficit disorder; FAS, fetal alcohol syndrome.

(CDC), more than 25% of AIDS cases are attributable to IV drug abuse. Not counted in this assessment are homosexuals who also are IV drug abusers. The CDC classifies these individuals only as homosexuals. IV drug use accounts for 52% of the AIDS cases in women (Amsel, 1990). Further complicating the picture is the long prodromal period possible between time of initial exposure to HIV and development of diagnosable symptoms. At special risk are minority populations, such as Puerto Ricans and African Americans, who have a proportionately higher incidence of AIDS in contrast with their numbers in the general population.

Chronic substance use suppresses the immune system. In particular, alcohol, amphetamines, and marijuana actively compromise the effectiveness of the body's immune system. Drug abuse contributes to the spread of AIDS in two ways:

1. Direct, through IV drug use with contaminated needles among drug abusers who share needles
2. Indirect, through "survival sex" in which teenagers and adults prostitute themselves to obtain the money to buy drugs (their anonymous and often multiple sex partners are frequently infected with the AIDS virus)

Prevention programs need to address high-risk sexual behaviors as well as drug abuse in a combined format because they are closely interrelated in women of childbearing age (Box 26–11).

AIDS in children of drug-abusing parents is a serious and growing threat to society. More than 50% of the infants born to women who test seropositive have the virus, and there is no known way to prevent maternal transmission to the fetus. Indirect or direct IV drug abuse is a major factor in the transmission of this fatal disease.

What do you think? What is your responsibility when you see a pregnant woman drinking an alcoholic beverage or smoking?

➤ *Check Your Reading*
7. What are the implications for women of having a substance use disorder?
8. What role does substance use play in pregnancy and neonatal care?
9. What are important considerations in the nursing care of adolescents with substance use disorders?

Box 26-11 ■ ■ ■ ■ ■
What Women Should Know About Pregnancy and AIDS

- 73% of AIDS cases are attributed to maternal transmission during pregnancy.
- A seropositive woman does not need to be sick with AIDS to transmit it to her fetus.
- 50% to 60% of children born to seropositive mothers will be infected.
- There is no way to prevent the fetus from becoming infected if the mother is infected.

Adapted from Mondanaro J. (1990). Community-based AIDS prevention interventions: Special issues of women intravenous drug users. In U.S. Department of Health and Human Services (Ed.), *AIDS and intravenous drug use: Future directions for community-based prevention research* (NIDA Research Monograph, p. 7893). Washington, DC: U.S. Department of Public Health and Human Services.

SUBSTANCE USE DISORDERS AND THE FAMILY

Chemical Dependency Is a Family Disease

The nature of the substance abuse disorders creates a psychodynamic force in the family leading to adaptive properties that influence how the family system functions. No one in close contact with a substance-dependent person can escape being touched by the disease process. Dependency on drugs or alcohol takes first priority, which means that little, if any, emotional support is available to family members. In response, family members develop defensive relating styles, conflict management, and rules in order to handle behaviors associated with the substance use disorder. The spouse generally is the most keenly aware of the pathological substance use pattern and its implications for family functioning. One woman described it as having her husband's mistress living in the house, so great was her husband's attachment to the bottle. His frequent visits to the basement to drink and returning with a lie to cover the time spent struck her as analogous to the way unfaithful spouses relate to their partners when they are involved in external relationships. Yet, although these behaviors would never be tolerated with an actual mistress, frequently they are endured with someone having equally heavy involvement with a psychoactive substance.

Anxiety, anger, and resentment are powerful emotions experienced by most family members coping with another family member abusing drugs. Anxiety in the spouse and children about excessive drug use in a family member creates its own set of problems. Each feels guilty, angry, and responsible for each other's response and has feelings associated with the identified patient. For example, the children may blame the mother for allowing their father to drink and abuse the family. The wife may resent the inability of the husband to be a good father. A child may feel that he or she is responsible for his or her father's unpredictable moods while he is under the influence of the psychoactive substance. In this family system, direct anger and grief are not expressed because of the changes in patterns of relating that occur due to the substance abusing member's behavior. Children often feel resentment at having to take the role of the parent when the parent cannot assume this role because of the disorder. The focus on the drug-taking behavior and patterns becomes as obsessive for the family as it does for the drug abuser. Although the reasons are different, the outcome is the same. There is little time for anything other than the incessant call of the psychoactive substance.

Without treatment, family members usually are unable to disengage themselves from the focus on the patient's drug-abusing behavior. Like the identified patient, they too give up their self-respect, often their possessions, and everything that is important to them in response to the addiction. In every story of a substance use disorder, there is a parallel family story with recurring themes of the family members' hopelessness and anger about the patient's unpredictability in emotional response, the lack of sensitivity the person under the influence of psychoactive drugs displays, and the sheer terror that those closest to the chemically dependent person experience, sometimes on a daily basis. Control is a constant underlying dynamic. The chemical-dependent substance user lacks control over the psychoactive agent; the family members seek to control the use of the drug. For this reason, the family members' behavior is often referred to as codependent.

Codependency

The term *codependency* was developed in the 1970s to describe a predictable pattern of behaviors in family members characterized by overfunctioning, lack of objectivity, powerlessness, and need to control another's behavior. Those closest to the patient try in every way possible to orchestrate a relationship that is meaningful. It is often experienced as a hopeless task accompanied by hypervigilance and feelings of intense loneliness, self-doubt, resentment, and anger, which preoccupy the individual with codependent behavior and influence his or her behavior. There is a wish to retaliate, generally with the knowledge that it will have no effect. According to Johnson (1990), the self-destructive patterns presented by the individual with substance use that are most likely to stimulate a strong desire to retaliate in the individual with codependent behavior include the following (p. 203):

1. Breaking family commitments, both major and minor
2. Spending more money than planned
3. Driving while intoxicated and getting arrested
4. Making inappropriate statements to friends, family, and coworkers
5. Arguing, fighting, and other antisocial actions

Although the family confronts the patient in anger about these breaches of contract or expectations, typically the confrontation fails to achieve its desired purpose of changing the addict's behavior. Reflex confrontations stemming from anger and resentment over behaviors suffered while under the influence increase the individual's painful feelings of shame and guilt, stimulating further substance use.

The need to rescue others, to make everything okay, and to not stir the waters to avoid stimulating further drug use and the wish to construct a world in which everything is predictable, and thus controllable, become defining characteristics for codependency. Ironically, these behavior patterns encourage the identified patient to continue the substance use by permitting this person to escape the consequences of his or her behavior and in many cases, by providing a legitimate rationale for downplaying the seriousness of the problem.

Enabling behaviors refer to actions designed to protect the chemically dependent person from the consequences of the dependency either by covering for the person or by denying his or her personal uneasiness about the addictive behavior. The behaviors represent an unspoken pact between the patient and family member to protect the patient from being embarrassed outside of the home by his or her behaviors related to substance use. This conspiracy of silence stems from the family's insecurity about themselves and a desire to protect their reputation in the community. It is not uncommon for family members to feel that if only they were different—more loving, a different personality, less angry, or more understanding—the chemically dependent person would stop using drugs. Guilt about their inability to be whatever it is they think they should be so that the person would not use drugs and shame about what is occurring within the family compel them to assume responsibility for controlling a living environment that is not controllable. The individual who is using enabling behavior patterns to cope unconsciously colludes with the family member who is abusing substances by allowing him or her to avoid taking responsibility for his or her actions. This happens because the substance-abusing individual is shielded from suffering the painful consequences of the dependency needed for recovery.

Recovery

In many instances, family members feel that unless the person with the substance use disorder seeks treatment, there is little purpose in engaging in treatment themselves. This is not true. Without external support, the family becomes so enmeshed in trying to control the dependency or in reacting reflexively to the behaviors of the person under the influence that they unconsciously enable the individual to deny the dependency.

The importance of a family focus should not be underestimated; the constructive support of the immediate family is identified as the single most important variable in preventing relapse. Often, affected family members enter treatment with the idea that the chemically dependent person is the problem in the family dynamics, and they see their role, as being of help to this person. Effective treatment of codependency requires the family members to understand their part in the family dynamics that revolve around the substance abuse. The primary goal in initial encounters with the family is to establish a therapeutic tone and to broaden the focus from the identified patient to include the entire family, particularly those who have power and influence.

Expected outcomes of codependency treatment are the reestablishment of personal boundaries, development of a strong sense of personal identity, and, in many instances, the restructuring of a life without a primary focus on substance use. Recovery from codependency begins when other family members begin to reorganize their lives in spite of, and not around, the problem. Group formats benefit the treatment of codependency, and there are many community resources (Al-Anon, Ephesians) available to help family members gain the proper perspective and knowledge of substance use disorders. These groups offer a safe place to explore feelings. People with similar issues guide and support skill development, identification and reinforcement of personal boundaries, and achievement of the balance needed for a satisfying, productive life. They assist each other in developing a healthy self-identity that does not ignore the existence of their life problem but rather helps them achieve the emotional detachment needed so that the responsibility for the substance abuse is returned to the chemically dependent family member.

Communication patterns in families coping with substance use disorders generally are negative and related to a number of family issues: (1) responsibility, (2) control, (3) adequacy, (4) self-esteem, and (5) trust. In many families, the person diagnosed with the disorder actually performs an important function by maintaining family homeostasis. Without the chemical dependence, family communication might be nonexistent. Discussions about the substance user's behavior form the content for most interactions. Abstinence frees the mind to engage in active dialogue with significant others, and it liberates the family from its constant vigilance over of the substance use. Often, however, there is nothing to take its place. This is where a problem arises.

For a significant period of time, the patient and the other family members have maintained a psychological distance from each other's worlds, and now each needs to reestablish emotional connections. Each individual needs to explore what is personally meaningful and to contribute to the development of a new family built around family strengths rather than a psychoactive substance. However, usually there is much anger and resentment, which need a safe repository. A safe repository could be in the form of a safe person, such as a therapist, who allows the person to vent his or her feelings and frustrations. Or it could take the form of physical activities, such as exercise, which allow the person to let off the physical manifestation of the anger. Moreover, the family dream of a meaningful family life will take time to cultivate. For those who have lived anesthetized with a psychoactive substance for a significant period of time, there has been little exposure to the types of values, skills, and attitudes required to live a meaningful life. Communication becomes the means by which families rediscover the possibilities of a life without psychoactive drugs. Once the psychoactive substance is no longer the center of discussion, families need help developing functional communication patterns.

Psychological treatment consists of helping families identify and correct dysfunctional communication patterns. Interventions build on family members' strengths, and each family member is expected to assume responsibility for modifying his or her part in the dysfunctional process. Family treatment often includes multifamily group support. Not all families enthusiastically embrace the idea of multifamily groups. The nurse can be an important resource in giving families permission to just listen until they feel comfortable participating. This simple intervention often is all that is needed to keep a family participating. The common bond of chemical dependence in the family serves as a powerful source of identification as families support each other's efforts to express powerful feelings and to develop effective coping strategies. Seeing oneself in relation to peers with similar experiences and hearing how others perceive them can destroy the tendency to see everything in one's own family as all good or all bad. The group format allows family members to test their ideas with other parents, spouses, and siblings rather than comparing themselves only in relation to their own family.

Treatment for Children

Children of chemically dependent parents experience long-lasting effects of substance use disorders even if they never ingest a psychoactive substance. Although they directly experience the effects of the disorder in the form of abuse or neglect, these children have an added disadvantage. They often have difficulty establishing normal behavioral standards for themselves because they lack the necessary role models and life experiences that could guide them appropriately. Normal emotions that should alert the child to danger, pleasure, and basic needs are overshadowed by the need to cope with the erratic and irrational behaviors of one or both parents. Instead, the child learns to suppress normal emotions and to control his or her inner conflict and chaos by pleasing others, staying out of the way, and repressing legitimate feelings of grief, anger, and resentment. These children learn mistrust, shame, and guilt instead of trust and self-confidence. The fear and emotional trauma of living in a dysfunctional home also manifests in childhood nightmares, perfectionism, behavioral problems, poor school performance, and passive withdrawal from life.

Children of drug-dependent parents frequently over-function or act out their distress. Having limited life experience, the child imagines that he or she is in some way responsible for the development of the chemical dependency. The child incorporates this information into his or her memory. There it lies dormant but is seen as an underlying dynamic as the child tries to please everyone, and it erupts from time to time in the form of panic attacks and depressive symptoms. What logically follows for the child from this faulty line of reasoning is that, if one creates the problem, it also is within one's power to fix the problem. Often, the youngster takes on responsibilities that should not be expected of a child to counteract feelings of helplessness. The child literally does not have a childhood experience, which further sabotages normal growth and development.

Many of these children doubt their own reality and do not realize until they leave home that their family life is different in critical and damaging ways. They avoid bringing other children home either because of the condition of the house, the unpredictability of the chemically dependent parent, or the wishes of the codependent parent to keep things at an even keel so as to avoid the possibility of stimulating drinking or abusive behavior. Al-Ateen and Al-Atot groups provide ongoing support for children and help reduce the feelings of isolation and family sabotage that children experience on a daily basis in chemically dependent families. School counselors are an invaluable resource for children coping with chemical dependency and dysfunctional behaviors in their families. As a nurse, you need to become acquainted with the professional services and community support opportunities available for children living in dysfunctional, chemically dependent households. The approach to the child needs to be proactive because the child's cry for help often is weak and indirect. Often, school or behavioral problems are the first indicator of severe dysfunction within the family. The child frequently does not request assistance. However, if it is offered, usually these children are highly receptive to understanding intervention.

Treatment for Adult Children of Alcoholics

Growing up in a dysfunctional home leads to significant problems in adulthood. So much emotional energy goes into hiding the family secret of addiction, helping maintain the false sense of normalcy, and squelching legitimate feelings that adult children of alcoholics (ACOAs) may have no memory of significant portions of their childhood. ACOAs are more likely to become substance abusers themselves, because this is the only life pattern they know, or to marry a chemically dependent person.

Often, they have trouble recognizing and expressing feelings in constructive ways. In varying degrees, they experience emotional overreactions or underreactions to stressful and emotional situations. It is hard for many ACOAs to trust their own reality or to consider their opinions valid. Growing up with a consistent pattern of unpredictable human responses keeps the developing child off balance, storing up memories that are reactivated in uncertain stressful situations as an adult. There is no solid base to draw from, with the result that previous maladaptive coping styles are carried into adult life, usually with limited awareness of how they restrict the development of intimacy and the normal give and take required of mature, adult relationships. For some, these attitudes are well ingrained because they have been passed on in the form of negative perspectives and feelings for generations. The repetitive intergenerational transmission of addictive behaviors and ways of responding to them occur without anyone's deliberate intent or awareness.

Adult children of alcoholics frequently complain that they feel as though they do not belong. Sudden outbursts or overreactions are remnants of a previous inability to make sense of a chaotic childhood superimposed on a current life event. Unfortunately, the spouse, coworker, or boss does not know the script and interprets the behavior negatively. Those who have grown up in a chemically dependent household often need to reconstruct new and different developmental memories that incorporate the reality of the dysfunctional family experiences, while developing a realistic and loving sense of self in relation to others. Usually, support or insight therapy is needed to achieve these objectives. Treatment focuses on identifying feelings and accepting their legitimate role in one's life, releasing anger, and separating feelings associated with past relationships from present relational circumstances. Guidelines for empowering adult children of alcoholics to try out new behaviors are presented in Box 26-12. Self-help groups designed to meet the needs of adult children of alcoholics are available in most communities.

Box 26–12 ■ ■ ■ ■ ■
Guidelines for Empowering Adult Children of Alcoholics

Analyze the appropriateness of an emotional response.

Feel the feelings.

Create your own reality as one that is supportive and nurturing.

Release shame-bound feelings by

Talking about them with a supportive person.

Claiming your emotions as your own and no longer governed by your parents' rules.

Cognitive restructuring.

Use positive self-talk to reestablish perspective.

Take actions that support your positive self-analysis.

Seek support from significant others to reinforce the new behaviors.

NURSING PROCESS APPLICATION

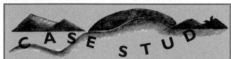

The Miller Family

As a case manager in the trauma unit of a local emergency department you are the nurse assigned to Sam Miller, a 49-year-old business executive, who sustained a fractured femur when he was in a motor vehicle accident yesterday. The emergency department report indicates that, at the time of the accident, Sam's blood alcohol level was 0.15 dl.

When you enter the room, you find his wife standing at the bedside. She communicates with you in short, terse sentences and appears to be unaffected by her husband's serious condition. While gathering a family history, you find that Sam has been drinking heavily (a 12-pack of beer or 2 L of wine daily for the past 10 to 15 years). He is currently on probation for driving under the influence. Susan, his wife of 28 years, tells you that she is aware that Sam drinks a lot but hopes that someday he will come to his senses and stop drinking. She tells you that he drinks daily and gets really drunk at least once or twice a week. Sam tells you, "My wife is exaggerating the amount I drink and I can quit drinking any time I want to; I have just been under a lot of pressure." You notice considerable tension between the couple. You find out that Sam and Susan have three children: Sarah, age 18 years; Trisha, age 16 years; and Judd, age 13 years. Trisha and Judd seem worried about their father, but Sarah tells you she is "fed up." She says, "I think my father is an alcoholic and I am tired of it; I wish he would stop drinking." You find that Sarah is an honor student, whereas Trisha and Judd are both experiencing difficulties in school. Trisha tells you she wants to run away.

ASSESSMENT	Assessment data are as follows:

Assessment data are as follows:
- Blood alcohol level on admission 0.15 dl (legal for intoxication in most states)
- Automobile accident related to excessive alcohol ingestion

- Minimization of alcoholism symptoms by patient and wife
- Tension and stress between couple
- Varying levels of denial among family members regarding father's drinking
- Inadequate understanding or knowledge of alcoholism among family members
- Verbalizations of anger and resentment by Sarah: "I'm fed up . . . I wish my father would stop drinking"
- School problems apparent for Trisha and Judd
- Trisha wants to run away
- Family members unable to relate to each other for mutual support, love, and affection

DSM-IV Diagnosis:	Alcohol Dependence (husband), Adjustment Disorder with Depressed Mood (wife)
Nursing Diagnosis:	Family Processes, Alcoholism, Altered related to long-term patterns of denial, rationalization, and enabling behaviors evidenced by behavioral problems in the children, marital discord, lack of knowledge of the disease process of alcohol dependence, and inability to relate to each other for mutual support, love, affection, and spiritual needs.

OUTCOME IDENTIFICATION, PLANNING, AND IMPLEMENTATION

Expected Outcome 1: By _____ the family will acknowledge the dysfunctional behavioral dynamics present in the family system.

Short-Term Goals	Nursing Interventions	Rationales
By _____ family members will admit the alcohol abuse problem of the patient to a trusted friend (minister, nurse, or member of a self-help group).	1. Assess the family members for factors that would keep them from accepting help, such as shame, guilt, or excessive denial. 2. Provide an opportunity for the family members to discuss their experiences of living with the disabling effects of alcoholism. 3. Listen; be genuine, and nonjudgmental. 4. Educate the family about the effects of alcoholism on the family.	1. Helps determine the best approach and types of referrals. 2–3. Assists you in joining with the family and validates their experience. 4. Encourages family members to have a realistic appraisal of their family dynamics and dispel myths and guilt.
By _____ the family members will strongly encourage the patient to enter a treatment facility.	1. Provide the family with a list of services and treatment options available. 2. Outline the benefits of a professional intervention or confrontation. 3. Assess the family's potential strength or desire to participate in an intervention or confrontation.	1–2. Ensures the family's continued support and helps them from returning to their previous state of denial. 3. To benefit the greatest from an intervention, family members need to be in agreement on the necessity for it.
By_____ the family members will recognize when their behavior protects (enables) the patient.	1. Define the term *enabling* for family members. 2. Encourage each family member to delineate at least one time when they enabled the patient. 3. Offer family members alternative choices to enabling and have them practice what they will say and do when a situation arises.	1–2. Reframing helping behavior as enabling behavior is often necessary. 3. Changing previously entrenched patterns of behavior requires practice and feedback. During times of anxiety, it is normal to return to previous ways of responding.

Expected Outcome 2: By_____ the parents will verbalize the need to resolve the discord in the marital relationship.

Short-Term Goal	Nursing Interventions	Rationales
By _____ the parents will openly acknowledge the long-term discord in their marriage with a trusted professional.	1. Encourage the couple to begin to talk about resentments and regrets that have occurred as a result of the alcoholism. 2. Have the patient and his wife each write out specific resentments that occurred as a result of the alcoholism. 3. Have the couple share these feelings in the presence of a therapist. 4. Teach the couple how to listen and attend to each other by not interrupting or defending while the other person is speaking. 5. Encourage marital counseling after discharge.	1. After many years of denial, it is important to begin to talk about feelings that have been buried. 2. Writing out the resentments and regrets before verbalization allows the couple to stay structured and specific rather than generalized (i.e., "You ruined my life"). 3–4. A professional would act as a mediator in this instance and will begin to teach the couple how to communicate without blaming, a common dynamic in alcoholic marriages. 5. To continue the support, this couple will need to change entrenched behaviors.

Expected Outcome 3: By _____ the family will acknowledge the need to relate to each other for their needs for mutual support, love, affection, and spirituality.

Short-Term Goals	Nursing Interventions	Rationales
By _____ the family will maintain appropriate roles with each other.	1. Continue to inform the family how roles have changed within their family system as a result of the alcoholism. 2. Have each family member identify which role they play in the family dynamics. 3. Assess individual family members' readiness for "letting go" of their roles in the enabling process.	1. Teaching may need to be repeated on the basis of individual family members' readiness to learn. 2–3. Helps family members to break through denial and to begin the grieving process.
By _____ the family members will be able to verbalize their support and caring for each other.	1. Encourage the family to identify what they need from each other. 2. Help family members realize that caring about each other is different than enabling or protecting.	1. Social and emotional isolation and denial of needs are common for alcoholic families. 2. Enabling behaviors are often intended to be caring behaviors.
By _____ the family will acknowledge the lack of spirituality in their daily lives and verbalize their need for spiritual nurturing.	1. Ascertain from each family member the degree of spiritual bankruptcy present. 2. Encourage family members to talk about their needs regarding spirituality and the presence of the God of their understanding in their lives.	1–2. Feeling hopeless and abandoned by God is not uncommon in alcoholic families.

Expected Outcome 4: By _____ the family will willingly attend support group meetings such as Alcoholics Anonymous, Al-Anon, and Al-Ateen.

Short-Term Goal	Nursing Interventions	Rationales
By _____ the family will agree to attend a support group meeting.	1. Encourage the mother to attend an Al-Anon meeting while the husband is still hospitalized.	1. In alcoholic families, once a crisis is over, it is not unusual to return to previous levels of denial.

2. If the wife is resistant to attending a meeting for herself, encourage her and the children to attend an open Alcoholics Anonymous (AA) meeting.
3. Assure the wife and children that anonymity is present at AA meetings.

2. Attending an open AA meeting will aid in breaking through denial that alcoholism affects all age and socio-economic groups.
3. Alcoholic families are often shame based and have concerns about being exposed.

Nursing Diagnosis: Denial, Ineffective related to a lifestyle of denial and rationalization evidenced by unrecognized guilt and shame, a knowledge deficit regarding the negative effects of alcohol abuse, and minimization of the symptoms of alcoholism.

OUTCOME IDENTIFICATION, PLANNING, AND IMPLEMENTATION

> **Expected Outcome 1:** By _____ the patient will admit that his drinking is out of control and his life has become unmanageable.

Short-Term Goals	Nursing Interventions	Rationales
By _____ the patient will willingly participate in a treatment program.	1. Approach the patient in a direct, genuine, nonjudgmental manner. 2. With a positive, supportive attitude, help the patient to see the need for treatment. 3. Encourage the patient to self-admit to an alcohol treatment program. 4. Assure the patient that alcohol dependence is a physiological problem and not a moral one.	1–2. Approach gains the trust of the patient to begin a therapeutic relation-ship and shows genuine concern for the patient. 3. Self-admittance is preferred be-cause the element of denial has been addressed to a certain degree. 4. Shows the patient that you are not judging his character; let him know that you believe he has an illness, not a moral problem.
By _____ the patient will verbalize the deleterious physiological and psycho-logical effects of excessive alcohol use.	1. Encourage the patient to compile a written list of the deleterious conse-quences of excessive alcohol use he has experienced in the past 10 years. 2. Have the patient present this list to a nurse on the unit and to his peer group.	1–2. Both of these interventions assist with breaking through the denial associ-ated with the illness.

> **Expected Outcome 2:** By _____ the patient will abstain from alcohol.

Short-Term Goals	Nursing Interventions	Rationales
By _____ the patient will verbalize all situations that could lead to a relapse.	1. Ask the patient to compile a list of situations that influenced excessive drinking (i.e., social situations, work-related affairs, after work). 2. Offer suggestions for engaging in these situations without drinking.	1–2. To help the patient avoid relapse, it is important to know what situations triggered excessive drinking in the past.
By _____ the patient and treatment team will draft a plan for prevention of relapse after discharge.	1. Encourage attendance at AA meetings while in treatment. 2. Help the patient to recognize his strengths and abilities. 3. Have the patient agree to attend AA and aftercare when discharged.	1–3. Sobriety is easier to maintain in a structured setting such as a treatment facility; a strong support group is neces-sary after discharge.

> **Expected Outcome 3:** By _____ the patient will acknowledge how the absence of a higher power has affected him on his life's journey.

Short-Term Goals	Nursing Interventions	Rationales
By _____ the patient will openly discuss any shame or guilt that he feels as a result of his drinking behavior.	1. Educate the patient about shame and guilt and how they fit into the cycle of abuse. 2. Encourage the patient to vent feelings of shame and guilt related to drinking.	1–2. Once the patient is sober, it is not uncommon to feel negative feelings that have been numbed for a long time. Venting these feelings in a safe place is very therapeutic.
By _____ the patient will admit that a power greater than himself will be able to help him maintain sobriety and heal broken relationships.	1. Encourage the patient to begin talking about the God of his understanding. 2. Inquire about any specific religious practices that would bring solace to the patient. 3. Ask the patient how he views his acceptance of the disease of alcoholism as part of his life's spiritual journey.	1–2. It is not unusual for an alcoholic to have abandoned all spiritual practices because of low self-esteem. 3. As the patient gains progress toward spiritual wholeness, he will be able to place his alcoholism in perspective.
By _____ the patient will engage in daily meditation to obtain spiritual nurturing and solace.	1. Encourage the patient to begin a process of daily meditation while in treatment. 2. Ask the patient whether there are any spiritual resources that you can provide for him.	1–2. To maintain sobriety, it is important for the alcoholic to abstain from mood-altering chemicals one day at a time; therefore, it is important to begin the practice of grounding oneself spiritually on a daily basis.

EVALUATION

Formative Evaluation: The family met many of the short-term goals. They were able to confront their father and help him get treatment, but they were unable to "let go" of their firmly entrenched roles in the family system. Susan and Sarah were able to nurture and support each other, but Trisha and Judd remained on the outside. Sam and Susan openly acknowledged their marital conflict and were willing to continue in marital therapy. Susan and the three children attended three open AA meetings. Sam met all of the short-term goals that were intended for him. He was able to talk about his need for spirituality. The three children and Susan, however, did not want to talk about a lack of spirituality in their lives.

Summative Evaluation: The family achieved each of the expected outcomes, except the need for relating to each other for mutual support, love, affection, and spirituality. The family was encouraged to continue with family therapy after discharge. Each individual family member had wounds to heal. They were encouraged to attend a 12-step support program and to find a sponsor within the support program to work with them individually. Family members do not heal at the same rate, and it is difficult to support other family members when you are not feeling supported yourself. Sam met each of the expected outcomes intended for him. He said, "I know I am an alcoholic and I am grateful that my higher power did not leave me. With the help of my higher power, my family's support, and my sponsor, I know I can stay sober."

Conclusions

Chemical dependency was identified as the nation's number one health problem in the late 1980s; funding for research related to drug abuse and treatment increased dramatically in the 1990s. Research initiatives in the 21st century reflect new possibilities for diagnosis and direction for treatment.

With the current focus on genome therapy, researchers will continue to look for genetic factors in the development of substance use disorders. Other research will search for cellular and biochemical explanations related to the effects of psychoactive drugs on the brain, especially those involved with the reinforcing properties of substance use dependence. For example, what is the effect of drug activity on the GABA neurotransmitter system, and what are the psychophysiological processes responsible for craving a psychoactive substance? Other important areas of research will center on understanding the interrelationships of the chronic effects of alcohol on the CNS and other organ systems.

Primary prevention strategies were developed when the National Institute on of Alcohol Abuse and Alcoholism established a prevention research branch to address strategies that might be effective in preventing drug problems (U.S. Department of Health and Human Services, 1990). Of particular concern are certain subpopulations vulnerable to substance use disorders with special treatment needs: adolescents, women, children, certain ethnic groups, the homeless, and the elderly, and so on. Due to the evolution of the Internet, an individual with substance abuse problems or his or her family members can now obtain information directly. The National Clearinghouse for Alcohol and Drug Information has set up a Website called "Prevline: Prevention Online" that is updated each month (see Additional Resources). This Website provides information on resources, referrals, the newest research, publications, and conferences related to substance abuse.

Relevant research questions related to primary prevention would include the following:

- What is the role of peer pressure on the drug-taking behaviors of high school and college students?
- What is the effect of parent skills training on the prevention of substance use disorders?
- What strategies of community intervention are most effective in meeting the specific prevention-treatment needs of Native Americans, women, and the homeless?

- What structural characteristics of the work situation enhance or prevent the development of substance use disorders?
- What is the relationship between life stressors and the development of substance use disorders?
- What is the role of social supports in the prevention of substance use disorders?

Research on secondary prevention of substance use disorders could focus on identifying the following:

- What type of treatment protocols are most effective in treating patients with different drug abuse topologies?
- What are the criteria for matching a chemically dependent person's need with appropriate treatment in different subpopulations (adolescent, women, maternal, elderly)?

Research related to tertiary prevention of substance use disorders could consider the following:

- What is the efficacy of using family (or behavioral) therapy approaches in the treatment of substance use disorders?
- What are the factors (personal, social, spiritual) most consistently related to recidivism in substance use disorders?

There is a need to develop better assessment tools for diagnosis. Improvement of current tools and formulation of more precise diagnostic tools for early detection of substance use disorders in general community and medical situations would enhance treatment initiatives. Developing better methods for the identification of persons at risk for the disorder also is warranted.

Key Points to Remember

- Psychoactive substances refer to any mind-altering drug capable of modifying a person's behavior.
- *Substance use disorder* is a medical term used to describe a predictable set of physical and psychological symptoms associated with the voluntary ingestion of a psychoactive substance.
- Current etiological models suggest a polygenic mode of transmission consisting of a dynamic interaction among physical, psychological, social, and situational factors.
- Common properties of substance use disorders are tolerance, physical and psychological dependence, reinforcing properties, concepts of relapse, and recovery.
- The DSM-IV distinguishes between substance abuse and substance dependence as the generic descriptors for all drug classifications.
- The primary drug classifications include alcohol, hypnotic sedatives, hallucinogens, narcotic analgesics, CNS stimulants, and volatile solvents.
- Persistent use of psychoactive drugs leads to physical

and emotional symptoms that in the extreme can cause death.
- Treatment for substance use disorders has an acute phase and a rehabilitative phase.
- The treatment goals for the acute phase relate to stabilizing the patient's medical status.
- Rehabilitation focuses on helping chemically dependent persons develop new coping skills needed for a life without drugs.
- Self-help groups (AA, Cocaine Anonymous, and Narcotics Anonymous) provide the fellowship and information chemically dependent persons and their families need for abstinence.
- Specific populations (women, infants, cultural groups, adolescents, elderly people) are at risk for the disorder or have special treatment needs.
- Substance use disorders affect the family as well as the identified patient.
- *Codependency* is a term used to describe maladaptive behaviors in family members that occur as a result of a personal response to substance use.

Learning Activities

1. Attend an open AA or Narcotics Anonymous meeting. Report on your experience to the class.
2. Write down everything you have heard about the cause of substance use disorders and how they should be treated. Include your own thoughts. Share your observations with your classmates. Have a class discussion about the paradoxes associated with substance use disorders.
3. Use the Internet to go to the information Website set up by the National Clearinghouse for Alcohol and Drug Information. Go to one link and investigate one publication for the workplace.

Critical Thinking Exercise

The school nurse had just arrived in her office when a high school junior raced into her office informing her that his classmate, John, had just collapsed outside the restroom. When she reached John's side, she observed a young man who appeared very sleepy with pinpoint pupils and who was breathing with depressed respirations. His pulse was 50 bpm, and he did not respond to her verbal questions. Several of the male students nearby told her that the patient and several other boys had just been in the restroom. Another student reported that John had fallen outside and banged his head against the door.

1. What evidence suggests that John's problem may be drug-related?
2. What other evidence do you need to support this point of view?
3. What are possible alternate explanations for these symptoms?

Because of his poor vital signs, the nurse made arrangements to have John admitted to the emergency department of the nearby hospital. Later that day, John's sister came into the nurse's office crying. She expressed great concern about her brother's behavior since their parent's divorce.

1. What other information would you want to know from John's sister?
2. Suggest alternative possibilities.
3. How would you check your assumptions about John's symptoms?

Additional Resources

National Clearinghouse for Alcohol and Drug Information (NCADI)

Prevline: Prevention Online
http://www.health.org/

The Website for the Center for Substance Abuse Prevention, Substance Abuse and Mental Health Services Administration, and Center for Substance Abuse Treatment.

National Institute on Alcohol Abuse and Alcoholism (NIAAA)

http://www.niaaa.nih.gov/

National Institute on Drug Abuse (NIDA)

http://www.nida.nih.gov/

Online AA Recovery Resources

http://www.recovery.org/aa/

Research Institute on Addictions

http://www.ria.org/

References

Alcoholics Anonymous. (1955). *Twelve steps.* New York: AA World Services.

Allen, K. (1998). Essential concepts of addiction for general nursing practice. *Nursing Clinics of North America, 33*(1), 1–13.

American Nurses Association. (1988). *Standards of addictions: Nursing practice with selected diagnoses and criteria.* Kansas City, MO: Author.

American Psychiatric Association. (1994). Substance-related disorders. In *Diagnostic and statistical manual of mental disorders* (4th ed., pp. 175–272). Washington, DC: Author.

American Psychiatric Association (1995). *Practice guideline for the treatment of patients with substance use disorders: Alcohol, cocaine, opioids.* Washington, DC: American Psychiatric Press.

American Psychiatric Association (1996). *Practice guideline for the treatment of patients with nicotine dependence.* Washington, DC: American Psychiatric Press.

Amsel, Z. (1990). Introducing the concept of "community prevention." In *AIDS and intravenous drug use: Future directions for community-based prevention research* (NIDA Research Monograph 93). Washington, DC: U.S. Department of Health and Human Services.

Arthur, D. (1997). Alcohol early intervention: A nursing model for screening and intervention strategies. *Australian New Zealand Mental Health Nursing, 6*(3), 93-101.

Brown, C., Pirmohamed, M., & Park, B. K. (1997). Nurses' confidence in caring for patients with alcohol-related problems. *Professional Nurse, 13*(2), 83-86.

Buskist, W., & Gerbing, D. (1990). *Psychology: Boundaries and frontiers.* Glenview, IL: Scott, Foresman.

Claassen, C. A., Gilfillan, S., Orsulak, P., Carmody, T. J., Battaglia, J., & Rush, A. J. (1997). Substance use among patients with a psychotic disorder in a psychiatric emergency room. *Psychiatric Services 48,* 353-358.

Crigger, N. (1998). Defying denial. *American Journal of Nursing, 98*(8), 20-21.

DuPont, R. I., & Gold, M. S. (1995). Withdrawal and reward: Implications for detoxification and relapse prevention. *Psychiatric Annals, 25*(11), 663-668.

Finnegan, L., & Kandall, S. (1992). Problems in pregnancy. In Lowenson J, Ruiz P, & Millman R (Eds.), *Substance abuse: A comprehensive textbook* (2nd ed.). Baltimore, MD: Williams & Wilkins.

Gafoor, M., & Rassool, G. H. (1998). The co-existence of psychiatric disorders and substance misuse: Working with dual diagnosis patients. *Journal of Advanced Nursing, 27,* 497-502.

Galanter, M., Castaneda, R., & Franco, H. (1991). Group therapy and self-help groups. In R. Frances & S. Miller (Eds.), *Clinical textbook of addictive disorders* (pp. 430-451). New York: Guilford Press.

Gerstein, D., & Harwood, H. (1990). *Treating drug problems* (Vol. 1). Washington, DC: National Academy Press.

Ghodse A. H. (1994). Combined use of drugs and alcohol. *Current Opinion in Psychiatry, 7,* 249-251.

Ghodse A. H. (1995). *Drugs and addictive behavior: A guide to treatment* (2nd ed.). Oxford: Blackwell Science.

Grinspoon, L. (1998). Addiction and the brain: Part I. *The Harvard Mental Health Letter, 14*(12), 1-3.

Gualtieri, T. (1990). The neuropharmacology of inadvertent drug effects in patients with traumatic brain injuries. *Journal of Head Trauma Rehabilitation, 5*(3), 32-40.

Haack, M. R. (1998). Treating acute withdrawal from alcohol and other drugs. *Nursing Clinics of North America, 33*(1), 75-92.

Helman, C. (1990). *Culture, health and illness: An introduction for health professionals* (2nd ed.). London: Wright.

Hughes, T. (1989). Models and perspectives of addiction: Implications for treatment. *Nursing Clinics of North America, 24*(1), 1-12.

Inteli-Health-Home to Johns Hopkins Health. (1998, May 13). Economic costs of alcohol and drug abuse estimated at $246 billion in the U.S.

Jaffe, J. H., & Martin, W. R. (1990). Opioid analgesics and antagonists. In A. Gilman, T. Rall, A. Nies, & P. Taylor (Eds.), *Goodman and Gilman's pharmacological basis of therapeutics* (8th ed., pp. 485-522). New York: Pergamon Press.

Jellinek, E. M. (1960). *The disease concept of alcoholism.* New Haven, CT: Hillhouse.

Johnson, V. (1990). *Intervention: How to help someone who doesn't want help.* Minneapolis, MN: Johnson Institute.

Kleber, H. (1990). The nosology of abuse and dependence. *Journal of Psychiatric Research, 24*(2), 57-64.

Leccese, A. (1991). *Drugs and society: Behavioral medicines and abusable drugs* (5th ed.). Englewood Cliffs, NJ: Prentice-Hall.

Levine, O. S., Vlahov, D., Koehler, J., Cohn, S., Spronk, A. M., & Nelson, K. E. (1995). Seroepidemiology of hepatitis B virus in a population of injecting drug users. *American Journal of Epidemiology, 142*(3), 326-341.

Markey, B. T. & Stone, J. B. (1997). An alcohol and drug education program for nurses. *AORN Journal, 66,* 845-853.

McCracken, A. L. (1998). Aging and alcohol. *Journal of Gerontological Nursing, 24*(4), 37-43.

Milkman, H., and Shaffer, H. (1985). *The addictions: Multidisciplinary perspectives and treatments.* Lexington, MA: Heath.

Miller, N., & Chappel, J. (1991). History of the disease concept. *Psychiatric Annals, 21,* 196-205.

Miller, N., Mahler, B., Belkin, M., & Gold, M. (1990). Psychiatric diagnosis in alcohol and drug dependence. *Annals of Clinical Psychiatry, 3*(1), 79-89.

Mondanaro, J. (1990). Community-based AIDS prevention interventions: Special issues of women intravenous drug users. In *AIDS and intravenous drug use: Future directions for community-based prevention research* (NIDA Research Monograph 93). Washington, DC: U.S. Department of Health and Human Services.

Muramoto M., & Leshau L. (1993). Adolescent substance abuse: Recognition and early intervention. *Primary Care, 20*(1), 141-152.

Mynatt, S. (1996). A model of contributing risk factors to chemical dependency in nurses. *Journal of Psychosocial Nursing and Mental Health Services, 34*(7), 13-22.

National Commission on Marijuana and Drug Abuse. (1973). *Drug use in America: Problem and perspective.* Washington, DC: U.S. Government Printing Office.

National Nurses Society on Addictions (NNSA), Drug and Alcohol Nurses Association (DANA), and American Nurses Association (ANA). (1987). *The care of clients with addiction: Dimensions of nursing practice.* Kansas City, MO: American Nurses Association.

Rosenberg, S. D., Drake, R. E., Wolford, G. L., et al. (1998). Dartmouth Assessment of Lifestyle Instrument (DALI): A substance use disorder screen for people with severe mental illness. *American Journal of Psychiatry, 155,* 232-238.

Rush, B. (1934). *Medical inquiries and observations upon the diseases of the mind.* New York: Doubleday.

Quinby, P., & Graham A. (1993). Substance abuse among women. *Primary Care 20*(1), 126-139.

Sander, W. (1997). Protocol for intervention and treatment of alcohol withdrawal. *Axone, 19*(1), 10-13.

Schuckit, M. A. (1995). A theory of alcohol and drug abuse: A genetic approach. In D. J. Lettieri, M. Sayers, & H. W. Pearson (Eds.), *Theories on drug abuse.* (NIDA Research Monograph 30). Washington, DC: U.S. Department of Health and Human Services.

Schuster, C., & Snyder, M. (1990). NIDA's medication development program-1989. In *Problems of drug dependence 1989.* (NIDA Research Monograph 95). Washington, DC: U.S. Department of Health and Human Services.

Stone, W., & Gottesman, I. (1993). A perspective on the search for the causes of alcoholism: Slow down the rush to genetic alcoholism. *Neurology, Psychiatry and Brain Research,* (1), 123-132.

Streissguth, A. P. (1986). Fetal alcohol syndrome: An overview and implications for patient management. In N. Estes & M. E. Heinemann (Eds.), *Alcoholism: Development, consequences, and interventions* (3rd ed.). St. Louis, MO: C. V. Mosby.

Streissguth, A. (1997). Fetal alcohol syndrome: What's new in alcohol and drugs? *The Brown University Department of Addiction Theory and Applications, 2*(6), 1-3.

Sullivan, J. (1995). *Nursing care of clients with substance abuse.* St. Louis, MO: Mosby-Year Book.

Tierney, J. A. (1997). Identification and treatment of alcohol abuse, dependence, and withdrawal. *Ohio Nurses Review, 72*(9), 3-7.

U.S. Department of Health and Human Services. (1990). *Healthy people 2000: National health promotion and disease prevention objectives.* (Publication No. [PHS] 91-50212). Washington, DC: U.S. Department of Health and Human Services.

Valliant, G. E. (1983). *The natural history of alcoholism: Causes, patterns and paths to recovery.* Cambridge, MA: Harvard University Press.

Wing, D. (1991). Goal setting and recovery from alcoholism. *Archives of Psychiatric Nursing, 5,* 178-184.

Wing, D. (1993). Applying the "Model of recovering alcoholics behavioral stages and goal setting" to nursing practice. *Archives of Psychiatric Nursing, 7,* 197-202.

Zacharias, S., Rodriguez-Garcia, A., Honz, N., & Hooper, C. (1998). Development of an alcohol withdrawal clinical pathway: An interdisciplinary process. *Journal of Nursing Care Quality, 12*(3), 9-18.

Suggested Readings

Alcoholics Anonymous. (1955). *12 Steps*. New York: AA World Services.

Allen, K. (1998). Essential concepts of addiction for general nursing practice. *Nursing Clinics of North America, 33*(1), 1-13.

American Nurses Association. (1988). *Standards of addictions: Nursing practice with selected diagnoses and criteria*. Kansas City, MO: Author.

American Psychiatric Association. (1994). Substance-related disorders. In *Diagnostic and statistical manual of mental disorders* (4th ed., pp. 175-272). Washington, DC: Author.

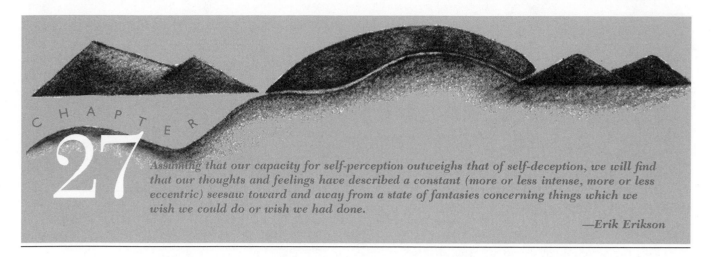

Assuming that our capacity for self-perception outweighs that of self-deception, we will find that our thoughts and feelings have described a constant (more or less intense, more or less eccentric) seesaw toward and away from a state of fantasies concerning things which we wish we could do or wish we had done.

—*Erik Erikson*

Behavioral Disorders

Learning Objectives

After studying this chapter, you should be able to:

1. Identify three factors that constitute a healthy personality.
2. Name three factors that identify an individual with a personality disorder.
3. Distinguish among the three clusters of personality disorders described in the *Diagnostic and Statistical Manual of Mental Disorders, Fourth Edition* (DSM-IV).
4. List three features and behavior patterns associated with each personality disorder.
5. For each personality disorder, identify two behaviors that affect the individual's relationships with family, friends, and caregivers.
6. Discuss three nursing diagnoses appropriate for each Axis II cluster.
7. Identify three patient outcomes appropriate for nursing diagnoses related to personality disorders.
8. Identify two interventions for each patient outcome.
9. Identify two medications useful when treating patients with personality disorders.
10. Discuss spiritual issues that affect patients with personality disorders.
11. Discuss spiritual issues that affect nurses who care for patients with personality disorders.

Key Terminology

Antisocial personality disorder
Avoidant personality disorder
Borderline personality disorder
Cluster A disorders

Cluster B disorders
Cluster C disorders
Dependent personality disorder
Histrionic personality disorder

Narcissistic personality disorder
Object constancy
Obsessive-compulsive personality disorder
Paranoid personality disorder

Personality disorder
Schizoid personality disorder
Schizotypal personality disorder
Splitting
Transitional objects

One of our greatest challenges in psychiatric nursing is in relating effectively to patients who are "difficult to work with." To face this challenge, it is necessary to study personality or behavioral disorders. As we journey with patients who have behavioral disorders, we sometimes see similar conduct in ourselves. This awareness can be not only frightening but also enlightening as we gain deeper understanding of our ability to relate to others and define our own sense of self.

A difficulty that arises when dealing with individuals with personality disorders is the tendency to judge or label unusual or dramatic conduct as abnormal rather than analyzing factors that cause the behavior. Judging patients interferes with forming therapeutic alliances. It increases the psychological and spiritual distress of the patient, and it leads to emotional frustration and spiritual distress for the nurse confronted with an inability to understand the "why" behind the patient's behavior and to respond to the patient in a loving manner.

Jeff's Story

Jeff is 40 years old, single, and living alone. He leads a quiet life and has no friends or associates. Jeff works as a mail sorter for the post office. He is known as a loner, rarely talking to his coworkers. He has never married, and his family states that he has never dated. His free time is spent alone building model airplanes, reading science fiction novels, and watching action movie videos. He has minimal interactions with anyone, including his parents and his brother.

He visits his family only when invited, usually during holidays such as Thanksgiving and Christmas. His mother states, "Jeff has always been quiet, to himself, doesn't need much, doesn't ask for much, and is a loner. I don't understand how he got like that, except maybe he is like his dad's brother who has schizophrenia. You know, I've never seen him angry, or happy, or emotional in any way, even if his football team wins a close game. He doesn't say much. I don't know what he even thinks about. I do know he takes care of his bills and is responsible for what he says he will do." ■

A HEALTHY PERSONALITY

How do you know when someone has a healthy personality? What is a personality disorder? Individuals with healthy personalities can

- Identify "self" as the total of strengths and weaknesses.
- Identify the types of interactions or thoughts that create joy, sadness, anger, love, hate, and other strong emotions.
- Relate to others without expecting others to meet all their needs.
- Define where they end and another person begins.

- Balance work and play.
- Express spirituality.
- Identify goals accomplished through discipline and creativity (Erikson, 1963; Maslow, 1968).

Janet's story, presented in Case Example 27–1, illustrates a woman with a healthy personality. Janet can receive love and trust from her family members and demonstrates these same qualities back to them.

■ CASE EXAMPLE 27–1
■ Janet's Story

Janet has very close relationships with her mother, her husband, and her two children. She can identify her strengths as a loving wife and as a mother who loves her children and encourages them to express their individuality. "My mother enjoyed my curiosity and ability to ask questions and learn new things. I know Mom is interested in fashion. I'm interested in music. We make a good pair. My daughter writes poetry. My son is like my husband, interested in woodwork." ■

What do you think? As you review the qualities of a healthy personality, which qualities describe you?

➤ *Check Your Reading*
1. Identify three behaviors necessary to a healthy personality.

PERSONALITY DISORDERS DEFINED

Personality disorders are listed on Axis II of the *Diagnostic and Statistical Manual of Mental Disorders, Fourth Edition* (DSM-IV). A personality disorder is defined as "an enduring pattern of inner experience and behavior that deviates markedly from the expectations of the individual's culture, is pervasive and inflexible, has an onset in adolescence or early adulthood, is stable over time, and leads to distress or impairment" (DSM-IV, 1994, p. 629).

You can ascertain these behaviors by observing how the individual relates to others. Watch the person's perception of surroundings and ability to solve problems. When assessing the patient for diagnosis, Westen (1997) found that a majority of clinicians make the diagnosis of a personality disorder by asking the patient to describe his interactions with others as well as observing the patient's behavior with the interviewer. Mansfield (1992) stated that personality disorders reflect deficiencies in how a person identifies feelings and in the ability to experience "self" as unique. The individual with a personality disorder does not look within to locate feelings or make decisions but instead looks outside the self for evaluations, directions, rules, or opinions.

PERSONALITY DEVELOPMENT: A VIEW FROM PSYCHOLOGY AND BIOLOGY

Understanding "why" something happens helps us accept difficult situations and improves our problem-solving. Such understanding is especially important when caring for individuals with personality disorders. If you can understand "why" a behavior pattern exists, you will be better prepared to develop expected outcomes and treatment interventions.

Margaret Mahler: Contributions to Object Relation Theory

To develop a model for the early phases of infant development, Margaret Mahler and her colleagues observed infants and their mothers. She distinguished the psychological birth of the infant (when the child has a beginning sense of being an individual, or self) from the biological birth. She theorized that the child passes through phases, or maturational events, to develop a separate and unique sense of being (Akhtar, 1992, 1995; Cauwels, 1992; Mahler, 1963, 1971, 1972a, 1972b). Mahler's phases follow:

1. *Autistic phase.* Mahler theorized that the neonate (1 to 2 months old) is encased in a self-absorbed barrier with no recognition of others.
2. *Symbiotic phase.* The infant (4 to 5 months old) begins to recognize the mother, becomes enmeshed with the mother's self, and perceives the mother as an extension of her own self.
3. *Separation-individuation phase.* The third phase is subdivided into four overlapping subphases.
   - *Differentiation subphase* (5 to 8 months). The child becomes aware of people other than the mother and can distinguish them. The child learns psychological separateness from the mother by beginning to explore both the body and the environment.
   - *Practicing subphase* (8 to 16 months). The child becomes more mobile, is able to crawl and toddle away from the mother, and checks in with the mother frequently.
   - *Rapprochement subphase* (16 to 25 months). The child increasingly differentiates self from mother and mother's environment; begins to learn that her separateness, autonomy, and motor abilities are limited; realizes that the self is no longer the center of the universe, and feels very small in a larger world. These feelings are exhibited by anxiety and ambivalent clinging and darting away from mother when she tries to confine or hold the child, who learns that the mother will be there for emotional support but is a separate being. The child begins to tolerate the mother's absence. The child who works through the conflicts in this subphase learns to deal with love and trusting of parents and how to view relationships with other people realistically.
   - *Object constancy subphase* (25 to 36 months). **Object constancy** is reached when one can evoke the memory of a significant other (or a parent, in the child's case), which assures the child that she is loved. During this subphase, the child learns to tolerate long separations from the mother by use of **transitional objects** (objects such as teddy bears, dolls, or blankets that remind the child of the mother). These objects are soothing to the child during times of stress or insecurity. Another task accomplished during this subphase is that the child learns to cope with intense emotions, such as ambivalence, frustration, and rage. The child forms a realistic view of self by internalizing a loving image and attitude of the mother and working through the powerful emotions of frustration and rage with the positive parental image intact.

Throughout the separation-individuation phase, the child has to work through conflicts between autonomy and dependence, as well as fears of engulfment and abandonment by the mother. The child learns that when the mother leaves, the absence is temporary, and the mother continues to exist even when the child cannot see her. The child also discovers that the mother will return (i.e., object constancy). During this phase, the child works through the tendency to see the mother as either all good, therefore meeting all needs, or all bad, not meeting needs.

Mahler and colleagues hypothesized that borderline personality disorder and other severe personality disorders developed during the rapprochement subphase of the separation-individuation phase of development. The cause of these disorders, these researchers suggest, is a mother who is either too emotionally distant from the child or excessively clinging to a child who needs to explore the environment.

W*hat do you think?* As you think about children you know, identify behaviors that are or were indicative of their movement through the phases identified by Mahler.

▶ *Check Your Reading*
2. What is the autistic phase of development described by Mahler?
3. Why did Mahler and associates identify the rapprochement subphase as an important stage in the development of borderline personality disorder?

The Biological View

Since the 1970s, biological studies have been performed on patients with an Axis I diagnosis. In the 1990s, some of these biological tests have been applied to people with Axis II personality disorders. Although this research is far from conclusive, it is useful in furthering knowledge about the biological etiology of personality disorders, assisting in the accurate labeling of the disorders, and promoting psychopharmacological agents to decrease symptoms. Research now focuses on cognitive-perceptual organization, affective regulation, impulse control, and anxiety and social inhibition (Kavoussi & Siever, 1991). Neuroanatomical research has recently reported using a PET scan to determine which regions of the brain are involved in brain activity that correlates with emotional responses such as happiness, sadness, and disgust in subjects who do not have a history of psychological problems (Reiman et al., 1997; Lane, Reiman, Ahern, Schartz, & Davidson, 1997). This research has later implications for individuals who have problems modulating their affect, such as patients with some Axis II disorders.

Genetics

Some reports (Coryell & Zimmerman, 1989; Mann, Stanley, McBride, & McEwan, 1986) of genetic and family studies suggest causal factors for the development of a personality disorder. Siever (1992) reported that schizotypal personality disorder is more prevalent in relatives of schizophrenic individuals than in relatives of patients with other psychiatric disorders. Genetic studies suggest that schizotypal traits occur more frequently than chronic schizophrenia in relatives of chronic schizophrenic patients. Schizotypal traits, therefore, may be a more common manifestation of the schizophrenogenic genotype than chronic schizophrenia. Some family studies suggest that paranoid personality disorder may be slightly more common in relatives of schizophrenic patients than in control subjects. More research is needed to determine what part of the etiology of personality disorders is genetic.

Neurotransmitters

Dopaminergic dysfunction, as measured by cerebrospinal fluid (CSF) and plasma levels of the dopamine metabolite homovanillic acid, has shown differences from the norm that correlate to psychotic symptoms in schizophrenia (Siever, 1985; Davidson & Davis, 1988). Siever and Davis (1991) demonstrated an increase in cerebrospinal and plasma homovanillic acid in preliminary studies of schizotypal patients. This finding correlates with positive schizotypal symptoms of magical thinking, illusions, and ideas of reference.

Several studies demonstrate serotonergic subsensitivity in impulsive behaviors of aggression and self-destruction (Brown & Linnoila, 1990). Brown et al. (1982) found that aggressive and suicidal behaviors in individuals with personality disorders correlated inversely with CSF levels of 5-hydroxyindoleacetic acid (5-HIAA), a major metabolite of serotonin. Some evidence links low levels of serotonin with suicidal behavior (Roy, 1989). Stanley and Stanley (1990) studied concentrations of serotonin and 5-HIAA in postmortem receptor-binding studies. They noted changes in both presynaptic and postsynaptic serotonergic binding sites in people who have been examined after suicide, as opposed to the postmortem studies of the control group. CSF 5-HIAA was tested in 193 neurologically normal newborn infants. It was demonstrated that there was a significantly lower level of 5-HIAA in the infants who have first-degree and second-degree relatives with antisocial personality disorder (Constantino, Morris, & Murphy, 1997).

Although some biological studies have been done on patients with panic disorder, they are not applicable to patients with cluster C personality disorders (described later in the chapter). More research is necessary to study the biological factors underlying the anxiety traits of patients with personality disorders.

Because many prison inmates are diagnosed with antisocial personality disorder, considerable research has focused on this population. Many of these people had attention deficit disorder in childhood. They also display a high rate of nonspecific EEG abnormalities. Their autonomic nervous systems are characterized by high arousal states, and the most recent research demonstrates that many of them have a depletion of serotonin and 5-HIAA. Such a deficiency has been linked to aggression in mammals.

What do you think? Do you think biology causes personality disorders or predisposes to personality disorders? If biology leads to predisposition, what factors increase the likelihood of the development of a personality disorder?

▶ *Check Your Reading*

4. What areas of study are currently being undertaken to understand the implications of biology in the etiology of personality disorders?
5. What have researchers found when studying 5-HIAA levels from individuals who have completed suicide?

DESCRIPTIONS OF PERSONALITY DISORDERS

The DSM-IV defines general diagnostic criteria for all personality disorders that specify that the person must demonstrate an enduring pattern of inner experiences and behavior that deviates from the person's cultural expectations. These patterns are evident in two or more of the following areas:

- *Cognition, or thought pattern:* The person has different ways of perceiving and interpreting self, others, and events in the environment.
- *Affect:* The person displays a range, intensity, lability, and appropriateness of emotional response different from those of others in the same cultural group.

- *Interpersonal functioning:* Individuals with personality disorders experience more difficulty socializing and maintaining friendships, work relationships, and marital relationships than others in their cultural group.
- *Impulse control:* People with personality disorders may be more impulsive, aggressive, or self-destructive than the norm.

These inflexible and enduring patterns are present across a broad range of personal and social situations. For example, a person may have the same problems with different bosses at several different work sites throughout a work history. This person probably is unable to recognize the pattern of inflexible behavior that was similar in each job. This inability leads to clinically significant distress in social, occupational, or other important areas of functioning. A person may have difficulty maintaining a friendship because the friend is expected to meet most of his emotional needs without reciprocity.

These behavioral and thought patterns exist over a long period. They generally begin in adolescence or early adulthood. They are not manifestations of any other psychiatric illness, nor are they due to direct physiological effects of a substance (such as alcohol or a medication) or a general medical condition (such as a head trauma).

> **W**hat do you think? Do you know anyone who displays difficult behaviors that do not change despite feedback? What is life like for that individual? What is it like being in a relationship with that individual?

> ► *Check Your Reading*
> 6. What is meant by "an enduring pattern of inner experience and behavior that deviates markedly from the expectations of the individual's culture"?
> 7. What are three behavioral or thought patterns exhibited by individuals with a personality disorder?

CLUSTERS OF BEHAVIORS

Personality disorders are grouped by common behavior patterns into three clusters on the Axis II part of the DSM-IV. Although the three clusters are useful in aiding clinicians with diagnosis of personality disorders, overlapping of behaviors points to the need for more research to differentiate one disorder from another. The first group, **cluster A disorders,** includes paranoid, schizoid, and schizotypal personality disorders. A common trait among patients with these disorders is that they often appear odd or eccentric. The second group, **cluster B disorders,** includes antisocial, borderline, histrionic, and narcissistic personality disorders. These patients typically exhibit dramatic, emotional, or erratic behaviors. The third group, **cluster C disorders,** includes dependent, avoidant, and obsessive-compulsive personality disorders. These patients characteristically display anxious or fearful behaviors.

Cluster A Personality Disorders

Paranoid Personality Disorder

The essential feature of a **paranoid personality disorder** is a pattern of mistrust and suspiciousness of others, beginning by early adulthood. The person with this disorder believes that others have malevolent motives for every interaction. In addition, people with this condition display at least four of the following:

- Suspicion that others are exploiting, harming, or deceiving them
- Preoccupation with doubts about the loyalty or trustworthiness of others
- Reluctance to confide in others, worry that others will later use this information against them
- Perception of hidden demeaning or threatening quality to the benevolent remarks made by others
- Grudges held against others who are perceived to be insulting or injurious
- Perception of attacks on character or reputation, with quick, angry reactions
- Suspicion regarding the fidelity of a spouse or sexual partner

Schizoid Personality Disorder

The essential feature of **schizoid personality disorder** is a pervasive pattern of detachment from social relationships and a restricted range of expression of emotions, particularly in interpersonal settings, beginning by early adulthood. Jeff, for example, manifests behavioral patterns consistent with this disorder. The person with a schizoid personality disorder displays at least four of the following:

- Lack of desire for or enjoyment of any close relationships, including being part of a family
- Consistent choice of solitary activities
- Little interest in a sexual relationship
- Little pleasure in any activities
- No close friends other than first-degree relatives
- Indifference to praise or criticism from others
- Emotional coldness or detachment and a flat affect

Schizotypal Personality Disorder

The essential feature of **schizotypal personality disorder** is a pervasive pattern of social and interpersonal deficits marked by acute discomfort with and a reduced capacity for close relationships. The condition begins by early adulthood. The person displays at least five of the behaviors identified in Medical Diagnoses and Related Nursing Diagnoses: Cluster A Personality Disorders.

> **W**hat do you think? Do you know anyone who typifies the cluster A personality disorders? How have you responded to this person? Knowing what you know about personality disorders, do you think you will respond differently in the future?

MEDICAL DIAGNOSES AND RELATED NURSING DIAGNOSES

Cluster A Personality Disorders

DSM-IV Diagnosis: Schizotypal Personality Disorder

A. A pervasive pattern of social and interpersonal deficits marked by acute discomfort with, and reduced capacity for, close relationships as well as by cognitive or perceptual distortions and eccentricities of behavior, beginning by early adulthood and present in a variety of contexts, as indicated by five (or more) of the following:

1. Ideas of reference (excluding delusions of reference).

2. Odd beliefs or magical thinking that influences behavior and is inconsistent with subcultural norms (e.g., superstitiousness, belief in clairvoyance, telepathy, or "sixth sense"; in children and adolescents, bizarre fantasies or preoccupations).

3. Unusual perceptual experiences, including bodily illusions.

4. Odd thinking and speech (e.g., vague, circumstantial, metaphorical, overelaborate, or stereotyped).

5. Suspiciousness or paranoid ideation.

6. Inappropriate or constricted affect.

7. Behavior or appearance that is odd, eccentric, or peculiar.

8. Lack of close friends or confidants other than first-degree relatives.

9. Excessive social anxiety that does not diminish with familiarity and tends to be associated with paranoid fears rather than negative judgments about self.

B. Does not occur exclusively during the course of Schizophrenia, a Mood Disorder With Psychotic Features, another Psychotic Disorder, or a Pervasive Developmental Disorder.

Note: If criteria are met prior to the onset of Schizophrenia, add "Premorbid," e.g., "Schizotypal Personality Disorder (Premorbid)."

Related Nursing Diagnosis	Definition	Example
Impaired Social Interaction	The state in which a person participates in an insufficient or excessive quantity or ineffective quality of social exchange	Impaired Social Interaction related to magical thinking and anxiety when in a social situation as evidenced by thoughts that the patient can feel a "sixth sense" when in a social environment, verbalizations regarding increased anxiety in a social setting, and statements that the patient experiences ideas of reference in social settings

Based on information from the *Diagnostic and Statistical Manual of Mental Disorders. Fourth Edition.* Copyright 1994 American Psychiatric Association. Nursing diagnoses and definitions from North American Nursing Diagnosis Association. (1999). *NANDA nursing diagnoses: Definitions and classification 1999-2000.* Philadelphia: NANDA.

► *Check Your Reading*

8. Describe two ways in which the schizotypal personality might be considered odd.

9. What is the essential feature or pattern of behavior for the individual with a paranoid personality disorder?

10. What is the essential feature or behavioral pattern for the individual with schizoid personality disorder?

Cluster B Personality Disorders

Antisocial Personality Disorder

The essential feature of **antisocial personality disorder** is a pervasive pattern of disregard for and violation of the rights of others. An individual with an antisocial personality disorder does not exhibit any sense of guilt and often is very manipulative. To make the diagnosis of antisocial personality disorder, the individual must be at least 18 years old and must have shown evidence of conduct disorder before the age of 15. Antisocial personality disorder—which used to be called psychopathic disorder, sociopathic disorder, or moral insanity—affects approximately 3% of American men and 1% of American women. These individuals do to not seek psychiatric treatment unless they also have an Axis I diagnosis or are remanded by the courts for evaluation of their mental status because of criminality or substance abuse. Much has been written about this disorder in the forensic literature.

The DSM-IV states that a diagnosis of antisocial personality disorder should be made if the person satisfies at least three of the behaviors identified in Medical Diagnoses and Related Nursing Diagnoses: Cluster B Personality Disorders.

MEDICAL DIAGNOSES AND RELATED NURSING DIAGNOSES

Cluster B Personality Disorders

DSM-IV Diagnosis: Antisocial Personality Disorder

Diagnostic Criteria

A. A pervasive pattern of disregard for and violation of the rights of others occurring since age 15 years, as indicated by three (or more) of the following:
   1. Failure to conform to social norms with respect to lawful behaviors as indicated by repeatedly performing acts that are grounds for arrest.
   2. Deceitfulness, as indicated by repeated lying, use of aliases, or conning others for personal profit or pleasure.
   3. Impulsivity or failure to plan ahead.
   4. Irritability and aggressiveness, as indicated by repeated physical fights or assaults.
   5. Reckless disregard for safety of self or others.
   6. Consistent irresponsibility, as indicated by repeated failure to sustain consistent work behavior or honor financial obligations.
   7. Lack of remorse, as indicated by being indifferent to or rationalizing having hurt, mistreated, or stolen from another.

B. The individual is at least age 18 years.

C. There is evidence of Conduct Disorder with onset before age 15 years.

D. The occurrence of antisocial behavior is not exclusively during the course of Schizophrenia or a Manic Episode.

Related Nursing Diagnoses	Definition	Example
Ineffective Individual Coping	Impairment of adaptive behaviors and problem-solving abilities of a person in meeting life's demands and roles	Ineffective Individual Coping related to lifestyle of defensive behaviors as evidenced by the patient's mistrust and suspicious statements directed toward others, aggressive behavior that is justified in the patient's mind as retaliatory, and blaming of others for own behavior
Ineffective Denial	The state of a conscious or unconscious attempt to disavow the knowledge or meaning of an event to reduce anxiety or fear, to the detriment of health	Ineffective Denial related to the patient's impaired ability to accept consequences for own behavior as evidenced by continuing the same pattern of rage and aggression, blaming others for own aggressive behavior, and refusing to acknowledge own contribution to arguments

Based on information from the *Diagnostic and Statistical Manual of Mental Disorders. Fourth Edition.* Copyright 1994 American Psychiatric Association. Nursing diagnoses and definitions from North American Nursing Diagnosis Association. (1999). *NANDA nursing diagnoses: Definitions and classification 1999–2000.* Philadelphia: NANDA.

Box continued on following page

MEDICAL DIAGNOSES AND RELATED NURSING DIAGNOSES

Cluster B Personality Disorders Continued

DSM-IV Diagnosis: Borderline Personality Disorder

Diagnostic Criteria

A. A pervasive pattern of instability of interpersonal relationships, self-image, and affects, and marked impulsivity beginning by early adulthood and present in a variety of contexts, as indicated by five (or more) of the following:

   1. Frantic efforts to avoid real or imagined abandonment. **Note:** Do not include suicidal or self-mutilating behavior covered in Criterion 5.

   2. A pattern of unstable and intense interpersonal relationships characterized by alternating between extremes of idealization and devaluation.

   3. Identity disturbance: markedly and persistently unstable self-image or sense of self.

   4. Impulsivity in at least two areas that are potentially self-damaging (e.g., spending, sex, substance abuse, reckless driving, binge eating). **Note:** Do not include suicidal or self-mutilating behavior covered in Criterion 5.

   5. Recurrent suicidal behavior, gestures, or threats, or self-mutilating behavior.

   6. Affective instability due to a marked reactivity of mood (e.g., intense episodic dysphoria, irritability, or anxiety usually lasting a few hours and only rarely more than a few days).

   7. Chronic feelings of emptiness.

   8. Inappropriate, intense anger or difficulty controlling anger (e.g., frequent displays of temper, constant anger, recurrent physical fights).

   9. Transient, stress-related paranoid ideation or severe dissociative symptoms.

Related Nursing Diagnoses	Definition	Example
Ineffective Individual Coping	Impairment of adaptive behaviors and problem-solving abilities of a person in meeting life's demands and roles	Ineffective Individual Coping related to inadequate psychological resources, poor self-esteem, and excessive negative thoughts about self as evidenced by impulsive alcohol consumption and sexual promiscuity, labile emotional states of anger and crying, and verbalization of feelings of being overwhelmed, alone, without support, and unable to identify the reasons for these feelings
Risk for Violence: Self-Directed	A state in which a person experiences behaviors that can be physically harmful to either self or others	Risk for Self-Directed Violence related to history of cutting self when highly emotional as evidenced by the patient's expressed fears of being abandoned by a significant other and sense of unreality
Self-Esteem Disturbance	Negative self-evaluation or feelings about self or self-capabilities, which may be directly or indirectly expressed	Self-Esteem Disturbance related to the patient's relationship problems with spouse as evidenced by the patient's describing self as unable to deal with conflict in the marriage, expressing guilt and feelings of shame about marital discord, and extreme sensitivity to criticism by spouse and other family members

MEDICAL DIAGNOSES AND RELATED NURSING DIAGNOSES

Cluster B Personality Disorders Continued

DSM-IV Diagnosis: Histrionic Personality Disorder

Diagnostic Criteria

A. A pervasive pattern of excessive emotionality and attention-seeking, beginning by early adulthood and present in a variety of contexts, as indicated by five (or more) of the following:

1. Is uncomfortable in situations in which he or she is not the center of attention.
2. Interaction with others is often characterized by inappropriate sexually seductive or provocative behavior.
3. Displays rapidly shifting and shallow expression of emotions.
4. Consistently uses physical appearance to draw attention to self.
5. Has a style of speech that is excessively impressionistic and lacking in detail.
6. Shows self-dramatization, theatricality, and exaggerated expression of emotion.
7. Is suggestible, that is, easily influenced by others or circumstances
8. Considers relationships to be more intimate than they actually are.

Related Nursing Diagnoses	Definition	Example
Self-Esteem Disturbance	Negative self-evaluation or feelings about self or self-capabilities, which may be directly or indirectly expressed	Self-Esteem Disturbance related to the patient's relationship problems with spouse as evidenced by the patient describing self as unable to deal with conflicts in the marriage, expressing guilt and feelings of shame about marital discord, and extreme sensitivity to criticism by spouse and other family members

Histrionic Personality Disorder

The essential feature of **histrionic personality disorder** is excessive emotionality and attention-seeking behavior, beginning by early adulthood. People with this disorder feel uncomfortable or unappreciated when they are not the center of attention and therefore behave in a manner to glean this attention. People with a histrionic personality disorder also display at least five of the behaviors identified in the DSM-IV.

Narcissistic Personality Disorder

The essential feature of **narcissistic personality disorder** is the pattern of grandiosity, need for admiration, and lack of empathy toward others, beginning by early adulthood. This tendency is manifested in five or more of the following:

• A grandiose sense of self-importance: achievements and talents are often exaggerated; the person often expects recognition as a superior performer without the commensurate achievements

• Preoccupation with fantasies of unlimited success, power, brilliance, beauty, or ideal love
• Belief that he or she is "special" and unique and can associate only with others who are also special and have a high status
• Need for an excessive amount of admiration
• An unrealistic sense of entitlement
• Interpersonal exploitation and taking advantage of others to meet personal goals
• Lack of empathy, as this individual is unwilling to recognize or identify with the feelings or needs of others
• Envy of others and belief that others are envious of him or her
• Arrogance and haughtiness in behavior and attitude

Borderline Personality Disorder

The essential feature of **borderline personality disorder** is a pervasive pattern of unstable interpersonal relationships, difficulty defining self and determining self-image, labile affects and mood, and marked impulsive behavior, beginning by early adulthood. This disorder is more pervasive in women than in men. In Case Example 27–2, Joanne demonstrates behavior patterns consistent with borderline personality disorder. The behavior of people with this disorder includes at least five of the behaviors identified in the DSM-IV.

People with borderline personality disorders frequently engage in a manipulative behavior referred to as **splitting,** which pits people against one another. Because of their tendency to view people as "all good" or "all bad," those with this disorder frequently are disillusioned when family, friends, or professional caregivers fail to be perfect. For instance, a hospitalized patient diagnosed with borderline personality disorder might tell one staff person that she is the best nurse, the only one who understands the patient, but at the same time the patient paints a negative picture of another staff member's behavior. If staff members are unaware of the patient's splitting behavior, contention and inconsistency in the patient's plan of treatment may develop.

■ CASE EXAMPLE 27–2
■ Joanne's Story

Joanne is 30 years old and has been married for 7 years to a man, Jack, who is quiet and passive. They have no children. Joanne is often impulsive, angry, emotional, and critical of others. She has a history of seeking revenge when angry. She is currently having an affair with a man she met at an Alcoholics Anonymous meeting. She feels "happy with Carlos" (her lover) and thinks her marriage with Jack is over. She is afraid to leave her husband because she feels Carlos, although fun, would never be able to support them financially.

Joanne does not work and perceives the work world as threatening and scary. Joanne has been clean and sober from alcohol and benzodiazepines for the last 7 months. She is going to Alcoholics Anonymous meetings to see Carlos, but she does not have a sponsor and does not feel comfortable discussing her issues publically.

Joanne has attempted suicide several times in her life. Two of the three overdose attempts were in response to termination of a relationship with a lover. She attempted suicide when, at age 16, she found her father with another woman. She told the therapist at the time, "If Mom leaves Dad, I'd be all alone. I was so upset by that prospect, I became overwhelmed with grief and took a razor to my wrist."

Joanne has had stormy relationships with women who tried to befriend her. "They were jealous of my talents, especially my sewing; they really did not want to be my friend; they really wanted to learn how to sew." Joanne is estranged from her family and discusses her anger at her mother and two sisters when asked why she has not maintained contact. Joanne also has a stormy relationship with God, fluctuating between intense love for Him and intense hatred. She feels alone much of the time. ■

What do you think? What do you think are effective ways to deal with splitting?

➤ *Check Your Reading*
11. State the essential feature demonstrated by the person with antisocial personality disorder and borderline personality disorder.
12. What common psychiatric problem often seen in the emergency department is part of the behavior exhibited by a person with borderline personality disorder?

Cluster C Personality Disorders

Avoidant Personality Disorder

The essential feature of **avoidant personality disorder** is a pervasive pattern of social inhibition, feelings of inadequacy, and hypersensitivity to negative evaluations from others, beginning by early adulthood. Individuals diagnosed with this personality disorder display at least four of the characteristics identified in the DSM-IV.

Dependent Personality Disorder

The essential feature of **dependent personality disorder** is the excessive need to be taken care of by others, which leads to submissive, clinging behavior and fear of separation, beginning by early adulthood. Individuals with a dependent personality disorder exhibit at least five of the characteristics identified in the DSM-IV. See Medical Diagnoses and Related Nursing Diagnoses: Cluster C Personality Disorders for avoidant and dependent personality disorders.

Obsessive-Compulsive Personality Disorder

The essential feature of **obsessive-compulsive personality disorder** is a preoccupation with orderliness and perfectionism developing by early adulthood. People with this disorder exert emotional as well as interpersonal control in relationships, at the expense of flexibility, openness, and efficiency. In Case Example 27–3, Martin demonstrates behavioral and emotional traits consistent with obsessive-compulsive personality disorder.

Additionally, people with this disorder exhibit at least four of the following behaviors:

- Preoccupation with details, rules, lists, order, organization, or schedules, to the extent that the major reason for an activity is lost
- Perfectionism that interferes with task completion. An example might be a student who has difficulty completing papers in a timely fashion because she expects herself to read every available reference. The student is demonstrating perfectionism that interferes with task completion.
- Excessive devotion to work and productivity to the exclusion of leisure activities and friendships
- Overconscientious, scrupulous, and inflexible belief system about morality, ethics, or values that is not part of the person's cultural or religious affiliation
- Inability to discard worn-out or worthless objects even

MEDICAL DIAGNOSES AND RELATED NURSING DIAGNOSES

Cluster C Personality Disorders

DSM-IV Diagnosis: Avoidant Personality Disorder

Diagnostic Criteria

A. A pervasive pattern of social inhibition, feelings of inadequacy, and hypersensitivity to negative evaluation, beginning by early adulthood and present in a variety of contexts, as indicated by four (or more) of the following:

1. Avoids occupational activities that involve significant interpersonal contact, because of fears of criticism, disapproval, or rejection.
2. Is unwilling to get involved with people unless certain of being liked.
3. Shows restraint within intimate relationships because of the fear of being shamed or ridiculed.
4. Is preoccupied with being criticized or rejected in social situations.
5. Is inhibited in new interpersonal situations because of feelings of inadequacy.
6. Views self as socially inept, personally unappealing, or inferior to others.
7. Is unusually reluctant to take personal risks or to engage in any new activities because they may prove embarrassing.

Related Nursing Diagnoses	Definition	Example
Anxiety	A vague, uneasy feeling whose source is often nonspecific or unknown to the individual	Anxiety related to fear that no one will accept the patient in a social setting as evidenced by preoccupation with potential embarrassing incidents that may occur, verbalizations of feelings of inferiority, fear, and apprehensiveness

Based on information from the *Diagnostic and Statistical Manual of Mental Disorders. Fourth Edition.* Copyright 1994 American Psychiatric Association. Nursing diagnoses and definitions from North American Nursing Diagnosis Association. (1999). *NANDA nursing diagnoses: Definitions and classification 1999-2000.* Philadelphia: NANDA.

Box continued on following page

when she has no reason (such as sentimental value) to hold on to these objects
• Reluctance to delegate tasks or to work with others unless they acquiesce to doing the assignment exactly as directed
• Hoarding money for the future and frugality when spending money on self or others
• Rigidity and stubborn thoughts and behavior

■ CASE EXAMPLE 27–3
■ Martin's Story

Martin is a 33-year-old computer programmer. He is known for being accurate, a perfectionist, and a person who is detail oriented. He often is critical of others as well as himself and believes that criticism "drives progress and competence." Martin spends most of his time at work because he is concerned about doing a superior job and because of the nature of his work (he says "one cannot do a half-baked job").

Martin has a girlfriend, Lilly, a nurse he met when he was working on a program for the local hospital's computer information department. Lilly claims that Martin is stingy with his time and financial resources; "He saves everything; he doesn't spend on himself either." Lilly complains that Martin and she have never had a vacation, as Martin can never see the "right" break in his work projects to get away. "I can barely get him to relax on a Saturday evening!"

Martin's subordinates say he "micromanages" their projects. His behavior causes resentment, and at times they "forget to do part of the project, because Martin will only do it over; let him do it in the first place!" Martin does not spend much time with his family. He feels out of place, as he views his siblings and parents as "emotionally charged." Martin feels the best way to deal with feelings is to think through the issues and "go on with life." Martin follows the rules of his religion but expresses no emotional commitment, nor does his spirituality seem to provide him with a sense of joy—only boundaries. ■

What do you think? Are there some occupations that are more suited to individuals who have cluster C personality disorders?

▶ *Check Your Reading*
13. State one characteristic of each of the cluster C personality disorders.

MEDICAL DIAGNOSES AND RELATED NURSING DIAGNOSES

Cluster C Personality Disorders Continued

DSM-IV Diagnosis: Dependent Personality
Disorder

Diagnostic Criteria

A. A pervasive and excessive need to be taken care of that leads to submissive and clinging behavior and fears of separation, beginning by early adulthood and present in a variety of contexts, as indicated by five (or more) of the following:

1. Has difficulty making everyday decisions without an excessive amount of advice and reassurance from others.

2. Needs others to assume responsibility for most major areas of his or her life.

3. Has difficulty expressing disagreement with others because of fear of loss of support or approval. **Note:** Do not include realistic fears of retribution.

4. Has difficulty initiating projects or doing things on his or her own (because of a lack of self-confidence in judgment or abilities rather than a lack of motivation or energy).

5. Goes to excessive lengths to obtain nurturance and support from others, to the point of volunteering to do things that are unpleasant.

6. Feels uncomfortable or helpless when alone because of exaggerated fears of being unable to care for himself or herself.

7. Urgently seeks another relationship as a source of care and support when a close relationship ends.

8. Is unrealistically preoccupied with fears of being left to take care of himself or herself.

Related Nursing Diagnosis	Definition	Example
Fear	Feeling of dread related to an identifiable source, which the person validates	Fear related to the anticipated loss of a parent as evidenced by increased questioning of the medical staff as to when the parent may die, hypervigilance about the parent's vital signs, refusal to leave the parent's side, and statements of concern regarding self-care after parent's death
Self-Esteem Disturbance	Negative self-evaluation or feelings about self or self-capabilities, which may be directly or indirectly expressed	Self-Esteem Disturbance related to relationship problems with spouse as evidenced by the patient describing self as unable to deal with conflict in the marriage, expressed guilt feelings and shame about marital discord, and extreme sensitivity to criticism by spouse and other family members
Personal Identity Disturbance	Inability to distinguish between self and nonself	Personal Identity Disturbance related to recent breakup of relationship with a significant other as evidenced by constant statements like "I'm nothing without him" and difficulty discussing self without mentioning the significant other as if he or she were part of self

NURSING PROCESS

Assessment

When working with patients who have personality disorders, the assessment must include questions regarding the patient's perception of self and others, expression of emotions, interaction with others, and patterns of relating, emotions, behavior, and thought. You need to determine whether these patterns are stable and occur over time. Examples of assessment questions appear in Box 27-1.

In addition to the questions that specifically identify a personality disorder, also assess the patient's spiritually to determine whether the patient is able to gain a sense of meaning out of life's experiences. Does the patient believe that life has purpose? Does the patient have a relationship with God? How does this relationship affect daily life? Does the patient experience comfort from spiritual beliefs? If so, what beliefs? Does the patient interpret failures and interpersonal difficulties according to a relationship or lack of relationship with God? Does spirituality assist the patient in dealing with life's difficulties? Is there anything that you might assist with in addressing spirituality for this patient?

Box 27-1 ■ ■ ■ ■ ■

Questions for Assessing Patients With Behavior Disorders

Thinking and Views of the World

Do you often find that you have different views of the world than most people? What are those ideas?

Suspiciousness

Do you ever think that others are trying to harm you in some way? Do you think that you are always the one getting the bad end of the bargain?

Affect—Anger

Are you often angry? What is your behavior like when you are angry? Do you become aggressive and at times get into physical fights? Do you ever feel like hurting or killing anyone? Have you ever been in trouble with the law?

Affect—Expression

Are you often very emotional? Has anyone ever told you that you are cold and do not show any emotions? Has anyone ever told you that you are seeking attention?

Impulsive Behavior

Do you ever become impulsive and maybe drink to excess, use illegal substances, or have sex on impulse with someone you do not know well?

Suicidal or Self-Mutilating Behavior

Have you ever been suicidal? Are you suicidal now? Have you ever hurt yourself by cutting or burning yourself? Do you do that now? When does this occur?

Relationships—Significant Other

Tell me about your relationships with others. Are you married, or do you have a significant other? What is that relationship like? Are you able to make decisions jointly? Do you often have arguments? What are these arguments about? Do you have any fears that your spouse or partner will have an affair? Do you ever think about having an affair?

Relationships—Family

What is your relationship like with your family? How do you get along with your children? How often do you see your parents and siblings? What is your relationship like with your parents and siblings?

Relationships—Work

How do you get along with your boss? Do you have any friends at work?

Relationships—Friends

Do you have any friends? How often do you visit with them? What activities do you do together?

Socialization

What types of socializing do you do? Do you enjoy these events, or do you become anxious and unable to participate comfortably?

Recurrent Patterns of Behavior

Do you find that you have had some of the same problems over the years? What have these problems been like? When did they start? Do you identify any patterns to these problems?

Diagnosis

The DSM-IV diagnoses suggest patterns in cognition, affect, interpersonal functioning, and impulse control that determine related nursing diagnoses. A patient with dependent personality disorder, for example, is likely to experience fear related to possible loss.

➤ *Check Your Reading*

14. State one question that you could ask a patient regarding his or her perception of self and others.
15. How would you determine that a patient demonstrated an enduring pattern of inflexible behavior?
16. Give one example of an assessment question that you might ask to determine the quality of a patient's relationships.

Outcome Identification

Expected outcomes are based on nursing diagnoses. Examples of outcomes and goals are listed in Table 27–1.

Planning

The planning phase of the nursing process consists of several parts: selecting the nursing interventions to meet the identified goals and collaborating with everyone involved in the patient's care to ensure consistency and commitment to the treatment plan. In planning interventions for the patient with a personality disorder, note that behaviors are stable and of long duration. Change does not occur overnight. Rather, it is gradual and characterized by an uneven course. Patience, forbearance, tolerance, and perseverance are prerequisites when you work with a patient who has a personality disorder.

➤ *Check Your Reading*

17. Identify one patient outcome for Case Examples 27–1 and 27–2.
18. When planning interventions for patients with personality disorders, what must you consider?

Implementation

Interventions for the patient with a personality disorder include counseling, which includes contracting with the patient for behavioral change and providing consistent limit-setting; health teaching regarding issues such as social skills, problem-solving, and risks of promiscuous behaviors; milieu therapy; and psychobiological interventions. Linehan (1993) devised a skill-based, cognitive-oriented program for patients with borderline personality disorder, called Dialectical Behavioral Therapy (DBT). Although Linehan uses a group approach to assist her patients; understanding skill building, as presented by Linehan, has assisted individuals with severe personality disorders to learn to cope with dysfunctional relationship and behavioral patterns.

Counseling and Health Teaching

Developing a therapeutic relationship with the patient is very challenging, sometimes exasperating, yet absolutely essential. These patients can change if they experience care in the context of a relationship with clear boundaries, defined and reinforced limits, and praise. You need to confront manipulation and deal with behavior matter-of-factly rather than punitively. Patients must know that they are valued. Box 27–2 lists general nursing strategies that are part of counseling the patient with a personality disorder.

Health teaching is an important strategy. Frequently, the patient does not know how to interact appropriately. Patients may misread social cues and respond in ways that increase their social isolation. Modeling desired behaviors provides concrete examples. The patient may be engaging in dangerous activities such as excessive alcohol intake, drug use, or promiscuous sexual behavior. Your teaching focuses not only on the risks associated with these behaviors but also on strategies to change these potentially destructive ways of being. Table 27–1 lists appropriate counseling and teaching interventions related to specific nursing diagnoses.

Milieu Therapy

When working with a person who has a personality disorder, you need to maintain not only a structure of activities but also your own personal and professional boundaries. Boundary maintenance is especially important with individuals having antisocial, borderline, histrionic, and narcissistic personality disorders (Smith, Taylor, Keys, & Gornto, 1997). Patients with these conditions may test your boundaries. For example, a patient might ask for a special favor or request that you bend the rules of the unit. Recognizing that the request may not be appropriate, you set a limit on the patient's behavior. If the limit-setting is done with respect and a rationale is offered, the effort may assist the patient to explore a lifelong behavioral pattern. The patient may become momentarily angered by your insistence on realistic boundaries. Patients need truth with empathy to begin to establish internal boundaries for themselves. If, however, limit-setting is perceived as punitive, rigid, or controlling, the patient will not learn from the experience and will repeat the behavior at another time.

Patients with some personality disorders, especially the individual with borderline personality disorder, experience abandonment anxiety when they are concerned that someone significant in their lives is leaving them. This is important to consider when the nurse establishes a therapeutic relationship with a patient. It is important to let the patient know when you are scheduled off duty or will be taking some time off for a vacation. Often, the patient may need something concrete to remind her that the nurse is returning to continue the therapeutic relationship. This item is known as a transitional object. Some examples of therapeutic transitional objects are an appointment card or a written assignment (written in the nurse's writing) (Cardasis, Hochman, & Silk, 1997; Gunderson, 1996).

Another important issue is the provision of safety, not only for the patient but also for other patients and staff members. The personality disorders most likely seen in inpatient settings include borderline, antisocial, and paranoid personality disorders. Individuals with these

T A B L E 2 7 – 1 Nursing Process Related to Findings Common in Personality Disorders

NURSING DIAGNOSIS	EXPECTED OUTCOMES	SHORT-TERM GOALS	INTERVENTIONS
Anxiety related to fear that no one will accept the patient in a social setting as evidenced by preoccupation with embarrassing incidents that may occur, verbalized feelings of inferiority in social settings, and signs of fear and apprehension	Patient will be able to recognize events that increase the feelings of apprehension and fear. Patient will experience less anxiety. Patient will be able accurately to interpret environmental stimuli in a social setting.	Patient will identify examples of embarrassing incidents and will plan methods to cope with these possible events. Assist the patient to interpret the environmental stimuli in the therapy room.	Ask the patient to pick another place, one with greater comfort. Ask the patient to interpret the environmental stimuli in that setting. Ask the patient to identify some of the similarities and differences in these environments. Ask the patient to compare similarities and differences between the comfortable setting and the social setting most feared. Teach the patient strategies such as deep breathing and relaxation techniques to decrease anxiety.
		Patient will be able to recognize events that increase the feelings of apprehension and fear.	Ask the patient to list several events in social settings that cause anxiety and fear. Discuss each incident to determine what the patient is thinking while experiencing anxiety. Teach the patient that negative thoughts increase feelings of anxiety and fear. Discuss other thoughts that could be used to assist the patient in feeling less anxious (e.g., use of positive affirmations). Discuss the benefits of spiritual interventions to decrease anxiety and fear.
		Patient will identify examples of embarrassing incidents and will plan methods to cope with these possible events.	Assist the patient in making a list of examples of embarrassing incidents feared in a social setting. Discuss how these incidents may occur. Discuss methods to avoid the embarrassing incidents. Discuss new ways to deal with embarrassing incidents that might occur. Teach the patient to recognize how negative thinking patterns may inflate perceptions of the incident. Use affirmations or prayer when these negative thought patterns occur.

Continued on following page

disorders have the potential to cause upheaval, disruption, and even violence on a unit. Dyckoff, Goldstein, and Schacht-Levine (1996) discussed using contracting with group of patients with borderline personality disor-der to reduce self-mutilating behavior. Using behavioral contracting is also useful with patients who demonstrate suicidal ideation and aggressive behavior (Marcus, 1995). Behavioral contracts provide a clear expectation of what

T A B L E   2 7 – 1   Nursing Process Related to Findings Common in Personality Disorders *Continued*

NURSING DIAGNOSIS	EXPECTED OUTCOMES	SHORT-TERM GOALS	INTERVENTIONS
Risk for Violence: Self-Directed related to history of cutting self when highly emotional as evidenced by patient's verbalization that she has been abandoned by her boyfriend and her verbalization that she is experiencing feelings of unreality	Patient will no longer self-mutilate.	Patient will be able to identify cues that usually occur before her self-mutiliating behavior. Patient will identify support systems that can assist her to prevent self-mutilating behavior.	Discuss how the patient self-mutilates, how long she has been doing this, and how she feels before and after cutting herself. Ask the patient to keep a journal and write her thoughts and feelings about subjects that are important to her emotionally. Ask her to include any thoughts or feelings that occur before self-mutilation. Discuss whether the patient becomes "spacey" or "numb" before cutting herself. Examine the patient's feelings of abandonment by her boyfriend. Help the patient identify being with another person as a way of decreasing the urge to self-mutilate. Help patient state that she can call a friend when feeling upset or "numb." Contract with the patient about going to a friend or family member's house when disturbed to defuse the intensity of the feelings. Encourage the patient to take a bath to sooth self and as a means of decreasing the urge to self-mutilate. Contract with the patient for safety so that the patient will call the nurse if she is unable to decrease the urge to self-mutilate.

types of behavioral patterns are unacceptable during times of stress and anxiety.

Psychobiological Interventions

Psychobiological interventions involve a collaborative relationship with a physician, nurse practitioner, or advanced practice psychiatric nurse specialist who may prescribe medications to help patients with personality disorders. The pharmacotherapeutic treatment of a patient with a personality disorder is symptomatic. Soloff, George, and Cornelius (1991) studied the use of psychotropic agents with patients diagnosed with borderline personality disorder, schizotypal personality disorder, and both disorders in a mixed presentation. The researchers found that haloperidol was helpful in improving global functioning; in decreasing schizotypal symptoms, depression, and hostility; and in improving impulse control. Unstable patients with borderline per-

sonality disorder demonstrated a strong response to amitriptyline for hostility and lack of impulse control, with a near significant effect on subjective feelings of depression (Soloff et al., 1991).

For patients demonstrating out-of-control or violent behavior, Keltner and Folks (1993) suggested either an oral anxiolytic or a medication from the sedative-hypnotic class. If the patient cannot take an oral agent, these clinicians recommended intravenous or intramuscular sedative-hypnotics, such as barbiturates, benzodiazepines such as diazepam, or antipsychotics such as haloperidol. Patients who exhibit agitated or psychotic behavior may respond to a neuroleptic medication.

Patients who demonstrate depression as well as a personality disorder may benefit from either a tricyclic antidepressant or a selective serotonin reuptake inhibitor (SSRI). The SSRIs are more expensive than the tricyclics, and the cost may be prohibitive to some patients. Monitor a patient on an antidepressant for suicidal

T A B L E 2 7 – 1 Nursing Process Related to Findings Common in Personality Disorders *Continued*

NURSING DIAGNOSIS	EXPECTED OUTCOMES	SHORT-TERM GOALS	INTERVENTIONS
Risk for Violence: Directed at Others related to patient's history of aggression, physical fights with others, and use of a weapon as evidenced by lack of remorse and verbalizations that he is justified in wanting to hurt his coworker for getting a raise and a promotion	Patient will not harm self or others.	Patient will identify alternatives to violence. Patient will give his gun to an exchange program (e.g., Guns for Money). The patient will identify other nonviolent behaviors that he can use when he feels like harming others.	Contract with the patient that he will use neither verbal nor physical threats while receiving treatment. Contract with the patient so that the patient will isolate himself in a safe room and try to determine other means of communicating his needs rather than verbal or physical aggression. In his next counseling session, discuss any verbally aggressive incidents with the patient. Locate an exchange program offered by the local police or a local business. If there is no program, have the patient agree to give any weapons to a significant person for safe keeping until he can locate a program. Discuss using a quiet but safe room to "cool off." Identify thought patterns that maintain the patient's anger. Discuss alternative thoughts the patient may use when he realizes he is ruminating about the situation that caused him to feel like harming someone. Assist the patient in thinking of new ways to voice his needs rather than using aggressive means.

ideation and the possibility of an overdose. The probability of completed suicide with an overdose of an SSRI is lower than that with a tricyclic; a tricyclic overdose could cause cardiac toxicity.

Your role is to monitor patients on medications for side effects and to teach patients about medications. This education assists in patient compliance. If the medications are an adjunct to psychotherapy, patients with personality disorders can become more functional.

What do you think? In the current managed care environment, how do you think a patient with a personality disorder fares with six to eight authorized visits?

➤ *Check Your Reading*

19. Give an example of counseling as a nursing intervention.
20. How can limit-setting encourage patient learning?

Evaluation

The evaluation stage of the nursing process helps you determine whether the patient has achieved the expected patient outcomes. The formative evaluation involves examining each short-term goal and comparing the patient's current thought pattern and behavior with the outcome criteria. For example, if the expected outcome is that the patient will determine other nonviolent behaviors that he can use when feeling like harming his coworkers, the current patient status might demonstrate that the patient has discussed with his boss going on a work detail or obtaining a transfer to another department. Or the patient might have chosen to stay away physically from his coworker, to prevent an aggressive act toward his coworker. If this patient decides on a strategy he can feel comfortable executing, he will successfully avoid an aggressive confrontation with his coworker. This process allows you to conclude in the summative evaluation that the expected outcome was achieved.

If, however, the formative evaluation demonstrates

Nursing Interventions Specific to Personality Disorder

What do you need to do to develop a relationship with a patient suffering with a personality disorder?

- Approach the patient with warmth and a quiet demeanor and without judging her behavioral patterns in a negative manner.
- Become aware of your own reactions to the patient's behavior; when feeling negative or very positive toward the patient, try to identify the behavioral pattern that generated the feeling inside of you. Evaluate whether you are reactive to this type of behavior and whether it would be in the patient's best therapeutic interests to receive direct feedback.
- Obtain clinical supervision to deal with the feelings toward the patient and discuss ways to approach the patient.
- Approach the patient with patience, persistence, consistency, flexibility, and trust.
- Present a direct and matter-of-fact approach; particularly when confronting the patient or providing limit-setting on a patient's behavior.
- Model appropriate problem-solving, interpersonal, and social skills.
- Reinforce appropriate behaviors; set clear limits when behaviors violate social or milieu norms.
- Encourage the patient to verbalize his or her feelings and thoughts.
- Encourage responsibility and accountability for his or her behavior.
- Establish clear and meaningful rules, regulations, and consequences.
- Contract for behavioral changes, such as prevention of aggressive and self-destructive behavioral patterns.

What do you need to assess regarding the patient's health status?

- Suicidal risk and self-destructive thoughts and behaviors.
- Aggressive and violent behavioral patterns.
- Impulsive behaviors, such as substance abuse, having several different sexual partners, shop lifting, reckless driving, binge eating.
- Use of substances (such as alcohol, marijuana, cocaine) to decrease anxiety or intense emotions.
- Affect responses, level of mood lability, anger, anxiety, apathy, denial of feelings, guilt, blame toward others, vengeful ideas or plans.
- Physiological responses, including gastrointestinal disturbances, appetite changes, self-mutilation, panic attacks.
- Cognitive responses, including repetitive thoughts about how difficult life is; self-blame; and blaming others. Are there suspicious thought patterns?
- Behavioral responses, including suicidal or self-mutilating behavior; aggressive behavior; impulsive behavior. Consistent difficulty relating to others.

- Response to and compliance with medication regiment and reasons for noncompliance; delayed effectiveness; side effects of the medications.
- Degree of social support.
- Knowledge level; ability and readiness to learn about the personality disorder and subsequent behavioral and thought patterns.
- Concurrent medical and psychiatric conditions.

What do you need to teach the patient and the patient's caregiver?

- Behavioral patterns that are part of the personality disorder so that the patient and family can begin to determine limits and realistic expectations.
- What to do when the patient exhibits suicidal ideation and may attempt suicide.
- What to do when the patient self-mutilates.
- What to do if the patient becomes angry and potentially violent.
- How to help the patient recognize his responsibility in his own day-to-day living.
- When to utilize community resources, such as the suicide hot line.
- When to call the therapist or take the patient to the emergency room for possible admission to an inpatient program.
- What symptoms the medications should decrease.

What skills will you want the patient and the caregiver to demonstrate?

- Ability to enter into a no-harm contract and remain safe.
- Ability to follow the medication and treatment plan.
- Ability to set limits that are based on therapeutic value rather than angry or negative feelings toward the patient.
- Ability on the part of the patient to give the rationale for the limits that are set by the therapist and family members.
- Ability on the part of the patient to identify some of his feelings as he relates to others.
- Ability on the part of the patient and caretakers to discuss realistic expectations of each other.
- Ability on the part of the patient to learn new coping patterns when feeling anxious or abandoned.

What other health professionals might need to be a part of this plan of care?

- Psychiatrist, advanced practice nurse psychotherapist, clinical social worker, or psychologist who is usually in charge of the overall treatment plan.
- Psychiatrist and an advanced practice nurse psychotherapist who is in charge of the medication management.
- Social worker to assist with access to community supports; insurance issues; access to entitlements; connection with community-based treatments.

B o x 2 7 – 2 ■ ■ ■ ■ ■
General Nursing Strategies Necessary in Counseling Patients With Personality Disorders

- Constant awareness of your own reactions to patient's behavior
- Supervision to deal with your feelings toward the patient
- Patience, persistence, consistency, flexibility, and trust
- A direct and matter-of-fact approach in confronting behavior
- Modeling appropriate problem-solving, interpersonal, and social skills
- Reinforcing appropriate behaviors
- Setting clear limits
- Encouraging verbal expression of feelings
- Encouraging responsibility and accountability
- Assisting the patient to delay gratification
- Establishing clear rules, regulations, and consequences
- Contracting for behavioral changes

that the short-term goals and expected outcomes were not accomplished, you are motivated to revisit the entire nursing process. Ask yourself whether the assessment was complete, the diagnoses accurate, and the plan adequate to achieve the identified outcomes. If not, modifications are made, and the process continues (Snapshot: Nursing Interventions Specific to Personality Disorder).

NURSING'S JOURNEY WITH PATIENTS WITH PERSONALITY DISORDERS

As you work with patients diagnosed with personality disorders, you may find yourself questioning your own skills, abilities, and limits of tolerance for difficult patients. Feelings of frustration are to be expected when you work with this population. Such feelings, however, need to be dealt with through supervision, if you are to remain a caring and holistic provider.

Your own spirituality can be affected when you work with patients who challenge your sense of competence. You may struggle with finding the answer to why you are not as effective as you would like to be with these patients. Talking about your own feelings, your frustrations, and your insecurities diffuses your tension and allows you to stay connected to the patient and maintain your own spiritual well-being. You may find that spiritual interventions such as prayer help you keep your perspective on healing. You are not responsible for a patient's healing. You are responsible for caring and providing the best that you have to offer. You can act as a healing presence and guide in a life troubled by personality disorder; you cannot accept responsibility for how the person chooses to conduct his or her journey (Ens, 1998).

NURSING PROCESS APPLICATION

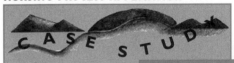

CASE STUDY

Nancy

Nancy, a 25-year-old single woman, is admitted to the inpatient psychiatric unit where you work because she recently lost her job and told her psychotherapist that she was going to kill herself. She lives alone in an apartment, has minimal support systems, and in the past few weeks began feeling suicidal and cut her wrists. She has exhibited self-mutilative behavior by cutting the top of her forearms. Nancy has two younger sisters. She reports that she was sexually abused by her father when she was in her teens and that her mother is a drug addict. Her parents divorced 15 years ago.

While taking her history, you find that Nancy has a long history of mental illness. When she was 13 years old, she was first admitted to an adolescent psychiatric unit and had two other admissions since that time. Nancy is visibly upset about this hospitalization and says to you "I am a failure; I can't do anything right."

Within a few days, the staff observes that the self-mutilation behavior has escalated; the verbalizations of suicide have also escalated. During a staff meeting you find that the unit manager and many of the nurses and the mental health technicians are very sympathetic with Nancy, while the psychiatrist and social workers and some of the nurses consider her behaviors manipulative.

The evening staff nurse reports that Nancy and one of the male patients, Jimmy, are spending all their free time together. Nancy tells you that she is in love with Jimmy, even though they have known each other for a short time. You also note that her emotions range widely within a span of a few moments, from being elated and laughing to crying hysterically.

ASSESSMENT	Assessment data are as follows:

- Suicidal ideation
- Self-mutilation behavior (cutting the tops of her forearms)
- Splitting behaviors evidenced by staff's reaction to patient
- Development of impulsive, intense relationship with male patient
- Minimal support system
- Emotional instability
- Verbalizations of failure

DIAGNOSIS	**DSM-IV Diagnosis:**	Borderline Personality Disorder
	Nursing Diagnosis:	Ineffective Individual Coping related to sudden loss of job and minimal support system as evidenced by staff-splitting behaviors, verbal manipulation, and self-destructive behavior

OUTCOME IDENTIFICATION, PLANNING, AND IMPLEMENTATION

Expected Outcome 1: By _____ the patient will be able to express a consistent, congruent response to staff with no evidence of splitting (idealizing or devaluing staff members).

Short-Term Goals	Nursing Interventions	Rationales
By _____ the patient will demonstrate significant reduction in extreme responses toward staff.	1. Convey an accepting attitude to the patient. Be honest and keep promises.	1. Trust is an issue for clients with borderline personality disorder; congruence in the nurse's behavior is of paramount importance.
	2. Gently challenge the patient's idealistic views with realistic responses.	2. Challenging the patient in a gentle manner will help correct distortions and decrease the incidence of splitting.
	3. Encourage the patient's participation in therapeutic groups.	3. In light of their inherent nature and purpose, groups decrease splitting because it will be confronted as the group works through the stages of group process.
By _____ the patient will express a realistic view of the staff and significant others in her life.	1. Challenge the patient's tendency to devalue others by setting firm limits similar to parents' need to set loving, firm limits for their children.	1–2. Patients often need assistance in the form of firm limit-setting to change an entrenched behavior.
	2. Encourage the patient to look for positive and negative features in staff and significant others.	
	3. Encourage the patient to share observations in a group setting.	3–4. Group formats can help the patient develop more constructive responses to significant others in her life.
	4. Teach the patient ways of centering self so that feedback can be nonthreatening.	

Expected Outcome 2: By _____ the patient will verbalize a desire to curtail manipulation as a way of getting needs met.

Short-Term Goals	Nursing Interventions	Rationales
By _____ the patient will express needs directly.	1. Give the patient support for direct, clear communication.	1. Patients are often rewarded for manipulative communication in their families of origin; positive support leads to an increase in positive behaviors.
	2. Assign the same staff members each shift and encourage all staff members to follow the treatment plan.	2. Consistent staff assignment will sharply decrease the patient's ability to split staff.

3. Do not argue, rationalize, or bargain with the patient.

4. Do not assume that all physical complaints are necessarily invalid.
5. Investigate any medical complaints; if they are invalid, redirect the patient.

6. Assure the patient that her needs will be met without her resorting to manipulation.

By _____ the patient will exhibit congruent verbal and nonverbal messages.

1. Have the patient practice clear, nonmanipulative communication with staff and group members.
2. Give the patient feedback regarding your observations.
3. Be consistent in your own verbal and nonverbal messages.
4. Praise the patient for engaging in behaviors that are free from manipulation and that indicate consideration and respect for others.

3. The patient may invite this behavior by her actions, but you are the professional and are expected to be an expert in clear, congruent communication.
4–5. The patient may have legitimate complaints, and they must be thoroughly evaluated, but continuing to engage in discussion regarding invalid complaints will negatively reward the patient.
6. This will reduce the incidence of manipulative behaviors.

1–2. Behaviors that are positively reinforced are likely to be repeated.

3. It is important for the nurse to provide mature role modeling.

Expected Outcome 3: By _____ the patient will verbalize a desire to continue on her life journey and cease verbalizations of self-destructive behavior.

Short-Term Goals	Nursing Interventions	Rationales
The patient will remain safe while in the hospital.	1. Assess degree of suicidality. 2. Implement suicide precautions—create a safe environment for the patient. 3. Formulate a short-term contract with the patient stating that she will not harm herself. 4. Renew contract as necessary. 5. Have the patient promise that she will seek out a staff member if the desire to harm herself arises.	1–2. Safety is a number-one priority for any patient with suicidal ideation. 3–4. Patients often are relieved to discuss suicidal feelings openly and feel supported by the strength of the staff member. Contracting to ask for assistance from a trusted staff member will decrease ambivalence and promote the decision to live rather than to die. 5. This action further supports the notion that the patient is a valued human being.
By _____ the patient will verbalize hope for her future.	1. Spend uninterrupted time with the patient and *listen* to her. 2. Encourage verbalization of honest feelings. 3. Ask the patient what has kept her from hurting herself in the past. 4. Encourage the patient to express any angry feelings and to get to the true source of her feelings.	1–2. Patients who have enough emotional pain to consider suicide benefit from uninterrupted time with a caring person. 3. This question assists the patient in remembering her strengths and support system. 4. Suicide and other self-destructive behaviors often are considered a result of anger turned inward.

Nursing Diagnosis: Risk for Self-Directed Violence related to history of sexual and emotional abuse as evidenced by cutting on forearms, inability to cope, and widely fluctuating emotions

OUTCOME IDENTIFICATION, PLANNING, AND IMPLEMENTATION

Expected Outcome 1: By _____ the patient will verbalize that her desire to self-mutilate has subsided.

Short-Term Goals	Nursing Interventions	Rationales
By _____ the patient will be able to identify and label positive and negative feelings.	1. Listen and encourage the patient to express her feelings openly and honestly. 2. Educate the patient that feelings are neither right nor wrong, good nor bad. 3. Encourage the patient to identify feelings of anxiety.	1–2. Patients often feel overloaded with all their feelings and need to learn ways to recognize basic feelings of sadness, happiness, pain, fear, and anger. 3. Self-mutilating behaviors often are accompanied by high levels of anxiety.
By _____ the patient will be able to connect the desire to self-mutilate with escalating anxiety levels.	1. Have the patient keep a journal of feelings or ask staff members for help when anxiety begins to escalate. 2. Encourage the patient to employ diversional measures such as journal-writing, walking, or anger work to deal with the desire to self-mutilate. 3. If the patient does engage in any form of self-mutilation, care for the wounds in a matter-of-fact manner. 4. Administer antianxiety medications as needed.	1–2. When the desire to self-mutilate occurs, engaging in some type of therapeutic activity is important. 3. Lack of attention to the maladaptive behavior may decrease its use as a coping mechanism. 4. Antianxiety medications are an appropriate short-term measure to deal with disabling anxiety and will foster patient compliance in the treatment plan.
By _____ the patient will be able demonstrate two new methods to reduce anxiety.	1. Teach at least four stress-reduction measures and have the patient demonstrate them. 2. Share the patient's accomplishments with other members of the team through the care plan.	1. The patient needs some alternative measures other than manipulation or self-mutilation for dealing with overwhelming feelings. 2. All staff members need to reinforce positive behaviors.

Expected Outcome 2: By _____ the patient will sign a contract not to engage in any further self-mutilating behavior.

Short-Term Goals	Nursing Interventions	Rationales
By _____ the patient will agree to talk to a staff member if the desire to self-mutilate arises.	1. Observe the patient's behavior frequently, but avoid appearing suspicious. 2. Secure a verbal contract from the patient indicating that she will talk to a staff member before engaging in any self-mutilating behavior. 3. Remove all dangerous objects from the patient's environment.	1–3. Patient safety is always a nursing priority. Verbal contracts support the patient's need to take positive action rather than engaging in a self-destructive act.
By _____ the patient will acknowledge the need to work through memories of childhood abuse to assist in decreasing painful repressed memories.	1. As the patient is ready, encourage her to share painful, repressed memories of abuse. 2. Remain nonjudgmental and nonreactive in your response to the patient when she is sharing. 3. Inform the patient that it is not necessary to recover every detail to feel better and that if remembering is more distressing than not remembering at this time, she should trust her own judgment.	1. Sharing painful memories often decreases anxiety. 2. Overreacting to the patient's pain, either positively or negatively, may affect her perception. 3. Always afford a patient the opportunity to maintain defenses; the patient must be psychologically ready to be vulnerable and should be allowed to learn to trust herself.

Nursing Diagnosis: Impaired Social Interaction related to disturbance of self-concept and absence of available significant others as evidenced by impulsive intense relationship with a male patient on the unit and a diminished ability to set personal boundaries

OUTCOME IDENTIFICATION, PLANNING, AND IMPLEMENTATION

> **Expected Outcome 1:** By _____ the patient will express feelings toward her male friend that are realistic, with the absence of intense emotions.

Short-Term Goal	Nursing Interventions	Rationales
By _____ the patient will demonstrate calm, consistent emotions when interacting with other patients.	1. Gently confront the patient's beliefs that intense feelings are a necessary part of a relationship. 2. Help the patient understand that intense, violent emotions are more harmful than beneficial to a relationship. 3. Teach the patient ways to increase the time between stimulus and response, such as counting to 10 or slow, deep breathing.	1–2. This patient grew up in a home in which emotions were particularly intense. She needs to know that relationships can thrive in the absence of intensity. 3. This will provide the patient with an opportunity to choose a different, more acceptable response. The patient will be able to set personal boundaries.

> **Expected Outcome 2:** By _____ the patient will be able to set personal boundaries.

Short-Term Goals	Nursing Interventions	Rationales
By _____ the patient will be able to verbalize the need for boundaries.	1. Educate the patient about personal boundaries. 2. Demonstrate how to set boundaries with the patient by maintaining a professional relationship.	1. Setting boundaries requires discipline and practice, and encouragement is needed. 2. Patients with borderline personality disorder frequently will encroach on the boundaries of professionals by asking for extra time or special favors.
By _____ the patient will be able to demonstrate setting boundaries on the unit (both with staff and with other patients).	1. Observe the patient's response in all group interaction on the unit and with her boyfriend. 2. Give the patient feedback about setting realistic boundaries with others.	1. It is not unusual for patients who are not used to setting boundaries to be very rigid with them initially. 2. Give realistic positive feedback for efforts to maintain boundaries.

> **Expected Outcome 3:** By _____ the patient will verbalize three community support systems that will be available to her at discharge.

Short-Term Goal	Nursing Interventions	Rationales
By _____ the patient will have contacted at least one community agency.	1. Have the patient talk with a social worker and her previous therapist to investigate suitable outpatient options. 2. Have the patient place the calls to the identified agencies and set up the appointments.	1. The patient will need help initially in knowing what is available in the community. 2. This will discourage dependence on the staff members.

EVALUATION

Formative Evaluation: Nancy met all of her short-term goals while in the hospital except in regard to her relationship with her boyfriend. He was discharged before her and came to see her every day. She said she was going to move in with him and that he was the "man of her dreams." On occasion, she continued to press the personal boundaries of staff members and showed little evidence of ability to set personal boundaries with her boyfriend.

With the help of group and individual therapy, Nancy stopped using manipulation to get her needs met and no longer engaged in staff-splitting behavior. With the help of anti-anxiety medication and staff support, Nancy stopped the self-mutilation. After 1 week of hospitalization, she no longer talked of suicide and began to express hope for the future. Nancy did acknowledge her need to work through her memories of childhood sexual abuse, and she contacted her previous therapist and set up an appointment before discharge.

Summative Evaluation: By discharge, Nancy had met all expected outcomes except those concerning her relationship with her boyfriend. Her feelings continued to be intense and unrealistic. She fantasized that he was going to take care of all of her problems. The treatment team was concerned that if the relationship began to falter, Nancy would be at risk for self-destructive behaviors again. They recommended she stay in weekly individual therapy.

Conclusions

Working with people with personality disorders is both challenging and rewarding. People who have personality disorders have significant relationship difficulties, including difficulty relating to the psychiatric nurse. Understanding the pattern of the person's behavior provides you insight into the best plan and intervention for the patient. The thoughts and behavior patterns of these patients are long standing. Therefore, you should expect change to occur slowly.

It is critical that you monitor your response to individuals with personality disorders. People with these disorders often are very angry, critical, manipulative, and distant in their interactions. If you react to these affective states emotionally, you may feel devalued and angry. When you intervene from an emotional foundation of anger and a sense of inadequacy, you fail to provide the patient with the opportunity for a different affiliation, a professional relationship based on empathy, problem-solving, and learning new ways of dealing with old issues.

Key Points to Remember

- A person with a healthy personality can relate to others even during periods of stress, frustration, and anger without devaluing the relationship. This person can describe self, identify likes and dislikes and strengths and weaknesses, and experience strong emotions such as joy, happiness, love, anger, and sadness.
- A person with a personality disorder has an enduring pattern of inner experience and behavior that is markedly different from those of that person's culture. This pattern is demonstrated in different ways of perceiving and interpreting self and others.
- In a person with a personality disorder, the range, intensity, lability, and appropriateness of emotional responses differs from the emotions expressed by most people.
- Individuals with personality disorders have problems relating to others, manifested by relationship difficulties at home, at work, and in the community.
- Impulse control is sometimes difficult for people with personality disorders, particularly those who have dramatic personality disorders.
- Mahler identified developmental tasks in relationship to the caretaker. She studied infants and mothers. Current discussions about the development of a personality disorder focus on Mahler's separation-individuation phase of development.
- Research currently is underway to understand the biological components of personality disorders. From that research, new treatment strategies may emerge.
- The DSM-IV has defined the personality disorders on Axis II. These have been separated into clusters of similar types of personality disorders. Cluster A includes odd or eccentric personality disorders such as paranoid, schizoid, and schizotypal personality disorders. Cluster B includes dramatic, emotional, or erratic behaviors exhibited by people with antisocial, borderline, histrionic, or narcissistic personality disorders. Cluster C includes anxious or fearful behavior manifested by people with dependent, avoidant, and obsessive-compulsive personality disorders.
- The nursing process is a cognitive structure that is helpful for preventing the nurse from becoming emotionally reactive to the behavior of a patient with a personality disorder.

Learning Activities

1. Read a novel involving characters who have personality disorders. Examples are Sylvia Plath's (1971) *The Bell Jar* and Judith Rossner's (1975) *Looking for Mr. Goodbar.* Such reading can provide you with insight into the perspective of a person with such a disorder.
2. Read a theoretical book such as Jerold Kreisman and Hal Straus's *I Hate You—Don't Leave Me: Under-* *standing the Borderline Personality* and Janice Cauwels' (1992) *Imbroglio: Rising to the Challenges of Borderline Personality Disorder.* These books provide understanding of the person with borderline personality disorder. They are written in language that is easy to understand and are helpful to share with patients to assist them in identifying with those having similar

behaviors, areas of distress, and the need for interventions promoting positive change.

3. Watch a movie such as *Shoot the Moon* (featuring a man who has borderline personality disorder and alcoholism and a stormy relationship with his wife) or *Fatal Attraction* (featuring a woman with borderline personality disorder who is having an affair with a married man). These stories are helpful in observing how a negative style of relating to others, extreme emotionality, and destructive and possessive behavior cause problems that are chaotic and destructive, both to the person with the disorder and to others.

4. Watch a daytime drama and identify characters who exhibit signs of personality disorders.

5. Search the Internet to obtain information about personality disorders. If you query a search engine for personality disorders, you will find many sites, including sites giving support to family members and individuals with Borderline Personality Disorder.

Critical Thinking Exercise

Jean is a 29-year-old graduate student in criminal justice. While visiting her Aunt McDougal, she slashed her left wrist several times. Frightened, her aunt rushed her to the local hospital's emergency department. There, the nurse's assessment of the lacerations showed several superficial wounds and a laceration that required two stitches. No arteries were punctured. During the interview, Jean told the nurse that she was upset with her psychotherapist and that she had left therapy after 10 years. She was convinced that her therapist's going on vacation was evidence that he did not care about her and was only interested in her money. After the lacerations were sutured, Jean was discharged.

1. What do you think the nurse assumed about Jean's behavior?

2. Suggest possible reasons why Jean was discharged.

3. What are alternative possibilities, besides suicide, to explain Jean's behavior?

When she arrived at her Aunt McDougal's home, she cried to her and said "Those doctors are just like the others, they don't believe me that I really want to die." Upset, Mrs. McDougal called a nurse therapist to talk to Jean. Mrs. McDougal was aware that this was not the first time Jean had attempted suicide. After the nurse therapist saw Jean, she spoke with Mrs. McDougal about her concerns.

1. Put yourself in the nurse therapist's place. What would you tell Mrs. McDougal?

2. What assumptions is Jean making about other people's responses to her cutting attempts?

3. What conclusions can you draw about Jean's behavior?

Additional Resources

Aggression

Listserve@maelstrom.stjohns.edu

Borderline Personality Disorder Support Group

Listserve@maelstrom.stjohns.edu

Cognitive Therapy for Personality Disorders

http://www.mhsource.com/edu/psytimes/p960241.html

Online Screening for Personality Disorders

http:www.med.nyu.edu/Psych/screens/pds.html

Personality and Personality Disorders

http://www.mentalhealth.com/mag1/p5h-per1.htm

References

Akhtar, S. (1992). *Broken structures. Severe personality disorders and their treatments.* Northvale, NJ: Aronson.

Akhtar, S. (1995). *Quest for answers: A primer of understanding and treating severe personality disorders.* Northvale, NJ: Aronson.

American Psychiatric Association. (1994). *Diagnostic and statistical manual of mental disorders* (4th ed.). Washington, DC: Author.

Brown, G. L., Ebert, M. H. M., Goyer, P. F., Jimerson, D. C., Klein, W. J., Barney, W. E., & Goodwin, F. K. (1982). Aggression, suicide and serotonin relationships to CSF amine metabolites. *American Journal of Psychiatry, 139,* 741-745.

Brown, G. L., & Linnoila, M. I. (1990). CSF serotonin metabolite (5-HIAA) studies in depression, impulsivity, and violence. *Journal of Clinical Psychiatry, 51* (Suppl.), 31-43.

Cardasis, W., Hochman, J. A., & Silk, K. R. (1997). Transitional objects and borderline personality disorder. *The American Journal of Psychiatry, 154,* 250-255.

Cauwels, J. M. (1992). *Imbroglio: Rising to the challenges of borderline personality disorder.* New York: Norton.

Constantino, J. N., Morris, J. A., & Murphy, D. L. (1997). CSF 5-HIAA and family history of antisocial personality disorder in newborns. *American Journal of Psychiatry, 154,* 1771–1773.

Coryell, W. H., & Zimmerman, M. B. A. (1989). Personality disorder in the families of depressed, schizophrenic, and never-ill probands. *American Journal of Psychiatry, 146,* 496–502.

Davidson, M., & Davis, K. L. (1988). A comparison of plasma HVA concentrations in schizophrenia patients and normal controls. *Archives of General Psychiatry, 45,* 564–567.

Dyckoff, D., Goldstein, L., & Schacht-Levine, L. (1996). The investigation of behavioral contracting in patients with borderline personality disorder. *Journal of the American Psychiatric Nurses Association, 2*(6), 71–75.

Ens, E. C. (1998). An analysis of the concept of countertransference. *Archives of Psychiatric Nursing, 12,* 273–281.

Erikson, E. H. (1963). *Childhood and society.* New York: Norton.

Gunderson, J. G. (1996). The borderline patient's intolerance of aloneness: Insecure attachments and therapist availability. *American Journal of Psychiatry, 153,* 752–758.

Kavoussi, R. J., & Siever, L. J. (1991). Biologic validators of personality disorders. In J. M. Oldham (Ed.), *Personality disorders: New perspectives on diagnostic validity.* Washington, DC: American Psychiatric Press.

Keltner, N. L., & Folks, D. G. (1993). *Psychotropic drugs.* St. Louis, MO: Mosby-Year Book.

Kreisman, J. J., & Straus, H. (1989). *I hate you—don't leave me: Understanding the borderline personality.* Los Angeles: Body Press.

Lane, R. D., Reiman, E. M., Ahern, G. L., Schartz, G. E., & Davidson, R. J. (1997). Neuroanatomical correlates of happiness, sadness, and disgust. *American Journal of Psychiatry, 154,* 926–933.

Linehan, M. (1993). *Skills training manual for treating borderline personality disorder.* New York: Guilford Press.

Mahler, M. S. (1963). Thoughts about development and individuation. *Psychoanalytic Study of the Child, 18,* 307–324.

Mahler, M. S. (1971). A study of the separation-individuation process and its possible application to borderline phenomena in the psychoanalytic situation. *Psychoanalytic Study of the Child, 26,* 403–424.

Mahler, M. S. (1972a). On the first three subphases of the separation-individuation process. *International Journal of Psychoanalysis, 53,* 333–338.

Mahler, M. S. (1972b). Rapprochement subphase of the separation-individuation process. *Psychoanalytic Quarterly, 41,* 487–506.

Mann, J. J., Stanley, M., McBride, P. A., & McEwen, B. S. (1986). Increased serotonin-2 and beta-adrenergic receptor binding in the frontal cortices of suicide victims. *Archives of General Psychiatry, 43,* 954–959.

Mansfield, P. (1992). *Split self split object: Understanding and treating borderline, narcissistic, and schizoid disorders.* Northvale, NJ: Aronson.

Marcus, P. (1995). *Psychiatric emergencies, module 3: Violence, aggression, and suicide.* St. Louis, MO: Mosby-Year Book.

Maslow, A. (1968). *Toward a psychology of being* (2nd ed.). Princeton, NJ: Norstrand Reinhold.

Plath, S. (1971). *The bell jar.* New York: Harper & Row.

Reiman, E. M., Lane, R. D., Ahern, G. L., Schwartz, G. E., Davidson, R. J., Friston, K. J., Yun, L., & Chen, K. (1997). Neuroanatomical correlates of externally and internally generated human emotion. *American Journal of Psychiatry, 154,* 918–925.

Rossner, J. (1975). *Looking for Mr. Goodbar.* New York: Pocket Books.

Roy, A. (1989). Suicide. In H. I. Kaplan, & B. J. Sudock (Eds.), *Comprehensive textbook of psychiatry* (5th ed.). Baltimore: Williams & Wilkins.

Siever, L. J. (1985). Biologic markers in schizotypal personality disorder. *Schizophrenic Bulletin, 11,* 564–575.

Siever, L. J. (1992). Schizophrenia spectrum personality disorders. In A. Tasman & M. B. Riba (Eds.), *American Psychiatric Press review of psychiatry* (Vol. 11). Washington, D.C.: American Psychiatric Press.

Siever, L. J., & Davis, K. L. (1991). A psychobiological perspective on the personality disorders. *American Journal of Psychiatry, 148,* 1647–1658.

Smith, L. L., Taylor, B. B., Keys, A. T., & Gornto, S. B. (1997). Nurse-patient boundaries crossing: How to recognize signs of professional sexual misconduct and intervene effectively. *American Journal of Nursing, 97*(12), 26–31.

Soloff, P. H., George, A., & Cornelius, J. (1991). Pharmacotherapy and borderline subtypes. In J. M. Oldham (Ed.), *Personality disorders: New perspectives on diagnostic validity.* Washington, DC: American Psychiatric Press.

Stanley, M., & Stanley, B. (1990, April). Postmortem evidence for serotonin's role in suicide. *Journal of Clinical Psychiatry, 51* (Suppl.), 22–27.

Westen, D. (1997). Divergences between clinical and research methods for assessing personality disorders: Implications for research and the evolution of Axis II. *American Journal of Psychiatry, 154,* 895–903.

Suggested Readings

Cardasis, W., Hochman, J. A., & Silk, K. R. (1997). Transitional objects and borderline personality disorder. *The American Journal of Psychiatry, 154,* 250–255.

Cauwels, J. M. (1992). *Imbroglio: Rising to the challenges of borderline personality disorder.* New York: Norton.

Ens, E. C. (1998, October). An analysis of the concept of countertransference. *Archives of Psychiatric Nursing, 12,* 273–281.

Gunderson, J. G. (1996). The borderline patient's intolerance of aloneness: Insecure attachments and therapist availability. *American Journal of Psychiatry, 153,* 752–758.

Houseman, C. (1990). The paranoid person: A biopsychosocial perspective. *Archives of Psychiatric Nursing, 5,* 176–181.

Linehan, M. (1993). *Skills training manual for treating borderline personality disorder.* New York: Guilford Press.

Marin, D., De Meo, M., Frances, A., Kocsis, J., & Mann, J. (1989, March). Biological models and treatments for personality disorders. *Psychiatric Annals, 19,* 143–146.

Valente, S. M. (1991, December). Deliberate self-injury management in a psychiatric setting. *Journal of Psychosocial Nursing, 29,* 19–25.

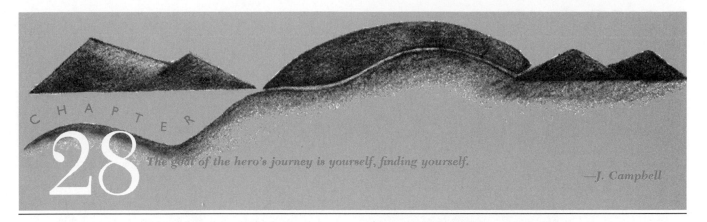

The goal of the hero's journey is yourself, finding yourself.

—*J. Campbell*

Dissociative Disorders

Learning Objectives

After studying this chapter, you should be able to:

1. Describe the behavior of dissociation along a continuum.

2. Identify two events in everyday life that are examples of dissociation.

3. Discuss three major categories of dissociative disorders, as described in *Diagnostic and Statistical Manual of Mental Disorders, Fourth Edition* (DSM-IV).

4. Describe two theories that explain dissociation disorders.

5. Specify one issue that is discussed for the controversy of the diagnosis of a dissociative disorder.

6. Relate three nursing interventions that assist in decreasing the severity of the patient's dissociation symptoms.

Key Terminology

Amnesia	Derealization	Fugue	Identity alteration
Childhood trauma	Dissociation continuum	Hypnosis	Identity confusion
Depersonalization	False memory syndrome		

When we perceive ourselves as being in a state of well-being, peaceful, and mentally healthy, there is a sense of unity of self as a human being with a basic personality. Our thoughts, feelings, and actions are connected and have a sense of continuity, most of the time. Thus, we have a perception of being integrated or whole. Persons with <u>dissociative disorders</u> experience gaps in memory, confusion, and, often, a sense of compartmentalization. This chapter focuses on some of the types of dissociative disorders, associated problematic behaviors, and nursing interventions.

The following example is based on the experiences of a woman manifesting a specific type of dissociative disorder.

 **Charlotte's Story**

A young woman appearing to be in her late 20s or early 30s was brought to the emergency department of a county hospital by police officers who had found her wandering the streets in the downtown area of a large city. The initial concern of the officers was prompted by the woman looking rather dazed and being unaccompanied in an area known for high crime activity. On questioning the woman about her activities, the officers were met with a blank stare and the woman's assertions that she was unaware not only of where she was but also of who she was. She voiced no objections when the police took her to the county hospital.

In the triage area, the woman was dubbed "Madame X" by an attendant who admitted to believing the patient was "faking" or was simply on some kind of drug. Interestingly, the label remained, and the patient seemed to like it, later introducing herself as Madame X to others on arriving on the psychiatric unit. During the assessment by the professional staff, the patient was alert and cooperative. Madame X claimed to have completely lost her memory for all details of her life. Although appearing quite perplexed, she did not give the impression of being distraught. After admission to the psychiatric unit, she appeared fairly comfortable in the milieu. After 2 days on the unit, Madame X was still amnesic. All of the physical findings and laboratory test results were within normal limits, and her drug screen was negative except for the presence of nicotine and caffeine. Because the patient appeared to be in excellent health and had not responded to verbal interventions, a consulting psychiatrist recommended an interview following administration of amobarbital sodium (Amytal Sodium). Madame X readily gave her consent to this procedure, and it was scheduled for the following day. The next morning, the patient's primary nurse accompanied her to the treatment room to offer support and a familiar face. During the interview, the patient responded openly to the questions posed by the psychiatrist. She revealed that her name was Charlotte S. and that she was 32 years old. For the past 4 years she had been living in a common-law relationship with a man several years older than she, about whom she had mixed feelings. Although he could be extremely physically and verbally abusive at times, there were other occasions when he was very "loving."

Charlotte remembered her childhood, adolescence, and young adulthood as being very deprived financially, socially, and emotionally. Her father had deserted the family when she was in the first grade, and she had been told many times by her mother that she was responsible for driving him away because she was such an evil girl who had been "shamed by God." The mother had multiple psychiatric hospitalizations over the years. Charlotte recalled no social support from relatives or others, describing herself as "alone" and "never good enough for anyone to care about." All of her relationships with men had been short-lived, but she had believed this latest one to be destined to last, admitting that she felt no significant anger about the physical, sexual, and verbal abuse she had tolerated from her "lover." About 5 days previously, he had announced that he no longer cared for her and had found another woman he preferred. He was planning to move out of the apartment they had shared for the past 4 years. "I remember feeling in a state of shock—like why was he doing this to me? I think I cried and begged him not to leave, but he did anyway and wouldn't even look at me. I kept hearing these

voices inside my head telling me how I was no good and everything was my fault. I think I left the apartment—maybe to look for him, but I don't remember much else about the police and the hospital."

Charlotte was suffering from a dissociative disorder referred to as *psychogenic amnesia*, most likely precipitated by what would be an event of devastating trauma to her—that of abandonment by someone whom she desperately wanted to believe cared about her. Both her recent and long-term memory were retrieved during the interview, and she experienced no lapses of memory while in the hospital. The major issues that emerged were a rather severe depression that had been dormant for many years, fueled by her low self-esteem.

THE CONCEPT OF DISSOCIATION

Although there was considerable interest in the concept of dissociation as a major defense mechanism in the 19th century, especially before the influence of Freud, concern about dissociative processes seemed to decrease between about 1920 and 1970 (Greaves, 1980).

As a concept for observation and scientific study, dissociation was first formulated by the French physician Pierre Janet (1907). He viewed dissociation as the primary phenomenon that explained the symptoms of hysteria, which typically involved somatic complaints and symptoms that were not supported by physical findings. With the dominant influence of Freudian theory in the latter part of the 19th and most of the 20th century, however, dissociation has been relegated to the position of a secondary defense mechanism to repression.

Freud (1962) viewed dissociation as simply a type of repression employed in the excision of threatening or unacceptable mental contents from conscious awareness. Although Janet pioneered the study of dissociative behaviors in the 1890s, there is debate about the validity of dissociative diagnosis in the literature (Cohen, Berzoff, & Elin, 1995). Opinions vary as to whether dissociation should always be classified as a psychopathological defense. In 1907, Janet first used the term dissociation as it is used today. Working primarily with "hysterical" female patients, who presented with myriad somatic symptoms expressed in a highly dramatic fashion, Janet asserted the mechanism always to be pathological. In Janet's practice, he discovered that his patients often possessed a multiplicity of *egos* or personalities that coexisted within individual women and that these personalities were able to function separately from each other. He described this phenomenon as a dissociative process, occurring because of a "weakening of the synthesizing power of the psyche" (Crabtree, 1992).

Other emerging authorities in the field, however, did not agree with him unanimously. For example, Taylor (1983), Prince (1907, 1914), and Myers (1903) all held that dissociation was a normal human function and that multiplicity, as described by Janet, was simply a fact of everyday life, to varying degrees. Indeed, Myers insisted in his writings in the 1880s and the 1890s that what is thought of as normal "consciousness" is only a small part of the human psyche. Both Myers and Taylor believed that the future of psychological research would be focused on exploring the parts of the human mind that are typically dissociated from our daily consciousness, which were considered the repository of the true richness of human nature.

> **W**hat do you think? Reread Charlotte's story. What is your reaction to her story? How would you respond to Charlotte?

> ➤ *Check Your Reading*
> 1. Who first coined the term *dissociation*?
> 2. How did Freud describe dissociation?

THE DISSOCIATION CONTINUUM

Some contemporary theorists view dissociation as a **continuum** that ranges from minor dissociations of everyday life, such as daydreaming, to the florid symptoms of identity alteration as experienced by Charlotte in the background story. As students in nursing school and other educational settings, most of us have probably experienced the pleasures of daydreaming to escape the drudgery of a boring lecture. Only when we were called on to answer a question were we jolted into the realization that we had a total lack of knowledge about the content presented in the last few minutes or even the last hour, even though we had been physically present in the classroom.

The argument for the adaptive value of dissociation has been promoted by several contemporary theorists, such as Braun and Sachs (1985), Kluft (1984), and Spiegel (1984). An idea central to the construct of dissociation as an adaptive entity is that it exists on a continuum and becomes maladaptive only when it surpasses certain limits in frequency or intensity or occurs in inappropriate contexts that may be harmful to the individual or others. Hilgard (1977) was instrumental in the modern era in advocating the existence of a dissociation continuum ranging from the normal to the pathological. He strongly promoted the idea that everyday life is full of small dissociations if we but look for them.

Merskey (1996) and Frankel (1996) wondered whether there is a scientific basis for the diagnosis of dissociative identity disorder. There is concern that the expectations of clinicians are influenced by the presentation of the symptoms and not by scientific evidence such as genetic or physiological studies to appropriately determine the diagnosis. This viewpoint may be reflected in clinician diagnostic practices. One clinician may evaluate a patient and label the clinical presentation as Dissociative Identity Disorder, whereas another may view the patient as having Borderline Personality Disor-

der, depending on the way the clinician interprets the criterion presented in the DSM-IV. The debate between clinicians can become heated, and more scientific investigation is needed to provide a diagnosis with good inter-rater reliability.

Putnam (1989) described dissociation as pathological when the individual's sense of consciousness, behavior, and identity is fragmented. Contrast this fragmentation of the sense of self with the temporary alteration in consciousness that occurs in daydreaming, "tuning out" of conversations, and "highway hypnosis." These examples on a continuum were supported by surveys conducted by Bernstein and Putnam (1986), using the Dissociative Experiences Scale (DES). The DES is a brief, self-administered questionnaire that asks one to estimate, by marking on a 100 mm line visual analog scale, the frequency with which specific dissociative experiences occur. The DES is shown in Box 28–1. This instrument has demonstrated a high degree of reliability and validity when scores of normal control subjects, people with occasional dissociative episodes, and patients with severe dissociative disorders were compared.

Vaillant (1986) classified dissociation as one of the "neurotic" defenses that are seen in adults under stress and are frequently used by obsessive-compulsive and hysterical persons. His definition of dissociation is

A temporary but drastic modification of character or sense of personal identity to avoid emotional distress; it includes fugue states and hysterical conversion reactions. (p. 25)

Sullivan placed much credence in the dissociative processes in development of the personality or the *self-system* (Marmer, 1994). Theoretically, the development of self-esteem begins in a fairly sequential pattern. What Sullivan referred to as the *good-me* evolved from positive appraisals by others, such as "Johnny is a good boy" or "Jenny is a smart girl." If the child hears genuine favorable comments often and is provided with tenderness and appreciation, these positive appraisals become a significant part of the sense of self. Conversely the *bad-me* reflects negative appraisals by others that are accompanied by increasing levels of anxiety. If barraged with comments such as "You're such a dummy" or "Why are you such a bad girl?" accompanied by varying degrees of rejection and other punishment, these views are also incorporated into one's sense of self. *Not-me* (not of me) is evidenced in *dissociated* behavior, which can be manifested in everyday lapses of consciousness (e.g., daydreaming) or in naturally occurring trance states; as can occur when one drives alone for long stretches on a road surrounded by monotonous terrain (previously referred to as "highway hypnosis"). Most of us have experienced the operation of not-me processes following a nightmare. When awakened, it may be difficult to determine who or where one is. The self-system usually responds quickly, however, and soon the person regains a normal state of consciousness. Viewed on a continuum, the not-me in a more pathological form is experienced in severe mental disorders, including, but not limited to, the dissociative disorders.

In much of the contemporary literature, dissociation is conceptualized as a post-traumatic defense, energized

Directions

This questionnaire consists of 28 questions about experiences that you may have in your daily life. We are interested in how often you have these experiences. It is important, however, that your answers show how often these experiences happen to you when you *are not* under the influence of alcohol or drugs. To answer the questions, please determine to what degree the experience described in the question applied to you and circle the number to show what percentage of the time you have the experience.

Example

0%   10   20   30   40   50   60   70   80   90   100%

1. Some people have the experience of driving a car and suddenly realizing they don't remember what has happened during all or part of the trip. Circle a number to show what percentage of the time this happens to you.

0%   10   20   30   40   50   60   70   80   90   100%

2. Some people find that sometimes they are listening to someone talk and they suddenly realize that they did not hear part or all of what was just said. Circle a number to show what percentage of the time this happens to you.

0%   10   20   30   40   50   60   70   80   90   100%

3. Some people have the experience of finding themselves in a place and having no idea how they got there. Circle a number to show what percentage of the time this happens to you.

0%   10   20   30   40   50   60   70   80   90   100%

4. Some people have the experience of finding themselves dressed in clothes that they don't remember putting on. Circle a number to show what percentage of the time this happens to you.

0%   10   20   30   40   50   60   70   80   90   100%

5. Some people have the experience of finding new things among their belongings that they do not remember buying. Circle a number to show what percentage of the time this happens to you.

0%   10   20   30   40   50   60   70   80   90   100%

6. Some people sometimes find that they are approached by people they do not know who call them by another name or insist that they have met them before. Circle a number to show what percentage of the time this happens to you.

0%   10   20   30   40   50   60   70   80   90   100%

7. Some people sometimes have the experience of feeling as though they are standing next to themselves or watching themselves do something and they actually see themselves as if they were looking at another person. Circle a number to show what percentage of the time this happens to you.

0%   10   20   30   40   50   60   70   80   90   100%

8. Some people are told that they sometimes do not recognize friends or family members. Circle a number to show what percentage of the time this happens to you.

0%   10   20   30   40   50   60   70   80   90   100%

9. Some people find that they have no memory for some important events in their lives (for example, a wedding or graduation). Circle a number to show what percentage of the time this happens to you.

0%   10   20   30   40   50   60   70   80   90   100%

10. Some people have the experience of being accused of lying when they do not think that they have lied. Circle a number to show what percentage of time this happens to you.

0%   10   20   30   40   50   60   70   80   90   100%

11. Some people have the experience of looking in a mirror and not recognizing themselves. Circle a number to show what percentage of the time this happens to you.

0%   10   20   30   40   50   60   70   80   90   100%

Box 28–1 ■ ■ ■ ■ ■
Dissociative Experience Scale *Continued*

12. Some people sometimes have the experience of feeling that other people, objects, and the world around them are not real. Circle a number to show what percentage of the time this happens to you.

0%   10   20   30   40   50   60   70   80   90   100%

13. Some people sometimes have the experience of feeling that their body does not seem to belong to them. Circle a number to show what percentage of the time this happens to you.

0%   10   20   30   40   50   60   70   80   90   100%

14. Some people have the experience of sometimes remembering a past event so vividly that they feel as if they were reliving that event. Circle a number to show what percentage of the time this happens to you.

0%   10   20   30   40   50   60   70   80   90   100%

15. Some people have the experience of not being sure whether things that they remember happening really did happen or whether they just dreamed them. Circle the number to show what percentage of the time this happens to you.

0%   10   20   30   40   50   60   70   80   90   100%

16. Some people have the experience of being in a familiar place but finding it strange and unfamiliar. Circle the number to show what percentage of the time this happens to you.

0%   10   20   30   40   50   60   70   80   90   100%

17. Some people find that they are watching television or a movie they become so absorbed in the story that they are unaware of other events happening around them. Circle the number to show what percentage of the time this happens to you.

0%   10   20   30   40   50   60   70   80   90   100%

18. Some people sometimes find that they become so involved in a fantasy or daydream that it feels as though it were really happening to them. Circle the number to show what percentage of the time this happens to you.

0%   10   20   30   40   50   60   70   80   90   100%

19. Some people find that they sometimes are able to ignore pain. Circle the number to show what percentage of the time this happens to you.

0%   10   20   30   40   50   60   70   80   90   100%

20. Some people find that they sometimes sit staring off into space, thinking of nothing. Circle the number to show what percentage of the time this happens to you.

0%   10   20   30   40   50   60   70   80   90   100%

21. Some people sometimes find that when they are alone they talk out loud to themselves. Circle the number to show what percentage of the time this happens to you.

0%   10   20   30   40   50   60   70   80   90   100%

22. Some people find that in one situation they may act so differently compared with another situation they feel almost as if they were two different people. Circle the number to show what percentage of the time this happens to you.

0%   10   20   30   40   50   60   70   80   90   100%

23. Some people sometimes find that in certain situations they are able to do things with amazing ease and spontaneity that would usually be difficult for them (for example, sports, work, social situations, etc.). Circle the number to show what percentage of the time this happens to you.

0%   10   20   30   40   50   60   70   80   90   100%

24. Some people sometimes find that they cannot remember whether they have done something or have just thought about doing that thing (for example, not knowing whether they have just mailed a letter or having just thought about mailing it). Circle the number to show what percentage of the time this happens to you.

0%   10   20   30   40   50   60   70   80   90   100%

Box continued on following page

B o x 2 8 – l ■ ■ ■ ■ ■
Dissociative Experience Scale *Continued*

25. Some people find evidence that they have done things that they do not remember doing. Circle a number to show what percentage of the time this happens to you.

| 0% | 10 | 20 | 30 | 40 | 50 | 60 | 70 | 80 | 90 | 100% |

26. Some people sometimes find writings, drawings, or notes among their belongings that they must have done but cannot remember doing. Circle the number to show what percentage of the time this happens to you.

| 0% | 10 | 20 | 30 | 40 | 50 | 60 | 70 | 80 | 90 | 100% |

27. Some people sometimes find that they hear voices inside their head that tell them to do things or comment on things that they are doing. Circle a number to show what percentage of the time this happens to you.

| 0% | 10 | 20 | 30 | 40 | 50 | 60 | 70 | 80 | 90 | 100% |

28. Some people sometimes feel as if they are looking at the world through a fog so that people and objects appear far away or unclear. Circle a number to show what percentage of the time this happens to you.

| 0% | 10 | 20 | 30 | 40 | 50 | 60 | 70 | 80 | 90 | 100% |

From Bernstein, E., & Putnam, F. W. (1986). Development of reliability and validity of a dissociative scale. *Journal of Nervous and Mental Disease, 174*(12), 727–735.

by the patient as protection from catastrophic trauma and pain. The tendency to detach oneself from memories, consciousness, and sense of identity is considered a natural response to repeated physical, verbal, and sexual abuse (Butler, Duran, Jasiukaitis, Koopman, & Spiegel, 1996). It is also a frequent response to other overwhelming traumas, including rape, combat, and other life-threatening situations (Steinberg, 1993). Because dissociative experiences occur within a number of psychiatric syndromes, including anxiety, mood disorders, and substance abuse disorders, it is essential that you have a conceptual understanding of dissociation in the journey with the patient, regardless of the path taken.

W*hat do you think?* What situations are you aware of in which dissociation would be a protective mechanism?

➤ *Check Your Reading*
3. Give one example of a minor dissociation associated with normal life.
4. What is the name of the scale used to determine the degree of dissociation experienced by an individual?
5. Identify at least two other psychiatric illnesses that may include dissociative experiences.

THE DETOUR OF PATHOLOGICAL DISSOCIATION

Steinberg (1993) noted that few topics in the mental health–mental illness spectrum have experienced as great a renewal of interest and investigation as the field of dissociation. A number of clinical reports and research studies in this area have accumulated. Also, the increased attention given to the range of childhood abuses resulting in cognitive and affective impairments

has provided impetus for the development of specialized treatment units for patients with dissociative disorders.

Although the dissociative disorders have historically been considered rare, understanding of the dissociation continuum has increased the numbers of patients diagnosed with these disorders (Butler et al., 1996; Cohen et al., 1995; Coons, Bowman, & Milstein, 1988; Franklin, 1990; Lewis, Yeager, Swica, Pincus, & Lewis, 1997; Putnam, 1989). If anything, the number of patients who have symptoms of these disorders is probably underreported because the symptoms frequently elude detection for two major reasons. First, dissociative manifestations may be indistinguishable from symptoms of other psychiatric syndromes, including those of the psychotic, mood, and anxiety disorders. Second, dissociative symptoms frequently are difficult for the patient to verbalize clearly because the patient is detached from his or her memories and sense of identity (Steinberg, 1993). As mentioned earlier, some clinicians will argue that owing to the lack of clarity, the dissociative diagnosis should not be made (Frankel, 1996).

The DSM-IV describes five symptoms considered a hallmark of dissociative disorders:

1. Amnesia
2. Derealization
3. Depersonalization
4. Identity confusion
5. Identity alteration

Variations of these behaviors can occur in persons with other mental health problems or in individuals subjected to overwhelming traumas.

Symptoms of Pathologic Dissociation

Amnesia

Amnesia is usually defined as memory loss related to personal data or events occurring during a specific period of time or even a loss of all past memories. Table 28–1 presents the characteristics of the five major types of amnesia. Some people with severe amnesia related to dissociative disorders frequently experience recurrent memory gaps. Other people are unable to remember their name, age, or activities occurring during specific hours, days, or longer periods of time. For example, a young woman in her 20s stated that her life was a "complete blank" between the ages of 9 and 12. It is crucial to distinguish between the description of amnesia given here and the amnesic behavior or syndrome attributed to specific pathophysiological factors, the most common of which is chronic heavy alcohol abuse. In the latter type, individuals often fabricate responses to questions, as if to deny any problems with their mental faculties. A careful observer, however, can usually note a pattern of vagueness to many responses to questions that call for dates or other historical details. With patients experiencing a dissociative amnesia, there is typically no attempt to cover up the memory loss. As one patient, a successful graphic artist with her own business, stated: "It's scary as hell to realize all of a sudden that today is Thursday, and I don't remember a thing since coming home from the office on Monday night. Where did those 2 days go? I look at my calendar and see that appointments were scheduled with clients.

T A B L E 2 8 – I	Types of Amnesia
TYPE	**CHARACTERISTICS**
Localized	Inability to recall events that occurred for a short period of time (a few hours to a few days); the most common type of amnesia. *Example:* Inability to recall events occurring during and following a burglary in one's home.
Generalized (global)	Loss of memory for a whole lifetime of experience, including one's personal identity; considered to be rare.
Selective (systematized)	Failure to recall some but not all events during a short period; continuous failure to recall specific events occurring after a specific time up to and including the present. The person forgets each successive event as it occurs, although is clearly alert and aware of what is happening at the time. *Example:* Not remembering anything about a burglary, but remembering when the police arrived.
Anterograde	Amnesia for short-term memory, although remote memory remains intact; present in blackouts; a common symptom of alcohol abuse; difficulty in learning new information.
Retrograde	Loss of memory about events that occurred before the amnesia-producing event.

Did I keep any of the appointments? I have no idea. Someone is going to notice that I 'space out' and think I'm going crazy. Maybe I am."

Derealization

Derealization occurs when objects in the external world take on a quality of unreality and estrangement. Thus, familiar people and places are perceived as unfamiliar or unreal. This symptom exists on a continuum from mild, brief feelings associated with anxiety to more severe manifestations, as in the example of Charlotte. Nothing about her surroundings was recognizable to her, although she had lived in the same city for a number of years. Other patients experiencing a high degree of derealization have described feeling that family members (e.g., a parent or spouse) were difficult to recognize as being their own. On the other end of the continuum, most of us have had temporary episodes of perceiving a familiar setting, such as a classroom or shopping mall, as being somewhat alien. This experience occurs most frequently when one's anxiety has shifted from moderate to severe, in which case we may be able to focus only on scattered details of the perceptual field (Butler et al., 1996). As one patient described it, "The neighborhood where I had lived for years looked like a two-dimensional stage set."

Depersonalization

Depersonalization is viewed as an alteration in the perception or experience of the self; one's usual sense of relatedness to the rest of the world is temporarily lost or changed. Some individuals describe feeling detached, being in a dream-like state, or feeling like outside observers of their own minds and bodies. Although *derealization* concerns perception of external objects, *depersonalization* is related more to the experience of self and is perhaps more limited in scope and possibly more distressing to the individual because the nature of one's existence is in question. One patient described feeling like a robot, experiencing his arms and legs as being mechanically controlled. Although he knew that this was not the case, the feeling persisted. Thus, reality testing is intact and people experiencing depersonalization are not delusional. Similar to derealization, depersonalization may be experienced in milder degrees when "normal" people are highly anxious or stressed in other ways. As another patient expressed the depersonalization experience for herself, "I'm sitting on the couch but I feel invisible—and yet I see myself from another part of the room. At least I think it's me, whatever me is. My body looks the same as it always did, and yet it doesn't seem to be a part of that 'me' I was talking about. If this isn't crazy, I don't know what is."

Identity Confusion

Identity confusion has been defined as a subjective sense of conflict, puzzlement, or uncertainty in relation to one's identity, usually accompanied by significant distress. Comments such as "I don't know who I am" are typical. Some patients arrive at clinics, hospitals, and emergency rooms claiming *global amnesia* or some other form of amnesia. If results of a medical and neurological work-up are negative, further assessment of the patient is necessary.

> Although Charlotte did not believe she had ever experienced a full-blown amnesic episode before, she later recalled that there seemed to be an ongoing inner struggle in which she doubted her identity. "It's like my insides are a boxing ring with two opponents. There's a fight going on and someone's going to get knocked out but I don't know which one. It's real scary sometimes."

Identity Alteration

Identity alteration is evidenced as an organized shift in one's personality, including the way one relates to others, character traits, knowledge, and preferences. Although similar to other dissociative symptoms, identity alteration usually occurs without the individual's awareness. It may be masked or overshadowed by more overt and commonly described symptoms such as anxiety and depression. Persons with what has traditionally been referred to as *multiple personality disorder* (dissociation identity disorder) undergo severe identity alteration. Additionally, they are often amnesic for their behavior or experiences during the altered identity state. This symptom can be assessed indirectly by questioning the patient about new objects in his or her possession, observing skills about which the patient was unaware, observing the patient's handwriting, and acquiring reports from others about the person's behavioral inconsistencies (Steinberg, 1993). One patient was noted to play the piano beautifully, particularly Chopin études, and kept a collection of musical scores. When she shifted periodically to an altered identity, she could do little more than "chopsticks" awkwardly with two fingers, claimed that she could not read music, and was totally uninterested in the piano. She would giggle in a child-like manner and insist, "We don't really like music that much."

Cause of Pathological Dissociation

According to Nemiah (1989), biological researchers attempted to define dissociative symptoms in terms of the ascending reticular activating system, thalamocortical projections, and other neurological pathways. Researchers have found structural changes in the brain regions involved in memory of individuals who have had psychological trauma. Several areas in the brain are involved with memory. The hippocampus and its adjacent cortex, the dorsal medial nucleus of the thalamus, and the amygdala are important to memory. The hippocampus initially stores the memory, and after several weeks the memory tracks are reorganized and stored in the adjacent areas. The amygdala is like an alarm system that integrates necessary information to elicit a stress response as needed. Psychological trauma can change these structures possibly because of high levels of glucocorticoids and other stress hormones (Burgess, Hartman, & Clements, 1995).

Bremner, Krystal, Charney, and Southwick (1996) compared the right hippocampal volume of patients with combat-related post-traumatic stress disorder to that of control subjects and found that those with post-traumatic stress disorder had a smaller volume in the hippocampus than the controls did. These authors also found the left hippocampal volume in 17 adult survivors of childhood physical and sexual abuse to be lower than in 17 comparison subjects who were matched by age and other demographic data (Bremner et al., 1996). This hippocampal change demonstrates deficits in free verbal recall measured by the Wechsler Memory Scale (Bremner et al., 1996). Epinephrine, adrenocorticotropic hormone, and glucocorticoids can affect memory and learning. Memory tracks may be altered by the increased release of these neurotransmitters as well as some neuropeptides. The physical changes in memory tracts should be pursued for future study as the sequelae of trauma and the role of dissociation are explored. As psychobiological research continues, it is imperative that nurses stay abreast of these activities. It is not inconceivable that, at some point, underlying brain mechanisms will be discovered that mediate certain types of dissociative symptoms.

Current views about dissociation tend to regard psychosocial factors as being the major causative elements of these disorders, particularly severely traumatic experiences occurring recently or in the past. An analysis of possible causative factors is included in the discussion of the specific disorders later in this chapter. See What Society Needs to Know: Dissociative Disorders.

Classification of Pathologic Dissociation

Currently the DSM-IV recognizes five dissociative disorders:

- Dissociative amnesia
- Dissociative fugue
- Depersonalization disorder
- Dissociative identity disorder (DID)
- Dissociative disorder not otherwise specified (DDNOS)

In the past, these disorders were classified as hysterical neuroses of the dissociative type. Memory disturbances often affect one's sense of identity, which may be manifested by changes in psychomotor behavior and affect. One or two of these functions may cease to work in concert or be integrated with the others. The behavior of some individuals experiencing this disintegrity of consciousness, memory, or identity appears bizarre. Other people, however, present themselves as alert, lucid, and generally appropriate. These same individuals may be totally unable to recall their names, addresses, or occupations.

WHAT SOCIETY NEEDS TO KNOW

Dissociative Disorders

What are dissociative disorders?

Dissociative disorders involve a temporary loss or disturbance of the ability to integrate memory, consciousness, identity, and sometimes motor behavior. Individuals who are diagnosed with a type of dissociative disorder will experience amnesia or memory loss that ranges from mild to severe and could include recent or past events. These disturbances can appear suddenly or gradually and can be chronic. Dissociative experiences appear on a continuum from daydreaming or "tuning out" to a complete fragmentation of self into a different personality.

What causes dissociative disorders?

In recent years, renewed interest in the study of dissociative disorders has been seen. Many current researchers are making a connection between dissociative experiences and repressed trauma or acute or long-term stress. Many mental health professionals consider the ability to detach oneself from memories, consciousness, and sense of identity to be a normal or natural response to repeated trauma or abuse.

How are dissociative disorders treated?

These conditions are treated with long-term psychotherapy. It is generally thought that it is better to allow memories to return when the person is psychologically ready, rather than to attempt to force or rush the return.

What is multiple personality disorder?

Once considered a rare condition, Multiple Personality Disorder (recently classified as Dissociative Identity Disorder) is now recognized as a more common entity. In this condition, patients have more than one distinct personality. They usually have a core personality, but the personality who goes to the doctor for treatment is often an alter or subpersonality. Changing from one personality to another can occur within seconds, or one personality may remain dominant for days. One common characteristic of patients diagnosed with this condition is that they were sexually abused as children. Most people diagnosed with this disorder are female, and their history may reveal suicide attempts, substance abuse, and self-mutilation.

Dissociative Amnesia

A person suffering from dissociative amnesia is plagued with the sudden inability to access information that has already been stored in one's memory bank. This inability is not caused by ordinary forgetfulness, and there is no evidence indicative of an underlying brain disorder (Kaplan, Sadlock, & Grebb, 1994). These individuals retain the capacity to learn new information; thus, they do not manifest what is termed *continuous amnesia*. Contrasted with patients with organically induced amnesias, who behave in a confused and disorganized manner, individuals with dissociative amnesia appear intact and coherent.

Dissociative amnesia is generally considered to be the most common type of dissociative disorder, occurring more frequently in women than in men. Often a thorough assessment uncovers a precipitating emotional trauma charged with conflict and painful feelings, as in the description at the beginning of this chapter. Charlotte's sudden abandonment by her lover triggered traumatic childhood conflicts related to being abandoned and unloved. This disorder generally begins abruptly, and patients are aware of their memory loss. Some people may be distraught about the memory loss; others may seem indifferent. Thus, during an initial assessment, it is important for nurses to evaluate the patient's affective state. As previously noted, most patients are alert before and after amnesia occurs. Some

report a slight clouding of consciousness, however, during the brief interval immediately surrounding the amnesic period.

The specific treatment varies with individual attributes, such as motivation and level of anxiety. If careful interviewing leads to no clues related to the traumatic precipitant and the patient remains amnesic, other approaches may be considered. As with Charlotte, amobarbital sodium given intravenously may facilitate recovery of memories. Other individuals may respond favorably to **hypnosis.** Once the buried memories are retrieved, psychotherapy may assist the person to cope with the painful feelings and depression that may follow (Dolan, 1991).

Dissociative Fugue

A person with dissociative **fugue** wanders, sometimes far from home, and may assume a completely new identity for an indefinite period of time—days, weeks, or longer. The individual's travel and behavior appear more purposeful than the confused wandering that may be seen in dissociative amnesia (American Psychiatric Association, 1994). As with other dissociative disorders, fugue states are considered rare in the general population. In contrast to the person with dissociative amnesia, the individual in a fugue is unaware of having forgotten anything. Following recovery, there is no recollection of activities that occurred during the fugue.

An interesting case illustrating psychogenic (dissociative) fugue occurred in New England during the 1880s (Case Example 28-1).

■ CASE EXAMPLE 28-1
■ Ansel Bourne's Story
■

On January 17, 1887, the Reverend Ansel Bourne withdrew over $500 from a bank in Providence, Rhode Island, with which to purchase a lot of land nearby. He left in a carriage that morning, did not return home that night, and nothing was heard of him for 2 months. On the morning of March 14, however, in Norristown, Pennsylvania, a man calling himself A. J. Brown, who had rented a small shop 6 weeks previously, stocked it with stationery, confectionery, fruit, and small articles and began to conduct business. He carried on his quiet trade without seeming eccentric or unnatural to anyone.

One day, however, he woke up in a fright. He called in the people of the house, urging them to tell him where he was. He claimed that he was Ansel Bourne, that he knew nothing about Norristown, and that he was totally ignorant about shopkeeping. The last thing he remembered—it seemed only yesterday—was drawing the money from the bank in Providence. He could not believe that 2 months had elapsed. After returning to Providence, he had complete amnesia for the 2 months of his absence. ■

This historic case of the Reverend Bourne is a fairly typical example of fugue episodes as they are reported in contemporary times. Some persons predisposed to fugue states have a history of heavy alcohol abuse, but this is certainly not always the case. Sometimes the fugue is less elaborate than that of Ansel Bourne's and may involve little more than brief, seemingly purposeful travel. In these instances, social contacts are usually minimal or avoided entirely. Reports of violent outbursts have been cited in reports of some persons; these outbursts are thought to be related to fear of unknown circumstances surrounding emergence from the fugue state. Unless the fugue is particularly prolonged, the most useful approach is to provide the patient with a safe, supportive environment with a low level of stimulation. Nurses can assume an especially important role by teaching nonprofessional staff and family members by modeling a "here and now" focus rather than probing behaviors that may precipitate agitation, leading to aggressive behavior.

Depersonalization Disorder

Depersonalization disorder is characterized by a recurrent or persistent change in the quality of self-awareness. One's own sense of reality may be temporarily lost. Some persons may describe themselves as being mechanical, detached from their bodies, or in a dream. These experiences are referred to as ego-dystonic, in that the individual realizes the bizarreness or unreality of the symptoms. As mentioned previously, depersonalization concerns feelings that one's own body or self is unreal or strange; derealization relates to the perception of objects in the external world as being in some way strange or unreal.

Persons experiencing this disorder usually seem to be markedly distressed and intact reality testing is maintained. The onset is rapid, but disappearance is usually gradual (American Psychiatric Association, 1994). It is currently believed that depersonalization disorder is associated with an array of precipitants, including psychological, neurological, and systemic diseases. Certain drugs, such as alcohol, barbiturates, benzodiazepines, scopolamine, and marijuana, among others, have been determined to be contributory. At this time, depersonalization is most often viewed as a *symptom* occurring in association with anxiety, depression, and schizophrenia. It is quite rare as a pure disorder (Kaplan et al., 1994).

Dissociative Identity Disorder

Considered one of the most controversial of all psychiatric disorders, dissociative identity disorder (DID) has achieved increasing notoriety in the past few years. Previously known as multiple personality disorder, DID is characterized by the existence of two or more personality states that can take full control of the person's behavior, accompanied by an inability to remember significant personal information. This inability of recall is too pervasive to be explained by ordinary forgetfulness. The new name highlights the failure of personality integration that is a central feature of this phenomenon in many patients. Although it is extremely difficult to obtain statistics about the prevalence of this disorder, it is believed to occur much more frequently than was previously thought. The majority of these patients report histories of severe trauma during childhood, including physical, sexual, and ritual cult abuse. Although DID is not usually diagnosed until adulthood, dissociative episodes are often initially experienced by patients at an early age. Lewis and colleagues (1997) obtained extensive histories from 12 individuals who had committed murder and were also diagnosed with DID. Each of these individuals had suffered severe abuse as children. Many exhibited trance behavior, several had fugue states, auditory hallucinations, and vivid imaginary companions and were described as being possessed as children. As adults, each of the individuals was described as having trances and time loss.

DID is considered the ultimate dissociative phenomenon that contains all the elements of the other disorders in this class. Patients with this syndrome manifest, on occasion, amnesia, fugue, and profound depersonalization. Without effective treatment, DID appears to be a lifelong process; however, it may present itself differently over a period of time (Kluft, 1985).

A number of cases of DID have been chronicled in the historical literature. *When Rabbit Howls* (Chase, 1987) is autobiographical and names the different personalities (alters), who were referred to as The Troops. The major character, Truddi, had been subjected to horrendous sexual abuse by her stepfather beginning at around 2 years of age. Many of the Troop members served protective functions for Truddi.

The best times growing up were when I was totally alone, at the rock in the back field of the second farmhouse. The rock was huge; it had a deep indentation in the middle, so deep you could barely see over the edge. I hated the snakes. They lay around on the rim of the rock, basking in the sun. Once you made it to the center of the rock, you kept an eye out for the snakes and any human being sneaking up on you from the house at the other end of the farm. (p. 83)

In this quote from *When Rabbit Howls,* Truddi's extreme hypervigilance is apparent. To relieve the frightened, exhausted child in her quest for a safe place, different Troop members (alters) would take over to protect her from the perpetrator. In Truddi's case, the melding of all personalities (integration) was not seen as a realistic goal of treatment.

Owing to the extreme complexity of this disorder, some cases may remain completely undetected, whereas others may be misdiagnosed. Nurses working in all settings need some knowledge of signs and symptoms manifested by patients with DID (Box 28–2). For example, many individuals present with complaints of physical problems that tend to be vague and unsupported by laboratory tests and other medical findings. Depression, mood swings, self-mutilative behavior, and suicidal ideation are often present in at least one personality. Additionally, sleep disturbances, similar to those noted in post-traumatic stress disorder are common and should always be included in the assessment interview (Putnam, 1989). Particularly significant are reports of "time loss," which some patients are reluctant to admit, along with fears of "going crazy." Phobic anxiety and substance abuse are not uncommon. Hallucinations (auditory, visual, and tactile) are often present and frequently denied initially. Auditory hallucinations often discuss the patient in the third person or may argue among themselves. In contrast to hallucinatory experiences in schizophrenia, these "voices" are heard within the patient's head and are heard clearly and distinctly (Coons, 1984). Additionally, many patients who have DID refer to themselves as "we" rather than "I."

Box 28–2 ■ ■ ■ ■ ■
Some Signs and Symptoms of Dissociative Identity Disorder

- Inconsistencies in accounts of elapsed time
- A history of several medical and psychiatric diagnoses
- Inconsistencies in physical behaviors, such as switching right-handedness or left-handedness, voice changes, or marked differences in clothing and hairstyles on different occasions
- Psychophysiological complaints, such as severe headaches, chest pain, or a fluctuation in pain threshold
- Hearing voices inside one's head talking to one another or to the person
- Reference to oneself as "we" rather than "I"

If the individual with DID requires hospitalization because of direct or indirect self-destructive behavior, milieu management is a critical factor in safe and therapeutic care (Stafford, 1993). The inability to trust others, frequency of self-mutilative episodes and suicidal ideation, and behavior patterns that are manipulative pose a challenge to the nurse. The novice nurse needs additional education and ongoing supervision to work effectively with these individuals. Many patients with DID also have an Axis II diagnosis of borderline personality disorder. This poses an additional challenge to the nurse to deal therapeutically with an individual who has difficulty relating to others, is often suicidal and angry, uses the unconscious defenses of splitting and projective identification, and has impulsive behavior patterns when experiencing abandonment anxiety. (Refer to Chapter 27 for more information on the nursing care of an individual with Borderline Personality Disorder).

Maintaining a safe environment is critical in the care of the patient with DID because these individuals frequently exhibit self-mutilative behavior, such as cutting or puncturing the skin with sharp objects, head banging, and a variety of other self-destructive behaviors. A discussion about self-mutilation and the nursing care of a patient who self-mutilates is given in Chapter 31. Before hospitalization, many DID patients have engaged in abuse of alcohol, other drugs, and illicit substances. (Dunn, Ryan, Paolo, & Van Fleet, 1995). Eating disorders are common. Individuals with DID often have a "favorite" nurse, until that nurse inadvertently displeases the patient in some way. At that point, the formerly trusted nurse is seen as "all bad" or as an enemy. Part of therapeutic nursing intervention is to maintain acceptance of the patient and to avoid taking rebuffs personally.

The nature of the traumas associated with DID poses an array of problems. Tessier (1992) avowed that we know exceedingly more about the physical, social, and psychological aftermath of childhood sexual abuse than we do of the spiritual consequences. She further asserts that our Western culture's norms of encouraging the victim to put the past behind one is destructive because healing cannot occur before the extensive damage to the spiritual part of the person is acknowledged. Thus, nurses, clergy, and other health professionals should focus on the healing aspects of treatment with caution. It is an essential part of the treatment to work through the anger and feelings of betrayal. Once the person has begun to explore the ramifications of the early child abuse has had on her life, the role of the perpetrator should be explored. As every case is unique, so is the extent of devastation to the human spirit. The decision to confront and forgive the perpetrator is a process that would seem best left to the victim as she traverses in the journey toward being a survivor.

Dissociative Disorders Not Otherwise Specified

The not-otherwise-specified (NOS) category is a residual one for disorders in which the primary feature is a dissociative syndrome that does not meet the criteria for one of the previously described types. Data from studies in which these patients were compared with persons diagnosed with DID (Briere & Runtz, 1990; Chu & Dill, 1990; Ross, Anderson, Heber, & Norton, 1990), however, have consistently supported the assertion that the dissociative disorders exist on a spectrum of increasing severity and complexity, with DID at the extreme end of the continuum. The most current research evidence supports the position that dissociative disorder not otherwise specified (DDNOS) is simply a milder variant of DID with less severe trauma and symptoms. From reviewed studies, it would appear that DID is the prototype human response to chronic, severe, **childhood trauma.**

> *What do you think about the following statement?* Dissociation is a gift from God to help us deal with overwhelming trauma and pain.

> ➤ *Check Your Reading*
> 6. What are the five hallmark symptoms of dissociative disorders?
> 7. Describe each of the five symptoms.
> 8. Describe the characteristics of the dissociative disorders.
> 9. Which dissociative disorder is considered to be the most controversial of all psychiatric disorders?

FALSE MEMORY SYNDROME

When providing therapy or psychological nursing support for any individual with psychological problems, it is important to recognize that there is an increased susceptibility to suggestions from others. The **false memory syndrome** can occur when a therapist suggests that an individual has been abused. The patient integrates these suggestions into his or her personal history and reacts as though this suggestion is reality. Yapko (1994) differentiated this from situations in which the patient reports to the therapist that he or she had been abused, based on actual knowledge of this incident; or when a patient independently remembers repressed memories; or when a therapist facilitates memory of a repressed state by use of therapeutic interventions, such as hypnotherapy, art therapy, and exploring cues in the environment that facilitate flashbacks. It is important to recognize that what we say can become another person's reality. To prevent false memory syndrome,

- Keep your professional boundaries clear.
- Interact with the patient by asking questions that are not leading in content, ask branching questions to assist the patient to clarify his or her problems areas.
- Support the patient to work through the issues he has identified at his or her own pace.
- Assist the patient to learn self-observation and self-soothing behaviors to assist in processing new information.

- Know the legal responsibility to report abuse.
- Understand physiological memory versus emotional reactivity to events in the current environment and how these events may affect past memory.
- Do not pressure a patient to provide a memory, even if the patient requests this (Calof, 1993; Gallop, Austin, McCay, Boyer, & Peternell-Taylor, 1997; Hall, 1996; Yapko, 1994).

> *What do you think?* When you listen to someone relate a story from your past, have you ever wondered if you really remember the event or whether the other person's memory becomes your reality? How do you understand this phenomenon?

> ➤ *Check Your Reading*
> 10. What is the false memory syndrome?
> 11. What two interventions will prevent the patient from experiencing the false memory syndrome?

NURSING PROCESS

Effective use of the nursing process with patients who have dissociation disorders requires a working knowledge of the continuum of dissociative experiences and the accompanying mild to severe symptoms.

Assessment

Assessment of the patient with a possible dissociative disorder uses strategies emphasized in Chapter 11 for evaluating mental status. Some of the specific assessment skills involve detection of dissociative symptoms, particularly those that relate to disturbances in memory, consciousness, and sense of identity. The nurse should be observant for any of the five cardinal symptoms of dissociative disorders: amnesia, derealization, depersonalization, identity confusion, and identity alteration. Although these symptoms may be present, to some degree, in many individuals under stress or with other psychiatric problems, they are particularly suggestive of a disturbance on the continuum of dissociative responses. Amnesia may be experienced in a global sense or to a milder degree, such as amnesia of activities surrounding one event, for instance an automobile accident. It is extremely important to listen carefully to the patient for subjective data, which typically take the form of a personal attribution statement in which the patient presents herself as a "nonknowing" person. The following examples are congruent with a dissociative state: "I don't know why I'm here." "The police brought me to the hospital."

Regardless of the setting, it is critical to assess the perception of reality of the individual who may be experiencing a dissociative episode. In dissociative amnesia states, the *objective data* are also critical. How upset does the patient appear? A careful physical assessment is essential because some persons' amnesia may have a specific pathophysiological cause. For example, transient global amnesia (TGA), often caused by transient ischemic attacks, migraine headaches, sedative-hypnotic drugs, or seizures, can mimic psychogenic (dissociative) amnesia. The personal identity of the patient with psychogenic amnesia is lost, however, whereas that of the individual with transient global amnesia is retained. Table 28–1 identifies the behaviors associated with various types of amnesia.

In the assessment of a patient who may be experiencing (or may have recently experienced) a fugue state, the situation becomes complex. These individuals are rarely brought to emergency departments or hospitals or to the attention of mental health professionals, because they typically do little to attract attention. Perhaps the most frequent reason for their entry into the system is an aggressive outburst against property or other persons.

Subjective data may be difficult to obtain because these patients are unaware that they have forgotten anything. Objective data should also include a thorough physical assessment because temporal lobe epilepsy may also involve episodes of travel, although a new identity is not assumed. Temporal lobe epilepsy seizures are not caused by psychosocial stress, as is often the case with dissociative fugues. Patients who have DID are more likely to be misdiagnosed as having other psychiatric disorders. As previously mentioned, depersonalization may occur as a symptom in numerous other psychiatric syndromes. It is sometimes the earliest presenting symptom of a person with a neurological disorder. Thus, symptoms of depersonalization should be observed carefully.

However the subjective and objective data are obtained, it is essential to remember that accurate problem identification and interventions depend on the quality of the data collected. Additionally, although nurses must be knowledgable about disease processes and specific disorders, the major purpose of the assessment phase is always to collect information needed to care for the patient in a holistic manner, regardless of the medical or psychiatric diagnosis.

Diagnosis

A critical analysis of the assessment data leads to clearer definitions of patient problems and decisions related to therapeutic nursing interventions. DSM-IV diagnoses for the patient with a dissociative disorder, and a related NANDA diagnosis, are presented in Medical Diagnoses and Related Nursing Diagnoses. Additional nursing diagnoses that may be appropriate for the patient with a dissociative disorder are as follows:

- Altered Role Performance
- Spiritual Distress
- Risk for Violence: Self-Directed
- Risk for Violence: Directed at Others
- Hopelessness
- Anxiety

Let us return to Charlotte, to see how the process of diagnosis worked in her case.

Charlotte was diagnosed as suffering from dissociative amnesia, according to the DSM-IV criteria. In reviewing the limited data initially obtained, however, it was apparent that many knowledge gaps existed regarding the unique nature of this person. For example, was she able to support herself financially? If not, was she motivated for vocational training? Did she have spiritual concerns? As mentioned previously, the most consistent message Charlotte had received from her mother was that she was a "bad" person, whose badness drove her father and others away. She had subsequently experienced disruptive, chaotic relations with others. Based on an appraisal of assessment data, her initial nursing diagnosis was Ineffective Individual Coping related to altered self-concept as evidenced by amnesia.

Outcome Identification

The primary expected outcome for a patient with a dissociative disorder is that the patient will develop new, more adaptive ways of coping with stress.

Planning

Based on the identified expected outcomes, the nurse and patient, working together with the interdisciplinary treatment team, jointly establish short-term goals, such as the following:

Expected Outcome
The patient will develop new, more adaptive ways of coping with stress.

Short-Term Goals
1. The patient will participate in life skills assessment group.
2. The patient will contact state agency regarding job training skills.
3. The patient will review transferable skills with a counselor.

The plan for Charlotte, and other patients diagnosed with a dissociative disorder, includes trying to establish rapport in a trusting relationship. This is considered especially important on Charlotte's arrival on the psychiatric unit. Although Charlotte's history was sketchy and there were no family or friends to provide additional data, the nursing staff were careful not to overwhelm the patient with questions she could not answer. She was initially engaged in occupational therapy and other milieu activities, based on the rationale that recall of the past might occur during activities that simulate life experiences.

MEDICAL DIAGNOSES AND RELATED NURSING DIAGNOSES

Dissociative Disorders

DSM-IV Diagnosis: Dissociative Amnesia

Diagnostic Criteria

A. The predominant disturbance is one or more episodes of inability to recall important personal information, usually of a traumatic or stressful nature, that is too extensive to be explained by ordinary forgetfulness.

B. The disturbance does not occur exclusively during the course of Dissociative Identity Disorder, Dissociative Fugue, Post-traumatic Stress Disorder, Acute Stress Disorder, or Somatization Disorder and is not due to the direct physiological effects of a substance (e.g., a drug of abuse, a medication) or a neurological or other general medical condition (e.g., Amnestic Disorder due to head trauma).

C. The symptoms cause clinically significant distress or impairment in social, occupational, or other important areas of functioning.

DSM-IV Diagnosis: Dissociative Fugue

Diagnostic Criteria

A. The predominant disturbance is sudden, unexpected travel away from home or one's customary place of work, with inability to recall one's past.

B. Confusion about personal identity or assumption of a new identity (partial or complete).

C. The disturbance does not occur exclusively during the course of Dissociative Identity Disorder and is not due to the direct physiological effects of a substance (e.g., a drug of abuse, a medication) or a general medical condition (e.g., temporal lobe epilepsy).

D. The symptoms cause clinically significant distress or impairment in social, occupational, or other important areas of functioning.

DSM-IV Diagnosis: Dissociative Identity Disorder

Diagnostic Criteria

A. The presence of two or more distinct identities or personality states (each with its own relatively enduring pattern of perceiving, relating to, and thinking about the environment and self).

B. At least two of these identities or personality states recurrently take control of the person's behavior.

C. Inability to recall important personal information that is too extensive to be explained by ordinary forgetfulness.

D. The disturbance is not due to the direct physiological effects of a substance (e.g., blackouts or chaotic behavior during Alcohol Intoxication) or a general medical condition (e.g., complex partial seizures). *Note:* In children, the symptoms are not attributable to imaginary playmates or other fantasy play.

DSM-IV Diagnosis: Depersonalization Disorder

Diagnostic Criteria

A. Persistent or recurrent experiences of feeling detached from, and as if one is an outside observer of, one's mental processes or body (e.g., feeling like one is in a dream).

B. During the depersonalization experience, reality testing remains intact.

C. The depersonalization causes clinically significant distress or impairment in social, occupational, or other important areas of functioning.

D. The depersonalization experience does not occur exclusively during the course of another mental disorder, such as Schizophrenia, Panic Disorder, Acute Stress Disorder, or another Dissociative Disorder, and is not due to the direct physiological effects of a substance (e.g., a drug of abuse, a medication) or a general medical condition (e.g., temporal lobe epilepsy).

DSM-IV Diagnosis: Dissociative Disorder Not Otherwise Specified

Related Nursing Diagnosis	Definition	Example
Ineffective Individual Coping	Impairment of adaptive behaviors and problem-solving abilities of a person in meeting life's demands and roles	Ineffective Individual Coping related to confusion about self

Based on information from the *Diagnostic and Statistical Manual of Mental Disorders. Fourth Edition.* Copyright 1994 American Psychiatric Association. Nursing diagnoses and definitions from North American Nursing Diagnosis Association. (1999). *NANDA nursing diagnoses: Definitions and classification 1999–2000.* Philadelphia: NANDA.

Nursing Interventions Specific to
Dissociative Disorder

What do you need to do to develop a relationship with a patient who has dissociative identity disorder?

- Understand that an individual with dissociative identity disorder has difficulty trusting others; approach the patient with a respectful attitude. Be consistent in your interventions to promote trust.
- Share time with the patient; taking care to respect the patient if he or she presents in an alternate personality.
- Avoid mocking the patient or judging the patient; this would violate the trust.
- Find ways to express hope with the patient by pointing out the patient's successes.
- Encourage the patient to discuss his or her thoughts and feelings; even if they do not make sense to the patient.
- Maintain therapeutic boundaries to provide a good therapeutic relationship.

What do you need to assess regarding the patient's health status?

- The patient should have a thorough neurological examination; including an EEG to rule out a temporal lobe seizure disorder or transient global amnesia.
- Evaluate patient's risk of self-harm by a suicide attempt or by self-mutilation.
- Utilize the Dissociative Experiences Scale to determine the patient's level of dissociative experience along the continuum.
- Physical responses include changes in heart rate, metabolism of medications, handwriting.
- Assess "loss of time" or subjective feelings of amnesia.
- Cognitive responses included thought pattern differences between personality states, depending on the personality's age and experience.
- Assess the patient for derealization.
- Behavior responses are different for each ego state; assess for inconsistent behavioral responses.
- Determine whether the patient is experiencing depersonalization.
- Assess the patient for identity confusion.
- Determine whether the patient is experiencing identity alteration.
- Assess the patient's social supports.
- Assess what the patient understands about his or her illness; assess his ability and readiness to learn.
- Determine whether the patient has any concurrent medical conditions.

What do you need to teach the patient and the patient's caregiver?

- The patient dissociated to maintain personal stability in the face of a crisis.
- Dissociation is something everyone experiences; teach the dissociation continuum.
- Assist the patient to learn new ways of coping when feeling self-destructive or a desire to self-mutilate.
- Assist the patient to understand that his or her experiences caused changes in the brain that make the patient more sensitive during times of high anxiety or intense depression.
- Discuss the role of psychopharmacological interventions.
- Discuss the importance of the therapeutic relationship as a safe relationship to discuss earlier experiences to gain meaning and understanding of how these events shape the here and now.
- The patient may demonstrate strong affect as he or she works through the past trauma; the therapeutic relationship assists the patient to deal with this strong affect and the earlier trauma.
- This working through and understanding earlier trauma takes time and can only be done in small increments to provide mastery of the intense emotional feelings.

What skills will you want the patient and caregiver to demonstrate?

- How to write a contract for safety and keep the environment around the patient safe.
- Identifying what increased the anxiety that precipitated the dissociation. This information can be gleaned by using a journal of thoughts, feelings, and daily events that stimulate feelings.
- Understanding of the medication regiment and the potential side effects of the medications.
- Understanding that the work in therapy takes time and is best thought of as rebuilding a building.

What other health professional might need to be a part of this plan of care?

- A psychiatrist who is familiar with dissociative disorders and understands the role of anxiety in these disorders. The psychiatrist can collaborate with an advanced psychiatric nurse to prescribe medications and determine the diagnosis. The psychiatrist is usually in charge of the overall treatment plan.
- Advanced psychiatric nurse practitioner or clinical specialist to provide intensive psychotherapy and to assist with medication monitoring.
- Social worker if the patient needs assistance with community resources.
- Art therapist to assist the patient to use art to understand her unconscious processes; particularly around the issues related to the trauma.
- Psychiatric occupational therapist to assist the patient with activities related to daily living and coping.

Because these treatment modalities did not seem to promote recall, the staff planned an amobarbital sodium interview. As Charlotte's life sketch was filled in with more details, the nursing staff formulated additional nursing diagnoses:
- Altered Role Performance related to chaotic style of living and lack of involvement in the pursuit of productive work and healthy relationships.
- Spiritual Distress related to feelings of being "evil" invoked by early childhood experiences related to abandonment by father and verbal abuse by mother.
- During and after participation in individual and group psychotherapy, Charlotte will assess her goals for a more satisfying lifestyle in relation to interpersonal and vocational experiences.
- Charlotte will begin to negate her self-perception of being "evil," "immoral," and "whorish" and will be able to point out one positive attribute about herself.
- Charlotte will report feeling a brightening in her mood, as evidenced by increased interaction with peers, social smiling, and normal sleep patterns.
- After participation in a psychoeducation group, Charlotte will state the major actions and potential side effects of her antidepressant medication.

The issues of implementation in Charlotte's care after her memory was regained involved
- Coordinating individual and group psychotherapy
- Administering the prescribed antidepressant medication and arranging a teaching session regarding both therapeutic and potential side effects of the drug
- Arranging for consultation with a hospital chaplain when this intervention was requested by the patient
- Providing opportunities in the milieu for Charlotte to experience success in completion of tasks and in interaction with peers

Because most patients with dissociative disorders have experienced physical and psychological trauma, it may be difficult to for the patient to establish rapport or trust with the nurse. If the patient is experiencing some form of amnesia, it is important to provide a safe, supportive environment and not pressure the patient for information. As with any other patient-nurse situation, the qualitative aspects of the relationship are of central importance: establishing rapport and developing trust. See Snapshot: Nursing Interventions Specific to Dissociative Disorders. ■

Evaluation

Evaluation of patient care occurs ideally throughout the nursing process. Treatment is considered effective when a patient not only regains memory for past events but also experiences an improved quality of life in interpersonal relationships and demonstrates an ability to plan for immediate and future needs. A necessary step is to look back at the goals to see if they were realistic under the circumstances. Should some modifications be made? Were the expected outcomes realistic based on the patient's clinical status and the therapeutic resources?

What do you think? If a patient has a history of trauma and abuse, why is it essential not to force the issue of forgiveness on the individual? What needs to occur before the individual can forgive the perpetrator?

► *Check Your Reading*
12. Identify four areas to be assessed in dissociative disorders.
13. Identify at least two nursing diagnoses appropriate to a patient with a dissociative disorder.
14. What is the most important outcome when working with a patient who has a dissociative disorder?
15. Identify at least two interventions used with a patient with a dissociative disorder.

NURSING PROCESS APPLICATION

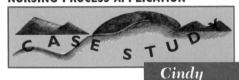

Cindy

Cindy is a 35-year-old file clerk who lives alone in an apartment in a major northern city. You are a home health nurse assigned to visit Cindy while she is recuperating from major abdominal surgery. On one of the visits, Cindy confides in you that she fears she is going insane. She tells you that for the past 2 years she has experienced increasingly frequent episodes of feeling "outside herself." Cindy says that during these episodes she feels like parts of her body are dead and she frequently loses her balance.

Cindy tells you that since her surgery she is experiencing these episodes more frequently, and each episode lasts 3 to 4 hours. She confides that you are the first person she has ever shared this information with and asks you to help her. She is markedly distressed and has difficulty sleeping. A mental status examination reveals that she is oriented to time, place, and person and has intact memory and good judgment. She tells you that she is concerned that she will lose her job if she does not get back to work soon. Cindy's parents were killed in an automobile accident when she was 14, and her only brother died of AIDS 3 years ago. She was raised as a Methodist but has not been to church since her parents were killed.

You refer Cindy to a psychiatrist, who diagnoses her with Depersonalization Disorder and asks you to continue seeing her once a week, to provide an assessment of her level of dissociation, to determine Cindy's safety to care for her wound, and because Cindy seems to trust you.

ASSESSMENT	Assessment data are as follows: • Persistent, recurrent feeling of being detached from self • Loss of balance during dissociative episode • Insomnia • No support system in place • History of trauma and loss • Fear of losing job and going insane • Marked distress

DIAGNOSIS	**DSM-IV Diagnosis:** Depersonalization disorder **Nursing Diagnosis 1:** Personal Identity Disturbance related to history of severe, traumatic interpersonal experiences and current stressor of severe illness evidenced by dissociative experiences, marked distress, insomnia, and fear of losing job.

OUTCOME IDENTIFICATION, PLANNING, AND IMPLEMENTATION

Expected Outcome 1: By _____ the patient will report a marked reduction in dissociative experiences.

Short-Term Goal	Nursing Interventions	Rationales
By _____ the patient will report one dissociative experience per week.	1. Continue to work on the trusting relationship that has been initiated. 2. Convey interest and caring. 3. Help the patient determine what is real and what is not real. Validate what is real and gently correct misperceptions. 4. Encourage the patient to limit her external environment. 5. Ask the patient to keep a record of any dissociative experiences she is having and share them with you at your next visit.	1–2. Trust is the basis of a therapeutic relationship and is especially important for a patient who is not grounded in reality. 3. As with a patient who is hallucinating, it is important not to reinforce what is not real. 4. This will foster psychological safety. 5. Actually recording the dissociative experiences aids in reinforcing reality.

Expected Outcome 2: By _____ the patient will verbalize absence of distress and fear of going insane.

Short-Term Goals	Nursing Interventions	Rationales
By _____ the patient will sleep at least 6 hours without interruption.	1. Educate the patient about the importance of sleep.	1. Dissociative experiences are known to occur more frequently when a patient is sleep deprived.

2. If the patient is unable to gain restful sleep via natural methods, consider sleeping medications until a pattern is established.
3. Have the patient keep a record of her sleep pattern.

2. If normal sleeping patterns have been interrupted for a long period of time, it is often necessary to intervene with medication.
3. Recording information helps the patient distinguish between reality and unreality.

By _____ the patient will report a significant reduction in anxiety.

1. Educate the patient about stress reduction measures such as meditation, writing, taking a warm bath, or talking to a friend.
2. Encourage the patient to try at least one new stress reduction measure each week.

1–2. Dissociative experiences are likely to be increased when the patient is anxious. Employing measures to reduce anxiety will aid in reducing the frequency of dissociation.

Nursing Diagnosis 2: Risk for Loneliness related to lack of support system, history of multiple losses, and the physical isolation necessitated by her current illness evidenced by lack of support system, marked distress, and fear of going insane.

OUTCOME IDENTIFICATION, PLANNING, AND IMPLEMENTATION

Expected Outcome 1: By _____ the patient will report a desire to rekindle a sense of spirituality.

Short-Term Goals	Nursing Interventions	Rationales
By _____ the patient will openly acknowledge her estrangement from the God of her understanding.	1. Encourage the patient to talk about her earlier relationship with God. 2. Offer to get the patient reading materials or to be available to listen. 3. Remain supportive and nonjudgmental if the patient describes anger toward God. 4. Ask the patient to describe times in her life when she found solace and comfort in her spiritual beliefs.	1–2. Being available to listen and to broach the subject of spirituality is an important part of healing for many patients with psychiatric conditions, especially when they have been spiritually bankrupt for a long time. 3. When patients have had multiple, profound losses, it is not unusual for them to be angry at God for "letting it happen." 4. This intervention shifts the focus and helps the patient get in touch with the self-nurturing aspect of a strong spiritual belief system.
By _____ the patient will report a desire to join a local church group.	1. Discuss with the patient the advantage of joining a church group. 2. Encourage the patient to be proactive in acknowledging her need for love and support and spirituality. 3. Honor the patient's initial reluctance in joining a group. 4. Continue to support growth, even though the patient may experience setbacks.	1–4. Even though the notion of joining a group may be appealing for many reasons, it is not unusual for patients to be reluctant. Framing this reluctance as fear rather than oppositional behavior will enable the nurse to continue to be supportive through any setbacks.

Expected Outcome 2: By _____ the patient will acknowledge the need to grieve the loss of her brother and her parents.

Short-Term Goals	Nursing Interventions	Rationales
By _____ the patient will discuss the anger and sadness related to the loss of her brother and parents.	1. Identify the functions that pent-up anger and sadness serve for the patient. 2. Explain the behaviors associated with normal grieving.	1–3. Knowledge of the acceptable feelings associated with normal grieving may aid in relieving some of the guilt and shame that inhibits resolution.

3. Encourage the expression of these feelings in a safe manner.
4. Encourage the expression of rage through participation in large motor activities, such as physical exercise, walking, or jogging.
5. Encourage the patient to also focus on the sad feelings that have been buried and convey to her that you are not uncomfortable with them.

4. This encourages the patient to be proactive and direct in processing negative feelings, in lieu of having them appear in a more pathological form.
5. Patients sometimes refuse to share their deepest feelings because they are trying to protect the nurse.

By _____ the patient will agree to pursue additional counseling for her issues surrounding loss.

1. Provide the patient with a list of grief groups available in the community.
2. Also provide the patient with a list of sliding scale community counseling centers.
3. Encourage the patient to continue on the path to good mental health.

1–2. Providing the patient with multiple options may make her feel more comfortable initially in individual therapy.

3. Patients who have been isolated for a long period of time need a strong patient advocate.

EVALUATION

Formative Evaluation. Cindy met each of the short-term goals. The dissociative episodes were dramatically reduced, and she reported being able to sleep. Within 2 months, she decided to contact the minister of the local Methodist church and begin attending services. This church also has a grief group, which Cindy will begin attending.

Summative Evaluation. All of the expected outcomes were also met. Within 3 months, Cindy reported no further dissociative experiences. She was close to completing her grief group and was attending church services on a regular basis. She told the nurse she was so grateful to feel whole again and to know she was not crazy.

Conclusions

A renewed interest in the phenomena of dissociation and dissociative disorders has undeniably occurred since the 1970s. A number of factors have contributed to this rebirth of interest. The suffering of many people from post-traumatic syndromes is one phenomenon that has increasingly called attention to the power of dissociative states. The plight of Vietnam veterans and, more recently, veterans of other international wars and disasters has called national attention to reactions of survivors, which typically include dissociative symptoms. Also in recent years, the concurrence among women of borderline psychopathology with dissociative symptoms and a history of incest has been increasingly noted (Gartner & Gartner, 1988). This finding serves as an additional factor contributing to heightened involvement in research and treatment of dissociative disorders. Finally, public awareness of severe child abuse, a major causative factor in chronic dissociative pathology, has dramatically increased within the past few years. It is imperative that professional nurses in all settings be attuned to detect dissociative symptoms and have a conceptual understanding of their mechanism. Otherwise, the symptoms may go unrecognized and untreated, and patients will be denied the care that they need to help them in their journey toward healing.

Key Points to Remember

- Persons with dissociative disorders experience gaps in memory, confusion, and often a sense of compartmentalization.

- Theorists have been divided as to whether dissociation is a pathological process or a part of normal human activity.

- Freud viewed dissociation as a form of the defense mechanism repression.
- Janet was the first theorist to use the term dissociation.
- Dissociation occurs along a continuum ranging from the mildest forms, which include daydreaming, to the most serious form, dissociative identity disorder.
- The DES is a scale that measures how frequently an individual experiences dissociation.
- Sullivan conceptualized dissociation as an expression of *not-me behavior*.
- Several theorists believe that further research is warranted prior to making a diagnosis of a dissociation disorder.
- Pathological dissociation has five hallmark symptoms: amnesia, derealization, depersonalization, identity confusion, and identity alteration.
- The DSM-IV recognizes five dissociative disorders: dissociative amnesia, dissociative fugue, depersonalization disorder, dissociative identity disorder, and dissociative disorder not otherwise specified.
- Assessment of dissociative disorders includes collecting data about memory, consciousness, and sense of identity, in addition to the five hallmark symptoms.
- There are several appropriate nursing diagnoses for patients with dissociative disorders. The most important, however, is Ineffective Individual Coping.
- Goals for a patient with a dissociative disorder include prevention of self harm, participating in individual and group psychotherapy, verbalization of self-concept, reduction of anxiety, improvement in mood, knowledge of medication, and improvement in coping skills.
- Implementation includes (1) preventing self-harm by providing a safe milieu and teaching the patient alternative coping skills when feeling overwhelmed or numb, (2) coordinating individual and group psychotherapy, (3) administering the prescribed antidepressant and/or antianxiety medication and arranging a teaching session regarding both therapeutic and potential side effects of the medications, (4) dealing with spiritual issues, and (5) providing opportunities in the milieu to decrease the patient's internal isolation.

Learning Activities

1. Complete the Dissociative Experiences Scale on yourself. What is your reaction to your score?
2. In the next week, try to be aware of the times you use dissociation as part of your normal activities of daily life.
3. Read *When Rabbit Howls* and discuss the patient's subjective experiences.

4. Obtain information about the False Memory Syndrome Foundation by using the Internet or by writing to 3401 Market Street, Suite 130, Philadelphia, PA 19104; 215 387-1865; http://advicom.net/~fitz/fmsf/
5. Obtain your local legal code about reporting child or elder abuse.
6. Use the Internet to visit a Web site about DID.

Critical Thinking Exercise

Molly is a 27-year-old black woman who was admitted to the dissociative disorder unit 2 weeks previously. She was diagnosed with dissociation identity disorder. During her stay on the unit, the nurses were able to assess at least 10 different personalities, or *alters*. Among these personalities were a destructive female, a frightened child, a seductive teenager, a soft-spoken young woman, and an angry male. At 7:30 PM, the nurse supervisor, Miss Yeager, responded to an emergency call about Molly. When Miss Yeager arrived on the unit, she saw Molly crouched in a fetal position hiding under a table in the dining room area. As soon as any staff members tried to touch her, she began to scream in a high-pitched shrill voice.

1. If you were Nurse Yeager, what would you need to know before you approached Molly?
2. What knowledge about multiple personality disorder would help you to determine your intervention?
3. Suggest possible interventions.

After about 45 minutes, the staff members were finally able to make some interventions that attended to Molly's needs. Then a nurse overheard two staff members talking about Molly. They were unhappy with Molly's manipulation of the staff and failure to take responsibility for her actions. Both of them were convinced that Molly was acting.

1. What assumptions have the two staff members made about dissociation identity disorder?
2. How might these assumptions affect their interactions with Molly?
3. What are possible ways they could test whether their assumptions are faulty?

Additional Resources

Child Abuse and Multiple Personality Disorder

http://wchat.on.ca/web/asarc/mpd.html

Dissociative Amnesia

http://www.cmhc.com/disorders/sx46.htm

Dissociative Fugue

http://www.cmhc.com/disorders/sx87.htm

Dissociative Identity Disorder (Multiple Personality Disorder)

http://www.sidran.org/didbr.html

Dissociative Identity Disorder: Symptoms and Treatment

http://www.cmhc.com/disorders/sx18.htm

Divided Hearts: DID/MPD Info and Support Web

http://www.dhearts.org/

References

American Psychiatric Association. (1994). *Diagnostic and statistical manual of mental disorders* (4th ed.). Washington, DC: Author.

Bernstein, E., & Putnam, F. W. (1986). Development of reliability and validity of a dissociation scale. *Journal of Nervous and Mental Disease, 174,* 727-735.

Braun, B. G., & Sachs, R. G. (1985). The development of personality disorder: Predisposing, precipitating, and perpetuating factors. In R. P. Kluft (Ed.), *The childhood antecedents of multiple personality.* Washington, DC: American Psychiatric Press.

Bremner, J. D., Krystal, J. H., Charney, D. S., & Southwick, S. M. (1996, July). Neural mechanisms in dissociative amnesia for childhood abuse: Relevance to the current controversy surrounding the "False Memory Syndrome." *American Journal of Psychiatry, 153* (7 Suppl.), 71-82.

Briere, J., & Runtz, M. (1990). Augmenting Hopkins SCL scales to measure dissociative symptoms: Data from two non-clinical samples. *Journal of Personality Assessment, 55,* 376-379.

Burgess, A. W., Hartman, C. R., & Clements, P. T., Jr. (1995). Biology of memory and childhood trauma. *Journal of Psychosocial Nursing and Mental Health Services, 33*(3), 16-26.

Butler, L. D., Duran, R. E. F., Jasiukaitis, P., Koopman, C., & Spiegel, D. (1996, July). Hypnotizability and traumatic experience: A diathesis-stress model of dissociative symptomatology. *American Journal of Psychiatry, 153* (7 suppl.), 42-63.

Calof, D. (1993, May). Facing the truth about false memory. *The Family Networker, 17* 38-41.

Chase, T. (1987). *When rabbit howls.* New York: E. P. Dutton.

Chu, J. A., & Dill, D. L. (1990). Dissociative symptoms in relation to childhood physical and sexual abuse. *American Journal of Psychiatry, 147,* 887-892.

Cohen, L., Berzoff, J., & Elin, M. (1995). *Dissociative identity disorder.* Northvale, NJ: Aronson.

Coons, P. M. (1984). The differential diagnosis of multiple personality: A comprehensive review. *Psychiatric Clinics of North America, 7,* 51-65.

Coons, P. M., Bowman, E., & Milstein, V. (1988). Multiple personality disorder: A clinical investigation of 50 cases. *Journal of Nervous and Mental Disease, 176,* 519-527.

Crabtree, A. (1992). Dissociation and memory: A two-hundred-year perspective. *Dissociation 5,* 150-154.

Dolan, Y. M. (1991). *Resolving sexual abuse: Solution-focused therapy and Ericksonian hypnosis for adult survivors.* New York: Norton.

Dunn, G., Ryan, J. J., Paolo, A. M., & Van Fleet, J. N. (1995). Co-morbidity of dissociative disorders among patients with substance use disorders. *Psychiatric Services, 46,* 153-156.

Frankel, F. H. (1996, July). Dissociation: The clinical realities. *American Journal of Psychiatry, 153* (7 Suppl.), 64-70.

Franklin, J. (1990). The diagnosis of multiple personality disorder based on subtle dissociative signs. *Journal of Nervous and Mental Disease, 178*(1), 4-14.

Freud, S. (1962). The neuro-psychoses of defense. In J. Strachey (Ed.), *Standard edition of the complete psychological works of Sigmund Freud* (Vol. 3). London: Hogarth Press.

Gallop, R., Austin, W., McCay, E., Boyer, M., & Peternell-Taylor, C. (1997). Nurses' views regarding false memory syndrome. *Archives of Psychiatric Nursing, 11,* 257-263.

Gartner, A., & Gartner, J. (1988). Borderline pathology in post-incest female adolescents. *Bulletin of the Menninger Clinic, 52,* 101-113.

Greaves, G. B. (1980). Multiple personality: 165 years after Mary Reynolds. *The Journal of Nervous and Mental Diseases, 168,* 577-596.

Hall, J. M. (1996). Delayed recall of childhood sexual abuse: Psychiatric nursing's responsibility to clients. *Archives of Psychiatric Nursing, 10,* 342-346.

Hilgard, E. R. (1977). *Divided consciousness: Multiple controls in human thought and action.* New York: John Wiley.

Janet, P. (1907). *The major symptoms of hysteria.* New York: Macmillan.

Kaplan, H. I., Sadlock, B. J., & Grebb, J. A. (1994). Dissociation disorders. In H. I. Kaplan & B. J. Sadlock (Eds.), *Synopsis of psychiatry* (6th ed.) Baltimore: Williams & Wilkins.

Kluft, R. P. (1984). Aspects of the treatment of multiple personality disorder. *Psychiatric Annals, 14*(3), 51-55.

Kluft, R. P. (1985). The natural history of multiple personality disorder. In Kluft, R. P. (Ed.), *The childhood antecedents of multiple personality disorder.* Washington, DC: American Psychiatric Press.

Lewis, D. O., Yeager, C. A., Swica, Y., Pincus, J. H., & Lewis, M. (1997). Objective documentation of child abuse and dissociation in 12 murderers with dissociative identity disorder. *American Journal of Psychiatry, 154,* 1703-1710.

Marmer, S. (1994). Theories of the mind and psychopathology. In R. E. Hales, S. C. Yudofsky, & J. A. Talbott (Eds.), *The American psychiatric textbook of psychiatry* (2nd ed.). Washington, DC: American Psychiatric Association Press.

Merskey, H. (1996). The manufacture of personalities: The production of multiple personality disorder. In L. Cohen, J. Berzoff, & M. Elin, (Eds.), *Dissociative identity disorder.* Northvale, NJ: Aronson.

Myers, T. (1903). *Human personality and its survival of bodily death* (Vol. 1 and 2). London: Longman, Green, and Co.

Nemiah, J. C. (1989). Dissociative disorders (hysterical neuroses, dissociative type). In H. P. Kaplan & B. J. Sadlock (Eds.), *Comprehensive textbook of psychiatry* (Vol. 1, 5th ed.). Baltimore: Williams & Wilkins.

Osborn, D. (1991). *Reflections on the art of living. A Joseph Campbell companion* (p. 154). New York: HarperCollins.

Prince, M. (1907). A symposium on the subconscious. *Journal of Abnormal Psychology, 2,* 67–80.

Prince, M. (1914). *The unconscious: The fundamentals of human personality, normal and abnormal.* New York: Macmillan.

Putnam, F. W. (1989). *Diagnosis and treatment of multiple personality disorder.* New York: Guilford Press.

Ross, C. A., Anderson, G., Heber, S., & Norton, G. R. (1990). Dissociation and abuse among multiple personality disorder patients, prostitutes, and exotic dancers. *Hospital and Community Psychiatry, 41,* 328–280.

Spiegel, D. (1984). Multiple personality as a post-traumatic stress disorder. *Psychiatric Clinics of North America, 7,* 101–110.

Stafford, L. L. (1993). Dissociation and multiple personality disorder: A challenge for psychosocial nurses. *Journal of Psychosocial Nursing and Mental Health Services, 31*(1), 15–20.

Steinberg, M. (1993). Advances in detecting dissociation. *Psychiatric Times, 10*(4), 20–23.

Taylor, E. (1983). *William James on exceptional mental states: The 1986 Lowell lectures.* New York: Scribner's.

Tessier, L. J. (1992). Women sexually abused as children: The spiritual consequences. *Second Opinion, 17*(3), 11–23.

Vaillant, G. (Ed.). (1986). *Empirical studies of ego mechanism and defense.* Washington, DC: American Psychiatric Press.

Yapko, M. (1994). *Suggestions of abuse: True and false memories of childhood sexual trauma.* New York: Simon and Schuster.

Suggested Readings

Coons, P. (1984). The differential diagnosis of multiple personality: A comprehensive review. *Psychiatric Clinics of North America, 1,* 51–65.

Dolan, Y. M. (1991). *Resolving sexual abuse: Solution-focused therapy and ericksonian hypnosis for adult survivors.* New York: Norton.

Herman, J. L. (1992). *Trauma and recovery.* New York: Basic Books.

Kaplan, H. I., Sadlock, B. J., & Grebb, J. A. (1994). Dissociation disorders. In H. I. Kaplan & B. J. Sadlock (Eds.), *Synopsis of psychiatry* (6th ed.). Baltimore: Williams & Wilkins.

O'Reilly-Knapp, M. (1996, October-December). From fragmentation to wholeness: An integrative approach with clients who dissociate. *Perspectives in Psychiatric Care, 32,* 5–11.

Putnam, F. W. (1989). *Diagnosis and treatment of multiple personality disorder.* New York: Guilford Press.

Stafford, L. L. (1993). Dissociation and multiple personality disorder: A challenge for psychosocial nurses. *Journal of Psychosocial Nursing and Mental Health Services, 31*(1), 15–20.

Yapko, M. (1994). *Suggestions of abuse: True and false memories of childhood sexual trauma.* New York: Simon and Schuster.

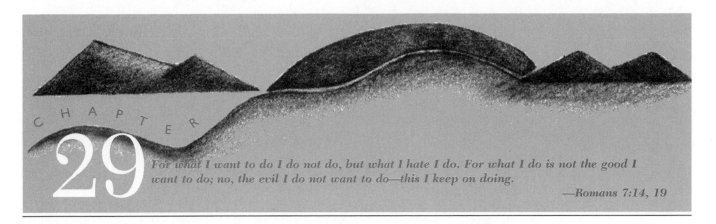

C H A P T E R

29

*For what I want to do I do not do, but what I hate I do. For what I do is not the good I
want to do; no, the evil I do not want to do—this I keep on doing.*

—*Romans 7:14, 19*

Psychosexual Disorders

Learning Objectives

After studying this chapter, you should be able to:

1. Discuss how sexuality changes across the life span.
2. Discuss the phases of the sexual response cycle.
3. Discuss abnormalities that occur across the phases of the sexual response cycle.
4. Describe the process for conducting a sexual assessment.
5. List and describe sexual deviations.
6. Discuss the spiritual aspects of normal and abnormal forms of sexual expression.
7. Apply the nursing process to patient situations in which there is either a sexual dysfunction or a sexual deviation.
8. Identify your own attitudes and biases about sexuality.

Key Terminology

Anorgasmia	Gender	Masochism	Sexual identity
Dyspareunia	Gender dysphoria	Orgasm	Sexual tension
Exhibitionism	Gender identity	Paraphilia	Sexuality
Fertility	Homosexuality	Pedophilia	Transsexualism
Fetishism	Human sexual response cycle	Premature ejaculation	Transvestic fetishism
Frotteurism	Impotence	Sadism	Vaginismus
Gay	Lesbian	Sex	Voyeurism

As we journey through life, each of us becomes increasingly aware of ourselves as sexual beings. This awareness is far broader than our recognition of lovemaking behaviors; it encompasses our views of ourselves as men and women, as mothers and fathers, as generative individuals who create and give to society in multiple ways. Our views are shaped by societal attitudes and mores, which seem to change with each generation. These shifting cultural pressures, however, are not the only determinant of sexual beliefs, attitudes, and behaviors. Parental views, spiritual and religious

teaching, socioeconomic status, and education all greatly affect our sexual behavior.

In our time, women's expressions of sensuality and sexuality have perhaps undergone the greatest transformation. Women are increasingly viewed by society as fully sexual beings who possess the right to say "no" to unwanted sexual advances. Courts have decided that married women can be victims of marital rape and their spouses punished accordingly. The whole issue of what constitutes consent to engage in sexual activity is brought to the courts with greater frequency.

Another issue that has undergone reconsideration is the diagnostic dilemma regarding whether homosexuality is an abnormal behavior or a variation of normal behavior. With the current epidemic of sexually transmitted diseases (STDs), the issue of sex education is more vital than ever, yet the debate continues over who should teach safer sex practices and at what age level.

These issues have an impact on psychiatric nursing. It belongs within the purview of all nurses to assess patients' sexual practices and be prepared to educate, dispel myths, assist with values clarification, refer to appropriate care providers when indicated, and share resources. Health promotion and disease prevention are key responsibilities for nurses. These actions alleviate or decrease patient illness and suffering and reduce health care costs. As a student of nursing, you are introduced to the complex issue of sexual behavior to facilitate thoughtful discussion of the topic and to develop personal belief systems that consider the broader perspective of sexual issues as they exist in contemporary society.

The goals of this chapter are to provide enough knowledge about normal and abnormal human sexuality for you to conduct a sexual assessment, to explain what is meant by human sexuality and the sexual response cycle, and to enable recognition of sexual dysfunctions that can occur at different stages of the cycle. You will be able to identify deviations from normal sexual behaviors and recognize nursing implications, formulate interventions, and state the rationale for planned therapeutic interventions. You will not be prepared to be a sex therapist.

To accomplish these goals, you must first explore personal sexual biases and knowledge deficits. You need to develop a degree of comfort when discussing sexual issues to put the patient at ease, thereby facilitating a candid dialogue. A basic knowledge of sexual anatomy and physiology, although essential, is insufficient for an appreciation of the complex nature of sexual development and behavior. Box 29-1 provides questions to encourage self-awareness about sexuality.

This chapter provides definitions of important terms, a review of the sexual response cycle and problems associated with a normal sexual response, an overview of the major sexual disorders, and an examination of the nurse's role in responding to sexual disorders through the modality of the nursing process. First, let's review John's story.

Box 29–1 ■ ■ ■ ■ ■
Questions to Encourage Sexual Self-Awareness

As you answer these questions, be aware of how you feel. Am I at ease? Uncomfortable? Embarrassed?

1. Am I comfortable being a woman (man)? When I consider my own sexuality, what do I mean? What behaviors and roles do I associate with my sexuality? Have I examined my own attitudes, feelings, and beliefs about sexual issues, such as:
   - Gender roles
   - Life cycle changes, including menstruation, pregnancy, and menopause
   - Sexually transmitted diseases, including AIDS
   - All forms of sexual activity, including masturbation/self-pleasure, homosexual activity, bisexual activity, fellatio, cunnilingus, anal intercourse, sexual activity with multiple partners, nonmarital sexual activity
   - Sexuality across the life cycle, that is, in children, adolescents, and the elderly
   - Sexuality in handicapped persons or in the mentally retarded
   - Lubrication, orgasm, ejaculation
   - Nudity (my own and others), touching my own body or another's body
   - Frequency of intercourse, positions for intercourse
   - Abortion, contraception
   - Talking about sexual issues with patients
2. As I look at my own attitudes, feelings, and beliefs, can I identify the sources of these? What part of my own attitudes, feelings, and beliefs can I attribute to my early upbringing? To my culture? To my religious beliefs? To my own sexual experiences?
3. Am I aware of what "turns me on" sexually? Conversely, what "turns me off" sexually?
4. Am I able to accept myself as a sexual human being? What about patients?
5. Am I willing to have my own beliefs challenged by learning accurate information regarding sexual issues?
6. Am I willing to increase my self-acceptance and my acceptance of others' sexuality?

John's Story

I call myself John, but maybe I should have chosen a less gender-specific name, like Chris. My appearance may confuse some people. It confuses me. I feel like I've spent my entire life trying to make the inner me match the outer me. Since I was young, I've felt this way, like somebody made a terrible mistake that I now have to try to correct. I was never like my sisters. They were sweet and delicate and played typical little girl games. I always knew that I was different... not a tomboy... but different—like I was molded into the wrong body. I felt that God had made a major mistake with me; he put me into the wrong body. My parents recognized that I wasn't like my sisters. Despite their best efforts to get me to conform, it never worked, so finally they gave up. I think I'm an embarrassment to them. They don't know how to explain me to their friends.

I feel like an outcast, never fitting into any group. For the past 3 years, I've dressed in male garments or unisex clothing. My hair is cut by a barber in a contemporary male style, and I drive a "macho" car. At the nursing home where I work, I do maintenance jobs such as washing and waxing floors. The nature of the job allows me to keep to myself, so I can avoid getting into personal conversations. After 3 years of hormone therapy, my appearance is more masculine, although my voice hasn't dropped as low as I had hoped it would. I'm more pleased with my outer appearance than I used to be, and I really feel great when someone addresses me as "mister" or "sir." Seeing myself undressed is still disturbing, and I can't go to places like the beach. My breasts are the biggest problem. I wear a binder all the time to try to get them as flat as possible.

Sex change surgery is extremely expensive, and it isn't easy to find surgeons who are experienced with the types of procedures involved. When you can find a surgeon, then you have to be able to convince him or her that you are not crazy for wanting to have these body-altering procedures because they are concerned that the person requesting the surgery will, at a later time, regret the decision. I don't ever expect to have a penis surgically constructed, but it would be nice to be able to stand at a urinal like other men, instead of using a stall. Penile construction involves a whole series of operations, and I could never afford them on my salary. I'm just hoping to find a surgeon who would be willing to remove my breasts. That would be enough to make me feel more like the man I was supposed to be. I'm not looking for surgery to make me attractive to females; for me, this isn't just "cosmetic" surgery. Loneliness is a problem—I admit that. And I would eventually like to have a relationship with a woman. But for now, my goal is simply to be more comfortable with me. ■

John's story provides a glimpse into the suffering experienced by an individual whose journey is marked by feeling as if she was born into the wrong body; she has the body of a woman, but the inner sense that she is a man. John suffers from gender dysphoria.

DEFINITIONS

Because there is considerable confusion regarding terms such as *sex, gender identity, gender, gender dysphoria, transsexualism, sexual identity,* and *homosexuality,* some definitions are presented (Stuntz, 1983).

The term **sex** refers to whether the person is anatomically male or female. This determination is based on the person's inherited biological endowment, that is, the vagina, ovaries, uterus, and 46XX karyotype or the penis, testicles, and 46XY karyotype.

Gender identity is the earliest acquisition of the basic sense of maleness or femaleness, which occurs normally during the first 18 months of life. It develops along with the sense of being a self separate from mother and all others. Gender identity thus is a part of self-identity, which in the normal course of personality development comes to include sexual identity. **Gender** refers to the person's psychological reaction to or sense of being male or female. A person has an inner conviction about being a boy or a girl, a man or a woman. Normally, sex and gender are the same, that is, "I have a vagina and I am a woman," or "I have a penis and I am a man." When sex and gender differ, however, the individual suffers from **gender dysphoria.** Such a person might have a physically normal female reproductive tract and yet have the "sense" that she is a male and might describe herself as "I am a man trapped in a woman's body." This is an example of the most extreme gender dysphoria, called **transsexualism.**

The identification of oneself as being male or female, the process of developing traits of masculinity or femininity, and the unfolding of the appropriate eroticism result in **sexual identity.** The majority of people develop a *heterosexual identity;* that is, they are sexually attracted to the opposite sex. A percentage of people in all cultures, however, develop a *homosexual identity,* wherein they express a sexual preference for people of the same gender. Homosexuals can be either *ego-syntonic,* in which the person is emotionally comfortable with his or her sexuality, or *ego-dystonic,* in which the person is emotionally distressed by the same-sex attraction. Homosexual men are frequently referred to as **gay** and homosexual women as **lesbian.**

In addition, some people are not exclusively heterosexual or homosexual but are attracted to members of both genders. These persons are bisexual in their sexual identity. Although sexual identity normally is believed to develop between the ages of 3 and 5 years, it is continually reworked and reinforced psychologically through adolescence and probably continues to develop in some measure throughout life. In the normal adult, the terms *gender identity* and *sexual identity* are synonymous; however, the gender-dysphoric person describes these terms as being at odds. Most such people describe their anatomy as being irrelevant to their sense of self (Stuntz, 1983).

What do you think? What factors have influenced your sense of yourself as a sexual being? If a fellow student revealed to you that he was bisexual, how would that affect your feelings for him as a nurse?

► *Check Your Reading*
1. Define the term *sex.*
2. What is the difference between sexual identity and gender identity?
3. What does it mean if an individual is gender-dysphoric?
4. To what does gender refer?

SEXUAL DEVELOPMENT ACROSS THE LIFE SPAN

Just as people are holistically physical, spiritual, and social beings, they are also sexual beings. Awareness and expression of sexuality change across the life span as the person grows and matures in all other domains. Sexuality encompasses the whole person. Physically, **sexuality** refers to appearance and physical expressions, such as kissing, hugging, embracing, fondling, and sexual intercourse. Socially, sexuality usually involves another person for full expression. Spiritually, sexuality includes a sense of connectedness and creativity. Table 29–1 illustrates the changes in sexual function, sexual self-concept, and sexual roles and relationships across the life span.

SEXUAL RESPONSE CYCLE

To evaluate sexual complaints in a scientific manner, you need knowledge of normal sexual functioning as well as

T A B L E 2 9 – 1 Stages of Human Psychosexual Development	
STAGE	**CHARACTERISTICS**
Prenatal	Chromosomal and hormonal factors influence the gender of the fetus.
	The gender of the fetus is determined by the 7th week.
Birth–2 y	Gender is assigned at birth.
	Societal influence reinforces the child's sexual identity.
	The infant is in the oral phase of development.
	Infants exhibit reflexive signs of sexual arousal.
	Physical affection toward the child is essential for normal psychosocial development.
2–5 y	The child is in the anal phase of development, characterized by learning sphincter control.
	The concept of privacy is manifested.
	Self-exploration of the genitals occurs.
	Awareness and mimicking of sex-role behaviors begins.
	Association between genitals and pleasure begins.
	The child has an attraction to the opposite-sex parent.
5–12 y	Sex play between age mates occurs.
	Curiosity about reproduction occurs.
	Friendships develop predominantly with same-sex age mates.
13–20 y	Sexual self-consciousness begins.
	There is an increase in sexual fantasy.
	Dating the opposite sex occurs.
	Concern about the physical changes of the body is evident.
	Menarche, breast enlargement, development of underarm and genital hair, and widening of the hips in females occur.
	Nocturnal emissions, broadening shoulders, increase in muscle mass, and development of body hair in males occur.
	Masturbation, petting, and intercourse occur.
Young adulthood	Individual is learning how to handle sexuality responsibly.
	Sexual experimentation and focus on sexual technique develop.
	Individual establishes long-term relationships.
	Pregnancy and childbearing are possible.
Middle adulthood	Self-acceptance is achieved.
	Performance anxiety decreases.
	Frequency of intercourse decreases.
	Hormonal changes—menopause occur.
	Secondary sex characteristics decrease.
	There is a change in erectile potential.
Late adulthood	Sexual activity is focused on intimacy rather than intercourse.
	Sexual accommodation is made for physical handicaps.
	Frequency of intercourse decreases.

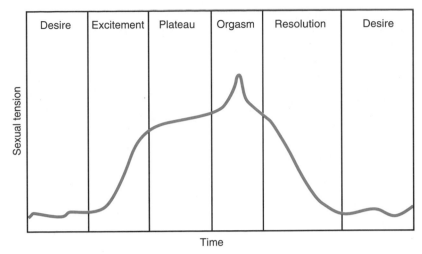

Figure 29-1
Stuntz's desire, excitement, plateau, orgasm, resolution, desire (DEPORD) model of the human sexual response cycle. (Redrawn from Stuntz, R. [1988]. Assessment of organic factors in sexual dysfunction. In R. Brown & J. Field [Eds.], *Treatment of sexual problems in individual and couples therapy* [pp. 188–201]. Dana Point, CA: PMA Publishing.)

deviations from the norm. Sexuality is a relational process that develops between two individuals of the same or opposite gender or between one person and his or her fantasy world. Physical and emotional intimacy is shared with the desire to relieve physical and emotional tension, in a manner that is described by most people as being supremely pleasurable.

One may think of "having sex" as being something like playing a violin. There are many parts of the violin, all of which must be in place and in working condition to allow the production of sound. That is, no music could be obtained without the neck, the pegs, the strings, the fingerboard, the sounding chamber with the "f"-shaped sound holes, and, of course, the bow. The similarities seem obvious. A woman interested in sexual activity must have the appropriate anatomy in working condition, normal hormones present in adequate amounts, a responsive and integrated nervous system, and, finally, to correspond with the "bow," an available and erect penis. Certainly, it is possible to produce excellent and intense sexual "music" without a partner and without relying either on the "bow" penis or the "violin" vagina, but for most individuals the truly soaring sensual experience requires the violin and the bow, the vagina and the penis.

Reproduction depends (in most cases) on the sexual act, which results in the pooling of male and female genetic material. This act of contributing genetic material toward the production of a fetus has been named sexual, and because of its overriding importance to the survival of the species, all societies have attempted to control sexual behavior in some manner. These societal constraints, sometimes in the form of religious dogma or moral teachings, introduce psychological tensions, which materially affect the manner of sexual expression and which, in turn, may produce symptoms of psychological illness. This is a more formal way of stating that beliefs, attitudes, and experience in regard to sexuality may influence the way people function and interact with other people.

An understanding of what is normal and expectable in the sexual response cycle is a prerequisite to recognizing what is "out of order." The research of Masters and Johnson (1970) provides an understanding of the sexual response cycle. Masters and Johnson are attributed with dividing the **human sexual response cycle** into four phases: excitement, plateau, orgasm, resolution. Kaplan (1979) later added the concept of a desire phase, which precedes the excitement phase and resumes following the end of the resolution phase.

Stuntz (1988) built on the antecedent work of Masters and Johnson and Kaplan to describe a model of the human sexual response cycle that he named the DEPORD (desire, excitement, plateau, orgasm, resolution, desire) model (Figure 29-1). The actual dimensions of sexual tension are difficult to measure empirically because there are few indicators other than self-report. Also, the total elapsed time of each phase of the cycle, as well as the cycle as a whole, varies with each person and with each sexual encounter. However, all complete normal human sexual response cycles pass consecutively through each of these phases; therefore, the model is consistent with, but not necessarily identical to, the sexual experiences of those people, men or women, whose sexual encounters involve normal response cycles. The DEPORD model, in general, is descriptive of the normal sexual response cycles of both men and women, although it is probable that sexual tension in women usually takes longer to rise through the excitement phase as well as longer to descend through the resolution phase.

Desire Phase

About 40% of the people applying to the Marriage Council of Philadelphia for help with their sexual problems described their difficulties as having to do with the desire for sexual activity (Leif, 1977). Many factors in one's life may affect the interest in sexual activity, including but not limited to age, both physical and emotional health, availability of a sexual partner, and the context of the individual's life (Chandraiah, Levenson, & Collins, 1991; Currier & Aponte, 1991; Dunning (1963; Williams, 1991). In fact, in a number of individuals, the lack of sexual desire is not a source of distress either to themselves or to their partners; in that situation, decreased or absent sexual desire would not be thought of as an illness. In general, however, hypoactive sexual desire is a ubiquitous and challenging disorder, associated with other psychiatric or medical conditions (Rosen & Leiblum, 1995).

Conversely, excessive sexual desire becomes a problem when this creates difficulties for the individual's partner or when such excessive desire drives that person to demand or force sexual compliance from unwilling partners.

The so-called male hormone testosterone (which is present in the circulation of both normal human women and men but in a much higher level in men) appears to be a prerequisite for sexual appetite in both men and women. Men who have lost the ability to produce testosterone describe the change in their sexual feelings in such terms as "I still have the basic inclination for sex but do not seem to have the energy to put it into effect." In some of these men, replacing their testosterone appears to restore their "sexual energy."

Testosterone appears to have a positive effect in increasing interest in sexual activity in women. A serendipitous finding confirmed this when postmenopausal women with breast cancer were given testosterone to slow the rate of the cancerous growth. Many of these women reported strong and unusual interest in sexual activity, including fantasies, dreams, and urges to become sexually involved, none of which they had entertained for many years prior. Although testosterone has been used frequently to increase sexual desire in postmenopausal women, there have been no well-designed treatment outcome studies, but there have been many case reports such as Ella's story (Case Example 29-1).

■ CASE EXAMPLE 29-1
■ Ella's Story

Ella is a 67-year-old woman, widowed many years, who has just been approached by a 75-year-old widower with a marriage proposal. Ella is concerned about the sexual implications of a marriage so late in life. She confided in her nurse practitioner, "I really haven't even thought about sex for so many years. I know Joe is just an old goat. He's always after me to take my clothes off." After discussing the possibility of a physiological cause for her lack of interest in sex, Ella's nurse practitioner gave her small doses of testosterone. Within a remarkably short time, Ella stopped talking about Joe as "an old goat" and began talking again about "how great life can be if you have the right partner." ■

There does not appear to be a direct relationship between the "female" hormone estrogen and sexual desire in women. A secondary effect, however, may be present in the requirement of estrogen for the maintenance of the normal vaginal distensibility and lubrication. If these functions are lost secondary to estrogen deficiency, as may occur in some postmenopausal women or in younger women who have had their ovaries removed, **dyspareunia** (painful coitus) and **vaginismus** (spasm of the vagina) may be the result. In addition to estrogen deficiency, there are other physical factors, such as vaginal infections and lesions to name a few, that can lead to dyspareunia and vaginismus. Once these occur, however, the causes then include a psychological anticipation of pain. At that point, the experience of painful coitus and the expectation of further coital discomfort may be hard to separate from the perceived lack of sexual desire. After all, no one, once burned, enjoys even the idea of putting their hand back on the hot stove.

In evaluating a patient with a sexual desire disorder, the physical assessment, including laboratory studies, would be performed before exploring psychological factors, such as emotional issues, life situation, and experiences (Alexander, 1993; Jensen, 1992; Leiblum, 1992; Patterson, 1993). The *Diagnostic and Statistical Manual of Mental Disorders, Fourth Edition* (DSM-IV) diagnostic criteria for desire phase disorders are shown in the box, Medical Diagnoses: Sexual Desire Disorders.

Excitement Phase

The excitement phase of the normal human sexual response cycle is that period of time during which sexual tension rises from the preceding level of sexual desire to the relatively high sexual tension levels that merge into the following plateau phase. Traditionally, penile erection and vaginal lubrication have been used as indicators of the presence or development of sexual excitement. If erection or lubrication does not occur in what, for that individual, is a sexually stimulating and appropriate situation, in that instance there has been an inhibition of sexual excitement, regardless of the causative factors. No other valid markers of sexual excitement occur except for the individual's self-report. For example, no physiological way exists to measure whether sexual excitement is experienced by a man who cannot obtain an erection or a woman who cannot become vaginally lubricated.

Finally, a few words about the difference in female and male sexual functioning. Pleasure aside, the female vagina can function purely as a physical receptacle for the erect male penis whether or not the woman feels sexual desire or excitement. This difference makes it possible for women to have intercourse without sexual feelings. The man must be able to demonstrate sexual excitement with a penile erection for him to be able to participate in coital activity. This is an absurdly simple but amazingly important difference in sexual functioning that is frequently overlooked or perhaps not fully appreciated. This difference is basic to the understanding of how men and women relate to each other sexually.

MEDICAL DIAGNOSES

Sexual Desire Disorders

DSM-IV Diagnosis:

Hypoactive Sexual Desire Disorder

Diagnostic Criteria

A. Persistent or recurrently deficient or absent sexual fantasies and desire for sexual activity.

B. The disturbance causes marked distress or interpersonal difficulty.

C. Occurrence not exclusively during the course of another Axis I disorder (other than a Sexual Dysfunction), such as Major Depression, and is not due exclusively to the direct physiological effects of a substance (drug of abuse or medication) or a general medical condition.

DSM-IV Diagnosis:

Sexual Aversion Disorder

Diagnostic Criteria

A. Persistent or recurrent extreme aversion to, and avoidance of all, or almost all, genital sexual contact with a sexual partner.

B. The disturbance causes marked distress or interpersonal difficulty.

C. Occurrence not exclusively during the course of another Axis I disorder (other than a Sexual Dysfunction), such as Obsessive-Compulsive Disorder or Major Depression.

Based on information from the *Diagnostic and Statistical Manual of Mental Disorders. Fourth Edition.* Copyright 1994 American Psychiatric Association.

The physiological changes that accompany the normal excitement phase are shown in Table 29-2. The DSM-IV diagnostic criteria for excitement phase disorders are shown in the box, Medical Diagnoses: Sexual Arousal Disorders.

Plateau Phase

As sexual tension continues to escalate, the plateau phase emerges out of the excitement phase at high levels of sexual tension. Sexual tension continues to increase but at a reduced rate until a level of orgasmic inevitability is reached, which marks the onset of the orgasmic phase. The plateau phase can be understood as a waiting period between the development of sexual excitement and the onset of orgasm, which most people perceive as extremely pleasurable and which sexually competent couples may wish to prolong until orgasm becomes inevitable. The physiological changes that accompany the normal plateau phase are shown in Box 29-2. The DSM-IV does not recognize any specific disorders or dysfunctions related primarily to the plateau phase.

Orgasm Phase

The orgasmic phase of the human sexual response cycle is attained only at high levels of sexual tension in both women and men. **Sexual tension** (also described as sexual arousal) is produced by a combination of mental activity, including thought, fantasy and dreams, and erotic stimulation of erogenous areas, which may be more or less specific for each individual. Most men require some penile stimulation and most women some clitoral stimulation, either directly or indirectly, to produce the high levels of sexual tension necessary for orgasm to occur. **Orgasm** may be described purely based on its physical characteristics as a neurophysiological event with accompanying release of erotic tension. Orgasm is considered by most individuals who have experienced that event as being the acme of pleasure. Comparisons have been made of orgasm descriptions made separately by women and by men. When references concerning the gender of the author or of the genitalia being stimulated are removed, it is impossible to determine whether the description was written by a man or by a woman. This suggests either that orgasm is not gender-specific, that is, that men and women enjoy a similar sensation, or that it is impossible to describe sensations accurately (Lawrence & Madakasira, 1992; Musher, 1990).

T A B L E 2 9 – 2 Physiological Changes Accompanying the Normal Excitement Phase	
CHANGES IN WOMEN	**CHANGES IN MEN**
Swelling of the vagina	Penile erection
Lubrication of the vagina	Nipple erection (two thirds of men)
Enlargement of the clitoris in diameter	
Nipple erection (two thirds of women) and darkening of the areolae	

MEDICAL DIAGNOSES

Sexual Arousal Disorders

DSM-IV Diagnosis:

Female Sexual Arousal Disorder

Diagnostic Criteria

A. Persistent or recurrent inability to attain or to maintain until completion of the sexual activity an adequate lubrication-swelling response of sexual excitement.

B. The disturbance causes marked distress or interpersonal difficulty.

C. The sexual dysfunction is not better accounted for by another Axis I disorder (except another Sexual Dysfunction) and is not due exclusively to the direct physiological effects of a substance (e.g., a drug of abuse, a medication) or a general medical condition.

DSM-IV Diagnosis:

Male Erectile Disorder

Diagnostic Criteria

A. Persistent or recurrent inability to attain or maintain an erection until completion of the sexual activity.

B. The disturbance causes marked distress or interpersonal difficulty.

C. The sexual dysfunction is not better accounted for by another Axis I disorder (except another Sexual Dysfunction) and is not due exclusively to the direct physiological effects of a substance (e.g., a drug of abuse, a medication) or a general medical condition.

Based on information from the *Diagnostic and Statistical Manual of Mental Disorders. Fourth Edition.* Copyright 1994 American Psychiatric Association.

There is at least one major gender difference concerning orgasm: most women who have experienced one orgasm may have repeated orgasms during the continuation of the same sexual activity. This occurrence depends on the maintenance of high levels of sexual tension through continued stimulation. Men, once they ejaculate as a part of their orgasm, go through a refractory period during which they cannot again ejaculate. The refractory period refers to the time required to produce another ejaculate and varies primarily according to age, with a young man measuring this refractory period in minutes, while an older man may require several hours. **Premature ejaculation** refers to the sudden release of semen with little or no penile stimulation. The inability to sustain high levels of sexual tension without ejaculating can seriously compromise the sexual act as a source of pleasure for both partners. Women, because they do not produce an ejaculate, do not have a comparable refractory period. The normal physiological changes occurring during the orgasm phase are shown in Table 29-3. The DSM-IV

diagnostic criteria for dysfunctions associated with the orgasm phase are shown in the box, Medical Diagnoses: Orgasmic Disorders.

Resolution Phase

During this phase, sexual tensions developed in prior phases subside to baseline levels presuming that sexual stimulation has ceased. The physiological changes that developed during the earlier phases of the response cycle now tend to dissipate. This is a period of psychological vulnerability and either may be a period of

Box 29-2 ■ ■ ■ ■ ■
Physiological Changes Accompanying the Normal Plateau Phase

- Increases in muscle tone, heart rate, blood pressure, and respiratory rate
- Appearance of a sex flush (in some people), which spreads across the upper body and face and resembles a measles rash without the itch

TABLE 29-3 Physiological Changes Accompanying the Normal Orgasm Phase	
CHANGES IN WOMEN	**CHANGES IN MEN**
A sudden surge of sexual tension	Pooling of seminal fluid in the proximal urethra caused by contractions of the prostate, seminal vesicles, and vas deferens
An equally sudden release of sexual tension	A sensation of ejaculatory inevitability
Simultaneous rhythmic contractions of the uterus, perivaginal muscles, and rectal muscles	Simultaneous contractions of the prostate, the perineal muscles, and the shaft of the penis propel a bolus of semen down the urethra

MEDICAL DIAGNOSES

Orgasmic Disorders

DSM-IV Diagnosis:

Female Orgasmic Disorder

Diagnostic Criteria

A. Persistent or recurrent delay in, or absence of, orgasm in a woman following a normal sexual excitement phase during sexual activity that the clinician judges to be adequate in focus, intensity, and duration. Some women are able to experience orgasm during noncoital clitoral stimulation but are unable to experience it during coitus in the absence of manual clitoral stimulation. In most of these women, this represents a normal variation of the female sexual response and does not justify the diagnosis. In some of these women, however, this does represent a psychological inhibition that justifies the diagnosis. This difficult judgment is assisted by a thorough sexual evaluation, which may even require a trial of treatment.

B. The disturbance causes marked distress or interpersonal difficulty.

C. The orgasmic dysfunction is not better accounted for by another Axis I disorder (except another Sexual Dysfunction) and is not due exclusively to the direct physiological effects of a substance (e.g., a drug of abuse, a medication) or a general medical condition.

DSM-IV Diagnosis:

Male Orgasmic Disorder

Diagnostic Criteria

A. Persistent or recurrent delay in, or absence of, orgasm in a man following a normal sexual excitement phase during sexual activity that the clinician, taking into account the person's age, judges to be adequate in focus, intensity, and duration.

B. The disturbance causes marked distress or interpersonal difficulty.

C. The orgasmic dysfunction is not better accounted for by another Axis I disorder (except another Sexual Dysfunction) and is not due exclusively to the direct physiological effects of a substance (e.g., a drug of abuse, a medication) or a general medical condition.

DSM-IV Diagnosis:

Premature Ejaculation

Diagnostic Criteria

A. Persistent or recurrent ejaculation with minimal sexual stimulation before, on, or shortly after penetration and before the person wishes it. The clinician must take into account factors that affect the duration of the excitement phase, such as age, novelty of the sexual partner or situation, and frequency of sexual activity.

B. The disturbance causes marked distress or interpersonal difficulty.

C. The premature ejaculation is not due exclusively to the direct effects of a substance (e.g., withdrawal from opioids).

Based on information from the *Diagnostic and Statistical Manual of Mental Disorders. Fourth Edition.* Copyright 1994 American Psychiatric Association.

---

pleasurable "afterglow" or may be described by some as being "uncomfortably emotionally exposed." With the restoration of normal physiological pulse, respiratory rate, and blood pressure, individuals frequently experience markedly increased perspiration. The DSM-IV does not recognize any specific resolution phase diagnoses.

What do you think? If you have never had vaginal (penile) intercourse, do you think you can be helpful to a patient who has an orgasmic disorder?

➤ *Check Your Reading*

5. What characterizes the desire phase?
6. What physiological changes occur during orgasm?
7. Define the plateau phase.
8. What are the dysfunctions that can occur during the desire phase?

SEXUAL DYSFUNCTIONS

A few of the sexual dysfunctions are discussed in detail.

Sexual Arousal Dysfunction

Erectile dysfunction is a common (affecting 10 to 20 million men in the United States) and multifactorial disease due to organic or psychological factors; erectile dysfunction strongly impairs the quality of life in a man

(Fabbri, Aversa, & Isidori, 1997). Men who experience erectile dysfunction may have feelings of embarrassment, guilt, or anxiety (Case Example 29-2). These psychological stressors may make it difficult for the individual to ask for help. Ego strength in men appears to be closely associated with the ability to perform sexually and to be attractive to the opposite sex. When a man decides to seek treatment for the complaint of erectile dysfunction, which may commonly be referred to as **impotence,** he may not know from which specialist he should seek treatment. If there is a family physician or medical generalist, he or she might be the first medical professional that the man consults. Other specialists that are sought out for the treatment of erectile dysfunction include urologists, psychiatrists, psychologists, and sex therapists. In many cases, patients who experience difficulties achieving and maintaining erections may already be in the care of a physician because many medical conditions and their treatments cause or contribute to erectile difficulties.

■ CASE EXAMPLE 29–2
■ Bill's Story

■ Bill is a 46-year-old unemployed salesman who was referred to the inpatient substance abuse program by his family physician. He is complaining of abdominal pain, loss of appetite, and low mood. A full health history revealed a pattern of heavy alcohol consumption over the past 4 years.

"I feel stressed out all the time," said Bill. "First it was job stress, then marital problems. Sales work was incredibly competitive; quotas and deadlines hung over me all the time. After work, I would wind down at the bar and then go home where I would have a few more drinks. After a while, our life really began to change. My wife said she felt left out, and the kids said I wasn't fun to be around anymore. When I tried to get close to my wife, I couldn't . . . you know . . . perform, and that made me feel even worse. I feel like such a loser. My wife thinks this program might save our marriage, but I'm afraid that I might not ever be the man I was." ■

As the nurse, you need to know how to assess a patient's complaint of impotence and should have a clear understanding of your educational role related to the sequelae of medical and surgical conditions in regard to sexual functioning. You have a primary responsibility to educate patients about medications and their side effects. For this reason, it is necessary to be informed about and comfortable with the topic of erectile dysfunction. The patient may not independently introduce the topic of sexual functioning, fearing the discomfort of the discussion. It is incumbent on you to ask questions about sexual functioning in a manner that allows the patient to speak candidly.

When a patient complains of impotence, a full assessment is carried out to determine the nature of the complaint. It is important to understand what the patient means when he says he is impotent. It is useful to have the patient explain what he is experiencing in his own words. If you do not understand the patient's vocabulary, it is important to encourage the patient to describe what happens or does not happen when he tries to perform sexually. Some patients equate impotence with infertility; therefore, it is important to clarify terms throughout the assessment, that is, explain the difference between impotence, which is the inability to achieve and maintain an erection adequate for intercourse, and fertility. **Fertility** refers to the viability of the sperm cells and their ability to reach and penetrate the ovum. The patient with erectile dysfunction can father a child through the aid of artificial insemination techniques, if treatment cannot restore functioning.

According to Greenblatt, Jungck, and Blum (1972), the incidence of impotence increases with age, with 50% of men reporting impotence by the age of 75. Kinsey's research found 27% of white men to be impotent by 75 years of age (Kinsey, Pomeroy, & Martin, as cited in Brown & Field, 1988). Other causes for impotence include medical illness, surgery, injury, anatomical defects, acute infection, medication side effects, and psychological causes. Davidson (1986) stated that there is an organic cause, particularly diabetes, to impotence seen in 50% of patients who have that complaint.

Organic causes include prescribed or illicit drug use; acute or chronic medical illness, such as diabetes, hypertension, cardiac disease, infection, or neurological disorders; surgical procedures; structural defects of the genitalia; and hormonal disturbances.

When assessing the complaint of impotence, there are several etiologic considerations. A sexual assessment tool, medical and psychiatric history, laboratory studies, and physical examination are used to identify the probable cause of the dysfunction. Treatment is guided by whether the cause is of an organic, psychological, or mixed type. Specific treatments for erectile dysfunction include vacuum erection devices, intracavernosal or intraurethral alprostadil injections, and penile implants (Koneneman, Mulhall, & Goldstein, 1997).

What do you think? If you have a male adolescent diabetic under your care, do you think it is appropriate to discuss the possibility of impotence as part of your diabetic teaching?

► **Check Your Reading**

9. Identify three causes of erectile dysfunction.
10. What is the difference between impotence and infertility?
11. What feelings are typically associated with erectile dysfunction?
12. Name three medical conditions associated with impotence.

Anorgasmia

■ **CASE EXAMPLE 29–3**
■ **Patricia's Story**

Patricia is a 25-year-old, married grade school teacher who has been admitted to an acute care psychiatric unit following an overdose of sedatives. On admission, she reported feeling depressed and generally unhappy with herself. Patricia and her husband of 3 years do not have children despite a shared desire to become parents. Patricia describes her husband as hard-working, loyal, and affectionate, yet Patricia says that she feels uncomfortable with the intimacy of marriage.

According to Patricia, the marriage was consummated on the wedding night, but Patricia was unable to achieve orgasm at that time or ever since, although she is able to achieve it with self-stimulation. Patricia's perceived inability to share herself intimately left her feeling like a failure as a wife. She increasingly avoided sexual activity, fabricating excuses when the opportunity for sexual intercourse presented itself.

Patricia never talked about her sexual concerns with her husband and had no close friends. Her mother, her closest relative, lives more than 200 miles away.

During the psychiatric assessment, Patricia revealed that she had come from a poor family and was an only child. To make ends meet, her mother worked as a store cashier in the evenings, while her father cared for her. Patricia's father was therefore the one to bathe her and to supervise other bedtime routines.

Patricia recalled that her father had started fondling her genitals while she was still a young child and proceeded to have intercourse with her when she was between the ages of 12 and 14 years old. Patricia says that she initially responded to this abuse with fear that she might be physically harmed. Later, her father threatened to abandon the family if Patricia shared their "secret."

The abuse stopped when Patricia's father was killed suddenly in a car accident. It was the father's insurance money that afforded Patricia the opportunity to go to college and pursue a teaching degree. Patricia never did tell her mother about her father's behavior, thinking that she might be blamed in some way.

As a young adult, Patricia began to feel an intrusive anger toward herself and both of her parents. Patricia hoped that by accepting a marriage proposal, she could get on with her life and put her past behind her. ■

In this story, Patricia would not have what Masters and Johnson (1970) termed *primary orgasmic dysfunction* but *secondary anorgasmia*. Patricia has experienced orgasm but in an inappropriate manner. The diagnosis of primary anorgasmia is used only when the patient has never experienced orgasm, either during intercourse of adequate duration or during masturbation.

Complaints of anorgasmia are not uncommon in patients with a history of sexual abuse. Maltz (1988) observed that incest is commonly identified by many therapists as the primary cause of a host of psychosocial problems, including sexual dysfunction. The degree of emotional distress and the form of the sexual dysfunction vary with the type of sexual abuse, that is to say, which body parts were fondled and whether there was penetration. Factors that affect the patient's resilience after the abuse include age, maturity, coping skills, personality traits, supportive relationships, the duration and frequency of abuse, and degree of violence. Therapy involves helping the patient to deal with guilt, anger, low self-esteem, helplessness, and trust. Treatment should also encompass all pertinent aspects of the family system and the roles of all family members within it, and intact boundaries must be created (DiGiorgio, 1998). Maltz (1988) believed that the final stage of treatment should focus on resolving the negative feelings directed at the abuser. She suggested that the patient confront the abuser directly, through face-to-face contact or by letter, or indirectly through an unmailed letter or in therapeutic role playing. Box 29–3 provides guidelines for helping a patient to disclose incest.

Anorgasmia is usually psychogenic in origin, although there can be a physiological basis, such as fatigue, acute illness, medication, decreased perineal musculature, or neurological and vascular conditions. Psychological factors that affect orgasmic potential include societal mores as they relate to women's sexual roles, family attitudes, childhood experiences, sex education or lack of it, and religious beliefs.

The evaluation of anorgasmia includes the patient's medical and psychiatric history, sexual history including current pattern of sexual functioning, physical examination, and laboratory studies. The sexual pattern of functioning includes questions about the use of foreplay before coitus and the duration of coitus. Women require a longer period of time to become fully aroused to achieve orgasm. Therefore, it is important to ascertain if one or both partners would benefit from sex education. The nonsexual aspects of the relationship with the sexual partner also affect the couple's ability to enjoy intimacy; therefore, the relationship itself should be explored. Discord or displeasure with a partner has a physiologically inhibiting quality. Likewise, unresolved psychological conflict may continue to intrude on sexual functioning.

Treatment of anorgasmia by trained professionals includes psychoanalysis, psychoanalytically oriented psychotherapy, and behavior modification. For patients who are diagnosed as having primary anorgasmia, masturbation therapy can be an effective adjunct to traditional modes of treatment. Cognitive therapies may be helpful, and in many cases, sex education is used to correct misinformation.

Sex education is in the domain of nursing and can take the form of didactic teaching, dispelling myths, facilitated discussion, charts, anatomical models, or other audiovisual aids. Other methods to assist the patient to cope with sexual dysfunction can take the form of values clarification, conflict resolution, role playing, communication skills, and, in some cases, relaxation techniques.

B o x   2 9 – 3 ■ ■ ■ ■ ■
Guidelines for Helping a Patient to Disclose Incest

Responding to Patient Needs During Counseling

Reassure the patient that
    You believe and do not blame the patient.
    The responsibility for incest belongs with the offender.
    The patient did the best she could to survive the circumstances.
    As a child, she was not in control of the situation.
    The details of the counseling will remain confidential.
    Victims of incest are "survivors" and recover from their victimization.
    Patients can get over their feelings of shame.
    Your feelings toward the patient will not change as a result of hearing about the incest.
Encourage and validate that
    The patient may temporarily feel worse about disclosure before starting to feel better.
    The patient has the right to feel anger and grief.
    The patient has the right to have positive feelings toward the offender.
    The patient did not deserve the abuse.
    The patient is making gains despite how small the gains seem.
    The patient is an important and intelligent person.
    You see the patient's coping mechanisms as "survivor skills" and adaptive.

Addressing Incest During Counseling

Elicit disclosure by
    Asking directly if sexual abuse occurred during childhood
    Using a structured questionnaire, such as an intake form, to receive a complete early sexual history
    Mentioning that the symptoms that the patient is describing have been related to histories of sexual abuse in other patients
    Defining incest for the patient
    Asking about best and worst experiences during childhood
    Being persistent in probing histories of sexual abuse
Once disclosure takes place
    Identify incest as a primary cause of the patient's difficulties.
    Acknowledge and validate the significance of the incest.
    Relate specific difficulties in adult life to coping skills developed to survive incest.
    Do not minimize incest even if it occurred infrequently.
    Encourage the patient to be fully aware of her own reactions to hearing about incest.

Reprinted from Josephson, F-B. (1987). Factors assisting female clients' disclosure of incest during counseling. *Journal of Counseling and Development, 65,* 475–478. © ACA. Reprinted with permission. No further reproduction authorized without written permission of the American Counseling Association.

The nurse also identifies the stage of psychosocial development in which the patient seems to be stalled. In the case of Patricia, childhood sexual abuse resulted in difficulties in trust. A review of Erikson's stages of psychosocial development may be helpful in understanding what the patient is experiencing (see Chapters 6 and 8). You reassure the patient that these psychological issues do not resolve overnight and may take patience over time to be resolved. You facilitate the patient's receptivity to exploring sexual issues and support the patient during periods of crisis. Increasing the patient's ability to cope with stress is a critical component of the nursing care plan. It is important to include both the patient and the partner in some, but not necessarily all, sessions because sexual functioning is a shared problem.

If you are providing care to the patient complaining of anorgasmia, you need to be a good listener. Sexual problems are usually difficult to discuss; the slow-paced interview allows time for the patient's story to unfold. Care of the anorgasmic patient involves sensitivity, emotional support, and encouragement. You can act as

a resource person by offering to make referrals to other health care professionals.

What do you think? You are caring for a mentally retarded patient who is sexually active. What do you see as your role in providing this patient with sex education?

► *Check Your Reading*
13. What is primary anorgasmia?
14. What is secondary anorgasmia?
15. What is the most common cause of primary orgasmia?
16. What are two interventions used to treat anorgasmia?

SEXUAL DISORDERS

People do not decide voluntarily what arouses them sexually. Rather, in maturing, they discover the nature of their own sexual orientation and interests. Individuals differ from one another in terms of

- The types of partners whom they find to be erotically appealing
- The types of behaviors that they find to be erotically stimulating

They also differ in intensity of sexual drive, in the degree of difficulty that they experience in trying to resist sexual temptations, and in their attitudes about whether or not such temptations should be resisted. The sexual disorders include many forms of **paraphilia,** a term used to identify repetitive or preferred sexual fantasies or behaviors that involve preference for use of a nonhuman object, repetitive sexual activity with humans involving real or simulated suffering or humiliation, and repetitive sexual activity with nonconsenting partners. Most paraphiliacs are men, and about 50% of those individuals develop the onset of their paraphilic arousal before age 18.

Paraphilia

There are eight distinct types of paraphilias (Table 29-4). The DSM-IV diagnostic criteria for paraphilias are shown in the box, Medical Diagnoses and Related Nursing Diagnoses: Paraphilias.

Cause

Case Example 29-4 illustrates how paraphilias manifested in two patients, Michael and Steve. There are a number of explanations for the causes of paraphilias (Brown, 1983). Various studies have implicated biological factors. These factors include abnormalities in the limbic system and temporal lobes of the brain. Abnormal levels of androgens have also been implicated. Kafka (1991) categorized sexual disorders of nonparaphilic men as well as paraphilic men as being reflective of sexual dysregulation disorders associated with a primary mood disorder. The psychoanalytic explanation is that

TABLE 29-4 Types of Paraphilias

TYPE OF PARAPHILIA	DEFINITION/CHARACTERISTICS
Exhibitionism	Characterized by recurrent, intense, sexual urges and sexually arousing fantasies involving the exposure of one's genitals to a stranger
Fetishism	Involves recurrent, intense sexual urges and sexually arousing fantasies involving the use of nonliving objects (e.g., bras, underpants, stockings)
Frotteurism	A recurrent preoccupation with intense sexual urges or fantasies involving touching or rubbing against a nonconsenting person
Pedophilia	Involves recurrent sexual urges and sexually arousing fantasies involving sexual activity with a prepubescent child
Masochism	Involves recurrent, intense sexual urges and sexually arousing fantasies involving the act (real or simulated) of being humiliated, beaten, bound, or otherwise made to suffer
Sadism	Involves recurrent, intense sexual urges and sexually arousing fantasies involving the act (real or simulated) of inflicting psychological or physical suffering (including humiliation) on someone else
Transvestic fetishism	A persistent association in a heterosexual man, lasting a total of at least 6 mo, between intense sexual arousal or desire and acts, fantasies, or other stimuli involving cross-dressing
Voyeurism	Involves recurrent, intense sexual urges and sexually arousing fantasies involving the act of observing unsuspecting people, usually strangers, who are naked, in the process of disrobing, or engaging in sexual activity
Paraphilia Not Otherwise Specified (NOS)	Paraphilias that do not meet the criteria for any of the specific categories
Telephone scatologia	A desire to place obscene phone calls
Necrophilia	A sexual attraction to corpses
Partialism	An exclusive sexual focus on parts of the body
Zoophilia	A sexual attraction to animals
Coprophilia	A sexual focus on feces
Klismaphilia	A sexual focus on enemas
Urophilia	A sexual focus on urine

Based on information from the *Diagnostic and Statistical Manual of Mental Disorders. Fourth Edition.* Copyright 1994 American Psychiatric Association.

MEDICAL DIAGNOSES AND RELATED NURSING DIAGNOSES

Paraphilias

DSM-IV Diagnosis:

Pedophilia

Diagnostic Criteria

A. Over a period of at least 6 months, recurrent, intense sexually arousing fantasies, sexual urges, or behaviors involving sexual activity with a prepubescent child or children (generally age 13 years or younger).

B. The fantasies, sexual urges, or behaviors cause clinically significant distress or impairment in social, occupational, or other important areas of functioning.

C. The person is at least 16 years old and at least 5 years older than the child or children in criterion A.

Related Nursing Diagnosis:

Altered Sexuality Patterns

Definition
The state in which an individual expresses concern regarding his or her sexuality.

Examples
Altered Sexuality Patterns related to conflict with preference of partner; knowledge/skill deficit about alternative responses to health-related transitions; altered body function or structure; illness or medical condition; lack of privacy; lack of significant other; ineffective or absent role models; conflicts with sexual orientation; fear of pregnancy or of acquiring a sexually transmitted disease; impaired relationship with a significant other.

Based on information from the *Diagnostic and Statistical Manual of Mental Disorders. Fourth Edition.* Copyright 1994. American Psychiatric Association. Nursing diagnoses and definitions from North American Nursing Diagnosis Association. (1994). *NANDA nursing diagnoses: Definitions and classification, 1995-1996.* Philadelphia: NANDA.

---

the individual failed to resolve the oedipal crisis and identifies with the parent of the opposite gender or selects an inappropriate object for libido focus. The behavioral model hypothesizes that whether the individual participates in paraphilic behavior or not depends on the type of reinforcement he or she receives following the behavior. The first act may be committed for a variety of reasons (e.g., modeling the paraphilic behavior of others, mimicking sexual behavior depicted in the media). But once the initial act has been committed, a conscious evaluation of the behavior occurs, and a decision is made of whether or not to repeat it. The last model to posit causative explanation is the transactional model of stress adaptation. This model suggests that the cause of paraphilias is most likely influenced by multiple factors.

■ **CASE EXAMPLE 29-4**
■ **The Stories of Two Paraphiliacs**

■ **Michael's Story**
Michael is a 26-year-old single white man who has reported an 8-year history of exhibitionistic behavior that increased at times of stress, anger, and depression. His sexual fantasies focus on power, dominance, and exposing himself. When Michael is not exposing himself, he spends hours driving around bus stops and masturbating while making verbal remarks to women waiting for buses.

Steve's Story
Steve is a 30-year-old single black man who has reported a compulsion that he has had since early adolescence: to view photographs of young boys between the ages of 11

and 15 and to masturbate while viewing these pictures. While masturbating, he would fantasize about oral-genital sexual activity as well as anal penetration. He also describes urges to rub against young boys while in swimming pools or at sporting events. He reports that he engages in these fantasies and behaviors at least four times a week or when the opportunity presents itself. ■

Treatment

The treatment is effected in line with the explanatory model for paraphilias being used. For example, a biological model might include blocking or decreasing the level of circulating androgens or treating the patient with an antidepressant such as fluoxetine (Prozac) or a mood stabilizer such as lithium (Kafka, 1991). The psychoanalytic model would assist the patient to identify unresolved conflicts and traumas from early childhood, thus resolving the anxiety that prevents him or her from forming appropriate sexual relationships. In the behaviorist model, the patient would be subjected to aversion techniques, such as the use of electric shock and chemical induction of nausea and vomiting in combination with exposure to photographs depicting the undesired behavior. These techniques have been successfully used to modify the undesirable behavior of the paraphiliac.

What do you think? Do you feel society needs to be informed of the whereabouts of sex offenders even though they have been rehabilitated?

➤ *Check Your Reading*
17. What is a paraphilia?
18. Name three of the eight different types of paraphilias.
19. State two possible causative explanations for the paraphilias.
20. What treatment is used for the paraphilias when the cause is considered to be physiological?

Gender Identity Disorder

Causality with respect to gender identity disorder (GID) is subdivisible into genetic, prenatal hormonal, postnatal, social, and postpubertal hormonal determinants, but there is as yet no comprehensive and detailed theory of causality (Money, 1994). Changes in the DSM-IV nomenclature include (1) adopting a single diagnosis of GID to apply to children, adolescents, and adults; (2) changes in the format of the criteria; and (3) placement in the section Sexual and Gender Identity Disorders (Bradley & Zucker, 1997). One study (Marantz & Coates, 1991) showed that 53% of mothers of boys with GID compared with only 6% of controls met the DSM-IV diagnosis of Borderline Personality Disorder or had symptoms of depression.

Children and adolescents with GIDs have four main characteristics (APA, 1994). First, the person has a strong and persistent cross-gender identification. This identification is not merely a desire for any perceived cultural advantages of being the other sex. In children, this cross-gender identification is manifested by four or more of the following:

1. A repeatedly stated desire to be, or insistence that he or she is, the opposite sex
2. In boys, a preference for cross-dressing or simulating female attire; in girls, an insistence on wearing only stereotypically masculine clothing
3. Strong, persistent preferences for cross-gender roles in make-believe play or persistent fantasies of being the opposite sex
4. An intense desire to participate in the stereotypical games and pastimes of the opposite sex
5. A strong preference for playmates of the opposite sex

In adolescents and adults, this cross-gender identification is manifested by statements of a desire to be the opposite sex, frequent masquerading as the opposite sex, a desire to live or be treated as the opposite sex, and the conviction that they have the typical feelings and reactions of the opposite sex.

Second, the person has persistent discomfort with her or his gender or a sense of inappropriateness in the gender role of that sex. In children, this persistent discomfort with one's sex is manifested by any of the following:

• In boys, assertions that their penis or testes are disgusting or will disappear or that it would be better not to have a penis; aversion to rough-and-tumble play;

and rejection of stereotypically male toys, games, and activities. (In a study of 275 boys and girls from 1978 through 1995, a male-to-female ratio of 6.6:1 was observed at a specialty clinic for gender identity disorders [Zucker, Bradley, & Sanikhani, 1997].)
• In girls, rejection of urinating in a sitting position, assertions that they will grow a penis, assertions that they do not want to grow breasts or menstruate, and marked aversion toward normative female clothing

This persistent discomfort with one's sex is manifested by preoccupation with getting rid of primary and secondary sex characteristics (e.g., requests for hormones, surgery, or other procedures to alter sexual characteristics physically to simulate the other sex) or by the belief that he or she was born the wrong sex.

Third, the disturbance is not concurrent with a physical intersex condition.

Finally, the disturbance causes clinically significant distress or impairment in social, occupational, or other important areas of functioning.

> **What do you think?** Do you believe it is immoral to have a sex change operation? Give your reasons. Why? Why not?

➤ *Check Your Reading*
21. Identify two characteristics of childhood GID.
22. Identify two characteristics of adolescent GID.
23. Identify two characteristics of adult GID.

HOMOSEXUALITY

Homosexuality is defined as sexual or erotic attraction to members of one's own sex. There are two types of homosexuality: obligatory and situational. In *obligatory homosexuality,* erotic and sexual desires are uniformly directed toward members of the same sex. In *situational homosexuality,* erotic and sexual desires are directed toward members of the same sex only in certain situations (e.g., long-term confinement in same-sex institutions, such as prison) (Saghir & Robins, as cited in Money & Mustapha, 1978).

Much controversy exists over whether homosexuality is a normal variant of human sexuality or whether it is a gender disorder. Although the percentage of people with a homosexual orientation in any population is difficult to determine, sexual activity between people of the same sex has occurred throughout history and across regional, national, social, and cultural boundaries. It occurs in animals as well as humans. Although homosexual expression of human sexuality has been considered normal and acceptable in various times, places, and cultures, it has nevertheless been considered inappropriate by much of society through the ages. Throughout history, religious leaders, legislators, and society at large have therefore sought to eliminate sexual activity between people of the same sex.

In 1974, the Board of Trustees of the American Psychiatric Association (APA) decided to label homosexuality a gender disorder only when the homosexuality is ego-dystonic. That is, homosexuality would be considered a gender disorder *only* when a person's sexual orientation causes him or her marked distress. Despite the APA's position, many people in psychiatry, biomedical science, religion, government, and society as a whole still have not come to terms with whether sexual activity between people of the same gender is a normal variant of human sexuality, a manifestation of a gender disorder, or a moral problem. Because of this, homosexuals are subjected to discrimination, stigmatization, and sometimes hate crimes.

A number of theories exist about why some people develop a homosexual orientation. Some medical researchers believe that intrauterine levels of sex steroids may play a role. They believe that the androgen levels to which a fetus is exposed in utero may affect not only the anatomical differentiation of males and females, but also psychosexual orientation. There is also some preliminary research to indicate a tendency for homosexual orientation to be inherited genetically.

Because the issue of homosexuality engenders such strong feelings and differing views in people, the nurse encounters a wide variety of approaches to helping patients with a homosexual orientation. For those mental health professionals who see sexual orientation as a normal variant of human sexuality, therapeutic efforts likely focus on helping patients to deal with the social stigma associated with homosexuality, helping patients foster healthy relationships, teaching patients how to avoid infection with HIV and other sexually transmitted organisms, and generally facilitating the efforts of patients to live emotionally satisfying lives.

Regardless of how a homosexual orientation develops and regardless of whether homosexuality is a normal variant or a gender disorder, many patients with a homosexual orientation come to therapy bearing a heavy load of pain. The person with a homosexual orientation frequently experiences profound shame and well-justified fears of stigmatization and hostility and sometimes even physical harm. As a nurse, it is vital that you demonstrate compassion in the face of such pain. Such compassion is at the core of a theistic world view, and it is the hallmark of the profession of mental health nursing.

> **What do you think?** One of the theories about the origin of homosexuality is that it results from a dominant, overbearing mother and a weak, passive father. What is your reaction to this theory?

> ➤ *Check Your Reading*
> 24. What is obligatory homosexuality?
> 25. What is situational homosexuality?
> 26. Discuss the biological theory of homosexuality.

27. What are the usual goals of treatment when homosexuals seek therapy?

OTHER SEXUAL PROBLEMS

Sexual problems can also result from head trauma, chromosomal abnormalities, and psychosis.

Sexual Problems Resulting From Head Trauma

Patients who have experienced head trauma with damage to the frontal lobe of the brain may display symptoms of promiscuity, poor judgment, inability to recognize triggers that set off sexual desires, and poor impulse control.

Sexual Problems Resulting From Chromosomal Abnormalities

Klinefelter's syndrome, a condition that is found on genetic examination, occurs in cases in which instead of the normal XY genetic coding for male gender, the patient has an extra X as his genetic make-up. These patients frequently present with immature genitalia and not uncommonly have schizophrenic symptoms.

Sexual Problems Resulting From Psychosis

Sexual functioning may be adversely affected any time there is a disturbance in an individual's ability to develop and maintain stable relationships. This is especially true for schizophrenic patients, who have difficulty coping with stress, a decrease in reality-based orientation to the world, and defense mechanisms that lead to withdrawn behavior (Case Example 29–5).

■ **CASE EXAMPLE 29–5**
■ **Josephine's Story**

Josephine has been admitted for inpatient psychiatric care after treatment on a medical unit for injuries sustained when she was struck by a car while running in the street. Josephine is well known to the staff and has had many previous admissions to stabilize her schizophrenia. Referral to a community mental health center had been only partially successful, in that Josephine did not return for treatment after the last discharge. She had been doing fairly well until 3 weeks before the automobile accident, when her purse containing her medication was stolen.

Instead of going to the health center to get a new prescription, she went to a bar and drank heavily. This pattern continued for 3 weeks, during which time the auditory hallucinations that Josephine had experienced in the past returned.

Josephine has been hearing a male voice telling her she was God's gift to men. These hallucinations, coupled with the effects of her heavy alcohol intake, led her into promiscuous behavior, soliciting sex with men in bars and proclaiming that she was doing "the Lord's work." Josephine's behavior put her in conflict with bar owners, and frequently she was asked to leave. On the night of the accident, after such an episode, Josephine ran out of the bar and into the street and was hit by a passing car. She fell to the pavement complaining of leg pain. An ambulance brought her to the hospital, and a radiograph showed that her leg was not broken. She was fully conscious and oriented but had no recall of the accident. The Mental Status Examination revealed auditory hallucinations consisting of commands to share herself with men and become "the mother of the Earth."

A review of Josephine's prior admissions showed that fluphenazine (Prolixin) was effective in controlling her symptoms of schizophrenia. A treatment plan was formulated to begin Josephine on oral fluphenazine and later change to fluphenazine (Prolixin Decanoate) (administered intramuscularly) to ensure better compliance. Hospital staff contacted the mental health center that would follow up on Josephine's progress, and the center approved of the plan. Josephine accepted the plan because she was afraid that she would come to harm again and because she trusted the staff.

The challenge to the nursing staff was to prevent Josephine from engaging in inappropriate sexual behavior while the hallucinations were still present. To facilitate this goal, female nurses cared for Josephine whenever possible. When male nurses had to care for Josephine, they set limits with her when she became seductive. Another intervention to reduce the risk of inappropriate sexual behavior was to place Josephine in a room closer to the nurse's station for closer monitoring. If these measures were not adequate, Josephine would be placed on close observation status (one nurse assigned to stay near Josephine at all times).

The policy on the unit was to have the hall monitored during the night so that patients did not have access to the rooms of other patients. In addition, all patients were informed on admission that visiting in the rooms of other patients was not allowed. The unit rule also stated that physical contact between patients was against policy and would result in discharge.

Because Josephine's sexually inappropriate behavior was driven by her command hallucinations, the staff expected that as the hallucinations resolved, the behavior would stop. Because compliance with an oral medication regimen had been a problem for Josephine, the staff expected that the change in the form of Josephine's medication would result in improved compliance.

Other issues of concern to the nurses were the patient's lack of "safer sex" practices, her lack of use of birth control, her lack of information about sex, and her need for screening for STDs. At a point when Josephine was able to hold a conversation free from the effects of her thought disorder, the staff initiated discussions with her about these issues. They provided Josephine with a referral to a gynecology clinic while she was still an inpatient.

The last issue of concern to the nurses was Josephine's self-esteem. As Josephine's symptoms abated, the behaviors that she had exhibited during her illness were a source of great embarrassment to her. The nurses responded to Josephine's embarrassment by being supportive, by being good listeners, and by encouraging her. The nurses frequently reminded Josephine that her behaviors were symptoms of an illness—not manifestations of a character weakness. ■

The schizophrenic patient's sexual drive may be altered only during the acute phase of illness or it may be of an ongoing nature. This could depend partially on the severity of the illness. In addition, patients with chronic schizophrenia have difficulty communicating their needs and concerns to others. For the schizophrenic patient, self-concept and ego strength deteriorate over time, further decreasing the patient's ability to develop or maintain intimate relationships.

Schizophrenia is not necessarily associated with sexual dysfunction or deviant sexual behavior, but the symptoms of schizophrenia and even the treatment with neuroleptic medications (Patterson, 1993) may make the patient vulnerable to disturbances in sexual functioning and often child-like and passive in relationships. The primary goal of the treatment team in the patient psychiatric setting is to control acute symptoms. Sometimes, the acute symptoms present as delusions. These delusions can be sexual in form, or they can be of a paranoid type that drives the patient away from meaningful relationships and produces a sexual problem from the resulting alienation. Delusions may also be of a grandiose nature in that the patient may believe himself or herself to be a great lover or have a "special mission" of a sexual nature.

Sexually inappropriate or dangerous behaviors that are of a delusional origin are noted during the initial psychiatric assessment. Even if the patient does not initially share these thoughts, they could emerge later in treatment as you develop rapport with the patient. Most patients respond to treatment with neuroleptic medications, and the inappropriate sexual behaviors resolve as the delusion subsides. Conversely, the patient who does not have delusions primarily of a sexual nature may, in the course of the hospitalization, be willing to discuss issues of daily living that might include relationships and sexuality. A third type of patient would be the schizophrenic who is admitted for control of acute symptoms but who additionally has a sexual problem that is not associated with the primary diagnosis. This problem may be detected by the patient's self-report, the physician's physical examination, or the nurse's assessment.

Some sexual problems require immediate interventions, such as alleviating the sexual symptoms caused by side effects of medications or controlling inappropriate sexual behavior. Other sexual problems are better managed through interventions as identified in the long-term goals (see the nursing process case study later in the chapter). These might include helping the schizophrenic to develop social skills that increase the probability of forming relationships. This may be accomplished by referring the patient to a psychosocial rehabilitation program. Some sexual problems can be remedied by achieving short-term goals that use education as a nursing intervention. Frequently, sexual myths and misinformation can be corrected, giving the patient almost instant relief from perceived problems. For instance, some people continue to believe that there is a connection between masturbation and becoming "crazy."

All patients can benefit from an assessment of their sexual knowledge. Sexual hygiene, methods of birth control, and sexual health are important issues, as is the patient's understanding of sexual anatomy and physiology. Although these topics may not be the initial focus of nursing interventions, they become important at some point in the course of the hospitalization. The nurse assesses the patient's sexual functioning and offers information when indicated. All patients on a psychiatric inpatient unit should be informed on admission about unit rules regarding personal contact between patients and between patients and staff. Limit-setting is done consistently, when indicated.

> **What do you think?** If your patient's sexual behavior is inappropriate according to social norms, do you have a role in helping the patient change this behavior?

➤ *Check Your Reading*

28. What is the connection between head trauma and sexual problems?
29. What impact does psychotic behavior have on sexuality?
30. What is Klinefelter's syndrome?

THE NURSE'S RESPONSE TO SEXUAL DISORDERS AND OTHER SEXUAL ISSUES

When making judgments regarding sexual behavior, it is important for the nurse to appreciate the state of mind that contributed to the individual's behavior. Inappropriate sexual behaviors can occur for a variety of reasons. For example, a person with schizophrenia may behave in a particular way in response to hallucinations, whereas the alcoholic's behavior may be a reflection of diminished judgment secondary to intoxication. A mentally retarded individual may become involved with a child (who may be of the same approximate mental age as he or she is) because of the lack of availability of adult partners and the lack of capacity to appreciate and understand fully the wrongful nature of his or her actions.

It is also important when discussing sexual deviations to differentiate between an individual's sexual orientation and interest and the individual's temperament and traits of character, such as kindness versus cruelty, caring versus uncaring, sensitivity versus insensitivity, conscientiousness versus lacking in conscience, and so on. Imagine the emotional and spiritual distress experienced by a pedophile who is unhappy with his sexual orientation. A person diagnosed with a sexual disorder may be a more concerned person dealing less than successfully with sexual temptations of a sort that are foreign to most individuals.

It is easy for a nonsmoker to argue that any smoker could stop if he or she really wanted to; in the case of the pregnant smoker, she should stop if not for her own sake, then surely for the sake of not damaging her unborn child. It is easy for a nonobese person to argue that successful dieting can be accomplished through will power alone. Similarly, it is easy for a person who is not tempted by inappropriate sexual thoughts or behaviors to argue that any sex offender could have stopped the behavior if he or she really wanted to and would simply determine to do so. When it comes to appetites or drives, such as hunger, thirst, pain, the need for sleep, or in the desire for sex, however, biological regulatory systems may exist that can cause an individual to experience desires to satisfy those hungers in ways that cannot be successfully resisted by will power alone. People can become so discomforted by cravings related to such appetites that they feel compelled to act in ways that diminish their discomfort.

When a person falls deeply in love with another person, be it a child or an adult, it becomes easy for that person to convince himself or herself that the relationship is good and healthy and not harmful or wrong. One of the major issues in trying to understand human behavior relates to where the line should be drawn between considering a person to be the passive product of life experiences and biological make-up and considering him or her (by virtue of having subjective consciousness) to be an active agent capable of transcending prior determinants.

NURSING PROCESS

Assessment

Caring for patients with sexual complaints requires of the nurse proficiency in the science as well as the art of the profession. Sexual issues are assessed scientifically by understanding the biological processes of the reproductive system. The manner in which you develop a helping relationship with the patient is more akin to an art in that it is tempered by compassion and empathy.

The sexual assessment includes both subjective and objective data. Many psychiatric hospitals use a nursing history tool that is biologically oriented but may have a few questions on sexual functioning. Health history questions pertaining to the reproductive system may be limited to menstrual history, parity, history of STDs, method of contraception, and questions regarding safer sex practices. There may be some vague questions about sexual functioning or sexual concerns. You may be uncomfortable exploring sexual issues with your patients for fear that you or the patient will be embarrassed or that you will not know what questions to ask or why you should ask them. Patients themselves may sense your discomfort with the topic, or they might also be uncomfortable when discussing sexual issues.

There are many tools available for conducting a sexual assessment that can supplement the basic health history, but forms and tools in themselves are impersonal and do not provide a good format for dialogue. An awareness of the content of a complete sexual assessment tool may, however, give you a fuller appreciation of the scope of questions to be asked and acquaint you with a conceptual framework.

Guidelines for Conducting a Sexual Assessment

The sexual history captures not only the patient's physiological functioning but also behavioral, emotional, and spiritual aspects of sexuality. It also includes cultural and religious beliefs in regard to sexual behavior and sexual knowledge base. During the assessment, both the nurse and the patient are free to ask questions and to clarify information. It is reasonable to defer lengthy sexual health assessment when acute psychiatric symptoms preclude a calm, thoughtful discussion. As symptoms subside and rapport is developed, the assessment may be resumed. With experience, you will be able to identify those patients who are at a greater risk for difficulties in sexual functioning. Key indicators of risk might include patients with a history of medical problems such as diabetes, multiple sclerosis, myocardial infarction, Parkinson's disease, epilepsy, or surgical procedures (Aass, Grunfeld, Kaalhus, & Fossa, 1993; Corney, Crowther, Everett, Howells, & Shepherd, 1993; Meyer-Bahlburg et al., 1993; Walbroehl, 1992); those requiring maintenance medications (Balon, Yeragani, Pohl, & Ramesh, 1993); or those who are experiencing relationship difficulties. Table 29–5 lists drugs known to have side effects that can disturb sexual function.

The initial sexual assessment may be a basic screening to detect areas of concern. It should be incorporated into the general physical assessment, which includes questions of a demographic nature, such as age, sex, marital status, religion, and educational level. The review of systems may reveal medical diagnoses that could have an impact on sexual functioning. The reproductive history is a logical place in history-taking to introduce nonthreatening questions of a sexual nature. In the psychiatric setting, many patients have illnesses that prevent them from developing relationships, yet they still have a need for sexual expression. If there appears to be an indication for a fuller assessment, you

TABLE 29–5 Drugs Known to Have Side Effects That Can Disturb Sexual Function

DRUG	EFFECT ON SEXUAL FUNCTION
Antianxiety	Decreased libido
Anticholinergics	Erectile dysfunction
Antidepressants	
Tricyclics	Decreased libido
MAOIs	Ejaculation difficulties Erectile dysfunction
Selective serotonin reuptake inhibitors	Decreased libido Erectile dysfunction
Antihistamines	Decreased libido Erectile dysfunction
Antihypertensives	
Diuretics	Erectile dysfunction
Centrally acting sympatholytics	Decreased libido Erectile dysfunction
Alpha- and beta-adrenergic blockers	Erectile dysfunction Ejaculation difficulties
Ganglion blockers	Erectile dysfunction Ejaculation difficulties
Sympathetic nerve terminal agents	Decreased libido Erectile dysfunction Ejaculation difficulties
Nonadrenergic vasodilators	Decreased libido Erectile dysfunction
Antipsychotics	
Phenothiazines	Decreased libido Erectile dysfunction Ejaculation difficulties
Butyrophenones	Erectile dysfunction Decreased libido
Narcotics	Decreased libido Erectile dysfunction Ejaculation difficulties
Cocaine	Decreased libido Ejaculation difficulties
Alcohol	Decreased libido Erectile dysfunction Ejaculation difficulties
Sedative-hypnotics	Decreased libido Erectile dysfunction Ejaculation difficulties
Marijuana	Decreased libido Erectile dysfunction
Amphetamines	Erectile dysfunction Ejaculation difficulties

MAOIs, monoamine oxidase inhibitors.
Data from *The Johns Hopkins Medical Journal,* 151(4), 1982; and *The Medical Letter,* 25(641), 73–76, 1983.

may want to use a complete sexual assessment tool as a reference from which to compile a more patient-specific interview. The complete assessment includes questions about the patient's family, relationship between the parents, acquisition of sexual information (both formal and informal), gender roles, toilet training history, and attitudes about sexuality and sexual expression.

An important issue to explore is the relationship of spirituality or religious belief to sexuality. An individual may experience acute spiritual distress related to his or her choice of sexual expression. This distress may originate in religious dogma or tenets of moral behavior. Imagine the spiritual distress of a prominent religious leader accused of being a pedophile. The significance and meaning of sexuality to the individual is far-reaching and is as important to understanding the individual's journey as the physical and psychological aspects of the assessment.

Settings for a Sexual Assessment

When the nurse conducts a sexual interview, she or he should provide a setting that allows for privacy and an absence of distractions. Although note-taking may be necessary for the beginner, it can be distracting to the patient and interrupt the flow of the interview. When necessary, it should be kept brief and unobtrusive. When you master the content of the sexual assessment, the questions flow in a logical sequence. You conduct the interview free from personal biases and judgmental attitudes that would impede open discussion of sexual issues. Body language communicates openness and receptivity. Good eye contact, relaxed posture, and friendly facial expressions facilitate the patient's comfort.

Conducting the Interview

First, the nurse introduces herself or himself to the patient and then explains the purpose of the sexual assessment. Inform the patient that confidentiality is strictly maintained. Questions should proceed from least intrusive to more intrusive. The interview should be efficient but not hurried. A directive approach guides the interviewee through a set of questions that can be used for data gathering that is less personal, whereas a less directive approach provides more information by allowing the patient to express feelings and beliefs

---

TABLE 29–6 Some Common Slang Expressions Related to Sexuality

MEDICAL TERM	SLANG EXPRESSION(S)
Breasts	Tits, sacks, front, headlights, knockers, boobs, bosom, bonkers, bust, jugs, buds
Climax	Come, go off, shoot cream, blast off
Clitoris	Bed fellow, little gem, badge of shame, gaiety, madness, narrow strip
Cunnilingus	Eating it, going down, eating pussy
Erection	Hard-on, stiff, bone, boner, hot rocks, lover's nuts
Fellatio	Going down, sucking, blowing, getting a blow job, giving head, cocksucking
Homosexual	*Male:* Fairy, fag, faggot, gay, queen, nellie, homo, swish, pervert, pansy, back door artist
	Female: Lez, sister, lesbo, dyke, bull dyke
Hymen	Cherry, membrane, maidenhead
Impotence	Couldn't get it up, couldn't get a hard-on
Intercourse, coitus	Make love, screw, fuck, get down, ball, make it, get laid, mess around, score, bang, jive, frig, get a piece, sleep with, get some tail, hook up
Masturbation	Jack off, jerk off, pocket pod, hand fuck, circle jerk, beat the meat, hand job
Menstruation	Curse, monthly period, devil's making ketchup, red-bearded cousin from the South, the flag's up, on the rag
Mutual oral-genital stimulation	Sixty-nine
Orgasm	Come, climax
Penis	Joystick, worm, dick, prick, stick, peter, rod, john, third leg, middle leg, joint, glans, cock, organ, thing
Pubic hair	Beaver, bush, pubes
Semen	Come, juice, egg white, gizzum
Sexual choice	Straight (heterosexual), gay (homosexual), AC-DC (bisexual)
Sexual desire	Horny, cold fish (decreased libido), nympho (increased libido)
Testes	Balls, nuts
Vagina	Pussy, hole, cunt, cat, pocketbook, treasure, twat, furburger, box, beaver, snatch, tunnel

Adapted from Green, R. (1975). *Human sexuality: A health practitioner's text.* Baltimore: Williams & Wilkins.

Box 29–4 ■ ■ ■ ■ ■
Patient Cues That May Indicate Concerns About Sexuality

Nonverbal Behaviors

- Showing discomfort through blushing, looking away, tight fists, fidgeting, crying
- Openly engaging in overt sexual behaviors, for example, touching own body parts, masturbating, exposing genitals, placing nurse's hand on genitals, making sexually suggestive sounds

Verbal Behaviors

- Telling sexually explicit jokes
- Making sexual comments about the nurse
- Asking inappropriate questions about the nurse's sexual activity
- Discussing sexual exploits
- Asking the nurse to perform sexual acts
- Expressing concern about relationship with partner
    "I don't feel the same about my partner."
    "My partner doesn't feel the same about me."
    "We're not as close."
    "Our relationship is changed."
    "My personal life has changed."
- Expressing concern that sexuality has been diminished, for example, feeling less of a man, less of a woman
    "I've lost my manhood."
    "I'm not as desirable as I once was."
- Expressing concern over lack of sexual desire
    "I'm not horny anymore."
    "My desire has changed."
    "I'm not the man/woman I used to be."
    "We don't click anymore."
- Expressing concern over sexual performance
    "I don't get wet."
    "I've lost my power."
    "Will I still be able to get hard?"
    "What will happen to my ability to perform?"
    "I can't perform like I used to."
- Expressing concern about one's love life
    "My love life has changed."
    "The spark has worn off."
- Expressing concern over the sexual impact of drugs, surgery, or some other medical issue
    "Will this drug interfere with my sex life?"
    "Will I still be able to perform sexually after surgery?"

tionship is maintained, and the patient learns a way of communicating that is less embarrassing. Table 29–6 presents some common slang expressions related to sexuality and their corresponding medical terms. You may find it helpful to share this information with patients.

Throughout the interview, it is important to note the patient's body language. Decreased eye contact, fidgeting, turning away from the interviewer, and hesitancy in answering questions may indicate an area of concern for the patient. Box 29–4 lists patient cues that may indicate concerns about sexuality.

At this point, you may choose to ask the patient if there is discomfort in the area of sexual functioning. Generally, it is more comfortable for the patient if you first ask questions in a general manner and then proceed to ask about the patient's specific experience. For example, "Some people who are prescribed this medication find it difficult to achieve an erection. Have you had this problem?" This type of question allows the patient to feel that he or she is not alone in what he or she is experiencing. Table 29–7 provides facilitative statements for the interviewer conducting a sexual assessment. Table 29–8 provides some interviewing dos and don'ts to follow when obtaining sexual information.

Diagnosis

A comprehensive sexual assessment reveals areas of sexual concern and dysfunction for the patient. These data are analyzed to determine the appropriate medical and nursing diagnoses. A sample nursing diagnosis might read: "Sexual Dysfunction related to marital problems evidenced in painful intercourse and inability to have orgasm."

Outcome Identification

The expected outcomes for a patient with a sexual problem vary with the medical and nursing diagnoses. The following are examples of expected outcomes for patients with sexual problems:

1. The patient will resolve marital difficulties and resume a satisfying sexual relationship with her spouse.
2. The patient will cease drinking and experience the ability to achieve an erection.
3. The patient will no longer experience pain while engaging in sexual intercourse.

Planning

Based on the identified expected outcomes, the nurse and patient, working together with the interdisciplinary team, jointly establish short-term goals, such as the following:

freely. Accepted medical terminology should be used when discussing sexual issues, but you must also know commonly used slang expressions to understand what the patient is saying. In the process of using medically correct terminology, the patient-nurse therapeutic rela-

TABLE 29–7 Facilitative Statements for the Interviewer Conducting a Sexual Assessment

PURPOSE	FACILITATIVE STATEMENT
To give a rationale for a question	As a nurse, I'm concerned about all aspects of your health. Many individuals have concern about sexual matters, especially when they are sick or when they are having other health problems.
To give statements of "generality" or "normality"	Most people are hesitant to discuss . . . Many people worry about feelings . . . Many people have concerns about . . .
To identify sexual dysfunction	Most people have difficulties sometime during their sexual relationships. What have yours been?
To obtain information	The degree to which unmarried persons have sexual outlets varies considerably. Some have sexual partners. Others have none. Some relieve sexual tension through masturbation. Others need no outlet at all. What has been your pattern?
To identify sexual myths	While growing up, most of us have heard some information or stories about sex that continue to puzzle us. Are there any that come to mind?
To identify feelings about masturbation	Many of us grown-ups have heard a variety of stories about masturbation and what problems it supposedly causes. This can cause worry even into adulthood. What have you heard?
To determine whether homosexuality is a source of conflict	Some say homosexuality is a mental disorder, others an emotional block, others a crime or sin. What is your attitude toward your homosexual orientation?
To identify an older person's concerns about sexual function	Many people, as they get older, believe or worry that this signals the end of their sex life. Much misinformation continues this myth. What is your understanding about sexuality during the later years? How has the passage of time affected your sexuality (sex life)?
To obtain and give information (miscellaneous areas)	Frequently people have questions about . . . What questions do you have about . . . What would you like to know about . . .
To close the history	Is there anything further in the area of sexuality that you would like to bring up now? I hope that if questions or concerns do come to mind in the future we'll be able to discuss them.

Adapted from Green, R. (1975). *Human sexuality: A health practitioner's text* (p. 89). Baltimore: Williams & Wilkins.

Expected Outcomes	Short-Term Goals
The patient will resolve marital difficulties and resume a satisfying sexual relationship with her spouse.	1. The patient will identify her feelings toward her spouse. 2. The patient will communicate her feelings toward her spouse, taking an "I" stance rather than a "blaming" stance. 3. The patient will participate in homework that focuses on small steps in achieving sexual satisfaction.
The patient will cease drinking and experience the ability to achieve an erection.	1. The patient will agree to attend Alcoholics Anonymous meetings. 2. The patient will work with a sponsor who will help him to remain sober. 3. The patient will not drink. 4. The patient will resume sexual activity.
The patient will no longer experience pain while engaging in sexual intercourse.	1. The patient will demonstrate relaxation exercises that she will use before sexual intercourse. 2. The patient will practice thought-stopping techniques to control her anticipatory fear that she will experience pain with sexual intercourse. 3. The patient will use a lubricant such as K-Y jelly before engaging in sexual intercourse.

Implementation

A decision tree is helpful for determining the appropriate course of treatment for a person with a sexual complaint, even if it will not be you who actually carries out the treatment (Figure 29-2). Although most nurses will never be sex therapists, all nurses need to know when and to whom to refer the patient with a sexual complaint. Depending on the nature of the problem, the patient may need a referral to such professionals as a marital counselor, psychiatrist, gynecologist, urologist, clinical nurse specialist, or pastoral counselor.

Many nursing interventions have already been discussed along with specific deviations. Appropriate strategies for intervening include milieu therapy, education, behavioral therapy, medication, and psychotherapy. Although psychotherapy alone has not been helpful in stopping the deviant sexual behavior, it does provide an adjunct support. Psychotherapy is used to assist the patient in identifying triggers that set off the inappropriate sexual behavior (Kaplan, 1975, 1979). Once the triggers have been identified, alternative coping skills are discussed. These alternative coping skills include thought blocking and thought changing. Snapshot: Nursing Interventions Specific to Psychosexual Dysfunction.

Covert sensitization, a behavioral technique, is a widely used procedure in the treatment of inappropriate sexual behaviors. Covert sensitization may act as a self-control technique whereby the individual uses the aversive cue to control the inappropriate behavior.

Medication is the last treatment intervention to be addressed. There is insufficient research and data to conclude that this intervention could be used independently as a treatment without the other interventions. The drug that is frequently used in treating sexual deviations, however, is medroxyprogesterone acetate (Depo-Provera). Medroxyprogesterone acetate, in both men and women, in sufficient quantity decreases sexual urges and assists in controlling the offending sexual behavior (Berlin, 1985).

Evaluation

Evaluation of expected outcomes and achievement of short-term goals relate to the level of control and personal satisfaction that is achieved. Acceptance of sexual dysfunction, such as impotence, as being a part of, but not necessarily the defining characteristic of, sexual behavior can result in greater satisfaction. The degree to which negative attitudes about sex are no longer problematic also is important.

What do you think? If you are treating a patient who confesses to pedophilia, what is your responsibility to the patient's spouse and children?

➤ *Check Your Reading*
31. Describe the setting for a sexual assessment.

TABLE 29-8 Do's and Don't's to Follow When Obtaining Sexual Information	
DO	**DON'T**
Obtain information about all areas of need	Focus only on sexuality
	Obtain information when others are present or take copious notes
Strive for an unhurried atmosphere	Check your watch, tap your foot
Maintain an attitude that is frank, open, warm, objective, empathetic	Project discomfort, become defensive
Use nondirective techniques when possible	Ask many direct questions
Have a prepared introduction to the stated purpose of interview	Be vague about the purpose of interview
Use appropriate vocabulary	Use street terms
"Check out" words to ensure that patient understands	Assume the patient understands what you're saying
Adjust the order of questions according to patient's needs	Follow a rigid form
Give the patient time to think and answer questions	Answer questions for the patient
Recognize signs of anxiety	Focus on getting information without recognizing patient's feelings
Give permission not to do something	Have preset expectations of the patient's sexual activity
Listen in an interested but matter-of-fact way	Overreact or underreact
Identify your attitudes, values, beliefs, and feelings	Project your concerns or problems onto the patient
Identify significant others	Assume that no one else is involved in the patient's sexual concerns
Identify philosophical and religious beliefs of the patient	Impose your moral judgments on the patient
Acknowledge when you don't have an answer to a question	Pretend you know when you don't

From *Human Sexuality: A Nursing Perspective* by Hogan, © 1980. Reprinted by permission of Prentice-Hall, Inc., Upper Saddle River, NJ.

SNAPSHOT

Nursing Interventions Specific to Psychosexual Dysfunction

What do you need to develop in a relationship with a patient who has a psychosexual dysfunction?
- Evaluate the severity of psychosexual dysfunction as described by the patient and the extent of current functioning.
- Approach the patient with acceptance and a willingness to listen and believe.
- Be caring, honest, empathetic, professional, and nonjudgmental.
- Speak slowly and clearly, and allow the patient time to respond.
- Use an indirect approach to allow for expression of feelings and beliefs.
- Explain the purpose of the sexual assessment and emphasize that confidentiality is strictly maintained.
- Provide emotional support during the sexual assessment, proceeding with least intrusive questions to more intrusive.
- Provide facilitative statements to encourage expression of feelings.
- Be aware of body language that reveals the patient's discomfort and indicates an area of concern for the patient.
- Provide an atmosphere of privacy.
- Provide information for further interventions and need for support of others.

What do you need to assess regarding the health status of a patient who has a psychosexual dysfunction?
- Observe for signs of difficulty concentrating, preoccupation, disinterest, or other cognitive symptoms.
- Observe for signs of detachment and withdrawal.
- Assess for risk of suicide or self-destructive thoughts.
- Assess for range of emotions: shock, blame, anger, rage, fear, shame, depression, anxiety, confusion.
- Assess for HIV risk, pregnancy, STDs, substance abuse, vital signs, concurrent medical problems.

What do you need to teach the patient, family, and caregiver?
- Medication management for core symptoms of depression, anxiety, panic, or sleep disturbance or medication management for psychosexual dysfunction

- Identification of high-stress, high-risk situations that might precipitate health or societal danger for the patient or others or pose a risk of incarceration for the patient's behaviors
- Coping skills
- Taking control of life and safety measures
- Encourage participation in a support group to understand that there are others who have experienced the same situation and to validate fears and feelings and resolve conflicts associated with the psychosexual dysfunction.
- Teach the use of relaxation skills in anxiety-arousing situations.
- Teach that the process of long-term healing involves recovery, avoidance, reconsideration, and adjustment.
- Instruct in the use of physical exercise to reduce tension in a nondestructive manner.
- Teach the patient to use spiritual guidance in times of self-doubt.

What skill do you want the patient or caregiver to demonstrate?
- Show positive coping skills.
- Practice relaxation techniques and stress management techniques under stressful conditions.
- Ability to express feelings and thoughts and not to self-isolate
- Ability to contract not to harm self or perform other self-destructive acts
- Ability to stop negative thoughts and obsessions; to think an action through
- Ability to take control of one's life
- Expression of feelings of anger, shame, fear, confusion, depression, and anxiety about future recovery and establishment of a relationship
- Establish caring, loving, sexual relationship with a significant other, even if the sexuality is adapted based on medical condition
- Increasing positive self-esteem and feelings about body image

What other health professionals might need to be part of this plan of care?
- Physicians, nurses, psychiatric social workers, clinical psychologists, sex therapists informed that the patient will need follow-up regarding the psychosexual dysfunction and the psychological trauma and physical problems surrounding it
- Police/Department of Child and Family Services for possible legal action against perpetrator (pedophilia, incest) or foster care of victims

STDs, sexually transmitted diseases.

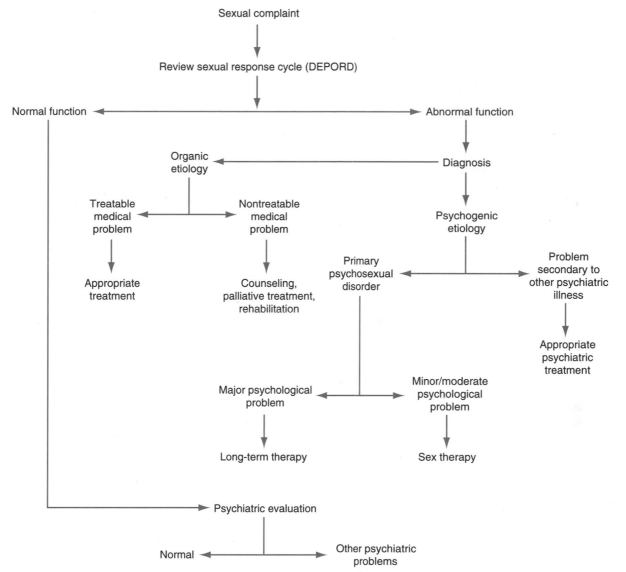

Figure 29-2
A decision tree used to help determine what interventions are appropriate for a patient with a sexual disorder.

32. Identify one nursing diagnosis for a sexual dysfunction.

33. What medication is used with sexual disorders such as pedophilia?

34. Identify two interventions used with patients with sexual disorders.

NURSING PROCESS APPLICATION

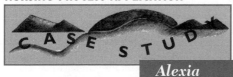

Alexia

Alexia is a senior in college who lives at home with her mother. Alexia's mother has been married twice and divorced twice; during Alexia's high school and college years, her mother has had numerous sexual partners, some of whom have lived with them for a time.

Until her high school senior prom, Alexia had remained a virgin. Then, on prom night, Alexia had her first sexual experience with her boyfriend of 9 months. Alexia enjoyed the experience, and she felt okay about it. She continued to have sexual relations with her boyfriend. Then, suddenly, he broke off the relationship. Alexia was devastated—depressed and desperately lonely. She felt as though she were the only teen in the world without a boyfriend.

Eager to replace that relationship, Alexia quickly resumed dating. She dated a number of young men. With her newfound freedom to engage in sexual relationships and her heightened interest in sex, Alexia readily had intercourse with the young men she dated. Although her much-longed-for romantic relationship never materialized, Alexia found the variety of sexual experiences exciting.

A week ago, however, Alexia noticed several small painful growths on her labia and several wartlike lesions near her anus. Concerned over these growths, she quickly overcame her anxiety and went to see her gynecologist. The gynecologist told Alexia that the labial lesions were genital herpes and that the warts were genital warts (condylomata acuminata). Those terms meant little to Alexia until the gynecologist told her that they were STDs. Alexia was stunned.

Still reeling with shock and embarrassment, Alexia began a course of treatment for the condition. The gynecologist dealt with the physical problem in a matter-of-fact manner, paying little attention to Alexia's emotional and spiritual reactions to the condition. Over the next few weeks, however, Alexia stopped dating. Soon, she even began to avoid talking with men, associating only with her girlfriends, to whom she expressed a total lack of interest in sex.

One of her friends suggested that she seek treatment at a Christian nurse-managed clinic. At first opposed to the idea because of her promiscuity, Alexia remembered the comfort she had early in life attending Sunday school. She agreed to go to a clinic and was seen on a weekly basis by a nurse clinical specialist in adult mental health.

ASSESSMENT

Assessment data are as follows:
- Presence of genital herpes and genital warts
- Shame and anxiety
- Lack of sexual desire
- Numerous sexual partners, lack of stable relationships
- Parental role model that did not model responsible sexuality

---

DIAGNOSIS

DSM-IV Diagnosis: Sexual Aversion Disorder

Nursing Diagnosis: Sexual Dysfunction related to the acute effects of two STDs as evidenced by withdrawal from relationships with men and lack of sexual desire

---

OUTCOME IDENTIFICATION, PLANNING, AND IMPLEMENTATION

> **Expected Outcome 1:** By _____ the patient will recognize the link between her search for meaningful relationships with men and her willingness to engage in sexual intercourse.

Short-Term Goals	Nursing Interventions	Rationales
By _____ the patient will discuss her feelings about her family situation.	1. Help Alexia to complete a family genogram. 2. Teach Alexia about family patterns—how behaviors and attitudes are transmitted from one generation to another, how events such as a divorce affect the whole family; teach her about family triangles. 3. Help Alexia to recognize the patterns of relationships in her family—in particular, the relationships Alexia's mother had with men.	1. A family genogram is a nonemotional method of diagramming and examining family patterns. 2–3. A family approach to Alexia's problem provides her with a way of analyzing and problem-solving about her own situation. By examining what has happened in her family, Alexia can understand her own behavior, not only as learned from the modeling of her mother but also as her own response to the intense anxiety and sense of loss that she must have felt within her family.

By _____ the patient will identify the impact of her family situation on her feelings and behaviors.	1. Encourage Alexia to identify and discuss her feelings about the divorce of her parents and the subsequent relationships her mother had with men.	1. By recognizing and discussing her own feelings, Alexia is taking the first step toward changing her own behavior. Unrecognized and unnamed feelings usually result in reactive and impulsive behaviors that are often self-destructive.
By _____ the patient will discuss the connection between her own lack of a stable, loving relationship with a father figure and her willingness to become intimately involved with many men.	1. Encourage Alexia to identify and discuss her feelings about the many losses she has experienced with men throughout her life. 2. Encourage Alexia to examine and discuss her own behaviors related to intimate relationships with men with what she observed and learned as a child growing up.	1–2. By understanding the deep losses that she experienced, Alexia is better able to understand her present behavior, to forgive herself, and to seek forgiveness from her God.
By _____ the patient will identify other alternatives to this pattern of behavior and relating to men.	1. Encourage Alexia to identify alternative ways of interacting with men in meaningful ways but without premature intimacy.	1. Identifying alternative modes of behaving before a situation presents itself is an empowering strategy. If Alexia waits to think through alternatives when she is confronted with the difficult situations, she may find that the old patterns of feeling and behaving overpower her ability to effectively problem solve.

Expected Outcome 2: By _____ the patient will identify practices and coping patterns that will help her to achieve meaningful relationships with men and will acknowledge restoration of sexual desire.

Short-Term Goals	Nursing Interventions	Rationales
By _____ the patient will identify the behaviors she currently exhibits when relating to men.	1. Encourage the patient that it is possible for her to change unhealthy patterns of behaving; just as she learned destructive patterns, she can relearn healthy patterns of relating. 2. Encourage the patient to role-play various scenarios in which she interacts with men. 3. Ask the patient to look at her behavior in these scenarios and to analyze her speech, her nonverbal behavior, her dress, and her feelings as she acts out these scenarios.	1. Patients are often discouraged about the prospects of changing patterns of behavior that seem deeply ingrained; encouragement provides hope for pursuing change. 2. By asking the patient to role-play, you are allowing her to see her own behaviors in a different and more objective way. 3. By asking her to identify each of her behaviors, you are putting her in charge of identifying her problematic behaviors and conveying confidence in her ability to find a solution to her problems.
By _____ the patient will examine these behaviors to determine which, if any, are sexually provocative behaviors or are behaviors that invite intimacy before a sound relationship has developed.	1. Ask the patient to analyze the responses to her behavior that she receives from men. Ask her if the responses she is receiving are sexual. Do the responses indicate a premature or inappropriate level of intimacy, given the stage of the relationship? 2. Ask the patient to categorize which of her own behaviors provoke these responses in men and which of her behaviors reinforce and encourage these responses in men.	1–2. By asking her to categorize her own behaviors, you are recognizing that not everything that she does needs to change. This is affirming to the patient. By asking her to examine the impact of her behaviors on men, you are affirming her responsibility and her role in the relationships that she develops; you are affirming her not as a victim but as someone who has the ability to take charge and to change.

By _____ the patient will examine behaviors that she needs to develop to really get to know and form meaningful relationships with men.

1. Explore alternative behaviors, ways of acting that are friendly and interested but with clear boundaries of sexual involvement.
2. Role-play various scenarios in which the patient tries out these new behaviors. Reanalyze the responses she receives.
3. Give homework assignments in which the patient keeps a journal of her interactions with men; ask her to analyze these interactions and to try out her new behaviors.

1. By establishing realistic boundaries, you are helping the patient to assume control over her body and sexual activities.
2. By role-playing different behaviors, you are allowing the patient to try out new ways of behaving in a safe, protected environment.
3. The journal entries keep the patient focused on the areas she is targeting for change; she is an active participant in the change—continually recording and evaluating her own responses.

By _____ the patient will identify strategies to cope with feelings that interfere with her development of meaningful relationships with men.

1. Ask the patient to keep a record of her feelings as she interacts with men. These recordings can be discussed within the therapy session to facilitate the patient's understanding of her own relationship patterns.

1. The ongoing recording and follow-up discussion of her feelings expand her awareness and understanding of her own patterns of behavior; greater understanding and awareness lead to greater control. The patient will state an understanding of her medical condition and its treatment and identify practices to prevent the contraction or spread of STDs.

Expected Outcome 3: By _____ the patient will state an understanding of her medical condition and its treatment and identify practices to prevent the contraction or spread of STDs.

Short-Term Goals	Nursing Interventions	Rationales
By _____ the patient will verbalize accurate information about her STDs and STDs in general.	1. Teach the patient the facts about STDs—the methods of contracting the diseases, the available treatments, and the risks. 2. Provide written information on this topic. 3. Assess the patient's understanding of the information presented.	1. People frequently have inadequate or inaccurate information about sexual issues. 2. Written information allows the patient to review the material in privacy. 3. It is important that you ask the patient to discuss the information you have presented. The patient may say that she understands or that she already knew the information to avoid the embarrassment of talking about a sensitive issue.
By _____ the patient will verbalize the risks of multiple sexual relationships and will state that condom use does not afford 100% protection against the risk of contracting all STDs.	1. The patient will verbalize an understanding that the only 100% guarantee of protection against STDs is abstinence from questionable sexual relationships, and that even protected sexual activity (sexual activity with the use of either a male or female condom) carries some risk of contracting STDs.	1. Patients frequently have inaccurate or inadequate information about the protection offered by condom use. If patients choose to engage in risky behavior, it is important that they have accurate information upon which to base their decisions.

Expected Outcome 4: By _____ the patient will state the meaning that she has found in the experience of having contracted STDs and will find spiritual comfort.

Short-Term Goals	Nursing Interventions	Rationales
By _____ the patient will verbalize the significance of the STDs on her life's journey.	1. Discuss the meaning of sexual expression.	1. Sexual expression is an intimate way of relating to another in a committed relationship. Sexual expression disconnected from a committed relationship often leaves the participants feeling used and unfulfilled.

2. Discuss the spiritual significance of sexuality.

2. Sexuality is an expression of our spirituality, in that sexuality transcends the individual and is creative. For many people, sexual intimacy outside of a marital relationship carries with it guilt and remorse for violation of religious beliefs.

By _____ the patient will use spiritual resources to alleviate the spiritual distress she is feeling.

1. Discuss with Alexia the spiritual resources (prayer, meditation, clerical counsel, reading of scripture or other inspirational materials) that might be helpful and supportive to her.
2. Ask how you might support Alexia in her efforts to attain comfort and consolation.

1. Alexia may find spiritual support and strength from these resources.

2. Offering the self is a caring therapeutic modality that shows support and help for the patient who is spiritually distressed.

EVALUATION

Formative Evaluation: Alexia met all of the short-term goals. She was able to examine her family situation, and she easily recognized that her pattern of relating to men was linked to her early family experiences and the behavior modeled by her mother. Alexia was able to identify that she engaged in a pattern of sexually flirtatious behavior and that she really never attempted to get to know a man before she had sex with him. She began to look at the behaviors she used to make friends with women and to transfer these behaviors to situations in which she found herself with men. Furthermore, Alexia became increasingly aware of her feelings of insecurity when she interacted with men and her overwhelming desire to be taken care of by them. She identified these feelings as being rooted in the many early losses she experienced. Alexia was knowledgeable about her own STDs as well as STDs in general. She sought the spiritual support of her clergyperson and found solace in prayer and scripture reading.

Summative Evaluation: Alexia met all of the expected outcomes. She developed friendships with two young men that involved social activities with groups of friends rather than sexual relationships. She expressed that "I feel like I am just learning how to be a friend to a guy." She was able to forgive herself for having STDs and to seek a committed relationship with a special person before engaging in sexual activity.

Conclusions

Sexuality is as much a part of who we are as our personality, our intelligence, and our physical appearance. Normal sexuality imbues our journeys with both creative and generative desires. When there are dysfunctions in sexuality, individual journeys can be painful. It is part of the nurse's role to understand and assess sexuality, to recognize when there are problems related to sexuality, to teach about it, and to offer empathy and concern to patients whose journeys are affected by sexual dysfunctions or disorders.

Key Points to Remember

- Sexual attitudes and behaviors are affected by multiple factors, including shifting cultural mores, religious teachings, parental role modeling, age, developmental stage, socioeconomic status, health, and education.
- It is essential for the nurse to examine personal attitudes and values concerning sexuality.
- The term *sex* refers to whether one is anatomically male or female.
- Gender identity refers to the earliest sense of maleness or femaleness had by an individual.
- Gender refers to the psychological reaction to or sense of being a male or female.
- Gender dysphoria refers to a sense of discomfort experienced when one's sex and gender differ.
- Transsexualism is the most common type of gender dysphoria.

- Sexual identity refers to the identification of oneself as male or female.
- Heterosexual identity means that the individual is attracted to individuals of the opposite sex.
- Homosexual identity means that the individual is attracted to individuals of the same sex.
- Sexual development continues over the life span.
- The sexual response cycle, according to Stuntz (1988), has six phases: desire, excitement, plateau, orgasm, resolution, and desire. Each phase is characterized by predictable behavioral and emotional responses.
- Dyspareunia refers to painful intercourse or coitus.
- The DSM-IV includes diagnostic criteria for disorders occurring during the various phases of the sexual response cycle.
- Erectile dysfunction can result from organic as well as psychogenic causes.
- Anorgasmia, or the inability to achieve an orgasm, is common in patients with a history of sexual abuse.
- The causes of anorgasmia include psychogenic trauma, medical problems, illness, medication, neurological conditions, and vascular conditions.
- Sexual disorders include paraphilias and gender identity disorders.
- There are many theories regarding the cause of homosexuality.

- Only when homosexuality is ego-dystonic is it considered to be a psychiatric illness.
- Head trauma that results in damage to the frontal lobe of the brain may result in promiscuous behavior, poor judgment, and poor impulse control.
- Klinefelter's syndrome is a genetic abnormality that produces sexual deviations.
- Psychoses can have an impact on sexual behavior and functioning.
- Sexual assessment must be holistic to understand fully the patient's situation.
- Sexual assessment collects data regarding medications that the patient is presently taking; many medications are associated with sexual dysfunction.
- A structured sexual assessment tool may assist the novice nurse to gather comprehensive sexual data.
- The setting for the sexual assessment should be private and quiet.
- The nurse needs to be aware of slang expressions used for sexual terms.
- Patients communicate nonverbally that they are uncomfortable with the sexual assessment.
- Interventions for sexual dysfunctions and disorders include medication, psychotherapy, behavioral therapy, teaching, and milieu therapy.

Learning Activities

1. Reflect on the sexual disorders presented in the chapter. What are your attitudes and beliefs about patients with paraphilias? Are you sympathetic? Do you believe they are in control and responsible for their behavior? What do you think society's view should be—punishment or treatment?
2. Complete the questions asked in Box 29–1. What do your answers tell you about yourself? Regarding sexuality, are you comfortable with your own sexuality? With that of others? Are you judgmental? Could you be helpful to someone who has a sexual disorder?
3. What factors have influenced your beliefs and values regarding sexuality?
4. What do you think is the impact of sexually explicit television, music videos, and movies on an individual's attitudes, values, and beliefs regarding sexuality?

Critical Thinking Exercise

Miss Jennifer Hines, a 24-year-old student nurse in her psychiatric nursing clinical experience, was assigned to Miss Gloria Thomas, a 27-year-old patient admitted with alcohol abuse. During one of the counseling interviews related to Miss Thomas' options when she left the detoxification unit, the patient told Miss Hines that she was gay and that she was sexually attracted to Miss Hines. When Miss Hines asked her why she felt this way, Miss Thomas said, "You must like me also, you treat me differently than you treat the other patients."

1. What assumptions is Miss Thomas making about Miss Hines' behaviors?
2. What evidence might suggest to Miss Thomas that her assumption is faulty?

3. What might happen if Miss Hines' response was different?

After Miss Thomas was discharged, she called Miss Hines at home to invite her to a party that she was having. She stated that a lot of Miss Hines' friends would be there.

1. Make sense of this information.
2. Consider alternate explanations.
3. What conclusions can be drawn about the nurse-patient relationship?

Additional Resources

American Psychological Association (APA)
http://www.apa.org/

Boston University Medical Center: Community Outreach Health Information System (COHIS)
http://gopher1.bu.edu/COHIS/index.html

Provides information about STDs.

CDC WONDER Public Health Database
http://www.cdc.gov/nchswww/datawh/cdcwond/cdcwond.htm

Provides information about STDs.

References

Aass, N., Grunfeld, B., Kaalhus, O., & Fossa, S. D. (1993). Pre- and post-treatment sexual life in testicular cancer patients: A descriptive investigation. *British Journal of Cancer, 67,* 1113-1117.

Alexander, B. (1993). Disorders of sexual desire: Diagnosis and treatment of decreased libido. *American Family Physician, 47,* 832-838.

American Psychiatric Association. (1994). *Diagnostic and statistical manual of mental disorders* (4th ed.). Washington, DC: Author.

Balon, R., Yeragani, V. K., Pohl, R., & Ramesh, C. (1993). Sexual dysfunction during antidepressant treatment. *Journal of Clinical Psychiatry, 54,* 209-212.

Berlin, F. S. (1985). Pedophilia: Medical castration and group counseling session help to modify this type of sexual behavior. *Medical Aspects of Human Sexuality, 19*(8), 79-88.

Bradley, S. J., & Zucker, K. J. (1997). Gender identity disorder. *Journal of the American Academy of Child and Adolescent Psychiatry, 36,* 872-880.

Brown, J. C. (1983). Paraphilias: Sadomasochism, fetishism, transvestism, and transsexuality. *British Journal of Psychiatry, 143,* 227-231.

Brown, R., & Field J. (Eds.). (1988). *Treatment of sexual problems in individual and couples therapy* (p. 236). Dana Point, CA: PMA Publishing Corp.

Chandraiah, S., Levenson, J. L., & Collins, J. B. (1991). Sexual dysfunction, social maladjustment, and psychiatric disorders in women seeking treatment in a premenstrual syndrome clinic. *International Journal of Psychiatry in Medicine, 21,* 189-204.

Corney, R. H., Crowther, M. E., Everett, H., Howells, A., & Shepherd, J. H. (1993). Psychosexual dysfunction in women with gynecological cancer following radical pelvic surgery. *British Journal of Obstetrics and Gynaecology, 100*(1), 73-78.

Currier, K. D., & Aponte, J. F. (1991). Sexual dysfunction in female adult children of alcoholics. *International Journal of Addiction, 26,* 195-201.

Davidson, J. (1986). Androgen replacement therapy in a wider context: Clinical and basic aspects. In L. Dennerstein & I. Fraser (Eds.), *Hormones and behavior* (p. 434). Amsterdam: Excerpta Medica.

DiGiorgio, M. J. (1998). Sibling incest: Treatment of the family and the offender. *Child Welfare, 77,* 335-346.

Dunning, P. (1963). Sexuality and women with diabetes. *Patient Education and Counseling, 21*(12), 5-14.

Fabbri, A., Aversa, A., & Isidori, A. (1997). Erectile dysfunction: An overview. *Human Repro Update, 3,* 455-466.

Greenblatt, R., Jungck, E., & Blum, H. (1972). Endocrinology of sexual behavior. *Medical Aspects of Human Sexuality, 6,* 110-131.

Jensen, S. B. (1992). Sexuality and chronic illness: A biopsychosocial approach. *Seminars in Neurology, 12,* 135-140.

Josephson, F.-B. (1987). Factors assisting female clients' disclosure of incest during counseling. *Journal of Counseling and Development, 65,* 475-478.

Kafka, M. P. (1991). Successful antidepressant treatment of non-paraphilic sexual addictions and paraphilias in men. *Journal of Clinical Psychiatry, 52*(2), 60-65.

Kaplan, H. S. (1975). *The illustrated manual of sex therapy.* New York: New York Times Book Co.

Kaplan, H. S. (1979). *Disorders of sexual desire and other new concepts and techniques in sex therapy.* New York: Brunner/Mazel.

Koneneman, K. S., Mulhall, J. P., & Goldstein, I. (1997). Sexual health for the man at mid-life: In-office workup. *Geriatrics, 52*(9), 76-78, 84-86.

Lawrence, J. S., & Madakasira, S. (1992). Evaluation and treatment of premature ejaculation: A critical review. *International Journal of Psychiatry in Medicine, 22*(1), 77-97.

Leiblum, S. R. (1992). The sexual difficulties of women. *Journal of the Medical Association of Georgia, 81,* 221-225.

Leif, H. (1977). What's new in sex research. *Medical Aspects of Human Sexuality, 7,* 94-95.

Maltz, W. (1988). Identifying and treating the sexual repercussions of incest: A couple approach. *Journal of Sex and Marital Therapy, 14,* 142-169.

Marantz, S., & Coates, S. (1991). Mothers of boys with gender identity disorder: A comparison of matched control. *Journal of the American Academy of Child and Adolescent Psychiatry, 30,* 310-315.

Masters, W. H., & Johnson, V. E. (1970). *Human sexual inadequacy.* Boston: Little, Brown.

Meyer-Bahlburg, H. F., Nostlinger, C., Exner, T. M., Ehrhardt, A. A., Gruen, R. S., Lorenz, G., Gorman, J. M., el-Sadr, W., & Sorrell, S. J. (1993). Sexual functioning in HIV and HIV injected drug-using women. *Journal of Sex and Marital Therapy, 19*(1), 56-68.

Money, J. (1994). The concept of gender identity disorder in childhood and adolescence after 39 years. *Journal of Sex and Marital Therapy, 20*(3), 163-177.

Musher, J. S. (1990). Anorgasmia with the use of fluoxetine [Letter]. *American Journal of Psychiatry, 147,* 948.

North American Nursing Diagnosis Association. (1994). *NANDA nursing diagnoses: Definitions and classification, 1995-1996.* Philadelphia: Author.

Patterson, W. M. (1993). Fluoxetine-induced sexual dysfunction [Letter]. *Journal of Clinical Psychiatry, 54*(2), 71.

Rosen, R. C., & Leiblum, S. R. (1995). Hypoactive sexual desire. *Psychiatric Clinics of North America, 18*(1), 107-121.

Saghir, M., & Robins, E. (1978). Male and female homosexuality. In J. Money & H. Mustapha (Eds.), *Handbook of Sexuality* (p. 1062). New York: Elsevier.

Stuntz, R. (1983). Gender dysphoria and dyssocial behavior. In L. B. Schlesinger & E. Revitch (Eds.), *Sexual dynamics of anti-social behavior* (pp. 88-89). Springfield, IL: Charles C Thomas.

Stuntz, R. (1988). Assessment of organic factors in sexual dysfunction. In R. Brown & J. Field (Eds.), *Treatment of sexual problems in individual and couples therapy* (pp. 188-201). Dana Point, CA: PMA Publishing Corp.

Walbroehl, G. S. (1992). Sexual concerns of the patient with pulmonary disease. *Postgraduate Medicine, 91,* 455-460.

Williams, W. (1991). Male sexuality. *Medical Journal of Australia, 155,* 101-104.

Zucker, K. J., Bradley, S. J., & Sanikhani, M. (1997). Sex differences in referral rates of children with gender identity disorder: Some hypotheses. *Journal of Abnormal Child Psychology, 25,* 217–227.

Suggested Readings

Dewis, M. E., & Thornton, N. G. (1989). Sexual dysfunction in multiple sclerosis. *Journal of Neuroscience Nursing, 21,* 175–179.

Dunning, P. (1993). Sexuality and women with diabetes. *Patient Education and Counseling, 21*(12), 5–14.

Green, R. (1975). *Human sexuality: A health practitioner's text.* Baltimore: Williams & Wilkins.

Hogan, R. (1980). *Human sexuality: A nursing perspective.* New York: Appleton-Century-Crofts.

Hook, M., Guevarra, J., Perce, M. K., & Scott-Sorenson, N. (1989). Critical care voices: Including sexual counseling in clinical practice. *Dimensions of Critical Care Nursing, 8,* 375.

Shell, J. A. (1990). Sexuality for patients with gynecologic cancer. *NAACOGS Clinical Issues in Perinatal and Women's Health Nursing, 1,* 479–494.

An eating disorder may be defined simply as an obsession with eating in the midst of an abundance of food. (Eating disorders rarely occur in countries where there is a scarcity of food supplies or among people who must worry where their next meal is coming from.)

—R. Epstein

Eating Disorders

Learning Objectives

After studying this chapter, you should be able to:

1. Discuss at least three important roles that food plays in life's journey.
2. Describe anorexia nervosa.
3. Describe bulimia nervosa.
4. Define binge eating disorder.
5. Define obesity.
6. Discuss the causes of eating disorders from a biological, psychological, socio-cultural, and spiritual perspective.
7. State at least four defining characteristics of anorexia nervosa, bulimia nervosa, and binge eating disorder.
8. Identify at least three factors you would assess in anorexia nervosa, bulimia nervosa, or binge eating disorder.
9. State at least three possible nursing diagnoses for a patient diagnosed with an eating disorder.
10. State at least two expected outcomes for a patient diagnosed with an eating disorder.
11. Discuss at least two treatment approaches for the patient with either anorexia nervosa or bulimia nervosa.
12. Discuss the psychiatric nurse's challenge when journeying with a patient with an eating disorder.

Key Terminology

Anorexia nervosa	Bingeing	Obesity	Purging
Binge eating disorder	Bulimia nervosa		

Carrie's Story

On the icy highway, Carrie applied the brake and the car spun forward, missing another vehicle by inches. She panicked, wrenched the wheel, and barely missed a truck coming from the opposite direction. A few seconds later Carrie managed to stop the car. With her hands shaking and her voice trembling, she turned to her friend and said, "I'm hungry."

"Hungry? Who thinks of food at a time like this?"

"I do," Carrie answered. "I think about food all the time." ■

From Billigmeier, S. (1991). *Inner eating*. Nashville, TN: Oliver Nelson.

THE ROLE OF FOOD

The journey marked by eating disorders begins with the role of food in our lives—a role that has always been and will always be a crucial one. Primarily, we need food for nourishment so that our bodies grow and develop during childhood years and remain healthy as we mature and age. In our journey, however, food plays other roles, roles that are worth pondering as we begin to understand eating disorders.

Food is often used as a reward or punishment for children's behaviors. Adults, too, use dinners out to court each other and to celebrate job promotions and birthdays. "Working lunches" are not only common but also, in some professions, the only way business is conducted. Holidays are distinguished from one another by the foods served: candy corn at Halloween, turkey on Thanksgiving, chocolates on Valentine's Day. Abstaining from food is an important practice of many of the world's religions on certain holy days. Additionally, Christian, Jewish, and Muslim observances such as Easter, Passover, and Ramadan are commemorated with special foods (Blackburn, Miller, & Chan, 1997).

Other than food's essential relationship to our health, the most important relationship, the one that wields the most power, is the one tied to our appearance. You need only to read a fashion magazine or watch television to be aware of the pressure placed on young women (and to a lesser degree, young men) to be thin. Many young people believe that they are defined by their weight and "can never be too thin." Anorexia nervosa and bulimia nervosa, both of which are characterized by disturbances in the person's perception of body shape and weight, may be young people's responses to this irrational pressure to be thin.

Food is used to meet other emotional needs, such as needs for comfort, security, and love. As Krueger (1997) states, "By its accumulation, as in obesity, it can shield one from the world. By its abstinence, as in Anorexia Nervosa, the illusion is created of needing no one or nothing" (p. 619). Table 30–1 provides an overview of the three formal eating disorders: Anorexia Nervosa, Bulimia Nervosa, and Binge Eating Disorder (newly

TABLE 30–1	Overview of the Three Types of Formal Eating Disorders
DISORDER	**CHARACTERISTICS**
Anorexia nervosa	Refusal to maintain a minimally normal body weight. The anorexic may control weight by either severely restricting caloric intake or engaging in a binge-purge cycle. Binge-purge eating occurs when a person eats a large amount of food over a short period of time and follows the eating with purging.
Bulimia nervosa	Characterized by repeated episodes of bingeing and purging through self-induced vomiting; misuse of laxatives, diuretics, or other medications; fasting; or excessive exercising. (Bingeing refers to overeating; purging refers to voluntarily vomiting or using methods to stimulate defecation.)
Binge eating disorder	Characterized by excessive intake of calories without effort to prevent weight gain. The person feels that he or she has no control over his or her eating. Behaviors include eating rapidly, eating until uncomfortably full, eating excessive amounts of food, and eating alone. The person feels guilty, disgusted, embarrassed, and depressed. It is important to be aware that not everyone who is obese engages in binge eating and not everyone who is diagnosed with a binge eating disorder is obese.

Based on information from the *Diagnostic and Statistical Manual of Mental Disorders. Fourth Edition.* Copyright 1994 American Psychiatric Association.

included in the *Diagnostic and Statistical Manual of Mental Disorders, Fourth Edition* [DSM-IV]. In addition, although not identified in the DSM-IV as a formal eating disorder, being overweight and obesity will be considered.

PREVALENCE

Anorexia nervosa and **bulimia nervosa** primarily affect white women, 12 to 22 years of age, in the middle and upper socioeconomic groups in industrialized countries such as the United States, Europe, Canada, Japan, Australia, and South Africa. Typical onset of anorexia nervosa is between 12 and 14 years of age and that of bulimia between 16 and 20 years of age. Males, representing between 0.4% and 10% of cases of anorexia nervosa and bulimia, fall into the same age group and cultures. Young women in Western cultures are vulnerable because of a shared emphasis on dieting, weight, and body shape. Current estimates place the prevalence of anorexia nervosa at 1% of American women and girls and of bulimia at 2% to 8% of adolescent and college women (Love & Seaton, 1991). Members of professions that emphasize physical appearance and rigid weight standards, such as dancers, flight attendants, athletes, actors, and models, are at especially high risk for eating disorders. In men, homosexuality or bisexuality appears to be an additional risk factor, especially for bulimia (Carlat, Camargo, & Herzog, 1997).

The incidence of **binge eating disorder** is less well researched, but there is considerable overlap with bulimia. Also, in samples drawn from weight control programs, nonpurge binge eating has been observed in 46% of obese participants (Allan, 1998). A greater percentage of men are affected by binge eating disorder than by anorexia or bulimia; the female-to-male ratio is approximately 3:2. Under the 1998 National Institutes of Health guidelines, 55% of the U.S. population is overweight (Brody, 1998). **Obesity,** defined as having a body mass index (BMI = kg/m^2) of at least 30 or a weight greater than or equal to 120% of ideal body weight, affects at least 30% of Americans (Solomon & Manson, 1997). Morbid obesity is defined as a BMI greater than 45.

RISKS

As nurses we need to be aware of eating disorders, not only because of their increasing frequency but also because of their potentially fatal outcomes. Even if a person recovers from the serious somatic changes caused by anorexia nervosa, it can lead to severe osteoporosis in later life as a result of amenorrhea (McGee, 1997). More urgently, it is reported to have a mortality rate of 5.9% to 23.8% (Neumarker, 1997).

Bulimia nervosa is also associated with life-threatening consequences, including severe electrolyte imbalances such as hypokalemia, which can lead to cardiac arrhythmias and cardiac arrest (Laraia & Stuart, 1990).

Obesity is also associated with multiple physical and psychological problems, among them diabetes mellitus, cardiovascular disease, osteoarthritis, breast cancer, sleep apnea, pulmonary embolism, and depression. Obesity has been called "the second leading cause of preventable death in the United States today" (Brody, 1998, p. F7).

HISTORICAL BACKGROUND

Evidence exists of problems in the regulation of food intake long before the 20th century. In 1st-century Rome, rooms called *vomitoria* were built expressly for guests to "heave the gorge" before returning to the banquet room at food orgies that were a common form of celebration. It was not until many centuries later, however, that any eating disorder was documented as an illness. Although Richard Morton in 1694 is credited with first naming the cause of anorexia as "arising in underlying sadness and anxious cares" (Patton, 1992, p. 281), not until the 1860s and 1870s did French and English physicians first describe several cases of an-

orexia. Louis-Victor Marce, in Paris, the first to define a disorder of "inappetency," recommended isolation from family and gradual refeeding as a treatment. Sir William Gull, a physician to England's Royal Family, called anorexia a disease separate from hysteria or biological eating problems. At the same time, Charles Lasègue, a French psychiatrist, saw anorexia as a form of rebellion in wealthy children who were stressed by all the dinner table rules and regulations. Lasègue further suggested that anorexia was connected with suffocating and manipulative parental love. The characteristics of anorexia, first cited in 1873, are still relevant (Box 30–1).

During the 1800s, the ideal woman was thought to be "perfectly" devout so that her spiritual beauty shone brightly. The ability to refuse food was viewed as an excellent form of self-discipline that translated into spiritual discipline—the mark of a devout, upper-class woman. (Thinness in the poor was viewed not as a symbol of restraint but rather as a reflection of a lower economic status in life.) "Thus, morally, spiritually, and socially it was considered desirable for Victorian women to refuse food, even before the dictates of 20th century fashion and advertising" (Epstein, 1990, p. 37).

At the turn of the century, Freud linked anorexia with emotional and sexual conflicts. Pierre Janet, a French psychiatrist in the early 1900s, agreed with Freud but connected this obsession to the spiritual issues of the Victorian age.

What *do you think?* Are you happy with your current weight?

► *Check Your Reading*

1. Identify three characteristics of anorexia nervosa.
2. Identify three roles that food plays in our lives.
3. Describe bulimia nervosa.
4. Describe binge eating disorder.
5. What are the life-threatening consequences of anorexia? Of bulimia? Of obesity?

CAUSES

Eating disorders share multifactorial causes, including biological factors, psychological factors, sociocultural factors, and spiritual factors. Each of these factors is discussed.

Box 30–1 ■ ■ ■ ■ ■
Characteristics of Anorexia Nervosa

- Refusal to eat
- Emaciation
- Amenorrhea
- Hypothermia
- Hyperactivity
- Hypotension

Biological Factors

It is clear that there is a strong biological component to eating disorders. At its most starkly simple, for example, obesity can be described as an equation: energy taken in − energy expended = energy stored. Humphries (1997) believed that anorexia may be caused, or at least perpetuated by, a zinc deficiency. But the greatest proportion of current research is on the genetics and the neurochemistry of eating disorders.

Genetic Factors

A person's genetic code influences metabolism, neuroendocrine and neurotransmitter functioning, and probably many other relevant variables. Although the evidence linking genetics directly with eating disorders is far from conclusive, some support exists for this link. For instance, twin studies demonstrate a higher incidence of eating disorders in monozygotic twins than in dizygotic twins. Furthermore, mothers and sisters of anorexics have a higher incidence of anorexia than sisters of controls. Major mood disorders such as depression and bipolar disorder seem to be prevalent in first-degree family members of anorexics (Kaplan & Sadock, 1991). Animal studies have found gene mutations related to thin sow syndrome and similar syndromes in goats and sheep (Treasure & Owen, 1997).

Neurochemical Factors

Role of Neurotransmitters and Brain Hormones

Researchers have found decreased levels of the neurotransmitters serotonin and norepinephrine in severe anorexics and bulimics, as well as increased levels of the brain hormone cortisol. These findings are similar to those in depressed people, and point to a fundamental problem in or near the hypothalamus, which regulates appetite. Serotonin is the specific neurotransmitter that seems most important in this process, involved in a feeling of fullness. Similar biochemical comparisons have been made between patients with eating disorders and those with obsessive-compulsive disorder (OCD), in whom the brain hormone vasopressin has also been noted to be low (Davis, Kaptein, Kaplan, Olmsted, & Woodside, 1998). Another chemical being investigated in laboratory animals is the hormone cholecystokinin, related to satiety. A variant of binge eating called "night-eating syndrome" is believed to be related to a phase delay in the brain's circadian rhythm (Stunkard, 1997).

Role of Endogenous Opioids

Another line of biological research into the cause of eating disorders focuses on the observation that binge eaters prefer concentrated sweets and other carbohydrates during periods of binging. This observation has led to the hypothesis that people who binge on sweets are deficient in endogenous opioid activity. Food with a high concentration of sugar stimulates β-endorphin activity and can lead to overeating (Mercer & Holder, 1997).

Elevated levels of endogenous opioids have been found in anorexic and bulimic patients; these appear to be released during dieting and also by exercise, reinforcing a "state of starvation dependence" (Marrazzi, Luby, Kinzie, Munjal, & Spector, 1997, p. 1741).

Psychological Factors

Current thinking favors psychological and personality factors as critical in the development of eating disorders. The journey marked by eating disorders has at its psychological base issues of coping, self-esteem, and perfectionism (Case Examples 30–1 and 30–2). "[T]he primary problem is not with food, but with issues of control, self-esteem, depression, difficulty with intimate relationships, and developmental expectations. The excessive regulation and usage of food and behaviors associated with these disorders are an expression of the individual's difficulties in those areas" (Riley, 1991, p. 715).

■ CASE EXAMPLE 30–1
■ Renee's Story

I have so many rules, I can't live with anyone. They couldn't stand it. Everything I do has to be perfect. I know some of the things I feel I have to do don't make sense, but I am compelled to do them and get very anxious if I am not allowed to do things my way. I have rules for everything: how I exercise, how I dress, how I clean, even how I study. I have got to have control of everything. ■

From Flood, M. (1989). Addictive eating disorders. *Nursing Clinics of North America, 24*(1), 48.

■ CASE EXAMPLE 30–2
■ Jennifer's Story

I feel helpless, worthless, that I can't control how someone responds to me. That's what brings me back to my body—to be destructive at least—to binge. It's a substitute for the things I can't get and want. I'm out of control. I take in something to feel better, then I feel more in control. ■

From Krueger, D. (1997). Food as self object in eating disordered patients. *The Psychoanalytic Review, 84*, 626.

Although multiple factors may be responsible for causing such emotional problems, the common outcome is that appetite comes to be driven by "external or psychological sources" (Hirsch, 1997, p. 116). By focusing attention on food, the patient's time is consumed, and this allows him or her to avoid making decisions and to reduce challenges. The person may become the center of the family's attention. Family dynamics, such as mother-child and parental relationships, as well as the role the eating-disordered person plays in the family, have an impact on the development and maintenance of the eating disorder. Other family problems, such as alcohol or substance abuse, rape, incest, verbal abuse, and neglect, are common in the backgrounds of people with eating disorders. Food, or refusal thereof, becomes the mechanism to deal with anger, hurt, and frustration.

The psychological characteristics of the anorexic include poor self-image, eagerness to please, all-or-nothing thinking, and extreme perfectionism. Curiously, as anorexics lose weight, fear of fatness increases. They lose the ability to read their own body signals. No conclusive explanation has been found for the grossly distorted body image that develops, but it appears not to be a sensory phenomenon (Szymanski & Seime, 1997). Another characteristic of anorexics is *alexithymia,* a difficulty in identifying and expressing one's feelings.

People with bulimia tend to be of normal weight but often feel tense and anxious before they binge. The **bingeing** episode brings a sense of relief. After the binge, the anxiety begins again to mount, until the individual purges. With **purging,** a release of tension occurs, as weight gain has once again been averted. See Home Care Clinical Practice Guidelines.

For nonpurging binge eaters, food becomes a companion, and bingeing gives the binger a temporary "lift" or "high" that she or he feels cannot be obtained through conventional means. In a study designed "as exploration of thoughts, moods and physiological sensations associated with binge eating in a non-purging population," 19 obese women were questioned. "While nearly half the participants reported awareness of being hungry before binging, when asked to rate the importance of hunger relative to other factors, it emerged as least important" (Arnow, Kenardy, & Agras, 1992, p. 163). The following quote describes a binger's response to stress (Billigmeier, 1991):

When you can't accomplish your too high goals, you eat. When things don't go right, you eat. When people don't do what they should, you eat. When events don't run smoothly, you eat. When people don't like your behavior, you eat. (p. 140)

See Home Care Clinical Practice Guidelines.

Sociocultural Factors

"It is difficult to watch television without being confronted by advertisements for both high-caloric foods as well as the latest diet plans. The social (and usually family) pressures are also contradictory: you must eat everything other people give you but you must not get fat" (Abraham & Llewellyn-Jones, 1997, p. 27).

■ CASE EXAMPLE 30–3
■ Veronica's Story

But thinness itself didn't matter to me as much as people's responses to it. . . . Every flattering comment was an affirmation of success. Since I came from a family which valued other people's opinion more than our own, I constantly sought the approval of others. . . . My thin figure gave me my only sense of worth. Until this time I never thought I could do anything well; staying thin was a major accomplishment. As much as I hated bulimia, I loved the self-esteem that being thin gave to me. ■

From Ault, M. (1990). I am a Christian bulimic. *Journal of Christian Nursing,* 7(1), 4–8.

There are numerous social and cultural factors that, paradoxically, contribute to both unhealthy underweight and unhealthy overweight. Beyond the inescapable presence of high-fat fast food and snacks, the sedentary American lifestyle, the bombardment of media images of thin people, and the glamorization of working out, there is also a pattern in Western culture of mind-body separation and deeply ambivalent attitudes toward all bodily functions.

Although the outward behavior of an anorexic woman may reflect the good little girl, her body is paying for every act of compliance by the brutality of starvation. The praise of initial weight loss makes the anorexic feel good and gives her something she desperately seeks: the attention and approval of others. The bulimic may be socially isolated because of the nature of the bingeing-purging ritual: there exists a deep fear of being rejected by others if it were to be discovered.

Compulsive overeaters may use food as a replacement for social relationships. In contrast to those who suffer with bulimia or anorexia, the compulsive overeater does not seem to have the same obsessive preoccupation with becoming fat. It is as if this extra weight provides the overeater with insulation from others, especially from the harmful words or abuse others might heap on him or her.

It is at times of transition and increased stress that people are most vulnerable to developing any of the eating disorders. Thus, adolescence is a critical period, as are times of other major changes or disruptions of routines and roles.

Spiritual Factors

Be perfect, therefore, as your heavenly Father is perfect. (Matthew 5:48)

You must be blameless before the Lord your God. (Deuteronomy 18:13)

From the Victorian age to the present, the journey marked by eating disorders has linked spiritual to perfectionist ideals. The aforementioned Bible verses actually refer to obedience to God rather than human efforts at living lives without error or flaw. The interpretation of these verses, however, may be distorted to focus on the person's need to be perfect. Such perfection includes total control of anger. For the eating-disordered person, it may involve suppression of all angry feelings.

If an anorexic sees perfection as a spiritual goal, he or she might—tragically—see weight loss as an act of devotion to God. Spirituality and asceticism have always

Home Care Clinical Practice Guidelines
ANOREXIA NERVOSA, BULIMIA NERVOSA, BINGE EATING DISORDER

Referral to a Psychiatric Home Care Program

Pre-Admission Screening
- Physical Examination
- Psychiatric Hx

Eligible
- Medical Clearance
- Not Suicidal
- No Self-mutilating behaviors
- Depression-Mild or Moderate
- No Psychosis
- Able to Contract
- Shows Gradual Improvement

Comprehensive Assessment Physical/Psychosocial/Spiritual
- Restore Addendum
- Depression Inventory
- Suicide Assessment Tool
- Psychosis Inventory
- Other assessment tools as appropriate

Ineligible (May Need In-Patient Treatment)
- Medical Complications
- Suicidal
- Self-mutilating behaviors
- Severe depression
- Psychotic behavior
- Inability to comply with treatment plan
- Inadequate response to treatments

Establish Plan of Care

Standards of Practice are based on the ANA Standards for Psychiatric & Mental Health Nursing

Areas marked ☑ are mandatory for diagnosis

Assessment

Health Status Assessment

Establish Measurable Outcomes

Cardiovascular
- ○ ☑ Temperature - notify physician if temp <96.8F (hypothermia)
- ○ ☑ Pulse - notify nurse or physician if pulse <40 per minute (bradycardia)
- ○ ☑ Systolic blood pressure - <70 mm/Hg (hypotensive)

Neurological/Psychological
- ○ ☑ Depression
- ○ ☑ Supression of feelings, esp. anger
- ○ ☑ Suicidal ideation
- ○ ☑ Disturbance body image
- ○ ☑ Disturbance self-esteem
- ○ ☑ Perfectionism
- ○ ☑ Obsession with body size/food
- ○ ☑ Sexual problems
- ○ ☑ Identity crisis
- ○ ☑ Lack of autonomy
- ○ ☑ Immaturity "black/white" thinking

Nutrition
- ○ ☑ Diet (food/fluids) Notify nurse or physician if severely dehydrated based on weight loss, i.e. (weight loss >20% of body wt over 3 mos)(serum potassium <2.5 mEq/L)

Hormonal
- ○ ☑ Notify nurse/MD if amenorrheic (without menstrual period)

Patient/Caregiver Education

Self Care Knowledge

Establish Measurable Outcomes

Medication Regimen
- ○ ☑ Demonstrates understanding of medication response, side effects, compliance and schedule if medication ordered by physician
- ○ ☑ Written materials provided
- ○ ☑ Home management

Family/Social support
- ○ Family demonstrates appropriate level of patient involvement in regimen (avoidance of power struggles)
- ○ Patient attends support groups (Overeaters Anonymous, peer support groups)
- ○ Family demonstrates ability to express frustration, fear and anger/feelings
- ○ Patient/family demonstrates understanding of Importance of structure in patient's day
- ○ Family demonstrates communication strategies to enhance patient's self-esteem, etc. and vice versa

Emotional/Spiritual
- ○ Patient/family demonstrate expression of feelings; supportive and non-judgmental approach
- ○ Patient demonstrates an understanding of developmental issues (girl to womanhood)
- ○ Spiritual interventions encouraged
- ○ Patient/family interaction encouraged
- ○ Empathetic approach
- ○ Demonstrates validation of the normalization of feelings
- ○ Home management
- ○ ☑ Written materials provided

Emergency Measures
- ○ Access 911/EMS
- ○ Access Restore nurse

Household Resources
- ○ Understands that the Anorexic's family: controlled, rigid, marked with less discord; Bulimic's family: marked with conflict, chaos, violence, substance abuse
- ○ Families involved with weight gain by Anorexia Nervosa pts is viewed as a strength

Lifestyle and Compliance
- ○ Engages in appropriate level of exercises daily
- ○ Eats a balanced diet
- ○ Engages in behavior modification (overeater) i.e., self-monitoring diary, limiting high carbohydrate foods in home; limiting unstructured time (Anorexic) has a peer/family member support her in goal-keeping (weight gained, exercise, vomiting)
- ○ Takes in fluid to restore electrolyte balance
- ○ Takes antidepressant medication (if ordered) w/o difficulty

Home Safety
- ○ Can maintain food intake without going to bathroom to vomit
- ○ Can maintain food intake without use of laxatives and other pills, i.e., amphetamines, diet pills to curb appetite or have frequent bowel movements. These will be removed from home

(Continued on next page)

Home care clinical practice guidelines: Anorexia nervosa, bulimia nervosa, binge eating disorder. (From Staff Builders Home Health Care, Staff Builders, Inc., 1983 Marcus Avenue, Lake Success, NY 11042-7011.)

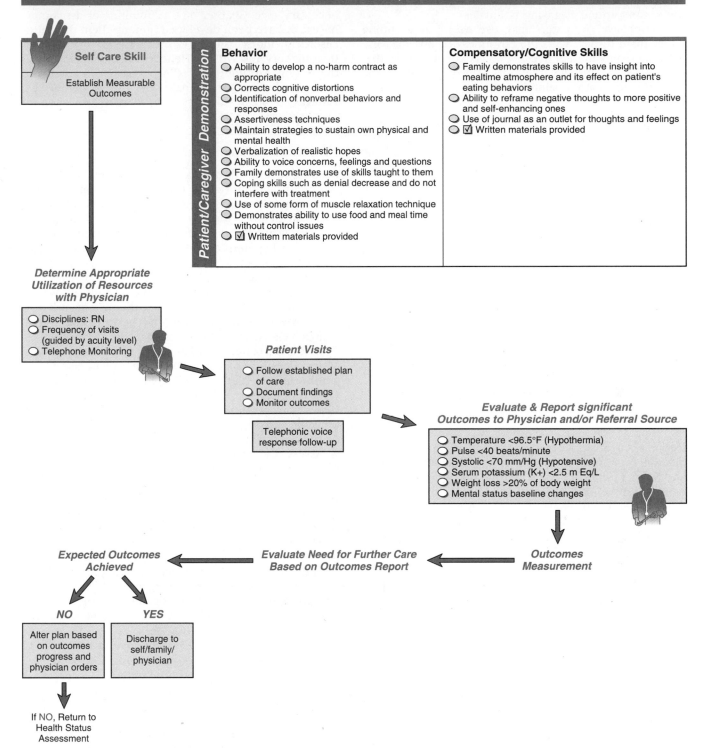

Home Care Clinical Practice Guidelines
ANOREXIA NERVOSA, BULIMIA NERVOSA, BINGE EATING DISORDER

Self Care Skill

Establish Measurable Outcomes

Patient/Caregiver Demonstration

Behavior
- ○ Ability to develop a no-harm contract as appropriate
- ○ Corrects cognitive distortions
- ○ Identification of nonverbal behaviors and responses
- ○ Assertiveness techniques
- ○ Maintain strategies to sustain own physical and mental health
- ○ Verbalization of realistic hopes
- ○ Ability to voice concerns, feelings and questions
- ○ Family demonstrates use of skills taught to them
- ○ Coping skills such as denial decrease and do not interfere with treatment
- ○ Use of some form of muscle relaxation technique
- ○ Demonstrates ability to use food and meal time without control issues
- ○ ☑ Writtem materials provided

Compensatory/Cognitive Skills
- ○ Family demonstrates skills to have insight into mealtime atmosphere and its effect on patient's eating behaviors
- ○ Ability to reframe negative thoughts to more positive and self-enhancing ones
- ○ Use of journal as an outlet for thoughts and feelings
- ○ ☑ Written materials provided

Determine Appropriate Utilization of Resources with Physician
- ○ Disciplines: RN
- ○ Frequency of visits (guided by acuity level)
- ○ Telephone Monitoring

Patient Visits
- ○ Follow established plan of care
- ○ Document findings
- ○ Monitor outcomes

Telephonic voice response follow-up

Evaluate & Report significant Outcomes to Physician and/or Referral Source
- ○ Temperature <96.5°F (Hypothermia)
- ○ Pulse <40 beats/minute
- ○ Systolic <70 mm/Hg (Hypotensive)
- ○ Serum potassium (K+) <2.5 m Eq/L
- ○ Weight loss >20% of body weight
- ○ Mental status baseline changes

Expected Outcomes Achieved ← **Evaluate Need for Further Care Based on Outcomes Report** ← **Outcomes Measurement**

NO

Alter plan based on outcomes progress and physician orders

YES

Discharge to self/family/ physician

If NO, Return to Health Status Assessment

had a strong relationship; self-starvation may be seen as an attempt "to transform oneself, through self-control, into a more worthy person" (Garrett, 1997, p. 265). Keeping this in mind helps the nurse remember that spiritual fulfillment and self-transformation can play an important part in recovery.

Because of the bulimic patient's need to purge, it has been equated in some patients to a spiritual cleansing of evil. The "evil" that lurks within may be seen as bad attitudes, impatience, or unhappiness with how her or his life's journey is unfolding. Anderson (1993) reported that many eating-disordered people he worked with felt the need to purify themselves of evil forces they believed lived within them. He also stated that, along with purging, some patients also cut themselves, describing the same spiritual cleansing rationales.

Compulsive overeaters may use eating as a coping mechanism to deal with the emptiness or absence of a spiritual reality in their lives. Food is expected to fill that emptiness. Because it cannot meet this expectation, the person is left with a painful void.

What do you think? Do you have your own theory about what causes anorexia? Bulimia? Obesity?

➤ *Check Your Reading*
6. What is the hypothesized role of serotonin in anorexia?
7. What evidence is there for a genetic link to eating disorders?
8. Cite one psychological issue that may be part of the cause of anorexia? Of bulimia? Of binge eating disorder?
9. Cite two possible family issues in eating disorders.
10. How do spiritual issues play into the cause of eating disorders?

RELATIONSHIP TO OTHER PSYCHIATRIC PROBLEMS

Depression is seen across the board in all eating disorders. A study by Walsh, Roose, Glassman, Gladis, and Sadik (1985) indicated lifetime prevalence of major depression at 71% for those with eating disorders. The long-term outcome is poor for as many as 40% of patients with eating disorders because of the co-occurrence of depression (Silverstone, 1992). Major depression or dysthymia is reported in as many as 50% to 75% of anorexics. OCD also is seen in up to 37% of anorexics (Thornton & Russell, 1997).

Bulimia has been seen with symptoms of mood lability, impulsivity, explosive interpersonal relationships, and self-mutilation (Hsu, 1990). Studies report that as many as 40% of these patients show signs of clinical depression: increased rates of anxiety (45%), substance abuse disorders (49%), and bipolar illness (12%). Bulimia also seems to have high co-incidence (as high as 60%) with borderline personality disorder. Binge eating disorder is also associated with increased rates of psychiatric illness, including major depression, panic disorder, and borderline and avoidant personality disorders (Yanovski, Nelson, Dubbert, & Spitzer, 1993).

NURSING PROCESS

Assessment

It is essential for the patient with an eating disorder to receive a comprehensive assessment, including physical, psychological, sociocultural, family, and spiritual assessment. A psychiatric history, a developmental history, and a history of substance abuse are also necessary (see Chapter 11). A number of assessment measures have been developed, among them the Eating Disorders Index (EDI) (Garner, 1991); the Bulimic Investigatory Test (BITE) (Henderson & Freeman, 1987); the Eating Attitudes Test (EAT) (Garner & Garfinkle, 1979); and the Questionnaire on Eating and Weight Patterns (Spitzer, Yanovski, & Marcus, as cited in Yanovski et al., 1993).

Physical Assessment

Because eating disorders are associated with high morbidity and mortality, the physical examination is extremely important. Begin by taking a full set of vital signs. Remember that the anorexic patient frequently has bradycardia, lowered body temperature, amenorrhea, and hypotension. It is important to assess how much the patient weighs, his or her normal as well as ideal body weight, how much he or she has gained or lost, and in what time frame the change in weight occurred. While you are weighing the patient, ask how he or she feels about his or her body: is the weight change related to mood or to external circumstances?

Assess the patient's eating habits. What is the pattern? Where does he or she eat? Does the patient fast or take amphetamines, diet pills, or caffeine pills to lose weight? Does the patient engage in binge-purge cycles of eating? If so, how does he or she feel about this pattern? Is bingeing and purging done in secret? How often does he or she engage in these behaviors?

Assess the patient's activity. Is the patient too sedentary? Or does the patient engage in excessive exercise? How does it make him or her feel? Is there a pattern to the patient's excessive exercise?

Assess for other physical signs of eating disorders. Anorexic patients frequently have significant hair loss; yellowish, dry, atrophic skin; lanugo; cessation of menses; cachexia; cyanosis of the extremities; and peripheral edema. Bulimic patients frequently display hoarseness, parotid gland enlargement (giving them a chipmunk appearance), tooth enamel erosion caused by regurgitation of stomach acid, scarred fingers, electrolyte imbalances, and dehydration.

Finally, assess the patient's elimination habits. Does the patient use laxatives or diuretics to lose weight? If so, how many are used and how often?

Psychological Assessment

Anorexic and bulimic patients have a core of psychological characteristics in common. These are shown in Box 30–2. The anorexic tends to use greater denial than the bulimic—not only denying hunger but also denying that there is a problem at all. The bulimic is usually aware of his or her problem and distressed about it. For the binge eater, body satisfaction appears to be a critical component of self-esteem. Overweight or obese female patients may be experiencing shame and other negative emotions, whereas male patients may be more likely to feel socially or physically inadequate.

Box 30-2 ■ ■ ■ ■ ■
Psychological Characteristics Common to People With Anorexia Nervosa and Bulimia Nervosa

- Low self-esteem
- Suppression of feelings, especially anger
- Perfectionism
- Reliance on schedules, lack of spontaneity
- Obsession with body size and food
- Sexual problems
- Identity crises
- Lack of autonomy
- Immaturity, "black-and-white" thinking
- Depression

Does the patient have a sense of hope? Are there potential strengths or coping skills the patient can be encouraged to develop?

Sociocultural Assessment

It is important to inquire about the patient's beliefs about what is normal weight and normal eating. Is there pressure on the patient to be thin? Does he or she feel that his or her acceptance and love are conditional, based on weight? How much has he or she integrated society's message that "you can never be too thin"? Or is there pressure in the household to overeat? Is the patient going through a difficult transition or role disruption? It is important to look at the quality and extent of the patient's support system. The anorexic tends to be introverted and isolated; the bulimic may appear extroverted, engaging in sexually promiscuous behaviors, drug use, stealing, and suicidal gestures. The obese patient is likely to be severely stigmatized, even ostracized.

Family Assessment

An assessment of family function often reveals significant differences between the anorexic and the bulimic. The family environment of the anorexic patient tends to be controlled and rigid, with little overt discord. The family environment of the bulimic patient may be conflictual and chaotic, with violence and substance abuse prevalent.

It is also important to assess the eating patterns of the family. Questions focusing on the family's approach to mealtimes might include the following:

Who plans the meals in your family?
Who cooks the meals in your family?
What are mealtimes like in your family?

Spiritual Assessment

Bordo (1997) described anorexia in terms of the "detachment of the body from the soul" (p. 110). In conducting a spiritual assessment, ask about the patient's view of himself or herself in relation to God. Is the patient active in a spiritual community? Does the patient feel that he or she is "not good enough"? Is there a need to strive for perfection? Does the patient use such rationalizations as "fasting makes me stronger"? Is the patient on a quest for the meaning of life?

Additional Areas to Assess

As you gather data from the patient and other reliable sources, include a variety of dimensions to help identify and clarify specific contributing factors for each patient. Love and Seaton (1991) listed the following dimensions as important aspects of the assessment:

- Alliance building
- Motivation for treatment
- Coping strategies

What do you think? Are there ways in which you can identify with an eating-disordered patient?

► Check Your Reading
11. What impact does anorexia have on blood pressure? On pulse?
12. Identify at least two areas in which anorexics and bulimics differ.
13. What would you want to know about a bulimic's eating patterns?
14. What impact might society's pressures have on individuals with eating disorders?

Diagnosis

Medical and nursing diagnoses for the patient with an eating disorder are shown in the box, Medical Diagnoses and Related Nursing Diagnoses: Eating Disorders.

Outcome Identification

Samples of expected outcomes for a patient with an eating disorder follow:

- The underweight patient will achieve and maintain his or her weight within normal parameters for his or her age and size.
- The patient's fluid and electrolyte balance will be within normal parameters; the patient will no longer engage in binge-purge eating.
- The patient will express an accurate appraisal of body size and body weight.

Planning

Sample short-term goals for a patient with an eating disorder follow.

MEDICAL DIAGNOSES AND RELATED NURSING DIAGNOSES

Eating Disorders

DSM-IV Diagnosis:

Anorexia Nervosa

Diagnostic Criteria

A. Refusal to maintain body weight at or above a minimally normal weight for age and height (e.g., weight loss leading to maintenance of body weight less than 85% of that expected; or failure to make expected weight gain during period of growth, leading to body weight less than 85% of that expected).

B. Intense fear of gaining weight or becoming fat, even though underweight.

C. Disturbance in the way in which one's body weight or shape is experienced, undue influence of body weight or shape on self-evaluation, or denial of the seriousness of the current low body weight.

D. In postmenarcheal females, amenorrhea, that is, the absence of at least three consecutive menstrual cycles. (A woman is considered to have amenorrhea if her periods occur only following hormone [e.g., estrogen] administration.)

Specify type:

Restricting Type: During the current episode of Anorexia Nervosa, the person has not regularly engaged in binge eating or purging behavior (i.e., self-induced vomiting or the misuse of laxatives, diuretics, or enemas).

Binge Eating Purging Type: During the current episode of Anorexia Nervosa, the person has regularly engaged in binge eating or purging behavior (i.e., self-induced vomiting or the misuse of laxatives, diuretics, or enemas).

DSM-IV Diagnosis:

Bulimia Nervosa

Diagnostic Criteria

A. Recurrent episodes of binge eating. An episode of binge eating is characterized by both of the following:

(1) Eating, in a discrete period of time (e.g., within any 2-h period), an amount of food that is definitely larger than most people would eat during a similar period of time and under similar circumstances.

(2) A sense of lack of control over eating during the episode (e.g., a feeling that one cannot stop eating or control what or how much one is eating).

B. Recurrent inappropriate compensatory behavior to prevent weight gain, such as self-induced vomiting; misuse of laxatives, diuretics, enemas, or other medications; fasting; or excessive exercise.

C. The binge eating and inappropriate compensatory behaviors both occur, on average, at least twice a week for 3 mo.

D. Self-evaluation is unduly influenced by body shape and weight.

E. The disturbance does not occur exclusively during episodes of Anorexia Nervosa.

Specify type:

Purging Type: During the current episode of Bulimia Nervosa, the person has regularly engaged in self-induced vomiting or the misuse of laxatives, diuretics, or enemas.

Nonpurging Type: During the current episode of Bulimia Nervosa, the person has used other inappropriate compensatory behaviors, such as fasting or excessive exercise, but has not regularly engaged in self-induced vomiting or the misuse of laxatives, diuretics, or enemas.

DSM-IV Diagnosis:

Binge Eating Disorder

Diagnostic Criteria

A. Recurrent episodes of binge eating. An episode of binge eating is characterized by both of the following:

(1) Eating, in a discrete period of time (e.g., within any 2-h period), an amount of food that is definitely larger than most people would eat in a similar period of time under similar circumstances.

(2) A sense of lack of control over eating during the episode (e.g., a feeling that one cannot stop eating or control what or how much one is eating).

B. The binge eating episodes are associated with three (or more) of the following:

(1) Eating much more rapidly than normal.

(2) Eating until feeling uncomfortably full.

(3) Eating large amounts of food when not feeling physically hungry.

(4) Eating alone because of being embarrassed by how much one is eating.

(5) Feeling disgusted with oneself, depressed, or guilty after overeating.

C. Marked distress regarding binge eating is present.

D. The binge eating occurs, on average, at least 2 d a week for 6 mo.

Note: The method of determining frequency differs from that used for Bulimia Nervosa; future research should address whether the preferred method of setting a frequency threshold is counting the number of days on which binges occur or counting the number of episodes of binge eating.

MEDICAL DIAGNOSES AND RELATED NURSING DIAGNOSES

Eating Disorders Continued

E. The binge eating is not associated with the regular use of inappropriate compensatory behaviors (e.g., purging, fasting, excessive exercise) and does not occur exclusively during the course of Anorexia Nervosa or Bulimia Nervosa.

Related Nursing Diagnoses:

Altered Nutrition: Less than Body Requirements

Definition
The state in which an individual experiences an intake of nutrients insufficient to meet metabolic needs.

Examples
Altered Nutrition: Less than Body Requirements related to insufficient intake of calories evidenced by weight 20% less than normal.

Body Image Disturbance: Disruption in the way one perceives one's body image; Body Image Disturbance related to fear of weight gain evidenced by preoccupation with being fat.

Fluid Volume Deficit: The state in which an individual experiences vascular, cellular, or intracellular dehydration; Fluid Volume Deficit related to purging activities evidenced by abnormal blood chemistry values.

Self Esteem Disturbance, negative self evaluation/feelings about self or self capabilities, which may be directly or indirectly expressed; Self Concept Disturbance: Self Esteem related to feelings of inadequacy evidenced by self-derogatory statements.

Based on information from the *Diagnostic and Statistical Manual of Mental Disorders. Fourth Edition.* Copyright 1994 American Psychiatric Association. Nursing diagnoses and definitions from North American Nursing Diagnosis Association. (1999). *NANDA nursing diagnoses: Definitions and classification, 1999–2000.* Philadelphia: NANDA.

Expected Outcome 1
The patient will achieve and maintain his or her weight within normal parameters for his or her age and size.

Short-Term Goals
- The patient will participate in treatment.
- The patient will acknowledge having an eating disorder.
- The patient will state the components of a balanced diet.
- The patient will eat a balanced diet.
- The patient's nutritional status will be stabilized.
- The patient will participate in an appropriate level of daily exercise.

Expected Outcome 2
The patient's fluid and electrolyte balance will be within normal parameters, and the patient will no longer engage in binge-purge eating.

Short-Term Goals
- The patient will agree to talk about urges to binge and purge.
- The patient's nutritional intake will restore normal fluid and electrolyte balance.
- The patient will discuss the destructive results of bingeing and purging.
- The patient will discuss alternatives to bingeing and purging.

- The patient will discuss feelings experienced before and after a binge-purge cycle.

Expected Outcome 3
The patient will express an accurate appraisal of body size and body weight.

Short-Term Goals
- The patient will accurately describe his or her body shape.
- The patient will accurately state his or her ideal body weight.
- The patient will identify the cognitive distortions that support an inaccurate appraisal of body image and weight.

The plan defines not only short-term goals but also the intensity of treatment. Whether treatment is offered in an outpatient or an inpatient setting depends on the severity of the patient's physical and psychiatric condition (see later in chapter). Regardless of the setting, the treatment team—which includes the patient and family—develops a treatment plan incorporating the appropriate expectations. The plan frequently includes a contract in which the patient agrees to specific goals. As a member of the team, it is essential for the nurse to engage the patient in a therapeutic alliance and to seek the patient's commitment to treatment.

*W*hat do you think? Are there any circumstances in which it is wrong to force an anorexic person to eat?

➤ *Check Your Reading*

15. Identify one expected outcome for an eating-disordered patient.
16. Identify one short-term goal to support the expected outcome that you identified in question 15.
17. Identify one nursing diagnosis that might be applied to an eating-disordered patient.

Implementation

There are several modalities of treatment for all eating disorders in both inpatient and outpatient settings:

1. Inpatient psychotherapy
   • Behavior modification
2. Outpatient psychotherapy
   • Individual and group therapies
   • Family therapy
3. Psychopharmacology
4. Spiritual aspects of care

Before caring for patients with eating disorders, however, it is essential for each of us to step back and evaluate our own ideas, values, opinions, and beliefs regarding people with eating disorders. The first step involves identifying beliefs and values regarding body shape and weight. Culture and society at large affect and subtly shape our thoughts and ideas. The question each of us must answer is, "Whose eyes am I looking through—my own or the eyes of society?" And further, "Am I making judgments about personal worth based on a person's body weight, shape, or size? Have I bought into cultural stereotypes, such as losing weight will solve all of life's problems or having a thin body will guarantee a happy-ever-after life?" The patient's sense of happiness, self-worth, and value as a human being are challenged if caregivers endorse such stereotypes. See the box, What Patients Need to Know: Eating Disorders.

As we care for overweight patients, it is important to realize that these people do not have more emotional problems than normal-weight people. Much of the emotional trauma they experience is most likely the result of prejudice and stigma and the cultural pressure to lose weight (Fontaine, 1991).

Nurses collectively must be willing to challenge these cultural stereotypes. This challenge begins with each nurse determining how to view a sense of human worth. Do we as nurses believe that "beauty is in the eye of the beholder" or are we too busy "judging the book by its cover"? Nurses stand at the door of opportunity; the question is, "Will we stand or walk through the door?" Nurses must be proactive when caring for patients with eating disorders. We must become leaders in this arena by "fostering a humane approach to body size" (Fontaine, 1991, p. 675).

Inpatient Psychotherapy

Anorexic patients are more likely to be seen on inpatient wards because the starvation state is life-threatening. If bulimia patients are hospitalized, it is usually for severe depression or suicidality. For instance, the following physical findings would warrant inpatient treatment:

1. Weight loss greater than 20% of body weight over 3 months
2. Heart rate less than 40 bpm
3. Temperature less than 36°C (96.8°F)
4. Systolic blood pressure less than 70 mmHg
5. Serum potassium less than 2.5 mEq/L
6. Severe dehydration

Psychiatric findings warranting inpatient treatment include

1. High risk for suicide
2. Self-mutilating behaviors
3. Severe depression
4. Inability to comply with treatment plan
5. Inadequate response to treatment
6. Psychotic behavior

Inpatient treatment provides the support, safety, physiological monitoring, and psychological care supportive of behavioral change offered by the 24-hour availability of nursing staff. The inpatient care of patients

WHAT PATIENTS NEED TO KNOW

Eating Disorders

Why do I need to sign a contract?

A contract is a written set of rules, consequences, and rewards to which both you and the treatment team have agreed. It can be renegotiated as progress is made. It serves as a guideline for identifying prohibited as well as desired behaviors. Items that are typically negotiated relate to meals; privileges such as television watching, radio playing, and trips off the unit; and weight gain.

What is healthy eating or "gentle" eating?

These are new behaviors to help you prepare and eat foods to achieve weight gain or weight stabilization goals. Some of the following eating behaviors are encouraged: eat food slowly, chew thoroughly, put utensils down between bites, do not eat while doing other activities, eat in a specific place at home (dining room), and sit down while eating at prescribed times.

WHAT PATIENTS AND FAMILIES NEED TO KNOW

Bulimia Nervosa

How is bulimia nervosa different from anorexia nervosa?

Bulimia is a separate and different condition from anorexia nervosa and compulsive eating. Most often the bulimic patient is normal weight or slightly overweight who binges and purges to maintain or lose weight. Also, anorexics who have lost their rigid control over fasting or not eating may purge as an attempt to gain some type of control. Sometimes, anorexics may have been bulimic before the onset of anorexia nervosa. It is estimated that bulimia may occur in as many as 40% of college women.

What is the binge-purge cycle?

This compulsive cycle is characterized by a total loss of control over food intake. The person consumes thousands of calories (binge) in foods that are high-calorie (candy bars) and high-carbohydrate (potato chips, cookies, cake), which she or he takes with lots of fluids (soft drinks, juices) and follows with a purge. The cycle may interfere with normal daily functioning to the same extent often seen with alcoholics or drug addicts. The bulimic becomes so preoccupied with binge-purge behavior that school, job, and relationships suffer as the patient becomes more isolated and depressed.

What are the different forms of purging?

There are various forms of purging, such as self-induced vomiting; using diuretics, laxatives, and enemas; or strict dieting or fasting. Excessive or vigorous exercise is also a form of purging, especially if it is done to prevent weight gain.

What can I do to stop the binge-purge cycle?

Seek professional help. It is difficult to stop the cycle. You have probably made promises to yourself every morning to stop bingeing and purging and then feel guilty when it happens. Having this sense of loss of control about eating may make you feel depressed and anxious. These are normal feelings when you feel powerless and unable to enjoy or take charge of your life.

with eating disorders requires interdisciplinary planning and collaboration to deal with the manipulation and "splitting" behaviors often displayed by the patients.

The patient contracts with the staff and participates in deciding goals (within safe parameters) as well as rewards for achievement of goals, such as gaining weight, exercising, or not vomiting. The anorexic patient in an inpatient setting must be closely monitored and may have peer as well as caregiver support to enhance his or her goal-keeping. For the bulimic or compulsive overeater, the plan may consist of keeping a daily self-monitoring diary, limiting amount of food per meal, limiting high-carbohydrate foods in the home, and limiting unstructured time. Behavior modification techniques are widely accepted as a form of treatment with eating-disordered patients. The key is to implement the behavior modification program in such a way that the patient is in control. Any struggles are then with the agreed-on plan, not with the caregivers. Control is essential for the patient with an eating disorder, so the success of treatment depends largely on this issue. (See Chapter 13 for other behavioral strategies.)

Outpatient Psychotherapy

The best approach to outpatient treatment is multifaceted and can include individual, family, nutritional, and group therapies (Hsu, 1990). Individual therapy may involve delving into the root issues of self-esteem, independence, sexuality, and perfectionism, as discussed earlier, or may be restricted to cognitive-behavioral strategies. (Cognitive therapy, discussed in Chapter 14, is an important modality in addressing the cognitive distortions that the patient holds regarding eating.) Some researchers suggest that families involved in family therapy be responsible for weight gain by anorexia nervosa patients, and this has shown signs of success (Dare, 1983). Accountability is part of group therapy or peer support groups that provide healthy interactions with others, helping to build self-esteem and feelings of worthiness so often lacking in patients with eating disorders. Garrett (1997) recommended as an adjunct the use of other processes such as meditation, music, art, and especially physical activities, for example, dancing, swimming, walking, and gardening.

Groups such as Overeaters Anonymous are helpful to many overweight and obese individuals. Because at least 95% of participants in weight loss programs involving dieting return to their initial weight within 5 years, and because wide fluctuations in weight are especially dangerous, weight maintenance, self-esteem enhancement, increased physical activity, and other lifestyle changes may be more realistic goals (Ciliska, 1998; Tanco, Linden, & Earle, 1998). See the box, What Patients and Families Need to Know: Bulimia Nervosa.

Psychopharmacology

Serotonin-related antidepressants such as fluoxetine (Prozac) have been shown to decrease depression and increase weight gain in anorexic patients as well as to decrease bulimic binge episodes by 50%. Therefore, the practitioner who has taken a thorough psychological and family history may be able to prescribe an antidepressant as an adjunct to addressing the patient's underlying problems. See the box, What Families Need to Know: Anorexia Nervosa.

Drugs that reduce appetite or increase satiety are called anorectics. The introduction of "fen-phen" (fenfluramine and phentermine) several years ago in the treatment of obesity generated an enormous amount of excitement. However, in September 1997, following the appearance of heart valve disease in a significant percentage of users, fenfluramine and a secondary form, dexfenfluramine, were withdrawn from the market. Clinical trials continue with these and related compounds. Other types of drugs used in obesity treatment (such as orlistat) interfere with digestion or absorption (Blackburn et al., 1997).

Spiritual Aspects of Care

The previously discussed interventions are considered traditional and provide an overall framework for caring for patients with eating disorders but do not represent a holistic approach to patient care. All people, whether or not they are practicing a particular formal religion, have a spiritual component (Carson, 1989). The person's spiritual nature must be considered as part of her or his total care, along with the physical and psychosocial components (Carson, 1989; Garrett, 1997).

Feeling out of control, unloved, or unaccepted can lead to hopelessness, helplessness, or lack of meaning in one's life. These feelings are reflective of spiritual distress. As a nurse committed to providing holistic care, you must address these spiritual issues with the eating-disordered patient. All the behavioral contracts, medications, and therapy will fail if the patient continues to feel unloved and unimportant. Garrett (1997), who urged us to place greater emphasis on recovery from anorexia and less on its etiology, wrote of the elements common to 32 people she studied who had recovered (p. 264):

1. Abandoning obsession with food and weight, concomitant with a critical understanding of social pressure
2. Having a sense that their lives were meaningful
3. Believing that they were worthwhile and that the different aspects of themselves were part of a whole person
4. Believing strongly that they would never return to self-starvation
5. Mentioning spirituality as a source of meaning

What do you think? Can an eating disorder ever be seen as a positive thing?

➤ *Check Your Reading*

18. Identify two physical and two psychiatric symptoms that would lead to inpatient treatment of an anorexic.
19. Identify two treatment interventions used with eating-disordered patients.
20. Identify one psychotropic medication used in the treatment of anorexia.

Evaluation

The plan of care needs to be continually evaluated to ensure that goals set are realistic and success adequately

---

WHAT FAMILIES NEED TO KNOW

Anorexia Nervosa

What do I need to know about anorexia nervosa?

Anorexia nervosa is a potentially life-threatening illness in which adolescent girls (or boys) literally starve themselves to death. These young people have an intense fear of becoming fat, relentlessly pursue thinness, and often have are deluded about their body image. The self-starvation is not only the absence of eating or the ingestion of low-calorie foods but also may involve purging, which includes behaviors such as inducing vomiting; taking diuretics, laxatives, or enemas; and excessively exercising to the point of exhaustion.

What should I do about cooking or preparing meals?

Often, anorexics have a personal "food list" of items they will eat. They will go to extreme lengths to avoid foods not on their list. You may begin noticing your adolescent hiding food, eating alone, or giving food to others or to household pets. Sometimes, the adolescent becomes involved with cooking rich, high-calorie meals for the family but will not even taste her or his own cooking.

What can I do to help my child?

Family therapy and intervention are key aspects to the long-term care and management of the anorexic patient. Understanding and family education are important aspects of gaining insight into what is happening within the family. Early recognition of self-starvation behavior is important. Medical treatment should be sought when a 10% to 15% weight loss occurs, rather than waiting longer, when the patient becomes more debilitated and dehydrated.

SNAPSHOT

Nursing Interventions Specific to Eating Disorder

What do you need to do to develop a relationship with a patient with an eating disorder?
- Examine your own feelings first. How do you feel toward your own body? How do you feel about fatness or thinness? Have you bought into societal's views that "you can't be too thin"? How will you deal with your feelings and attitudes when you interact with the patient?
- Approach the patient with empathy and compassion.
- Avoid anything that implies that the patient's worth as an individual is linked to weight.

What do you need to assess regarding the patient's health status?
- Weight loss greater than 30% over 3 months
- Heart rate less than 40 bpm
- Temperature less than 96.8°F (36°C)
- Systolic blood pressure less than 70 mmHg
- Serum potassium less than 2.5 mEq/L
- Severe dehydration
- Suicidality
- Self-mutilating behaviors
- Severe depression
- Inability to comply with treatment plan
- Inadequate response to treatment
- Psychotic behavior
- Patient's medications

What do you need to teach the patient and the patient's caregiver or significant other?
- Management of medication issues
- Use of cognitive-behavioral techniques to deal with anxiety that may contribute to bingeing and purging
- Importance of self-esteem
- Importance of stress management
- Importance of family involvement
- Importance of patient exerting appropriate control

What skills do you want the patient and patient's caregiver or significant other to demonstrate?
- Behavior modification strategies
- Self-esteem enhancement activities
- Stress management techniques, such as use of music, art, meditation, and physical activities
- Use of peer support groups such as Overeaters Anonymous
- Medication management
- Spiritual well-being activities

What other health professionals might need to be a part of this plan of care?
- Physician and psychiatrist to manage the physical as well as the psychiatric aspects of care
- Social worker to assist patient with access to community resources
- Psychiatric nurses in community settings, including home care and community mental health centers, who may monitor the therapy issues over time

measured. The formative evaluation looks at short-term goals initially set for a patient with an eating disorder to see if these goals need to be modified. Perhaps the goals did not include a focus on decreasing the anxiety experienced by the patient before mealtime. Modifying the plan might include teaching the patient relaxation techniques to make mealtimes more pleasurable. The summative evaluation examines the patient's physical, emotional, and spiritual state as treatment ends. The summative evaluation answers the following questions:

1. Has the patient gained or lost weight (depending on the goal)?
2. Is the patient's fluid and electrolyte balance restored?
3. Is the patient articulating a normal body image?
4. Is the patient feeling as if his or her life matters? Is he or she feeling loved?

See Snapshot: Nursing Interventions Specific to Eating Disorder.

NURSING PROCESS APPLICATION

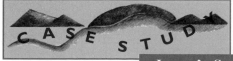
CASE STUDY

Jenny's Story

Jenny, a 13-year-old girl, has been admitted to a psychiatric unit. According to her parents, her normal weight is 100 lb and she has rapidly lost 20 lb over the past month on a strict diet. During the admission interview, her mother states that she is very proud of Jenny, especially when she finishes first in her competitive gymnastic program. Jenny believes that losing weight will help her improve her skills, so that she can attain a better score and stay at the top at the next regional gymnastics meet. Jenny's mother says that she is a "straight 'A' student in school" and the "perfect, obedient" child. Lately, her parents say, they are exasperated with her dieting and refusal to eat even her favorite foods. On admission, Jenny's weight is 80 lb, and her height is 5 ft, 5 in. Her mother reports that Jenny started her menses at age 11, but has not had a period for the past year.

Jenny remains quiet and withdrawn, glaring at her parents while avoiding eye contact with the nurse. The nurse notes that her skin is cool and slightly yellow, with a fine covering of lanugo. Her mother states that Jenny often tells her gymnastics coach she is fat.

ASSESSMENT   Assessment data are as follows:
- Emaciated, sallow skin color
- 20% body weight loss
- Amenorrhea for the past 12 months
- Appearance of lanugo
- Overachiever; "perfect, obedient" child

DIAGNOSIS   **DSM-IV Diagnosis:**   Anorexia Nervosa

Nursing Diagnosis: Altered Nutrition: Less than Body Requirements related to self-starvation behaviors as evidenced by 20-lb weight loss, amenorrhea, lanugo, and emaciated appearance

---

OUTCOME IDENTIFICATION, PLANNING, AND IMPLEMENTATION

> **Expected Outcome 1:** By _____ the patient's weight will be within safe limits.

Short-Term Goal	Nursing Interventions	Rationales
By _____ the patient will establish a minimum weekly weight gain (0.5 to 1.5 kg/wk).	1. Provide nutrition consultation to facilitate weight gain.	1. Medical and nutritional management is needed to provide for a safe regimen of weight gain in the patient's debilitated state. The patient is more likely to eat foods she has chosen.
	2. Initiate eating contract that specifies three meals per day to be eaten with other patients and staff.	2. Contract negotiation fosters the patient's independence and provides for positive reinforcement of appropriate eating behavior.
	3. Observe patient during and after eating, noting any rituals or signs of purging.	3. During early hospitalization, some deception as well as a need to feel in control of the environment and food intake occurs. Purging may occur as a response to weight gain.
	4. Maintain a regular weighing schedule (usually one to three times per week) with the patient in lightweight clothing. In extreme obsession cases, you may need to weigh the patient with her back to the scale (to prevent patient from knowing actual weight).	4. Limited weighing focuses on the issue of trust and minimizes the patient's obsessing about weight gain or loss. The patient will demonstrate minimal complications from nutritional imbalances.

> **Expected Outcome 2:** By _____ the patient's weight will be within normal limits.

Short-Term Goal	Nursing Interventions	Rationales
By _____ the patient will exhibit minimal adverse side effects caused by the refeeding schedule.	1. Begin the refeeding schedule slowly. 2. Check laboratory values.	1–2. The patient is at risk for arrhythmias, bradycardia, hypotension, electrolyte imbalance (especially hypokalemia), and hypothermia.

3. Monitor vital signs and observe for adverse side effects to refeeding.

3. Other problems may occur with too rapid weight gain, including congestive heart failure, abdominal discomfort, edema, and gastric dilation. Monitor for edema and abdominal distention.

Nursing Diagnosis: Body Image Disturbance related to inaccurate perception of self and dysfunctional family system as evidenced by statements of being fat despite thinness, emaciated appearance, and controlling behavior of parents

OUTCOME IDENTIFICATION, PLANNING, AND IMPLEMENTATION

Expected Outcome 1: By _____ the patient will establish a more realistic body image.

Short-Term Goal	Nursing Interventions	Rationales
By _____ the patient will have a realistic perception of her body image.	1. Explore need to excel at gymnastics and possible feelings of inadequacy. 2. When unrealistic statements are made with regard to body size, gently confront patient with reality. 3. Assist the patient to identify manageable goals related to gymnastics and self. 4. Encourage acceptance of shortcomings as well as strengths.	1. Feelings of inadequacy, loneliness, or need to be perfect within the family system need to be examined. 2–4. Self-deprecating comments and an inability to see self as someone unique and distinct within the family are important. Often, the patient feels helpless in family situations and finds comfort in control of eating behavior because parents may not control this aspect of life.

Expected Outcome 2: By _____ the patient will verbalize feelings and acknowledge self by taking responsibility for actions.

Short-Term Goal	Nursing Interventions	Rationales
By _____ the patient will verbalize feelings with nurse and members on the unit.	1. Make encouraging comments. 2. Listen nonjudgmentally and without criticism. 3. Avoid overreacting when patient has deceived staff, for example, hiding food or purging.	1. Therapeutic communication and unconditional positive regard promote feelings of trust, which are necessary before the patient will verbalize feelings. 2–3. Patients often come from rigid family environments in which the parents (usually the mother) make all their decisions and expect them to be perfect in everything they do.

EVALUATION

Formative Evaluation: Jenny did not meet her weekly weight gain goals for her first 2 weeks of hospitalization. She would hide food and secretly purge. The contract was renegotiated and the expectations of weight gain were reduced to weight maintenance for 1 week, to which she agreed. During that time, Jenny was able to talk about the expectations of weight gain, which made her feel powerless and helpless, plus the feelings of fullness in her stomach. She was beginning to understand the family dynamics and needed unhurried, unconditional acceptance by the nurse during the early phase of her treatment. A supportive, forgiving atmosphere was the important milieu setting for Jenny to work on her family and spiritual needs.

Summative Evaluation: By discharge, Jenny had gained 15 lb and was feeling in better control of her own life. She decided to take a short break from gymnastics until she could rebuild her strength. Her mother was upset that she would not make the gymnastic competition. Jenny was able to express her feelings to her mother about the pressure she felt. She was beginning to feel more in touch with who she really was, a young beautiful child of God who did not have to prove anything to be accepted in His love. Jenny had not mentioned how "fat she was" during her last

3 weeks of hospitalization. An outpatient family therapy program was negotiated. Jenny and her parents agreed to attend. Jenny also began to be involved with the youth group at her church.

Conclusions

Eating disorders stem from a variety of cultural, physiological, and psychological factors and are a form of addiction, similar to alcoholism or drug abuse. Behavioral changes necessary to conquer this addiction, however, are not found in abstinence or avoidance. Rather, the patient with an eating disorder must redefine her or his relationship with food and explore the reasons she or he has turned to food to solve problems. Ferraro (1990, p. 188), herself a recovering bulimic, urged us, as nurses, to "invest the time and effort required to maintain our own

health," to care for ourselves in order to care for others. Never underestimate the importance of your part in the recovery process. In the words of Halek (1997):

The role of the nurse in the treatment of eating disorders requires a wide range of skills and confidence in managing high levels of anxiety. For many patients, the nurse is the key professional involved in their care and is in a position to offer significant treatment and support to individuals who suffer these distressing problems. (p. 63)

Key Points to Remember

- Food plays several important roles in our lives: to provide nutrition; to reward achievement, to punish misbehaviors; and to comfort, support, and express love. Also, it is intricately tied to our impressions of ourselves in terms of body image and self-esteem.
- Anorexia nervosa and bulimia primarily affect young, white women in the middle to upper socioeconomic groups in Western countries.
- Eating disorders are associated with significant medical consequences, including life-threatening conditions.
- Problems with food regulation have a historical basis.
- Anorexia nervosa is a disorder characterized by the refusal to maintain a normal body weight; this is done through strict dieting or engaging in a food binge-purge cycle.
- Bulimia nervosa is characterized by repeated episodes of bingeing and purging.
- Binge eating disorder is characterized by excessive intake of calories.

- The cause of eating disorders is believed to be multifactorial with significant roles played by biological, psychological, sociocultural, and spiritual issues.
- There is a significant co-occurrence of psychiatric problems, such as depression, OCD, panic disorder, and personality disorders, along with eating disorders.
- The assessment for eating disorders must include a comprehensive physical examination along with a focus on mental status and family, psychological, sociocultural, and spiritual issues.
- There are many nursing diagnoses appropriate to the eating disorders, including Nutrition, Alteration in: Less than Body Requirements, Fluid Volume Deficit, and Self Concept Disturbance in Body Image: Self Esteem.
- The identified outcomes focus on restoring nutritional and fluid and electrolyte balance as well as achieving normal weight.
- The nursing interventions focus on various modes of therapy in either an inpatient or an outpatient setting, psychopharmacology, and spiritual support.

Learning Activities

1. Reflect on the following questions in your journal: What do I think about weight? Do I link my own self-worth with my weight? Do I link the value of others to their weight? Do I give preferential treatment to people whose appearance is more pleasing to me? How much is my thinking affected by social stereotypes about weight and body shape?

2. Watch television one night and keep track of how many commercials or television programs extoll the

value of thinness and the desirability of fast food. What impact does this have on young people's attitudes toward food? Toward diet? Toward what is good and desirable in relationship to body size and shape?

3. Survey one fashion magazine. How many advertisements do you see that promote the idea that a woman's or man's self-worth is tied to outward appearance? When you look at advertisements showing slim models, how do you react?

Critical Thinking Exercise

Terri Mader, a 5-ft, 9 in., 16-year-old high school swimmer, was admitted to the eating disorder unit weighing 98 lb. Her father was her swim coach and traveled with her to meets, while her mother, an executive, stayed home to care for her brother who was 13 years old. She was referred to the eating disorder unit by the physician who examined her following a fainting episode before her last swim meet when she lost consciousness for several minutes. She told the referring physician that she had been taking laxatives to keep her weight down.

1. What assumptions do you think Terri is operating under?
2. What evidence suggests that she may be anorexic?
3. What other possibilities might explain Terri's behavior?

One week following admission, Terri asked the nurse for her as needed laxative. The nurse, aware of her abuse of laxatives, refused to give it to her. One hour later, her attending psychiatrist called the nurse on the unit stating, "I just received a call from my patient that you will not give her medication. I order you to give it to her now."

1. What is the psychiatrist's point of view?
2. Give an alternative viewpoint of the situation.
3. What conclusions might be drawn about the relationships among the nurse, the patient, and the psychiatrist?

Additional Resources

American Academy of Child and Adolescent Psychiatry (AACAP)
http://www.aacap.org/

American Psychiatric Association (APA)
http://www.psych.org

Eating Disorders Shared Awareness (EDSA)
http://www.eating-disorder.com

This Webpage lists two Websites:
Mirror Mirror (Canada) and Something Fishy (United States), both related to eating disorders.

The Renfrew Center
http://www.renfrew.org

References

Abraham, S., & Llewellyn-Jones, D. (1997). *Eating disorders: The facts* (4th ed.). Oxford, England: Oxford University Press.

Allan, J. D. (1998). New directions in the study of overweight [editorial]. *Western Journal of Nursing Research 20*(1), 7-13.

American Psychiatric Association (1994). *Diagnostic and statistical manual of mental disorders* (4th ed.). Washington, DC: Author.

Anderson, N. T. (1993). *Released from bondage.* Nashville, TN: Thomas Nelson.

Arnow, B., Kenardy, J., & Agras, W. S. (1992). Binge eating among the obese: A descriptive study. *Journal of Behavioral Medicine, 15,* 161-163.

Ault, M. (1990). I am a Christian bulimic. *Journal of Christian Nursing, 7*(1), 4-8.

Blackburn, G. L., Miller, D., & Chan, S. (1997). Pharmaceutical treatment of obesity. *Nursing Clinics of North America, 32,* 831-848.

Billigmeier, S. (1991). *Inner eating.* Nashville, TN: Oliver Nelson.

Bordo, S. (1997). Anorexia nervosa: Psychopathology as the crystallization of culture. In M. M. Gergen & S. N. Davis (Eds.), *Toward a new psychology of gender.* New York: Routledge.

Brody, J. (1998, June 9). New guide puts most Americans on the fat side. *The New York Times,* p. F7.

Carlat, D. J., Camargo, C. A., Jr., & Herzog, D. B. (1997). Eating disorders in males: A report on 130 patients. *American Journal of Psychiatry, 154,* 1127-1132.

Carson, V. B. (1989). *Spiritual dimensions of nursing practice,* Philadelphia: W. B. Saunders.

Ciliska, D. (1998). Evaluation of two nondieting interventions for obese women. *Western Journal of Nursing Research, 20*(1), 119-130.

Dare, C. (1983). Family therapy for families containing an anorectic youngster. In D. E. Redfern (Ed.), *Understanding anorexia nervosa and bulimia.* Columbus, OH: Ross Laboratories.

Davis, C., Kaptein, S., Kaplan, A. S., Olmsted, M. P., Woodside, D. B. (1998). Obsessionality and anorexia nervosa: The moderating influence of exercise. *Psychosomatic Medicine, 60,* 192-197.

Epstein, R. (1990). *Eating habits and disorders.* New York: Chelsea House.

Ferraro, A. R. (1990). Bulimia: A look from within. *Pediatric Nursing, 16,* 187-191.

Flood, M. (1989). Addictive eating disorders. *Nursing Clinics of North America, 24*(1), 45-53.

Fontaine, K. L. (1991). The conspiracy of culture. *Nursing Clinics of North America, 24*(1), 669-676.

Garner, D. M. (1991). *EDI-2: Eating disorder inventory 2. Professional manual.* Odessa, FL: Psychological Assessment Resources.

Garner, D. M., & Garfinkle, P. E. (1979). Eating attitudes test: An index of symptoms of anorexia nervosa. *Psychological Medicine, 9,* 273-279.

Garrett, C. J. (1997). Recovery from anorexia nervosa: A sociological perspective. *International Journal of Eating Disorders, 21,* 261-272.

Halek, C. (1997). Eating disorders: The role of the nurse. *Nursing Times, 93*(28), 63-66.

Henderson, M., Freeman, C. P. (1987). A self rating scale for bulimia: The BITE. *British Journal of Psychiatry, 150*(1), 18-24.

Hirsch, J. (1997). The coming of genetics in the control of ingestion. *Appetite, 29*(2), 115-117.

Hsu, L. K. G. (1990). *Eating disorders.* New York: Guilford Press.

Humphries, L. L. (1997). Stress and eating disorders. In T. W. Miller (Ed.), *Clinical disorders and stressful life events.* Madison, CT: International University Press.

Kaplan, H. I., & Sadock, B. J. (1991). *Synopsis of psychiatry* (6th ed.). Baltimore: Williams & Wilkins.

Krueger, D. (1997). Food as self object. *The Psychoanalytic Review, 84,* 617-630.

Laraia, M. T., & Stuart, G. W. (1990). Bulimia: A review of nutritional and health behaviors. *Journal of Child and Adolescent Psychiatry, 3,* 91-96.

Love, C. C., & Seaton, H. (1991). Eating disorders: Highlights of nursing assessment and therapeutics. *Nursing Clinics of North America, 26,* 677-680.

Marrazzi, M. A., Luby, I. & E. D., Kinzie, J., Munjal, D., Spector, S. (1997). Endogenous codeine and morphine in anorexia and bulimia nervosa. *Life Sciences, 60,* 1741-1747.

McGee, C. (1997). Secondary amenorrhea leading to osteoporosis: Incidence and prevention. *Nurse Practitioner: American Journal of Primary Health Care, 22*(5), 38, 41-45, 48 passim.

Mercer, M. E., & Holder, M. D. (1997). Food cravings, endogenous opioid peptides and food intake: A review. *Appetite, 29,* 325-352.

Neumarker, K.-J. (1997). Mortality and sudden death in anorexia nervosa. *International Journal of Eating Disorders, 21,* 205-212.

Patton, G. C. (1992). Eating disorders: Antecedents, evolution and course. *Annals of Medicine, 24,* 281-285.

Riley, E. A. (1991). Eating disorders as addictive behavior: Integrating 12-step programs into treatment planning. *Nursing Clinics of North America, 26,* 715-718.

Silverstone, P. H. (1992). Is chronic low self-esteem the cause of eating disorders? *Medical Hypotheses, 39,* 311-315.

Solomon, C. G., & Manson, J. E. (1997). Obesity and mortality: A review of the epidemiological data. *American Journal of Clinical Nutrition, 66* (Suppl. 4), 1044S-1050S.

Stunkard, A. (1997). Eating disorders in the last 25 years. *Appetite, 29,* 181-190.

Szymanski, L. A., & Seime, R. J. (1997). A re-examination of body image distortion: Evidence against a sensory explanation. *International Journal of Eating Disorders, 21,* 175-180.

Tanco, S., Linden, W., & Earle, T. (1998). Well-being and morbid obesity in women: A controlled therapy evaluation. *International Journal of Eating Disorders, 23,* 325-339.

Thornton, C., & Russell, J. (1997). Obsessive compulsive comorbidity in the dieting disorders. *International Journal of Eating Disorders, 21,* 83-87.

Treasure, J. L., & Owen, J. B. (1997). Intriguing links between animal behavior and anorexia nervosa. *International Journal of Eating Disorders, 21,* 307-311.

Walsh, B. T., Roose, S. P., Glassman, A. H., Gladis, M., & Sadik, C. (1985). Bulimia and depression. *Psychosomatic Medicine, 47,* 123-131.

Yanovski, S. Z., Nelson, J. E., Dubbert, B. K., & Spitzer, R. L. (1993). Association of binge eating disorder and psychiatric comorbidity in obese subjects. *American Journal of Psychiatry, 150,* 1472-1479.

Suggested Readings

Ferraro, A. R. (1990). Bulimia: A look from within. *Pediatric Nursing, 16,* 187-191.

Flood, M. (1989). Addictive eating disorders. *Nursing Clinics of North America, 24,* 45-53.

Fontaine, K. L. (1991). The conspiracy of culture. *Nursing Clinics of North America, 26,* 669-675.

Garrett, C. J. (1997). Recovery from anorexia nervosa: A sociological perspective. *International Journal of Eating Disorders, 21,* 261-272.

White, J. H. (1992). Women and eating disorders, Part I: Significance and sociocultural risk factors. *Health Care for Women International, 13,* 301-362.

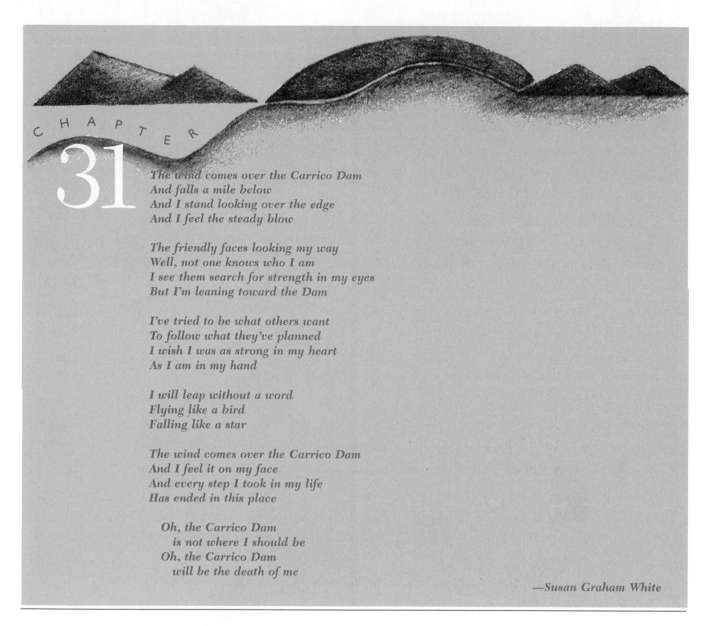

The wind comes over the Carrico Dam
And falls a mile below
And I stand looking over the edge
And I feel the steady blow

The friendly faces looking my way
Well, not one knows who I am
I see them search for strength in my eyes
But I'm leaning toward the Dam

I've tried to be what others want
To follow what they've planned
I wish I was as strong in my heart
As I am in my hand

I will leap without a word
Flying like a bird
Falling like a star

The wind comes over the Carrico Dam
And I feel it on my face
And every step I took in my life
Has ended in this place

Oh, the Carrico Dam
is not where I should be
Oh, the Carrico Dam
will be the death of me

—Susan Graham White

Suicide

Learning Objectives

After studying this chapter, you should be able to:

1. Discuss one fact related to the history of suicide.

2. Describe three examples of the theoretical foundations for the study of suicidal behavior.

3. List five questions used to assess the level of lethality of a patient's suicide potential.

4. Identify two clinical variables that influence a patient's suicidal behavior.

5. List two symptoms that are present when a patient is at risk for self-mutilation.

6. Identify three behavior patterns that would indicate that a patient is at risk for a lethal suicidal attempt.

7. Identify two nursing interventions for a patient who exhibits self-mutilative behavior.

8. Discuss three nursing interventions for a patient who has made a serious suicide attempt.

9. Identify two methods to help you with your own feelings, beliefs, and behaviors resulting from working with suicidal or self-mutilating patients.

10. Discuss two reasons for continuing to evaluate the nursing care provided for suicidal patients.

Key Terminology

Alexithymia	Every-15-minute checks	Life balance	Suicidal ideation
Completed suicide	Indirect self-destructive	One-to-one supervision	Suicide
Direct self-destructive	behavior	Parasuicidal behavior	Suicide attempt
behavior	Level of lethality	Self-mutilation	Suicide gesture

Life is an unpredictable and even hazardous journey. Sometimes the journey is smooth, happy, and trouble-free. Other times it feels as if we hit every pothole, run into every fallen branch and are forced to detour because of a blocked path. All of us face choices about how we will cope with the hazards of the roadway. Although some of these choices are made consciously and others unconsciously; all choices depend on our individual coping style, our faith in our ability to change, our world view, and our skill in maintaining a life balance.

The term **life balance** refers to the interaction among the physical, psychological, social, and spiritual variables in each of our lives that keeps us feeling well and that allows us to believe that life is generally good and worth continuing. An important component of life balance is the spiritual component. For example, a person with a theistic world view is likely to believe that physical life is a precious gift from the Creator and that it is not ours to terminate at will. Also consistent with a theistic world view is the perspective that physical life is only a part of life and that there is a spiritual afterlife.

When a person's life balance becomes so seriously disturbed that he or she loses the belief that the journey has meaning and is worth continuing, the person may engage in suicidal behavior. Suicidal behavior may be a desperate person's last message—that life's journey is unbearable and that the person sees ending physical life as the only way to end the pain.

 ### Charles Thomas's Story

Charles Thomas is a 55-year-old white married man who had been relatively free of physical and emotional problems most of his adult life. He always prided himself on his ability to handle whatever problems he encountered, until the day he was seen in the emergency department for a psychiatric evaluation at the recommendation of his internist.

In the emergency department, Mr. Thomas related the following story to the psychiatric liaison nurse: "I own my own business—in fact I have run it by myself for 25 years. Over the last 5 years I've tried to get my wife interested in learning the business, so she could take part in it with me, but she hasn't been interested. Eventually, I wanted my son to take over the business."

Problems Begin to Mount

"Then, 2 years ago, I started having problems with my youngest son. He started to use drugs and even ended up arrested a few times for stealing. During the past year, I started to have financial problems with my business; I was forced to lay off one of my employees. God knows how hard that was for me! My daughter is away at college; my oldest son is married and lives out of state."

Feeling Alone

"For the first time in my life, I felt alone. I knew that, because of his drug problems, I couldn't count on my youngest son to help with the business. My wife didn't seem to understand that I needed help. I felt myself becoming more and more overwhelmed and depressed."

Crisis

"Now I worry all the time about losing my business, even though my accountant keeps assuring me that it's fine. This morning I told my wife that I couldn't go on; I told her that I wanted to die. I know I must have frightened her. She immediately called my doctor, who told her to bring me here for evaluation. To tell you the truth, I was too tired and worn out to even resist."

Assessing the Scope of the Problem

The psychiatric liaison nurse noted that Mr. Thomas was tearful. He said that he had not been able to sleep for the past week. He felt that he had no support from his family and stated that he did not want to go on with his life. Mr. Thomas told the nurse that he felt he was a total failure, both in running his business and in taking care of his family, and that he felt hopeless about making any changes in his situation.

Mr. Thomas said that he could not concentrate and was losing or forgetting things he needed to do at work. He was experiencing a lack of drive and energy; he was withdrawn and had begun to isolate himself from his friends and family, and he no longer enjoyed activities that he used to find pleasurable, including sex. He related that his appetite was poor; in the past 6 weeks, he has lost 20 lb.

A Suicide Plan Revealed

Mr. Thomas also admitted to the psychiatric liaison nurse that he had formulated a suicide plan: he had been practicing how to knot a strong rope that he had bought to hang himself. He had checked his insurance policy to see what coverage his family would receive on his death, but then he had begun to wonder whether his family would receive any of the money if he were to hang himself.

Crisis Averted, Healing Begun

When he began to realize the seriousness of his thoughts, he decided to talk to his wife one more time before implementing his plan. That was when she called the family internist for help.

After a full psychiatric evaluation, Mr. Thomas was diagnosed as having major depression with suicidal ideation and was hospitalized to prevent suicide as well as to begin treatment for the depression.

This chapter helps you to explore why people like Charles Thomas attempt and often successfully complete suicide; what factors influence a person's decision to take his or her own life; the influence of maintaining a positive life balance on the risk of suicide; and what you can do to help prevent suicides.

DEFINITIONS RELATED TO SUICIDE

When we think of the term **suicide,** we usually think of a conscious attempt to kill oneself. Suicidal behavior, however, occurs on a continuum, so some important terms related to suicide are defined here:

- Indirect self-destructive behavior
- Direct self-destructive behavior
- Suicide attempt (suicide gesture)
- Suicidal ideation
- Parasuicidal behavior
- Completed suicide
- Lethality of suicide threat

Indirect self-destructive behavior refers to activities that are potentially detrimental to a person's physical, psychological, social, and spiritual well-being. These behaviors may result in death but without the person's conscious intent or awareness. Examples of these behaviors include anorexia, bulimia with purging, use of alcohol or other drugs of abuse, and engaging in unprotected sex with multiple partners.

Direct self-destructive behavior involves activities that signal that a person intends to cause self-harm or death. The person has an awareness of the desired outcome, with a cognitive component of a self-destructive plan. Examples of self-destructive behaviors include wrist slashing, self-mutilation, buying a gun and munitions for the purpose of ending life, and taking an overdose of prescribed medications.

A **suicide attempt** or **suicide gesture** is the use of direct self-destructive behavior for the express purpose of killing oneself. **Parasuicidal behaviors** are those actions that are intentionally self-injurious, such as cutting the wrists or taking a nonlethal overdose of drugs (Kreitman, 1977; Linehan, 1993). The term **suicidal ideation** refers to a person's thoughts about suicide. The term **completed suicide** refers to willful, self-inflicted, life-threatening acts that result in death. Finally, the term **level of lethality** of suicide threat refers to the seriousness of a suicide threat—the degree to which it is likely to result in death.

What do you think? What are your thoughts and feelings about suicide threats? Should they be taken seriously?

➤ *Check Your Reading*
1. Define the concept of life balance.
2. What is indirect self-destructive behavior?
3. How is indirect self-destructive behavior different from direct self-destructive behavior?
4. How does suicidal behavior relate to indirect and direct self-destructive behavior?

EPIDEMIOLOGY OF SUICIDE

Suicide is not something unique to 20th century life; there have always been people who out of hopelessness have committed suicide to end the pain of living. The attitude of society toward suicide has ranged from mild disapproval to outright condemnation. St. Thomas Aquinas (1225–1274) argued against suicide by claiming that suicide was a violation of love—love of self, neighbor, and society. He stated that committing suicide represented a breach of God's sovereignty over us. St. Thomas Aquinas described suicide in terms of theft; suicide steals God's gift of life and so misappropriates the property that rightfully belongs to God.

In the United States, there has been public debate as to whether there are some situations in which suicide is acceptable. For instance, a Michigan physician, Dr. Kevorkian, has assisted people who are terminally ill to commit suicide. These assisted suicides challenged the Michigan law that governs this practice. The Hemlock Society publishes literature on the "how to's" of completing a suicide. There are Web sites on the Internet that discuss how to attempt suicide, as well as those that offer suggestions of hope to prevent such an action. In 1994, Oregon state passed a bill that allows physicians and pharmacists to prescribe and dispense lethal doses of a pain medication to terminally ill patients who choose to end their lives.

PREVALENCE OF SUICIDE

The American Association of Suicidology reports the most current statistics on suicide on its Internet Web page [http://sun1.iusb.edu/~jmcintos/AAS.linkspg.html]. The statistics for 1995 ranked suicide as the ninth leading cause of death in the United States, with 11.9 persons per every 100,000 population completing a suicidal act (Anderson, Kochanek, & Murphy, 1997; McIntosh, 1997). Busch, Clark, Fawcett, and Kravitz (1993) reported that of the 30,000 suicides that occur in the United States each year, 5% to 6% take place in an inpatient psychiatric hospital. These statistics are, at best, estimates of suicides, however. Sometimes physicians, coroners, and police are reluctant to cite a death as a suicide because of variances in criteria that would indicate a completed suicide. It is likely that some deaths that are the result of "accidents" such as drowning, car wrecks, gunshot wounds, drug abuse, and self-poisoning may actually be suicides but are missed in the count. According to Durkheim, the term *suicide* should be applied to all cases of death that result either directly or indirectly from the positive or negative acts of the victim himself and in which the victim knows the consequences of the acts (Durkheim, 1951).

Suicide ends all kinds of human journeys; it is not bounded by culture, age, class, religion, or socioeconomic status. Although women tend to make more suicide attempts than men, more men complete the suicidal act (McIntosh, 1997).

White men constitute the highest risk group for completing suicide, followed by Native Americans, blacks, Hispanics, and Asians. More men who complete suicide are single, followed by widowed, separated, and divorced men (Forster, 1994; McIntosh, 1997). Table 31-1 presents statistics on completed suicides by age group, and Table 31-2 summarizes the myths and realities of suicide.

TABLE 31–1 Completed Suicides by Age Group

AGE GROUP (Y)	COMPLETED SUICIDES (%)
15–24	13.3
25–34	15.4
35–44	15.4
45–54	14.6
55–64	13.3
65–74	15.8
75–84*	20.7
85 and older	21.6

*The age group most at risk according to this study are people who are between 75 and 84 years old.

From Anderson, R.N., Kochanek, K.D., & Murphy, S.L. (1997). Advance report of final mortality statistics, 1995. *Mortality Vital Statistics Report, 45*(11, Suppl 2). Hyattsville, MD: National Center for Health Statistics.

> **What do you think?** Should physician-assisted suicide be legalized throughout the country?

➤ *Check Your Reading*
5. What is the ninth leading cause of death in the United States?
6. Who makes more suicidal gestures, men or women?
7. Who is more likely to complete a suicidal act, a single white man, a Hispanic woman, or an adolescent Asian?

SUICIDE AS A SYMPTOM OF PSYCHIATRIC ILLNESS

Suicide is one of the outcomes of untreated depression. From 15% to 20% of all patients diagnosed with major depression complete suicide. Additionally, patients with psychotic depression have a high risk for completing suicide. This is due to the combination of symptoms, including

- Depression
- Delusions
- Guilt
- Paranoid thoughts
- Social withdrawal
- Hopelessness and feelings of worthlessness

Psychotic patients have a tendency to withdraw from seeking adequate psychiatric intervention and often use violent methods to commit suicide (Forster, 1994). Estimates are that between 10% and 13% of individuals with schizophrenia die from suicide (Torrey, 1995). The patients with schizophrenia who are more likely to attempt suicide are those with more severe symptoms, frequent hospitalizations, poor social functioning, symptoms of depression with a sense of hopelessness, and those who have substance abuse. Patients who have both positive and negative symptoms of psychosis as well as those who do not respond to neuroleptics or the atypical antipsychotics are at high risk for a suicidal gesture or completion (Meltzer & Okayli, 1995).

Wolfersdorf, Hole, Steiner, and Keller (1990) identified a suicidal depressive syndrome. They describe patients with major depression to be at the highest risk, especially those patients who have feelings of worthlessness, anxiety, depressive delusions, sleep disturbances, and a history of past suicidal behavior. William's story illustrates the potential for a suicide attempt resulting from a major depression (Case Example 31-1).

■ CASE EXAMPLE 31–1
■ William's Story

William had a history of dysthymia, a long-term depression. He had been placed on fluoxetine HCl (Prozac) 20 mg twice a day. During the course of treatment, he was laid off from work. He became depressed, he was unable to get out of bed in the morning, his energy had

TABLE 31–2 Myths and Realities of Suicide

MYTH	REALITY
Only psychotic people commit suicide.	Suicide can be a choice made by a sane and moral person.
Suicidal persons are fully intent on dying.	Most persons who think about suicide have mixed feelings about dying.
Suicide is an impulsive act.	The suicide act may be impulsive, but usually suicide has been carefully thought out.
The chance of suicide lessens as depression gets better.	When a person's depression is lifting, he or she has more energy to carry out a previously considered suicide plan.
Suicide can be an inherited trait.	Although alcoholism and depression are most likely genetic, and having a relative who has committed suicide is a risk factor, no known genetic markers for suicide exist.
Most suicidal persons give no warning.	About 75% of people who attempt or commit suicide give definite clues about their intent.
If you suspect suicidal ideation, do not bring the subject up; it might make the person kill himself or herself.	Open talking is most often a relief to the suicidal person. Talking actually decreases the risk of suicide.
All nonwhite persons have a lower suicide rate than whites.	Except for young African-American men, all nonwhites have a lower suicide rate than whites.
Professionals such as doctors, lawyers, dentists, police officers, and air traffic controllers have a low suicide rate.	Professionals such as those listed have a higher suicide rate than the general population.
People who are psychotic have the greatest chance of killing themselves among those with psychiatric illnesses.	Although risk increases with psychosis, among people with serious mental illness, those with alcoholism and depression are most at risk for suicide.
Only people with serious problems, mental illness, or physical illness think about suicide.	At one time or another, almost everyone contemplates suicide.
People who just want attention use suicide threats to manipulate others.	*All* suicide threats should be taken seriously. Even if a suicide threat is manipulative, the person may inadvertently commit suicide.
People who go from "rags to riches" are less likely to commit suicide than those who lose their money.	People with a sudden change in fortune (success, riches, acclaim) are also at risk for suicide.

decreased, and he had difficulty concentrating. Often, he would feel like yelling about being laid off; other times, he felt tearful. He felt no one understood how much work meant to him; it did not just pay bills, it gave a purpose to his life. William was afraid to share his feelings of loss with his girlfriend, for fear she would leave him. He felt his parents would be critical. He had not told his therapist how depressed he felt because he was afraid he would be hospitalized, as he was when he was younger. William's depression became worse; he began to question the value of his life. He started to plan for what he could do to end his life and therefore his misery. His girlfriend noticed he had become more preoccupied; he did not call her as often as he used to. She asked him to "level with her, as she felt scared she was going to lose him." He did tell her he was feeling hopeless and a burden. She encouraged him to tell his therapist how he was feeling so he could get better. ■

Several other psychiatric disorders are associated with suicidal behavior, such as bipolar disorder, schizophrenia, and substance abuse disorders. Patients who have bipolar disorder are at risk for suicide when they are depressed. The symptoms of suicidal ideation are particularly important to note when the depressive symptoms

in the mania are severe (Strakowski, McElroy, Keck, & West, 1996). This suggests that all bipolar patients can be at risk for suicidal potential, regardless of affective state. Schizophrenic patients have a 9% to 12.9% rate of completed suicide (Meltzer Okayli, 1995). Many of these patients experience hopelessness about the chronicity of their illness and do not always communicate their suicidal intent or plan. Because of these factors, they are at high risk and require a thorough assessment. Another psychiatric disorder often associated with completed suicide is alcohol and substance abuse. Alcohol is associated with 25% to 50% of all completed suicides (Forster, 1994). The risk increases dramatically when the patient suffers from major depression along with alcoholism (Cornelius et al., 1995).

Patients who have personality disorders are also at risk for suicidal attempts and completed suicide. Individuals with Borderline Personality Disorder have a high rate of attempted suicide. A criterion for diagnosis of Borderline Personality Disorder in the *Diagnostic and Statistical Manual of Mental Disorders, Fourth Edition* (DSM-IV) (1994) is "recurrent suicidal behavior, gestures, or threats, or self-mutilating behavior." Brodsky, Malone, Ellis, Dulit, and Mann (1997) suggested that the target symptom in Borderline Personality Disorder is impulsivity as well as an association between childhood abuse and self-destructive behaviors. These are important factors to keep in mind when assessing a patient for level of lethality. Asking direct questions about early childhood abuse and impulsive behavior, including parasuicidal behavior or other self-destructive acts, is important to prevent possible future suicidal gestures or completion. In a study examining individuals who had completed suicide and had an Axis II diagnosis of a personality disorder; the authors determined that 95% of the individuals had a depressive disorder, substance abuse, or both along with the personality disorder diagnosis (Isometsä et al., 1996).

Self-mutilation, or intentional self-destructive behavior that destroys or alters body tissue, occurs in an estimated 24% to 40% of psychiatric patients and approximately 750 per 100,000 of the general population (Favazza, 1987). Self-mutilating behavior has a different psychological intention than a suicidal gesture. Patients who self-mutilate often have a history of being neglected as well as sexually and physically abused as children (Barstow, 1995; Goodwin, 1989; Herman, 1992).

Self-mutilation often occurs when patients have **alexithymia,** or the inability to identify and put words to the experience of emotional feelings. In 1972, Sifnoes described alexithymia, using the Greek *a* for lack, *lexis* for word, and *thymos* for feeling (Sifnoes, 1972). Alexithymia as a disturbance in affective and cognitive functioning in which emotions are experienced mostly in physical form (American Psychiatric Association [APA], 1984). Patients with alexithymia identify body sensations as emotional feelings. These individuals use actions to express emotions. People who have alexithymia have a disturbed communication style in which the emotional and the symbolic functions are strained. Their fantasy life is impoverished, and their interpretation of life's events is concrete and literal (Wheeler & Broad, 1994). Often when patients self-mutilate, they are angry, lonely, scared, and fearful of abandonment. Sifnoes (1996) noted that the development of alexithymia is often found in individuals who have a history of childhood psychological trauma because of the physiological changes in the brain due to the trauma.

Van der Kolk (1987) discussed an animal model in which self-mutilation was observed. Using Harlow's work with monkeys, which studied monkeys' reactions to receiving "nurturing" from a wire monkey as opposed to a mother monkey, responses were observed regarding issues such as separation from mother and peers, the effect on socialization, and parenting future generations. The monkeys that were separated from the mother monkey during the 1st year of life demonstrated abnormal social and sexual behavior. These monkeys did not mate, and if a female monkey in this group was artificially inseminated, she mutilated or killed her babies. Young monkeys who were removed from their mothers demonstrated socially withdrawn or aggressive behaviors. These monkeys developed self-destructive and self-stimulating behaviors such as huddling, self-clasping, self-sucking, and self-biting. Animal behavior, particularly primate behavior, can assist in understanding human behavior. If monkeys self-mutilate in reaction to a separation from their mothers, self-mutilation behaviors observed in humans may also be tied to early deprivation.

> **What do you think?** If physician-assisted suicide were legalized across the country, what impact would that have on the suicide risk of people diagnosed with major depression?

> ► *Check Your Reading*
>   8. Why do you need to do a suicide assessment on a patient who is diagnosed with schizophrenia?
>   9. What is the relationship between alcohol use, depression, and suicide?
>   10. Why do some patients self-mutilate?

CAUSE OF SUICIDE

No one theory adequately explains suicidal or self-destructive behavior or guides clinical practice. Biological, psychological, sociocultural, and spiritual factors may all contribute to self-injury.

Physical Factors

Biological studies have found that neurotransmitters, such as dopamine, serotonin, and endogenous opioids, influence self-injury, but the actions of these biochemical agents are poorly understood. There is some evidence to indicate that low levels of serotonin are present in some people who have attempted suicide (Roy, 1989). Stanley and Stanley (1990) studied concentrations of serotonin and 5-HIAA (a serotonin metabolite) in postmortem receptor binding studies. They noted changes in both presynaptic and postsynaptic serotoninergic binding sites in the brains of individuals who have completed suicide and have been examined postmortem as opposed to the postmortem studies of the control group.

The relationship between self-injury and the endogenous opioids was discovered serendipitously. Naloxone, a blocker of opioid effects, was administered to several developmentally delayed patients, and the incidence of self-injury decreased significantly (Favazza, 1989).

Psychological Factors

Psychological theories suggest that self-destructive behavior may have its roots or beginnings in early interpersonal trauma. These theories focus on the role of aggression and the inner world of the suicidal person.

According to Freud (1964), the act of suicide represents a conflict between the instincts for life and death. Suicide apparently occurs when the wish for death predominates, and the patient no longer is able to maintain a life balance on his or her journey. Menninger (1938) suggested that the individual turns aggression that is intended for others inward against the self. According to Adams (1985), the "aggression turned inward" theory may be a way of understanding suicide as well as other self-destructive behaviors, such as self-mutilation, eating disorders, and smoking, and other indirect self-destructive behaviors, such as self-neglect, compulsive gambling, alcohol and drug abuse, selling drugs, and taking other extreme risks.

Some common psychological antecedents to self-destructive behaviors are depression; eating disorders; drug and alcohol dependency or abuse; bipolar disorder; personality disorders, such as borderline personality disorder, narcissistic personality disorder, antisocial personality disorder, and histrionic personality disorder; cognitive mental disorders; and psychoses, particularly with command hallucinations; feeling despairful; cultural expectations; and religious rites (Barstow, 1995).

■ CASE EXAMPLE 31–2
■ Mary's Story

Mary often feels lonely, isolated, and depressed because she believes no one cares for her. She frequents a local bar in an effort to meet an available man. Mary usually drinks a few beers and then hard liquor as the night progresses. She flirts with several men and sometimes goes home with one of them. She wakes up feeling alone and scared and often has a hangover. Her sense of self is negative; she says she is "a lowlife." Mary's problems with low self-esteem, difficulty relating to others, and aloneness are not solved by her current behavioral pattern. Her actions lead only to self-defeat and worsening feelings about the self, with greater dissatisfaction. Mary's despair increases, and, along with it, the risk for suicidal behavior also increases. ■

According to Beck (1963), hopelessness and negative expectations are psychological variables that may be used to predict suicide. He stated that hopelessness plays a critical role in suicide and is illustrated in the sequence of events that leads a depressed person to commit suicide. The person believes there is no way out, believes that the existing problems are insoluble ones, and anticipates disastrous outcomes (Beck, 1967). In a 10-year prospective follow-up study looking at the relationship between hopelessness and suicide, 165 patients were hospitalized with suicide ideation. Out of 11 patients who committed suicide, 10 (90.9%) had scored nine or greater on the Beck Hopelessness Scale. One patient (9.1%), who ultimately committed suicide, had scored lower than a nine (Beck, Steer, Kovacs, & Garrison, 1985).

People with a diminished capacity to cope are at increased risk for suicidal behavior. Folkman and Lazarus (1984) defined coping as thoughts and actions that are flexible, solve problems, and reduce stress. The more flexible and varied an individual's coping repertoire is, the better able the person is to deal successfully with the challenges that appear in every life's journey. It is important to note, however, that even the best coping skills can be taxed to their limit by too many stressors at one time or stressors that are too intense and demanding. Rickelman and Houfek (1995) identified several thought processes that are often present in individuals who are at high risk for completed suicide: cognitive rigidity, dichotomous thought pattern, and an attributional style of hopelessness and depression.

Social Factors

The social and cultural context in which a person lives also influences the expression of suicidality (Adams, 1985). Durkheim (1951) described four types of suicide that are integrally linked to the quality of community life:

- Egotistical
- Anomic
- Fatalistic
- Altruistic

In an *egotistical suicide,* a person's ties to the community are too loose or tenuous, the person is not invested in maintaining his or her relationship with the community, the person has no close relationships, and the person does not respond to the usual social constraints on behavior.

In an *anomic suicide,* the individual experiences the aloneness or estrangement that occurs as a result of a precipitous deterioration in his or her relationship with society (e.g., loss of a job, a close friend, a parent).

In a *fatalistic suicide,* the person feels that he or she is excessively regulated; there is no personal freedom or hope for obtaining it.

In *altruistic suicide,* rules or customs demand suicide under certain situations; in these situations, self-inflicted death is viewed as honorable. Altruistic suicides may be seen in time of war, such as the kamikaze attacks by Japanese pilots on U.S. ships in World War II.

Racism is also linked with suicide. Durkheim (1951) suggested that any group that is denied society's usual privileges and rights experiences an increased risk for alienation and anomic suicide. Studies of black populations indicate that there has been a dramatic increase in the suicide rate in young black men (Davis, 1982).

Spiritual Factors

In a theistic world view, our spirits are seen as eternal. There are times in each of our lives, however, when we deny the existence of our spirit, when we refuse to rely on our spirit, and when we seem to ignore the importance of our spirit to our overall health and well-being. It is essential to assess each patient's spirituality to assist the patient to recognize and use spirituality to maintain a positive life balance and improve coping skills.

According to Vanzant (1992),

spirit is the life essence which is covered and protected by the skeletal frame we call the body. . . . Spirit has only one purpose and mission, which was determined by God at the time of creation. . . . Everything that has life, can create life, nurtures life or serves a purpose in life, is spirit. (p. 55)

Frankl (1964) was acutely aware of the importance of spirit operating in people as he observed his own behavior and responses and those of fellow prisoners during his confinement in a Nazi concentration camp. He observed that spirit was intricately tied to meaning and purpose in life as well as hope. Frankl observed that when people find life meaningless and without purpose and God seems distant and uncaring, there is no reason to live. He believed that suffering is a requisite ingredient of living; and that finding meaning in that suffering is an important ingredient for survival. Frankl wrote that if a person succeeds in discovering a "why" for the suffering, he or she will continue to grow despite all indignities (Frankl, 1964).

Frankl (1964) also viewed hope as an expression of a healthy spirit and a prerequisite to survival. Conversely, Frankl believed that hopelessness, an expression of a depleted spirit, could be fatal. Frankl cited the case of a prisoner who pinned his hopes on being rescued from the concentration camp on a certain date. When it became clear that the rescue operation would not occur on the expected date, the man died within a matter of hours.

Nurses are in an extraordinary position to encourage patients to reestablish their purposes in life, to renew their hopes, and to tap into their own spirituality. Some patients may have lost their faith in God or have felt an alienation from their own values or from other people. These people experience life as no longer having any meaning or purpose, and they may find it too painful to continue. In essence, these people have lost hope. It is possible through a comprehensive nursing assessment and intervention that hope can be restored; patients may feel a sense of connectedness to their own values, to themselves, to their God, and to others.

> **What do you think?** How would you go about encouraging hope in a patient who expressed suicidal ideation?

➤ Check Your Reading

11. Explain the aggression turned inward theory.
12. Why does this theory provide a way of understanding suicide as well as other self-destructive behaviors, such as self-mutilation?
13. How does the social and cultural context in which a person lives contribute to an understanding of suicidal behavior?
14. What is meant by the spirit of life, and how does that relate to understanding life's purpose?

DYNAMICS OF SUICIDE

The suicide of a patient, the premature end of a journey, is perhaps the most devastating experience in the practice of psychiatry and psychiatric nursing. Through the act of suicide, the individual communicates his or her final message to others. The person may view suicide as a way to escape life's suffering and a way to get away from situations that are viewed as intolerable, such as the loss of a spouse, a difficult relationship,

chronic major psychiatric symptoms of hallucinations or flashbacks of early abuse, the loss of a series of jobs, or a terminal illness. Different people meet adversity with their own styles of coping, depending on personal problem-solving skills, self-esteem, ability to relate to others, and defense mechanisms. A person who has a poorly integrated personality may respond to stress by committing suicide.

As a result of studying suicide notes and conducting discussions with people who have attempted suicide, many theorists have begun to understand the emotional components of suicide. Suicidal patients characterize their emotional states as feeling

- Intense anger
- Devastating depression
- Profound feelings of hopelessness
- A loss of life's meaning and purpose

Often the suicidal person expresses ambivalence about completing the act; while wishing to be dead, this individual sometimes has a desire to be saved or rescued. Mintz (1971) stated,

> [I]t is a clinical fact that the suicidal person is usually highly ambivalent about committing suicide. None would seek help if this were not true. (p. 62)

This ambivalence provides the opportunity to intervene and attempt to convince despairing people that suicide is not the answer.

Shneidman (1996) identified what he calls the Ten Commonalities of Suicide

- The Common purpose of suicide is to seek a solution.
- The Common goal of suicide is cessation of consciousness.
- The Common stimulus of suicide is unbearable psychological pain.
- The Common stressor in suicide is frustrated psychological needs.
- The Common emotion in suicide is hopelessness-helplessness.
- The Common cognitive state in suicide is ambivalence.
- The Common perceptual state in suicide is constriction.
- The Common action in suicide is escape.
- The Common interpersonal act in suicide is communication of intention.
- The Common pattern in suicide is consistency of lifelong styles.

From Schneidman, E. S. (1996). The suicidal mind. New York: Oxford University Press.

NURSING PROCESS

When providing care for the suicidal patient and the patient's family, you can use your knowledge of the epidemiology, cause, and dynamics of suicidal behavior as a guide. This knowledge has an impact on the effectiveness of the nursing process.

Assessment

To perform a comprehensive assessment, you must focus on the physical, psychological, social, and spiritual domains that represent the foundation of human functioning (Cardell & Horton-Deutsch, 1994). An important consideration is to determine the patient's positive or negative life balance. This is assessed by observing the patient's adaptive or maladaptive behavior when the patient is confronted with a problem. Does the patient use positive physical, psychological, social, and spiritual means of examining the problem to determine healthful options, or is the patient using negative physical, psychological, social, or spiritual options toward problem-solving? See Chapter 11 for in-depth assessment information.

SEVERITY INDEX FOR RISK OF SUICIDE

Another consideration is whether or not the patient is in a high-risk group for suicide (Box 31-1). Box 31-2 identifies questions to ask and observations to make when assessing a person's risk of suicide. Box 31-3 provides clues to suicidal ideation.

Green, Katz, and Marcus (1995) identified a severity index useful in assessment of risk. The severity of the patient's condition is conceptualized as a continuum ranging from *no suicidal ideation* to a *severe level of suicidal risk*. Using the severity index assists you in planning the intensity and type of care the patient requires to prevent a suicidal gesture (Figure 31-1).

Box 31-1 ■ ■ ■ ■ ■
Groups at High Risk for Suicide

- People with a family history of suicide
- People with a previous history of having attempted suicide
- Psychotic patients, especially those with command auditory hallucinations
- Depressed people (including those who are terminally ill)
- People who are overwhelmed or under great stress
- Patients with personality disorders, such as schizoid, schizotypal, histrionic, borderline, and antisocial
- People addicted to alcohol or other drugs
- People who experience extreme guilt and shame
- Patients with persistent flashbacks
- Adolescents who suffer with a major depression or have friends or family members who have completed suicide
- People with early-stage organic brain syndrome or AIDS dementia

Box 31-2 ■ ■ ■ ■ ■
Questions to Ask and Observations to Make When Assessing a Person's Risk of Suicide

Questions to Ask

- How much are you thinking about suicide or harming yourself?
- Do you have a plan? (If yes: "Could you tell me about your plan?")
- Have you ever attempted to harm yourself before? (If yes: "Could you describe what happened?")
- Do you have any idea what might have triggered your thoughts about harming yourself?

Observations to Make

- Is there a weapon or a method available to the patient?
- Observe the verbal and nonverbal clues that the patient is giving about her plan to commit suicide or to do self-harm. Is the patient feeling as though she is a burden that her family would do better without? Has she given away valuable items? Has she checked her will or life insurance policy?
- Does the patient comprehend his degree of risk for suicide or self-harm? Does he verbalize a fear of being alone?
- What is the level of knowledge of the patient or significant other about depression (or any otherpsychiatric or physical disorder the patient may have) and about suicidal ideation?
- Assess the patient for abuse of alcohol or other drugs.
- Assess the patient's ability to function in her roles at work, at home, and in the community. How does the patient view her purpose in life?
- Determine the patient's ability to interact with others. Can the patient ask for help when feeling overwhelmed? Is the patient isolated from others?
- How supportive and available to the patient are the family or significant other(s)?
- Does the patient feel abandoned? Does the patient make statements of loss?
- Is the patient experiencing rage?
- Determine the patient's degree of depression and anxiety.

From Green, E., Katz, J., & Marcus, P. (1995). Practice guidelines for suicide/self harm prevention. In E. Green & J. Katz (Eds.), *Clinical practice guidelines for the adult patient* (pp. 250-1–250-21). St. Louis, MO: Mosby–Year Book.

ASSESSMENT OF THE PHYSICAL DOMAIN

It is helpful to determine whether the patient has any signs or symptoms of a physical illness. Does the patient focus on body sensations, particularly if she has chronic

Box 31–3 ■ ■ ■ ■ ■
Clues to Suicidal Ideation

Direct Statements

· "I can't take it anymore."
· "Life isn't worth living anymore."
· "I wish I were dead."
· "Everyone would be better off if I died."

Indirect Statements

· "It's okay now, soon everything will be fine."
· "Things will never work out."
· "I won't be a problem much longer."
· "Nothing feels good to me anymore, and probably never will."
· "How can I give my body to medical science?"

Behaviors

· Giving away prized possessions
· Writing farewell notes
· Making out a will
· Putting personal things in order

Physical Clues

· Headaches
· Muscle aches
· Trouble sleeping
· Constipation
· Change in appetite
· Weight loss

Emotional Clues

· Social withdrawal
· Feelings of hopelessness
· Feelings of helplessness
· Confusion
· Irritability
· Feeling exhausted

pain? Does the patient experience the pain as more excruciating when overwhelmed with emotional issues? Is the patient experiencing the neurovegetative signs of depression, such as difficulty concentrating, changes in appetite, decreases in energy, decreases in libido, or changes in sleep pattern? You might want to ask the following:

· What are your thoughts about your illness? What impact has this illness had on your life?
· How would you describe your pain? Are there times when the pain is more difficult to handle?
· Have you noticed changes in your concentration?

Your appetite? Your energy level? Your interest in sex? Your need for sleep?

ASSESSMENT OF THE EMOTIONAL DOMAIN

When a patient is experiencing suicidal thoughts, he is also having problems in the emotional domain and is usually experiencing feelings of despair and hopelessness. These feelings are expressed through a suicide plan (Sanger, Thomas, & Whitney, 1988). To assess the emotional domain thoroughly, you must ask the patient directly: "Have you ever had, or are you now having, thoughts of hurting yourself?" Box 31–4 offers suggestions for talking to a patient who has suicidal ideation.

If the patient answers in the affirmative, you continue to inquire about the presence of a plan and the lethality of the plan. *Lethality* refers to seriousness of the suicide threat, including the means that the patient plans to use to commit the suicide and the availability of those means. You might ask, "Do you have a plan? If so, could you describe it to me? Do you have a weapon? Is it readily available to you?" If the patient responds, "I do not really have a plan. . . . I just think that life would be better if I were gone. And besides . . . my religion strictly forbids suicide," the patient is experiencing suicidal ideation, does not have a lethal plan, and is experiencing strong religious constraints against committing suicide. Your nursing response would affirm the patient's religious constraints and encourage the patient to write and sign a no-harm contract stating that he or she will not harm himself or herself.

If the patient responds, "I think about suicide all the time. . . . It scares me so much I don't want to be alone. I have a loaded gun in the drawer of my bedside table. So far I haven't had the courage to use it . . . but I think it's just a matter of time. Things seem so hopeless. I really believe that everyone would be better off if I were dead," the response indicates the presence not only of serious and persistent suicidal ideation but also of a highly lethal plan. The patient knows exactly how she will commit suicide and has the weapon available to her. In this case, the patient requires inpatient care to ensure her safety.

You must also determine whether the patient has a history of a previous suicide attempt or attempts or if anyone in the patient's family has ever attempted or completed a suicide gesture (Cugino et al., 1992). You need to inquire, "Have you written a suicidal note? What does the note say? Where is the note? What do you think will happen when you die? Have you given any thought about what will happen to your family and friends when they learn of your suicide?" You need to determine whether the patient is depressed and how the patient views the depression. Does the patient express hope for the future? Has the patient told anyone about his or her suicidal thoughts or plans? Does the patient see himself or herself as having any worth or value?

ASSESSMENT OF THE COGNITIVE DOMAIN

Implementing a suicidal gesture is part of the cognitive domain. To assess the cognitive domain. To assess the

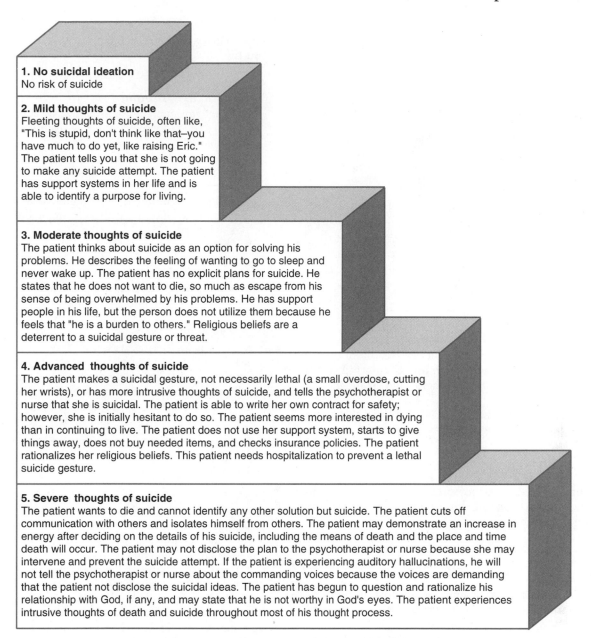

1. No suicidal ideation
No risk of suicide

2. Mild thoughts of suicide
Fleeting thoughts of suicide, often like, "This is stupid, don't think like that–you have much to do yet, like raising Eric." The patient tells you that she is not going to make any suicide attempt. The patient has support systems in her life and is able to identify a purpose for living.

3. Moderate thoughts of suicide
The patient thinks about suicide as an option for solving his problems. He describes the feeling of wanting to go to sleep and never wake up. The patient has no explicit plans for suicide. He states that he does not want to die, so much as escape from his sense of being overwhelmed by his problems. He has support people in his life, but the person does not utilize them because he feels that "he is a burden to others." Religious beliefs are a deterrent to a suicidal gesture or threat.

4. Advanced thoughts of suicide
The patient makes a suicidal gesture, not necessarily lethal (a small overdose, cutting her wrists), or has more intrusive thoughts of suicide, and tells the psychotherapist or nurse that she is suicidal. The patient is able to write her own contract for safety; however, she is initially hesitant to do so. The patient seems more interested in dying than in continuing to live. The patient does not use her support system, starts to give things away, does not buy needed items, and checks insurance policies. The patient rationalizes her religious beliefs. This patient needs hospitalization to prevent a lethal suicide gesture.

5. Severe thoughts of suicide
The patient wants to die and cannot identify any other solution but suicide. The patient cuts off communication with others and isolates himself from others. The patient may demonstrate an increase in energy after deciding on the details of his suicide, including the means of death and the place and time death will occur. The patient may not disclose the plan to the psychotherapist or nurse because she may intervene and prevent the suicide attempt. If the patient is experiencing auditory hallucinations, he will not tell the psychotherapist or nurse about the commanding voices because the voices are demanding that the patient not disclose the suicidal ideas. The patient has begun to question and rationalize his relationship with God, if any, and may state that he is not worthy in God's eyes. The patient experiences intrusive thoughts of death and suicide throughout most of his thought process.

Figure 31–1
Severity index for suicide risk. (Data from Green, E., Katz, J., & Marcus, P. [1995]. Practice guidelines for suicide/self harm prevention. In E. Green & J. Katz [Eds.], *Clinical practice guidelines for the adult patient* [pp. 250-1–250-21]. St. Louis, MO: Mosby–Year Book.)

cognitive domain, it is important to determine how often the patient thinks about suicide or a suicide plan:

- Is the patient preoccupied with himself?
- What is the patient's view of the problems that are overwhelming her?
- Does the patient have insight into these problem areas or her behavior?
- Is the patient's judgment clouded with intrusive thoughts of suicide?
- Does the patient experience voices telling him to commit suicide (command auditory hallucinations?) Is the patient able to tell you about these hallucinations, or is the patient being directed by these auditory hallucinations not to talk to others?
- Does the patient focus on negative themes to the exclusion of other, more positive thoughts?

ASSESSMENT OF THE SOCIAL DOMAIN
Often people who are suicidal feel a lack of social support. You should assess the social domain to determine the patient's perception of her support network.

- Is the patient interacting with family, friends, boss, and coworkers in the usual manner?

Box 31-4 ■ ■ ■ ■ ■

Suggestions for Talking to a Patient Who Has Suicidal Ideation

- · Ask: "How are you feeling?"
- · Ask: "Are you still having thoughts about hurting yourself?"
- · Ask: "Have your thoughts changed?"
- · Ask: "Do you have a plan to hurt yourself?"
- · Ask: "If you have a plan, would you tell me about it?"
- · Never say: "You shouldn't feel that way." Instead say: "It must be painful to feel that way."
- · If you are unsure what to say, continue to listen in attentive silence, encouraging the patient to speak by using open-ended statements such as, "And then what happened?" "Uh huh . . ." "Tell me more about . . ."

- • If the patient is in a hospital or a day treatment center or partial hospitalization program, is this individual participating with patient peers and staff in the milieu?
- • Has the patient eliminated social activities that were once a pleasurable and meaningful part of life?

ASSESSMENT OF THE SPIRITUAL DOMAIN

According to Green and coworkers (1995), when you assess the spiritual domain, it is important to ask the following questions:

- • What is the patient's relationship with a deity or higher power?
- • Does the patient have a sense of purpose in life?
- • Does the patient have hope that his or her problems will have a meaningful resolution?
- • Has the patient begun to question the role of his or her spiritual beliefs in light of the current crisis?
- • Is the patient angry with God, or does the patient feel that God is angry with him or her?
- • Does the patient believe that God is using the current difficulties as a means of punishment?
- • Is the patient connected with his faith community, either through a spiritual leader or through members of his religious group?
- • Does the patient experience meaning through participation in religious rites, rituals, and other religiously oriented activities?

What do you think? A common myth is that if you ask a person directly about suicidal thinking it will put the idea into the person's mind. How would you respond to someone who told you this?

➤ *Check Your Reading*

15. What questions would you ask a patient to determine whether there is a risk in the physical domain?
16. What questions in the emotional domain give information about the lethality of the patient's suicidal plan?
17. What questions in the cognitive domain are helpful to determine the extent of the patient's suicidal plan?
18. Why are the questions in the social domain important to determining the patient's level of suicidal ideation?
19. What three indicators are present when a patient has severe thoughts of suicide?

Diagnosis

The next step in providing care is to identify the appropriate medical and nursing diagnoses. Case Example 31-3 illustrates a patient for whom Risk for Self-Mutilation would be an appropriate nursing diagnosis.

■ CASE EXAMPLE 31-3
■ Janice's Story

Janice is a recovering alcoholic currently in therapy to explore issues related to a history of childhood sexual molestation. During the course of therapy, Janice revealed to her mother that her father's best friend sexually molested her. Janice's mother did not display the emotion that Janice expected after the disclosure. Janice became emotional and then cut herself with a sharp knife. She claimed she felt relief. While exploring this incident in therapy, she remembered that she has been cutting herself since her adolescence. She began to explore whether there might be a correlation between her tendency toward self-mutilation and her history of sexual abuse.

An appropriate nursing diagnosis for Janice is Risk for Self-Mutilation related to unresolved grief, inability to express feelings, fears of abandonment, and fears that her mother will be unsupportive as evidenced by Janice's past self-mutilative behaviors when experiencing these same reactions.

For Charles Thomas, the patient we met at the beginning of the chapter, an appropriate nursing diagnosis might be Risk for Violence: Self-Directed related to numerous perceived failures, feelings of abandonment by his significant others, depressed mood, and feelings of hopelessness as evidenced by verbalizations of suicidal thoughts to his wife.

Outcome Identification

The expected outcomes for a patient with a nursing diagnosis of Risk for Violence: Self-Directed or Risk for Self-Mutilation are as follows:

- The patient will remain free from self-harm while maintaining the highest degree of autonomy that is possible.
- The patient will not exhibit suicidal or self-mutilative behaviors.

Planning

When planning care for a suicidal patient, it is important to take into account the following factors:

- Patient's past and present history of emotional and physical illnesses
- Patient's life experiences
- Patient's cultural, ethical, and religious or spiritual background

Based on the identified expected outcomes for the patient at risk for suicide or self-mutilation, the nurse, the patient, and the interdisciplinary care team jointly establish short-term goals, such as the following:

Expected Outcomes

The patient will remain free from self-harm while maintaining the highest degree of autonomy that is possible.

Short-Term Goals

- The patient will write and sign a no-harm contract.
- The patient will agree to talk to a staff member if he experiences a change in suicidal thinking.

Expected Outcomes

The patient will not exhibit suicidal or self-mutilative behaviors.

Short-Term Goals

- The patient will participate in the unit activities.
- The patient will discuss his self-destructive feelings rather than act on them.
- The patient will participate in efforts to understand the crises that lead to his suicidal or self-mutilative behaviors.
- The patient will turn over to the staff any objects that could be used to harm himself.

Return now to the case of Charles Thomas, to see how care planning worked in his case.

To address Mr. Thomas's diagnosis of Risk for Violence: Self-Directed, Mr. Thomas's nurse, working together as part of the interdisciplinary care team and together with the patient, established the following expected outcome: "Mr. Thomas will remain free from self-harm while maintaining the highest degree of autonomy that is possible." Specific short-term goals related to this expected outcome were as follows:
- Mr. Thomas will remain free from harm while in the hospital.
- Mr. Thomas will seek out staff for support if he feels an increase in the urge to harm himself.
- Mr. Thomas will contract for safety with the nursing staff as a means of demonstrating impulse control.

➤ *Check Your Reading*

20. Identify a nursing diagnosis that might be appropriate for a patient who has threatened to slash his or her wrists.
21. Identify two expected outcomes for the patient who is at risk for self-mutilation or suicide.
22. State a short-term goal for a patient whose expected outcome is that he or she "will remain free from self-harm while maintaining the highest degree of autonomy that is possible."

Implementation

Once you have identified short-term goals for the patient at risk for suicide or self-mutilation, you are ready to plan appropriate interventions to help the patient meet his or her goals. The following strategies should be part of the plan of care for any patient at risk for suicide or self-harm.

HANDLE SUICIDE THREATS AS EMERGENCIES

Consider any case of attempted suicide a serious psychiatric emergency. Conduct a full assessment to determine the appropriate interventions. Does the patient require inpatient care, a 23-hour bed in the psychiatric emergency area, or is outpatient care adequate, such as a partial hospitalization or multiple visits to the outpatient therapist? If the patient is stable enough to go home, with whom should the patient go home? Sometimes patients deny suicidal ideation to gain the freedom to go home to make a more serious suicide attempt or to please a family member or staff person. Therefore, assess the patient's level of potential for parasuicidal behavior by repeatedly asking questions about contemplating a suicidal gesture in several different ways during your interaction with the patient.

In your interview, include questions about future plans, including plans for the day of the evaluation, plans for the next few days, plans for the weekend, and longer-term plans. If the patient is unable to make future plans, assess this issue further. If the patient cannot engage in problem-solving, including not being able to structure time effectively for meaningful activity, this is a signal that the patient may require a hospital stay to support him in problem-solving to deal with the factors that caused the suicidal ideation.

Determine the Patient's Level of Lethality. It is important to determine the patient's level of lethality to plan the most appropriate intervention (Box 31–5). This assessment helps the interdisciplinary team in an inpatient or partial hospital setting to ascertain whether the patient should be on a "suicide watch."

There are two types of suicide watches: *every-15-minute checks* and *one-to-one supervision*. For instance, if the patient demonstrates less lethal thoughts of suicide, with no explicit plan, and is still able to engage in problem-solving, every-15-minute checks would be appropriate.

In **every-15-minute checks,** a staff member checks on the patient every 15 minutes to ensure patient safety. Also, the patient takes an active part in the suicide watch by agreeing in writing, in the form of a no-harm contract (Figure 31–2) to inform the staff if he or she has any changes in suicidal ideation. If the patient can write his or her own no-harm contract, the patient experiences increased ownership of impulse control. While awake on every-15-minute checks, the patient is responsible for notifying staff members of changes in suicidal ideation.

Box 31–5 ■ ■ ■ ■ ■
Determining the Suicidal Patient's Level of Lethality

- How specific are the details of the plan? Has the person worked out the specifics? Where? How? When?
- How lethal is the proposed method? High-risk methods include using a gun, jumping, hanging, poisoning with carbon monoxide, and engineering an automobile accident. Examples of low-risk methods are slashing the wrists, inhaling house gas, and ingesting pills.
- Are the means available? A person who says that he will shoot himself and has a loaded gun in a bedside stand is in grave danger of committing suicide. Likewise, a person who states he will jump to his death and has access to a high building is at serious risk.
- Is the person psychotic? People who are psychotic are at high risk regardless of the specificity of the details, lethality of method, and availability of means. Their impulse control, judgment, and thinking are so impaired that they are at risk.

If the patient has a suicide plan, has been thinking about a note that he or she wants to leave behind, has a means to carry out the suicide plan, has no plans for the future, and is hesitant to write a no-harm contract or will not sign a no-harm contract, one-to-one supervision is the most appropriate intervention. In **one-to-one supervision,** staff members monitor the patient constantly, without interruption, until the patient presents a less lethal suicide risk.

For any patient on a suicide watch, observe the patient to see whether he or she experiences a reduction in suicidal ideation and an increase in problem-solving ability. If you determine that the patient feels more in control of his or her impulses and the issues related to his or her problem areas, consult the other members of the interdisciplinary team, including the attending psychotherapist or psychiatrist, before reducing the level of suicide watch. If the patient seems to be feeling more depressed and hopeless, continue to determine the level of suicidal lethality and consult the interdisciplinary team, including the attending psychotherapist or psychiatrist. Placing the patient on a more restrictive suicide watch may be appropriate.

To reduce a patient's risk, remove the patient from any immediate danger to a physically safe environment and remove all harmful objects, including drugs. Assign the patient to a room that is easily accessible and can be observed closely.

IDENTIFY THE UNDERLYING CRISIS

Try to identify the crisis that led to the episode of suicide or self-harm, and help the patient identify options for dealing with the issues behind the crisis (Badger, 1995). If the patient cannot identify any options, hospitalization is indicated to prevent a suicide attempt. Ask the patient with a history of suicide attempts if this crisis is similar to others in the past when she felt suicidal. Hospitalization is indicated in this situation as well. Patients with a history of suicide attempts often repeat such behavior as a means of problem-solving. During each session with a hospitalized patient, discuss options for dealing with the underlying issues.

Ask the Patient to Sign a No-Harm Contract. Ask the patient to sign—or, ideally, to write and sign—a no-harm contract. Milieu therapy, individual psychotherapy, family psychotherapy, problem-solving groups, art therapy, and movement therapy are important aspects of an inpatient hospital stay for helping prevent the patient from carrying out suicidal impulses. During each therapy session, evaluate the degree to which the patient is complying with the contract and the degree of suicidal intent.

Engage the Patient's Support Network. If the patient identifies a key support person, ask the patient to contact this person, to tell him or her about the seriousness of the problem, and to request support. If the patient cannot identify any support network, hospitalization is indicated. If the patient is hesitant to involve a support person, hospitalization is also appropriate.

I, _____ , promise not to harm myself for the next

24 hours. I commit myself to tell the nursing staff of any change in my thinking regarding the

infliction of self-harm. That is, I will tell them of any increase in the frequency or intensity of thoughts

about injuring myself, or any change in the seriousness of my potential plan for harming myself.

I will cooperate with the staff to preserve my own well-being.

SIGNED: _____

WITNESSED: _____

DATE: _____

Figure 31–2
A sample no-harm contract.

When a patient is suicidal, he feels totally alone and worthless. A supportive friend or family member can reinforce the patient's worth. It is important to encourage the patient to allow support people to be integrated into treatment (Mullis & Byers, 1987).

Monitor Your Own Feelings. It is important that you continually assess your own feelings about suicide and suicidal ideation in patients. If you find that you tend to discount the suicidal threats of patients as acting out, attention-seeking, or manipulation, you may miss a potentially lethal suicide threat. If you have such thoughts about patients with suicidal ideation or patients who self-mutilate, seek clinical supervision to help you understand the patient's desperation.

When there are several suicidal or self-mutilative patients on the unit at the same time, a staff meeting to discuss each patient's care and the feelings of staff members about the behavior of the patients may be helpful (Gallop, 1992). Staff members who maintain a positive life balance by integrating work, play, spiritual beliefs, and exercise in their lives are better equipped to deal with patients who are chronically depressed and hopeless about the quality of their lives (Badger, 1995).

Return now to the story of Charles Thomas, to see how the mental health team intervened to help him meet his short-term goals.

A thorough assessment to determine Mr. Thomas's suicidal intent reveals that Mr. Thomas has advanced suicidal ideation. Members of the nursing staff therefore encourage Mr. Thomas to write a no-harm contract in his own words, and they ask Mr. Thomas to seek them out every 15 minutes to demonstrate a commitment that he would not harm himself. While Mr. Thomas is on 15-minute checks, the nursing staff members assess Mr. Thomas's level of safety.

During his hospitalization, Mr. Thomas is encouraged to attend all milieu groups to increase his repertoire of options for problem-solving and to increase his level of social interaction. The nursing staff also request an evaluation for antidepressant medications to help Mr. Thomas feel more energetic, sleep better, have a better appetite, concentrate for longer periods, and feel an increase in libido. After a psychiatrist prescribes an antidepressant medication for Mr. Thomas, the nursing staff members begin to teach him about the role that medication will play in his recovery. They monitor side effects and medication compliance.

Once Mr. Thomas's condition improves, he begins attending a stress reduction group that is co-led by the staff occupational therapist, and the nursing staff teach him relaxation exercises to use when business worries intrude on his thoughts. ■

➤ *Check Your Reading*

23. What are the indications for hospitalization for a patient with suicidal ideas?
24. When is it appropriate to use every-15-minute checks?

25. When is it appropriate to place a patient on one-to-one supervision?
26. How can you avoid becoming drained by patients who are suicidal or self-mutilate?

Evaluation

As we implement care for the patient who uses self-injury or suicide to problem-solve, it becomes important to evaluate the process of this care. The formative evaluation provides us with information about the patient's progress as well as information about the deficiencies and reasons the patient may not have benefitted from the implementation of the plan. Questions for further clinical research in nursing can grow out of a thorough summative evaluation as we explore more effective ways to deliver nursing care to the suicidal patient.

One issue that is important to examine during the evaluation phase of the nursing process is when the plan of care is not working (Case Example 31-4). See Snapshot: Nursing Interventions Specific to Suicide.

■ CASE EXAMPLE 31-4
■ Anne's Story

Anne continued to cut herself no matter what the members of the nursing staff did. The staff members were feeling demoralized. "We have tried everything—what else can we do? She just keeps cutting!" The case was reviewed by a nurse from another unit who was not familiar with Anne but who was interested in providing nursing care to patients who self-mutilate. The nurse from the other unit asked the staff if they had worked with Anne to determine thoughts she may have before self-mutilating. This nurse provided the nursing staff with several questions that may assist Anne to learn if she dissociates before self-mutilating. Does she use the self-mutilation to punish herself or to deal with overwhelming feelings? The nurses on the unit felt better after the consultation because they now had a new direction in which to proceed. ■

Another example that points out the need for an ongoing evaluation of care would be a patient whose suicidal ideation is lethal, and the nursing staff members fail to recognize the seriousness of this ideation. In this situation, the formative evaluation identifies the deficiencies in the care that was given (Case Example 31-5).

■ CASE EXAMPLE 31-5
■ John's Story

John had been hospitalized for 2 days after he came to the emergency department reporting feeling suicidal. He is well known to the staff and frequently comes through the emergency department for a brief hospitalization after telling the staff members there that he is suicidal. The psychiatric nursing staff members feel John abuses the system, as he is a known alcoholic and drug abuser who manipulates a hospital stay by saying he is suicidal. This time John left the hospital and within 24 hours shot himself in the head with a hand gun. The members of psychiatric staff were upset: some sad, some angry, some questioning their care. After evaluating the overall care, the deficit cited was that the staff members did not perform an in-depth suicidal evaluation before John's discharge. One nurse claimed, "He looked like his usual self—I thought he was just going to get his booze and he'd be back." Another nurse asked, "How do we know when someone is being manipulative?" ■

In Case Example 31-5, the nursing staff's belief that they knew the patient's next move got in the way of a comprehensive evaluation that may have prevented John's suicide. Evaluating the care delivered to the patient on a routine basis decreases mistakes or omissions made owing to predictions of the patient's behavior based on the nurses' emotional response to the patient's behavior. In the practice of psychiatric nursing, it is important to monitor any emotional response you may have toward a patient's behavior to prevent nursing judgment errors. Because hospital stays are short, evaluations of the patient care need to be done daily and communicated during change of shift reports.

The evaluation stage in the nursing process provides opportunities for new strategies in providing comprehensive care. If the nursing staff members become stuck in an intervention cycle that is not successful, a peer review by a nurse who is interested in the patient's problem may be helpful. Receiving clinical supervision from a certified clinical specialist also assists the nursing team to determine patient outcomes and interventions that are within the patient's capacity. Additionally, using the current literature to assist with planning and implementation of the nursing care is helpful.

➤ *Check Your Reading*
27. When is it appropriate to evaluate the nursing care of a patient who is suicidal or self-mutilating?
28. How often should this evaluation take place?
29. What can you do when the nursing interventions are not helping the patient achieve the desired patient outcomes?

Nursing Interventions Specific to Suicide

What do you need to do to develop a relationship with a patient who is suicidal?

- Approach the patient in a nonjudgmental way to encourage disclosure of the intent to do self harm.
- Assess the individual by asking several questions about the patient's physical, emotional, cognitive, social, and spiritual status. This will provide information about the patient's level of hopelessness and isolation as well as the suicidal risk potential.
- Share time with the patient, particularly if the patient is a high risk of suicide and is placed on one-to-one suicide watch. This decreases the patient's isolation and can promote problem-solving of the initial crisis that led the patient to feel suicidal.
- Avoid sarcasm, feelings that the patient is "attention seeking" or "manipulating." Patients who express suicidal ideation are feeling overwhelmed and need assistance to problem-solve.
- Find ways to assist the patient to find hope in the crisis without negating the emotional pain that the patient is experiencing.
- Encourage the patient to discuss his/her view of the problems and feelings that these issues raise.

What do you need to assess regarding the patient's health status?

- Patients who have chronic illnesses, such as multiple sclerosis, cancer, and AIDS often have suicidal ideation and may make a parasuicidal attempt.
- Assess whether there are brain changes, such as organic changes in the frontal or temporal lobe, that can contribute to behavior that is disinhibited; the patient may therefore not have impulse control.
- Measure level of lethality and determine the patient's stage of suicidal risk (none to severe).
- Determine whether the patient is compliant with the prescribed medication regiment.
- Determine whether the patient is manifesting depression.
- Determine whether the patient is abusing substances.
- Has the patient ever made a parasuicide attempt? Is there a family history of parasuicidal behavior or completed suicide?
- What is the patient's cognitive style? Is there dichotomous thinking, where the patient thinks of issues as being only "good or bad." Is the patient rigid? Are the thoughts negative, devoid of hope? Does the patient view himself or herself as a burden or as worthless? Does the patient think the problems cannot be solved without committing suicide?
- Does the patient have a support network?
- Does the patient have a spiritual base?
- Can the patient mobilize his or her emotional resources to do problem-solving?

What do you need to teach the patient and the patient's caregiver?

- Suicidal ideation is a symptom of being stuck in a crisis.
- With crisis intervention that is goal-directed, steps can be taken to deal with the crisis at hand.
- Medications can ease the depressed symptoms, lower the level of anxiety, reduce the hallucinations, or prevent withdrawal symptoms. The patient needs to take the medications as directed to facilitate the reduction of the symptoms.
- Hospitalization can be used to provide a safe environment to begin work on the issues at hand while preventing impulsive, self-distructive behavior.
- A partial hospitalization program may be a follow-up to a short-term hospitalization stay to continue to provide an environment that is structured and oriented toward problem-solving.
- Outpatient psychotherapy is necessary to support the problem-solving effort to prevent further suicidal behavior while dealing with the issues.
- Suicidal ideation is not "attention seeking" or "manipulative behavior"; it is a symptom that is indicative of the individual's feeling psychologically overwhelmed. Immediate crisis intervention and follow-up will prevent a suicidal gesture.

What skills will you want the patient or caregiver to demonstrate?

- Listen to the patient if he or she is making suicidal statements and seek immediate treatment.
- Teach the patient and family members about the stages of suicidal ideation.
- Use the psychiatric emergency department if the patient determines that he or she is feeling overwhelming urges to die.
- Contact the therapist or a clergy person if the patient is having suicidal ideation.

What other health professionals might need to be a part of this plan of care?

- A physician, a psychiatrist, and the primary care physician who is in charge of the overall treatment plan, including medication management.
- A social worker who will assist with community resources.
- A nurse psychotherapist (clinical specialist or psychiatric nurse practitioner) who may be the primary therapist and in some states prescribes medications for the patient.
- A psychiatric occupational therapist to assist the patient with problem-solving skills, such as structuring the patient's day, and to assist with stress-reduction exercises.

NURSING PROCESS APPLICATION

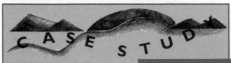

Mark

You are a psychiatric clinical nurse specialist working in the emergency department of a large metropolitan hospital in the Southwest. The staff nurse asks you to consult with Mark, a 23-year-old male who attempted suicide last evening, and his mother, Jane, a 49-year-old elementary school teacher. When you arrive, Mark is unconscious, and his mother tells you that he took a bottle of over-the-counter sleeping pills and drank a large quantity of alcohol. She is distressed but seems to be coping well. On interviewing her, you find that Mark has a long history of problems, and this episode is not a complete surprise to her. Mark's parents divorced when he was 18 years old. His two older sisters are both in college and doing well. His father is a recovering alcoholic who has remarried. Mark quit school at age 15 and has not been able to cope with life in an effective manner since that time.

Jane has an active support group and a strong spiritual base. She tells you that she is concerned that Mark will never mature to adulthood because he has made so many poor choices in his life. You discover that he has a criminal record for unauthorized use of a vehicle when he was 18. Jane tells you that she feels guilty because she did not encourage Mark to go to church and receive the sacraments of First Communion and Confirmation when he was a young boy.

When Mark awakens from his semicomatose state the next day, he tells you that he was concerned that his girlfriend was pregnant and felt life was not worth living anymore. He says, "I don't think there is a God or anyone who loves me; everyone would be better off if I were dead." As soon as he is recovered physically, Mark is moved to the psychiatric unit.

ASSESSMENT

Assessment data are as follows:
- Serious suicide attempt
- Poor coping skills
- Hopelessness
- History of criminal activity
- Verbalizations of despair regarding perceived loss of God's love and family support
- Supportive mother
- Lack of attainment of educational goals or job training skills

---

DIAGNOSIS

DSM-IV Diagnosis: Major Depressive Disorder, Single Episode, Severe without Psychotic Features

Nursing Diagnosis 1: Risk for Violence: Self-directed related to feelings of worthlessness and hopelessness as evidenced by serious suicide attempt, poor coping skills, and history of criminal activity.

OUTCOME IDENTIFICATION, PLANNING, AND IMPLEMENTATION

> **Expected Outcome 1:** By _____ the patient will no longer verbalize thoughts of suicide or self-destruction.

Short-Term Goals	Nursing Interventions	Rationales
By _____ the patient will seek out staff members when feeling the urge to harm himself.	1. Determine appropriate level of suicide precautions. 2. Assess the patient's level of suicidal potential and reassess daily. 3. Initiate suicide precautions as warranted by current level of suicidality. 4. Convey warmth and unconditional acceptance of the patient.	1–3. Providing a safe environment for the patient is a number-one priority. 4. This conveys the message to the patient that he is a worthwhile person.

5. Monitor closely for any changes in mood or temperament.

5. Once medications are beginning to take effect, the patient may have enough energy to take his life.

By _____ the patient will make a short-term verbal contract not to harm himself.

1. Initiate a 24-hour no-harm contract with the patient by assisting him in writing a contract stating that he will not harm himself.
2. Be caring but firm in requesting the contract.
3. Involve the patient in as much of the treatment planning as possible.

1–2. Discussing suicidal feelings with a caring person provides the patient with a sense of security and provides some relief that the professional will be able to protect him from his negative feelings.

3. Assists in making the patient more responsible for his health and well-being.

Expected Outcome 2: By _____ the patient will demonstrate three new coping mechanisms.

Short-Term Goal	Nursing Interventions	Rationales
By _____ the patient will verbalize at least four alternative ways of coping with stress.	1. Educate the patient about ways to reduce stress, such as meditation, guided imagery, engaging in physical activity, and keeping a journal. 2. Remain an active listener and spend time with the patient. 3. Encourage the patient to express any feelings he may be experiencing, such as anger, fear, disappointment. This can assist with problem-solving.	1. The patient needs to develop skills that will replace the tendency to turn to self-destructive behavior for relief. 2. The patient may feel shame about the suicide attempt and may have difficulty sharing honestly. 3. Self-destructive behavior is often seen as anger turned inward. Understanding intense emotions in a productive way can be very therapeutic.

Expected Outcome 3: By _____ the patient will be connected with two outside community resources for assistance with any suicidal ideation after discharge.

Short-Term Goal	Nursing Interventions	Rationales
By _____ the patient will contact an outside agency for support upon discharge.	1. As soon as the patient is physically able, provide him with a list of outside agencies. 2. Continue to encourage the patient. 3. Consider a family therapy session with the patient's mother. 4. Clarify the relationship between the patient and his girlfriend.	1–2. Increasing the patient's support system will lessen the tendency toward suicidal behavior. Social isolation always increases the risk of suicide. 3. The mother wants to be supportive and will need assistance in this process. An attempted suicide is a very traumatic event. 4. The possibility of the girlfriend's pregnancy was the trigger event for the suicide attempt and should not be overlooked at this time.

Nursing Diagnosis 2: Spiritual Distress related to perception of loss of God's love and support from nuclear family as evidenced by suicide attempt, verbalizations of lack of spiritual presence, and hopelessness.

OUTCOME IDENTIFICATION, PLANNING, AND IMPLEMENTATION

Expected Outcome 1: By _____ the patient will improve overall spiritual well-being.

Short-Term Goals	Nursing Interventions	Rationales
By _____ the patient will make positive statements about his life.	1. Engage in active listening and convey a caring, genuine attitude.	1. Attempting suicide is indicative of low self-worth; this patient needs to know that he is a worthwhile human being.

2. Provide examples from literature, the bible, and life experiences of people who have overcome great difficulties.

3. Encourage and accept verbalization of all feelings; gently help patient access intense feeling states.
4. Encourage the patient to remember a time in his life when he felt nurtured, loved, and accepted.

2. Helps the patient see that much can be learned from experiencing hardships, and many others have overcome great personal tragedy and have a stronger spiritual self because of it.
3. Depressed persons often bury feelings, especially anger, and need encouragement to verbalize them.
4. Enables the patient to shift the focus from negative thought patterns to more positive thinking.

By _____ the patient will articulate a belief system he finds acceptable.

1. Provide spiritual reading material consistent with the patient's spiritual beliefs.
2. Offer to pray with or for the patient.
3. Use guided imagery, prayer, and/or music to aid in healing past hurts.

4. Encourage the patient to try new religious exercises gradually and more than one time.

1–2. These interventions assure the patient of your continued caring and concern and interest in his spiritual growth.

3. Getting in touch with one's spiritual self can be accomplished in many ways.
4. Spiritual well-being or distress will vary from day to day. Letting the patient know this is normal will keep him from getting discouraged the patient will develop a support system with a church or self-help group.

By _____ the patient will initiate a healthy relationship with a person who has a well-developed sense of spirituality.

1. Educate the patient about healthy relationships.
2. Use role-playing to prepare the patient for new relationships.
3. Explore with the patient the negative aspects of previous relationships.
4. Observe the patient in therapy groups and gently give the patient feedback about your observations.

5. Ask the patient to talk about three adults he knows who have a well-developed sense of spirituality.
6. Encourage the patient to contact one of these persons for support after he is discharged.

1–3. This patient has a long history of difficult relationships.

4. The patient may be unaware of how his actions and reactions invite negative or undesirable behavior in others.
5. This exercise helps provide the patient with role models.

6. Supports the patient in becoming assertive in meeting his spiritual goals.

By _____ the patient will participate in group activities at a church or self-help group.

1. Encourage participation in prayer, social, and athletic groups while in the hospital.
2. Remain an advocate for the patient and do not be discouraged by setbacks.

1. These groups foster learning about oneself in relationship to others.

2. This patient has a long history of setbacks, and expecting perfection in following the treatment plan would be self-defeating. This could increase the patient's "all or nothing" thinking patterns.

Expected Outcome 2: By _____ the patient will find a job, engage in job training skills, or begin an educational program.

Short-Term Goals	Nursing Interventions	Rationales
By _____ the patient will articulate goals in life.	1. Support the patient in exploring both short-term and long-term goals. 2. Give the patient feedback about the realistic completion of his goals.	1. This patient has a history of impulsive activity. Setting goals will give the patient some hope for the future. 2. If goals are too global, the patient will experience failure again.

| By _____ the patient will obtain a job or educational counseling. | 1. Refer the patient to a vocational counselor or social worker.

2. Remain an advocate for the patient in this process. | 1. Becoming successful in a job that uses his natural talents will foster self-esteem.
2. Suicidal, depressed patients have a high degree of negativity and need a great amount of support. |

EVALUATION

Formative Evaluation: Mark met all of the short-term goals except initiating a healthy relationship with a person who has a well-developed sense of spirituality. He did not contact anyone while he was in the hospital and had difficulty in identifying three people whom he knew who had a strong sense of spirituality. Prior to hospitalization, Mark was isolated socially except for his relationship with his girlfriend. Mark did agree to return for aftercare therapy groups at the hospital and to participate in individual therapy. He was able to write a no-harm contract, and did follow through when he began to feel hopeless at one point during the hospital stay. He also contacted the local rehabilitation agency to begin working on vocational training. Mark said that his real dream was to go to college, but did not think that was realistic right now.

Summative Evaluation: Mark met all of the expected outcomes regarding suicidal behavior but was still having difficult outcomes related to spiritual distress. His overall sense of spiritual well-being was dramatically improved by discharge, but he continued to experience difficulty with finding a support system. He says that he grew up feeling that he did not "fit in." The staff recommended that Mark remain in outpatient therapy and aftercare for at least 3 months because he remains vulnerable to returning thoughts of suicide.

Conclusions

Providing nursing care for a patient who is suicidal is a complex issue. The idea that someone wants to end his or her life generates feelings in the nurse that need to be acknowledged to provide care that is thoughtful. A suicidal patient may not disclose suicidal feelings and thoughts in order to complete the act. When a patient is successful in committing suicide, the nursing staff have to evaluate the care delivered without blaming one another.

The key to providing comprehensive care to the patient who is suicidal is to perform an in-depth assessment regularly until the patient has a decrease in suicidal ideation. Determining whether the patient is not at risk for suicide or a severe suicidal risk using the continuum described in the chapter can guide whether the patient requires hospitalization, every-15-minute checks, or one-to-one supervisions. Questions that relate to the patient's ability to control his or her impulses to commit suicide are important in determining the intensity of care. Asking the patient to write his or her own contract for safety and placing that document in the chart is helpful in deciding whether the patient is joining with the care team to prevent a suicidal gesture. Assisting the patient to think through other options to problem-solve the crisis that was perceived as overwhelming and precipitated the suicidal thoughts can provide hope for the patient. Encouraging the patient to use his or her support system can reinforce the patient's value to others and may decrease the feelings of isolation. Assisting the patient to think through his or her spiritual beliefs by providing linkages with clergy and church members may assist the patient to use this powerful mechanism to regain a sense of purpose.

It is important to assist the patient to understand the depression or other psychiatric illness that may have played a part in the feelings of wanting to die. By providing psychoeducation about the illness and the treatment, the nurse is promoting hope for a future.

Patients who self-mutilate have different psychodynamics than suicidal patients. Some patients have symptoms of self-mutilation and are *moderately* to *severely suicidal*. It is important to assess the patient who self-mutilates for suicidal ideation as well as dissociation, rage reactions, alexithymia, and feelings of worthlessness and shame. Patients who self-mutilate often have difficulty relating to others and are socially isolated. It is important to assist the patient to link the act of self-mutilation with causal factors by assisting him or her in identifying the thoughts that preceded the action. The patient who self-mutilates often feels shame about the self-injury. By providing the patient with appropriate medical care for the injury and a thoughtful approach for exploring the psychodynamics, the nurse can help the patient reduce this self-mutilating behavior. It is important that the nurse not behave in a punitive manner to teach the patient that this behavior is unacceptable. This would further alienate the patient and is countertherapeutic.

The nursing care of this population of patients is potentially draining for the nurse. It is important to be aware of your own feelings about the patient and to receive clinical supervision or time away from the patient if you are feeling overwhelmed by your negative feelings toward the patient. Maintaining your own positive life balance is a worthy investment for your own mental health, especially when working with patients who are suicidal or who self-mutilate.

Key Points to Remember

- The National Center for Health Statistics in 1990–1991 ranked suicide as the ninth cause of death in the United States, with 11.9 persons per every 100,000 population completing a suicidal act. Of the suicides that occur in the United States, 5% to 6% take place in an inpatient psychiatric hospital.
- Suicidal ideation and completion are not bounded by culture, age, class, religion, or socioeconomic status. Women tend to make more suicide attempts than men; however, more men complete the suicidal attempt. White men are the highest risk group for completing suicide, especially if the man is single and between the ages 75 and 84 years old.
- Suicide is one of the outcomes of untreated depression. There are several other psychiatric disorders that are associated with suicidal behavior, such as bipolar disorder, schizophrenia, personality disorders, such as borderline personality disorder and antisocial personality disorder, and substance abuse disorders.
- Self-injury or intentional self-destructive behavior that destroys or alters body tissue occurs in an estimated 24% to 40% of psychiatric patients. Self-mutilating behavior has a different psychological intention than a suicidal gesture. Patients who self-mutilate often have a history of child abuse, sexual abuse, and neglect. Self-mutilation often occurs when patients have alexithymia, or the inability to identify and put words to the experience of emotional feelings.
- There is no one theory that adequately explains suicidal or self-destructive behavior or can guide clinical practice. Biological, psychological, sociocultural, and spiritual factors may all contribute to self-injury.
- A comprehensive suicide assessment must include the physical, emotional, cognitive, social, and spiritual domains that represent the foundation of human functioning. An assessment also includes evaluating the patient to determine whether he is in the high-risk group.
- Patients who pose a threat to themselves through the use of a suicidal gesture or self-mutilation have an *at risk for* nursing diagnosis.
- A severity index can be used when determining the nursing diagnosis and plan for a patient who is suicidal. This severity index is conceptualized as a continuum of the patient with *no suicidal ideation* to a patient with a *severe level of suicidal risk*. This information can assist the nurse in planning what type of care the patient requires to prevent a suicidal gesture.
- The overall goal for the patient is to protect the patient from self-harm while helping him or her maintain the highest degree of autonomy that is possible, with a predicted outcome that the patient will no longer display suicidal or self-mutilative behavior.
- If a patient is successful in committing suicide, the nursing staff have to evaluate the care delivered without blaming one another.

Learning Activities

1. Role-play performing a suicide assessment interview. During this exercise, instruct the "patient" to play varying levels of suicidal lethality. The "nurse" determines the nursing care of the "patient," who then responds to the planning and implementation by getting better or more suicidal. During this role-playing exercise, the "patient" shares with the "nurse" why he or she got better or worse.
2. Attend a support group for suicide survivors in the community. Write your thoughts and feelings about this experience.
3. Use the Internet to find two sites relating to suicide: one for prevention and one that is instructive to the reader in terms of how to commit suicide. Patients who are suicidal and have access to the Internet may use the "how to" site as a justification for their own suicidal attempt.

Critical Thinking Exercise

Jane Bayer, school nurse, is one of four members of the high school crisis team that evaluates high-risk students for potential self-destructive behaviors. Today the student under review is Peter. Peter lives with his parents and two sisters. He has a 3.8 grade-point average and has just been accepted to Harvard University as a chemistry major. He has come to the attention of the team because of an incident in gym class during which he "accidentally" cut his wrists. At that time, the nurse was told by Peter that his parents were getting a divorce and that his father was not sure he could afford to pay Peter's college tuition.

1. What clinical assumptions can you make about Peter's behavior?
2. How would the team assess Peter to check their assumptions?
3. What further evidence would you need to make a treatment determination?

The team decided to call Peter in to talk to him about his plans. Peter told the team that he was looking forward to college and had bought a new car and a new computer that he had lent to his girlfriend. He seemed in very high spirits and thought that the team was overreacting to his sisters' call to the counselor about his moodiness.

1. Do you have evidence that suggests that the team needs to act immediately?

2. If the team decided that an immediate intervention was needed, what else could happen as a result?

3. What could happen if an intervention was not taken?

Additional Resources

American Association of Suicidology
http://www.suicidology.org

Grief and Loss Resource Center
http://www.rockies.net/~spirit/grief/grief.html

The Samaritans
http://www.samaritans.org.uk
or http://www.mhnet.org/samaritans

References

Adams, K. S. (1985). Attempted suicide. *Psychiatry Clinics of North America, 8,* 183-203.

American Psychiatric Association. (1984). *The American Psychiatric Association's psychiatric glossary.* Washington, DC: American Psychiatric Press.

American Psychiatric Association. (1994). *The diagnostic and statistical manual of mental disorders* (4th ed.). Washington, DC: American Psychiatric Press.

Anderson, R. N., Kochanek, K. D., & Murphy, S. L. (1997). Advance report of final mortality statistics, 1995. *Mortality Vital Statistics Report, 45*(11, Suppl 2), Hyattsville, MD: National Center for Health Statistics.

Badger, J. (1995). Reaching out to the suicidal patient. *American Journal of Nursing, 95,* 24-32.

Barstow, D. (1995). Self-injury and self-mutilation: Nursing approaches. *Journal of Psychosocial Nursing and Mental Health Services, 33,* 19-22.

Beck, A. T. (1967). *Depression: Clinical, experimental and theoretical aspects.* New York: Harper Row.

Beck, A. T., Brown, G., Berchick, R. J., Stewart, B. L., & Steer, R. A. (1990). Relationship between hopelessness and ultimate suicide: A replication with psychiatric outpatients. *American Journal of Psychiatry, 147,* 190-195.

Beck, A. T., Steer, R. A., Kovacs, M., & Garrison, B. (1985). Hopelessness and eventual suicide: A 10-year prospective study of patients hospitalized with suicidal ideation. *American Journal of Psychiatry, 142,* 559-563.

Brodsky, B. S., Malone, K. M., Ellis, S. P., Dulit, R. A., & Mann, J. J. (1997). Characteristics of Borderline Personality Disorder associated with suicidal behavior. *American Journal of Psychiatry, 154,* 1715-1719.

Busch, K. A., Clark, D. C., Fawcett, J., & Kravitz, H. M. (1993). Clinical features of inpatient suicide. *Psychiatric Annals, 23,* 256-262.

Cardell, R., & Horton-Deutsch, S. (1994). A model for assessment of inpatient suicide potential. *Archives of Psychiatric Nursing, 8,* 316-372.

Cornelius, J. R., Salloum, I. S., Mezzich, J., Cornelius, M., Fabrega, H., Ehler, J. G., Ulrich, R. F., Thase, M. E., & Mann, J. J. (1995). Disproportionate suicidality in patients with comorbid major depression and alcoholism. *American Journal of Psychiatry, 152,* 358-363.

Cugino, A., Markovich, E. I., Rosenblatt, S., Jarjoura, D., Blend, D., & Whittier, F. C. (1992). Searching for a pattern: Repeat suicide attempts. *Journal of Psychosocial Nursing, 30,* 23-25.

Davis, R. (1982). Black suicide and social support system: An overview and some implications for mental health practitioners. *Phylon, 43,* 304-314.

Durkheim, E. (1951). *Suicide.* Glencoe, IL: Free Press.

Favazza, A. R. (1987). *Bodies under siege: Self mutilation in culture and psychiatry.* Baltimore: Johns Hopkins University Press.

Favazza, A. R. (1989). Why patients mutilate themselves. *Hospital and Community Psychiatry, 40,* 137-145.

Folkman, S., & Lazarus, R. (1984). *Stress, appraisal, and coping.* New York: Springer.

Forster, P. (1994). Accurate assessment of short-term suicide risk in a crisis. *Psychiatric Annals, 24,* 571-578.

Frankl, V. E. (1964). *Man's search for meaning.* New York: Washington Square Press.

Freud, S. (1964). New introductory lectures on psychoanalysis: Lecture XXII. In *Anxiety and instinctual life.* London: Hogarth.

Gallop, R. (1992). Self-destructive and impulsive behavior in the patient with a borderline personality disorder: Rethinking hospital treatment and management. *Archives of Psychiatric Nursing, 6,* 178-182.

Goodwin, J. M. (1989). *Sexual abuse: Incest victims and their families* (2nd ed.). Chicago: Year Book Medical.

Green, E., Katz, J., & Marcus, P. (1995). Practice guidelines for suicide/self harm prevention. In E. Green & J. Katz (Eds.), *Clinical practice guidelines for the adult patient* (pp. 250-1-250-21). St. Louis, MO: Mosby-Year Book.

Herman, J. L. (1992). *Trauma and recovery.* New York: Basic Books.

Isometsä, E. T., Henriksson, M., Heikkinen, M. E., Aro, H. M., Marttunen, M. J., Kuoppasalmi, K. I., & Lönnqvist, J. K. (1996). Suicide among subjects with personality disorders. *American Journal of Psychiatry, 153,* 667-673.

Kreitman, N. (1977). *Parasuicide.* Chichester, England: Wiley.

Linehan, M. M. (1993). *Cognitive-behavioral treatment of Borderline Personality Disorder.* New York: The Guilford Press.

McIntosh, J. L. U.S.A. suicide 1995 official final data [AAS Web site]. 1997. Available at: http:///www.suicidology.org. Accessed June 22, 1999.

Meltzer, H. Y., & Okayli, G. (1995). Reduction of suicidality during Clozapine treatment of neuroleptic-resistant schizophrenia: Impact of risk-benefit assessment. *American Journal of Psychiatry, 152,* 183-190.

Menninger, A. (1938). *Man against himself.* Orlando, FL: Harcourt Brace.

Mintz, R. S. (1971). Basic considerations in the psychotherapy of the depressed patient. *American Journal of Psychotherapy, 2,* 56-72.

Mullis, M. R., & Byers, P. H. (1987). Social support in suicidal inpatients. *Journal of Psychosocial Nursing, 25,* 16-19.

Rickelman, B.L., & Houfek, J.F. (1995) Toward an interactional model of suicidal behaviors: Cognitive rigidity, attributional style, stress, hopelessness, and depression. *Archives of Psychiatric Nursing, 9,* 156-168.

Roy, A. (1989). Suicide. In H. I. Kaplan & B. J. Sadock (Eds.), *Comprehensive textbook of psychiatry* (5th ed.). Baltimore: Williams & Wilkins.

Sanger, E., Thomas, M. D., & Whitney, J. D. (1988). A guide for nursing assessment of the psychiatric inpatient. *Archives of Psychiatric Nursing, 2,* 334-338.

Shneidman, E. S. (1996). *The suicidal mind.* New York: Oxford University Press.

Sifnoes, P. E. (1972). *Short-term psychotherapy and emotional crisis.* Cambridge, MA: Harvard University Press.

Sifneos, P. E. (1996). Alexithymia: Past and present. *American Journal of Psychiatry, 153 (7 suppl.),* 137-141.

Stanley, M., & Stanley, B. (1990). Postmortem evidence for serotonin's role in suicide. *Journal of Clinical Psychiatry, 51,* 22-28.

Strakowski, S. M., McElroy, S. L., Keck, P. E., & West, S. A. (1996). Suicidality among patients with mixed and manic bipolar disorder. *American Journal of Psychiatry, 153,* 674-676.

Torrey, E. F. (1995). *Surviving schizophrenia: A manual for families, consumers, and providers* (3rd ed.). New York: HarperCollins.

U.S. Department of Health and Human Services, National Center for Health Statistics. (1992). *Vital statistics report, 40, 1990-1991.* Hyattsville, MD: Public Health Service.

Van der Kolk, B. A. (1987). *Psychological trauma.* Washington, DC: American Psychiatric Press.

Vanzant, I. (1992). *Tapping the power within.* New York: Harlem River Press.

Wheeler, K., & Broad, R. D. (1994). Alexithymia and overeating. *Perspectives in Psychiatric Care, 30,* 7-10.

White, S. G. (1990). Carrico Dam [Hazlewood]. On *Journeys* [cassette]. Washington, DC.

Wolfersdorf, M., Hole, G., Steiner, B., & Keller, F. (1990). Suicide risk in suicidal versus nonsuicidal depressed patients. *Crisis, 11,* 85-97.

Suggested Readings

Badger, J. (1995). Reaching out to the suicidal patient. *American Journal of Nursing, 95,* 24-32.

Buchanan, D. M. (1991). Suicide: A conceptual model for an avoidable death. *Archives of Psychiatric Nursing, 5,* 341-349.

Cardell, R., & Horton-Deutsch, S. (1994). A model for assessment of inpatient suicide potential. *Archives of Psychiatric Nursing, 8,* 366-372.

Linehan, M. M. (1993). *Cognitive-behavioral treatment of Borderline Personality Disorder.* New York: Guilford Press.

Plath, S. (1996). *The bell jar.* New York: HarperCollins.

Rickelman, B. L., & Houfek, J. F. (1995). Toward an interactional model of suicidal behaviors: Cognitive rigidity, attributional style, stress, hopelessness, and depression. *Archives of Psychiatric Nursing, 9,* 156-168.

Roy, A. (1989). Suicide. In H. I. Kaplan & B. J. Sadock (Eds.), *Comprehensive textbook of psychiatry* (5th ed.). Baltimore: Williams & Wilkins.

Shneidman, E. S. (1996). *The suicidal mind.* New York: Oxford University Press.

C H A P T E R

32

For this is the great error of our day, that physicians separate mind from body.

—Socrates

Psychophysiological Disorders

Learning Objectives

After studying this chapter, you should be able to:

1. Recognize the impact of psychophysiological illness on routine health care.
2. Describe the contributions that Descartes, Cannon, and Selye have made to the recognition of the stress response.
3. Describe an interactive model of stress and physical illness.
4. Describe the components of a complete psychophysiological and spiritual assessment.
5. List the five pain-producing structures of the back.
6. List the factors contributing to the poor description of most pelvic pain.
7. Describe the two major psychophysiological theories related to development of hypertension.
8. Describe the role of serotonin and norepinephrine in the development of a migraine headache.
9. Identify the physical and psychological factors that contribute to the development of temporomandibular disorder.
10. Describe the common characteristics of somatoform disorders.
11. List the differentiating characteristics of each of the seven somatoform disorders.
12. Identify expected outcomes of working with a patient diagnosed with a psychophysiological disorder.
13. Identify expected outcomes of working with family members of a patient diagnosed with a psychophysiological disorder.
14. Describe the use of the nursing process in the holistic care of a patient with low back pain.
15. Describe the holistic treatment of each of the psychophysiological illnesses discussed.
16. Identify how research has clarified the relationships among the physical, psychological, and spiritual components of health.

Portions of this chapter are from the previous edition chapter contributed by Frances B. Wimbush, PhD, RN.

Key Terminology

Body Dysmorphic Disorder
Chronic back pain
Chronic pelvic pain
Conversion Disorder
Hypertension
Hypochondriasis

La belle indifférence
Migraine headache
Pain Disorder
Primary gain
Psychophysiological
  assessment

Psychophysiological illness
Secondary gain
Somatization Disorder
Somatoform Disorder Not
  Otherwise Specified

Somatoform Disorders
Temporomandibular disorder
Undifferentiated Somatoform
  Disorder

It has been estimated that as many as 70% to 80% of all visits to internists and family practice physicians are made by people suffering from **psychophysiological illness.** Unexplained complaints of chest pain, abdominal pain, fatigue, shortness of breath, back pain, headache, anxiety, and depression comprise about 25% of all primary care visits, and an organic cause can be found in only 16% of these patients (Kroenke, 1991). Increasingly, we recognize the psychological dimension of these illnesses; clearly, psychological issues interrelate with the body in such an intimate manner that we cannot separate one from the other and still do justice to alleviating the patient's problem.

We have been much slower to recognize the importance of the spiritual dimension. No research looks at the role that spiritual distress plays in the etiology of psychophysiological illnesses or at the role of spiritual well-being in the healing of patients diagnosed with these illnesses. Although the research to support the role of spirituality is lacking, to ignore the spiritual component is a disservice to our patients. Patients suffering with these illnesses need care that addresses physical, psychological, spiritual, cognitive, and social issues; anything less brings them only partial healing or relief.

In this chapter, the nurse is introduced to the most prevalent psychophysiological illnesses: chronic pain (back and pelvic), hypertension, migraines, and **temporomandibular disorder** (TMD). In addition, you are presented with information about the seven types of somatoform disorders: body dysmorphic disorder, conversion disorder, hypochondriasis, somatization disorder, pain disorder, undifferentiated somatoform disorder, and somatoform disorder not otherwise specified. Each diagnosis is discussed in holistic terms, beginning with the epidemiology and progressing through the etiology, psychological and spiritual factors, and treatment. The nursing process is applied to the journey of Monica, a young woman who suffers from chronic back pain. Some of the contributing factors of Monica's story are generic to all psychophysiological illnesses.

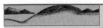

Monica's Story

I am a 28-year-old woman with a master's degree in math. My car was hit in the rear when I was driving to work on a snowy afternoon 2 years ago. My initial diagnosis was acute muscle spasm of the back and neck. I was seen by my internist, who prescribed cyclobenzaprine HCl (Flexeril) and hot compresses and told me to rest. I followed the treatment and returned to work as a computer programmer 3 days after my injury. I could not sit without discomfort. I was sleeping poorly and had no appetite.

The Problem Escalates

I continued to have shooting pain in my back and arms. I could not stand, sit, or lie down for more than 30 minutes without experiencing increased pain. I also lost 6 lb. I went back to my internist, and he discontinued the cyclobenzaprine and ordered propoxyphene napsylate–acetaminophen (Darvocet) for pain. With this drug, I could manage to sit at my computer for almost a complete day, but I continued to lose weight and could not sleep.

My parents, who lived out of state, insisted that I come home for a visit. This entailed a 6-hour car ride. I complied with their wishes, although I knew I could not sit still for more than a few hours without experiencing increased pain. I arrived at my parents in acute distress. I had never told them about the accident, and I did not tell them during the visit. I slept on a pull-out bed, which was very soft and did not support my back and neck. When I left my parents, I was in excruciating pain; after I got home, I called my doctor, who prescribed Fiorinal with Codeine. This did little to relieve my pain during the day, but I began to sleep a little better.

Surgery Becomes an Option

I could not work the following week because of muscle spasms in my back. I called my doctor multiple times because of the pain. He insisted that I now consult an orthopedic surgeon. The surgeon diagnosed me as having facet injury and recommended extensive surgery. My husband was pressuring me to have the surgery because we had not been able to be intimate since before the accident because of my back and neck pain.

I wanted a second opinion before surgery. The second physician suggested I try physical therapy and counseling before surgery. I felt it was important to try the more conservative treatment before resorting to surgery. I chose a certified specialist in adult psychiatric nursing for my counselor. When I talked to her on the phone, she encouraged me to begin a holistic approach to my problems. She said that I needed to deal with the components of my life that contribute directly to my physical pain and my inability to recover from the accident.

A Psychophysiological Approach

I see my counselor once a week, and I go to physical therapy three times a week. In therapy, I have learned to control my pain with deep breathing and imagery. I practice every day. I take deep breaths and imagine myself at my grandfather's farm. I pretend to go there as I did as a child. I walk through the fields and visit with the animals. It was a safe, secure place for me, and now I revisit it in my mind daily. I have stopped taking the Fiorinal with Codeine, and I just take two to four ibuprofen a day to help ease the muscle spasms. The physical therapist has taught me to do stretching exercises, and I do them daily also.

A New Approach to Life

In counseling, I also have learned to accept myself as a person who has been in an accident and now has pain. I have told my boss that I cannot do overtime for now and that I must stretch every hour. I find that I am more productive when I rest. This was a hard lesson for me—I felt like I was giving up and allowing my pain to rule my life. I also have been more honest with my parents and my husband. My parents just cannot seem to understand that I cannot drive to their house and that they will have to visit me. They call me selfish and refuse to visit. It's difficult not seeing my parents; even though they are in good health, they have never been to my home. I am learning in counseling that always doing what another person wants is "codependent behavior." My husband has been more understanding. He has learned to listen to me, and we have been able to resume a different but in some ways more satisfactory sexual relationship.

My injury will be with me the rest of my life. It has taught me a valuable lesson in taking care of myself and being honest about my feelings. Spiritually, I have developed a very strong personal connection with God. I am learning to depend on Him. I realize that I can still be a good person without overfunctioning in my relationships. I also feel I am taking better care of myself. This injury has taught me to ask for the things I need. I wish my back would just be better, but it is not; however, I can live a full, healthy life if I allow myself. ■

HISTORICAL OVERVIEW

Mechanistic View

The modern medical model is based on the philosophy of René Descartes. In 1632, Descartes described the human body as a machine that operates on scientific principles. This mechanistic view of the body split the mind and spirit from the body (Descartes, 1967). Even today, many health care practitioners treat the patient's body and not the whole person.

Theory of Homeostasis

Claude Bernard's (1957) theory of homeostasis described the body as a self-regulating machine that is kept in balance through feedback from one organ to another. Bernard's model has made explorations about the links among mind, body, and spirit in health and illness almost impossible to consider. Viewing the body as a machine, it is impossible to consider how the lifestyle, emotions, and spirituality affect this machine that is the person and contribute to health and illness.

Psychophysiology describes an illness as an interaction between the mind, body, and spirit. Almost all physical problems are affected by the mind and spirit. Stress is generally accepted to play a part in most illnesses.

Theory of Stress

The theory of stress and how it affects the body began with the work of Walter Cannon (1929). Cannon elucidated the body's capacity to fight or flee during stress. The "fight or flight" response is a sympathetic nervous system reaction that causes the release of epinephrine and norepinephrine to most major organ systems. This response is adaptive for a short period of time and mobilizes the body for intense exertion. However, these responses can be maladaptive and lead to disease if they continue for a prolonged period.

Hans Selye (1956) described the general adaptation syndrome (GAS). Selye reported a triad of pathological consequences to prolonged stress: adrenal gland enlargement, thymus involution, and gastrointestinal ulceration. Current research indicates that Selye's GAS was not completely correct. In a series of classic studies, Mason (1968, 1971) refined the stress response and demonstrated that it is more specific than originally described by Selye.

A stress is a stimulus that is perceived by the person. To be viewed as stressful, this stimulus must be perceived consciously or unconsciously as a threat to the person. The person also must feel that the demand made by the stress is beyond his or her ability to cope. This threat sets off a series of physiological responses. Repeated and prolonged episodes of arousal in the absence of active movement toward resolution of the conflict set up the pathway for physical illness (Girdano, Everly, & Dusek, 1997; Sterling & Eyer, 1981). Figure 32–1 presents an overview of the factors that affect the relationship between stress and physical illness.

Factors within the person (age, sex, socioeconomic status, occupation, education, and fitness) all interact to decrease or increase this response. Behaviors of the person also modify the stress response (smoking, alcohol, drug use and abuse, eating habits, and exercise).

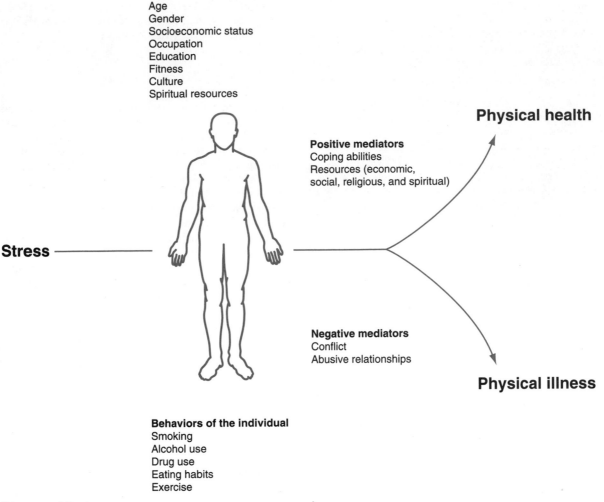

Factors within the individual
Age
Gender
Socioeconomic status
Occupation
Education
Fitness
Culture
Spiritual resources

Physical health

Positive mediators
Coping abilities
Resources (economic,
social, religious, and spiritual)

Stress

Negative mediators
Conflict
Abusive relationships

Physical illness

Behaviors of the individual
Smoking
Alcohol use
Drug use
Eating habits
Exercise

Figure 32-1
An overview of the factors that affect the relationship between stress and physical illness.

Mediating factors diminish (coping, economic resources, and social support) or attenuate (unresolved conflict and abusive relationships) the person's responsiveness. The person's coping abilities, spiritual support, and economic resources, as well as "people" resources such as family and friends, modify reactivity. Unresolved conflict and abusive relationships intensify reactivity.

Psychophysiological disorders are conditions that are thought to be a result of excessive arousal, maladaptive coping, and chronic distress. Stress may act as a catalyst for a disease already present in the body or accelerate the progression of an illness. Stress leads to a person's diminished capacity to defend against and recover from illness with a rapid response.

> **W**hat do you think? What factors influence your response to stress?

➤ *Check Your Reading*
1. What does the theory of homeostasis say about the body?
2. What is GAS?
3. Identify two factors within the person that either decrease or increase the individual's responsivity to stress.
4. Identify two mediating factors that diminish or attenuate responsivity to stress.

DIAGNOSIS

Diagnosis begins with a multifaceted **psychophysiological assessment.** The clinical history is focused on the whole person, the person's story, not just the physical symptom. A careful social, educational, occupational, spiritual, and family history can elucidate the relationships among the person's presenting problem and the rest of her or his life.

Use of Psychometric Instruments

The use of psychometric instruments can answer specific questions regarding the psychological status of the patient. The instruments selected for review here are only a small number of those available for use.

State-Trait Anxiety Inventory

The State-Trait Anxiety Inventory (STAI) (Speilberger, Gorsuch, & Lushene, 1970) is a 40-item tool that contains self-report scales for measuring two different types of anxiety: state and trait. The STAI-Trait Anxiety Scale contains 20 statements that ask respondents to describe how they usually feel. The scale also contains 20 items but asks for a description of how the respondent feels at a specific point in time. The STAI is a popular tool for assessing anxiety; it is convenient, reliable, grounded in psychological theory, and able to be used in many contexts.

Beck Depression Inventory

The Beck Depression Inventory (BDI) (Beck, 1972) is an instrument that approximates clinical judgments of depression. The inventory is composed of 21 multiple-choice items that reflect specific behavioral signs of depression. The behavioral signs are weighted in severity from 0 to 3. The BDI is widely used in both research and clinical situations.

Coping Strategies Questionnaire

The Coping Strategies Questionnaire (CSQ) is a 48-question checklist in which subjects report the degree to which they use six cognitive and two behavioral coping strategies. The CSQ also contains two additional categories related to the subjective ability to control and decrease pain. This instrument is widely used to assess patients' coping with pain.

Derogatis Stress Profile

The Derogatis Stress Profile (DSP) is a 77-question tool that provides assessment under decreasingly specific aspects: 11 dimensions, three domains, and an overall global stress score. The domains are environment, personality mediators, and emotional response. The dimensions are domestic, vocational, health, time pressure, driven behavior, attitude, posture, role definition, relaxation potential, anxiety, depression, and hostility (corresponding to the three domains listed previously). The DSP is a useful tool for evaluating the general stress a patient is under and the various stresses a patient experiences (Derogatis, 1995).

Life Experience Survey

Sarason, Johnson, and Siegel (1978) developed the Life Experience Survey (LES) to measure a person's assessment of life stresses experienced during the preceding year. The LES is a 57-item self-report inventory. The respondent is asked to identify which events were experienced during the past year, whether the event was viewed as positive or negative on a seven-point scale, and what was the perceived impact of the event rated on a seven-point scale. A higher score on the LES is indicative of increasing life stress.

Symptom Check List 90

The Symptom Check List (SCL) 90 (revised) is a 90-item self-report symptom inventory (Derogatis, 1977). Each item is rated on a five-point scale from "not at all" to "extremely." The responses are then interpreted along nine symptom severity dimensions: somatization, obsessive-compulsive, interpersonal sensitivity, depression, anxiety, hostility, phobic anxiety, paranoid ideation, and psychoticism. Scoring requires adding specific items for each of the nine dimensions to obtain distress scores. This test briefly evaluates a broad range of symptoms. It can serve as a screening tool and guide the practitioner to further evaluation.

Sickness Impact Profile

The Sickness Impact Profile may be used to assess quality of life. It consists of 136 questions assessing 12 categories involved in daily living and indicates an individual's perception of his or her ability to perform these activities. It is scored by scaling within the categories, and also has an overall score. The 12 categories assessed are (physical dimension) ambulation, mobility, body care and movement; (psychosocial dimension) social interaction, communication, alertness, behavior, sleep and rest, eating, work, home management, and recreation and pastimes (Gilson et al., 1975).

Sarason Social Support Questionnaire

The Sarason Social Support Questionnaire (SSQ-6) (Sarason, Sarason, & Shearin, 1986, 1987) consists of six items, each of which presents a given set of circumstances that require social support. The tool then asks on whom the respondent could rely in that situation and how satisfied they are with that support. The number of supports are quantified. In addition, the individual's satisfaction with support is measured by the use of a six-point scale.

Spiritual Well-Being Scale

Most psychophysiological assessments do not include the spiritual dimension. This is a serious oversight leading to an incomplete database. Ellison's (1983) Spiritual Well-Being Scale could appropriately be used, along with additional interview questions, to assess spiritual health. The instrument consists of two subscales, the Religious Well-Being and the Existential Well-Being subscales. The religious scale measures the individual's well-being in relationship to God; the existential scale measures the individual's well-being in relationship to a personal sense of life's meaning and significance. Each of the subscales has 10 items rated on a Likert scale of 0 to 6.

Other Psychometric Instruments

Many other specific tools can be used to evaluate the various psychophysiological disorders. The McGill Pain Questionnaire is standard for the evaluation of chronic pain. Visual analogue scales and pain drawings are frequently used for a subjective evaluation of chronic pain. Diaries often are important to document the patient's symptoms and drug use.

Use of Measures of the Stress Response

The final aspect of assessment is a psychophysiological measurement of the stress response. The measurement of temperature, heart rate, and blood pressure (BP) responses during a discussion of a stressful event provides documentation of physiological reactivity. Twenty-four-hour monitoring of heart rate and BP along with keeping of a diary of daily events contributes an overview of cardiovascular reactivity.

> **What do you think?** What is your response to the significance given to psychometric testing for psychophysiological disorders?

> ➤ *Check Your Reading*
> 5. Why does the assessment include the use of psychometric instruments?
> 6. What is the LES used to evaluate?
> 7. What are the two components of the Spiritual Well-Being Scale?
> 8. How does measuring physiological reactivity contribute to your assessment?

CHRONIC BACK PAIN

An estimated 60% to 80% of Americans experience low back pain at least once in their life, and the majority resolve this pain in fewer than 2 months (Rowlingson, 1993). Monica in the opening story is one of the 10% to 40% of all patients with back injuries who go on to develop a chronic pain disorder (Waddell, 1996). **Chronic back pain** is defined as pain that persists for more than 6 months and results in the need for long-term treatment. A total of 1% to 2% of low back pain is caused by disk herniation. Postural and muscular low back pain account for 80% to 90% of all complaints. Chronic back pain imposes not only the physical impact of the pain but also the emotional, spiritual, and occupational effects. For this reason, this physical disorder has significant implications as a mental health issue.

In a holistic approach to chronic back pain, the definition of pain is made by the patient. The patient describes where the pain is, what exacerbates the pain, and what relieves it. Although no anatomical or physiological basis for the pain which the patient describes may be known, the pain is accepted as described by the patient. The inability to define the precise cause of the patient's pain may be due to our poor understanding of the mechanisms of pain development (Burckhardt,

1990). Low back pain and disability need to be treated concurrently because the most effective method of pain alleviation is to return the patient to his or her normal routine. Both patient and practitioner must be involved in maintaining the patient's treatment in order to effectively treat this illness (Waddell, 1996).

Source

We do know that five pain-producing structures exist in the lower back (Box 32–1). Under normal circumstances, the anterior spinal column with its vertebrae and disks performs the weight-bearing functions of the body. Trauma, dysfunction, or degeneration of the anterior spinal column triggers pain, which causes increased curvature in the lumbar lordotic region. Reflex muscle spasm then occurs in an attempt to stop the motion and decrease irritation of the tissues. These spasms shift the spine and move the weight-bearing functions to the more delicate posterior elements. The facet joints are stressed, the alignment is distorted, and more pain and muscle spasm occur (Rowlingson, 1993).

Specific Diagnoses

Many specific diagnoses for low back pain reflect the area of dysfunction. Posterior facet syndrome is caused by a rotational strain on both the facet joints and the anulus fibrosus of the intervertebral disk. Myofascial syndrome and piriformis syndrome are caused by spasms and changes in the muscles of the lower back. These syndromes can progress into facet-disk pain, with sustained contractions of the muscles. Sacroiliac syndrome is a common chronic condition in which the exact pathological lesion is obscure, but the lesion involves the muscles and joint of the lower back and hip. As the diagnostic procedures for low back pain are further refined, more specific diagnoses will evolve.

Psychological and Spiritual Responses

Depression, significant spiritual distress, and even drug abuse, are common concurrent issues with chronic back pain and may contribute to the person's assuming a sick role. The loss of occupational and family roles may contribute to the person's depression and sense of despair. Spiritually, the patient may wonder "Why did God

Box 32–1 ■ ■ ■ ■ ■
Pain-Producing Structures in the Lower Back

Posterior longitudinal ligaments
Interspinous ligaments
Nerve roots and dorsal coverings
Facet joints
Deep muscles

let this happen to me?" "Why doesn't He make me better?" and "Does He have a purpose for my suffering?" The answers to these questions contribute to his or her ability to accept and cope with the chronic back pain. Sometimes, the excessive use of pain medications, including narcotic analgesics, results in drug abuse. Alcohol is frequently consumed in greater quantities in an effort to reduce the pain. Withdrawal from pain medication or alcohol can complicate the treatment process.

Treatment

The treatment of chronic back pain emphasizes management of the pain and the accompanying dysfunction. Most low back pain is, and should be, treated by primary care professionals. These patients do not need to be referred to specialists (Waddell, 1996). Three broad categories of treatment exist: medical management, cognitive-behavioral treatments, and spiritual intervention. The goal of treatment is control of pain and resumption of activities (Box 32–2). The patient must be a partner in the planning of care.

Medical Treatment

Aspirin and other nonsteroidal antiinflammatory drugs (NSAIDs) help to decrease the inflammation and should be recommended or prescribed. Muscle relaxants reduce the reflex muscle spasms. Tricyclic antidepressants decrease the underlying depression and promote sleep. Physical therapy is essential to learn how to stretch and relax the back.

Cognitive-Behavioral Treatment

Cognitive-behavioral treatments include biofeedback, relaxation, exercise, and diet. These techniques can be used to help decrease anxiety and muscle spasm (Rowlingson, 1993). Exercise and weight loss are important components in reducing low back pain. Daily stretching and muscle toning exercises strengthen the muscles and decrease pain. Resumption of normal activities is critically important to recovery (Waddell, 1996). Losing weight, especially in the abdominal region, decreases the strain on the back.

Spiritual Intervention

Spiritual intervention includes encouraging the patient to use spiritual resources that have been meaningful in the past and to consider trying new ones. Asking the patient about the meaning of the pain in her or his life is a way to focus the patient on the important spiritual task of providing an acceptance of the new limitations imposed by this chronic illness. The goal of helping the patient to cope with chronic pain is related to the patient's perseverance in maintaining a positive mental outlook.

Box 32–2 ■ ■ ■ ■ ■
An Overview of Chronic Back Pain

Characteristics

Affects 40% of the population

Treatment

Medical
  Aspirin
  Nonsteroidal antiinflammatory drugs
  Muscle relaxants
  Tricyclic antidepressants
Cognitive-behavioral
  Biofeedback
  Relaxation
  Diet
  Physical therapy and exercise
Spiritual
  Helping others
  Inspirational reading
  Journaling
  Music
  Meditation
  Prayer

What do you think? How does knowing about chronic back pain fit in with your notion of psychiatric nursing?

➤ *Check Your Reading*

9. Name one reason why depression often accompanies low back pain.
10. What are included in cognitive-behavioral treatments?

CHRONIC PELVIC PAIN

Chronic pelvic pain is defined as nonmenstrual pelvic pain of greater than 6 months' duration. It may be intermittent or continuous. Chronic pelvic pain is a major diagnosis for women, accounting for 10% of outpatient visits and up to 25% of diagnostic laparoscopies. It is the third most common indication for hysterectomy and accounts for approximately 75,000 hysterectomies annually. The average age of patients with chronic pelvic pain is 30 years (Hillis, Marchbanks, & Peterson, 1995).

Diagnosis

Traditionally, the diagnostic laparoscopic procedure has been used to evaluate the patient with chronic pelvic pain. It has been assumed that if all visible intrapelvic abnormalities have been excluded by laparoscopy, the cause of the pain is psychogenic. A substantial body of controlled investigations shows that the laparoscopic examination, although it can identify the presence of adhesions and endometriosis, cannot differentiate which patients will experience pelvic pain (Hodgkiss & Watson, 1994).

The Nature of the Pain

The pain experienced by women who suffer from chronic pelvic pain is poorly localized because the parenchyma of the internal pelvic organs do not contain pain receptors. The arterial walls in the peritoneum are richly innervated. Pain from the pelvic organs often is perceived at a site far from the source. Pain from the fundus of the uterus is perceived as lower midline abdominal pain. Pain from the ovaries only occurs when stretching of the surrounding peritoneum and vascular structures occurs. Therefore, the description of pelvic pain can be vague and seemingly anatomically incorrect (Hodgkiss & Watson, 1994).

Psychological and Spiritual Responses

Studies have documented that patients whose journey is complicated by chronic pelvic pain are significantly more likely to develop depression, somatization, substance abuse, and sexual dysfunction. Sexual abuse is significantly correlated with chronic pelvic pain (Walker et al., 1995). All of these psychological complications carry a high rate of spiritual distress as well.

Individuals with chronic pelvic pain have a tendency to "doctor shop" in an effort to obtain relief from their pain. The use of analgesic drugs to control pain over an extended period contributes to the risk of drug addiction or dependency.

Treatment

A comprehensive, multidisciplinary approach that addresses the physiological aspects of the pain as well as the psychological and spiritual needs of the patient is necessary.

Medical Treatment

Medications traditionally prescribed include hormones and NSAIDs. Frequently, these women have had several surgeries. About 30% of all chronic pelvic pain patients have already undergone a complete abdominal hysterectomy. After a hysterectomy, 40% of women continue to experience long-term pain (Hillis et al., 1995). Conservative surgical approaches may be considered to relieve pain. These include removal of endometrial implants and presacral neurectomies and lysis of adhesions (Kames, Rapkin, Naliboff, Afifi, & Ferrer-Brechner, 1990).

Psychological and Spiritual Care

The psychological and spiritual components of a comprehensive treatment approach include stress management, relaxation, cognitive therapy, spiritual support, and sex education. The treatment focuses on all aspects of the person's life, including family, social life, spiritual life, occupation, and sexual functioning. The treatment for patients with chronic pelvic pain must be supportive and empathetic (Kames et al., 1990).

Psychological treatment, stress management, and relaxation help women cope with chronic pain. Education concerning the relationship between past abuse and current pain helps women psychologically connect the multifaceted issues they experience. Support groups are another important component to healing (Box 32-3).

> **What do you think?** What do you see as your role in helping a woman who has a history of being sexually abused and who is currently suffering with chronic pelvic pain?

➤ *Check Your Reading*
11. Define chronic pelvic pain.
12. Name two of the psychiatric disorders that are commonly associated with chronic pelvic pain.
13. What does the treatment for chronic pelvic pain include?

HYPERTENSION

Hypertension is a multifactorial psychophysiological illness. The most consistent and profound response during stress is elevation of BP (Timo et al., 1997). Hypertension is a life-threatening disorder and a significant risk factor for the development of coronary artery disease and cerebral vascular disease. More than 16 million Americans have high BP. Hypertension is twice as frequent among blacks as whites (Alexander et al., 1996). Black women have an incidence of hypertension four and a half times higher than that of white women. The incidence of hypertension is greater for men than

Box 32-3 ■ ■ ■ ■ ■
An Overview of Chronic Pelvic Pain

Treatment

Medical
    Medications
    Hormones
    Nonsteroidal antiinflammatory drugs
Psychological
    Stress management
    Relaxation
    Cognitive therapy
    Sexual education

women until women reach menopausal age, when women surpass men (American Heart Association [AHA], 1992).

Hypertension is defined by the World Health Organization as chronically elevated BP exceeding 160/95 mmHg. Borderline hypertension is defined as BP above 140/90 mmHg. The risk of developing fatal or nonfatal end-organ damage is correlated with the amount of rise in blood pressure over 160/95 mmHg (AHA, 1992).

Causes

Physiological Causes

The cause of essential hypertension is unknown, and the pathophysiological mechanisms vary among individuals. High BP may result from increased cardiac output, increased peripheral resistance, and increased blood volume due to decreased sodium and water excretion (Guyton, 1996). Multiple behavioral, psychological, social, dietary, and other factors influence BP and contribute to the development of essential hypertension (Alexander et al., 1996).

Two major psychophysiological theories relate behavioral factors to the development of essential hypertension: the hyperreactivity theory and the symptom specificity theory. The hyperreactivity theory states that excessive reactivity in BP to all environmental stimuli initiates and maintains essential hypertension. The symptom specificity theory states that a consistent reactivity in BP to specific environmental stressors initiates and maintains essential hypertension. Increased cardiovascular reactivity is seen in children of hypertensive parents and in borderline hypertensive persons. This provides support for the theory that increased reactivity is a precursor to essential hypertension (Fredrickson, 1991).

Psychological and Social Causes

Socioeconomic status and stressors, including poverty, low occupational and educational status, and high stress levels, are related to essential hypertension (Alexander et al., 1996). Anger, both suppressed and expressed, is positively related to hypertension (Niaura & Goldstein, 1992). Verbal communication also is related to increased BP reactivity or hypertension. Talking for 2 minutes increases BP from 10% to 50% above resting baseline, and the higher the resting BP, the greater the increase during talking. The faster an individual speaks, the greater the increase in BP (Thomas & Friedmann, 1994). Speaking to a person of perceived higher status causes significantly greater increases in BP than speaking to a person of the same status (Long, Lynch, Machira, Thomas, & Malinow, 1982).

Treatment

The medical management of hypertension has been refined (Box 32-4). The use of pharmacological agents

Box 32-4 ■ ■ ■ ■ ■
An Overview of Hypertension

Characteristics

Gender
  Male
  Female (postmenopausal)
Culture: Blacks twice as likely to get hypertension as whites
Course: Chronic blood pressure greater than 160/95 mmHg

Treatment

Medical: Pharmacological agents
Psychosocial
  Behavior modification
  Relaxation
  Biofeedback
  Diet and exercise
Spiritual
  Helping others
  Inspirational reading
  Journaling
  Music
  Meditation
  Prayer

to reduce BP is generally accepted. For further discussion of drug treatment of hypertension, see general medical-surgical and pharmacology texts.

Dietary interventions include weight reduction, alcohol and caffeine limitation, low-salt diets, and fat and cholesterol reduction. Moderate to excessive use of alcohol is related to increased hypertension. Exercise has been demonstrated to reduce BP. In general, a healthy diet low in fats and salt and a consistent exercise regimen are beneficial in reducing BP (Alexander et al., 1996).

Behavioral and psychological treatments of hypertension include psychotherapy, relaxation, and biofeedback. Biofeedback and relaxation seem to be most effective when combined with pharmacological treatment. These behavioral interventions may permit reduction of medication dose and may decrease end-organ damage (Walton, Pugh, Gelderloos, & Macrae, 1995).

What do you think? How might spiritual distress relate to chronic hypertension?

➤ *Check Your Reading*

14. What does the hyperreactivity theory say about hypertension?
15. What is the relationship of anger to hypertension?
16. What is the effect of speech on BP?
17. Name two of the behavioral and psychological approaches to the treatment of hypertension.

MIGRAINE

Approximately 16 to 18 million people suffer from **migraine headaches** throughout their life journeys. Diagnosis of a migraine rests on the presence of characteristic symptoms in the patient's history. Migraine headaches usually begin in adolescence, although they may begin in childhood. They rarely begin after age 40. Four times as many women as men are treated for migraines. The migraine headache presents with a pulsating quality that is usually, but not always, unilateral. The headache lasts from 2 hours to days. Migraines occur most frequently on awakening but may occur at any time of day. Diamond and Dalessio (1986) reported that migraines are more common on weekends and during vacations; however, this finding was refuted by Morrison (1990). On average, migraines occur one to three times a month and are recurrent.

Symptoms

The prodrome is the period of time preceding the migraine that occurs hours to days before the headache. The prodrome may include subtle symptoms (e.g., change in mood, irritability, or fatigue) or specific symptoms (e.g., blurring of vision, increased sensitivity to sound, or inability to tolerate bright lights). If the patient with migraines learns to recognize his or her specific prodrome pattern, the ability to abort the migraine will increase. Patients suffering with migraines usually have low blood pressure and high heart rates. Their extremities generally are vasoconstricted, causing them to have cold hands and feet. During the migraine, they experience vasodilatation, and their hands, feet, and body become warm. Anorexia, nausea, vomiting, and diarrhea usually accompany the migraine, along with increased urinary frequency. Often, these patients experience increased sensitivity to light, sound, movement, and smell. They complain of tenderness and sometimes swelling on the side of the skull where the headache is experienced. After the headache leaves, patients may feel either euphoric or depressed. Feelings of fatigue may last several days after the headache.

Classification

Migraines are divided into two types: migraine with aura and migraine without aura (International Headache Society, 1988). An aura is a group of neurological symptoms that precedes the headache by 5 to 20 minutes. The most common symptoms of the aura are visual disturbances (Saper, Silverstein, Gordon, & Hamel, 1993). Once the aura begins, the physiological pattern of the migraine is initiated.

Precipitants

Migraines can be precipitated by many factors, including the menstrual cycle, stress, physical activity, caffeine, certain foods, and alcohol. Some women have migraines only during menstruation. Migraines usually decrease or cease after menopause. During pregnancy, migraines usually stop.

Migraines occur after periods of stress when the person relaxes (Benedittis, Lorenzetti, & Pieri, 1990). This may account for the association of migraines with weekends and vacations. Variations in sleeping patterns, hot weather, and humidity also may precipitate a migraine. Chronic use of daily headache medicines may cause rebound headaches.

Mechanism

The precise mechanisms involved in the production of migraine headaches are still under investigation. Vascular, neural, and biochemical factors are involved in migraines. For instance, metabolic factors such as estrogen, tyramine, and tyrosine play a role in many migraine headaches. These factors, in combination with internal and external stress, initiate a cascade of physiological changes (vascular and neural) that produce the headache. The aura is produced by a cortical vasospasm or a spreading depression of neural activity. Pain is inhibited during the aura. After the aura fades, a vasodilation occurs. This eliminates the pain inhibition, and the migraine headache pain begins (Olsen, 1991; Welch, 1987).

Vascular Factors

During a migraine headache, scalp vessels dilate. The aura of the migraine is caused by vasospasm followed by a reactive vasodilation during the headache. The dilation is associated with increased blood vessel permeability and the release of bradykinin and proteolytic enzymes. However, recent evidence shows that the decrease in cerebral blood flow is insufficient to cause neural ischemia and that the subsequent increase in blood flow does not always correlate with the onset of the headache. Increased platelet adhesiveness occurs during a migraine. The increased platelet activity could contribute to the impaired circulation during the migraine (Hilton & Cummings, 1972). Free fatty acids mobilized by norepinephrine may activate the platelets to release serotonin. Bradykinin, histamine, and other polypeptides may act in concert with serotonin in increasing the vascular wall sensitivity to pain.

Neural Factors

Neural theories of migraines propose that the decreased cerebral blood flow in migraines is a consequence of decreased metabolic demands and spreading depression of cortical neural activity. It is still unknown whether vascular or neural mechanisms are the primary causal factor in migraines.

Biochemical Factors

Biochemicals such as serotonin and norepinephrine are the mediators of neural transmission and vascular reactivity. Serotonin levels fall during a migraine. Serotonin promotes platelet aggregation (Dalsgaard-Nielsen & Genefke, 1974; Jarman et al., 1991).

Norepinephrine levels rise during a migraine, causing vasoconstriction in the peripheral vascular bed. Patients with migraines have elevated sympathetic activity and higher norepinephrine levels when compared with people without headaches. The rise may be a response to the physiological stress of the migraine and may be a consequence rather than a precipitating factor.

Other Factors

Of all patients with migraines, 75% have a first-degree relative with migraines. The personality of migraine patients has been described as hard-working, hard-driving, and perfectionistic. Symptoms of depression with insomnia, anorexia, constipation, lack of libido, and feelings of hopelessness are frequently reported.

Foods and beverages that cause vasodilation are associated with migraine headaches. Alcoholic beverages, processed foods containing nitrates, and monosodium glutamate are common triggers. Hard cheeses, beer, and red wine are high in tyramine, which may trigger migraine headaches. Phenylethylamine in chocolate may provoke a headache. Caffeine in food and drinks also may cause vasoconstriction and precipitate a migraine (Saper et al., 1993).

Treatment

Many drugs are used for the prevention and treatment of migraine headaches. Pharmacology texts provide further information regarding drug treatment of migraines.

The most widely used nonpharmacological treatment is relaxation training combined with thermal biofeedback. A metaanalysis evaluating the use of propranolol and the effectiveness of biofeedback and relaxation training concluded that these two different treatments have similar results. Both treatments were associated with a 45% decrease in headaches (Holroyd & Penzien, 1990).

A patient with migraines is encouraged to avoid foods and beverages that might trigger a headache (Saper et al., 1993) and to engage in daily exercise as a preventive strategy for migraines. Exercise causes vasodilation, which reduces the risk of developing a migraine. See Box 32–5 for an overview of management of migraine headaches.

What do you think? Do you or does anyone you know suffer with migraines? If so, what impact does having migraines have on one's life?

➤ *Check Your Reading*

18. Name two precipitants of migraine headaches.

Box 32–5 ■■■■■
An Overview of Migraines

Characteristics

Onset between adolescence and age 40 years
Affects women more frequently than men
Pulsating pain
Pain lasts 2 hours to days
Pain occurs on awakening
Relative with history of migraine
Symptoms of depression and despair
Insomnia, anorexia, constipation

Symptoms

Premigraine
  Prodrome
    Low blood pressure and high heart rate
    Cold hands and feet
During migraine
  Extremities become warm
  Nausea, vomiting, diarrhea
  Sensitivity to light, sound, smell, and movement
  Tenderness on skull
Postmigraine
  Feeling of euphoria or depression
  Fatigue

Treatment

Medical: Multiple pharmacological agents
Psychological
  Relaxation with biofeedback
  Stress management
Spiritual
  Helping others
  Inspirational reading
  Journaling
  Meditation
  Prayer

19. What happens to levels of serotonin during a migraine?
20. What happens to levels of norepinephrine during a migraine?
21. What is the most widely used nonpharmacological treatment for migraine headaches?
22. Name two foods that are associated with migraines.

TEMPOROMANDIBULAR DISORDER

TMD has been defined as chronic or intermittent pain in the face, neck, or ears that is the result of a problem in the mandibular area caused by a variety of joint, muscular, nerve, and dental problems. Symptoms can occur alone or together. A great deal of research has documented that TMD is stress-related (Jones, Rollman, & Brooke, 1997).

Several theories have attempted to explain the cause of TMD. Early theories suggested a displacement of the condyle within the temporomandibular joint. This later was demonstrated to be anatomically impossible. Currently, it is proposed that most of the pain associated with TMD does not come from the joint but from the muscles of mastication. Stress leads to clenching the jaw, and grinding or bruxing teeth and has been found to be the origin of the pain associated with TMD (Katzburg, Westesson, Tallents, & Drake, 1996). Another cause of TMD is removal of upper and lower molars, which can result in misalignment of the jaw, placing a strain or pressure on the mandibular joint. The patient complains of clicks or pain. However, a significant number of patients with mandibular joint pain have normal temporomandibular joints. In addition, patients with molars removed and misalignment of the jaw do not always report pain (Dolwick, 1995).

It is estimated that between 50% and 60% of the general population have experienced one or more of the symptoms of TMD. Women report TMD more frequently than do men, and the symptoms seem to increase with age. TMD frequently is first reported in people in their 30s and 40s (Buxbaum & Myslinski, 1993).

As previously mentioned, a great deal of research has documented that TMD is stress-related (Jones, Rollman, & Brooke, 1997; Rudy, Turk, Kubinski, & Zaki, 1995). In a study of 34 patients experiencing chronic TMD, 50% suffered from major depression and 15% suffered from Posttraumatic Stress Disorder.

In assessing the patient for TMD pain and dysfunction, the health care professional cannot assume that it is the result of only mechanical or neuromuscular problems because sufficient research data suggest that stress also is a factor.

The conservative approach to treating TMD has been found to be the most effective in the majority of cases. The objective of treatment is to rest the joint and relax the muscles. This can be accomplished through the use of local heat; soft diet; NSAIDs; muscle-relaxing drugs; joint exercises; and behavioral, relaxation, and biofeedback therapy. Patients with TMD often benefit from dental appliances (occlusal therapy), which have as their goal the realignment of the joint and the restoration of the normal range of movement of the jaw. Surgical procedures should be avoided in most circumstances except acute injury (Curran et al., 1995). For those patients not responding to standard treatment, appropriate cognitive-behavioral counseling, biofeedback, and the use of spiritual resources are critical to their improvement (Turk, Rudy, Kubinski, Zaki, & Greco, 1996), as noted in Box 32–6.

Box 32–6 ■ ■ ■ ■ ■
An Overview of Temporomandibular Disorder

Characteristics

Affects women more frequently than men
Onset between 30 and 40 years of age
History of depression or stress

Signs and Symptoms

Clenching jaw
Grinding teeth
Misalignment of jaw
Normal joint or some dysfunction

Treatment

Physical
    Dental appliances
    Antiinflammatory drugs
    Muscle relaxants
    Physical therapy
    Soft diet
Psychological
    Behavior modification
    Relaxation therapy
    Biofeedback
Spiritual
    Helping others
    Inspirational reading
    Journaling
    Music
    Meditation
    Prayer

What do you think? What are your thoughts about the significant correlation between depression and TMD?

➤ *Check Your Reading*
23. What is TMD?
24. What is the relationship between stress and TMD?
25. Name two of the treatment approaches used with TMD.

SOMATOFORM DISORDERS

Somatoform disorders are defined as a group of disorders in which the person presents with physical symptoms suggesting a physiological etiology. However, after an in-depth assessment and diagnostic testing, no organic disease or physiological abnormalities are found. Because no positive evidence of physical problems is able to be identified, the presumption is made that the physical problems of substance abuse or of mental disorders (e.g., anxiety attacks) are psychological in origin. A variety of physical symptoms are not under the control of the patient. This group of disorders is so widespread that it may involve 30% to 40% of the medical patients seen in general and family practice settings (Fava, 1992). Somatoform disorders are classified as psychiatric disorders.

Under the heading of Somatoform Disorders, the *Diagnostic and Statistical Manual of Mental Disorders,* Fourth Edition (DSM-IV) (American Psychiatric Association [APA], 1994) lists several distinct and yet possibly related disorders. The seven disorders listed are Body Dysmorphic Disorder, Conversion Disorder, Hypochondriasis, Somatization Disorder, Pain Disorder, Undifferentiated Somatoform Disorder, and Somatoform Disorder Not Otherwise Specified.

They differ from the DSM-IV category Psychological Factors Affecting Medical Conditions because no medical conditions exist in a somatoform disorder. The new DSM-IV category Psychological Factors Affecting Medical Conditions may be useful with patients experiencing psychophysiological disorders. The essential feature of this condition is the presence of one or more specific psychological or behavioral features that negatively affect a general medical condition. It could be used in a patient with low back pain who insists on doing activities that aggravate the pain. Persons with Somatoform Disorders may submit to unnecessary or unwarranted surgical procedures. In addition, because the health care providers are looking for the organic cause of specific symptoms, true pathology may be overlooked. The possibility exists among this group of patients of psychoactive substance abuse because of overuse of prescribed medications.

Many of these patients report a history of avoiding social or occupational activities. Often an obsessive-compulsive personality trait or depression is seen in these patients. These patients experience spiritual distress. They are likely to resist referral for mental health care. The intensity of the symptoms often decreases with support from a concerned health care provider (Box 32-7).

Body Dysmorphic Disorder (Dysmorphophobia)

Body Dysmorphic Disorder is the preoccupation with an imagined flaw in appearance in a normal-appearing person. These patients most frequently focus on a facial defect and less commonly are concerned about physical deformity in other parts of their bodies. The patients may focus on this defect for many hours a day, and these thoughts may dominate their lives with resulting impairment in social work roles. The social isolation and

Box 32–7 ■ ■ ■ ■ ■
An Overview of the Somatoform Disorders

Physical symptoms with no disease or abnormalities
Physical symptoms worsen during crisis
"Physician-shopping"
Unwarranted surgical procedures
Substance abuse
Avoidance of social or work activities
Obsessive-compulsive or depressive personality
Refusing referral for mental health care
Symptoms not intentional (not under conscious control)

depression related to their physical appearance may lead to repeated hospitalizations, suicide attempts, and completed suicides. The key to the identification of a Body Dysmorphic Disorder is the patient's *excessive* concern over the perceived physical defect. Individuals with this problem present as early as the teen years through the 20s. These patients often seek plastic surgery, which will not correct the distorted ideation. No familial pattern or predisposing factors have been identified. It is reported equally in males and females. Body Dysmorphic Disorder is a chronic condition that usually persists for several years. The diagnostic criteria for Body Dysmorphic Disorder are given in Medical Diagnoses and Related Nursing Diagnoses: Body Dysmorphic Disorder.

Conversion Disorder

Conversion Disorder is the presentation of an alteration or loss of a sensory-motor function that is not the result of a physiological disorder. Conversion disorders develop in response to a catastrophic event such as threat of loss or harm, which results in the development of physical symptoms. The resulting symptoms lead to serious deficits in functioning. Although conversion disorders are rarely reported today, this was a common diagnosis 20 years ago. The most common conversion symptoms include paralysis, seizure, disturbance in coordination, or blindness. However, these patients may present with the complete array of neurological symptoms.

The symptoms experienced by the patient are serious but not intentionally produced. The key to the identification of a conversion disorder is that the person appears calm although the symptoms are serious. This calmness and relative lack of concern is referred to as *la belle indifférence.* The patient may also present his or her symptoms in a dramatic manner.

Adolescence and early adulthood is the most common age of onset, although a conversion disorder may appear at any age. Conversion disorder is more common in women than in men, and some data suggest a familial

MEDICAL DIAGNOSES AND RELATED NURSING DIAGNOSES

Body Dysmorphic Disorder

DSM-IV Diagnosis: Body Dysmorphic Disorder

Diagnostic Criteria

A. Preoccupation with an imagined defect in appearance. If a slight physical anomaly is present, the person's concern is markedly excessive.

B. The preoccupation causes clinically significant distress or impairment in social, occupational, or other important areas of functioning.

C. The preoccupation is not better accounted for by another mental disorder (e.g., dissatisfaction with body shape and size in Anorexia Nervosa).

Related Nursing Diagnoses	Definition	Example
Body Image Disturbance	The person experiences or is at risk to experience an alteration in how one perceives one's body. The person expresses (verbally or nonverbally) a negative response to a perceived change in structure or function of the body.	A person has obsessive concern over a small freckle.
Self Esteem, Chronic Low	A person experiences long-standing negative self-evaluation about his or her appearance or capabilities. The person expresses shame or guilt, feels unable to deal with new events or situations, rejects positive feedback, and exaggerates negative feedback about self.	A man who refuses to accept a compliment related to his appearance.

Based on information from the *Diagnostic and Statistical Manual of Mental Disorders. Fourth Edition.* Copyright 1994 American Psychiatric Association. Nursing diagnoses and definitions from North American Nursing Diagnosis Association. (1999). *NANDA nursing diagnoses: Definitions and classification, 1999-2000.* Philadelphia: NANDA.

pattern. Commonly, a predisposing physical illness with similar symptoms has occurred either in the patient or in someone who is close to that person (APA, 1994). It has been reported more frequently in rural populations and in people with lower socioeconomic and educational status.

People who experience a conversion disorder derive **primary gain,** that is, the stress they experienced from the trauma is no longer felt; **secondary gain** also is derived; because of the conversion symptoms, the person no longer has to participate in distasteful or stressful activities, for example, a soldier who develops paralysis of his arm can no longer hold a gun and is therefore removed from combat. The diagnostic criteria for conversion disorder are given in Medical Diagnoses and Related Nursing Diagnoses: Conversion Disorder.

Hypochondriasis

Hypochondriasis has four major criteria:

1. The patient is preoccupied with bodily functions (frequently focusing on heartbeat, breathing, or digestion, or on a minor physical ailment such as a small scratch or cough).

2. The patient interprets the symptoms as indicative of a serious illness.

3. A comprehensive physical examination finds no evidence of a physical disorder.

4. The fear of having a serious illness continues despite medical reassurance that this is not the case.

The beliefs are not delusional, in that the patient can acknowledge the possibility that he or she is exaggerating the extent of the disease or that disease may not be present (APA, 1994). This concern, however, causes clinically significant problems and negatively affects social and work roles.

Hypochondriasis most commonly occurs between the ages of 20 and 30, although it may appear at any age. It is equally common in males and females, and no familial pattern exists. Predisposing factors include stress and past experience with the presenting symptoms. Usually hypochondriasis is chronic, with remission and exacerbation of the symptoms. The problem must be present for at least 6 months and is not better accounted for by other mental or somatoform disorders. It is most important in the diagnosis that the early stages of a medical condition not be overlooked. Physician-shopping is common because patients cannot get the answer they want. These patients resist referral to mental health practitioners (APA, 1994). The diagnostic criteria for hypochondriasis are given in Medical Diagnoses and Related Nursing Diagnoses: Hypochondriasis.

Somatization Disorder

Somatization Disorder is the presentation of many physical complaints that occur with no identified organic basis for the complaints. The identification of somatization must include four pain symptoms in differing sites or functions. The distinction between somatization and conversion disorders is based mainly on the number of signs and symptoms; somatization disorder includes multiple physical symptoms in several body

MEDICAL DIAGNOSES AND RELATED NURSING DIAGNOSES

Conversion Disorder

DSM-IV Diagnosis: Conversion Disorder

Diagnostic Criteria

A. One or more symptoms or deficits affecting voluntary motor or sensory function suggest a neurological or other general medical condition.

B. Psychological factors are judged to be associated with the symptom or deficit because the initiation or exacerbation of the symptom or deficit is preceded by conflicts or other stressors.

C. The symptom or deficit is not intentionally produced or feigned (as in Factitious Disorder or Malingering).

D. The symptom or deficit cannot, after appropriate investigation, be fully explained by a general medical condition, by the direct effects of a substance, or as a culturally sanctioned behavior or experience.

E. The symptom or deficit causes clinically significant distress or impairment in social, occupational, or other important areas of functioning or warrants medical evaluation.

F. The symptom or deficit is not limited to pain or sexual dysfunction, does not occur exclusively during the course of Somatization Disorder, and is not better accounted for by another mental disorder.

Specify type of symptom or deficit:
With Motor Symptom or Deficit
With Sensory Symptom or Deficit
With Seizures or Convulsions
With Mixed Presentation

Related Nursing Diagnoses	Definition	Example
Physical Mobility, Impaired	The person experiences limitations of physical movement but is not immobile. The person has decreased ability to move purposefully, decreased muscle strength or control.	A person who is depressed or who has experienced a traumatic event.
Individual Coping, Ineffective	The person is not able to manage internal or environmental stressors adequately because of inadequate resources (psychological, behavioral, or cognitive). The person is able to state that he or she cannot cope with the situation, uses defense mechanisms inappropriately, and is not able to meet expectations of his or her life roles.	When a person has difficulty adapting to stressful events, the usual coping mechanisms that have been successful in past similar situations may be ineffective.

Based on information from the *Diagnostic and Statistical Manual of Mental Disorders. Fourth Edition.* Copyright 1994 American Psychiatric Association. Nursing diagnoses and definitions from North American Nursing Diagnosis Association. (1999). *NANDA nursing diagnoses: Definitions and classification, 1999-2000.* Philadelphia: NANDA.

MEDICAL DIAGNOSES AND RELATED NURSING DIAGNOSES

Hypochondriasis

DSM-IV Diagnosis: Hypochondriasis

Diagnostic Criteria

A. Preoccupation with fears of having, or the idea that one has, a serious disease based on the person's misinterpretation of bodily symptoms.

B. The preoccupation persists despite appropriate medical evaluation and reassurance.

C. The belief in Criterion A is not of delusional intensity (as in Delusional Disorder, Somatic Type) and is not restricted to a circumscribed concern about appearance (as in Body Dysmorphic Disorder).

D. The preoccupation causes clinically significant distress or impairment in social, occupational, or other important areas of functioning.

E. The preoccupation is not better accounted for by Generalized Anxiety Disorder, Obsessive-Compulsive Disorder, Panic Disorder, a Major Depressive Episode, Separation Anxiety, or another Somatoform Disorder.

Specify if:

   With Poor Insight: If, for most of the time during the current episode, the person does not recognize that the concern about having a serious illness is excessive or unreasonable.

Related Nursing Diagnoses	Definition	Example
Fear	A feeling of physiological or emotional disruption related to an identifiable source that is perceived as dangerous. The person has feelings of apprehension, behaviors of avoidance, and deficits in attention, performance, or control.	The person may feel that he or she is critically ill and will die.
Role Performance, Altered	The person experiences a disruption in how he or she perceives his or her life roles. There is a conflict within the person related to his or her ability to carry out one or more of life's roles (social, work, family).	The person is so preoccupied with his or her perception of having a serious disease that he or she is not able to perform his or her role as parent, spouse, church member.

Based on information from the *Diagnostic and Statistical Manual of Mental Disorders. Fourth Edition.* Copyright 1994 American Psychiatric Association. Nursing diagnoses and definitions from North American Nursing Diagnosis Association. (1999). *NANDA nursing diagnoses: Definitions and classification, 1999-2000.* Philadelphia: NANDA.

systems. The most frequent complaints are pseudoneurological, gastrointestinal, female reproductive, psychosexual, pain, and cardiopulmonary. Many of these patients are anxious or depressed (APA, 1994).

Symptoms of somatization disorders begin during the teen years and occasionally in the 20s. Menstrual difficulties are often one of the earliest complaints in females. Younger patients may present a variety of initial complaints such as abdominal pain, depression, headaches, or seizures. This diagnosis is rare in males. A familial tendency can be seen with somatization disorders. Somatization disorder is a chronic problem; the patient's symptoms vary in seriousness, but it is rare for a year to pass without the patient seeking medical attention (APA, 1994). The diagnostic criteria for somatization disorder are given in Medical Diagnoses and Related Nursing Diagnoses: Somatization Disorder.

Pain Disorder

The patient with **Pain Disorder** is preoccupied with pain when no physical findings account for the pain or for its intensity. Psychological factors play a definite role in the beginning or worsening of pain. This pain is not voluntarily produced, and the diagnosis is not appropriate if the pain is better accounted for by another mental disorder. Pain Disorder usually begins during the 30s and 40s, although it can occur at any age. This diagnosis occurs more frequently in females, particularly with headache and musculoskeletal pain, and some evidence of a familial pattern has been found (APA, 1994).

The patient reports a history of excessive analgesic use with no pain relief and frequently requests surgery. It is not unusual for a patient to have adopted the lifestyle of an invalid. Patients who are also depressed or who have pain related to terminal illness are at increased risk for suicide attempts. The patient with pain disorder resists the possibility that psychological factors may be involved in the complaints of pain and may spend considerable time and energy searching for care.

In many patients, the DSM-IV diagnosis of Major Depression is also appropriate (APA, 1994). The diagnostic criteria for Pain Disorder are given in Medical Diagnoses and Related Nursing Diagnoses: Pain Disorder.

MEDICAL DIAGNOSES AND RELATED NURSING DIAGNOSES

Somatization Disorder

DMS-IV Diagnosis: Somatization Disorder

Diagnostic Criteria

A. A history of many physical complaints beginning before age 30 years that occurred over a period of several years and resulted in treatment being sought or significant impairment in social, occupational, or other important areas of functioning.

B. Each of the following criteria must have been met, with individual symptoms occurring at any time during the course of the disturbance:

(1) *Four pain symptoms:* A history of pain related to at least four different sites or functions (e.g., head, abdomen, back, joints, extremities, chest, rectum, during menstruation, during sexual intercourse, or during urination).

(2) *Two gastrointestinal symptoms:* A history of at least two gastrointestinal symptoms other than pain (e.g., nausea, bloating, vomiting other than during pregnancy, diarrhea, or intolerance of several different foods).

(3) *One sexual symptom:* A history of at least one sexual or reproductive symptom other than pain (e.g., sexual indifference, erectile or ejaculatory dysfunction, irregular menses, excessive menstrual bleeding, vomiting throughout pregnancy).

(4) *One pseudoneurological symptom:* A history of

at least one symptom or deficit suggesting a neurological condition not limited to pain (conversion symptoms such as impaired coordination or balance, paralysis or localized weakness, difficulty swallowing or lump in throat, aphonia, urinary retention, hallucinations, loss of touch or pain sensation, double vision, blindness, deafness, seizures; dissociative symptoms such as amnesia; or loss of consciousness other than fainting).

C. Either (1) or (2):

(1) After appropriate investigation, each of the symptoms in Criterion B cannot be fully explained by a known general medical condition or the direct effects of a substance (e.g., a drug of abuse, a medication).

(2) When a related general medical condition is present, the physical complaints or resulting social or occupational impairment are in excess of what would be expected from the history, physical examination, or laboratory findings.

D. The symptoms are not intentionally produced or feigned (as in Factitious Disorder or Malingering).

Related Nursing Diagnoses	Definition	Example
Pain, Chronic	A person experiences pain that is intermittent or persistent and lasts for more than 6 months. The person may be angered, frustrated, or depressed because of the situation.	A person demonstrates depressive behaviors because he or she is not able to be free of pain.
Management of Therapeutic Regimen, Ineffective	The patient experiences difficulty integrating a program of treatment into his or her daily life because he or she does not receive relief. The patient may state that he or she would like to incorporate the regimen but has difficulty doing so. He or she may choose inappropriate methods for meeting the treatment regimen.	Because of frustration due to no relief from multiple symptoms, physician-shopping occurs and different regimens are used.

Based on information from the *Diagnostic and Statistical Manual of Mental Disorders. Fourth Edition.* Copyright 1994 American Psychiatric Association. Nursing diagnoses and definitions from North American Nursing Diagnosis Association. (1999). *NANDA nursing diagnoses: Definitions and classification, 1999–2000.* Philadelphia: NANDA.

MEDICAL DIAGNOSES AND RELATED NURSING DIAGNOSES

Pain Disorder

DSM-IV Diagnosis: Pain Disorder

Diagnostic Criteria

A. Pain in one or more anatomical sites is the predominant focus of the clinical presentation and is of sufficient severity to warrant clinical attention.

B. The pain causes clinically significant distress or impairment in social, occupational, or other important areas of functioning.

C. Psychological factors are judged to have an important role in the onset, severity, exacerbation, or maintenance of the pain.

D. The symptom or deficit is not intentionally produced or feigned (as in Factitious Disorder or Malingering).

E. The pain is not better accounted for by a Mood, Anxiety, or Psychotic Disorder and does not meet criteria for Dyspareunia.

Code as follows:

Pain Disorder Associated With Psychological Factors: Psychological factors are judged to have the major role in the onset, severity, exacerbation, or maintenance of the pain. (If a general medical condition is present, it does not have a major role in the onset, severity, exacerbation, or maintenance of the pain.) This type of Pain Disorder is not diagnosed if criteria are also met for Somatization Disorder.

Specify if:

Acute: Duration of less than 6 months.

Chronic: Duration of 6 months or longer.

Pain Disorder Associated With Both Psychological Factors and a General Medical Condition: Both psychological factors and a general medical condition are judged to have important roles in the onset, severity, exacerbation, or maintenance of the pain. The associated general medical condition or anatomical site of the pain (see below) is coded on Axis III.

Specify if:

Acute: Duration of less than 6 months.

Chronic: Duration of 6 months or longer.

Note: The following is not considered to be a mental disorder and is included here to facilitate differential diagnosis.

Pain Disorder Associated With a General Medical Condition: A general medical condition has a major role in the onset, severity, exacerbation, or maintenance of the pain. (If psychological factors are present, they are not judged to have a major role in the onset, severity, exacerbation, or maintenance of the pain.) The diagnostic code for the pain is selected based on the associated general medical condition if one has been established or on the anatomical location of the pain if the underlying general medical condition is not yet clearly established—for example, low back, sciatic, pelvic, headache, facial, chest, joint, bone, abdominal, breast, renal, ear, eye, throat, tooth, and urinary.

Related Nursing Diagnoses	Definition	Example
Chronic Pain	See Somatization	The person has significant pain that lasts longer than 6 months (chronic back pain).
Role Performance, Altered	See Hypochondriasis	Because of the pain, the person must take several breaks during the work day to change position and exercise.

Based on information from the *Diagnostic and Statistical Manual of Mental Disorders. Fourth Edition.* Copyright 1994 American Psychiatric Association. Nursing diagnoses and definitions from North American Nursing Diagnosis Association. (1999). *NANDA nursing diagnoses: Definitions and classification, 1999-2000.* Philadelphia: NANDA.

Somatoform Disorder Not Otherwise Specified

Somatoform Disorder Not Otherwise Specified includes disorders with somatoform symptoms that do not meet the criteria for any specific Somatoform Disorder. Some of these disorders are pseudocyesis, which is a false belief accompanied by physical signs of pregnancy; a disorder with nonpsychotic hypochondriacal symp-

toms of less than 6 months' duration; and a disorder involving unexplained physical complaints, such as fatigue or body weakness of less than 6 months' duration that are not due to another mental disorder (APA, 1994).

Undifferentiated Somatoform Disorder

Undifferentiated Somatoform Disorder is when the patient's symptoms and physical findings do not meet the description of Somatoform Disorder. The patient has fewer physical complaints or symptoms, and the symptoms are not voluntarily produced. The symptoms are unlike the multiple exaggerated complaints seen in somatoform disorders. As in many of the somatoform disorders, the symptoms cannot be explained by physical abnormalities after medical examination and are thought to be psychological in origin. In addition, the patient's complaints occur without the diagnosis of another somatoform or psychotic disorder. No data suggest that this diagnosis is more common in one gender or has common predisposing factors or familial tendencies. Many patients with this disorder are anxious and depressed, but they have fewer physical and social limitations than those with Somatoform Disorder. The course of the disease is variable (APA, 1994). The diagnostic criteria for Undifferentiated Somatoform Disorder are given in Medical Diagnoses and Related Nursing Diagnoses: Undifferentiated Somatoform Disorder.

Treatment

Treatment of somatoform disorders traditionally has been limited to insight-oriented psychotherapy; the success of this approach has been limited. Therefore, a holistic framework is more appropriate in conditions in which it is difficult to ascertain a physiological basis. Although patients usually resist suggestions that they may have psychological reasons for these disorders, they respond to a caring environment in which they are respected and not dismissed as "crazy" or "neurotic." When the clinician seriously considers the patient's expressions of pain, other symptoms, and in fact the patient's whole story, the clinician is providing holistic care. In such cases, the patient and the health care provider are more likely to engage and begin effective work toward recovery (Cohen, 1986; Corbin, Hanson, Hopp, & Whitley, 1988; Goldberg, Novack, & Gask, 1992). Table 32–1 summarizes important characteristics of somatoform disorders.

What do you think? After reading this information on somatoform disorders, what would you say to someone who commented that someone's illness is "all in his or her head"?

MEDICAL DIAGNOSES AND RELATED NURSING DIAGNOSES

Undifferentiated Somatoform Disorder

DSM-IV Diagnosis: Undifferentiated Somatoform Disorder

Diagnostic Criteria
A. One or more physical complaints (e.g., fatigue, loss of appetite, gastrointestinal or urinary complaints).
B. Either (1) or (2):
   (1) After appropriate investigation, the symptoms cannot be fully explained by a known general medical condition or the direct effects of a substance (e.g., a drug of abuse, a medication).
   (2) When a related general medical condition is present, the physical complaints or resulting social and occupational impairments are in excess of what would be expected from the history, physical examination, or laboratory findings.

C. The symptoms cause clinically significant distress or impairment in social, occupational, or other important areas of functioning.
D. The duration of the disturbance is at least 6 months.
E. The disturbance is not better accounted for by another mental disorder (e.g., another Somatoform Disorder, Sexual Dysfunction, Mood Disorder, Anxiety Disorder, Sleep Disorder, or Psychotic Disorder).
F. The symptom is not intentionally produced or feigned (as in Factitious Disorder or Malingering).

Related Nursing Diagnoses	Definition	Example
Role Performance, Altered	See Hypochondriasis	Because of excessive fatigue, a mother is unable to care for her children.
Ineffective Individual Coping	See Conversion Disorder	Mechanisms used in past situations do not help the person adjust in this situation.

Based on information from the *Diagnostic and Statistical Manual of Mental Disorders. Fourth Edition.* Copyright 1994 American Psychiatric Association. Nursing diagnoses and definitions from North American Nursing Diagnosis Association. (1999). *NANDA nursing diagnoses: Definitions and classification, 1999-2000.* Philadelphia: NANDA.

TABLE 32-1 Important Characteristics of the Somatoform Disorders

DISORDER	DESCRIPTION	AGE	GENDER	PREDISPOSING FACTORS
Body Dysmorphic Disorder	Excessive attention to imagined flaws in appearance, usually on an exposed body part	Teens to 30s	No gender differences	None
Conversion Disorder	The person is calm while experiencing symptoms such as paralysis, seizures, or blindness	Teens to early adulthood	More frequent in females	Catastrophic event (war or disaster); the person may have been exposed to a disease with similar symptoms.
Hypochondriasis	Preoccupation with body function (heart rate, breathing); the person is convinced that he or she has a serious illness but can acknowledge that he or she may be exaggerating.	20 to 30	No gender differences	Stress and past experience with symptoms
Somatization Disorder	Expression of several symptoms in several body systems	Teens to 20	More common in females than in males	Menstrual difficulties, abdominal pain, depression, headache
Pain Disorder	Preoccupation with pain with no real physical cause identified	Any age	More common in females than in males	History of use of analgesics. The patient typically denies the possibility of psychological involvement. Major depression may be present.
Undifferentiated Somatoform Disorder	Fewer physical symptoms than above; no physical cause can be found.	None identified	No gender differences	None identified
Somatoform Disorder Not Otherwise Specified	Somatoform symptoms that do not meet the criteria for any specific somatoform disorder	None identified	No gender differences	None identified

➤ *Check Your Reading*

26. What does *la belle indifférence* mean? In what somatoform disorder is this symptom commonly seen?
27. What is a Conversion Disorder?
28. What are the characteristics of Somatoform Disorder?
29. What is Body Dysmorphic Disorder?

NURSING PROCESS

The focus of care for patients with psychophysiological disorders is holistic, taking into account physical, psychosocial, and spiritual sources for the behavior that is being demonstrated.

Assessment

Assess the whole person—mind, body, and spirit—rather than just the signs and symptoms of the disease. Keep in mind that multiple causes for the presenting signs and symptoms may exist. Understanding this helps the nurse to perform a comprehensive assessment in which he or she collects physical, psychosocial, and spiritual data about the patient and family that may have an impact on the patient's care.

Diagnosis

Specific nursing diagnoses are based on the assessment of the patient and her or his presenting behaviors. Although two patients may have the same psychophysiological illness and display similar signs and symptoms, the nursing diagnoses for these two patients may be quite different because of the uniqueness of each patient (Carpenito, 1993).

When developing nursing diagnoses for patients with psychophysiological disorders, it also is important that the diagnoses describe not only the patient's physiological problems but also his or her psychosocial and spiritual problems. Nursing diagnoses for patients with psychophysiological problems therefore truly run the gamut from A (activity intolerance) through S (social isolation). For example, for the patient with chronic back pain, appropriate diagnostic labels addressing physical problems might include Pain and Fatigue. Likewise, appropriate diagnostic labels addressing psychosocial and spiritual problems might include Anxiety, Knowledge Deficit, Self Esteem Disturbance, and Altered Role Performance.

Spirituality is a significant aspect of any chronic illness, because of its wearing and relentless nature (Carpenito, 1993). The spiritual components of the patient's life should be thoroughly reviewed.

Let us look now at how a specific diagnostic label, Ineffective Individual Coping (a label that could well apply in any psychophysiological disorder), might apply to the 28-year-old woman, Monica, with chronic back pain:

Ineffective Individual Coping related to frequent and intense pain, as evidenced by weight loss, fatigue, and poor judgment related to decisions or activities

Outcome Identification

The expected outcomes for a particular patient depend on the specific psychophysiological illness and nursing diagnoses. For the patient with chronic back pain whose diagnosis we just examined, an appropriate expected outcome might be as follows:

The patient will experience significant relief and improved management of pain from her back pain.

Planning

The short-term goals for a particular patient depend on her or his medical diagnosis, her or his nursing diagnoses, and the expected outcomes flowing from those diagnoses. For our patient with back pain, short-term goals might be as follows:

Expected Outcome
The patient will experience significant relief and improved management of pain related to back pain.

Short-Term Goals
- The patient will verbalize feelings of stress, fear, or anger.
- The patient will express her feelings in a nondestructive manner.
- The patient will verbalize the connection between stress and pain.
- The patient will participate in the treatment program designed to decrease or control the chronic back pain.

- The patient will use problem-solving to identify positive alternative coping strategies.
- The patient will demonstrate alternative coping strategies for dealing with pain, stress, and emotional problems.
- The patient will verbalize an understanding of the relationships among stress, lifestyle issues, exercise, and the occurrence of back pain.
- The patient will verbalize an understanding of the relationship between spirituality and physical health.
- The patient will develop plans for follow-up therapy to maintain and continue her progress.

Implementation

Direct your nursing interventions first toward the patient and second, toward the patient's family. For our patient with chronic back pain and a nursing diagnosis of Ineffective Individual Coping related to frequent and intense pain, the interventions used to meet the short-term goals with the patient would include

- Focusing care on both physical problems and psychosocial and spiritual problems.
- Discussing with the patient the relationships among physical, psychosocial, and spiritual issues.
- Asking the patient about her perceptions of the back pain. How does she understand this back pain? What does she think causes her pain? What does she think will help the pain?
- Asking the patient to identify goals for the care she is receiving. Enlist the full engagement of the patient in the healing process by using open-ended questions, encouragement, and active listening.
- Helping the patient to complete a stress inventory of her lifestyle, support systems, dependency needs, expression of emotions, and spiritual supports. Encourage the patient to identify areas where change is needed.
- Discussing with the patient the results of the stress inventory. The patient may be unaccustomed to making links between lifestyle issues, sources of stress and satisfaction, spiritual resources, and the development of physical symptoms.
- Providing positive feedback when the patient begins to express her feelings about emotional issues.
- Role-playing to build the patient's confidence in her abilities to express her feelings verbally, especially with her parents.
- Teaching the patient stress management strategies, such as meditation, thought-stopping techniques, deep breathing and relaxation, and rehearsal of stressful interpersonal situations. All these strategies are effective at managing and defusing stress; the more effective the patient is at managing stress, the less she will express the stress somatically.
- Gradually making the link between emotions and physical expressions. Positively reinforce the patient's growing awareness of this link.
- Teaching the patient the use of the problem-solving approach. The patient may never have learned a

logical, step-by-step approach to dealing with problems.

- Teaching the patient about the importance of lifestyle changes in managing stress. Good nutrition, eliminating caffeine and alcohol from the diet, regular exercise, and adequate rest are essential parts of this teaching.
- Teaching the patient about the significance of spirituality in healing; the importance of finding balance in meeting physical, emotional, and spiritual needs; and the importance of finding time for God (however the individual defines God) and spiritual practices.
- Teaching the patient about the importance of follow-up treatment to serve as a check on progress made and to help her modify strategies that need fine-tuning.

For this same patient, the family interventions used to meet the short-term goals would include

- Teaching the family the concept of psychophysiological illness and the relationship between stress and physical signs and symptoms.
- Involving the family in teaching stress management techniques. Family members can be a powerful support if they are knowledgeable about what is helpful to the patient.
- Involving the family in teaching about lifestyle issues. Again, the support of a family in changing diet, exercise, and rest patterns can make the difference between success and failure.
- Talking with the family or significant other to determine whether they are communicating that only physical symptoms are acceptable, and that verbal expression of feelings is unacceptable. If this is the message being received by the patient, the patient's continued improvement is in question.

Evaluation

Evaluation involves returning to the expected outcomes and short-term goals. Looking at the short-term goals is the formative aspect of the evaluation and tells the nurse whether the plan is on the right track. If the short-term goals are not being met, review the interventions and the assessment data to determine whether the assessment was complete and whether the interventions were appropriate and adequate. For instance, the nurse caring for our patient with chronic back pain might evaluate that the patient experienced difficulty in verbalizing the relationship between stress and physical symptoms. During the teaching intervention, the nurse observed that the patient was a very concrete learner. This was not part of the initial data assessment. The nurse then modified the intervention to use a different teaching technique. Apply this process to every short-term goal and make appropriate modifications.

The summative evaluation focuses on the expected outcomes. In the example that we have been using, the nurse caring for the patient with back pain would ask, "Is the patient experiencing significant relief and improved management of the pain from chronic back pain?" If the answer is yes, then the nurse can conclude that the plan was effective; if the answer is no, then the nurse reviews the whole process, from assessment to interventions, to determine the appropriate modifications. See Snapshot: Nursing Interventions Specific to a Psychophysiological Disorder.

➤ *Check Your Reading*
30. What are the three areas to assess in patients with psychophysiological illnesses?

NURSING PROCESS APPLICATION

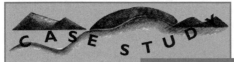

Monica

The case study approach for outcome identification planning and implementation in Monica's case might read as follows.

ASSESSMENT

Assessment data are as follows:
- Chronic back and neck pain described as increasingly intolerable since auto accident
- Guarded body movements
- Fatigue and feelings of despair in life situation
- Social withdrawal from usual activities and friends
- Pain increases with stress
- Spiritual distress results from her emotional and physical problems

DIAGNOSIS

DSM-IV Diagnosis: Chronic Pain

Nursing Diagnosis: Chronic Pain related to back and neck injury for past 2 years as evidenced by statements of pain and guarded body movements

OUTCOME IDENTIFICATION, PLANNING, AND IMPLEMENTATION

> **Expected Outcome 1:** By _____ the patient will achieve a satisfactory measure of pain control and engage in activities of daily living without preoccupation of pain.

Short-Term Goals	Nursing Interventions	Rationales
By _____ the patient will accept some pain and learn how to cope more effectively with it.	1. Acknowledge and validate patient's experience of pain.	1. All pain experiences are real. Pain always has a cause, either physical or psychological in origin.
	2. Encourage the patient to identify situations that influence the occurrence and severity of pain.	2. Pain assessment is paramount to understanding the nature of pain. Pain is individualized—personal meanings and situations that evoke emotional responses influence the expression of pain.
	3. Involve the patient in setting goals for establishing pain management.	3. Involving the patient increases her feelings of autonomy and control by her participating actively in her pain-control program.
	4. Provide for adequate rest.	4. Fatigue will increase the patient's perception of pain. The patient will use noninvasive pain relief measures, including diversional and recreational activities.
By _____ the patient will use two noninvasive pain relief measures.	1. Teach the patient ways to manage pain such as biofeedback, relaxation, meditation, skin stimulation (heat or cold), massage, imagery, music, and recreational and diversional activities (e.g., crafts, painting).	1. This encourages the patient to take responsibility for treatment of pain and allows her the opportunity to select which noninvasive method works best.
	2. Give positive feedback on efforts to share feelings and to use pain relief measures.	2. Encouragement helps the patient receive support.

Nursing Diagnosis: Spiritual Distress related to chronic neck and back pain as evidenced by withdrawal from social functions, church activities, and friends, along with feelings of despair

OUTCOME IDENTIFICATION, PLANNING, AND IMPLEMENTATION

> **Expected Outcome 1:** By _____ the patient will participate in social and recreational functions that add positive quality to her life.

Short-Term Goal	Nursing Interventions	Rationales
By _____ the patient will look forward to pleasurable, social activities as a time out from pain.	1. Explore with the patient the specific meaning the pain has in her life.	1. Support the patient's endeavors to find meaning and understanding in her pain suffering.
	2. Encourage the patient to experience life, endure some pain, and to learn ways to move beyond the pain experience.	2. Hopefully, this will add quality to the patient's life situation, prevent despair, and help her cope more effectively.
	3. Provide reassurance to both patient and family as she works through issues and finds meaning in her pain.	3. Supportive therapy is important during this time and assists both the patient and her family to cope.
	4. Provide activities the patient can do with others and enlarge her support system.	4. This will provide her the opportunity to be with others and experience pleasure and prevent a sense of aloneness.
	5. Encourage participation in social church functions.	5. Choosing activities that build on the patient's interests and personal strengths fosters greater participation.

EVALUATION

Formative Evaluation: Monica achieved all of the short-term goals. She began to understand that her unresolved issues with her family contributed to her back pain experience. She found that church groups and meditation were helpful therapies to deal with her pain.

Summative Evaluation: Monica achieved all of the expected outcomes through outpatient counseling. She became active in her church and her husband reported they were beginning to make contact with their old set of friends. She still experienced back pain but was able to use relaxation, meditation, and imagery to respond and deal with the pain at work and at home, which strengthened her self-esteem and promoted a more satisfying life. Support from her husband helped her recovery.

SNAPSHOT

Nursing Interventions Specific to Psychophysiological Disorder

What do you need to do to develop a relationship with a patient suffering from a psychophysiological disorder?
- Approach the patient with understanding and acceptance that the patient's symptoms are real.
- Convey to the patient that the problem (symptoms) are not "all in his (or her) mind."
- Address the issues the patient brings up with honest, clear answers.
- Find ways of supporting the patient's view without denying the mind-body connection.
- Encourage the patient to identify things that make the patient's symptoms worse.
- Encourage the patient to identify things that make the patient feel better.
- Support the patient's efforts to develop healthy life habits.

What do you need to assess regarding the patient's health status?
- Identify destructive behaviors (affective and behavioral) that make the physical symptoms worse.
- Identify if the patient is responding with self-isolation, blaming, guilt, anger, hopelessness, fear, and depression. These may be evaluated and quantified using a standard tool, such as the Beck Depression Inventory, Derogatis Stress Profile, or Holmes-Rahe Life Event Inventory.
- Identify physiological changes, including increasing frequency and severity of symptoms, weight loss, sleeplessness, fatigue, and development of new symptoms.
- Identify cognitive responses: self-blame, rumination over the past (past surgeries, medical treatments), and inability to make decisions.

- Measure vital signs, including heart rate, blood pressure, and hand temperature (these measurements should ideally be made during periods of stress and relaxation).
- Determine response to and compliance with treatment regimen, including determination, exercise, and medication.
- Identify degree of social support.
- Identify knowledge level and readiness to learn.
- Past history of condition.

What do you need to teach the patient and/or the patient's caregiver?
- Mind-body connection with development of symptoms
- Stress physiology and its relationship to symptoms
- Relaxation physiology and alleviation of symptoms
- Importance of determination and exercise to maintain health
- Importance of mind-body-spirit balance

What skills will you want the patient and/or caregiver to demonstrate?
- Deep breathing
- Relaxation techniques
- Ability to use thought-stopping techniques to deal with negative thoughts
- Ability to identify and ask for support
- Ability to relate daily activities to symptoms

What other health professionals might need to be a part of this plan of care?
- Primary care physician and/or psychiatrist who is usually in charge of the overall treatment plan including medication management
- Physical therapist to teach exercises to decrease pain and increase mobility

Conclusions

Psychophysiological disorders are the underlying cause of the majority of visits to internists and family practice physicians. Because psychological and spiritual components affect the patient's physical symptoms, it is important that this group of patients be treated in a holistic manner. Many illnesses belong to this diagnostic category; the chapter presents only the most prevalent. Nurses need to remember that there are multiple causes for presenting symptoms.

Key Points to Remember

- René Descartes viewed the body as a machine, totally separate from mind and soul.
- Walter Cannon was the first to identify the body's capacity to fight or flee during stress.
- Hans Selye described the general adaptation syndrome.
- Stress is a stimulus perceived by the person as a threat that exceeds his or her coping abilities.
- An interaction occurs among stress, factors within the patient, behaviors of the patient, and mediators that influence the development of illness.
- Multiple psychometric instruments are used to assess the psychological functioning of the patient.
- A psychophysiological measurement of stress response is obtained through temperature, heart rate, and blood pressure responses during the discussion of a stressful event.
- Chronic back pain can originate in five pain-producing structures in the lower back.
- Treatment for chronic back pain includes the use of medications as well as cognitive-behavioral treatments.
- Chronic pelvic pain is highly correlated with depression, somatization, substance abuse, sexual dysfunction, and sexual abuse.
- Treatment of chronic pelvic pain includes medications as well as stress management, relaxation, cognitive therapy, and sexual education.
- Essential hypertension is a life-threatening disorder with multifactorial causes.
- The cause of hypertension is unknown, but it is known that factors such as stress, poverty, anger, talking, and educational status can adversely affect blood pressure.
- The hyperreactivity theory states that excessive reactivity in blood pressure to all environmental stimuli initiates and maintains essential hypertension.
- The symptom specificity theory states that a consistent reactivity in blood pressure to specific environmental stressors initiates and maintains essential hypertension.
- Treatment for hypertension includes medication, behavioral and psychological interventions, and lifestyle changes.
- Migraine headaches produce pain that can be incapacitating.
- A prodrome is the period preceding the migraine and occurs hours to days before the headache. The prodrome includes many symptoms, for example, change in mood, irritability, fatigue, blurring of vision, and increased sensitivity to sound.
- Migraines are divided into two types: migraine with aura and migraine without aura.
- An aura is a group of neurological symptoms that precede a headache by 5 to 20 minutes.
- Migraines can be precipitated by stress, caffeine, certain foods, and alcohol, as well as by the menstrual cycle.
- Serotonin plays a role in migraine headaches; serotonin falls during a migraine and promotes platelet aggregation that may contribute to the decrease in cerebral blood flow during a headache.
- Norepinephrine levels rise during a migraine, causing vasoconstriction in the peripheral vascular bed.
- Treatment of migraine headaches includes medications as well as relaxation training combined with thermal biofeedback.
- Temporomandibular disorder (TMD) is defined as chronic or intermittent pain in the face, neck, and/or ears that is the result of a problem in the mandible joint caused by a variety of muscular, nerve, or dental problems.
- TMD has a strong stress component in its etiology.
- The treatment of TMD includes medication, joint exercises, relaxation training, and biofeedback therapy.

Learning Activities

1. Keep a lifestyle journal for a week. Write down your activity, how you are feeling about doing the activity, and any bodily responses you have to doing this activity.
2. Review your journal. Did your bodily responses correspond with physical problems you might have? For example, did you feel tightness in your head? If so, are you prone to headaches? What feelings were being expressed through your pain?
3. Pay attention to what mediates or lessens your body's response to stress. Do you use any strategies that could be generalized to dealing with stress in a healthy manner?
4. Review the guidelines for relaxation, controlled breathing, and guided imagery that appear in Chapter 23. Practice these over the next week while you monitor your body's response to stress. Note any change. If a change occurs, note what it is.

Critical Thinking Exercise

Veronica is a 10th grader at Barton High. She visits the nurse's office weekly with somatic complaints such as stomach aches, menstrual cramps, headaches, and sore throat. She tells the nurse that she lives with her father and uncle. Most of the time she visits the nurse during the second class period, gym class. The gym teacher is concerned that Veronica is trying to avoid gym. When Veronica does go to gym class, she refuses to shower with the other girls. In consulting the nurse, the gym teacher has requested that Veronica be returned to class as soon as possible when she sees the nurse. She wonders if Veronica might have some other problem.

1. What does the gym teacher seem to be assuming?
2. Give an alternative viewpoint that could be plausible and fits the facts.

3. Under what assumptions do you think Veronica is operating?

After 1 month, the nurse asks Veronica why she visits the office so frequently. Veronica starts to cry, stating that she does not like to exercise because it hurts her back. The nurse makes an appointment with the doctor to examine Veronica's back. On the day of the appointment, Veronica is absent.

1. What can the nurse infer from Veronica's behavior?
2. Make sense of the data.
3. What conclusions, if any, can you draw from the given evidence?

Additional Resources

Buros Institute of Mental Measurements
http://www.unl.edu/buros/

Georgetown University's Web page with medical links
http://www.dml.georgetown.edu/hsintresources.html

Internet Mental Health
http://www.mentalhealth.com/

Temporomandibular disorders
http://www.nidr.nih.gov/news/pubs/tmd/menu.htm

References

Alexander, C. N., Schneider, R. H., Staggers, F., Sheppard, W., Clayborne, B. M., Rainforth, M., Salerno, J., Kondwani, K., Smith, S., Walton, K., & Egan, B. (1996). Trial of stress reduction for hypertension in older African Americans, Part II: Sex and risk subgroup analysis. *Hypertension 28*, 228-232.

American Heart Association. (1992). *1993 Heart and stroke facts statistics*. Dallas, TX: Author.

American Psychiatric Association. (1994). *Diagnostic and statistical manual of mental disorders* (4th ed.). Washington, DC: Author.

Beck, A. (1972). *Depression: Causes and treatment*. Philadelphia: University of Pennsylvania Press.

Benedittis, G., Lorenzetti, A., Pieri, A. (1990). The role of stressful life events in the onset of chronic primary headache. *Pain, 40,* 65-75.

Bernard, C. (1957). *An introduction to the study of experimental medicine*. New York: Dover Publications.

Burckhardt, C. (1990). Chronic pain. *Nursing Clinics of North America, 25,* 863-870.

Buxbaum, J., & Myslinski, N. (1993). Headache associated with temporomandibular dysfunction. In C. Tollison & R. Kunkel (Eds.), *Headache diagnosis and treatment*. Baltimore: Williams & Wilkins.

Cannon, W. (1929). *Bodily changes in pain, hunger, fear and rage: An account of recent research into the function of emotional excitement* (2nd ed.). New York: Appleton.

Carpenito, L. (1993). *Nursing diagnosis: Application to clinical practice* (5th ed.). Philadelphia: J. B. Lippincott.

Carson, V. B. (1989). *Spiritual dimensions of nursing practice*. Philadelphia: W. B. Saunders.

Cohen, S. (1986, June 15). Somatoform disorders: Symptoms and psychiatric implications. *Hospital Practice*, 165-198.

Corbin, L. J., Hanson, R. W., Hopp, S. A., & Whitley, A. C. (1988).

Somatoform disorders. How to reduce overutilization of health care services. *Journal of Psychosocial Nursing and Mental Health Services, 26*(9), 31-34.

Curran, S. L., Sherman, J. J., Cunningham, L. L., Okeson, J. P., Reid, K. I., & Carlson, C. R. (1995). Physical and sexual abuse among orofacial pain patients: Linkages with pain and psychologic distress. *Journal of Orofacial Pain 9,* 340-345.

Dalsgaard-Nielsen, T., & Genefke, I. K. (1974). Serotonin (5-hydroxytryptamine) release and uptake in platelets from healthy persons and migrainous patients in attack-free intervals. *Headache, 14,* 26-32.

Derogatis, L. (1977). *SCL-90-R*. Baltimore: Johns Hopkins University Press.

Derogatis, L. (1995). *The Derogatis Stress Profile (DSP): A summary report*. Towson, MD: Clinical Psychometric Research.

Descartes, R. (1967). *Philosophic works of Descartes* (Vol. 2). (E. Haldane & G. Ross, Trans.). Oxford, England: Oxford University Press.

Diamond, S., & Dalessio, D. (1986). *The practicing physician's approach to headache* (4th ed.). Baltimore: Williams & Wilkins.

Dolwick, M. F. (1995). Intra-articular disc displacement, Part I: Its questionable role in temporomandibular joint pathology. *Journal of Oral Maxillofacial Surgery, 53,* 1069-1072.

Ellison, C. W. (1983). Spiritual well-being: Conceptualization and measurement. *Journal of Psychology and Theology, 11*(4), 330-340.

Fava, G. (1992). The concept of psychosomatic disorder. *Psychotherapy Psychosomatic, 58,* 112.

Fredrickson, M. (1991). Psychophysiological theories on sympathetic nervous system reactivity in the development of essential hypertension. *Scandinavian Journal of Psychology, 32,* 254-274.

Gilson, B. S., Gilson, J. S., Bergner, M., Bobbitt, R. A., Kressel, S., Pollard, W. E., & Vesselago, M. (1975). The Sickness Impact Profile: Development of an Outcome Measure of Health Care. *American Journal of Public Health, 65,* 1304-1310.

Girdano, D., Everly, G., Jr., & Dusek, D. (Eds). (1997). *Controlling stress and tension: A holistic approach* (5th ed.). Boston: Allyn and Bacon.

Goldberg, R., Novack, D., & Gask, L. (1992). The recognition and management of somatization. *Psychosomatics, 33,* 55-61.

Guyton, A. (1996). *Textbook of medical physiology* (9th ed.). Philadelphia: W. B. Saunders.

Hillis, S. D., Marchbanks, P. A., & Peterson, H. B. (1995). The effectiveness of hysterectomy for chronic pelvic pain. *Obstetrics and Gynecology, 86,* 246-250.

Hilton, B. P., & Cummings, J. N. (1972). 5-Hydroxytryptamine levels and platelet aggregation responses in subjects with acute migraine headache. *Journal of Neurology, Neurosurgery and Psychiatry, 35,* 505-509.

Hodgkiss, A. D., & Watson, J. P. (1994). Psychiatric morbidity and illness behaviour in women with chronic pelvic pain. *Journal of Psychosomatic Research, 38,* 3-9.

Holroyd, K., & Penzien, D. (1990). Pharmacological versus nonpharmacological prophylaxis of recurrent migraine headache: A meta-analytic review of clinical trials. *Pain, 42,* 1-13.

International Headache Society. (1988). Classification and criteria for headache disorders, cranial neuralgias and facial pain. *Cephalalgia, 8*(Suppl. 7), 1-96.

Jarman, J., Fernandez, M., Glover, V., Steiner, T. J., Clifford-Rose, F., & Sandler, M. (1991). Platelet 3H-imipramine binding in migraine and tension headache in relation to depression. *Journal of Psychiatric Research, 24,* 205-211.

Jenkins, C., Zyzanski, S., & Roseman, R. (1970). *Jenkins activity survey manual.* New York: Psychological Corp.

Jones, D. A., Rollman, G. B., & Brooke, R. I. (1997). The Cortisol response to psychological stress in temporomandibular dysfunction. *Pain, 72,* 171-182.

Kames, L., Rapkin, A., Naliboff, B., Afifi, S., & Ferrer-Brechner, T. (1990). Effectiveness of an interdisciplinary pain management program for the treatment of chronic pelvic pain. *Pain, 41,* 41-46.

Katzberg, R. W., Westesson, P., Tallents, R. H., & Drake, C. (1996). Anatomic disorders of the temporomandibular joint disc in asymptomatic subjects. *Journal of Oral and Maxillofacial Surgery, 54,* 147-153.

Kroenke, K. (1991). Symptoms in medical patients: An untended field. *American Journal of Medicine, 92* (Suppl. 1A), 3S-6S.

Long, J., Lynch, J., Machira, N., Thomas, S., & Malinow, K. (1982). The effect of status on blood pressure during verbal communication. *Journal of Behavioral Medicine, 5,* 165-172.

Mason, J. (1968). A review of psychoendocrine research on the sympathetic-adrenal medullary system. *Psychosomatic Medicine, 30,* 631-653.

Mason, J. (1971). An evaluation of the concept of nonspecificity in stress theory. *Journal of Psychiatric Research, 8,* 323-333.

Morrison, D. P. (1990). Occupational stress in migraine: Is weekend headache a myth or reality? *Cephalalgia, 10,* 189-193.

Niaura, R., & Goldstein, M. (1992). Psychological factors affecting physical conditions: Cardiovascular disease literature review, part II. *Psychosomatics, 33,* 146-155.

North American Nursing Diagnosis Association. (1999). *NANDA nursing diagnoses: Definitions and classifications, 1999-2000.* Philadelphia: NANDA.

Olsen, J. (Ed.). (1991). *Migraine and other headaches: The vascular mechanisms.* New York: Raven Press.

Rowlingson, J. (1993). Low back pain. In C. Warfield (Ed.), *The principles and practices of pain management* (pp. 129-140). New York: McGraw-Hill.

Rudy, T. E., Turk, D. C., Kubinski, J. A., & Zaki, H. S. (1995). Differential treatment responses of TMD patients as a function of psychological characteristics. *Pain, 61,* 103-112.

Saper, J., Silverstein, S., Gordon, C., & Hamel, R. (1993). *The handbook of headache management.* Baltimore: Williams & Wilkins.

Sarason, I., Johnson, J., & Siegel, J. (1978). Assessing the impact of life changes. *Journal of Consulting and Clinical Psychology, 46,* 932-946.

Sarason, I., Sarason, B., & Shearin, E. (1986). Social support as an individual difference variable: Its stability, origins and relational aspects. *Journal Personality and Social Psychology, 50,* 845-855.

Sarason, I., Sarason, B., & Shearin, E. (1987). A brief measure of social support: Practical and theoretical implications. *Journal of Social and Personal Relations, 4,* 497-510.

Selye, H. (1956). *Stress of life.* New York: McGraw-Hill.

Speilberger, C., Gorsuch, R., & Lushene, R. (1970). *The State-Trait Anxiety Inventory Manual.* Palo Alto, CA: Consulting Psychologists Press.

Sterling, P., & Eyer, J. (1981). Biological basis of stress-related mortality. *Social Science and Medicine, 153,* 3-42.

Thomas, S., & Friedman, E. (1994). Cardiovascular responses during verbal communication: Effect of rate of verbalization in blood pressure and heart rate responses of Type-A and Type-B cardiac patients. *Journal of Cardiovascular Nursing, 9*(1), 16-26.

Timo, M., Lippi, G., Venanzi, S., Gentili, S., Quintaliani, G., Verdura, C., Monarca, C., Saronio, P., & Timo, F. (1997). Blood pressure trend and cardiovascular events in nuns in a secluded order: A 30-year follow-up study. *Blood Pressure, 6*(2), 81-87.

Turk, D. C., Rudy, T. E., Kubinski, J. A., Zaki, H. S., & Greco, C. M. (1996). Dysfunctional patients with temporomandibular disorders: Evaluating the efficacy of a tailored treatment protocol. *Journal of Consulting and Clinical Psychology, 64,* 139-146.

Waddell, G. (1996). Keynote address for primary care forum on low back pain: A twentieth century health care enigma. *Spine, 21*(24), 2820-2825.

Walker, E. A., Katon, W. J., Hansom, J., Harrop-Griffiths, J., Holm, L., Jones, M. L., Hickok, L. R., & Russo, J. (1995). Psychiatric diagnoses and sexual victimization in women with chronic pelvic pain. *Psychosomatics, 36*(6), 531-540.

Walton, K. G., Pugh, N. D. C., Gelderloos, P., & Macrae, P. (1995). Stress reduction and preventing hypertension: Preliminary support for a psychoneuroendocrine mechanism. *Journal of Alternative and Complementary Medicine, 1,* 263-283.

Weil, A. (1995). *Spontaneous healing.* New York: Random House.

Welch, K. M. A. (1987). Migraine: A biobehavioral disorder. *Archives of Neurology, 44:*323-327.

White, P. (1993). Pain management. In C. Warfield (Ed.), *The principles and practices of pain management* (pp. 27-39). New York: McGraw-Hill.

Suggested Readings

Burckhardt, C. (1990). Chronic pain. *Nursing Clinics of North America, 25,* 863-870.

Lowery, B. (1987). Stress research: Some theoretical and methodological issues. *Image: Journal of Nursing Scholarship, 19,* 42-46.

Reiter, R., Shakern, L., Gambone, J., and Milburn, A. (1991). Correlation between sexual abuse and somatization and nonsomatic chronic pelvic pain. *American Journal of Obstetrics and Gynecology, 165,* 104-109.

Rowlingson, J. (1993). Low back pain. In C. Warfield (Ed.), *The principles and practices of pain management* (pp 129-140). New York: McGraw-Hill.

Saper, J., Silverstein, S., Gordon, C., and Hamel, R. (1993). *The handbook of headache management.* Baltimore: Williams & Wilkins.

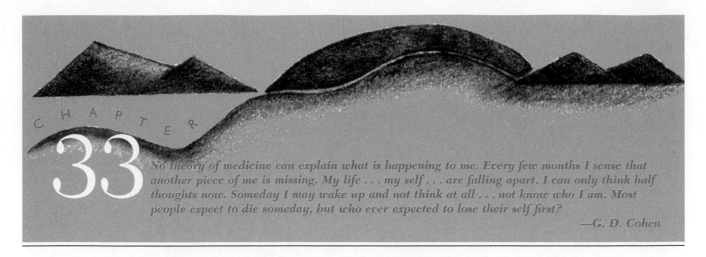

C H A P T E R

33

No theory of medicine can explain what is happening to me. Every few months I sense that another piece of me is missing. My life . . . my self . . . are falling apart. I can only think half thoughts now. Someday I may wake up and not think at all . . . not know who I am. Most people expect to die someday, but who ever expected to lose their self first?

—G. D. Cohen

Cognitive Disorders

Learning Objectives

After studying this chapter, you should be able to:

1. Characterize the historical perspective of cognitive disorders.
2. Identify the defining characteristics of acute cognitive disorders (delirium).
3. Describe the treatment and nursing care of acute cognitive disorder.
4. Contrast the different types of dementia as chronic cognitive disorders.
5. Identify the defining characteristics of dementia.
6. Describe current theories related to the cause of Alzheimer's disease.
7. Apply the nursing process at different stages of dementia.
8. Describe family caregiver issues and related nursing interventions to support the caregiver.
9. Identify legal and ethical issues related to the care of patients with cognitive disorders.

Key Terminology

Acetylcholine
Advance directives
Agnosia
Alcohol-induced persisting amnestic disorder
Alzheimer's disease
Anomia
Aphasia
Apraxia
Ataxia

Brain stem
Catastrophic reactions
Conservatorship
Creutzfeldt-Jakob disease
Crystallized intelligence
Delirium
Dementia
Disorientation
Durable power of attorney
Dysphagia

Emotional disinhibition
Ginkgo biloba
Global memory loss
Huntington's disease
Korsakoff's syndrome
Lewy body dementia
Limbic system
Normal-pressure hydrocephalus

Parkinson's disease
Pick's disease
Plasticity
Pseudodementia
Remote memory
Short-term memory
Sundown syndrome
Vascular dementia

The clarity and purpose of each individual's personal journey depends on an individual's ability to reflect on its meaning. Cognition represents a fundamental human feature that distinguishes living from existing. This mental capacity has a distinctive, personalized impact on the individual's physical, psychological, social, and spiritual conduct of life. For example, the ability to "remember" the connections between related actions and how to initiate them depends on cognitive processing. Moreover, this cognitive processing has a direct relationship to activities of daily living. Although primarily an intellectual and perceptual process, cognition is closely integrated with an individual's emotional and spiritual values. When human beings can no longer understand facts or connect the appropriate feelings to events, they have trouble responding to the complexity of life's many challenges. Profound disturbances in cognitive processing either cloud or destroy the meaning of the journey. The labyrinth of current knowledge about cognitive disorders requires a compassionate understanding of the patient and family from both a medical and a human perspective. Nursing interventions involve three therapeutic goals: protecting patient dignity, preserving functional status, and promoting quality of life for cognitively impaired patients.

Francis's Story

For over 30 years, Francis was a well-known corporate attorney who took pride in his ability to cite relevant law cases from memory. The first signs of his failing memory came when he could no longer connect the appropriate citation with his current law cases. An avid pinochle player, Francis gradually forgot how to play cards. Other subtle signs were present long before he received the official diagnosis. For example, when he visited his daughter, he occasionally turned to the cellar door instead of the bathroom. His family attributed his behavior to benign forgetting and unfamiliarity with a new setting, but elusive personality changes alarmed Mrs. Michaels. Francis would get angry over simple things. His outbursts, however, were transitory and episodic. It was hard to pinpoint the meaning of his emotional blankness around issues he would once have had strong opinions about.

Francis was a quiet man, so only Mrs. Michaels had a true awareness of his growing deficits in communication. In simple social situations, his speech seemed normal. Other people didn't seem to notice the personality change. Without validation from her husband or others, Mrs. Michaels had trouble trusting her own judgment and growing fear of changes in her husband's behavior. She would get angry with him but was unsure when her anger did not produce familiar responses. Francis now had two responses, both out of character with his past decisive and collaborative behavior in the marriage. He would get angry and frustrated, or he would withdraw emotionally. It pained Mrs. Michaels to see her husband, with whom she had a close relationship and on whom she depended for major decisions affecting every aspect of their lives, unable to connect at any meaningful level with her. At times he was more lucid, and the "old Francis" seemed to emerge, but these times grew fewer, gradually replaced with confusion and growing agitation.

Francis's Diagnosis

Francis received the medical diagnosis of dementia in the summer of 1997, after laboratory studies and a CT scan failed to reveal other causes. In some ways, his wife was relieved to have his condition labeled. The physician advised Mrs. Michaels to seek legal advice regarding an advance directive, estate planning, protection of financial assets, and a durable power of attorney. Again she had trouble accepting the need to take these actions. After all, her husband was a lawyer himself. She felt her husband would be insulted by the suggestion of going to an outside lawyer, and indeed he was. As the physician explained, however, unless the family attended to legal matters while Francis still knew what he was signing, the document would not hold up legally. In such instances, the family needs to have the patient declared mentally incompetent by a court, and for most families this is an extremely painful alternative.

Francis was still driving and resisted giving up his car keys. His wife was reluctant to force the issue because she felt sad for him. Moreover, her previous pattern of relating to him was through acquiescence, and she couldn't bring herself to cross him. In some ways, taking the actions needed to stop his driving also acknowledged a painful reality she was not quite willing to accept. Finally, the possibility of his being involved in an accident or hurting himself or others because of his condition motivated her to take the necessary steps. Mrs. Michaels introduced the topic of driving and legal alternatives when her husband seemed less agitated, and in time she achieved the necessary cooperation.

Francis wanted to do more than he was capable of doing, and he became frustrated when he was unable to accomplish simple tasks. He blamed his wife for his inability to find things. Mrs. Michaels could see he was responding to his failing abilities rather than attacking her reliability. Her love for him and her sadness about his condition allowed her to accept his outbursts without retaliation, but his behavior affected the way she felt about herself. Fortunately, Francis did not seem fully aware that his accomplishments were much more modest than before, although his limitations were painfully obvious to Mrs. Michaels. He could still enjoy simple family and commonplace social interactions, but he became agitated in unfamiliar social situations. Uncomplicated excursions to see a parade or a birthday party would bring delight; activities that demanded a complex social response served to frustrate or silence him.

Francis's Progressing Disease

As the disease progressed to the middle stage, Francis lost the power to express his thoughts and feelings verbally. This loss was the worse part for his wife. Later, she would comment that there were two deaths she experienced with Francis: the death of communication with the person she knew as her husband and his actual death. The first death was the worst.

As Francis became nonverbal, touch became an important vehicle of communication. When he became agitated, sitting quietly with him and holding his hand seemed to calm him. Mrs. Michaels found that praying with him was a form of communication they could still share. The familiar prayers were an automatic rather than recent memory, and he seemed to find comfort in remembering them.

Care in the middle stages was constant and intense because Francis was unable to complete even the simplest activities of daily living without massive external support. His table manners disintegrated. He either stared at his food or grabbed it with his hand, shoving it into his mouth. Mealtime required constant supervision to make sure that Francis ate properly and to prevent his choking. Francis needed full assistance with dressing, and he could no longer bathe himself. Incontinence and mobility became issues that required consistent attention. In many ways, however, coping with the physical care was easier than responding to the growing emotional dependence and lack of communication. Francis followed his wife everywhere, allowing no more than 12 inches between them. To Francis, Mrs. Michaels represented his only security in an increasingly alien world, although he no longer seemed to know who she was or how she fit into his life. Reconciling the "before" and "now" portraits of Francis was particularly painful but even more so was her growing inability to connect with him as a person.

Caring for Francis day in and day out was physically and emotionally wearing. Mrs. Michaels coped with the problem by engaging a nurse's aide to come in the evening to bathe and put him to bed. The aide could get up at night with him if he wandered, and Mrs. Michaels could finally get the sleep she needed. With the help of the aide and the support of her adult children, Mrs. Michaels kept her husband at home until he died 4 years later. Caring for him at home was her choice, and she had the financial means to accomplish it. It is not every family's choice or realistic option.

Francis's Death

Toward the end of his life, Francis had trouble swallowing, and he experienced significant weight loss. Only the physical shell of the man remained, a frail shadow of his former physical body. He could no longer even respond with the interactive ability of a young infant. There were few connections between Francis and his environment. He responded to music and prayer but to little else. Finally, Francis found release through death from the imprisonment of a mind that no longer served him as a source of information. His wife experienced sadness and relief but also a significant void. Her total caregiving, consuming every moment of her life for so many years, had left little time for the development of other relationships. Now, her role as caregiver suddenly terminated. The void left an empty hole in the fabric of her life that required time to "reweave." ■

HISTORICAL PERSPECTIVES ON COGNITIVE DYSFUNCTION

Greek philosophers early recognized the power of the mind as the conductor and regulator of human behavior (see Chapter 7). In ancient times, the mind, commonly acknowledged as the center of thought and emotion, was subdivided into different regions in the brain. Their biological aspects, however, were not well described until the 19th century.

Understanding of Dementia

Dementia was the first identified psychiatric disorder, described by an Egyptian prince in 3000 BC (Mack, Forman, Brown, & Frances, 1994). A few centuries later, Hippocrates included phrenitis as one of six types of mental disorders. This disorder presented as "an acute mental disturbance with fever" (Mack et al., 1994, p. 516). Today, similar symptoms would be classified as febrile delirium.

In the 18th century, dementia was described as "a disease consisting in a paralysis of the spirit characterized by abolition of the reasoning faculty; . . . abolition may follow: (1) damage to the brain caused by excessive usage, congenital causes, or old age; (2) failure of the spirit; (3) small volume of the brain; (4) violent blows to the head causing brain damage; (5) incurable diseases, such as epilepsy, or exposure to venoms" (Diderot & d'Alembert, 1765, cited in Berrios, 1994, p. 6). Today, we would call the "abolition of the reasoning faculty" and "failure of the spirit" the loss of self.

By the 19th century, most clinicians thought of dementia as the product of "brain softening" resulting in cognitive impairment. They believed that cerebral arteriosclerotic hardening of the arteries, together with biological risk factors such as syphilis, alcohol, hypertension, and the aging process, caused dementia (Berrios, 1994). Even in the earlier parts of the 20th century, cognitive disorders traditionally have been thought of as "senility," a common and perhaps standard part of the aging process. In fact, the word *senile* derives from the Latin, *senilis*, meaning "pertaining to old age."

In 1907, Alois Alzheimer presented his findings of

presenile dementia based on observations of a 51-year-old woman with severe memory loss. His work represented the first definitive description of dementia as an organic behavioral syndrome. Alzheimer was intrigued that a woman so young could have such profound memory loss, and he followed the course of her dementia until she died at the age of 56. Alzheimer proposed that her symptoms were consistent with a diagnosis of progressive neurological dysfunction. He described symptoms related to cognitive impairment, delusional thinking, and hallucinations. Over time, his patient became mute and was bedridden. On autopsy, Alzheimer found concrete evidence of neuritic plaques and neurofibrillary tangles in the woman's brain. He described his observations: "Scattered through the entire cortex, especially in the upper layers, one found miliary foci that were caused by the deposition of a peculiar substance in the cerebral cortex" (Alzheimer, 1987, p. 79). The substance Alzheimer found in his patient's brain is referred to today as β-amyloid protein.

Today, it is clear that the lesions Alzheimer originally described early in the 20th century are consistent with the distinctive structural and biochemical changes in the brains of patients with Alzheimer's disease. This scientific understanding accounts for the prevailing classification of cognitive disorders as organic behavioral syndromes and the current research on their neurological and biological markers. Contemporary research has established that the brain operates as a biological unit, with each of its three principal regions—cerebral cortex, limbic system, and **brain stem**—responsible for different functions.

The cerebral cortex is commonly associated with cognitive processes, the limbic system with emotional processes, and the brain stem with basic life processes such as breathing and temperature regulation. A wide variety of lesions, as well as structural and metabolic disturbances in the brain, can cause significant changes in cognitive and behavioral functioning. Some of these determinants are reversible, and others are not, at least within our current scope of knowledge.

BRAIN FUNCTION AND COGNITIVE DISORDERS

Normal Brain Functioning

The central nervous system (CNS) carries messages from the brain to different areas of the body, which act in concert to negotiate life tasks effectively. When the physiological changes in brain tissue associated with cognitive disorders occur, the brain can no longer send messages, despite having an intact CNS. It is as if the telephone is off the hook. All of the structural elements are still in place, but the connection between the wiring and phone receiver is broken. Messages can be neither transmitted nor received until the "phone connection" is restored.

The brain has a certain amount of **plasticity,** so that when one area of the brain is damaged, other areas can reorganize and partially compensate for the injury. For example, as the brain struggles with a small cerebral vascular accident, other parts of the brain can take over the functions of the damaged area. Unfortunately the progressive degeneration of brain tissue associated with Alzheimer's disease and loss of acetylcholine, a neurotransmitter, eliminates plasticity (see Chapter 7 for a more detailed explanation of the neurotransmitter and a more complete discussion of neurophysiology).

Regions of the Brain

Cognitive disorders affect one or more of the brain regions, most typically the cerebral cortex and then the limbic system. As the disease progresses, global involvement occurs in all three regions, resulting in profound neurovegetative signs and symptoms and eventual death.

Cerebral Cortex

The cerebral cortex, often referred to as the information-processing center of the brain, receives, retrieves, and processes information that becomes the basis for making decisions. Voluntary motor functions occur under the direction of the cerebral cortex. Memory, recall, visuospatial functions, and the ability to calculate and construct complex data into a meaningful whole are associated with higher cortical functioning. Damage to the cerebral cortex results in language impairment. Complex cortical functions in the brain regulate the integrated mental activities involved in perception, thinking, speaking, comprehension, and listening. They play an important role in communication, allowing a person to understand and respond verbally and nonverbally to another person's communication. With loss of communication ability, the individual's capacity to make sense of the journey or to share its meaning with another is lost.

When damage is localized, it is more indicative of vascular dementia. Two areas of the brain, named after the investigators who discovered them, are particularly important in language deficits. These deficits may occur as a primary diagnosis or may be superimposed on a multiinfarct or dementia of the Alzheimer's type. In 1865, a French physician, Paul Broca, discovered that damage to the left frontal lobe resulted in an impaired use of expressive language. When damage occurs in this region of the brain (causing Broca's aphasia), an individual struggles to form words without much success. Interestingly, patients who have an inability to formulate the same words in intentional meaningful sentences can sing familiar songs with ease (Box 33-1).

In 1874, a German researcher, Carl Wernicke, described damage to the left temporal lobe resulting in a person's inability to understand language and to use words in a meaningful way. Left temporal lobe damage is known as Wernicke's aphasia, or receptive aphasia. Here the normal connections allowing the patient to understand and respond appropriately to verbal messages are lost. Sentence structure is no longer connected to symbolic meanings, so that although a person tries to

Box 33-1 ■ ■ ■ ■ ■

Language Deficits Associated With Cerebral Cortex Damage That Can Accompany a Cognitive Disorder

	Broca's Aphasia	Wernicke's Aphasia
Area of brain affected	Left frontal lobe	Left temporal lobe
Resultant deficit	Impaired expressive language	Impaired receptive language
Characteristics	Difficulty forming words or meaningful sentences	Impaired ability to understand and respond to verbal messages

communicate through words, the message expressed is meaningless babble. Often the listener's inability to make sense of patients' messages becomes so frustrating to patients that they stop talking.

From a behavioral perspective, the higher cortical functions act together as a highly complex conceptual organizer of information. They allow people to gather and interpret data about their world, to make observations, to problem solve, and to draw valid conclusions. Human beings rely on their ability to think (cognition) in a variety of interrelated ways. First, cognitive processes integrate and connect the self with human experience by acting as the bridge between reality and its personalized meaning. When the connections are broken, cognitive deficits directly affect a person's ability to complete behavioral tasks. The capacity to process perceptual data cognitively and make sense of it directly influences an individual's reasoning skills and the appropriateness of judgments. Resourceful living typically reveals an individual's ability to make clear decisions about what is occurring and to plan for the future. Dementia gradually robs an individual of cognitive processing abilities, and others must act on behalf of the patient.

Limbic System

The **limbic system** regulates emotional arousal, memory, and basic drives such as aggression, food, and sex. Patients with damage to the limbic system display significant personality alterations. They have little control over the expression of their emotions. Some become apathetic and emotionally disengage from their environment. Others become emotionally labile, with episodic crying, laughing, and anger appearing with close approximation. These rapid changes in emotions are seemingly unrelated, in many cases, to external stimuli. The patient with limbic system involvement displays little control over sexual and anger expression. This lack of discretion is called emotional disinhibition. The patient may appear physically able. Those unfamiliar with the behavioral changes associated with cognitive impairment may not realize that the patient has a cognitive deficit governing his or her emotional responses.

Multiple Causes

Cognitive disorders originate from multiple causes. For this reason, current thinking considers cognitive disor-

ders a syndrome rather than a specific disease. Jacques (1992) defined a syndrome as "a characteristic pattern of clinical features—the symptoms and signs—which can be caused by one or other of a number of illnesses" (p. 2). The customary clinical features of a behavioral syndrome help define the nature of the deficit and point to its central pathology. General agreement exists about the nature of cognitive impairment regardless of cause.

Delirium is the name given to the acute forms of cognitive dysfunction resulting from secondary changes in brain metabolism. *Dementia* is the term used to describe cognitive disorders that are chronic. Acute cognitive disorders represent a separate category that is quite distinct from chronic forms, rather than both being viewed on a continuum of cognitive dysfunction. The *Diagnostic and Statistical Manual of Mental Disorders, Fourth Edition* (DSM-IV) (American Psychiatric Association [APA], 1994) criteria describe the basic defining characteristics of both acute and chronic cognitive disorders, each as a streamlined unit, with delirium due to multiple causes and dementia due to multiple causes. The intent of the current nomenclature is to classify each as an explicit syndrome of behaviors rather than as a single disease.

Acute cognitive disorders (delirium) can occur as a primary syndrome; as the corollary of excessive use of alcohol; and as a result of a host of structural, metabolic, and infectious causes. Delirium can be superimposed on chronic cognitive disorders, increasing the confusion and cognitive impairment the individual already suffers. It is important to distinguish between the dementia already present and that imposed by a delirium to facilitate prompt diagnosis and correction of new problems that could threaten optimal function of the patient.

What do you think? Have you known anyone with a cognitive disorder? What do you think would be your greatest challenge in providing care for such a patient? What if the person was a loved one?

► *Check Your Reading*
1. How would you describe the differences between Wernicke's aphasia and Broca's aphasia?
2. Why would the nurse consider dementia a syndrome?

ACUTE COGNITIVE DISORDERS: DELIRIUM

Delirium represents a group of acute cognitive disorders directly attributable to diagnosable neurological, metabolic, and toxic conditions that influence brain function. Although extreme confusion is a key symptom, the precise presentation of symptoms varies, reflecting the specific underlying physical disturbance (Box 33-2).

Some patients become stuporous; others become agitated. In most cases, the patient's presenting behavior is bizarre and dramatic. Delirious patients also can experience significant perceptual changes, such as hallucinations, illusions, and disorientation. Hallucinations, when they occur, typically are visual. A patient may report having "night visitors" or seeing a vision of a deceased family member. Illusions take the visual form of misinterpreting staff as police or a piece of medical equipment as a lethal weapon. Shadows on the wall appear as monsters. **Disorientation,** defined as an inability to know who one is, where one is, or what the time or date is, is a common occurrence. In contrast to patients with psychotic disorders, most delirious patients are oriented to person; they know their names. But they experience difficulty with time and date, and they have trouble identifying their current circumstances appropriately. See What Families Need to Know: Delirium.

Nursing Care for Delirium

Delirium represents a state of acute physical and psychological urgency. Accurate assessment is perhaps the most critical element of effective nursing care; it can mean the difference between life and death. Typically, delirious patients present in the emergency room in a state of acute confusion and usually not of their own volition (Batt, 1989).

Emergency Triage

Emergency medical triage of the delirious patient is a primary nursing intervention. Patients with suspected delirium should receive treatment as a medical emergency first and then from a psychiatric treatment perspective. Autonomic symptoms, such as elevated blood pressure, tachycardia, fever, excessive perspiration, and constricted pupils, provide evidence of an acute medical emergency. Prompt stabilization of cardiopulmonary disorders is a priority.

Besides assessment for emergency physical conditions, evaluation of the patient's mental status is critical. Patients with acute cognitive impairment often are a danger to themselves or others. The threat they pose depends on the nature of the cognitive deficit and its underlying pathology, particularly if drug induced. Until proved otherwise, suicide or homicide potential is always a possibility with delirious patients. (See Chapters 11 and 31 for further detail on assessment and treatment.) With these patients, you must decide quickly whether the patient's symptoms warrant immediate physical or psychological intervention or a combination of modalities.

Establishing the Diagnosis

Once the nurse addresses the emergency aspects of the patient's condition, the next step is to confirm the diagnosis of delirium through patient history, observation of symptoms, and laboratory and other diagnostic tests. Patients with delirium rarely are good historians. Even with periods of relative lucidity, delirious patients are unable to give accurate, coherent information because the psychoactive substance, infection, imbalance, or injury

Box 33-2 ■■■■■
Common Features of Delirium

Reduced ability to maintain attention to external stimuli (e.g., questions must be repeated because attention wanders) and to shift attention appropriately to new external stimuli (e.g., perseverates answer to previous question)

Disorganized thinking, as indicated by rambling, irrelevant, or incoherent speech

At least two of the following:

Reduced level of consciousness (e.g., difficulty keeping awake during examination)

Perceptual disturbances: misinterpretations, illusions, or hallucinations

Disturbance of sleep-wake cycle with insomnia or daytime sleepiness

Increased or decreased psychomotor activity

Disorientation to time, place, or person

Memory impairment (e.g., inability to learn new material, such as the names of several unrelated objects after 5 minutes, or to remember past events, such as history of current episode of illness)

Clinical features develop over a short period of time (usually hours to days) and tend to fluctuate over the course of a day

Either of the following:

Evidence from the history, physical examination, or laboratory tests of a specific organic factor (or factors) judged to be causatively related to the disturbance

In the absence of such evidence, a presumed organic factor if the disturbance cannot be accounted for by any nonorganic mental disorder (e.g., manic episode accounting for agitation and sleep disturbance)

Based on information from the *Diagnostic and Statistical Manual of Mental Disorders. Fourth Edition.* Copyright 1994 American Psychiatric Association.

WHAT FAMILIES NEED TO KNOW

Delirium

What is delirium?

Delirium is an acute, reversible problem that can be frightening, as extreme confusion leads to symptoms that are bizarre and dramatic. Many different causes of delirium exist including most physical illnesses, medications, drugs, or alcohol. In young adults and children, delirium is more often associated with drug toxicity, head trauma, infection, and brain tumor.

What does delirium look like?

Hallucinations, delusions, disorientation, and extreme anxiety may occur, which can lead to the possibility of the person harming himself or herself or others. These symptoms appear quite suddenly, and once the cause is treated, the symptoms subside as rapidly as they occurred.

What should I do?

It is most important to remember that seeking medical attention is of an urgent nature when delirious symptoms appear. Take your loved one or family member immediately to an emergency care setting. The sooner medical intervention occurs, the quicker the cause can be determined and the symptoms treated. Your quick response in this type of emergency can literally mean life or death for the delirious patient.

remains operative in their brains. Typically, direct patient interviews are postponed until the delirium symptoms have cleared. When the patient is the only available informant, having the same interviewer and keeping careful notes are important. These patients may appear cognitively intact during one interview and quite confused at a second interview the same day. Comparison data are essential to the development of an accurate diagnosis and appropriate treatment. Usually, seeking information from the person accompanying the patient elicits the most accurate data during the assessment and acute treatment phase.

Obtaining a complete history, particularly that of symptom onset and behavioral change, is essential to developing an appropriate treatment plan. Those in close contact with the patient usually can report a distinct change in behavior. Critical data include identification of precipitating factors, such as medications the

TABLE 33–1 Differential Diagnosis of Delirium and Dementia

FEATURE	DELIRIUM	DEMENTIA
Onset	Acute, often at night	Insidious
Course	Fluctuating, with lucid intervals during the day; worse at night	Stable over the course of the day
Duration	Hours to weeks	Months or years
Awareness	Reduced	Clear
Alertness	Abnormally low or high	Usually normal
Attention	Lacks direction and selectivity; distractibility; fluctuation over the course of the day	Relatively unaffected
Orientation	Usually impaired for time; tendency to mistake unfamiliar for familiar places and persons	Often impaired
Memory	Immediate and recent impaired	Recent and remote impaired
Thinking	Disorganized	Impoverished
Perception	Illusions and hallucinations, usually visual and common	Often absent
Speech	Incoherent, hesitant, slow, or rapid	Difficulty in finding words
Sleep-wake cycle	Always disrupted	Fragmented sleep
Physical illness or drug toxicity	Either or both present	Often absent, especially in Alzheimer's disease

From Lipowski, Z. (1990). *Delirium: Acute confusional states* (p. 192). New York: Oxford University Press.

patient currently is taking; blows to the head or falls; drug use, particularly as it relates to the past few days; recent illness; recent intrusive procedures (e.g., root canal); and changes in environment. If the patient has suffered a recent blow to the head, the area needs to be identified. Two of the most common causes of delirium in adults in long-term care settings are respiratory infection (pneumonia) and urinary tract infection. Information about past treatment for emotional and physical illness is important, and you need to document history of drug use, including polydrug use (e.g., cocaine and benzodiazepines). Abrupt withdrawal from alcohol, barbiturates, or benzodiazepines can lead to episodic symptoms of delirium. Moreover, the cross-tolerance effects of past drug abuse can influence the choice of medication to reduce delirium symptoms. The agitation, explosive anger, and clouded consciousness associated with other psychiatric disorders such as bipolar disorder and psychosis can mimic delirium. Thus, data about past psychiatric treatment can be helpful in establishing a differential diagnosis of delirium rather than mania or psychosis. Table 33-1 summarizes differences in the differential diagnosis of delirium and dementia.

Observation of individuals with suspected delirium reveals a characteristic constellation of behavioral symptoms. Patients may appear stuporous or in a state of high agitation; there can be a rapid shift between the two states. Memory for immediate and recent events is difficult to elicit (Marachlewski, 1994). The patient's speech may be incoherent, rambling, and at complete odds with reality. Seriously affected patients may indicate visceral effects, such as the sensation of bugs crawling under their skin. Patients also may demonstrate a compulsive reflex, picking at bed covers or clothing (Foreman & Zane, 1996; Haller & Binder, 1995).

Other observations relate to the patterning of symptoms. With delirium, symptoms present a distinctive configuration. Symptoms appear suddenly, often beginning at night, and they present a fluctuating course of symptom exacerbation and remission. Florid cognitive symptoms and explicit behavior changes noted over a short period suggest a delirium rather than dementia. The cognitive symptoms, although intense, usually last no more than a few hours or days and rarely longer than a month. Once the underlying pathology is recognized, the symptoms can be reversed quickly and dramatically.

Finding the cause of the delirium obviously forms the foundation for decisions about primary treatment. Delirium in the elderly is particularly important to assess because these patients are less likely to be substance abusers and may have underlying dementia. Keith (1994) suggested that "delirium is frequently superimposed on dementia in up to 40% of hospitalized demented patients and complicating the differential diagnosis of the two conditions, which are by no means mutually exclusive" (p. 42).

Virtually anything that disrupts the body's normal balance can trigger delirium in the elderly (Table 33-2). Possible causes include congestive heart failure, malnutrition, dehydration, diabetes, hypoxia affecting cerebral blood flow, pneumonia, and hypokalemia. Drug toxicity, particularly with anticholinergic or arrhythmia drugs, is particularly dangerous in the elderly because of

TABLE 33-2 Common Causes of Delirium	
CONDITION	**MANIFESTATIONS**
Vascular insufficiency	Thrombosis or embolism, transient ischemic attacks, hypoxia
Cerebral vascular accident	Subdural hematoma, intracranial hemorrhage, ruptured aneurysm
Tumors	Primary malignant, metastatic, benign
Electrolyte imbalances	Hyper/hypokalemia, chloremia, natremia, glycemia
Fluid volume depletion	Diuretics, inadequate fluid intake
Postsurgery, intensive care unit psychosis	Physiological or psychological stress
Infections	Viral, bacterial, meningitis, brain abscess
Drug toxicity	Virtually any drug, steroids, digitalis, beta-blockers, anticholinergics, amphetamines
Drug withdrawal	Barbiturates, alcohol, benzodiazepines, hypnotic sedatives
Nutritional deficiencies	Vitamin B_{12}, niacin, thiamine

the slower metabolic rate that allows medication build-up in these patients (Table 33-3). Patients with premorbid organic brain disease are at highest risk for the development of anticholinergic symptoms, characterized by confusion, agitation, visual hallucinations, disorientation, incoherence, stupor, and bizarre behavior.

Delirium in the young is associated most frequently with drug toxicity, head trauma, infection, and brain tumors. The violent behaviors associated with delirium are particularly dangerous with young adults having drug toxicity or head trauma. These patients have greater physical capacity to harm themselves and others. In young adults presenting with violent behavior, organic brain disease should be considered until it is ruled out.

Determination of underlying pathology causing the delirium requires a thorough physical assessment, appropriate laboratory tests, and other diagnostic assessments, such as MRI, angiogram, and CT scan. Table 33-4 lists common laboratory tests and their clinical applications. Testing should be completed as quickly as possible because the data become the basis for treatment decisions. For example, patients can achieve symptom relief quickly with the discontinuation or dose reduction of the drug responsible for the delirium. Sometimes, restoration of fluid or electrolyte balance clears the delirium. Immediate blood and toxicologic screening tests can save an individual's life and often mandate the prompt need for surgery, gastric lavage, intubation, or transfer to the intensive care unit. Fever suggests an infectious origin, whereas abnormally elevated pulse

TABLE 33-3 Underlying Mechanisms of Medication-Induced Mental Changes

MECHANISM OF ACTION	MEDICATION EXAMPLES
Anticholinergic interactions	Atropine
	Scopolamine
	Antihistamines
	Antipsychotics
	Antidepressants
	Antispasmodics
	Antiparkinsonian agents
Decreased cerebral blood flow	Antihypertensives
	Antipsychotics
Depression of respiratory center	Central nervous system depressants
Fluid and electrolyte alterations	Diuretics
	Alcohol
	Laxatives
Altered thermoregulation	Alcohol
	Psychotropics
	Narcotics
Acidosis	Diuretics
	Alcohol
	Nicotinic acid
Hypoglycemia	Hypoglycemics
	Alcohol
	Propranolol
Hormonal disturbances	Thyroid extract
	Corticosteroids

From Miller, C. A. (1995). *Nursing care of older adults: Theory and practice* (2nd ed., p. 441). Philadelphia: J. B. Lippincott.

and blood pressure suggest drug withdrawal. Tests such as the Glasgow Coma Scale and CT scan of the head can reveal subdural hematomas. Other common tests used in differential diagnosis include MRI, PET scan, and angiogram.

Patient Care Guidelines

The first nursing interventions involve ensuring the patient's safety and stabilizing the patient medically. Once the patient's physical condition is secure, nursing interventions are oriented toward behavior and symptom reduction. No single nursing intervention is equally effective in all cases. Instead, nursing interventions are specifically tailored to meet the needs of the individual patient and the specific demands of the situation (McCracken, 1994).

Most delirium patients respond best to one-to-one clinical supervision from a single caregiver because the ability to shift attention from one person to another in a meaningful way diminishes in direct proportion to the brain pathology. Establishing eye contact and identifying the purpose of the interview offer a significant landmark when sensory input threatens the patient's security.

Patients with acute confusional states lack the concentration needed to follow a discussion. Expecting them to follow a complicated conversation increases their anxiety as well as the caregivers'. Instead, one directive at a time, delivered in calm, yet decisive tones, provides the structure a patient needs when the objective world does not make sense. Additionally, nurses may have to identify themselves at regular intervals, orienting the patient to the setting and what will happen next. Lack of environmental cues increases anxiety, whereas information needed for familiarization with the environment calms the anxious patient. As the patient's condition improves, the level of intervention lessens to adapt to the patient's growing awareness and responsiveness to environmental cues.

The nurse also may choose to limit the number of people present. Patients with acute cognitive deficits overreact to almost any stimulus. Asking those who seem to agitate the patient to leave for a short time can go a long way in reducing patient frustration. If this is done tactfully, most significant others are grateful that you have taken charge of the situation. Explaining that patients with delirium act irrationally toward those they care about helps soften the perception of rejection.

Containing Patient Anxiety

Delirious patients are acutely anxious, and their tension level is contagious. Staff and other patients often have difficulty maintaining calm around the patient in an acute confusional state. Yet what the patient needs most are clear boundaries and someone to take charge of the situation. Staff attitude is important. All personnel involved with the patient should have a thorough understanding of delirium, which allows them to maintain a nonanxious presence and a consistent approach. Using a minimum of simple, concrete words spoken in a calm, low, but authoritative voice can calm patients much more easily than trying to reason with them.

Reducing Environmental Stimuli

Inadvertent actions taken by others, even if totally unrelated to the patient, are sources of distraction. Environmental noises often increase agitation. Ideally, you will have the option of placing the delirious patient in a quiet room, with the door closed, apart from the mainstream of activity. This measure helps reduce sensory incitement. If this is not possible, the patient needs to have the curtains drawn around the bed. Lighting is important because a poorly lit room, glare, and reflections can stimulate illusions and other perceptual distortions. Because many patients are both physically and emotionally exhausted from the effects of their delirium, a quiet environment provides a needed respite. Decreasing environmental stimuli has a complementary therapeutic effect in that it expands the patient's cognitive functioning capacity.

Minimizing Perceptual Distortions

Spatial-perceptual distortions found in acute confusional states often lead to significant misinterpretations of people, space, objects, or directives. For example, patients may misinterpret nurses moving toward them as huge malevolent persons out to kill them. Remember that delirious patients typically have limited ability to interpret accurately and respond to environmental, physical, or emotional stimuli because of neurobiochemical changes in the brain. Repeated orientation and basic explanation of activities help to reduce misperceptions (Hill, Risby, & Morgan, 1992).

Giving Medication

Medication may be necessary if the patient is combative or extremely difficult to manage. Preferably, it is given before the patient is ready to hurt someone. Indications for immediate medication to manage anxiety include suspiciousness, combative gestures, intense anger, threats, and threatening body language. If the patient is highly agitated, small doses of a high-potency neuroleptic, such as haloperidol, are administered, generally in doses of 0.25 to 5.0 mg intramuscularly, to reduce tension. These neuroleptics have fewer cardiotoxic, sedative, and anticholinergic side effects than the low-potency neuroleptics. Moreover, these medications are less likely to decrease the seizure threshold than lower-potency neuroleptics, and they tend to have a lessened adverse effect on the patient's cognitive functioning. Repeat administration of the antipsychotic medication is appropriate after 30 minutes, when indicated. The addition of a benzodiazepine (lorazepam) is helpful if previous treatment with the antipsychotic medication proves ineffective. When administering medications, supervise the medication administration when it is taken orally to en-sure that the medication is swallowed. You need to record the patient's response to the medication and to report any adverse effects.

Eliminating Causative Factors

Elimination of the causal factors is central to the nursing management of patients with delirium. Following identification of the cause, appropriate medication, nutrition, and electrolyte support are aimed at restoring the patient to premorbid functioning and providing for the comfort and safety of the patient. Because causative agents vary, so does the treatment. Obviously, antibiotics for patients with infectious disorders, such as meningitis or encephalitis, are appropriate. Correction of malnutrition, dehydration, electrolyte imbalance, and vitamin deficiencies can reduce the severity and continuation of delirium symptoms related to these contingencies. If medication toxicity is suspected—for example, steroids, lithium, or digitalis toxicity—the implicated drug should be discontinued immediately. Some drug toxicities, such as barbiturates, require gradual discontinuance. They cannot be withdrawn precipitously without significant adverse effects. Such patients must be weaned gradually from drugs. They are given titrated doses of the drug until the symptoms are brought under control, and then the drug is gradually removed.

Patients who require immediate stabilization with medication exhibiting cross-tolerance behaviors typically receive benzodiazepines to minimize withdrawal symptoms. For example, the acute symptoms of alcohol

TABLE 33–4 Suggested Laboratory Tests for Patients Presenting With Cognitive Disorders

TEST	CLINICAL APPLICATION
Complete blood count, white blood cell count with differential, sedimentation rate	Presence of infection
Blood chemistry, blood urea nitrogen, creatinine	Renal failure
Glucose	Diabetes, hypoglycemia
Triiodothyronine, thyroxine, thyroid-stimulating hormone	Thyroid disease
Electrolytes (Na$^+$, K$^+$, Ca^{2+}, Cl$^-$, PO$_4^{3-}$)	Electrolyte imbalance
Serum folate level	Liver disease or failure
Vitamin B$_{12}$ level	Nutritional deficits
Ratio of serum alanine aminotransferase to serum aspartate aminotransferase	Liver disease or failure
Venereal Disease Research Laboratory, rapid plasma reagin	Syphilis
Drug blood levels	Drug toxicity for therapeutic drugs (e.g., steroids, digitalis toxicity) or nonprescribed drugs (e.g., barbiturates, cocaine, phenodiazepines, alcohol)
Urinalysis, glucose, acetone	Urinary tract infection, diabetes
Albumin	Renal failure
Porphyria screen	Renal failure
Leukocytes	Infection
Urine toxicology (barbiturates, phenodiazepines, cocaine)	Drug toxicity
Chest radiograph	Presence of infection
CT, PET, MRI	Brain tumor, subdural hematoma, brain hemorrhage, infection

withdrawal respond well to temporary administration of a benzodiazepine. Virtually all of the drugs in this classification are useful in reducing the seizures and the acute confusional states associated with alcohol withdrawal. The most frequently used, however, are chlordiazepoxide, diazepam, oxazepam, and lorazepam. (See Chapter 26 for more information on cross-tolerance.)

When making treatment decisions, it is important to realize that several contributing factors can coexist in creating the patient's delirium.

Managing Aggressive Behavior

The primary treatment goal in the management of aggressive behavior is to prevent its escalation into actual violence toward self, others, or objects in the environment. In addition to using medication for tension relief, staff attitude is critical. Close but relaxed supervision is a key strategy in preventing the escalation of aggressive behavior among patients with cognitive changes. Sometimes the use of a "sitter," a paraprofessional to stay with the patient, is an excellent alternative to restraints and a cost-effective way of providing close supervision. Moving the patient out of the area into a quiet, nonstimulating environment is crucial because delirious patients lack the capacity to do this on their own. If the patient is expressing anger toward a particular staff member, it may be appropriate to have another staff member be the primary contact. The same holds true for family members. Also, if a specific object (e.g., a photograph on the wall or a television set) triggers a hostile reaction, remove the object from the patient's environment.

The way in which staff approach patients and the number of demands placed on them affects physical and verbal aggression. For example, approaching the patient from the side with arms at one's side and using the patient's name with simple directives is less threatening than quick or random movements.

SNAPSHOT

Nursing Interventions Specific to Delirium

What do you need to do to develop a relationship with a patient suffering with delirium?

- Facilitate medical stabilization of the patient to reduce symptoms and behaviors.
- Have a professional nurse assigned to the patient.
- Establish eye contact and speak in a calm manner.
- Provide simple explanations of procedures and activities.
- Encourage verbalization of feelings.
- Minimize environmental distractions and stimuli.

What do you need to assess regarding the patient's health status?

- History of onset of symptoms, characteristics
- Precipitating factors, including use of new medication, increased stress, recent accident
- Patient's usual behaviors and functional ability
- Known medical diagnoses
- Prescription and over-the-counter medications used or recently discontinued
- Physiological responses, including vital signs, appetite and weight changes, fatigue, urinary output, constipation, diarrhea, pain, fever, changes in quality of respirations, sleep-wake cycle, psychomotor activity
- Level of consciousness
- Cognitive responses, including confusion, or problems with concentration, memory, or speech
- Behavioral responses, including agitation, aggression, angry outbursts, crying, poor grooming, inattention to self-care, deficits in instrumental and other activities of daily living
- Use of alcohol

What do you need to teach the patient and/or patient's caregiver?

- Reversible, treatable nature of condition
- Symptoms to identify and report
- Behaviors that could indicate increasing agitation or potential aggressive behaviors, and describe strategies to prevent and manage these situations
- Measures to protect themselves and the patient from patient's aggressive behaviors
- Importance of simple instructions and consistency in caregiving activities
- Follow-up care that is required

What skills do you want the patient and/or caregiver to demonstrate?

- Compliance with treatment plan
- Ability to fulfill self-care demands
- Prevention or avoidance of factors that could increase symptoms and behaviors
- Reduction of environmental stimuli
- Recognition of medication side effects

What other professionals may be part of the plan?

- Physician or medical specialists, depending on underlying cause
- Psychiatrist

Providing patients with choices is a useful intervention as long as the patient is not combative, threatening, suspicious, or intensely angry, and the choices do not compromise the rights of others. Statements such as "I'd like to ask you to come with me to the room down the hall where we can talk about this with less distraction," said in a quiet, firm voice is more effective than a sudden show of force. When needed, however, a calm but decisive show of force, delivered verbally with uncomplicated direct language, often decreases patient anxiety and encourages cooperation. Never turn your back to a delirious patient, and never try to subdue a patient without sufficient personnel.

In the event of escalating aggression, staff members need to act decisively and deliberately, with physical force if necessary. One person explains the purpose of each movement in advance, in a composed voice. Seclusion and restraints need application with compassion and respect for the patient's dignity as a human being. Chapter 35 also provides more guidelines for anticipating and handling violent behavior.

Follow-Up Care

Many patients lack insight related to an association among lifestyle factors, drug abuse, past hospitalizations for mental illness, past trauma, and current circumstances, even after the immediate medical condition has stabilized. Nevertheless, including patients in treatment planning, to whatever extent possible once their symptoms are under control, usually is beneficial. Follow-up referral for treatment of drug abuse or medication monitoring can prevent further episodes of delirium. See Snapshot: Nursing Interventions Specific to Delirium.

> **W***hat do you think?* Knowing what you know about delirium, how would you respond to someone who said a psychiatric nurse only "talks" to patients?

➤ *Check Your Reading*
3. How would you describe the common characteristics of delirium?
4. Why is an accurate diagnosis so important?
5. What interventions would the nurse use to contain the delirium patient's anxiety?
6. What medication is the most useful with delirium patients? Why?

NURSING PROCESS APPLICATION

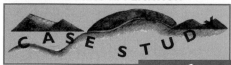

Randy

Randy is a 17-year-old high school senior who is admitted into the intensive care unit after smoking crack cocaine at a friend's party. He is delirious and confused as to how he ended up in the emergency department. His friends report that he had smoked two to three rocks of crack during the evening. They became alarmed when they found him in the shower with all of his clothes on with the shower running. As he sat in the shower, he was formulating sentences using nonsensical terms while crying and laughing. He became combative when his friends tried to take him out of the shower. They called 911 for assistance.

ASSESSMENT	Assessment data are as follows:
	• Delirious and confused
	• Impaired cognition
	• Combative
	• Rapid mood swings

DIAGNOSIS

DSM-IV Diagnosis: Delirium

Nursing Diagnosis: Acute Confusion related to delirium as evidenced by use of nonsensical terms, fluctuations in mood, agitation, and impaired cognition

OUTCOME IDENTIFICATION, PLANNING, AND IMPLEMENTATION

Expected Outcome 1: By _____ the patient will have safely detoxified from crack.

Short-Term Goals	Nursing Interventions	Rationales
By _____ the patient will have safely detoxified from crack.	1. Monitor vital signs. 2. Check level of consciousness. 3. Decrease environmental stimuli. 4. Administer medications as ordered.	1–3. Detoxification can lead to alterations in normal vital signs; it is especially important to monitor for cardiac arrhythmias and seizure activity. 4. Medications typically ordered are antipsychotics, sedatives, antiarrhythmics, and anticonvulsants. Psychotropic medication can decrease symptoms and agitated behavior.
By _____ the patient will have a premorbid level of cognitive functioning.	1. Encourage Randy to do as much as possible for himself after detoxification phase. 2. Provide orientation to environment, present new information slowly. 3. Talk to Randy about mutual areas of interest (i.e., friends at school, sports, hobbies).	1. Active participation in his own care assists the patient to maintain self-esteem and independence, which are important developmental issues for an adolescent. 2–3. After a period of acute confusion, a slow process of orientation will support memory and orientation for the patient.
By _____ the patient will demonstrate socially acceptable behavior.	1. Discuss with Randy the crack episode. Determine if this was one-time experimentation or a pattern of abuse. 2. Encourage Randy to ventilate his feelings, especially any shame or embarrassment over drug use. 3. Refer Randy to drug rehabilitation program.	1–3. Early assessment and intervention are important components in planning nursing care for an adolescent using drugs. 2. Shame and guilt accompany actions that are socially unacceptable (e.g., taking a shower with all your clothes on).
By _____ the patient will participate in activities and with others at a socially acceptable level.	1. Encourage Randy to participate in unit activities. 2. Assess level of confusion and watch for return to normal functioning.	1. Participation in unit activities is a socially acceptable type of behavior that encourages a sense of belongingness. 2. Delirium confusion is marked by an acute onset and usually is temporary once the underlying cause is treated (e.g., drug use).

EVALUATION

Formative Evaluation: Randy met each of the short-term goals. He was a very pleasant adolescent and participated readily in the therapeutic milieu. He admitted to a one-time experimentation with crack, stating that everyone was trying it, and he wanted to "see what it was like."

Summative Evaluation: Randy achieved all of the expected outcomes. He decided to attend an outpatient support group that supported a "just say no" attitude toward drugs. He verbalized on several occasions how lucky he was to have survived his drug experimenting and how fortunate he was to have friends who promptly sought medical help for him.

CHRONIC COGNITIVE DISORDERS: DEMENTIA

Edwards (1993) defined **dementia,** the term used for chronic cognitive disorders, as "a set of conditions, medically diagnosed, and leading to recognized and measurable behavioral changes in an individual" (p. 6). By contrast with delirium, which responds to treatment, dementia is a degenerative neurological disorder that invariably worsens and always ends in death. There is no known cure.

Chronic cognitive disorders have a slow insidious onset, with gradual deterioration of cognitive, mental, and physical neurological systems (Alafuzoff, 1992). The conditions comprising the chronic cognitive disorder classification include primary dementia, dementia with extrapyramidal symptoms, dementia caused by brain lesions, dementia associated with other conditions, and pseudodementia. Common features of dementia, encompassing all chronic cognitive disorders, regardless of cause, are presented in Box 33–3. Distinguishing among the different types (Box 33–4) can be important for diagnosis. All patients need a comprehensive neurological assessment to rule out reversible causes of dementia, to provide treatment direction, and to establish parameters for families regarding genetic implications. For example, treatment of underlying hypertension can

Box 33-3 ■■■■■
Common Features of Dementia

Impairment in short-term and long-term memory

One of the following:

Impairment in abstract thinking: Inability to find similarities and differences between related words, trouble defining related words

Impaired judgment: Inability to make plans, hiding money, giving money or possessions away, accusing spouse of infidelity, acting out sexually

Disturbances of higher cortical functioning: Aphasia (disturbance in language), apraxia (inability to carry out motor activities), agnosia (failure to recognize objects or people), constructional difficulty (inability to copy figures or assemble blocks or put things together in a logical way)

Personality: Changes or inappropriate accentuation of personality traits

Known organic cause or determination that the disorder is not a mental disorder

Based on information from the *Diagnostic and Statistical Manual of Mental Disorders. Fourth Edition.* Copyright 1994 American Psychiatric Association.

offset further insults to brain tissue in some cases, whereas this would not be the case for the Alzheimer's disease patient. Familial Alzheimer's and Huntington's disease raise questions in first-degree relatives about their chances of contracting the disorder and are important determinants of future family genetic decisions. See What Families Need to Know: Dementia.

Primary Dementia

Alzheimer's Disease

Clinicians consider **Alzheimer's disease** a primary dementia because the syndrome occurs with distinctive brain lesions and without any known physiological basis. The disorder is classified as a neurological brain disease with multifactorial causes (Giacobini & Barton, 1997; O'Brien, 1994). Alzheimer's disease affects more than 4 million people, making it the most common neuropsychiatric illness in the elderly. The actual course of the disorder follows a predictable pattern of early, middle, and late stages, each displaying characteristic behaviors and requiring a different focus of treatment. Figure 33-1 illustrates the stages of Alzheimer's disease. Yi, Abraham, and Holroyd (1994) referred to the early stage as the amnestic stage, the middle stage as the dementia stage, and the late stage as the vegetative stage.

Morphologically, Alzheimer's disease patients develop neurofibrillary tangles and neuritic plaques, which take up space in the brain as lesions, replacing normal tissue in the cell body of the neuron (Edwards, 1993). There is a global decline in cortical functioning, particularly during the middle stages, that affects not only cognitive functioning but also the voluntary exercise of bodily functions. As the disease progresses, patients lose control over their bladder and bowel functions and later over swallowing. Other signs of increased neurological deficit appear as an inability to walk. Seizures are common. Death inevitably occurs as a result of neurological complications imposed by the brain lesions.

Alzheimer's disease represents the clinical prototype for chronic cognitive disorders (Berrios, 1994). It is the most common form of dementia, and the care given to dementia patients regardless of cause is essentially the same, particularly in the middle and late stages of the disorder. Although classified as a single disorder, Yi and coworkers (1994) suggested that Alzheimer's disease represents a syndrome of related disorders with multiple origins.

The cognitive symptoms of dementia involve serious memory impairment and significant alterations in language, perceptual acuity, ability to abstract, ability to problem solve, and ability to make appropriate judgments. Patients ultimately experience **global memory loss** (loss of all memory), and **aphasia** (loss of meaningful verbal communication). Noncognitive behavioral symptoms can be just as profound. They include significant personality changes, purposeless movements, agitation and aggression, overreaction to situations, irritating behavior, and emotional disinhibition. Medical terms related to the neurological, language, and behavioral deficits found with dementia are presented in Table 33-5.

Box 33-4 ■■■■■
Types of Dementias

Primary Dementia

Alzheimer's disease
Pick's disease
Creutzfeldt-Jakob disease
Lewy body dementia

Dementia With Extrapyramidal Symptoms

Huntington's disease

Dementia Due to Brain Lesions

Vascular dementia

Dementia Associated With Other Physical Conditions

Normal-pressure hydrocephalus
Alcohol-induced persisting amnestic disorders
AIDS dementia complex
Parkinson's disease
Multiple sclerosis

WHAT FAMILIES NEED TO KNOW

Dementia

How do I know if my family member has dementia?

Some of the early signs family members notice are a change in cognitive functioning or personality. Short-term memory impairment occurs with a noticeable loss of the ability to remember activities of daily living, including carrying on a meaningful conversation. The most disturbing and troubling symptoms are related to personality changes. A lower frustration level, a lack of interest, and a decreased attention span are among the early changes noted. Restlessness and rapid mood changes may occur, followed by periods of blank facial expression. In the early stage, the patient may be aware that something is wrong with his or her mind and how it's working.

What can I do to help?

No known cures for dementia exist. Learning about the disease process and caregiving measures to promote optimal function are important. Also beneficial is obtaining assistance and support for family members and caregivers. The Alzheimer's Association is an excellent source of education and support. Most cities have local chapters and may provide a hotline for assistance.

Pick's Disease

This type of dementia occurs most often between the ages of 40 and 60, striking less than 1% of the population. Although the symptoms of **Pick's disease** resemble Alzheimer's disease in many ways, the changes in the brain differ. With Pick's disease, there is a characteristic shrinkage of brain tissue, particularly in the frontal and temporal lobes. Consequently, behavioral changes inconsistent with the level of cognitive deficit (language, memory, visuospatial skills) are early diagnostic signs (Keith, 1994). Emotional disinhibition, evidenced in hypersexuality and exhibitionism, can appear as a dominant behavioral symptom. Patients with Pick's disease typically display greater emotional apathy, irritability, or mood disturbance. Patients with this disorder may exhibit excessive ritualistic picking, scratching, licking, or sucking. Diagnosis of Pick's disease is based on results of

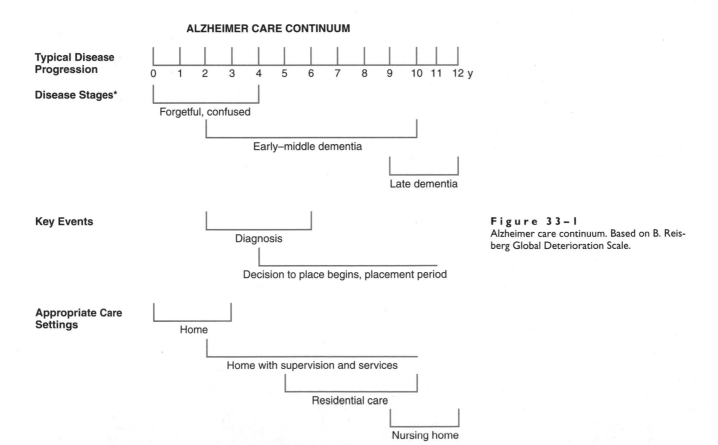

Figure 33-1

Alzheimer care continuum. Based on B. Reisberg Global Deterioration Scale.

TABLE 33-5 Terms Related to Neurological Deficits Found in Dementia

TERM	DEFINITION
Agnosia	Inability to recognize mirror image, familiar others, or everyday objects
Agraphia	Inability to write
Apraxia	Inability to carry out purposeful motor functions, despite intact structural musculature and sensory functions
Akathisia	Extreme motor restlessness and inability to remain seated
Anomia	Difficulty in associating the right word with an object
Aphasia	Inability to communicate verbally and/or understand verbal communication. *Receptive* aphasia refers to being unable to comprehend what one has heard; *expressive* aphasia refers to being unable to express oneself verbally, despite understanding the message; *global* aphasia refers to a combination of the two, that is, the patient can neither comprehend messages nor verbally respond
Ataxia	Difficulty walking; impaired fine motor coordination
Carphologia/floccillation	Purposeless picking at bedcovers or clothes
Constructional difficulty	Inability to put objects together, or to copy complex figures
Dysarthria	Slurred speech, difficulty in articulating words
Dysphagia	Difficulty swallowing
Echolalia	Repeating words or questions without being able to respond appropriately
Formication	Illogical sensation of bugs crawling under one's skin
Mutism	Patient does not communicate verbally despite intact physical structural ability to speak
Paraphasia	Substituting a word or describing rather than naming an object

CT imaging. There is no known cure for the disorder, and most of these patients die within 6 years of diagnosis (Edwards, 1994).

Creutzfeldt-Jakob Disease

Creutzfeldt-Jakob disease is an extremely rare brain disorder that causes dementia, occurring in approximately 1 of every million people (Edwards, 1994). The cause of the disorder is a slow-acting virus that has existed in the patient's body long before it manifests itself symptomatically. Symptoms are more varied than with Alzheimer's disease. They include psychotic behavior; loss of muscular function; and muscle spasms, seizures, and visual symptoms beyond memory loss. These patients show heightened emotional lability, and behavioral reactions can appear quite extreme (Edwards, 1994). Again, there is no known cure for the disorder, and patients typically die within a year of diagnosis.

Dementia of the Lewy Body Type

Lewy body dementia is a chronic cognitive disorder associated with subcortical pathology and the presence of Lewy body substance formation in the cerebral cortex. Similar to Alzheimer's disease, abnormal brain matter is found at autopsy. Although the Lewy body substance appears with senile neuritic plaques, the customary neurofibrillary tangles associated with Alzheimer's disease are scant or absent. Current findings suggest that dementia identified with this cause may be much more prevalent than originally suspected (Keith, 1994).

Consistent with a diagnosis of Lewy body dementia is a greater fluctuation of cognitive impairment with episodic periods of confusion and lucid intervals, similar to that seen with delirium. In contrast to the patient with delirium, however, the fluctuating symptom pattern persists over a significant period. Eventually the symptom pattern presents with the sustained serious neurological deficits associated with end-stage dementia. These patients show a toxic effect to neuroleptic medications, reacting with profound rigidity and immobility, and the course of their disease is more rapid than that seen with Alzheimer's disease. They are more likely to experience paranoid delusions, vivid hallucinations, unexplained falls, and transient disturbances in consciousness (Keith, 1994).

Dementia With Extrapyramidal Symptoms

Huntington's disease, also known as Huntington's chorea and St. Vitus' dance because of its characteristic involuntary jerking movements, is a genetically inherited progressive neurological disease and is transmitted as an autosomal dominant trait (Keith, 1994). If one parent has the disorder, there is a 50% probability of it occurring in the child. Although the disease is present at birth, the symptoms manifest themselves in affected adults between the ages of 35 to 45.

Many but not all patients with the disorder eventually develop dementia. Huntington's disease affects reasoning abilities. Individuals with the disorder become poor problem solvers, typically displaying impoverished judgment. Patients gradually lose their ability to converse intelligently and later to speak. Emotional disinhibition and aggressive behavior are common symptoms (Keith, 1994). Patients with Huntington's disease are at risk for suicide because of the depression often associated with the disorder and the knowledge that most of them have about the course of their disease. This disorder also presents with marked disturbances in motor abilities, particularly with abnormal random movements of the extremities and lower part of the body. Although the disorder can be diagnosed early, there is no cure. The prognosis is for a vegetative existence, and early death.

Dementia due to Brain Lesions

Anything that takes up space in the brain (subdural hematoma, intracranial neoplasm, aneurysm, benign cysts) can create cognitive changes. With a brain lesion, the patient initially presents with a sudden onset of symptoms and with a focal presentation of signs and symptoms related to the precise area of damaged brain tissue. Well-localized signs and symptoms always warrant CT scan and MRI and sometimes cerebral angiography to rule out possible brain lesions as part of the assessment protocol.

Vascular Dementia

The second most common chronic cognitive disorder, **vascular dementia,** is a broad term used to describe dementia symptoms secondary to vascular disease of which there are many varieties. Multiinfarct dementia occurs most often. Consequently, many people refer to all types of vascular dementia as multiinfarct dementia when, in fact, there are many other subtypes. Multiinfarct dementia is associated with small cerebral vascular accidents (strokes), which cause cell destruction and death of brain tissue. Although a major stroke can represent a life-threatening event resulting in paralysis, coma, and death, smaller infarcts can affect speech, thought patterns, memory, and behavior. Cerebral emboli, more common with atherosclerosis, create a similar symptom pattern (Dutherie & Glatt, 1988; Kase, 1986).

Brain imaging via a CT scan or MRI pinpoints the affected area and the extent of brain damage. Neurological examination includes level of consciousness, sensory evaluation, reflexes, and pain perception to verify the diagnosis. The degree of recovery from each infarct varies greatly, with some patients responding to medication and stabilizing at a relatively high level of cognitive functioning. Others show little or no recovery.

Risk factors for the development of multiinfarct dementia include hyperlipidemia, diabetes mellitus, cigarette smoking, and excessive alcohol consumption. Differential diagnosis is important, as treatment depends entirely on control of risk factors and specific therapy aimed at the cause (Abrams, Beers, & Berkow, 1995).

Any type of vascular impairment can destroy brain tissue. For example, a blood clot can block a cerebral artery, cutting off the supply of oxygen to the brain. A ruptured blood vessel in the brain can result in a hemorrhagic stroke. Brain tissue in the affected area dies within a few minutes of oxygen deprivation. From that point forward, the parts of the body controlled by those brain cells can no longer function properly.

There is little question that an accurate diagnosis and prompt treatment to minimize permanent brain damage are essential components of effective nursing care. With vascular dementia, the onset is more abrupt, and the patient displays a fluctuating course of symptom development. There is likely to be evidence of focal neurological signs and symptoms. Vascular dementia presents with a distinctive progression pattern. It manifests a less rapid and more stepwise mental decline than other forms of dementia. The progression of behavioral symptoms tends to plateau after each infarct, with each episode creating a deeper level of dysfunction (Hamdy, Turnbull, Clark, & Lancaster, 1994). As the number of vascular insults increases, so does the level of cognitive deficit. Dementing signs and symptoms appear as patchy rather than global dysfunction. There is less evidence of the inclusive cortical dysfunction characteristic of Alzheimer's disease. Many of these patients retain intact functioning in some areas of daily self-care, while displaying significant deficits in others until the disorder is well advanced. Death often occurs from cardiac rather than neurological causes.

Another type of vascular dementia is called Binswanger's disease, named for Otto Binswanger, who originally described it in 1894 as a chronic, progressive encephalitis. It is associated with persistent severe hypertension and systemic vascular disease. It presents as a degenerative subcortical vascular disorder with symptoms of dementia, focal neurological signs and symptoms, and significant motor deficits, including pseudobulbar palsy. The patient experiences aphasia, hemiplegia, and sensory disturbances consistent with subcortical infarctions involving the basal ganglia and thalamus. Diagnosis by CT scan and MRI is correlated with a decrease in the density of hemispheric white matter and significantly enlarged ventricles (Albert & Lafleche, 1991).

Dementia Associated With Other Physical Conditions

Normal-Pressure Hydrocephalus

Normal-pressure hydrocephalus is a reversible form of dementia that accounts for about 10% of cases. It occurs in elderly patients, as the brain atrophies, and additional fluid forms to fill the spaces in the ventricles. The patient typically presents with a triad of symptoms: memory loss, physical gait disturbances, and urinary incontinence. An early appearance of problems with gait or urinary incontinence suggests a differential diagnosis of normal-pressure hydrocephalus. Dementia symptoms can be completely reversed or significantly diminished with ventricle shunts inserted in the brain. Under sterile conditions, the surgeon inserts a plastic tube in the brain to reroute the fluid into the jugular vein. It is a procedure with significant risk to patients, but it offers them a temporary opportunity to reduce the impact of symptoms. Over time, the symptoms of dementia return and usually become permanent.

Alcohol-Induced Persisting Amnestic Disorders

Chronic use of alcohol can result in loss of brain cells and dementia. Without proper nutrition to provide needed vitamins, "slow starvation of brain cells may result" (Edwards, 1994, p. 69), and the person can develop dementia. **Alcohol-induced persisting amnestic disorder,** or **Korsakoff's syndrome,** occurs because of a thiamine deficiency. The deficiency affects cortical functioning. If a person drinks enough over a significant period, there is brain cell destruction, accompanied by significant deficits in recent and remote memory. By contrast with the dementia associated with Alzheimer's disease, in which the progression is consistently downhill, the Korsakoff patient demonstrates fluctuation in symptoms and changes in personality. The symptoms are more compatible with the pathophysiological changes secondary to excessive alcohol abuse. Such patients may demonstrate consistent difficulty with abstract thinking and calculations and impaired judgment. They do not, however, show the progressive intellectual deterioration associated with the diffuse neurological signs of Alzheimer's disease or the stepwise progression of a multiinfarct dementia.

AIDS Dementia Complex

AIDS dementia complex is a behavioral syndrome that can appear as an isolated symptom set or with other CNS complications of the AIDS virus. Symptoms reflect global cognitive impairment. Patients have **ataxia** (lack of motor coordination), memory disturbances, and an inability to concentrate. Typically, motor problems precede other cognitive symptoms. Once begun, however, the course of the syndrome can be rapid, "characterized by severe dementia with mutism that occurs within a few weeks or months, or it can be a milder, less precipitous one that lasts many months or longer than a year" (Hamdy et al., 1994, p. 55). Typically, the patient loses memory for recent events and is unable to carry out activities of daily living without considerable assistance (Harvath, Patsdaughter, Bumbalo, & McCann, 1995).

One in 10 persons with AIDS is over 50 years of age—a fact that is little known among nurses. AIDS in the elderly can present as dementia and can be mistaken for Alzheimer's disease or other chronic illnesses. It is important that nurses recognize the ways that AIDS dementia presents in the elderly. Usually, the onset is rapid, frequently accompanied by extrapyramidal symptoms, ataxia, leg tremors, peripheral neuropathy progressing to weakness, and abnormal reflexes such as a positive Babinski sign. Patients may experience difficulty concentrating, lack interest in daily activities, and exhibit withdrawal. The confusion and other cognitive difficulties may wax and wane. Additionally, the aphasia seen in Alzheimer's disease is usually absent in AIDS dementia. These clinical differences between Alzheimer's disease and AIDS dementia stem in part from the differences in pathology. Alzheimer's disease predominantly involves the cerebral cortex; AIDS dementia predominantly involves subcortical structures (Whipple, 1996).

Parkinson's Disease

The development of **Parkinson's disease** appears to be associated with a deficiency of dopamine, a neurotransmitter in the brain needed for controlling complex muscle function. Parkinson's disease can produce dementia symptoms, particularly if the disorder develops later in life.

Dementia symptoms occur in approximately 30% to 40% of patients with Parkinson's disease, and more subtle cognitive changes are noted in an additional 40% (Cummings, 1988; Keith, 1994). For this reason, these patients need to have a good neurological assessment at regular intervals. Another reason for a good differential diagnosis of signs and symptoms associated with dementia is the higher-than-normal incidence of depression in Parkinson patients. Depressive symptoms respond to antidepressant medication.

The disease itself typically appears in middle adulthood (ages 45 to 65), and progressive neurological deterioration occurs over many years. Typically, the dementia associated with Parkinson's disease takes the form of a marked difficulty with language function and abstract thinking rather than significant memory loss (Edwards, 1994). Patients experience dysarthria and impaired ability to retrieve information. Although less able to process information, they typically do not seem to have the same level of aphasia and agnosia experienced by Alzheimer's patients. Parkinson's disease and Alzheimer's disease can occur together, thus complicating the diagnostic picture (Keith, 1994).

Multiple Sclerosis

Patients with advanced multiple sclerosis can demonstrate dementia symptoms secondary to multiple sclerosis. The course of the disease is quite similar to that of Parkinson's disease but is related to CNS demyelination (Absher & Cummings, 1994). Additionally, significant personality alterations appear, typically apathy or mood swings. Patients do not display the behavioral problems associated with other forms of dementia.

Depressive Disorder

Depressive disorder in the elderly frequently presents with symptoms characteristic of irreversible dementia. Some people call this a reversible dementia, or **pseudodementia,** because although the symptoms are similar, the disorder is treatable. In reality, depression in the elderly is neither a reversible nor a pseudo form of dementia. It is a mood disorder presenting with marked vegetative symptoms and acute confusion that mimic the chronic cognitive disorder. It is treatable in many cases with appropriate antidepressants (Alexopoulos & Abrams, 1991).

There are several important differences that can aid the clinician in making a differential diagnosis. There are significant differences in the patient's history and in the way patients express themselves about their symptoms.

Answers to assessment questions reflect a personal or family history of depressive disorder. The patient expresses feelings of worthlessness, hopelessness, or anhedonia. A rapid onset, particularly if associated with a life event or situation, suggests a differential diagnosis of depressive disorder. Usually the depressed patient recognizes that something is wrong with concentration or memory. The dementia patient typically does not display a similar awareness. These patients sense that there is something wrong, but they seem less concerned and are unable to pinpoint the nature of their difficulty—for example, in concentrating.

Depression can be a clinical feature superimposed on early dementia because the signs and symptoms of chronic cognitive disorders tell only one part of the dementia story: Inevitably the human story line of dementia is about loss. Personal losses suffered with chronic cognitive disorders are profound, multidimensional, and progressive for patients even in the early stage. Antidepressant medications can relieve depressive symptoms, although they cannot retard the progression of the neurological symptoms. Both the Geriatric Depression Scale (see Chapter 21) and the Mini-Mental State Examination (Figure 33-2) are helpful tools in distinguishing whether or not the patient is depressed, demented, or both. If the patient is depressed and receives effective treatment, the scores on both the Geriatric Depression Scale as well as the Mini-Mental State Examination improve. If the patient is depressed and demented, treatment for depression only improves the score on the depression inventory. See Figure 33-3 for a decision tree regarding the differential diagnosis of dementia and depression.

An additional consideration when working with patients with dementia (with or without depression) is the possibility of clinical depression in the caregiver. Research supports that depression is common among caregivers, particularly those with limited options and sources of social support (Farran, Horton-Deutsch, Fiedler, & Scott, 1997; Farran, Horton-Deutsche, Loukissa, & Johnson, 1998). As the story of the journey clouded by cognitive disorder unfolds, everyone involved in the journey encounters with shattering clarity the meaning of person, the challenge of compassion, and the limits of medical knowledge. The recognition of the losses involved—self, role, value, dignity, and personal meaning for the victim and loss of freedom and status for the caregiver—is inevitable.

What do you think? Since a great deal of caregiving responsibility falls to family members, should family members be compensated for providing nursing care? As society's demographics continue to change, with a greater proportion of the entire population falling in the "old-old" category, how should we provide for the mental and physical needs of this group? Is it realistic to rely so heavily on family members? How could society better support the caregiver? How do you see psychiatric nursing playing a role in meeting the growing needs for care in this population?

> *Check Your Reading*

7. What would be the first nursing action in the treatment of delirium? Why is this action important?
8. What are the differences between delirium and dementia?
9. What are the primary differences between Alzheimer's disease and vascular dementia?

Incidence and Prevalence of Dementia

Alzheimer's disease, the most common cause of dementia, accounts for 60% to 80% of dementia cases (Weiler, 1994). Treatment costs range from $80 to $90 billion a year (Hamdy et al., 1994). The disorder is age-related because the prevalence and incidence of the disorder increase sharply with age. These data are consistent worldwide (Rocca, 1994). Alzheimer's disease, however, is not a normal process of aging. Healthy older adults do not experience profound cognitive deficits as they age. They may demonstrate a gradual decline in recall and recognition memory, but healthy older adults retain **crystallized intelligence,** found in the individual's commonsense judgments, creativity, and wisdom (Amaducci, Falcini, & Lippi, 1992; Bennett & Evans, 1992).

The incidence of dementia is on the increase. People are living longer, and past the age of 70, the frequency of a dementia diagnosis jumps substantially. Moreover, the elderly represent the most rapidly growing segment of the population in the United States. By the year 2050, approximately 67 million Americans will be age 65 or older, and of this number, approximately 14 million will develop dementia.

Dementia affects women more often than men. Other demographic variables, such as occupation, marital status, or living arrangements, do not appear greatly to affect the development of the disorder.

Speculation About Causes of Dementia

Theories about the causes of dementia of the Alzheimer type are many and varied. To date, however, researchers have been unable to pinpoint the precise cause of dementia. Currently, there is no known therapeutic treatment to stop the progression of neurological deficit symptoms. Common causation theories include the following speculations.

Genes

Certain family genograms demonstrate a high familial incidence, with specific clinical features of early onset and rapid progression in a larger-than-normal percentage of first-degree relatives (Breitner & Folstein, 1984). In these families, more than 50% of clinically diagnosed dementia patients have at least one first-degree relative with the disorder. Evidence of a genetic abnormality on chromosome 14 is associated with the disorder. Genetic mapping may provide some clues to familial occurrence in Alzheimer's disease (Goate, 1997).

THE ANNOTATED MINI MENTAL STATE EXAMINATION (AMMSE)

MiniMental LLC

NAME OF SUBJECT _____ Age _____

NAME OF EXAMINER _____ Years of School Completed _____

Approach the patient with respect and encouragement.
Ask: Do you have any trouble with your memory? ☐ Yes ☐ No
May I ask you some questions about your memory? ☐ Yes ☐ No

Date of Examination _____

SCORE	ITEM

5 ( ) **TIME ORIENTATION**

Ask:

What is the year_____(1), season _____(1),

month of the year_____(1), date_____(1),

day of the week _____(1) ?

5 ( ) **PLACE ORIENTATION**

Ask:

Where are we now? What is the state_____(1), city_____(1),

part of the city_____(1), building_____(1),

floor of the building_____(1)?

3 ( ) **REGISTRATION OF THREE WORDS**

Say: Listen carefully. I am going to say three words. You say them back after I stop.

Ready? Here they are... PONY (wait 1 second), QUARTER (wait 1 second), ORANGE (wait one

second). What were those words?

_____(1)

_____(1)

_____(1)

Give 1 point for each correct answer, then repeat them until the patient learns all three.

5 ( ) **SERIAL 7 s AS A TEST OF ATTENTION AND CALCULATION**

Ask: Subtract 7 from 100 and continue to subtract 7 from each subsequent remainder

until I tell you to stop. What is 100 take away 7 ?_____(1)

Say:

Keep Going. _____(1),_____(1),

_____(1),_____(1),

3 ( ) **RECALL OF THREE WORDS**

Ask:

What were those three words I asked you to remember?

Give one point for each correct answer._____(1),

_____(1), _____(1),

2 ( ) **NAMING**

Ask:

What is this? (show pencil) _____(1). What is this? (show watch)_____(1).

For more
information or
additional copies
of this exam,
call (617)587-4215

© 1975, 1998 MiniMental LLC

O V E R

Figure 33–2
"MINI-MENTAL STATE." A PRACTICAL METHOD FOR GRADING THE COGNITIVE STATE OF PATIENTS FOR THE CLINICIAN. *Journal of Psychiatric Research,* 12(3):189–198, 1975. © 1975, 1998. MiniMental LLC.

Illustration continued on following page

MiniMental LLC

1 ( )   REPETITION

Say:

Now I am going to ask you to repeat what I say. Ready? No ifs, ands, or buts.

Now you say that. _____ (1)

3 ( )   COMPREHENSION

Say:

Listen carefully because I am going to ask you to do something:

Take this paper in your left hand (1), fold it in half (1), and put it on the floor. (1)

1 ( )   READING

Say:

Please read the following and do what it says, but do not say it aloud.   (1)

Close your eyes

1 ( )   WRITING

Say:

Please write a sentence. If patient does not respond, say: Write about the weather. (1)

_____

_____

1 ( )   DRAWING

Say: Please copy this design.

TOTAL SCORE _____   Assess level of consciousness along a continuum

Alert	Drowsy	Stupor	Coma

	YES	NO
Cooperative:	☐	☐
Depressed:	☐	☐
Anxious:	☐	☐
Poor Vision:	☐	☐
Poor Hearing:	☐	☐
Native Language:		

	YES	NO
Deterioration from previous level of functioning:	☐	☐
Family History of Dementia:	☐	☐
Head Trauma:	☐	☐
Stroke:	☐	☐
Alcohol Abuse:	☐	☐
Thyroid Disease:	☐	☐

FUNCTION BY PROXY

Please record date when patient was last able to perform the following tasks.
Ask caregiver if patient independently handles:

	YES	NO	DATE
Money/Bills:	☐	☐	_____
Medication:	☐	☐	_____
Transportation:	☐	☐	_____
Telephone:	☐	☐	_____

F i g u r e   3 3 – 2 *Continued*

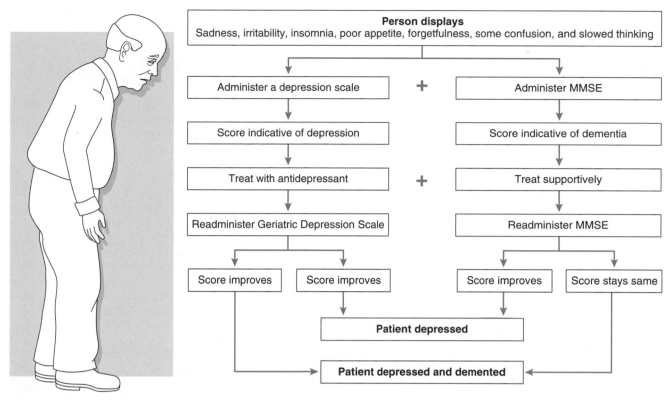

Person displays
Sadness, irritability, insomnia, poor appetite, forgetfulness, some confusion, and slowed thinking

Administer a depression scale	+	Administer MMSE
Score indicative of depression		Score indicative of dementia
Treat with antidepressant	+	Treat supportively
Readminister Geriatric Depression Scale		Readminister MMSE

| Score improves | Score improves | | Score improves | Score stays same |

Patient depressed

Patient depressed and demented

Figure 33–3
Dementia, depression, or both? . . . That is the question. MMSE, Mini-Mental State Examination.

Specific gene mutations have been identified in people who develop Alzheimer's disease (Snowden, 1997). The *ApoE4* gene on chromosome 19 has been identified in nearly two thirds of all people who develop late-life Alzheimer's disease. Genes on chromosomes 14 and 21 have been linked with the form of Alzheimer's disease that develops in midlife.

One of the strongest arguments for a genetic formulation of the disorder is its connection with Down's syndrome. Scientists have identified gene sites on chromosome 21 for the amyloid protein precursor of Alzheimer's disease. Alzheimer's disease is more prevalent in families with Down's syndrome. Of patients with Down's syndrome who live much past the age of 35, a large percentage develop symptoms of dementia (Edwards, 1994).

Decreased Acetylcholine

The role of acetylcholine in the development of dementia has been studied extensively (Hamdy et al., 1994; Nordberg, 1992). **Acetylcholine** is a neurotransmitter judged essential in message transmission by "carrying the electrical impulse across the synapse from the axon of one cell to the dendrite of another" (Edwards, 1993, p. 69). Abnormally low levels of the neurotransmitter have been found in the brain tissue of patients with dementia. Researchers had hoped that by giving dementia patients lecithin, a food substance containing choline, the precursor of acetylcholine, and hydrogine, a medication with similar properties, they might be able to stimulate memory and retard memory loss. Attempts to treat

patients clinically using this drug have, however, proved uneventful, despite clear evidence that a significant loss of the transmitter occurs with dementia.

Donepezil is a drug that improves cognition and the patient's ability to function (Friedhoff, 1998). For 24 weeks, 473 patients with mild to moderately severe Alzheimer's dementia received placebo, or 5 mg or 10 mg of donepezil. Eighty percent of patients receiving donepezil showed improved cognitive function or no decline while they were taking the drug. The 10-mg dose was shown to be the most optimal dose, with maximal benefits and good tolerability. The drug seems to block the chemical breakdown of acetycholine and thereby increases levels of acetylcholine in the brain.

The drug tacrine hydrochloride, known by the trade name Cognex and developed by Parke Davis, was the first drug marketed for use with patients with early dementia. It works by inhibiting the breakdown of acetylcholine. Although this drug does not modify the overall progression of the disorder, it appears to have a delaying effect on the memory loss in the beginning stages in some patients. The predominant potential side effect is liver toxicity. Careful weekly monitoring of aspartate transaminase for liver toxicity should accompany administration of this drug. Other relevant side effects include gastrointestinal distress ranging from nausea to diarrhea and abdominal pain.

β-Amyloid

β-amyloid is a protein fragment found in plaques in the areas of the brain associated with memory. It is unclear if the increased β-amyloid is a result or cause of dementia, but it is known that this protein fragment can form channels that allow excess calcium to enter nerve cells, thereby promoting cell deterioration (Berg, 1998; Tokarski, 1996).

Ministrokes

A long-term study of nuns that assessed their physical and cognitive functions annually and then performed postmortem brain examination for the presence of plaques characteristic of Alzheimer's disease showed that the women who had manifest symptoms of dementia in cognitive testing had suffered small strokes that often were undetected during their lives (Snowden, 1997). The researchers concluded that many of the language and memory changes associated with these small strokes are mislabeled as normal aging, thereby delaying or omitting treatment.

Estrogen

Although the research to date has been limited, there is some evidence that there is a decreased risk of women developing dementia if they are estrogen users (Yaffe, 1998).

Slow-Acting Virus

Some researchers believed that a slow-acting virus created the neurofibrillary tangles in the brain associated with dementia, but reports of studies designed to isolate the virus or to replicate the symptoms in animals have failed to verify an association (Rocca, 1994).

Increased Aluminum

Elevated trace levels of aluminum have been found in the brain tissues of Alzheimer's victims, a finding that has led to a research focus on the role of aluminum in the causation of the disease. However, people with elevated levels of aluminum, such as persons with cancer of the digestive tract who cannot metabolize this metal, do not develop dementia (Cooke & Gould, 1991).

Care of the Dementia Patient

The staging of dementia is important because the symptoms and related levels of nursing care differ so dramatically in each stage. Care begins as supportive for the patient and educative for the family in the early stage. In the middle stage, nursing care is largely oriented toward behavior management. The nurse or primary caregiver provides total care for patients in the late stage. These stages in the course of a dementing illness, although fluctuating in duration, are so consistent that they provide a suitable framework for considering the comprehensive care of the dementia patient from diagnosis to death (Holthaus, 1997).

Three goals, referred to as the 3 "P's" (protecting, preserving, promoting) govern the care of the dementia patient from initial diagnosis to death (Table 33–6).

Protecting the Dignity of the Patient

Patients with dementia lose all defining characteristics of self, but they should never have to lose their right to dignity as unique human beings. Although some are quite basic, there are many ways in which the nurse can protect the dignity of the patient. Referring to the patient by name each time you enter the room acknowledges the patient as a person. Avoid calling the patient "honey," "baby," or "sweetie," and hence recognize the person with dementia as an adult, not a child, even though behaviors are not those of an adult.

Related to acknowledging the patient's name is recognizing the patient's presence, even when the individual is unable to participate fully in the discussion. More often than not, health care conversations take place in the presence of the dementia patient, but they occur almost as if the patient were not physically present. The staff talk to the family without ever looking at or verbally acknowledging the patient's presence. Regardless of the patient's mental condition, the nurse can protect the

TABLE 33–6 Goals for Care of the Patient With Cognitive Disorders: The Three P's

GOAL	RELATED INTERVENTION
Protecting the dignity of the patient	Referring to the patient by name Individualizing nursing actions Incorporating cultural practices Providing privacy
Preserving functional status	Providing a structured environment Working from the patient's strengths Encouraging socialization Providing boards and cues for reality orientation Establishing and adhering to caregiving routines
Promoting quality of life	Stating advance directives Supporting losses Encouraging family interaction

person's dignity with a simple introduction. Identifying the purpose of the consultation in simple words places the patient as part of the conversation and provides important orienting cues. Modest eye contact and body movements that include the patient in the conversation can occur with little effort, without distracting from the information given to family members (Danner, Beck, Heacock, & Modlin, 1993).

Responding to communication efforts, rather than dismissing them as irrelevant or correcting them as untrue, recognizes the patient's attempt to connect through words. For example, one patient consistently greeted his nurse with "Hi, Sally, how are the kids?" In this situation, an appropriate response might be "Mr. Jones, tell me about Sally. It sounds like she was someone special in your life." A little later, the nurse might add, "I think I may remind you of someone else, but my name is Mrs. Allen, and I will be your nurse for the day." Making an issue of the patient's confusion through direct confrontation and immediate correction of a cognitive error rarely is useful. Entering the patient's life and stating the person's name at the beginning of the conversation fosters social bonding.

Individualized physical and socially oriented nursing actions that acknowledge the unique humanness of the dementia patient concurrently reinforce the patient's dignity. For example, considering the patient's cultural standards and religious preferences in planning care can answer fundamental social and spiritual needs. Individualizing basic nursing actions can be as simple as providing the patient with privacy for intimate examinations, toileting, bathing, and dressing. That the patient is unaware of nakedness is unimportant. Even if the patient cannot fully appreciate your efforts, the family usually is grateful for respect shown a dementing relative's personhood. You are often an innocent but important role model of respect for family and ancillary personnel taking care of the patient. Nursing actions to show respect take little additional time or skill. Yet each time you confirm the value of the dementia patient as a person through words, actions, and touch, caring in the true sense of the word occurs.

Preserving Functional Status

Preserving functional status is particularly important during the early stage because cognitive deficits are mild. Again the interventions are simple caring actions that require only time, patience, and imagination. Most people, including dementia patients, perform more effectively when they are acting on their personal strengths and preferences. Detailed information about previous functioning, behavior, likes, and dislikes provides a baseline for choosing nursing interventions that best support the patient's independent functioning. Dementia patients frequently have difficulty staying involved with daily activities and taking charge of their lives without cues even in the early stage. Although they continue to participate in planned activities, these patients frequently need some assistance with structuring their free time. They also may need reminders to complete tasks and verbal cues on how to accomplish them.

Once the patient enters the late stage of dementia and assumes a vegetative state, little functional ability remains. You can still, however, support the little that is left. For example, offering the patient juices, using the patient's hand to guide a spoon, and stroking the throat while telling the patient to swallow fulfill this function.

Personal strengths of individual and collective family members also are important to assess and reinforce because the patient's quality of care ultimately depends on the family's investment. These can include a strong faith, a loving relationship with the patient, financial resources, and a good sense of humor. Each of these personal assets can lend resiliency to the caregiving role and ultimately benefit the patient.

Promoting Quality of Life

It is not easy to watch a person deteriorate neurologically and change from a functional adult to a vegetative state, unable to communicate and incapable of even simple personal care. Quality-of-life issues begin to emerge with diagnosis, and the family must move quickly on the patient's behalf to maximize quality of life later. For example, financial and legal planning should be enacted early, when patients are still aware of what their decisions mean. Eventually, the patient will lose the mental capacity to handle money matters, make decisions about property, and implement advance directives legally. Advise patients to protect assets through a **durable power of attorney,** which designates a decision maker, and to initiate **advance directives,** which describe a patient's wishes, early in the disease process, when patients know what they are signing. Nurses have a significant advocacy role in encouraging patients and families to discuss the future need for these documents and to do so before someone needs them—this can be too late. Additionally, the Patient Self-Determination Act of 1990 requires facilities that receive Medicare funding to inform patients about their rights to make advance directives. Having these documents can prevent later problems (High, 1992; Hirsch, 1990; Levine & Lawlor, 1991).

Throughout the illness, professional and family caregivers can provide for the patient's quality of life by anticipating and responding to patient distress in a compassionate, knowledgeable manner. Education and emotional support for family members helps caregivers take the necessary actions to enhance the quality of the patient's life and their own lives.

Quality of life becomes particularly important in the late stage of dementia, creating significant ethical dilemmas for many families. Family members often are in a quandary about whether to provide nutrition and hydration when the patient can no longer function as a human being. Use of intravenous lines to support hydration is a question when the quality of life is so limited. The desirability of prolonging life is a common source of conflict. Ideally, these decisions related to care are made before the need presents itself because discontinuance of extraordinary measures is difficult once they are initiated. Hospice services can provide significant comfort and family support during the terminal stages of the illness. Pointing this resource out may be necessary because many families do not think of a hospice as a resource for the dementia patient.

Implementation: Individualizing Care for Specific Stages

Early Stages of Dementia

Nursing care of patients in the early stage typically takes place in the home, unless the patient is admitted for diagnostic studies or another reason. (See Chapter 15 for more on home health assessment.) The nurse's role is primarily educational when he or she is called for other medical reasons or at a community health presentation. Care in the early stage centers on the following critical care issues:

1. Obtaining a differential diagnosis
2. Family education
3. Patient safety
4. Conservation of functional ability
5. Legal protection

Differential Diagnosis

Obtaining an accurate differential diagnosis of dementia is essential. Alzheimer's disease is basically a rule-out disorder; that is, the diagnosis is made after family history, laboratory tests, and brain imaging eliminate other disorders with similar cognitive deficits from active consideration. A differential diagnosis to rule out toxic or metabolic causes is extremely important. Some forms of dementia are reversible or controllable with medication and it is a disservice to patients to rob them of their optimal function by not treating conditions when possible.

Sources of information needed to make a differential diagnosis of dementia include a full neurological assessment, laboratory tests to rule out metabolic factors (see Table 33-4), family history of the patient's past behavior and symptom progression, Mini-Mental State Examination, and functional assessment of activities of daily living. A CT scan identifies structural deficits. Brain imaging with PET provides the clinician with information about changes in the metabolic activity and neurochemical characteristics associated with dementia.

If medical test findings fail to account for the cognitive changes, the differential diagnosis is Alzheimer's disease. Typically, testing of patients in the early stage reveals a normal EEG, CT, and MRI (Holcomb, Links, & Smith, 1989). Findings from laboratory tests are within normal range. Guidelines for a multidisciplinary psychiatric assessment are presented in Table 33-7. Extensive psychotherapy is not indicated in the care of dementia patients, but supportive interventions may help alleviate depressive symptoms in the early stage.

Nursing diagnoses are expressed in functional terms and reflect the patient's ability to meet basic needs. Sample nursing diagnoses describing the patient may include

- Altered Thought Processes related to dementia
- Impaired Physical Mobility related to compromised cortical functioning
- Alteration in Nutrition, less than body requirements, related to neurological deficits in swallowing

---

TABLE 33–7 Psychiatric Assessment of the Patient With Alzheimer's Disease

Purpose	• Assessment of primary and secondary psychiatric manifestations of Alzheimer's disease and differential diagnosis from psychosis, depression, anxiety, and phobias • Behavioral disturbances • Rule out delirium • Assess needs and strengths of patient, caregiver, and family • Treatment planning • Educate caregivers
Areas assessed	• Family history (dementing illness, psychiatric disease, neurologic disease, substance abuse) • Social history (education, past level of functioning per occupational history, close relationships, current living situation) • Medical history (all past and present medical illnesses; past surgeries; past trauma, especially head; allergies; medication) • Psychiatric history (psychotic illness, depressive illness, other psychiatric illnesses, psychiatric symptoms, past and current treatments, hospitalizations, suicide, violence) • Present illness (length of cognitive loss, other presenting problems, physical symptoms, functional deficits, psychiatric symptoms) • Mental status (appearance, behavior, speech, mood, hallucinations, delusions, anxiety, phobias, cognition). For delirium: medical evaluation; for behavioral disturbances: environment
Process	• History of patient, caregiver, family • Mental status examination • Medication review
Sources of information	• Patient, caregiver, and family • Past medical and psychiatric records • Multidisciplinary team

From Abraham, I., Holroyd, S., Snustad, D., Manning, C., Brashear, H. R., Diamond, P., & Thompson-Heisterman, A. (1994). Multidisciplinary assessment of patients with Alzheimer's disease. *Nursing Clinics of North America, 29*(1), 120.

- Ineffective Individual Coping related to cognitive deficits
- Self Care Deficit related to cognitive deficits around bathing, grooming, eating
- Altered Role Performance

Nursing diagnoses involving the family may include

- Ineffective Family Coping related to care of the dementia patient
- Knowledge Deficit related to the disease and care of the dementia patient
- Spiritual Distress related to caregiver burden associated with dementia
- Caregiver Role Strain related to 24-hour care
- Social Isolation related to 24-hour care of the dementia patient
- Altered Role Performance
- Powerlessness related to the diagnosis of a terminal illness

Because dementia is basically a rule-out disorder, an accurate history of past performance and functioning is of primary importance. Family members can provide invaluable insight into changes from past performance and the impact of the patient's current behaviors. Box 33-5 summarizes behaviors characteristic of the early stage.

Ask questions about past psychiatric history, particularly depression and chemical dependence, head trauma, and recent stressful events. Data about sleeping and eating patterns, level of supervision required, availability of care, and financial resources help the clinician understand the nature and depth of the cognitive deficit. Box 33-6 is an assessment guide outlining areas of psychosocial concern with potential behavioral descriptors. You can use this guide or a similar format to develop and document baseline behavioral data from the assessment interview.

Appearance

Although few changes in physical characteristics are visible to the casual observer, the family may have noticed a distinct change in the patient's attention to dress and cleanliness. Lack of interest in hygiene is common. A problem less frequently talked about involves the cleanliness of patients living alone. With dementia, the sense of smell diminishes, so the patient may have a strong urine smell from not bathing or wiping correctly without being aware of it. Most patients, even in the early stage, may need gentle encouragement to shower daily and to use good oral hygiene.

Memory Deficits

Memory impairment during the early stages involves the storage and retrieval of new information. The patient's recent memory loss is not a simple forgetting of objects such as a pocketbook or an appointment. Rather it is for common activities of daily living that the individual was able to recall without any difficulty. **Short-term memory** (immediate and recent memory) for things that happened that day, or even a few minutes ago, is impaired, whereas in most instances **remote memory** for events in the past is preserved. Thus, these patients typically can recall what happened 10 years ago but cannot tell the interviewer what they just had for breakfast or whether it was raining yesterday.

Learning new information is no longer possible because the short-term memory required to process and synthesize new information misses a meaningful connection with the current situation (Hamdy et al., 1994). Memory loss creates demonstrable problems with initiating and sustaining conversations. Patients evidence constructional difficulty and cannot put discrete pieces of data or objects together in a meaningful whole (Abraham, Fox, & Cohen, 1992).

Personality Changes

Ironically, often the personality changes accompanying memory loss rather than the loss itself cause family members to seek a definitive diagnosis for their relative. Common personality changes involve low tolerance for normal frustration and oversensitivity to the remarks of others. Family members complain of their relative's lack of initiative, decreased attention span, and diminished emotional presence. They describe declining self-awareness as: "He just doesn't seem interested anymore." "He seems to get angry over things that never bothered him before." "She just seems so self-absorbed, not at all like her old self."

Emotional lability and restlessness are other characteristic behaviors. A patient with dementia can go from tears to laughter, from silence to boisterous talking, all in a matter of minutes. A patient may deny an emotional state or feeling reaction to a situation, even with direct confrontation. Moreover, the patient's facial expression may show little response to change, although agitated and clenched body language frequently speaks volumes. Some patients sit for long periods with a blank stare. When spoken to, there seems to be a delayed reaction before the patient responds. Rumination about a variety of subjects is common.

Box 33-5 ■ ■ ■ ■ ■
Behavior Patterns Found in the Early Stage

Initial variance according to which part of the brain is most affected
Forgetfulness
Trouble concentrating, carrying on an in-depth conversation
Trouble coping with everyday events, particularly unstructured
Change in personality, most commonly apathy, irritability, or sudden temper outbursts
Language disturbance
Limited problem solving ability; ability to learn new things is more difficult

Box 33-6 ■ ■ ■ ■ ■

Nursing Assessment Guide for Developing Behavioral Assessments for Dementia Patients

Category	Behavioral Descriptors
Appearance (hygiene, physical characteristics, cleanliness, dress)	Neat/disheveled appearance, poor/good physical hygiene, cachectic/normal body weight, erect/stooped/listing posture, weakness in arms/legs, gross/fine tremors
Memory deficits (recent and remote memory, orientation, intellectual judgment, insight)	Memory loss (assess immediate, recent, and remote), visuospatial skills, appropriate/inappropriate problem solving, knowledge of current events, confabulation, presence of visual/auditory hallucinations, delusions, thought blocking, orientation to person/place/time, misinterpretation of visual/auditory/olfactory stimuli, ability to engage in tasks requiring multiple skill knowledge
Personality changes (mood and emotions expressed)	Appropriate/inappropriate, bland, flat, dull, sad, fearful facial expression; labile, dull, angry, euphoric, limited, agitated, suspicious, cooperative, appropriate/inappropriate expression of feeling; personality changes noted by family; overreaction/underreaction to situations, distractibility, appropriate/inappropriate judgment (give specific example); makes lewd remarks, exposes self, openly masturbates, touches people inappropriately
Psychomotor functioning (motor activity, human response to situation)	Lack of precision in voluntary movements, hyperactive, pacing, slowed movements, repetitive or nondirective gestures; disturbance in sleep patterns, difficulty walking, seizures, loses balance, night walking, aimless/goal-directed actions, sundown syndrome
Communication ability (ability to communicate verbally and in writing)	Delayed/blocked verbal communication, mutism, inability to grasp meaning of spoken/written word, perseveration, inability to find words, difficulty writing words and signing name
Nutrition and elimination	Nutrition above/below nutritional requirements; refuses food, sits and stares at food, "cheeks" food without swallowing, tries to eat inedible objects/spoiled food; difficulty with swallowing, choking; incontinence (specify bladder, bowel); smears feces, urinates/defecates in inappropriate places

Other personality changes involve patient judgments about critical matters, hoarding, or giving away assets. The affected individual does not seem as aware of the risks involved or the consequences of certain life decisions related to money and other assets. Not uncommonly, patients with an undiagnosed dementia appear in the psychiatrist's office seeking marital therapy because the spouse feels a husband (wife) is becoming increasingly irresponsible and not attending to previous obligations, such as payment of bills.

Other factors, such as delirium, depression, and unfamiliar environments, can account for some personality changes, and these need to be accounted for before attributing them to the dementia. For example, more than a few patients in the early stage are aware that there is something wrong with their minds. When the Alzheimer's patient clutches his or her head, and asks "What is wrong with me," or makes statements such as "I wish I were dead" or "I want to go home," these are all poignant indications of the anguish of experiencing a world that is slipping out of view. As the disease progresses, patients become less acutely aware of most

things in their world, including the meaning of their illness. Initially, however, awareness is common, and the nurse needs to monitor patients showing depressive ideation closely. Any attempt, gesture, or specific plan of suicide is cause for alarm. Antidepressant medication, carefully monitored, can provide a significantly higher quality of life for many patients in the early stage. See Box 33-7 for poem "Away."

Communication Difficulty

Communication difficulties appear early in the disorder, occurring as one or more of the language problems identified in Table 33-8. Suggested nursing interventions are provided related to each type of deficit. Some patients handle their problem with word finding and comprehension by filling in the blanks with new data that may or may not make sense. Others become silent rather than expose their deficit. For many patients, the language deficits in dementia begin with thought blocking, a difficulty in finding the right words to express a complete thought or to describe an object (Lee, 1991).

Box 33-7 ■ ■ ■ ■ ■
Away

> I cannot say, and I will not say
> That he is dead, he is just away.
> With a cheery smile, and a wave of his hand,
> He has wandered into an unknown land.
> And left us dreaming how very fair
> It must be since he lingers there.
> And you—O you, who the wildest yearn
> For the old-time step and the glad return—
> Think of him fairing on, as dear
> In the love of there as the love of here;
> Think of him still as the same, I say:
> He is not dead—he is just away!
> —James Whitcomb Riley (1849–1916),
> American poet

Compounding the language problem is a concurrent reduction in the flow of ideas.

Superficial conversations usually fail to reveal thought blocking. Only when the conversation progresses to a deeper level requiring abstract thinking and complex problem solving does the difficulty emerge. This is both good and bad. It is good in the sense that the individual responds appropriately and continues to receive the social support from others. It is bad in the sense that other people are not always aware of the patient's problems until well into the conversation, thus creating embarrassment for the patient and the involved listener, as Case Example 33-1 shows.

■ **CASE EXAMPLE 33-1**
■ **Bill's Story**

■
■ Bill Clarke is a dementia patient who appears friendly and
■ physically fit. His wife took him to the podiatrist, and as he
■ was waiting for his turn, a Red Cross worker struck up a
■ conversation with him. "Isn't it wonderful that Dr.
■ Magothy has set up his new podiatry practice here?" she
said. And Bill replied, "Yes, it is wonderful. We can never have too many." Encouraged by his response, the Red Cross worker continued her conversation, "And isn't it terrible about the damage the tornado caused last month?" To which Bill replied, "Yes, it is wonderful. We can never have too many." The worker looked at him with an odd expression, as she realized that he was responding automatically but had little comprehension of the meaning of his words. ■

Even in the early stage, difficulty in naming familiar objects (**anomia**) is a problem for many patients. The words may still be available to the patient, but their meaning undergoes subtle modification. For example, Francis Michaels had been able to remember his law case citations without prompting. In the early stages of the disease, he was able to use the cues from his wife and look up the citations to continue his law practice. His previous reputation for legal excellence and semblance of similar functioning initially prompted his clients to overlook what was increasingly obvious to his family— that Francis was no longer able to fully comprehend what he was reading. Labeling common objects, placing clothing and utensils in sequential order, periodically explaining television commentary, and saying the name of visitors as they enter the room are all strategies to help the patient with object name recognition.

Conversation is particularly difficult for the patient if there are several people talking or the conversation requires sudden shifts to a different topic. Patients may have difficulty understanding complex statements made by others, or they may fail to comprehend issues entirely. Transitions from one subject to another are less fluid. Simple nursing actions can help the patient maintain focus on the conversation by, for example, providing logical links through words and spacing the concrete verbal, visual, and tactile prompts needed to comprehend basic messages. Using multiple communication modalities in the delivery of a message also helps patients to grasp ideas. For example, using written words or pictures to complement the spoken word, touch to emphasize a point, or looking in the direction of the

TABLE 33-8 Communication Problems and Nursing Interventions in the Early Stage

PATIENT PROBLEM	NURSING INTERVENTION
Problem finding words	Supply missing words, name objects, post printed signs for common word objects
Difficulty with comprehension	Use simple concrete words, one thought at a time; use names instead of pronouns
Communication anxiety increases in crowds	Limit number of people present during an interview
Shortened attention span	Use short session rather than long ones; gauge interactions by observing patient behavior
Delayed verbal response	Allow for additional processing time; restate message using the same words if necessary; reinforce all attempts at communication
Increasing agitation	Use eye contact, a calm reassuring voice, and patient observation to diffuse the situation; give reassurance, acceptance, and full attention to patient needs
Tells the same story repetitively	Ask the patient to expand on a small part of the story, thank the patient for sharing, and move to a different topic; identify and use the underlying theme

object described can assist patients in continuing a social conversation.

Because long-term memory is not affected in the early stages, conversations focused on the past have meaning to both the patient and the caregiver. Patients have an easier time expressing connected thoughts about the past. Speech is more spontaneous because the patient does not have to "think" about the interrelationships in the story. Content relationships already are present and are logically assembled in long-term memory. Thus, patients find it easier to describe a past feeling from memory than to identify their present emotional state. Comprehension of verbal messages increases with the use of simple language, presenting one idea at a time, and using the same words with repetitive instructions.

Psychomotor Functioning

When the nurse focuses on the patient's abilities rather than disabilities and designs interventions to support strengths and compensate for behavioral losses, patients often can respond on a higher level. Being able to perform simple tasks gives the patient a sense of mastery.

The ability to handle gadgets and to carry out coordinated purposeful movements, actions so automatic for most people, fade in the course of dementia, despite the patient's ownership of intact skeletal, motor, and sensory body systems. Referred to as **apraxia,** the patient's motor deficit is more apparent with new or more complex tasks and consequently may be dismissed as an unfamiliarity with the task requirements. More automatic motor activities, such as dressing, eating, and walking, show less decline until the patient has moved into the middle stages of the disease. As tasks requiring complicated, purposeful movements become increasingly difficult for patients to maneuver, the patient's behavioral response turns into anger or passivity. Either response provides a dilemma. It saddens the caregiver to watch the person give up and sit with a dejected posture, uninterested and uninvolved—without hope. Handling the anger without retaliating is difficult because of the amount of attention and repetition required for task completion. The incessant nature of the demand with such a limited outcome tries the patience of even the most dedicated caregiver.

The inability to complete simple tasks is not the fault of the patient. In the early stage, the patient sincerely wants to help but cannot complete coordinated tasks without verbal prompts and constant attention. Yet the semiinvolvement and understanding of part, but not all, of the steps needed for task completion is bewildering for the family caregiver, as Case Example 33–2 illustrates.

■ CASE EXAMPLE 33–2
■ Betty's Story

■ My sister Betty tries to do many things around the
house—set the table, wash the dishes, dust the furniture,
and little things like that. She is always eager to help, but
she gets confused and doesn't finish anything. That's what
gets me so upset. I get so frustrated sometimes that I want

to lash out. For example, she will get the silverware out of the drawer, walk to the table, pick up the napkins, and walk back to the drawer with both silverware and napkins. I know that Alzheimer's is causing her to act this way, but little things happen like this every day. Because on the surface she seems like her normal self, I often forget she doesn't have a brain that is fully working. ■

The family needs education and emotional support to surmount these difficulties. Practical strategies help the caregiver to respond properly to the patient's constant desire to be involved and equally persistent need for supervision to complete even simple tasks. Suggestions that could be offered to the caregiver include:

1. Avoid tasks involving multiple or concurrent steps. Simple tasks with well-defined sequential steps are more appropriate.
2. Offer praise to encourage cooperation and reduce anxiety.
3. Model desirable behaviors to provide additional cues.
4. Use distraction and postponement to dissipate agitation and anger.
5. Remain calm to avoid having the patient sense the caregiver's frustration, which could negatively affect the patient's function.

Nutrition and Elimination

A final area of concern is the patient's nutritional status and elimination patterns. Many patients begin to have eating difficulties even in the early stage. Their table manners become lax, and sometimes they forget they have just eaten or fail to know when it is mealtime without prompting. Caregivers need to assume responsibility for ensuring adequate nutritional intake. Elimination habits are important pieces of data. Having knowledge of the patient's normal elimination patterns during the early stage helps the caregiver time bathroom breaks later on when the patient needs assistance. Boxes 33–8 and 33–9 provide helpful tips for responding with nutritional and elimination challenges.

Family Education

In the early stage, family members provide most of the care for patients, with episodic support from the nurse and the intermittent use of adult day care centers. For months, even years, patients can remain independent with minimal assistance. Most patients in the early stage can communicate their needs, at least on a superficial level, and they seem normal to others. In fact, the spouse of a dementia patient who looked older than her husband was asked by an attorney with some embarrassment, "I know this is an unusual question, but which one of you is the Alzheimer's patient?" (Zarit, Orr, & Zarit, 1985).

Education of the family begins as soon as the diagnosis is confirmed. Immediate family members play an important role in the care of the dementia patient, first as informants, then as patient advocates, and finally as the primary caregiver and patient supporter. Legal issues

Box 33–8 ■■■■■
Measures to Facilitate Eating

- Present food that is attractive, colorful, and flavorful.
- Involve patient in food preparation.
- Serve one course at a time.
- Check temperature of food; patient may lack judgment when something is too hot.
- Serve familiar foods.
- Make mealtime a routine.
- Substitute healthy foods for sweets and "junk food."
- Provide healthy finger-food snacks like graham crackers.
- Use plastic tablecloths or placemats for easier clean-up.
- Use sturdy plastic dishes and cups for minimum breakage.
- Use contrasting dishes and tablecloth to make dishes easier to distinguish from the background.
- Allow the patient to continue feeding self by using finger foods.

and care decisions related to a dementia diagnosis make it imperative that the family understand the diagnosis and its implications for care early in the course of the disease. An excellent educational resource guide is *The Thirty-Six Hour Day,* a compilation of family experiences with the disorder at different stages, written by Mace and Rabins (1991). Although other books also offer help, this book remains the definitive resource for family caregivers.

Support groups for family members of dementia patients offer an ongoing, practical socioeducational re-

Box 33–9 ■■■■■
Measures to Facilitate Toileting

- Use incontinence products (i.e., pads).
- Place plastic over chair or other furniture being used.
- Verbally remind patient or take patient to bathroom every hour or so.
- Place a portable commode in the patient's bedroom if the bathroom is too far away.
- Use easy-to-remove clothing (i.e., those with Velcro closures, or two-piece exercise suit).
- Install handrails and grab bars anchored to studs next to toilet.
- Provide a toilet seat raised with arms if the seat is too low.
- Try using a colored, padded toilet seat to call attention to toilet.
- Remove toilet seat cover.

source—even in the early stage. They offer a safe place to explore such specific issues as:

1. "Should the patient stop driving?"
2. "Should you tell other people of the diagnosis, particularly coworkers, or adult children?"
3. "Should the patient wear an ID bracelet or carry a card indicating a dementia diagnosis?"
4. "How do I handle my spouse's sexual desires when I don't feel as though it is an adult relationship anymore?"

Coaching family members to use all of the senses and past memories in talking with patients typically helps them feel more comfortable and increases the chance of patient participation in conversation. Part of the coaching process is supportive, but it also has an educational format (Kuhlman, Wilson, Hutchinson, & Wallhagen, 1991). Helpful guidelines to understanding the symptoms and effects of memory loss on patient behavior include the following:

1. The reduced animation found in the patient's facial expression and physical movements is part of the disease process, not a reflection on the social interaction.
2. There may be noticeable pauses in the conversation and a sharp reduction in spontaneous speech.
3. Keep conversation simple and straightforward.
4. The patient's speech may be difficult to understand, and it is appropriate to provide an educated guess about what the patient is trying to say.
5. Overconcern about minor matters and repetition indicate a need for additional reassurances from the family caregiver.
6. Touch is an important form of communication when words no longer provide connections.
7. Sharing important moments from the past with the patient provides a bridge to connection even if the patient does not seem to respond.

Safety Issues

Safety issues become the responsibility of the caregiver early in the disorder. A safe environment allows the dementia patient both physical freedom and a sense of security. These patients need a physical environment that provides room to pace. It is important to avoid the use of scatter rugs that may lead to falls, to mark clearly changes in floor elevations, and to wipe up floor spills promptly because the patient will not notice these. In addition to their cognitive inability to correct their missteps, these patients are subject to the same sensory losses that make falls in the elderly more problematic.

Safety in the home is a challenge. The dementia patient typically wants to engage in normal activities but does not always register how this should be accomplished. Patients turn on the stove and forget it is on or use a sharp instrument in an inappropriate way. Simple strategies to protect the patient include cleaning up spills, keeping sharp instruments out of reach, monitoring patients who wander, taking the knobs off the stove, and locking up toxic substances. Although the temptation exists to reprimand patients in the hope of influencing future behavior, this response rarely has a productive result even though the patient may understand what the caregiver is saying. The patient's recent memory retrieval loss does not permit learning transfer to a new situation.

Interpersonal safety is a necessary requirement for effective functioning in the early stage. Dementia patients cope with their environment best when they have a consistent and predictable daily social routine. Nurses can help family members develop and maintain a daily routine that the patient can count on for security. Changes should be avoided whenever possible. When the patient's circumstances require a significant alteration, as in a move to a nursing home, including familiar objects, such as pictures, scrapbooks, religious articles, or a favorite throw, makes the transition easier.

Safety also entails taking responsibility for ensuring the safety of others who may be inadvertently endangered by the patient with memory loss. Of considerable concern is the dementia patient's wish to drive. Family members find it difficult to take this last vestige of independence away from the patient, particularly when the individual can go to familiar places without any apparent difficulty. Although restricting the patient's driving is not easy, it is absolutely essential because these patients have difficulty with their reasoning and constructional abilities. Explaining to families that they are acting on the patient's behalf helps with guilt feelings. Box 33-10 provides environmental safety issues (Donnelly & Karlinsky, 1990).

Conservation of Functional Ability

Many simple nursing strategies can help patients maintain existing function for as long as possible. Each patient presents a unique blend of behaviors and attitudes, some of which are easier to handle than others in the early stage. Nursing interventions need to be flexible, geared to the individualized needs of the patient, and adapted to fluctuations in behavior. As Case Example 33-3 shows, normalizing tasks that the patient can accomplish and providing verbal or written cues help patients perform activities that otherwise would not be possible.

■ **CASE EXAMPLE 33–3**
■ **Reba's Story**

■ Reba Jordan could not remember how to make a sandwich, which distressed her greatly. Rather than simply making the sandwich herself, her daughter took all of the ingredients out of the refrigerator and placed them on the counter. Mother and daughter then proceeded to make the sandwich as a joint fun activity. The daughter named each ingredient when the time came to use it, and her mother handed it to her. The activity became a shared experience in which both could participate and enjoy their time with each other. ■

Previously learned and familiar material lingers and remains intact for longer periods. It follows that interventions recognizing and using patient strengths around

Box 33–10 ■ ■ ■ ■ ■
Measures to Facilitate Environmental Safety

- Maintain consistent lighting throughout rooms, hallways, or entryways.
- Paint a handrail or use reflector tape if the hallway or stairs are dark.
- Install lights in dark closets.
- Keep the furniture in the same place.
- Use decals on glass doors that are difficult to see.
- Mark the edges of stairs with black tape.
- Keep small pets out of walkways.
- Check the lawn and grounds for places that a person may trip, fall, or become otherwise injured (e.g., uneven surfaces or walkways, holes in the lawn, fallen branches, thorny bushes, cracked pavement, hoses, or a low clothesline).
- Ensure that clothing fits properly—not too long or trailing on the floor.
- Use well-fitting shoes.
- Avoid use of extension cords and unplug appliances not in use.
- Keep temperature of water heater set at 120°F to avoid scalding.
- Place signs that say "Do Not Touch" or "Stop, Very Hot" on appliances, such as oven, coffee maker, toaster, crock pots, irons.
- Place all medications out of reach.
- Install a secure gate and a light switch at the top and bottom of stairs.
- Use a night-light.
- Keep a flashlight, light switch, or lamp beside the bed.
- Use recliners and furniture that provide assistance to get up.

automatic learned activities are more likely to be successful and to foster self-confidence. When the patient requires structural cues or guidance, you need to assess how much should be given and what areas the patient can handle. By providing cues and assisting only to the point at which the patient can take over, the patient can stay functional for a longer period.

Early-stage dementia patients often cannot execute complex tasks requiring memory and visuospatial skills, such as dialing a telephone or making a meal unassisted. With verbal cues and minimal assistance, they can continue to perform these activities. For example, many phone systems have a built-in memory for frequently called phone numbers. A card placed next to the phone with a single-digit number and the person's name can permit independent phone use, whereas trying to remember the person's phone number and dialing sequential digits are beyond the patient's cognitive capability.

Participating in activities within his or her scope of cognitive ability enhances the patient's self-esteem. Simple activities that patients in the early stage can do without significant difficulty include polishing silver, watering plants, folding laundry, washing windows, and sorting socks. Music, rhythm, and hand-clapping make use of gross and fine motor abilities and generally are enjoyed by dementia patients. Such activities offer an opportunity for socialization without a heavy demand for interaction—something beyond the patient's capability. Familiar recordings such as country or religious music encourage patient participation even more because they stimulate automatic memories. Physically focused activities, such as tossing balls, Frisbees, beanbags, or balloons to others, help patients drain off excess energy and provide a social outlet.

Excessive anxiety decreases cognitive functioning in all individuals, but the dementia patient has more limited cognitive ability to work with in responding appropriately to complex life situations. Persistent worry and overconcern about simple life issues are common occurrences. Cognitively confused patients benefit from repeated orientation to their setting. Rules and unit policies should be identified in simple, easily understandable terms. Orienting cues, such as seasonal pictures, calendars, clocks, large-print signs identifying different rooms, and printed patient names, serve as important reminders to patients in the early stage. Some hospital units print the patient's name on the door in large letters. Others place a picture of the patient when he or she was younger to stimulate recognition. All of these interventions help decrease anxiety. Patience, understanding, and frequent reassurance also can help the patient cope with the issues of the moment.

Judgments and Decision-Making

Cognitive limitations also mean that the patient may exercise poor judgment or become combative when unable to meet real or perceived expectations. At the same time, caregivers need to realize that dementia patients may have "some impaired cognitive skills, but also retain some decision-making skills" (Weiler, 1994, p. 36) during the early stage. Whenever possible, these patients should be encouraged to make their own decisions. Although it is sometimes difficult to distinguish when to support and when to limit the patient's decision-making powers, choices provide a sense of purpose and feeling in control. Issues that do not compromise the safety or well-being of self and others can be left to the patient's discretion, for example, which food to eat first or where to go next.

Related to the capacity to make decisions on one's own behalf is the issue of advance directives and durable power of attorney. Legal definitions of competency come into play in understanding the needs of the Alzheimer's patient and the balance between the rights of the patient and the needs of the family. Issues of competency become important with the signing of legal documents, such as wills, living wills, informed consent, and power of attorney. In legal terms, *competent* is used to describe individuals who have reached the age of 18 and are able to act on their own behalf. *Incompetent* is a legal term used to describe individuals who have had their cases reviewed in a court proceeding and have been declared incompetent by the judge or jury to manage their own affairs.

A diagnosis of dementia does not automatically mean that a person is legally incompetent. In the early stages of the disease, the patient may not be fully capable of understanding or meeting all of his or her health care needs but often is capable of handling affairs with assistance. Patients are considered competent as long as they retain their decision-making capacity. Legal matters should be handled with the dementia patient during the early stages of the disorder, when the individual is still able to understand the process of decision-making involved in durable power of attorney.

Most patients and their families appreciate a frank discussion and advance directives. Open discussion gives dementia patients the opportunity to ask questions and to take charge of their lives to whatever extent is possible. By including the family in the process of developing advance directives most responsive to an individual patient's needs early on, when the patient clearly expresses wishes, most family members feel more confident during the late stages of the disease.

Support for Social Functioning

Supporting social functional ability is an art. Because most patients with mild or moderate cognitive deficits are treated at home for financial and personal reasons, creating social occasions in the home should be a consistent effort. Most patients respond more effectively in a familiar environment, surrounded by their customary furnishings. Activities need not be elaborate or long-lived. In the home, providing simple opportunities for socialization requires only the imagination and a little time. Uncomplicated social activities provide needed stimulation for the patient. An uncomplicated game, listening to music, group exercise, going for a walk, and pointing out flowers or trees are relevant examples. Regularly receiving a greeting or a kind word is important to the patient as a human acknowledgment. It helps decrease the patient's feelings of loneliness and anxiety.

One-to-one interactions work better than group activities. Visiting with a group provides too many simultaneous demands. Moreover, people avoid dementia patients because their behavior seems eccentric. This nonacceptance heightens the sense of social isolation for the patient and supportive others in social situations.

Reeves (1993) proposed a nursing intervention designed to support the patient's individuality and use the patient's ability to remember things in the past to enhance self-esteem. It involves making a display book with the patient and family entitled "This Is Your Life." The book highlights past and present family pictures displayed in chronological order. It includes data about the patient's interests, hobbies, and past achievements. Creating an individualized display book stimulates memories and reinforces the patient's sense of self. The photographs act as a stimulant to conversation about the life story and help the staff to see the patient as a real person. Additionally, the nurse can encourage patients to display personal items in their rooms. Mementos provide security for the patient and serve as a topic of conversation for professional caregivers providing direct physical care. For families who visit infrequently, suggest the making of a videotape.

Adult Day Care Centers

Intermittent and regular respite extends the family's ability to provide a meaningful environment for the patient. Support existing social skills with referrals to adult day care programs, in which the patient has multiple opportunities for socialization. Adult day care centers for the cognitively disabled are increasing in popularity as a realistic solution for mild and moderate cognitive deficits. Established in the community as an outpatient alternative to nursing home placement, some day care centers are private pay, and others are partially or wholly subsidized by public funds. The patient is brought on a regular basis to a treatment center with a structured program for patients with cognitive impairment. Appropriate stimuli provide the patient with opportunities for personal expression, exercise, and support of remaining functioning.

Adult day care programs typically operate on a half-day or full-day schedule of activities, offered every day or on selected days of the week. Participation offers several benefits. Most significantly, adult day care programs for the cognitively impaired provide structured activities specifically geared to the patient's developmental needs. Time spent away from the primary caregiver in a supervised social setting also provides respite for the caregiver, which allows for a better attitude toward the patient. Having the patient in a safe, structured, and stimulating environment relieves family anxiety about the stress of providing 24-hour care and guilt related to resentment about the unrelenting "call to care." Thus, adult day care programs allow the patient to stay at home longer, often with considerable cost savings to the family and community.

Respite Care

Another form of respite care involves overnight stays in a nursing home setting or a specified block of time in which a trained caregiver comes to the home. Respite provides at least a limited time away from the patient for rest and rejuvenation. Family members use it to catch up on errands, to visit old friends, and to take vacations. You often need to remind the family of the need to take time off: "You can't give from an empty cupboard." Because many family members become so involved, it is hard for them to see the wisdom of the intervention (Grollman & Kosik, 1997; Hay, 1998).

Medical Treatment

Regular medical evaluation is important to monitor the progress of the disease and identify related problems. Routine examinations at 6-month intervals usually are sufficient to allow changes in cognitive function to be detected. Of course, new or significant changes in symptoms warrant more immediate attention.

As mentioned earlier, donepezil is approved for use with early dementia, and some patients in the early stage benefit from antidepressant medications. The latter prove useful in clearing the cognitive symptoms associated with depression that may complicate the overall picture. Most patients do not require other psychotropic drugs during the early stage. Many need them in the middle stages to reduce agitation and induce sleep. As with all medications in the elderly, metabolic build-up should be monitored carefully.

When conventional medicine is unable to offer treatment that cures or controls a disease, patients and their caregivers often explore alternative and complementary therapies as a means of symptom management, comfort, and hope. For these individuals, using a treatment of questionable value may seem superior to taking no action at all. Not surprisingly, more than half of persons with dementias and their caregivers use a variety of alternative and complementary therapies ranging from magnetic therapies to homeopathic remedies to fasting regimens (Coleman, Fowler, & Williams, 1995). Although many of the alternative and complementary therapies used have little hard evidence supporting their value, some research is beginning to demonstrate their effectiveness. One popular example is the herb **ginkgo biloba,** which has been shown to improve memory, attention, and social function in persons with early Alzheimer's disease due to its ability to increase blood flow in small vessels (LeBars, Katz, Berman, Freedman, & Schatzberg, 1997). The growing research findings related to alternative and complementary therapies that is becoming available and consumers' significant interest and use of these treatments challenges nurses to keep current of new findings. Without robbing patients and their caregivers of hope (and perhaps some benefit through the placebo effect), nurses need to assist in separating fact from fad and protect patients from harm from the use of unsafe or useless practices.

Middle Stage of Dementia

In the middle stage, cognitive decline is more rapid and noticeable. Marked dependency and disability become apparent. Box 33–11 lists behavior symptoms common to the middle stage of dementia.

Disorientation

Disorientation, the lack of connection to time and place, becomes a consistent feature in the middle stage. Although orientation to self typically remains intact for a longer time than place and time, patients often cannot recognize themselves in the mirror (**agnosia**), identify significant people in their lives, or describe their relationship to significant others.

Another form of disorientation is the wish to be transported to a different time and place. Not uncommonly, patients ask plaintively to "go home" or mistake people in their current environment for those in their past life. Understanding that "going home" frequently refers to longing for their more emotionally satisfying

Box 33–11 ▪▪▪▪▪
Behavior Symptoms Common in the Middle Stages of Dementia

Trouble eating
Child-like behavior
Inability to perform self-care activities unassisted
Trouble communicating and following directions
Emotional disinhibition
Bowel and bladder incontinence
Wandering, so that patient cannot be left alone
Pacing and agitation
Visual hallucinations
Difficulty recognizing family and friends
Meaningless words and actions
Catastrophic reactions
Sundown syndrome

past allows you to ask questions about the patient's earlier life. In many instances, this intervention not only stops the rumination momentarily but also reduces the patients' sense of loneliness and fear by anchoring them in a safer time. Gently stroking the patient's hand or arm, reassuring the patient that he or she is safe and you will protect them helps, as does distraction. If the patient lacks the ability to speak, the caregiver can employ touch and use a photograph, memento in the patient's room, or a family fact from the chart to encourage the patient. Patients sometimes talk as if someone important to them who has died still lives. Asking the patient to talk about significant people in his or her past is much more helpful than providing the reality orientation that the person has died. Providing the "facts of the situation" sometimes causes the patient to grieve the loss as if it is occurring in the present (Burgener, Shimer, & Murrell, 1993).

Reality validation of past life experience is far more effective than reality orientation, which serves only to confuse the patient more in some cases. When coupled with frequent environmental orientation prompts, gentle encouragement, patience, and touch, the intervention is quite effective with many middle-stage dementia patients (Davidson & Stern, 1991).

Self-Care

Most self-care and activities of daily living are now beyond the patient's ability to complete. The coordinated efforts required for dressing, bathing, and eating do not fit together in the patient's mind. However, although the patient's mind is dementing rapidly, the patient, at least initially, can still complete activities of daily living with significant caregiver assistance. Step-by-step prompting, using the same simple words repetitively, combining the words with touch, and filling in difficult spots make patient task achievement possible. For example, touching the patient's leg and saying, "Now lift this leg and put it in the pants," provide the multisensory cues to complete a task the patient could not accomplish otherwise. You can offer similar combined cues for performance of other simple tasks, such as bathing and eating. These simple nursing actions to help patients preserve remaining function also serve to enhance the patient's self-esteem and social participation. Over time, the patient's capacity to participate diminishes, and total care is necessary.

Distinct neurological deficits in the middle stage directly alter the functioning of many body systems. Voluntary control of physical functions diminishes, leaving the patient with loss of control first over bowels and bladder and later with the inability to swallow (**dysphagia**). Physical movements increasingly become reflexive, rather than purposeful. Although the patient's skeletal and muscular systems demonstrate normal function potential, the neurobiological connections sending messages from the brain to the muscles are permanently disconnected. Consequently the patient becomes unable to perform voluntarily even the most routine, purposeful actions. Physical impairment also may include unsteadiness in gait and a listing posture, with the patient's upper torso tilted toward one side when walking. Falls are common, and the patient needs careful supervision at this point in the disease.

Marked psychomotor agitation and retardation are common. Restlessness, agitation, and aimless pacing replace normal motion. Whether the nervous energy takes the form of pacing, repetitively sitting down and getting up, or following primary caregivers wherever they go, the seemingly pointless and constant pattern is unnerving and exhausting to watch. Of all the behaviors these patients demonstrate, this is one of the most troublesome. Table 33–9 provides guidelines for understanding the meaning of selected patient behaviors in the middle stage.

As the patient enters the middle stage, the level of nursing care takes a sharp shift from compensatory support to behavior management and physical intervention. Quality care of the dementia patient requires flexibility, patience, and creativity. The patient's behavioral symptoms provide steady but highly unpredictable challenges for caregiving strategies. What worked well in coping with yesterday may not work at all today. Moreover the care required characteristically is much more intense, physically draining, and never completed. The patient in the middle stage requires close supervision and assistance with most aspects of self-care, nutrition, and elimination.

Communication

Even simple communication in the middle stage becomes more complicated as the connections involved in thought processing are increasingly extinguished. Responses tend to be in the form of one word, a "yes" or "no" answer that may or may not bear any relationship to the question. Because the patient can no longer verbally communicate personal needs or problems, you must anticipate most patient needs and respond to them with little or no patient input. From the patient's perspective, narrowed communication translates into a frightening and lonely existence. Anyone who works with these patients cannot help but wonder if the "diminished presence" is solely a function of the cognitive disorder or also a reflection of their "giving up" because they can no longer understand what is happening or communicate their needs to others. It is important for nursing staff to try to determine the significance of specific behaviors. For instance, agitation can be due to constipation, fatigue, or misperception of the environment. Recognizing that the patient is limited in expressing needs, the nurse must be sensitive to covert problems communicated through behaviors.

Agitation

Persistent restlessness, irritability over small things, striking out at the air, and aimless pacing are agitated behaviors common to patients in middle-stage dementia. Assessment of a physical cause for the agitation is the first approach. If there is no evidence of a physiological cause, such as fecal impaction, infection, or fatigue, survey the environment for the presence of possible irritants or sensory overload, both frequent causes. Like young children, agitation and irritability increase when the patient is tired or hungry.

The goal of nursing interventions is to minimize any factors maintaining the behavior. Simple distraction—for example, "I'd like you to show me a picture in the day room" or "I'd like you to help me set the table"—often stops the behavior, at least momentarily. Approaching the patient with a low-key, calm approach tends to soothe the patient. A snack or simple activity can distract the patient and significantly reduce tension. High-stimuli situations should be avoided, and small doses of high-potency medications can be quite effective in interrupting agitated behaviors. Stroking the patient's arm and encouraging the individual to remain seated while talking slowly in a calm voice can reduce the penetrating agitation in some patients (Deutsch & Rovner, 1991).

TABLE 33–9 Common Behavior Management Problems With Related Nursing Strategies in the Middle Stages of Dementia

BEHAVIOR	POSSIBLE MEANINGS	SUGGESTED INTERVENTION
Wandering	Limited awareness of environmental stimuli Boredom Feelings of being lost	Redirect patient with word cues and word signs. Provide sensory stimulation. Reorient patient frequently. Increase safety monitoring. Use Medic-Alert bracelet.
Rummaging	Lack of control over environment Searching for a sense of security	Give patient something to do. Use distraction (a glass of juice, a look out the window). Give reassurance. Make a busy box with safe rummaging items. Ask family members to bring in expendable, familiar items.
Incontinence	Difficulty with finding bathroom Inability to remove clothing Limited awareness of stimulus to use toilet	Take patient to bathroom at frequent intervals. Praise for performance. Overlook accidents. Simplify clothing to facilitate removal. Use one-step orienting commands ("Slip pants down to your knees"). Change soiled or wet clothing immediately. Note normal times of elimination and toilet. Watch for possible signs (pulling at clothing, increased agitation). Turn light on in bathroom. Use bedside commode at night.
Difficulty following directions	Too much sensory input Complex task	Provide step-by-step instructions. Repetitively provide information on time, place, person, schedule, and routine. Use signs, color coding, written word plus signs, calendars, large-number clocks to facilitate recognition.
Profound memory loss	Cognitive impairment, anxiety, grief	Try to focus on the feelings behind the behavior and affirm these in words and actions. Note times and patterns of behaviors to detect environmental antecedents that can be modified.

Screaming

A variant of agitation in dementia patients is screaming and loud repetition of single words or phrases. Screaming can represent boredom, or it can be a way of getting the caregiver's attention. Loud and incessant talking, however, rattles those who hear it, and because this behavior consists often of an unintelligible shrieking sound, it is unnerving. Again it is helpful to realize that the patient typically does not scream intentionally. In fact, most patients are unaware that they are speaking or annoying others. Screaming, similar to other behaviors, is an effort to communicate. Good baseline data can assist you in providing the most effective response. By observing when the screaming occurs, for example, you might determine whether the patient is tired, hungry, or in need of attention, allowing you to respond more appropriately to the patient's underlying needs rather than to the screaming behaviors. Soft music or television sometimes quiets the patient.

Eating Difficulty

Eating becomes a problem during the middle stages of dementia, manifesting itself in a variety of ways. Aesthetically, these patients typically display grossly inappropriate table manners. Eating can become a problem nutritionally for patients who overeat or undereat with little recognition of what they are doing. Progressive neurological deficits make it physiologically harder to swallow and increase the possibility of aspiration. Moreover, patients "forget" how to get food to their mouths, to chew, and to swallow. Mealtime becomes a supervised experience.

You can use a variety of strategies to encourage good eating habits. Mirroring the eating process by picking up the fork, encouraging the patient to follow suit, and providing verbal prompts such as, "John, pick up your spoon," as you mirror the action are effective in helping patients eat more easily. Reminding patients verbally to chew and to swallow also helps. Most patients need to have their food cut up, and some may need food pureed. Following small bites with a drink also helps the patient swallow. The caregiver or nurse needs to use words and careful manipulation of the food materials to help patients avoid taking in large portions without chewing or swallowing.

Dining with the dementia patient in a community dining room is a challenge. Many patients are quite disruptive, taking food from other patients' trays, pocketing food items, and shoving food in their mouths without chewing. These patients may call out or throw and push food away onto other residents' trays. Some patients eat spoiled food, stashed at an earlier time or taken from the garbage. Their cognitive and perceptual deficits make it impossible for them to recognize food as such. If you try to assist, these patients may grab at your hands or clench their jaws to prevent intake. Because many of them can no longer smell, they may not realize the food is bad. Some patients try to eat inedible materials such as styrofoam cups, plastic tableware, plants, dirt, and paper napkins. For this reason, plastic knives, forks, and spoons should not be used because some patients may bite down on the utensil and swallow it.

Simplifying the number and presentation of food items can reduce the effort for the patient. Some patients do better having one food item at a time, rather than facing the full meal. Opening milk cartons, cutting up meat into small bite-size pieces, and presenting one eating utensil at a time seem to help focus patients on their meal. Usually, spoons work best. Alternating foods provides variety and makes undesired foods more appealing. Here you need to allow time and to practice patience because patients in the middle stage of dementia have a tendency to start and stop eating many times during a meal. This can be nerve-racking unless you understand that the behavior is not under the patient's voluntary control. If the patient seems unable to use utensils, nutritional finger foods such as cheese squares, finger sandwiches, or fruit chunks can supply needed nutrients without agitating the patient.

Combativeness

Research has demonstrated a connection between impaired cognition and aggression. Understand that aggression exhibited by dementia patients is quite different from hostile acts demonstrated by patients with a psychiatric disorder, such as antisocial personality disorder. The dementia patient has neither a deliberate wish to harm another person nor a criminal intent. Aggressive actions typically occur as brief outbursts, most often as a random response to the environment. Frequently the aggressive behavior of the Alzheimer's patient diminishes as the disease progresses because the patient becomes less involved with the environment and simultaneously more feeble.

Catastrophic Reactions

Catastrophic reactions have some characteristics in common with combativeness, but they are less likely to be attacks on other people. More frequently, a **catastrophic reaction** resembles in form and intent the temper tantrum of a 2-year-old. These behaviors represent overreactions to stimuli in the environment and typically occur as brief episodes of heightened anger and frustration. During a catastrophic reaction, the patient may strike out at the caregiver, cry, scream, and appear extremely agitated. Like a 2-year-old, the dementia patient seems to have limited awareness of the consequences of the outburst or its impact on others.

Understanding that these patients have lost the capacity to express their needs in simple ways that might reduce their frustration helps you to be more compassionate. With a limited way to respond to anxiety, these patients turn to physical aggression as a way of making their needs known to others. Their immediate familiar caregiver is the recipient of the aggressive act, as with the toddler. Catastrophic reactions often occur when the caregiver is offering genuine assistance, which makes the outburst even more troubling. A possible explanation is that the caregiver's actions remind the patients of things they can no longer do for themselves.

Box 33–12 ■ ■ ■ ■ ■
Measures to Deal With Agitated or Destructive Behavior

- Avoid clutter.
- Reduce unnecessary stimulation.
- Simplify tasks or activities.
- Have a list of emergency numbers by the telephone.
- Reduce unnecessary sound.
- Remove unsteady furniture or pieces with sharp edges.
- Secure windows.
- Block large areas of breakable glass.
- Take knobs off stove and other appliances if possible.
- Make sure medications are out of reach and securely stored.
- Keep childproof covers over electrical outlets.
- Place locks on drawers and cupboards.
- Remove all hazardous materials—matches, lighters, poisonous flowers or plants.
- Supervise smokers and use self-extinguishing ashtrays.
- Check smoke detectors and keep a fire extinguisher handy.

The best treatment is prevention. Simplifying the environment helps make the situation more manageable. Many activities of daily living that precipitate a catastrophic reaction are tolerated without incident at a different time of day. Picking the most desirable time for morning care may involve moving the activity to the afternoon. Distraction is particularly effective as an intervention strategy. For example, the nurse might say, "Betty, we can come back to this, but I would like to show you (name something) over here." Touching and moving the patient to a different location also help. Involvement in other activities, particularly those containing large motor movement, diverts the patient's attention and rechannels nonproductive energy. Reducing choices, eliminating or breaking down tasks that are too complex into smaller components, and responding to questions that overwhelm the patient are strategies to offset the potential for a catastrophic reaction (Anton & Casey, 1994; Chrisman, 1991). Box 33-12 details measures to deal with agitated and destructive behavior.

Sundown Syndrome

Sundown syndrome, or sundowning (Evans, 1991), describes an increased confusion and agitation noted in many dementia patients occurring during the late afternoon and early evening hours. It also has been known to occur first thing in the morning in some isolated cases. Treatment of this diurnal pattern consists of keeping the patient active during the earlier parts of the day and planning the patient's day so that stimuli are reduced during the period traditionally associated with sundowning. Medications are helpful adjuncts to treatment, but for maximum effectiveness, they need to be given at the beginning of the episode, not after the agitation has become full-blown. Administration of low doses of antipsychotic medication (haloperidol) or a benzodiazepine (lorazepam) around 4:00 PM helps reduce the incidence of sundowning. Box 33-13 provides measures to deal with the hallucinations, illusions, and delusions that are characteristic of dementia, particularly in sundown syndrome (Flint, 1991).

Emotional Disinhibition

Patients with dementia sometimes exhibit inappropriate behaviors in the form of touching others in sexually inappropriate ways, disrobing in public areas, or making sexually explicit comments referred to as **emotional disinhibition.** Patients exhibiting sexual behaviors toward others, masturbating in public, or disrobing obviously cannot be permitted to do this because of the consequences to themselves and others. Handling the problem, however, is important. Understanding the patient as having the social skills of a very young child can help you respond compassionately, as Case Example 33-4 illustrates. Patients who undress may feel too warm or may simply need to go to the bathroom. Depending on the situation, you can offer the opportunity for toileting or lead the patient to a room and help with redressing.

Box 33–13 ■ ■ ■ ■ ■
Measures to Deal With Hallucinations, Illusions, and Delusions

- Make sure environment is not too stimulating.
- Maintain adequate lighting to decrease shadows.
- Look for sources of glare (magazine pages, tabletops, etc.). Reduce glare from the sun (close blinds) and from objects (use frosted bulbs, nonglare wax).
- Keep background noises at a minimum.
- Avoid changing furniture and wall hangings.
- Remove or cover mirrors if they cause confusion or frighten the person.
- When talking to the patient, give him or her something to hold onto (e.g., your hand, a stuffed animal).
- Avoid television programs that are violent or disturbing.
- Make sure you have an exit if the patient is aggressive.

■ Jack O'Donnell was in the hospital suffering from vascular dementia and a diabetic crisis. He pinched the nurse's rear end as she came closer to the bed, saying, "I've been away from home a long time." Before his illness, Jack would never have made such a comment. The nurse, recognizing emotional disinhibition as a symptom of dementia, was able to pat his arm and say to him, "It must be hard to feel like you are alone," and change the subject. Had she taken his action as a personal attack and his statement verbatim, her nonunderstanding could have worsened Jack's cognitive impairment. From that point forward, she also made sure that she was not in a position where a similar incident might occur. ■

Sleep Disturbances

With dementia, there is a characteristic reversal of the sleep-wake cycle so that the patient is sleepy during the day and awake at night (Vitiello, Bliwise, & Prinz, 1992). Many patients wake up spontaneously throughout the night and become night-walkers, much to the consternation of the caregiver who must get up and make sure that the patient gets safely back to bed. When patients wander at night, they are quite likely to get into trouble, partially because of the darkened environment. Patients who climb into bed with other patients in nursing homes or stand in the doorways of other patients' rooms are causes of anxiety. At home, patients may turn on the stove or attempt to leave the house.

Several nursing interventions help reduce the incidence of night-walking. First, the caregiver needs to keep the patient active during the day. Engaging in simple, stimulating activities during the day helps the patient work off excess energy. Avoiding stimulant intake, such as coffee, tea, coke, or cigarettes, near bedtime and offering a small snack in the early evening help keep the patient relaxed. If diuretics are used, it is important to use them early in the day. Patients often get up to go to the bathroom at night and, once up, begin their travels. Should the patient arise during the night, you can instruct the caregiver to guide the patient to the bathroom but to limit conversation at this time. Allowing the patient to become fully alert makes it harder to get him or her back to sleep. Careful use of medication may offset negative symptoms influencing sleep onset and duration (Heim, 1986; Holmberg, 1997; Young, Muir-Nash, & Ninos, 1988).

Repetitive Behaviors

Repetitive behaviors that serve no functional purpose also are a persistent element of the middle stage. They are particularly distressing to the caregiver because logical responses do not stop the repetitive flow. Typical behaviors can include asking the same question or performing the same task over and over again or following the caregiver. Understanding that repetition helps create

security for the dementia patient in a world that no longer makes sense helps make responding in a different way possible. Providing a supportive, nonthreatening structural environment offsets the insecurity that cognitive disorders create. Distraction, touch, calm words, ignoring the behavior, or redirecting the conversation often helps break the repetitive words momentarily.

At least equally disconcerting is the patient's need to follow the caregiver wherever the caregiver goes. As one individual expressed it, "I can't even go to the bathroom by myself. There he is, and I feel guilty shutting him out." This phenomenon, although wearing under any circumstances, becomes a little more tolerable when caregivers can realize that these patients are simply trying to maintain their bearings in an increasingly unfamiliar environment. By staying close to the familiar caregiver, the patient feels some degree of safety and security.

Use of Restraints

Restraints are useful only as a last resort and then only for specific short periods. Each time patients are restrained, even for a good reason, they lose a part of their personal freedom, their sense of themselves as people, and they become more confused.

Physically, patients in restraints are more prone to develop contractures and decubitus formation because the restraints severely restrict their voluntary movements. If restraints are continued once the patient is asleep, the head of the bed should be elevated to prevent aspiration. Being restrained can increase the patient's restlessness, as the patient struggles for freedom from the restraints.

Today there are a variety of restraint alternatives available. Restraint systems such as wedge cushions used in wheelchairs; geri-chairs with trays; reclining chairs; low beds with mesh side rails; and the use of alarms for wheelchairs and beds all promote safety while minimizing or totally removing the dehumanizing aspects of vest and wrist or ankle restraints. In addition, vest restraints, used in the bed or wheelchair, can help the patient maintain an upright position and prevent unnecessary falls. Bilateral wrist and ankle restraints should be used only as a last resort, for example, for intravenous infusion and should be applied for the shortest time possible, to prevent contracture and decubitus formation. Their use requires careful monitoring. When physical restraints become necessary, they should be applied with compassion and with the patient's comfort in mind. Sometimes, placing the patient in a wheelchair or geri-chair with a vest restraint near the nurses' station allows the patient to feel social without being tied up like an animal. The stimulation of seeing people without needing to do very much socially has a calming effect.

Nursing staff should obtain a physician's order that specifies the type and duration of use for restraints.

Spiritual Needs

Providing for the spiritual needs of patients and families is a critical nursing concern. As memory for current

Box 33–14 ■ ■ ■ ■ ■
Caregiver's Prayer

O God, grant us the wisdom and serenity to be good caregivers to our families and friends. Help us to see clearly what would help, when it would help, and how best to give help.

Teach us patience, and we will bring love to the task. Guide us away from our panic, and toward our compassion, that we may continue to build happy memories with our families.

Help us to be creative, caring, and faithful to Your guidance. Forgive us when we lose our patience, and grant us strength and peace.

From Eddy Alzheimer's Services, 220 Burdett Avenue, Troy, NY 12180; 518-272-1792.

events fades, the recollection of religious music, Scripture passages, and worship rituals continues to be a hold on reality for the Alzheimer's patient. Boxes 33–14 and 33–15 include a caregiver's and a patient's prayer, respectively.

Legal Issues

Once patients reach the middle stage of dementia, most are no longer legally competent to handle their own affairs. If the durable power of attorney has not been established earlier, it is too late. Another legal procedure, referred to **conservatorship,** involves the court appointment of a legal guardian to handle the patient's personal affairs. The conservator has legal power over the patient's finances but none over the actual patient. To make legal decisions about the person, a guardian is needed. This person can make decisions for the patient, including nursing home placement. Guardianship is a complex legal process through which one person or entity (guardian) acquires legal responsibility for another person (ward) who is unable to care for his or her affairs because of mental or physical incapacity. At times, the guardian is granted limited decision-making. It is important to review a copy of the court document to understand the conditions of conservatorship and guardianship rather than rely on the verbal descriptions offered by the family or significant others.

End Stage of Dementia

Alzheimer's disease is a terminal disorder, always ending in death. Box 33–16 presents behaviors associated with the final stage, often referred to as the vegetative stage. Typically, there is a significant weight loss related to the patient's growing inability to swallow. The patient looks cachectic, with sunken facial features. Communication with the outside world ceases. If not bedridden, the patient has a slow and unsteady gait. Sleep patterns increase, and it is difficult to help the patient maintain any sort of mobility. Many patients assume a fetal position and have contractures caused by immobility.

Changes in respiration (Cheyne-Stokes respirations) and vital signs, seizures, and decreased urine volume signal body system shutdown before death. Some patients refuse food by clenching the jaw, spitting food out, or turning the head away from the caregiver. Other patients may bite down on a spoon or fork (for this reason, plastic should not be used) or will not close their mouth and chew. Many patients enter a coma during the last few weeks or months, demonstrating twitching and seizure-like activity but little other responsiveness to the environment. Death usually occurs from secondary neurological complications of the disorder. Frequent complications include aspiration pneumonia, systemic infection associated with tissue immobility, dehydration, and

Box 33–15 ■ ■ ■ ■ ■
Patient's Prayer

O God, the trouble with having a memory problem is the frustration and fear I feel every day. I can never be quite sure that I have done and said the right things. I have memories—happy memories of my family and my youth, of beautiful days with my loved ones, of my education and of my faith. Help me to preserve those.

The two things I want never to forget are gratitude and love; I am grateful to those who love and help me—my family, my caregivers, and you, my God.

From Eddy Alzheimer's Services, 220 Burdett Avenue, Troy, NY 12180; 518-272-1792.

Box 33–16 ■ ■ ■ ■ ■
Symptoms in the End Stage of Dementia

Global loss of memory, long-term as well as short-term memory
Significant weight loss
Verbal communication limited to guttural sounds or mutism
Loss of voluntary bladder and bowel control
Extreme difficulty swallowing
Bedridden state
Other signs of profound neurological loss, such as blindness or seizure
Cheyne-Stokes breathing
Fetal position
Contractures, pressure ulcers, systemic infection, pneumonia

Box 33-17 ■ ■ ■ ■ ■
Guidelines for Encouraging Eating in End-Stage Dementia

Use the patient's name and describe what you are doing.

Give fluids slowly and allow additional time. Use words, such as "Swallow it now, Dan" as an extrasensory cue.

Use frequent, small offerings rather than expecting the patient to take large quantities.

Provide liquids, soup, and juices. Juices and clear liquids are generally tolerated better than water.

Stroke the throat to stimulate swallowing reflexes.

Provide frequent mouth care because of mouth breathing and general dehydration. Use lemon water or treated swabs to stimulate saliva. Petroleum jelly or other lip preparation can keep the lips moist.

What do you think? Knowing what you now know about Alzheimer's disease, would you want to be told if you had this diagnosis? How would knowing change your journey? Do you support assisted suicide in Alzheimer's patients? Does our health care system support the kind and amount of "caring" required by patients with Alzheimer's disease and their caregivers? Are there deficits in the system that make assisted suicide an appealing option for individuals and families? How do your views about assisted suicide fit into your spiritual world view?

► *Check Your Reading*
10. What does sundowning mean? How can the nurse reduce its effects?
11. What guidelines should the nurse follow in deciding to apply restraints to dementia patients?
12. What is the role of the nurse in the care of the patient during the end stage of dementia?

starvation because the patient is no longer able to swallow.

Nursing interventions center on keeping the patient comfortable, nourished, and hydrated. Methods for providing nutritive support include spoon feeding, intravenous infusion of fluids and electrolytes, and tube feeding. Fluid intake is critical, particularly when the patient refuses food. Fruit juices seem to be better tolerated than plain water. High-protein nutritional supplements such as Ensure are regularly offered. Guidelines for stimulating oral intake are presented in Box 33-17. Regular skin care, range of motion exercises, and frequent turning of the patient help offset the effects of serious immobility. You can help family members assume partial responsibility for these activities if they are so inclined. Sometimes providing acts of comfort for their loved one is supportive to the family. Another overlooked activity is saying a meaningful goodbye, even if the patient does not seem to register it. Encourage the patient to "let go," pray with the patient, or gently stroke an exposed body part.

You can provide for the spiritual needs of the patient by asking the family's wishes for a priest, rabbi, or minister and arranging for a visit as indicated. If the patient is to have an autopsy, the family may wish to fill out the appropriate papers beforehand because time is a critical factor in handling brain tissue examinations. Handling funeral arrangements before the actual death also is helpful for families who wish this intervention. Above all, continue to protect the dignity of the patient and family and provide for the highest quality of life possible for the patient. When the patient actually dies, you can be helpful by acknowledging the void the caregiver is likely to experience and providing referrals if needed. See Snapshot: Nursing Interventions Specific to Dementia.

ISSUES FOR FAMILY MEMBERS

Dementia is a story of family deprivation for many families and of courage for those who willingly accompany the patient during this part of the journey. Chronic cognitive disorders ravish the hearts of the victim's family, who watch a once strong personality gradually but inevitably and completely lose its defining characteristics. The loss of a person to dementia leaves little to hold onto for security or understanding. All that is known is that dementia patients, as the family knew them, are irrevocably lost. They know that their relative will get worse and will die and that the time from diagnosis to death can last several (up to 19) years, with an average of 7 or 8 years. No other conclusions can be drawn. In addition to the loss of a partner, a parent, or a sibling, the diagnosis usually creates significant alterations in lifestyle and may affect financial and estate planning. A major shift in role responsibilities is unavoidable for concerned family members (Dickson & Ranseen, 1990; Kuhlman et al., 1991).

Dementia is a "family disease" in that the dementia patient loses the ability to care for self, prompting others to step in, often with significant role reversal. Caring for the patient can affect the health and well-being of those who must provide it 24 hours a day, 7 days a week. Painful issues such as putting a loved one in a nursing home, quality of life, and making end-of-life decisions for the patient create stress and guilt for many family members.

Financial matters often are of considerable concern, as the care of many dementia patients is not reimbursable by a significant number of private and public insurance programs. Families need help with accessing community resources and planning financial contingencies

Nursing Interventions Specific to Dementia

What do you need to do to develop a relationship with a patient suffering with a dementia?
- Provide consistency in caregivers and caregiving activities.
- Introduce self and provide basic explanation of activities.
- Use simple, one-stage directions.
- Control environmental stimuli.
- Use touch therapeutically.
- Reorient patient as needed.

What do you need to assess regarding the patient's health status?
- Cognition including abstract thinking, judgment, orientation, reasoning ability, personality changes, short- and long-term memory
- History of illness: onset, pattern of progression, symptoms
- Medical history, current health conditions
- Diagnostic tests that have been completed, including CT scans, blood analysis, electroencephalogram
- Family history
- Social history
- Occupational history
- Physiological responses, including vital signs, appetite and weight changes, continence, gait, sleep-wake cycle, activity, output
- Behavioral responses, including wandering, agitation, aggression, anxiety, depression, suicide risk, inability to perform instrumental and other activities of daily living
- Factors that affect behavior
- Medications
- Alternative and complementary therapies used, including herbs, special diets, fasting, energy work, magnets, and other devices
- Family support
- Caregiver: health status, competency, support, respite
- Safety of environment

What do you need to teach the patient and/or patient's caregiver?
- Nature and expected progress of disease
- Use of memory triggers
- Establishment of schedule for basic activities, including bathing, toileting, meals, naps
- Monitoring of intake and output, weight, skin status
- Recognition of nonverbal indications of needs and problems
- Use of redirection and distraction to reduce behaviors
- Identification of new symptoms or changes
- Physical and mental activities
- Environmental modifications to promote orientation and function, including signs, color coding, clocks, control of sensory stimuli
- Safety measures, including alarms on exits, cessation of driving, securing poisonous substances, safe clothing and shoes, use of Medic-Alert bracelet, having recent photo of patient available
- Legal issues that should be addressed, including advance directives, durable power of attorney
- Sources of information and support
- Community resources for caregiving assistance and respite

What skills do you want the patient and/or caregiver to demonstrate?
- Ability to comply with treatment plan
- Ability to satisfy self-care requirements
- Ability to identify and report changes in status
- Use of resources for support and caregiver assistance

What other professionals might need to be part of the plan of care?
- Physician, psychiatrist
- Occupational therapist
- Physical therapist
- Social worker
- Recreational therapist
- Nursing assistant, home health aide
- Attorney
- Clergy

to provide for the care of their relative without impoverishing the caregiver. Support groups sponsored by the Alzheimer's Association are particularly useful informational resources in this regard.

Abuse of Dementia Patients

Dementia, for some patients, is a troubled narrative, with accounts of abuse and neglect. The overwhelming burdens of caregiving can be responsible for many episodes of abuse of dementia patients. A smaller number of families abandon their demented relative to the ravages of the disease with little compassion or understanding.

Abuse of the elderly, similar to other forms of abuse, typically occurs in secret. The reasons for abuse vary. For some, the patient's behavior is annoying. Sometimes the designated caregiver resents being given or acquiring the care responsibility and takes it out on the patient. Other families keep a dementing patient in substandard living conditions without appropriate supervision or adequate stimulation, for none other than financial reasons. In many instances, the patient does not suffer active abuse but rather neglect as the patient's needs increase (Abraham, Onega, Chalifoux, & Maes, 1994).

All cases of actual or suspected abuse of the dementia patient should be reported to the appropriate state agency; in some states, the local police department is contacted to investigate the situation. Nurses should become familiar with the abuse reporting laws in their specific states (see Chapter 35 for more in-depth discussion of abuse).

Characteristics of Family Care

The family should be considered an integral part of the treatment team from the moment of diagnosis. Families assume the bulk of responsibility for the care of cognitively impaired elderly individuals, with the most common caregiver being the spouse or daughter. Women still constitute the largest cohort of caregivers to the frail elderly, and their needs are just beginning to emerge as the focus of research studies (Wykle, 1994).

Most dementia patients do not require skilled nursing care until the disease is well advanced. Even then it is not always reimbursable because so much of the care involves basic custodial functions not covered by insurance. Yet care must be given consistently because without it, the patient would not be able to perform simple activities of living. Eventually, all dementia patients symptomatically present as a danger to self, if not others. Fortunately, efforts of the Alzheimer's Association, American Association of Retired Persons, and the Gray Panthers have resulted in laws protecting the assets of caregivers seeking to provide adequate care for a relative with dementia.

In many cases, the primary caregiver and other family members are hidden patients (Kahana, Biegel, & Wykle, 1994), with significant health care needs obscured from view by the more pressing needs of the patient. Some are related to care of the patient. Concurrently, many older caregivers have physical and emotional needs apart from their caregiving role that receive little attention because of preoccupation with their relative's profound functional disability. The multidimensional needs of caregivers are found in common concerns expressed by family members in a 10-year support group (Table 33–10). The list of concerns and level of responsibility are only the tip of the iceberg in thinking about family needs associated with dementia. In fact, Stepworth (1994) suggests that "caregivers as an aggregate are an underserved population that is at high risk for mental and physical health difficulties" (p. 7).

Referral to support groups and allowing time to work with the family around legal, medication, and behavioral issues is extremely important. Many issues that one would not ordinarily think of plague the caregiver of patients with chronic cognitive disorders. These include parental rights expected by the patient when an adult parent is no longer capable of providing care for the adolescent or young adult, how to deal with cognitive judgments and decisions that do not make sense, and how to be supportive without being controlling.

Friends, particularly if the dementia patient is younger (40s or 50s), might abandon the family because they simply do not know how to handle the situation. Spouses experience discomfort, with the sense of no longer being married but not being divorced or widowed either. Fortunately, a number of community resources are available for family members at low or no cost because of the current emphasis on dementia and family support.

Family and environmental obstacles to preserving function in the dementia patient require careful appraisal. For example, the work schedule of the designated caregiver may preclude giving the proper attention to the patient. Lack of financial resources, other family obligations, role reversals, and other conflicts have a negative impact on potential support. The patient picks up on the family tension but lacks the cognitive skills to respond appropriately. Unable to relate in words, these patients respond in the only way they can—through acting out their frustration or anxiety. Nurses can help family members understand that many

TABLE 33–10 Common Concerns of Family Members Facing Dementia	
PHASE OF DEMENTIA	**FAMILY CONCERN**
Early stage	Setting limits, especially with driving
	Having patience with the patient
	Handling legal and financial matters on behalf of or for the patient
	Social isolation
	Sexual requests common with marriage partners
	Role reversals
Middle stage	Dealing with anger and frustration, without feeling guilty
	Handling the patient's bowel elimination accidents
	Coping with the never-ending constancy of caregiving
	Having personal time alone or to spend with friends
	Coping with the constant requests for assistance
	Managing the patient's excessive talking, pacing, and restlessness
	Responding to unintelligible or difficult-to-understand communication
	Strains in family relationships
	Coping with competing demands on time
	Lack of assistance or appreciation from other family members (extended, immediate)
	Need for respite
Late stage	Nursing home and other care decisions
	Quality-of-life and end-of-life decisions
	Autopsy and funeral home decisions
After death	Restructuring a life without caregiving
	Finding new meanings

of the difficult behaviors displayed by the patient are reactions to the environment. The behaviors represent an attempt to communicate even though their meaning is not readily understandable.

Knowledge deficits also can impair the family's ability to respond with the acceptance and understanding a dementia patient needs so desperately. You need to assess the family's knowledge of the disorder. The family needs instruction in the best ways to reduce negative behaviors. There seems to be a direct correlation between the patient's level of agitation and demands and the caregiver's sense of burden.

Support for expression of negative emotions and fear about the future should be ongoing. Many caregivers feel guilty because they are angry about the major disruption in their lives. Sadness about the patient's condition and the projected outcome of the disease leave many feeling helpless and ineffective. Families need to know that it is okay to feel angry and bewildered about their lives being turned upside down, with seemingly no purpose. They need reassurance that their feelings of helplessness are real but not their fault. They often need support and understanding in making difficult decisions about the dementia patient's future, without having the patient's input. Here, support groups for family members can be invaluable in helping caregivers vent frustrations, learn about the nature of the disease, and develop new ways to help their relative conserve optimal functioning.

Support Groups

Support groups are a protected, supportive place and space in time, where the caregiver can turn for needed nurturance. Family members learn what to expect and get excellent tips on how to make things go more easily. Support groups provide a place for the caregiver to laugh (something they do not do very often) to cry, to get angry, and to get needed support to make difficult decisions. Whether the family decides to go the nursing home route or to keep the patient at home, to extend a patient's life through tube feeding or to withdraw extraordinary measures, the group supports the caregiver's right to choose.

Support groups encourage the caregiver to express feelings about the patient and the burden of caregiving in a safe environment, where people understand and accept the feelings. Feelings of guilt, anger, and resentment are commonly experienced emotions, and it is important that the caregiver realize that they are normal responses to a highly abnormal situation. Group members also help members anticipate the next step in the dementia process, provide useful networking contacts, and sometimes swap equipment. Even if the family member normally is not a "group person," the information obtained through the support group can be quite useful. In contrast to group psychotherapy, there is no pressure on group members to participate actively. They can listen and derive significant benefits.

▶ *Check Your Reading*

13. In what ways are support groups helpful in the treatment of dementia patients and their families?
14. What are some of the common concerns of family caregivers at different stages of dementia?

NURSING PROCESS APPLICATION

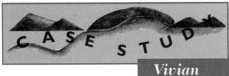

Vivian

Vivian, age 87, has been diagnosed with Alzheimer's disease. Her oldest daughter, diagnosed with terminal cancer, had been her primary caretaker, and now a shift of burden of responsibility has moved to the youngest daughter who lives in another state. Vivian spent 2 months living with her youngest daughter, Helen, who herself was 68 years old and suffering from gout, hypertension, and edema of the lower extremities. Helen and her husband found it extremely difficult to cope with Vivian's mental confusion and disorientation when moving about the house. During her times of confusion, Vivian would forget names and become agitated and verbally abusive. Helen noted that Vivian would turn on the stove and then forget to turn it off. Vivian remained angry and upset with her oldest daughter, stating that there was nothing wrong with her and she did not need any help.

Before Vivian's placement in an adult semiassistive home care setting, she was found wandering outside Helen's home. She had hidden her morning medications and dentures under a pillow. On admission she has flat affect, is sullen and withdrawn, and reports that Helen is not giving her medications.

ASSESSMENT Assessment data are as follows:
  • Decline in cognitive function

- Forgetful; memory impairment
- Impaired judgment
- Confusion

DIAGNOSIS

DSM-IV Diagnosis: Dementia, Alzheimer's Disease

Nursing Diagnosis: Chronic Confusion related to altered cerebral functioning as evidenced by memory loss, decline in cognitive functioning, and impaired judgment

---

OUTCOME IDENTIFICATION, PLANNING, AND IMPLEMENTATION

Expected Outcome 1: By _____ the patient will function at an optimal level, given the increasing degree of memory and cognitive loss.

Short-Term Goal	Nursing Interventions	Rationales
By _____ the patient will be less confused and maintain contact with reality.	1. Orient to time, place, and person. 2. Break down complex tasks (e.g., dressing, eating) into simple, individual steps. 3. Be consistent with approach; preferable to have the same staff work with patient. 4. Put calendar, clock, and activity schedule in patient's room and throughout home. 5. Use familiar objects brought in from the patient's home environment (i.e., favorite pictures, bedspread, drapes). 6. Speak slowly and calmly (while facing person); use simple phrases and words. 7. Plan few activities in the evening when patient is more apt to become confused.	1–2. Alzheimer's disease leads to altered cognitive function. As the disease progresses, patients are unable to recognize their limitations. Consistent orientation is needed when short-term memory is impaired. 3–5. Environmental stimuli are misinterpreted, leading to reality distortions along with misidentification of close relatives and poor insight. Use of own objects maintains familiarity. Sameness and repetition lessen confusion. 6. Impaired cognitive status may make it difficult to comprehend abstract concepts or lengthy sentences. Facing the person provides the maximum amount of verbal and nonverbal communication to transpire. 7. Sundowning (increased confusion and agitation) occurs most often in the late afternoon and early evening hours.

Expected Outcome 2: By _____ the patient will communicate effectively with others.

Short-Term Goal	Nursing Interventions	Rationales
By _____ the patient will communicate with others.	1. Encourage reminiscing and talk to patient about familiar and meaningful things. 2. Provide group activities (e.g., singing, dancing, crafts) that are simple and familiar to perform.	1. Long-term memory fades slower than short-term memory. Reminiscing helps the patient by distracting from present condition and allows him or her to reexperience the joys and accomplishments of the past. 2. Group activities increase socialization and minimize feelings of alienation and despair.

Nursing Diagnosis: High Risk for Injury related to altered cerebral functioning as evidenced by wandering and forgetting to turn off the stove

Expected Outcome 3: By _____ the patient will remain safe in the assistive nursing home.

Short-Term Goals	Nursing Interventions	Rationales
By _____ the patient will not wander outside of the assistive home care protective boundary.	1. Check on Vivian's status at regular intervals. Set alarm doors on alert mode. 2. Spend short, frequent intervals with Vivian. 3. Play soft music on the radio. 4. Encourage use of bathroom before retiring. 5. Maintain Vivian's activity level during the day. 6. Discourage naps or keep at a minimum.	1–2. Monitoring and supervision of patient can prevent threats to safety. 3. Soft music provides orientation and produces a calming effect on patient. 4. This may decrease need to get up in the night to use the bathroom and may prevent incontinence. 5. Regular activity maintains muscle tone and promotes a normal sleep pattern. 6. Napping can interfere with normal sleep pattern and lead to restless, wandering behavior at night.
By _____ the patient will not cook in the kitchen unless assisted by staff.	1. Supervise any cooking in the kitchen. 2. May need to remove knobs from kitchen stove. 3. Cap electrical outlets.	1–3. Cognitively impaired patients are unable to make safe judgments about seemingly routine habits.

EVALUATION

Formative Evaluation: Vivian met each of the short-term goals. She was easily distracted from using the kitchen when offered craft projects of making flower arrangements. She readily communicated with her roommate and enjoyed talking about the good old times when she lived on a farm.

Summative Evaluation: Vivian achieved each of the expected outcomes. All of the expected outcomes were continued as a part of her ongoing plan of care. Over a 1-month period, as Vivian became accustomed to her new setting, less wandering behavior was noted, probably due to an increase in her socialization-type activities, which she thoroughly enjoyed. Overall, she seemed to adjust to her environment. Less confusion was noted by her family when they visited.

Conclusions

Cognitive disorders rob the minds of their victims and the hearts of their families. In the 21st century, cognitive disorders are likely to achieve an even greater research focus as the graying of America forces clinicians and researchers to grapple with their understanding and treatment.

Dementia, in many instances, is a story of family courage. Family members who assume the burden of care for dementia patients encounter personal demands that call for constant involvement and caring. The care is emotionally, physically, and often spiritually draining. Yet many families, knowing all of these contingencies, choose to care for their demented relative in a compassionate manner for the rest of the journey. They make personal sacrifices that their relative can never acknowledge. This they do on a daily basis. Their caring actions on behalf of another human being are heroic yet are inconspicuous and undervalued by society. Even the patient cannot thank them for their efforts.

Key Points to Remember

- Delirium is the name given to the acute forms of cognitive disorders. The disorder represents an acute confusional state, characterized by an abrupt onset, fluctuation in level of consciousness, disorientation, and an identifiable physical cause.
- Emergency triage of the delirious patient is a first-order assessment, followed by psychiatric intervention.
- Reducing environmental stimuli, frequent orientation to surroundings, and staff attitude are important dimensions of effective care with the delirious patient.

- Dementia is a chronic cognitive disorder. The disorder represents a progressive neurological disorder, characterized by memory loss, changes in personality, and deficits in communication and constructional ability.
- Vascular dementia presents with a stepwise progression, not the steady decline of Alzheimer's disease.
- Alzheimer's disease is basically a rule-out disorder.
- Patient history is one of the most important sources of information in Alzheimer's disease.
- Symptoms in the early stage concern memory loss, personality changes, and psychomotor deficits. They are mild, and the patient usually can function independently.
- Protecting patient dignity, preserving patient func-

tioning, and promoting quality of life are the three goals of patient care with patients suffering from dementia.
- Care in the early stage centers on providing compensatory care for the patient and education for the family.
- In the middle stage of dementia, the primary emphasis of care is on behavior management of difficult patient behaviors associated with global neurological deficits.
- The end stage of dementia is characterized by a global loss of function and neurological deficits of a magnitude that eventually lead to death as a result of primary or secondary factors. Pneumonia and systemic infection are common causes of death.

Learning Activities

1. Interview a family caregiver in your community. Ask the caregiver's perspective on caring for dementia patients. Ask what has been the hardest part of the experience. What has been the most rewarding part of the experience?
2. To avoid duplication, this exercise can be done in small groups and the results shared with the larger group. Find out about the day care programs and religious and social services that caregivers can use in your community. Use the Yellow Pages, and call the

different programs. Find out eligibility requirements, payment schedules, and criteria for expulsion from the program. Report on how easy it is to access these services and any other information you think might be helpful in securing appropriate services for the Alzheimer's patient and family caregivers.
3. Attend an Alzheimer's support group in your community and report on some of the concerns expressed at the meeting.

Critical Thinking Exercise

Nurse Carlson has been the primary nurse for Mrs. Anne Holmes, an 85-year-old dementia patient, since her arrival 3 weeks ago at Bailey's Nursing Home. Today, Anne has been asking frequently to "go home" to talk to her husband. Nurse Carlson is aware that Mrs. Holmes' husband died 9 months ago. She approaches Mrs. Holmes and asks her to tell her about her memories with her husband.

1. What assumptions can you make about Nurse Carlson's understanding of patients with dementia?

2. If Nurse Carlson had used a reality orientation approach with Mrs. Holmes, what might have resulted?

3. What is an alternative to the above approaches?

The following day, Mrs. Holmes' daughter called the nurses' station to ask what people were telling her mother. She reported that her mother had just told her in their phone conversation that she and her nurse had had a wonderful talk about her husband yesterday.

Suggest a response to the daughter that would make sense of the situation. Consider an alternative response(s) and the possible results or consequences. What conclusion(s), if any, can be drawn about the daughter's behavior?

Additional Resources

Alzheimer's Association

919 North Michigan Avenue
Suite 1000
Chicago, IL 60611
800-272-3900
http://www.alz.org
Provides a 24-hour hotline, free publications, and information about local chapters. *Worship Services for People With Alzheimer's Disease and Their Families: A Handbook* is also available through this organization.

American Association of Retired Persons (AARP)

601 E Street, NW
Washington, DC 20049
Advocacy group for elderly; also provides (for a reasonable fee) training materials associated with reminiscence therapy.

National Institute on Aging (NIA)

Public Information Office
Federal Building
Room 5C27
Building 3
9000 Rockville Parkway
Bethesda, MD 20892
http://www.nih.gov/nia
Alzheimer's Disease Education and Reference Center (ADEAR) is available through NIA.

References

Abraham, I., Fox, J., & Cohen, B. (1992). Integrating the bio into the biopsychosocial: Understanding and treating biological phenomena in psychiatric-mental health nursing. *Archives of Psychiatric Nursing, 4*, 242-259.

Abraham, I., Holroyd, S., Snustad, D., Manning, C., Brashear, H. R., Diamond, P., & Thompson-Heisterman, A. (1994). Multidisciplinary assessment of patients with Alzheimer's disease. *Nursing Clinics of North America, 29*(1), 113-127.

Abraham, I., Onega, L., Chalifoux, Z., & Maes, M. J. (1994). Care environments for patients with Alzheimer's disease. *Nursing Clinics of North America, 29*(1), 157-170.

Abrams, W. B., Beers, M. H., & Berkow, R. (1995). *Merck Manual of Geriatrics* (2nd ed., 1186-1187). Whitehouse Station, NJ: Merck Research Laboratories.

Absher, J., & Cummings, J. (1994). Cognitive and noncognitive aspects of dementia syndromes: An overview. In A. Burns & R. Levy (Eds.), *Dementia*. London: Chapman & Hall.

Alafuzoff, I. (1992). The pathology of dementias: An overview. *Acta Neurologia Scandanavia, 138*(Suppl.), 8.

Albert, M. S., & Lafleche, G. (1991). Neuroimaging in Alzheimer's disease. *Psychiatric Clinics of North America, 14*, 443-459.

Alexopoulos, G. S., & Abrams, R. C. (1991). Depression in Alzheimer's disease. *Psychiatric Clinics of North America, 14*, 327-340.

Alzheimer, A. (1987). About a particular case of cerebral cortex. *Journal of Alzheimer's Disease and Related Disorders Association, 1*, 79-85.

Amaducci, L., Falcini, M., & Lippi, A. (1992). Descriptive epidemiology and risk factors for Alzheimer's disease. *Acta Neurologia Scandanavia, 138*(Suppl.), 21-25.

American Psychiatric Association (1994). *Diagnostic and Statistical Manual of Mental Disorders* (4th ed.). Washington, DC: American Psychiatric Association.

Anton, C., & Casey, D. (1994). Clinical paths at Norton Psychiatric Clinic. In P. Spath (Ed.), *Clinical paths: Tools for outcome management*. Washington, DC: American Hospital Association.

Batt, I. (1989). Managing delirium. *Journal of Psychosocial Nursing, 27*, 22-24.

Bennett, D., & Evans, D. (1992). Alzheimer's disease. *Disease Monographs, 38*, 1-64.

Berg, L. (1998). Alzheimer's can be diagnosed in the very early stages. *Archives of Neurology, 55*(3), 301-322.

Berrios, G. E. (1994). Dementia: Historical overview. In A. Burns & R. Levy (Eds.). *Dementia*. London: Chapman & Hall.

Breitner, J., & Folstein, M. (1984). Familial Alzheimer dementia: A prevalent disorder with specific clinical features. *Psychology of Medicine, 14*, 63-80.

Burgener, S., Shimer, R., & Murrell, L. (1993). Expressions of individuality in cognitively impaired elders. *Journal of Gerontological Nursing, 19*, 13-21.

Chandra, V., Kokmen, E., Schoenberg, B., Beard, C. M. (1989). Head trauma with loss of consciousness as a risk factor for Alzheimer's disease. *Neurology, 41*, 1576-1578.

Chrisman, M. (1991). Agitated behavior in the cognitively impaired elderly. *Journal of Gerontological Nursing, 17*(12), 9-13.

Cohen, G. D. (1990). Alzheimer's disease: Clinical update. *Hospital and Community Psychiatry, 41*, 496-497.

Coleman, L. M., Fowler, L. L., Williams, M. E. (1995). Use of unproven therapies by people with Alzheimer's disease. *Journal of the American Geriatric Society, 43*, 747-750.

Cooke, K., & Gould, M. H. (1991). The health effects of aluminum: A review. *Journal of Research in Social Health, 111*(5), 163-168.

Cummings, J. (1988). Intellectual impairment in Parkinson's disease: Clinical, pathologic, and biochemical correlates. *Journal of Geriatric Psychiatry Neurology, 1*, 24-36.

Danner, C., Beck, C., Heacock, P., & Modlin, T. (1993). Cognitively impaired elders: Using research findings to improve nursing care. *Journal of Gerontological Nursing, 19*, 5-11.

Davidson, M., & Stern, R. (1991). The treatment of cognitive impairment in Alzheimer's disease: Beyond the cholinergic approach. *Psychiatric Clinics of North America, 14*, 461-482.

Deutsch, L., & Rovner, B. (1991). Agitation and other noncognitive abnormalities in Alzheimer's disease. *Psychiatric Clinics of North America, 14*, 341-351.

Dickson, L., & Ranseen, J. (1990). An update on selected organic mental syndromes. *Hospital and Community Psychiatry, 41*, 290-300.

Donnelly, R., & Karlinsky, H. (1990). The impact of Alzheimer's disease on driving ability: A review. *Journal of Geriatric Psychiatry and Neurology, 3*(2), 67–72.

Dutherie, E., & Glatt, S. (1988). Understanding and treating multi-infarct dementia. *Clinical Geriatric Medicine, 4*(4), 749–766.

Edwards, A. (1993). *Dementia: Perspectives on individual differences.* New York: Plenum Press.

Edwards, A. (1994). *When memory fails: Helping the Alzheimer's and dementia patient.* New York: Plenum Press.

Evans, L. (1991). The sundown syndrome: A nursing management problem. In W. Chenitz, J. Stone, & S. Salisbury (Eds.), *Clinical gerontological nursing: A guide to advanced practice.* Philadelphia: W. B. Saunders.

Farran, C. J., Horton-Deutsch, S. L., Fiedler, R., & Scott, C. (1997). Psychiatric home care for the elderly. *Home Health Care Services Quarterly, 16*(12), 77–92.

Farran, C. J., Horton-Deutsch, S. L., Loukissa, D., & Johnson, L. (1998). Psychiatric home care of elderly persons with depression: Unmet caregiver needs. *Home Health Care Services Quarterly, 16*(4), 57–74.

Flint, A. (1991). Delusions in dementia: A review. *Journal of Neuropsychiatry and Clinical Neuroscience, 3*, 121–130.

Foreman, M. D., & Zane, D. (1996). Nursing strategies for acute confusion in elders. *American Journal of Nursing, 96*(4), 44–51.

Friedhoff, L. (1998). Donepezil improves Alzheimer's patients' ability to function. *Neurology, 50*(1), 12–18.

Giacobini E., & Barton, J. M. (1997). *Alzheimer's disease: From molecular biology to therapy.* Portland, OR: Birkhauser.

Goate, A. M. (1997). Molecular genetics of Alzheimer's disease. *Geriatrics, 52* (Suppl. 2), S9–S12.

Grollman, E. A., & Kosik, K. S. (1997). *When Someone You Love Has Alzheimer's: The Caregiver's Journey.* Boston, MA: Beacon Press.

Haller, E., & Binder, R. (1995). Delirium, dementia and amnestic disorders. In H. Goldman (Ed.), *Review of general psychiatry.* Norwalk, CT: Appleton & Lange.

Hamdy, R., Turnbull, J., Clark, W., & Lancaster, M. (1994). *Alzheimer's disease: A handbook for caregivers* (2nd ed.). St. Louis, MO: C. V. Mosby.

Harvath, T., Patsdaughter, C., Bumbalo, J., & McCann, M. (1995). Dementia-related behaviors in Alzheimer's disease and AIDS. *Journal of Psychosocial Nursing, 33*(1), 35–38.

Hay, J. (1998). *Alzheimer's and dementia: Questions you have . . . answers you need.* New York: Peoples Medical Society.

Heim, K. M. (1986). Wandering behavior. *Journal of Gerontological Nursing, 12*, 4.

High, D. M. (1992). Research with Alzheimer's disease subjects: Informed consent and proxy decision making. *Journal of the American Geriatric Society, 40*, 950–957.

Hill, C., Risby, E., & Morgan, N. (1992). Cognitive deficits in delirium: Assessment over time. *Psychopharmacology Bulletin, 28*, 401–407.

Hirsch, H. (1990). Legal and ethical considerations in dealing with Alzheimer's disease. *Legal Medicine*, 261–326.

Holcomb, H., Links, J., & Smith, C. (1989). Positron emission tomography: Measuring the metabolic and neurochemical characteristics of the living human nervous system. In N. Andreason (Ed.), *Brain imaging: Applications in psychiatry.* Washington, DC: American Psychiatric Press.

Holmberg, S. (1997). Evaluation of a clinical intervention for wanderers on a geriatric unit. *Archives of Psychiatric Nursing, 11*(21), 160–165.

Holthaus, J. (1997). I-FAAD (Instrument for Affirming Alzheimer's Disease): Understanding and affirming stage specific cognitive decline. *American Journal of Alzheimer's Disease, 12*, 167–170.

Jacques, A. (1992). *Understanding dementia* (2nd ed.). Edinburgh, Scotland: Churchill Livingstone.

Kahana, E., Biegel, D., & Wykle, M. (Eds.) (1994). *Family caregiving across the life span.* Thousand Oaks, CA: Sage Publications.

Kase, C. (1986). Multi-infarct dementia: A real entity? *Journal of the American Geriatric Society, 34*, 482–484.

Keith, I. (1994). The differential diagnosis of dementia. In A. Burns & R. Levy (Eds.), *Dementia,* London: Chapman & Hall.

Kuhlman, G., Wilson, H. S., Hutchinson, S. A., & Wallhagen, M. (1991). Alzheimer's disease and family caregiving: Critical synthesis of the literature and research agenda. *Nursing Research, 40,* 331–337.

LeBars, P. L., Katz, M. M., Berman, N., Freedman, A. M., & Schatzberg, A. F. (1997). A placebo-controlled, double-blind, randomized trial of an extract of ginkgo biloba for dementia. *Journal of the American Medical Association, 278*, 1327–1332.

Lee, V. (1991). Language changes and Alzheimer's disease: A literature review. *Journal of Gerontological Nursing, 17*, 16–20.

Levine, J., & Lawlor, B. (1991). Family counseling and legal issues in Alzheimer's disease. *Psychiatric Clinics of North America, 14*, 385–386.

Mace, N., & Rabins, P. (1991). *The thirty-six hour day.* Baltimore: Johns Hopkins University Press.

Mack, A., Forman, L., Brown, R., & Frances, A. (1994). A brief history of psychiatric classification: From the ancients to DSM-IV. *Psychiatric Clinics of North America, 17*(3), 515–523.

Marachlewski, M. (1994). Anticholinergic syndrome. *Journal of Psychosocial Nursing, 32*(9), 22–24.

McCracken, A. (1994). Special care units: Meeting the needs of cognitively impaired patients. *Journal of Gerontological Nursing, 20*, 41–44.

Nordberg, A. (1992). Biological markers and the cholinergic hypothesis in Alzheimer's disease. *Acta Neurologia Scandinavia, 138* (Suppl.), 54.

Reeves, C. (1993). Home from home: Practical aspects of caring for the confused elderly in a nursing home. In Wilcock, G. (Ed.), *The management of Alzheimer's disease* (pp. 133–149). Petersfield, England: Wrightston Biomedical Publishing Ltd.

Rocca, W. (1994). Frequency, distribution, and risk factors for Alzheimer's disease. *Nursing Clinics of North America, 29*, 101–111.

Snowden, D. (1997). New gene for late-onset Alzheimer's disease. *Journal of the American Medical Association, 277*(10), 837–840.

Stepworth, D. (1994). Telephone counseling interventions with caregivers of elders. *Journal of Psychosocial Nursing, 32*(3), 7–11.

Tokarski, C. (1996). New shades of Alzheimer's research. *Provider, 22*(5), 75.

Vitiello, M., Bliwise, D., & Prinz, P. (1992). Sleep in Alzheimer's disease and the sundown syndrome. *Neurology, 42*(Suppl. 7), 83–93.

Weiler, K. (1994). Legal aspects of nursing documentation for the Alzheimer's patient. *Journal of Gerontological Nursing, 20*(4), 31–40.

Whipple, B. (1996). The overlooked epidemic: HIV in older adults. *American Journal of Nursing, 96*(2), 23–28.

Wykle, M. (1994). The physical and mental health of women care-givers of older adults. *Journal of Psychosocial Nursing, 32*(3), 41–44.

Yaffe, K. (1998). Estrogen therapy in postmenopausal women: Effects on cognitive function and dementia. *Journal of the American Medical Association, 279*(9), 688–695.

Yi, E., Abraham, I., & Holroyd, S. (1994). Alzheimer's disease and nursing: New scientific and clinical insights. *Nursing Clinics of North America, 29*(1), 85–99.

Young, S., Muir-Nash, J., & Ninos, M. (1988). Managing nocturnal wandering behavior. *Journal of Gerontological Nursing, 14*, 6.

Zarit, S., Orr, N., & Zarit, J. (1985). The burden victims of Alzheimer's disease: Families under stress. New York: University Press.

Suggested Readings

Blanchard, F., & Hess, T. M. (1996). *Perspectives on cognitive changes in adulthood and aging.* New York: McGraw-Hill.

Brawley, E. C. (1997). *Designing for Alzheimer's disease: Strategies for creating better care environments.* New York: John Wiley.

Cohen, D., & Eisendorfer, C. (1986). *The loss of self.* New York: NAL Penguin.

Cutler, N. R., & Sramek, J. J. (1996). *Understanding Alzheimer's disease.* Jackson: University Press of Mississippi.

Esiri, M. M. (Ed.). (1997). *Neuropathology of dementia.* Cambridge, England: Cambridge University Press.

Glickenstein, J. K. (1997). *Therapeutic interventions in Alzheimer's disease: A Program of functional skills for activities of daily living and communication* (2nd ed.). Gaithersburg, MD: Aspen.

Gwyther, L. P. (1997). *"Home is where I remember things": A curriculum for home and community Alzheimer's care.* Durham, NC: Duke University Medical Center.

Keck, D. (1996). *Forgetting whose we are: Alzheimer's disease and the love of God.* Nashville: Abingdon.

Kovach, R. C. (Ed.). (1997). *Late stage dementia care: A basic guide.* Washington, DC: Taylor & Francis.

Mace, N., & Rabins, P. (1991). *The thirty-six hour day.* Baltimore: Johns Hopkins University Press.

Quinn, M. J., & Tomita, S. K. (1997). *Elder abuse and neglect* (2nd ed.). New York: Springer.

Stehman, J. M. (Ed.). (1996). *Handbook of dementia care.* Baltimore: Johns Hopkins University Press.

U.S. Department of Health and Human Services. (1996). *Recognition and initial assessment of Alzheimer's disease and related dementias.* Rockville, MD: Author.

Weiner, M. F. (1996). *Dementias: Diagnosis, management, and research* (2nd ed.). Washington, DC: American Psychiatric Press.

Yi, E., Abraham, I., & Holroyd, S. (1994). Alzheimer's disease and nursing: New scientific and clinical insights. *Nursing Clinics of North America, 29*(1), 85-99.

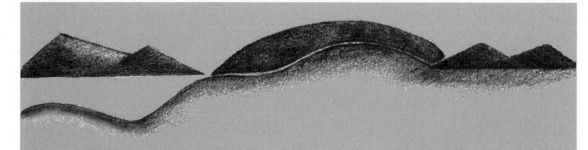

VI The Journey and Society

Traveler's Log

For years I struggled to practice holistic nursing in the field of psychiatric rehabilitation; I yearned to effectively define and enact the ideologies of the mental health nurse in a tertiary care setting. Although I believe that I ultimately achieved this goal, I felt a need to go beyond the practice modality that I had constructed.

My primary reason for change related to an emerging understanding that many of the nurses I worked with could not comprehend the value of the nursing role in psychiatric rehabilitation. Thus, their tendency was to move on to an acute psychiatric placement or to move out of the field of psychiatric nursing at the earliest possible opportunity.

I realized that if I intended to affect any improvements in the nursing care of seriously mentally ill people, then I myself needed further education. Thus, my call to university. I felt a sense of urgency—I wanted to learn; I wanted to share my "self" and my learning with other psychiatric and mental health nurses who were, or who would potentially be, experiencing professional confusion. This began my journey to the place where I now find myself—a nurse educator.

I lived and continue to live out a passion for the field of psychiatric rehabilitation. I can only trust that if the road I am traveling is blocked for me, my energies and resources will still be channeled into a means of living my life to its fullest potential—service to those who are chronically and persistently mentally ill.

—Judith Buchanan, RN, MHSc

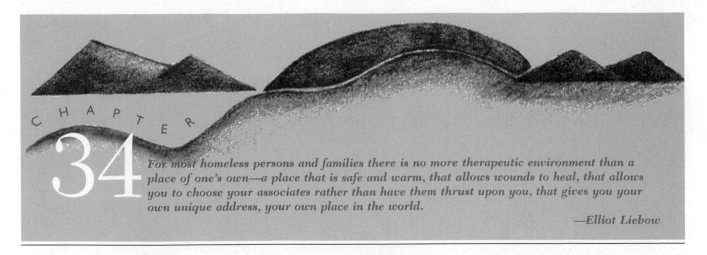

C H A P T E R

34

For most homeless persons and families there is no more therapeutic environment than a place of one's own—a place that is safe and warm, that allows wounds to heal, that allows you to choose your associates rather than have them thrust upon you, that gives you your own unique address, your own place in the world.

—Elliot Liebow

Poverty and Homelessness

Learning Objectives

After studying this chapter, you should be able to:

1. Describe the structural and personal precipitants of homelessness.
2. Identify social and personal attitudes toward the homeless.
3. Identify populations at risk for homelessness.
4. Examine personal values and biases with regard to homeless individuals.
5. Develop an individual approach using the nursing process with homeless patients.

Key Terminology

Admission diversion	Homelessness	Single-room occupancy units	Social margin
Deinstitutionalization	Learned helplessness	Social disaffiliation	Unemployment rate
Gentrification	Poverty		

Nurses encounter the poor and homeless in many settings including emergency departments, walk-in clinics, inpatient units, shelters, soup kitchens, and churches. Nurses may walk around the homeless congregated near heating grates outside a health care facility or come face to face with the economically disadvantaged within a wide variety of health care settings. Nursing, because of its holistic focus on people, is uniquely qualified to have a major impact on the poor and the homeless. Most nurses are motivated by caring, the essential component in the roles of clinician, educator, advocate, and team member. To engage and assist the homeless and the poor, the nurse relies on the nursing process to assess real and potential problems, intervene effectively, and evaluate results.

Within the boundaries of a professional relationship,

nurses are privileged to participate in patients' unique journeys. The nurse is most effective with vulnerable patients when she or he establishes relationships that accommodate the patient's history; current life conditions; and physical, mental, and spiritual strengths and weaknesses. Remember that poverty and homelessness can result from chronic personal trauma, acute personal disaster, or long-set family and community patterns making escape from such distress difficult (Lynch, Kaplan, & Salonen, 1997). The poor and homeless are not faceless. The first step in nursing care is an appreciation of the humanity and individuality of each patient.

Robert is a formerly homeless man eager to share his story "so folks will know how it is." A self-aware man, his recovery program has taught him to speak unflinchingly of his struggle to conquer the self-destructive behaviors that led to his experience with homelessness.

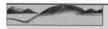
Robert's Story

I lived with my mother until I was 19 years old. We had a strong family, and I was learning to lay brick for a trade. But even then I was playing with drugs on the weekends. Not too much, I never missed work, and I still had money in my pocket. But me and my friends, we were experimenting just the same.

I met my wife around the same time. She was 4 years older than me but had gotten married when she was 14. Because of that, she already had six little kids. My mother went through some stress because she thought it was crazy for a 19-year-old to take on six kids, but I loved my wife so we got together. We never actually got married—I guess you could say we were common-law married. We had two more kids of our own while we were together.

Robert's Drug Habit

I worked steady as a bricklayer for years. I'm 51 years old now, and my life didn't fall apart until 7 years ago. But while I was working and raising my family, I got more and more into using drugs. I tried everything that came out a few times, but my drug of choice was heroin. They call it "drug of choice" because it's how I preferred to get high. I didn't care for cocaine, although I did snort it a couple of times. I didn't like alcohol either, but I got my wife started drinking. She wanted to be able to feel like I felt. I see now that I did her no favor, but we were stupid back then.

Seven years ago, things went bad for me. All these years, I had gotten into little scrapes with the law, but nothing too serious. I prided myself on not being willing to rip off my family to support my drug habit. Somehow, I started doing things I never thought I could do. I'd get a paycheck on Friday, shoot it up over the weekend, be broke on Monday. I was stealing things to sell to buy drugs, including stealing things from my own kids. I'm still ashamed of ripping off my son's VCR. The addiction took over my life, and I gave up everything for it. Remember, I had a steady job, nice wife, eight kids, and a home by this time. But there were dark parts of me inside that I couldn't face, so I self-medicated. I couldn't get honest, so I would get high. I was still working, but you can see I was way out of control at home. My wife and kids had a meeting. They decided that I had to get out of the house until I could get straight. It was a shock to me, but they said I could come back as soon as I was clean. If my addiction hadn't been so strong, I'm sure that their ultimatum would have killed me.

So what did I do the first night? I was lost, in another world. Me, homeless? I would have said it was impossible except that it was true.

Life in a Homeless Shelter

The first night, I went to Jefferson Shelter [name changed]. It was hell when I look back—toilets not working right, rats and bugs in the building, too many guys—but I didn't have a choice. I didn't make a reservation, if you know what I mean. They put us out at 7:00 in the morning every day, no matter what—if it was snowing, raining, if you were sick. It was all too bad. I didn't know what to do those first few days. I wasn't working for that stretch, so I just followed the crowd. First, we went to a soup kitchen and waited in a long line to get breakfast. Then after that, the men walked to a church nearby to get breakfast again. At least it was something to do. It was strange to feel like I had too much time on my hands.

I was in overnight shelters for 3 years while I was using heroin heavy. I look back now, and it was lost time. Can you believe I still worked? I sure didn't have any money to show for it, but I kept up my trade. While I was working one day, I hurt my back. I was laying some mortar, and I must have turned my back and then had bad pain. It was hard to walk, but believe it or not, I walked and worked. I guess the heroin did me some good!

To make a long story short, one day after my back injury, I got very sick. I was coughing and weak, so I went to the doctor at the clinic. She said I had pneumonia and needed to stay in bed to get better. The only place I could stay in bed was at the infirmary at the H.O.P.E. Shelter [name changed]. The H.O.P.E. Shelter is the Ritz of the city because you actually live there for 24 hours a day. Also, the infirmary has nurses to take care of you, and when you get better, they get you a bed upstairs in the main shelter. It was a way out of the overnight shelters, and I was so sick I needed to be taken care of. So I went to the infirmary.

The rules in the infirmary were very strict. No drugs or alcohol in the building, or you were barred for life. When I got better from my pneumonia, I stayed out 3 nights in a row and was discharged against my will. But by then I had been hooked up with the drug rehab program at the shelter.

Rehabilitation

The rehab program has one of the best success rates in the city. It's run by recovering alcoholics and addicts, and they don't cut you any slack. If you're not serious about recovery, they make you leave and you need to reapply to get back in. Beds are limited, so I didn't want to mess up. The inpatient program lasts a year, and then the outpatient program goes on for as long as you want. I guess I was finally sick and tired of being sick and tired, so I entered the program.

The program helped me come back to sanity. It was tough, and I went off the heroin cold turkey. I got support but also a lot of confrontation. Little by little, I got back my self-respect. I was still a homeless man, though.

I never realized that people could see you on the street and actually look through you. Man, that is cold! I was ashamed of being homeless, so I would get a defensive attitude. When I was using, I didn't care what people thought of me. When I was clean, it hurt. I felt like I was some bug that people wanted to squash.

I was clean and working my program aggressively for 3 years. I got promoted in the program to be hall monitor and was doing good. In the program, you can't work for a year. When it was time to go back to the world, I felt strong. I think I got cocky, though, because 7 months ago, I relapsed. I overdosed on heroin and was found unconscious in the bathroom at the shelter. Not only was it humiliating, but I was barred from the shelter for life. I really blew it.

I used heroin again for 2 months and went back to my life in overnight shelters. But, thank God, I had folks who believed in me—my friends in the program, my doctor, and my nurses. They encouraged me to get back into recovery. Five months ago, I did. I knew I couldn't keep hiding from myself. It is hard work, but I'm trying to stay honest with myself.

I now live in an apartment with my son. I work full time, and I go to two meetings a day. I've been up and I've been down, but I see how powerful the addiction is in my life. I need to fight every day to stay clean.

Tell people that homeless folks are just folks. Some are crazy; some are high; some are just down on their luck. It's scary and lonely out there. I'm an old man, but I can truthfully say I was in bad shape when I was homeless.

I live my life day to day now. My family and I are trying to work out our differences. Seven years is a long time to be out there, you know. Did I tell you I have 20 grandkids now? I want to be a grandfather they can be proud of. ■

WHAT POVERTY IS

Poverty in its most general definition is the lack of resources for a reasonably comfortable lifestyle. Although we typically associate poverty with a shortage of money and other material goods, people can be spiritually, psychologically, and socially disadvantaged, as well (Baier, Murray, North, Lato, & Eskew, 1996). We may all know people who live in big houses and drive nice cars but have no relationship with God, no sense of peace or well-being, and no friends or support networks. In 1995, material poverty was a fact of life for 13.8% of the American population (U.S. Bureau of the Census, 1997). This translates to a family of four living on $15,569 per year or less. Consider that many country club memberships cost more than that. Poverty is linked to increased death rates at younger ages (Waitzman & Smith, 1998), as well as to detrimental physical and psychosocial health habits across the life span (Lynch et al., 1997).

Herth (1996) identified that inner resources such as hope can be detrimentally affected by traits associated with poverty, such as decreased energy, constant loss, lack of hope in others, and a lessened sense of personhood. In terms of health care access, Goetchens (1986) linked poverty with longer waits for service, increased exposure to multiple providers, and treatment

with less dignity and respect in general. Poverty clearly renders individuals more vulnerable to "falling through the cracks" of society. One disastrous result of such vulnerability is the phenemenon of homelessness.

WHAT HOMELESSNESS IS

Homelessness is not a new phenomenon but a long-standing global problem that gained increased prominence in the United States since the 1970s. Blau (1992) identified five major periods within the history of homelessness. The first, in the preindustrial period, was highlighted by an absolute scarcity of adequate housing.

The second period of homelessness occurred during the early industrial period, in the late 18th to early 19th centuries. Rural workers in France and England often were temporarily homeless when they journeyed to cities to find factory jobs. This transitional homelessness usually was due to lack of immediate employment, insufficient income, or paucity of housing. Although difficult, it seems to have been a sort of rite of passage for some.

The third phase of homelessness started with the colonization of the undeveloped world (Asia, South America, and Africa) and still exists today. To find work, large groups of homeless workers congregate in metropolitan areas of primitively industrialized countries. Because this system of industrialization favors cheap labor over the welfare of workers, laborers must settle for temporary or poorly paid jobs. Employers and governments make little investment in providing for the shelter of workers who are easily replaced by other, less demanding workers.

The fourth period of homelessness, coinciding with the era of modern industrialization, shifts our focus to the United States. Blau (1992) described sharp increases in the number of homeless people during periods of unregulated capitalism (in the late 19th century as well as in the 1920s and during the Depression). These spurts of unregulated capitalism created a sharply divided economy with dramatic class and income distinctions in the population. Interestingly, homelessness essentially vanished during times of prosperity or war. Blau (1992) characterized homelessness during this phase as highly responsive to the variations in business cycles.

The fifth upsurge of homelessness started in the early 1980s with deindustrialization and a shift to a service economy. Contemporary social factors have promoted increased homelessness. These include an increase in low-paying jobs, cutbacks in low-cost housing, and reductions in social welfare programs.

The study of **homelessness** has been hampered by the lack of a standardized definition of the term (Bachrach, 1992). In 1998, the National Coalition for the Homeless was unable to provide an estimate of how many homeless people live in the United States, partially because there are so many variations on not having a stable residence. Advocates for street dwellers and shelter residents coined the word "homeless" in the late 1970s to protect undomiciled people from stigma and stereotyping. In 1987, the federal government defined *homelessness* as the absence of "fixed, regular, and adequate nighttime residence" or the need to use shelters, institutions, or public or private places not designed for regular sleeping accommodations as a primary nighttime residence (Stewart B. McKinney Homelessness Assistance Act of 1987, p. 10). Yet homelessness is a problem more complex than the lack of a place to live (Bachrach, 1992).

Homelessness can be defined differently depending on whether the affected population is the "old homeless" or the "new homeless." The *old homeless* match Blau's fourth period of homelessness, during times of economic hardship. These people included tramps, hoboes, and skid row dwellers whose numbers surged during the Depression. Schubert (1935) described tramps and hoboes as young men who left home to escape economically depressed hometowns and traveled from place to place to find jobs. Skid row dwellers were primarily older white alcoholic men living in run-down urban areas around railroad tracks and trucking companies. These people would find casual employment as needed and often had needs met by religious missions dedicated to the salvation and support of skid row residents. Interestingly, these people generally had some kind of stable shelter in flophouse motels, private homes, or mission dormitories. Had any of these people attempted to live on the street, they would have been taken to jail. Furthermore, skid row residents were concentrated in urban areas and were avoided and ignored (Rossi, 1990).

The face of homelessness changed in the late 1970s and early 1980s with the appearance of the new homeless. The *new homeless* consisted of men, women, and children literally without shelter, as evidenced by the sight of people sleeping on steam grates, in abandoned cars, or in cardboard boxes. Contemporary homelessness is characterized by a lack of permanent and reasonable shelter. Its precipitating factors are

- Extreme poverty
- Social isolation
- Estrangement from networks of family or friends
- Exhaustion of last-ditch resources aimed at maintaining domiciled status

The reality of homelessness is overwhelming. Nurses function most effectively when they understand the population to be served.

What do you think? Someone says to you, "No one needs to be homeless in the United States; they want to live that way." How would you respond?

▶ *Check Your Reading*
1. Define poverty.
2. Define homelessness.
3. Compare and contrast the old homeless and the new homeless.

WHO THE POOR AND HOMELESS ARE

We can no longer be lulled into the insular belief that poverty and homelessness happen only to certain groups within the population. As advocates and educators, nurses have a particular responsibility to maintain awareness of those affected by poverty, homelessness, and the risk of both. Statistics prove that single men compose the largest group of homeless people in the United States. Lindblom (1991) pointed out that single, unattached men make up approximately 70% of the adult homeless population. Similarly, Carter, Green, Green, and Dufour (1994) found that 73% of adult homeless patients using a free clinic in Georgia were men. Marin (1991) encouraged sensitivity to the plight of homeless men, pointing out that these men are viewed unsympathetically because of social values deriding male neediness and vulnerability. No one can dismiss the tragedy of homelessness for single men. These men are, in a sense, remnants of the "old homeless," traditionally represented by unattached men. However, they do not fit the profile of the "new homeless" who are victims of the deindustrialization of society.

The Chronic Mentally Ill

Review for yourself the number of tasks, personal encounters, and readjustments you make each day to maintain your lifestyle. Imagine being constantly challenged by a debilitating and exhausting emotional illness and having no place to call home. This is the challenge facing chronically mentally ill, homeless people on a daily basis.

The numbers of the homeless mentally ill are difficult to ascertain because this population is poorly measured. Widely varying estimates of the prevalence of mental illness among the homeless range from 10% to 85% (Rossi, 1990), but most sources agree that approximately one third of the homeless population has some mental illness (Dennis, Buckner, Lipton, & Levine, 1991; Federal Task Force on Homelessness and Severe Mental Illness, 1992). Mental illnesses affecting the homeless include but are not limited to schizoid personality disorder, anxiety disorders, depressive disorder, and bipolar disorder (Wallsten, 1992). The incredible stress of homelessness is in itself a predisposing factor for emotional distress.

The mentally ill generally display poor interpersonal skills, inadequate problem solving strategies, disorganized or psychotic thinking, and a global inability to tend to their own needs. Baier, Murray, North, Lato, and Eskew (1996) found that mentally ill people tended to be homeless longer than others in a research sample, and often stayed out of shelters. Extreme physical deprivation confounds the picture by making differentiation of psychological and somatic symptoms difficult (Bachrach, 1992). The consequence of severe mental illness can be the inability to find or maintain employment, to develop trusting relationships, to preserve housing arrangements, or to meet physical and psychological health needs (Federal Task Force on Homelessness and Severe Mental Illness, 1992). The incidence of attempted suicide is high across all groups within the adult homeless population (Interagency Council on the Homeless, 1990).

The influx of the chronically mentally ill into the homeless population generally is credited to the policy of **deinstitutionalization.** Based on a civil liberties philosophy stating that institutions provided inhumane care for the mentally ill, deinstitutionalization mandated that scores of patients be released from state mental hospitals. Advocates of deinstitutionalization believed that patients could be absorbed by community mental health centers (Bachrach, 1992). Neuroleptic medications had facilitated symptom management so the mentally ill appeared healthier. Although intended as a compassionate solution to harsh institutional conditions, deinstitutionalization released patients before adequate supports could be established in the community. Funds for state hospitals were not transferred to community mental health centers. Many patients never received a complete assessment of their needs.

Although imperfect, institutions provided structure, social context, food, clothing, and medical services to their residents. On their own, chronically mentally ill individuals have difficulty accessing bureaucratic systems. The burden of outreach and support for these patients therefore fell on understaffed, unfunded, and unprepared community mental health clinics. These conditions have conspired to create a chaotic environment in which many chronically mentally ill patients have essentially been left to their own devices.

Deinstitutionalization also has led to admission diversion. **Admission diversion** is a gatekeeping tactic that limits access to state mental hospitals (Bachrach, 1992). Although civil rights of the mentally ill are protected, some people who try to use inpatient mental health services have been discouraged from doing so. The strategy has contributed further to the number of chronically mentally ill people left homeless.

Substance Abusers

The problem of substance abuse contributes to factors that may lead to homelessness. Between 35% and 40% of the homeless are estimated to have alcohol and/or drug problems (Fischer & Breakey, 1990; Interagency Council on the Homeless, 1990; Lindblom, 1991). Alcohol abuse, drug addiction, and mental health problems also share a high coincidence. Statistics demonstrate that approximately one quarter of homeless drug and alcohol abusers have a history of mental hospital stays, and one half of the chronically mentally ill homeless abuse alcohol or drugs (Interagency Council on the Homeless, 1990). The National Coalition for the Homeless (1997) associates mental illness and substance abuse with increased difficulty finding permanent housing to escape homelessness.

Consider the impact of chemical dependence on one's life. The networks of family and friends often are broken as alcohol or drug use becomes a prominent feature of daily existence. Substance abusers may display erratic, impulsive, or antisocial behavior while intoxicated or high. Fischer and Breakey (1990) found that alcoholics were more likely to come from dysfunctional families, not graduate from high school, and have fewer job skills, all of which adversely affect the capacity to find or maintain work. Those abusing illicit drugs run a high risk of arrest and legal conflicts. Not only is possession of the drug and associated paraphernalia illegal but also support of the drug habit may require further illegal activities such as drug dealing, theft, or prostitution (Fischer & Breakey, 1990).

The physical toll exacted by substance abuse is devastating. Alcoholics treated at homeless shelter medical clinics demonstrate grossly inflated incidences of liver disease, seizure disorders, hypertension, nutritional and gastrointestinal disorders, and severe trauma (Fischer & Breakey, 1990). The chemically dependent have an increased capacity for high-risk behaviors ranging from physical fights to prostitution. Unsafe sexual practices lead to increased risk of sexually transmitted disease, including exposure to HIV.

What do you think? What is our responsibility as a society to the homeless?

➤ *Check Your Reading*
4. How does chronic mental illness predispose a patient to homelessness?
5. How are social ties jeopardized for homeless substance abusers?

Women

The appearance of women living in public shelters or on the streets has provided disconcerting evidence that homelessness is an increasingly universal phenomenon (Liebow, 1993). Many researchers identify women as a fast-growing subgroup among the homeless (Milburn & D'Ercole, 1991; Warren, Menke, Clement, & Wagner, 1992), but reasons for this trend are varied. The Interagency Council on the Homeless (1990) reported that women head 80% of homeless families, are younger than other homeless people, and have fewer supportive friends and relatives, lower employment rates, and less education. Eighty percent of homeless women with children belong to a minority group (Interagency Council on the Homeless, 1990). Milburn and D'Ercole (1991) listed housing instability, poverty, work problems, unemployment, and victimization as primary risk factors for homelessness in women.

Poverty is a major stressor leading to female homelessness. Before losing their homes, 82% of homeless women with children lived below the poverty line (Milburn & D'Ercole, 1991). In 1997, the U.S. Bureau of the Census reported that women without high school diplomas earned an average of $16,666 per year. The daily struggle of trying to provide for one's needs as well as the needs of one's children on such meager funds is psychologically exhausting. Psychological exhaustion and crisis-oriented lifestyles are strongly associated with homeless women (Warren et al., 1992).

Vulnerability to victimization is another predominant cause of homelessness in women. Homeless women are rarely married, experience more loss of social support than homeless men, and report familial abuse (spouse or child) as a major precursor to homelessness (Milburn & D'Ercole, 1991). Experiences of abuse often lead to social isolation, which predisposes people to homelessness. Jackson and McSwane (1992) found that the pregnancy rate in homeless women was twice that in the domiciled population because of limited access to birth control and a high incidence of rape. Pregnancy, however, may boost the self-esteem of homeless women who feel otherwise powerless in American mainstream society.

Children

Children sadly remind us of the grim reality of poverty and homelessness. They are innocent victims, doomed to live on the street or in shelters. Shelters are large, loud, harshly lit places with little privacy and few safe places to play. In 1997, the U.S. Bureau of the Census estimated that 20% of all American children lived below poverty level, with dramatically higher rates for black (41.5%) and Hispanic (34.3%) children. The impact of homelessness on children is profound and long-lasting (Ziesemer, Marcoux, & Maxwell, 1994).

Children have joined the ranks of the homeless either as members of homeless families or runaways, "throwaway" children, or "unaccompanied youths." Families often become homeless as a result of eviction, parental loss of employment or benefits, or abuse in the extended family (Milburn & D'Ercole, 1991). Runaway children generally are thought to have homes they can return to if they so desire (Interagency Council on the Homeless, 1990). Most, however, cannot return home because of family conflict. *Throwaway children* are abandoned by their families because of economic hardship or parental drug addiction. Although some throwaway children are literally abandoned, others live in such deprivation that their health and welfare are seriously undermined. *Unaccompanied youths* usually are boys between the ages of 12 and 18 years who have no accompanying parent and no home. These children often are failed by a shelter system that does not accept unaccompanied children and refers these youths to runaway homes where their special needs go unmet (Interagency Council on the Homeless, 1990).

Children living in poverty and hardship often are candidates for foster care. Yet foster care situations are prime launching sites into homelessness, as many children run away from foster homes before reaching emancipation at age 18 (Lindblom, 1991).

Infant mortality for the homeless is 25 deaths per 1000 live births, as compared with 12 deaths per 1000 births for nonhomeless babies. Homeless children are at increased risk for hunger, poor nutrition, compromised physical health, developmental delays, psychological problems, and educational underachievement (Rafferty & Shinn, 1991). They typically have immunization delays, are at increased risk for lead poisoning, and have a high incidence of iron deficiencies related to inadequate nutrition. In addition, homeless children display language delays, difficulties with personal and social tasks, shortened attention spans, depression, anxiety, behavioral problems, poor scores on standardized math and reading tests, and poor school attendance (Rafferty & Shinn, 1991; Ziesemer et al., 1994). The list of actual and potential problems for homeless children can be overwhelming. Nurses in community health, obstetrical, emergency department, mental health, and school settings are frequently the first health professionals to make contact with these children. The loss of one's home and the shock of adjusting to life in a shelter—or on the street—produces psychological trauma in all homeless people (Goodman, Saxe, & Harvey, 1991). The impact of such trauma in early life has yet to be measured.

The Elderly

In 1995, 14.8% of people 65 years old and older in the United States lived below the poverty level (U.S. Bureau of the Census, 1997). Estimates of the elderly homeless population range from 3% (Interagency Council on the Homeless, 1990) to 6% (Wallsten, 1992). The lower percentage of the homeless elderly may be attributed to Social Security and other entitlements that provide income to obtain some kind of housing (Interagency Council on the Homeless, 1990). Wallsten (1992) suggested, however, that the actual number of the elderly homeless is underestimated because the elderly avoid shelters where they may be mugged, treated unkindly, or referred for institutionalization. Factors specific to the elderly, such as the threat of senility, need for special transportation, and vulnerability to attack by younger people, make homelessness particularly difficult for the older person (Damrosch & Strasser, 1988).

The trauma and extraordinary stress of homelessness seem to be borne out by mortality data related to the so-called longer-term homeless. The average age of death among those enduring extended periods of homelessness is in the early 50s. According to the Interagency Council on the Homeless (1990), "Because of special available benefits, persons over 65 rarely become homeless; and because of the harsh conditions of homelessness, few long-term homeless persons ever reach 65" (p. 37).

Immigrants, Illegal Aliens, and Minorities

People living in developing countries who come to the United States often have hopes of finding new opportunities. Unfortunately, their hopes frequently are dashed when they encounter a strange culture with an incredibly bureaucratic system. Often immigrants are simply baffled by paperwork and clearances, and illegal aliens may be innocent victims of government quotas. Employment and housing are critical problems for this group, rendering them vulnerable to abusive working conditions (if work is found) and to living with many others in inadequate housing. When multiple stresses build, the immigrant may become homeless as a casualty of an overloaded system.

Minorities in general are overrepresented in the poor (U.S. Bureau of the Census, 1997) and homeless (Burt, 1992) populations. Blacks consistently have composed approximately 40% of the homeless population (Interagency Council on the Homeless, 1994). In 1990, the National American Indian Housing Council estimated that 25% of the Native Americans in the United States lived in cars, makeshift shelters, tents, or substandard housing. More than 80% of homeless women with children are nonwhite (Interagency Council on the Homeless, 1990). Poverty and unequal opportunities for minorities and noncitizens are amplified in the homeless population.

> **W**hat do you think? Nursing has a history of reaching out to the poor and disenfranchised. What special role might nurses play to assist the homeless and poor?

> ▶ *Check Your Reading*
> 6. What factors make the chronically mentally ill vulnerable to homelessness?
> 7. How does homelessness affect children's long-range chances to succeed?
> 8. Why do the elderly homeless avoid public shelters?
> 9. List factors that make immigrants and illegal aliens vulnerable to homelessness.

FACTORS LEADING TO HOMELESSNESS

Becoming homeless is a journey rather than a discrete event. The socioeconomic aspects of the journey include the withdrawal of financial support from educational and advocacy government programs, increased poverty, chronic unemployment, limited low-income housing, deinstitutionalization, and a "burn-out" syndrome in which upper- and middle-class sympathy for the homeless is waning. Personal factors such as chronic mental illness, drug and alcohol abuse, family violence, physical infirmity, estrangement from kin and friendship support systems, poor tolerance for frustration, and difficulty developing and maintaining trust also are implicated in the journey to homelessness.

Homelessness most often is caused by loss or lack of employment and independent residence and social margin. The **social margin** is composed of the group of family members, friends, and associates who offer emergency assistance and support in the wake of

personal disaster. Although you may wonder why anybody is homeless in America, some researchers puzzle over why all extremely poor individuals do not become homeless. Recognizing that homelessness occurs with the collision of socioeconomic and personal factors can help you understand why people travel different journeys.

Structural Causes of Homelessness

Unemployment

In 1989 the Urban Institute found that approximately 75% of homeless adults were unemployed. In 1997, the U.S. Bureau of the Census found that 31.6% to 63.9% of unemployed Americans lived below poverty level. Rossi (1990) defined the **unemployment rate** as a measure of the percentage of people in the work force who are out of jobs, yet unemployed people not seeking employment are not counted. Defining unemployment to include only job seekers was originally a way of eliminating the retired, the disabled, and women staying at home. It was not intended to avoid counting persons out of work for long periods of time too discouraged to continue job searches. As the need for unskilled and low-skilled laborers continues to dwindle with advancing technology, many people have become "discouraged workers."

The psychological sequelae of being unemployed range from mild to crippling. Consider the benefits of employment, which Smith (1987) cited as social contacts, time structure, social status, personal identity clarification, and a regular schedule. Warr (1987) identified nine effects of unemployment on emotional well-being (Box 34-1). Your awareness of the detrimental results of unemployment can enhance your sensitivity to the plight of the homeless unemployed.

Box 34-1 ■ ■ ■ ■ ■
Effects of Unemployment

1. Decreased income—the most devastating effect
2. Constricted world, with no need to go out into the world to interact
3. Loss of "traction" or momentum to achieve
4. Loss of flexibility in decision-making
5. Loss of satisfaction with new job-related skill development
6. Increasingly uncertain future
7. Discrimination experienced in society, with patient rejected more and experiencing embarrassment
8. Deterioration of quality and nature of interpersonal contacts
9. Diminished social status and position

From Warr, P. (1987). *Work, employment, and mental health.* New York: Oxford University Press, by permission of Oxford University Press.

Inadequate Low-Cost Housing

All homeless people lack a residence, even a substandard place to live. Between 1970 and 1983, an overall effort was made to renovate properties occupied by the very poor, primarily **single-room occupancy units** (SROs) (Interagency Council on the Homeless, 1990). Although often substandard, SROs offered inexpensive housing to a large segment of young and middle-aged single people ineligible for public housing or federal housing entitlements (Interagency Council on the Homeless, 1990). The dissolution of SROs contributed significantly to homelessness.

Many SROs were destroyed or converted to other uses in an effort to revive major cities through **gentrification,** the conversion of low-cost properties to higher-rent housing. A result was the eviction of impoverished people unable to live in improved, more expensive quarters. Other low-cost housing has been lost to arson or to abandonment by investors, who can invest more profitably in other real estate.

Lindblom (1991) also highlighted the deficiency of supported housing for the mentally ill, the drug-dependent or alcohol-dependent, and otherwise compromised indigent people. He pointed out the difficulty of developing any new low-cost housing, especially for disadvantaged populations. Many inhabitants of upper- and middle-class neighborhoods block construction of low-cost housing in the vicinity of their homes to avoid "contamination" of the neighborhood and declines in property values. This is the so-called "not in my back yard" (NIMBY) phenomenon.

Shortage of Social Services

Social service programs developed in the 1960s during the so-called War on Poverty. Programs designed to educate, train, and financially assist the poor received substantial federal and state government support. The growing economic concerns of the 1970s and 1980s, particularly the budget deficit and the focus of the Reagan administration on decreasing peoples' dependence on the government, led to widespread voter rejection of social welfare programs. Budget cutbacks caused services provided by these social welfare programs to be slashed. The federal government cut training and job program spending by 70% between 1981 and 1990. Twenty-five percent of young people have been eliminated from summer job programs. Blau (1992) noted that five programs providing income to the financially marginal—Aid to Families with Dependent Children, Social Security, disability benefits, unemployment insurance, and food stamps—either lost funds or saw the number of recipients limited. The Balanced Budget Act of 1997 and welfare reform have not eased the plight of the poor; increasingly more responsibility is placed on states to create their own social safety net for the most vulnerable in society.

Income security programs awaken conflicting feelings for many people. Concern for the needy may be offset by suspicion about welfare recipients who abuse the system and by stereotypes associated with the unemployed. Racial and gender stereotypes are called into play, as are attitudes toward the aging and the young. Many social programs provide support, even if minimal, to the elderly, children, women, and minorities. Who fills in for what the government cannot provide? Advocates for the poor and homeless, churches, individuals, and service clubs contribute as they can, but needs remain overwhelming.

> **What do you think?** What can be done to provide affordable housing and jobs while at the same time not creating dependence on the system?

➤ *Check Your Reading*
10. List effects of unemployment and inadequate social service support on psychological well-being.

Personal Causes of Unemployment

Overwhelmed Families

The 1990s brought much talk of "family values" and the devastating breakdown occurring in families. Some advocates of limiting social benefits argue that families provide the ultimate safety net for members lacking financial and emotional resources. If a family member is mentally ill or substance abusing, however, family resources may dwindle over time. Imagine trying to cope with a chronically schizophrenic son who responds to auditory hallucinations, speaks in neologisms, dresses bizarrely, and might disappear without warning for months at a time. A supportive family may be unduly stressed by an unexpected familial illness or loss of a job. How would you feel if you and your 70-year-old spouse were barely making ends meet with Social Security and your daughter, her husband, and their three children needed to move in after becoming unemployed?

If intact, families of prehomeless and homeless people often are stretched to the breaking point. Not only have chronically mentally ill people been deinstitutionalized but the institutionalization of family members who need comprehensive support is now also difficult. Involuntary commitment requires a person to be harmful to self or others, and many chronically mentally ill people needing care do not meet this criterion. Inpatient substance abuse programs may have long waiting lists and often require some form of detoxification before admission. As one mother of a homeless chronically alcoholic son in Washington, D.C. said wearily, "We've run out of ideas, and we don't have enough money. It kills his father to see him like this, but it will kill me to have him home."

The family cannot be expected to take over where government policies have left huge gaps. Some families cut off contact with a troubled member to avoid being saddled with a commitment that family members cannot take on. Families that do take on their mentally ill, drug-abusing, or violent member find little community support. Programs to meet treatment needs often do not exist, and neighbors may justifiably have concerns.

Expecting families to be the sole providers of economic and emotional support for family members requiring comprehensive services is unreasonable.

Reilly (1993) researched frequently occurring patterns within families of origin of homeless individuals. A summary of dysfunctional dynamics includes physical, psychological, or sexual abuse and neglect; physical abandonment; familial alcohol and drug abuse; and isolation from communities and other family members. With this level of family distress, a homeless person has essentially no family to turn to in times of needs. A family so internally broken cannot provide a haven when a person is threatened by external stresses.

Social Disaffiliation

Social disaffiliation is estrangement from connective bonds that tie people to social support networks and provide a psychological sense of safety, security, and trust (Goodman et al., 1991). Even the threat of homelessness may precipitate actual or perceived abandonment and leave a person isolated, distrustful, and lonely.

Awareness of these dynamics should help you understand behaviors the homeless may demonstrate. Building trust with a disaffiliated patient requires tremendous time and perseverance. Often, homeless individuals have been rejected as "losers" or have been blamed for their fate. These reactions from formerly supportive others reinforce feelings of isolation and hamper the homeless person's ability to form relationships (Goodman et al., 1991).

Learned Helplessness

Learned helplessness is the fixed belief that a person's actions will have no influence or impact on the course of life (Seligman, 1975). Learned helplessness is associated with profound depression and is most likely to occur when people feel personally responsible for their adverse circumstances, believe the situation to be long-term, and credit global rather than specific factors for causing their problems (Goodman et al., 1991).

The belief that one has no control over one's life may be realistic. Homelessness does attack one's sense of competence and independence. Rossi (1990) pointed out too that the extreme poverty that precedes homelessness is linked with depression and hopelessness, which often intensify with the deprivation of homelessness. Herth (1996) emphasized the healing nature of hope on the ability of homeless families to survive and overcome the trauma of displacement. Creating an interdependent nurse-patient relationship with someone who perceives himself or herself to be helpless is a challenge. You need to address the patient's needs while simultaneously guarding against rescuing him or her and fostering passive dependence. Long-ingrained patterns require much time to change. You can provide support and hope that such growth is possible.

> **What do you think?** How could you as a nurse respond to "learned helplessness"?

➤ *Check Your Reading*
11. What is the impact of family dysfunction on homelessness?
12. Define social disaffiliation.
13. How can learned helplessness affect the nurse-patient relationship?

ATTITUDES TOWARD THE HOMELESS

As human beings, nurses are vulnerable to preconceived ideas and attitudes about the homeless. You therefore need to clarify your own values about poverty, homelessness, mental illness, substance abuse, and other factors related to this population. If you hold a bias or unwitting prejudice, you may need to seek supervision from another nurse to approach patients openly. As an advocate, you also have the opportunity to assess others for preconceived ideas and attitudes.

Distancing

People who are made uncomfortable by the homeless avoid anxiety by creating interpersonal barriers. Such barriers are erected by creating and maintaining myths about the homeless and by promoting fear of personal involvement. Myths about the homeless abound: "They could all work if they wanted to." "They're crazy and dangerous." "I'll catch fleas if I touch one of them." "They'll drink up any money I give them anyway." You can debunk myths by educating the public about the realities of homelessness. You also should be aware of any feelings of distance from patients and seek help from colleagues in exploring those feelings.

Disgust and Disdain

Disgust and disdain for the homeless often are based on a cursory assessment. Personal hygiene may be compromised in homeless persons, but an appreciation of living conditions in shelters or on the street might foster empathy. Disdain is a contemptuous rejection of the homeless person as being unworthy of regard. Disgust and disdain are blocks to building mutual relationships and may serve a protective function for the holders of these attitudes. Your role as educator and advocate is called into service to examine and challenge these feelings.

Moral Superiority

Moral superiority goes hand in hand with fear, disgust, and a sense of one's precedence over the other. Homelessness is not a sign of a personal defect or weak character. An attitude of moral superiority indicates a perception of an unequal power between people. This stance precludes honest communication, sharing, or understanding the homeless person's circumstances. Be particularly sensitive in detecting any personal sense of moral superiority when working with the homeless.

Guilt

Guilt is a useful feeling when it motivates us to correct a wrong. If it is misdirected, however, guilt may be crippling and prevent action rather than promote it. Seeing homeless men, women, and children on the street touches a chord within us. That chord should promote responsibility rather than guilt. Taking responsibility for using our own time, money, and effort to intervene one-on-one is more useful than feeling a global sense of guilt about all homeless people. As an educator, you can reframe homelessness as a situation for empathy and caring rather than guilt.

Fear

Homeless people are just people like the rest of us. This knowledge should ease fears of the homeless as a group and help to challenge the fear that some experience as a knee-jerk reaction. It is naive and potentially dangerous, however, to disregard fear completely. Be attentive to fear as a sign of possible peril and educate others to be respectful of those feelings. Just as people with homes can be antisocial and otherwise risky, homeless people can be dangerous as well.

> **What do you think?** What are your feelings and attitudes toward the homeless?

> ➤ *Check Your Reading*
> 14. How do preconceived ideas and attitudes affect the nurse-patient relationship?

NURSING PROCESS

The nursing process offers an organized approach to working with homeless people. A sense of structure and pacing can be particularly helpful when you must practice in a potentially chaotic environment. Having a systematic guide to approaching interventions with the homeless may lessen your anxiety and communicate professional competence to the patients themselves.

Assessing Homeless Patients

Because homelessness is a multidimensional state of being, assessment should be multidimensional. Physical assessment skills are put to good use as the nurse seeks to uncover any somatic deficits or dysfunction. Unusual behavior may have roots in a physical cause; for example, a confused patient may be intoxicated, hypo- or hyperglycemic, or suffering from a head injury. The goal of the psychosocial assessment, however, should be to reveal and support the patient's positive coping skills.

A psychosocial assessment should be approached with flexibility, sensitivity, and a willingness to go at the patient's pace. Cowger (1994) devised an assessment tool for social workers, which is easily modified for nursing (Table 34–1). Cowger stated that an emphasis on the patient's dysfunction may make that the focus of the assessment, which in turn leads to self-fulfilling prophecies and increases the patient's dependence on the nurse. An assessment focused on patient strengths empowers him or her to take control of his or her life and adopt new solutions to old problems. Therefore, a nursing assessment based on identifying and maximizing patient strengths is also an initial intervention.

Interventions for the Homeless

Interventions for the homeless must be realistic and focused on the patient's priorities. The plan should include not only goals but also concrete steps designed to meet the objectives. For example, it is not enough to plan that a homeless patient will meet a clinic appointment. You must strategize with the patient to find transportation to the clinic, to devise a way to communicate the patient's needs to the clinic's staff (referrals or advance phone calls are helpful), and to design a plan for learning the results of the evaluation. If the clinic appointment is not a priority for the patient, it may be missed as other needs take precedence. The most effective planning is done with flexibility, patience, and a willingness to reschedule activities when necessary.

Meeting emotional and spiritual needs is more difficult than planning to meet physical needs. You may have only sporadic contact with a homeless person and lack the time to develop a long-term relationship that would allow you to respond to his or her emotional and spiritual needs. You therefore need to plan to make the most of short interactions and to communicate caring, respect, compassion, and a belief in the homeless person's innate worth and dignity.

Strategies Directed at Changing the System

First, interventions include actions to address the systemwide issues that lead to homelessness as well as actions that directly serve the homeless person. Proactive interventions involve trying to prevent homelessness in the first place. Historically, nurses have championed the cause of the economically and socially disadvantaged through advocacy, education, and political involvement.

Advocacy means championing the cause of the homeless. Hodnicki (1990) believed that nurses, as homeless advocates, could write about health issues for community newspapers, consult with legislators on health concerns, and coordinate coalitions of public and private enterprises to support and assist the homeless. Financial contributions, volunteering in literacy programs, and voting for elected officials sympathetic to the homeless are also means of advocacy.

TABLE 34–1 Strengths-Focused Assessment Guidelines

Emphasize the Patient's Understanding of the Facts
Focus the assessment on the patient's view of the situation, the meaning the patient assigns to the situation, and the patient's related feelings or emotions.

Example: With a newly homeless alcoholic, tailor questions to elicit the patient's understanding of alcohol use, its relation to homelessness, and how the person feels about it.

Believe the Patient
Assume the patient is trustworthy and is telling the truth.

Example: If the patient has an obvious impairment such as inebriation or psychosis, believe the patient's feeling content and reexplore the facts when symptoms are controlled.

Discover What the Patient Wants
Focus on what the patient wants and expects from the nurse and on what resolution the patient wants or expects in the current problem situation.

Example: If a homeless patient wants the nurse to obtain free medications and sees them as a solution to depression, then the nurse can plan interventions around the patient's motivation.

Move the Assessment Toward Personal and Environmental Strengths
Steer the assessment toward identifying possibilities and existing strengths rather than obstacles.

Example: A homeless patient who will accept antipsychotic medication from only one nurse can be viewed as capable of forming some trust and rapport rather than as noncompliant and uncooperative.

Do Multidimensional Assessment of Strengths
Identify the patient's interpersonal skills, emotional strengths, ability to think clearly, and motivation. Uncover any external supports the patient may have, such as family, friends, religious affiliations, or community groups.

Example: A homeless mother without a supportive family may have perseverance, intelligence, and tentative links with a church support group.

Use the Assessment to Discover the Patient's Uniqueness
Center the assessment around the patient's unique self and response to the problem. Norms are useful only in confirming that the patient is an individual.

Example: If most patients are distressed by homelessness and your patient claims not to be, accept your patient's novel reaction and use that for information.

Use Language the Patient Understands
Assessments should be done in clear, self-explanatory English (or whatever language the patient best understands). The assessment must be accessible and useful for both patient and nurse.

Example: Write down patient statements verbatim and avoid translating them into nursing jargon.

Make Assessment a Mutual Activity Between Patient and Nurse
Ensure that the assessment is open and shared between patient and nurse. Allow the patient to "own" the assessment by stressing the importance of understanding his or her wants and needs.

Example: Pace the assessment to allow time for the patient to ask questions, clarify feelings, and stress important points.

Reach a Mutual Agreement on the Assessment
The nurse should do the assessment in open association with the patient.

Example: Write down information and share it with the patient to check accuracy and confirm goals. The patient can be given a copy of the assessment to keep.

Avoid Blame and Blaming
Blaming the patient for the situation is disrespectful, leads nowhere, and supports a deficit-centered style of assessment. Nurses must refrain from judging and should maintain open minds about the host of possible causes in any situation.

Example: A homeless alcoholic may not view chemical dependence as detrimental. The nurse uses this as information rather blaming the patient for being homeless.

Avoid Cause-and-Effect Thinking
Avoid cause-and-effect thinking, which leads to blaming. Don't forget that each problem is multilayered and consists of a complex set of actions and dynamics.

Example: A homeless crack addict who has lost a job may have lost it because of cutbacks rather than because of addiction.

Assess, Don't Diagnose
Nursing diagnosis is understood as a way of labeling a deficit or dysfunction. Maintain the focus on mutual exploration of the patient's coping skills, relationship patterns, and style of negotiating the world.

Example: Nonsensical or difficult-to-understand answers given by the patient will still provide information without taking away his or her right to share a personal story in a dignified manner.

Nursing modification based on Cowger, C. D. (1994). Assessing client strengths. Clinical assessment for client empowerment. *Social Work, 39*(3), 262–268. Copyright 1994, National Association of Social Workers, Inc., Social Work.

SNAPSHOT

Nursing Interventions Specific to Poverty and Homelessness

What do you need to do to develop a relationship with a patient who is poor and homeless?

- Build trust. This is an arduous task with the homeless, which is also constrained by time limits.
- A long-term relationship is most effective to build the patient's confidence. The homeless are often accustomed to being overlooked, ignored, or treated in an overly familiar or in disrespectful ways.
- Address the adult patient as "Mr.," "Mrs.," or "Miss" until invited to do otherwise.
- Remember to use the person's name.
- Be careful to assess the patient's educational level and communicate information in terms that he or she understands. Beware of stereotypes—homeless people can have PhDs or virtually no education at all.
- Be consistent.
- Avoid making promises that are impossible to deliver.
- Find concrete ways to help, which is very effective in building interpersonal bridges.

What do you need to assess regarding the patient's health status?

- General medical status
- Nutritional status
- Ability to obtain, store, and take medications
- Psychiatric status
- Access to safety, that is, a shelter
- Use of drugs and alcohol
- Spiritual health

What do you need to teach the patient?

- Medication issues; reason for taking; side effects and how to deal with them; untoward-effects; warnings; importance of adhering to medication schedule

- How to store medication and keep it safe
- Disease process; causes of depression; course of disease; and treatments
- Nutrition issues; review community resources (e.g., soup kitchens' availability, schedule, any eligibility requirements)
- Emergency measures—where to go for emergency medical or social services supports
- Importance of social support and strategies to obtain it
- Maintaining safety—ways to minimize vulnerability on the street
- Importance of emotional support and the value of interpersonal connections
- Importance of spiritual behaviors, such as prayer

What skills do you want the patient to demonstrate?

- Ability to access available community resources and supports for shelter, medical care, and food
- Ability to enter into a no-harm contract and remain safe
- Ability to follow medication and treatment plan
- Ability to use thought-stopping techniques and other cognitive strategies to deal with distorted thinking patterns
- Ability to perform personal care
- Ability to identify and express feelings
- Coping skills
- Relaxation techniques

What other health care professionals might need to be a part of this plan of care?

- Physician (i.e., psychiatrist and/or primary care physician) who is usually in charge of the overall treatment plan, including medication management
- Social worker to assist with access to community supports; insurance issues; access to entitlements; connection with community-based treatments

---

Second, education, both of self and others, is an important strategy for change. Nurses need to learn about the problems of the homeless in their cities or towns. Where do they live? What are the problems? Where do their children go to school? What resources are available?

Nurses also need to share their knowledge about the homeless with professional associates, family, friends, and other patients. Nurses have the power to dispel many of the myths surrounding homelessness. Inaccurate information about the homeless promotes distance

and blocks the development of cooperative efforts between the homeless and the domiciled to address problems.

Third, political involvement is a critical strategy. Voting is an essential way to influence the political process, but nurses also need to communicate opinions and questions to legislators. Letters to legislators influence votes. Nurses need to find constructive ways to protest political decisions with which they feel dissatisfied.

Protesting homelessness is also important. People

living on the streets is a national tragedy. Political involvement also may mean helping the homeless to register as voters or simply objecting to citizens being victimized. Remember that the poor feel powerless and unimportant. You need to speak for underprivileged adults and children.

Interventions With Homeless People

Direct interventions with the homeless are the basis of nurse-patient relationships in this population. Learn about the multidimensional needs of the homeless and be prepared to individualize care. See the snapshot of nursing interventions that summarizes strategies for relationship building, health status assessment, and teaching self-care information and self-care skills.

Strategies for Nurse Self-Care

An axiom in psychiatry states that the therapist can take the patient only as far as the therapist has gone. An appropriate variation of this axiom for working with the homeless might be, "Nurses can care for the homeless only as well as they care for themselves." Being with the homeless is emotionally draining and often painful. You therefore must care for yourself physically, emotionally, and spiritually if you wish to continue caring for others. A support group of other nurses and professionals working with the homeless can be an important source of substance and perspective. Interventions to enhance your own self-care are also essential when working with the homeless population.

Recognizing one's own limits is very important. Homelessness is tragic, and the tragedy is intensified when patients stop being a faceless group and become personally familiar. Practice within appropriate personal and professional boundaries to avoid being overwhelmed and frustrated.

Another strategy for self-care is maintaining the balance between work and rest and recreation. To work with the homeless, you must feel refreshed. Recreational activities and sufficient time to relax help you maintain an even outlook.

Evaluating Interventions

Recognize that working with the homeless presents tremendous challenges, so that evaluation of care requires realistic expectations. Some homeless people are well motivated to change and eagerly accept any suggestion or gesture of help. Others are noncompliant, antisocial, entrenched, actively substance abusing, or engaged in acting-out behaviors. The measurement of progress may not be in achieving objective outcomes but in making infinitesimal steps in relationship building.

Patient noncompliance may be a frequent outcome of well-planned interventions. Noncompliance may be a temporary setback or a long-established stance, but you should avoid personalizing the patient's failure to follow through. Focusing the evaluation on what the patient has achieved rather than on how the patient has failed is a helpful way to frame the final step of the nursing process. A patient who takes medication once a day instead of twice a day is still halfway there.

What do you think? The tragedy of homelessness could be overwhelming. What can you do as an individual nurse to effect change?

► *Check Your Reading*
15. How does relationship building enhance work with the poor or homeless patient?
16. What is the value of consistency with the poor or homeless patient?
17. How does the nurse care for herself or himself while working with the poor and homeless?

NURSING PROCESS APPLICATION

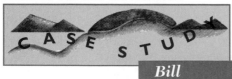

Bill

While working as a case manager in the emergency department, you are introduced to Bill, a 54-year-old man who has lived on the streets for the past 5 years. Before that, he lived with his mother, who is now dead. He is in the emergency department because he was beaten by a group of gang members. His affect is restricted, and you notice that he does not seem to trust you. When you ask Bill if he has any friends, he tells you that he does not and that he prefers to be alone. He does admit to having an older sister, Ann, but tells you he only talks to her at Christmas and is not interested in having a relationship with her. On further interviewing, you find that he has never had an intimate relationship and receives little pleasure from any hobbies or interests. He tells you that he did like working on the computer when he was living with his mother but says "I will never be able to take care of myself or have anything."

ASSESSMENT	Assessment data are as follows: • Homeless adult male • Multiple bruises and lacerations • Verbalizations of inability to exert any influence in current life situation • Restricted affect • Mistrust of health professionals • Receives little pleasure from social interaction • Enjoys solitary activities
DIAGNOSIS	**DSM-IV Diagnosis:** Schizoid Personality Disorder **Nursing Diagnosis:** Powerlessness related to lack of support system since mother's death evidenced by reality of current living situation (homeless), verbalizations of despair and apathy.

OUTCOME IDENTIFICATION, PLANNING, AND IMPLEMENTATION

> **Expected Outcome 1:** By discharge the patient will be able to be an active participant in effectively managing his life.

Short-Term Goals	Nursing Interventions	Rationales
By _____ the patient will participate in a decision regarding his care.	1. Encourage the patient to express needs and wants about care while in the hospital. 2. Allow the patient to establish self-care routines. 3. Provide positive feedback for decisions that are made by the patient.	1–2. Providing the patient with simple choices will increase his feelings of self-control. 3. Unrealistic goals set by the patient could lead to failure and increase feelings of powerlessness.

> **Expected Outcome 2:** By _____ patient will verbalize a desire to exert some control over his life.

Short-Term Goals	Nursing Interventions	Rationales
By _____ the patient will request help making decisions regarding his discharge plans.	1. Take time to establish a trusting relationship with the patient. 2. Encourage the patient to consider some type of group home as a transition to living alone. 3. Remain a patient advocate throughout this process. 4. Tell the patient that you believe he can have a quality life and that you believe in him.	1. The patient has a long history of not trusting. 2. Attempting independent living prior to job training and necessary therapy may lead to failure. 3–4. Nurses often take the place of family and friends as the sole support system for the patient.

> **Expected Outcome 3:** By _____ the patient will verbalize statements of hope for the future.

Short-Term Goals	Nursing Interventions	Rationales
By _____ the patient will verbalize hope and meaning in his existence.	1. Encourage the patient to express negative feelings of hopelessness, despondency, and alienation. 2. Help the patient to identify some positive aspects of his life, such as a sister who is living in the same locale and his computer skills.	1. This allows the patient an opportunity to ventilate feelings that have been pent up for a long time. 2–3. Feeling powerlessness does not promote an honest appraisal of one's situation.

3.   Help the patient identify behaviors that promote hopelessness and power-lessness, such as isolation.

4.   Encourage the patient to discuss how spiritual beliefs have affected him.

5.   Offer to provide some spiritually based readings for the patient.

4–5.   It is not unusual for homeless persons to feel abandoned by God. Finding a relationship with the God of their understanding often restores hope.

EVALUATION

Formative Evaluation: Bill was able to participate in limited decision-making regarding his self-care and did ask for help from the staff members in regard to living arrangements after discharge. He did acknowledge that his world fell apart after his mother died, and he acknowledged the tremendous impact of her death. He initiated a phone call to his sister and stated that he looked forward to having a relationship with her.

Summative Evaluation: Bill partially met the expected outcomes. The case manager felt that Bill would need more support before he could effectively manage his life. Bill did begin to verbalize statements of hope for the future, however. He stated, "I am looking forward to learning more about computers and to getting a job so I can support myself." He stated that he was never really abandoned by God and expressed a desire to attend a church service.

Conclusions

The journey that takes people to poverty and homeless-ness is complex and painful. Nurses have an important role to play in working with the poor and homeless as clinicians, advocates, educators, and fellow human beings. The approach taken by the individual nurse must have personal meaning. This story provides one example:

It was a chilly, overcast day when the horseman spied the little sparrow lying on its back in the middle of the road. Reining in his mount, he looked down and inquired of the fragile creature, "Why are you lying upside down like that?" "I heard the heavens are going to fall today," replied the bird. The horseman laughed, "And I suppose your spindly legs can hold up the heavens?"

"One does what one can," said the little sparrow.

Key Points to Remember

- Poverty and homelessness result from a complex set of personal and structural factors.
- Homelessness has existed throughout history.
- A standardized definition of homelessness hampers the study of the phenomenon.
- The face of homelessness changed from tramps, hoboes, and skid row dwellers to the new homeless in the 1970s, 1980s, and beyond.
- Deinstitutionalization is the civil rights–based action that released thousands of chronically mentally ill inpatients to community mental health centers unpre-pared to handle them.
- Admission diversion is a gatekeeping tactic that limits access to state mental hospitals by restricting admis-sion criteria.
- Eighty percent of homeless families are headed by single women.
- Homeless children suffer long-term detrimental ef-fects resulting from poor physical and mental health, inadequate nutrition, early trauma, and educational underachievement.
- Throwaway children are literally abandoned because of poverty and parental drug addiction.

- Homeless substance abusers suffer from a myriad of physical illnesses that impede efforts to escape from homelessness.
- Immigrants and illegal aliens are vulnerable to homelessness because of complicated bureaucratic structures.
- Minorities are overrepresented in the homeless population.
- Homelessness primarily is still an urban problem but has appeared in rural areas because of the rural economic crunch.
- Unemployment results as a shift from a goods-based to a service-based economy, which requires better-educated workers and eliminates less-skilled positions.
- Gentrification is the destruction of low-cost properties to make room for higher-rent housing units.
- Dysfunctional family dynamics exist in the families of origin of many homeless individuals.
- Healthy families can be overwhelmed by the needs of a chronically mentally ill, unemployed, or substance-abusing member and may be unable to provide shelter and support.

- Social disaffiliation is the profound estrangement of an individual from a known social support network.
- Learned helplessness is a phenomenon in which individuals feel powerless in their own lives and become passive and indifferent as a result.
- Preconceived ideas and attitudes toward the homeless block the building of meaningful relationships.
- Nursing assessment based on identifying and maxi-mizing the strengths of the patient is an important initial intervention.
- Planning care for the poor and homeless must be mutually determined and reality based.
- Nursing interventions for the poor and homeless include political, direct, and self-care strategies.
- Evaluation of nursing interventions should focus on patient success rather than on patient failure.

Learning Activities

1. List any attitudes or preconceived ideas you have about the poor and the homeless. Explain the experience or exposure you have had that led you to develop your attitudes or ideas.
2. Discuss your list with your classmates. How many attitudes or preconceived ideas did you identify? Did identifying your attitudes and ideas help you to view them differently? Did any other students provide feedback to challenge your attitude or preconceived idea?
3. If you were working with a poor or homeless patient, what would you consider important in establishing a relationship with the patient? What strategies would you employ to encourage compliance?

Critical Thinking Exercise

Jane Smith, RN, is a nurse at a busy clinic in the suburbs. One day a mother brings in her five children to see the doctor. Jane notes that the family is dressed in multiple layers of older clothing, and that the mother doesn't have current immunization records on three of the children. Although the mother seems genuinely caring with the children, one of Jane's colleagues notes during the physical examination that the children are unbathed and two of them have body lice. Jane notices the oldest child taking Band-Aids from an examination room drawer, which he explains are for his mother's blistered feet.

1. What assumptions would you make about this family?
2. How would you explain your assumptions to Jane?

3. How would you approach this family based on your assumptions?

The doctor takes Jane aside and asks her to call Child Protective Services. He explains to Jane that poor people don't live in the suburbs, so he is concerned that the mother is neglecting her children.

4. What information can Jane provide to the doctor to enhance his knowledge about poverty and homelessness?
5. How could Jane find resources to help this family? How would she go about building a relationship with the mother? What approaches could she use to work with the children?

Additional Resources

The Homeless Handbook
http://www.infoxchange.net.au/hhb

Homeless Home Page
http://csf.colorado.edu/homeless/index.html

Homes for the Homeless
http://198.68.10.253/hfh/opendoor.html

National Coalition for the Homeless
http://nch.ari.net/

References

Bachrach, L. (1992). What we know about homelessness among mentally ill persons: An analytical review and commentary. *Hospital and Community Psychiatry, 43,* 453–464.

Baier, M., Murray, R., North C., Lato, M., & Eskew, C. (1996). Comparison of completers and noncompleters in a transitional residential program for homeless mentally ill. *Issues in Mental Health Nursing, 17,* 337–352.

Blau, J. (1992). *The visible poor: Homelessness in the United States.* New York: Oxford University Press.

Burt, M. (1992). *Over the edge.* New York: Russell Sage.

Carter, K. F., Green, R. D., Green, L., & Dufour, L. T. (1994). Health needs of homeless patients accessing nursing care at a free clinic. *Journal of Community Health Nursing, 11*(3), 134-147.

Cowger, C. D. (1994). Assessing patient strengths: Clinical assessment for patient empowerment. *Social Work, 34,* 262-267.

Damrosch, S., & Strasser, J. A. (1988). The homeless elderly in America. *Journal of Gerontological Nursing, 14*(10), 26-29.

Dennis, D. L., Buckner, J. C., Lipton, F. R., & Levine, I. S. (1991). A decade of research and services for homeless mentally ill persons: Where do we stand? *American Psychologist, 46,* 1129-1138.

Federal Task Force on Homelessness and Severe Mental Illness. (1992). Outcasts on main street. Washington, DC: Author.

Fischer, P. J., & Breakey, W. R. (1990). The epidemiology of alcohol, drug, and mental disorders among homeless persons. *American Psychologist, 46,* 1115-1128.

Goetchens, J. (1986). The cries of the poor are the voice of God. Washington, DC: Columbia Road Health Services.

Goodman, L., Saxe, L., & Harvey, M. (1991). Homelessness as psychological trauma: Broadening perspectives. *American Psychologist, 46,* 1219-1225.

Herth, K. (1996). Hope from the perspective of homeless families. *Journal of Advanced Nursing, 24,* 743-753.

Hodnicki, D. R. (1990). Homelessness: Health-care implications. *Journal of Community Health Nursing, 7*(2), 59-67.

Interagency Council on the Homeless. (1990). *The 1990 annual report of the Interagency Council on the Homeless.* Washington, DC: Author.

Interagency Council on the Homeless. (1994). *Priority: Home! The federal plan to break the cycle of homelessness.* Washington, DC: Author.

Jackson, M. P., & McSwane, D. Z. (1992). Homelessness as a determinant of health. *Public Health Nursing, 9,* 185-192.

Liebow, E. (1993). *Tell them who I am: The lives of homeless women.* New York: Free Press.

Lindblom, E. (1991). *Toward a comprehensive homelessness prevention strategy.* Fannie Mae Annual Housing Conference, Washington, DC.

Lynch, J.W., Kaplan, G.A., & Salonen, J.T. (1997). Why do poor people behave poorly? Variation in adult health behaviors and psychosocial characteristics by stages of the socioeconomic lifecourse. *Social Science and Medicine, 44,* 809-819.

Marin, P. (1991, July 8). Why are the homeless mainly single men? *The Nation,* 46-50.

Milburn, N., & D'Ercole, A. (1991). Homeless women: Moving toward a comprehensive model. *American Psychologist, 46,* 1161-1169.

National Coalition for the Homeless. (1997). *Homelessness in America: Unabated and increasing.* Washington, DC: Author.

Rafferty, Y., & Shinn, M. (1991). The impact of homelessness on children. *American Psychologist, 46,* 1170-1179.

Reilly, F. (1993). Experience of family among homeless individuals. *Issues in Mental Health Nursing, 14,* 309-321.

Rossi, P. (1990). The old homeless and the new homeless in historical perspective. *American Psychologist, 45,* 945-959.

Schubert, H. J. P. (1935). *Twenty thousand transients: A year's sample of those who apply for aid in a northern city.* Buffalo, NY: Emergency Relief Bureau.

Seligman, M. E. P. (1975). *Helplessness: On depression, development, and death.* San Francisco: Freeman.

Smith, R. (1987). *Unemployment and health: A disaster and challenge.* Oxford: Oxford University Press.

U.S. Bureau of the Census. (1997). *Statistical abstract of the United States* (117th ed., pp. 474-479). Washington, DC: U.S. Government Printing Office.

Waitzman, N. J., & Smith, K. R. (1998). Phantom of the area: Poverty-area residence and mortality in the United States. *American Journal of Public Health, 88,* 973-976.

Wallsten, S. M. (1992). Geriatric mental health: A portrait of homelessness. *Journal of Psychosocial Nursing, 30*(9), 20-24.

Warr, P. (1987). Work, employment, and mental health. New York: Oxford University Press.

Warren, B. J., Menke, E. M., Clement, J., & Wagner, J. (1992). The mental health of African-American and Caucasian-American women who are homeless. *Journal of Psychosocial Nursing, 30*(11), 27-30.

Ziesemer, C., Marcoux, L., & Marwell, B. E. (1994). Homeless children: Are they different from other low income children. *Social Work, 34,* 658-668.

Suggested Readings

Berck, J. (1992). *No place to be: Voices of homeless children.* Boston: Houghton Mifflin.

Herth, K. (1996). Hope from the perspective of homeless families. *Journal of Advanced Nursing, 24,* 743-753.

Liebow, E. (1993). *Tell them who I am. The lives of homeless women.* New York: Free Press.

Morse, G. A., Calsyn, R. J., Miller J., Rosenberg, P., West L., & Gilliland, J. (1996). Outreach to homeless mentally ill people: Conceptual and clinical considerations. *Community Mental Health Journal, 32,* 261-273.

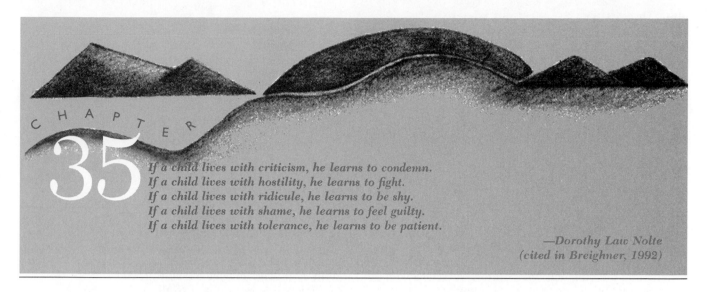

35

If a child lives with criticism, he learns to condemn.
If a child lives with hostility, he learns to fight.
If a child lives with ridicule, he learns to be shy.
If a child lives with shame, he learns to feel guilty.
If a child lives with tolerance, he learns to be patient.

—Dorothy Law Nolte
(cited in Breighner, 1992)

Violence

Learning Objectives

After studying this chapter, you should be able to:

1. Appreciate the scope of violence in American society.
2. Define terms such as violence, abuse, neglect, and sexual abuse.
3. Discuss some of the key characteristics of family violence and abuse.
4. Discuss the hostage response, which is characteristic of victims of any interpersonal violence.
5. Describe the various types of family victimization, including sibling violence and parents as victims.
6. Discuss at least three causes of family violence.
7. Describe the perpetrator of abuse.
8. Describe the victim of abuse.
9. Describe the cycle of abuse.
10. Describe the long-term effects of childhood psychological and emotional abuse.
11. Identify predictors of violence in psychiatric and other patients.
12. Discuss predisposing characteristics of violent persons.
13. Discuss the overall direct and indirect effects of violence in society on the person.
14. Describe nursing's role in violence prevention from a primary, secondary, and tertiary perspective.
15. Describe the long-term effects of child abuse.
16. Apply the nursing process to a case study in which spousal abuse is present.
17. Apply the nursing process to a case study in which child abuse is present.
18. Apply the nursing process to a case study in which elder abuse is present.
19. Apply the nursing process to a case study in which a psychiatric patient becomes violent.

Key Terminology

Abuse	Elder abuse	Instrumental violence	Sexual abuse
Battered-child syndrome	Emotional abuse	Mutual combat model	Spousal abuse
Battering syndrome	Enabler	Neglect	Violence
Child abuse	Expressive violence	Restraints	Wife-battering model
Cycle of abuse	Hostage response	Seclusion	

Almost daily, in newspapers, on television, and on radio, we are confronted with stories of random violence, workplace violence, stranger violence. We are horrified and frightened. We fear that we will be touched by the violence. We comfort ourselves with the thought that violence occurs "somewhere out there," somewhere we are not. Read Joyce's story and think about how many other women live with violence or the threat of violence as an everyday occurrence.

 **Joyce's Story**

I did not, and even today, do not think of my husband, Lou, as a violent man. He wouldn't always be violent when he was upset. I guess that's what unsettled me the most. I could never exactly figure what it was that would set him off. He hit me for the first time shortly after we were married. He couldn't find his cufflinks. Since I unpacked everything, he tore into me. He hit me with the back of his hand and sent me across the room. He was full of apologies the next day, and more than a year went by before he hit me again. I don't really remember what set him off that time. But soon the time between the hitting was down to months, then weeks. I did everything I could think to please him. But I just couldn't think of everything. I remember once when I yelled at him, he came back at me and said, "I guess things are getting too easy around here." Then he slapped and punched me. I started to go a little crazy. I just couldn't think of everything. All the time he was around I felt like I was walking on a tightrope. Just one little slip and I knew I might get it. When he did hit me, I was relieved. At least I didn't have to be so tense anymore. ■

From *Intimate violence: The definitive study of the causes and consequences of abuse in the American family.* Published by Simon & Schuster. Copyright 1988 by Richard J. Gelles and Murray A. Straus.

FAMILY VIOLENCE, ABUSE, AND THE JOURNEY

Joyce's denial of her husband's violence kept her in a dangerous situation. Denial prevents people as well as society from facing up to the truth and the need for change. Increasingly, our denial is shattered by incidents of violence that take place in schools and even in hospital settings. Across the United States, emergency departments are being equipped with metal detectors to search visitors and patients for weapons. Nurses in settings other than psychiatry are being trained to deal with aggressive behavior (Selby, 1992).

Violence is not limited to the random and senseless murders that occur on the streets of the United States. Violence affects families—women, children, and elders. Atrocities are committed against friends and neighbors, by someone in the family, by one or more of the persons supposed to love, protect, and cherish them. These acts of betrayal, violence, and sometimes murder usually take place in the home, the one place we should be assured a safe haven from the stresses of the world. The violence that occurs in our homes is not a private matter to be dealt with and handled by those most intimately involved. Rather, violence is a public matter. We are all affected. When we turn away from the brokenness, pain, and suffering of others; when we allow ourselves to be immune to the screams, bruises, and cuts of a child; when we ignore the blackened eyes and the bruised belly of a pregnant woman; when we deny that elders are abused by their children—then we give tacit approval to acts of violence that are fundamentally wrong.

As Gelles and Straus (1988) stated in their comprehensive research into intimate violence, "People are not for hitting" (p. ii). The victims of abuse do not need criticism or pity. What they need is the support and intervention of a society both shocked and appalled at what is transpiring behind closed doors. Our outrage must be operationalized into strategies that change attitudes encouraging violence, that offer refuge and places of healing for victims, and that offer both consequences for violent acts and treatment for abusers.

One of the difficulties in estimating the extent of family violence is in defining the term *violence*. For example, is parental spanking of a child an act of child abuse or discipline? Can a husband who forces his wife to perform oral sex be found guilty of a crime, or is he just an insensitive, mean individual? Figure 35-1 illustrates that all acts of physical and sexual violence are issues of power and control.

Terms Describing Violence

Gelles and Straus (1988) as well as others who have written about family violence generally support a definition of **violence** that includes any acts (from a pinch or a slap to murder) carried out with the intention of causing physical pain or injury to another person.

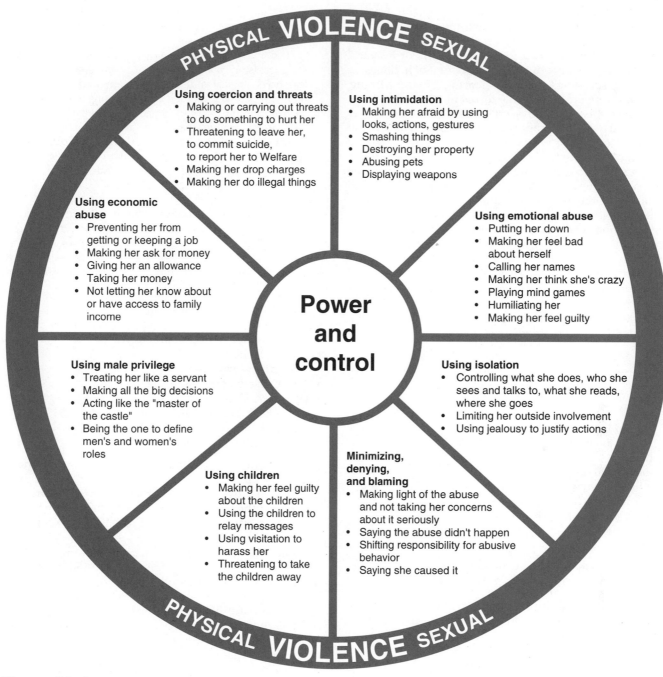

PHYSICAL VIOLENCE SEXUAL

Using coercion and threats
- Making or carrying out threats to do something to hurt her
- Threatening to leave her, to commit suicide, to report her to Welfare
- Making her drop charges
- Making her do illegal things

Using intimidation
- Making her afraid by using looks, actions, gestures
- Smashing things
- Destroying her property
- Abusing pets
- Displaying weapons

Using economic abuse
- Preventing her from getting or keeping a job
- Making her ask for money
- Giving her an allowance
- Taking her money
- Not letting her know about or have access to family income

Using emotional abuse
- Putting her down
- Making her feel bad about herself
- Calling her names
- Making her think she's crazy
- Playing mind games
- Humiliating her
- Making her feel guilty

Power and control

Using male privilege
- Treating her like a servant
- Making all the big decisions
- Acting like the "master of the castle"
- Being the one to define men's and women's roles

Using isolation
- Controlling what she does, who she sees and talks to, what she reads, where she goes
- Limiting her outside involvement
- Using jealousy to justify actions

Using children
- Making her feel guilty about the children
- Using the children to relay messages
- Using visitation to harass her
- Threatening to take the children away

Minimizing, denying, and blaming
- Making light of the abuse and not taking her concerns about it seriously
- Saying the abuse didn't happen
- Shifting responsibility for abusive behavior
- Saying she caused it

PHYSICAL VIOLENCE SEXUAL

Figure 35–1
All acts of physical and sexual violence are issues of power and control. (Redrawn from the Domestic Abuse Intervention Project, 204 West Fourth Street, Duluth, MN 55806.)

Abuse is more difficult to define. The term has been politicized, and it is not clinical or scientific. Therefore, definition of abuse varies greatly across individuals. In 1974, however, the National Center on Child Abuse and Neglect (Child Abuse Prevention and Treatment Act, 1974) defined **child abuse** as follows:

The physical or mental injury, sexual abuse, negligent treatment, or maltreatment of a child under the age of 18 by a person who is responsible for the child's welfare under circumstances which indicate that the child's health or welfare is harmed or threatened thereby.

Gil (1975) broadened this formal definition by including

any acts of commission or omission by a parent or an individual, an institution, or by society as a whole which deprive a child of equal rights and liberty, and/or interfere with or constrain the child's ability to achieve his or her optimal developmental potential. (p. 345)

These definitions of abuse focus on children. We should not, however, be limited to children when we consider abuse. Clearly, adults can be victims of abuse as well.

The National Center on Child Abuse and Neglect introduced the concepts of mental injury, sexual abuse, and neglect as dimensions of abuse. Examining the specifics of abuse poses a formidable task. For instance, how do we define **emotional abuse?** Such things as belittling, scorning, ignoring, tearing down, harping, and criticizing are all possible forms of emotional abuse. Emotional abuse can be overt as well as subtle. Gelles and Straus (1988) reported that one woman, on repeated occasions, was subjected to her husband showing her gifts he had purchased for his girlfriend. The husband told his wife that he would return home after delivering the gifts. These behaviors continued while the family was on welfare.

Repeated attacks on a person's self-esteem can leave deep, lasting scars. Victims of physical abuse frequently say that the physical scars of family violence fade, but the pain from emotional wounds continues to fester beneath the surface forever. The signs of emotional abuse are not as easily recognized as the bruises, cuts, and scars from physical abuse. Instead, emotional abuse becomes apparent when we hear the stories of victims. Consider Tracy's comments in Case Example 35–1.

■ CASE EXAMPLE 35–1
■ Tracy's Story

He rarely says a kind word to me. He is always critical. The food is too cold or it's too hot. The kids are too noisy. The house is a mess. I am a mess. He says I spend too much money and then complains that I look like I got dressed in a used-clothing store. He says I am too fat or too skinny. No matter what I do he says it isn't any good. He tells me I am lucky he married me because no one else would have me. ■

From *Intimate violence: The definitive study of the causes and consequences of abuse in the american family.* Published by Simon & Schuster. Copyright 1988 by Richard J. Gelles and Murray A. Straus.

Emotional abuse in childhood may also extend into emotional abuse of the adult child by the hypercritical, unloving, frustrated, or conflicted parent, as shown by Art, a 30-year-old single man diagnosed with depression with paranoid ideation (Case Example 35–2).

■ CASE EXAMPLE 35–2
■ Art's Story

Recently released from a psychiatric inpatient unit, Art has returned home to live with his biological mother and stepfather. His healthy younger brother lives elsewhere in his own apartment. Art has been seriously and persistently mentally ill most of his life, with depression that began in early adolescence.

When the home health psychiatric nurse makes an initial assessment visit, Art's mother voices her rage toward the patient and states she doesn't want him living in her home. Art's brother stops by and starts to taunt the patient until he realizes a nurse, that is, an "outsider," is present, and the patient tells the nurse he lives in the cellar (which he does).

The initial psychiatric nursing assessment reveals a lifelong history of physical abuse, combined with relentless psychological and emotional abuse perpetuated by both the patient's mother and his younger brother, who have no insight into the impact their behaviors have on the patient or into their own psychopathology, that is, their need to mistreat, target, and abuse the patient. The stepfather, an attorney, acts as if Art does not exist, and they do not talk to each other. Art eats all of his meals alone in his room in the cellar. ■

The ramifications of childhood physical, sexual, emotional or psychological abuse are long-term and far reaching (Bryant & Range, 1995; Chabrol, Talmon, Peresson, & Alengrin, 1995; Dutton, van-Ginkel, & Starzomski, 1995; Botsis, Plutchik, Kotler, & Van Praag, 1995) and may include

- Diminished self-esteem
- Depression
- Problems with social competency
- Submissiveness
- Generally anxious trait
- Anger or rage control problems
- Hypersensitivity to criticism
- Social alienation or withdrawal
- Emotional numbing
- Shame and guilt-prone traits

In addition to the child who is the victim of abuse, the family processes and operational rules become distorted and dysfunctional for all family members. For example, other family members (including other children who may or may not be abused) become keepers of terrible family secrets.

Sometimes other family members ignore, deny, or repress the abuse in a facade of normality. Sometimes, as in Art's story, the abused child is further tormented by being made the butt of family jokes, as family members coalesce around blaming, punishing, and mocking the child victim, who has been singled out to occupy the victim role (for whatever reason). Such dysfunctional families are quite toxic, and if the victimized child survives to adulthood, he or she may distance themselves both emotionally and geographically from the abusers (Forward, 1989).

In some dysfunctional, toxic families, child abusers may never change, may never hear the message, may deny the abuse, may accuse the victim of being crazy or of lying, and so forth. In other words, they never change. Some toxic parents may continue the emotional abuse of the adult child until the adult child, to survive emotionally or psychologically, must sever the relationship (Forward, 1989).

When nurses assess increasingly frail or failing elderly patients with adult children who are physically or emotionally distanced, they must avoid making value judgments because they can seldom access or ever truly know all that occurred within someone else's family system, and some patients and their children take their family secrets to their graves. These realities are part of the complexities and the reason why it is often so difficult to identify and intervene in the often hidden phenomenon of intrafamilial abuse. However, from a psychiatric nursing perspective, you must also bear in mind that interlocking, interdependent psychopathology among family members can still be worked with, ameliorated or resolved, even after the death of an involved family member, through a variety of therapeutic interventions.

How do we define **neglect?** Generally, neglect represents acts of omission rather than a physical act of commission. Parents may fail to provide the basic necessities for their children or on a more passive level may be emotionally unavailable to their children, leaving them isolated in a harsh world. Acts of neglect include failing to seek and follow through with medical care for a sick child. In areas of neglect, the dilemma is whether the neglect is purposeful or comes from lack of adequate financial and material resources to care properly for children.

Finally, what about sexual abuse? Kempe, Silverman, Steele, Droegmueller, and Silver (1962) defined **sexual abuse** as

the involvement of dependent and developmentally immature children and adolescents in sexual activities that they do not fully comprehend, to which they are unable to give informed consent, or that violate social taboos of family roles. (p. 107)

This definition has not been without detractors. Some say the definition is so broad as to allow social scientists to define even excessive hugging as abuse. Others would like to see sexual abuse of children limited to only forced sexual intercourse. Finkelhor and Yllö (1985) suggested that sexual abuse refers to activities involving the genitals that are for the gratification of at least one person.

Until the 1970s, sexual abuse of children remained largely hidden. Two attitudes promoted secrecy. The first was the powerful taboo against adults having sex with children that exists not only in American society but also in other societies. The second attitude is that Americans are generally unwilling to discuss sexuality openly. By the late 1970s, however, an explosion of official reports of child sexual abuse caused a general concern for the welfare of children.

W*hat do you think?* Have you ever cared for a patient who was a victim of abuse of any kind? If so, what was your role in assisting that individual? Did you directly confront the abuse issue?

➤ *Check Your Reading*
1. Define violence.
2. Define sexual abuse.
3. Define neglect.
4. Discuss the long-term effects of childhood abuse.

Extent of Violence and Abuse

National statistics provide an incomplete picture of the incidence and extent of family violence and abuse. Data from the National Crime Survey conducted by the Department of Justice, in which 60,000 households throughout the United States were surveyed, usually reflect violence that victims are willing to label as criminal and report to authorities. In addition, the Federal Bureau of Investigation (FBI) compiles data about eight categories of crimes reported to the police. Included are data regarding homicide, rape, robbery, aggravated assault, burglary, larceny, motor-vehicle theft, and arson. Crimes that originate out of family violence, such as nonaggravated assault, are not reported to the FBI, and information about the relationship between the victim and the offender is collected only for homicide. Despite the limitations of the data, they do provide some insights regarding the extent of family violence. For instance, consider the following statistics:

1. About 20% of all murder victims in the United States are related to their assailants. In about one third of these situations, the victim is a woman killed by either her husband or boyfriend (Attorney General's Task Force on Family Violence, 1984).

2. Most crimes committed by relatives (57%) are committed by spouses or ex-spouses. In about 25% of situations in which the spouse or ex-spouse is the assailant, victims reported that they had been attacked at least three other times in the previous 6 months (Klaus & Rand, 1989).

3. Between 1.8 and 2.9 million women are battered yearly. In fact, battering is the single most common cause of injury to women, exceeding mugging, motor-vehicle accidents, and occupational injuries combined, as noted in the report *Battered Women and Criminal Justice* (1987) (cited in Landes, Foster, & Siegel, 1991).

4. The cost of absenteeism from work as a result of assaults on women results in an economic loss to the United States of millions of dollars every year, plus many more millions spent on medical bills (Berger, 1990).

5. Pregnancy offers no immunity against violence. Eight percent of all pregnant women are assaulted by their husbands or boyfriends during pregnancy. These assaults inflict both physical and psychological harm on the mother-to-be. Some also injure or kill the fetus (Koop, 1987-88).

6. More than 2 million reported cases of child abuse occur at the hands of parents, grandparents, guardians, or others. In addition, there may be another 1 million cases of child abuse that go unreported. Between 2000 and 5000 children die every year as a result of their injuries (Landes et al., 1991; Saltman, 1986).

7. Almost as many adolescents are mistreated as younger children. Approximately 42% of abused children are between the ages of 12 and 17 (Saltman, 1986).

8. Incest—the act of sexual intercourse between closely related family members—is the most common form of adolescent sexual abuse. Incest is estimated to

occur in about 14% of all families. The common perpetrators include fathers, stepfathers, uncles, and brothers. In some cases, a father sexually abuses all of his daughters throughout their preadolescent and adolescent years (Saltman, 1986).

9. **Elder abuse** is the abuse of parents and grandparents by children and grandchildren. It is estimated to claim between 500,000 and 1 million victims yearly. The House Select Committee on Aging estimates that only one in every six cases is reported (Saltman, 1986).

No data are available regarding the extent of emotional abuse. Survey results yielding data regarding incidence of physical abuse, however, indicate that physical and emotional abuse go hand in hand. Thus, we know that there are no fewer victims of emotional abuse than there are victims of physical abuse. The true incidence of emotional abuse probably far exceeds that of physical violence. Little research has been done on emotional abuse, perhaps because so many of us are guilty of an occasional or even frequent verbal barrage against a loved one that the behavior is too close or too common to allow for objective study. Gelles and Straus (1988) contended that emotional abuse is not a case of "there but for the grace of God go I"; rather, it is that we know the enemy, and it is ourselves.

CHARACTERISTICS OF THE JOURNEY MARKED BY FAMILY VIOLENCE AND ABUSE

The problems of family violence and abuse are not limited to a particular socioeconomic group. Violence occurs at all levels of society and in all parts of the United States. Even the "best" families produce victims, perpetrators, and **enablers** of violent behavior, but there are certain key characteristics of family violence.

Family violence is the only crime in which the victim always knows the identity of the offender. Moreover the perpetrators of family violence do not see their acts as crimes, nor do they see their victims as such. Family violence is usually accompanied by a certain amount of brainwashing. Abused children come to believe that they deserve the severe beatings they receive because they are bad and uncontrollable. Abused wives become convinced that they are failures in carrying out their responsibilities as wives and mothers. Sexually abused children are told that their perpetrator's actions are normal signs of affection. In truth, the victim assumes responsibility for the crime.

Responses of Victims

This assumption of responsibility, characteristic of a generalized **hostage response,** is common to victims of any form of interpersonal violence (Tilden & Shepherd, 1987). Victims tend to blame themselves for the abuse and develop a sense of being unworthy of help, a fear of not being believed, a skepticism regarding the motiva-

tions of others, and, in the case of chronic abuse, a persistent irrational belief that each attack will be the last. Abused wives typically say, "If only I had. . . ." Children might say, "I deserved that beating to keep me in line." Sexual abuse victims are likely to think, "I must have led him on." Each of the victims harbors the hope that the abuse will stop if they act differently.

The victim feels shame, guilt, and embarrassment. These feelings form a cloak of silence that prohibits the victim from seeking outside help. Victims find it difficult to believe that outsiders could possibly understand or identify with the humiliation that is part of their lives. This appraisal of society's response increases the feelings of hopelessness and isolation experienced by victims.

The spiritual distress is almost unfathomable as the victim becomes increasingly hopeless and despairing. Some victims, seeking help from their organized faith, have experienced more blame as they are told to be "better wives" and to "forgive and forget." It becomes difficult for victims to pray and to believe in a loving and powerful God when the reality of their lives is so out of control and frightening and when the clergy people they speak to imply the abuse is somehow their fault or only offer platitudes.

Because of fears of reprisal from their abuser, victims are hesitant to seek help from the criminal justice system. In addition, victims are immobilized by the belief that they are economically and emotionally dependent on the abuser. They fear that by reporting the violence the family will be torn apart.

It is common for victims to believe that violence and abuse are natural parts of family life. The long-term effects of violence and abuse are depression, suicidal ideation, low self-esteem, anxiety, and impaired relationships outside of the family (Perry & Daugherty, 1995). Family violence tends to be repeated and to grow worse over time. Therefore, early intervention is needed to prevent abuse from occurring and to deal with it once it has occurred.

What do you think? What kind of early intervention is needed to prevent abuse from occurring?

▶ *Check Your Reading*

5. What are the characteristics of the hostage response?
6. What are the spiritual issues of abuse?
7. How does brainwashing fit in with abuse?
8. What are the usual feelings experienced by victims of abuse?
9. Why don't victims of abuse seek help from the criminal justice system?

Forms of Victimization

A common assumption is that women and children are the only victims of family violence or that if they are not the only victims, they are at least the most common victims. Neither of these views is correct. Hidden victims make up a significant part of the problem of family violence. The most common form of family violence is between siblings. The most overlooked may be the violence directed at parents by adolescent children. These forms of victimization have received far less attention as social problems.

Sibling Violence and Abuse

Sibling violence is not new. The Bible recounts the story of Cain and Abel, a story of intense sibling rivalry that eventually led to the death of Abel at his brother's hands. Sibling conflict is such a common aspect of family relations that many people accept it as the norm. American families have a set of expectations that maintain that "boys will be boys" and "kids will fight." These attitudes may actually encourage sibling conflict.

Most cases of sibling conflict involve slaps, pushes, kicks, bites, and punches. Significant numbers of siblings, however, face brothers or sisters who pose a more lethal threat because they have guns or knives. Emotional abuse may exist, with or without physical abuse.

Parents as Victims

Another form of abuse is physical violence perpetrated by children, usually adolescents, against their parents. This form of violence seldom comes to public attention unless the child kills or maims the parent. Parent victims find little support in the community and virtually no services to help them. Parents fear that if they reveal how they are victimized at home, they will be publicly victimized as well by being blamed for their child's behavior. They feel ashamed, guilty, and embarrassed and, as a result, suffer from anxiety and depression. Terrified of their violent children and afraid that they will be publicly blamed for their children's behavior, they remain prisoners at home. Parents create a wall of denial that serves to give license to the child's violence and to perpetrate this form of hidden intimate violence.

Elders as Victims

"Honor thy father and thy mother," one of the Ten Commandments, has taken on greater significance with today's increasing life span (Janz, 1990). Yet five types of elder abuse exist (Landes et al., 1991, p. 41):

1. *Physical:* "I know I push her sometimes, but she is always there," a daughter explaining the repeated bruising of her mother.

2. *Financial:* "My grandsons only come to see me at the beginning of the month. They take my social security check to the corner store and cash it for me. Sometimes they don't come right back, and when they do, most of the money is gone. So I have to make do for the rest of the month."

3. *Psychological:* "My son gets so frustrated with me,

I guess I move too slow for him, and I am a burden. . . . but he yells at me, tells me he wishes that I would die. . . . I know he doesn't mean it."

4. *Sexual:* "It started when my grandson had to help me in the bathroom. He started to touch me. . . . I didn't like it, but I was too embarrassed to say anything."

5. *Self-abuse or self-neglect:* "She was brought to the hospital by paramedics. She was confused, dehydrated, and had a maggot-infested leg and weighed about 60 lb. She was bruised all over her body and had a gash on her face. 'I don't want to get anyone in trouble,' she said. Efforts to find out who had done these things to her were futile. Two weeks after being brought to the hospital, she died, and her daughter could not be located."

What do you think? What factors promote silence on the part of the elderly person who is abused by a family member?

➤ *Check Your Reading*
10. What is sibling abuse?
11. What is the wall of denial that maintains the secrecy of a parent as a victim?
12. Give an example of psychological abuse directed against an elder.
13. Why don't parents who are victims get help from the community?

CAUSES OF FAMILY VIOLENCE AND ABUSE

In their seminal work on family violence, Gelles and Straus (1988) contended that people who hit family members do so because they can get away with it. This proposition is based on three beliefs. The first is that there are few, if any, costs for being violent at home. The second belief is that American society lacks effective social controls to deal with domestic violence. The third belief is that certain social and family structures reduce social controls and, in doing so, reduce the costs and increase the rewards of being violent.

Few Costs of Family Violence

Most people who abuse family members are able to control their temper when they are confronted with situations that make them angry outside the home. An abusive husband is usually not abusive to his secretary. An abusive father would not dream of hitting someone else's child who happened to annoy him. Why? These people share the unconscious knowledge that potential costs and punishments await them if they engage in violent behavior. This recognition is enough to restrain most people.

Violence that occurs within the home results in few costs for the perpetrator. The abusive husband may be encouraged by police to leave the home situation "just to cool down." The abusive father may be reported to an overwhelmed social service department that makes a cursory investigation and dismisses the charge as unfounded.

Gelles and Straus (1988) contended that the social exchange theory provides an explanation for the proposition that people who hit family members do so because they can. The social exchange theory asserts that human interaction is regulated by the pursuit of rewards and the avoidance of punishments and costs. When one individual provides services to another, the other is obliged to render a reward in some way. As long as the exchange is reciprocal, the relationship continues. Without reciprocity, the interaction is broken off because the first person realizes all the costs and no benefits.

Family dynamics add an important twist to the normal assumptions of social exchange theory. With no reciprocity in the exchange of services and rewards, it is not so easy to break off interaction. Divorce is always an option but never an easy one. Divorce carries with it decisions regarding children, distribution of property, living space, and financial resources. Yet even with the difficulties in seeking a divorce, it is possible to become an ex-spouse; it is never possible to become an ex-parent. Children are seldom able to respond equitably with rewards for what parents provide. Some parents, unable to break off the relationship with their children, respond to being asked to give more with anger, frustration, and resentment. Conflict is a common response; violence may be involved. Social exchange theory suggests that people engage in violence against family members only when the costs of violence do not outweigh the rewards. Although our society has standard costs for violence, these costs are rarely paid by those who are violent in the home.

Absence of Effective Social Controls

A number of factors contribute to the lack of consequences for the perpetrators of domestic violence. Police tend to respond slowly to calls about violence in the home. This tendency can be explained by three factors. First, domestic violence poses a threat to the police officer. Every year, significant numbers of officers are killed responding to domestic disturbances. Second, police officers are not traditionally rewarded for how well they handle domestic violence. Instead, rewards are given for good police work involving robberies and drug trafficking. Consequently, responding to domestic calls receives a low priority among law enforcement officers. Third, the police officer may be an abusing spouse and not inclined personally to be responsive to the needs of the victims.

Even when the police are called to a home, arrests are not common. Child abuse usually is handled as a child welfare matter and not as a criminal justice matter. In unusual cases when arrests are made, chances are that no additional costs will be paid by the abuser. The criminal justice system does not want to bear responsibility for breaking up families, despite the reality that the infrastructure of the family has already been clearly

broken and only a facade of togetherness exists (if even that facade exists). Wives who press charges are frequently counseled to drop them. The argument presented to wives places them in a no-win situation. A representative of the court system may argue, "If we put him in jail, he'll lose his job, and you will have to go on welfare. Why don't you go home and "kiss and make up?" This same line of reasoning is used when fathers batter their children. When the mother is the perpetrator of the abuse, judges are even more hesitant about placing them behind bars for fear of further damaging the children. Clearly the criminal justice system holds little threat for the person who is violent against loved ones. The lack of real cost may even encourage further violence.

Some women seek restraining orders in the hope of keeping their husbands away. All too frequently, the restraining order serves to fuel the anger and violence that the wife is trying desperately to avoid (Draucker, 1997). Few other costs exist. Presumably, public knowledge of a person's violence at home could lead to a loss of social or economic status. In reality, however, such a loss seldom occurs.

Family and Social Structures That Support Violence

The social and family structures that are most important in reducing the cost of family violence include (1) social attitudes about family violence; (2) the high value placed on the right to privacy within the home; and (3) the structural inequality that exists within the modern family.

Social Attitudes

Violence may be woven into the American character. Certainly, we do not have to delve far or deep into our history to find many examples of violence. Reading a newspaper or listening to the evening news provides us with daily reminders of the violent nature of our society.

We legitimize violence. This legitimization can be seen in the public outcries for retribution in statements such as "blow them to smithereens" following public awareness of crimes committed abroad against Americans and perceived abuses of American interests. Violence is common in cartoons, television shows, movies, and even in children's fairy tales and nursery rhymes.

During the 1960s, the U.S. Commission on the Causes and Prevention of Violence conducted a survey focusing on attitudes about public as well as private, or family, violence. This survey revealed the following (Stark & McEvoy, 1970):

- 25% of men and 17% of women stated that there were some circumstances in which spouse-to-spouse violence was warranted and appropriate.
- 86% of those surveyed stated that "strong discipline" was necessary in the rearing of children.

• 70% of the respondents indicated that it was necessary for young boys to engage in fistfights as part of growing into manhood.

Fifteen years after the U.S. Commission on the Causes and Prevention of Violence survey was conducted, Gelles and Straus (1988) asked a national sample of more than 2000 subjects two questions that focused on attitudes about violence between family members. The responses revealed that 25% of wives and 33% of husbands believed that slapping between spouses was sometimes necessary, normal, and good. More than 70% of the respondents believed that slapping a 12-year-old child was necessary, normal, or good.

Parent-to-child violence is so common that most Americans consider physical discipline an essential part of parenting. In the Gelles and Straus national survey, the *absence* of physical punishment, not the hitting of children, was considered deviant.

Society closes its eyes and ears to family violence even when the violence escalates beyond what society tolerates as normal within families. Neighbors might report violence to the police but seldom become personally involved both because of fear for their own safety and because violence is a "family matter." Society tends to deny that many of the violent acts that occur between family members are "really violent." Instead the true nature of these acts is hidden behind euphemisms such as "domestic disturbance" or "family matter." Box 35-1 identifies many of the societal myths that support abuse.

Value of Privacy

Factors such as industrialization, urbanization, and modernization have caused the family to evolve from a public institution to a private one. As the family became increasingly private, it also became isolated from social control. The audience for violence is typically limited to husband, wife, and one or two children. This privacy shelters offenders and victims from public eyes and social sanctions and affords a shielded setting for private violence. In families in which abuse is the norm, the abuser increasingly limits and controls the amount of time victims can socialize outside of the family. In the notorious 1987 case in which 6-year-old Lisa Steinberg was found unconscious in the apartment of Hedda Nussbaum and Joel Steinberg, Steinberg's abuse was directed at both Lisa and Hedda. For years, he systematically cut Hedda off from all outside contacts, including her job and her family (Ferrato, 1991).

Structural Inequality of the Family

Many areas of family inequality support violent and abusive behavior. First is inequality of size. Most husbands are larger and stronger than their wives and certainly larger than their children; most mothers are larger and stronger than young children. Size is important. Surveys have shown that mothers who typically hit

their children engage in less physical discipline as the children enter into adolescent years, not because of fewer conflicts between mother and child but because the adolescent's larger size poses a risk of retaliatory violence directed toward the mother.

Beyond physical inequality are social and economic inequality. Men typically enjoy greater social and economic status than do women. This greater status translates into power within the family. Husbands can hit their wives without fear of economic or social costs. Likewise, parents control the economic and social resources of their children. Wives put up with an occasional beating rather than deal with the costs of trying to survive outside the home without money, credit, or work experience. Viewing violence within an unequal family structure makes it clear that all violence is really an abuse of power in which the stronger person takes advantage of the weaker.

Wives and children have historically been regarded as the legal property of the husband and father. This view not only allowed a man's violent behavior but also encouraged it as a way of controlling and keeping his possessions "in line." Although those laws have long since been abolished in favor of recognizing the worth of women and children, attitudes do not die just because laws change. The attitude that husbands have the right to discipline their wives and children and the family and social structures that support violent behavior serve to stack the cards against the victims of domestic violence and abuse. In no other social situation in which violence plays a factor do the victims have to weigh losing their homes and financial security against the costs of being physically assaulted.

What do you think? What impact does television violence have on the violence that occurs within families?

➤ *Check Your Reading*
14. How does the value placed on privacy support violence?
15. How does the structural inequality of the family support violence?
16. When Gelles and Straus state that violence continues because the abusers can get away with it, what do they mean?

Characteristics of Abusers

Social and cultural factors that allow abusers to hit family members are not the total explanation for violence. Many couples never engage in violent physical exchanges; some parents abhor hitting their children. What other factors predispose some people to become violent? Some researchers have focused on the role of biology, including neurophysiology, neurotransmitters, genetics, and the presence of a psychiatric disorder. Others have focused on the personal characteristics of abusers, the role of alcohol and drugs, and abuse as mutual combat.

Box 35-1 ■ ■ ■ ■ ■
Myths Surrounding Domestic Violence and the Facts Concerning These Myths

Myth	Fact
Violence among family members is a private matter.	Violence is a public concern. It is costly to society in multiple ways, including lost productivity and health care costs. The long-term costs of damaged lives is inestimable.
The abuse cannot be that terrible, or the woman would leave.	The ties that bind women to abusive men are complex. The woman may be financially dependent on the man and afraid that she will not be able to manage on her own.
Women who remain in abusive relationships tend to become helpless.	Sometimes abused women seem to be placating and passive toward their abuser. These behaviors must be viewed in the context of the constant fear in which the woman lives. Placating, passive behavior represents an effort to avoid future violence. Many women have the courage and will eventually leave even though the odds are stacked against them.
Alcohol and drugs cause abuse.	The use of alcohol and drugs only gives the abuser an excuse for violence; they do not cause violent behavior.
Abuse occurs more in lower socioeconomic groups.	Battering takes place just as often among middle and upper classes. This myth is maintained by racial bias. Many women in middle and upper classes may go to greater lengths to conceal their injuries. Health care providers are less likely to suspect abuse in a middle-class or upper-class woman.
Batterers are uneducated men who cannot cope in the world.	Many batterers are successful professionals—physicians, attorneys, public officials, clergymen, college professors. They share a common characteristic of being unusually dependent on their partners.
Battered wives will never change.	Most women who leave abusive relationships are careful not to marry another batterer, if they remarry at all.
Battering men will never change.	Some men are shocked into confronting their problems when their partners leave them or when they serve prison sentences. Behavioral therapy can teach battering men how to express aggression appropriately and how to negotiate with rather than coerce women.
Families should be kept together at all costs.	Children develop severe emotional problems from living with a batterer. They improve dramatically when they are removed from the situation when their mother moves out.

Data from King, M. C., & Ryan, J. (1989). Abused women: Dispelling myths and encouraging intervention. *Nurse Practitioner, 14*(5), 47-58; and Collier, J. A. (1987, May). When you suspect your patient is a battered wife. *RN*, 22-25.

Biological Factors and Violence

In addition to the social factors that support violence, researchers continue to look to the brain for explanations of violent behavior. The results of biological research are not conclusive but seem to indicate a higher incidence of violence in persons with partial complex seizures. This research has focused on the role of the limbic system in episodic dyscontrol. Monroe (1970) argued for the validity of this theory by pointing out the effectiveness of anticonvulsant regimens in limiting or eliminating episodic dyscontrol (Tardiff, 1989).

Nocturnal wandering with episodic violence as part of the nocturnal wandering behavior pattern has been reported by Schenck and Mahowald (1995), Guilleminault, Moscovitch, and Leger, (1995), and Moldofsky, Gilbert, Lue, and MacLean (1995). Many of these nocturnal wanderer patients had multiple episodes of serious violence. The findings of these studies vary: One patient improved with clonazepam; others were found to have temporal lobe abnormalities; some had concomitant drug abuse disorders.

Volkow and colleagues (1995) studied abnormal brain glucose metabolism and found lower metabolic values in violent psychiatric patients in certain brain regions than controls, which was hypothesized to have contributed to the subjects' violent behaviors.

Kaerkkaeinen and coworkers (1995) studied urinary excretion of bufotenin in paranoid violent patients but the results were inconclusive. Dabbs, Carr, Frady, and Riad, (1995) found higher levels of testosterone in violent criminals.

Other researchers have focused attention on the role of the neurotransmitters in violent behavior. For instance, increased levels of norepinephrine and dopamine are associated with violence and aggression. Additionally, decreased levels of serotonin are associated with impulsivity. Pihl and coworkers (1995) found that lowered tryptophan levels and alcohol ingestion were associated with increased aggression. Results supported the theory that low serotonin levels may be involved in the etiology of aggression, and that persons with low brain serotonin levels may be particularly susceptible to alcohol-induced violence.

Genetics may also play a part in violent behavior, but the research is equivocal. A number of studies of prison populations have shown a disproportionate number of XYY men, but other researchers have failed to show a relationship between this genetic abnormality and violence. Kraus (1995) studied a male serial killer who had multiple preexisting factors, including antisocial personality disorder, abnormally elevated urinary chemical kryptopyrroles, abnormal chromosomal patterns, and brain injuries. Kraus argues that this case shows that criminal tendencies have biological origins. Tardiff (1989) looked at subjects who had been adopted and found that the crimes of the subjects were more related to their alcohol use than their genetics, although there was support for the thesis that nonviolent petty property crime has a genetic basis.

Presence of Psychiatric Illness

One of the myths about psychiatric patients is that they are all wild, violent, and out of control. Although this myth is not true, some diagnoses carry an association between violence and the symptoms of the illness. For instance, Andreason and Black (1995) noted that "patients with schizophrenia, mania, mental retardation, and brain disorders are more likely to become violent. . . . In the hospital psychotic disorders are more likely to lead to violence than nonpsychotic disorders"

(p. 521). Within the psychotic group, those driven by their delusions were more likely to commit seriously violent acts.

Patients experiencing psychotic symptoms, however, are not the only perpetrators of violence. Borderline and antisocial personality disorders as well as childhood and adolescent diagnoses and substance abuse are all correlated with increased rates of violent and assaultive behaviors (Copel, 1996).

> **What do you think?** How have your attitudes toward psychiatric nursing been influenced by the myth that most psychiatric patients are violent?

➤ Check Your Reading

17. What is the relationship between psychiatric problems and incidents of violence?
18. How is the limbic system implicated in explanations of the cause of violence?
19. How do delusions and hallucinations relate to acts of violence?
20. What neurotransmitters are implicated in violent behavior?
21. What does research suggest regarding the role of genetics in violent behavior?

Personal Characteristics of Abusers

Personal factors such as low self-esteem, immaturity, extreme dependence, and insecurity certainly contribute to abuse. The hate-filled man releases his hostility by beating his wife. The frustrated mother lashes out at her young children. The rebellious adolescent expresses anger by beating up younger siblings. For a brief moment, the violent behavior provides the abuser with a false sense of power.

Some people hit others to relieve pent-up anger and then justify their actions as necessary. Violence is used to control. Parents use it to control children. Men use it to control women. Some abusers beat down their victims until the victim will do anything just to prevent further violence. The measure of control gained by the abuser temporarily boosts self-esteem.

The violence may follow disappointments in the work setting. Abusive men, unable to fulfill the masculine ideals of American society and feeling desperate and hopeless about their social situation, may choose to vent their anger and frustration at their wives and children.

Men who abuse their wives often say that their violence was caused by their wives' infidelity, by threats to separate or seek a divorce, or by other external incidents (Stamp & Sabourin, 1995). The violence is a desperate means for the man to control his wife. The couple may be locked in a sequence of actions and reactions that lead to tragic consequences (Berger, 1990). Box 35-2 details the similarities among abusive men.

Box 35-2 ■ ■ ■ ■ ■
Ways to Spot a Potential Batterer

There are ways to spot a potential batterer, but often we don't see the warning signs. Here is a list to watch for. Please share these characteristics with friends and family members in dating relationships.

· *He comes on too strong.* Beware of the man who loves you instantly and wants to see you all the time. He is responding to his own fantasies, not the real you.

· *He has very traditional ideas about men's and women's roles.* Watch out for the man who thinks a woman should stay at home, take care of her husband, and follow orders.

· *He believes in using force or violence to solve problems.* If he overreacts to little problems, such as not being able to find a parking space, that's a bad sign. Other signals include throwing things, punching walls, and being cruel to animals when he is angry.

· *He thinks poorly of himself.* Batterers are insecure people with low self-esteem, but they may act tough to cover up these feelings of inferiority.

· *He is jealous.* He keeps tabs on you and wants to know where you are at all times. He is jealous not only of other men but also of your friends and family.

· *He is self-centered.* The man who thinks only of fulfilling his own needs is a bad risk.

· *He has extreme highs and extreme lows in his moods.* His mood swings are like Dr. Jekyll and Mr. Hyde.

· *He blames others when things don't work out.* Anything bad that happens to him is someone else's fault. He will eventually start blaming you when things go wrong.

· *He is a product of a violent family.* Children from violent homes often grow up thinking that violence is normal, acceptable behavior.

· *He behaves badly toward others.* Even if he is kind to you now, the way he functions with the rest of the world may be the way he ultimately functions with you.

· *He treats you roughly at times.* Abuse during dating is a *guarantee* of later, more violent abuse. Even playful wrestling or tickling to the point at which you're frightened or have been hurt may suggest an abusive nature. Do not think that marriage will change him for the better; it will almost certainly change him for the worse.

· *He makes you feel scared or threatened.* Are you afraid to break up with him because he might hurt you? Do you change your life to keep from making him angry? If so, you are being abused and should seek help.

Alcohol and Drugs

Sometimes abusers use alcohol or drugs as an excuse for their violence. The truth, however, is that alcohol and drugs are only factors in abuse. Someone who is violent will be violent with or without drinking and drug use. Drinking to excess and using drugs provides a time-out from the rules of society and gives a convenient excuse for violent behavior.

A drunk usually denies responsibility for actions. American society feeds into that denial by offering excuses for the violence stemming from drinking. The person was not in control, could not think rationally, and had fewer inhibitions. American culture tends to minimize aggression that comes with drunkenness.

Not only does heavy drinking afford an occasion for violence to occur but also it can lead to problems with alcohol among women who are abused. Alcoholism among women is a growing problem, and the largest precipitating cause is believed to be spouse abuse (Berger, 1990). Box 35-3 details the myths regarding the relationship between alcohol and abuse.

Abuse as Mutual Combat

Gage's (1991) alternative view of spousal abuse suggests a continuum along which abusive relationships occur

(Table 35-1). There are two continua along which violence occurs. The first is characterized by what Straus and Gelles (1988) call **expressive violence,** in which the goal is to cause pain or injury to the other. This type of violence is also referred to as "mutual combat or conjugal violence." The second is characterized by **instrumental violence,** in which the goal is to control the behavior of the other.

Expressive violence results from intense emotional upheaval combined with poor impulse control. Each partner plays a role (although not necessarily an equal role) in the escalation of this type of violence. Each partner feels victimized by the other. The roles of victim and perpetrator are blurred and may fluctuate with the circumstances. The partners share responsibility for the eruption of violence. This view of violence is consistent with a **mutual combat model** because violence is not congruent with the value systems of the participants, they usually express genuine remorse after incidents of violence, and the possibility for constructive change is favorable.

Instrumental violence is used to exploit and control another person. In cases of instrumental violence, the roles of victim and perpetrator are clearly defined, and the man is almost always the perpetrator. Any expression of remorse is usually shallow and is itself a form of manipulation directed toward meeting the needs of the perpetrator rather than a genuine concern for the victim. This form of violence is consistent with the

Box 35–3 ■ ■ ■ ■ ■
Domestic Violence and Alcohol Abuse—Debunking the Myths

Myth	Fact
Battering is a direct result of alcohol abuse.	Battering is a socially learned behavior and is not a direct result of substance abuse.
Most abuse occurs at the hands of alcohol abusers.	Many men who batter do not abuse alcohol; many alcoholic men do not batter their female partners. Alcohol use may provide the excuse for battering; however, batterers also engage in violent behavior toward their female partners when they are cold sober.
Treatment for alcohol use also cures battering behavior.	Alcoholism and battering require separate treatment. The first priority even before treatment is protection of the woman.
Women who abuse alcohol are more likely to be abused.	Some women have alcohol abuse problems and they are also abused; other women turn to substance abuse in response to the battering.
A woman's substance abuse is a direct cause of violent behavior in her partner.	A woman's substance abuse problems in no way relate to the cause of the battering she receives.

wife-battering model. There is usually little motivation for change when instrumental violence is the norm.

Neidig, Friedman, and Collins (1984) contended that, without intervention, many couples progress from the expressive to the instrumental end of the violence continuum.

Role of Religion and Spirituality in Violence

There has been no research examining the relationship between violence and spirituality or religion, but we may assume that a person who is victimized suffers spiritually. For instance, the woman or child victim might wonder, "Why has God forsaken me?" "I must really deserve this treatment. Even God doesn't care about me." These feelings may be intensified if the woman is encouraged by a church member or leader to "try harder to please your husband," or is asked "what did you do to make him angry?" She may be counseled to "obey your husband no matter what because that is what God commands." Such advice is destructive to the woman and only adds to the pain and difficulty of her situation. Furthermore, it is a distortion of a theistic and a scriptural view of life. There is *absolutely no*

TABLE 35–1 Expressive Versus Instrumental Violence

EXPRESSIVE VIOLENCE	INSTRUMENTAL VIOLENCE
Violence that is primarily an expression of emotion (e.g., anger, jealousy)	Violence that is used primarily as an instrument to achieve a goal
Mutual and reciprocal violence; victim and perpetrator roles not fixed	Unilateral violence; victim and perpetrator roles fixed
Violence in context of escalating conflict	Violence as deliberate effort to punish or control
Sequential, gradual, predictable progression to violence	Relatively sudden and rapid progression to violence
Mutual conflict, stress, frustration, and anger precede violent incident	Little provocation for violent incident
Genuine remorse and sorrow follow incident; violence inconsistent with values; belief that violence will be controlled	Shallow remorse and sorrow follow incident; violence consistent with values; feelings of resignation and hopelessness
Unpredictable; high potential for escalation and "accidental" injury	Potential for violent retaliation, homicide or suicide
Relatively benign psychological consequences	Serious psychological consequences: helplessness, depression, low self-esteem, external locus of control
Brief, skill-building therapy with couples	Long-term therapy with individuals; separation; legal sanctions
Termed *mutual combat, spouse abuse, conjugal violence*	Termed *battering*

Published in RN. Copyright © 1987 Medical Economics, Montvale, NJ. Reprinted by permission. Modified from Collier, J. A. (1987, May). When you suspect your patient is a battered wife. RN, 22–25.

Box 35–4 ■ ■ ■ ■ ■
Position Statement on Physical Violence Against Women

The American Nurses Association (ANA) supports education of nurses, health care providers, and women in skills necessary for prevention of violence against women; assessment of women in health care institutions and community settings; and research on violence against women. ANA believes there is a need to increase awareness of the health problem of violence against women as well as reduce injuries and psychological misery associated with this crime. ANA believes health care professionals must be educated as to their role in the assessment, intervention, and prevention of physical violence against women. Further, ANA supports the Year 2000 Health Objectives, which cite the surveillance, prevention, and intervention for violent behavior as a priority issue for the nation.

Physical violence against women is behavior intended to inflict harm and includes slapping, kicking, choking, punching, pushing, use of objects as weapons, forced sexual activity, and injury or death from a weapon. Physical violence is by definition assault and it is a crime. Ninety-five percent of serious assaults by a spouse or intimate partner are men battering women. Abuse is the leading cause of injury to women, and homicide a major cause of traumatic death to women.

Physical violence against women is pervasive and cuts across all ethnic, racial, religious, and socioeconomic groups. Based on national survey results, 1.8 million women are beaten by their husbands each year. Stated another way, one of every eight husbands assaults his wife at least once during a given year. Abuse during courtship and cohabiting relationships affects between 16% and 23% of all dating relationships. The FBI estimates that one in two women will be physically assaulted by her male partner during her lifetime. Frequently physical abuse begins during pregnancy with 25% to 30% of pregnant women reporting abuse prior to or during pregnancy. Pregnant women reporting abuse are more likely to deliver a low-birth-weight infant.

Injuries to women sustained from abuse include contusions, concussions, lacerations, fractures, and gunshot wounds. Emergency room records document that 22% to 35% of women presenting any complaint are there because of symptoms related to physical abuse. Some 1000 women are killed each year by their male partner, almost always following years of physical abuse. The economic costs of interpersonal violence are high, especially if a weapon is involved.

The lifetime cost of firearm deaths and injuries is estimated at $23 billion in 1990 with more than 80% of the medical care costs borne by public funds. During the same year, injuries caused by interpersonal violence requiring hospitalization cost an estimated $80 billion. Because most physical violence between intimate partners goes underreported, the economic costs are grossly underrepresented.

There is a need to:
· Increase awareness of and sensitivity to the health problem of physical violence against women.
· Reduce intentional injuries and the associated economic costs and psychological misery.
· Heighten awareness of health professionals as to their role in the assessment, intervention, and prevention of physical violence against women.

The American College of Obstetricians and Gynecologists, the Surgeon General, and the Centers for Disease Control and Prevention have forwarded recommendations that all women be routinely screened for physical abuse and offered counseling, education, advocacy, and appropriate referrals. The Year 2000 Health Objectives cite the surveillance, prevention, and intervention for violent behavior as a priority issue for the nation.

Therefore, the ANA supports:
· Routine education of all nurses and health care providers in the skills necessary to prevent violence against women
· Routine assessment and documentation for physical abuse of all women in any health care institution or community setting
· Targeted assessment of women at increased risk of abuse including pregnant women and women presenting in emergency rooms
· Education of all women as to the cycle of violence, the potential for homicide, and community resources for primary, secondary, and tertiary prevention and care
· Inclusion of the topic of violence against women in all undergraduate nursing curriculums
· Education of school-age children and adolescents in public schools about relationships without violence and community resources for help
· Research on violence against women, including the development and evaluation of nursing models for preventive assessment, intervention, and treatment for abused women, their children, and perpetrators of violence

Courtesy of the American Nurses Association, Washington, D.C.

justification within Scripture for a husband to beat his wife. In fact, Scripture commands husbands to love their wives as their own bodies.

In considering the spirituality of the abuser, we can only speculate that the abuser does not experience spiritual well-being. Abusing another and exerting coercive power is inconsistent with spiritual wellness and antithetical to loving others as ourselves.

> **W**hat do you think? How do your own religious and spiritual beliefs influence your attitudes toward violence and abuse?

➤ *Check Your Reading*

22. Identify three characteristics of abusive men.
23. Identify two myths regarding the role of alcohol and abuse.
24. State three ways that alcohol is linked to violence.
25. What is the difference between expressive and instrumental violence?
26. Describe the mutual combat model.

NURSING PROCESS WITH ABUSED WOMEN

The American Nurses Association (ANA) has issued a position statement on physical violence against women, the most common form of **spousal abuse.** The ANA supports the Year 2000 Health Objectives, which cite surveillance, prevention, and intervention for violent behavior as a priority issue for the United States. The ANA's position statement is shown in Box 35-4.

Assessment

The statistics regarding the incidence of abuse toward women are frightening. In 1980, one in three women was estimated to have experienced intentional injury at the hands of a male partner (Straus et al., 1980). Moreover, many of these women were abused while pregnant. In fact, a national telephone survey of more than 6000 households revealed that the risk of pregnant women having experienced abuse during the previous year was almost 61% greater than the risk to women who were not pregnant (Straus & Gelles, 1988). Approximately 8% to 11% of pregnant women are abused during their pregnancies (Helton et al., 1987; Hillard, 1985).

Many women who are abused seek medical treatment (Moss & Taylor, 1991). Some come to emergency departments seeking treatment for an acute injury; others may present at medical or mental health clinics as part of scheduled or unscheduled appointments. A pregnant woman may present at an emergency department requesting that a nurse or physician check to see if her baby is all right. Usually the presenting complaint is not abuse. Instead the woman may present with injuries that are several days old and offer vague and incomplete histories regarding the nature of the injury. See Box 35-5 for general indicators of abuse.

It is incumbent on nurses and physicians to conduct assessments that are nonjudgmental and gentle but also direct in approach (Parker & McFarlane, 1991). Figure 35-2 displays an appropriate abuse assessment screen. Figure 35-3 shows the CSR Abuse Index, and Box 35-6 includes questions for assessing emotional abuse.

The assessment is conducted in a private setting, with assurances of confidentiality. Sometimes it is essential that you intervene between the woman and her partner. The man may have accompanied her into a health facility for treatment and fully intends to stay by her side at all times. To ensure that privacy is maintained and the woman has a safety zone in which to speak outside the hearing of her partner, you may need to make a statement to the male partner, such as "This part of the examination is done in private. You must remain outside." Such a statement establishes patient privacy as a protocol of the agency, maximizes the woman's opportunity to talk, and minimizes the influence exerted by the man to maintain silence about the abuse.

> **W**hat do you think? How would you respond in a situation where the woman's partner refuses to leave the examining room?

Box 35–5 ■ ■ ■ ■ ■
General Indicators of Abuse*

- Significant behavioral or psychological changes in a pregnant woman
- Miscarriage
- Numerous health problems, from physical injuries to psychological complaints to somatic disturbances
- Bruises, visible or covered with makeup or clothes (e.g., long sleeves or high collars), such as bruises around the woman's neck
- Other physical signs, such as broken ribs, back or spine injuries, or soft tissue injuries on the woman's torso or extremities
- Reasons given for the woman's injury or injuries do not match the physical evidence (e.g., claims of being accident prone)
- Psychological complaints, including anxiety, depression, sleep disturbances, or impaired decision making
- Suicidal thoughts or attempts
- Feelings of worthlessness
- Somatic complaints, such as frequent headaches, gastrointestinal distress, heart palpitations, or dizziness
- Presence of an over-protective man
- Feels the need to account for every hour of the day to her mate

*All of these symptoms and complaints have many other causes; however, they may be related to domestic abuse.
Data from Moss, V. A. (1996). Abuse of women: Its effect in the workplace and what employers can do to help. *Surgical Services Management, 2*(10):34-36.

1. Have you ever been emotionally or physically abused by your partner or someone important to you?

☐ Yes   ☐ No

2. Within the last year, have you been hit, slapped, kicked, or otherwise physically hurt by someone?

☐ Yes   ☐ No

If yes, by whom? _____

Number of times _____

3. Since you've been pregnant, have you been hit, slapped, kicked, or otherwise physically hurt by someone?

☐ Yes   ☐ No

If yes, by whom? _____

Number of times _____

Mark the area of injury on the body map at right.

4. Within the last year, has anyone forced you to have sexual activities?

☐ Yes   ☐ No

If yes, who? _____

Number of times _____

5. Are you afraid of your partner or anyone you listed above?

☐ Yes   ☐ No

Figure 35–2
Abuse assessment screen. (Developed by the Nursing Research Consortium on Violence and Abuse, 1989. Redrawn from Parker, B., & MacFarlane, J. [1991]. Identifying and helping battered pregnant women. *Maternal Child Nursing, 16*, 162.)

► *Check Your Reading*

27. Identify three general indicators of abuse.
28. Why is it important for the nurse to ask the woman direct questions about the possibility of abuse?
29. What is the usual presenting complaint of the pregnant woman who has been abused?

Interviewing

You may find it difficult to ask questions that allow abused women to discuss the violence openly. Many abused women have commented that when they sought treatment for their injuries, no one ever asked them if the injury was the result of abuse. Feeling ashamed and guilty, the woman is unlikely to volunteer this information unless the care provider asks for it and is willing to listen in a nonjudgmental, accepting manner. Box 35-7 includes sample assessment questions to facilitate the process.

Documentation

It is imperative that you thoroughly document the assessment process. Clinical records may be used as evidence if the woman decides to seek legal redress. Comprehensive documentation also alerts the next care provider who may intervene to deal with vague, poorly defined injuries. The use of a body map allows the specific injuries to be diagrammed and information about the injuries noted. If the woman consents, photographs are also taken. Sometimes it is beneficial for the woman to return the next day for more photos, so that the full extent of bruising and swelling is evident.

The pictures are signed and dated and sealed in an envelope or container with any other evidence, such as clothing. The envelope or container is stored in a safe place. The woman needs to sign a release-of-information form, so that a court may request the records. This evidence may prove useful if she attempts to substantiate charges of continued abuse. Even if she is not ready to prosecute at this time, she may be ready at a later time.

If the woman does not admit to being beaten, you cannot note abuse in the chart, but you can write, "The explanation of the patient's injuries is inappropriate," or "The patient's description of the circumstances surrounding the infliction of her injuries is inconsistent with the injury pattern." If the woman states that her injuries were the result of abuse, it is imperative for you to document accordingly. For example, write, "Patient states she was beaten up by her husband" (Moss & Taylor, 1991).

You must recognize that the abused woman may feel embarrassment, shame, and even responsibility for the

DIRECTIONS: For each question, indicate the number from the designated scale that best describes your relationship with your partner.

Questions #1 to #14

3—FREQUENTLY   2—SOMETIMES   1—RARELY   0—NEVER

_____ 1. Continually monitors your time and makes you account for every minute?

_____ 2. Accuses you of having affairs with other men or acts suspicious of you?

_____ 3. Is rude to your friends?

_____ 4. Discourages you from starting friendships with other women?

_____ 5. Is critical of things such as cooking, clothes, or appearance?

_____ 6. Demands a strict account of how you spend money?

_____ 7. Moods change radically, from very calm to very angry, or vice versa?

_____ 8. Is disturbed by your working or by the thought of your working?

_____ 9. Becomes angry more easily when he drinks?

_____ 10. Pressures you for sex much more often than you like?

_____ 11. Becomes angry if you do not want to go along with his request for sex?

_____ 12. Quarrels over financial matters?

_____ 13. Quarrels about having children or raising them?

_____ 14. Strikes you with his hand or feet (slaps, punches, kicks)?

Questions #15 to #26

6—FREQUENTLY   5—SOMETIMES   4—RARELY   0—NEVER

_____ 15. Has he ever struck you with an object?

_____ 16. Has he ever threatened you with an object or weapon?

_____ 17. Has he ever threatened to kill either you or himself?

_____ 18. Does he give you visible injuries (such as welts, bruises, cuts)?

_____ 19. Have you ever had to receive first aid because his violence to you resulted in injuries?

_____ 20. Have you ever had to seek professional aid for any injury at a medical clinic, doctor's office, or hospital emergency department?

_____ 21. Has he ever hurt you sexually or made you have intercourse against your will?

_____ 22. Is he ever violent toward children?

_____ 23. Is he ever violent toward other people outside your home and family?

_____ 24. Does he ever throw objects or break things when he is angry?

_____ 25. Has he ever been in trouble with the police?

_____ 26. Have you ever called the police or tried to call them because you felt you or members of your family were in danger?

_____ TOTAL

To score responses, simply add up the points for each question. This sum is the ABUSE INDEX SCORE. To get some idea of how abusive your partner is, compare your index score with the following chart:

92–120	Dangerously abusive
35–91	Seriously abusive
13–34	Moderately abusive
0–12	Nonabusive

If at all possible, your partner should complete a CSR Abuse Index form. The difference in the results should be discussed with the program counselor. Does your partner grossly underestimate that he is abusive? If so, why?

Figure 35–3
The CSR Abuse Index. (From *The Family Secret* by William Stacey and Anson Shupe. Copyright © 1983 by William Stacey and Anson Shupe. Reprinted by permission of Beacon Press, Boston.)

Box 35-6 ■ ■ ■ ■ ■
Emotional Abuse Checklist

Keeping You Away From Other People

- Does your partner get angry when you talk on the phone?
- Does he open your mail?
- Does he keep you from seeing friends?
- Is he angry when you are just a little late getting home?
- Does he want you home when he is home?

Always on Your Mind

- Do you worry about what he will think about your make-up? Or how you dress?
- Do you ask him whom you can see or where you can go?
- Are you careful of what you say so that he will not get upset?
- Do you feel you are "walking on eggshells"?

Putting You Down: Humiliation

- Does he call you names like "stupid," "bitch," or "whore"?
- Does he tell you what is "wrong" with you in front of other people?
- Has he made you do things that make you feel ashamed?
- Does he say that no one else would want you or love you?

Threats

- Does he threaten to leave you?

- Has he said he will go crazy or kill himself if you leave?
- Does he say he will hit you or beat you if you don't obey?

Feeling Sick and Tired

- Does he keep you up late asking you about men in your past?
- Do you work so hard to please him that you feel worn out?
- Do you feel sick, yet you are not sure what is wrong?
- Are you unable to do things you used to do easily?

Small Demands

- Does he demand that dinner be served right on the minute?
- Does he insist that the house look just so?
- Do you have to report how you spend every dollar?

Sweet Talk and Threats

- After he has been mean, does he act sweet and loving?
- After he has hit you, does he give you a present or take you out?
- When you decide to leave, does he give you hope for change?

---

abuse. The abuse victim may use denial as a coping mechanism. Even if she reports abuse, there is a tendency to minimize its frequency and severity. The woman may believe that others will not define her problem as seriously as she does, and minimizing the event makes her feel less alienated from others. To respond to these feelings, establish rapport through concern, interest expressed in the woman's story, and an expressed desire to assist the woman.

Determining the Woman's Safety

Initially, you are interested in determining whether the woman is safe, as females are most often the homicide victim (Wilson, Johnson, & Daly, 1995). Keeping in mind that the frequency and severity of violence usually escalate over time, recognize that the risk for a lethal outcome is a frightening reality (Case Example 35–3). The risk of homicide is increased in the presence of the following factors (Campbell, 1986; Parker & McFarlane, 1991):

- A handgun in the home
- Substance abuse
- Extreme jealousy
- Battering during pregnancy

The battered woman's risk of being killed by her partner is greater if she leaves him or makes it clear to him that she is ending the relationship.

■ CASE EXAMPLE 35-3
■ Kate's Story

Kate was hiding from her boyfriend, who'd hurt her several times. He tracked her down by tricking one of her children into giving him the address. He broke through the front door and went after Kate, shoving her against cupboards, breaking her nose, kicking and punching her, breaking her ribs, and blackening her eyes. While the boyfriend splattered Kate's blood across the kitchen, her deaf and mute daughter watched in silent terror. ■

From Ferrato, D. (1991). *Living with the enemy* (p. 61). New York: Aperture.

Box 35-7 ■ ■ ■ ■ ■

Sample Assessment Questions
in Determining Abuse

- Has somebody hurt you?
- Are you safe at home?
- Your partner seems to frighten you. Has he hurt you?
- Can you tell me about any times during your relationship when you and your partner have had physical fights?
- Is your present relationship one in which you are hurt?
- Do you feel that your partner controls your life too much?
- The injuries that you have remind me of injuries that I have seen on other women who have been hurt or abused. Did anyone hurt you?
- It is routine for me to ask all women patients if they are presently in a relationship with someone who is abusing them. Are you in such a relationship?

Data from King, M. C., & Ryan, J. (1989). Abused women: Dispelling myths and encouraging intervention. *Nurse Practitioner, 14*(5), 47-58; and Moss, V. A., & Taylor, W. K. (1991). Domestic violence. *AORN Journal, 53,* 1158-1164.

Campbell (1986) developed an instrument to use in assessing the potential for homicide (Figure 35-4).

What do you think? How would you describe the nurse's role with a victim of spousal abuse?

▶ *Check Your Reading*

30. Identify three situations that increase the woman's risk of being murdered at the hands of her abuser.
31. What is the significance of taking pictures of the woman's injuries? Why would you want her to return the next day for more pictures?
32. If the woman's explanation of her injuries is not consistent with what you observe, how would you document this inconsistency?

Cycle of Abuse

The **cycle of abuse** usually occurs in three predictable stages:

1. Increasing tension
2. Explosion of anger
3. Loving reconciliation (the honeymoon phase)

The first stage is one of increasing tension. The batterer becomes displeased over things that his victim has done. These things can be either real or imagined, minor or trivial. The event that precipitates an angry outburst may be that his mate burned his toast or "talked back."

The batterer reacts to this perceived insult with verbal abuse or slapping his partner. In an effort to minimize his anger, the woman may attempt to appease him or move out of his way. Her passivity actually fuels his lack of self-control. His verbal barrages last increasingly longer. The slaps get harder. He blankets her with his physical presence as he looks for signs of resistance.

The second stage occurs with an explosion of anger. The abuser, no longer exercising any self-control, releases his tension in an outburst of physical violence that can result in serious injury or even death. The abuser may use his fists, he may throw his mate across a room, he may burn her with cigarettes or scald her with hot liquids, he may break her arms, or he may force sexual acts on her. The form of abuse may vary, but it is always out of proportion to the woman's perceived offense.

Women who have experienced severe beatings do not always seek medical care immediately. They may try to hide the beatings and convince themselves that they are not really hurt.

The third stage, that of loving reconciliation, frequently referred to as the honeymoon phase, occurs as the abuser apologizes and makes amends. He appears to be contrite and promises that he will control himself from now on. He also believes that he has taught her such a lesson that he will never be forced to strike her again. Even in his contrite mode, he is able to blame the woman for the event.

Wanting desperately to believe that this man who presents himself as loving and contrite is really what her partner is like, the woman may decide to stay and give him another chance. She believes he loves her and needs her.

There are other reasons for taking him back. The woman may feel trapped in this relationship because of lack of a support system or lack of economic resources or job skills. She may be too ashamed to tell her family. Or she may fear retaliation from her spouse if she should leave.

Regardless of why she stays, tension starts to build once the reconciliation is over, and the cycle begins again. Figure 35-5 illustrates the cycle of violence.

Sexual Abuse

In addition to the beatings that abused women suffer, many are also subjected to rape and other forms of sexual abuse (Weingourt, 1990). This form of abuse is typically not reported unless the woman is specifically asked about it (Gelles, 1977) (for a discussion of rape, refer to Chapter 36).

In a study conducted by Weingourt (1990), a convenience sample of 53 women was interviewed at a major medical center in New England. The focus of the research was marital and cohabitant relationships. The women were being treated for a primary depressive or anxiety disorder; women with psychotic behavior were excluded from the study. Data were collected by means of a semistructured interview protocol. Each woman was asked, "Have you ever felt as if you were being pressured or forced to have sexual relations with a man when you really didn't want to?"

As a result of research conducted after killings, several risk factors have been associated with homicides (murders) of both batterers and battered women. We cannot predict what will happen in your case. However, we would like you to be aware of the danger of homicide in situations of severe battering, and we would like you to see how many of the risk factors apply to your situation. (The "he" in the questions refers to your husband, partner, ex-husband, ex-partner, or whoever is currently physically hurting you.)

Please circle Yes or No for each question below.

1. Has the physical violence increased in frequency over the past year?	Yes	No
2. Has the physical violence increased in severity over the past year, or has a weapon or threat with a weapon been used?	Yes	No
3. Does he ever try to choke you?	Yes	No
4. Is there a gun in the house?	Yes	No
5. Has he ever forced you into sex when you did not wish to do so?	Yes	No
6. Does he use drugs ("uppers" or amphetamines, speed, angel dust, cocaine, "crack," heroin, mixtures, or other street drugs)?	Yes	No
7. Does he threaten to kill you, or do you believe he is capable of killing you?	Yes	No
8. Is he drunk every day or almost every day? (In terms of quantity of alcohol)	Yes	No
9. Does he control most of your daily activities? For instance, does he tell you who you can be friends with, how much money you can take shopping, or when you can take the car?	Yes	No
10. Have you ever been beaten by him while you were pregnant? (If never pregnant by him, check here: _____ .)	Yes	No
11. Is he violently and consistently jealous of you? (For instance, does he say, "If I can't have you, no one can.")	Yes	No
12. Have you ever threatened or tried suicide?	Yes	No
13. Has he ever threatened or tried suicide?	Yes	No
14. Is he violent toward your children?	Yes	No
15. Is he violent outside the home?	Yes	No

Total Yes answers _____

THANK YOU. PLEASE TALK TO YOUR NURSE, ADVOCATE, OR COUNSELOR ABOUT WHAT THE DANGER ASSESSMENT MEANS IN YOUR SITUATION.

Figure 35–4

Danger assessment. (Reprinted with permission from Campbell, J. *Advances in Nursing Science*, Nursing assessment for risk of homicide in battered women, vol. 8[36–51], 45. © 1986, Aspen Publishers, Inc.)

The analysis of the 53 interviews revealed that 17 (32%) of the women had been raped by their husbands, and 16 (32%) had been raped and battered by their husbands. Two women reported being battered but not raped, and 18 denied abuse of any kind in their marital relationships. Therefore, 33 (62%) of the women being treated for depression and anxiety had been raped by their husbands. In addition, all but two of the women reported that the rape had occurred more than twice.

This study did not use a nonclinical sample, but the results can be compared with other studies that relied on nonclinical samples. Russell (1982) reported that 14% of her married sample had been raped by their spouses.

Frieze (1983) reported that 34% of her sample of battered women had experienced marital rape, whereas only 7% of her nonbattered group had similar experiences.

A comparison of these results with the results of Weingourt's (1990) sample demonstrates that the incidence of marital rape in the clinical sample is at least twice as high as that of the nonclinical sample. In 33 (62%) of the interviews, the women identified marital rape. Seventeen (51%) of the women who were raped reported no other form of violence, whereas 16 (48%) reported physical and sexual abuse. This finding tends to challenge Frieze's (1983) conclusion that marital rape is typically linked with battering and tends to support Russell's (1982) conclusion that rape may be the only form of abuse experienced by women and must be separately investigated.

Weingourt's (1990) data also revealed a significant relationship between child sexual abuse and wife rape. Twenty-four women out of the 33 who had been raped reported being sexually abused as children, whereas only 8 out of the 20 nonraped wives had been sexually molested as children.

The clinical ramifications of these findings suggest that wife rape is a significant negative factor in the lives of clinically depressed and anxious women and is closely linked with a history of having experienced child abuse. The comments made by the women indicated high levels of self-deprecation, feelings of worthlessness and helplessness, negative feelings toward men and marriage, and feelings of shame about sex (Weingourt, 1990).

W̲hat do you think? Should abuse be considered when assessing every depressed woman?

➤ *Check Your Reading*

33. What is the cycle of abuse?
34. What happens in the honeymoon phase of the cycle of abuse?
35. What does research suggest about the relationship between depression or anxiety and sexual abuse?
36. What does research suggest about the relationship between child abuse and wife rape?
37. Identify three of the feelings commonly expressed by women who have been raped within their marriages.

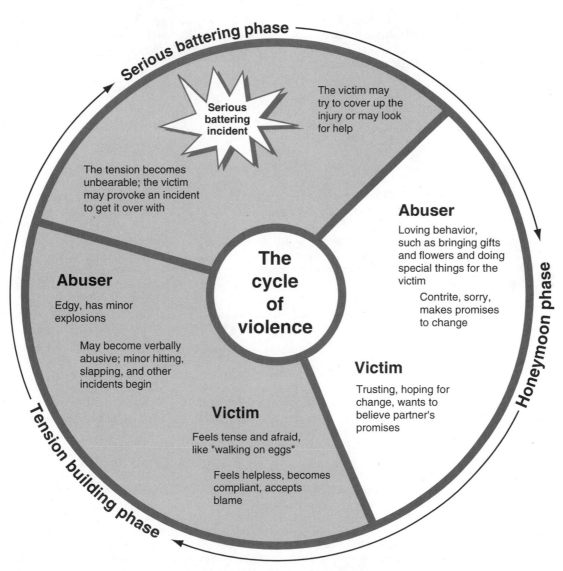

Figure 35–5
The cycle of violence. (Redrawn from YWCA of Annapolis and Anne Arundel County, 1517 Ritchie Highway, Arnold, MD 21012.)

Diagnosis

The analysis of the assessment data leads to a long list of potential nursing diagnoses as well as potential *Diagnostic and Statistical Manual of Mental Disorders, Fourth Edition* (DSM-IV) (American Psychiatric Association [APA], 1994) diagnoses. See Medical Diagnoses and Related Nursing Diagnoses for Violence.

Outcome Identification

The development of goals with the abused woman is a mutual, collaborative process between you and the patient. You must avoid imposing goals on the woman. For instance, you may believe that the most important objective is for the woman to terminate the relationship with her partner. This may be the expected outcome for the woman, but she may be unable to consider it. You must respect the woman's timing and right to choose what is best for her. Additionally, goals are affected by the setting in which you have contact with the woman. When you care for an abused woman in an emergency department, you are concerned with her immediate safety, whereas if you are working as a psychiatric nurse in a counseling relationship with an abused woman, you might focus more on the long-term psychological effects of abuse.

MEDICAL DIAGNOSES AND RELATED NURSING DIAGNOSES

Violence

DSM-IV Diagnoses: Adjustment Disorder With Anxiety, Adjustment Disorder With Depressed Mood, Major Depressive Disorder (see Chapter 25), Dysthymic Disorder, Generalized Anxiety Disorder (see Chapter 23), Alcohol Dependence (see Chapter 26), Alcohol Abuse (see Chapter 26), Other Substance-Related Disorders (see Chapter 26)

Related Nursing Diagnoses	Definition	Example
Anxiety	A vague, uneasy feeling whose source is often nonspecific or unknown to the individual	Anxiety related to unpredictable and dangerous behavior of a partner as evidenced by fearful comments
Ineffective Individual Coping	Impairment of adaptive behaviors and problem solving abilities of a person in meeting life's demands and roles	Ineffective Individual Coping related to living in a violent situation as evidenced by use of alcohol to deal with an unbearable situation
Altered Family Processes	The state in which a family that normally functions effectively experiences a dysfunction	Altered Family Processes related to tension, fear, and violence as evidenced by acting-out behaviors of children and fear of wife
Fear	Feeling of dread related to an identifiable source, which the person validates	Fear related to the constant threat of physical harm as evidenced by comments related to history of old injuries
Spiritual Distress	Disruption in the life principle, which pervades a person's entire being and which integrates and transcends one's biological and psychosocial nature	Spiritual Distress related to feelings of abandonment by God as evidenced by comments that prayers are unanswered
Hopelessness	A subjective state in which a person sees limited or no alternatives or personal choices available and is unable to mobilize energy on own behalf	Hopelessness related to the belief that the cycle of abuse cannot be broken as evidenced by comments that none of the suggested measures will change current circumstances

Based on information from the *Diagnostic and Statistical Manual of Mental Disorders, Fourth Edition.* Copyright 1994 American Psychiatric Association. Nursing Diagnoses and definitions from North American Nursing Diagnosis Association. (1999). *NANDA nursing diagnoses: Definitions and classification 1999–2000.* Philadelphia: NANDA.

Planning

Keeping the woman's goals and the practice setting in mind, identify goals that might include the following:

- The woman will be able to identify a place of safety should she decide to leave her partner.
- The woman will be able to discuss freely the abusive incident.
- The woman will experience caring and concern from nurses and other health care providers.
- On a self-rating scale, the patient will express feelings of increased self-esteem.
- On a self-rating scale (or a standardized depression scale), the patient will rate her mood as less depressed.
- On a self-rating scale (or a standardized anxiety scale), the patient will rate her mood as less anxious.
- The woman will be able to verbalize a plan to leave her partner.
- The woman will abstain from substance abuse.
- The woman will be able to discover meaning from her experiences and experience spiritual well-being as she moves toward physical and emotional healing and wholeness.

> ➤ *Check Your Reading*
> 38. Identify at least two potential nursing diagnoses associated with abuse.
> 39. Identify two expected outcomes of working with an abused woman.
> 40. Identify two short-term goals for working with an abused woman.

Implementation

Nursing's responses to abuse are best analyzed by looking at the three levels of prevention: primary, secondary, and tertiary. Two general caveats regarding interventions, however, affect all levels of prevention. The first is the need to treat the woman with the utmost respect and dignity and avoid blaming her for what has happened. Victim blaming has been implicated in the development of the **battering syndrome** characterized by unsuccessful help seeking, vague physical complaints, and serious psychosocial problems such as substance abuse (Burgess, 1985; Campbell & Sheridan, 1989). Campbell and Sheridan warned that women who receive negative care or are blamed for their situation are at increased risk for a number of consequences:

1. Killing their abusers
2. Being killed by their abusers
3. Committing suicide
4. Losing their unborn children

A second caveat permeating all interventions is that the woman must receive necessary information about local shelters and the national hotline number for shelter and battering information. This information may be essential to her own safety and that of her children when and if she decides to leave her partner.

Primary Prevention

Your nursing role is that of a community educator on the problems of battering, the cycle of abuse, risk factors that place a woman at risk for battering, and available community resources and services for women who are at risk for or are experiencing battering. Education is essential in preventing abuse. Nurses must work to heighten the public's awareness of the extent and seriousness of battering.

Your educational role extends to the law enforcement and legislative communities as well. These groups must examine practices and laws that encourage or provide tacit approval or indifference to the plight of abused women. Letter writing, petitions, and lobbying are effective interventions to change attitudes and practices at the societal level and to increase funding for community resources to serve abused women. Nurses have been particularly effective in the areas of community education, lobbying, and national policy. For instance, Burgess (1985) devoted her career to conducting research on violence, rape, and the science of victimology. She was appointed to serve on the 1983 U.S. Attorney General's Task Force on Family Violence.

Secondary Prevention

The second level of intervention includes all the screening activities within the community: focusing on formal abuse assessment of women who seek care in emergency departments; informal referrals among concerned friends and family members; and referrals for abuse by health providers in other settings, such as mental health clinics, women's health clinics, and drug treatment centers. Figure 35–6 provides safety planning information that you could give to a woman during a screening or counseling session. Many shelters include a 24-hour hotline, telephone or walk-in crisis counseling, and information and referral services for nonresidents of the shelter.

Tertiary Prevention

The third level of intervention usually occurs when the woman seeks medical care at an emergency department, a drug treatment center, physician's office or clinic, or a mental health facility. The woman's help-seeking behavior takes various forms. She might seek treatment for injuries incurred during an acute battering incident, substance abuse, vague physical symptoms, or emotional difficulties.

Campbell and Sheridan (1989) identified a three-part focus for the nurse in an emergency department who intervenes to deal with life-threatening, health-threatening, and health-related problems. Table 35–2 identifies these problems and the appropriate interventions.

What is the psychiatric nurse's role with the abused woman who seeks therapy? Usually the woman does not openly seek therapy to deal with the effects of abuse but presents herself with depression or extreme anxiety. You must screen the woman for abuse and respond

Whether you leave or stay, you will be safer if you have an escape plan

Where can you go for safety? The best choice is to the home of someone who cares for you—someone who will support you no matter what you do. This might be a good friend or a relative. If you do not have this kind of person in your life, or if it is unsafe to go there, think about a motel (if you can afford it) or a shelter for battered women.

Practice getting to a safe place from your house when you are not under stress. Plan for a quick getaway day or night. Find excuses to go outdoors that will not make your abusive partner suspicious; for example, walking the dog or taking out the garbage.

When you need to escape, pretend you are going to do one of those tasks. Once outside, just keep going. Get into the car and drive off quickly, or keep walking until you get to a phone. Call for help.

If you have children, make plans for taking them. Prepare older children to go to a neighbor's house if you cannot get away. They can call the police. Police officers may help you leave with younger children. If you must leave without the children, go back for them with the police, or pick them up at school or a babysitter's when your partner is not around.

PREPARATION

1. Identify some behaviors or circumstances leading up to an explosive situation; for example, chemical or alcohol use, stress, sex, and holidays.

2. How have you protected yourself and your children from being hurt in this past? What has worked? What has been unsafe?

3. What supports do you have available? Friends? Family? Neighbors? Church? Counselors?

4. Are you familiar with the legal protection available to you?

5. Are you familiar with medical services available to you?

SAFETY PLAN CHECKLIST

_____ 1. Access to important phone numbers—police, friends, shelters, hotline

_____ 2. Access to transportation—money for the bus, extra set of car keys, taxi phone numbers

_____ 3. Important papers organized and ready to take in the event of sudden flight—Social Security card, legal papers, food coupons, driver's license, children's birth certificates

_____ 4. Access to money—cash, checkbook, savings account number, credit cards

_____ 5. Clothes—prepacked suitcase for you and your children

Figure 35–6
Safety-planning information that you could give to a woman during a screening or counseling session.

appropriately. The following five strategies may be useful in assisting the woman in breaking out of the cycle of abuse:

1. Guiding the woman toward examining her feelings
2. Helping the woman to look at her situation realistically
3. Supporting the woman during the decision-making process
4. Supporting the woman through any crises
5. Providing the woman with the opportunities to express her anger and to work through her depression

Specific facilitative and inhibitive nursing responses are shown in Box 35–8.

Tertiary prevention also involves long-term therapy, counseling, and rehabilitation offered to battered women, their children, and the batterer.

Therapeutic rituals may be substituted for violent rituals, wherein both the woman and the batterer learn new behaviors (Shami, 1995). Another approach is to assist the female victim in learning how to shift the balance of power within the marital dyad (Wileman, 1995). However, these therapeutic interventions should only be attempted when it has been unequivocally determined that the situation is sufficiently safe for such interventions to be attempted, and where the batterer is motivated and has some insight into the inappropriate-

ness of his violent behaviors. The primary consideration must be for the safety of the woman.

Many women and their children seek refuge in shelters, where they are assured physical safety, their basic material needs are met, and they find the much needed emotional support that allows healing to begin.

Shelters do not provide long-term solutions to the problems of abuse. They do provide a safe place for women to begin to make plans for the future. More than 50% of shelter residents return to their mates for varying lengths of time. Many women return to the shelter many times before finally deciding to leave their partner permanently. Box 35–9 includes information given to women seeking shelter at Maryland's House of Ruth.

Shelter staff assist abused women to develop problem solving skills. Crisis intervention is provided, and referrals are made for long-term counseling, including marital counseling. Figure 35–7 illustrates a model of nonviolence presented to residents as an alternative to the violence that has characterized their lives. Residents are encouraged to practice self-sufficient behaviors while residing in the shelter. They share in the daily chores of meal preparation, caring for children, laundry, and cleaning. Special attention is paid to the needs of children who have also been victimized either by being abused or by witnessing their mothers' abuse.

Nurses play important roles in shelters both in salaried and volunteer positions. The nurse's role includes

- Assessing health status of the residents
- Intervening to meet the health needs of residents
- Developing and coordinating programs designed to address the developmental and health needs of children
- Serving as a resource to shelter staff regarding access to other community services
- Offering support and guidance to the residents
- Serving as a health teacher on important topics such as prevention of sexually transmitted diseases, use of birth control methods, risks of cigarette smoking, nutrition, use of prescription medications, child care and development, and stress reduction
- Serving on the advisory board of the shelter that

evaluates and develops programs, reviews policies, and educates the community at large

Nursing faculty have used shelters as clinical placements for students. Such placements offer valuable learning experiences to nursing students and additional nursing resources to the shelter residents and staff. In other areas, nurses are managing employee assistance programs to reach out to abused nurses.

However, it must be pointed out that in the case of abused women, including abused nurses, the batterer may threaten to come into the workplace and beat or kill the woman there. Such threats, when reported to the employer or nurse manager, must be responded to quickly and firmly, using the organizational policies and procedures for processing such threats. It is essential not to dismiss such threats or to take them lightly, as some violent batterers are capable of entering the workplace and murdering the woman there.

T A B L E 3 5 – 2 Appropriate Interventions With an Abused Woman in an Emergency Situation

PROBLEMS	INTERVENTION
Life-Threatening Issues	
Physical injuries	Initiate body map detailing old and new injuries. Take photographs of injuries. Notify police if a serious injury (e.g., wound from weapon, head injury) to explain options to woman. Radiographic body map of old and new fractures.
Suicide risk	Psychiatric admission. Homicide risk assessment. Assist woman to assess her risk, explore possibility of having neighbors call police when they hear sounds of fighting. Teach woman to monitor frequency and severity of beatings. Initiate restraining order procedures. Discuss disarming gun or having police impound gun. Make sure woman has a safe place to go.
Health-Threatening Issues	
Sexual abuse	Allow freedom to discuss. Assure the woman of normality of her response to partner's behavior. Examine for vaginal and anal injury. Assess for sexually transmitted diseases. Collect evidence of rape. Explore contraceptive concerns.
Substance abuse	Discuss with the woman and make appropriate referral.
Depression	Refer to support group and/or mental health facility. Psychiatric admission if symptoms are severe enough or in presence of suicide intent.
Health-Related Issues	
Low self-esteem	Help the woman identify strengths. Let her know her reactions and feelings are normal. Refer to support group.
Support systems	Refer to the community nurse. Explore ways of expanding support system. Refer to supportive professionals.
Concern for children	Explore effects of abuse on the children. Explore adequacy of the children's health care.
Legal concerns	Explain the laws related to child abuse (make sure this is done by police if present). Show the woman her records.
	Discuss confidentiality and explain future access. Refer the woman to police for restraining order or arrest, and refer her to legal aid for divorce.
Alternative residency (family or shelter)	Refer the woman to shelter hotline. National Domestic Violence Hotline for shelter and battering information is 800-333-SAFE (7233).
	Initiate calls if the woman desires.
	Provide privacy and phone for the woman to initiate contact.
Obtaining belongings	Shelter hotline has suggestions.
Transportation	Police often will help.

Modified from Campbell, J. C., & Sheridan, D. J. (1989). Emergency nursing interventions with battered women. *Journal of Emergency Nursing, 15*(1), 14–15.

What do you think? Do you know anyone who stays in an abusive relationship? What are the reasons for staying? Do you have a helping role with this person? If so, what is the nature of that role?

➤ *Check Your Reading*

41. Give at least two nursing interventions aimed at primary prevention.
42. Give at least two nursing interventions aimed at secondary prevention.
43. Give at least two nursing interventions aimed at tertiary prevention.
44. Identify at least three potential roles for nurses working in shelters for abused women.
45. What is the battering syndrome?

Box 35–8 ■ ■ ■ ■ ■

Facilitative and Inhibitive Nurse Responses to the Abused Woman

Facilitative Responses

· Asking the woman if abuse is occurring
· Identifying behavior as abusive
· Acknowledging seriousness of abuse
· Expressing belief in the woman's story
· Acknowledging that the woman does not deserve the abuse
· Being directive in exploring resources
· Telling the man to stop the abuse
· Aiding the woman to consider full range of available options
· Avoiding telling the woman what to do
· Aiding the woman to evaluate her own strengths
· Suggesting tangible resources, such as a shelter or financial aid
· Offering support groups with other abused women
· Listening actively and empathically

Inhibitive Responses

· Demonstrating anger or irritation with the woman
· Blaming the woman
· Advising the woman to accept battering as better than nothing
· Withholding help until the woman leaves her abuser
· Aligning with the abuser
· Not responding to abuse after disclosure
· Advising the woman to leave her abuser

Modified from Limandri, B. (1987). The therapeutic relationship with abused women. *Journal of Psychosocial Nursing, 25*(2), 9–16.

Evaluation

The evaluation of nursing care is a formative and summative process. The formative evaluation is ongoing. The nurse who comes to know a woman better gains a greater appreciation of the woman's story, the processes she uses for decision-making, and the dilemmas facing her. This greater knowledge adds in the assessment and leads to mutual modification of goals, plans, and interventions.

The summative evaluation at the termination of the relationship is dictated by the mutually established goals and by the setting where the relationship between the nurse and the woman occurs. For instance, it would be unrealistic for a nurse in an emergency department to expect to see a woman permanently leave her abusing partner. A more realistic goal would be to make sure that the woman's immediate safety is ensured. In a longer-term relationship with an abused woman, however, you might assist the woman to work toward a permanent dissolution of the abusive relationship. The woman may be ready to leave her partner if the answer to the following questions is "yes":

· Has she begun to develop concrete plans about income, shelter, legal aid, and so on?
· Does she no longer worry about him but instead focuses on her own needs?
· Does she recognize abuse as a pattern rather than isolated incidents?

➤ *Check Your Reading*

46. What is important in a summative evaluation of nursing care for an abused woman?
47. Identify what is important in conducting a formative evaluation of the nursing care provided to an abused woman.

NURSING PROCESS WITH ABUSED CHILDREN

· Vernon. Two years old. Death due to fractures of the ribs and multiple tears of the liver, pancreas, and mesentery. The mother and her lover are on drugs. The mother says her lover beat the child.
· Sally. Five years old. Second-degree and third-degree burns on her hands and palms. Mother says the child's father punished her for being naughty by holding her hands over the stove.
· Anne. Five years old. Dead on arrival when brought to hospital by mother and police. Death attributed to overdose of methadone. Mother admits to being an addict and says she left the drug "lying around" (Fontana, 1983, pp. 48–49).

The stories go on and on. In 1962, Kempe and coworkers coined the term **battered-child syndrome** to describe the serious pattern of injuries frequently resulting in deaths in some of the children they were treating. These researchers undertook a nationwide survey of hospitals and law enforcement agencies in an

Box 35-9 ▪ ▪ ▪ ▪ ▪
Maryland Legal Remedies for Battered Women

Criminal Remedies

- *Police protection:* The police must respond to domestic disturbance calls in the same manner that they respond to all other calls for assistance. Police may arrest a person if the officer has an arrest warrant. Police may arrest on the scene without a warrant in all cases in which a crime was committed or attempted in the presence of an officer. Police may also arrest on the scene if the crime was not committed in their presence, if a weapon was used, and/or great bodily harm resulted. Police may also arrest without a warrant if the officer has probable cause to believe that the person battered his spouse or other family member with whom the person resides and there is evidence of physical injury and unless the person is immediately arrested he may not be apprehended or may cause injury or damage property or tamper with or dispose of evidence, if a report is made to the police within 48 hours of the incident.

- *Police accompaniment:* The police are required by law to accompany the battered woman back to the family home to retrieve clothes and personal belongings for the immediate use of her and her children. Use of this law is technically limited to married women but is routinely extended to unmarried women. Police usually cooperate with this law, but the officer's attitude may vary.

- *Criminal prosecution:* Any battered woman can bring criminal charges against her assailant. To do so she must obtain a police report number and request a court commissioner to issue either a warrant or a summons for her violent partner. The most common disposition of criminal charges is either probation or probation before judgment. Batterers are rarely incarcerated, and this generally occurs when they have an extensive violent criminal record.

Civil Remedies

- *Protection provided through the Domestic Violence Act:* Effective October 1, 1992, the *protection order* available to battered women has been changed. The new law in Maryland allows victims of abuse to receive protection, child support, and other financial support. The abuser can also receive counseling. *Abuse* is defined as an act that causes serious bodily harm or that places one in fear of imminent serious bodily harm. Assault and battery, sexual offenses, false imprisonment, and the abuse of a child or vulnerable adult also constitute abuse. If you have experienced any of this in your relationship with your partner, legal protection is available.

To be entitled to receive assistance under the new law, any one of the following must apply:
- You must be married to, separated from, or divorced from the abuser.
- If you are not married to the abuser but have a sexual relationship with him currently or in the past, you must have lived with the abuser for at least 90 days within the past year.
- You must be related to the abuser by blood, marriage, or adoption.
- You must be a parent, stepparent, child, or stepchild of the abuser and have lived with the abuser for at least 90 days within the past year.
- You must have children in common with the abuser, even if you are not married to him and don't live with him (the children must be biological or adopted).
- You must be an adult who is physically or mentally disabled (unable to provide his or her daily needs).
- If a child is being abused in the home, the following persons can ask the court for protection for the child: a blood relative of the child, an adoptive parent, a state's Attorney, or the department of social services in the county where the child lives.

There is a two-step process that you must follow to get a protection order against your abuser. You must go to the District Court or circuit court in your city or town and complete the paperwork provided by them detailing the incidence of abuse and your fear. If you are eligible for the ex-parte the judge can order protection from the abuser for up to 7 days and also give you temporary custody of the children. A hearing will then be scheduled in which you and the abuser appear before a judge to state your case. It is at this time that you can receive additional protection from the abuser. The judge can order your abuser out of your home for up to 200 days. He can also order other measures to protect you and your children.

For assistance in filing an ex-parte, the House of Ruth has an advocate available at the District Court of Baltimore City, Fayette and Gay Streets, room #303 (385-2263) from 8:30 to 12:30 Monday through Friday to provide you with support and assistance in going through this process.

For more information on legal options for battered women in Maryland, call the House of Ruth domestic violence legal clinic at 410-554-8463 or 410-554-8464.

From Maryland Legal Remedies for Battered Women from the House of Ruth, 2201 Argonne Drive, Baltimore, MD 21218.

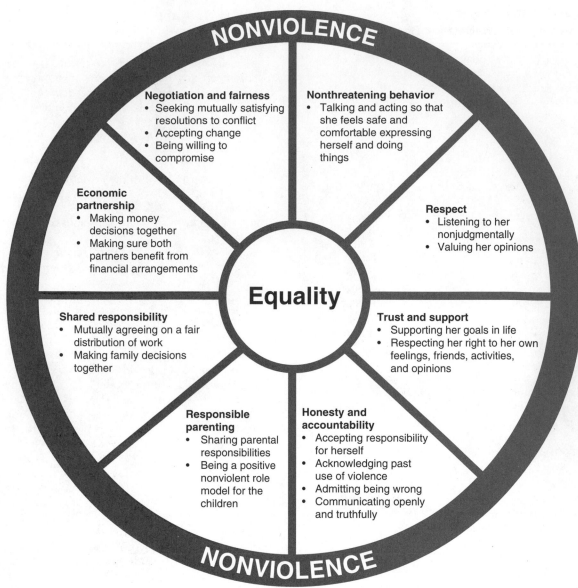

Figure 35-7
A model of nonviolence. (Redrawn from the Domestic Abuse Intervention Project, 204 West Fourth Street, Duluth, MN 55806.)

attempt to determine how many cases of physical abuse were reported in a year. The results were published in the *Journal of the American Medical Association.* Seventy-one major hospitals had reported a total of 302 patients with battered-child syndrome. Thirty-three of these children had died, and 85 had sustained permanent brain damage. Furthermore, 77 district attorneys had reported encountering 447 cases of child abuse (Fontana, 1983).

Kempe's landmark research served to raise the consciousness of physicians in the United States. Physicians began to look beyond the vague and incredulous explanations provided by parents about their child's injury. They began to look at radiographs showing evidence of old fractures, bruises in various stages of resolution, and unexplainable scars to tell them the stories of abuse that the child was too young or too frightened to tell.

The estimated incidence of child abuse exceeds those 1962 figures by at least 5000-fold. More than 2 million cases of child abuse are reported yearly; perhaps as many as 1 million cases go unreported. The numbers are staggering and almost incomprehensible. So are the ways in which adults abuse children. Children are bashed, lashed, beaten, flayed, stomped, suffocated, strangled, gut-punched, choked with rags, beaten with cords and wires, poisoned, sliced, ripped, steamed, fried, boiled, and dismembered. Adults use every conceivable weapon, including fists, belt buckles, straps, hairbrushes, lamp cords, sticks, baseball bats, rulers, shoes and boots, lead or iron pipes, bottles, brick walls, bicycle chains, pokers, knives, scissors, chemicals, lighted cigarettes, boiling water, steaming radiators, open gas flames, and drugs.

Many children seen today are likely to have serious injuries resulting from sudden explosive acts of violence, often precipitated by the child's crying, feeding behaviors, or toilet-training problems.

What do you think? As you read about stories of child abuse, what do you think is society's role in responding to these horrific stories? What should it be?

➤ *Check Your Reading*
48. What is the battered-child syndrome?
49. Who focused the nation on the plight of abused children?
50. What do the radiographs of battered children usually show?

Assessment

Not all children are at equal risk for the battering syndrome. Box 35-10 shows the risk factors for child abuse. Prompt identification and assessment of the abused child is essential to intervene and prevent some of the long-term consequences of abuse. Although most abused children do not grow into delinquent adolescents or even abusive adults, the risk is considerably higher for these children. They are also at risk for school problems, psychological adjustment difficulties, failed marriages, loss of productivity, and general psychopathology (McCloskey, Figueredo, & Koss, 1995).

Identification of the abused child begins with a complete history and physical examination. During the history-taking, note whether the history seems adequate or is lacking in comprehensiveness. Does the history come from one of the parents? If not, where are the parents? Are there any discrepancies or contradictions in the history? Has there been a delay in seeking treatment for the child's injuries?

Parents are interviewed about the child's social and medical history. Do the parents report past injuries? Are their explanations believable? Are the bruises in

Box 35–10 ■ ■ ■ ■ ■
Risk Factors for Child Abuse

- The child is physically, mentally, or emotionally impaired.
- The family is experiencing high levels of stress.
- One or both parents' childhood histories include substance abuse, depression, isolation, or abuse.
- One or both parents use or abuse alcohol or drugs.
- Society generally accepts parental right to use corporal punishment to discipline children.

places that are normally points of contact in a fall or accident? In some communities, hospitals are linked by a networked database that allows identification of children who have been taken to many different facilities for emergency care. If the child requires inpatient admission, the reaction of the parents is carefully observed and documented.

If abuse is suspected, the parents need to be informed regarding the suspicions of the health care team. Any suspicions of child abuse *must be reported to the child protective authorities.* Reporting is not a matter of judgment or choice; it is a matter of law. Health professionals are required to report their suspicions and are protected against litigation if their suspicions are found to be ungrounded. When making a report to the child protective authorities, document date, time, name and title or position of the person you spoke with; the information you gave to that person; and their response, for example: "Someone will investigate the reported abuse within _____ days." It is essential to document these points, as protective service agencies vary in their responsiveness to reported abuse, and staff capabilities and professional judgment in these agencies may also be highly variable. It is also useful to inform the party to whom you make the formal report that you are documenting the contact, your conversation, and their response to the information you have imparted.

The child should also be interviewed. The feasibility of interviewing the child depends on the child's age and physical condition. Figure 35–8 shows the TRIADS checklist a useful form in assessing for child abuse (Burgess, Hartman, & Kelley, 1990). This form can be used to guide the interview with the child. TRIADS is an acronym that encompasses the dimensions of child abuse:

- *T*ypes of abuse (physical, sexual, or psychological)
- *R*ole of the offender (intrafamilial or extrafamilial)
- *I*ntensity of the abuse (age when abuse began, number of times abused, and numbers of offenders involved)
- *A*utonomic response of the child: (1) numbness that may be manifested in depression, anger, hostility, or defiance; or (2) rebelliousness or hyperarousal manifested in night terrors, stomach aches, startle reflex, avoidance behaviors, crying, or enuresis
- *D*uration of the abuse (over what period has the abuse taken place)
- *S*tyle of the offender (whether the activities to the child were sudden or spontaneous; repetitively patterned; or ritualistic and ceremonial)

Comprehensive documentation is essential in cases in which child abuse is suspected. This documentation consists of the results of the physical examination, including radiographs and other specialized tests used for dating injuries, the history and interview, and photographs taken.

➤ *Check Your Reading*
51. What must you do if you suspect child abuse?

I. TYPE OF ABUSE

Physically Abusive Acts (check all that apply)

_____ 1. Bit, cut, punched

_____ 2. Deprived of meals

_____ 3. Physically restrained, tied up

_____ 4. Witnessing physical violence

Sexually Abusive Acts

_____ 5. Touching/fondling of breasts

_____ 6. Touching/fondling of genitals

_____ 7. Placing of finger into victim's vagina or rectum

_____ 8. Oral-genital sexual activity

_____ 9. Placement of penis into victim's vagina

_____ 10. Placement of penis into victim's rectum

_____ 11. Placement of object into victim's vagina

_____ 12. Placement of object into victim's rectum

_____ 13. Taking sexualized pictures of victim (e.g., naked)

_____ 14. Sexual acts with other victims

_____ 15. Witnessing sexual acts

Psychologically Abusive Acts and Threats

_____ 16. Being called derogatory names

_____ 17. Being told he or she was the cause of the abuse

_____ 18. Threatened not to tell about the abuse

_____ 19. Threatened he or she would be killed

_____ 20. Threatened parents would be killed

_____ 21. Threatened siblings would be killed

_____ 22. Threatened with loss of parents' love

_____ 23. Witnessing psychological abuse to others

Ritual Use of Any of the Following

_____ 24. Special table or altar

_____ 25. Sex involving unusual practices

_____ 26. Imitations and reversals of the Roman Catholic Mass

_____ 27. Excretions (e.g., semen, urine, feces, blood)

_____ 28. Circle

_____ 29. Chants or songs, especially with names of demons

_____ 30. Animals or insects

_____ 31. Robes or masks

_____ 32. Torches, candles, or darkness

_____ 33. Drugs or potions

_____ 34. Dismemberment or cannibalism

II. ROLE RELATIONSHIP OF VICTIM TO OFFENDER

_____ 35. Intrafamilial (biological)

_____ 36. Intrafamilial (step)

_____ 37. Extrafamilial, acquaintance

_____ 38. Extrafamilial, authority figure to child

_____ 39. Extrafamilial, caretaker to child

_____ 40. Extrafamilial, stranger

_____ 41. Age of offender

_____ 42. Male offender

_____ 43. Female offender

Figure 35–8
The TRIADS checklist for assessing child abuse. (From Burgess, A. W., Hartman, C. R., & Kelley, S. J. [1990]. Assessing child abuse: The TRIADS checklist. *Journal of Psychosocial Nursing and Mental Health Services, 28*[4], 13, 14.)

III. INTENSITY OF ABUSE

_____ 44. Age of victim when abuse began
_____ 45. Age of victim when abuse ended
_____ 46. Sex of child (M or F)
_____ 47. Multiple offenders
_____ 48. Multiple victims

Please estimate how many times abuse occurred.

_____ 49. 1 time
_____ 50. 5 to 10 times
_____ 51. 11 to 20 times
_____ 52. More than 20 times

IV. AUTONOMIC RESPONSE OF THE CHILD

_____ 53. Hyperaroused state   (describe): _____
_____ 54. Numbed state   (describe): _____
_____ 55. Frightened by threats: no   somewhat   very   extremely
_____ 56. Has continuing fears: no   somewhat   very   extremely

V. DURATION OF ABUSE

For what length of time did the abuse occur?

_____ 57. Less than 1 month
_____ 58. 1 to 6 months
_____ 59. 6 to 11 months
_____ 60. 1 to 2 years
_____ 61. 3 to 5 years
_____ 62. More than 5 years

VI. STYLE OF ABUSE

_____ 63. Single abusive incident: blitz
_____ 64. Multiple abusive incidents: patterned
_____ 65. Ritualistic abuse

Figure 35-8 *Continued*

52. What would you include in your nursing documentation regarding contact with a child protective agency and why?
53. What is the TRIADS checklist?
54. Identify two future problems that abused children are at greater risk for developing.

Diagnosis

The analysis of child abuse is generally done by a team of health care providers consisting of a physician, nurse, and social worker. They examine the assessment data and determine the answers to two questions:

1. Is the history consistent with the observed injury or injuries?
2. Could the child have received any of these injuries in the manner described?

The conclusions of this team may be presented in legal proceedings to determine whether the child should be removed from the custody of care providers.

Burgess and colleagues (1990) suggested that the analysis of the TRIADS checklist provides useful direction for intervention. For instance, if the child has been subjected to either patterned or ritualized sexual abuse, there is overwhelming arousal of the child's autonomic nervous system—so much so that the child's innate protective system is totally disrupted. The child's symptoms can be grouped under sensory, perceptual-cognitive, and interpersonal disruptions leading to the following potential nursing diagnoses:

• Sensory/Perceptual Alterations, hyperactivity, related to living in constant fear of abuse and evidenced by the mother's report that the child is difficult to manage and always on the "move"
• Sensory/Perceptual Alterations, nightmares, related to recurring thoughts and fears of being abused as evidenced by the child's waking up during the night crying and frightened and the child's verbalizations regarding content of nightmares
• Sensory/Perceptual Alterations, startle response, related to living in constant fear of abuse as evidenced by the child's quick startle response to any stimuli

- Sensory/Perceptual Alterations, internal and external cues that produce intrusion of images and auditory and kinesthetic information, related to the trauma as evidenced by the child's description of auditory and kinesthetic hallucinations
- Altered Thought Processes related to a sense of guilt and responsibility about the cause, predictability, and future concerns about abuse as evidenced by the child's verbalizations of personal blame
- Powerlessness related to the inability to assert and protect self and to repeated violations of personal boundaries by abuser as evidenced by the child's fearfulness when anyone touches the child
- Fear related to repeated incidents of abuse as evidenced by the child's withdrawal from others
- Altered Sexuality Patterns related to acting out actions previously directed toward self by abuser as evidenced by the child's sexually precocious verbalizations and acting-out behaviors

Outcome Identification

Some communities have done a better job than others in establishing home-based, family-centered interventions. The expected outcomes of such home-based programs are to

1. Decrease the stress in the home by providing many nontraditional child services including homemaker service, respite care, transportation, emergency child care, and vocational counseling
2. Assist the parents to learn alternative coping responses to deal with children
3. Improve communication patterns and methods of problem solving and to provide therapy for the parents and child(ren)
4. Children removed from a home need ongoing support and therapy. Burgess and coworkers (1990) suggested that the goals of therapy include
   - Desensitizing the child to the sensory and perceptual cognitive cues associated with the abuse
   - Assisting the child to master relaxation techniques to correct the sensory overload
   - Assisting the child to learn cognitive strategies to deal with the distress related to the trauma experience
   - Assisting the child to develop healthy relationships that allow the development of trust and empathy

Planning

The planning phase of care for the battered child revolves around whether the child remains in the home or not. Courts are reluctant to remove children from homes and efforts are made to keep families together.

What do you think? Occasionally, a child's death will be reported in the media. On investigation, it is learned that this child was well known to the child protection authorities and the child's family was frequently monitored for child abuse. When such situations occur what do you think of the court's approach to do everything to keep families together?

► *Check Your Reading*

55. State one expected outcome of nursing interventions with an abused child.
56. State two short-term goals of nursing interventions with an abused child.

Implementation

Primary Prevention

The primary level of intervention involves increasing community sensitivity to the issue of child abuse. You might be involved in education about the incidence of child abuse, the long-term sequelae to child abuse, and each community member's responsibility to report suspected cases of abuse. Primary prevention includes lobbying efforts to increase funding and resources that support educational efforts in this area.

Secondary Prevention

Secondary prevention involves identifying the child at risk and referring the child for appropriate treatment. It also involves the maintenance of 24-hour hotlines that allow potential abusers to defuse their angry and violent impulses.

Tertiary Prevention

The tertiary level of prevention involves intervening with the abused child as well as with the abuser. Recognize that for the cycle of abuse to stop, both the victim and the perpetrator need help. You may work directly with the abuser to examine patterns of abuse and alternative ways of responding, or you may refer the abuser to a mental health clinic or specific therapy group designed to deal with the problems of the perpetrator of abuse.

Abused children usually require long-term therapeutic support in the following areas:

- Providing corrective emotional experiences that allow the development of trust and empathy
- Teaching cognitive strategies such as thought-stopping, clarification, reframing beliefs, and linking stress directly to the trauma of abuse
- Role playing focused to teach the child to discriminate threatening exploitive behavior from safe behavior in others
- Desensitizing the fearful child to involvement with others
- Training in empathy skills
- Teaching relaxation
- Using psychopharmacological aids in achieving relaxation

Hartman and Burgess (1988) suggested a model that explains how the experience of abuse is processed by the child. This model, shown in Figure 35–9 includes four phases. The first looks at the characteristics of the child before the incident occurs. The second phase examines how the child processes the experience. The third focuses on what happens when and if the child discloses the experience. The fourth phase deals with the postabuse outcome.

➤ *Check Your Reading*

57. State one nursing intervention aimed at primary prevention.
58. State one nursing intervention aimed at secondary prevention.
59. Identify two areas of focus in long-term therapy with abused children.

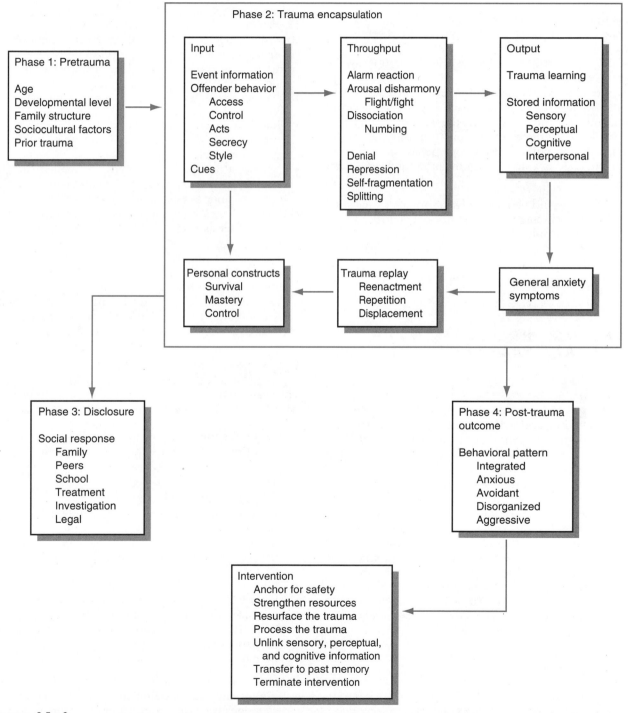

Figure 35-9

Information processing in victims. (Redrawn from Hartman, C. R., & Burgess, A. W. Information processing of trauma. *Journal of Interpersonal Violence,* 3[4], pp. 443–457, copyright © 1988 by Sage Publications. Reprinted by permission of Sage Publications, Inc.)

Evaluation

The evaluation of care for the abused child focuses on both formative and summative issues. The formative outcomes include the following questions:

- Is the abuser open to receiving assistance?
- Does the abuser remain involved in a therapeutic relationship?
- Is there abatement of the abuse to the child?

The summative evaluation focuses on the following questions:

- Has the cycle of abuse been broken?
- Is the abuser seeking help to change the responses to the child?
- Is the child still being physically, emotionally, or sexually abused?
- Is there evidence that the long-term consequences to abuse are abating (e.g., the child is performing better academically and socially in the school setting, the child is no longer acting out sexually aggressive behavior, the child's delinquent behavior is decreasing, the child is able to form meaningful friendships).

➤ *Check Your Reading*
60. What would be included in a formative evaluation of the nursing care of an abused child?
61. What would be included in the summative evaluation of the nursing care of an abused child?
62. What behaviors would indicate that the long-term consequences of child abuse were abating?

NURSING PROCESS WITH AN ABUSED ELDER

Assessment

The five types of elder abuse are physical, psychological, sexual, financial, and self-neglect. Frequently, they are seen in emergency departments with injuries that do not fit the description given by the caregiver. Other times, the abuse and neglect come to the attention of neighbors or community and home care nurses who have occasion to enter the elderly person's home and observe the living conditions. Others may observe the elderly person being psychologically abused by an elderly spouse or an adult child or grandchild. Financial abuse may come to the attention of others when the elderly person is unable to pay bills or buy groceries, medication, or other necessary items (Thobaben, 1993).

A study conducted by Fulmer and Ashley (1989) identified nine neglect indicators that strongly suggest that an elder is being neglected:

1. Poor hygiene
2. Poor nutrition
3. Poor skin integrity
4. Contractures
5. Urine burns or excoriation
6. Pressure ulcers
7. Dehydration
8. Impaction
9. Malnutrition

Fulmer and Ashley also suggest that the decision tree in Figure 35–10 be used in deciding whether or not a particular indicator points to neglect.

➤ *Check Your Reading*
63. What are the five types of elder abuse?
64. Identify at least four indicators of elder abuse.

Diagnosis

The analysis of data when an elderly person is being abused or neglected leads to nursing diagnoses that cover the gamut of physical, psychological, social, and spiritual issues that nurses are responsible to treat, including PTSD with dementia (McCartney & Severson, 1997). Possible nursing diagnoses might include

- Fluid Volume Deficit related to inadequate fluid consumption evidenced by poor skin turgor and imbalance in electrolytes
- Colonic Constipation related to inadequate fluid intake, lack of exercise, and inadequate nutritional intake of fiber as evidenced by impaction
- Pain related to injury sustained when pushed by son or daughter as evidenced by massive bruising on left side
- Spiritual Distress related to sense of isolation and betrayal by son or daughter as evidenced by verbalizations that "God has forgotten me"
- Nutrition, Less than Body Requirements, related to lack of money to buy adequate groceries as evidenced by loss of weight of 10 pounds in last 2 months

Outcome Identification

There are two expected outcomes for an elderly person who is abused or neglected. These long-term goals are

- Provide for the safety of the elder.
- Break the cycle of abuse and mistreatment.

Planning

Short-term goals for an abused elder might include the following:

- The patient will have normal fluid and electrolyte balance.
- The patient's injuries will heal completely.
- The patient will consume adequate calories for age, body size, and energy requirements.
- The patient will feel secure in his or her environment.
- The patient will be free from violence.
- The patient will experience spiritual well-being.

➤ *Check Your Reading*
65. Identify expected outcomes of nursing interventions with an abused elder.
66. Identify two short-term goals for an abused elder.

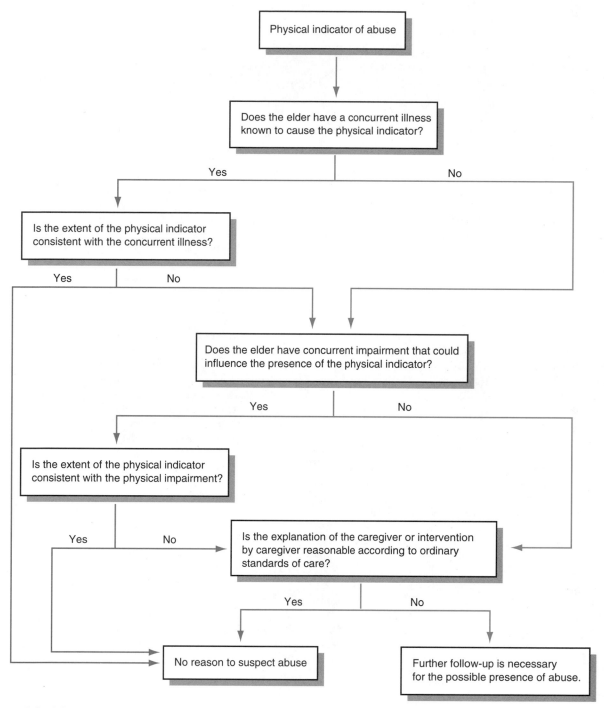

Figure 35–10
Clinical indicators of elder abuse. (Redrawn from Fulmer, T. T., & Ashley, J. [1989]. Clinical indicators of elder abuse. *Applied Nursing Research, 2*[4], 161–167.)

Implementation

Fulmer (1989) suggested that intervention in cases in which elder abuse is suspected requires a multidisciplinary approach. This process allows a particular nurse or case manager to obtain a variety of opinions about a given case and make appropriate decisions when planning care with an elderly person.

A key consideration when intervening is whether the elderly person is in immediate danger. If so, emergency action is taken to remove the elder. The nurse must consider whether anyone else in the environment is in danger. Are health care providers or protective service case workers who go into the home to intervene in danger? The goal is to protect the elderly person and anyone else from harm.

Box 35–11 ▪ ▪ ▪ ▪ ▪
Toward Prevention: Some Do's and Don't's

Toward Prevention . . . for Individuals

Do's

· Stay sociable as you age; maintain and increase your network of friends and acquaintances.
· Keep in contact with old friends and neighbors if you move in with a relative or to a new address.
· Develop a "buddy system" with a friend outside the home. Plan for at least a weekly contact and share openly with this person.
· Ask friends to visit you at home; even a brief visit can allow observations of your well-being.
· Accept new opportunities for activities. They can bring new friends.
· Participate in community activities as long as you are able.
· Volunteer or become a member or officer of an organization. Participate regularly.
· Have your own telephone; post and open your own mail. If your mail is being intercepted, discuss the problem with postal authorities.
· Stay organized. Keep your belongings neat and orderly. Make sure others are aware that you know where everything is kept.
· Take care of your personal needs. Keep regular medical, dental, barber, hairdresser, and other personal appointments.
· Arrange to have your Social Security or pension check deposited directly to a bank account.
· Get legal advice about arrangements you can make now for possible future disability, including powers of attorney, guardianships, or conservatorships.
· Keep records, accounts, and property available for examination by someone you trust as well as by the person you or the court has designated to manage your affairs.
· Review your will periodically.
· Give up control of your property or assets only when *you* decide you cannot manage them.
· Ask for help when you need it. Discuss your plans with your attorney, physician, or family members.

Don't's

· Don't live with a person who has a background of violent behavior or alcohol or drug abuse.
· Don't leave your home unattended. Notify police if you are going to be away for a long period. Don't leave messages on the door while you are away.
· Don't leave cash, jewelry, or prized possessions lying about.
· Don't accept personal care in return for transfer or assignments of your property or assets unless a lawyer, advocate, or another trusted person acts as a witness to the transaction.
· Don't sign a document unless someone you trust has reviewed it.
· Don't allow anyone else to keep details of your finances or property management from you.

Toward Prevention . . . for Families

Do's

· Maintain close ties with aging relatives and friends. Keep abreast of changes in their health and ability to live independently.
· Discuss an older relative's wishes regarding health care, terminal medical care alternatives, home care in the case of incapacitation, and disposition of his or her personal assets.
· Find sources of help and use them. Chore services, housekeeping, home-delivered meals, senior recreation, day care, respite care, and transportation assistance are available in many communities.
· With the older person's consent, become familiar with his or her financial records, bank accounts, will, safe deposit boxes, insurance, debts, and sources of income before he or she becomes incapacitated. Talk and plan together now about how these affairs should be handled.
· Anticipate potential incapacitation by planning as a family who will take responsibility, such as power of attorney or in-home caregiving if an aging relative becomes incapacitated.
· Closely examine your family's ability to provide long-term, in-home care for a frail and increasingly dependent relative. Consider the family's physical limits.
· Plan how your own needs will be met when your responsibility for the dependent older relative increases.
· Explore alternative sources of care, including nursing homes or other relatives' homes, in case your situation changes.
· Discuss your plans with friends, neighbors, and other sources of support before your responsibilities become a burden. Ask for their understanding and emotional support—you may need them.
· Familiarize family members with emergency response agencies and services available in case of sudden need.

Don't's

· Don't offer personal home care unless you thoroughly understand and can meet the responsibilities and costs involved.
· Don't wait until a frail older person has moved in with you to examine his or her needs. You need to consider access, safety, containment, and special needs. (Do you need a first-floor bathroom, bedroom, or entry ramp? Will carpets or stairs become barriers? Do you need a fenced yard to prevent the loved one from wandering away? Does your kitchen allow you to prepare special diets or store medications properly? Can you move the person safely in case of fire?)
· Don't assume that poor interpersonal relationships between you or other members of the household and the older person involved will disappear.

Box 35–11 ■ ■ ■ ■ ■

Toward Prevention: Some Do's and Don't's *Continued*

- Don't expect irritating habits or problems (e.g., alcohol abuse) to stop or be controlled once the dependent person moves into your home.
- Don't ignore your limitations and overextend yourself. Passive neglect could result.
- Don't hamper the older person's independence or intrude unnecessarily on his or her privacy. Provide a private telephone if you can and make other changes if possible.
- Don't label your efforts a failure if home care is not possible and you must seek an alternative.

Toward Prevention . . . for Communities

Do's

- Develop new ways to provide direct assistance to caregiving families. Improve crisis response to help families that face the difficult decision to discontinue home care.
- Through public awareness programs, advocate the cause of caregiving families and the needs of victims of mistreatment.
- Ask other community groups to become more involved in aging service programs, including those at nursing homes or senior citizen housing projects. Their involvement can lead to improved facilities and services.
- Encourage both public and private employers to help caregiving families, especially those with caregivers nearing or beyond retirement age, with fixed incomes and increasing health problems.
- Publicize available support services and professionals available to caregivers, such as senior day care centers, chore services, companions, and housekeeping services. Caregivers may not know about them.
- Give public agency employees basic training in responses and case management. They can be trained to recognize some of the causes of neglect or abuse of older persons and can help in support roles.
- Provide training for community gatekeepers and service workers—primary care physicians, public health and social workers, law enforcement officers,

transportation and utility workers, postal employees, and others—to help them recognize at-risk situations and take appropriate action.
- Expand Neighborhood Watch programs and similar community groups to include training on home care of the frail elderly, identification of the signs of mistreatment, and how to provide assistance or initiate preventive actions to reduce such victimization.
- Open your eyes and ears to the possibility that mistreatment is occurring. Become aware of individuals who are at risk. Develop procedures for investigation, public education, and public support of assistance to troubled families.
- Recognize that many forms of mistreatment or abuse are crimes. Volunteers can help victims file formal complaints, seek compensation for losses, seek prosecution of guilty parties, and give the victim assistance subsequent to prosecution. Prosecution can result in sentencing, diversion, training, counseling, or other types of family assistance services as alternatives to criminal sanctions. Urge public support of agencies to provide the necessary services.

Don't's

- Don't ignore family caregivers of dependent elderly. They are significant parts of the community. Community services can try to involve isolated people in appropriate services or self-help programs. Those at risk, or living in isolation, simply may lack knowledge or information and may welcome community outreach.
- Don't assume that gerontology is a study confined to universities and hospitals. Begin to educate the entire community about aging. (This should be as common in public education as information about child care.)
- Don't sensationalize stories of abuse of older persons. Instead, try to arouse public interest in techniques and strategies to prevent abuse.
- Don't start a major intervention just because an older person is alone or is said to be eccentric. The goal is to seek the least intrusive alternative.

Adapted from American Association of Retired Persons (1987). *Domestic mistreatment of the elderly: Towards prevention—some do's and don'ts* (Pamphlet). In T. T. Fulmer. (1989). Mistreatment of elders: Assessment, diagnosis, and intervention. *Nursing Clinics of North America, 24,* 707–716. © 1987, American Association of Retired Persons. Reprinted with permission.

In an effort to break the cycle of abuse, the second expected outcome, consideration must be given to the family considered as the patient, mandatory reporting laws, and long-term follow-up of high-risk and mistreated elders, with resolution as the goal (Penhale & Kingston, 1997). The family in the role of patient is an essential consideration. In cases of elder abuse, there is usually more than one person in the family unit in need of psychosocial or health intervention. For instance, if

an elderly woman is being abused by an alcoholic daughter, both mother and daughter need treatment.

You must be familiar with mandatory reporting laws in your state. Every Congress since 1974 has supported legislation that prevents harm to elders and treats the elderly, prompting states to pass elder abuse protection statutes. Box 35–11 developed by the American Association of Retired Persons (AARP), includes prevention tips for the elderly person, for families, and for communities.

Evaluation

The evaluation of nursing care for an elderly person who has been abused or neglected includes a formative and a summative aspect. Formative evaluation is ongoing and addresses the database, nursing diagnoses, plan, and achievement of short-term goals. The formative evaluation address the following questions:

- Is the patient safe?
- Are the patient's injuries healing?
- Has a normal balance been reestablished for nutrition and fluid needs?
- Is the patient adequately cared for?
- Is the patient feeling secure?
- Is the patient feeling spiritually well?
- Are the patient's caregivers receiving help?

The summative evaluation focuses on the safety of the elder and whether the cycle of abuse or mistreatment has ended.

➤ *Check Your Reading*

67. Why is a multidisciplinary approach the best when dealing with potential elder abuse?
68. Identify three questions that you would want answered in evaluating the care provided to an abused elder.

NURSING PROCESS AND VIOLENT PATIENTS

As violence in society has increased, so too has violence in hospital settings (Morrison, 1993). According to Distasio (1994), 65% of psychiatric staff members are assaulted by psychiatric patients. The prediction of who will erupt into violent behavior is the focus of a great deal of psychiatric research, with some progress being made in our ability to predict who among the mentally ill will become violent (Fulwiler, Grossman, Forbes, & Ruthazer, 1997; Crowner, Peric, Stepcic, & Ventura, 1995).

Linaker and Busch (1995) found that violent episodes in psychiatric patients were preceded by six behaviors: confusion, irritability, boisterousness, physical threats, verbal threats, and attacks on objects (these behaviors should be assessed by the nurse as the escalation stage of impending violence). Morrison (1993) cited five myths about violence in psychiatric settings that need to be debunked (Box 35-12).

Assessment

Distasio (1994) identified violence as a three-stage process. Figure 35-11 illustrates this violence continuum: the calm, or baseline, stage; the preassaultive stage, which can last for brief periods or for more extended periods; and the violent act or the assaultive acute excitement stage. Distasio (1994) also reports that intervention is possible during the preassaultive stage before the violence is impelled into action.

There are four key predictors of violence: diagnosis, history, legal status on admission, and presence or absence of dementia. The following psychiatric diagnoses are associated with violent behavior (Bjorkly, 1995; Grossman et al, 1995; Nestor, Haycock, Doiron, Kelly, & Kelly, 1995).

- Psychosis
- Bipolar disorder
- Mania
- Paranoia
- Dementia
- Substance abuse
- Personality disorders

Box 35-12 ◼ ◼ ◼ ◼ ◼
Commonly Held Myths About Violence in Psychiatric Settings

1. *The person with a mental illness who strikes out is viewed as out of control or impulsive.* Most incidents of violence are deliberate and chosen to get what the patient wants.
2. *Using a punching bag when angry decreases aggression and violence.* Social learning theory indicates that using a punching bag reinforces the likelihood that aggression will be repeated or will escalate to actual physical violence. Patients should be encouraged to talk over their anger with those involved. Appropriate limits must be set on the patient's behavior. Patients must be held responsible for their behavior. Negotiated contracts and brief time-outs are effective strategies in dealing with violence.
3. *For psychiatric nursing staff, doing a good job means helping patients regain control to ensure a safe environment.* Patients who have a coercive interactional style tend to use violence in settings in which the focus is on control.
4. *Aggression and violence occur when staff are inconsistent or are in conflict.* Research conducted on this relationship shows that only about 8% of patient violence is related to staff inconsistencies.
5. *The clinician who is afraid is most often the victim of assault.* When studying violence, two patterns have been found for the patient's choice of victim. Either patients assaulted other men, or they assaulted vulnerable others. It is generally the staff member without peer support who is the most vulnerable. Frequently, this staff member does not support the overuse of physical restraints and is "set up" by other staff for assaults from patients.

From Morrison, E. F. (1993). Toward a better understanding of violence in psychiatric settings: Debunking the myths. *Archives of Psychiatric Nursing, 7*, 328–335.

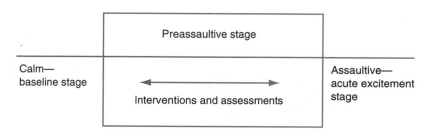

Figure 35-11
Violence continuum and stages. (Adapted with permission from Distasio, C. Violence in health care: Institutional strategies to cope with the phenomenon. *Health Care Supervisor, 12*[4], 1–34. © 1994, Aspen Publishers, Inc.)

Hillbrand (1995) found that self-destructiveness and suicide attempts prior to hospitalization correlated with the highest incidence of aggression against others in a hospitalized sample of 103 male forensic inpatients during a 3-year period. Friday (1995) presented striking evidence that violence has a psychological impact on children and young adults in the United States, particularly those in underserved communities, and discussed the implications of learning a pattern of behavior that routinely includes lifelong violence as part of one's environment and community.

A history of assaultive or violent behavior is an excellent predictor of future assaultive or violent behavior. When staff are aware of this aspect of the patient's history, violence is assumed to be a possibility in caring for this patient. Patients with a known history of violent behavior should never be underestimated.

Patients who are committed to a psychiatric facility by the court system are more prone to violent behaviors than patients who are admitted voluntarily. Involuntarily committed patients are frequently angry about having been committed, are not compliant with medications or other aspects of the treatment plan, and are usually hostile to staff members.

Patients with dementia often exhibit poor behavioral control. This dyscontrol is associated with hitting, punching, pinching, biting, and other aggressive acts. Staff caring for demented patients must exercise excellent judgment to maintain safety for themselves and others (Cahill, Stuart, Laraia, & Arana, 1991).

Usually it is possible to assess behaviors which indicate that the patient's behavior is escalating. These behaviors include the following (Distasio, 1994):

- Affective changes such as labile mood swings and inappropriate reactions.
- Pressured speech, response to hallucinations, intrusiveness, negative verbalizations, muttering to self.
- Motor agitation and inability to be still; pacing.
- Sudden changes in level of consciousness, confusion, increased disorientation.
- Reddened face, flaring nostrils, clenched fists, gritted teeth, glaring, angry facial expressions.

What do you think? Have you ever encountered violence in the clinical setting? If so, what did you do? What would you do to protect yourself and others from a violent patient?

➤ *Check Your Reading*
69. Identify four behaviors that should alert you to a patient's increasing agitation.
70. What are the four predictors of patient violence?
71. Why is it not an appropriate intervention to suggest that the patient defuse anger by using a punching bag?
72. Identify two myths that surround the issue of patient violence.

Diagnosis

The nursing diagnosis most appropriate in the situation of a potentially violent patient is Risk for Injury directed at others related to having limits placed on personal behavior and evidenced by pacing, muttering obscenities, and clenched fists (North American Nursing Diagnosis Association, 1999).

Outcome Identification

The expected outcomes of intervening with an angry and potentially explosive patient include

- The patient will refrain from violence.
- The patient will use nonviolent strategies to deal with anger.
- No one will get hurt.

Planning

The short-term goals for an angry and potentially explosive patient include the following:

- The patient will demonstrate greater calm.
- The patient's behavior will not escalate to the assaultive stage.
- The patient will experience a decrease in stress.

Implementation

When considering interventions to prevent or to deal with patient violence, nurses need to focus on the stages that occur across the violence continuum. These include the preassaultive stage, the assaultive stage, and the postassaultive stage, when the patient returns to baseline behaviors.

Preassaultive Stage of the Violence Continuum

Multiple interventions exist to deescalate violence. Staff require training in both verbal techniques of deescalation and physical techniques to restrain without harm so that they are prepared to respond to violent behavior (Patterson, Leadbetter, & McComish, 1997). Appropriate training is effective in decreasing injuries to patients as well as staff members, and can help them identify staff characteristics that increase the risk of assault (Lanza, Kayne, Hicks, & Milner, 1991).

Verbal interventions can be effective during the escalation stage when the patient is becoming more agitated. Stevenson (1991) identified eight broad areas involved in intervention.

ANALYSIS OF PATIENT AND SITUATION

As soon as you begin to determine exactly what the patient feels is needed, you have begun to intervene. During this process, you are attempting to hear the patient's feelings and concerns. If you already know the patient well, this time initially spent listening and attending to the patient's concerns may allow you accurately to determine the problem and a suitable solution. If you do not know the patient well, your role is primarily an observer, gathering sufficient information with which to plan an intervention.

Initially, you want to encourage the patient to go to a place that is quiet and safe. Frequently, this goal can be accomplished by telling the patient that you are concerned and want to listen. The patient needs the reassurance that people are interested and willing to help. It is essential during this beginning stage to acknowledge the patient's needs regardless of whether the expressed needs are rational or irrational, possible or impossible to meet. Clearly and simply state your expectations for the patient's behavior: "I expect that you will stay in control." Offer medication as needed, if it is available and appropriate.

USE OF VERBAL TECHNIQUES OF DEESCALATION

You need to be an excellent listener and able to respond to the patient in a therapeutic manner. The goal is to convey to the patient that you are calm, controlled, open, nonthreatening, and caring. You should maintain a relaxed poise. This may prove a challenge to the nurse who is feeling fear. Maintaining a calm exterior when your interior is in an upheaval requires considerable self-discipline.

The best stance is to accept your feelings of anxiety and fear. If you accept them and still continue trying to help the escalating patient, you will gain increased comfort and proficiency in dealing with these kinds of uncomfortable situations. In addition, patients, who are very sensitive to what is going on around them during their hyperaroused, escalating state, will undoubtedly be aware of your fears, but will still relate to you because they will sense that you are genuine and they are important enough for you to persist in your efforts to assist them in regaining self-control.

RESPECT FOR THE PATIENT'S PERSONAL SPACE

The personal space of the patient is an important consideration. If the patient is sitting, you should sit. Having your eyes on the same level as the patient's eyes decreases the sense of intimidation and gives the patient the message that you are communicating as equals. Allow the patient enough personal space, large enough so that the patient does not perceive you as intrusive but not so much that you and the patient cannot talk in a normal voice (Dill, Dill, Sibey, & Brende 1997). Persons who are poised for violence need up to four times more space than they would normally require.

The patient may invade your space with verbal abuse and use of profanity. You cannot take the patient's words personally or respond in kind. It is also important not to end the conversation because of the patient's verbal abusiveness or forbid the patient from communicating in this way. Abusive language may be the only way that the patient can express feelings.

INTERACTION WITH THE PATIENT

When you speak to the patient, your voice should be low and calm. Never respond to the patient with yelling, but continue to model controlled behavior. Using open-ended statements, such as "You think people are always unkind to you?" is more effective than asking, "What is wrong with you?" It is important to avoid ending statements with "Okay?" This may create ambivalence in the patient and give the erroneous impression that choices exist. Your interaction with the patient should not sound punitive, threatening, accusatory, or challenging. It is better to find out what is behind the patient's feelings and behaviors.

Honestly verbalize the patient's options. Encourage the patient to assume responsibility for the choices made. This approach decreases the sense of powerlessness that often precipitates violence. Do not, however, offer options that are not possible. Discovering that you have promised something you cannot deliver only increases the patient's anger. If the patient is unable to make a choice, acknowledge the patient's decision-making difficulty: "You seem too upset to make a decision right now. I will make the decision for you now."

AWARENESS OF POSTURE AND BODY LANGUAGE

Pay attention to your posture and body language while interacting with the patient. Body language needs to be congruent with the words spoken and the tone of your voice. Slouching sometimes conveys ease and relaxation, whereas arms folded across the chest denotes being closed and unwilling to listen to another person's ideas. Sometimes a gentle touch may be helpful, but *do not touch the patient if you are unsure about its appropriateness.* It is best to ask the patient, "Would it be okay if I touched your hand? I would like to comfort you." Without the patient's permission, given verbally or through body language, touching may be perceived as threatening and intrusive.

INVESTMENT OF TIME IN THE PROCESS

When you begin a verbal intervention, have a time frame in mind. The amount of time needed varies with the patient and the particular situation—depressed, suicidal, or frightened patients may require more time; manipulative patients should be given less time. According to Stevenson (1991), 8 to 10 minutes is usually sufficient initially; if progress is being made, the time can be extended. Limits need to be firmly yet gently set regarding time, informing the patient that there will be no further discussion of the matter. Once these limits have been set, see that they are consistently enforced.

ATTENTION TO THE ENVIRONMENT

Not only is it important to attend to the verbal techniques of deescalation but also the environment in which this occurs is critical. A quiet place, but one that is visible to staff, is most beneficial in helping a patient regain control. Staff should know who is working with the patient and for how long, so that uninterrupted time is allowed.

ASSURANCE OF THE NURSE'S SAFETY

If you are going to communicate in a calm manner, you must feel safe. There are some basic considerations for ensuring your safety. First, avoid wearing dangling earrings or necklaces. The patient may become focused on these, and serious injury is possible if the patient were to grab at them. If you are wearing such jewelry, take it off before going to deal with an agitated patient. Second, having enough staff for back-up is essential. Although you do not want to appear overly threatening, do not handle potential violence without this back-up. Only one person should talk to the patient, but staff need to maintain an unobtrusive presence in case the situation escalates.

Third, always know the layout of the area. The placement of furniture and the presence of obstacles or hazards are important to prevent injury if the patient requires **restraints.** Fourth, make sure that you are not standing directly in front of the patient or in front of the doorway; this position could be perceived as confrontational. It is better to stand off to the side and encourage the patient to have a seat.

Fifth, if you are interviewing a patient who begins to escalate, provide feedback to the patient about what you observe: "You seem to be very upset." Such an observation allows the feeling to be explored and may deescalate the situation. If the patient's behavior continues to escalate, end the interview and assure the patient that the staff will provide for the patient's as well as everyone else's safety. Sixth, avoid confrontation with the patient either through verbal means or through a show of force with security guards. Verbal confrontation and processing of the incident must occur when the patient is calm. The show of force by security guards

may serve to escalate the patient's behavior; therefore, security personnel are better kept in the background until they are needed to assist (Rosenthal, Edwards, Rosenthal, & Ackerman, 1992).

Assaultive Stage of the Violence Continuum

If the verbal deescalation techniques fail to calm the patient and the patient progresses to the assaultive or excitement phase, the staff must respond quickly. Generally a team approach of about five staff members is advisable, but the team may need to be larger if the patient requires it. One leader speaks to the patient and instructs members of the team.

Each team member is trained in the correct use of physical restraining maneuvers as well as the use of physical restraints. The team is organized before approaching the patient so that each team member is clear regarding individual responsibility for limb-securing assignments. Before approaching the patient, the team is prepared with the correct number and size of restraints and medication, if ordered. The team leader explains to the patient in a matter-of-fact manner exactly what the team is about to do and why. The team remains calm and acts to restrain the patient physically as quickly as possible and escort the patient to the locked seclusion room. If restraints are to be used, the patient is informed at this point of the team's intent and the reason for the team's actions. Sometimes, the patient is ready to cooperate and lies down on the bed with arms at each side. The patient is then restrained with either four-point or two-point restraints.

Once the patient is restrained, the nurse might administer an intramuscular injection of a benzodiazepine, a major tranquilizer, barbiturate, or antihistamine, depending on the physician's order. Your role in administering an intramuscular injection to an agitated patient is to provide an explanation to the patient for the medication and to make sure that the patient is properly restrained so that the medication can be safely administered. Note that chemical restraint (i.e., use of a medication to sedate a patient) is considered to be the most restrictive intervention, even more restrictive than mechanical restraints. Throughout this time, the team leader must continue to relate to the patient in a calm, steady voice, communicating decisiveness, consistency, and control.

While the patient is restrained and in **seclusion,** staff must closely monitor the patient to determine the patient's ability to reintegrate into the unit activities. Reintegration is gradual and is geared to the patient's ability to handle increasing amounts of stimulation. If the reintegration proves to be too much for the patient, resulting in increased agitation, the patient is returned to the room or another quiet area.

Generally a structured reintegration is the best approach. For instance, reintegration can begin by reducing a patient in four-point restraints to two-point restraints. Once the patient no longer requires restraints or once the patient no longer requires the locked seclusion room, the patient may be given specified time-out periods to leave the room and move slowly into the milieu of the unit. The time-out periods are gradually increased until the patient is able to maintain control within the unit.

Postassaultive Stage of the Violence Continuum

Once the patient no longer requires seclusion and restraints, the staff should process the incident with the patient as well as among themselves. Processing with the patient is an important part of the therapeutic process. Discussing what has occurred allows the patient to learn from the situation, to identify the stressors that precipitated the out-of-control behavior, and to plan alternative ways of responding to these stressors in the future.

Return to Baseline

The staff processing is critical for a number of reasons. First, a review is necessary to ensure that quality care was provided to the patient. The staff need to examine critically their responses to the patient. Questions to be answered include the following:

1. "Could we have done anything that would have prevented the violence?"
2. "If the answer is "yes," then what could have been done, and why wasn't it done in this situation?"
3. "Did the team respond as a team? Were team members acting according to the policies and procedures of the unit? If not, why not?"
4. "How do staff members feel about this patient? About this situation?" Feelings of fear and anger must be discussed and handled. Otherwise the patient may be dealt with in a punitive and nontherapeutic manner. Employee morale, productivity, use of sick leave time, transfer requests, and absenteeism are all affected by patient violence, especially if a staff member has been injured. Staff members must feel supported by their peers as well as by the organizational policies and procedures established to maintain a safe environment.
5. "Is there a need for additional staff education regarding how to respond to violent patients?"

➤ *Check Your Reading*
73. Why is verbal intervention so important during the preassaultive stage of the violence continuum?
74. Why is a team approach critical when dealing with a violent patient?
75. Identify three issues that you need to consider to protect yourself when you intervene with an agitated patient.

Documenting a Violent Episode

There are a number of areas that you must document in situations in which violence was either averted or actually occurred:

- The assessment of behaviors that occurred during the preassaultive stage
- The nursing interventions and the patient's responses
- An evaluation of the interventions used
- A detailed description of the patient's behaviors during the preassaultive and assaultive stage
- All nursing interventions used to defuse the crisis
- The patient's responses to those interventions
- How the patient was reintegrated into the unit milieu

Evaluation

The evaluation of the nursing care provided to a patient who is either potentially violent or who becomes violent is a critical step in the nursing process. It is necessary to evaluate the nursing staff's ability to avert violence whenever possible through deescalation techniques and to deal with violence in a manner that minimizes the chance of injury to both the patient and the staff. The evaluation is also important in determining whether factors inherent in the nurse-patient interactions or within the environment actually promote anger and violence. For instance, are staff interacting in a punitive and arbitrary manner without respect for patients' rights? When limit-setting is necessary, is it done in a respectful way? Are privacy needs of patients being respected? Is the unit overcrowded? Does the unit provide a healthy balance between structured time and quiet time? An evaluation of this type provides vital information about the quality of care, the adequacy of unit and organizational policies relating to safety, and the need for continuing staff education in the management of aggressive behavior.

What do you think? Should nurses be required to take courses in personal defense?

➤ *Check Your Reading*
76. What do you document in the the preassaultive stage?
77. What do you document in the handling of a violent episode?
78. Identify two areas of information provided in the evaluation of care for a patient who became violent.
79. Why is it important to look at the environment when evaluating care for a patient who became violent?

NURSING PROCESS APPLICATION

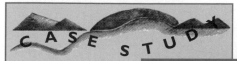

Rhonda

Rhonda, a 27-year-old mother of three preschool children, has had frequent emergency department visits for bruises, contusions, and two broken fingers. She relates that her husband has a fiery temper just like her father's and that he gets real mad when the children don't pick up their toys and behave. Rhonda confides that she is afraid that she will take her anger out on the children. She states that out of fearing for the children's safety, she will try to divert her husband's anger at the children to her. She has voiced the desire to get out of the abusive relationship but admits having few marketable skills and that the cost of supporting three children would not allow them to survive on a minimum-wage income.

ASSESSMENT

Assessment data are as follows:
- Contusions, bruises, broken fingers
- Unsafe home environment
- Few marketable skills
- Feelings of hopelessness and powerlessness

DIAGNOSIS

DSM-IV Diagnosis: Adjustment Disorder with Anxiety

Nursing Diagnosis: Powerlessness related to inability to control violent home situation as evidenced by physical injury and feelings of dissatisfaction over present life situation.

OUTCOME IDENTIFICATION, PLANNING, AND IMPLEMENTATION

> **Expected Outcome 1:** By _____ the patient will experience support, caring, and concern from staff and friends.

Short-Term Goals	Nursing Interventions	Rationales
By _____ the patient will experience a safe, supportive environment.	1. Reassure the patient of her safety. 2. Determine and make arrangements for safety of the children. Can they stay with a relative, or does the child protective services need to be contacted? 3. Explore effects of abuse on children and adequacy of their health care.	1–2. Safety is the primary goal for both the patient and children when abuse occurs. 3. It is important to be an advocate not only for the abused mother but also for the children.
By _____ the patient will have dealt with any life-threatening or physical injuries.	1. Take photos; initiate body map detailing old and new injuries. 2. Conduct assessment in private, being especially attentive of a nonjudgmental and gentle approach.	1. Documentation of injuries is an important legal function. The medical record may be used as evidence in legal litigation. 2. This type of approach maintains the patient's self-esteem.
By _____ the patient will experience comfort and power from other sources.	1. Encourage the patient to seek comfort from religious sources, that is, clergy, praying. 2. Provide privacy and support for any other additional measures, such as meditation or visual imagery.	1–2. Spiritual distress is very real for the abused. Often, it becomes difficult for them to pray or feel that God is a loving, powerful force in their lives.

Nursing Diagnosis: Risk for Violence: Directed at Others related to abusive environment as evidenced by outbursts of anger from her husband.

OUTCOME IDENTIFICATION, PLANNING, AND IMPLEMENTATION

> **Expected Outcome 1:** By _____ the patient will verbalize a plan to leave her partner and the abusive family situation.

Short-Term Goal	Nursing Interventions	Rationales
By _____ the patient will identify two strategies to break out of the cycle of abuse.	1. Provide educational information regarding the cycle of abuse. 2. Provide numbers and addresses for local shelters and the national and local hotline numbers for shelter and battering information. 3. Provide opportunities for the patient to control decisions about the plan of care, that is, arrange for social work to give information about financial alternatives. 4. Encourage the patient to express feelings such as anger, depression, and anxiety.	1–2. The role of education as primary prevention is important. Awareness of risk factors, cycle of abuse, and problems associated with battering are essential to be discussed with the patient. 3. Encouraging decision-making increases the patient's self-esteem and feelings of being in control of her life situation. 4. Expression of feelings provides opportunity for the patient to come to terms with the situation and work through feelings in a supportive atmosphere.

> **Expected Outcome 2:** By _____ the patient and her children will have a plan of safety and escape whether they leave or stay.

Short-Term Goal	Nursing Interventions	Rationales
By _____ the patient will have identified the components of a safety plan checklist.	1. Administer the TRIADS checklist and Campbell's danger assessment. 2. Review the components of safety planning for both the patient and her children. 3. Provide information about police protection and specific legal remedies for the patient.	1. Accurate assessment of the family situation is imperative for early intervention, so that both the patient and her children are assured physical safety. 2–3. Safety planning includes a plan to escape and information about police and legal protection.

EVALUATION

Formative Evaluation: Rhonda was able to meet all of her short-term goals, although she had the most difficulty in determining how she was going to separate herself from her husband and manage her affairs financially. Social work was helpful in presenting information on Aid for Dependent Children and various battered women and family shelters. Her children were placed in a program that provides for long-term therapeutic support in dealing with the violent family environment.

Summative Evaluation: Rhonda achieved all of the expected outcomes, including the decision to not take herself or her children back into the abusive environment. She and her children sought protection in a battered family's shelter. With assistance from the social worker and public attorney, she brought criminal charges against her husband, which involved issuing a warrant and restraining order. Other avenues of support, which the attorney explained to her are entitled to battered women under the Domestic Violence Act (1992), included financial and child support and placement of her husband into a counseling program that provides rehabilitation and services to the violent partner. Emotionally, Rhonda felt more powerful in making decisions to care for both herself and children. She told her nurse she felt like God had finally answered her prayers.

See the snapshot view of nursing interventions that facilitate the care and handling of a violent patient.

SNAPSHOT

Nursing Interventions Specific to Violence

What do you need to do to develop a relationship with a patient who exhibits violent or threatening behaviors?

- Examine your own feelings first. How does this patient, or other violent patients, make you feel and how will you manage your own feelings when you interact with the patient?
- Approach the patient with empathy and compassion, recognizing that the violent-prone or violent patient is in emotional pain also and that all behavior, including violence and threats, has meaning.
- Demonstrate respect for the patient by calling the patient by his or her proper name, unless and until the patient gives you permission or asks you to address him or her by another name.
- Approach the patient unhurriedly and with a calm and calming demeanor.
- Identify yourself and inform the patient that you will be there for the patient to talk with if he or she so desires.
- Be authentic.
- Respect the patient's private space and do not touch the patient or behave intrusively, for example, keep a comfortable, arm's length distance between yourself and the patient at minimum.
- Look the patient in the eye when speaking to him or her, but do not stare or do anything else that would suggest a confrontational or challenging attitude on your part.
- Remember that the violent patient is a human being and often, he or she is also frightened of the violent behaviors and the inability to self-control.

What do you need to assess regarding the patient's health status?

(*Tip:* Ask the most sensitive questions very gently and last, so that if the patient ends the interview abruptly, you will still have accessed other data.)

- Suicidal, homicidal, or other destructive thoughts.
- Ask the patient how he or she handles anger, disappointment, rejection, and the like.
- Response to frustration, for example, yelling, breaking or throwing inanimate objects, hitting people, punching holes in walls.
- Ask the patient how long he or she has been troubled by violent or threatening behaviors. For example, How did it start? When did it start?

- Assess for transgenerational familial violence (who, what, when, why, outcome?).
- Delusions (e.g., others in his or her environment are impersonating family members or significant others and therefore must be killed)
- How does the patient express his or her anger?
- Identify the patient's patterns of abusive or violent behaviors.
- How does the patient feel about his or her violent behaviors? Are they seen as wrong? As inappropriate?
- Does the patient think that his or her rage, anger, and violent or threatening behaviors are proportionate to the provocation?
- Is the patient a drug or alcohol (or both) abuser?
- What is the patient's physical health status?
- Assess the patient for any coexisting medical conditions.
- Assess the patient's medications.
- Assess the patient's compliance with the medication regimen.
- Obtain the patient's vital signs.
- When performing the physical assessment, observe for bruises, lacerations, healed wounds, etc., which may have been inflicted by others who were previously involved in altercations with the patient.
- What is the patient's nutritional status?
- Assess the patient's hygiene and overall physical conditions. Does the patient take care of himself or herself, or is there evidence of self-neglect or other self-destructive behaviors?
- What is the patient's physical response to frustration (e.g. sweating, reddened face, pacing, fist clenching)?
- What kind of social support system does the patient have, if any?
- What is the patient's understanding of why he or she is in the mental health system?
- What are the patient's feelings about his or her violent or threatening behaviors?
- Is the patient motivated to learn how to better manage his or her unacceptable behaviors?
- Does the patient have the ability and readiness to learn to change his or her violent behaviors?
- What is the patient's experience with the criminal justice system, that is, has the patient ever been arrested? Convicted? Incarcerated?
- Is the patient a court-ordered psychiatric referral?

What do you need to teach the patient and/or the patient's caregiver/significant other?

- How to avoid triggering the patient's violent or threatening behaviors.
- How to recognize escalation and impending violence early.
- Verbal deescalation

Continued on following page

SNAPSHOT

Nursing Interventions Specific to Violence *Continued*

- Removal of self and others from around the patient as a safety measure when necessary
- Medication purpose, side effects, interactive and cumulative effects, food and drug interactions, adverse reactions, and so forth
- Importance of compliance with the medication regimen
- Relationship between medication and behavioral control
- Steps the patient can take when he or she gets angry and begins to feel loss of control
- Stress management exercises and techniques
- Maintaining safety
- Emergency measures and interventions
- Avoidance of self-blame in caregivers if or when patient loses control, that is, nothing justifies violence and they did not provoke the patient's out-of-control behaviors
- Spiritual well-being as part of the healing process for both the patient and his or her family and significant others (if the latter are still in the patient's support system)

What skills will you want the patient and/or caregiver to demonstrate?

- Ability to use stress management techniques effectively
- Compliance with the medication regimen
- Ability to adhere to the plan of care
- Ability to identify and verbalize feelings
- Ability to use thought-stopping techniques and other cognitive strategies to deal with distorted thinking that may precede violent episodes
- Ability to remove oneself from a situation to avoid loss of control, that is, taking a time out
- Ability to structure day-to-day time and activities
- Coping skills and safety measures

What other health professionals might need to be a part of this plan of care?

- Physician or psychiatrist who will be responsible for the overall plan of care
- Social worker to assist the patient in access to community resources
- Parole or probation officer to ensure that the patient maintains compliance with any court-ordered psychiatric treatment (this is also a good motivator to remain in treatment for some violent patients).

Conclusions

Violence is a growing problem in the United States. We read about it daily in our newspapers; we see the graphic pictures on the covers of popular magazines; and we are inundated with the details of drive-by shootings and other random acts of violence in our television news broadcasts. The problem is not limited to streets and ghettos but reaches into our homes, our workplaces, our places of worship. Wives are battered by husbands, children are battered by parents, and grandparents are battered by grandchildren. We should not be surprised that the violence has spilled over to health care facilities and is a major concern for health care providers in emergency departments as well as in psychiatric settings. *Violence is a public health problem,* and its direct and indirect effects on each of us is profound:

- Lifestyle changes; people are less trusting of anyone outside their immediate family circle; avoidance of nighttime or after-dark activities.
- More apprehension about those with mental illness.
- More fearfulness of the homeless, with little, if any, distinction between the mentally ill homeless and other homeless.
- Frequent fearful thoughts about violence and ways to avoid becoming a victim of violence.
- Fear of random violence, (e.g., drive-by shootings).
- Fear of one-time stranger violence (e.g., robbery, rape, burglary).
- Fear of workplace violence, regardless of the workplace setting.

Nursing's role extends beyond that of direct caregiver (Glass, 1997). Nurses have a responsibility to the community to provide education, to lobby legislators to change laws that support violence, and to lend their support to activities that reach out to the victims of violence. Professionally, nurses need to show care, concern, and support for colleagues who are the victims of violence. They need greater involvement in community and professional associations that facilitate participation in the legislative process. Nurses must continue to practice ethically and function as patient advocates. Finally, they must lend their support and participation to the health care agendas of their state nursing associations and ANA's grassroots political groups, which are in the forefront of nursing advocacy associations for programs, laws, and methods to intervene in the escalating cycle of violence.

Key Points to Remember

- Violence includes any acts carried out with the intention of causing physical pain or injury to another person.
- Abuse is difficult to define. Gil (1975) defined it to mean any acts of commission or omission by a parent or a person, an institution, or society as a whole that deprive a child of equal rights and liberty or interfere with or constrain the child's ability to achieve optimal developmental potential.
- Neglect represents acts of omission rather than a physical act of commission.
- Sexual abuse is the involvement of dependent and developmentally immature children and adolescents in sexual activities that they do not fully comprehend, to which they are unable to give informed consent, or that violate social taboos of family roles.
- The extent of violence in families is great. About 2 million women are abused every year; about 20% of all murder victims are related to their assailants.
- Most crimes committed by relatives are committed by spouses or ex-spouses. Pregnancy offers no immunity against violence.
- More than 2 million children are abused every year.
- About as many adolescents are mistreated as younger children.
- Incest is estimated to occur in about 14% of all families.
- Approximately 500,000 to 1 million elders are abused yearly.
- Family violence is usually accompanied by brainwashing of the victims.
- Victims frequently assume responsibility for the abuse; this process is called the hostage response.
- Victims of family abuse frequently experience shame, guilt, embarrassment, and extreme spiritual distress.
- Family violence tends to be repeated and grow worse over time.
- Other forms of victimization include sibling violence and abuse, abuse of parents by children, and elder abuse.
- Contributing causes to family violence include few costs for family violence, absence of effective social controls, inequality in the family structure, social attitudes that support violence, value of privacy, biological factors, psychiatric illness, personal characteristics of the abuser, alcohol and drugs, and abuse as mutual combat.
- Two types of violence between spouses are instrumental violence and expressive violence.
- Sometimes abused women are further abused spiritually by people who distort Scripture and religion.
- The American Nurses Association has taken an official position against violence.
- There are a number of assessment screens for assessing the abused woman.
- The interview of the abused woman must be gentle and direct.
- Pregnant women who have been abused generally present at emergency departments expressing concern over the health of the baby.
- Documentation is critical when a woman has been abused. Nursing notes may be subpoenaed if the woman presses charges against her assailant. Document all evidence of injury, use a body map to show the location of injury, and take pictures of injuries.
- It is vitally important when assessing an abused woman to determine her safety.
- The cycle of abuse includes a period of increasing tension; followed by an explosion of anger; followed by the honeymoon, or reconciliation, phase.
- Sexual abuse is another area to assess for in working with women.
- When working with an abused woman, avoid anything that sounds like blaming her for her situation.
- Primary prevention with battered women includes education of the community regarding the risks of abuse.
- Secondary prevention with battered women includes screening activities that occur within the community.
- Tertiary prevention with battered women includes emergency treatment, counseling, and the work that goes on in shelters.
- The battered-child syndrome was identified in 1962 by Kempe and colleagues to describe the serious pattern of injuries frequently resulting in death in some of the children they were seeing.
- Whenever you suspect child abuse, you must report it to the child protective authorities.
- The TRIADS checklist is an excellent form for assessing child abuse.
- The interventions used in cases of child abuse also include primary, secondary, and tertiary prevention.
- Five types of elder abuse are physical, psychological, financial, sexual, and self-neglect.
- Fulmer and Ashley (1989) have identified nine neglect indicators for elder abuse: poor hygiene, poor nutrition, poor skin integrity, contractures, urine burns, pressure ulcers, dehydration, impaction, and malnutrition.
- Intervention in cases of elder abuse is best done by a multidisciplinary team that focuses on making sure the elder is safe, ensuring the environment is safe for the elder, and working with the family.
- As violence increases in society, it is also increasing in the health care system.
- Violence occurs along a continuum moving from the baseline stage, to the preassaultive stage, to the assaultive–acute excitement stage.
- Four key predictors of violence are diagnosis, history, legal status on admission, and presence or absence of dementia.
- During the preassaultive stage of violence, verbal deescalation can be effective.
- The assaultive stage requires a crisis team approach involving seclusion, mechanical restraints, and use of medication.

- During the postassaultive stage, the patient is gradually reintegrated into the unit; the incident is processed both with the patient and with the staff.

- Evaluation of the nursing care provided to a patient who became violent may suggest the need for staff continuing education and revision of unit policies and procedures.

Learning Activities

1. Watch the made-for-television movie *The Burning Bed*, with Farrah Fawcett. What factors supported the violence that was directed toward the character played by Fawcett? What led to her killing her spouse? What does the movie suggest to you about society's response to abused women?
2. Find out what facilities are available for abused women in your community. Take a field trip to a shelter for abused women and find out how the shelter operates. What services do they offer? Who pays for those services? Who goes there for help? What can you do to help in the problem of violence against women and children?
3. Call the child protective services and inquire about procedures for handling a report of potential child abuse.
4. Find out about the laws in your state regarding your role in reporting elder abuse.
5. Find out if your local prison or criminal justice system has a rehabilitation program for violent offenders. If so, ask if the program permits outsiders to visit as a learning experience, for example, groups that visit and talk with inmates enrolled in the program about their personal life experiences, events that led to their incarceration, their thinking about the actions and behaviors that resulted in their incarceration, and actions they are taking to change their behaviors.

Critical Thinking Exercise

Bill Bains, a 35-year-old dual diagnosis patient was admitted by the court system 10 days ago, following an incident in which he drove his car through the neighbor's front porch. Before the car incident, Bill had just been told by his wife that she was not interested in a man who could not keep a job. He had recently been fired from his job as assistant police chief in their small town. The staff members were concerned that Bill was suicidal and attempted to delay his discharge as long as possible. Finally, Bill's physician, Dr. Yu, suggested to him that the team would review his case and consider his discharge. Pacing the hall with his suitcase in tow, Bill waited for the team's approval of his discharge. At 10:00 AM, Dr. Yu told Bill that the team wanted him to wait 1 more day.

1. What evidence might suggest Bill's potential for violence?

2. What assumptions do you think Bill is operating under?

3. What possible reactions might Bill have?

As Dr. Yu was informing Bill of the team's decision, Nurse Roberts was on the phone calling a code blue (a silent emergency code for an assault team). Bill turned to Dr. Yu and shouted, "You S.O.B., you lied to me!" Pushing the doctor, he bolted out of his room and yelled, "I've got to get out of here and find a job." Nurse Roberts standing near Bill's room, said to Bill, "Can you listen to what the team decided?"

1. How might Bill respond to Nurse Roberts' words?
2. Evaluate Nurse Roberts' response based on your evaluation of Bill's violence potential.
3. Consider alternate reactions; what else could happen as a result?

Additional Resources

Minnesota Center Against Violence and Abuse (MINCAVA)

http://www.mincava.umn.edu

National Domestic Violence Hotline

800-333-7233 (SAFE)

Pacific Center for Violence Prevention

http://www.pcvp.org/

SafetyNet Domestic Violence Resources

http://home.cybergrrl.com/dv/

Sexual Assault Information Page

http://www.cs.utk.edu/~bartley/saInfoPage.html

References

Andreason, N., & Black, D. (1995). Suicide and violent behavior. In N. Andreason & D. Black (Eds.), *Introductory textbook of psychiatry* (2nd ed.). Washington, DC: American Psychiatric Press.

Attorney General's Task Force on Family Violence. (1984). *Final report*. Washington, DC: U.S. Department of Justice.

American Psychiatric Association. (1994). Diagnostic and statistical manual of mental disorders (4th ed.). Washington, DC: Author.

Berger, G. (1990). *Violence and the family*. New York: Franklin Watts.

Bjorkly, S. (1995). Trauma and violence: The role of early abuse in the aggressive behavior of two violent psychotic women. *Bulletin of the Menninger Clinic, 59*, 205-220.

Botsis, A., Plutchik, R., Kotler, M., & Van Praag, H. M. (1995). Parental loss and family violence as correlates of suicide and violence risk. *Suicide and Life Threatening Behavior, 25*, 253-260.

Brennan, W. (1997). Pressure . . . violence and aggression in the workplace. *Nursing Times, (93)(43)*, 29-32.

Breighner, J. (1992, May 27). Your child learns [giving great comfort]. *The Catholic Review*, p. 15.

Bryant, S., & Range, L. (1995). Suicidality in college women who were sexually and physically abused and physically punished by parents. *Violence and Victims, 10*, 195-201.

Burgess, A. (1985). Advancing the science of victimology. *Journal of Psychosocial Nursing, 23*(1), 35-38.

Burgess, A. W., Hartman, C. R., & Kelley, S. J. (1990). Assessing child abuse: The TRIADS checklist. *Journal of Psychosocial Nursing and Mental Health Services, 28*(4), 6-14.

Cahill, C. D., Stuart, G. W., Laraia, M. T., & Arana, G. (1991). Inpatient management of violent behavior: Nursing prevention and intervention. *Issues in Mental Health Nursing, 12*, 239-252.

Campbell, J. C. (1986). Nursing assessment for risk of homicide with battered women. *Advances in Nursing Science, 8*(4), 36-51.

Campbell, J. C., & Sheridan, D. J. (1989). Emergency nursing interventions with battered women. *Journal of Emergency Nursing, 15*(1), 12-17.

Chabrol, H., Talmon, N., Peresson, G., & Alengrin, D. (1995). Psychopatholog of victims of aggression. *Medicine and Law, 14*, 631-633.

Child Abuse Prevention and Treatment Act of 1974, Pub. L. No. 93-247.

Collier, J. A. (1987, May). When you suspect your patient is a battered wife. *RN*, 22-25.

Copel, L. (1996). *Nurse's clinical guide to psychiatric and mental health care*. Springhouse, PA: Springhouse Corporation.

Crowner, M., Peric, G., Stepcic, F., & Ventura, F. (1995). Psychiatric patients' explanations for assaults. *Psychiatric services, 10*, 614-615.

Dabbs, J., Carr, T., Frady, R., & Riad, J. (1995). Testosterone, crime and misbehavior among 692 male prison inmates. *Personality and Individual Differences, 18*, 627-633.

Dill, B., Dill, J. E., Sibcy, G. A., & Brende, J. (1997). The registered nurse's role in the office treatment of patients with histories of abuse: A proposed treatment model. *Gastroenterology Nursing, 20*, 162-167.

Distasio, C. (1994). Violence in health care: Institutional strategies to cope with the phenomenon. *Health Care Supervisor, 12*(4), 1-34.

Draucker, C. (1997). Impact of violence in the lives of women: Restriction and resolve. *Issues in Mental Health Nursing, 18*, 559-586.

Dutton, D., van-Ginkel, C., & Starzomski, A. (1995). The role of shame and guilt in the intergenerational transmission of abusiveness. *Violence and Victims, 10*(2), 121-131.

Ferrato, D. (1991). *Living with the enemy*. New York: Aperture.

Finkelhor, D., & Yllö, K. (1985). License to rape: Sexual abuse of wives. New York: Holt, Rinehart & Winston.

Frieze, I. H. (1983). Investigating the causes and consequences of marital rape. *Journal of Women in Culture and Society, 8*, 532-553.

Fontana, J. V. (1983). *Somewhere a child is crying*. New York: Mentor.

Forward, S. (1989). *Toxic parents*. New York: Bantam Books.

Friday, J. (1995). The psychological impact of violence in underserved communities. *Journal of Health Care for the Poor and Underserved, 6*, 353-359.

Fulmer, T. T. (1989). Mistreatment of elders: Assessment, diagnosis, and intervention. *Nursing Clinics of North America, 24*, 707-716.

Fulmer, T. T., & Ashley, J. (1989). Clinical indicators of elder neglect. *Applied Nursing Research, 2*, 161-167.

Fulwiler, C., Grossman, H., Forbes, C., & Ruthazer, R. (1997). Early-onset substance abuse and community violence by outpatients with chronic mental illness. *Psychiatric Services, 48*, 1181-1185.

Gage, R. B. (1991). Examining the dynamics of spouse abuse: An alternative view. *Nurse Practitioner, 16*(4), 11-16.

Gelles, R. J. (1977). Power, sex and violence: The case of marital rape. *Family Coordinator, 26*, 335-347.

Gelles, R. J., & Straus, M. A. (1988). *Intimate violence*. New York: Simon and Schuster.

Gil, D. (1975). Unraveling child abuse. *American Journal of Orthopsychiatry, 45*, 346-356.

Glass, C. (1997). Domestic violence: Personally challenging the nursing profession. *Lamp, 54*(2), 4-6.

Grossman, L., Haywood, T., Cavanaugh, J., Davis, J., & Lewis, D. (1995). State psychiatric hospital patients with past arrests for violent crimes. *Psychiatric Services, 46*, 790-795.

Guilleminault, C., Moscovitch, A., & Leger, D. (1995). Forensic sleep medicine: Nocturnal wandering and violence. *Sleep, 18*, 735-748.

Hartman, C. R., & Burgess, A. W. (1988). Information processing of trauma. *Journal of Interpersonal Violence, 3*, 443-457.

Helton, A., McFarlane, J., Anderson, E. T. (1987). Battered and pregnant: A prevalence study. *American Journal of Public Health, 77*, 1337-1339.

Hillard, P. J. (1985). Physical abuse in pregnancy. *Obstetrics and Gynecology, 66*, 185-190.

Hillbrand, M. (1995). Aggression against self and aggression against others in violent psychiatric patients. *Journal of Consulting and Clinical Psychology, 63*, 668-671.

Janz, M. (1990, September/October). Clues to elder abuse. *Geriatric Nursing*, 220-222.

Kaerkkaeinen, J., Raeisaenen, M., Huttunen, J., Kallio, E., Naukkarinen, H., & Virkkunen, M. (1995). Urinary excretion of bufotenin (*N, N*-dimethyl-5-hydroxytryptamine) is increased in suspicious violent offenders: A confirmatory study. *Psychiatry Research, 58*, 145-152.

Kempe, C. H., Silverman, F. N., Steele, B. F., Droegmueller, W., & Silver, H. K. (1962). The battered-child syndrome. *Journal of the American Medical Association, 181*, 105-112.

Klaus, P., & Rand, M. R. (1989). *Family violence. Bureau of Justice Statistics Special Report*. Washington, DC: U.S. Department of Justice.

Koop, C. E. (1987-88). Family violence "appalling." *The Washington COFO Memo, Coalition of Family Organizations, 7*(4), 1.

Kraus, R. (1995). An enigmatic personality: Case report of a serial killer. *Journal of Orthomolecular Medicine, 10*(1), 11-24.

Landes, A., Foster, C. D., & Siegel, M. A. (1991). *Domestic violence: No longer behind the curtains*. Wylie, TX: Information Plus.

Lanza, M. L., Kayne, H. L., Hicks, C., & Milner, J. (1991). Nursing staff characteristics related to patient assault. *Issues in Mental Health Nursing, 12*, 253-265.

Linaker, O., & Busch, I. Predictors of imminent violence in psychiatric inpatients. (1995). *Acta Psychiatrica Scandinavica, 92*, 250-254.

McCartney, J., & Severson, K. (1997). Sexual violence, post-traumatic stress disorder and dementia. *Journal of the American Geriatrics Society, 45*(1), 76-78.

McCloskey, L., Figueredo, A., & Koss, M. (1995). The effects of systemic family violence on children's mental health. *Child Development, 68*, 1239-1261.

Menuck, M. (1983). Clinical aspects of dangerous behavior. *Journal of Psychiatry and Law, 11*, 227-304.

Moldofsky, H., Gilbert, R., Lue, F., & MacLean, A. (1995). Violence, sleep, nocturnal wandering: Sleep-related violence. *Forensic Sleep Medicine 18*, 731-739.

Monroe, R. R. (1970). *Episodic behavioral disorders* (p. 25). Cambridge, MA: Harvard University Press.

Morrison, E. (1993). Toward a better understanding of violence in psychiatric settings: Debunking the myths. *Archives of General Psychiatry, 7*, 328-335.

Moss, V. A., & Taylor, W. K. (1991). Domestic violence. *AORN Journal, 53*, 1158-1164.

Neidig, P. H., Friedman, D. H., & Collins, B. S. (1984). *The violence continuum: A conceptual model of spouse abuse with clinical implications.* Unpublished manuscript.

Nestor, P., Haycock, J., Doiron, S., Kelly, J., & Kelly, D. (1995). Lethal violence and psychosis: A clinical profile. *Bulletin of the American Academy of Psychiatry and the Law, 23,* 331-341.

North American Nursing Diagnosis Association. (1999). *NANDA nursing diagnoses: Definitions and classification 1999-2000.* Philadelphia: Author.

Parker, B., & McFarlane, J. (1991). Identifying and helping battered pregnant women. *Maternal Child Nursing, 16,* 161-164.

Patterson, B., Leadbetter, D., & McComish, A. (1997). De-escalation in the management of aggression and violence. *Nursing Times, 93*(36), 58-61.

Penhale, B., & Kingston, P. (1997). Elder abuse, mental health and later life: Steps towards an understanding. *Aging and Mental Health, 1,* 296-304.

Perry, O., & Daugherty, T. (1995). Trait anxiety of college males who witnessed murder or injury as a child. *College Student Journal, 29,* 243-245.

Pihl, R., Young, S., Harden, P., Plotnick, S. T., Chamberlain, B., & Erwin, F. (1995). Acute effect of altered tryptophan levels and alcohol on aggression in normal human males. *Psychopharmacology, 119,* 353-360.

Risk for violence, self-directed or directed at others (NANDA). (1996). In *Nursing diagnosis: Definitions and classification, 1997-1998.* Philadelphia: NANDA.

Rosenthal, T. L., Edwards, N. B., Rosenthal, R. H., & Ackerman, B. J. (1992). Hospital violence: Site, severity and nurses' preventive training. *Issues in Mental Health Nursing, 13,* 349-356.

Russell, D. E. H. (1982). *Rape in marriage.* New York: Macmillan.

Saltman, J. (1986). *The many faces of family violence* [Pamphlet 635, p. 4]. New York: Public Affairs Pamphlets.

Schenck, C., & Mahowald, M. (1995). A polysomnographically documented case of adult somnambulism with long-distance automobile driving and frequent nocturnal violence: Parasomnia with continuing danger as a noninsane automatism? *Sleep, 18,* 765-772.

Selby, T. L. (1992, April). Nurses face growing risk of violence and abuse. *The American Nurse, 3.*

Shami, M. (1995). Using rituals in couple therapy in cases of wife battering. *Journal of Family Therapy, 17,* 383-395.

Stamp, G., & Sabourin, T. (1995). Accounting for violence: An analysis of male spousal abuse narratives. *Journal of Applied Communication Research, 23,* 284-307.

Stark, R., & McEvoy, J. (1970). Middle-class violence. *Psychology Today, 4*(11), 52-54, 110-112.

Stevenson, S. (1991). Heading off violence with verbal de-escalation. *Journal of Psychosocial Nursing and Mental Health Nursing, 29*(9), 6-10.

Straus, M. A., & Gelles, R. J. (1988). Societal change and change in family violence from 1975 to 1985 as revealed by two national surveys. *Journal of Marriage and Family, 48,* 465-479.

Straus, M. A., Gelles, R. J., & Steinmetz, S. K. (1980). *Behind closed doors: Violence in the American family.* New York: Anchor Books.

Tardiff, K. (1989). The current state of psychiatry in the treatment of violent patients. *Archives of General Psychiatry, 49,* 493-499.

Thobaben, M. (1993). Elder abuse. *Home Healthcare Nurse, 6*(4), 37-38.

Tilden, V. P., & Shephard, P. (1987). Battered women: The shadow side of families. *Holistic Nurse Practitioner, 1*(2), 25-32.

Volkow, N., Tancredi, L., Grant, C., Gillespie, H., Valentine, A., Mullani, N., Wang, G., & Hollister, L. (1995). Brain glucose metabolism in violent psychiatric patients: A preliminary study. *Psychiatry Research, 61,* 243-253.

Weingourt, R. (1990). Wife rape in a sample of psychiatric patients. *Image: Journal of Nursing Scholarship, 22*(3), 144-147.

Whitehorn, D., & Nowlan, M. (1997). Towards an aggression-free health care environment. *Canadian Nurse, 93*(3), 24-26.

Whittington, R. (1997). Violence to nurses: Prevalence and risk factors. *Nursing Standard, 12*(5), 49-56.

Wileman, R., & Wileman, B. (1995). Toward balancing power in domestic violence relationships. *Australian and New Zealand Journal of Family Therapy, 16,* 165-176.

Wilson, M., Johnson, H., & Daly, M. (1995). Lethal and nonlethal Violence against wives. *Canadian Journal of Criminology, 37,* 331-361.

Suggested Readings

Bain, E. (1997). Safe Nursing: A call to nursing educators for the next millennium. *Massachusetts Nurse, 67*(4), 3, 7.

Bai, Y., Liu, C., & Lin, C. (1997). Risk factors for parasuicide among psychiatric inpatients. *Psychiatric Services, 48,* 1201-1203.

Clarke, P., Pendry, N., & Kim, Y. (1997). Patterns of violence in homeless women. *Western Journal of Nursing Research, 19* 490-500.

Distasio, C. (1994). Violence in health care: Institutional strategies to cope with the phenomenon. *Health Care Supervisor, 12*(4), 1-34.

Elliott, P. (1997). Violence in health care: What nurse managers need to know. *Nursing Inquiry, 4,* 257-261.

Everett, L. W. (1990). A family violence shelter as a place for psychiatric-mental health nursing students. *Nurse Educator, 15*(3), 67.

Ferrato, D. (1991). *Living with the enemy.* New York: Aperture.

Harris, G., & Rice, M. (1997). Risk appraisal and management of violent behavior. *Psychiatric Services, 48,* 1168-1176.

Hunter, K. (1997). Violence prevention in the home health setting. *Home Healthcare Nurse, 15,* 353-359.

Hurlebaus, A., & Link, S. (1997). The effects of an aggressive behavior management program on nurses' levels of knowledge, confidence, and safety. *Journal of Nursing Staff Development, 13,* 260-265.

Moss, V. A., & Taylor, W. K. (1991). Domestic violence. *AORN Journal, 53,* 1158-1164.

Murray, M. G., & Snyder, J. C. (1991). When staff are assaulted. *Journal of Psychosocial Nursing and Mental Health Nursing, 29*(7), 24-29.

Otiniano, M., Herrera, C., Hardman, M. (1997). Abuse of Hispanic elders: A case study review. *Clinical Gerontologist, 18*(1), 39-43.

Rad, J. P., Stern, A. L., Wolfe, J., & Ouimette, P. C. (1997). Use of a screening instrument in women's health care: Detecting relationships among victimization history, psychological distress, and medical complaints. *Women and Health, 25*(3), 1-17.

Shea, M., Mahoney, M., & Lacey, J. (1997). Breaking through the barrier to domestic violence intervention. *American Journal of Nursing, 97*(6), 26-34.

Tardiff, K., Marzuk, P. M., Leon, A. C., & Portera, L. (1997). A prospective study of violence by psychiatric patients after hospital discharge. *Psychiatric Services, 48,* 678-681.

Thobaben, M. (1993). Elder abuse. *Home Healthcare Nurse, 6*(4), 37-38.

Ward, S. (1997). Violence is not dignity, excellence, service, or justice. *Surgical Services Management, 3*(7), 6.

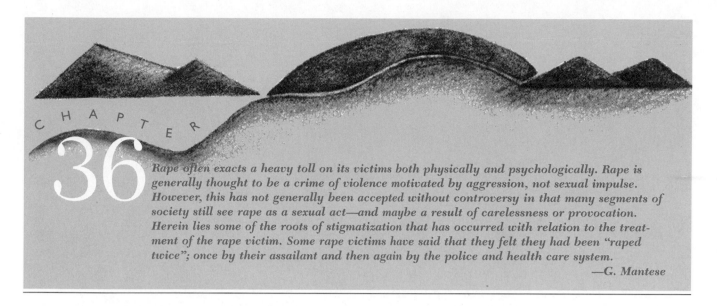

Rape

Learning Objectives

After studying this chapter, you should be able to:

1. Describe the types of sexual assault and identify their risk factors.
2. Describe the expected short-term and long-term reactions of victims of sexual assault.
3. Define and describe Rape-Trauma Syndrome.
4. Describe the nurse's role with the victim of sexual assault.
5. Describe nursing research to promote the development of legislation aimed at helping victims of sexual assault.
6. Describe an innovative nurse examiner program that was developed to meet the forensic and supportive clinical needs of victims of sexual assault.
7. Identify expected outcomes and short-term goals for patients who have experienced rape.
8. Apply the nursing process to a patient situation in which Rape-Trauma Syndrome is the nursing diagnosis.

Key Terminology

Acute Stress Disorder	Posttraumatic Stress Disorder	Sexual assault	Sexual harassment
Attempted rape	Rape	Sexual coercion	Sexual imposition
Evidence	Rape-Trauma Syndrome	Sexual contact	

Rape is a devastating act with far-reaching and often long-lasting consequences. It is an act of violence in which the perpetrator violates the personhood of the survivor while exerting absolute control. This heinous act has been with us since the beginning of recorded history. Rape played a prominent role in Greek mythology. The Bible chronicles historical incidents of rape.

More recently, during the Bosnian war, women and children were being raped as the world looked on in horror at the level of atrocities that were being committed (Weaver, 1993).

The outcomes of this violent act show similarities to the story of Persephone, which follows, who though sad and resistant to being taken by force, eventually is able to seek and receive the pity of her captor, returning to earth and the birth of spring. If only each survivor were able to recover from this trauma of rape and be reborn. But even Persephone is doomed to relive forever her journey to the dark underworld, where she had been swept away against her will to become the "mate" and thus sexual partner of the powerful male ruler of the kingdom of the dead (Tomaino, 1991).

Persephone's Story

Persephone, young, beautiful, and innocent daughter of harvest goddess Demeter in the ancient Greek legend, wanders alone to the shade of forest trees in a meadow by the sea to pick flowers. She is suddenly swept up by the strong arm of Hades, king of the underworld, and forced to be his mate. She cries out and resists her kidnapper but is unable to escape his strong, forceful attack. Kept in the underworld against her will, she refuses to eat or drink and withers and grows very sad. Finally, Hades takes pity on her and allows her to return to her family on earth but not before she eats four pomegranate seeds. When Persephone returns to earth, the flowers sprout and spring returns. However, because she has eaten these seeds of the forbidden fruit of the underworld, she is destined always to return to Hades for 4 months in the year, and the season of winter is born. ■

The story of Persephone is an allegory shielding the reader from the true terror of the person being raped. A first-person account graphically recounts the horror and powerlessness of a rape victim.

Jane's Story

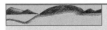

I got raped about 3 years ago about this time of year. At the time I was married and living with my husband in a rather dangerous part of town. One night we had been attending a community meeting together . . . at the meeting I felt he was putting me down and ignoring what I had to say and so I left by myself. . . .

I was still very angry when I left and got on the subway. I was preoccupied with my anger at my husband, and I wasn't noticing what was going on around me. So when I got off the train, I didn't notice the fact that a man was following me. In the neighborhood where I was living, it was rather dark and we rarely saw any police. I just got off the train and I was walking along with my head down and thinking and not noticing footsteps behind me until I got to my house. I got to my house and went into the entryway. This man suddenly appeared and slipped through the door behind me. He had a gun. At that point he said (he looked sort of excitable), "Do what I tell you, I won't hurt you."

He made me leave the building and took me down the block and across the street. While he was taking me there—with this gun on me—a car passed and there were people around the block and nobody noticed anything. Even if I could have attracted attention, I had no confidence that anybody would help me and that people would just mind their own business. If I tried to call out to somebody, I would end up getting shot.

This man made me go behind a building, and as we were going behind the building, there were people in lighted apartments with windows open and I didn't call out to them. They could hear us going around the building, but nobody noticed or nobody decided to mind anybody's else's business. Nobody came to investigate or anything.

And . . . um . . . he . . . um. So, the man . . . um. He forced me to take off my lower clothing; he forced me to have intercourse with him behind this building. Before the actual rape took place, I was frantically trying to talk him out of it by saying things. "You don't want me." Like, you know, he was white. "I'm ugly, I'm black, and you don't want me. . . ."

After the rape I didn't feel anything. I was trying to think like he was thinking so that he would let me go and not kill me . . . because he certainly had the power to do that . . . he had hurt me and he had promised he wouldn't . . . so, it was real weird, like he was real chummy and started talking to me, offering me a cigarette and telling me that he had just gotten out of jail and he hadn't had a woman for so long that he couldn't wait. I was acting as though I was real concerned for him because he had this gun, right?

And, okay, we were having this discussion and the chummy thing about the cigarettes afterward, but every once in a while he would say, "Are you going to tell anybody?" and he still had the gun. "You're not going to tell anybody, are you?" and like these threats in between this friendly conversation. And so I said, "No, I'm not going to tell anybody. No, I'll certainly not." I told him I wouldn't even tell my husband because my husband would kill me. And no, I wouldn't do that, I wouldn't tell anybody. And so he finally believed me and we got back onto the street and he disappeared. ■

Although there is certainly no "typical" rape survivor, Jane's story illustrates the surprise, shock, horror, bargaining for one's life, and potential for shame that are characteristic of the journey marked by rape. The remainder of this chapter explores not only these reactions but also the nurse's role in caring for rape survivors, definitions of rape and related terms, incidence and demographics of rape, types of rape, the impact of nursing research, the Rape-Trauma Syndrome, and the application of the nursing process to a patient who has been raped.

THE ROLE OF NURSES IN THE JOURNEY MARKED BY RAPE

Rape is one of the fastest-growing violent crimes reported in the United States. Victims of this crime are cared for by both psychiatric nurses and nurses in a variety of clinical settings. Rape survivors typically enter the health care delivery system through the emergency department but may also be seen in pediatric units, intensive care units, medical-surgical units, ambulatory care facilities, physician's offices, women's clinics, psychiatric settings, or in the community. Nurses may play a significant role in providing treatment for rape survivors as well as their families as they try to make sense of what has happened and attempt to get their journey back on course.

Emergency Department Nurses

The nurse in the emergency department frequently has the first caring contact with the rape survivor. The emergency department nurse, or specially trained rape team nurse, is responsible for providing emotional support and physical treatment for possible sequelae of the trauma, including prophylactic treatment for potential sexually transmitted disease and pregnancy. The nurse also participates in ensuring the accurate collection of **evidence,** such as pictures of injuries and semen samples, which are used to prosecute the perpetrator of the crime (Holloway & Swan, 1993).

Psychiatric, Community, and Ambulatory Care Nurses

Nurses who work within the community, in ambulatory care, or in mental health settings often see rape survivors who are struggling to recover from the trauma. The nurse provides continued caring through counseling, support, and referral to support groups for rape survivors. It is important that nurses within all clinical settings are knowledgeable about the possible long-term psychological sequelae of the rape experience on the patient's journey. Nurses need to understand normal and abnormal coping patterns and to be able to teach about these issues (Ruckman, 1992). In addition, increasing public awareness of rape through community teaching activities allows nurses to become active in rape prevention and to influence public policy.

What do you think? Have you ever known anyone who was raped? What was that person's experience in the aftermath of the rape? What happened to that person in the hospital?

➤ *Check Your Reading*
1. What is unique about the emergency department nurse in relation to the rape survivor?
2. Identify two of the services provided to rape survivors by nurses working in the community and in ambulatory care settings.
3. What is the nurse's role in collecting evidence from a rape survivor?

DEFINITION OF RAPE AND RELATED TERMS

The legal definition of rape differs from state to state, which leads to much confusion and ambiguity. Today the terms criminal sexual conduct, **sexual assault,** and rape can be used interchangeably. They refer to any type of sexual contact without consent between two or more people, regardless of their sex or marital status. Sexual contact may involve the sex organs of one or both, including any degree of penetration, no matter how slight, of the vagina or anus by a penis, hand, or object (Ledray, 1994). **Rape** within the scope of this chapter refers to any forced sex act with lack of adult consent. In this expanded definition, men are included as rape survivors.

Related to rape are other forms of sexual victimization. These are different from sexual intercourse and penetration, yet they produce common sequelae and long-lasting damage to the survivor.

For example, **attempted rape** involves force or threat of force to have sexual intercourse against the person's consent. It differs from rape only in that penetration has not occurred. Threat or actual force is present, so that the intended victim may actually fear for her or his life.

Sexual harassment involves nonconsensual sexual activity obtained from a person through abuse of a power relationship, such as a teacher or boss.

Sexual imposition involves the use of actual force or threat of harm to obtain sexual favors, for example, kissing or petting.

Sexual contact involves the nonconsensual touching of the intimate body parts of a person, such as breasts or buttocks.

Sexual coercion refers to ostensibly consensual intercourse that occurs subsequent to intense verbal coercion, including emotional pressure, threats to end the relationship, or false promises (Koss & Harvey, 1987).

It is likely that these different types of sexual victimization result in traumatic aftereffects, in that attitudes toward men, sexuality, and intimate relationships are influenced. The overall traumatic impact of sexual victimization depends on the survivor's past experiences, perception of the experience, and the trauma itself (Hall, Hirschman, Graham, & Zaragoza, 1993).

What do you think? As you read these very formal definitions of different types of sexual victimization, can you identify with any of them? Have you ever experienced any of them? If so, what was your reaction?

➤ *Check Your Reading*
4. Define rape.
5. Define sexual harassment.
6. What is the difference between sexual contact and sexual coercion?

DEMOGRAPHICS OF RAPE

A typical rape survivor does not exist. Of the reported survivors, 93% are female, 5% to 10% are male, and 90% of perpetrators are male. Although one can be raped at any age (Tyra, 1993), women between the ages of 16 and 19 are at the greatest risk. It is projected that one of every six women is raped sometime in her lifetime. Nonwhite women are likely to be raped at a younger age, between ages 12 and 19, whereas white women are at highest risk between 20 and 34. As Brownmiller (1975) pointed out, rape can be a crime of opportunity. Women who live in urban lower-class neighborhoods having high rates of crime and juvenile delinquency are subject to the greatest risk. Black, teenage, urban lower-class girls are the group of women who run the greatest risk of being assaulted. Twenty-nine percent of women are raped in their own home and 28% are raped in their car. Only 2% are raped in the street (Ledray, 1994).

Male victims of rape have great difficulty reporting the crime because of stigmatization, fear of being ridiculed or not believed, shame, wanting to forget, fear for their lives, or they see no point in reporting it. Twenty-three percent report fearing for their lives if they report (King & Woolett, 1997). Rapes can occur anywhere, not just in the stereotypical prisons or in isolated living situations. Sixty-five percent of men reporting rape state that it occurred in their home or the home of their assailant. Thirty percent had been assaulted by a member of their family and 25% report being assaulted by more than one person (usually three persons) (King & Woolett, 1997). The motivating factor of the perpetrator is not one of homosexual attack because of sexual desire resulting from deprivation but that of violence and domination. Some rapists who define themselves as heterosexual rape both men and women. Table 36–1 provides profiles of types of rapists.

➤ *Check Your Reading*
7. Why are black, teenage, urban, lower-class girls at greatest risk for sexual assault?
8. What is the motivating factor when men rape other men?

INCIDENCE OF RAPE

Rape affects the lives of thousands of people each year. The statistics on rape in the United States alone are alarming. It has been estimated that a rape is reported every minute of every day. One out of every four women born in the United States will be raped at some point in her life (Ledray, 1994). The number of reported rapes increased dramatically during the 1970s, with a 59% rise from 1970 to 1977 alone. The increase of reported rapes

was likely the result of a more responsive legal system as well as the establishment of rape crisis centers across the United States. Between 1978 and 1987, there was a 34.8% increase in reported cases of rape, compared with an increase of 2.8% in murders. This increase in reported rapes was higher than for any other violent crime except aggravated assault, which had a 49.6% increase (Mantese et al., 1991).

These statistics are even more alarming because only one out of every five rapes is actually reported. The most frequent reason (39%) for not reporting rape is the woman's own feelings of guilt for somehow causing the rape. Other reasons include being too embarrassed to tell anyone (35%), fear of police response (23%), and feared retribution from the assailant (19%), whose parting words often were "If you tell anyone . . . I'll rape your daughter next" or "I'll kill you the next time." Another 19% believed that reporting the rape would do no good (Ledray, 1990).

> **W**hat do you think? Do you know anyone who was raped and did not report the crime? What were the reasons for not reporting the rape? How has the individual coped with the aftermath of the crime?

➤ *Check Your Reading*
9. State three reasons why women do not report being raped.
10. Identify two possible reasons why rape statistics have increased so dramatically.

TYPES OF RAPE

Marital Rape

The basis for marital immunity appears to have been the opinion published in 1736 by then chief justice of England, Matthew Hale. It was his view that "the husband cannot be guilty of a rape committed by himself upon his lawful wife, for by their mutual matrimonial consent and contract the wife hath given up herself in this kind unto the husband which she cannot retract" (Trevelyan, 1991, p. 40).

Clearly the law today has moved from viewing a woman as the property of her husband to viewing her as an equal partner in the marriage. In 1965, the Law Commission (United Kingdom) was set up by statute to promote reform of the law and pointed out that a husband's right to sexual intercourse was not now enforceable by the courts. It argued that "a woman, like a man is entitled on any particular occasion to decide whether or not to have sexual intercourse, outside or inside marriage" (Trevelyan, 1991, p. 36). A husband has no immunity from conviction for indecent assault. Therefore, a wife who has been raped by her husband can take him to court. There continues to be some differing interpretations of this law, and conflicting decisions have been rendered by different judges.

TABLE 36-1 Profiles of Types of Rapists

TYPE	INCIDENCE (%)	CHARACTERISTICS
Power—assurance	80%	Rape to resolve doubts about manhood and feelings of sexual inadequacy Select victims their own age Rape close to home Talk and use little force even though they carry a weapon for control Low self-esteem Average intelligence Low achievers Loners Nonathletic Degrade women and don't trust them Seldom have a relationship with a woman
Power—assertive	10–12%	Act out anger and induce fear in victim Threatening and threaten to kill Degrade the victim Use profanity Often use obscene, threatening phone calls Expose themselves Outgoing, social, self-confident, smart, athletic, well dressed Often drive a flashy car Like traditional masculine activities and sports Appear to like women Meet people in singles bars Healthy sexual appetite that is not easily satisfied They want the woman to fight them during sex Multiple orifice assault Attacks are sporadic with no set pattern Intelligent and often able to evade police Become more violent with each rape
Anger—retaliation	5%	Express anger against women Target older women in their 60s and 70s Kick and beat victims violently, leave bruises Rape near their homes Rape infrequently, usually once a year Rape is spontaneous Rape day or night, and usually as a result of a fight with a woman They are not drunk during rape, but drink before and after Explosive temper, impulsive Hate women and are usually divorced Unable to keep a job
Anger—excitation	2%	Terrify victim Most dangerous; victims are found murdered Keep the victim alive for days before killing Plan for months before picking victim Elaborate torture setting in home Con their victim into going home with them Keep elaborate records of their victims—names, dates, pictures, details Often outdoorsmen; collect and know guns and knives Intelligent No prior arrest record Have big dogs Victims can be women but are often men Easy to prosecute once caught because of the files they keep

From: RECOVERING FROM RAPE, 2nd Edition by Linda E. Ledray, © 1994 by Linda E. Ledray. Reprinted by permission of Henry Holt and Company, LLC.

As of 1990, there remain only seven states in the United States that still have spousal exclusion laws against a wife claiming marital rape. It is important to remember that even though a wife can now report marital rape in 43 of the 50 states in the United States, most will not or cannot (Ledray, 1994). Research has shown that women who experience significant depressive symptoms, anxiety, panic disorders, and present clinically with these issues or somatic equivalents should be assessed for potential abuse by their husbands. This might be the only chance that many marital rape situations will be addressed or discovered (Thelen, 1998; Weingourt, 1990).

> *What do you think?* Knowing these facts about marital rape, how should this knowledge inform your nursing practice with women?

> ► *Check Your Reading*
> 11. What is marital rape?
> 12. What has supported marital rape as an accepted practice?
> 13. What is the relationship between marital rape and depression and anxiety in women?

Date and Acquaintance Rape

Growing in recognition, but still often unreported, is the phenomenon of date and acquaintance rape. Approximately 75% of all rapes are date or acquaintance rape (Anglin, Spears, & Hutson, 1997). Investigations indicate that up to 78% of interviewed women had experienced some form of sexually assaultive date behavior, with 15% of the sample reporting date rape (Linton, 1987). Women rarely report rapes when they know their attackers and especially if they were on a date. Date rape refers to forced sexual contact within the context of what could be construed as a date or the preliminaries of what could lead to a date. Victims of date rape are often impaired by the use of drugs or alcohol making them easier targets. The illegal use of flunitrazepam (Rohypnol) has recently been found to be used in many date or acquaintance rape cases. Flunitrazepam, a benzodiazepine, rapidly dissolves and once in solution is colorless, odorless, and tasteless. It can cause drowsiness, impaired motor skills, and anterograde amnesia. Because of the anterograde amnesia it is often difficult to obtain an accurate history of events (Anglin et al., 1997). Acquaintance rape includes situations in which the victim has met the assailant prior to the assault and has seen him on several occasions but does not know him well.

Failure to report such rapes may reflect in part the cultural value that under certain circumstances it is acceptable for a man to coerce or force a woman to have sex. The rape survivor is often "blamed" by herself or others for having been provocative or even naive.

Some rape survivors continue to date the person who raped them, confusing their boyfriend's force with love and affection. Some rape survivors come from dysfunctional families and may not see forced sex as unusual. Others may have their first sexual experience this way and so have no way of knowing if this behavior is unusual or not. Rape is traumatic, whether it happens to girls, women, men, or boys, but it can be especially devastating to adolescents who are forming their own identities and sexual patterns in this developmental stage (Ellis, 1991; Kennedy, 1993; Sawyer, Desmond, & Lucke, 1993; King and Woolett, 1997).

As a result of public exposure of this problem, especially on college campuses, colleges across the United States are sponsoring antirape seminars and establishing counseling centers to raise awareness of rape as a potentially significant problem. Nurses need to be aware of this type of rape because the survivors may present for treatment in a variety of settings.

> *What do you think?* Should nursing take a more proactive response in the preventive activities directed toward date rape?

Office Rape

Office rape has recently been identified as a new form of rape and is receiving national attention especially in relation to sexual harassment suits. Office rape is upsetting in that women often have much to lose. They are forced, coerced, or intimidated into performing sexual acts for fear of losing their job or status. The woman feels confusion, guilt, shame, and self-blame for participating when the guilt rests with the person in position of authority who abused his power. Survivors need to be encouraged to act in their own self-interest, report the incidents, and follow up with legal actions as necessary.

> ► *Check Your Reading*
> 14. What is date rape?
> 15. Why is date rape so dangerous for adolescents?

NURSING PROCESS

When the rape survivor presents for initial treatment after the trauma, she is first informed of personal rights. The nurse functions as a patient advocate to ensure that these rights are explained and supported. Box 36–1 summarizes the rights of people who have been raped.

Assessment

The assessment focuses not only on a physical examination but also on emotional, spiritual, cognitive, and social assessment. Legal evidence is collected in addition to the routine nursing responsibilities.

Box 36–1 ■ ■ ■ ■ ■
Rights of People Who Have Been Raped

The right to have contact with a rape crisis advocate

The right to decide how family or friends are notified

The right to notify their personal physician

The right to have gentle, sensitive treatment and confidentiality ensured

The right to have all tests and consents explained

The right to have follow-up referrals for counseling and, if necessary, medical treatment

Physical Assessment and Collection of Medicolegal Evidence

It is important for the nurse involved in the initial assessment following a rape to be familiar with any local reporting regulations or procedures to ensure that the examination is completed and the evidence is collected in the proper legal or forensic method. For example, in some jurisdictions, there may be state-issued evidence collection kits with specific procedures to be followed. The kit is used when the evidence may be used potentially to prosecute the perpetrator. These evidence collection kits ensure that certain specimens are collected uniformly from each survivor. The kits are then sealed so that all evidence collected is not tampered with. The use of these kits allows for more consistency in the type of evidence collected and ensures the chain of evidence is carefully followed (Aiken, 1993).

There are five essential components that are addressed in the forensic examination by any treating facility for the rape survivor (Ledray & Arndt, 1994):

1. Treatment and documentation of injuries, as well as evidence of force
2. Treatment and evaluation of sexually transmitted diseases
3. Pregnancy risk evaluation and prevention
4. Arrangements for follow-up counseling
5. Collection of evidence following protocols

The rape survivor receives a thorough physical assessment. Particular note is made of evidence of trauma, that is, contusions, lacerations, and so forth. If the police were involved, they may recommend a police photographer be called for legal documentation before treatment is initiated. Vaginal, oral, and anal examinations are performed with the woman's permission to determine need for treatment and to obtain documentation for legal proceedings.

In this initial assessment, the nurse acts as patient advocate, providing privacy, supporting and explaining all aspects of this procedure, assisting with the collection of evidence, assuring the patient of her safety, and recognizing the significance of all these details to the patient's journey. The evidence collection usually involves some special training because it is imperative to ensure that proper legal procedures are followed. The physical assessment must be documented carefully, to assist with possible prosecution of the perpetrator. In 53 cases associated with women pressing charges against the assailant, evidence of trauma was significantly associated with a successful prosecution (Aiken, 1993; Rambow, Adkinson, Frost, & Peterson, 1992).

You need to assess the type of assault, including the time, place, and circumstances of the assault. Ask the patient to describe what occurred. For instance, you might gently ask the patient specifics about the attack. Box 36–2 provides sample questions that you might ask.

What do you think? If you were working in an emergency department, how would you

Box 36–2 ■ ■ ■ ■ ■
Sample Assessment Questions for Rape Survivors

"Could you describe what the attacker did to you?"
"Were you fondled?"
"Did the attacker perform oral sex on you? Did the attacker force you to perform oral sex?"
"Did the attacker attempt vaginal intercourse with you? Was there penetration?"
"Did the attacker attempt rectal intercourse with you? Was there penetration?"
"Did the attacker experience an ejaculation? Did it happen on your body or inside of your body?"

approach a woman who presented for treatment following a rape?

➤ *Check Your Reading*
16. What are the five essential components of the forensic examination?
17. What is included in the physical assessment of a rape survivor?
18. What is the purpose of police photographs of a rape survivor?

Assessment of Mental State

The rape survivor's mental status is assessed for cognitive, behavioral, and affective changes. The person may seem confused, may be unable to respond verbally, and may have alterations in psychomotor functioning, all of which can be normal reactions to a devastating event. Make careful note of all behaviors, emotions, and cognition, including subjective and objective data. A persistent pattern of fear and anxiety is one of the most common and well-documented reactions to sexual assault. Initial reactions during the assault itself may be predictive of later problems. Survivors almost always report fearing for their lives during a sexual assault. Being under the total domination of a threatening, unpredictable person is a terrifying experience, whether or not weapons are used or overt life-threatening statements are made (Calhoun & Atkeson, 1991; Ruckman, 1992).

In the past few years, hospitals throughout the United States have successfully developed treatment protocols specific to the rape survivor, usually emphasizing evidence collection. Hospital staff and the police have also become educated to dispel the long-held beliefs and myths about rape survivors. One of the most common myths is that the attacker was overcome with sexual desire. Sometimes myths have interfered with the survivor's receiving supportive care and the reassurance so essential during the emergency room examination and subsequent interviews (Responding to Rape, 1992). Box 36–3 lists the common myths about rape.

➤ *Check Your Reading*

19. What are some of the common feelings reported by rape survivors?
20. Name at least four myths associated with rape.

Assessment of Spiritual State

Survivors of rape usually ask "Why me?" In attempting to answer this question, they may conclude that they were responsible for the attack. They may accept the myths about rape as if they were truths and act on them accordingly, heaping greater pain and suffering on themselves. They may feel guilty and even sinful if they have concluded that they dressed "too flirtatiously" or were "overly friendly" or "led the attacker on." Such conclusions are, of course, erroneous because no matter how someone dresses or behaves, no one asks to be hurt or violated in the way that rape does. The feelings of guilt and perhaps sinfulness are religious issues. These feelings may isolate the victim from God and the support that a relationship with God may offer. You need to assess these spiritual concerns because significant spiritual distress could block healing.

What *do you think?* How might personal religious and/or spiritual beliefs affect a victim's response to having been raped? How might these same beliefs influence the attitudes of police officers and health care providers toward the victim?

➤ *Check Your Reading*

21. What is the impact of guilt on the patient's spirituality?

Box 36–3 ■ ■ ■ ■ ■
Common Myths About Rape

Women "ask" to be raped by the provocative dress that they wear, the seductive behaviors that they display, and the places that they frequent.
Most rapists are oversexed.
Most rapes are committed by strangers.
Rape is usually an impulsive act, done without planning.
Only females get raped.
Rape is a sexual act.
It is dangerous for a person to try to get away from the attacker.
Rapes usually take place in dark, secluded places.
A healthy woman should be able to "fight off" the attack of an unarmed man.
Only promiscuous women get raped.
Women mean "yes" when they say "no."

22. What factors would make the patient experience guilt?

Assessment of Family Response

Because the support of family and the patient's significant other can be critical to healing, the nurse must assess their level of understanding as well as their feelings about rape. This is possible if the patient is accompanied to the treatment center by family or a significant other. Observe the family or significant other with the patient to determine their feelings toward the patient. Also, ask them the following questions:

1. "What do you understand about the crime of rape?"
2. "Tell me what you know about the survivor's responses to being raped."
3. "Tell me what you know about the myths that surround rape."
4. "How are you feeling now?"

Your observations of nonverbal behavior and the answers that the family or significant other give provide you with a foundation from which to intervene in a supportive manner.

What *do you think?* The rape victim says to you, "My family must never know about this." How would you respond?

➤ *Check Your Reading*

23. Identify at least two reasons why the nurse assesses families or the patient's significant other in relation to their understanding of and feelings about rape.

Diagnosis

The most appropriate *Diagnostic and Statistical Manual of Mental Disorders,* Fourth Edition (DSM-IV) (American Psychiatric Association, 1994) diagnosis for a patient who has been raped is either **Posttraumatic Stress Disorder** or **Acute Stress Disorder,** both of which relate to anxiety- and stress-related behavioral symptoms associated with a traumatic event (see Chapter 23 for DSM-IV criteria for Acute Stress Disorder). The main North American Nursing Diagnosis Association diagnosis for the person who has been raped is Rape-Trauma Syndrome, which describes both the acute and the long-term effects of being raped. There may be other appropriate nursing diagnoses depending on the results of the physical and mental examinations and the survivor's needs. Burgess and Holmstrom's (1974) description of the rape-trauma syndrome divides the reaction into an acute phase, lasting from a few days to several weeks, and a long-term reorganization phase, which may last for years. DSM-IV diagnoses for rape survivors and the related nursing diagnoses are shown in Medical Diagnoses and Related Nursing Diagnoses: Rape.

MEDICAL DIAGNOSES AND RELATED NURSING DIAGNOSES

Rape

DSM-IV Diagnosis: Posttraumatic Stress Disorder

Diagnostic Criteria

A. The preson has been exposed to a traumatic event in which both of the following were present:

(1) The person experienced, witnessed, or was confronted with an event or events that involved actual or threatened death or serious injury, or a threat to the physical integrity of self or others.

(2) The person's response involved intense fear, helplessness, or horror.

Note: In children, this may be expressed instead by disorganized or agitated behavior.

B. The traumatic event is persistently reexperienced in one (or more) of the following ways:

(1) Recurrent and intrusive distressing recollections of the event, including images, thoughts, or perceptions.

Note: In young children, repetitive play may occur in which themes or aspects of the trauma are expressed.

(2) Recurrent distressing dreams of the event.

Note: In children, there may be frightening dreams without recognizable content.

(3) Acting or feeling as if the traumatic event were recurring (includes a sense of reliving the experience, illusions, hallucinations, and dissociative flashback episodes, including those that occur on awakening or when intoxicated).

Note: In young children, trauma-specific reenactment may occur.

(4) Intense psychological distress at exposure to internal or external cues that symbolize or resemble an aspect of the traumatic event.

(5) Physiological reactivity on exposure to internal or external cues that symbolize or resemble an aspect of the traumatic event.

C. Persistent avoidance of stimuli associated with the trauma and numbing of general responsiveness (not present before the trauma), as indicated by three (or more) of the following:

(1) Efforts to avoid thoughts, feelings, or conversations associated with the trauma.

(2) Efforts to avoid activities, places, or people that arouse recollections of the trauma.

(3) Inability to recall an important aspect of the trauma.

(4) Markedly diminished interest or participation in significant activities.

(5) Feeling of detachment or estrangement from others.

(6) Restricted range of affect (e.g., unable to have loving feelings).

(7) Sense of a foreshortened future (e.g., does not expect to have a career, marriage, children, or a normal life span).

D. Persistent symptoms of increased arousal (not present before the trauma), as indicated by two (or more) of the following:

(1) Difficulty falling or staying asleep.

(2) Irritability or outbursts of anger.

(3) Difficulty concentrating.

(4) Hypervigilance.

(5) Exaggerated startle response.

E. Duration of the disturbance (symptoms in Criteria B, C, and D) is more than 1 month.

F. The disturbance causes clinically significant distress or impairment in social, occupational, or other important areas of functioning.

Related Nursing Diagnosis

Rape-Trauma Syndrome

Definition

The state in which an individual experiences a forced, violent sexual assault (vaginal or anal penetration) against her or his will and without her or his consent. The trauma syndrome that develops from this attack or attempted attack includes an acute phase of disorganization of the victim and family's lifestyle and a long-term process of reorganization of lifestyle.

Example

Rape-Trauma Syndrome related to rape as evidenced by emotional reactions, physical trauma, genitourinary trauma, and spiritual distress.

Based on information from the *Diagnostic and Statistical Manual of Mental Disorders. Fourth Edition.* Copyright 1994 American Psychiatric Association. Nursing diagnosis and definition from North American Nursing Diagnosis Association. (1999). *NANDA nursing diagnoses: Definitions and classification, 1999-2000.* Philadelphia: NANDA.

Burgess, a professor of nursing, and Holmstrom, a professor of sociology, first coined the term rape-trauma syndrome in 1974. Their initial work analyzed the responses of 92 adult rape survivors treated at Boston City Hospital between 1972 and 1974 and identified an acute stress reaction to the life-threatening forcible rape that they had just experienced (Block, 1990). The women ranged in age from 17 to 73, worked at a variety of occupations, and represented a variety of ethnic classes and social backgrounds. The rape survivors ranged in physical attractiveness from plain to very pretty and were dressed in a wide range of styles. Interviews were conducted within 30 minutes after the woman had been admitted to the hospital, and telephone and in-home follow-up visits were conducted for a year (Burgess & Holmstrom, 1974).

Rape-Trauma Syndrome includes both the acute-phase and the long-term reorganization process that occurs as a result of forcible rape or attempted forcible rape. The behavioral, somatic, and psychological reactions are a part of a syndrome that is an acute stress reaction to a life-threatening situation.

Inherent in the definition is the concept that although rape is primarily a sexual act, it should be properly considered an act of violence with sex used as the weapon (Burgess & Holmstrom, 1974). Viewing the rape survivor as a victim of violence might lead to more compassionate, more objective, and less judgmental responses. Both health care providers and the criminal justice system stigmatize rape survivors in a manner that is not afforded any other victim of violent crime (Aguilera, 1990). It is not surprising then that the survivor of rape experiences a syndrome with specific symptoms.

> **W**hat do you think? The statement that rape is more a crime of power than lust refers to the violent nature of rape. What are your reactions to that statement?

> ➤ *Check Your Reading*
> 24. What are the two probable DSM-IV diagnoses for a patient who has been raped?
> 25. What are the two phases of the Rape-Trauma Syndrome?
> 26. What are the manifestations of Rape-Trauma Syndrome?

Disorganization (Acute) Phase

The two-phase reaction of the syndrome begins with an acute phase, in which there is a great deal of disorganization in the person's lifestyle resulting from the rape.

IMPACT REACTION
In the immediate hours following the attack, the person may experience an extremely wide range of emotions. Feelings of fear as well as shock or disbelief may predominate. In Burgess and Holmstrom's initial study (1974), two emotional styles were described:

- The expressed style, in which emotion was outwardly expressed through crying, smiling, sobbing, restlessness, or tenseness.
- The controlled style, in which feelings were not outwardly displayed, and the person appeared calm, composed, and subdued.

SOMATIC REACTIONS
In the weeks immediately following the incident, rape survivors describe a number of somatic reactions. If the person has suffered physical trauma, general soreness, bruising, and other physical complaints of injury are apparent. If the person was forced to have oral sex, irritation and trauma to the throat are frequently reported. Sleep pattern disturbances are common, with either inability to sleep or inability to fall back asleep once awakened. Rape survivors often become nauseated just thinking of the rape and frequently have decreased appetite. Gynecological symptoms are usually present, for example, vaginal discharge, burning on urination, or itching (Burgess & Holmstrom, 1974). Current research shows through colposcopic examination that trauma can occur in 1 or more of 11 anatomical sites and that multiple sites (3 or more) are generally involved in 94% of women tested. Most of the trauma occurs as an entry injury, with insertion or attempts at insertion (Slaughter, Brown, Crowley, & Peck, 1997). Other studies have shown a correlation between sexual assault victims and women presenting to physicians with gastrointestinal problems. These women have been shown to have more medical symptoms and higher somatization scores (Leserman et al., 1996). In general, the symptoms appear to be both directly related to the physical trauma sustained and partly generated by the emotional trauma.

EMOTIONAL REACTIONS
In the days and weeks after the rape, survivors continue to express a wide range of emotions: fear, humiliation, embarrassment, anger, and self-blame. A fear for their lives is the most pervasive emotion, which is expressed in a variety of ways. Some are hysterical and cry a great deal; others withdraw and refuse to talk with anyone. During the days and weeks that follow the original assault, rape survivors commonly experience nervousness, nightmares, inability to concentrate, startle responses, and other manifestations of anxiety. These responses tend to decrease over time, but sometimes spontaneous recovery reaches a limit beyond which there can be little improvement without professional intervention (Calhoun & Atkeson, 1991).

Depressive symptoms, including crying spells; sleep and appetite disturbances; fatigue; suicidal ideation; and feelings of guilt, worthlessness, hopelessness, and spiritual distress, are common in the first few weeks following an assault. Depression is more common in women than men, and some women may have had problems with depression before the assault. Frank, Turner, Stewart, Jacob, and West (1981) studied the relationship between past psychiatric symptoms and women's response to sexual assault. The researchers' results were inconclusive but suggested that women with a history of psychiatric problems, including but not limited to depression, represent a group at high risk for sexual assault and that women with a history of psychiatric problems are at risk for particularly severe reactions to sexual assault. Additionally, the researchers discovered a strong relationship between certain aspects of a person's prior psychiatric history and response to rape, which suggests that although assessment of current state is important, information about the rape survivor's past psychiatric history is also valuable to the clinician. Rape survivors with a history of psychotropic drug treatment, suicidal ideation, and suicide attempts seem to be especially likely to experience a severe reaction following a rape (Frank et al., 1981).

Another common response was to seek support from family members not normally seen daily; in Burgess's study, 48 of 92 women made special trips home, which often meant traveling to another city. The women did not always tell family why they were contacting them for support, and deciding whether or not to tell family often was difficult (Burgess & Holmstrom, 1974). Continuing nightmares and dreams are especially disturbing during this phase.

Reorganization Phase

In Burgess and Holmstrom's study (1974), the coping and reorganization process began at different times for individual survivors, based somewhat on their ego strength, social support networks, and the way others treated them as victims. In Frank and coworkers' study (1981), the impact of the trauma was affected somewhat by the survivor's previous contact with mental health professionals and previous psychiatric history. In general, survivors did not experience all the same symptoms in the same sequence; what was consistent were the two phases: the acute phase of disorganization and the mild to moderate symptoms experienced in the reorganization process.

The nurse in a variety of settings may come in contact with rape survivors who may be in the reorganization phase; for example, women may come to a community clinic seeking treatment for an apparently unrelated problem. These women may appear to have made an outward adjustment; they are back at their jobs; and relationships on the surface appear relatively normal. This is positive and should be supported. Despite seeming outwardly adjusted, however, these women may experience a variety of subtle but troubling symptoms. Rape may have long-term effects on behavior. Survivors may have prolonged depressions and unexplained crying spells. It is not uncommon for nightmares to persist. Burgess and Holmstrom (1974) reported that nearly 50% of the women they studied changed residence within a relatively short period of time after the rape, generally to ensure safety and facilitate functioning in a normal style.

Some rape survivors develop new phobias as a defensive reaction to the rape. Often the link between the circumstances of the rape and the phobic behavior is clear: A woman attacked in her bed is afraid of being indoors; a woman attacked while walking to her car from the grocery store may become fearful of leaving her home to do errands. Almost all women fear being alone. A woman who has been raped by her husband has an especially difficult time in readjustment, needing to interact with her attacker and perhaps pretending to her family and to herself that the rape did not occur. Often, women experience a crisis in their sexual life following a rape. Box 36–4 summarizes the responses characteristic of the two phases of the Rape-Trauma Syndrome.

Box 36–4 ■ ■ ■ ■ ■
Responses Characteristic of Rape-Trauma Syndrome

Acute Phase

Fear
Denial
Anger
Guilt
Anxiety
Self-blame
Tension
Embarassment
Crying
Shock or disbelief
Masked feelings
Somatic reactions
Calmness
Composure

Reorganization Phase

Increased motor activity
Outward composure
Denial of feelings
Sexual problems
Nightmares and other sleep disturbances
Anxiety
Prolonged symptoms of depression
Phobias

What do you think? Because the response to rape occurs in different phases, what kind of anticipatory guidance would you provide a woman who had recently been raped?

▶ *Check Your Reading*

27. Describe the patient's behavior in the impact stage.
28. State at least four somatic concerns that are common in the acute phase of Rape-Trauma syndrome.
29. Describe two common emotional reactions that occur during the acute phase of Rape-Trauma Syndrome.
30. What happens during the reorganization phase of Rape-Trauma Syndrome?

Outcome Identification

The expected outcomes for a patient with the nursing diagnosis of Rape-Trauma Syndrome include

• The patient will demonstrate decreased anxiety, fear, and guilt.

- The patient will experience physical healing.
- The patient will establish an adequate balance of rest, sleep, and activity.
- The patient will verbalize feelings about the rape.
- The patient will be able to find meaning in the trauma and to find spiritual comfort.
- The patient will participate in treatment programs.

Planning

Based on the identified expected outcomes, you and the patient, working together with the interdisciplinary team, jointly establish short-term goals, such as the following.

Expected Outcome
The patient will demonstrate decreased anxiety, fear, and guilt.

Short-Term Goals
- The patient will verbalize feelings of anxiety, fear, and guilt.
- The patient will recognize that she did not cause the rape.
- The patient will verbalize strategies for keeping safe.

Expected Outcome
The patient will experience physical healing.

Short-Term Goals
- The patient will express the resolution of physical irritations such as sore throat, vaginal itching and burning, and bruises.

Expected Outcome
The patient will establish an adequate balance of rest, sleep, and activity.

Short-Term Goals
- The patient will sleep through the night and feel rested.
- The patient will experience decreasing frequency of nightmares.
- The patient will resume normal eating and will regain any lost weight.

Expected Outcome
The patient will verbalize feelings about the rape.

Short-Term Goals
- The patient will verbalize the details of the rape experience.
- The patient will freely express feelings about the rape experience.

Expected Outcome
The patient will be able to find meaning in the trauma and to find spiritual comfort.

Short-Term Goals
- The patient will verbalize the significance of this experience to her life's journey.
- The patient will use spiritual resources (e.g., prayer, meditation, Scripture reading, pastoral counseling) to seek comfort for the trauma.

Expected Outcome
The patient will participate in the treatment program.

Short-Term Goals
- The patient will make and keep appointments for follow-up treatment. The patient will follow through with treatment suggestions.

The plan takes into account whether or not the patient is in the acute disorganization phase or in the reorganization phase of Rape-Trauma Syndrome. Progressive hospitals have planned ahead for the treatment of rape victims and have established protocols to provide care in a comprehensive, caring, sensitive manner. Such hospitals frequently have hired employees, either nurses or counselors, who are trained to meet the needs of the rape survivor.

Disorganization (Acute) Phase

The initial plan involves identifying the person who will work closely with the patient within the hospital setting. Depending on the organization system of the hospital's emergency department, either a nurse or rape crisis worker acts as patient advocate. The counselor's role varies depending on the counselor's skill and background, the philosophy of the center, and the needs of the survivor. Ideally, the plan provides the woman with access to a supportive person who facilitates and guides the initial stages of her journey into the health care system. This nurse and other members of the health care team, including a physician with special training in gynecology and forensics related to the rape examination, need to establish quickly physical and mental status priorities that require immediate attention. Often the immediate care of the rape survivor falls to the generalist nurse in the emergency department, who may have conflicting treatment priorities due to managing a busy patient load. This person may assist in the forensic examination but does not always have the special training to provide the empathetic counseling and support that the victim needs. At the very least, this nurse can provide the privacy the rape survivor needs. This patient needs to be triaged as an emergency and taken to a private area. The patient cannot shower or douche prior to physical examination if she plans to prosecute. If oral penetration is a factor, she cannot take anything by mouth, as this also will destroy the evidence. After the physical examination, the patient should be allowed to shower. Some hospitals provide clean underwear. Prophylactic measures to prevent the possibility of pregnancy and sexually transmitted diseases are often given.

The initial planning must also address the long-term issues that the patient will encounter in her continuing journey. Therefore, a comprehensive initial plan includes anticipatory guidance for the long-term consequences of rape and options to respond to these consequences.

Reorganization Phase

The long-term plan for rape survivors provides for continuing support and counseling. The time for this continuing support varies with the individual. Some recover quickly, others spend years struggling to heal from the trauma inflicted by the attack. In the next section, interventions are described that address both the needs during the acute phase and the continuing need to support the victim struggling to reorganize.

➤ *Check Your Reading*

31. Identify at least three expected outcomes for a rape survivor.
32. Identify at least three short-term goals for nursing care of a rape survivor.
33. Identify two ways in which the initial plan differs from the long-term plan.

Implementation

Disorganization (Acute) Phase: Crisis Intervention

In Chapter 13, you learned about the Aguilera model of intervention known as crisis intervention. Crisis intervention is the ideal means of helping rape survivors. Rape is a sudden, overwhelming experience in which usual coping mechanisms can be inadequate. With rapid, skillful intervention, development of serious long-term disabilities may be prevented and new coping patterns may emerge that can help the individual function at a higher level of equilibrium than before the crisis (Aguilera, 1990). The nurse who encounters and intervenes with a rape survivor at any phase of disintegration or reorganization should be mindful of both crisis intervention theory and the Rape-Trauma Syndrome. One of the most effective intervention models exists in Minneapolis, Minnesota—the Sexual Assault Resource Service (SARS). This model focuses on providing care not only during the acute phase following the rape but also during the long-term healing process of the Rape-Trauma Syndrome.

Reorganization Phase

A number of intervention models in the United States are devoted solely to the care of the rape survivor; these models use sexual assault nurse examiners (Jezierski, 1992; Scott, 1992).

THE SEXUAL ASSAULT RESOURCE SERVICE MODEL

SARS in Minnesota provides care to rape survivors immediately after the attack as well as follow-up care. Since

September 1977, nurses trained in both mental health and gynecology have provided primary care to rape survivors in Minneapolis through SARS, which was originally begun as a research demonstration treatment program funded through the National Institute of Mental Health. This program began as a result of concern of nurses working in the obstetrics-gynecology clinic at Hennepin County Medical Center, where rape survivors were referred for follow-up care. Before the program's inception, 75% of survivors never returned for follow-up to the clinic, a fact disturbing to the nurses who realized they were not adequately meeting their patients' needs (Ledray, 1992). Now as a result of the program's success, survivors are seen at five private hospitals as well as in the county hospital, and service has been expanded to treat males and children as well.

SARS is staffed by professional, salaried, trained nurses who are on call 24 hours a day, 7 days a week, to see rape survivors who come to the center or who are brought to the emergency department. The SARS staff have identified seven components of care important to provide during the initial crisis period. Research conducted has confirmed that women who received this crisis support recovered more quickly than those who did not (Ledray, 1992).

1. *Providing emotional support.* The rape survivor is shown an attitude of positive regard and given the support to express anxieties and fears freely without fear of criticism.

2. *Responding to the patient as normal.* The patient is seen as a normal healthy individual who is reacting to a serious life crisis. The woman is reassured that her response to the rape, whether or not she fought or struggled, was the right thing to do, recognizing her survival as paramount. Rape survivors are told that their confusion and disorganization are normal responses to a traumatic event and that frequent shifts in feelings are often experienced by others after being raped.

3. *Maintaining a nonjudgmental attitude.* The counselor must be nonjudgmental not only to the behavioral response of the survivor but also in judging the event to be a rape. Survivors have often been subject to the myths and prejudices of police and treatment staff, who may subtly or overtly convey to the woman that "she asked for it" or that the rape is "faked" to achieve some sort of secondary gain or attention. This blaming response of the caregiver can compound the survivor's response and prolong the inability to cope with the event.

4. *Helping the patient regain control.* It is critical to help the patient regain control of her body, self, and situation. The physical assault of the rape results in a tremendous loss of power and control, and unfortunately, in many more traditional situations, experiences with the police, medical staff, and the courts can reinforce loss of control. Acting as a patient advocate and guide through the maze of physical examinations, treatment options, and legal alternatives, the nurse can assist the survivor to make informed decisions and help her to regain a sense of control.

5. *Communicating separateness from the event.* The woman must know that she is separate from the event; "the victim is not a raped woman; she is a woman who has been raped" (Ledray, 1990). Women who have been raped often express that they feel "dirty." Separating themselves from the event assists them in the task of regaining some self-esteem.

6. *Helping the patient find support.* It is important to identify for the rape survivor someone within her social support network who can handle the knowledge about the rape. Survivors are often hesitant to talk with family or friends because of feelings of guilt or embarrassment or fear of rejection. Rape survivors need to be gently supported to understand that others may respond to the rape event in a less than sensitive manner, based on their personal inability to deal with the reality of the rape.

7. *Ensuring personal safety.* Finally, the nurse can help the rape survivor to identify those factors that can ensure her personal safety and make her less vulnerable. Not only are external factors relating to safety discussed but also the fears and concerns that often continue long after the life-threatening event has occurred (Ledray, 1990). Box 36–5 provides tips for prevention of sexual assault.

B o x 3 6 – 5 ■ ■ ■ ■ ■
Tips for Prevention of Sexual Assault

At Home

- Your obvious hiding places for keys are just as obvious to your attacker. Consider leaving a key with a trusted neighbor.
- *Everyone* should use only initials and last names on mailboxes and phone listings.
- Be prepared to enter your house without complications. Have your keys in hand when you reach the door.
- If a window or door has been forced or broken while you were absent, *do not enter.* Go to your neighbor's house and call the police.
- Install the proper deadbolt locks and a door viewer, and *remember to use them.*
- Make sure that all windows are properly secured.
- Install good interior and exterior lighting for protection. Use timers for additional security while you are away.
- Instruct all family members not to answer the door automatically. Before unlocking the door, they should use the door viewer and require identification from all delivery and repair persons as well as police officers.
- Never let strangers inside your house to use the phone. Keep the door locked and offer to make the call for them. Also, remember not to reveal that you are home alone. Do not leave messages on the outside of your door advertising your absence.
- If you live in an apartment, avoid going to the basement laundry room alone.
- Trim bushes and shrubbery so no one can hide in or behind them, especially if they are close to doors or windows.
- Keep emergency phone numbers handy by each phone.
- Take a self-defense course to help rebuild an internal sense of security.
- Vary your routine each day, because over 70% of rapes are planned.

In Your Car

- Always lock your car doors when driving or parked.
- Be mindful of suspicious activity, and always park in lighted areas.
- Always have keys in hand when entering your car.
- Do not stop for stranded motorists. Call for assistance at the nearest police station or phone booth.
- Never leave your house keys attached to car keys at service stations or parking lots.
- Keep your car in good running order, and always have enough gas.
- Keep your car in gear while halted in traffic to make a quick getaway.
- Never pick up hitchhikers.

When Walking

- If you must carry a purse, don't dangle it by your side.
- Don't carry large sums of cash or extra credit cards.
- Always be aware of your surroundings and note any suspicious characters. Try to walk with a "buddy."
- Stay in well-lighted areas and avoid shortcuts.
- If a driver stops to ask questions, avoid getting close to the car.
- If someone threatens or harasses you, attract attention to yourself by screaming, yelling, whistling, or activating a hand-held siren device.
- Don't depend entirely on tear gas, pepper spray, or other sprays for protection. The wind may sabotage your defense.
- Dress comfortably and wear shoes that you can run or move quickly in.
- Don't hitchhike.

SNAPSHOT

Nursing Interventions Specific to Rape

What do you need to develop a relationship with a patient who has experienced rape?
- Evaluate the severity of response to the traumatic event and the extent of current functioning.
- Approach the patient with acceptance and willingness to listen and believe.
- Be caring, honest, empathetic, and professional.
- Speak slowly, clearly, and allow the patient time to respond.
- Explain all procedures for the emergency medical examination.
- Prepare the victim for questions that might later be asked by police.
- Provide physical and emotional support during any procedure.
- Provide an atmosphere of privacy.
- Provide information for further interventions and need for supportive others.

What do you need to assess regarding the health status of a patient who has just been raped?
- Observe for signs of difficulty concentrating, preoccupation, disinterest, or other cognitive symptoms.
- Observe for signs of detachment and withdrawal.
- Assess for risk of suicide or self-destructive thoughts.
- Assess for range of emotions: shock, disbelief, blame, anger, rage, fear, depression, anxiety, confusion.
- Assess for physical trauma: bruising, lacerations, bleeding, pregnancy, sexually transmitted diseases, body systems, alcohol or drug use, vital signs, concurrent medical conditions.
- Perform rape assessment and evidence collection per policy and law.

What do you need to teach the patient and/or family or caregiver?
- Medication management for core symptoms of depression, anxiety, panic, and sleep disturbance
- Identification of situations to avoid that might precipitate distress and memories and elimination of those experiences or reminders
- Teaching the patient to stay in the present and avoid or minimize becoming overwhelmed by the memories of the traumatic experience
- Coping skills

- Taking control of life and safety measures
- Encourage participation in a support group to understand that there are others who have experienced the same situation and to validate fears, feelings, and resolve conflicts associated with the traumatic event
- Teach that there are four phases in long-term adjustment (recovery, avoidance, reconsideration, and adjustment) to understand that there is a process of healing
- Teach to use relaxation skills in anxiety-arousing situations
- Instruct to use physical exercise to reduce tension in a nondestructive manner
- Remind the patient that it is not her fault

What skills do you want the patient and/or family or caregiver to demonstrate?
- Ability of supportive others to listen to the "story" and not blame themselves or the victim
- Show positive coping skills
- Practice relaxation techniques and stress management techniques under stressful conditions
- Ability to express feelings and thoughts and not self-isolate
- Ability to contract not to harm self or perform other self-destructive acts
- Ability to stop negative thoughts and obsessions, to think through an action plan
- Application of locks, change in routine, taking control of life in a positive and safe manner
- Ability to take control of emotions and not let them dominate
- Expression of feelings of anger, denial, blame, shock, fear, confusion, anxiety, future relationships
- Establish caring, loving, sexual relationship again with a significant other
- Talking with friends and others about the rape in a positive way
- Becoming socially involved with people you trust
- Increasing positive self-esteem and feelings about body image

What other health professionals might need to be part of this plan of care?
- Physician, emergency room doctor, gynecologist, nurse practitioner in the emergency room for rape examination and after for follow-up regarding trauma and other physical problems
- Rape crisis counselor or therapist for emergency room intervention, advocacy, and aftercare support
- Police for evidence collection and possible further legal actions

FAMILY SUPPORT AND EDUCATION

The support and understanding of the patient's significant other and family is conducive to the healing process. If the patient is accompanied by a family member, ask the patient's permission about whether or not she wants the family involved in the teaching and support. If the patient is agreeable, actively engage the family in the interventions. For instance, the family needs to know about:

- The myths that surround rape
- The range of normal responses to the trauma
- The characteristics of the Rape-Trauma Syndrome
- The need for long-term support from the family and perhaps from a professional source

Some family members also may need help from a professional source to work through their own feelings about the rape. See Snapshot: Nursing Interventions Specific to Rape.

Evaluation

Evaluating the outcome of the nursing interventions depends on reviewing the short-term goals leading to the expected outcomes. In any crisis, the goal focuses on assisting the individual to restore equilibrium and to prevent serious long-term disability. The answers to the following questions provide important information for evaluation.

- Is the patient less anxious, fearful, and guilty?
- Have the physical injuries healed?
- Has the patient reestablished balance in rest, sleep, and activity patterns?
- Can the patient verbalize feelings about the rape?
- Is the patient able to fit the rape into the pattern of her life?
- Is the patient experiencing spiritual well-being?
- Is the patient able to use meaningful spiritual interventions for comfort?
- Has the patient participated in follow-up treatment?

The person who has been raped reaches a critical juncture in the journey of life. The assault violates the person's sense of personal safety, sexuality, and self-esteem. Effective nursing care can play a significant role in the healing of the patient who has been raped.

What do you think? What would be your skills in working with a rape survivor?

➤ Check Your Reading
34. What is SARS?
35. Identify at least three components of effective counseling with rape survivors.
36. Identify at least five safety practices for women that decrease the risk of being raped.
37. What is involved in family support and education?

NURSING PROCESS APPLICATION

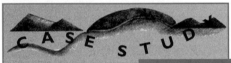

Mary

Mary is transported by the police to the emergency department of the local hospital. The initial information is taken by a staff nurse who obtains Mary's signed authorization for treatment. A physician examines Mary's wrist and proceeds to stitch up the laceration.

You are a psychiatric liaison nurse called to the emergency department to provide support to Mary. You take Mary into a private setting, assure Mary that she is safe, and gently ask her to recount her story.

I awoke tonight gagged [illegible] hands pinned down by someone wearing leather gloves and holding a razor to my throa[t] [illegible] wasn't quite sure I was awake. The main thing I can remember wanting was the light. I was able to notice the time because I had a luminous dial watch on. I had this terrible feeling of being in the middle of a nightmare that seemed more realistic than ordinary and I couldn't make it stop. I was trying to establish if there was really a person there. When I struggled, I got my wrist cut and then I realized that I was risking my life and that I'd better hold still and let the man have intercourse with me. He was very fast. He didn't have any clothes on the bottom half of his body. He didn't say much and I couldn't see his face because he had a ski mask on. He ran out the window still not wearing any clothes. I got up and turned on the lights after I got my wrists untied. I felt numb. I tried to leave the apartment after about 45 minutes and then I realized that I didn't have any cash because the man had stolen my purse. I had a fear of going outside my building because I realized he could be nearby. I realized that the man had been in my apartment for some time and that he must have had a flashlight because he gagged me with my own dish towel. It was then that I thought to call the police, not because I had been raped but because I wanted to get out of my apartment.

Mary is tearful and anxious and states, "I feel so dirty" and "I was so scared." As you continue to spend time with Mary, you review her legal rights and assure her that throughout the examination process you will remain with her. As you talk with Mary, you are formulating the following nursing care plan.

ASSESSMENT	Assessment data are as follows:

- Laceration on wrist
- Crying
- Verbalization of fear of the perpetrator: "I'm so scared"
- Verbalization about the rape
- Verbalization of self-denigrating comments: "I feel so dirty"
- Evidence of bruising on inner thighs and perineal area

DIAGNOSIS

DSM-IV Diagnosis: Posttraumatic Stress Disorder

Nursing Diagnosis: Rape-Trauma Syndrome related to rape as evidenced by verbalizations of sexual attack, crying, anxiety, laceration on wrist, and comments about feelings of fear and self-denigration.

OUTCOME IDENTIFICATION, PLANNING, AND IMPLEMENTATION

Expected Outcome 1: By _____ the patient will demonstrate decreased anxiety, fear, and guilt.

Short-Term Goals	Nursing Interventions	Rationales
By _____ the patient will verbalize feelings of anxiety.	1. Stay with the patient. 2. Provide privacy. 3. Listen attentively to the patient's story. 4. Display empathy. 5. Explain what will happen to the patient during the medicolegal examination. 6. Obtain signed consent for the examination. 7. Document all physical and emotional data (including verbatim accounts of what the patient said). 8. Document laboratory test results and whether any pictures of the patient's injuries were taken.	1–3. Your manner conveys respect and a safe environment that allows for free expression of feelings. 4–5. Explaining what will happen decreases anticipatory anxiety and increases a sense of personal control. 6. Signed consent is part of the legal protocol. 7–8. Comprehensive documentation is needed for medical and legal follow-up.
By _____ the patient will verbalize an understanding of Rape-Trauma Syndrome.	1. Explain to the patient the normal reactions of rape survivors during the acute phase as well as during the reorganization phase.	1. Anticipatory guidance lowers anxiety and increases a patient's sense of being in control.
By _____ the patient will verbalize strategies for keeping safe.	1. Teach the patient strategies to minimize risk at home, in her car, and on the street. 2. Provide a written teaching guide of these strategies. 3. Arrange for the patient to go home with a family member or support person.	1–3. Knowing that there are concrete steps to take to maximize safety and minimize risk gives the patient a sense of control and decreases fear and anxiety. The written guide allows the patient to review the strategies when anxiety lessens.

Expected Outcome 2: By _____ the patient will experience decreased physical symptoms.

Short-Term Goal	Nursing Interventions	Rationales
By _____ the patient will express decreased discomfort from her physical injuries.	1. Treat the patient's physical injuries. 2. Instruct the patient to manage her injuries at home.	1–2. Taking care of physical injuries validates the patient's worth, provides comfort, and allows for collection of physical evidence to be used for prosecution of the perpetrator.

Expected Outcome 3: By _____ the patient will verbalize her feelings about the rape.

Short-Term Goal	Nursing Interventions	Rationales
By _____ the patient will verbalize the details of the experience and will verbalize her feelings about the rape experience.	1. Gently inquire about what happened. 2. Encourage the patient's free expression. 3. Remain neutral and empathetic.	1–3. Verbalization decreases feelings of guilt, anxiety, and isolation and allows for validation from others that the rape was as serious as the patient perceives it to be.

Expected Outcome 4: By _____ the patient will find meaning in the trauma and find spiritual comfort.

Short-Term Goals	Nursing Interventions	Rationales
By _____ the patient will verbalize the significance of the rape on her life's journey.	1. Ask the patient what she thinks this event means to her life. 2. Explain to the patient the importance of trying to find significance in all of life's experiences, even the most painful and difficult ones.	1–2. Initially the patient may not be able to verbalize the meaning and significance of the event, but your questions will encourage her in the process of finding meaning.
By _____ the patient will use spiritual resources to seek comfort and to relieve the distress she is feeling.	1. Ask the patient if she has spiritual resources (such as prayer, Bible reading, and meditation) that are meaningful to her. 2. Ask if there is something you can do to respond to her spiritual distress (i.e., pray with or for her).	1. Encouraging the patient to use spiritual resources draws on an important source of strength. 2. Offering to meet spiritual needs can be a loving and compassionate intervention to someone who is feeling traumatized and unable to meet her own spiritual needs.

Expected Outcome 5: By _____ the patient will participate in the treatment program.

Short-Term Goal	Nursing Interventions	Rationales
By _____ the patient will keep follow-up appointments.	1. Give the patient the results of her physical examination. 2. Provide information about physical and emotional follow-up. 3. Provide appointments or referrals.	1–3. These interventions encourage the patient to be part of decision-making and help the patient to deal with the long-term reorganization phase of recovery.

EVALUATION

Formative Evaluation: Mary met each of the short-term goals except that she was not able to use spiritual resources in her healing. She stated that she was just "too angry at God" for allowing the rape to happen to her and that at this time she was not ready to turn to God or anything remotely related to God.

Summative Evaluation: Mary achieved each of the expected outcomes except that she did not find meaning in her trauma or find spiritual comfort. For most of the expected outcomes, the nursing care plan was adequate, appropriate, efficient, and effective. To help Mary find meaning in her trauma and help her to find spiritual comfort, the nurse gathered additional spiritual assessment data and discovered that for some time Mary has suffered from spiritual distress related to other unresolved losses in her life. Mary says, "I know that I am going to have to deal with my anger toward God at some point . . . but I am just not ready to do it now." The nurse therefore modified the plan of care to accept Mary's feelings and to encourage her to pursue this area when she believes she is ready.

Conclusions

Rape, an act of violence, dramatically alters the survivor's journey. The attack itself frequently results in physical injury, including lacerations and bruises. The most significant impact, however, is on the emotional and spiritual aspects of the survivor's journey. As if the rape were not traumatic enough, sometimes the survivor is blamed and stigmatized by society, health care workers, the legal system, and loved ones, who hold her responsible for the rape.

Rape-Trauma Syndrome, a NANDA diagnosis describing the survivor's response to rape, identifies an acute reaction of disorganization followed by long-term reorganization. The survivor experiences a wide array of reactions that involve somatic complaints, affective lability, cognitive problems, and spiritual distress. The nurse plays an important role in responding to the rape survivor, both in the immediate aftermath of the rape and during the long-term process of healing.

Key Points to Remember

- The nurse may encounter the rape survivor in a variety of health care settings and so must be knowledgeable about the possible long-term psychological sequelae of the experience. This knowledge assists in understanding normal and abnormal coping patterns, in developing appropriate teaching and support, and in making referrals.
- Although there is no "typical" rape survivor, young women between the ages of 12 and 34 are at most risk. It is estimated that one of six women is raped at one time in their lives.
- Some people assume that sexual assault is motivated by sexual desire. It isn't. It is a violent crime, a hostile attack, that attempts to hurt, humiliate, and control the victim.
- Sexual assault includes all forms of sexual contact carried out against the will and without the consent of the survivor. It can affect both men and women. These assaults can include both the actual use of force and the threat of force on the survivor or another person.
- Date rape, referring to forced sexual contact within the context of what could be construed as a date, is a growing problem on college campuses.

- Rape-Trauma Syndrome, as originally identified by Burgess and Holmstrom (1974), is the acute-phase and the long-term reorganization process that occurs as a result of forcible rape or attempted forcible rape. The behavioral, somatic, and psychological reactions are part of a syndrome that is an acute stress reaction to a life-threatening situation.
- The rape survivor's initial contact with the health care system may be a forensic examination. The sexual assault nurse clinician, or examiner, a specially trained nursing professional as exemplified by Ledray's (1994) program in Minneapolis, can provide comprehensive care to the sexual assault survivor. In other areas, statewide protocols and evidence collection kits have been developed. The forensic examination should include treatment and documentation of injuries, treatment and evaluation of sexually transmitted diseases, pregnancy risk evaluation and prevention, crisis intervention, and arrangements for follow-up counseling. This also includes the collection of medicolegal evidence while maintaining the proper chain of evidence.

Learning Activities

1. Look in your local telephone directory and see if there are any rape crisis centers in your community. If there are, call and talk to one of the counselors. Ask about the types of services that are provided. What are the major issues confronting the person who is healing from the trauma of rape?
2. Take an informal survey of your family and friends. Ask them what they think about rape. Take note of how many people's thinking is affected by myths that surround the issue of rape.

3. Call up your state legislator and ask for copies of laws pertaining to rape. Ask about your state's position on marital rape.
4. Visit the emergency department of your local hospital. Inquire regarding what services are provided for rape survivors. Do they provide rape counselors or psychiatric nurses? What procedures do they have in place to gather evidence to be used for a legal examination?

Critical Thinking Exercise

Karen Polk, a 26-year-old paralegal, decided to work late to finish some extra work. As she was getting into her car in the parking lot at 10:00 PM, a man with a knife told her that he would kill her if she resisted. At knifepoint Karen was raped. Bruised and frightened, she was unable to move or scream. At 11:00 PM, a jogger saw her lying on the ground near her car and called the police. Karen was taken by the police to the emergency department at a nearby hospital.

1. What assumptions do you have about who is to blame?
2. What evidence led you to this point of view?
3. If you were the nurse in the emergency department, what would you say to Karen?

Nurse Abbott met Karen at the door of the emergency department. She stayed with her while the doctor examined her. Nurse Abbott allowed Karen to talk as much as she needed to. As Karen talked, she shook her head saying, "I shouldn't have worked late. Please don't call my mother, she will have a heart attack." Nurse Abbott responded, "We'll do whatever is needed to keep you safe."

1. What other types of reactions would you expect to see with rape survivors?
2. Consider alternate responses that Nurse Abbott might use.
3. What conclusion(s) can you draw about Nurse Abbott's clinical abilities?

Additional Resources

Minnesota Center Against Violence and Abuse (MINCAVA)

http://www.mincava.umn.edu

MINCAVA offers information and resources about violence and all kinds of abuse. MINCAVA also offers links to other related resources.

Sexual Assault Information Page

http://www.cs.utk.edu/~bartley/saInfoPage.html

References

Aiken, M. M. (1993). False allegation: A concept in the context of rape. *Journal of Psychosocial Nursing and Mental Health Services, 31*(11), 15-20.

Aguilera, D. (1990). *Crisis intervention: Theory and methodology.* St. Louis: C. V. Mosby.

American Psychiatric Association. (1994). *Diagnostic and statistical manual of mental disorders* (4th ed.). Washington, DC: Author.

Anglin, D., Spears, K., & Hutson, H. (1997). Flunitrazepam and its involvement in date or acquaintance rape. *Academy of Emergency Medicine 4*(4), 323-326.

Block, A. (1990). Rape-Trauma Syndrome as scientific expert testimony. *Archives of Sexual Behavior, 19*(54), 309-323.

Brownmiller, S. (1975). *Against our will: Men, women, and rape.* New York: Simon and Shuster.

Burgess, A., & Holmstrom, L. (1974). Rape-trauma syndrome. *American Journal of Psychiatry, 131*(9), 981-985.

Calhoun, K., & Atkeson, B. (1991). *Treatment of rape victims: Facilitating psychosocial adjustment.* New York: Pergamon Press.

Davis, L., & Brody, E. (1979). *Rape and older women: A guide to prevention and protection.* Washington, DC: U.S. Department of Health, Education, and Welfare, Public Health Service, National Institute of Mental Health.

Ellis, G. M. (1991). Acquaintance rape. *Perspectives in Psychiatric Care, 30*(1), 11-16.

Frank, E., Turner, S. M., Stewart, B. D., Jacob, M., & West, D. (1981). Past psychiatric symptoms and the response to sexual assault. *Comprehensive Psychiatry, 22*(5), 479-487.

Hall, G. C. N., Hirschman, R., Graham, J. R., & Zaragoza, M. S. (1993). *Sexual aggression: Issues in etiology, assessment, and treatment.* Bristol, PA: Taylor and Francis.

Holloway, M., & Swan, A. (1993). A & E management of sexual assault. *Nursing Standard, 7*(45), 31-35.

Jezierski, M. (1992). Sexual assault nurse examiner: A role with lifetime impact. *Journal of Emergency Nursing, 18*(2), 177-179.

Kennedy, P. H. (1993). Sexual abuse within adult intimate relationships. *Clinical Issues in Perinatal and Women's Health Nursing, 4*(3), 391-401.

King, M., & Woolett, E. (1997). Sexually assaulted males: 115 men consulting a counseling service. *Archives of Sexual Behavior, 26*(6), 579-588.

Koss, M., & Harvey, M. (1987). *The rape victim: Clinical and community approaches to treatment.* Lexington, MA: Stephen Greene Press.

Ledray, L. (1990). Counseling rape victims: The nursing challenge. *Perspectives in Psychiatric Care, 26*(2), 21-27.

Ledray, L. (1992). The sexual assault nurse clinician: A fifteen year experience in Minneapolis. *Journal of Emergency Nursing, 18*(3), 217-222.

Ledray, L. (1994). *Recovering from rape* (2nd ed.). New York: Henry Holt.

Ledray, L., & Arndt, S. (1994). Examining the sexual assault victim: A new model for nursing care. *Journal of Psychosocial Nursing, 32*(2), 7-12.

Leserman, J., Drossman, D., Li, Z., Toomey, T., Nachman, G., & Glogau, L. (1996). Sexual and physical abuse history in gastroenterology practice: How types of abuse impact health status. *Psychosomatic Medicine 53*(1), 4-15.

Linton, M. A. (1987). Date rape and sexual aggression in dating situations: Incidence and risk factors. *Journal of Counseling Psychology, 34*(2), 186-196.

Mantese, G., Mantese, V., Mantese, T., Mantese, J., Mantese, M. L., & Essique, C. (1991). Medical and legal aspects of rape and resistance. *Journal of Legal Medicine, 12,* 58-84.

North American Nursing Diagnosis Association. (1999). *NANDA nursing diagnoses: Definitions and classification, 1999-2000.* Philadelphia: NANDA.

Rambow, B., Adkinson, C., Frost, T., & Peterson, G. (1992). Female sexual assault: Medical and legal implications. *Annals of Emergency Medicine, 21*(6), 78-82.

Responding to rape and sexual attack. (1992). *Nursing Standard, 5*(18), 31.

Ruckman, L. M. (1992). Rape: How to begin the healing. *American Journal of Nursing, 92*(9), 48-51.

Sawyer, R. G., Desmond, S. M., & Lucke, G. M. (1993). Sexual communication and the college student: Implications for date rape. *Health Values: Achieving High Level Wellness, 17*(4), 11-20.

Scott, V. (1992). More information on SANE's in Houston . . . sexual assault nurse examiners. *Journal of Emergency Nursing, 18*(2), 95.

Slaughter, L., Brown, C, Crowley, S., & Peck, R. (1997). Patterns of genital injury in female sexual assault victims. *American Journal of Obstetrics and Gynecology, 176*(3), 609-616.

Thelen, M. H. (1998). Fear of intimacy and attachment among rape survivors. *Behavior Modification 22*(1), 108-116.

Tomaino, S. (1971). *Persephone: Bringer of spring* (pp. 32-36). New York: Crowell.

Trevelyan, J. (1991). Marital rape. *Nursing Times, 87*(13), 40-41.

Tyra, P. A. (1993). Older women: Victims of rape. *Journal of Gerontological Nursing, 19*(5), 36-37.

Weaver, K. (1993). A city under siege. *Nursing Standard, 7*(49), 18-20.

Weingourt, L. (1990). Wife rape in a sample of psychiatric patients. *Image: The Journal of Nursing Scholarship, 22*(3), 144-147.

Suggested Readings

Aiken, M. M. (1993). False allegation: A concept in the context of rape. *Journal of Psychosocial Nursing and Mental Health Services, 31*(11), 15-20.

Burgess, A., & Holstrom, L. (1974). Rape-trauma syndrome. *American Journal of Psychiatry, 131*(9), 981-985.

Davis, L., & Brody, E. (1979). *Rape and older women: A guide to prevention and protection.* Washington, DC: U.S. Department of Health, Education, and Welfare, Public Health Service, National Institute of Mental Health.

Ledray, L. (1990). Counseling rape victims: The nursing challenge. *Perspectives in Psychiatric Care, 26*(2), 21-27.

Ruckman, L. M. (1992). Rape: How to begin the healing. *American Journal of Nursing, 92*(9), 48-51.

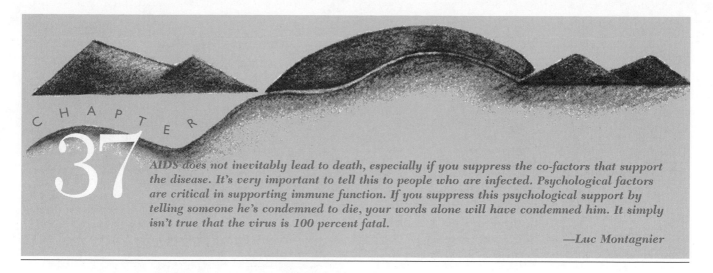

AIDS does not inevitably lead to death, especially if you suppress the co-factors that support the disease. It's very important to tell this to people who are infected. Psychological factors are critical in supporting immune function. If you suppress this psychological support by telling someone he's condemned to die, your words alone will have condemned him. It simply isn't true that the virus is 100 percent fatal.

—Luc Montagnier

AIDS/HIV

Learning Objectives

After studying this chapter, you should be able to:

1. Define terms such as AIDS, AIDS-dementia complex (ADC), and HIV-positive.
2. Discuss the nature of AIDS as a holistic disease.
3. Identify three psychological responses to AIDS.
4. Identify three spiritual responses to AIDS.
5. Describe compassion fatigue.
6. Discuss the significance of compassion fatigue on professionals as well as on nonprofessionals caring for people with AIDS.
7. Discuss the psychiatric sequelae of AIDS.
8. Discuss at least three strategies for differentiating depression from ADC.
9. Discuss the implications of AIDS for family members.
10. Discuss the two paths available to nurses faced with the AIDS crisis.
11. Apply the nursing process to a patient with AIDS.

Key Terminology

AIDS	HIV	Safer sex
AIDS-dementia complex	HIV-positive	Worried well
Compassion fatigue		

The journey involving **AIDS** exacts a high toll from patients and caregivers alike. AIDS is a terrible disease. But it is important to keep in focus, as this chapter's initial quote exhorts us to do, that maintaining a positive outlook and hope are essential ingredients to maintaining quality of life through the journey marked by AIDS. Reading this chapter will help you to appreci-ate the psychological and spiritual concomitants of AIDS as well as the nature of your role in responding to these issues.

The following excerpt from *Thanksgiving: An AIDS Journal* (Cox, 1990) provides a glimpse into the inner world of Elizabeth Cox as she stood by watching and caring for her husband as he fought against AIDS.

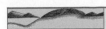

Keith's Story

This morning Keith went to see Dr. Davis about the sores in his mouth. Dr. Davis said that they looked like herpes. They have been very painful and debilitating for about five days now. I am terrible with this kind of health problem when it comes to sympathy for Keith—I seem to have no patience. He is uncomfortable enough to be miserable but it isn't serious enough for me to switch into my Florence Nightingale role. Hearing Keith moan about his mouth reminds me that he is sick and that this disease isn't going away. He is too uncomfortable for me to leave Luke with him for any length of time. Lots of feelings of being trapped and I hate them.

Constantly worrying about Keith. He is so white and thin. He went off ribavirin two weeks ago because he couldn't tolerate it. He is starting a lesser dose tomorrow. The plan is two weeks on, two weeks off. I don't understand how it can be good for him if it takes away his appetite and keeps him from sleeping.

Keith is on so many drugs. Or on and off them. If they don't have to be kept in the refrigerator, Keith keeps them in a plastic cosmetics bag. Diphenhydramine, naltrexone, tetracycline, metronidazole, lidocaine, dapsone, Zovirax, triamcinolone cream, Mycelex.

Timelessness. Marooned in the present. No way of planning for the future. Like living in a vacuum. I feel it is killing us. Hot and sticky outside. Uncomfortable inside: Keith says air conditioning makes him cough and his skin itch. In any case the air conditioner in the bedroom is broken. It makes a terrible sound and blows hot air.

Time has stopped and it makes me panic. I cannot sleep. I walk into Luke's room and remember another time I felt that everything had stopped. We were waiting for Luke to be born. He was two weeks overdue. I couldn't sleep at night; I was too uncomfortable. I tossed and turned and periodically lumbered to the bathroom. I knew I was disturbing Keith, he often joked or complained about my fitfulness, but I was too miserable to care. One night Keith turned to me and said, "Would it help if I read to you?" I was touched: Keith hardly ever read. I handed him the collection of stories by Colette by my side of the bed and he took the book, sat up in bed, and read, slowly and carefully, occasionally putting his hand on my belly or stroking my hair. I don't remember the story; I remember watching him read. He finished the story at dawn. I said I still didn't feel sleepy but felt so incredibly tired. Maybe a beer would help. So we shared a beer and watched the sun come up. We held hands. It didn't matter that it was morning; we were waiting for something that transcended the limits of night and day. We watched the dawn and then fell asleep. I am haunted by the thought that we are waiting now, waiting for something equally monumental. And now there is no pregnant belly to watch move.

Last night Keith said to me, "It is a very strong instinct, the feeling that you want to reach a resolution. Dying is a temptation. You and Luke keep reminding me that dying is not the solution...but it never goes away."

I worry about Keith's depression. I am bitchy, angry, aggressive, hostile. But Keith seems to be beyond that. He is so angry he is silent and withdrawn. When his father was noncommittal and almost uninterested in helping us out financially (his uncle never responded), it was as if Keith had been stabbed and now he has retired to lick his wounds. But it seems to me that his wounds are not healing naturally. He is trying to heal them with determination. And it is just too exhausting.

Thanksgiving: An AIDS journal (p. 6). © Copyright 1990 by Elizabeth Cox, reprinted by permission of Wylie, Aitken & Stone, Inc.

AIDS has been recognized in the United States since 1981. During that year, the pattern of unexpected illness and deaths in the homosexual population was attributed to AIDS. Since then, most of the research interest and monies have been focused on discovering a cure and better treatments for the disease. The focus has been on the physical aspects of the disease. Little interest has been given to the emotional, psychological, and spiritual aspects of AIDS. Yet, as Dr. Montagnier's quote indicates, these issues are essential to maintaining a healthy immune system.

A shift in thinking from purely "curing" to "caring" is beginning to occur. Such a shift requires a transformation of thinking for many. The tools are no longer pharmacological preparations and miracles of medical technology. The tools include the self to communicate acceptance of the sufferer, to provide support through the dying process, to educate about the disease and its course, to explore ways to improve quality if not duration of life, and to provide existential support as the sufferer struggles to find meaning and purpose in his or her life (Belcher, Dettmore, & Holzmer, 1989; Carson, 1989; Carson, 1990; Carson, 1993; Carson & Green, 1992; Carson, Soeken, Shanty, & Terry, 1990). Caring, as described, contains both psychological and spiritual elements.

PSYCHOLOGICAL PROBLEMS ASSOCIATED WITH AIDS

The psychological problems most often associated with **HIV** infection can be graphed on a continuum, moving from the problems of those whose behaviors place them at low risk for the infection to the problems of those whose behaviors are highly risky and to those who are infected. Figure 37–1 illustrates the continuum of HIV-related psychiatric problems.

The first group of people with whom we are concerned have either no risk or little risk for the infection. People at low risk include

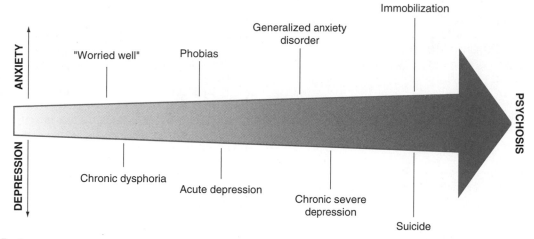

Figure 37-1
The continuum of HIV-related psychiatric problems. (From Ostrow, D. G. [1986]. A psychiatric overview of AIDS. *International Journal of Neuroscience, 32,* 647–659.)

- Those who have been involved in monogamous relationships since 1978
- Those who have engaged only in **safer sex,** such as mutual masturbation and sex with condoms
- Those who are not sexually active
- Those who have only household, social, and work-place contact with HIV-infected people.

People who fall into this level of risk and who have HIV-related psychosocial problems are called the **worried well.**

The next group includes those who are at moderate risk for the infection but are presently negative for HIV. The people who fall into this risk category include

- Heterosexuals with multiple sexual partners
- Health care workers with accidental needlesticks or with significant exposure to blood of **HIV-positive** (serum positive for HIV) people

The third and fourth groups engage in the same high-risk behaviors; however, the third group is not infected and the fourth group is HIV-positive. People at high risk include

- Men who engage in same-sex relations
- People who use intravenous (IV) drugs and share needles
- People who engage in bisexual behavior or those with a bisexual sexual partner
- People who engage in sexual contact with an intravenous drug user
- Infants born to intravenous drug-using mothers
- Sexual partners of HIV-infected people
- Hemophiliacs
- People who received blood transfusions before 1985

The psychological reactions differ for each of these groups.

The worried well generally display symptoms of anxiety. They feel angry and concerned about their chances of becoming infected and may experience sexual difficulty. They may even develop symptoms similar to those of HIV-positive people (e.g., fatigue, weight loss, and diarrhea).

People who are at both moderate and high risk for HIV infection but who are not infected are subject to all the concerns of the worried well, with some significant additions. These people may experience immediate relief when the results of a blood test to determine the presence of HIV are negative. But in the face of risky behaviors, fears persist regarding the accuracy of the test and whether the inevitable has only been postponed. The person is faced with choices regarding future sexual behaviors and how to deal with sensitive issues such as practicing safer sex. They may experience guilt over former sexual practices and IV drug use. They fear disclosing their risk to partners who themselves are at low risk. Pathological denial is also a mechanism used by the HIV-negative person who is at risk. Such individuals block the reality of their risky behaviors and continue with such behaviors as if everything were OK (Taylor & Robertson, 1994; Wenger, Kusseling, Beck, & Shapiro, 1994).

The psychological problems of the fourth group, those who are HIV infected, can be categorized into two types:

1. *Functional,* which usually involves an adjustment disorder with depression or anxiety as the predominant symptom
2. *Organic brain syndrome,* which includes major depression, dementia, and delirium

The spiritual issues of AIDS, having to do with finding meaning and purpose in life, dealing with possible guilt over lifestyle choices, and resolving a relationship with God or a higher power, present concurrently with the aforementioned psychosocial and psychiatric problems (Carson, 1990; Carson & Green, 1992; Kendall, 1994).

What do you think? What have you observed regarding society's attitudes toward AIDS and individuals infected with HIV?

► *Check Your Reading*
1. What are the spiritual issues of a person diagnosed with AIDS?
2. What are the three psychological reactions to AIDS?
3. Who are the worried well?
4. Identify three risk factors for acquiring AIDS.

AIDS: THE DISEASE

Etiology

HIV, a retrovirus that attacks specific components of the immune system, is the etiological agent of AIDS. The transmission of AIDS occurs through the exchange of body fluids, particularly blood and semen. HIV has an affinity for the T helper (T) cells and inserts its genetic material into the host chromosome. The role of the T cell is to regulate the functioning of other components of the immune system. HIV produces a progressive decline in the numbers of T cells, causing the immune system to lose the stimulus to "turn on" in response to invaders; this leaves the person susceptible to many diseases.

Solomon, Temoshok, O'Leary, and Zich (1987) strongly suggested that a complete understanding of AIDS must proceed from a perspective combining biological, psychological, and social factors. Carson (1990) suggested that the spiritual component is also essential to understanding the disease progression. In a study of 100 HIV-infected people, Carson and Green (1992) and Carson (1993) demonstrated a significant relationship between hardiness and spiritual well-being. Individuals who were both hardy and spiritually well demonstrated a high degree of participation in prayer, vitamin use, and support to other people with AIDS. This suggests that physical, psychological, social, and spiritual changes associated with AIDS may contribute to the disease's progression. The change in immunological functioning caused by HIV affects other bodily systems as well. For instance, the immunosuppression that occurs with HIV opens the door to opportunistic infections such as toxoplasmosis and to neoplasms such as Kaposi's sarcoma.

In December 1997, 641,086 people in the United States were reported to the Centers for Disease Control and Prevention (CDC), having been diagnosed with AIDS. The majority of these people continue to be men, although the number of women facing this disease increases steadily. From January 1996 to December 1997, the number of U.S. women with AIDS rose to 13,105 cases. This excludes pediatric cases. The cumulative total of women with AIDS in this country reached 98,468 by the end of 1997. The cumulative total of men reported to the CDC as having AIDS by late 1997 was more than five times that amount, reaching 534,532 cases. People in their 30s seem to be the group with the largest incidence of AIDS (CDC, 1997).

Children are not immune to the effects of AIDS on the U.S. population. As of the beginning of 1995, 6209 cases of AIDS were reported in children younger than 13 years of age. By December 1997, that number reached slightly more than 8000. Perinatally acquired AIDS declined during the 1990s, due to successful attempts to promote voluntary prenatal HIV testing and because of the use of zidovudine (AZT) by pregnant, HIV-positive women.

AIDS-related deaths were found to have decreased by more than 25% in the years 1995 through 1998. The decline may be attributed to the increasing use of combination antiretroviral therapy, including the use of protease inhibitors. Nonetheless, deaths occurring from the disease had reached close to 400,000 in this country as of December 1997, with 1% of that total being the deaths of children.

Although in the United States the largest groups of AIDS sufferers are homosexual men and IV drug users, the disease does not affect only these groups. The virus does not have an affinity for individuals with a specific sexual preference; rather, it has an affinity for a specific environment in which it can best thrive. HIV is a fragile group of cells that dies quickly once outside of the body. It requires an extremely warm medium with a specific pH level to remain alive. It finds that medium primarily in blood and semen and, to a lesser extent, in all body fluids.

What do you think? Are there things that should be done that are currently not being done to address the problem of AIDS?

► *Check Your Reading*
5. What group has been most affected by AIDS?
6. Why is the spiritual component important in our focus on AIDS?
7. What type of virus causes AIDS?
8. What are the three modes of HIV transmission?

Mode of Transmission

Because HIV is spread through the exchange of blood and semen, the virus is transmitted primarily through sexual activity, blood exposure, and childbirth. Although the most risky sexual activity is receptive anal intercourse, vaginal and oral intercourse also are risky. At present, most cases of HIV infection have occurred in men who engage in homosexual anal intercourse. However, HIV can also be transmitted through heterosexual or lesbian sexual activities.

Blood contains an even higher concentration of HIV than does semen. IV drug use with a shared needle is the most common method of blood exposure transmission. In addition, clotting factors (given to hemophiliacs) that were derived from blood transfusions between 1978 and 1985 have been implicated in blood exposure to HIV.

Several health care workers have been reported to have become infected with HIV through accidental needlestick injuries or through blood contact on nonintact skin and mucous membranes.

Perinatal transmission—transmission from mother to child—can occur in utero; however, as noted earlier, the incidence is on the decrease (CDC, 1997). See What Society Needs to Know: AIDS.

Prevention

Currently, no known cure exists for AIDS. Although intensive research is being directed toward the discovery of a cure, the thrust of public health programs is prevention through education. Former U.S. Surgeon General C. Everett Koop was instrumental in waging an intensive AIDS education campaign aimed at all Americans but especially at those engaging in risky behaviors, such as IV drug use and casual and unprotected sexual contact. The educational efforts have two purposes: to provide information about ways to stop the spread of the virus and to decrease the epidemic of fear.

Prevention can be accomplished by avoiding risky behaviors through

- Safer sex practices (e.g., using condoms and not exchanging body fluids)
- Disinfection of dirty needles and syringes that were used to inject street drugs

For health care workers, prevention can be accomplished through

- Use of universal precautions with all patients, including the use of barrier methods (e.g., gloves and eye shields) to prevent the patient's blood and body fluids from contacting the provider's skin or mucous membranes
- No capping of used needles
- Disposal of used needles in puncture-proof containers

Education to deal with the epidemic of fear focuses on the fact that AIDS is only spread through exchange of blood or body fluids. This means that social, household, and workplace contact can continue unchanged. It is safe to talk to an HIV-infected person; hug, touch, eat meals together; and use the same bathroom facilities with no fear of contagion (American Foundation for AIDS Research, 1996; Aruffo, Thompson, Gottleib, & Dobbins, 1995).

A study by Baldwin and Baldwin (1988) examined the effectiveness of AIDS education in reducing risk-taking behavior among college students. The results of this study were not encouraging. Although students were knowledgeable about AIDS and a few worried about either contracting the disease or their risk, this did not greatly motivate cautious behavior. Knowledgeable students were no more inclined to avoid risky behaviors than were less knowledgeable students. Although students with more accurate knowledge were inclined to have had fewer vaginal intercourse partners in the

WHAT SOCIETY NEEDS TO KNOW

AIDS

What types of contact are OK and safe in caring for a person with AIDS?

The HIV infection most often is transmitted through intimate sexual contact; however, contact with blood and other body fluids may result in transmission of the infection. Authorities say that casual, nonintimate contact is safe. Studies have been conducted of noninfected people who share household utensils, towels, linens, and toilet facilities with infected people, and the noninfected people show no evidence of HIV transmission. Authorities also say that it is highly improbable that AIDS can be transmitted by an insect bite. Touching the person with AIDS on the arm or hand and avoiding the use of unnecessary protective clothing are important ways of expressing your care. It is important to remember that AIDS is a largely preventable disease because of its mode of viral transmission and the fragile nature of the virus. Although abstinence from sexual intercourse is the only certain way of preventing the transmission of AIDS, the consistent use of latex condoms and a spermicide containing nonoxynol 9 can significantly

reduce the likelihood of HIV transmission. Education about safe health practices is important for both patient and family.

The person with AIDS is immunosuppressed and is at increased risk of developing opportunistic infections. People with normally benign infections such as colds or flu should therefore temporarily avoid contact with the person with AIDS. Intermittent acute infections interspersed with periods of wellness characterize the course of AIDS.

What community resources are available for people with AIDS?

The following is a partial list of community resources:
- Public Health Service AIDS Hotline: 800-337-AIDS
- American Public Health Association *Special Initiatives on AIDS* series: American Public Health Association Publication Sales, Department 5037, Washington, DC 20061-5037
- National Gay Task Force Crisis Line: 800-221-9044

previous 3 months, the effect of knowledge was small. For every point increase in knowledge score, only a 0.03 decline in the number of partners was seen. Also, having more knowledge did not reduce casual sexual relationships or increase the use of condoms.

Students who assessed themselves to be at risk had more sexual partners than nonworriers. Although students who worried about contracting the disease reported using condoms more than students who did not worry, the worriers did not decrease the number of sexual encounters in which they engaged. In fact, the frequency of casual sexual relationships was greater in the worrying group than in the nonworrying group. Factors that correlated with more cautious behavior were gender (females were more cautious than males), the use of seatbelts, and older age at the time of first sexual intercourse experience (the younger the student was when he or she became sexually active, the more partners he or she had experienced, and the more he or she engaged in casual sex).

The researchers concluded that AIDS education that focuses on cognitive-emotional factors alone is insufficient to change behavior. They suggested a much broader socialization program that aimed at making young people more aware of and responsible regarding risks of social problems such as alcohol and drug abuse, unwanted pregnancies, driving without seatbelts, sexually transmitted diseases (STDs), and AIDS transmission. Effective AIDS education must address more than the cognitive domain; it must be directed to the whole person. Other studies have documented the inadequacy of cognitive knowledge to change behaviors (McLean et al., 1994; Ridge, Plummer, & Minichiello, 1994; Seal & Agostenelli, 1994).

What do you think? What helps you change bad or risky behaviors? How do we incorporate other approaches in addition to cognitive training in our educational processes?

➤ *Check Your Reading*

9. Describe universal precautions for health care workers.
10. Identify the two-pronged focus of public education with regard to AIDS.
11. Why is a cognitive approach to AIDS education insufficient?

PSYCHOLOGICAL, SOCIAL, AND SPIRITUAL IMPLICATIONS OF AIDS

This section deals with the psychological, social, and spiritual implications of AIDS and includes vignettes from the story of W. Carole Chenitz, a nurse who died of AIDS in February 1992. These vignettes, which are excerpts from a chapter entitled "Living With AIDS" in a book called *HIV/AIDS: A Guide to Nursing Care* (Chen-

itz, 1992), are a poignant window into the impact of AIDS on a woman, nurse, and mother.

Stigma of AIDS

The reaction of society to AIDS has been so negative and fear-laden that people diagnosed as HIV-positive become the recipients of society's emotional baggage in regard to the disease. As Carole Chenitz (1992) wrote,

We were afraid that if people found out that I had AIDS, Kimberly would be ostracized by her classmates. So we decided to wait. Kim felt comfortable with this, since many of her classmates had made negative comments about gays and people with AIDS. While we were sure that the overwhelming majority of people in our community would respond with concern and compassion, we were afraid about the one or two who would react from unbridled fear. (p. 452)

People with AIDS can be expected to experience the same shock, denial, fear, anger, acceptance, and resignation that Kübler-Ross (1975) described as part of the dying process. (See Chapter 21 for further discussion of reaction to loss.) However, the reaction to AIDS is further complicated by factors not present in other terminal illnesses. Tibesar (1986) noted that the transmissible, terminal, and stigmatizing characteristics of AIDS place an unusual burden on those infected. Because the disease has been linked with homosexual intercourse and IV drug use, it has been approached from a moralistic view.

Kayal (1985) discussed what happens when the etiology of a disease is framed in moral language and the illness in question affects individuals who have been "religiously stigmatized and legally proscribed minorities" (p. 218). The afflicted are blamed for their illness. This is exactly what has happened with AIDS.

It is worthwhile to read a quote from Kevin Cahill (1983), an internationally known parasitologist:

When a fatal infection had struck down veterans attending an American Legion convention, health professionals across the country joined in the search for a solution. When women using tampons became ill with toxic shock syndrome, medical societies and research centers immediately focused their enormous talents on that problem. But when the victims were drug addicts, and poor Haitian refugees and homosexual men, their plight did not, somehow, seem as significant to those expected to speak for the health professions. No major research programs were announced, and until it became clear that the disease could spread to the general population through blood transfusions, organized medicine seemed a part of the conspiracy of silence. (p. 2)

Kayal (1985) asserted that AIDS has been so tied to a lifestyle that is viewed by many as sinful, hedonistic, or perverted that society has failed to respond to the suffering of people with AIDS. This failure to respond has characterized more than just the medical system. The response of government, families, churches, and other social institutions has been too little too late (Shilts, 1987).

The present epidemic of AIDS challenges American society to examine its attitudes about sexuality—specifically, homosexuality. Some contend that AIDS is a just punishment for sexual activity that they view as immoral, and even that AIDS is God's response to immoral behavior. People who hold this view claim to know the mind of God, which may lend them a degree of credibility; however, this view increases the social alienation of people with AIDS. Murphy (1988) argued against the idea of AIDS being a just punishment, noting the disproportion between the impact of the activity and a punishment as devastating as AIDS. After all, said Murphy, if AIDS is a just punishment for a particular sexual behavior, why are child abusers not afflicted with an even greater punishment?

Regardless of why AIDS occurred or how or why a particular person contracted the infection, both a theistic perspective and the high standards of professional nursing call for compassion rather than judgment.

Isolation of People With AIDS

American society is further challenged to examine persistent attitudes about the ministrations of comfort and compassion, acceptance of individual differences, and society's responsibility to deal with the suffering of its young. As Carole Chenitz (1992) wrote:

Not only did the emotional needs I had go unrecognized, but no one touched me. No one in the hospital staff took my hand, rubbed my back, gave me support, or did any of the comfort and care measures that we nurses pride ourselves on. I will never forget how I felt.... I was unclean, untouchable, undesirable, a patient with a disgusting disease. If you get too close, you may get it, too. (p. 452)

These are not challenges to be addressed easily or without pain, and their debate continues without resolution in government, schools, places of business, and families.

In her book, *AIDS: The Ultimate Challenge,* Elizabeth Kübler-Ross (1987) spoke to the challenge facing America in the care of people with AIDS:

Since we can no longer deny that AIDS is a life threatening illness that will eventually involve millions of people and decimate large portions of our human population, it is our choice to grow and learn from it, to either help people with this dread disease or abandon them. It is our choice to live up to this ultimate challenge or to perish. (p. 13)

Some individuals and organizations have exemplified a positive response to the challenge of AIDS and have reached out with compassion and willingness to care for people with the disease. In San Francisco, the Shanti project is such an example. Shanti is a community organization that uses a peer counseling model to work with people with AIDS, their significant others, and their family members. The counselor's job is to empathize with patients without judging them and to work collaboratively with other health care providers regarding ways to approach certain people with the disease (McCaffrey, 1987). There have been other cases where the response to the AIDS challenge has been far from compassionate.

What happens to the person with AIDS who is caught in this societal struggle? Sometimes he or she is left to deal with the illness in isolation. The homosexual person with AIDS frequently bears the brunt of society's homophobia—irrational fear, intolerance, and dread of any person believed to be homosexual. The homosexual person with AIDS is rejected, condemned, and ostracized. Homophobia can seriously harm a homosexual person's self-image. Murphy (1986) quoted a young gay man, who in the midst of a counseling session in which the counselor was attempting to assure the young man of God's love said, "How can God love me? I am one of His mistakes" (p. 39).

"Crisis of Knowing"

The crisis of AIDS for the person with the disease begins with the diagnosis. As Carole Chenitz (1992) wrote:

Two years ago I donated blood during a blood drive. Ninety days later, on a cold, gray northern California day, I received a certified, registered letter. It was my day to work the evening shift, as I did every Monday. This enabled me to conduct a seminar for the nurses and to facilitate a multifamily therapy group on the substance abuse inpatient unit. The letter was from the blood bank, informing me that I was HIV-positive. My heart stopped as I read the letter. "How can this happen? There must be some mistake. Oh my God, I'm going to die!" I was scared. I felt that I had just walked through a warp in time and space. I was now on the other side of the pale seeing myself and my life as if it belonged to someone else. I felt each breath would be my last. Waves of pain, fear, and sadness washed over me. "What am I going to do? Who can I talk to? What about my children?" (p. 437)

For many, the diagnosis brings people the knowledge that even though they feel fine, they are HIV-positive. Feeling as if he or she is carrying a time bomb ticking away the minutes and days of life, the person with AIDS is faced with questions that are not easy to answer. "How do I tell others that I am HIV-positive? What do I tell them about how I became HIV-positive?" This may mean "coming out" with honesty about a lifestyle characterized by IV drug use or homosexuality. Figure 37-2 illustrates the spectrum of social responses to AIDS.

Because these are such difficult issues to face, the initial "telling" of the diagnosis must be done by a professional knowledgeable about the course of AIDS—someone who can provide accurate information that the person can hear and comprehend. This professional must also possess counseling skills. The incidence of suicide among newly diagnosed AIDS patients is significant enough to warrant every safeguard against this happening. The incidence of suicidal crisis, suicide attempts, and completed suicides is high in AIDS patients.

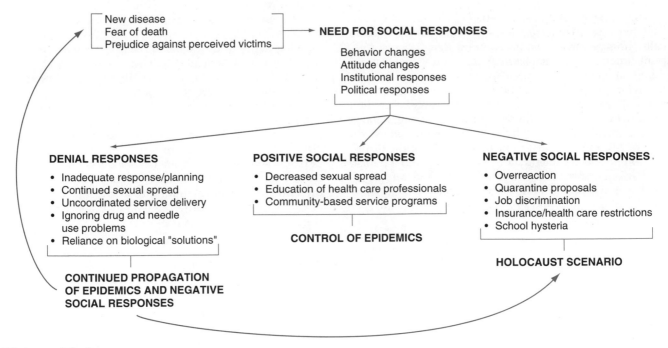

Figure 37-2
The spectrum of social responses to AIDS. (From Ostrow, D. G. [1988]. Models for understanding the psychiatric consequences of AIDS. In T. P. Bridge, A. F. Mirsky, & F. K. Goodwin [Eds.], *Psychological, neuropsychiatric, and substance abuse aspects of AIDS* [Vol. 44, pp. 85–94]. New York: Raven Press.)

For people with AIDS or those who are HIV-positive, the diagnosis precipitates a crisis of such magnitude that it can totally overwhelm their psychological defenses. AIDS not only presents the possibility of death but also generates fears regarding disfigurement, changes in role, body function, and self-esteem.

Loss of Social Support

The loss of social support is one of the many losses experienced by people with AIDS. As they become increasingly more debilitated by the disease process, they find themselves more alone in their efforts to cope. Some people with AIDS rely on denial to block the pain of confronting what their ultimate future will probably hold. Many throw themselves into a frenzy of activity as if by keeping active they can stop the disease from progressing. This denial has both healthy and unhealthy implications. It allows a semblance of hope and the ability to plan for a future that may not occur, but the denial may block the reflection about needed lifestyle changes that could result in a healthier immune system.

Process of Dying of AIDS

Death is another issue confronting the person with AIDS. As Chenitz (1992) wrote

Like many people with AIDS, I am not afraid of death, I am afraid of dying. The dying process and how that will

be handled is of great concern to me. Everyone is going to die. Death is a part of life. However, AIDS brings with it a terribly painful, often humiliating dying process and that terrifies me. (p. 454)

Younger people have greater difficulty coping with terminal illness because the prospect of dying disrupts many hopes, plans, and expectations. Some fear leaving dependent children.

The fear of death is heightened by the exacerbations of the illness, negative reactions to the treatments, and the perception of increasing losses. For instance, a 35-year-old actor, who had suffered severe weight loss and had Kaposi's lesions on his face, was fearful of losing future auditions for television commercials. His fear was not just for the immediate loss of financial security but also for the ultimate loss of his self-image (Moynihan, Christ, & Gallo-Silver, 1987).

Existential Issues and AIDS

Tibesar (1986) noted the importance of facing existential issues as the person with AIDS increasingly contemplates his or her own death as a reality. As Carole Chenitz (1992) wrote

It was still a shock to me that my life was evolving this way. Initially I was too sick to think about my life and my goals. Later when my energy was so low, loss of work wasn't difficult to bear, since I couldn't do it anyway. However, the loss of who I was and what I had done my entire adult life hit after several months: I wasn't a nurse anymore. I still had a license, but I would never practice nursing again. All of the articles published, papers presented, book chapters written, grants developed, and classes taught didn't matter now. It was gone. If I were to survive, I would need to develop new skills. I would have to learn to accept my new life. I needed to learn to relax. Maybe I could salvage something from my old life, but I wasn't sure what. (p. 451)

These issues, which are psychosocial as well as spiritual in nature, include the following (Tibesar, 1986):

- *Self-identity:* characterized by questions such as "Who am I now? Am I still the same person even though my body fails me daily? Does anyone still love me for who I am?"
- *Meaning of life:* characterized by questions such as "Is there some value to my suffering and loss? Has my life been important?"
- *Adversity:* characterized by statements such as "Is life always so cruel? Can there be anything worse than an unfair death?"
- *Fate:* exemplified by statements like "Why has this happened to me? Why must I be deprived of the life I love?"
- *Stigma:* characterized by statements such as "Is this a punishment for being who I am?"
- *Relationships:* characterized by fears such as "Will my friends and family reject me? Will my lover leave me?"
- *Productivity:* characterized by statements such as "I've lost my job. I feel so weak, and I'm fatigued doing the slightest tasks. Am I of any use to anyone?"
- *Heritage:* characterized by concerns such as "What can I leave behind? How will people remember me?"

Coming to grips with these existential issues frequently is complicated by unresolved conflicts and concerns over life choices, such as IV drug use, or guilt over sexual activities that exposed the person to HIV. Further complicating this existential quest may be low self-esteem, social isolation and alienation, and public discrimination and condemnation.

The spiritual issues facing the person with AIDS may be greatly affected by whether he or she is homosexual or bisexual or whether AIDS was contracted through IV drug use or a blood transfusion. The gay person with AIDS frequently is faced with a church that reacts by blocking the meeting of his or her existential, spiritual needs. Fortunato (1987) claimed that because much of Western religion has been terrified of sexuality in general, it is completely put off by those whose sexuality is remarkable in its difference. Gay people may need to go beyond the mainline traditional church, regardless of denomination, to seek spiritual support.

The spiritual needs of the IV drug user may be at the heart of his or her dependence on drugs and may partially explain the success of the many 12-step recovery programs (e.g., Narcotics Anonymous) that have, at their core, a reliance on a higher power to overcome the addictive behavior. Leech (1977) contended that much drug use is an attempt to fill a spiritual void regarding a sense of inner, spiritual meaning in the lives of drug users. Life seems empty, directionless, and filled with pain. Drug use may be one attempt to anesthetize a gnawing spiritual distress.

Still another spiritual scenario concerns the person who has contracted AIDS through a tainted blood transfusion. The sense of unfairness and anger regarding this situation may lead to spiritual despair and alienation from God. This is illustrated by a quote from Kimberly Bergalis, who contracted AIDS from her dentist. Bergalis (Hilts, 1991), consumed with anger about her plight, wrote

My life has been sheer hell. Who do I blame? I blame Dr. Acer and every single one of you bastards. Dr. Acer was infected and had full-blown AIDS and you stood by not doing anything about it. You are all just as guilty as he was. You've ruined my life and my family's. (p. 11)

W*hat do you think?* If you had AIDS, how would you want to be told?

➤ *Check Your Reading*
12. What is the crisis of knowing for the person newly diagnosed as HIV-positive?
13. Describe at least four of the existential issues confronted by the person with AIDS.
14. Why are AIDS patients so stigmatized?

PSYCHIATRIC IMPLICATIONS OF AIDS

The psychiatric implications of AIDS are significant. In a 1998 study of psychiatric care in a new AIDS nursing home, 423 of the first 675 patients admitted were seen for psychiatric consultation. The patients ranged in age from 22 to 70 years. Most were coping with multiple losses of health, fitness, homes, careers, loved ones, strength, and functional capacity. All had multiple and severe medical illnesses. Of the 423 patients evaluated, 422 (99.8%) had one or more psychiatric disorders; 351 (83%) had diagnoses of dementia; 349 (82.5%) were substance abusers; 276 (65%) had psychiatric diagnoses other than cognitive or substance abuse, and 61 (14.4%) had delirium. These patients were younger, more medically and psychiatrically ill, on more complex medical regimens, and had a higher prevalence of both dementia and substance abuse than those in a separate study of geriatric nursing homes (Cohen, 1998).

Depression

Given the nature of AIDS, it is no surprise that depression is a common response to the diagnosis. In one study that involved a retrospective chart review of 52 hospitalized AIDS patients, 83% of the patients exhibited affective mood disturbance. Characteristically, the patients were sad and withdrawn, expressed low self-esteem and hopelessness, and displayed psychomotor retardation (Atkinson, Capadini, Levine, & Price, 1996; Perry & Markowitz, 1986).

Etiology

The organic depression that is sometimes seen in AIDS patients may be due to brain lesions within the limbic system. Because expressions of emotion are regulated in the limbic system, a limbic system infection also may result in mood disturbances. This relationship between depression and neurochemical disturbances in AIDS patients is a tentative explanation open to considerably more research (Michels & Marzuk, 1993; Morris, 1996; Pert, Ruff, Ruscetti, Ferrar, & Hill, 1988).

The adjustment disorder with depressed mood reported in people with AIDS may be a response to the multiple losses associated with role, body image, and social support, coupled with fear of death and feelings of helplessness. Untreated, this depression can further erode the patient's immune system and decrease his or her interest in engaging in health-promoting behaviors. In the opening story, Keith's journey with AIDS was punctuated with an adjustment disorder with depressive symptoms.

Treatment

Depression is treated with a variety of antidepressant medications to deal with the sadness and apathy. In addition, a psychostimulant such as methylphenidate HCl (Ritalin) may be added to deal with fatigue and weakness. Supportive therapy also is used to assist the patient to deal with the many issues that seem to go hand in hand with AIDS, such as issues of loss, self-esteem, guilt, isolation, and anger.

AIDS-Dementia Complex

AIDS-dementia complex (ADC), also referred to in the American Psychiatric Association's (1994) *Diagnostic and Statistical Manual, Fourth Edition* (DSM-IV) as dementia due to HIV disease, is a major complication of HIV infection occurring in 70% to 90% of all AIDS patients (Michels & Marazuk, 1993; Portegies, 1994; Rosenberg, McLaulin, Bennett, & Mathisen, 1996). Symptoms of ADC may appear in the absence of other symptoms of AIDS. This fact has led researchers to consider ADC to be a direct consequence of HIV infection. Belinda Mason, a young woman who contracted AIDS through a tainted blood transfusion during emergency surgery, illustrated the impact of ADC in the following quote (Hilts, 1991):

Sometimes I forget what I'm saying in the middle of a sentence. I am constantly confronted with the obvious losses in my life, but one of the greatest is the diminishing of my intellect; I used to have a razor-sharp tongue and I could use my hillbilly wisdom, fly by the seat of my pants. That used to define who I was; now AIDS has consumed my identity. (p. 11)

Etiology

Several explanatory hypotheses regarding the etiology of ADC exist. The first has to do with how HIV gets into the brain. It has been suggested that monocytes may transport HIV into the central nervous system (CNS) (Rosenberg et al., 1996). The monocyte, a circulating white blood cell, triggers an immune response by engulfing invader cells and delivering these cells to other components of the immune system. Monocytes possess a migratory ability that allows them to travel throughout the body to remove foreign particles. When a monocyte enters a tissue, it is called a macrophage. HIV binds to the CD4 receptor found on the surface of the monocyte as well as on that of the T cell. Unlike the T cell, however, the monocyte is not killed by the HIV and may serve as a reservoir for the virus.

HIV has been found in macrophages recovered from the brain tissue of some persons with ADC. Monocytes have the ability to cross the blood-brain barrier and may be the transport mechanism for HIV into the CNS. Because not all studies have replicated this finding, there may be another mechanism by which HIV is transported into the CNS. Once HIV enters the CNS, the exact mechanism of inducing cognitive, behavioral, and sensorimotor changes is unknown.

Neurodiagnostic Findings

CT reveals cerebral atrophy with ventricular enlargement. MRI has been shown to be more sensitive in displaying the characteristic white matter pallor. EEGs show mild slowing of brain wave activity, but it is nonspecific. White blood cells are found in cerebrospinal fluid (CSF) in 20% of ADC patients, and elevated protein levels are present in 60% of ADC patients. The presence of HIV in the CSF of most patients with ADC may serve as a marker of neurological involvement.

Symptoms

In the early stages of ADC, the symptoms are difficult to distinguish from a functional adjustment depressive reaction to the diagnosis. Initially, the patient may present with apathy, withdrawal, loss of interest in social activities, impaired memory, decreased ability to concentrate, decreased libido, ataxia, subtle difficulties in coordination, erratic and impulsive behavior, agitation, confusion, increased sensitivity to alcohol and prescribed medications, and hallucinations. Patients may need to make lists to be able to carry out activities of daily living (ADLs). They may lose their train of thought in midsentence. The changes in cognitive functioning and problem-solving affect their abilities to think abstractly. They may display difficulty transferring learned information to new situations.

These patients may exhibit impaired impulse control and emotional lability, characterized by agitation, combativeness, and panic attacks. Safety and self-care issues are major nursing concerns regarding the patient with ADC.

CNS abnormalities become more profound as the disease progresses. The primary symptoms are moderate to severe global cognitive impairment and psychomotor retardation. Characteristically, patients may stare vacantly, display little spontaneous verbal or motor activity, and as death approaches, lapse into a mute state. Paradoxically, some patients display the exact opposite behavior and become restless and agitated. Incontinence of urine and feces also is common (Horvath, 1994; Kosmyna, Whipple, & Scura, 1996).

Treatment

The treatment of ADC may include the use of low-dose antipsychotics such as haloperidol (Haldol) to decrease confusion, disorganization, and agitation. Psychostimulants such as methylphenidate and antidepressants such as fluoxetine HCl (Prozac) are used to treat the fatigue, weakness, and apathy.

What do you think? How would you deal with teaching safer sex practices to a patient who is suffering from ADC? What ethical issues does this suggest?

➤ *Check Your Reading*

15. What is ADC?
16. What does neurodiagnostic testing reveal in regard to ADC?
17. What medications are used to treat depression associated with AIDS?
18. Give two ways that cognitive functioning is impaired in ADC.

CAREGIVERS OF PEOPLE WITH AIDS

In any comprehensive discussion of AIDS, the needs of the caregivers of people with AIDS must be addressed. Just as AIDS dictates a challenging journey for the patients themselves, so the caregivers are faced with their own journey of psychological and spiritual adjustment. The initial story focusing on Elizabeth Cox's experiences illustrates the daily struggle faced by the care provider. The stigmatizing effect of AIDS on patients is also experienced by caregivers, whether they are family members, lovers, or friends. Not only are they confronted with the intense pain of their own grief but also they may be faced with society's reactions of fear, homophobia, and moral self-righteousness, as well as isolation and rejection (Flaskerud & Tabura, 1998; Roth, Siegel, & Black, 1994; Theis, Cohen, Forrest, & Zelewsky, 1997; Turner, Pearlin, & Mullan, 1998). In addition, the caregiver frequently is dealing with his or her own feelings of shock, denial, and anger at first learning that a daughter, son, spouse, parent, lover, or friend is either homosexual, bisexual, or an IV drug user. Similar feelings surround the realization that the loved one has contracted the disease. Spiritually, caregivers contend with feelings about God's role in the disease, God's availability as a support, and the meaning that their loved one's illness holds for them.

Ross and Clark-Alexander (1998) reported that mothers who provide care for children with HIV/AIDS scored significantly lower than alternative caregivers in coping styles; the mothers used more passive and emotive coping than the alternative caregivers. The researchers concluded that nurses must be particularly aware of the importance of providing interventions for these mother-caregivers to assist them in coping, thereby decreasing their stress and improving the quality of their lives.

The bereavement following the death of a lover from AIDS is complicated by the fact that the significance of the lost relationship is totally discounted by society. Individuals facing such loss experience feelings of isolation and disconnectedness, emotional confusion, and denial of their own vulnerability (Sowell, Bramlett, Gueldner, Gritzmacher, & Martin, 1991). Let us look back and continue with our initial story.

Elizabeth Cox's journey included the challenge of integrating the facts about her husband's past homosexual activity into her sense that she knew him. The diagnosis of AIDS in Keith left her shocked and dismayed but also with an overwhelming sense of betrayal. The fact of AIDS did not fit in with her knowledge of who Keith was. Fortunately for Keith, Elizabeth successfully dealt with her sense of betrayal. Her decision to stand by Keith's side as he battled AIDS was supported by the love she had for him. However, she still struggled with how to tell people about what was wrong with Keith, who to tell, and then how to deal with the reactions of others once they were told. Spiritually, Elizabeth found meaning and purpose in her journey through the writing of her journal, which she hoped would help others faced with a similar walk.

In addition to the psychological and spiritual adjustments that can be overwhelming to the caregiver, the whole spectrum of physical care must also be dealt with. AIDS in its full-blown stage is a debilitating disease that wastes once-robust bodies with relentless diarrhea and vomiting, unsightly lesions, cognitive deficits, and overwhelming weakness. Many of those who die with AIDS are young. This fact holds a special poignancy for caregivers. The care requirements of such a disease are demanding (Hays, Magee, & Chauncey, 1994).

Nurses who provide much of the hospital-based care for AIDS patients are not immune to the demands of the caring role. In a survey conducted by *Nursing 88* (Brennan, 1988) of 346 nurses from 15 institutions, their responses reflected how AIDS had spread over the preceding years—1983 to 1988. On the average, respondents had cared for a total of 44 people with AIDS. However, most of the nurses reported having cared for more than half that number in 1987 and 1988. At the time of the survey, most of the nurses were caring for at least 10 AIDS patients.

When asked how they felt about caring for AIDS patients, 73% of the nurses responded that they were concerned for their own safety. About half (47%) reported feeling frustrated at their patients' poor prognoses. Others (19%) reported feeling angry about having to care for people with AIDS. Their anger was directed at the disease itself, hospital and government authorities, and the patients, some of whom the nurses held responsible for their illness.

When asked about their families' reactions to their caring for people with AIDS, 80% responded that their relatives were concerned about their (the nurses') safety. The responses to the query "What is your overall reaction to caring for people with people with AIDS?" were mixed. Many (41%) expressed ambivalence; more than one third of the nurses disliked caring for AIDS patients, either moderately (23%) or intensely (14%). However, some nurses responded that they enjoyed taking care of people with AIDS, moderately (10%) or very much (11%). These nurses identified the work as challenging and rewarding. One nurse said, "If nurses don't take care of the AIDS patients, who will?" (Brennan et al., 1988).

Nurses and other caregivers are subject to what Poliandro (1991) called **compassion fatigue.** This is a result of chronic stress and occurs before burnout. The signs of compassion fatigue are shown in Box 37–1. The needs of the patients are so great that the caregiver may find that, increasingly, the needs of the patient come first and his or her own needs come last. Poliandro suggested four rules for caregivers for preventing compassion fatigue (Box 37–2).

Support groups, where caregivers can express their feelings associated with the caregiving role, provide a mechanism for preventing physical and emotional exhaustion. These groups have proved beneficial to nurses as well as to nonprofessional caregivers. The caregiver is allowed to talk about feelings of frustration, of being overwhelmed, of the difficulty in maintaining the semblance of being "strong and in control," and of the pain of loss. The group is usually structured in a way that the caregiver receives affirmation, suggestions for dealing with concrete problems, a sense of connectedness with caregivers who are struggling with similar

Box 37–1 ■ ■ ■ ■ ■
Signs of Compassion Fatigue

> If you experience these symptoms when caring for people with AIDS, it is time to take measures to relieve the stress in your life.
> · Withdrawal from others
> · Inappropriate anger, hostility, or general irritation
> · Reluctance to cooperate with coworkers or to participate on the health care team
> · Inability to enjoy life
> · Sense of being overwhelmed by endless tasks, both at home and on the job
> · Chronic fatigue
> · Feeling of isolation
> · Rigid approach to problems
> · Constant sense of pressure
> · Sense that your work has become rote, routine

Modified with permission from Cassidy, J. (1991). Compassion fatigue. *HEALTH PROGRESS*, Jan-Feb, p. 55.

Box 37–2 ■ ■ ■ ■ ■
Rules for Preventing Compassion Fatigue

> 1. Give to yourself just as you take care of others.
> 2. Allow yourself to feel good about what you do. Feeling good about yourself makes you a more effective caregiver.
> 3. It is part of your professional duty to see to your own daily replenishment.
> 4. Set realistic limits for yourself and others. This ensures that you will be able to continue to care for others.

Modified with permission from Cassidy, J. (1991). Compassion fatigue. *HEALTH PROGRESS*, Jan-Feb, p. 54.

issues, and encouragement to care for and nurture self (Scanlon & Packard, 1991).

W*hat do you think?* If you were caring for an AIDS patient, what would your role and responsibility be toward that patient's caregivers?

➤ *Check Your Reading*
19. What is compassion fatigue?
20. Give three characteristics of compassion fatigue.
21. Give two strategies for prevention of compassion fatigue.

NURSING AND AIDS

The nursing profession is faced with its own journey in dealing with AIDS. Nurses are part of society as a whole and as such are subject to the same fears and stereotypes as others. What sets nurses apart is the expectation, society's and their own, not only that they will provide care but also that they will care (Byrne & Murphy, 1993; McCann, 1997). The AIDS journey for nursing offers a path of avoidance and a path of care. The path of avoidance is taken by nurses who would rather not confront AIDS. This is exemplified in Chenitz's (1992) observation of nursing care during her first admission for pneumocystis pneumonia:

That is, they cared more about whether all of the rules were complied with, whether I had the blanket I needed when I rang the call bell, whether my bed was neat and clean, whether I had the oxygen at the proper setting, and not at all about how I was. I was a case, not a person. Shocked and emotionally distraught about my AIDS diagnosis, this dispassionate care fed my sense of unreality. I was in a living nightmare. (p. 445)

As time goes on and the number of AIDS patients increases, the path of avoidance will become increasingly more difficult to choose.

The path of care includes research, education, and direct care; many nurses have chosen to walk this path. A review of nursing literature for the period of 1987 to

1998 revealed thousands of articles related to AIDS. These articles, focusing on research, education, and care issues, reflected the commitment of nursing to take this journey. In a 1991 article in the *American Journal of Nursing,* Meyer stated, "HIV disease has challenged nurses' competence, courage, and compassion—and they've risen to meet that challenge" (p. 26). Many nurses have confronted their own fears and anxieties and have decided to rise above their feelings to care for people with AIDS. Nursing stands in the forefront in the care of people with AIDS. The disease is one that places high demands for compassionate and skilled care (Peloquin, 1990; Sherman, 1996). The nurse, armed with a holistic approach to patient care, is the best equipped of the health team members to respond to these demands. The following quote from Chenitz (1992) illustrates the impact that a caring approach can have on the person with AIDS:

All the nurses on this unit were like that (compassionate). They loved being nurses, and they defined nursing as caring, compassionate, loving, nonjudgmental care. They cleaned, bathed, touched, started IV's, helped me to the commode and gave me medicine with great efficiency, but what really mattered is that they did it with compassion. I felt my sense of dignity return, the dignity I felt in their care. The unit was a healing place where I knew I would live and be okay. I got a glimmer that there is life after AIDS. (p. 444)

Psychiatric Nursing and AIDS

Psychiatric nurses are involved in the care of AIDS patients in many service settings. Nurses who function in a psychiatric consultation-liaison capacity are confronted with the demands of AIDS in general inpatient units in which patients are treated for the opportunistic infections that are the hallmark of AIDS. Psychiatric nurses also are confronted with caring for people with AIDS in psychiatric inpatient units, community mental health centers, and the home. Both physical and psychiatric care is being provided in all of these arenas. A brief description of the nurse's role in each of these settings is followed by an examination of the nursing process with AIDS patients.

Psychiatric Consultation–Liaison Nursing and AIDS

Again, let's focus on the initial story.

Keith fell ill on a trip to England and was hospitalized for treatment of *Pneumocystis carinii* pneumonia. Although no psychiatric consultation–liaison nurse was available, a staff counselor worked with Keith and his wife, attempting to support them as they dealt with the magnitude and terror associated with the diagnosis. ■

In the United States, providing support could well be the role of the psychiatric consultation–liaison nurse who is part of the support system when a patient first receives the diagnosis of AIDS. The role draws on knowledge of crisis intervention to help the patient and family in practical problem-solving and decision-making.

The psychiatric consultation–liaison nurse may be part of the discharge planning team and, as such, needs to be familiar with community resources. For instance, the nurse may provide information related to the availability of support groups; self-help groups; counseling about financial, legal, and social matters; psychiatric counseling; and buddy systems, in which individuals in the community assist with shopping, transportation, and other necessities of life.

The psychiatric consultation–liaison nurse may be part of nursing's initial assessment of organic mental disorders and may be the stimulus for an in-depth neuropsychiatric evaluation. Perry and Markowitz (1986) reported that in several studies, a review of nursing notes in both medical and psychiatric settings revealed that nurses documented discrete neuropsychological symptoms such as "unable to remember my name" or "somewhat disoriented" yet made no request for neurological or psychiatric evaluations. Perry and Markowitz concluded that nurses' lack of knowledge regarding the neuropsychiatric complications of AIDS led them to attribute unusual behaviors to hostility and psychopathology.

Another aspect of the psychiatric consultation–liaison nurse's role in working with AIDS patients is to assist the medical nurses to cope with their own feelings about this type of care. A psychiatric consultation–liaison nurse might conduct a staff support group in which nurses can express their feelings. Still another role involves supporting the family, friends, and significant others who are faced with their own grief.

Psychiatric Inpatient Nursing and AIDS

The most common psychiatric problems associated with AIDS—adjustment disorder with depression as the major symptom and an organic mental disorder—already have been discussed. However, these diagnoses could possibly lead to an inpatient psychiatric stay. The presence of a person with AIDS on an inpatient psychiatric unit presents nursing with challenges.

For instance, a psychotic patient who has an AIDS-related syndrome raises some really tough nursing issues. Simple procedures such as using universal precautions become complex and time consuming with a psychotic patient. How do you explain wearing gloves to a psychotic patient, who may already be dealing with delusional and hallucinatory ideation regarding feelings of guilt, worthlessness, and shame? Whenever nursing staff members implement universal precautions, they must provide a clear explanation to each patient. They must assess each patient thereafter for countertherapeutic effects. They also must intervene therapeutically to minimize anxiety and other feelings triggered by universal precautions.

Polk-Walker (1989) discussed a case scenario that illustrates the problems of treating a patient who is both psychotic and diagnosed with AIDS (Case Example 37–1). This example raises issues concerning safety as well as resource allocation. Psychiatric facilities may be faced with making decisions regarding the needs of many patients compared with the needs of a few. In the future, AIDS patients may find that admission to a psychiatric unit is difficult and that early transfers or discharges become the norm.

■ CASE EXAMPLE 37–1
■ Sherri's Story

■ Sherri is a young IV drug abuser who was transferred to a psychiatric hospital from a local hospital, where she had just given birth. In addition to being HIV-positive, Sherri was paranoid and verbally and physically assaultive at the time of admission. She was placed in a single room with private bathroom facilities. However, she was allowed to freely walk the unit. Although universal body fluid precautions were standard hospital procedure, the staff could not maintain the isolation of Sherri's body fluids because she continually removed her sanitary napkin and sat in patient chairs, thereby contaminating patient-care areas. Various options, including seclusion, were discussed and dismissed. The treatment team decided to place this patient on one-to-one supervision for the remainder of her hospital stay. However, the use of one-to-one intervention represented a significant expenditure of nursing resources. In addition, the one-to-one intervention exacerbated the patient's paranoia, requiring more intensive psychotherapeutic intervention. ■

The inpatient psychiatric nurse must confront other issues as well. For instance, ethical concerns regarding who should receive information regarding the patient's HIV antibody status become important. The rights of the patient to confidentiality compared with the need to know by other patients, staff members, and medical facilities staff members must be examined. The doctor is allowed to disclose information regarding a patient's positive antibody test to the rest of the staff members because the entire staff is considered one treatment unit. However, the legality of disclosure of AIDS antibody testing to outpatient facilities is not clear (Binder, 1987; Harding, Gray, & Neal, 1993).

Binder (1987) cited two examples that vividly illustrate the ethical and legal quagmire surrounding the issue of confidentiality with AIDS patients. The first case involved a 22-year-old with a diagnosis of paranoid schizophrenia who suddenly bit a patient who was HIV-positive. In the second case, a 23-year-old bisexual man was admitted for depression and suicidal ideation and requested an HIV antibody screening. The test result was positive yet he refused to tell his girlfriend with whom he was having an active sexual relationship. In both of these cases, the law protected the patient's right to confidentiality. However, according to the Tarasoff decision, clinicians are required to warn potential victims of violence (Kadzielski, 1991). The question that arises is whether the Tarasoff decision can be extended to cover other types of life-threatening risks (see Chapter 5).

Community Mental Health Nursing and AIDS

People with AIDS receive most of their care outside of hospitals. This fact, coupled with the devastating emotional toll exacted by the disease on patients, family members, and caregivers, creates a tremendous vacuum of need that can be filled with the services of community mental health nurses. The interventions most likely to be provided include crisis intervention; support and bereavement groups; individual, family, couples, and group psychotherapy; case management; and community education and consultation.

The recognition of HIV as a community mental health problem has stimulated the development of training programs designed to prepare community mental health professionals to deal with the problems associated with HIV. The training programs usually target the needs of individual patients with AIDS as well as present strategies for safeguarding the community's health in relation to HIV (Knox & Gaies, 1990).

Psychiatric Home Care and AIDS

Increasingly, people with AIDS are receiving skilled nursing care in their homes. Economics is one of the primary driving forces that support this move. In the mid-1980s, the first study on costs of the care of people with AIDS was conducted. The CDC estimated the costs at approximately $150,000 per patient. This estimate was determined from inpatient costs. In 1989, estimates were between $23,000 and $55,000 for the cost of AIDS health care (AIDS epidemic, 1989, p. 152). These conservative estimates were based on home care, community support, outpatient therapies, and hospice care, with little emphasis on inpatient care. Neither of these studies included the costs for drug therapy. The treatment of a disease such as cancer has been shown to be more effective with the use of multiple drug combinations of chemotherapy, as well as the use of treatments that are multimodal in nature (i.e, surgery, chemotherapy, and radiation in the treatment of breast cancer). The same has been found for the treatment of AIDS. Combination therapies are a success and many include multiple drugs. Among these are found the highly effective HIV protease inhibitors (Flexnor, 1998).

With several new antiretroviral drugs approved in the United States by 1999, clinicians use a variety of 2-, 3-, even 4-drug combinations to treat HIV infection. Protease inhibitor therapy is a recent advance in the treatment of AIDS. In cases in which it is used with nucleoside analogues or nonnucleoside reverse transcriptase inhibitors, the AIDS plasma viral loads decrease, CD4 cell counts increase as disease progression drops, and life is prolonged. These advantages do not come without a price. There are side effects and there are monetary costs. Protease inhibitors themselves are expensive, with an annual wholesale price ranging from $4320 to $8010 per patient in 1998 (Flexnor, 1998). Combination drug regimens can cost about $10,000 per year. These estimates climb as each year passes. They point to the known fact that the most cost-effective methods of treatment are community-based and home-based.

Most home care to the person with AIDS is provided by medical-surgical and hospice nurses. However, as more home care agencies develop a psychiatric service component, increasingly the psychiatric home care nurse also is involved in this care. The psychiatric home care nurse is confronted not only with the patient's feelings of depression, social isolation, stigmatization, helplessness, and grieving but also with the caregiver's similar feelings that must be dealt with to teach the caregiver how to care for the person with AIDS. People with AIDS who display the neuropsychiatric complications associated with ADC present safety and support challenges to nurses as well as to nonprofessional care providers.

Although home care is preferable to inpatient care, it is not without difficulties (Carney, 1990). These difficulties range from social to medical to personal, and they have an additional impact on the patient's feelings of depression. The social difficulties revolve around returning to a community setting where neighbors, acquaintances, landlords, and others are terrified of the disease and therefore terrified of association with the person with AIDS. Consequently, many people with AIDS have encountered housing problems when fearful landlords initiated eviction proceedings based on vague pretexts.

As a result of rejection by family and friends, the person with AIDS may be alone at home without any support except that offered by home care staff. Families and friends do not always rally around to offer love and support to the person with AIDS. It seems that in periods of crisis, families either pull together or become more alienated. Many parents who have a son or daughter with AIDS are confronted with the dual realizations that their child engaged in either a homosexual or an IV drug-using lifestyle and that their loved one is dying. Adjustments to these facts may prove too much for the coping abilities of family members, and they may retreat from contact with the person with AIDS.

Some communities have intricate social support systems in place to assist the person with AIDS in meeting many daily needs. The psychiatric home care nurse must be knowledgeable about the available community services. For instance, in San Francisco, a group of volunteers delivers meals to homebound people with AIDS who are too weak to prepare their own meals. Baltimore has a volunteer "buddy" system, in which the person with AIDS is assisted with transportation and obtaining housing, clothing, food, and other necessities of life. Other communities have little social support available to the person with AIDS.

> **W***hat do you think?* Who should bear the cost of AIDS care?

► *Check Your Reading*

22. What are the two paths available to nurses facing the crisis of AIDS?

23. Give an example of an appropriate nursing intervention for a psychiatric consultation–liaison nurse.
24. Give an example of an appropriate nursing intervention for an inpatient psychiatric nurse.
25. Give an example of an appropriate nursing intervention for a community mental health nurse.

NURSING PROCESS

The nursing process is applied to the care of the person with AIDS in a fashion similar to the care of other patients.

Assessment

The assessment of the person with AIDS uses the strategies suggested in Chapter 11 for evaluating mental status. Specific assessment skills focus on determining the degree of depression. For instance, you might use a standardized depression scale, such as the Beck Depression Scale (see Chapter 25), for this purpose. Slowed cognitive and sensorimotor functions are revealed with neuropsychological tests. For instance, the Mini-Mental State Examination (MMSE) (see Chapter 33) would be used as part of a dementia assessment providing specifics regarding short-term memory, attention, and fine motor skills. Patients with ADC perform poorly on tests that require rapid fine motor movements, sustained attention and concentration, and cognitive flexibility. A thorough mental status examination is necessary with special attention to performance in "serial sevens" and other tasks requiring sequencing. Asking patients to repeat a list of numbers provides information regarding short-term memory. Individuals with unaffected cognition can remember five to seven numbers. Scores of four or less suggest memory impairment and a need to provide the patient with verbal or written cues to assist in the completion of routine tasks. Because anxiety and educational level can affect patients' performance on this test, the results must be interpreted with caution.

Gait ataxia or slowing of rapid movements may be one of the clearest signs of neurological damage, especially in the early stages of ADC. Suspected sensory deficit should be further assessed by asking the patient to identify numbers "written" on his or her fingertips with a capped pen while his or her eyes are closed. If the patient is unable to do this accurately, this suggests the need to attend to safety issues. For instance, it becomes essential for someone to check the water temperature before a patient bathes or showers.

Swanson, Cronin-Stubbs, and Colletti (1990) identified strategies to assess for upper extremity functioning. Patients can be asked to alternately supinate and pronate their hands. If a patient has difficulty initiating this movement, frontal lobe damage is suggested. Clumsiness or inability to maintain the movements may suggest basal ganglia damage. Upper extremity motor deficits may benefit from assistive devices and from occupational therapy.

MEDICAL DIAGNOSES AND RELATED NURSING DIAGNOSES

AIDS

DSM-IV Diagnosis: Adjustment Disorder

Diagnostic Criteria

A. The development of emotional or behavioral symptoms in response to identifiable stressor(s) occurring within 3 months of the onset of the stressor(s).

B. These symptoms or behaviors are clinically significant as evidenced by either of the following:

    1. Marked distress that is in excess of what would be expected from exposure to the stressor

    2. Significant impairment in social or occupational (academic) functioning

C. The stress-related disturbance does not meet the criteria for another specific Axis I disorder and is not merely an exacerbation of a preexisting Axis I or Axis II disorder.

D. The symptoms do not represent Bereavement.

E. Once the stressor (or its consequences) has terminated, the symptoms do not persist for more than an additional 6 months.

Specify if:

Acute: If the disturbance lasts less than 6 months

Chronic: If the disturbance lasts for 6 months or longer

Adjustment Disorders are coded based on the subtype, which is selected according to the predominant symptoms.

The specific stressor(s) can be specified on Axis IV.

309.0 With Depressed Mood

309.24 With Anxiety

309.28 With Mixed Anxiety and Depressed Mood

309.3 With Disturbance of Conduct

309.4 With Mixed Disturbance of Emotions and Conduct

309.9 Unspecified

Related Nursing Diagnoses	Definition	Example
Risk for Violence: Self-Directed	A state in which a person experiences behaviors that can be physically harmful to the self	Risk for Violence: Self-Directed related to feelings of hopelessness secondary to diagnosis of AIDS, as evidenced by suicidal ideation
Ineffective Individual Coping	Impairment of adaptive behaviors and problem-solving abilities of a person in meeting life's demands and roles	Ineffective Individual Coping related to new diagnosis of AIDS, as evidenced by verbalizations of hopelessness and suicidal ideation
Spiritual Distress	Disruption in the life principle that pervades a person's entire being and that integrates and transcends one's biological and psychological nature	Spiritual Distress related to feelings of guilt about lifestyle as evidenced by verbalizations that God will punish him
Hopelessness	A subjective state in which a person sees limited or no alternatives or personal choices available and is unable to mobilize energy on own behalf	Hopelessness related to belief that the person has no reason for living once diagnosed with AIDS, as evidenced by suicidal ideation
Anticipatory Grieving	Intellectual and emotional responses and behaviors by which people work through the process of modifying self-concept based on the perception of potential loss	Anticipatory grieving related to awareness of many losses associated with diagnosis of AIDS, as evidenced by sad affect and verbalization that he has lost so much already

Based on information from the *Diagnostic and Statistical Manual of Mental Disorders. Fourth Edition.* Copyright 1994 American Psychiatric Association. Nursing diagnoses and definitions from North American Nursing Diagnosis Association. (1999). *NANDA nursing diagnoses: Definitions and classification 1999-2000.* Philadelphia: NANDA.

Abstract thinking, a higher neuropsychological function, can be assessed by asking patients to explain the meaning of common proverbs, such as "People who live in glass houses shouldn't throw stones." The inability to explain the proverb or the provision of a literal, concrete answer may indicate the patient's impaired ability to abstract. This limits the patient's ability to learn new behaviors, such as practicing safer sex, and to problem solve. Problem-solving ability can be evaluated by providing a patient with a hypothetical situation, such as "What would you do if you were in a theater and saw a fire?" Asymptomatic patients perform better on tests of memory, motor coordination, and general intellectual functioning than do patients who have progressed farther in the disease process.

Differentiating Depression From Dementia

The differentiation between depression and ADC is not an obvious one; however, because the treatment for each is different, it is an important distinction to make. Both psychiatric complications are behaviorally displayed through apathy and psychomotor retardation. Depressed individuals usually express feelings of hopelessness and worthlessness during interviews. They may admit to suicidal ideation. They usually present with a sad and morose affect. These behaviors are not typical of the ADC patient.

Further differentiation can be made through neuropsychological tests that distinguish between depression and dementia. Individuals with dementia experience difficulty drawing; this is not true of the depressed person. Asking patients to draw simple figures such as squares or triangles may be telling in determining whether the patient is depressed or not. Another test to differentiate depression from dementia involves asking patients to generate a list of words beginning with a specific letter of the alphabet. Demented persons will be unable to produce more than a few words, whereas this task will pose no challenge to the depressed individual (Swanson et al., 1990).

> **W***hat do you think?* How would you provide education to an HIV-positive individual who asked you if it was okay to engage in sexual activity? In providing this education, what personal feelings would you have to confront?

➤ *Check Your Reading*
26. Give two ways to differentiate between depression and ADC.

27. Why would you use a standardized assessment scale such as the Montgomery-Asburg Depression Scale?
28. What information would the Mini-Mental State Examination provide?

Diagnosis

The analysis of the assessment data leads to decisions regarding the nature of the patient's problems and provides direction for your interventions. For example, Jim is newly diagnosed with AIDS. He has *Pneumocystis carinii* pneumonia. He is devastated with the diagnosis and despondent. He states that he wishes he were dead and he is sure that AIDS is a punishment from God for his homosexual lifestyle. Jim comments that everyone has deserted him except his significant other. Jim's family has totally disowned him.

Part of the assessment involved administering a standardized depression inventory; Jim's score indicated serious depression. His score of 29 on the Mini-Mental State Examination indicated no cognitive deficit. This data, combined with observations of sad affect, verbalizations of hopelessness, psychomotor retardation, Jim's isolation from his family, his sense of guilt, and suicidal ideation point to the medical and nursing diagnoses shown in the box entitled Medical Diagnoses and Related Nursing Diagnoses: AIDS.

Outcome Identification

The expected outcomes for a patient such as Jim diagnosed with AIDS might include

- The patient will remain free from harm.
- The patient will demonstrate effective coping skills in dealing with the diagnosis of AIDS.
- The patient will resolve his guilt feelings and experience the forgiveness of God.
- The patient will express hope in being able to find meaning in the remainder of his life.
- The patient will resolve the grief feelings associated with his many actual and anticipated losses.

Planning

The plan for Jim involves carrying out any medically ordered treatment and establishing goals that improve his coping, relieve his sense of spiritual distress, reduce his hopelessness, and support him in his grieving. Appropriate short-term goals include the following.

Expected Outcomes	Short-Term Goals
The patient will remain free from harm.	1. Within 2 weeks of taking antidepressant medication, the patient will have an improvement in his score on the Montgomery-Asburg Scale.

The patient will demonstrate effective coping skills in dealing with the diagnosis of AIDS.

2.   After attending two medication group sessions, Jim will state the major action of his antidepressant medication and at least four side effects and strategies for managing them.
3.   After participating in individual psychotherapy, Jim will exhibit a brightening in his mood, as evidenced by smiling, spontaneous verbalizations, attention to appearance, and a statement that he has no suicidal ideation.

1.   After participating in individual psychotherapy, Jim will express hope and, through self-appraisal, will evaluate his mood to be improved.
2.   After participating in individual psychotherapy, Jim will state a willingness to participate in AIDS support groups as a way to bolster his own coping skills.

The patient will resolve his guilt feelings and experience the forgiveness of God.

1.   As a result of talking to the nurse and clergy about his feelings of spiritual distress, Jim will verbalize a feeling of peace about this issue and a sense of meaning and order to the experience.

The patient will express hope in being able to find meaning in the remainder of his life.

1.   After participating in several educational groups addressing the issue of living with AIDS, Jim will verbalize that life can still have significance—in fact, even more significance—with a diagnosis of AIDS.

The patient will resolve the grief feelings associated with his many actual and anticipated losses.

1.   After participating in an educational group emphasizing strategies for coping with AIDS, Jim will express knowledge about the grieving process and greater confidence in his ability to deal with the losses related to AIDS.

Implementation

Implementation of nursing care for the person with AIDS must be truly holistic. As Chenitz (1992) wrote

Compassion, assurance, and competence is what I need from health care providers. You have not failed me if I die. You have failed me if I die alone, frightened, in pain or distress. It is enlightened help with the dying that I need. I want help to maintain my dignity, keep me pain free, and allow my family and friends to be there. Too often today this type of treatment is not available. Why not? This is nursing care, and for this we are responsible. (p. 455)

Examining the issues of implementation involved in Jim's care includes specific interventions, such as

- Administering the antidepressant medication
- Assigning Jim to a medication teaching group
- Assigning Jim to a nurse psychotherapist with whom he will meet for individual sessions
- Assigning Jim to an AIDS educational group
- Contacting a clergy person of Jim's choice or, if Jim has no preference, contacting the clergy person assigned to the institution where Jim is admitted
- Ensuring that Jim's individual treatment plan includes spiritual interventions such as talking about Jim's guilt and his feelings that God will punish him, assisting Jim to create some order and meaning out of his present situation, possibly praying with Jim, and informing him about chapel services.

More important than the specific interventions used with Jim is the overall quality of the relationships that are developed with Jim. He cries out for acceptance, affirmation, and reassurance that hope exists and that he is worthy of such hope. These needs cannot be met in the mechanized or rote manner implied in a step-by-step list of interventions but in relationships in which Jim's basic sense of worth is unconditionally affirmed without judgment or qualification (Carson, 1990; Carson et al., 1990).

Evaluation

The care of a patient diagnosed with AIDS, such as Jim, requires ongoing evaluation. This formative evaluation looks at the patient's day-to-day responses to the nursing interventions and identifies any new assessment data as well as any additional nursing diagnoses not identified in the initial plan of care.

The summative evaluation of care is specified in the expected outcomes and the short-term goals. If the criteria for goal achievement are not met, the data are reexamined to determine the answers to questions such as

- Was the assessment adequate?
- Does additional assessment data need to be incorporated?
- Were the goals appropriate?
- Was the intervention appropriate?
- Was the specified time frame for achieving the goal appropriate?

The answers to these questions give direction to possible modifications of the plan of care.

NURSING PROCESS APPLICATION

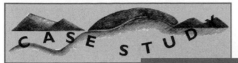

Tony

Tony is a 25-year-old homosexual man who was diagnosed as being HIV-positive a year ago. At that time, he was spending many of his free evenings in gay bars. Since his diagnosis, he has stopped going to gay bars and has tended to spend his free time watching television or taking his dog Sparky for walks in the park. Tony is employed as an assistant grocery store manager and is well liked by his employees. Recently, however, he has missed work because of infections associated with AIDS. His coworkers suspect the diagnosis and are beginning to avoid him. Tony feels isolated and extremely lonely. His family members, who live in another state, are not aware of his diagnosis, sexual orientation, or lifestyle.

ASSESSMENT	Assessment data are as follows: • Feeling isolated and lonely • Increasing work absences • Cut off from family members, both emotionally and geographically • Deteriorating medical condition
DIAGNOSIS	**DSM-IV Diagnosis:** Adjustment Disorder with depressive symptoms and AIDS **Nursing Diagnosis:** Anticipatory Grieving related to decreased quality of life and near-certain death as evidenced by loss of health status and awareness of losses associated with AIDS.

OUTCOME IDENTIFICATION, PLANNING, AND IMPLEMENTATION

Expected Outcome 1: By _____ the patient will express his feelings, concerns, and fears about having AIDS.

Short-Term Goal	Nursing Interventions	Rationales
By _____ the patient will express his grief to the health care team.	1. Provide and support anticipatory grief responses. 2. Acknowledge the stage of grief Tony is experiencing (denial, anger, bargaining, depression, or acceptance). 3. Listen to Tony's perceptions about his diagnosis of AIDS by using therapeutic communication skills, active listening, silence, and acknowledgment.	1–2. Grief is a normal response to all types of loss. Strong feelings are evoked when dealing with issues of AIDS and death. 3. Any type of meaningful loss (e.g., loss of parent, body part, role, or functioning) will precipitate a reaction that will follow the general stages or patterns of the grief response.

Expected Outcome 2: By _____ the patient will make decisions about his care and the near-certain loss of his life.

Short-Term Goal	Nursing Interventions	Rationales
By _____ the patient will examine the loss within a spiritual context.	1. Help Tony to identify those aspects of AIDS that he can control—informed consent, advanced directives—and those specific aspects that are distressing and uncontrollable.	1–2. The diagnosis of AIDS can strip the patient of a sense of meaning and purpose in life. A disease with a grave prognosis, AIDS challenges coping and adaptive behavior. Being informed and

2. Keep Tony informed of his condition, prescribed treatments, medications, therapies, and test results.

educated about the disease helps patients to cope.

Nursing Diagnosis: Social Isolation related to lack of family support and to the stigma and societal nonacceptance and fear of the disease as evidenced by changes in work friendships.

OUTCOME IDENTIFICATION, PLANNING, AND IMPLEMENTATION

Expected Outcome 1: By _____ the patient will explore contact with and seek assistance from family, friends, clergy members, and community resources.

Short-Term Goals	Nursing Interventions	Rationales
By _____ the patient will verbalize his fears of rejection related to telling his parents about his illness.	1. Support Tony in all endeavors to initiate contact with family and friends. 2. Provide education about AIDS to Tony's family and friends.	1. Support encourages the patient to verbalize needs and initiate actions. 2. Often, people withdraw out of fear of contracting AIDS from the patient. Education assists in alleviating this ignorance and reduces the fear of transmission.
By _____ the patient will identify behaviors that increase meaningful relationships.	1. Introduce Tony to the various types of support and outreach groups for people with AIDS. 2. Ask Tony whether he participates in, or is interested in participating in, a religious group or activity; if so, contact an appropriate group or institution that has programs supportive of people with AIDS.	1–2. Community support through self-help groups and religious institutions can help patients cope with not only emotional and social issues but also spiritual issues.

EVALUATION

Formative Evaluation: Tony met each of the short-term goals. In therapy, Tony was encouraged to express his feelings and to take as much time as needed to forgive himself for not taking appropriate precautions to avoid contracting and transmitting AIDS, so that he could move on. Tony also talked with other homosexual patients who were cut off from their families, and this helped him considerably in dealing with his emotional pain and fears of reaching out and asking for help. Tony had a great deal of difficulty in calling his parents to tell them of his diagnosis. When he did tell them about the diagnosis, they asked about how he contracted the disease. After years of keeping his sexual orientation a secret from his family, Tony finally admitted to them that he lived a homosexual lifestyle. To his utter surprise, Tony's parents said that they loved him unconditionally, regardless of his lifestyle. Tony told them how ashamed he felt about not taking precautions to protect himself during sexual relations.

Summative Evaluation: Tony met each of the expected outcomes, except for showing interest in religious activities; Tony said that he wasn't ready to deal with "all that stuff." The staff respected his wishes. Tony did, however, reach out to a local AIDS support group and attended meetings regularly after discharge. The staff arranged for a member of the support group to visit Tony before discharge to establish a support network. Tony did finally call his parents, and to his surprise they caught the next flight to be with him. Tony stated that in his meetings with his parents, he felt accepted and loved for who he is. See Snapshot: Nursing Interventions Specific to AIDS-Related Depression.

SNAPSHOT

Nursing Interventions Specific to AIDS-Related Depression

What do you need to do to develop a relationship with a patient diagnosed with AIDS?

- Approach the patient with warmth, a quiet demeanor, and acceptance.
- Share time with the patient, even if he or she talks little or not at all.
- Be honest, empathetic, and compassionate.
- Avoid lighthearted or too forceful an approach.
- Speak slowly and allow the patient time to respond.
- Address the patient by his or her preferred name (don't assume it is okay to use the patient's first name until you ask), talk with the patient, and listen carefully to what he or she shares.
- Find ways to express hope without negating the pain experienced by the patient.
- Encourage the patient to identify and discuss feelings.

What do you need to assess regarding the patient's health status?

- Suicidal risk or self-destructive thoughts
- Affective responses, including anger, anxiety, apathy, bitterness, denial of feelings, guilt, despondency, irritability, helplessness, and hopelessness (All of these responses may be evaluated and quantified using a standardized depression inventory such as the Beck Depression Scale, the Zung Self Report Depression Index, or the Hamilton Depression Inventory.)
- Physiological responses, including gastrointestinal disturbances, appetite changes, constipation, fatigue, sexual disturbances, sleep disturbances, weight changes, headache, and menstrual changes
- Cognitive responses, including confusion, slowed thinking, indecisiveness, problems with concentration, self-blame, and pessimism (Differentiate between depression and dementia.)
- Behavioral responses, including isolation and withdrawal; crying; agitation; alcoholism; drug addiction; slowed activity; poor personal hygiene; underachievement; and inability to perform instrumental activities of daily living such as cooking, balancing a checkbook, budgeting money, and structuring time
- Vital signs, including sitting and standing blood pressure if the patient is taking medication that leads to orthostatic hypotension
- Weight, especially if the patient is experiencing changes in appetite

- Response to and compliance with medication regimen and reasons behind noncompliance and delayed effectiveness
- Degree of social support
- Knowledge level and ability and readiness to learn
- Concurrent medical conditions

What do you need to teach the patient and the patient's caregiver?

- Medication issues: reasons for taking the medication, side effects and how to deal with them, untoward effects, warnings, and importance of adhering to a medication schedule
- Disease process, causes of depression as part of AIDS diagnosis, course of disease, and treatments
- Nutrition issues
- Emergency measures
- Importance of social support and strategies to obtain it
- Maintaining safety
- Lifestyle and compliance issues such as benefits of exercise and stress management
- Importance of emotional support
- Importance of achieving spiritual well-being

What skills will you want the patient and/or caregiver to demonstrate?

- Ability to enter into a no-harm contract and remain safe
- Ability to follow medication and treatment plan
- Ability to use thought-stopping techniques and other cognitive strategies to deal with distorted thinking patterns
- Ability to perform personal care
- Ability to identify and express feelings
- Coping skills
- Relaxation techniques

What other health professionals might need to be a part of this plan of care?

- Physician: to be in charge of the overall treatment plan including medication management; usually a psychiatrist or a primary care physician
- Social Worker: to assist with access to community supports, insurance issues, access to entitlements, and connection with community-based treatments
- Psychiatric Occupational Therapist: to assist the patient with instrumental activities of daily living such as time management, cooking, and budgeting
- Nursing Assistant or Home Health Aide: to assist patient with personal hygiene and grooming, if necessary

Conclusions

Increasingly, the care of the person with AIDS is extending into the psychiatric arena. AIDS is a terrible disease that exacts an enormous psychological and spiritual toll on people with AIDS, family members, caregivers, and others. The disease taxes coping responses to the limit and beyond. The level of support required to assist patients and others who deal with AIDS demands skilled interventions and an integrated team effort among mental health professionals, including psychiatric nurses.

The crisis initiated by an HIV-related infection is of such magnitude as to lead people to commit suicide at alarming rates. The existential and spiritual crisis that follows the diagnosis of AIDS can strip the person of a sense of meaning, purpose, and worth, or the spiritual comfort that is possible with a relationship to God, leaving the person spiritually and emotionally naked and vulnerable.

The psychiatric problems of adjustment disorder with depressed mood, AIDS-related dementia (dementia due to HIV disease), and major depressive episode necessitate active treatment and are not illnesses that can be managed by the patient alone or by a single caregiver, no matter how concerned and involved he or she is.

Psychiatric nurses therefore have a major role to play in the care of the person with AIDS. Psychiatric nurses encounter these patients in the general hospital population, in psychiatric units, in the community, and in the home. In all of these sites, the nursing process provides the framework for approaching care in a systematic manner; the interventions of crisis intervention, psychological and spiritual support, and education are the tools needed to assist the person with AIDS in coping with the disease.

Key Points to Remember

- AIDS is a terrible disease; it affects individuals in a holistic manner.
- The psychological reactions to AIDS vary from those who are the worried well to those with psychiatric disorders such as major depression.
- The spiritual implications of AIDS include feelings of guilt for lifestyle choices; a sense of hopelessness and despair; existential crises; and alienation from God.
- AIDS has been recognized since 1981.
- Since 1981, almost a half million cases of full-blown AIDS have been reported.
- Most cases of AIDS are among homosexual and bisexual men and IV drug users. However, the incidence of cases among women and children is increasing.
- AIDS is preventable through practicing sexual absti-

nence, practicing safer sex, avoiding IV drug use, avoiding sharing needles, and avoiding the exchange of body fluids.
- AIDS is not spread through casual contact.
- The most common psychiatric sequelae of AIDS are adjustment disorder with either feelings of depression or anxiety, major depression, and ADC.
- AIDS patients endure isolation, stigma, and feelings of worthlessness.
- Caregivers of AIDS patients can experience compassion fatigue.
- Assessment of an AIDS patient differentiates between depression and dementia.
- The nursing process offers a systematic way to provide holistic care for people with AIDS.

Learning Activities

1. Read an excerpt from Elizabeth Cox's book, *Thanksgiving: An AIDS Journal*. Write your reflections in your journal. If you were in Elizabeth's place, how do you think that you would react?
2. Find out what supports are available for AIDS patients in your community and your state.
3. The following diseases are either caused or exacerbated by lifestyle choices:
   - AIDS
   - Herpes
   - Congestive heart failure

- Diabetes
- Substance abuse disorder

Why is it that some of these diseases provoke stigma and moral indignation and others do not?
4. Reflect on your thoughts, feelings, and attitudes about AIDS. Would your responses facilitate or hinder your caring for a patient with AIDS?
5. What does the following statement mean to you: "Rather than consider AIDS a terrible physical disease, it has been couched in terms of immorality and religious imperatives."

Critical Thinking Exercises

Roy Jefferson, a 29-year-old AIDS patient, was admitted to the inpatient psychiatric unit with extreme anxiety and depression following a doctor's appointment in which he

learned that his T cells were dangerously low. Roy, since being diagnosed as being HIV-positive 4 years ago, had turned his life around. No longer sexually active, he had stopped abusing drugs and was experiencing relatively good health. Part of his rehabilitation included being a spokesman for a local AIDS association to educate others about the disease.

1. What assumptions do you have about people who are HIV-positive?
2. Consider the psychiatric nurse's role in comparison to the role of the nurse in another setting.
3. What effect might your assumptions have on your clinical comfort with AIDS patients?

Following an interview with Roy, Bruce, a nursing student, informed his teacher that he had asked Roy to speak to the group of student nurses about his course of illness. The teacher wanted to know the purpose of the meeting and was told that it was an intervention strategy to allow Roy to resume a previous level of functioning.

1. What assumptions can you make about Bruce's point of view concerning AIDS patients?
2. How would you check your assumptions?
3. Consider alternate interventions.

Additional Resources

APA Online

http://www.psych.org/
Information about the American Psychiatric Association.

Boston University Medical Center: Community Outreach Health Information System

http://web.bu.edu/cohis

U.S. Department of Health and Human Services (HHS)

http://www.os.dhhs.gov/

References

AIDS epidemic causes financial drain on return in hospitals. (1989). *AIDS Alert, 4,* 152.

American Foundation for AIDS Research. (1996). HIV/AIDS. *Educator, 7*(1), 2-8.

American Psychiatric Association. (1994). *Diagnostic and statistical manual of mental disorders* (4th ed.). Washington, DC: Author.

Aruffo, J. F., Thompson, R. G., Gottlieb, A. A., & Dobbins, W. N. (1995). An AIDS training program for rural mental health providers. *Psychiatric Services, 46*(1), 79-81.

Atkinson, J. H., Capadini, L., Levine, J. F., & Price, R. W. (1996). Dementia, depression and quality of life. *Patient Care, 30*(9), 131-140, 143.

Baldwin, J. D., & Baldwin, J. I. (1988). Factors affecting AIDS-related sexual risk-taking behavior among college students. *The Journal of Sex Research, 25,* 181-196.

Belcher, A., Dettmore, D., & Holzmer, S. (1989). Spirituality and sense of well-being in persons with AIDS. *Holistic Nursing Practice, 3*(4), 16-25.

Binder, R. (1987). AIDS antibody tests on inpatient psychiatric units. *American Journal of Psychiatry, 144,* 176-180.

Brennan, L. (1988). The battle against AIDS: A report from the nursing front. *Nursing '88, 18*(4), 60-64.

Byrne, V., & Murphy, J. (1993). Are we preparing future nurses to care for individuals with AIDS? *Journal of Nursing Education, 32*(2), 84-86.

Cahill, K. (1983). *The AIDS epidemic* (p. 2). New York: St. Martin's Press.

Carney, K. L. (1990). AIDS care comes home. *Home Healthcare Nurse, 8*(2), 32-37.

Carson, V. (1989). *Spiritual dimensions of nursing practice.* Philadelphia: W. B. Saunders.

Carson, V. (1990). Spirituality and spiritual direction: Important issues to the person with AIDS. *The Journal of Christian Healing, 12*(3), 37.

Carson, V. (1993). Prayer, meditation, exercise, and vitamin use: Behaviors of the hardy individual who is HIV+, diagnosed with ARC or AIDS. *Journal of the Association of Nurses in AIDS Care, 4*(3), 18-28.

Carson, V., & Green, H. (1992). The relationship of spiritual well-being and hardiness in the AIDS patient. *Journal of Professional Nursing, 8,* 209-220.

Carson, V., Soeken, K. L., Shanty, J., & Terry, L. (1990). Hope and spiritual well-being: Essentials for living with AIDS. *Perspectives in Psychiatric Care, 26*(2), 28-34.

Centers for Disease Control and Prevention. (1997). *HIV/AIDS Surveillance Report, 9*(2), 1-43.

Chenitz, W. C. (1992). Living with AIDS. In J. H. Flaskerud & P. J. Ungvarski (Eds.), *HIV/AIDS: A guide to nursing care* (pp. 440-460). Philadelphia: W. B. Saunders.

Cohen, M. A. (1998). Psychiatric care in a nursing home. *Psychosomatics, 39,* 154-161.

Cox, E. (1990). *Thanksgiving: An AIDS journal.* New York: Harper & Row.

Flaskerud, J. H., & Tabora, A. (1998). Health problems of low-income female caregivers of adults with HIV/AIDS. *Health Care Women International, 19*(1), 23-36.

Flexnor, C. (1998). HIV protease inhibitors. *The New England Journal of Medicine, 338,* 1281-1291.

Fortunato, J. (1987). *AIDS: The spiritual dilemma.* San Francisco: Harper & Row.

Harding, A. K., Gray, L. A., & Neal, M. (1993). Confidentiality limits with clients who have HIV: A review of ethical and legal guidelines and professional policies. *Journal of Counseling Developments, 71,* 297-305.

Harvath, T. A. (1994). Interpretation and management of dementia related behavior problems. *Clinical Nursing Research, 3*(1), 7-26.

Hays, R. B., Magee, R. H., & Chauncey, S. (1994). *AIDS Care, 6,* 393-397.

Hilts, P. J. (1991, August 4). Patient's letter begs Bush to fight stigma of AIDS. *The Sun,* pp. 1A, 11A.

Kadzielski, M. (1991). Recent cases interpret the Tarasoff duty to warn. *Health Progress, 2,* 15-16.

Kayal, P. M. (1985). "Morals," medicine, and the AIDS epidemic. *Journal of Religion and Health, 24,* 218-237.

Kendall, J. (1994). Wellness spirituality in homosexual men with HIV infection. *Journal of the Association of Nurses in AIDS Care, 5*(4), 28-34.

Knox, M. D., & Gaies, J. S. (1990). The HIV tutorial for community mental health professionals. *Community Mental Health Journal, 26,* 559-566.

Kübler-Ross, E. (1975). *Death: The final stage of growth.* Englewood Cliffs, NJ: Prentice-Hall.

Kübler-Ross, E. (1987). *AIDS: The ultimate challenge.* New York: Macmillan.

Leech, K. (1977). *Soul friend.* San Francisco: Harper & Row.

McCaffrey, E. A. (1987). Counseling AIDS patients. *AIDS Patient Care, 1*(2), 26-28.

McCann, T. V. (1997). Willingness to provide care and treatment for patients with HIV/AIDS. *Journal of Advanced Nursing, 25,* 1033-1039.

McLean, J., Bouton, M., Brookes, M., Lakhani, D., Fitzpatrick, R., Dawson, J., McKechnie, R., & Hart, G. (1994). Regular partners and risky behavior: Why do gay men have unprotected intercourse? *AIDS Care, 6,* 331-341.

Meyer, C. (1991). Nursing and AIDS: A decade of caring. *American Journal of Nursing, 91*(12), 26-31.

Michels, R., & Marzuk, P. M. (1993). Psychiatric aspects of HIV infection. *The New England Journal of Medicine, 329,* 634-638.

Morris, N. J. (1996). Depression and HIV+ disease: A critical review. *Journal of American Psychiatric Nurses Association, 2,* 154-163.

Moynihan, R. T., Christ, G. H., & Gallo-Silver, L. (1987, April 8-10). *Psychosocial, spiritual, and bereavement issues in the treatment of terminally ill people with AIDS.* Paper presented at Care of Terminally Ill Persons with AIDS, Ottawa, Canada.

Murphy, P. (1986, March/April). Pastoral care and persons with AIDS. *The American Journal of Hospice Care,* 38-40.

Murphy, T. (1988). Is AIDS a just punishment? *Journal of Medical Ethics, 14,* 154-160.

Peloquin, S. M. (1990). AIDS: Toward a compassionate response. *The American Journal of Occupational Therapy, 44,* 271-278.

Perry, S., & Markowitz, J. (1986). Psychiatric interventions for AIDS-spectrum disorders. *Hospital and Community Psychiatry, 37,* 1001-1006.

Pert, C. B., Ruff, M. R., Ruscetti, F., Ferrar, W., & Hill, J. (1988). HIV receptors in the brain and peptides that block viral activity. In T. P. Bridge, A. F. Mirsky, & F. K. Goodwin (Eds.), *Psychological, neuropsychiatric and substance abuse aspects of AIDS* (pp. 73-83). New York: Raven.

Poliandro, E. (1991, January/February). Compassion fatigue. *Health Progress,* 54-55, 64.

Polk-Walker, G. C. (1989). Treatment of AIDS in a psychiatric setting. *Perspectives in Psychiatric Care, 25*(2), 9-13.

Portegies, P. (1994). AIDS dementia complex: A review. *Journal for AIDS, 7,* 538-549.

Ridge, D. T., Plummer, D. C., & Minichiello, V. (1994). Young gay men and HIV: Running the risk? *AIDS Care, 6,* 371-378.

Ross, M. A., & Clark-Alexander, B. (1998). Caregivers of children with HIV/AIDS: Quality of life and coping styles. *Journal of the Association of Nurses in AIDS Care, 9*(1), 58-65.

Rosenberg, D. M., McLaulin, B., Bennett, M., & Mathisen, K. (1996). Diagnosing HIV dementia: A retrospective analysis. *Journal of the Association of Nurses in AIDS Care, 7*(6), 57-66.

Roth, J., Siegel, R., & Black S. (1994). Identifying the mental health needs of children living in families with AIDS or HIV infection. *Community Mental Health, 30,* 581-593.

Scanlon, C., & Packard, M. (1991, January/February). Seeing to one's self. *Health Progress,* 50-53.

Seal, D. W., & Agostenelli, G. (1994). Individual differences associated with high-risk sexual behavior: Implications for intervention programmes. *AIDS Care, 6,* 393-397.

Sherman, D. W. (1996). Nurses' willingness to care for AIDS patients in spirituality, social support, and death anxiety. *Image: Journal of Nursing Scholarship, 28,* 205-213.

Shilts, R. (1987). *And the band played on: Politics, people, and the AIDS epidemic.* New York: St. Martin's Press.

Solomon, G. F., Temoshok, L., O'Leary, M., & Zich, J. (1987). A psychoneuroimmunological perspective on AIDS research: Questions, preliminary findings, and suggestions. *Journal of Applied Psychology, 17,* 286-308.

Sowell, R. L., Bramlett, M. H., Gueldner, S. H., Gritzmacher, D., & Martin, G. (1991). The lived experience of survival and bereavement following the death of a lover from AIDS. *Image: Journal of Nursing Scholarship, 23,* 89-94.

Swanson, B., Cronin-Stubbs, D., & Colletti, M. A. (1990). Dementia and depression in persons with AIDS: Causes and care. *Journal of Psychosocial Nursing, 28*(10), 33-39.

Taylor, I., & Robertson, A. (1994). The health needs of gay men: A discussion of the literature and implications for nursing. *Journal of Advanced Nursing, 20,* 85-89.

Theis, S. L., Cohen, F. L., Forrest, J., & Zelewsky, M. (1997). Needs assessment of caregivers of people with HIV/AIDS. *Journal of the Association of Nurses in AIDS Care, 8*(3), 76-84.

Tibesar, L. J. (1986). Pastoral care: Helping patients on an inward journey. *Health Progress, 67*(4), 41-47.

Turner, H. A., Pearlin, L. I., & Mullan, J. T. (1998). Sources and determinants of social support for caregivers of persons with AIDS. *Journal of Health and Social Behavior, 39,* 137-151.

Wenger, N. S., Kusseling, F. S., Beck, K., & Shapiro, M. F. (1994). *AIDS Care, 6,* 399-405.

Suggested Readings

Carson, V. (1990). Spirituality and spiritual direction: Important issues to the person with AIDS. *The Journal of Christian Healing, 12*(3), 37.

Carson, V. (1993). Prayer, meditation, exercise, and vitamin use: Behaviors of the hardy individual who is HIV+, diagnosed with ARC or AIDS. *Journal of the Association of Nurses in AIDS Care, 4*(3), 18-28.

Carson, V., & Green, H. (1992). The relationship of spiritual well-being and hardiness in the AIDS patient. *Journal of Professional Nursing, 8,* 209-220.

Carson, V., Soeken, K. L., Shanty, J., & Terry, L. (1990). Hope and spiritual well-being: Essentials for living with AIDS. *Perspectives in Psychiatric Care, 26*(2), 28-34.

Chenitz, W. C. (1992). Living with AIDS. In J. H. Flaskerud & P. J. Ungvarski (Eds.), *HIV/AIDS: A guide to nursing care* (pp. 440-460). Philadelphia: W. B. Saunders.

Cox, E. (1990). *Thanksgiving: An AIDS journal.* New York: Harper & Row.

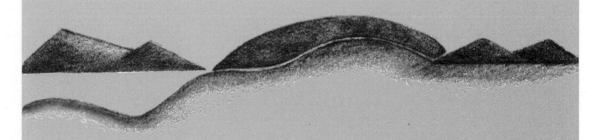

VII The Journey Forward

Traveler's Log

What is it like to be in private practice? No 2 days are the same. Here is a typical day.

8:00 AM   The office manager says a patient called on schedule and reported that a planned medication change had gone well.

8:15 AM   Review laboratory reports that have just arrived via fax. The results are concerning. The patient is on Cytomel and needs a dosage adjustment. I call the patient and discuss changes in her life since her last appointment and the dosage change. I then call the new prescription in to her local pharmacy.

8:30 AM   Compile results of last week's neuropsychological testing. I summarize my findings and type a report for an attorney assisting a patient with an insurance claim.

11:00 AM Conduct a new patient intake. The patient was requesting a second opinion on the need for a stomach stapling. She is morbidly obese. The intake reveals a 25-year history of abuse. She is able to reach catharsis for the first time. We set follow-up visits. I feel optimistic regarding her prognosis.

1:00 PM   Male patient with severe schizophrenia I have been following for 5 years. He had been on a high dose of risperidone and developed side effects exacerbated by cough medicine with codeine. I evaluated a dangerous interaction with the P450 liver enzyme system and decreased his risperidone dose by 75%. He is doing much better on a greatly reduced dose.

2:00 PM   Psychotherapy session with a male patient I recently diagnosed with borderline personality disorder. He is 50 years old and just beginning to address many long-standing issues. I never cease to be amazed how many years some people can wait before being able to confront the angst in their lives.

3:00 PM   Medication check for a man with bipolar disorder hospitalized several months ago. He is back to work full time and doing well. A delightful visit.

3:45 PM   Visit from a favorite drug rep. He leaves samples, videotapes, and cookies!

4:00 PM   Scheduled psychotherapy session with a 52-year-old woman with schizoaffective disorder who has just been weaned off clonazepam, which she was on for 14 years. She looks 10 years younger and is joking and enjoying life for the first time since she was 33.

5:00 PM   Psychotherapy session with 19-year-old woman with bipolar disorder who has just moved in with her boyfriend. He is monitoring her medications and adjusting her dosages for her.

6:00 PM   Return telephone calls from the day.

7:00 PM   Go home, eat dinner, and read the mail. It has been another rewarding day. What a joyous way to practice nursing.

—Mary Moller, RN, APRN, MSN

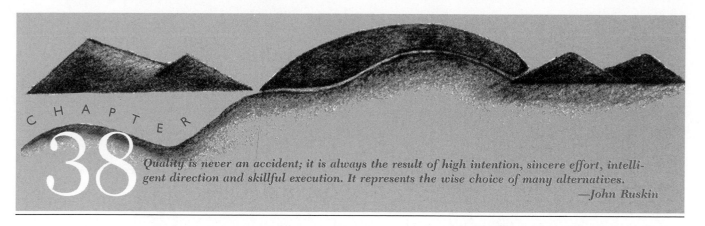

Quality is never an accident; it is always the result of high intention, sincere effort, intelligent direction and skillful execution. It represents the wise choice of many alternatives.

—*John Ruskin*

Research, Outcomes, and Quality Improvement

Learning Objectives

After studying this chapter, you should be able to:

1. Describe the psychiatric nurse's role in continuous quality improvement and nursing research.
2. Explain the process of continuous quality improvement.
3. Specify the relevance of research as an integral part of quality psychiatric nursing practice.
4. Apply two research methods when identifying an area in psychiatric nursing practice in need of improvement.
5. Discuss the trend toward interdisciplinary management of mental health care.
6. Identify critical pathways as an interdisciplinary methodology in psychiatric nursing.

Key Terminology

Benchmarking
Brainstorming
Cause-and-effect diagram
Clinical indicator
Clinical pathways
Collaborative practice

Continuous quality improvement
Critical pathways
Decision matrix
Informational privacy
Informed consent

Outcome-based quality improvement
Performance improvement
Performance indicator
Qualitative research
Quantitative research

Sentinel event
Strategic planning
Survey
Total quality management
Trend chart
Triangulation

As the nursing profession grows, it evolves. Changes occurred in the 1990s that led nursing into team membership yet built the profession's autonomy through the leadership role nursing assumed in the process of improvement. Hospitals and affiliated psychiatric programs and services are required to have a **total quality management** (TQM) program to satisfy the Joint Commission on Accreditation of Healthcare Organizations (JCAHO) and other regulatory agencies that monitor and evaluate quality of services. The success and measurement of interventions is determined through nursing research. This chapter integrates both TQM and selected nursing research techniques into a practical guide. The goal of psychiatric nursing interventions is measurable improvements or outcomes. Nurses want validation of effectiveness. They want evidence that their practices are sound and if not, they want to change or improve.

QUEST FOR QUALITY

Continuous quality improvement (CQI) incorporates the philosophy of TQM. This synonym is an approach to the continuous study and improvement of the processes of providing health care services to meet the needs of individuals and others (JCAHO, 1998).

A systems approach is the basis of CQI. The patient's treatment needs are viewed as an ongoing process, not as a narrow distinction between inpatient or outpatient services. The patient is also viewed as a consumer. The system reviews its response to patient needs and expectations. **Performance improvement** (PI) studies functions and processes to increase the probability of achieving desired outcomes and better meet the needs of individual patients and other users of the service. Interdisciplinary collaboration is now the standard for psychiatric teams. Each of the disciplines has a role to play in CQI. The different services must work together to effectively provide care just as a jigsaw puzzle is not complete if even the smallest part is missing.

Continuous quality improvement (CQI) has many applications to psychiatric nursing practice. As we move through the 21st century, more and more evidence-based practice will be used. Studying CQI will give the basic nursing student one way to explore management accountability, teamwork, continuous improvements in work processes, customer orientation, and statistical analysis.

> **W***hat do you think?* As a nursing student, what role do you play in the PI process?

> ➤ *Check Your Reading*
> 1. What is one characteristic of PI and CQI?
> 2. Name at least one driving force behind the TQM/CQI movement.
> 3. In what ways does the traditional multidisciplinary psychiatric team need to change to incorporate a CQI approach fully?

EVOLUTION OF TOTAL QUALITY MANAGEMENT

Historical Influences

The quest for quality in health care has been evolving over a number of decades. Historically, physicians functioned independently, and it was the individual practitioner's responsibility first "to do no harm," as stated in the Hippocratic oath, and to provide the best care possible. During the Crimean war, Florence Nightingale started keeping mortality statistics to identify unacceptable standards (Nielsen, 1992). With the development of hospitals and the emergence of nursing, medical specialty practices, and ancillary health care services, the responsibility and accountability for quality health care came to include a variety of providers and the institutions in which health care professionals work.

Joint Commission on Accreditation of Healthcare Organizations

Federal regulation of hospitals significantly increased as a result of the Social Security Act of 1965, which created Medicare and Medicaid and established conditions of participation for hospitals. In 1972, amendments to the Social Security Act required professional standards review organizations and quality assurance (QA) standards for health care providers. The evolution of JCAHO is chronicled in the *Guide to Quality Assurance* (1988). In 1972, JCAHO published a manual on hospital accreditation, and the American Hospital Association developed a patient bill of rights and a QA program for medical care in hospitals. In 1975, JCAHO published the quality of professional services standard. This was replaced in 1979 with a chapter on QA. Further amendments to Title VI of Social Security, the enactment of the Consolidated Omnibus Budget Reconciliation Act in 1985, and the Omnibus Budget Reconciliation Acts of 1986, 1987, 1989, and 1990 expanded the demand for hospital monitoring and the evaluation of the quality, efficiency, and costs of care.

Focus on Inspection and Individual Performance

Initially, the focus of professional, accrediting, and regulatory groups was on inspection and individual performance to improve the quality of care. The approach was problem-oriented and focused on meeting minimal standards. The term used at this basic level was QA. As health care costs began to spiral upward, however, increasing attention focused on cost containment and improved efficiency in health care. In traditional nursing QA, the full spectrum of services and the flow of patient care were not addressed. Only those processes and interventions within nursing's scope of concern were considered. The quality improvement (QI) approach encourages interdisciplinary analysis and problem-solving without assignment of blame to specific disciplines or individuals. The result is a more holistic approach to patient care. Quality monitoring ensures that accredited organizations follow standards that produce quality results.

The 10-Step Process

During the 1980s, JCAHO moved from a problem-focused approach to systematic monitoring and evaluation. To facilitate this process, JCAHO published the *Ten-Step Model for the Monitoring and Evaluation Process* in 1985. The model was modified in 1991 to incorporate the CQI approach. Box 38–1 lists the 10 steps.

This 10-step process is used to identify patterns of care that do not meet the established standards and that need improvement. The highest priority for monitoring and evaluation are high-volume, high-risk, or problem-prone aspects of care. Data are collected over a series of cases or events. Data are then analyzed to identify specific patterns or trends that indicate a need for improvement. When the threshold, a preestablished level, is reached, a more intensive evaluation is triggered.

The weakness in the earlier monitoring and evaluation approach was that it followed the organizational structure and focused on intradepartmental issues rather than patient care improvement. Problems related to the integration of services from a number of departments and services often require interdepartmental analysis and problem-solving.

Nursing has traditionally focused on aspects of nursing care such as the quality and timeliness of nursing assessments, nursing care plans, and specific nursing interventions (e.g., use of locked-door seclusion and restraints, as needed medication, and medication errors). Although these are important aspects of care, they are only part of quality-based health care. The goal is to focus on quality measurements such as nurse performance and organizational measures that explore processes and integration of services.

What do you think? How do you think consumers of nursing care measure quality?

➤ *Check Your Reading*
4. Describe nursing's traditional approach to QA.
5. Name at least 4 steps in the Joint Commission's 10-step process.

History of Continuous Quality Improvement

The movement from quality control to QA and now to CQI began in industry. In the 1920s and 1930s, American manufacturing and engineering industries began using TQM to improve the quality of their goods and services. W. Edwards Deming's principles and work on statistical QC led Japan's post–World War I economy to go from severe economic problems to becoming a leader in the world markets.

Impact of Deming and Juran on Continuous Quality Improvement

Two of the leading experts on quality control, Deming and Joseph Juran, worked with Japanese companies to develop strategies for improving the quality of products and services. They recognized the need for a management approach to QI and the need to involve staff members at all levels in the QI process. Deming and Juran built on the theoretical work done in the 1920s by the Bell Telephone Laboratories quality engineering group. Walter Shewhart, a member of this group, had identified the need for statistical analysis in evaluating quality. Shewhart recognized that some minor variation in quality would always occur over time. The real issue, Shewhart proposed, is to determine when this variation is statistically significant (Juran, 1988).

Applying this principle, Deming studied the Japanese approach to industrial application of QI and developed his famous 14 points of QI shown in Box 38–2. Deming stressed that it is important for managers to understand that most people want to do a good job and that most quality problems are systems problems unrelated to individual performance. Resolving systems problems requires a coordinated management approach and teamwork. Rather than focusing on finding the "bad apples," it is important to develop the overall competency of all employees.

Definition of Quality

Deming, Juran, and other leaders in the quest for quality recognized the importance of defining terms, particularly *quality*. A typical problem is that personal definitions vary. Hospital administrators may look at services provided, census reports, financial statements, physician satisfaction, and patient complaints to develop a definition of quality. Physicians may judge quality according to the types of medical equipment and facilities available; working relationships with hospital administrators, nurses, and other personnel; the reliability and response time for obtaining laboratory results; the drugs in the pharmacy's formulary; and patient responses to the treatment provided. Nurses may define quality according to their working conditions and relationships with other staff, cleanliness or the units, time spent in direct patient care, and practice standards. Patients may define quality according to their improved health; treatment by physicians, nurses, and other hospital staff; ease of registration; respect for confidentiality; the hospital meal menu; and billing problems.

Juran (1992) noted that *quality* has multiple meanings but cited two critical definitions: "[Q]uality is product satisfaction" (p. 7) and "quality is freedom from deficiencies" (p. 510). He developed a universal way of total quality thinking known as the *quality trilogy:* planning, control, and improvement. Crosby (1979) defined *quality* as conforming to requirements and

Box 38-2 ■ ■ ■ ■ ■
Deming's 14 Points of Quality Improvement

1. Create, publish, and disseminate to all employees a statement of the aims and purposes of the organization. The management must demonstrate constant commitment to this statement.
2. Learn the new philosophy—top management and everybody.
3. Understand the purpose of inspection: to improve processes and reduce cost.
4. End the practice of rewarding business based on price tag alone.
5. Improve, constantly and forever, the system of production and service.
6. Institute training.
7. Teach and institute leadership.
8. Drive out fear. Create trust. Create a climate for innovation.
9. Optimize the efforts of teams, groups, and staff areas toward the aims and purposes of the organization.
10. Eliminate exhortations for the work force.
11a. Eliminate numerical quotas for production. Instead, learn and institute methods for improvement.
11b. Eliminate management by objective. Instead, learn the capabilities of processes and how to improve them.
12. Remove barriers that rob people of pride of workmanship.
13. Encourage education and self-improvement for everyone.
14. Take action to accomplish the transformation.

focused on lack of defects. Deming (1986) stated that "quality should be aimed at the needs of the consumer, present and future" (p. 5). Organizations need to recognize that they have both internal and external customers and that these customers are integral to defining quality. Internal customers are departments or individuals dependent on the services provided or the processes performed by another department.

Total quality requires participation by everyone: all units and all employees, workers, and management of the organization. All the leaders in the quality revolution agree that it is the responsibility of management to define quality and to ensure that all employees know that definition. Quality improvement focuses on minimizing variation. Crosby (1984) noted that "[T]he system for causing quality is prevention, not appraisal." (p. 73). Deming and Juran realized that there were no quick fixes or overnight solutions to quality problems.

Implementation of a QI program takes years, not weeks or months. Organizations must make a long-term commitment to quality. The first step is to recognize your customers and their needs. Once an organization has identified current and potential customers, internal and external, a mission statement can be developed and planning begun.

What do you think? How do you measure quality?

➤ *Check Your Reading*

6. What was Deming's contribution to the development of CQI?
7. How did Juran define quality?
8. Identify at least 5 of the items in Deming's 14 points of QI.

CONCEPTS OF CONTINUOUS QUALITY IMPROVEMENT AND HEALTH CARE

The implementation of a CQI program requires a systematic approach on the part of the organization.

Mission, Goals, Objectives, and Philosophy

The first step for an organization moving toward a program of CQI involves the development of a mission statement, a philosophy to guide the organization's future, and goals and objectives to guide its daily operations. Therefore, the mission, goals, and objectives, and philosophy should reflect

- Purpose of the organization (i.e., to provide quality patient care services)
- Organization's commitment to quality improvement (as reflected by definition and as evidenced at all levels)
- System of values and beliefs that ensures quality improvement (excellence through standards of practice and performance)
- Patient care delivery system conducive to quality improvement (e.g., primary nursing, case management, collaborative practice)
- System to quantify results
- Organizational commitment and leadership as essential components in CQI
- Organization's shared purpose in CQI
- Organization's focus on customers in CQI
- Organization's long-term commitment to CQI

The organizational commitment to CQI, however, must be operationalized throughout the organization.

Strategic Planning

Like all organizations, health care organizations must have some guiding force that moves them from point A to point B. Most organizations, including those involved in health care, call this guiding force **strategic planning.** Strategic planning helps all involved look 3 to 5 years ahead by using current and projected environmental changes and trends. It is within this strategic plan that the foundation for quality improvement is laid.

CQI places great emphasis on planning for quality and the need for continuous feedback so that corrections can be made. The Deming quality cycle (Figure 38–1) emphasizes the ongoing nature of this process. Activities included under the *plan* portion of the cycle are determining improvement goals and targets and determining methods to reach these goals. The *do* portion of the cycle includes providing education and training and implementing work. *Study* refers to reviewing the results and evaluating the effects of implementation. *Act* requires that appropriate action be taken. CQI is based on the continuous cycle of these four processes.

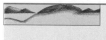

Beginning the Process—One Unit's Experience

The JCAHO *1995 Accreditation Manual for Healthcare* arrived on the psychiatric unit. Pat took this opportunity to move her staff members into active involvement in CQI and PI. Quoting from the manual, she explained that the focus for their unit would be to examine the systems and processes used to deliver care while continuing to recognize the importance of the competence of individual staff members.

To improve the quality of the care they gave and to prepare for the upcoming JCAHO survey, the unit would be developing performance indicators. These would be used to measure the degree of accomplishment of objectives and show outcomes to quantify progress toward the attainment of goals. Teams would be needed to direct and plan the preparation for the survey. Pat was introducing the concepts and would provide guidance to the groups who would be making decisions based on the systems, processes, and performance indicators on which the staff members

agreed. The unit would be working as part of an interdisciplinary team, and the agency would be part of a statewide and national project. Collaborative decision making would be used to validate which indicators would be selected for validation of the system's effectiveness for quality patient care. All staff members would be involved in the team process.

Pat used her group leadership skills to ask key questions that needed to be answered. Who is involved in the care we provide? How can we tell if everyone is satisfied? What do we really want to accomplish with our care? Is our unit appropriately staffed and equipped? Are our patients benefitting from being hospitalized? The staff all contributed their own questions and a beginning fact-finding strategy emerged. This would be their chance to prove they were doing a good job or improve so they would be.

Data collection needed planning and could be done in a variety of ways. The unit chose to develop a survey to solicit opinions from all patients and people involved in their care. They focused on defining the problem first. This step is key to successful research; if the step is skipped in the rush to find solutions it causes many failures.

The process would take time, but the psychiatric unit staff members were starting 3 years before the survey and were eager to prove their success. Pat ended her presentation by encouraging everyone to keep the list of topics they developed and think about other topics that could be added before beginning the data collection.

At the completion of the task, the unit members had clearly identified their customers and determined their customers' needs, wants, and expectations.

Collecting and Organizing Data

Tools used by quality teams help them analyze problems, set priorities, facilitate decision-making, generate solutions, and document progress. Table 38–1 lists and defines CQI terms. The JCAHO manual includes the steps to prepare for the accreditation survey. The complete process as well as a description of the survey is included in the manual.

These tools can be illustrated in the case study involving the psychiatric unit. The group can use multivoting to identify their unit's *s*trengths, *w*eaknesses, *o*pportunities, and *t*hreats (SWOT analysis). New ideas and solutions can be generated with **brainstorming,** the ideas prioritized through the multivoting process, and a flow chart developed that displays the entire process. The group members can then use a **cause-and-effect diagram** or Pareto diagram to identify factors contributing to the problem or causing a certain effect (e.g., noncompliance, substance abuse, recidivism). Asking repetitive "Why?" questions is one way of uncovering root causes and avoiding mistakenly interpreting an effect as a cause.

Once a team decides on the root cause of a problem,

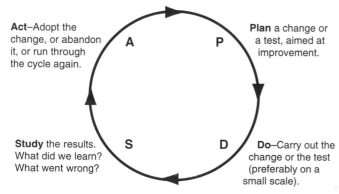

Act–Adopt the change, or abandon it, or run through the cycle again.

Plan a change or a test, aimed at improvement.

Study the results. What did we learn? What went wrong?

Do–Carry out the change or the test (preferably on a small scale).

Figure 38–1
The Deming quality cycle. (Redrawn from *The New Economics for Industry, Government, Education* by W. Edwards Deming by permission of MIT and The W. Edwards Deming Institute. Published by MIT, Center for Advanced Educational Services, Cambridge, MA 02139. Copyright 1993 by The W. Edwards Deming Institute.)

T A B L E 3 8 – 1 Continuous Quality Improvement Tools	
TERM	**DEFINITION**
Brainstorming	Method used to generate ideas without criticism or judgment. Team members are asked to quickly list or call out all the ideas that they think of related to a specific problem or topic, without first filtering or evaluating the ideas.
Multivoting	This is used once the brainstorming has been completed to determine whether all or only a few of the ideas noted will be explored. Multivoting is a process of setting priorities or narrowing the field of possibilities.
Idea logs	These are logs of good ideas that surface but may not be relevant to the task at hand. Use of the log prevents the team from being distracted from its main task, yet allows the group to return to that idea at a later time.
Storyboards	Graphic representations of proposals or process stories used to document and communicate the activities and progress of the group.
Flow charts	Graphic displays of all the steps and decision points in a process that help a team see the "big picture."
Cause-and-effect diagrams	Representations of the various factors that might contribute to a problem.
Pareto diagrams	These diagrams use the Pareto principle, which says that in any group of things that contribute to a common effect a relatively few contributors account for most of the effect. These diagrams help the team members to focus on the "vital few" rather than the "trivial many." They help identify those factors most significant in causing a certain effect.
Decision matrix	A listing of all pertinent criteria that is followed by an evaluation of different alternatives according to specified criteria.
SWOT analysis	A multivoting method that allows for assessing an idea as a strength, a weakness, or an opportunity for improvement.

a **decision matrix** can help them determine the best solution. A decision matrix allows the team to list all the pertinent data and then evaluate different alternatives according to specified criteria. This effort helps the team select the best solution. For difficult situations, flow charting, displaying the process from admission to discharge to readmission, might reveal some important information about where the system may be breaking down. For instance, it might show that problems occurring within the first 3 days after discharge lead to noncompliance or that support is adequate but structure is insufficient. The idea is that looking at the process in its entirety can provide valuable information that would otherwise not be brought forth. Storyboards provide easy-to-follow explanations that serve as useful educational tools.

The tools can be used in a variety of ways. At times, their use is mandated as in the occurrence of a **sentinel event.** Beginning in late 1995, several major hospital errors, such as wrong side surgery and medication errors causing deaths, led JCAHO to the conclusion that something more was needed to reduce the risk of these serious problems. Their policy on sentinel events (JCAHO, 1998) requires accredited organizations to report serious outcomes such as unanticipated death or major loss of function. The event must be listed even if the outcome was not death in some cases. For behavioral health, the suicide of a patient in a setting where the patient receives around-the-clock care (e.g., hospital, residential treatment center, crisis stabilization center) is a sentinel event. The incident is researched and a root cause analysis produced. The acceptable

analysis focuses on systems and processes not individual performance. As in all quality improvement, the analysis looks first at the specific case and then expands to organizational causes.

*W**hat do you think?*** Does the focus on systems and processes rather than individuals decrease individual accountability?

▶ *Check Your Reading*
9. What is the purpose of the mission to CQI?
10. Explain the strategic planning process.
11. List four CQI tools.

Earl's Dilemma

After the meeting, Pat was reviewing her notes when Earl, the senior case manager, came in. "That was a good meeting. We came up with some good ideas to explore, but now that I've had some time to think I have another." Pat looked up and responded, "I could tell something was bothering you and hoped you'd share it."

"I'm really concerned about our rehospitalization rates," Earl said. "I work hard at getting a discharge plan in place and then the patients leave and don't follow what they've agreed to. Take Barbara, for instance. She's been in and out of our unit five times in the past 6 months. She comes in hallucinating, paranoid, and malnourished because she won't take her medicines and doesn't eat once she goes home. Her drinking is a problem too. I looked at her last blood work and she's really beginning to show liver problems. When she drinks, she's even harder to handle. Last month she came in through the emergency department because she got into a fight at a bar and her 'boyfriend' broke her arm. I know she has rights, but I wonder about the ethics of using the system with someone who hasn't the capacity to change. Today, the police brought her into the emergency department about 2 hours ago on an emergency petition. She was threatening to kill herself because she couldn't make the voices stop. I had hoped this new medicine would help. She just needs closer supervision. This time maybe I can get her into a supervised living arrangement. The landlord is not going to allow her back in her apartment because of all the noise complaints. As her case manager, I don't feel much satisfaction."

"I know how frustrating it can be for you," Pat said. "We get patients stable only to have them leave and boomerang right back. Is this something you want to study and improve?"

"Yes," Earl replied. "In the past all we've done is chart audits to show what mistakes we've made: how many medication errors or missed orders. I'm not saying that's not important, but what I'd really like to do is have more patient success. PI seems to just fix the little problems but doesn't touch the real issues," Earl complained. "We need PI indicators that will show better patient outcomes. Can this be an outcome we can achieve?"

"I think that would be wonderful," said Pat. "We can use Barbara as a case study to identify all the areas, people, and processes involved, and then see if we can make a difference. We can ask all the departments to help us brainstorm. I'm sure other units have patients who return time and again," Pat continued. "The chart audits we do are still necessary. The data we collect helps us solve problems and provide better care. It's not just a matter of finding fault. We try to make improvements that will help everybody. Your idea for a case study is just what we need to start identifying indicators to add the new outcome piece. I'll let you present this at the next meeting. I'm sure all of us would like to show we make a difference with our most important people—our patients."

Establishing Quality Teams

Everyone is involved with quality improvement in behavioral health care. Teams selected by managers plan the process and monitor progress. Effective teams represent all disciplines and involve both clinical and nonclinical people. The teams may be divided into patient care and management teams (Schuler, 1994). The quality council has the task of identifying the specific needs for improvement—the quality projects. For each project, a quality team or circle has responsibility for resolving the problem successfully. The members of the team may be drawn from all levels of the management hierarchy and from different departments or levels of care. The team collects data, diagnoses the causes of the problems, stimulates the development and implementation of remedies, and establishes controls to "hold" the gains.

Developing a quality team in Barbara's case might help identify key factors that affect her noncompliance and keep her coming back to the hospital. The quality team might be composed of the inpatient treatment team: physician, nurse, counselor, and social worker. In Barbara's case, the team might bring in people outside the organization (with her consent) who will be involved in her care after discharge.

The quality team might determine that Barbara would be more likely to comply with her medication regimen if she had a home visit by a psychiatric home care nurse for the first 3 days after discharge. The team might also identify some of the stressors that trigger crisis in Barbara's life in conjunction with a significant other, and the home care nurse can develop a plan to diminish these.

Decision Analysis

Traditionally, health care organizations have used hierarchical decision models based on hospital structure organized around functional areas or disciplines. Quality teams need to include all areas or disciplines involved in a given process or provision of a service. These teams need to be empowered to participate in the decision-making processes that affect their projects.

The process of integrative decision-making requires education and training of participants. It also requires the support of administration. Managers may fear that this process will undermine their authority, but they need to be trained to recognize how this process actually facilitates their ability to resolve problems that affect their areas but fall outside their purview. They need to recognize that the barriers between departments are one of the primary causes of system problems.

Quality teams also need to use decision analysis in assessing and evaluating treatment processes and outcomes. Coleman (1989) described diagnostic probabilities for patients with suicidal ideation. She stated that decisional analysis can improve indicator development because it can assist in determining which decisions are most likely to be appropriate, thereby making indicators based on those decisions more likely to be valid and useful. Participation in the quality improvement process requires that all employees, regardless of discipline or area, be trained in problem-solving and decision-making.

Monitoring and Evaluating Care and Service

Important aspects of care and service are those with the highest priority and greatest significance in determining outcomes. The JCAHO guidelines recommend that organizations concentrate on aspects of care or service that are high volume, high risk, or problem prone. Fauman (1990) noted that determining which aspects of psychiatric care to monitor and how to monitor them has proved difficult for many clinicians. Difficulties exist in

- Determining which aspects of care and service are most important
- Determining ways to measure and quantify clinical aspects of care
- Determining appropriate indicators to monitor these aspects of care and service
- Allocating the time and resources required for monitoring
- Trying to change treatment outcomes when many factors over which clinicians have limited or no control influence the outcomes

Defining the activities in behavioral terms helps the team quantify and measure them. Schroeder and Katz (1992) reported on sets of universal and specialty aspects of care identified at the Third Annual Conference on Nursing Quality Assurance. Some of the universal aspects of care most applicable to nursing were as follows:

- Knowledge deficit
- Hygiene
- Safety
- Psychosocial issues and emotional support
- Patient and family education
- Medication administration
- Patient satisfaction
- Management of violent behavior

Aspects of care identified by the mental health nursing group included the following:

- Therapeutic groups
- Hallucination and psychosis
- Multidisciplinary treatment
- Withdrawal
- Electroconvulsive therapy
- Suicide precautions

Some additional aspects of care pertinent to psychiatry are

- Discharge planning
- Crisis management of ambulatory patients
- Special treatment procedures such as seclusion, restraints, and patient rights

Standards of Care and Practice

For each identified aspect of care or practice, it is important to determine standards. Kirk and Hoesing (1991) stated that standards are needed to

- Provide direction
- Reach agreement on expectations
- Monitor and evaluate results (e.g., did results meet the standard, not meet the standard, or exceed the standard?)
- Guide organizations, people, and patients to obtain optimal results

External organizations such as the JCAHO, the Health Care Financing Administration (HCFA), federal and state regulatory organizations, the American Nurses Association (ANA), specialty boards, and licensing or certification groups establish some standards. Internally, a department or a discipline can develop standards. Nursing is working as a discipline to define standards of practice for nurses as part of the health care team. Standards of practice such as these are broad statements of the work of a discipline. Standards of care may be developed by an organization to outline processes and desired outcomes for patient care. Some standards of care are written by a single discipline, but interdisciplinary standards of care are becoming more common (Mason, 1999, p. 17).

Considerable attention is currently focused on clinical practice guidelines. There are examples of four clinical practice guidelines from psychiatric home care throughout the book. These are valuable in facilitating health care delivery and improving patient outcomes. Guidelines or standards of practice represent appropriate evaluation and treatment based on the state-of-the-art in medicine and nursing. Standards of care or practice allow us to compare an organization to the state-of-the-art in medicine and nursing. These standards change as knowledge and technology increase.

The ANA published the first standards of psychiatric and mental health nursing in 1973. These were revised in 1982 and again in 1994 (ANA, 1994). The Society for Education and Research in Psychiatric–Mental Health Nursing (SERPN) was established to maintain quality in the specialty. In 1996, SERPN established standards for basic preparation for entry into psychiatric practice. Their requirements are found in Box 38-3.

Competence and Quality

Quality care in mental health nursing depends on the availability of qualified, competent staff. Assuring competence is an expectation of CQI. Competency tests are routinely administered to validate the skills of nurses before they are hired. Physical and mental health assessment skills are essential; missing a patient's physical or mental health problem delays recovery of health and return to function and increases company costs. The biological basis for mental health problems requires a comprehensive understanding of neuroscience in order

Box 38-3 ■ ■ ■ ■ ■
Basic Preparation for Psychiatric Practice

Knowledge

- Biological and psychological theories of mental health and mental illness
- Psychotherapeutic modalities
- Substance abuse and dual diagnoses
- Care of populations at risk
- Community as milieu as a therapeutic modality
- Cultural and spiritual implications of nursing care
- Family dynamics in mental health and illness
- Psychopharmacology
- Legal and ethical factors, including documentation specific to the care of those with a mental illness

Skills

- Comprehensive biopsychosocial and spiritual assessment
- Interdisciplinary collaboration
- Identification and coordination of relevant resources for patients and families
- Use of psychiatric diagnosis classification system
- Therapeutic communication
- Therapeutic use of self
- Psychoeducation with patients and families
- Administering and monitoring psychopharmacological agents

Data from Society for Education and Research in Psychiatric and Mental Health Nursing. (1997). *Primary mental health and advanced practice psychiatric nursing.* Pensacola, FL: SERPN.

frequency of data collection. Data may be available through medical records, management information systems, logs, or other databases. Use of computer systems facilitates the collection, organization, and display of data. Automation may also be more cost-effective in the long-term. Adequate sample sizes are determined through statistical methods. Most nurses are not expected to do the statistical analysis. Data in large studies are entered into computers by data entry personnel. Nurses need to collect and organize the data in a manner that facilitates the entry. In large studies, computers are used for display and communication of the results. The computer printout identifies patterns or trends in an easy-to-follow **trend chart.** Specific attention is paid to trends or patterns in the data. The quality team analyzes the data to identify any potential for improvement. If there is such potential, the quality team facilitates the development and implementation of a plan to improve the process or service. Follow-up is then required to maintain the gains and to assess the effectiveness of actions.

Barbara's story describes the all-too-frequent plight of patients with a psychiatric illness as well as the feelings of frustration of the staff members working with them. Many nurses, when confronted with CQI, react with the same level of frustration expressed by Earl. They view PI activities as having limited value. For success with CQI, Pat will need to win over her staff members and let go of much of her traditional managerial oversight.

to explain the disease process to patients and caregivers. Medication teaching and management requires psychopharmacology knowledge. Mental health nurses need to keep current in physical assessment and stay knowledgeable about diseases. Just as the medical profession is adding primary care providers, in home care, Medicare expects psychiatric nurses to handle the physical problems of the psychiatric patient as well as the mental health needs. Insurers, researchers, and physicians are requesting mental health evaluations for their patients when expected outcomes are not achieved. More advanced practice nurses in mental health are being prepared as psychiatric nurse practitioners than clinical nurse specialists to ensure competency in both physical and psychiatric assessment and intervention.

Reporting of Data

In developing a monitoring system, the quality team must agree on the information needed and on the

TOTAL QUALITY IMPROVEMENT AS A TEAM EFFORT

Improving performance through CQI requires nursing participation because nurses are involved in all aspects of patient care. Nurse managers support, coach, and train their staff in the quality improvement process. Professional nurses pride themselves on the care they give; CQI lets everyone from nursing assistants to transporters and dietary workers share in the activities. Successful programs increase access to care and make quality care more affordable. The staff members "own the process," but they are energized by the results, the feedback, and the management support. To make the system work, the unit needs to move from retrospective to concurrent review, from an individual to a team approach, with continuous improvements focused on work processes, customer orientation, and statistical analysis.

It took Rita Lautz and Katherine Lynn (1995) 3 years of using CQI to restructure the delivery of care on their psychiatric unit. Successful changes included a shift in work roles for both managers and clinicians. They devised a new skill mix that upgraded nursing assistants with training to become psychiatric counselors and redesigned the assignment system for psychiatric care. Those functions required by licensing and accreditation standards remained solely within the registered nurse role. Decentralized management decision-making and the use of quality teams promoted active staff participation. A business unit tracked the new design's budget needs and resource production. Active problem-solving, conflict resolution, and decision-making using consensual validation became the role of staff councils, which included staff nurses with demonstrated leadership skills and expertise in psychiatric nursing. Nurses in this setting reported CQI offers autonomy, investment satisfaction, and job satisfaction resulting in lower staff turnover and satisfied patients and staff members.

Psychiatry has long used the multidisciplinary approach to treatment planning. Treatment teams regularly include a psychiatrist, a nurse, a social worker, and a recreation or occupational therapist. In some cases, psychologists or other professionals participate in treatment planning and therapy. Treatment teams have resulted in greater coordination and integration of patient care on inpatient units, but these teams usually have limited participation and input from crisis intervention services counselors, outpatient therapists, home health nurses, social workers, group home supervisors, and others who have a significant role in the patient's treatment.

In Barbara's story, focusing only on traditional nursing care limits the impact on the course of her illness or treatment. The problem of multiple hospitalizations needs to be assessed by the entire treatment team, which includes psychiatrists, nursing staff members, psychiatric technicians, nursing assistants, social workers, occupational and recreational therapists, and others. Barbara needs to be involved from the beginning, and follow-up must be arranged after patient discharge. This requires close coordination among crisis intervention services, inpatient staff members, outpatient providers, and community providers.

Patient Response and Outcomes

Increasing attention is being paid to treatment outcomes in psychiatry, particularly with the expansion of managed care. Psychiatric services are being forced to define their treatment goals and interventions better to achieve these goals. Goals need to be defined in behavioral terms, and psychiatry programs must be able to demonstrate effectiveness in the utilization management of services and the achievement of positive patient outcomes based on these goals.

One way to demonstrate quality and effectiveness of services is to monitor whether or not critical treatment

objectives are achieved. Quality teams can focus on analysis of the treatment process to develop critical paths and outcome data that are valid and reliable. Assessing the quality of services means focusing on patient responses and outcomes. Documenting clinical outcomes provides a way to monitor results. Using the assessments and treatment plans, we can review the problems, goals, and interventions to evaluate patient outcomes.

Outcome-Based Quality Improvement

Regulating bodies such as Medicare continually search for validation of care effectiveness. Regulation provides for action by public entities to improve function, correct failure, and control entry and continuation of service by health care providers and organizations (Donaldson, 1998). Just as Earl wished for a better outcome for Barbara, the Colorado Center for Health Policy and Research in Denver sought to measure better outcomes for home care patients. The center conducted a pilot study of Medicare and non-Medicare home health patients including those with chronic mental or behavioral problems. The results of this study were used for a national project called the Outcome and Assessment Information Set (OASIS) (Koch, 1997). This systematic approach to collecting outcome-related data is used by home health agencies to improve and maintain quality using outcome findings.

The outcome process is assessed in three ways. First, an examination is done of how the care is delivered: environment, staff members' qualifications, equipment, and technical devices. These are defined as *structural measures of quality.* Second, how the care is planned and provided, comprehensiveness of assessments, and adequacy of care planning are reviewed. As in other quality models, these are process measures of quality. Finally, the focus is on exploring what happens to the health of patients after care. This is the outcome measure and is the primary focus.

Outcomes are the most important quality measure. In addition to payers, many accrediting bodies, including JCAHO and the National League for Nursing (NLN), have become outcome oriented. Additionally, consumer groups, such as the American Association of Retired Persons (AARP) and the National Alliance for the Mentally Ill (NAMI) are lobbying for improved patient care. Health care quality became such an important issue that President Clinton formed an advisory commission on consumer protection and quality in the health care industry. In 1998, they proposed a consumer bill of rights in an attempt to legislate quality. Outcomes help everyone measure quality.

Patient outcomes are central to CQI. As a monitor, they can be used to highlight what works and does not work for patient welfare. Unlike chart audits that are detail specific, outcomes are broader based. Only unusually good or bad outcomes trigger an examination of the care provided. Outcomes measurement is a team-centered activity with a specific two-stage process; outcomes are first defined and then measured.

There are different types of outcomes. Those that focus on patients reflect a change in health status over time. This is measured between two points during care. Shaughnessy and Crisler (1995) broadly defined health status as physiological, functional, cognitive, emotional, and behavioral health. The change must come from within the patient and not be the result of external control, such as an in-home counselor providing transportation to a partial hospitalization program. Outcomes may be positive, negative, or validate maintenance of the same level. Change can occur as a result of disease progression or care provided.

Defining and Choosing Outcomes

Confusion exists over what are and are not outcomes. Critical pathways, care planning, treatment regimens, cost, utilization and assessments are not outcomes (Shaughnessy & Crisler, 1995). All of these items are either processes that are done directly for the patient or that are used to evaluate the care needs or care provided for the patient or services provided to the patient. *Goals* are expected outcomes, and they are periodically evaluated for goal attainment; goals can be patient focused or system focused such as those measured in **outcome-based quality improvement** (OBQI).

Patient goals are individual. One patient's goals may not be attainable by all patients with that illness. Only by examining health status over time can outcomes be assessed or measured. Although outcomes that validate goal achievement are still a basic part of evaluating the patient's response to a specific intervention, these outcomes are not useful for OBQI because they are generally subjective and refer only to a short portion of care. Some examples of OBQI outcomes include compliance with treatment regimens, stabilization in pain interfering with activity for a designated period after discharge, and hospitalization and rehospitalization rates. Hospital admission is an outcome that typically reflects a substantial change in patient health status over time. Hospitalization and rehospitalization rates are global outcomes that can be used to compare all patients regardless of illness or care delivery method.

Elizabeth's Story

Mrs. Elizabeth Williams, a recently widowed, frail southerner, sat passively through the psychiatric admission process. This visit occurred shortly after her spouse of 60 years died after a long illness. She gave monosyllabic responses to most questions and was selectively mute to many. Her hair appeared dull and matted. The home environment was cluttered, with old papers, dirty clothes, and dishes piled throughout the house. She looked thin; her clothes hung on her small frame. The admission assessment weight showed a 30-lb weight loss since her last physician visit 4 months earlier. Her arms and legs were bruised after several falls while trying to walk to the bathroom. She felt weak and had no interest in eating or taking care of herself. Elizabeth admitted to feeling sad and depressed for several months. Confusion clouded her recall of dates and her medical history. She stated she felt exhausted much of the time and spent most of her day in bed. At her daughter's insistence and to avoid being hospitalized, she reluctantly agreed to have a nurse visit her at home. Fran, the home care nurse, completed the assessments including suicidal ideation. Elizabeth assured Fran that she would never take her own life, but she hoped God would take her to join her husband soon. Admission discharge planning included possibly seeking a higher level of care.

Elizabeth was admitted to home care with a diagnosis of major depression. At this point, her activity of daily living bathing skill was rated as "unable to use the tub or shower." Jeanette, the social worker, visited to see if Elizabeth would accept a higher level of care, but she adamantly refused to consider moving. After gradually building trust and gaining compliance with an antidepressant, Fran convinced her to allow a home care aide to prepare a meal and to help her with bathing. Elizabeth needed a great amount of assistance and physical therapy to rebuild her atrophied muscles. Lola, the home care aide, tenderly cared for Elizabeth's physical needs and slowly encouraged her to be more active. Using cognitive structured approaches; in-home exercises; and closely monitoring the advancement of a low dose of an antidepressant, Elizabeth gradually improved. She started dressing herself, then fixing her own meals, and finally showering and walking independently. She resumed attending the local senior center and playing bridge. She confessed to Fran at her last visit, "I truly wanted to die. Now I feel so much better. I promise to take my medicine so I'll stay well. I want to help with my new grandchild who'll be born in the spring." Discharge ratings showed improvement in all categories to independence. ■

All patients with depression may not achieve such dramatic improvements, but all patients can be rated and compared using outcomes. The outcomes illustrated in Elizabeth's story are part of on-going data set collection being conducted by the HCFA. OASIS proposes outcome-based quality improvement for agencies participating in Medicare. As Koch (1997) wrote,

For the first time in the history of the Medicare home care program, agency efforts to meet Medicare's regulatory requirements will closely "mirror" efforts to meet JCAHO

or Community Healthcare Accreditation Program (CHAP) accreditation requirements. This is truly a step forward in promoting quality services. (p. 34)

OASIS is an example of a partnership between a regulatory body and providers. HCFA uses OASIS information to facilitate interdisciplinary care and coordination of services. Agencies can use the data item results to compare their agency's performance to all others and maintain an effective, data-driven, OBQI program. (See the section later, on benchmarking performance.)

The OASIS data items were developed to measure patient outcomes in home health care. Data is collected from patients at admission and discharge and every 60 days if the patient remains under care. OASIS provides a tool for collecting data to measure outcomes. Outcome measures in addition to ambulation and locomotion and bathing include transferring, management of oral medications, housekeeping, pain interfering with activity, dyspnea, confusion, discharge to independent living, acute care hospitalization, behavioral problem frequency, and nursing home admission (Shaughnessy & Crisler, 1995).

Nurse's Role in Outcome Research

Nursing literature is replete with outcome studies. Reading the studies builds a better understanding of the strategies that psychiatric nurses are using to improve care for the mentally ill. Reading journals is one way of maintaining competence and staying current with patient care options. An article by Sallah (1997) detailed the process used by a group of British forensic psychiatric nurses to build consensus for mentally ill disordered offenders. The group's efforts produced common guidelines for the treatment, care, and management of mentally disordered offenders. This study is beneficial to all mental health providers because the management of aggressive and self-injurious behavior is a common concern.

Carmen Berrios and William Jacobowitz (1998) sought a solution to the use of restraints and seclusion for mentally ill children who were in danger of harming themselves. The positive results obtained from the pilot study on therapeutic holding led to the implementation of therapeutic holds as an initial standards modality or managing aggressive pediatric patients. Reading the article provides enough detail for most nurses to follow the directions and safely employ the techniques. The article uses clear diagrams and indicates those patients who benefit and those who should be excluded.

Patient and outcome measure selection are other ways that psychiatric nurses can be involved in the research process. Nursing research provides the tools necessary to collect data, monitor progress, and evaluate success or need for improvement to obtain positive outcomes. Basic statistics and nursing research techniques taught at the baccalaureate level provide many of the skills required for CQI and PI tasks. Nursing's contribution through research is discussed later in this chapter.

W*hat do you think?* In what CQI and PI tasks have you observed nurses participating?

► *Check Your Reading*
12. List three benefits of team involvement in CQI.
13. Differentiate a goal from an outcome in CQI.
14. Define OASIS.

Statistical Analysis and Display of Data

Because externally reported measures of quality health care are intended to inform or lead to action, proposers of such measures have a responsibility to ensure that the results of the measures are meaningful, scientifically sound, and interpretable. (McGlynn, 1998, p. 470)

Statistical analysis is designed to measure the identified variables. Outcomes historically measured death, disability, dissatisfaction, illness, and pain (Lohr, 1988). Recently, measures called *health-related quality of life* added the patient's perceived dimensions of physical, social, and role functioning, mental health, and overall health perceptions to the clinical assessments (Mitchell, Ferketich, Jennings, & American Academy of Nursing Experts Panel on Quality Care, 1998). Client satisfaction continues as part of quality improvement when used as one outcome variable measured by managed mental health care organizations (Ingram & Chung, 1997).

In recognition that some variation in quality is inevitable, Shewhart proposed that it is necessary to be able to determine when variation is significant (cited in Juran, 1988). CQI is the process of minimizing variation and increasing conformance to standards. To assess and evaluate the data collected in the monitoring and evaluation process, team members must have a basic understanding of statistical concepts, such as sampling techniques, validity, reliability, sensitivity, the nature of variables, frequency distributions, and standard deviation. It is also important to become familiar with some of the types of graphic displays used to communicate results. These include pie charts, bar charts, histograms, scatter diagrams, cumulative frequency curves, and frequency distributions.

Outcome measurement uses a rating scale for documenting patient status. A score of 0 is the most optimistic: the higher the number, the lower the person's function. Nurses have published research using outcomes assessed by rating scales (Forbes, 1998; Resnick, 1998a; Rockwood, Stolee, Howard, & Mallery, 1996). Nurses who employ the scale need training to establish inter-rater reliability. The large OASIS sample showstest-retest reliability, the stability of the instrument over repeated administrations (Polit & Hungler, 1995).

Benchmarking Performance

Another feature of quality management is **benchmark- ing.** A benchmark is defined as a standard or reference by which others can be measured or judged. Purchasers and consumers of behavioral health services lack sufficient information to make informed selections among health plans and providers. Benchmarking allows comparison across health plans and providers based on their quality and performance outcomes. Currently, cost seems to be the only easily obtainable information. Many other factors are equally important, including professional training and expertise of staff, ease of access into the system, provision of most appropriate provider, and type of treatment. The danger for consumers without this information is that cost alone may be used in selecting these important services.

Behavioral health care organizations started collaboratively collecting data in an organized way to document the degree to which their services are effective. Using benchmark data from each other allows the development of accountable reports that can be used for marketing, quality improvement, and political action. (Kramer & Trabin, 1997). Members agree to use the same methods for data collection and analysis and abide by the agreed principles of confidentiality and data privacy.

This benchmarking activity produces a report card for similar types of behavioral health care organizations. These report cards can show an organization to be excellent, fair, or in need of improvement. The risks and costs are great. Areas most often measured include access to care, appropriateness of care, quality of care, patient clinical and functional outcomes achieved, prevention services, and, for some, patient and customer satisfaction.

In 1997, there were four national behavioral benchmarking studies in process. The American Managed Behavioral Healthcare Association studied 20 indicators in a sample selected to measure the areas listed earlier for mental health and substance abuse treatment coverage for approximately 100 million people. The National Committee for Quality Assurance accredits health maintenance organizations (HMOs). Their Health Employment Data Information Set (HEDIS) includes indicators for managed behavioral health care. Consumer satisfaction with managed care for publicly funded programs is the major focus of the Mental Health Statistics Improvement Program. In 1998, NAMI **surveyed** managed care organizations and consumers to determine best practices for consumer satisfaction and concluded that most of the managed care organizations were seriously deficient in the provision of psychiatric care (Hall & Beineke, 1998).

In health care, management can use the principles of benchmarking to compare their organization to similar health care organizations, focusing on such outcomes as cost, length of stay, mortality rates, readmission rates, and patient satisfaction. Benchmarking documented psychiatric nurses' greater risk of occupational injury (Love & Hunter, 1996); the diagnoses and frequency of home mental health care (Ohlund, 1997); the role of nurses in primary mental health and advanced practice psychiatric nursing (SERPN, 1997), and demographic and psychosocial characteristics of patients receiving psychiatric home care as well as outcomes on health status, self-care knowledge, and self-care skill in a sample of more than 700 patients (Carson, Alonzo, & Alva, in press).

> Using benchmarking in Barbara's case would help to review successful treatment modalities used in other similar facilities. The CQI leader might look at how leading competitors handle recidivism in noncompliant patients. ■

In March 1998, JCAHO adopted the nationwide benchmarking process whimsically titled ORYX. This initiative was designed as a way for acute care hospitals to provide opportunities for benchmarking and for performance comparisons by participating groups. Participants collect and submit data about 32 performance measures. Once the data is standardized, JCAHO will publicly release the data. After January 1, 2000, failure to meet the ORYX requirements will result in an automatic special recommendation, which would affect the agency's accreditation status. The deficient area must be addressed and an acceptable report written and submitted to resolve the deficiency. The Joint Commission believes that such a system will, in the long run, save more money than it costs. "Ultimately, in the increasingly competitive health care market, only those companies that can quantitatively prove they are efficient in providing excellent service and outcomes at low cost will survive," according to JCAHO's associate director of home care accreditation for the western region, Darryl Rich, PharmD (Kaplan, 1998, p. 21). The OASIS Medicare program is a set of performance measures and not a performance measurement system like ORYX. Many agencies are incorporating both requirements in the selection of a performance measurement system. As of October 26, 1998, there were 68 approved home care systems, including Behavioral Pathway Systems and Mental Health Outcomes Management System. A complete list is available from JCAHO's Website (available at oryx@jcaho.org).

Clinical Indicators

Standards are integrated with aspects of care by using indicators. JCAHO defined a **clinical indicator** as a quantitative measure that can be used to monitor and evaluate the quality of important aspects of care and practice (JCAHO, 1995). Indicators serve as screens that identify or direct attention to specific performance issues that require more intense review (Box 38–4).

Box 38-4 ■ ■ ■ ■ ■
Guidelines for Developing Quality Indicators

For each indicator, it is necessary to
- Define all terms that may be ambiguous or require clarification for collection purposes.
- Indicate whether it is a sentinel event or a rate-based indicator. All sentinel events require further investigation, but rate-based indicators require further assessment only if the occurrence rate shows a significant trend, exceeds predetermined thresholds, or differs substantially from benchmarks. Examples of sentinel events in psychiatry are patient self-injury, suicide, or use of seclusion or restraints. Some rate-based indicators are against medical advice, elopements, and transfers to medicine.
- State whether the indicator addresses a process or an outcome of care or service.
- Provide rationale for the use of the indicator.
- Provide a description of indicator population.
- List the specific data elements that will be collected.
- Describe underlying factors that may influence the indicator's rate or activity.
- Reference the indicator to existing databases.

To prepare for ORYX, the Maryland Hospital Association (MHA) is conducting a quality indicator project assessing psychiatric care indicators. One important aspect of care identified in psychiatry is the use of special treatment procedures such as seclusion. The standard is that designated special treatment procedures require clinical justification. Using standards of care and standards of practice, indicators for the use of seclusion can be developed. Box 38-5 lists data elements to examine for this indicator. By collecting data about all occurrences of seclusion, it is then possible to determine if all the applicable standards of care and practice are being maintained. Every hospital participating in the MHA indicator study trained their behavioral health staff members to use an established data collection protocol. MHA is providing regular reports to all participating hospitals on the incidence of the indicator's use with all the patients in the study thus allowing each hospital to benchmark their rates of seclusion to the rates in comparable facilities.

The process of selecting and measuring indicators is not easy. Staff members must be actively involved and educated to the process. Precision is critical to accuracy. MHA is attempting to control all these variables in their QI project. The study is designed to help providers of mental health and substance abuse services provide clients and payers with program and outcome evaluation.

Extensive written materials and multiple training sessions prepared the participants for the task of documenting the care to collect the outcome measurement data. To assure quality and acceptable submission of reports, the MHA regularly tests the participants with

situations to be analyzed and rated. Feedback and correct answers are provided. A typical scenario might ask whether a patient should be included or excluded by age or length of stay and whether or not talking a patient into taking medication constitutes the use of involuntary restraint. For adolescents, nurses are expected to differentiate between a time out and use of seclusion using the duration of the intervention as the differentiating factor. According to Nell Wood, the Director of the QI project,

The project has an unofficial motto: "It's not the data, it's what you do with it." Data by itself is powerless. But sharing that data and the comparative data that go along with it on a regular basis with leadership, department managers, and clinicians facilitates a better understanding of the agency's performance and the "why" behind that performance. That's when it becomes a truly powerful tool. (personal communication, January 13, 1999)

What do you think? Is benchmarking data used by most consumers to make health care decisions?

➤ *Check Your Reading*
15. Define benchmarking.
16. Explain the consequences of not meeting the ORYX requirement.
17. List three psychiatric indicators.

Box 38-5 ■ ■ ■ ■ ■
Possible Data Elements for Seclusion as a Clinical Indicator

- Rationale for using seclusion is clearly stated in the record.
- Seclusion was used to prevent patient from injuring self or others or to prevent serious disruption to the therapeutic environment.
- Rationale for using seclusion addresses the inadequacy of less restrictive techniques.
- There is a written order for restraint or seclusion that is time-limited and does not exceed 24 hours.
- Clinical assessment of the patient before and during the period of seclusion is documented in the record.
- Physician's oral order is obtained within 1 hour if seclusion is implemented on an emergency basis by nursing staff members.
- As needed orders are not used to authorize the use of seclusion.
- Patient is observed at least every 15 minutes, and observations of behavior are documented in the record.
- Door to the seclusion room is opened at least once an hour, and the patient is checked and offered use of the toilet.

ROLE OF NURSING IN THE CONTINUOUS QUALITY IMPROVEMENT PROCESS

The primary role of nursing in the CQI process is to help provide an environment that facilitates it. Successful CQI depends on managerial participation, a collective responsibility approach, flexible objectives, and continuous improvement (McLaughlin & Kaluzny, 1990).

Nursing practice must concentrate less on individual development and responsibility and more on collective development and responsibility. Nurses must look at practice as it fits within specific processes and understand how nursing processes affect patient care delivery and the quality of care provided by the system. CQI concentrates on changing the system so that the conditions likely to result in problems are less likely to occur. This process treats the root cause of the problem rather than a symptom. Nursing, as an integral part of the hospital, must develop a culture and environment conducive to developing CQI programs that fit these standards. The JCAHO revised standards are based on the concepts shown in Box 38-6. For nursing, a new culture requires the following processes:

- Strategic planning
- Collaborative practice
- Identification of important aspects of care
- Indicators and standards of excellence through performance

Planning and Collaboration

In strategic planning, nursing executive leadership becomes instrumental in the success or a nursing CQI process. The first step involves ensuring that all CQI initiatives are based on the organization's strategic plan, mission, goals and objectives, and philosophy (Figure 38-2). The nursing administration commitment to the CQI process must reflect

- A pursuit toward meeting the nursing quality goal.
- Demonstrated commitment to CQI principles.
- A rigorous training program for all employees.
- An environment conducive to teamwork, creativity, and risk-taking.

The second process for creating a nursing CQI program is **collaborative practice.** Here, all involved in a specific process work together as a multifunctional team to improve the quality of care provided the patient. Collaboration could potentially include housekeeping, dietary, radiology, medicine, nursing, and other functions. As indicated by the potential composition of a team, team members need not be from the clinical arena only. Collaboration is understood to imply that the individuals share a common goal and desire to affect the situation at hand positively. Without collaboration, traditional boundaries and barriers are not successfully overcome, and the ability to study processes and systems diminishes.

Collaboration has been shown to improve patient care and enhance patient outcomes. Yet despite its known value, collaboration remains difficult to promote among health care providers. Some resist its integration into their practices, thinking that it is "easier to do it myself." Still, CQI can be achieved only through successful collaboration. The trend of integrating health care systems in the mid- to late 1990s created more than 300 groups (Coile, 1997). It is difficult for large organizations to develop and implement QI projects in which there are multiple hospitals and staffs. A system-level team consisting of professionals with expertise on the subject to be improved and QI process experts have been effective in determining outcomes to improve and in identifying the processes likely to produce improvements.

Collaboration has not been the traditional method of communicating patient care needs between nurses and physicians. Physicians have traditionally assumed the power in any decision-making process regarding patient care and patient outcomes. Successful collaboration depends on mutual respect. All team members must be

Box 38-6 ■ ■ ■ ■ ■

Joint Commission on the Accreditation of Healthcare Organizations Revised Standards Concepts

- A hospital can improve patient care quality—that is, increase the probability of desired outcomes, including patient satisfaction, by assessing and improving those governance, managerial, clinical, and support processes that most affect patient outcomes.
- Some of these processes are carried out by medical, nursing, and other clinicians; some by governing body members; some by managers; and some by support personnel. Some are carried out jointly by more than one of these groups.
- Whether carried out by one or more groups, the processes must be coordinated and integrated. Coordination and integration require the attention of the managerial and clinical leaders of the hospital.
- Most governance, managerial, medical, nursing, and other clinical and support staff members are both motivated and competent to carry out the process well. Therefore, the opportunities to improve the process—and thus improve patient outcomes—are much more frequent than are mistakes and errors. Consequently, without shirking its responsibility to address serious problems involving deficits in knowledge or skills, the hospital's principal goal should be to help everyone improve the process in which he or she is involved.

Data from Joint Commission on Accreditation of Healthcare Organizations. (1995). *1995 accreditation manual for healthcare.* Oakbrook Terrace, IL: JCAHO.

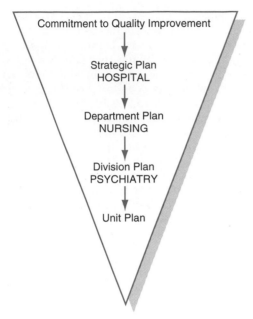

Figure 38–2
The flow of quality improvement, from commitment to unit plan.

clear about their professional focus and contribute to the group process. Members must be willing to collaborate and accept the group's decisions. Group process is not always easy and some conflict is expected (Megel, Elrod, & Rausch, 1996).

Nurse as Clinician

The journey of health care in the future will be collaborative, with patient and professional travelers embarking on a jointly traveled interdisciplinary path. Collaborative models of care make the patient a partner in the treatment process. Instead of viewing the individual components of health care delivery separately, collaborative models use an integrated approach to identify critical treatment outcomes and determine the treatment process required to meet those outcomes. Key to a collaborative model is the organization, coordination, and integration of all health-related activities into a comprehensive, holistic treatment approach.

Other hospital departments affect both the cost of services provided and the quality of the patient's journey. The availability of medical records can facilitate emergency services, admission procedures, and greater integration and coordination of services among different levels of care. Delays in obtaining laboratory results or consultations can result in longer patient stays with increased costs. If the physician prescribes medications not included on the pharmacy formulary, there may be delays in obtaining the medication or the physician may need to substitute other, less effective medications. Scheduling problems in ambulatory services can prevent patients from following through with outpatient care and cause patient dissatisfaction. Billing problems can mean delays in payment for the hospital services and

generate patient complaints. The lack of transportation, food, and medication in the home can quickly lead to rehospitalization. Resolution of these kinds of problems requires problem-solving teams with members from all departments and services including community-based providers who can provide in-home assessments and supervision.

To facilitate the journey, interdisciplinary health care teams make the necessary "travel arrangements." Written interdisciplinary clinical care plans, referred to as critical pathways, clinical decision-making trees, or care mapping directs travelers toward the desired destination and documents their progress. As health care accountability becomes more and more of an issue, interdisciplinary case management of symptoms and integrated reporting mechanisms are likely to replace discipline-specific treatment protocols and reporting measures. Research findings need to be replicated and put into practice to make them relevant. Clinical nurses incorporate the findings and give feedback to the researchers on their own success with the proposed methods. The more times an intervention is successful, the greater the value to the patient and the credibility of the nursing profession.

Role of Case Management in Collaborative Models

Psychiatric nurses have a unique opportunity to develop their role as case manager into a "power position" in the health care system. The case manager operates from a position of power because he or she is able to negotiate cross-professional goals that are directly linked to how dollars are spent. Case management paradigms support a collaborative interdisciplinary health care model with a "new" emphasis on "care and doing *with* the person rather than cure and doing *to* the person" (Phillips, 1995, p. 4). Case management legitimizes the nurse's caring role in psychiatric nursing, prompting greater ownership of the caring that nurses have always provided patients. Shared responsibility in health care decision-making will make outcome research and the development of interdisciplinary collaborative models a prominent feature of mental health care as we move into the future.

> **W**hat do you think? Look at the practice patterns in the facility where you are assigned. Is there evidence of collaborative practice? If so, what impact does such practice have on patient outcomes? If there is no evidence of collaboration, what impact does this lack have on patient outcomes? Should nursing students be involved in a collaborative approach?

► *Check Your Reading*
18. What do we mean by collaborative models of health care delivery?

19. How do critical pathways enhance and support the design and goals of collaborative models?
20. In what way does case management support collaborative health care?

Diagnosis-Specific Criteria and Critical Pathways

Critical pathways, or **clinical pathways,** are diagnosis-specific or procedure-specific guidelines for the management and treatment of patients. For each diagnosis, expectations of types of services and timeliness of services are being developed. The guidelines identify key functions and services needed and time frames for these activities. For example, a critical path for a diagnosis of bipolar disorder, mixed state, would establish for each day of hospitalization the services and activities expected to take place.

Critical Pathways

The focus on outcomes led health care providers to search out a process for monitoring and tracking patient care to determine them. Critical pathways, clinical pathways, and clinical practice guidelines are all similar. "A clinical pathway is a proactive multidisciplinary set of daily prescriptions and outcomes for the care of a specified patient population from preadmission to postdischarge" (Graybeal, 1993, p. 42). The terms *pathway* and *map* describes how the tool provides a visual display of the patient's treatment and response to care. The pathway is a diagram of the care from the beginning of treatment until discharge.

There are many benefits to using critical pathways to direct mental health care. The care of the patient remains goal- and outcome-focused. Each step of the care is preplanned to follow a logical progression. Multiple care providers can follow the guidelines and achieve desired outcomes. The pathways eliminate redundancy and help staff remain focused on the expected outcomes timeline. Critical pathways include guidelines for documentation that assist with staff orientation and decrease unnecessary documentation. The care is based on standards that are evident to all providers. The tool evaluates the actual care according to the standard. Patient and family education are built in components of clinical practice guidelines. Differences or variations among patients and providers can be used to determine the best practices or areas for improvement (Mark & Garet, 1997).

Each critical pathway represents a detailed written care plan for all levels of patient care related to a particular medical diagnosis. It identifies every aspect of the patient's care and defines who is accountable for the care, when the care will be delivered, and how. The plan includes the coordination of all patient activities. It specifies time estimates for procedures, tests, and treatment completion. Patient activities are ordered sequentially, and the plan identifies potential problems that might arise. This information becomes a part of a flow chart that provides a graphic representation of the interdisciplinary health care prescribed for the patient. Figure 38-3 provides a sample critical pathway.

The development and use of critical pathways to plan and organize patient care have several advantages. First, the method, when properly implemented, promotes a more coordinated approach to health care delivery and results in reduced hospital and patient costs. Collaboration about the disorder and choices about intervention lead to greater consistency of approach among diverse practitioners. Developing the critical pathway forces various disciplines to discuss their differences and their overlaps in function. The result is an expedient care plan that all disciplines own and agree to implement. Outcome data are essential at the beginning of a clinical pathway study; as modifications are made, outcome data provide the evidence of success or areas to improve. Symptom reduction in behavioral health care is listed as one of the elements of the ORYX initiative's performance measurement system. Diseases such as schizophrenia and bipolar illness can be tracked for symptom improvement with the use of clinical pathways (Mark & Garet, 1997).

Some mental health nurses believe critical pathways, care maps, and clinical decision-making trees depersonalize the care they give. They complain that there is little time to address other needs. Nurses need to recognize the tremendous opportunity for collaboration these clinical practice guidelines provide. Opportunities exist for nurses to quantitatively prove the benefits of the care we provide and win greater respect from all members of the health care team. As health care professionals, nurses share in the responsibility of "doing the right things rights" (Gray, 1997, p. 20). The guidelines do not replace the clinical judgment of the nurse; however, they do provide valuable information for making informed clinical decisions. The mental health nurse of the future has an important role in on-going evaluation and refinement of these clinical guidelines to ensure they remain appropriate for our patient care (Bailey, Litaker, & Mion, 1998).

> **W***hat do you think?* Follow a critical pathway when providing care for a mentally ill patient. Identify the pros and cons of using the tools from your personal experience.

> ➤ *Check Your Reading*
> 21. What role do standards of practice play in a CQI model?

PATIENT SATISFACTION COMPARED WITH PATIENT NEEDS

The transition from traditional QA to CQI made including the patient in care a necessity rather than an option. Patients are no longer willing to accept the services provided them without question; instead, patients are demanding quality care provided in a

THE UNION MEMORIAL HOSPITAL
NURSING SERVICE DEPARTMENT
INITIATION OF INPATIENT LITHIUM
PLAN OF CARE

EXPECTED LOS _____ DAYS
(LOS DEPENDENT ON DIAGNOSIS)
DATE POC REVIEWED BY MD _____

DATE	DAY 1	DAY 2	DAY 3	DAY 4	DAY 5	DAY 6	DAY 7	DAY 8
CONSULTS	Med consult if indicated. Consider diet consult.							
TESTS	Thyroid function test, BUN, serum creatinine (or within 7 days pre-admission). Baseline pregnancy test if indicated. Consider 24-hr urine for creatine clearance		Lithium level (± q2–3 days)	Check lithium results				
ACTIVITY	Dependent on condition.							
TREATMENTS	Baseline vital signs, weight, I&O. Assess for lithium toxicity (nausea, vomiting, diarrhea, tremors, muscle twitching, edema) & therapeutic effects qd.							
MEDS	Lithium (dose per MD order).		Reevaluate for ↑ + q3 days.					
DIET	Maintain pre-hospital diet unless contraindicated. Maintain adequate fluid intake (min. 32 oz/day).							

				On discharge: Follow-up evaluation discharge plan
DISCHARGE PLANNING	Assess for compliance/discharge needs/referrals.	Initiate/implement discharge plan. Refer to PHP, OPD, HHC, NBC if indicated.		
TEACHING	Baseline med. teaching	Offer lithium teaching booklet. Refer to med/illness teaching group.	Reinforce med/illness teaching qd (reason, dosage, time, side effects). Teach warning signs of illness qd. Teach expected results of med qd (mild transient edema, increased urination).	

ADMISSION DATE ____   DAYS IN ROUTINE BED ____   DISCHARGE DATE ____   DAYS IN ICU ____

Figure 38-3
An example of a clinical pathway. (Courtesy of The Union Memorial Hospital, Baltimore, MD.)

cost-effective manner. Patient satisfaction is directly proportional to the organization's ability to meet his or her needs, wants, and desires.

Patient satisfaction traditionally focused on the patient's assessment of services provided. In the past, however, health care organizations frequently developed patient care service goals without ever asking patients what was important to them. Today, health care organizations have changed this approach to focus on patient involvement, as dictated by the philosophy of CQI. Patient-provider interactions now play an important part in the patient's perception of the services. Patient dissatisfaction encourages him or her to seek the same services from another provider. Perception is important because the patient's perception of having needs, wants, and desires met results in satisfaction.

The patient's perception in the actual production process is paramount in most health care services. The patient must participate in the delivery of care, cooperating with even the most painful of procedures. (Wilson, 1991, p. 11)

The process of assessing patient's needs, wants, and desires and incorporating them into the organization's QI plan depend on several components, according to Black (1992, p. 320):

- A commitment to addressing patient satisfaction issues at all levels of the organization
- Monitoring and analyzing trends of patient complaints
- Incorporating patient satisfaction and dissatisfaction as components of the QI program
- Developing and continually maintaining a "guest relations" type program
- Actively soliciting patient opinions and perceptions

Organizational Commitment

Organizational commitment to patient satisfaction must be reflected in the organization's strategic plan and operationalized throughout the organization at all levels. The nursing division's QI plan must include a commitment to meeting the needs, wants, and desires of its patients.

Monitoring and Analyzing Trends

Monitoring patient complaints is paramount in the process of continuously improving patient care. The level of patient satisfaction is frequently reflected in the complaints voiced by the patient or the patient's family. This monitoring device has become so important that many regulatory and licensing agencies have enacted legal requirements that an individual be specifically identified and dedicated to this function in both psychiatry and medicine. Analyzing trends in patients' complaints allows for changes in the systems that will be responsive to meeting patient needs and improving patient satisfaction.

Focus on Satisfaction and Dissatisfaction

The QI model implies an organization should look at both: "It is just as important to look at patient satisfaction as at patient dissatisfaction" (Black, 1992, p. 321). Survey research has been used to determine patient satisfaction with clinical nurse specialists in psychiatric-mental health nursing (Baradell, 1995). The study found that the more clinical improvements the patient reported, the more satisfied they were with the care provided. This information is valuable in planning patient satisfaction queries and patient care. When nurses at admission begin care with a needs assessment and mutual goal planning, the patient is actively involved and can measure progress. Providing the patient with positive feedback describing gains leads to satisfaction.

Patient satisfaction and dissatisfaction have far-reaching effects. State regulators use these measures when interviewing patients before accrediting agencies for Medicare-reimbursed care. All Medicare patients in home care must be educated about how to report problems or complaints both directly to the agency and to the state, if a satisfactory resolution is not attained. Published satisfaction survey results of hospitals, HMOs, doctors, and other health care agencies influence the patient customer base. Good results are widely advertised; conversely, those committed to QI quickly address patient dissatisfaction. Written patient satisfaction feedback, for example, a thank-you note, may be required for salary increases. Management's constructive feedback to nurses on their performance promotes pride and a positive sense of self that is critical for job satisfaction in psychiatric nursing. This is especially important for nurses caring for chronically mentally ill patients who may have little capacity to thank the nurse themselves. All praise, letters, telephone calls, and so forth, should be shared with the individual nurse. Good results should be cause for celebration. Many agencies have bulletin boards with letters and patient comments posted for all to see. Having comment cards and pens available increases the likelihood of receiving feedback.

Satisfaction measurement is universal in health care settings committed to CQI. All departments of the agency, from dietary to finance, have customers. Patient satisfaction measures need to include all areas, not just the nursing care. These departments should also evaluate how they get along with the other areas of the institution. Employee satisfaction with the agency and management needs to be conducted regularly with the results publicized and discussed and improvements planned and completed based on the feedback. Patient satisfaction is an on-going measure of CQI. The survey instrument is a good example of the use of combined research methods.

Guest Relations

The business industry incorporated the concept of guest relations many years ago and found it to be effective in increasing customer satisfaction. Health care is now beginning to incorporate guest relations in its strategic plan. The guest relations concept can be operationalized, for instance, in a "patient-first" program. Patient-first programs usually emphasize behaviors such as caring and compassion, courtesy, respect, dignity, and "the patient is always right." This area has become so important that organizations are incorporating the concept into job descriptions and performance standards.

Guest relations programs are important because patients frequently use the "halo effect" when rating hospital services; for example, the nurse is not caring and compassionate; therefore, the hospital is not caring and compassionate. Because this effect happens all too frequently, employees must be aware of guest relations.

Patient Feedback

Health care providers have traditionally failed to place enough emphasis on the impact of patients' perceptions on their level of satisfaction. Therefore, organizations have been remiss in developing effective patient feedback systems. Feedback systems are essential if organizations are to develop services responsive to patient needs. Feedback systems allow an organization to

- Determine what is important to the patient.
- Determine if the organization is meeting patient needs.
- Determine how to improve services presently provided.
- Communicate to the patient, and say "thanks" for the feedback.

Many methods have been used to assess patient satisfaction and obtain patient feedback in general. These include suggestion boxes, patient surveys such as Gallup polls, informal interviews by senior management, and interviews at the time of discharge. Organizations have employed people to filter complaints as well as feedback. In some organizations, these individuals are referred to as patient representatives and in others as patient advocates. The titles are not important, but their roles are.

Patients' Rights

One of the most important rights that any individual has is the right to receive quality medical care regardless of race, creed, nationality, economic status, or illness. Unfortunately, obtaining this right has been a long struggle for many. To ensure that all individuals are treated ethically in relation to the majority, civil laws have been enacted to further ensure that the rights of all individuals are protected.

Although the concept of health care rights has always been somewhat controversial, this is even truer in mental health care. In recent years, special attention has been focused on the rights of the mentally ill. Many federal, state, local, professional, and health regulatory agencies and organizations have enacted laws and standards that help ensure that the rights of the mentally ill are upheld (Box 38-7). In 1973, the American Hospital Association issued a patients' bill of rights, which has been used in many hospitals throughout the United States. In 1980, Congress passed the Mental Health Systems Act (MHSA), which created rights for the mentally ill. In 1983, JCAHO developed policy statements on the rights of the mentally ill. The importance of patients' rights and the protection of those rights are also found in the *Code for Nurses With Interpretive Statements* (ANA, 1985). This code explicitly defines your professional responsibility to ensure and uphold these rights (see Chapter 5).

JCAHO dedicated an entire section of the *1995 Accreditation Manual for Healthcare* (1995) to patient rights. This section of the manual stresses that organizational policies and procedures must describe the mechanisms by which the patient's rights are protected and exercised. Box 38-8 lists patient rights.

Local organizations such as community mental health centers (CMHCs), in conjunction with federal and state agencies, have developed standards that ensure that the rights of mentally ill patients are not violated. These organizations have become the gatekeepers, ensuring quality health care. Their mission is to develop standards that ensure the mentally ill have access not only to health care but also to "quality" health care and to develop a mechanism by which to address their concerns without repercussions.

Any QI program developed in psychiatry, like other disciplines, must take into account the rights of the mentally ill patient, especially the right to quality care. Involving the patient in care and assessing the needs, wants, and desires of the patient are important in implementing a process that ensures these needs will be met.

Box 38-7 ■ ■ ■ ■ ■
Laws and Standards Upholding Patients' Rights

1973	The American Hospital Association issued a patients' bill of rights.
1976	The American Nurses Association defined the nurse's professional responsibility to ensure and uphold patients' rights in the *Code for Nurses*.
1980	Congress passed the Mental Health Systems Act, which mandated rights for the mentally ill.
1983	Joint Commission on the Accreditation of Healthcare Organizations developed policy statements on the rights of the mentally ill.

Box 38-8 ■ ■ ■ ■ ■
Joint Commission on the Accreditation of Healthcare Organizations
Patients' Rights

- The right of the patient to the hospital's reasonable response to his or her request and needs for treatment or services, within the hospital's capacity, its stated mission, and applicable law and regulations
- The right of the patient to considerate and respectful care
- The right of the patient, in collaboration with his or her physician, to make decisions involving his or her health care
- The right of the patient to information at the time of admission about the hospital's mechanism for the initiation, review, and, when possible, resolution of patient complaints concerning the quality of care
- The right of the patient to the information necessary to enable him or her to make treatment decisions that reflect his or her wishes

Data from Joint Commission of Healthcare Organizations. (1995). *1995 accreditation manual for healthcare.* Oakbrook Terrace, IL: JCAHO.

W*hat do you think?* Why is it important to have formal statements of patients' rights?

➤ *Check Your Reading*
22. Why is patient involvement a necessity in a CQI model?
23. Give one reason why it is important to monitor and analyze trends in patient complaints.
24. Give two reasons why patient feedback systems are important.
25. What is the most important right that any patient has?

CREATING SOLUTIONS

Nursing leaders such as Peplau, Paterson, Zdrad, and Parse developed conceptual models and nursing theory relevant to psychiatric nursing practice. Other theoretical insights are drawn from the social and biological sciences. But we must be willing to explore new frontiers of knowledge and skill in collaborating with other health professionals and health care consumers. Peplau argued that "The 21st century is quite likely to be the century of the professional nurse" (cited in Huch, 1995, p. 40). This will only be true if nurses take advantage of the opportunities offered by changes in the health care delivery system.

Why is research so important to nursing? The printed word (books and journals) provides access to new knowledge, which in turn is the first step in the process of transforming practice.

If psychiatric nurses wish to be recognized for what they do, they must validate their contributions through solid contributions to the body of nursing research. Nurses must design, implement, and evaluate patient care studies that demonstrate the effectiveness of their interventions. Without a research base that psychiatric nurses can claim as their own, the voices of those closest to the patient remain unheard. Without a clear and united voice as professionals, nurses cannot hope to be recognized as peers in health care. Research that integrates ideas from different disciplines can help advance models that will make a difference in health care delivery in a time of tightened resources.

Research findings and generalizations are important for making critical clinical judgments and affecting policy decisions. It is not the findings of a single study or even a body of related studies that directly affect policy. Rather, it is the concepts and theoretical perspectives developed through social science research that permeate every aspect of policy-making. As a body of knowledge emerges, it accumulates and combines with data derived from other sources to define and redefine issues. Solid research acts as a supportive rationale for recommending certain policies over others. In doing research, the nurse may assume the combined role of researcher, teacher, and advocate in developing interdisciplinary health care policies that directly and indirectly affect nursing care.

Nurse as Researcher

Every practicing nurse has a part to play in nursing research, whether as an investigator, a user of the outcomes, a data collector, or someone identifying problem areas requiring research. Although nurses generally obtain advanced graduate education to develop an appropriate research design and conduct a relevant data analysis, the process of performance improvement transforms all staff members into researchers through on-going participation in the process. The search for quality supports clinical research experimentation and application. Collaboration between and among health care staff members, inpatient, outpatient, and community settings, academia, and business is commonplace. Government and private funding sources now look for such partnerships as criteria for awarding grant money for research. Specific populations are also targeted for study. For 1999, the National Institute of Mental Health (NIMH) priority groups (www.nimh.nih.gov) included

- Alcohol and drug abuse
- Schizophrenia
- Chronic mentally ill homeless
- Demonstration projects for least restrictive environments for institutionalized mentally ill patients

Psychiatric nursing organizations seek practice-based content for presentations at their conferences. Psychiatric and other nursing and health care journals are publishing articles and sections about research that works and similar topics. Good research studies have relevance, a practical focus that permits them to be realistically implemented, and writing that is clear but not overly technical.

Funding for research continues to be a limiting force to knowledge expansion. Designing, implementing, evaluating, and disseminating the results of research is expensive and time-consuming. In clinical practice situations in which research is carried out, the nurse most often is involved as a data collector or as the one who performs the research protocol under the direction of the principal investigator. Therefore, although not the initiator of research, the nurse is essential in ensuring that the data are accurate and the study is valid. If for any reason, data are inaccurately measured or not recorded properly, a specimen is lost, or a part of the protocol is missed, the mistake needs to be honestly and quickly reported so that the error can be incorporated in the analysis. Otherwise, the validity of the study stands in jeopardy.

Staff nurses also may play a primary role in identifying research questions. The clinically based nurse who works with the mentally ill on a daily basis probably has more opportunity to identify questions related to patient care than do researchers, who traditionally work in nonclinical settings. That nurse is constantly asking about the significance of a patient behavior, the best response in a particular situation, or the basis for using one treatment approach rather than another. Any of these reflections may yield productive research questions that could have a significant impact on the diagnosis and treatment of psychiatric symptoms.

The staff nurse also facilitates others' research. The nurse can act as a role model for others in the carefulness and seriousness with which data collection is approached. Nurses sometimes have opportunities in their own institutions and at external research conferences to attend meetings at which the results of research are reported. These conferences offer the chance to participate in discussions about the implementation of research findings and, most valuable of all, to work with members of other disciplines caring for the mentally ill. Psychiatry is more advanced than any other discipline in understanding that its subject matter is interdisciplinary and that most of the work done in the psychiatric setting can be accomplished by a variety of specially trained health professionals.

By taking a more active role in the research process, the nurse can assume responsibility for enhancing research protocols. An energetic investment in research carries with it not only a better understanding of mental illness and how its deviations twist and torture many lives but also the responsibility to search vigorously for the answers that will allow us to diminish suffering. By valuing the research process and participating in that process, we can offer other travelers the possibility of fuller and happier lives.

Associated Legal and Ethical Responsibilities

In addition to assuming greater responsibility for the actual conduct of research, nurses often need to be advocates and teachers in implementing their legal and ethical responsibilities in the research process. As the person most often present in the patient's therapeutic environment, the nurse plays an important role in protecting the patient's right to self-determination in matters of informational privacy, informed consent, and truth-telling. Managing this role becomes a truly awesome responsibility when a patient lacks the cognitive ability to understand fully the nature of consent.

Informational Privacy

Informational privacy is a term describing a person's right to have full control over any personal information used in research studies. Scanlon and Fibison (1995) identified the key elements associated with informational privacy, which are listed in Box 38-9. Nurses have an added obligation to make sure that mentally ill patients' right to informational privacy is honored. Patients frequently are neither aware of potential difficulties nor able to act fully on their own behalf. The nurse must ensure that

- The patient understands the type of information sought and agrees to it.
- The patient is given the opportunity to correct errors in the data.
- The data are reported on a group rather than on an individual basis.
- Nothing of a personal nature that could result in harm to or discrimination against a patient is disclosed.

Issues regarding storage of information, access to it or to the patient by people other than the investigator, and procedures for ensuring the anonymity also need to receive attention. Having well-defined policies and

---

B o x 3 8 – 9 ■ ■ ■ ■ ■
Key Elements of Informational Privacy

- Only relevant personal information should be collected.
- Rationale for collecting the information should exist.
- Informed consent must be obtained before disclosure of information to others.
- Information gathered for one purpose should not be used for another purpose without informed consent from the patient.

From Scanlon, C., & Fibison, W. (1995). *Managing genetic information: Implications for nursing practice.* Washington, DC: American Nurses Association.

procedures for protecting the patient's right to informational privacy helps prevent inopportune disclosure.

The attempt to collect beginning data on millions of home health care patients for OASIS by HCFA was halted on March 23, 1999, after concerns about informational privacy came to light. The OASIS data collection included questions about mental state and psychiatric symptoms, their frequency, and their severity. Janlon Goldman, director of the Health Privacy Project at Georgetown University, called for a delay of the project until privacy issues have been resolved. "Unfortunately, the applicable law here—the Privacy Act of 1974—extends very little assurance that the collected identifiable data will be handled confidently and securely" (cited in O'Harrow, 1999, p. A5).

Informed Consent

Informed consent is another legal and ethical concern with mentally ill patients. Although health care providers in all research settings are charged with full disclosure of facts and potential risks of engaging in the study before a patient signs the consent form, the decision-making abilities of the mentally ill often are not fully intact. Consequently, the nurse may need to carefully consider the words used to convey the information needed for informed consent so that the patient readily and completely understands. Often, more than one session is needed. In the case of an incompetent patient, the person acting on the patient's behalf or designated as the patient's guardian must have the complete information needed for informed consent that the patient normally would receive.

Informed consent involves the presentation of the data in Box 38-10, with sufficient opportunity for the person to ask questions and to have them honestly answered before making a decision about engaging in a study. Furthermore, the person must retain the option to withdraw from study participation without penalty at any time. Documentation of informed consent usually is a requirement for conducting research. The form for consent is submitted for review as part of the research proposal to the Institutional Review Board for Human Subjects before research begins.

Truth-Telling

Truth-telling is providing a person with full disclosure of all known facts related to the purpose of the data collection and research on request during and after research completion. However, information management or research outcomes can have a number of implications for the patient, and some or these can be disturbing. Although nurses have an obligation to inform patients of sensitive information on request, Scanlon and Fibison (1995) noted that this requirement can create a dilemma for the nurse as part of the interdisciplinary health care team.

The nurse may at times be confronted with conflicts in the area of truth-telling, in part because the nurse does not interact with the patient in isolation but rather as a part of a team. A patient may ask the nurse directly for information that someone else has decided the

patient should not have. This experience of being "caught in the middle" can be stressful for the nurse and can compromise professional integrity. Nurses should seek opportunities within the team to arrive at more honest and direct ways of managing information (Scanlon & Fibison, 1995).

Research Models in the 21st Century

CQI drives nursing and health care to change. The nursing profession no longer blindly accepts interventions. The evidence of the effectiveness of what we do must be based on results from well-designed research studies (Gray, 1997). Populations need health care that is appropriate, is beneficial, and can be delivered at reasonable costs. Clinical studies continue, especially in clinical settings. Clinical pathways, clinical guidelines, or protocols are ways to integrate evidence into practice. Psychiatric nursing students should review these tools and compare the risks and benefits of following them for themselves. As Hildegard Peplau said,

It would be a grave mistake to say that we know all that we must know or that we must stop the development of finding out more in order to get in and work with disciplines in terms of what we should do, which is the main point of interdisciplinary work . . . unless you are going to be involved in doing the research for them. If you go empty handed to the interdisciplinary team you go gravely disadvantaged, and you are then very vulnerable to being put in the position of hand maiden instead of colleague. (cited in Huch, 1995, pp. 40–41)

The evidence gained throughout the 1990s, the decade of the brain, demonstrated how research models used in psychiatric nursing in the 21st century will continue to be biologically based. Significant research findings occurred in the 1990s related to abnormalities in the brain structure and function in patients suffering from major mood disorders, schizophrenia, and Alzheimer's disease (Blanchard & Neale, 1994; Bornstein, Schwartzkopf, Olson, & Nasrallah, 1993; Keefe, 1995). Cognitive deficits are now known to predict the onset of Alzheimer's disease.

Box 38–10 ■ ■ ■ ■ ■

Essential Information Required for Informed Consent

- Purpose of the study
- Benefits and risks of participation
- Measures to ensure confidentiality
- Option to withdraw from the study
- Third-party access to research information
- Publication of research findings
- Secondary use of individual data by the same investigator in other subsequent studies

Depression became a focus for all health care settings following the publication of the guidelines for *Depression in Primary Care* (Agency for Health Care Policy and Research, 1993b). Depression is now known to be a common sequelae following myocardial infarction and stroke. Patients with progressively debilitating conditions, including Parkinson's disease, Alzheimer's disease, chronic obstructive pulmonary disease, macular degeneration, and hearing loss are at high risk for depression (Hays, Wells, & Sherborne, 1995; Sturm & Wells, 1995). Significant numbers of depressed patients were found in nursing homes. These findings extended the need for psychiatric interventions in areas other than the mental health units and created increased demand for nurses with both medical-surgical and psychiatric nursing experience.

The 21st century will see a demand for collaboration that will expand the role of advanced psychiatric nursing. More collaborative research involving psychiatric nursing, geriatric nursing, and others is expected as more holistic care is delivered. Research on cost containment and reduction will continue as the need for services increases. Research focusing on prevention of mental illness, including gene research, will increase in the future, with the hope that more diseases will be eradicated and others shortened.

Quantitative Research Methods

Most QI is based on the rational scientific model known as **quantitative research.** This is most common and well-established model of clinical research in health care and psychiatric nursing. Quantitative researchers depend on explicit numbers and facts to explain their findings. A study uses structured techniques to explain the relationship between or among variables. Paper and pencil instruments, such as checklists, questionnaires, and scales are used to measure objective changes; a variety of statistical procedures reveal the results. A large sample provides the required numbers of responses to determine statistical significance. Quantitative studies require deductive reasoning skills.

The advantages of using quantitative studies are many. Well-designed deductive studies can be replicated by other researchers. Quantitative data provide the concrete numerical information needed to support external funding of research projects and treatment protocols. Objective data about the efficacy of treatment related to days lost from work, cost of care, length of time in the hospital, and so on provide the rationale for making needed changes in the delivery of psychiatric nursing care.

Qualitative Research Methods

Qualitative research, also used in psychiatric nursing, is sometimes referred to as a phenomenological approach. With this methodology, the researcher uses inductive reasoning, drawing from descriptions of individual experiences to create a narrative about its meaning.

This relational methodology is particularly consistent with Peplau's (1952) observation that the nurse-patient relationship represents the crux of psychiatric nursing.

Qualitative methodologies take a holistic approach to the study of phenomena and seek to look effectively at the whole person, not just at discrete variables—at the unspoken meanings as well as the articulated facts. Qualitative methodologies include direct quotations, paraphrased descriptions, and summaries of predominant and recurring themes.

Qualitative research considers the subject's views as the key element in understanding human reality. Thus, the data are always contextually bound. Understanding does not flow from a simple quantitative assessment of the individual's social or psychological reality. For example, with a qualitative approach, the researcher would ask the subject to describe his or her social support system. By contrast, quantitative research would use a written instrument such as the Global Assessment of Functioning Scale to measure the individual's level of function (Goldman, Skodol, & Lave, 1992). The information from each would be important. They might complement each other, but the reported findings are likely to be quite different in many ways.

Quantitative research begins with established hypotheses and seeks to prove their validity; qualitative methodologies seek to describe experiences and to generate hypotheses through logical inference. Qualitative research employs dialogue with subjects. The researcher asks selected subjects to describe an action or experience in their own words. The interview process is collaborative and informal.

Triangulation

Triangulation in research refers to the use of multiple methods, both quantitative and qualitative, to gather research data. For example, the researcher might use observation, written assessment tests, and structured interviews to obtain information about a person's depression. Triangulation is particularly useful in complex studies with many possible or interacting variables. When multiple methods of analysis are used, it is critical to compare and contrast the findings and offer explanations for unexpected or conflicting results. Although quantitative findings such as test results may be identical, using qualitative methods, it is possible to identify other areas that would impact the outcome and success of the intervention. Both quantitative and qualitative studies are acceptable to accrediting bodies.

National Center for Nursing Research

A major opportunity to help bridge the gap between research and clinical practice occurred with the establishment of the National Center for Nursing Research at the National Institutes or Health. The National Center for Nursing Research holds special promise for increasing research efforts critical to nursing practice and research initiatives in the 21st century. Planned initiatives at the

National Center for Nursing Research are presented in Box 38–11.

Two other resources for enhancing clinical effectiveness through research methods are the National Institutes of Health (NIH) consensus development conferences and the Agency for Health Care Policy and Research. These ongoing efforts produce practical information useful to providing patient care. The guidelines and decisions demonstrate the best of collaborative practice for gaining consensus and improving patient outcomes.

> **W**hat do you think? How do you think you can presently support research? What clinical questions intrigue you? How would you go about obtaining answers to those questions?

➤ **Check Your Reading**

26. How does the nurse protect the patient's right to self-determination through the principles of informational privacy and informed consent?
27. How would you describe the differences between quantitative and qualitative research methodologies?
28. Why is research important to the development of psychiatric nursing and the role of the nurse in the 21st century?

FUTURE TRENDS

The millennium symbolizes many things: changes in our lives, the passing of an age, beginnings, endings, and so much more. For each one of us, the millennium is an indicator about our own lives, the passage of time, and our place in history. (Porter-O'Grady, 1998, p. 5)

All aspects of nursing and health care will be influenced by the advancement of technology (Brown, 1998). Health care research and information is available to all through the Internet. JCAHO, NIMH, Sigma Theta Tau, and many other professional organizations can be contacted online through their Web sites. Laptop computers simplify data collection and analysis. Computers automatically track patient progress, reduce paperwork, and eliminate duplicate documentation thus saving time for more patient contact.

Psychiatric nurses need to develop computer competence and to research ways to use technology to improve practice and patient outcomes. Computer access and use is beginning to be a marketing and recruitment tool for many agencies. With the demand for nurses growing, increased computer productivity may become a requirement. Advanced practice nurses in all clinical specialties need to be mentors to their colleagues, develop realistic research agendas, and manage initiatives that integrate research findings into clinical practice.

Box 38–11 ■ ■ ■ ■ ■

Planned Initiatives at the National Center for Nursing Research

- Developing a research agenda identifying research initiatives that combine scientific rigor with societal relevance
- Targeting nursing research priorities determined by the nursing scientific community as most likely to influence nursing practice
- Funding research programs capable of generating multiple interlocking studies that build on and support one another
- Developing a cohort or nurse scientists through postdoctoral and individual career development study opportunities for midcareer and senior-level nursing scientists
- Generating strategies to enhance interdisciplinary collaboration and cofunding of interdisciplinary research projects
- Establishing an intramural research program at the National Center for Nursing Research at the National Institutes of Health, related to both basic and clinical research initiatives

Data from National Institute for Nursing Research. (http://www.gov/ninr).

Conclusions

The 21st century presents the profession of nursing with its greatest challenge—work efficiently and effectively to keep costs down and improve successful patient outcomes. Psychiatric nurses are expected to do more for more patients. Computers eliminate much of the redundancy that has kept nurses away from the patient. To be acknowledged as equal members of the health care team, nurses must maintain comprehensive, up-to-date knowledge about the nature and treatment of mental illness. They must be articulate and willing to share professional insights, taking a leadership role in the development of research questions and other activities that demonstrate clinical competence. Research defines the best possible practices and technology facilitates the transmission of the knowledge to the nurse and from the nurse to the patient.

CQI will be maintained in order to assure quality care. As nursing outcomes prove the effectiveness and cost-saving benefits of our interventions, we will move into partnerships with other services and close alliances will result. Critical pathways and care maps will continue to efficiently direct care. The incidence of hospitalization for mental illness will decrease through continued gene research, pharmacological studies, and nursing intervention studies. Research will build the evidence that mental health nursing needs to maintain its position as a profession. Mental health and psychiatric nurses will be found more in outpatient, community, and other practices than in hospitals.

Mental health is an integral component of holistic care

requiring the expertise of child, adolescent, adult, and gerontologic mental health nurses. The future for the specialty is exciting; nurses now, more than ever, need to build their own knowledge and keep informed to prepare for the demands and rewards of the years ahead.

Key Points to Remember

- The journey of psychiatric nursing in the 21st century is collaborative, outcome driven, fiscally controlled, and researched based.
- Continuous improvement will drive nursing to change and adapt, adding new knowledge to enable the process.
- Psychiatric nurses in the 21st century are expected to provide holistic care and must be educationally and clinically prepared to do so.
- Outcomes demonstrate the effectiveness of mental health care to patients, providers, insurers, and the public.
- Every practicing nurse has a part to play in nursing research, whether as an investigator, a user of the research outcomes, a data collector, or someone who identifies problems requiring research.
- Despite the requirements for outcomes of care, nurses have legal and ethical responsibility for maintaining patient rights and confidentiality.
- The model of health care delivery in psychiatric nursing is becoming more resource driven and biologically based than has been the case.

- The neurosciences will continue to play an increasingly important role as an essential framework for considering the etiology of major mental disorders.
- Quantitative research represents a decontextualized data-based type of information that is useful in comparing treatment approaches and developing appropriate medication protocols.
- Qualitative research uses inductive reasoning, drawing from descriptions of individual experience to create a narrative about its meaning.
- An interdisciplinary health care team needs an integrated approach to documentation of care. Outcome achievement and critical pathways serve this purpose.
- Advanced practice nurses in the psychiatric field need to take leadership roles in mentoring their colleagues, developing realistic research agendas, and managing initiatives that integrate research findings into clinical practice.

Learning Activities

1. A newly admitted psychiatric patient is found dead. A brief suicide note is found on the desk next to the curtain rod where he hung himself. Create a chart showing the event and possible root causes and solutions to prevent a similar occurrence in the future.
2. Using the definition of quality and the standards for psychiatric mental health nursing, decide whether quality care is being provided at your clinical site. Prepare one suggestion for performance improvement.
3. Working with a partner or group, design two patient

satisfaction tools that incorporate questions about the structure, processes, and outcomes of care at your clinical site. Use open-ended questions and an interview format for one, a rating scale or other quantitative tool for the other. Obtain patient and agency permission and be sure to maintain confidentiality and respect for patient rights. Administer each tool to four patients and discuss the results with others in your group. Include an analysis of your own satisfaction with the assignment, and the ease or difficulty of the data collection, and rate the value of the information obtained.

Critical Thinking Exercises

1. Once you begin to practice psychiatric nursing after graduation, you will be expected to participate in performance improvement. After reading the content in this chapter, identify three alternative solutions for Barbara that would change her rehospitalization rate and maintain her rights. Should Earl, the case manager, feel responsible for Barbara's failure? If not, why not?

2. Think about a problem or an issue you have observed on the psychiatric unit or during a home visit with a mentally ill patient. Identify a research question you might want to ask about this problem or issue. Defend your rationale for choosing it. Specify the methodology you think would best address your research question.

Additional Resources

Agency for Health Care Policy and Research
http://www.ahcpr.gov/clinic

American Academy of Child and Adolescent Psychiatry
http://www.aacap.org

Joint Commission on Accreditation of Healthcare Organizations
http://www.jcaho.org/

Oryx: The next evolution in accreditation: Questions and answers about the Joint Commission's planned integration of performance measures into the accreditation process.

Mental Health Infosource
http://mhsource.com

National Institute of Mental Health
http://www.nimh.nih.gov/

National Institute of Nursing Research
http://www.nih.gov/ninr

References

Agency For Health Care Policy and Research. (1993a). Clinical practice guideline: Depression in primary care. *Detection and diagnosis* (Vol. 1). (AHCPR Publication No. 93-0550). Washington, DC: U.S. Government Printing Office.

Agency For Health Care Policy and Research. (1993b). Clinical practice guideline: Depression in primary care. *Treatment of major depression* (Vol. 2). (AHCPR Publication No. 93-0551). Washington, DC: U.S. Government Printing Office.

American Nurses Association. (1985). *Code for nurses with interpretive statements.* Washington, DC: American Nurses Association.

American Nurses Association. (1994). *Statement on psychiatric-mental health clinical nursing practice and standards of psychiatric-mental health clinical nursing practice.* Washington, DC: American Nurses Publishing.

Bailey, D. A., Litaker, D. G., & Mion, L. C. (1998). Developing better critical paths in healthcare: Combining "best practices" and the quantitative approach. *Journal of Nursing Administration, 28*(1), 21-26.

Baradell, J. G. (1995). Clinical outcomes and satisfaction of patients of clinical nurse specialists in psychiatric-mental health nursing. *Archives of Psychiatric Nursing, 9,* 240-250.

Berrios, C. D., & Jacobowitz, W. H. (1998). Therapeutic holding: Outcomes of a pilot study. *Journal of Psychosocial Nursing, 36*(8), 14-18.

Black, M. K. (1992). The consumer: Product of our efforts. In C. G. Meisenheimer (Ed.), *Improving quality: A guide to effective program.* Rockville, MD: Aspen.

Blanchard, J., & Neale, J. (1994). The neuropsychological signature of schizophrenia: Generalized or differential deficit? *American Journal of Psychiatry, 151,* 40-48.

Bornstein, R., Schwarzkopf, Olson, S., & Nasrallah, H. (1993). Third ventricle enlargement and neurophysiological deficit in schizophrenia. *Biological Psychiatry, 31,* 954-961.

Brown, B. (1998). 10 trends for the new year. *Nursing Management, 29*(12), 33-36.

Carson, V. B., Alonzo, & Alva. (in press). Clinical outcomes in psychiatric home care. *Home Care Provider.*

Coile, R. Jr. (1997). Top trends for managed care: 1997-2000. *Russ Coile's Health Trends, 9*(2), 5-8.

Coleman, R. L. (1989). The use of decision analysis in quality assessment. *Quality Review Bulletin, 15,* 383-391.

Crosby, P. B. (1979). *Quality is free.* New York: McGraw-Hill.

Crosby, P. B. (1984). *Quality without tears.* New York: McGraw-Hill.

Deming, W. E. (1993). *The new economics for industry.* Cambridge, MA: MIT.

Deming, W. E. (1986). *Out of the crisis.* Cambridge, MA: Massachusetts Institute of Technology.

Donaldson, M. S. (1998). Accountability for quality in managed care. *The Journal on Quality Improvement, 24,* 711-725.

Fauman, M. A. (1990). Monitoring the quality of psychiatric care. *Psychiatric Clinics of North America, 13*(1), 73-88.

Forbes, D. (1998). Goal attainment scaling: A responsive measure of client outcomes. *Journal of Gerontological Nursing, 24*(12), 34-40.

Goldman, H. H., Skodol, A. E., & Lave, T. R. (1992). Revising axis V for DSM-IV: A review of measures of social functioning. *American Journal of Psychiatry, 149,* 1148-1156.

Gray, J. A. M. (1997). *Evidence-based healthcare: How to make health policy and management decisions.* New York: Churchill Livingstone.

Graybeal, K. (1993). Clinical pathway development: The Overlake model. *Nursing Management, 24*(4), 42-46.

Hall, L. L., & Beineke, R. (1998, summer). Consumer and family views of managed care. *Managed Behavioral Healthcare: A Current Reality and Future Potential, 78,* 77-85.

Hays, R. D., Wells, K. B., & Sherborne, C. D. (1995). Functioning and well-being outcomes of patients with depression compared with chronic general medical Illnesses. *Archives of General Psychiatry, 52,* 11-19.

Huch, M. (1995). Nursing and the next millennium. *Nursing Science Quarterly, 8*(1), 38-44.

Ingram, B., & Chung, R. (1997). Client satisfaction data and quality improvement planning in managed mental health care organizations. *Health Care Management Review, 22*(3), 40-52.

Joint Commission on Accreditation of Healthcare Organizations. (1985). *Ten-step model for the monitoring and evaluation process.* Oakbrook Terrace, IL: JCAHO.

Joint Commission on Accreditation of Healthcare Organizations. (1988). *Guide to quality assurance.* Oakbrook Terrace, IL: JCAHO.

Joint Commission on Accreditation of Healthcare Organizations. (1995). *1995 accreditation manual for healthcare.* Oakbrook Terrace, IL: JCAHO.

Joint Commission on Accreditation of Healthcare Organizations. (1998). *Using performance measurement to improve outcomes in behavioral health care.* Oakbrook Terrace, IL: JCAHO.

Juran, J. M. (1988). *Juran on planning for quality.* New York: Free Press.

Juran, J. M. (1992). *Juran on quality by design.* New York: Free Press.

Kaplan, L. K. (Ed.). (1998). Tough questions about ORYX: Is ORYX a four-letter word? *Infusion, 5*(2), 18-23.

Keefe, R. (1995). The contribution of neuropsychology to psychiatry. *American Journal of Psychiatry, 152*(1), 6-13.

Kirk, R., & Hoesing, H. (1991). *The nurses' guide to common sense quality management.* West Dundee, IL: S-N Publications

Koch, L. A. (1997). Using Oasis to reach OBQI. *Caring, 16*(8), 34-46.

Kramer, T., & Trabin, T. (1997). *Performance indicator measurement in behavioral healthcare: Data capture methods, cost-effectiveness, and emerging standards.* Portola Valley, CA: Institute for Behavioral Healthcare.

Lautz, R. J., & Lynn, K. (1995). Productivity and peerage. *Nursing Management, 26*(10), 57-59.

Lohr, K. N. (1988). Outcome measurements: Concepts and questions. *Inquiry, 25*(1), 37-50.

Love, C. C., & Hunter, M. E. (1996). Violence in public sector psychiatric hospitals: Benchmarking nursing staff injury rates. *Journal of Psychosocial Nursing, 34*(95), 30-34.

Mark, H., & Garet, D. E. (1997). Interpreting profiling data in behavioral health care for a continuous quality improvement cycle. *The Joint Commission Journal on Quality Improvement 23,* 521-528.

Mason, K. (1999). Standards of care: Policies, procedures and practice guidelines. *Advance for Nurses, 1*(6), 17.

McGlynn, E. A. (1998). Choosing and evaluating clinical performance measures. *The Joint Commission Journal on Quality Improvement, 24,* 470-479.

McLaughlin, C. P., & Kaluzny, A. D. (1990). Total quality management in health: Making it work. *Health Care Management Review, 15*(3), 7-14.

Megel, M. E., Elrod, M. E., & Rausch, A. K. (1996). Conflicts experienced by quality assurance/improvement professionals: A Delphi study. *Journal of Nursing Care Quality, 10*(2), 75-82.

Mitchell, P. H., Ferketich, S., Jennings, B. M., & American Academy of Nursing Expert Panel on Quality Health Care. (1998). Quality health outcomes model. *Image: Journal of Nursing Scholarship, 30*(1), 43-46.

Nielsen, P. A. (1992). Quality of care: Discovering a modified practice theory. *Journal of Nursing Quality Care, 6*(2), 63-76.

O'Harrow, R. Jr. (1999, April 1). Under fire, U.S. amends plan to collect health care data. *The Washington Post,* A5.

Ohlund, G. (1997). *Psychiatric home care benchmarking study.* La Jolla, CA: Ohlund and Associates.

Peplau, H. (1952). *Interpersonal relations in nursing.* New York: Putnam.

Phillips, J. (1995). Nursing theory based research for advanced nursing practice. *Advances in Nursing Science, 8*(1), 4-5.

Polit, D. E., & Hungler, B. P. (1995). *Nursing research: Principles and methods* (5th ed.). Philadelphia: J. B. Lippincott.

Porter-O'Grady, T. (1998). Signposts for the next century. *Nursing Management, 29*(12), 5.

Resnick, B. (1998a). Efficacy of beliefs in geriatric rehabilitation. *Journal of Gerontological Nursing, 24*(7), 34-44.

Rockwood, K., Stolee, P., Howard, K., & Mallery, L. (1996). Use of goal attainment scale to measure treatment effects in an anti-dementia drug trial. *Neuroepidemiology, 15,* 330-338.

Sallah, D. (1997). A shared attempt towards provision of quality and effective care: A consensus conference on the outcomes of care for mentally disordered offenders. *Psychiatric Care, 4,* 202-210.

Scanlon, C., & Fibison, W. (1995). *Managing genetic information: Implications for nursing practice.* Washington, DC: American Nurses Association.

Schroeder, P., & Katz, J. (1992). Seeking consensus on important aspects of nursing care. *Quality Review Bulletin, 18*(2), 63-65.

Schuler, H. J. (1994). Quality management. In R. Spitzer-Lehmann (Ed.), *Nursing management desk reference.* (pp. 504-518). Philadelphia: W. B. Saunders.

Shaughnessy, P. W., & Crisler, K. S. (1995). *Outcome-based quality improvement: A manual for home care agencies on how to use outcomes.* Washington DC: National Association for Home Care.

Society for Education and Research in Psychiatric-Mental Health Nursing. (1996). *Educational preparation for psychiatric-mental health nursing practice.* Pensacola, FL: Society for Education and Research in Psychiatric-Mental Health Nursing.

Society for Education and Research in Psychiatric and Mental Health Nursing. (1997). *Primary mental health and advanced practice psychiatric nursing.* Pensacola, FL: SERPN.

Sturm, R., & Wells, K. B. (1995). How can care for depression become more cost effective? *Journal of the American Medical Association, 273,* 51-58.

Wilson, C. K. (1991). A climate for excellence an impossible dream? In P. Schroeder (Ed.), *The encyclopedia of nursing care quality issues and strategies for quality care.* Rockville, MD: Aspen.

Suggested Readings

Bailey, D. A., Litaker, D. G., & Mion, L. C. (1998). Developing better critical paths in healthcare: Combining "best practices" and the quantitative approach. *Journal of Nursing Administration, 28*(1), 21-26.

Barrell, L. M., Merwin, E. I., & Poster, E. C. (1997). Patient outcomes used by advanced practice psychiatric nurses to evaluate effectiveness of practice. *Archives of Psychiatric Nursing, 11,* 184-197.

D'Arco, S. H., & Hargreaves, M. (1995). Needlestick injuries: A multidisciplinary concern. *Nursing Clinics of North America, 30*(1), 61-76.

Guiliamo, K., & Poirier, C. (1991). Nursing care management: Critical pathways to desirable outcomes. *Nursing Management, 22*(3), 52-55.

Huch, M. (1995). Nursing and the next millennium. *Nursing Science Quarterly, 8*(1), 38-44.

Joint Commission on Accreditation of Healthcare Organizations. (1997). *Guide to performance improvement in behavioral health Care.* Oakbrook Terrace, IL: JCAHO.

Joint Commission on Accreditation of Healthcare Organizations. (1998). *Using performance measurement to improve outcomes in behavioral health care.* Oakbrook Terrace, IL: JCAHO.

McEwen, M. (1994). Promoting interdisciplinary collaboration. *Nursing and Health Care, 15,* 304-307.

Mohr, W., & Fantuzzo, J. (1998). The challenge of creating thoughtful research agendas. *Archives of Psychiatric Nursing, 12*(1), 3-11.

Newman, M. (1994). Into the 21st century. *Nursing Science Quarterly, 7*(1), 44-45.

Sasala, D. B., & Jasovsky, D. A. (1998). Using a hospitalwide performance improvement process for patient education documentation. *Joint commission Journal on Quality Improvement 24,* 313-322.

Van Manen, M. (1990). *Researching lived experience.* Albany, NY: State University of New York.

Zonsius Klingelsmith, M., & Murphy, M. (1995). Use of total quality management sparks staff nurse participation in continuous quality improvement. *Nursing Clinics of North America, 30*(1), 112.

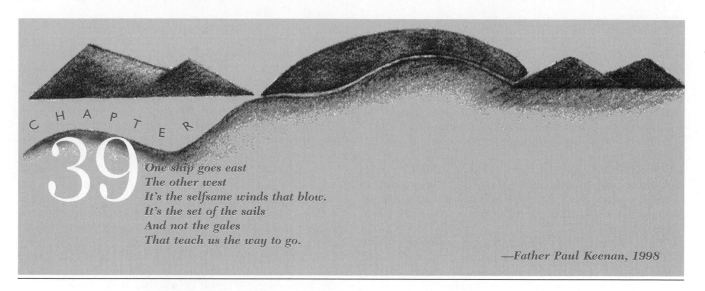

*One ship goes east
The other west
It's the selfsame winds that blow.
It's the set of the sails
And not the gales
That teach us the way to go.*

—*Father Paul Keenan, 1998*

Skills Needed for the Forward Journey

Learning Objectives

After studying this chapter, you should be able to:

1. Discuss the trends within the mental health care system that will influence psychiatric nursing.

2. Discuss at least three skills that the psychiatric nurse may need in order to function within the mental health care system of the future.

3. Discuss the importance of "setting your sails" if psychiatric nursing is to make a difference in the mental health care system of the future.

Dear Student:

This chapter is different from those that have gone before. In a sense, it is a send off to you as you continue your journey in nursing. Although a few of you will remain in psychiatric nursing and explore the richness of this specialty, more than likely most of you will move on to other nursing specialties. Regardless of where your journey takes you, this letter has significance to you. By reading this textbook, you and I (as well as the other contributors) have journeyed together for a time. We have tried to impart to you our love of psychiatric nursing; the breadth and depth of the specialty; and the application of the specialty, not only to the care of the seriously and persistently mentally ill but also to your entire journey. We have tried to take you beyond nursing as a job and a career, and pointed you to nursing as a ministry, a calling, and an art—as Florence Nightingale said:

Nursing is an art, and if it is to be made an art, it requires as exclusive a devotion, as hard a preparation, as any painter's or sculptor's work. For what is having to do with dead canvas, or cold marble compared with having to do

with the living body, the temple of God's spirit. (cited in Baly, 1991, p. 68)

We have tried to integrate the most current findings in biological psychiatry with your personal communication and relationship skills. We have tried to show you that nursing is more than "doing to" or "for" another; it is also being present to another person spiritually and assisting that person as he or she makes sense out of life. We have tried to convey to you the power of the individual's story as he or she struggles with illness and moves toward health.

You may be aware that there are plenty of doomsayers regarding the future of psychiatric nursing, in fact, all of nursing. Discussion about the state of psychiatric nursing includes the following observations of trends:

- The present focus on integrated curricula in nursing schools does not provide students with a valid perspective on psychiatric nursing; therefore, nursing students are disinclined to choose this specialty.

- Nursing lacks a critical mass of outcome research that demonstrates the value of psychiatric nursing.

- Current leaders in psychiatric nursing are, to put it bluntly, getting old. Many of these nurses were educated with funds provided in the 1960s and early 1970s by the National Institute of Mental Health. These funds were eliminated during the Reagan administration. This lack of financial support has curtailed the number of younger nurses coming into the specialty.
- The patient population cared for by psychiatric nurses is not a population with whom everyone wants to work—both psychiatric patients and nurses continue to be viewed through the stigma that surrounds psychiatric illness.
- Much of health care is focused on business and the "bottom line" rather than the care and the caring aspects of what we do. This is discouraging to nurses, many of whom have left the profession.
- Hospital-based employment opportunities are diminishing. As competition for the health care dollar increases, many health care facilities increase their profit margins by downsizing their nursing staff. The nursing staff members are frequently viewed not as a necessity but as the facility's biggest expense. In their place, hospitals are hiring cheaper, unlicensed staffers to take over the responsibilities once held by nurses. This trend is seen not only in acute medical surgical hospitals but also in psychiatric facilities, where psychiatric nurses are being replaced by technicians.
- Within facilities in which nurses are still providing care, the cost-cutting measures have resulted in fewer nurses while increasing the responsibilities of each nurse. Where ratios were once 1 nurse to 5 patients, now 1 nurse cares for 10 patients—an alarming trend in psychiatry, in which the reason for admission has narrowed to be: "assessed dangerousness to self or others" (Cook, 1999).

Certainly, these trends are appalling; in fact, they are frightening enough to make prospective and even current nurses rethink their career choices. However, such a response is short sighted, lacking hope, narrow, and unfocused. This is not the first period in the history of nursing that we have faced and weathered challenging circumstances (see Chapter 2). In many ways, this is the best of times and the worst of times. Opportunities abound for those who set their sails and do not let the gale winds of the health care system blow them off course. You have to be absolutely clear as to why you are becoming a nurse, and you must keep that clarity with you always as you make patient care decisions and career choices. You must believe that you make a difference. If you find that you are no longer making a difference, you must reset your sails, and focus on what you can accomplish today—not the "if onlys" of the past or the "what ifs" of the future—on the power of today and what you can do to make a difference in the present (Jones, 1997).

The opportunities for psychiatric nurses are no longer limited to hospital settings; there is a need for psychiatric nurses in community mental health centers, home care, homeless clinics and shelters, nursing homes, assisted living facilities, schools, industry, and managed care organizations. There is certainly no lack of patients for whom psychiatric nurses can provide care. According to the 1994 National Co-Morbidity Study (cited in Boivin, 1999), almost 50% of the American population have a lifetime prevalence of developing a psychiatric disorder. The needs of the seriously and persistently mentally ill are still largely unmet, and psychiatric nurses with their wholistic perspective are in a unique position to meet those needs. In addition, there are countless individuals who are able to function at home, work, and school but are overwhelmed by the demands and fast pace of today's world. They too could benefit from the mental health interventions provided by psychiatric nurses (Boivin, 1999).

But what skills are needed to turn today's obstacles into challenges? What kind of changes are required of the profession? Will we be able to make these changes and survive? I, for one, am hopeful that we can and will.

It is clear that there must be fundamental changes in nursing school curricula, where faculty are faced with finding the right balance between maintaining the humanistic focus (so long the hallmark of psychiatric-mental health nursing) and responding to the changing needs of the health care marketplace. Mohr and Naylor (1998) reported on the University of Pennsylvania School of Nursing's attempts to find this balance. Table 39-1 shows the core content, the psychiatric-mental health content, and the psychiatric-mental health competencies adopted by this faculty.

In addition to changes in psychiatric-mental health curricula, there is a need for nurses to expand their knowledge and comfort in the business arena. Learning the language of business is becoming a necessity, not a luxury. Nurses are rising to this challenge not because they are selling out to greed and the worship of the dollar but because they are savvy enough to know that by couching patient welfare issues in the language of business, their effectiveness as patient advocates increases exponentially.

Psychiatric nurses must also step up their efforts to get their leaders involved in outcome research and quality improvement. In some arenas, the clinical and cost effectiveness of the psychiatric nurse is a well-kept secret. A review of the bodies of literature produced by social workers, psychologists, and psychiatric nurses finds that, by comparison, psychiatric nurses have produced a limited amount of definitive outcome research. We are just not as effective at communicating that we make a difference. The newly opened doors of community-based and home-based services provide psychiatric nurses with leadership opportunities not only in program development and implementation but also in outcome research that demonstrates quality.

Psychiatric nurses have mistakenly avoided involvement in physical care. Yet this is one of our strengths and our differentiating characteristic from other mental health providers. Rather than deny our medical background, we should celebrate it. Our grounding in the workings of the body provides us with a unique perspective unmatched by any other mental health provider except the psychiatrist. In addition to our knowledge of psychopathology, we understand and can teach about

TABLE 39–1 Core Content, Psychiatric Mental Health Content, and Competencies

CORE CONTENT	HEALTH COURSE CONTENT	PSYCHIATRIC–MENTAL COMPETENCIES
Growth and development along the lifespan; child and adolescent development	Age-appropriate care for psychiatric clients; recognition of major child/ adolescent disorders	Plan and implement age-appropriate care. Articulate interventions that might be used with children/adolescents. Contrast child and adolescent needs and interventions with those of adults.
Neuroanatomy, neurophysiology, neuroendocrinology, neuroimmunology	Neurocognitive alterations in mental illness, neurobiologic alterations in mental illness, stress management	Demonstrate basic assessment skills to include a. sensory perception, cognitive deficits b. information processing resulting in alterations of behavior and social functioning and biopsychoneuro-immunologic changes
Diagnostic thinking; inductive, deductive, and retroductive reasoning; syntactical thinking	Major psychiatric diagnostic classifications per *Diagnostic and Statistical Manual of Mental Disorders, Fourth Edition,* mental health alterations and nursing diagnosis, client in context	Identify symptoms of each category. Describe what data are present and demonstrate how conclusions reached.
Basic management principles; case management	Referral processes, expected outcomes of psychiatric treatment	Ability to participate in case management and management of psychiatric care, plan for a continuum of care, mobilize resources to provide safety, structure, and support for the mentally ill.
Critical pathways	Critical pathways related to major mental illness	Implement critical pathways related to patients with major mental illnesses.
Interdisciplinary roles	Roles of various mental health care providers, including roles of psychiatric nurses with various levels of education	Demonstrate ability to work with various members of the interdisciplinary team.
Health care promotion and illness prevention	Smoking cessation principles; exercise, endorphins, enkephalins, nutritional aspects of mental health; principles of sobriety	Plan and facilitate a mental health promotion plan for a client with serious mental illness.
Community health	Community mental health; community support initiative; at-risk populations; social policy regarding care of mentally ill	Participate in delegating care and making appropriate referrals for psychiatric patients. Identify at-risk populations and major policy governing mentally ill.
Ethical and legal principles; values clarification	1. Nurse practice acts 2. Standards of practice for psychiatric–mental health nursing 3. Confidentiality 4. Least restrictive treatment	Clarify personal values continuously regarding mental illness. Facilitate others to clarify values and attitudes related to self and mental illness.
Person as consumer, family/significant other	Principles of collaborative relationships with individuals, and families and consumer and advocacy groups; competency vs. deficiency paradigms	Demonstrate ability to partner with individuals and families in developing and implementing care plans for psychiatric patients.
Basic pharmacology	Major psychotropic agents for identified psychiatric illness that include a. action and expected effects b. side effects and toxicity c. potential interactions with other medications	Evaluate effects of medication on patients, including symptoms, side effects, toxicity, and potential interactions with other medications or substances. Teach patients and families medication management. Evaluate outcomes of medications.
Principles of learning and learning theories	Psychoeducational approaches to working with individuals, families, and consumers	Demonstrate ability to develop and implement a teaching project related to mental health–illness issues.

Table continued on following page

TABLE 39–1 Core Content, Psychiatric Mental Health Content, and Competencies *Continued*

CORE CONTENT	HEALTH COURSE CONTENT	PSYCHIATRIC–MENTAL COMPETENCIES
Communication theory and skills	Therapeutic use of self a. understanding, using, and controlling affective responses b. integrating affective and cognitive responses with appropriate interventions c. continuing clarification and maintenance of professional boundaries d. evaluating interventions with psychiatric clients	Demonstrate therapeutic use of self.
Stress and crisis; crisis intervention; violence	Stress-crisis continuum; principles of anger and aggression; crisis intervention with psychiatric clients	Assess seven levels of stress-crisis for intervention strategy. Assess potential violence; intervene in acute agitation.
Cultural and ethnic differences; spiritual needs	Compare and contrast psychiatric symptoms and cultural and spiritual self-expression	Provide culturally and spiritually competent care that meets client needs.
Conceptual models; theories	Recognition of how conceptual models and theories provide frameworks for practice	Articulate a model or theory of practice. Provide a rationale for the interventions chosen by relating it to a model or theory.
Chronic illness	Symptom management in seriously and persistently mentally ill; relapse care/prevention	Establish therapeutic relationship with seriously and persistently mentally ill patients.
Advocacy	Consumer advocacy groups	Observe functioning of advocacy groups. Become acquainted with support groups and articulate their role.
Concepts of risk and screening	Risk factors, screening, and referral related to psychiatric illness and social problems: a. suicide/homicide b. substance abuse c. violence/abuse	Screen for substance use/abuse. Screen for victim violence/abuse. Screen for suicide and homicide.
Group process	Therapeutic factors in group intervention	Demonstrate beginning group participation/leadership skills.
History (from demonology to biology); development of the psychosocial and sociocultural points of view	Mental illness through the ages; ideas carried over through history, ideas carried over through the arts; normal and abnormal behavior through the eyes of the scientist	Trace the nature and scope of thinking about psychopathology. Trace the progress that has been made in the understanding of human behavior.

From Mohr, W. K., & Naylor, M. D. (1998). Creating a curriculum for the 21st century. *Nursing Outlook, 46*(5), 206–211.
Adapted from 1996 guidelines published for Psychiatric Mental Health Curriculum generalist preparation by the Society for Education and Research in Psychiatric Nursing.

medications; we monitor the physical effects of medications; and we are knowledgeable and can intervene regarding issues of nutrition, exercise, and sleep that influence psychiatric symptomatology. Patients become ill in a wholistic manner and deserve to be treated in a wholistic manner. This does not eliminate the need for specialists, but it places a demand on psychiatric nurses to broaden their diagnostic and intervention paradigm to consider nonpsychiatric causes for behaviors that present as psychiatric symptoms. This broad perspective is essential as the health care system strives to contain costs. Across the country, schools of nursing are beginning to respond to this need through master's degree programs that integrate skills of the nurse practitioner with those of the psychiatric clinical nurse specialist.

The political and policy arena offers other challenges for psychiatric nurses. It is essential that as individuals and as a group we stand up and make our voices heard in the political and policymaking processes. We cannot passively accept decisions imposed upon our profession by legislators, insurance companies, other mental health providers, or the courts. Our voices must continue to argue for the needs of the disenfranchised patients for whom we provide care and to present cogent arguments regarding the importance of psychiatric nursing to the mental health system.

An example of an effective response to a policy change occurred in Maryland over the years 1997 through 1999. The care of patients receiving Maryland Medicaid was shifted from state administration to the control of two managed behavioral health companies. In establishing the guidelines for care under the new organization, Maryland Health Partners, psychiatric home care nurses were not recognized as providers. This occurred despite the fact that they had been providing needed care to the seriously and persistently mentally ill for many years and there was no alternative service for these patients. When the regulations were published in summer 1997, the directors of psychiatric home care programs from across the state met to plan strategy. The strategy included

- Organizing and forming Behavioral Home Health Nurses Association
- Developing a position paper that was sent to officials within the legislature, Maryland Health Partners, and the Department of Mental Health
- Lobbying selected state representatives with a known reputation for favoring nurses
- Lobbying other nursing groups
- Networking at Nurses' Night at the State Legislature
- Developing and implementing an educational program for the case managers who made the day-to-day decisions about patients
- Developing and submitting a paper to the Home Health Nurses Association detailing the advocacy efforts made on behalf of a vulnerable population

These efforts required the combined talents of many psychiatric nurses. The results were that the regulations were rewritten and home-based psychiatric nursing was recognized as a valuable part of the psychiatric continuum. Behavioral Home Health Nurses Association continues its efforts as other issues arise that threaten psychiatric home care nurses and, ultimately, the patients that they serve.

The example just given leads to the discussion of another skill increasingly needed by psychiatric nurses, and that is collaboration. The members of the Behavioral Home Health Nurses Association were not able to change anything by themselves. Their efforts included state legislators, other nurses and nursing groups, and even psychiatrists. We are not alone within the mental health care system, and we must reach out in partnership toward other players in the system.

Another skill needed, or perhaps it is a personal attribute, is flexibility in the face of change. None of us knows where our journeys will lead us, but we can be certain that those journeys will traverse new territories and demand different responses and skills. Change is frightening to people—psychiatric nurses are no exception—yet there are times when we must move away from our comfort zone, try new things, and change. The following poem provides a positive perspective on change (Jones, 1997):

> *Expanding . . . contracting . . .*
> *Breathing out . . . breathing in . . . .*
> *Life is about change*
> *In the midst of constancy.*
> *We go to the Fair. We watch horses run.*
> *And in the midst of our laughter*
> *And whispered fears*
> *Sits a statue*

> *At the foot of your stairs*
> *Who seems to have it all together.*
> *And yet somehow*
> *She envies us—*
> *Our laughter*
> *And our chaos*
> *As we run*
> *Up the stairs . . . .*
> *To*
> *Meet, embrace and dance again*
> *With "change."*

The last skill I want to discuss with you is the need to develop the mind-set of a lifelong learner. I used to think that once I obtained my master's degree, I would know everything there was to know about psychiatric nursing. Was I surprised to find out that the coursework for a master's degree certainly focused my knowledge but in no way provided me with all the facts that I needed. Instead, it helped me to develop the tools and thinking skills necessary to continue the exploration. And this revelation was even more true in the process of obtaining a doctorate. Learning can never be confined to a certain time in life or a designated place. As long as we remain open we continue to learn, grow, and develop. Within the textbook we have tried to point out other sources of information: professional journals, colleagues, the Internet, community resources, and the stories of patients and families. Seek these sources out and allow your journey to twist and turn because you are learning and changing.

I want to end this letter to you in the way that many of the chapters have begun and that is with a story. Nancy Shoemaker, a contributor to this book, wrote her story about why she became a psychiatric nurse. Nancy is a perfect example of someone who set her sails and moves forward in uncharted seas embracing the change that confronts her.

Nancy's Story

I am one of those people who always knew that I wanted to be a nurse. From my earliest childhood fantasy and throughout my career spanning more than 25 years, I have never wanted to be anything else. Of course, according to my family, I didn't turn out to be a "real nurse," that is, one with a white uniform and a white cap. I chose psychiatric nursing right from the start because early in my clinical studies, I realized that I mainly wanted to talk to patients. I needed to hear their stories, their particular questions, and their needs so that I could find out the answers and teach them what they needed to know (or find the right resource).

I learned that if I approached any patient—regardless of age, gender, cultural background, or diagnosis—with an attitude of respect and genuine caring, I could get the patient to communicate with me. So I embarked on a lifelong quest to learn about people, find out the problems and seek new solutions with every patient, and learn about myself at the same time. By listening to feedback from my patients, I learned about my own strengths and weaknesses. For example, I know that I talk too fast and tend to be impatient, but I am a sincere idealist who perseveres to solve any problem long after others have given up.

My passion for psychiatric nursing has never wavered; I have never felt burned out or doubted my role as a nurse. But I have learned that I require certain supports in my work environment in order to thrive. In my first job, I was blessed with a caring, professional, multidisciplinary team experience. I believe these elements are necessary to provide excellent patient care: staff members who care about patients, mental health professionals with appropriate credentials, and professionals from multiple specialties who provide a comprehensive view of the patient and treatment.

I have carried that model with me as a yardstick to measure every other work setting. In order to work to my fullest potential, I require a leader and a few peers who share my vision for seeking excellent patient care. Working with others to foster the highest quality of patient care provides me with continuous indirect rewards, in addition to the direct pleasure of seeing improvement in patients and families.

In today's tumultuous era of health care, it is more challenging than ever for the nurse to deliver excellent patient care. New communication systems are being developed, old criteria are being replaced, standards are being revised, and everything is going faster. Looks like there is a lot to learn... ■

God speed on your journey.

With Warmest Regards,

Verna Benner Carson, PhD, RN, CS-P

References

Baly, M. (Ed). (1991). *As Miss Nightingale said . . . : Florence Nightingale through her sayings—a Victorian perspective.* London: Scutari Press.

Boivin, J. (1999, January). Psychiatric nursing: In search of a new generation. *Nursing Spectrum,* 4.

Cook, J. H. (1999, December–January). Nursing a headache. *Working Woman,* 16.

Jones, L. B. (1997). *Jesus in blue jeans: A practical guide to everyday spirituality.* New York: Hyperion.

Keenan, P. (1998). *Good news for bad days: Living a soulful life.* New York: Warner Books.

Mohr, W. K., & Naylor, M. D. (1998). Creating a curriculum for the 21st century. *Nursing Outlook, 46,* 206–211.

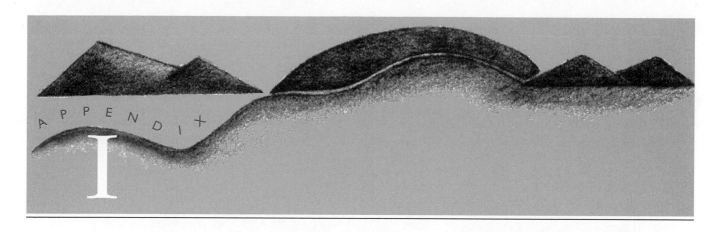

Standard Patient and Family Curriculum With Sample Teaching Tools

I. Patient education overview
  A. Purpose
  B. Introduction of instructor and participants
  C. Role of the participants
  D. Rights and responsibilities
  E. Expectations regarding participation, assignments, acceptable behavior
  F. Role of the instructor
  G. Topics for the different sessions
  H. Any materials (as necessary)
  I. Participant questions

II. Definition of mental illness
  A. Definition
  B. Overview of types of mental disorders
    1. Schizophrenia (see Patient Education: Schizophrenia)
    2. Other psychotic disorders
    3. Depressive disorder
    4. Anxiety disorder
    5. Bipolar disorder
    6. Cognitive disorders
    7. Personality disorder
    8. Substance use disorder
  C. Major symptoms experienced
    1. Behavioral symptoms
    2. Thought disturbances
    3. Perceptual disturbances
    4. Mood and emotional disturbances
  D. Variability of experiences
    1. Range of responses
    2. Participant responses
  E. Diagnostic procedures
    1. Physical examination
    2. Psychiatric examination
    3. Psychological tests
    4. Psychosocial assessment

  F. Treatment approaches
    1. Medical
    2. Medication
    3. Psychotherapies
    4. Educational
  G. Participant questions

III. Medications
  A. What each participant should know
    1. Name and type of medication
    2. Dosage and administration schedule
    3. Actions and side effects
    4. Special instructions
  B. Categories of major psychotropic medications
    1. Antipsychotic drugs (see Patient Education: Medications—Let's Check Your Learning)
    2. Antidepressant drugs
    3. Antianxiety agents
    4. Mood stabilizers
    5. Medications to treat side effects
  C. General principles of taking medications
    1. Rules
    2. Proper storage
    3. Cautions
  D. Importance of adhering to medication regimens
  E. Hazards of substance abuse
  F. Participant discussion of different experiences with medications
  G. Participant questions

IV. Monitoring mental illness
  A. Concept of illness
    1. Acute versus chronic nature
    2. Cyclic dynamics
    3. Relapse

PATIENT EDUCATION

Schizophrenia

What is schizophrenia?

Although no one knows the exact cause of schizophrenia, there are some things that we do know. First, schizophrenia is a brain disease; the brain chemicals do not work correctly. Second, there are things that can make a person more likely to get schizophrenia, such as developments before birth, trauma early in life, excessive stress, and inheritance. Third, schizophrenia does seem to run in families. It is not inherited like brown eyes but it does seem to be related to genetics.

Will I ever get better?

Although no two people with schizophrenia have the same experiences, there are many people with schizophrenia who function quite well. The illness is a chronic one and never goes away. But it is possible to learn about the illness and how you respond to it, and take charge of it. For instance, you may learn that when you are under a lot of stress, you have a recurrence of your schizophrenia symptoms. Over time, you can learn to recognize stress before you get sick and take action to reduce its impact on you.

What are the different types of schizophrenia?

There are five different types of schizophrenia. They are (1) paranoid, which is characterized by extreme suspiciousness, ideas about personal greatness (called delusions of grandeur), ideas about people trying to harm you (delusions of persecution), and hearing voices that no one else hears (called auditory hallucinations); (2) catatonic, which is characterized by a rigid, strange, or waxy (easily bendable) posture and negativity; (3) disorganized, which is characterized by no facial expressions, silly behavior, and incoherent communication; (4) undifferentiated, which is characterized by symptoms found in more than one type of schizophrenia; and (5) residual, which is characterized by lack of motivation and withdrawal without any of the strange perceptual symptoms such as hallucinations or delusions.

How can the doctor be sure that I have schizophrenia?

You have to have the symptoms of one of the types of schizophrenia for at least 6 months before the diagnosis of schizophrenia is made.

What can I do to keep myself well?

Actually, there are a lot of things that you can do. First, take your medication just as it is prescribed. If you have side effects that bother you, tell your nurse or doctor. Sometimes, the dose can be adjusted; sometimes, another medication of the same type will work better; sometimes, there is a simple but practical solution to the side effects (such as sucking on sugar-free candy to deal with a dry mouth). Whatever you do, don't just stop. If you do that, the symptoms will surely return. The next thing you can do is to learn as much as you can about how you react to the disease. Try to figure out what brings on the symptoms. It is stress and worry? Is it not getting enough sleep? The better you understand how you respond to the illness, the better able you will be to make healthy choices that will keep you well. Some other important things for you to do include eating a balanced diet, getting enough exercise, being around people who love you, working at something that is important to you, staying spiritually well, learning ways to cope with stress, structuring your time, and learning ways to distract yourself when hallucinations bother you.

What happens if the symptoms come back?

Unfortunately, the periodic return of symptoms is just what makes an illness chronic. But it is not the end of the world if symptoms return. If you are able to recognize the signs early enough, you may be able to prevent a relapse. This is an area in which your family and friends can help. Sometimes, they will see the warning signs before you do and can help you get the needed help.

What I need to know

Answer true or false to the next five items.
1. I have schizophrenia because I am a bad person.
   ❏ Yes   ❏ No
2. Hallucinations are hearing, seeing, smelling, tasting, or feeling things that no one else hears, sees, smells, tastes, or feels.
   ❏ Yes   ❏ No
3. A delusion is a belief that is not based on facts.
   ❏ Yes   ❏ No
4. Schizophrenia is caused by cancer.
   ❏ Yes   ❏ No
5. Schizophrenia is a brain disease.
   ❏ Yes   ❏ No

Choose the correct answer.
6. I have
   a. Paranoid schizophrenia
   b. Catatonic schizophrenia
   c. Disorganized schizophrenia
   d. Residual schizophrenia
   e. Undifferential schizophrenia

PATIENT EDUCATION

Schizophrenia Continued

7. Schizophrenia is
   a. Curable
   b. Chronic
   c. Contagious
   d. Catching
8. My symptoms include
   a. Suspicious thoughts
   b. Changes in my posture
   c. Silly behavior
   d. No motivation

9. I can learn to stay well by
   a. Managing my stress
   b. Eating organic foods
   c. Avoiding all medications
   d. Using alcohol and drugs
10. Learning about my illness
   a. Allows me to treat myself
   b. Gives me more to worry about
   c. Increases my control of the illness
   d. Leads to my cure

Carson, V. B. (1999). *Restore Family Behavioral Health Program*. New York: Staff Builders.

B. Symptoms
  1. Meaning of symptoms
  2. Recognizing symptoms
  3. Self-monitoring
  4. Individual symptom list
  5. Signs of relapse
C. Response needed
  1. Communication of concern
  2. Communication with family and support people
  3. Communication with health care provider
  4. Decrease of environmental stress
  5. Active positive response to seek assistance
D. Participant exchange about the meaning of mental illness as a chronic disorder
E. Participant discussion of experiences related to different symptoms
F. Participant questions

V. Coping and managing stress
  A. Definition of stress and coping
  B. Stress response
    1. Physiological effects
    2. Psychological effects
    3. Behavioral effects
    4. Sociological effects
  C. Stress and mental illness
  D. Reducing stress
    1. Lifestyle factors
    2. Environmental factors
    3. Relaxation techniques
    4. Cognitive coping techniques
  E. Developing individualized techniques to manage stress
  F. Participant discussion of stress management experiences
  G. Participant questions

PATIENT EDUCATION

Atypical Antipsychotic Medications

There are two kinds of antipsychotics: traditional and atypical. You are taking an atypical antipsychotic medicine. It is used to calm you, to stop delusions (beliefs that only you have), and to stop hallucinations (hearing, seeing, feeling, or smelling things that are not there). These medications are used in several diseases, including
- Schizophrenia
- Bipolar disorder or manic-depressive disorder
- Tourette's syndrome
- Dementia
- Other medical conditions that produce agitation, delusions, and hallucinations

The atypical antipsychotics include
- Clozaril (trade name)
- Clozapine (chemical or generic name)

- Risperdal (trade name)
- Risperidone (chemical or generic name)
- Zyprexa (trade name)
- Olanzapine (chemical or generic name)

The Name and Dose of Your Medication

You are taking _____ .
The dose is _____ mg _____ times a day. Do not stop taking your medication without your doctor's supervision; this will make your symptoms return.

If you forget to take your medicine but remember within 2 to 3 hours, take it. If it has been longer than 2 to 3 hours, skip the missed dose and take the remaining doses as scheduled. DO NOT DOUBLE UP.

PATIENT EDUCATION

Atypical Antipsychotic Medications Continued

Side Effects of Atypical Antipsychotic Medication

The following table lists possible side effects of these drugs and ways to deal with these side effects if you should be bothered by them. Please remember to let your nurse know about any symptoms that are new or that bother you. Your nurse will be able to help you with these.

Side Effect	*What to Do*
You feel dizzy	Drink plenty of fluids (6 to 8 12-ounce glasses of water every day). Change positions slowly, especially when you are standing up from a sitting or lying down position.
You are sleepy and feel groggy.	This will get better. Be patient and avoid activities that require fast thinking.
You are constipated.	Drinking more fluids, including prune juice, should help; eat bulk foods and exercise.
Your mouth is dry.	Suck on sugarless hard candy or chewing gum. Make sure you take good care of your teeth.
Your mouth is full of spit or saliva.	This will get better. Until it improves, carry tissues with you to wipe away the extra spit.

Side Effect	*What to Do*
You feel your heart racing. You have a seizure.	Stop taking the medication, and call the doctor immediately.
You feel like you have the flu, your throat is sore, you feel weak and feverish, you might have sores in your mouth (especially with clozapine).	Stop taking the clozapine (if that is the name of your medicine) and call your doctor immediately.

Warnings for Atypical Antipsychotic Medications

- Tell your doctor if you are pregnant or planning a pregnancy.
- Do not drive or operate machinery until you know how you will react to this medicine.
- Do not drink alcohol while taking this medicine.
- Keep all your appointments with your doctor and the laboratory so that your response to the medicine can be checked (for clozapine). Your doctor may need to change the amount of medicine you are taking, especially the first few weeks.
- Tell your doctor and nurse ALL the medications you are taking.
- Do not stop taking your medication without your doctor's approval. The dosage should be slowly decreased.
- Do not share your medication with other people.
- If you have an upset stomach and need an antacid, take it 2 hours before or after this medication.
- During the summer when it is hot and you are sweating more, increase the amount of fluid that you drink.

From Carson, V. B. (1999). *Restore Family Behavioral Health Program*. New York: Staff Builders.

VI. Communication and relationship skills
A. Definition of communication and relationship
B. Types of communication
  1. Verbal
  2. Nonverbal
C. Styles of communication
  1. Direct
  2. Indirect
  3. Active
  4. Passive
  5. Assertive
  6. Aggressive
D. Relating communication style to situation
E. Conversations
  1. Initiating interactions
  2. Topics
  3. Roles
F. Effective communication
  1. Principles
  2. Communication techniques
G. Role of communication in relating to others
H. Interpersonal interactions
  1. Social versus therapeutic relationship
  2. Phases of a relationship
I. Participant practice in effective communications and relating to others
J. Participant questions

PATIENT EDUCATION

Medications

Let's Check Your Learning

1. What medication are you taking?
2. Your medication is called a(n)
   a. Traditional antipsychotic
   b. Atypical antipsychotic
   c. Antidepressant
   d. Antianxiety
3. Your medication helps control
   a. Sadness
   b. Abnormal movements
   c. Hallucinations
   d. Dry mouth
4. What is the dose of your medication?
5. You should have taken your medication 2½ hours ago. You should
   a. Double up on your dose; take remaining doses as scheduled.
   b. Forget about that day's doses; start over the next day.
   c. Take the dose and take remaining doses as scheduled.
6. If your mouth is dry, you should
   a. Drink lots of prune juice
   b. Suck on sugarless candy
   c. Spit more
   d. Stop taking your medicine
7. If you feel constipated, you should
   a. Stop taking your medicine
   b. Drink at least 8 glasses of fluid a day

   c. Eat sugarless candy
   d. Change positions slowly
8. If you feel dizzy, you should
   a. Drink a glass of prune juice
   b. Eat sugarless candy
   c. Stop taking your medicine
   d. Change positions slowly
9. Your medicine helps with delusions, which are
   a. Beliefs that are not based on facts
   b. Strange sensations—like hearing voices or seeing things—that others do not share
   c. Unusual body movements
   d. A desire to withdraw from others
10. If you feel sleepy, you should
    a. Stop taking the medicine.
    b. Avoid activities that require concentration.
    c. Make yourself concentrate on fine details.
    d. Sleep until you feel rested.
11. If you taking clozapine and you feel like you have the flu-like achy muscles, fever, weakness, and sore throat, you should
    a. Stop taking the medicine; call your doctor immediately.
    b. Drink lots of fluid, go to bed, and rest.
    c. Take Tylenol, drink fluid, and eat bulk foods.
    d. Take Tylenol and change positions slowly.
12. If you are taking clozapine, how often must you have your blood drawn?

From Carson, V. B. (1999). *Restore Family Behavioral Health Program.* New York: Staff Builders.

VII. Interactions with family and support network representatives
   A. Roles of family members and support network representatives
   B. Effects of patient's mental illness on others
   C. Effects of temperament on coping with patient's mental illness
   D. Rights and responsibilities of family members and support network representatives
   E. Role of members in assisting management, treatment, and rehabilitation of the patient
      1. Gaining access to services
      2. Monitoring
      3. Medication management
      4. Partnership for care
   F. Communication with family members and others
   G. Participant practice and role-play of interactions with family members and support network representative

VIII. Community resources
   A. Identification of available resources
   B. Access to resources
      1. Procedures
      2. Strategies
   C. Categories of resources
      1. Housing and shelter
      2. Food
      3. Income
      4. Health care
      5. Rehabilitation
      6. Leisure activities
   D. List potential resources
      1. Social Security income
      2. Social Security disability income
      3. Public housing
      4. Private groups (e.g., Salvation Army, National Alliance for the Mentally Ill)
      5. Department of mental health (local and state)

6. Subsidized living residences
7. Medicare or Medicaid
8. Hospitals and clinics
9. Hotlines
10. Vocational rehabilitation services
E. Participant discussion about experiences with community resources

1. Positive
2. Negative and how resolved
F. Participant questions
IX. Detailed investigation of specific diagnoses of mental illness (as appropriate for participants or group)

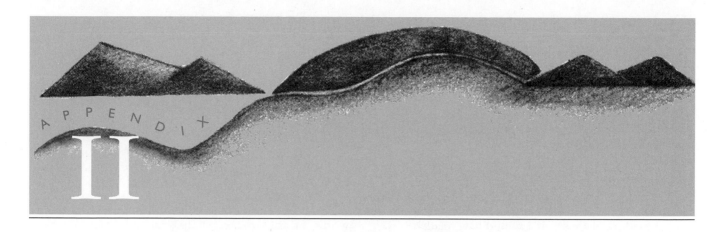

Spiritual Interventions Appropriate for Psychiatric Patients

DEFINITIONS OF AND DIFFERENTIATION BETWEEN SPIRITUALITY AND RELIGION

Spirituality is a broad term—one that is elusive to define but incredibly important to understand so that spiritual needs receive the attention that they deserve. Many people confuse spirituality and religion. These are certainly related terms, but it is worthwhile to differentiate them; both are important to psychiatric patients.

Spirituality is of the heart, it relates to experiences and the meanings we ascribe to those experiences, it is the way we align ourselves with God or the Divine. It is the recognition of the spirit within us and the commitment to make choices, to develop attitudes, and to behave in ways consistent with that presence. Spirituality usually involves relationships and feelings of connectedness to and a sense of responsibility for the well-being of others and the world around us.

Conversely, *religions* are "human-made"; they provide structure, rules and consequences, rituals, symbolism, and a way to worship that shapes our relationship to the Divine. For many individuals, religion provides the most important expression of their spirituality. For others, religion is irrelevant to their lives. And still others use religion to meet needs other than those that are spiritual, such as social needs and needs for belonging and affirmation. The following discussion provides you with guidelines for meeting both the spiritual as well as the religious needs of your psychiatric patients.

INTERVENTIONS TO MEET SPIRITUAL NEEDS

There are two general categories of interventions, ministry of action and ministry of word. Both of these categories refer more to the kind of person you are and your willingness to enter into a relationship with openness, genuineness, vulnerability, and true compassion than to specific concrete tasks or strategies.

Ministry of Action

Ministry of action refers to the "way you do what you do." Some questions to ask yourself about the way you do what you do include

1. Do I listen and hear not only the words that the individual uses but also the feelings expressed by the words and the message that lies under the surface of the words?

2. Am I willing to respond to the hidden messages that individuals convey?

3. Do I really accept people as they are, even when they act in ways that are not lovable? Do I judge others harshly and hastily without looking below the surface for the "whys and wherefores" of their behaviors?

4. Do I really care about what happens to others? Do I communicate that care in the little things that I do as I go about doing my assigned task? Do I go out of my way for others? Am I gentle when I provide physical ministrations to people?

1131

5. Are my words gentle? Are those words uttered with a sense of concern for the effect they may have on the listener? Am I thoughtful about the words that I choose, recognizing the power they hold to build up another person's sense of worth or to add injury to an already wounded individual?

6. Am I able to be present with others and attempt to fully enter into their experiences and their pain? Or do I build a protective wall between myself and others that allows me to avoid being touched by their pain?

7. Do I support others as they make decisions? Am I able to accept their decisions even when they are in conflict with decisions that I would have made?

8. Do I revere the uniqueness of the other person? Am I able to see beyond troubling behaviors and disordered thinking to the wonder of who that person really is?

9. Do my actions and my attitudes communicate hope in the person's ability to change? Or do my actions and attitudes communicate hopelessness and cynicism about the person's future?

10. Do I accept that everyone's spiritual journey is unique? Do I recognize that although I may be privileged to participate in another's journey, it is neither my responsibility nor my right to dictate the direction of that journey?

Ministry of the Word

Ministry of the word refers to the specific verbal interventions that focus on spiritual issues. When we verbally acknowledge the importance of spirituality or religion, we are not only giving the patient permission to discuss these issues but also giving credibility to the patient's beliefs and practices. Some examples of verbal interventions include the following:

1. Asking about spiritual matters in our initial assessment of a patient and in our ongoing interactions with the patient is important. Questions that validate the importance of the spiritual to the patient's healing include the following:

- What do you think God's role is in your illness?
- What is God's role in your healing?
- How does your spirituality or relationship to God help you or hinder you as you go through each day?
- What do you hope for?
- What supports your hope?
- How can I support your beliefs?
- What did that experience mean to you?
- What have you learned from this experience?

2. Asking about the place of prayer in the patient's life may provide a powerful intervention for you and other health professionals. Prayer is communication with the Divine; it serves the same purpose that all communication does and that is to provide a bridge or link to the one to whom we are communicating. Prayer may take many forms: some people use formalized prayers such as the Lord's Prayer spoken by Christians, others quietly meditate, still others engage in conversa- tional monologue with God. Regardless of the form prayer takes, it is important for you to be aware that as a form of communication, prayer may be negatively affected by illness. People who are suffering and in pain often have difficulty praying. They may feel cut off or estranged from God just because they are un- able to communicate. What can you do? You can always offer to pray *for* them. You can also ask if they would like you to pray *with* them. Two caveats are in order here. First, always ask—never assume this is what the patient wants. Remember, your focus is on meeting the patient's needs and not your own. Second, the words of your prayer should not be based on your faith tradition, which might increase the patient's anxiety and concern. The prayer should be either in a form that the patient is comfortable with or generic enough so as to reestablish that communication bridge between the patient and the Divine. For instance, if you are Christian and you are praying for a Jewish patient, your prayer can be addressed "Dear God" or "Dear Father of Abraham [Isaac, Jacob]." If the patient is delusional or hallucinating and desires prayer, you address the underlying theme of the delusion or hallucination. For instance, if a patient is expressing a delusional belief that the Federal Bureau of Investigation (FBI) has wiretapped the inpatient unit, you would not pray that God destroy the FBI. Rather, you would pray: "Dear God, please ease my patient's fear and give him peace of mind."

3. Share your own perspective from the "I" posi- tion, never from the perspective of evangelizing or persuading the patient to accept your beliefs. Remem- ber, as caregivers we are in a position of power in relationship to patients. It is important not only that we recognize the unequal power distribution between us and our patients but also that we *never impose our beliefs on patients.* The guidelines regarding the appropriateness of self-disclosure provided in Chapter 10 are also appropriate when it comes to sharing our spirituality or our religious beliefs. This sharing is never in the form of telling the patient "You should be- lieve this" or "You should do this "; rather, the sharing takes the following form: "I find that this belief or practice is helpful in my life" or "I have come to believe. . . ."

INTERVENTIONS TO MEET RELIGIOUS NEEDS

Religion, with its beliefs, rituals, and communal experi- ence, serves as a vehicle for the expression of a person's spirituality. Most people satisfy their spiritual needs through a particular religious tradition. Ideally, religion provides an atmosphere for spiritual development. It is not necessary for you to become an expert on the practices of all religions. Rather, you need to be an expert at *inquiring* about the practices that are meaningful and important to your patient, and, to the best of your ability, incorporating, facilitating, or allowing those practices within the context of the care you are providing.

Theistic Religions

Tables A-1 through A-5 provide specific information regarding the practices of various theistic faiths. See Chapter 1 for discussion of different world views.

T A B L E A – I Jewish Beliefs and Practices Affecting Health Care	
RELIGIOUS GROUP	**BELIEFS AND PRACTICES**
Observant Jews (Orthodox Judaism and some Conservative Jewish groups)	*Birth:* For observant Jews, babies are named by the father. Male children are named 8 days after birth, when ritual circumcision is done. A mohel performs the circumcision. Circumcision may be postponed if the infant is in poor health. Female babies are usually named during the reading of the Holy Torah. Nurses need to be sensitive to the wishes of the parents when caring for babies who have not yet been named. *Care of women:* A woman is considered to be in a ritual state of impurity whenever blood is coming from her uterus, such as during menstrual periods and after the birth of a child. During this time, her husband will not have physical contact with her. When this time is completed, she will bathe herself in a pool called a *mikvah.* Nurses need to be aware of this practice and be sensitive to the husband and wife because the husband will not touch his wife. He cannot assist her in moving in the bed, so the nurse will have to do this. An Orthodox Jewish man will not touch any women other than his wife, daughters, and mother. Home health care workers need to be aware of these practices. *Dietary rules:* (1) Kosher dietary laws include the following: No mixing of milk and meat at a meal; no consumption of food or any derivative thereof from animals not slaughtered in accordance with Jewish law; use of separate cooking utensils for meat and milk products; if a client requires milk and meat products for a meal, the dairy foods should be served first, followed later by the meat. (2) During Yom Kippur (Day of Atonement), a 24-hour fast is required, but exceptions are made for those who cannot fast because of medical reasons. (3) During Passover, no leavened products are eaten. (4) May say benediction of thanksgiving before meals and grace at the end of the meal. Time and a quiet environment should be provided for this. *Sabbath:* Observed from sunset Friday until sunset Saturday, Orthodox law prohibits riding in a car, smoking, turning lights on and off, handling money, and using television and telephone. Nurses need to be aware of this when caring for observant Jews at home and in the hospital. Medical or surgical treatments should be postponed if possible. *Death:* Judaism defines death as occurring when respiration and circulation are irreversibly stopped and no movement is apparent. (1) Euthanasia is strictly forbidden by Orthodox Jews, who advocate the strict use of life-support measures. (2) Prior to death, Jewish faith indicates that visiting of the person by family and friends is a religious duty. The Torah and Psalms may be read and prayers recited. A witness needs to be present when a person prays for health so that if death occurs God will protect the family and the spirit will be committed to God. Extraneous talking and conversation about death are not encouraged unless initiated by the patient or visitors. In Judaism, the belief is that people should have someone with them when the soul leaves the body, so family and/or friends should be allowed to stay with patients. After death, the body should be left alone until buried, usually within 24 hours. (3) When death occurs, the body should be untouched for 8 to 30 minutes. Medical personnel should not touch or wash the body but allow only an Orthodox person or the Jewish Burial Society to care for the body. Handling of a corpse on the Sabbath is forbidden to Jewish persons. If need be, the nursing staff may provide routine care of the body, wearing gloves. Water in the room should be emptied, and the family may request that mirrors be covered to symbolize that a death has occurred. (4) Orthodox Jews and some Conservative Jews do not approve of autopsies. If an autopsy must be done, all body parts must remain with the body. (5) For Orthodox Jews, the body must be buried within 24 hours. No flowers are permitted. A fetus must be buried. (6) A 7-day mourning period is required by the immediate family. They must stay at home except for Sabbath worship. (7) Organs or other body parts such as amputated limbs must be made available for burial for Orthodox Jews, since they believe that all of the body must be returned to earth. *Birth control and abortion:* Artificial methods of birth control are not encouraged. Vasectomy is not allowed. Abortion may be performed only to save the mother's life. *Organ transplant:* Donor organ transplants generally are not permitted by Orthodox Jews but may be allowed with rabbinical consent. *Shaving:* The beard is regarded as a mark of piety among observant Jews. For the very Orthodox, shaving should not be done with a razor but with scissors or electric razor, since a blade should not contact the skin. *Head covering:* Orthodox men wear skull caps at all times, and women cover their hair after marriage. Some Orthodox women wear wigs as a mark of piety. Conservative Jews cover their heads only during acts of worship and prayer. *Prayer:* Praying directly to God, including a prayer of confession, is required for Orthodox Jews. Nurses should provide quiet time for prayer.

Table continued on following page

TABLE A–1 Jewish Beliefs and Practices Affecting Health Care *Continued*	
RELIGIOUS GROUP	**BELIEFS AND PRACTICES**
Reform Jews	*Birth:* Reform Jews may or may not adhere to the practices referred to for observant Jews. They favor ritual circumcision, but it is not imperative. *Care of women:* Reform Jews do not observe the rules against touching. *Dietary rules:* Reform Jews usually do not observe kosher dietary restrictions. *Sabbath:* Usually worship in temples on Friday evenings. No strict rules. *Death:* Advocate use of life support without heroic measures. Allow for cremation but suggest that ashes be buried in a Jewish cemetery. *Organ transplants:* Donation or transplantation of organs allowed with permission of a rabbi. *Head coverings:* Generally pray without wearing skull caps.

From Carson, V. B. (1989). *Spiritual dimensions of nursing practice.* Philadelphia: W. B. Saunders. Based on data compiled from Gershan, J. A. (1985). Judaic ethical beliefs and customs regarding death and dying. *Critical Care Nurse, 5,* 32–34; Kertzer Rabbi, M. N. (1978). *What is a Jew?* (4th ed.). New York: Collier Books; McAteer, J. (Ed.). (1975). Religion: Recognizing your patient's spiritual needs. *Nursing Update, 6*(1), 3–9; Pumphrey, J. (1977). Recognizing your patient's spiritual needs. *Nursing 77, 7,* 64–70; Sauer, M. (1987, August 18). Personal communication; and Whaley, L. F., & Wong, D. L. (1987). *Nursing care of infants and children* (3rd ed.). St. Louis, MO: C. V. Mosby.

TABLE A–2 Roman Catholic and Eastern Orthodox Beliefs and Practices Affecting Health Care	
RELIGIOUS GROUP	**BELIEFS AND PRACTICES**
Roman Catholic	*Birth:* Since Roman Catholics believe that unbaptized children are cut off from heaven, infant baptism is mandatory. For newborns with a grave prognosis, stillborns, and all aborted fetuses (unless evidence of tissue necrosis and prolonged death are present), emergency baptism is required. The nurse calls a priest to perform the baptism unless the death might occur before the priest arrives. In that case, anyone can baptize by pouring warm water on the infant's head and saying, "I baptize you in the name of the Father, of the Son, and of the Holy Spirit." All information about the baptism is recorded on the chart, and the priest and family notified. *Holy Eucharist:* For clients and health care givers who are to receive communion, abstinence from solid food and alcohol is required for 15 minutes (if possible) prior to reception of the consecrated wafer. Medicine, water, and nonalcoholic drinks are permitted at any time. If a client is in danger of death, the fast is waived since the reception of the Eucharist at this time is very important. *Anointing of the sick:* The priest uses oil to anoint the forehead and hands and, if desired, the affected area. The rite may be performed on any who are ill and desire it. Persons receiving the sacrament seek complete healing and strength to endure suffering. Prior to 1963, this sacrament was only given to persons at time of imminent death, so the nurse must be sensitive to the meaning this has for the client. If possible, the nurse calls a priest before the client is unconscious but may also call when there is sudden death, since the sacrament may also be given shortly after death. The nurse records on the care plan that this sacrament has been administered. *Dietary habits:* Obligatory fasting is excused during hospitalization. However, if there are no health restrictions, some Catholics may still observe the following guidelines: (1) Anyone 14 years or older must abstain from eating meat on Ash Wednesday and all Fridays during Lent. Some older Catholics may still abstain from meat on all Fridays of the year. (2) In addition to abstinence from meat, persons 21 to 59 years of age must limit themselves to one full meal and two light meals on Ash Wednesday and Good Friday. (3) Eastern Rite Catholics are stricter about fasting and fast more frequently than Western Rite Catholics, so it is important for the nurse to know if a client is Eastern or Western. *Death:* Each Roman Catholic should participate in the anointing of the sick as well as the Eucharist and penance before death. The body should not be shrouded until after these sacraments are performed. All body parts that retain human quality must be appropriately buried or cremated. *Birth control:* Prohibited except for abstinence or natural family planning. Referral to a priest for questions about this can be of great help. Nurses can teach the techniques of natural family planning if they are familiar with them; otherwise, this should be referred to the physician or to a support group of the church that instructs couples in this method of birth control. Sterilization is prohibited unless there is an overriding medical reason. *Organ donation:* Donation and transplantation of organs are acceptable as long as the donor is not harmed and is not deprived of life. *Religious objects:* Rosary prayers are said using rosary beads. Medals bearing the images of saints, relics, statues, and scapulars are important objects that may be pinned to a hospital gown or pillow or be at the bedside. Extreme care should be taken not to lose these objects, since they have special meaning to the client.

TABLE A–2 Roman Catholic and Eastern Orthodox Beliefs and Practices Affecting Health Care
Continued

RELIGIOUS GROUP	BELIEFS AND PRACTICES
Eastern Orthodox	*Birth:* The child must be baptized within 40 days after birth. If sprinkling or immersion into water is not possible, baptism is performed by moving the baby in the air in the sign of the cross. An ordained priest or a deacon must be notified for this. *Holy Eucharist:* The priest is notified if the client desires this sacrament. *Anointing of the sick:* The priest conducts this in the hospital room. *Dietary habits:* Fasting from meat and dairy products is required on Wednesday and Friday during Lent and on other holy days. Hospital clients are exempt if fasting is detrimental to health. *Special days:* Christmas is celebrated on January 7 and New Year's on January 14. This is important to the care of a client who is hospitalized on these days. *Death:* Last rites are obligatory. This is handled by an ordained priest who is notified by the nurse while the client is conscious. The Russian Orthodox Church does not encourage autopsy or organ donation. Euthanasia, even for the terminally ill, is discouraged, as is cremation. *Birth control:* This as well as abortion is not permitted.

From Carson, V. B. (1989). *Spiritual dimensions of nursing practice.* Philadelphia: W. B. Saunders. Based on data compiled from Hendricks, D. W. (1975). What is a Catholic? In L. Rosten (Ed.), *Religions in America.* New York: Simon and Schuster; McAteer, J. (Ed.). (1975). Religion: Recognizing your patient's spiritual needs. *Nursing Update, 6*(1), 3–9; O'Brien, W. J. (1987, August 25). Personal communication; Pumphrey, J. (1977). Recognizing your patient's spiritual needs. *Nursing 77, 7,* 64–70; and Whaley, L. F., & Wong, D. L. (1987). *Nursing care of infants and children* (3rd ed.). St. Louis, MO: C. V. Mosby.

TABLE A–3 Various Protestant Beliefs and Practices Affecting Health Care

RELIGIOUS GROUP	BELIEFS AND PRACTICES
Assemblies of God (Pentecostal)	*Baptism:* Water baptism by complete immersion is practiced when an individual has received Jesus Christ as Savior and Lord based on Acts 2:38. *Holy Communion:* Notify clergy if the client desires. *Anointing of the sick:* Members believe in divine healing through prayer and the laying on of hands. Clergy is notified if client or family desires this. *Dietary habits:* Abstinence from alcohol, tobacco, and all illegal drugs is strongly encouraged. *Death:* No special practices. *Other practices:* Faith in God and in the health care providers is encouraged. Members pray for divine intervention in health matters. Nurses should encourage and allow time for prayer. Members may speak in "tongues" during prayer.
Baptist (over 27 different groups in the United States)	*Baptism:* Do not practice infant baptism. *Holy Communion:* Clergy should be notified if the client desires. *Dietary habits:* Total abstinence from alcohol is expected. *Death:* No general service is provided, but the clergy does minister through counseling, prayer, and Scripture as requested by the client or family, and the client is encouraged to believe in Jesus Christ as Savior and Lord. *Other practices:* The Bible is held to be the word of God, so the nurse should either allow quiet time for Scripture reading or offer to read to the client.
Christian Church (Disciples of Christ)	*Baptism:* Do not practice infant baptism but have dedication service. Believers are baptized by immersion. *Holy Communion:* Open communion is celebrated each Sunday and is a central part of worship services. The nurse notifies the clergy if the client desires it, or the clergy may suggest it. *Death:* No special practices. *Other practices:* Church elders as well as clergy may be notified to assist with meeting the client's spiritual needs.
Church of the Brethren	*Baptism:* Do not practice infant baptism but have dedication service. *Holy Communion:* Usually received within church, but clergy will give it in the hospital when requested. *Anointing of the sick:* Practiced for physical healing as well as spiritual uplift and held in high regard by the church. The clergy is notified if the client or family desire. *Death:* The clergy is notified for counsel and prayer.
Church of the Nazarene	*Baptism:* Parents have the choice of baptism or dedication for their infant. Emphasis is on the believer's baptism, which is regarded as a symbol of the New Covenant in Jesus Christ. *Holy Communion:* Pastor will administer if the client wishes. *Dietary habits:* The use of alcohol and tobacco is forbidden. *Death:* Cremation is permitted, and term stillborn infants are buried. *Other practices:* Believe in divine healing but not to the exclusion of medical treatment. Clients may desire quiet time for prayer.

Table continued on following page

RELIGIOUS GROUP	BELIEFS AND PRACTICES
Episcopal (Anglican)	*Baptism:* Infant baptism is practiced and is considered urgent if the infant is critically ill. The priest is notified to administer the sacrament. Lay persons may baptize in an emergency. *Holy Communion:* The priest is notified if the client wishes to receive this sacrament. *Anointing of the sick:* Priest may administer this rite when death is imminent, but it is not considered mandatory. *Dietary habits:* Some clients may abstain from meat on Fridays. Others may fast before receiving the Eucharist, but fasting is not mandatory. *Death:* No special practices. *Other practices:* Confession of sins to a priest is optional; if the client desires this, the clergy should be notified.
Lutheran (10 different branches)	*Baptism:* Baptize only living infants any time, but usually 6 to 8 weeks after birth. Adults are also baptized, and modes of baptism as appropriate include sprinkling, pouring, or immersion. *Holy Communion:* Notify the clergy if the client desires this sacrament. Clergy may also inquire about the client's desire. *Anointing of the sick:* The client may request an anointing and blessing from the minister when the prognosis is poor. *Death:* A service of Commendation of the Dying is used at the client's or family's request.
Mennonite (12 different groups)	*Baptism:* No infant baptism, but the child may be dedicated if requested by the parents. *Holy Communion:* Served twice a year, with foot washing as part of ceremony. *Dietary habits:* Abstinence from alcohol is urged for all. *Death:* Prayer is important at time of crisis, so contacting a minister is important. *Other practices:* Women may wear head coverings during hospitalization. Anointing with oil is administered in harmony with James 5:14 when requested.
Methodist (over 20 different groups)	*Baptism:* Notify the clergy if the parent desires baptism for a sick infant. *Holy Communion:* Notify the clergy if a client requests it prior to surgery or another health crisis. *Anointing of the sick:* If requested, the clergy will come to spray and sprinkle the client with olive oil. *Death:* Scripture reading and prayer are important at this time. *Other practices:* Donation of one's body or part of the body at death is encouraged.
Presbyterian (10 different groups)	*Baptism:* Infant baptism is practiced by pouring or sprinkling. Immersion is also practiced at times for adults. *Holy Communion:* Given when appropriate and convenient, at the hospitalized client's request. *Death:* Notify a local pastor or elder for prayer and Scripture reading if desired by the family or client.
Quaker (Friends)	*Baptism and Holy Communion:* Since Friends have no creed there is a diversity of personal beliefs, one of which is that outward sacraments are usually not necessary since there is the ministry of the Spirit inwardly in such areas as baptism and communion. A few Friends baptize with water. *Death:* Believe that the present life is part of God's kingdom and generally have no ceremony as a rite of passage from this life to the next. Personal beliefs and wishes need to be ascertained, and the nurse can then act upon the client's wishes. *Other practices:* The name of the Quaker infant is recorded in official record books at the local meeting.
Salvation Army	*Baptism:* No particular ceremony, but they do have an Infant Dedication ceremony. *Holy Communion:* No particular ceremony. *Death:* Notify the local officer in charge of the Army Corps for any soldier (member) who needs assistance. *Other practices:* The Bible is seen as the only rule for one's faith, so the Scriptures should be made available to a client. The Army has many of its own social welfare centers, with hospitals and homes where unwed mothers are cared for and outpatient services provided. No medical or surgical procedures are opposed, except for abortion on demand.
Seventh-Day Adventist	*Baptism:* No infant baptism is practiced, but have dedication services. *Holy Communion:* Although this is not required of hospitalized clients, the clergy is notified if the client desires. *Anointing of the sick:* The clergy are contacted for prayer and anointing with oil. *Dietary habits:* Since the body is viewed as the temple of the Holy Spirit, healthy living is essential. Therefore the use of alcohol, tobacco, coffee, and tea and the promiscuous use of drugs are prohibited. Some are vegetarians, and most avoid pork. *Special days:* The Sabbath is observed on Saturday. *Death:* No special procedures. *Other related practices:* Use of hypnotism is opposed by some. Persons of homosexual or lesbian orientation are ministered to in the hope of correction of these practices, which are believed to be wrong. A Bible should always be available for Scripture reading.
United Church of Christ	*Baptism:* Practice infant and adult baptism. Three modes are used as appropriate: pouring, sprinkling, and immersion. *Holy Communion:* Clergy is notified if the client desires to receive this sacrament. *Death:* If the client desires counsel or prayer, notify the clergy.

From Carson, V. B. (1989). *Spiritual dimensions of nursing practice.* Philadelphia: W. B. Saunders. Based on data compiled from Bingman, S. F. (1987, August). Personal communication; McAteer, J. (Ed.). (1975). Religion: Recognizing your patient's spiritual needs. *Nursing Update, 6*(1), 3–9; and Pumphrey, J. (1977). Recognizing your patient's spiritual needs. *Nursing 77, 7,* 64–70.

TABLE A-4 Islamic and Muslim Beliefs and Practices Affecting Health Care

RELIGIOUS GROUP	BELIEFS AND PRACTICES
Islam	*Birth:* A baby is bathed immediately after birth, before giving it to the mother. The father (or mother if the father is not available) then whispers the call to prayer in the child's ears so that the first sounds it hears are about the Muslim faith. Circumcision is culturally recommended before puberty. A baby born prematurely but at least 130 days gestation is given the same treatment as any other infant. *Dietary habits:* No pork is allowed, nor alcoholic beverages. All *halal* (permissible) meat must be blessed and killed in a special way. This is called *zabihah* (correctly slaughtered). *Death:* Prior to death, family members ask to be present so that they can read the Koran and pray with the client. An Imam may come if requested by the client or family but is not required. Clients must face Mecca and confess their sins and beg forgiveness in the presence of their family. If the family is unavailable, any practicing Muslim can provide support to the client. After death, Muslims prefer that the family wash, prepare, and place the body in a position facing Mecca. If necessary, the health care providers may perform these procedures as long as they wear gloves. Burial is performed as soon as possible. Cremation is forbidden. Autopsy is also prohibited except for legal reasons, and then no body part is to be removed. Donation of body parts or organs is not allowed, since according to culturally developed law persons do not own their body. *Abortion and birth control:* Abortion is forbidden, and many conservative Muslims do not encourage the use of contraceptives since this interferes with God's purpose. Others feel that a woman should only have as many children as her husband can afford. Contraception is permitted by Islamic law. *Personal devotions:* At prayer time, washing is required, even by those who are sick. A client on bed rest may require assistance with this task before prayer. Provision of privacy is important during prayer. *Religious objects:* The Koran must not be touched by anyone ritually unclean, and nothing should be placed on top of it. Some Muslims wear *taviz*, a black string on which words of the Koran are attached. These should not be removed and must remain dry. Certain items of jewelry such as bangles may have religious significance and should not be removed unnecessarily. *Care of women:* Since women are not allowed to sign consent forms or make a decision regarding family planning, the husband needs to be present. Women are very modest and frequently wear clothes that cover all of the body. During a medical examination, the woman's modesty should be respected as much as possible. Muslim women prefer female doctors. For 40 days after giving birth and also during menstruation, a woman is exempt from prayer since this is a time of cleansing for her.
American Muslim Mission	*Baptism:* No baptism is practiced. *Dietary habits:* In addition to refusing pork, many will not eat traditional black American foods such as corn bread and collard greens. *Death:* The family is contacted before any care of the deceased is performed. There are special procedures for washing and shrouding the body. *Other practices:* Quiet time is necessary to permit prayer. Members are encouraged to use black physicians for health care. Since these clients do not smoke, their request for a nonsmoking roommate should be honored.

From Carson, V. B. (1989). *Spiritual dimensions of nursing practice.* Philadelphia: W. B. Saunders. Based on data compiled from Henley, A., & Clayton, J. (1982). Religion of the Muslims. *Health Social Service Journal, 92,* 918–919; McAteer, J. (Ed.). (1975). Religion: Recognizing your patient's spiritual needs. *Nursing Update, 6*(1), 3–9; Mead, F. S., & Hill, S. S. (1985). *Handbook of denominations in the United States* (8th ed.). Nashville, TN: Abingdon Press; Peterson, W. J. (1982). *Those curious new cults in the 80s.* New Canaan, CT: Keats; Pumphrey, J. (1977). Recognizing your patient's spiritual needs. *Nursing 77, 7,* 64–70; and Rahim, A. (1987, August 7). Personal communication.

TABLE A-5 Christian Science, Jehovah's Witnesses, Church of Jesus Christ of Latter-Day Saints, Unitarian Universalist, and Unification Church Beliefs and Practices Affecting Health Care

RELIGIOUS GROUP	BELIEFS AND PRACTICES
Christian Science	*Birth:* Use physician or nurse midwife during childbirth. No baptism ceremony. *Dietary habits:* Since alcohol and tobacco are considered drugs, they are not used. Coffee and tea are often declined. *Death:* Autopsy is usually declined unless required by law. Donation of organs is unlikely, but is an individual decision. *Other practices:* Do not normally seek medical care, since they approach health care in a different, primarily spiritual, framework. They commonly utilize the services of a surgeon to set a bone but decline drugs and, in general, other medical or surgical procedures. Hypnotism and psychotherapy are also declined. Family planning is left to the family. They seek exemption from vaccinations but obey legal requirements. Report infectious diseases and obey public health quarantines. Nonmedical care facilities are maintained for those needing nursing assistance in the course of a healing. *The Christian Science Journal* lists available Christian Science nurses. When a Christian Science believer is in the hospital, the nurse should allow and encourage time for prayer and study. Clients may request that a Christian Science practitioner be notified to come.

Table continued on following page

T A B L E A – 5 Christian Science, Jehovah's Witnesses, Church of Jesus Christ of Latter-Day Saints, Unitarian Universalist, and Unification Church Beliefs and Practices Affecting Health Care *Continued*

RELIGIOUS GROUP	BELIEFS AND PRACTICES
Jehovah's Witnesses	*Baptism:* No infant baptism is practiced. Baptism by complete immersion of adults is done as a symbol of dedication to Jehovah, since Jesus was baptized. *Dietary habits:* Use of alcohol and tobacco is discouraged, since these harm the physical body. *Death:* Autopsy is a private matter to be decided by the persons involved. Burial and cremation are acceptable. *Birth control and abortion:* Use of birth control is a personal decision. Abortion is opposed based on Exodus 21:22–23. *Organ transplants:* Use of organ transplant is a private decision and if used must be cleansed with a nonblood solution. *Blood Transfusions:* Blood transfusions violate God's laws and are therefore not allowed. Clients do respect physicians and will accept alternatives to blood transfusions. These might include use of nonblood plasma expanders, careful surgical techniques to decrease blood loss, use of autologous transfusions, and autotransfusion through use of a heart-lung machine. Nurses should check unconscious clients for Medic Alert cards that state that the person does not want a transfusion. Since Jehovah's Witnesses are prepared to die rather than break God's law, nurses need to be sensitive to the spiritual as well as the physical needs of the client.
Church of Jesus Christ of Latter-Day Saints	*Baptism:* If a child over the age of 8 is very ill, whether baptized or unbaptized, a member of the church's priesthood should be called. *Holy Communion:* A hospitalized client may desire to have a member of the church priesthood administer this sacrament. *Anointing of the sick:* Mormons frequently are anointed and given a blessing before going to the hospital and after admission by laying on of hands. *Dietary habits:* Abstinence from the use of tobacco; beverages with caffeine such as cola, coffee, and tea; alcohol and other substances considered injurious. Mormons eat meat but encourage the intake of fruits, grains, and herbs. *Death:* Prefer burial of the body. A church elder should be notified to assist the family. If need be, the elder will assist the funeral director in dressing the body in special clothes and will give other help as needed. *Birth control and abortion:* Abortion is opposed except when the life of the mother is in danger. Only natural means of birth control are recommended. Artificial means can be used when the health of the woman is at stake (including emotional health). *Personal care:* Cleanliness is very important to Mormons. A sacred undergarment may be worn at all times by Mormons and should only be removed in emergency situations. *Other practices:* Allowing quiet time for prayer and the reading of the sacred writings is important. The church maintains a welfare system to assist those in need. Families are of great importance, so visiting should be encouraged.
Unitarian Universalist Association	*Baptism:* Infant baptism is unnecessary and if used at all is without trinitarian formula. Usually dedicate their children. *Death:* Cremation is often preferred to burial. *Other practices:* Use of birth control is advocated as part of responsible parenting. Strong support for a woman's right to choice regarding abortion is maintained. Unitarian Universalists advocate donation of body parts for research and transplants.
Unification Church	*Baptism:* No baptism. *Special days:* Sunday mornings are used to honor Reverend and Mrs. Moon as the true parents, and members get up at 5:00 A.M., bow before a picture of the Moons three times, and vow to do what is needed to help the Reverend accomplish his mission on earth. *Death:* Believe that after death one's place of destiny will depend on his or her spirit's quality of life and goodness while on earth. In the afterlife, one will have the same aspirations and feelings as before death. Hell is not a concern, since it will not be a place as heaven grows in size. Persons who leave the Unification Church are warned that Satan may try to possess them. *Other practices:* All marriages must be solemnized by Reverend Moon in order to be part of the perfect family and have salvation. The church supplies its faithful members with life's necessities. Members may use occult practices to have spiritual and psychic experiences.

From Carson, V. B. (1989). *Spiritual dimensions of nursing practice.* Philadelphia: W. B. Saunders. Based on data compiled from Chworowsky, K. M., & Raible, C. G. (1975). What is a Unitarian/Universalist? In L. Rosten (Ed.), *Religions in America.* New York: Simon and Schuster; Durst, M. (1984). *To bigotry, no sanction.* Chicago: Regnery Gateway; Evans, R. L. (1975). What is a Mormon? In L. Rosten (Ed.), *Religions in America.* New York: Simon and Schuster; Henschel, M. G. (1975). What is a Jehovah's Witness? In L. Rosten (Ed.), *Religions in America.* New York: Simon and Schuster; John, D. (1962). *The Christian Science way of life.* Englewood Cliffs, NJ: Prentice-Hall; Jones, I. H. (1984). Bearing witness. *Nursing Times,* 80, 47–48; McAteer, J. (Ed.). (1975). Religion: Recognizing your patient's spiritual needs. *Nursing Update,* 6(1), 3–9; McDowell, J., & Stewart, D. (1982). *Handbook of today's religions—understanding the cults.* San Bernardino, CA: Here's Life; Pumphrey, J. (1977). Recognizing your patient's spiritual needs. *Nursing 77,* 7, 64–70; Richards, F. (1977). What they believe and why: Roman Catholics, Jehovah's Witnesses, and Christian Scientists. *Nursing Monitor,* 144, 65–66; Sontag, F. (1977). *Sun Myung Moon and the Unification Church.* Nashville, TN: Abingdon Press; and Stokes, J. B. (1975). What is a Christian Scientist? In L. Rosten (Ed.), *Religions in America.* New York: Simon and Schuster.

Nontheistic Religions

Many of the religions practiced in the Far East are nontheistic. Buddhism is *pantheistic* (believing everything is god). Other religions, such as Hinduism, are *polytheistic* (believing in many gods). The beliefs, practices, and rituals are not as easily classified and categorized as they are for the theistic faiths (Van Voorst, 1994). For this reason, it is absolutely essential that you ask the Buddhist patient what practices, beliefs, and rituals are important to him or her. This holds true for the Hindu patient, the Native American patient, and any patients with whose belief systems you are unfamiliar.

References

Carson, V. B. (1989). *Spiritual dimensions of nursing practice.* W. B. Saunders, Philadelphia.

Van Voorst, R. E. (1994). *Anthology of world scriptures.* Belmont, CA: Wadsworth.

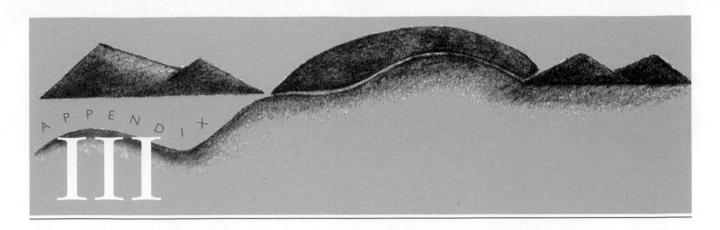

DSM-IV Classification

NOS = Not Otherwise Specified.

An *x* appearing in a diagnostic code indicates that a specific code number is required.

An ellipsis (. . .) is used in the names of certain disorders to indicate that the name of a specific mental disorder or general medical condition should be inserted when recording the name (e.g., 293.0 Delirium due to Hypothyroidism).

Numbers in parentheses are page numbers.*

If criteria are currently met, one of the following severity specifiers may be noted after the diagnosis:

Mild
Moderate
Severe

If criteria are no longer met, one of the following specifiers may be noted:

In Partial Remission
In Full Remission
Prior History

Disorders Usually First Diagnosed in Infancy, Childhood, or Adolescence (37)

MENTAL RETARDATION (39)
Note: These are coded on Axis II.
317	Mild Mental Retardation (41)	
318.0	Moderate Mental Retardation (41)	
318.1	Severe Mental Retardation (41)	
318.2	Profound Mental Retardation (41)	
319	Mental Retardation. Severity Unspecified (42)	

---

*Refers to page numbers in DSM-IV.
Based on information from the *Diagnostic and Statistical Manual of Mental Disorders. Fourth Edition.* Copyright 1994 American Psychiatric Association.

LEARNING DISORDERS (46)
315.00	Reading Disorder (48)
315.1	Mathematics Disorder (50)
315.2	Disorder of Written Expression (51)
315.9	Learning Disorder NOS (53)

MOTOR SKILLS DISORDER
315.4	Developmental Coordination Disorder (53)

COMMUNICATION DISORDERS (55)
315.31	Expressive Language Disorder (55)
315.31	Mixed Receptive-Expressive Language Disorder (58)
315.39	Phonological Disorder (61)
307.0	Stuttering (63)
307.9	Communication Disorder NOS (65)

PERVASIVE DEVELOPMENTAL DISORDERS (65)
299.00	Autistic Disorder (66)
299.80	Rett's Disorder (71)
299.10	Childhood Disintegrative Disorder (73)
299.80	Asperger's Disorder (75)
299.80	Pervasive Developmental Disorder NOS (77)

ATTENTION-DEFICIT AND DISRUPTIVE BEHAVIOR DISORDERS (78)
314.xx	Attention-Deficit/Hyperactivity Disorder (78)
.01	Combined Type
.00	Predominantly Inattentive Type
.01	Predominantly Hyperactive-Impulsive Type
314.9	Attention-Deficit/Hyperactivity Disorder NOS (85)
312.8	Conduct Disorder (85)
	Specify type: Childhood-Onset Type/ Adolescent-Onset Type
313.81	Oppositional Defiant Disorder (91)
312.9	Disruptive Behavior Disorder NOS (94)

FEEDING AND EATING DISORDERS OF INFANCY OR EARLY CHILDHOOD (94)

307.52	Pica (95)
307.53	Rumination Disorder (96)
307.59	Feeding Disorder of Infancy or Early Childhood (98)

TIC DISORDERS (100)

307.23	Tourette's Disorder (101)
307.22	Chronic Motor or Vocal Tic Disorder (103)
307.21	Transient Tic Disorder (104)
	Specify if: **Single Episode/Recurrent**
307.20	Tic Disorder NOS (105)

ELIMINATION DISORDERS (106)

——.—	Encopresis (106)
787.6	With Constipation and Overflow Incontinence
307.7	Without Constipation and Overflow Incontinence
307.6	Enuresis (Not Due to a General Medical Condition (108)
	Specify type: **Nocturnal Only/Diurnal Only/Nocturnal and Diurnal**

OTHER DISORDERS OF INFANCY, CHILDHOOD, OR ADOLESCENCE

309.21	Separation Anxiety Disorder (110)
	Specify if: **Early Onset**
313.23	Selective Mutism (114)
313.89	Reactive Attachment Disorder of Infancy or Early Childhood (116)
	Specify if: **Inhibited Type/Disinhibited Type**
307.3	Stereotypic Movement Disorder (118)
	Specify if: **With Self-Injurious Behavior**
313.9	Disorder of Infancy, Childhood, or Adolescence NOS (121)

Delirium, Dementia, and Amnestic and Other Cognitive Disorders (123)

DELIRIUM (124)

293.0	Delirium Due to . . . *[Indicate the General Medical Condition]* (127)
——.—	Substance Intoxication Delirium (129) *(refer to Substance-Related Disorders for substance-specific codes)*
——.—	Substance Withdrawal Delirium (129) *(refer to Substance-Related Disorders for substance-specific codes)*
——.—	Delirium Due to Multiple Etiologies *(code each of the specific etiologies)* (132)
780.09	Delirium NOS (133)

DEMENTIA (133)

290.xx	Dementia of the Alzheimer's Type, With Early Onset *(also code 331.0 Alzheimer's disease on Axis III)* (139)

.10	Uncomplicated
.11	With Delirium
.12	With Delusions
.13	With Depressed Mood
	Specify if: **With Behavioral Disturbance**
290.xx	Dementia of the Alzheimer's Type, With Late Onset *(also code 331.0 Alzheimer's disease on Axis III)* (139)
.0	Uncomplicated
.3	With Delirium
.20	With Delusions
.21	With Depressed Mood
	Specify if: **With Behavioral Disturbance**
290.xx	Vascular Dementia (143)
.40	Uncomplicated
.41	With Delirium
.42	With Delusions
.43	With Depressed Mood
	Specify if: **With Behavioral Disturbance**
294.9	Dementia Due to HIV Disease *(also code 043.1 HIV infection affecting central nervous system on Axis III)* (148)
294.1	Dementia Due to Head Trauma *(also code 854.00 head injury on Axis III)* (148)
294.1	Dementia Due to Parkinson's Disease *(also code 332.0 Parkinson's disease on Axis III)* (148)
294.1	Dementia Due to Huntington's Disease *(also code 333.4 Huntington's disease on Axis III)* (149)
290.10	Dementia Due to Pick's Disease *(also code 331.1 Pick's disease on Axis III)* (149)
290.10	Dementia Due to Creutzfeldt-Jakob Disease *(also code 046.1 Creutzfeldt-Jakob disease on Axis III)* (150)
294.1	Dementia Due to . . . *[Indicate the General Medical Condition not listed above]* *(also code the general medical condition on Axis III)* (151)
——.—	Substance-Induced Persisting Dementia *(refer to Substance-Related Disorders for substance-specific codes)* (152)
——.—	Dementia Due to Multiple Etiologies *(code each of the specific etiologies)* (154)
294.8	Dementia NOS (155)

AMNESTIC DISORDERS (156)

294.0	Amnestic Disorder Due to . . . *[Indicate the General Medical Condition]* (158)
	Specify if: **Transient/Chronic**
——.—	Substance-Induced Persisting Amnestic Disorder *(refer to Substance-Related Disorders for substance-specific codes)* (161)
294.8	Amnestic Disorders NOS (163)

OTHER COGNITIVE DISORDERS (163)

294.9	Cognitive Disorder NOS (163)

Mental Disorders Due to a General Medical Condition Not Elsewhere Classified (165)

293.89   Catatonic Disorder Due to . . . *[Indicate the General Medical Condition]* (169)
310.1   Personality Change Due to . . . *[Indicate the General Medical Condition]* (171)
          Specify type: Labile Type/Disinhibited Type/Aggressive Type/Apathetic Type/Paranoid Type/Other Type/Combined Type/Unspecified Type
293.9   Mental Disorder NOS Due to . . . *[Indicate the General Medical Condition]* (174)

Substance-Related Disorders (175)

[a]*The following specifiers may be applied to Substance Dependence:*

With Physiological Dependence/Without Physiological Dependence
Early Full Remission/Early Partial Remission
Sustained Full Remission/Sustained Partial Remission
On Agonist Therapy/In a Controlled Environment

The following specifiers apply to Substance-Induced Disorders as noted:
   [I]With Onset During Intoxication
   [W]With Onset During Withdrawal

ALCOHOL-RELATED DISORDERS (194)
Alcohol Use Disorders
303.90   Alcohol Dependence[a] (195)
305.00   Alcohol Abuse (196)

Alcohol-Induced Disorders
303.00   Alcohol Intoxication (196)
291.8   Alcohol Withdrawal (197)
          Specify if: With Perceptual Disturbances
291.0   Alcohol Intoxication Delirium (129)
291.0   Alcohol Withdrawal Delirium (129)
291.2   Alcohol-Induced Persisting Dementia (152)
291.1   Alcohol-Induced Persisting Amnestic Disorder (161)
291.x   Alcohol-Induced Psychotic Disorder (310)
    .5   With Delusions[I, W]
    .3   With Hallucinations[I, W]
291.8   Alcohol-Induced Mood Disorder[I, W] (370)
291.8   Alcohol-Induced Anxiety Disorder[I, W] (439)
291.8   Alcohol-Induced Sexual Dysfunction[I] (519)
291.8   Alcohol-Induced Sleep Disorder[I, W] (601)
291.9   Alcohol-Related Disorder NOS (240)

AMPHETAMINE (OR AMPHETAMINE-LIKE)–RELATED DISORDERS (204)
Amphetamine Use Disorders
304.40   Amphetamine Dependence[a] (206)
305.70   Amphetamine Abuse (206)

Amphetamine-Induced Disorders
292.89   Amphetamine Intoxication (207)
          Specify if: With Perceptual Disturbances
292.0   Amphetamine Withdrawal (208)
292.81   Amphetamine Intoxication Delirium (129)
292.xx   Amphetamine-Induced Psychotic Disorder (310)
    .11   With Delusions[I]
    .12   With Hallucinations[I]
292.84   Amphetamine-Induced Mood Disorder[I, W] (370)
292.89   Amphetamine-Induced Anxiety Disorder[I] (439)
292.89   Amphetamine-Induced Sexual Dysfunction[I] (519)
292.89   Amphetamine-Induced Sleep Disorder[I, W] (601)
292.9   Amphetamine-Related Disorder NOS (211)

CAFFEINE-RELATED DISORDERS (212)
Caffeine-Induced Disorders
305.90   Caffeine Intoxication (212)
292.89   Caffeine-Induced Anxiety Disorder[I] (439)
292.89   Caffeine-Induced Sleep Disorder[I] (601)
292.9   Caffeine-Related Disorder NOS (215)

CANNABIS-RELATED DISORDERS (215)
Cannabis Use Disorders
304.30   Cannabis Dependence[a] (216)
305.20   Cannabis Abuse (217)

Cannabis-Induced Disorders
292.89   Cannabis Intoxication (217)
          Specify if: With Perceptual Disturbances
292.81   Cannabis Intoxication Delirium (129)
292.xx   Cannabis-Induced Psychotic Disorder (310)
    .11   With Delusions[I]
    .12   With Hallucinations[I]
292.89   Cannabis-Induced Anxiety Disorder[I] (439)
292.9   Cannabis-Related Disorder NOS (221)

COCAINE-RELATED DISORDERS (221)
Cocaine Use Disorders
304.20   Cocaine Dependence[a] (222)
305.60   Cocaine Abuse (223)

Cocaine-Induced Disorders
292.89   Cocaine Intoxication (223)
          Specify if: With Perceptual Disturbances
292.0   Cocaine Withdrawal (225)
292.81   Cocaine Intoxication Delirium (129)
292.xx   Cocaine-Induced Psychotic Disorder (310)
    .11   With Delusions[I]
    .12   With Hallucinations[I]
292.84   Cocaine-Induced Mood Disorder[I, W] (370)
292.89   Cocaine-Induced Anxiety Disorder[I, W] (439)
292.89   Cocaine-Induced Sexual Dysfunction[I] (519)
292.89   Cocaine-Induced Sleep Disorder[I, W] (601)
292.9   Cocaine-Related Disorder NOS (229)

HALLUCINOGEN-RELATED DISORDERS (229)
Hallucinogen Use Disorders
304.50   Hallucinogen Dependence[a] (230)
305.30   Hallucinogen Abuse (231)

Hallucinogen-Induced Disorders
292.89   Hallucinogen Intoxication (232)
292.89   Hallucinogen Persisting Perception
            Disorder (Flashbacks) (233)
292.81   Hallucinogen Intoxication Delirium (129)
292.xx   Hallucinogen-Induced Psychotic Disorder
            (310)
   .11   With Delusions[I]
   .12   With Hallucinations[I]
292.84   Hallucinogen-Induced Mood Disorder[I]
            (370)
292.89   Hallucinogen-Induced Anxiety Disorder[I]
            (439)
292.9   Hallucinogen-Related Disorder NOS
            (236)

INHALANT-RELATED DISORDERS (236)
Inhalant Use Disorders
304.60   Inhalant Dependence[a] (238)
305.90   Inhalant Abuse (238)

Inhalant-Induced Disorders
292.89   Inhalant Intoxication (239)
292.81   Inhalant Intoxication Delirium (129)
292.82   Inhalant-Induced Persisting Dementia
            (152)
292.xx   Inhalant-Induced Psychotic Disorder (310)
   .11   With Delusions[I]
   .12   With Hallucinations[I]
292.84   Inhalant-Induced Mood Disorder[I] (370)
292.89   Inhalant-Induced Anxiety Disorder[I] (439)
292.9   Inhalant-Related Disorder NOS (242)

NICOTINE-RELATED DISORDERS (242)
Nicotine Use Disorder
305.10   Nicotine Dependence[a] (243)

Nicotine-Induced Disorder
292.0   Nicotine Withdrawal (244)
292.9   Nicotine-Related Disorder NOS (247)

OPIOID-RELATED DISORDERS (247)
Opioid Use Disorders
304.00   Opioid Dependence[a] (248)
305.50   Opioid Abuse (249)

Opioid-Induced Disorders
292.89   Opioid Intoxication (249)
            Specify if: With Perceptual Disturbances
292.0   Opioid Withdrawal (250)
292.81   Opioid Intoxication Delirium (129)
292.xx   Opioid-Induced Psychotic Disorder (310)
   .11   With Delusions[I]
   .12   With Hallucinations[I]
292.84   Opioid-Induced Mood Disorder[I] (370)
292.89   Opioid-Induced Sexual Dysfunction[I] (519)

292.89   Opioid-Induced Sleep Disorder[I, W] (601)
292.9   Opioid-Related Disorder NOS (255)

**PHENCYCLIDINE (OR
PHENCYCLIDINE-LIKE)–RELATED
DISORDERS** (255)
Phencyclidine Use Disorders
304.90   Phencyclidine Dependence[a] (256)
305.90   Phencyclidine Abuse (257)

Phencyclidine-Induced Disorders
292.89   Phencyclidine Intoxication (257)
            Specify if: With Perceptual Disturbances
292.81   Phencyclidine Intoxication Delirium (129)
292.xx   Phencyclidine-Induced Psychotic Disorder
            (310)
   .11   With Delusions[I]
   .12   With Hallucinations[I]
292.84   Phencyclidine-Induced Mood Disorder[I]
            (370)
292.89   Phencyclidine-Induced Anxiety Disorder[I]
            (439)
292.9   Phencyclidine-Related Disorder NOS (261)

**SEDATIVE-, HYPNOTIC-, OR ANXIOLYTIC-
RELATED DISORDERS** (261)
Sedative, Hypnotic, or Anxiolytic Use Disorders
304.10   Sedative, Hypnotic, or Anxiolytic
            Dependence[a] (262)
305.40   Sedative, Hypnotic, or Anxiolytic Abuse
            (263)

**Sedative-, Hypnotic-, or Anxiolytic-Induced
Disorders**
292.89   Sedative, Hypnotic, or Anxiolytic
            Intoxication (263)
292.0   Sedative, Hypnotic, or Anxiolytic
            Withdrawal (264)
            Specify if: With Perceptual Disturbances
292.81   Sedative, Hypnotic, or Anxiolytic
            Intoxication Delirium (129)
292.81   Sedative, Hypnotic, or Anxiolytic
            Withdrawal Delirium (129)
292.82   Sedative-, Hypnotic-, or Anxiolytic-Induced
            Persisting Dementia (152)
292.83   Sedative-, Hypnotic-, or Anxiolytic-Induced
            Persisting Amnestic Disorder (161)
292.xx   Sedative-, Hypnotic-, or Anxiolytic-Induced
            Psychotic Disorder (310)
   .11   With Delusions[I, W]
   .12   With Hallucinations[I, W]
292.84   Sedative-, Hypnotic-, or Anxiolytic-Induced
            Mood Disorder[I, W] (370)
292.89   Sedative-, Hypnotic-, or Anxiolytic-Induced
            Anxiety Disorder[W] (439)
292.89   Sedative-, Hypnotic-, or Anxiolytic-Induced
            Sexual Dysfunction[I] (519)
292.89   Sedative-, Hypnotic-, or Anxiolytic-Induced
            Sleep Disorder[I, W] (601)
292.9   Sedative-, Hypnotic-, or Anxiolytic-Related
            Disorder NOS (269)

POLYSUBSTANCE-RELATED DISORDER
304.80   Polysubstance Dependence[a] (270)

OTHER (OR UNKNOWN) SUBSTANCE-RELATED DISORDERS (270)
Other (or Unknown) Substance Use Disorders
304.90   Other (or Unknown) Substance Dependence[a] (176)
305.90   Other (or Unknown) Substance Abuse (182)

Other (or Unknown) Substance-Induced Disorders
292.89   Other (or Unknown) Substance Intoxication (183)
            Specify if: With Perceptual Disturbances
292.0   Other (or Unknown) Substance Withdrawal (184)
            Specify if: With Perceptual Disturbances
292.81   Other (or Unknown) Substance-Induced Delirium (129)
292.82   Other (or Unknown) Substance-Induced Persisting Dementia (152)
292.83   Other (or Unknown) Substance-Induced Persisting Amnestic Disorder (161)
292.xx   Other (or Unknown) Substance-Induced Psychotic Disorder (310)
   .11   With Delusions[I, W]
   .12   With Hallucinations[I, W]
292.84   Other (or Unknown) Substance-Induced Mood Disorder[I, W] (370)
292.89   Other (or Unknown) Substance-Induced Anxiety Disorder[I, W] (439)
292.89   Other (or Unknown) Substance-Induced Sexual Dysfunction (519)
292.89   Other (or Unknown) Substance-Induced Sleep Disorder[I, W] (601)
292.9   Other (or Unknown) Substance-Related Disorder NOS (272)

Schizophrenia and Other Psychotic Disorders (273)

295.xx   Schizophrenia (274)
The following Classification of Longitudinal Course applies to all subtypes of Schizophrenia:

Episodic With Interepisode Residual Symptoms (*specify if:* With Prominent Negative Symptoms)
Episodic with No Interepisode Residual Symptoms
Continuous (*specify if:* With Prominent Negative Symptoms)
Single Episode in Partial Remission (*specify if:* With Prominent Negative Symptoms)
Single Episode in Full Remission Other or Unspecified Pattern

   .30   Paranoid Type (287)
   .10   Disorganized Type (287)
   .20   Catatonic Type (288)
   .90   Undifferentiated Type (289)
   .60   Residual Type (289)

295.40   Schizophreniform Disorder (290)
            Specify if: Without Good Prognostic Features/With Good Prognostic Features
295.70   Schizoaffective Disorder (292)
            Specify type: Bipolar Type/Depressive Type
297.1   Delusional Disorder (296)
            Specify type: Erotomanic Type/Grandiose Type/Jealous Type/Persecutory Type/Somatic Type/Mixed Type/Unspecified Type
298.8   Brief Psychotic Disorder (302)
            Specify if: With Marked Stressor(s)/Without Marked Stressor(s)/With Postpartum Onset
297.3   Shared Psychotic Disorder (305)
293.xx   Psychotic Disorder Due to . . . *[Indicate the General Medical Condition]* (306)
   .81   With Delusions
   .82   With Hallucinations
——.—   Substance-Induced Psychotic Disorder (*refer to Substance-Related Disorders for substance-specific codes*) (310)
            Specify if: With Onset During Intoxication/With Onset During Withdrawal
298.9   Psychotic Disorder NOS (315)

Mood Disorders (317)

Code current state of Major Depressive Disorder or Bipolar I Disorder in fifth digit:

1 = Mild
2 = Moderate
3 = Severe Without Psychotic Features
4 = Severe With Psychotic Features
    Specify: Mood-Congruent Psychotic Features/Mood-Incongruent Psychotic Features
5 = In Partial Remission
6 = In Full Remission
0 = Unspecified

The following specifiers apply (for current or most recent episode) to Mood Disorders as noted:

[a]Severity/Psychotic/Remission Specifiers
[b]Chronic
[c]With Catatonic Features
[d]With Melancholic Features
[e]With Atypical Features
[f]With Postpartum Onset

The following specifiers apply to Mood Disorders as noted:

[g]With or Without Full Interepisode Recovery
[h]With Seasonal Pattern
[i]With Rapid Cycling

DEPRESSIVE DISORDERS
296.xx   Major Depressive Disorder (339)

.2x   Single Episode[a, b, c, d, e, f]
.3x   Recurrent[a, b, c, d, e, f, g, h]
300.4   Dysthymic Disorder (345)
         Specify if: Early Onset/Late Onset
         Specify: With Atypical Features
311   Depressive Disorder NOS (350)

BIPOLAR DISORDERS

296.xx   Bipolar I Disorder (350)
.0x   Single Manic Episode[a, c, f]
         Specify if: Mixed
.40   Most Recent Episode Hypomanic[g, h, i]
.4x   Most Recent Episode Manic[a, c, f, g, h, i]
.6x   Most Recent Episode Mixed[a, c, f, g, h, i]
.5x   Most Recent Episode
         Depressed[a, b, c, d, e, f, g, h, i]
.7   Most Recent Episode Unspecified[g, h, i]
296.89   Bipolar II Disorder[a, b, c, d, e, f, g, h, i] (359)
         Specify (current or most recent episode):
         Hypomanic/Depressed
301.13   Cyclothymic Disorder (363)
296.80   Bipolar Disorder NOS (366)
293.83   Mood Disorder Due to . . . *[Indicate the
         General Medical Condition]* (366)
         Specify type: With Depressive Features/
         With Major Depressive–Like Episode/With
         Manic Features/With Mixed Features
—.—   Substance-Induced Mood Disorder *(refer
         to Substance-Related Disorders for
         substance-specific codes)* (370)
         Specify type: With Depressive Features/
         With Manic Features/With Mixed Features
         Specify if: With Onset During
         Intoxication/With Onset During
         Withdrawal
296.90   Mood Disorder NOS (375)

Anxiety Disorders (393)

300.01   Panic Disorder Without Agoraphobia (397)
300.21   Panic Disorder With Agoraphobia (397)
300.22   Agoraphobia Without History of Panic
         Disorder (403)
300.29   Specific Phobia (405)
         Specify type: Animal Type/Natural
         Environment Type/Blood-Injection-Injury
         Type/Situational Type/Other Type
300.23   Social Phobia (411)
         Specify if: Generalized
300.3   Obsessive-Compulsive Disorder (417)
         Specify if: With Poor Insight
309.81   Posttraumatic Stress Disorder (424)
         Specify if: Acute/Chronic
         Specify if: With Delayed Onset
308.3   Acute Stress Disorder (429)
300.02   Generalized Anxiety Disorder (432)
293.89   Anxiety Disorder Due to . . . *[Indicate the
         General Medical Condition]* (436)
         Specify if: With Generalized Anxiety/With
         Panic Attacks/With Obsessive-Compulsive
         Symptoms

—.—   Substance-Induced Anxiety Disorder *(refer
         to Substance-Related Disorders for
         substance-specific codes)* (439)
         Specify if: With Generalized Anxiety/With
         Panic Attacks/With Obsessive-Compulsive
         Symptoms/With Phobic Symptoms
         Specify if: With Onset During
         Intoxication/With Onset During
         Withdrawal
300.00   Anxiety Disorder NOS (444)

Somatoform Disorders (445)

300.81   Somatization Disorder (446)
300.81   Undifferentiated Somatoform Disorder
         (450)
300.11   Conversion Disorder (452)
         Specify type: With Motor Symptom or
         Deficit/With Sensory Symptom or Deficit
         With Seizures or Convulsions/With Mixed
         Presentation
307.xx   Pain Disorder (458)
.80   Associated With Psychological Factors
.89   Associated With Both Psychological
         Factors and a General Medical
         Condition
         Specify if: Acute/Chronic
300.7   Hypochondriasis (462)
         Specify if: With Poor Insight
300.7   Body Dysmorphic Disorder (466)
300.81   Somatoform Disorder NOS (468)

Factitious Disorders (471)

300.xx   Factitious Disorder (471)
.16   With Predominantly Psychological Signs
         and Symptoms
.19   With Predominantly Physical Signs and
         Symptoms
.19   With Combined Psychological and
         Physical Signs and Symptoms
300.19   Factitious Disorder NOS (475)

Dissociative Disorders (477)

300.12   Dissociative Amnesia (478)
300.13   Dissociative Fugue (481)
300.14   Dissociative Identity Disorder (484)
300.6   Depersonalization Disorder (488)
300.15   Dissociative Disorder NOS (490)

Sexual and Gender Identity Disorders (493)

SEXUAL DYSFUNCTIONS (493)
*The following specifiers apply to all primary Sexual
Dysfunctions:*

Lifelong Type/Acquired Type
Generalized Type/Situational Type
Due to Psychological Factors/Due to Combined Factors

Sexual Desire Disorders

302.71	Hypoactive Sexual Desire Disorder (496)
302.79	Sexual Aversion Disorder (499)

Sexual Arousal Disorders

302.72	Female Sexual Arousal Disorder (500)
302.72	Male Erectile Disorder (502)

Orgasmic Disorders

302.73	Female Orgasmic Disorder (505)
302.74	Male Orgasmic Disorder (507)
302.75	Premature Ejaculation (509)

Sexual Pain Disorders

302.76	Dyspareunia (Not Due to a General Medical Condition) (511)
306.51	Vaginismus (Not Due to a General Medical Condition) (513)

Sexual Dysfunction Due to a General Medical Condition (515)

625.8	Female Hypoactive Sexual Desire Disorder Due to . . . *[Indicate the General Medical Condition]* (515)
608.89	Male Hypoactive Sexual Desire Disorder Due to . . . *[Indicate the General Medical Condition]* (515)
607.84	Male Erectile Disorder Due to . . . *[Indicate the General Medical Condition]* (515)
625.0	Female Dyspareunia Due to . . . *[Indicate the General Medical Condition]* (515)
608.89	Male Dyspareunia Due to . . . *[Indicate the General Medical Condition]* (515)
625.8	Other Female Sexual Dysfunction Due to . . . *[Indicate the General Medical Condition]* (515)
608.89	Other Male Sexual Dysfunction Due to . . . *[Indicate the General Medical Condition]* (515)
———.—	Substance-Induced Sexual Dysfunction *(refer to Substance-Related Disorders for substance-specific codes)* (519) *Specify if:* With Impaired Desire/With Impaired Arousal/With Impaired Orgasm/With Sexual Pain *Specify if:* With Onset During Intoxication
302.70	Sexual Dysfunction NOS (522)

PARAPHILIAS (522)

302.4	Exhibitionism (525)
302.81	Fetishism (526)
302.89	Frotteurism (527)
302.2	Pedophilia (527) *Specify if:* Sexually Attracted to Males/Sexually Attracted to Females/Sexually Attracted to Both *Specify if:* Limited to Incest

Specify type: Exclusive Type/Nonexclusive Type

302.83	Sexual Masochism (529)
302.84	Sexual Sadism (530)
302.3	Transvestic Fetishism (530) *Specify if:* With Gender Dysphoria
302.82	Voyeurism (532)
302.9	Paraphilia NOA (532)

GENDER IDENTITY DISORDERS (532)

302.xx	Gender Identity Disorder (532)
.6	In Children
.85	In Adolescents or Adults *Specify if:* Sexually Attracted to Males/Sexually Attracted to Females/Sexually Attracted to Both/Sexually Attracted to Neither
302.6	Gender Identity Disorder NOS (538)
302.9	Sexual Disorder NOS (538)

Eating Disorders (539)

307.1	Anorexia Nervosa (539) *Specify type:* Restricting Type, Binge-Eating/Purging Type
306.51	Bulimia Nervosa (545) *Specify type:* Purging Type/Nonpurging Type
307.50	Eating Disorder NOS (550)

Sleep Disorders (551)

PRIMARY SLEEP DISORDERS (553)
Dyssomnias (553)

307.42	Primary Insomnia (553)
307.44	Primary Hypersomnia (557) *Specify if:* Recurrent
347	Narcolepsy (562)
780.59	Breathing-Related Sleep Disorder (567)
307.45	Circadian Rhythm Sleep Disorder (573) *Specify type:* Delayed Sleep Phase Type/Jet Lag Type/Shift Work Type/Unspecified Type
307.47	Dyssomnia NOS (579)

Parasomnias (579)

307.47	Nightmare Disorder (580)
307.46	Sleep Terror Disorder (583)
307.46	Sleepwalking Disorder (587)
307.47	Parasomnia NOS (592)

SLEEP DISORDERS RELATED TO ANOTHER MENTAL DISORDER (592)

307.42	Insomnia Related to . . . *[Indicate the Axis I or Axis II Disorder]* (592)
307.44	Hypersomnia Related to . . . *[Indicate the Axis I or Axis II Disorder]* (592)

OTHER SLEEP DISORDERS

780.xx	Sleep Disorder Due to . . . *[Indicate the General Medical Condition]* (597)
.52	Insomnia Type
.54	Hypersomnia Type
.59	Parasomnia Type
.59	Mixed Type
——.—	Substance-Induced Sleep Disorder *(refer to Substance-Related Disorders for substance-specific codes)* (601)

Specify type: Insomnia Type/Hypersomnia Type/Parasomnia Type/Mixed Type
Specify if: With Onset During Intoxication/With Onset During Withdrawal

Impulse-Control Disorders Not Elsewhere Classified (609)

312.34	Intermittent Explosive Disorder (609)
312.32	Kleptomania (612)
312.33	Pyromania (614)
312.31	Pathological Gambling (615)
312.39	Trichotillomania (618)
312.30	Impulse-Control Disorder NOS (621)

Adjustment Disorders (623)

309.xx	Adjustment Disorder (623)
.0	With Depressed Mood
.24	With Anxiety
.28	With Mixed Anxiety and Depressed Mood
.3	With Disturbance of Conduct
.4	With Mixed Disturbance of Emotions and Conduct
.9	Unspecified

Specify if: Acute/Chronic

Personality Disorders (629)

Note: These are coded on Axis II.

301.0	Paranoid Personality Disorder (634)
301.20	Schizoid Personality Disorder (638)
301.22	Schizotypal Personality Disorder (641)
301.7	Antisocial Personality Disorder (645)
301.83	Borderline Personality Disorder (650)
301.50	Histrionic Personality Disorder (655)
301.81	Narcissistic Personality Disorder (658)
301.82	Avoidant Personality Disorder (662)
301.6	Dependent Personality Disorder (665)
301.4	Obsessive-Compulsive Personality Disorder (669)
301.9	Personality Disorder NOS (673)

Other Conditions That May Be a Focus of Clinical Attention (675)

PSYCHOLOGICAL FACTORS AFFECTING MEDICAL CONDITION (675)

316	. . . *[Specified Psychological Factor]* Affecting . . . *[Indicate the General Medical Condition]* (675)

Choose name based on nature of factors:
Mental Disorder Affecting Medical Condition
Psychological Symptoms Affecting Medical Condition
Personality Traits or Coping Style Affecting Medical Condition
Maladaptive Health Behaviors Affecting Medical Condition
Stress-Related Physiological Response Affecting Medical Condition
Other or Unspecified Psychological Factors Affecting Medical Condition

MEDICATION-INDUCED MOVEMENT DISORDERS (678)

332.1	Neuroleptic-Induced Parkinsonism (679)
333.92	Neuroleptic Malignant Syndrome (679)
333.7	Neuroleptic-Induced Acute Dystonia (679)
333.99	Neuroleptic-Induced Acute Akathisia (679)
333.82	Neuroleptic-Induced Tardive Dyskinesia (679)
333.1	Medication-Induced Postural Tremor (680)
333.90	Medication-Induced Movement Disorder NOS (680)

OTHER MEDICATION-INDUCED DISORDER

995.2	Adverse Effects of Medication NOS (680)

RELATIONAL PROBLEMS (680)

V61.9	Relational Problem Related to a Mental Disorder or General Medical Condition (681)
V61.20	Parent-Child Relational Problem (681)
V61.1	Partner Relational Problem (681)
V61.8	Sibling Relational Problem (681)
V62.81	Relational Problem NOS (681)

PROBLEMS RELATED TO ABUSE OR NEGLECT (682)

V61.21	Physical Abuse of Child (682) *(code 995.5 if focus of attention is on victim)*
V61.21	Sexual Abuse of Child (682) *(code 995.5 if focus of attention is on victim)*
V61.21	Neglect of Child (682) *(code 995.5 if focus of attention is on victim)*
V61.1	Physical Abuse of Adult (682) *(code 995.81 if focus of attention is on victim)*

V61.1   Sexual Abuse of Adult (682) *(code 995.81 if focus of attention is on victim)*

ADDITIONAL CONDITIONS THAT MAY BE A FOCUS OF CLINICAL ATTENTION (683)

V15.81   Noncompliance With Treatment (683)
V65.2   Malingering (683)
V71.01   Adult Antisocial Behavior (683)
V71.02   Child or Adolescent Antisocial Behavior (684)
V62.89   Borderline Intellectual Functioning (684)
         Note: *This is coded on Axis II.*
780.9   Age-Related Cognitive Decline (684)
V62.82   Bereavement (684)
V62.3   Academic Problem (685)
V62.2   Occupational Problem (685)
313.82   Identity Problem (685)
V62.89   Religious or Spiritual Problem (685)
V62.4   Acculturation Problem (685)
V62.89   Phase of Life Problem (685)

Additional Codes

300.9   Unspecified Mental Disorder (nonpsychotic) (687)

V71.09   No Diagnosis or Condition on Axis I (687)
799.9   Diagnosis or Condition Deferred on Axis I (687)
V71.09   No Diagnosis on Axis II (687)
799.9   Diagnosis Deferred on Axis II (687)

Multiaxial System

Axis I   Clinical Disorders
            Other Conditions That May Be a Focus of Clinical Attention
Axis II   Personality Disorders
            Mental Retardation
Axis III   General Medical Conditions
Axis IV   Psychosocial and Environmental Problems
Axis V   Global Assessment of Functioning

Index

Note: Page numbers in *italics* refer to illustrations; page numbers followed by (t) refer to tables; and page numbers followed by (b) refer to boxes.